Joseph
399-4721

M. Wilson - 545-3396

J. J. Bailey Jr

THE PRINCIPLES AND PRACTICE OF MEDICINE

Twentieth Edition

THE PRINCIPLES AND

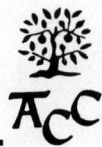

APPLETON-CENTURY-CROFTS/New York

PRACTICE OF MEDICINE

Twentieth Edition

A. McGEHEE HARVEY, M.D., D.Sc. (Hon.)
Eli K. Marshall, Jr. Professor of Medicine and
Director Emeritus of the Department of
Medicine, The Johns Hopkins University
School of Medicine; Physician-in-Chief
Emeritus, The Johns Hopkins Hospital,
Baltimore, Maryland

RICHARD J. JOHNS, M.D.
Professor of Medicine, Massey Professor of
Biomedical Engineering and Director of the
Department of Biomedical Engineering, The
Johns Hopkins University School of Medicine,
Baltimore, Maryland

VICTOR A. McKUSICK, M.D., D.Sc. (Hon.)
William Osler Professor of Medicine and
Director of the Department of Medicine, The
Johns Hopkins University School of Medicine;
Physician-in-Chief, The Johns Hopkins
Hospital, Baltimore, Maryland

ALBERT H. OWENS, Jr., M.D.
Professor of Medicine, Professor of Oncology
and Director of the Oncology Center, The
Johns Hopkins University School of Medicine,
Baltimore, Maryland

RICHARD S. ROSS, M.D.
Professor of Medicine, Dean of the Medical
Faculty and Vice President for Medicine, The
Johns Hopkins University School of Medicine,
Baltimore, Maryland

LIBRARY OF CONGRESS CATALOGING IN PUBLICATION DATA
Main entry under title:
The Principles and practice of medicine.
    Based on The principles and practice of medicine,
    by Sir W. Osler.
    Bibliography: p.
    Includes index.
    1.   Internal medicine. I. Harvey, Abner McGehee,
    1911–   II. Osler, William, Sir, Bart., 1849–1919.
Principles and practice of medicine.
RC46.P89   1980   616′.026   79-23358
ISBN 0-8385-7930-2

Cover Design: A Good Thing, Inc.
Text Design: Alan Gold
Index: Philip James

PRINTED IN THE UNITED STATES OF AMERICA

THIS volume is dedicated to the physicians of the Medical Service of the past for their precept and guidance, to our colleagues of today for their support and encouragement, and to the students, our colleagues of tomorrow, for their stimulation and criticism.

CONTRIBUTORS*

STEPHEN C. ACHUFF
Assistant Professor of Medicine

ARNOLD E. ANDERSEN
Assistant Professor of Psychiatry

FRANK C. ARNETT, JR.
Assistant Professor of Medicine

WILMOT C. BALL, JR.
Associate Professor of Medicine
Joint Appointment in Environmental Health
  Science

THEODORE M. BAYLESS
Associate Professor of Medicine

LEWIS C. BECKER
Associate Professor of Medicine

WILLIAM R. BELL
Associate Professor of Medicine
Assistant Professor of Radiology

EUGENE R. BLEECKER
Assistant Professor of Medicine

TURNER BLEDSOE
Formerly Associate Professor of Medicine
Presently Vice President for Health Affairs,
  Maine Medical Center

HAYDEN G. BRAINE
Assistant Professor of Oncology
Instructor in Medicine

E. JAMES BRITT
Instructor in Medicine

BERNADINE H. BULKLEY
Associate Professor of Medicine
Assistant Professor of Pathology

TURNER E. BYNUM
Assistant Professor of Medicine

JOHN L. CAMERON
Professor of Surgery

REX B. CONN, JR.
Formerly Professor of Laboratory Medicine
Presently Professor of Pathology and
  Laboratory Medicine, Emory University

JOSEPH T. COYLE
Associate Professor of Pharmacology &
  Experimental Therapy
Associate Professor of Psychiatry

PETER E. DANS
Associate Professor of Medicine

CATHERINE DeANGELIS
Associate Professor of Pediatrics

MAHLON R. DeLONG
Assistant Professor of Neurology
Assistant Professor of Physiology

DANIEL B. DRACHMAN
Professor of Neurology

THOMAS P. DUFFY
Formerly Assistant Professor of Medicine
Presently Associate Professor of Medicine,
  Yale University

JOHN T. FLAHERTY
Assistant Professor of Medicine

NICHOLAS J. FORTUIN
Associate Professor of Medicine

GIRAUD V. FOSTER
Associate Professor of Physiology
Associate Professor of Medicine

IRWIN M. FREEDBERG
Professor of Dermatology

BARRY GORDON
Assistant Professor of Neurology

GARETH M. GREEN
Professor of Environmental Health Science
Joint Appointment in Department of
  Medicine

H. LEON GREENE
Assistant Professor of Medicine
Assistant Professor of Radiology

ROBERT I. GREGERMAN
Associate Professor of Medicine

JOHN W. GRIFFIN
Assistant Professor of Neurology

LAWRENCE S. C. GRIFFITH
Associate Professor of Medicine
Assistant Professor of Radiology

HUBERT T. GURLEY
Assistant Professor of Emergency Medicine
Assistant Professor of Medicine

A. McGEHEE HARVEY
Eli K. Marshall, Jr. Professor of Medicine

THOMAS R. HENDRIX
Professor of Medicine

LAWRENCE W. HIRST
Instructor in Ophthalmology

T. H. HSU
Associate Professor of Medicine
Assistant Professor of Radiology

RICHARD L. HUMPHREY
Assistant Professor of Oncology
Assistant Professor of Medicine
Assistant Professor of Microbiology

J. O'NEAL HUMPHRIES
Formerly Robert L. Levy Professor of
  Cardiology
Professor of Medicine
Presently Professor of Medicine, University
  of South Carolina School of Medicine

*Unless otherwise indicated, faculty appointments are at The Johns Hopkins University School of Medicine, Baltimore, Maryland.

JOHN B. IMBODEN
Associate Professor of Psychiatry
Instructor in Medicine

CAROL J. JOHNS
Associate Professor of Medicine (on leave)
Acting President, Wellesley College

RICHARD J. JOHNS
Massey Professor of Biomedical
    Engineering
Professor of Medicine

LAWRENCE M. LICHTENSTEIN
Professor of Medicine
Associate Professor of Microbiology

PAUL S. LIETMAN
Wellcome Associate Professor of Clinical
    Pharmacology
Associate Professor of Medicine
Associate Professor of Pediatrics
Associate Professor of Pharmacology and
    Experimental Therapeutics

JAMES J. LIPSKY
Assistant Professor of Medicine
Assistant Professor of Pharmacology and
    Experimental Therapeutics

WILLIS C. MADDREY
Associate Professor of Medicine

JOHN J. MANN
Assistant Professor of Medicine

SIMEON MARGOLIS
Professor of Medicine
Associate Professor of Physiological
    Chemistry

GUY M. McKHANN
Kennedy Professor of Neurology

VICTOR A. McKUSICK
William Osler Professor of Medicine
Joint Appointment in Biology
Joint Appointment in Epidemiology

HAROLD A. MENKES
Associate Professor of Medicine
Joint Appointment in Environmental Health
    Science

JON K. MEYER
Associate Professor of Psychiatry
Assistant Professor of Surgery

NEIL R. MILLER
Assistant Professor of Ophthalmology
Assistant Professor of Neurology
Instructor in Neurosurgery

WILLIAM E. MITCH
Formerly Associate Professor of
    Pharmacology and Experimental
    Therapeutics
Formerly Associate Professor of Medicine
Presently Associate Professor of Medicine,
    Harvard University

PATRICK A. MURPHY
Associate Professor of Medicine
Associate Professor of Microbiology

HAROLD H. NEWBALL
Assistant Professor of Medicine

DAVID S. NEWCOMBE
Associate Professor of Environmental
    Health Science
Joint Appointment in Medicine

ERNST F. L. NIEDERMEYER
Associate Professor of Neurological
    Surgery
Associate Professor of Neurology

PHILIP S. NORMAN
Professor of Medicine

ALBERT H. OWENS, JR.
Professor of Oncology
Professor of Medicine

ARNALL PATZ
Professor of Ophthalmology

NATHANIEL F. PIERCE
Associate Professor of Medicine

THOMAS J. PREZIOSI
Associate Professor of Neurology

THADDEUS E. PROUT
Associate Professor of Medicine

PHILIP R. REID
Assistant Professor of Medicine
Assistant Professor of Pharmacology and
    Experimental Therapeutics

RICHARD S. ROSS
Professor of Medicine

R. PATTERSON RUSSELL
Associate Professor of Medicine

R. BRADLEY SACK
Associate Professor of Medicine
Associate Professor of Microbiology
Joint Appointment in Pathobiology

DANIEL G. SAPIR
Associate Professor of Medicine

MARVIN M. SCHUSTER
Professor of Medicine
Assistant Professor of Psychiatry

LYLE SENSENBRENNER
Associate Professor of Oncology
Associate Professor of Medicine

THOMAS W. SIMPSON
Associate Professor of Pathobiology
Joint Appointment in Department of
    Medicine
Joint Appointment in Health Services
    Administration

KIM SOLEZ
Assistant Professor of Pathology
Assistant Professor of Medicine

WILLIAM G. SPEED III
Associate Professor of Medicine

JERRY L. SPIVAK
Associate Professor of Medicine

MARY BETTY STEVENS
Associate Professor of Medicine

WARREN R. SUMMER
Associate Professor of Medicine
Associate Professor of Anesthesiology
Joint Appointment in Environmental Health
    Science

JIMMIE T. SYLVESTER
Assistant Professor of Medicine
Assistant Professor of Anesthesiology
Joint Appointment in Environmental Health
    Science

PETER B. TERRY
Assistant Professor of Medicine
Joint Appointment in Environmental Health
    Science

ALEXANDER S. TOWNES
Formerly Associate Professor of Medicine
Presently Professor of Medicine, University
    of Tennessee School of Medicine

JOHN E. A. TYSON
Formerly Associate Professor of
    Gynecology and Obstetrics
Presently Professor of Obstetrics,
    Gynecology and Reproductive Science,
    University of Manitoba

JOHN C. URBAITIS
Assistant Professor of Psychiatry

W. GORDON WALKER
Professor of Medicine

PATRICK C. WALSH
Professor of Urology

KO-PEN WANG
Assistant Professor of Medicine
Assistant Professor of Laryngology and
    Otology

LARRY WATERBURY
Assistant Professor of Medicine
Assistant Professor of Oncology

MYRON L. WEISFELDT
Professor of Medicine

JAMES L. WEISS
Assistant Professor of Medicine

ANDREW WHELTON
Associate Professor of Medicine

PAUL K. WHELTON
Assistant Professor of Medicine

ROBERT I. WHITE, JR.
Professor of Radiology
Assistant Professor of Medicine

G. MELVILLE WILLIAMS
Professor of Transplantation Surgery

ROBERT A. WISE
Fellow in Environmental Physiology
Fellow in Medicine

THOMAS N. WISE
Assistant Professor of Psychiatry
Assistant Professor of Medicine

DAVID S. ZEE
Associate Professor of Neurology
Associate Professor of Ophthalmology

PHILIP D. ZIEVE
Professor of Medicine

THOMAS M. ZIZIC
Assistant Professor of Medicine

CONTENTS

SECTION FIVE   Pulmonary Disease
Gareth M. Green (Section Editor)

SECTION SIXTEEN   Psychiatry in Medicine
           John B. Imboden (Section Editor)

SECTION NINETEEN   Special Topics in Medicine
Richard J. Johns (Section Editor)

PREFACE

IN THE 20TH EDITION, the majority of the sections have been completely revised, whereas a few have undergone minor revisions and the factual information and the bibliography brought up to date. A new chapter on Age Related Problems has been added to Section 19: Special Topics in Medicine, and the chapter on Adolescent Medicine has been moved to this section.

Since the last edition was published in 1976, several of the authors have taken new positions in other medical schools. In view of the fact that the basic theme of this textbook has been the approach to medical practice as exemplified by the staff of a single Department of Medicine, these authors have been replaced by others who still remain or have more recently come to Johns Hopkins. The only exceptions are four authors who left after this revision was in preparation: Turner Bledsoe, Thomas P. Duffy, J. O'Neal Humphries, and Alexander Townes.

We extend our deepest appreciation to our former colleagues and welcome the new contributors. These include: Stephen C. Achuff, Arnold E. Andersen, Frank C. Arnett, Jr., Lewis C. Becker, Eugene R. Bleecker, Hayden G. Braine, E. James Britt, Bernadine H. Bulkley, Turner E. Bynum, Joseph T. Coyle, Peter E. Dans, Catherine DeAngelis, John T. Flaherty, Giraud V. Foster, Irwin M. Freedberg, Barry Gordon, Gareth M. Green, Robert I. Gregerman, John W. Griffin, Hubert T. Gurley, Lawrence W. Hirst, T. H. Hsu, James J. Lipsky, Neil R. Miller, William E. Mitch, Harold H. Newball, David S. Newcombe, Arnall Patz, Lyle Sensenbrenner, Kim Solez, Jerry L. Spivak, Jimmie T. Sylvester, Peter B. Terry, John E. A. Tyson, Patrick C. Walsh, Ko-Pen Wang, James L. Weiss, Paul K. Whelton, G. Melville Williams, and Robert A. Wise.

We also wish to thank all of our colleagues who have offered constructive criticism and whose advice in editing the various sections has been of great help.

Again, our deepest appreciation goes to the various secretaries who have been so helpful in the recording of this volume.

THE EDITORS

PREFACE TO THE SEVENTEENTH EDITION

IN 1892 THE FIRST EDITION of Sir William Osler's textbook was published, in which he covered single-handedly the entire field of medicine. His book was well received both as a scientific work and as a contribution to literature. When the time came for the seventh edition, he wrote the following in a letter to Dr. Lewellys Barker: "This new edition will not be a very serious revision, as they will not break up the plates, but in the next edition we can do as we like. It would be very nice if you and Thayer came in with me as joint authors. It would be possible, I think, to arrange to have the work kept up as a Johns Hopkins Textbook of Medicine." This never came about. After Dr. Osler's death, the textbook was edited by Dr. Thomas McCrae until the completion of the twelfth edition in 1935. After the death of Dr. McCrae, Dr. Henry Christian continued as editor through the sixteenth and last edition published in 1947.

This current revision was conceived as a Johns Hopkins Textbook of Medicine as proposed by Osler. There was hesitancy to assume this task in view of the several excellent, comprehensive textbooks of medicine already available. However, it was decided that there was a need for a different type of textbook, one which would complement the existent encyclopedic texts. This text emphasizes clinical problems rather than disease entities. It attempts to describe and define the way in which the experienced physician approaches the solution and management of such problems.

This is clearly not a revision of Dr. Osler's great book. Nor is it the product of a single author. Rather, it is the product of a single department in which the preservation of a heritage of clinical excellence has been a major goal. We hope this volume reflects the tradition of excellence which this Department of Medicine received from Dr. Osler.

THE EDITORS

FOREWORD

IN THE PRACTICE OF MEDICINE the physician is confronted by three basic questions:

1. What is the matter with the patient?
2. What can I do for him?
3. What will be the outcome?

A fourth question, Why did it happen? will also arise in the mind of the inquiring physician who feels that each patient affords an opportunity and imposes a responsibility to contribute to a better understanding of causation and prevention.

The usual textbook of medicine does not prepare the practitioner to deal systematically with these questions. Its focus is upon the disease rather than the patient. It presents its subject matter in a series of essays each devoted to a description—as simple and straightforward as possible—of the disease entity. Some general information may be provided but rarely is sufficient emphasis placed upon the confusing complexities which arise in the day-to-day investigation and management of clinical problems.

The answer to the first of the questions enumerated above is the key to the answers to the second and third. The first question is the only one that requires an analytical approach, and obviously the analysis must begin with a study of the patient and must continue to be focused upon him until a solution is reached.

It is our purpose to produce a book which is built around the patient rather than the disease—the patient and the problems which he presents in diagnosis, management, and prognosis. Consideration will be given to the methods employed in acquiring factual data, the discriminating use of ancillary diagnostic techniques, and the systematic analysis of the accumulated information. This book also presents the essential information necessary for an understanding of the basic mechanisms involved in the various manifestations of disease, the important features of the natural history of the major diseases, the principles involved in the management of the patient, and the estimation of the probable outcome. In order to devote more space to the sequential steps which should be taken by the physician seeking the answers to his three basic questions, we have avoided as far as possible duplication of the type of presentation so successfully employed in texts already available. Since much of the material contained in current texts is to be sacrificed, the physician may have to turn elsewhere to fill the gaps in his knowledge of the subject in hand. To meet this need for quick access to more detailed information on specific topics, particular attention has been devoted to the selection and cross-indexing of the bibliography.

THE EDITORS

THE PRINCIPLES AND PRACTICE OF MEDICINE

Twentieth Edition

SECTION ONE
The Approach to the Patient*

To those who have chosen a career in medicine there can be no better basic motto than to strive to be a person with technical skill, broad scientific knowledge and wisdom, and with those personal characteristics of warmth and humility which serve to cement the art with the science of medicine. Such a person exemplifies the inscription on the statue of Edward Livingston Trudeau: "To cure sometimes, to relieve often, to comfort always."

Every student and practitioner of medicine should familiarize himself with the classic essay on *The Care of the Patient* by Francis Peabody.[1]

> The practice of medicine in its broadest sense includes the whole relationship of the physician with his patient. It is an art, based to an increasing extent on the medical sciences but comprising much that still remains outside the realm of any science. The art of medicine and the science of medicine are not antagonistic but supplementary to each other. There is no more contradiction between the science of medicine and the art of medicine than between the science of aeronautics and the art of flying. Good practice presupposes an understanding of the sciences which contribute to the structure of modern medicine, but it is obvious that sound professional training should include a much broader equipment.
>
> The treatment of disease may be entirely impersonal; the care of a patient must be completely personal. The significance of the intimate personal relationship between physician and patient cannot be too strongly emphasized, for in an extraordinarily large number of cases both diagnosis and treatment are directly dependent on it, and failure of the young physician to establish this relationship accounts for much of his ineffectiveness in the care of patients.
>
> What is spoken of as a "clinical picture" is not just a photograph of a man sick in bed; it is an impressionistic painting of the patient surrounded by his home, his work, his relations, his friends, his joys, sorrows, hopes, and fears.
>
> Thus, the physician who attempts to take care of a patient while he neglects those factors which contribute to the emotional life of this patient is as unscientific as the investigator who neglects to control all the conditions which may affect his experiment. The good physician knows his patients through and through and his knowledge is bought dearly. Time, sympathy and understanding must be lavishly dispensed but the reward is to be found in that personal bond which forms the greatest satisfaction of the practice of medicine. One of the essential qualities of the clinician is interest in humanity, for the secret of the care of the patient is in caring for the patient.

These beautifully expressed thoughts about the physician and his relationship to the patient are even more important to emphasize today than when they were written over 50 years ago. Medicine has become, and will continue to become, much more a science, not less, so that the physician of tomorrow will have to be more a scientist, not less. Nevertheless, the art of medicine remains, and the physician must continue to be wise and understanding with a deep respect for the patient as a human being. The secret of success in the care *of* the patient is still in caring *for* the patient.

CHAPTER 1

Clinical Information and Clinical Problem Solving
RICHARD J. JOHNS

The kind of patient care described by Peabody[1] in the introduction is the goal of all conscientious physicians. The effectiveness of patient care depends upon a number of factors, but two of the principal determinants of concern of physicians are 1) the quality of the diagnostic management; and 2) the quality of therapeutic management. Diagnostic management of a patient encompasses all of the steps which lead

---

* Contributors to this section in previous editions included Rex B. Conn, Martin W. Donner, John B. Imboden, Louis C. Lasagna, Robert E. Miller, Anthony J. Reading, Roger C. Sanders, Philip A. Tumulty, and Henry N. Wagner, Jr.

from the patient's complaints to a clear understanding of the patient's problems. Therapeutic management of a patient encompasses all of the measures directed toward correcting or alleviating the patient's problems. Taken together, these activities, diagnostic and therapeutic management, can be considered to be two aspects of clinical problem solving.

All textbooks have limitations. This is evident when one attempts to teach the basic precepts of medical practice by the written word alone. Attitudes, values, and professional integrity are acquired principally through precept and experience rather than by didactic means. That is why clinical teaching must go on around the bedside as well as through books. The fact that these aspects of the practice of medicine may often seem neglected in textbooks is in no way intended to deemphasize their importance. It is simply an acknowledgment of a reality: that much of the burden for imparting these precepts falls more heavily on clinical teachers than on textbooks. Wherever such material can be meaningfully rendered into print, we have attempted to include it in this book.

This initial chapter is designed to give the reader a summary overview of this process of solving a patient's clinical problem. The subsequent chapters address the process in more detail: the collection and the evaluation of clinical information, the ways in which information is analyzed and synthesized, and the basis of clinical decision making. The final chapter is devoted to the difficult issues in patient management.

CLINICAL PROBLEM SOLVING

Experienced clinicians approach and solve the problems of their patients with apparent ease. The novice, in contrast, may have difficulty eliciting even the basic information about the patient's problem. This paradox has led some to ascribe this skill in problem solving to "experience," to the "art of medicine," clinical "insight," or "judgment." To be sure, problem-solving ability improves with experience, and there are important humanistic elements in obtaining clinical information which are artful. Nevertheless, such formulations are not instructive to the novice who wishes to learn these skills or to the practitioner who wishes to improve his clinical ability.

Clinical problem solving is neither an arcane art nor a mysterious process. It is a method which parallels the scientific problem-solving process, as will be described below. It is a method that can be both taught and learned. It requires both knowledge and skill, and these skills can be refined only through practice.

Clinical problem solving is the cornerstone of clinical medicine.

THE SCIENTIFIC METHOD

This analytic process by which clinical information leads to the diagnosis is closely akin to the scientific method—the process whereby experimentation leads to the discovery of new knowledge.

As shown in Figure 1-1, the experiment yields data. Through analysis of these data and an extraction of meaning from them, an hypothesis is formulated which will explain the observed facts. The process does not stop at that point. The scientist then designs a further experiment which will test (support or refute) the current hypothesis. The scientist may also have formulated alternative hypotheses and will design an experiment to distinguish between them.

In the clinical setting, the experimental procedure may be the interrogation of the patient, the examination of the patient, or the performance of some laboratory test (Fig. 1-2). The resulting information is analyzed by differential diagnosis (consideration of all reasonable possibilities) to yield a tentative hypothesis (tentative diagnosis or diagnoses). These, in turn, prompt the clinician to ask further questions, make further observations, or order tests which will support, refute, or distinguish between the diagnoses under consideration. Figure 1-2 also illustrates the cyclic or iterative nature of this process.

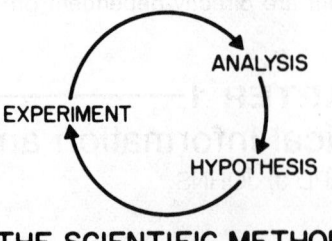

THE SCIENTIFIC METHOD

FIGURE 1-1. This illustrates the recursive nature of the scientific method in which the analysis of experimental data leads to the formulation of an hypothesis. This hypothesis, in turn, suggests further experimental studies which will test the hypothesis.

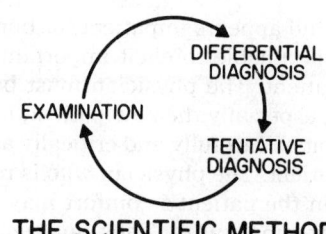

THE SCIENTIFIC METHOD IN THE CLINICAL SETTING

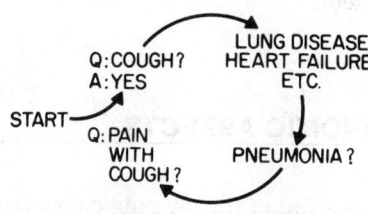

CLINICAL EXAMPLE

FIGURE 1–2. This shows the clear parallel between the general scientific method (Fig. 1–1) and the scientific method applied in the clinical setting. In the upper illustration experimental data are obtained through examination; analysis of these data is called differential diagnosis; the formulation of an hypothesis is stated as a tentative diagnosis. This tentative diagnosis, or hypothesis, is tested by obtaining further data through further examination. The clinical example shown in the lower portion is drawn from history taking.

The discussion of these similarities is not mere pedantry. It leads to a number of practical points:

1. The collection and analysis of clinical information is essentially the application of the scientific method to the solution of a clinical problem.

2. These methods can be taught and learned; it is not an art in which one is either gifted or not. Proficiency can be improved by consciously considering the meaning of each piece of information as it is received.

3. It is a rapidly iterative process. The cycle is repeated *within* the time interval of asking a few questions or physical observations. This explains the mystery of why the novice fails to ask the key question or seek the key physical finding.

4. It is an ongoing process. There are no irrefutable hypotheses, only unrefuted hypotheses. In clinical terms, the physician should not arrive at a diagnosis and abandon any further consideration of alternative explanations. He must remain alert for information which does

not fit with his current hypothesis and for sources of new information which might make him alter his considerations. When uncertain, he should continue to seek ways of testing the tentative diagnosis.

5. Consideration of a diagnosis that can neither be confirmed nor excluded fails to advance the decision-making process. This is directly parallel to a scientific hypothesis that cannot be tested.

6. Finally, clinical problem solving is as sensitive to flawed or missing information as are scientific experiments. A major difference lies in the fact that often clinical decisions must be made on what is acknowledged to be incomplete evidence.

In summary, the diagnostic process is a dynamic one which begins with the initial contact with the patient. Each piece of information obtained from or about the patient prompts the physician to consider new hypotheses and to test or to discard others. Studies indicate that skilled physicians may consider 15 or 20 diagnostic possibilities during the initial contact with the patient, but they rarely have more than 5 or 6 possibilities under active consideration at any one time.

Many students are taught that differential diagnosis is limited to an orderly, formal consideration of all of the diagnostic possibilities which is performed only after all of the clinical information has been acquired. This is a counterproductive notion. A review of the diagnostic possibilities at that point is helpful, but it is the rapid iteration of the diagnostic process throughout the encounter with the patient that enables the physician to obtain the information that will lead him to the appropriate conclusion.

INFORMATION *VERSUS* DATA

Clinical information can be obtained from the patient himself through dialogue (the history) or through observation (the physical examination). Information may also be obtained from laboratory or radiographic examinations. These sources of information (dialogue, observation, the laboratory) are quite separate and distinct. These distinctions, however, obscure the similar way in which the experienced physician uses clinical data whatever their source.

In each instance this collection of clinical information is not simply data collection. Data are a group of facts, whereas information implies the communication of knowledge. Thus, clinical information imparts meaning; it is meaningful data, not just an ensemble of facts. Furthermore, information may prompt the physician to take certain actions, actions which include seeking further information.

This distinction between data and information can be exemplified. A patient complains of weakness and breathlessness and is found to have a blood pressure of 135/80 mm Hg. The information content of this datum, 135/80, is usually taken to be that this patient's blood pressure is normal. However, the information, or the meaning of this, is quite different if last week the data included a blood pressure of 190/110 mm Hg. Now, the physician knows the patient was hypertensive and is presently normotensive. This prompts the collection of more information regarding the possibility of recent myocardial infarction, blood loss, and the like.

This distinction between data and information explains one of the mysteries of history taking. For example, the complete novice can ask all the "usual" questions and record the patient's answers with fidelity. Such an interview (data collection) may not impart much knowledge about the patient's problem even when these data are subsequently reviewed by an expert. The communication of clinical information imparts meaning to the experienced interviewer which guides and directs his further dialogue with the patient. Thus, each datum communicates information to the experienced person. From this it is apparent that some important analysis occurs during the course of the collection of clinical information. Analysis is not simply a separate, subsequent event.

This leads to the following dicta: 1) The experienced clinician weighs each piece of clinical data as he elicits it for its meaning, for its information content. 2) He also analyzes it in the context of other information about the patient to determine if there is still more information which should be acquired. 3) The collection and analysis of clinical information proceed in parallel, not as separate, sequential steps.

HUMANISTIC ASPECTS

None of the foregoing emphasis on the scientific aspects of the collection and analysis of clinical information should be interpreted as deprecation of the importance of the humanistic aspects of dealing with patients. Indeed, disregard of these aspects can even prevent the collection of clinical information. The physician who appears impatient, or bored, or insensitive may be unable to elicit important information from the patient. The physician must be aware that the patient, especially the new patient, is scrutinizing him every bit as carefully and critically as he is examining the patient. The physician who is rough and uninterested in the patient's comfort may be unable to feel an abdominal mass. Thus, inattention to these important aspects may defeat the whole purpose of clinical information analysis—the solution of a patient's problem.

ECONOMIC ASPECTS

A major complaint of the lay public concerning modern medical care is its "excessive" cost. Many believe that the clinical problem-solving process, both diagnostic and therapeutic, is too costly. Yet the individual patient insists upon and is entitled to high quality medical care. Are these positions antithetical?

The direct answer is that these are not antithetical views. Every physician has as a part of his responsibility to his patients the obligation not to waste clinical resources. Irrelevant or redundant laboratory data do not improve the quality of care, but they do contribute substantially to the cost of care. This topic will be addressed later in this section when discussing the prudent use of ancillary studies in diagnostic management and in discussing prudent therapeutic management. It will also be addressed throughout the book in outlining the optimum sequence in the diagnostic management of specific clinical problems. Inept sequences are a major source of waste. For example, when dealing with the problem of anemia it is wasteful and pointless to obtain serum iron, folate, and B_{12} determinations simultaneously before determining whether the patient's red cells are normocytic, macrocytic, or microcytic. We shall outline a series of questions that a clinician can ask when selecting ancillary tests and procedures in the investigation of a problem in which he is not experienced (Chap. 2).

Other aspects contributing needlessly to the expense of hospital medical care include 1) hospitalizing patients for problems that can readily be managed on an ambulatory basis; 2) failing to use effectively the time during which the patient is hospitalized; and 3) failing to plan in advance for the patient's discharge from hospital. These, too, are items of expense that detract from rather than contribute to the quality of care given to the patient.

SUMMARY

This chapter supports the view that the collection and analysis of clinical information, whatever its source, is the cornerstone of patient care. The skills involved can be taught and learned. The approach is similar to any scientific problem-solving endeavor, but the ef- fective physician must have an understanding of the humanistic elements involved in the care of the sick.

In the subsequent chapters of this section the various ways of acquiring and analyzing clinical in- formation will be discussed. Furthermore, attention will be given to the use of this information in the diag- nostic and therapeutic management of patients.

CHAPTER 2
The Collection and Evaluation of Clinical Information
RICHARD J. JOHNS

Clinical information encompasses information ob- tained by conversing with the patient and his rela- tives (the history), information obtained by observing and examining the patient (the physical examina- tion), as well as information obtained through labora- tory examinations of the patient or specimens ob- tained from the patient (laboratory tests), and from special procedures such as endoscopy. Different tech- niques are required for the collection and evaluation of these different kinds of information. Before dis- cussing these specific examples, we should consider certain common features which influence the selec- tion of what information should be obtained and how it should be evaluated whatever its source.

ATTRIBUTES OF CLINICAL INFORMATION

It is neither possible nor desirable to obtain *all* clini- cal information on *every* patient. As a consequence, there must be some selectivity in choosing what in- formation to obtain. How does one make this deci- sion? A number of attributes of clinical information are important in making this selective judgment. These include the information's 1) accuracy, 2) preci- sion, 3) variance, 4) specificity, 5) sensitivity, 6) valid- ity, 7) risk, 8) cost, and 9) benefit. For example, the wise physician would not choose to obtain informa- tion of dubious validity, particularly if its collection is associated with some risk.

Physicians are accustomed to think that these at- tributes apply only to laboratory tests. They apply to all types of clinical information, including historical facts and physical findings as well. Does the absence of a history of rheumatic fever exclude the possibility of rheumatic mitral insufficiency? Does a lid-lag spe- cifically mean hyperthyroidism? Is a liver edge palpa- ble 1 cm below the costal margin normal? These questions are as amenable to assessment as the ques- tion: Does a fasting blood glucose concentration of 124 mg/dl mean diabetes mellitus?

A clear understanding of these attributes is fun- damental to the selection and evaluation of all kinds of clinical information. In the discussion which fol- lows, we shall draw upon nonlaboratory examples wherever possible to emphasize the breadth of appli- cability of these concepts.

ACCURACY
Accuracy is the measure of how closely the given piece of clinical information represents the correct and true state. The usual examples drawn from clini- cal chemistry indicate that the accuracy of blood glu- cose concentrations are assessed by analyzing repli- cates of an authentic glucose standard. The test is deemed to be accurate if there is close agreement be- tween the observed and the true value.

This concept of accuracy is equally applicable to historical information.[14] When asking about alcohol consumption, the patient may indicate he drinks only one or two cocktails before dinner. This is accurate information if it reflects the true state. It is not accu- rate if he in fact has two cocktails before lunch, three before dinner, and several more drinks after dinner. Thus, if a piece of information is of particular impor- tance (or if there is reason to question its accuracy), the physician should take steps to authenticate it be- fore using it in his analysis of a problem. This princi- ple of authentication applies to historical information and physical findings as well as to laboratory tests and special procedures.

PRECISION

Precision is a measure of the reproducibility of a piece of information. A common measure of precision is to note the variability, or variance, in the results when the observation is repeated on replicates or on successive occasions. Blood pressure measurements by auscultation may be consistent and reproducible in a hypotensive patient, but they may not accurately reflect the true intra-arterial pressure. In this example the measurement would be precise, but inaccurate. It is a common error to consider information which is highly reproducible (precise) to be accurate. Precise information may or may not be accurate. (It is not possible to have information which is accurate, but imprecise.)

VARIANCE

The variability in observations, including clinical observations, come from several sources.[24] Some are attributable to the observational method itself, some to the observer, and some to the feature being observed. A simple example—determining the location of the liver edge by palpation—can illustrate these points.

Suppose one observer reports the liver edge to be two fingerbreadths below the right costal margin and another reports it to be 4 cm below. One source of variance stems from using a variable unit of measurement of size, distance, and the like (fingerbreadths, hen's eggs, golf balls); this source of variance is easily avoided. Apart from this, there is variance from quantizing: On one occasion a 3.5 cm measurement might be rounded up to 4 cm and on another down to 3 cm. Even greater variance can be introduced by the methodology. Was the measurement made with the patient fully supine? Was it in full inspiration? These all contribute to the *variance of the method*.

There may be differences in the way the observer performs the measurement from time to time which leads to *intraobserver variance*. There are also differences between the way different observers perform the measurement, *interobserver variance*.

Still another kind of variance relates to differences in the location of the liver edge from one person to another. This kind of variance of an attribute will be discussed in the context of normality and the normal range.

DIAGNOSTIC SPECIFICITY AND SENSITIVITY[7,9,11,35]

The specificity of clinical information and its sensitivity are important in assessing its meaning, yet these terms are often only vaguely or imperfectly understood. Specificity and sensitivity relate to the infer-

---

TABLE 2–1
Relationship Between Findings and Conditions

Condition	Finding	
	Positive	Negative
Present	True positive (TP)	False negative (FN)
Absent	False positive (FP)	True negative (TN)

---

ences which may be drawn about the patient's *condition* based upon the presence or absence of a certain *finding*. The condition may be a disease, e.g., diabetes mellitus, or an abnormality, e.g., pulmonary consolidation, and the finding may be a laboratory test result, historical fact, or physical finding.

Table 2–1 indicates the four possible relationships between a finding and a condition. It would be ideal if a positive finding were invariably associated with the condition; this would be perfect specificity. It would also be ideal if a negative finding invariably meant that the condition were absent; that would be perfect sensitivity. Unfortunately, such perfection rarely obtains, and there are falsely positive findings (the condition is actually absent) and falsely negative findings (the condition is actually present).

The clinician must have some insight into the likelihood that a positive finding is a true positive or a false positive when interpreting a finding. Similarly, a negative finding must be interpreted in view of the likelihood that it is a false negative. Furthermore, the choice of a procedure which is highly specific or is very sensitive will depend upon whether the objective is to confirm (rule in) the condition or exclude its presence (rule out). Table 2–2 summarizes the differences between specificity and sensitivity.

Specificity

Egophony over the right lower lobe is a finding which has a high degree of specificity for the condition, pulmonary consolidation of the right lower lobe. As can be seen in Table 2–2, this positive finding is useful in ruling in pulmonary consolidation. The reason that it is useful is that most positive findings are true positives (FP $\ll$ TP), and it is highly specific (FP $\ll$ TN). The absence of egophony, however, cannot be used to exclude the presence of consolidation.

An example of specific test is the finding of *M. tuberculosis* on sputum culture. It is highly predictive

TABLE 2-2
Properties of Specific and Sensitive Findings

	Specific Test or Finding	Sensitive Test or Finding
Purpose or utility	To confirm the presence of the disease or condition (rule in) by means of a *positive* result	To exclude the presence of the disease or condition (rule out) by means of a *negative* result
Designed to maximize	The fraction of positive results (TP + FP) which are true positives (TP), or	The fraction of negative results (TN + FN) which are true negatives (TN), or
Predictive value	$\dfrac{TP}{TP\ +\ FP}$	$\dfrac{TN}{TN\ +\ FN}$
Indeterminate result	When negative, condition may or may not be present	When positive, condition may or may not be present

of the presence of the condition, active pulmonary tuberculosis. Again, the failure to culture tubercle bacilli in the sputum does not exclude the possibility of active pulmonary disease.

Sensitivity

Stiffness of the neck is a sensitive test for acute meningitis. This means that if there is no evidence of stiffness of the neck, it is unlikely that the patient has an acute meningitis. As shown in Table 2–2, most negative findings are true negatives, there are very few false negatives, i.e., patients with acute meningitis who have no stiffness of the neck.

Nuchal rigidity is certainly not a specific test for acute meningitis, for most positives are *not* true positives. Indeed, its predictive value is poor since most patients with stiff necks do not have acute meningitis, but have some other condition.

The analogous sensitive test would be the tuberculin skin test. A negative test result makes active tuberculosis unlikely, but a positive test is not necessarily associated with active disease.

Logical and Strategic Errors

The chief logical errors have already been mentioned and illustrated in Table 2–2. A negative specific finding does not exclude the condition, and a positive sensitive test does not necessarily mean the condition is present.

Strategic errors are also possible. The first kind of strategic error is to fail to weigh the consequences of being wrong. For example, the consequences of failing to treat acute bacterial meningitis are grave. Accordingly, in a patient with fever, headache, and mental confusion one would pursue the diagnosis of meningitis with a specific test, such as lumbar puncture, even if there were no stiffness of the neck. Where the cost of error is high, even a slight risk of a false negative result is unacceptable.

Similarly, it is a strategic error to embark upon a risky diagnostic or therapeutic venture based upon a solitary positive specific finding, especially if there is no collateral evidence to support it.

Finally, there is the problem which arises from screening patient populations for conditions with a low prevalence. Let us assume the use of a highly specific test for a certain kind of cancer has a specificity of 0.98. This is equivalent to having only 2 percent false positives among those not having the condition. If this test is applied to a population whose prevalence of this cancer is 100 per 100,000, we would expect approximately 100 true positives and 2,000 false positives per 100,000. Thus, among those having positive tests, only 5 percent would have cancer and 95 percent would not. All of these patients would be subjected to the anguish and to the expense and perhaps risk of having further examinations to determine whether their test was truly or falsely positive. In this example the benefit to the 5 percent may outweigh the discomfiture to the 95 percent. If, however, the test has only slightly less specificity, say 0.90, the expected false positive would be 99 percent of all positives.

The two key points are that the physician must have some notion of 1) the prevalence of the condition *in the population being screened* (not some other population); and 2) the specificity of the test or finding being used. The implication of the first point is that a screening procedure that is appropriate for patients consulting a cardiologist may be totally inappropriate when applied to patients consulting a general practitioner. For example, the prevalence of coronary artery disease would be much higher in the former group.

RISK, COST, AND BENEFIT

Risks and costs relate to the *collection* of clinical information, not to the information itself. The benefits, if any, accrue from the *use* to which the information is put, not from simply possessing the information. Consideration of risks, costs, and benefits are important in determining what clinical information to collect. As will be shown, these considerations are not limited to high-risk or high-cost decisions, nor should consideration be limited to those interested in medical ethics (risk *vs.* benefit) or medical economics (cost *vs.* benefit).

Benefits from clinical information may be diagnostic, therapeutic, or prognostic. Since the collection of information is almost always associated with some cost, and perhaps even some minimal risk, there is no merit in collecting a piece of clinical information if it is of no benefit to the patient.

There are three common problems concerning benefit. First, there is the problem of clinical information obtained by habit. For example, there may be reason to repeat a patient's white blood cell count, but was the differential count beneficial or was it simply requested by habit? Is 12 months the appropriate interval for a "check-up" for an asymptomatic, apparently disease-free person? What information should be collected in such a "check-up"? Even acknowledging that sometimes it is cheaper and more efficient to collect certain information than it is to decide whether or not to obtain it, we should periodically pause to question the benefit of some of our "routine procedures."

Second, physicians sometimes fail to distinguish between clinical interest and patient benefit. It may be of considerable interest to repeat a liver biopsy on a patient with hepatitis, but it is not justifiable unless the information would alter the patient's management. A good test is to ask, "What would I do differently if the result is A *vs.* B *vs.* C?" If the course of action is the same whatever the result, there is usually no clinical benefit from possessing the information.

This issue of clinical interest should not be confused with clinical investigation. In that latter circumstance it may be justified to obtain information that is of no benefit to the patient (if the legal and ethical requirements are met). The justification is based on the fact that a nontrivial question has been asked and that the information being sought will contribute to the answer.

The third problem is the most difficult, the notion of marginal benefit. This issue arises most often in obtaining information to exclude a diagnostic possibility. Take the case of a patient for whom there is reason to suspect infective endocarditis. There is clearly potential benefit from obtaining several blood cultures. If the first five cultures are negative, what is

the benefit (the marginal, or incremental, benefit) of obtaining one more? If ten are negative, what is the benefit of obtaining one more? Since the patient may *not* have infective endocarditis, and since in some patients *with* endocarditis the bacteria cannot be demonstrated on culture, when should one stop collecting information? Put another way, the probable benefit from collecting additional information is steadily decreasing. Similar questions may arise in seeking the site of occult gastrointestinal bleeding, or seeking the primary site of a metastatic carcinoma. In each, the issue is how far to go in the face of negative results and a declining marginal benefit. In the example of suspected endocarditis there are data to suggest the prudent course, but in most instances we have no data on marginal benefit.[27,28,34]

Risk assessment in medicine is not an exact science, and assessment of risk *vs.* benefit, or risk/benefit ratio is even less exact, since benefit must also be quantified. The difficulties in assessing risk are several: 1) The probability of a given untoward outcome is often not known. 2) There are difficulties in weighing the severity of unfavorable outcomes. (Which is worse, a 0.1 probability of thrombocytopenia or a 0.0001 probability of respiratory arrest?) 3) There are important variations in risk factors among different patients with different diseases. This ability to balance risks *vs.* benefits, although poorly understood, is generally done conscientiously and comfortably. A common shortcoming, as mentioned before, results from undertaking procedures which have low (but not zero) risk and no benefit.

Physicians are primarily concerned with the benefits of clinical information. While they are also concerned with the associated risks, they are often much less concerned about the costs. Concerns about costs usually focus on high-cost tests and procedures and extend to being certain that they are clinically indicated. It is appropriate that cost not be considered to be a deterrent to obtaining needed information. Nonetheless, more attention should be given to the total cost of the high volume, low-cost tests that may be of no benefit to the patient. These are the tests and studies ordered by habit which were mentioned before.

EVALUATION

NORMALITY

In the assessment of clinical information, the most common evaluation is to determine whether a given finding is normal or abnormal. The term "normal" is subject to varied interpretations.* In the context of clinical decision making, we shall define a normal finding as one which is innocuous and warrants no diagnostic or therapeutic action. An abnormal finding, then, is one that is not innocuous and may warrant action. Such evaluations of normality are not limited to comparing the patient's fasting blood glucose with the "normal range" of blood glucose. Similar evaluations are performed on historical information: How many tampons per day represent a normal menstrual flow *vs.* menorrhagia? Similar issues are raised in assessing physical findings such as retinal arteriolar narrowing, pallor of mucous membranes, obesity, and findings that imply abnormality.

In principle, assessment of normality is straightforward. One compares the given observation in the patient with similar observations in a group of comparable persons known to be normal and free of disease. This implies that we know 1) the normal group is normal and disease-free, 2) that they are comparable to the patient (age, sex, ethnic origin, and the like), 3) the range of variation with the normal group, and 4) the criteria for defining abnormality.

In practice, we usually do not have valid information on these points. The control group may be a nonrandom sample of apparently healthy persons. Their age and sex distribution may not be known. The assessment of range and limits of normality may be based on statistical assumptions that are unproven or invalid.[16]

Fortunately, many clinical observations are either clearly normal or abnormal, and there is no difficulty in making the decision. In some instances the patient's findings are borderline, and the aforementioned problems arise. A brief example will serve to illustrate them.

It is relatively simple to obtain an accurate measurement of a patient's body weight. Having obtained this information, how do you determine if the patient's weight is normal or if he is overweight? When the patient is grossly overweight, the answer is obvious and no refined comparison is needed. Indeed, one need not have weighed the patient. In less obvious

instances one must have data on body weight of normal subjects and a criterion for abnormality.

The usual approach to this problem is to consult a table listing average weight and range by height, sex, and body build. For example, adult males with a height of 5 feet 11 inches and medium build are listed as having an average weight of 158 pounds and a normal range of 144 to 179. Thus, if the patient weighed 180 pounds he would be evaluated as being slightly overweight. These commonly used tables, however, are not data obtained from surveying a sample of normal population. They are derived from life insurance information and reflect the average body weight associated with the minimum mortality.[25] These ideal weights probably form a better basis for comparison than population-derived norms, for independent measures suggest our population is overweight and as a consequence population means are higher than the ideal weight.

Body weight also illustrates the added information content of individual norms or individual time trends. A weight of 180 pounds today has additional meaning if the patient weighed 190 pounds 2 months ago. That is, a weight gain, or loss, has greater value than knowing the weight at one point in time.

In summary, each piece of clinical information should prompt the question, "Is this normal or abnormal?" In making this evaluation, knowledge is required of the range observed in normal subjects and that these subjects are comparable to the patient. Finally, additional information can be gleaned from comparing current and past observations in the same individual, since in many instances the variance in a given person is far less than the variance in the population, and time trends may provide added insights.

CLINICAL IMPORT

Once it is established that a finding is abnormal, there is a second level of evaluation which occurs almost imperceptibly. How important is this abnormal finding? Some findings are always important, that is, they require explanation. The history of hematemesis, the finding of a hard lymph node, and an elevated serum calcium concentration are always important. Other clinical information may be conditionally important. For example, the history of a nosebleed may be important in the context of a bleeding disorder, but otherwise inconsequential. Finding a broken tooth may be important in the context of a patient with a pulmonary abscess (possible aspiration), but otherwise trivial.

Information that is either intrinsically or conditionally important must be carefully verified. The

---

* Murphy[11] points out that "normal serum cholesterol level" may mean: 1) a bell-shaped probability distribution of cholesterol values; 2) the most representative cholesterol value as defined by a mean; 3) the most commonly encountered cholesterol values as defined by a range. This is the usual "laboratory normal range"; 4) cholesterol values most suited for reproduction and survival; 5) cholesterol values unlikely to cause harm; 6) a committee's consensus, that is, "approved" cholesterol values; and 7) the ideal cholesterol value.

next chapter emphasizes the analysis which important clinical findings demand. When a patient states he has been "spitting up blood," it is essential that you determine whether he coughed up blood, vomited blood, or simply expectorated blood from a nosebleed.

CONVERSING WITH PATIENTS AND OBTAINING A HISTORY

GENERAL CONSIDERATIONS

Vital clinical information is derived from conversation with the patient. This process, often called "history taking," is not simply a question and answer session, it is a dialogue. The physician must listen with care to what the patient is saying, he must interpret what the patient is trying to say, and he must be attuned to what the patient does not say—topics and issues the patient avoids.

The principal complaint which patients make about "modern scientific medicine" is the failure of physicians to communicate with them adequately. A physician should recognize this and be aware that his conversations with the patient can accomplish a great deal of good. He should also realize that ill-conceived or misinterpreted conversations can result in great, even irreparable, harm to the patient.

This section is first concerned with the information-gathering aspects of conversing with patients. Finally, some of the other aspects of communicating with patients (explaining, answering questions, counseling) are discussed.

OBTAINING THE HISTORY[5,6,10,12]

History taking involves several distinct elements. One aspect involves the elicitation of straightforward factual information, e.g., "Does anyone in your family have diabetes?" If provision is made for further explanation of the question, the expert, the novice, or even a simple questionnaire can obtain this type of information with equal facility.

A second aspect involves branching to other questions depending upon the patient's response to an earlier question. Here, one sees differences between the expert and the novice. For example, when asked whether he has headaches, the patient may reply, "occasionally." The novice may simply record "occasional headaches," but the more experienced clinician will want to explore further the nature of these headaches—are they caused by emotional tension, hypertension, sinusitis, or brain tumor? He will

ask questions in an attempt to distinguish between these possibilities. Thus, the skilled physician will analyze the historical data while acquiring them. Furthermore, he will act on this analysis in order to ask other questions that develop the data further. The physician traverses the cycle shown in Figure 1–2 with each response.

A third aspect relates to the rich and relatively unstructured information about the patient's complaint, the history of his present illness. Obtaining this information embodies the elements discussed above, but it also requires flexibility, analysis, interpretation, assessment of nuances and nonverbal communication. In these areas the expert clinician excels.

Finally, it must be emphasized that taking a history is not an isolated, circumscribed procedure. Further historical information may be gathered during the physical examination, upon examining laboratory results, or later in the course of the patient's illness. For example, finding a murmur of mitral stenosis demands questioning the patient again about sore throats, manifestations of rheumatic fever, and congestive failure. Similarly, finding an apical infiltrate on chest film requires reexploration of symptoms referable to tuberculosis.

Practical Considerations

Since the initial taking of a history is usually the physician's introduction to the patient, it is important that this relationship get off to a good start. Some practical considerations to successful history taking are described in the following paragraphs.

1. Make the patient comfortable, both physically and mentally. A few moments spent in friendly conversation will allow the patient to settle down before proceeding to the business at hand.

2. Make certain the patient knows who you are and understands your role in his care. With team approaches to patient care there is increasing opportunity for confusion which leads to uncertainty and resentment.

3. In general, interview the patient alone. At times, a parent or spouse may insist upon being present. Try to avoid this, but do not force the issue against strong opposition. On the other hand, family members may be a source of valuable information which should be sought at an appropriate time. This is obvious when the patient is unable to communicate adequately because of the nature of his illness or its severity. In other instances, the family may possess information not known by the patient, or which he is unwilling to disclose (for example, failure to take prescribed medications, personality deterioration, change in appearance, and alcoholism).

4. Give the patient the conviction that he has a warm and understanding listener and adequate time in which to tell his whole story. The patient must feel that the physician has no distracting concerns or commitments. Avoid writing detailed notes while the patient is talking. The atmosphere should be one of thoughtful conversation, not the dictation of a diary.

5. Meaningful questions cannot be asked without an understanding of the general nature of the patient's problem. Hence, at the outset afford the patient enough time to express in his own terms, without interruption, his basic reasons for visiting you. Otherwise, questioning of the patient will be routine, haphazard, and unrevealing.

6. The sequence in which the history is obtained is dictated by the specific circumstances. Thus, if the patient is severely ill, infirm, or emotionally upset, it is wise to inquire about the present illness before reviewing the past health and the family history. Since the patient is most interested in his current problem, this sequence which begins with the present illness is generally preferable.

7. Assure the patient that you appreciate that he may have forgotten much of his past history, and not to be concerned if he has. This is of particular importance when talking to elderly patients who may feel inadequate and embarrassed by their difficulties with memory.

8. Encourage the patient to use his own words, and not simply to recite diagnoses and interpretations of other physicians.

9. Never make the patient feel inadequate, dull, or distraught. If a particular line of questioning makes the patient embarrassed or anxious, move on to another topic without pressing too far at the time of the initial encounter. However, it is wise to explore that topic later once rapport has been established, for such behavior may indicate significant information lies in that area.

10. Do not spend so much time and effort extracting specific details about less consequential points in the history that the patient's temper and the physician's energies are exhausted before the crucial items are reached.

11. As a corollary, do not let the patient's narrative bog down in needless detail or drift off into irrelevancies. The reminder must be gentle, "I believe you were telling me about . . . " lest the patient feel he has been chastised.

12. The patient must be requestioned as the illness proceeds and new information evolves. Neglect of this important point is a common cause of failure to make a correct diagnosis. Requestioning may also be necessary because the patient is too ill, tired, confused, or frightened at the time of the initial interview.

Begin at the Beginning

It is essential to delineate the exact manner in which the illness began. What were the precise circumstances of its onset? Where was the patient? What was he doing? One must be certain that the patient is actually starting his story at the beginning. Patients often date the onset of their illness by some dramatic occurrence, forgetting to tell the events which led up to it. These are frequently highly significant. Thus, the insidious onset of fatigue and mild weight loss may give important insight into the nature of an acute upper abdominal pain which started 6 months later. The physician must push the patient's recall back to the earliest beginnings of his illness. It may be helpful to ask the question, "Are you certain your health was entirely normal before this particular symptom began?" Often a reference to a date or season will prompt recollection. For example, "Were you feeling perfectly well last Christmas?"

Chronic, Recurrent Illness

When dealing with a complicated illness in which the basic pattern is recurrence of episodes of similar manifestations (e.g., fever and joint pains), one should acquire a detailed account of typical episodes. Often the initial and the most recent episodes are the most revealing and give insight into changes which may have occurred over time.

Importance of Details

Patients sometimes tell small details about their illnesses which are disregarded by the physician because at the time they do not seem pertinent to the rest of the story. For example, a patient insisted that he got chills, fever, and jaundice each time he took a cathartic, and only then. This detail did not make much sense and was ignored. Search for the usual causes of intermittent fever were unrevealing until the patient was given a cathartic and subsequently developed a temperature of 105° F, chills, and jaundice. He was later found to have diverticulitis of the colon with abscess formation. Cathartics precipitated acute episodes by showering his liver with septic emboli.

Avoid Bias

In taking a medical history, the physician must weigh and analyze the information as it is being acquired. As mentioned before, this formulation and testing of hypotheses as to what may be the cause of the patient's illness is a major element in the gathering of meaningful information. The physician must discipline himself, however, to avoid bias. He must not disregard or ignore information that does not fit with a current hypothesis that he has under consideration. Furthermore, he should not ask leading questions in a manner that makes it difficult for the patient to disagree. "You do find that greasy foods give you indigestion, don't you?" The history should be an unbiased statement of *all* the facts presented by the patient.

Be Critical

Do not accept uncritically such expressions as "arthritis," "eczema," "pneumonia," or "indigestion." An episode of "pneumonia" may, in reality, have been a pulmonary infarction, or "indigestion" may have been coronary insufficiency. Acquire the details and interpret the facts. Do not simply record the patient's own diagnosis; do not be biased by other physician's diagnoses. Conservative skepticism is a desirable trait.

Similarly, be cautious in evaluating such major symptoms as fever, weight loss, hemoptysis, hematemesis, black stools, chills, convulsions, hematuria, pain, and lapse of consciousness. These are often heralds of serious underlying disease and demand explanation.

Quantify Symptoms

Whenever possible, have the patient quantify his symptoms in simple terms. Thus, sputum production can be expressed in terms of cups, diarrhea in number of stools, dyspnea in flights of stairs, and orthopnea in number of pillows required for comfort in sleeping. Such manifestations take on increased significance when thus quantified.

Environmental Factors

Inquire whether the present illness was associated with alterations in the patient's environment. This could include any incident, such as going on a picnic in the country or getting a job in a slaughterhouse. Has anyone or anything (such as a dog or a pet bird) in the patient's home or work environment been ill in the recent past? Have any of the patient's relatives ever had a similar illness?

Drugs

If possible, list all the drugs the patient may have been taking, with the approximate dates on which they were administered. Describe any untoward reactions that the patient may have had to these agents. Delineate what effect, if any, they may have had upon the manifestations of the illness. Thus, in the differential diagnosis of acute polyarthritis it is important to know that adequate salicylate therapy failed to affect the degree of joint involvement.

It is often difficult to get an accurate history of drug usage, even when a drug reaction is suspected. Patients often regard as "drugs" only those medications that are expensive, prescribed, or given by injection. They may not realize that you want to know about *all* tablets, capsules, pills, and liquids. Commonly overlooked, but potentially important agents are sedatives, laxatives, tonics, "nerve medicines," "vitamins," birth control pills, and menstrual cramp remedies.

Other Information Sources

Valuable information contained in the records of previous hospitalizations is often allowed to lie fallow. A telephone call to a former physician, hospital history room, or corner drugstore may answer a perplexing problem. Thus, finding a coin lesion on a 10-year-old chest film may be the deciding factor in excluding cancer as its cause. A patient suspected of having ingested poison may be found, when the druggist is called, to have taken a harmless substance. Failure to explore these ancillary sources of information is a common and serious shortcoming.

Evaluate the Person

It is as important to understand the person afflicted by the disease as it is to understand the disease afflicting the person. Information about both are obtained at the same time. The patient's attitude, demeanor, and appearance all give the perceptive physician insights into the patient as does the way in which the patient relates to the physician.

The patient should be given an opportunity to discuss the way in which the illness has affected him. This permits the physician to evaluate the patient's reaction to the illness. Direct questions may be helpful: "How has all this affected you—your family, your job, your finances, your pursuit of pleasures?" "Has this illness gotten you down?"

It is also important to explore the patient's perception of his illness: "What do you make of this?" "What do you think is wrong?" "Do you feel you are getting better or worse?" "What is especially worrisome to you?" Quite often the physician is surprised to learn of the patient's misapprehensions. For example, it is important to know whether a worried patient with back pain is concerned about having cancer or about losing his job.

Only if the physician understands the patient can he deal with him effectively. In this regard, empathy is a useful diagnostic tool—by putting oneself in the patient's position one can be guided to areas which are of concern to the patient.

Encourage Communication

At the conclusion of the interview, it is helpful to say in an unhurried way, "Is there anything more you want to tell me . . . about anything at all?" Explain to the patient that you hope he will regard your office as a place in which he can feel free to discuss fully any and all matters which may be of concern to him.

PAIN AS A SYMPTOM

Pain merits special consideration since it is frequently the predominant or only clinical manifestation of a wide variety of disease processes. Pain serves to illustrate the proper analysis of an aspect of the patient's history, because, being a subjective manifestation of disease, it can be evaluated only through careful questioning of the patient. Carefully assessed, it stands preeminent among the manifestations of disease which lead to proper diagnosis.

Clinical Aspects

Several types of pain can be distinguished clinically.

Superficial pain derived from injury to skin and superficial somatic structures has two components. There is the sharp, pricking sensation which elicits a startle response, withdrawal, and tachycardia. The second, slower, aching component may persist for extended periods after the initial injury. These pains are felt superficially and can be localized with precision. In most instances the lesion producing the superficial pain is readily apparent. There are, however, two general exceptions. The first is pain caused by nerve or nerve root involvement, e.g., arm pain with cervical disc disease. The second is superficial pain referred from a deeper structure, e.g., wrist pain as a manifestation of angina pectoris.

Visceral pain is dull or aching; it is associated with quiescence, slowing of the pulse, often with some fall in blood pressure, and sweating and nausea. This last manifestation is responsible for the common designation of "sickening" when referring to deep pain. These vasovagal responses may be associated with all of the major visceral pain syndromes (angina pectoris; biliary, renal, and bowel colic; bladder pain; pancreatitis; peptic ulcer), especially when the pain is severe. These responses can also occur with injury to muscle, fascia, periosteum, or arteries.

Deep pain is often poorly localized and is felt to arise from an area beneath the surface rather than from a point. Vague localization and misleading re-

ferral of deep pain are two important problems in analyzing pain, e.g., diaphragmatic peritonitis produces pain referred to the shoulder.

Factors that alter pain perception are of clinical importance. It is clear that in the heat of an athletic event or of physical combat, a serious injury may be sustained without experiencing any pain whatsoever. Pain may not be perceived until the danger and excitement are over. In contrast, fear, anxiety, and apprehension all serve to heighten the perception of pain. These factors are of importance not only in evaluating pain, but also in alleviating pain. A different phenomenon is exhibited by patients with frontal lobe lesions. They perceive the pain, but it induces no emotional response. In contrast, there are some patients who hyperreact to pain.

Pain should always be methodically analyzed as follows: localization, radiation, character, exacerbating and ameliorating factors, associated phenomena, and time relationships. These will be discussed in turn.

Sequential Steps in the Analysis of Pain

LOCALIZATION. It is essential that the patient localize the point of origin of his discomfort as precisely as possible. The localization of pain is usually obvious when the lesion is superficial, but with deep pain the patient may confuse the area of radiation with its point of origin, and, hence, mislead the physician. It is best to request that the patient indicate with his index finger the area from which the discomfort seems to stem, and then to indicate the extent of diffusion of the pain around this point. Ask the patient to describe the depth at which the pain seems to be located. The pattern of pain arising from any given structure may be extremely variable. Thus, the pain of angina pectoris may be felt substernally, in the interscapular area, in the shoulder, down the arms, in the wrist or fingers, or in the neck or jaw.

RADIATION. It is also imperative that the patient trace with his finger the pattern of radiation of his distress in response to the question, "Where does your pain move?" It should be emphasized again that, when the point of origin of the pain is silent, the area of radiation may be assumed to be the site of origin. For example, angina pectoris may be present only as a peculiar sensation he gets in the left hand when he hurries for the bus, or a peptic ulcer may be mistaken for an orthopedic condition because the patient has recurrent severe pain in the midback.

CHARACTER. Questions to elicit information about pain must be carefully phrased. Patients are frequently unfamiliar with pain as an experience in life, and their concept of what the word "pain" connotes may be very limited. To some it may simply mean the sensation they had when they slammed a door on a finger or when they burned themselves in the kitchen. Many patients, therefore, will not be aware that they are experiencing what the physician calls pain. It is well to avoid use of the narrow question "Do you have pain?" and to employ broader expressions such as "distress" "discomfort," or "unpleasant feelings." Some patients, for a variety of personal reasons, such as fear, shame, or denial, will conceal their true symptoms.

In describing the quality of a pain, the patient's choice of words will be colored by both his vocabulary and his interpretation of what is happening. However, there are certain basic characteristics which may serve to guide the physician in his effort to identify the source of pain. For example, anginal pain may be described as "crushing," "squeezing," "burning," "searing," "tight," "constricting," "heavy," or "cutting off of breath," but basically it has a midline component and is steady without appreciable fluctuation. The pain of a peptic ulcer may be "gnawing," "burning," "eating," "hungry," "tight-fisted," or "like a dull toothache," but it is also steady and is localized below the surface of the abdomen. "Bloated," "distended," or "dyspeptic" feelings are the hallmarks of gallbladder disease. The pain of gallstones or of renal colic is paroxysmal in severity, but it also has a steady component, in contrast to the truly colicky pain associated with obstruction of a hollow viscus such as the gut. Special questioning may be required to bring out the fact that the patient is having true colic. "Does it grab and let go intermittently?" "Is it like the sensation you have when you urgently need to move your bowels, but are unable to do so?" A tearing pain may be described by the patient with a dissecting aneurysm. A throbbing pain suggests that arterial pulsation is an important factor, while a very sharp, burning, transitory pain is more characteristic of a nerve root origin.

PRECIPITATING AND AGGRAVATING FACTORS. Extract from the patient a detailed description of the exact setting in which his pain occurs. A general description will not suffice. The particulars of the story frequently supply the key. Precisely what was the patient doing when he got the pain? What were the specific circumstances surrounding the occurrence of the pain? What factors seem to precipitate or exaggerate the pain? Is it affected by activity, coughing, breathing, eating, time of day, etc.? If the pain is episodic, ask the patient to describe a typical spell in full detail.

Lack of clear-cut answers to this kind of probing is sometimes an indication of functional illness, although one has to be careful, since some important organic diseases may be characterized initially by a vague discomfort which is hard to put into words. Carcinomatosis, for example, frequently presents such symptoms.

FACTORS BRINGING RELIEF. Again, one must insist upon a complete listing of all factors that seem to diminish the discomfort. These factors generally will have to be suggested to the patient by the physician, so that no important categories are omitted.

One cannot discount any of the factors which the patient claims play a role in his discomfort, even though they may sound inconsequential, or even bizarre. The diagnosis may be overlooked because the physician concludes that what the patient says does not make sense. The key to the diagnosis may be contained in the very peculiarity of the patient's story. It is prudent to accept the patient's story at face value. It is an error to censor the patient's account to accommodate one's own thinking.

In order to evaluate the character of a patient's pain and related changes, it is essential that the observer be familiar with whatever medications the patient has been receiving. Drugs may ameliorate or alter the key symptoms or manifestations of an illness. Thus, morphine may profoundly change the pain and muscle spasm associated with a ruptured appendix. Drugs may also induce symptoms or changes which have nothing to do with the underlying disease process. For example, the development of polyarthritis following acute tonsillitis may suggest rheumatic fever, when it is, in fact, caused by allergy to the penicillin used to treat the tonsillitis.

Dependency upon drugs of various sorts may significantly color the patient's description of his symptoms and make the differential diagnosis of chronic or recurrent discomfort particularly difficult.

ASSOCIATED PHENOMENA. In this category are included all of the clinical manifestations associated with the patient's pain, such as anxiety, dyspnea, sweating, nausea, and vomiting. The physician must insist upon an unabridged listing, and he must act as the prompter.

TIME RELATIONSHIPS. The average duration of discomfort has important significance in understanding its source. The pain of angina pectoris lasts for only a few minutes and is relieved by the immobility that it imposes on the patient. The intermittent pain of intestinal colic and its causative peristaltic overactivity lasts only a few seconds. On the other hand, the discomfort of a peptic ulcer may last an hour or more, unless some food or an alkali is taken.

The frequency and specific time at which a pain occurs are also of importance. Epigastric pain that occurs daily with a constant relationship to meals is characteristic of a peptic ulcer, while the pain of gall-bladder disease comes at unexpected times and is independent of eating or exercise. The pain of hypertrophic arthritis is most severe during the period of early activity after a night's sleep. Peptic ulceration is one of the few conditions that cause chronic, recurrent abdominal discomfort at night. Nocturnal intensification of skeletal pain is frequently observed in metastatic carcinoma, and repetitive episodes of chest discomfort at night would suggest angina decubitus or hiatus hernia. Environmental factors, at home or on the job, should be investigated because of the role that they often play.

It is helpful to ask, "Have you ever previously had a pain at all similar to this one?" Patients have a way of describing an episode of pain as a unique experience. The physician is thus misled into thinking it is an acute and newly formed process, only to discover to his chagrin that this illness can be traced to one of several similar episodes dating back many years. Since the knowledge that an episode of pain is part of a recurrent process vitally affects one's thinking about the nature of the pain, this point must be pursued forcefully.

OTHER COMMUNICATION

To this point emphasis has been on obtaining information *from* patients. Of equal importance is the ability to impart information *to* patients. This is fundamental to obtaining the patient's confidence and cooperation in both diagnostic and therapeutic management. It is a key element in fostering patient satisfaction. There are special features involving both the special nature of the doctor–patient relationship and the special attitudes of people who are sick which merit discussion.

Stated negatively, poor communication between physician and patient is an important cause of the increasing frequency of malpractice suits. The physician who is hurried in his explanations is often assumed to be hurried in his judgments. Failure to understand and cope with a patient's unrealistic expectations can lead to disappointment, anger, and litigation even when the outcome is as good as could reasonably be expected. Hasty dismissal of realistic patient concerns by hearty and unwarranted reassurances can lead to the development of unrealistic expectations.

Physicians must be aware of the nature of the psychological relationship which usually exists between a patient and his doctor. The patient goes to a physician because he expects to trust and believe in him. Frequently, this belief and trust is amazingly uncritical and naive. What the physician says is regarded as infallible, even though the patient may actually know very little about his physician's qualifications.

Conversely, patients can lack confidence and trust in a physician over aspects that are unrelated to professional competence. For example, the physician's attire or demeanor may not fit with the patient's expectations of how a physician should dress or act. Physicians who choose to ignore such expectations are no less competent clinicians, but they do create problems for themselves in establishing this mutual trust which is so important.

Thus, in conversing with patients, certain general principles can be set forth to guide the physician:

1. Avoid careless, haphazard conversation, and give considered thought to everything the patient is told. The passing mention that the patient has a slight heart murmur serves no useful purpose, and will likely produce needless worry.

2. At the outset, assay the intellectual, emotional, and social capacities of the patient, and pitch the content of the conversation accordingly. It is important to avoid a patronizing air, whatever the patient's intellectual level.

3. Be certain you understand the patient's question and its implications to him before attempting to answer it. For example, an ulcer patient may ask, "Why am I still having pain?" He may not be interested in an explanation of the pathophysiology; he may really mean, "Does it mean that my ulcer is not healing, or do I have cancer?"

4. Employ simple expressions that are easily understood. Terms that are often misinterpreted are "tumor" (interpreted as cancer), "functional" (malingering), "chronic" (hopeless), and "nervous" (psychotic).

5. Never frighten the patient, but foster optimism, self-confidence, and security. Not frightening the patient does not mean that he is to be misled, because only the truth will sustain the patient's faith. However, he should be told the truth in a manner which creates understanding of his problem, dissipates fear, and leads to confidence in the future. Sometimes it is the physician's responsibility to soften the truth in order that it will accomplish this.

6. By thoughtfulness, thoroughness, and personal dignity, increase the patient's confidence.

OUTLINE OF THE HISTORY

It is essential that the physician have a firmly established habit pattern in what was described as the fact-gathering aspect of history taking. This includes the family history, the history of past illnesses, the review of systems, and personal and social matters. The advantages of a rote pattern are 1) no intellectual effort is devoted to what topic is next, and full attention can be devoted to interpreting the meaning of each response; and 2) it is much less likely that a topic will be overlooked.

There are a variety of outlines or formats for recording the patient's history. There may be personal or institutional preferences for one or another.[18,32,33] It is essential, however, to adopt one format and adhere to it until it becomes a habit.

THE PHYSICAL EXAMINATION

There are aspects of the patient's illness that are revealed only by physical examination. Inadequacies in the appraisal of these aspects cannot be corrected by excellence in the history or by generous selection of laboratory studies.

Physical examination is often considered only as an initial appraisal of the patient. However, the other areas in which it provides essential information should also be recognized. In the diagnostic process (Chap. 3), it is important that the patient be reexamined periodically. New signs may have developed or physical signs may be sought and discovered on the basis of ancillary findings. Furthermore, changes in physical signs may provide crucial information on the course of the illness or on the patient's response to therapy. It is essential, therefore, to consider the physical examination as a continuing, dynamic process which is carried out, not at just one point in time, but throughout the period of observation of the patient.

Proficiency in physical examination depends upon three related factors:

1. Thoroughness in the routine examination
2. Skill in techniques of physical examination
3. Understanding the sequential logic used in the examining process

The importance of thoroughness is obvious. Unless the skin is carefully inspected, the physician will not discover a melanoma on the patient's back. Similarly, if he does not have sufficient skill in auscultation, he will miss the diastolic rumble of mitral stenosis.

The importance of the third factor, understanding the logic involved, is more subtle. A novice may be as thorough as an expert on routine examination, and as skilled in techniques of examination, yet he may be unable to extract as much information from a physical examination as the expert can. The proficiency of the expert is related to his ability to branch out from his routine examination. This branching is similar to that described in history taking. For example, upon finding signs of pulmonary consolidation, the expert will consider the possibility of pulmonary infarction, and he will measure and compare the circumferences of the patient's legs. These actions are based in part upon greater experience and in part upon the habit of analyzing the meaning of each physical finding and searching for others that may be related.

This section is designed to supplement and extend, rather than to supplant, standard texts on physical diagnosis. In keeping with the format of this book, much of the specific information on physical signs and their interpretation is presented in relation to the relevant clinical problem. The areas to be emphasized here are: 1) the thorough examination; 2) the practical considerations in examining patients; and finally, 3) the sequential logic used in physical examination.

THE THOROUGH EXAMINATION

There is often confusion between thoroughness and completeness. It is neither possible nor desirable to perform a complete examination. A succussion splash need not be sought in every patient, nor should every patient be subjected to caloric vestibular stimulation. However, there are occasions when it is essential to branch off the mainstream of the examination into a special routine. In one of these special routines, it may be important to listen for a bruit over the popliteal artery, or in another to perform vestibular stimulation tests. The recognition of these occasions will be discussed in a later section.

The thorough routine examination contains certain elements which should never be omitted. They will be discussed below. The necessity for diligence in performing these examinations is illustrated by the case of a woman whose chills, fever, and lung abscesses were a diagnostic problem until the pelvic examination (which was deferred because she was "too sick") was performed. Examination revealed a soft cervix and a boggy, tender uterus. Upon further questioning she acknowledged having induced an abortion. Pelvic thrombophlebitis was producing septic emboli. Although thoroughness is important in all areas, there are some in which it is essential.

Areas in Which Physical Examination Is Indispensable

As mentioned initially, there are some abnormalities which, if missed, can never come to the physician's attention. As a consequence, the physician must exercise particular diligence in performing these portions of the examination. For example, a testicular nodule will not be revealed except by careful palpation, while a routine chest x-ray will readily reveal cardiac enlargement. Nevertheless, some physicians will, in error, examine the genitalia in a cursory fashion, but percuss the heart borders with meticulous care.

Table 2–3 lists some of the physical findings which provide information not obtained by other means. A few of those meriting special attention will be discussed in more detail.

Of equal importance is the realization that physical examination has certain shortcomings. For example, if the physician suspects a mediastinal mass on the basis of venous congestion limited to the head and arms, he should percuss the width of the mediastinum, but he should not rely upon negative findings. He should obtain x-ray studies, for only the grossest of lesions can be detected by percussion. Table 2–4 lists the areas in which other techniques should be employed to supplement physical examination.

SEVERITY OF ILLNESS. The most important single observation to make about a patient is to determine the severity of his illness, for the answer often indicates what must be done for the patient, and how rapidly. In a sense, this is an interpretation, a judgment, rather than an observation. Yet there are patients who are only slightly pallid, slightly restless, and slightly sweaty, but who appear severely ill to the experienced observer. The ability to recognize this poorly defined picture of severe illness comes largely with experience. It is, however, good practice to ask

---TABLE 2–4---
Findings Best Defined by Techniques Other Than Physical Examination

Masses (lung, mediastinum, retroperitoneal space, intracranial, nasopharyngeal, intrahepatic)
Intraocular pressure, visual fields
Cardiac size
Cardiac arrhythmias
Lesions within the gastrointestinal tract
Diminished alveolar ventilation

oneself at the outset of the examination: How sick is the patient?

Fortunately for the less experienced observer, severe illness is often accompanied by alterations in the vital signs: temperature, pulse rate, respiratory rate, and blood pressure. Certain pitfalls should be kept in mind in considering the vital signs. Oral temperatures may be erroneously low with mouth breathing, drinking of cool liquids, and shock. An elevated thermometer reading in the presence of a cool skin may indicate failure to shake down the thermometer, fever together with shock, or factitious fever. Errors in peripheral pulse rate measurements often arise in tachyarrhythmias where each heartbeat does not produce a systolic ejection. Respiratory rate measurement may be inaccurate, especially in periodic breathing. Furthermore, a normal rate need not indicate adequate ventilation. A previously hypertensive patient with shock may have normal blood pressure, and there may be variation in the blood pressure in the limbs with coarctation or dissecting aneurysm of the aorta.

Some additional findings should alert the physician to the urgency of the problem. These are listed in Table 2–5. Some of these manifestations may be produced by less ominous causes, e.g., increased intracranial pressure caused by pseudotumor cerebri, but the findings must be taken seriously until it is proven that the condition is benign.

GENERAL OBSERVATION. Quite apart from indicating the severity of the patient's illness, the general appearance of the patient gives information about his personality, distress, and reaction to his disease. This information can be obtained only by observation, yet all too often the physician pushes ahead with the specific aspects of physical examination without stopping to ask, "Is there anything unusual about this patient's attitude, mental status, appearance, or body build?"

Certain precise information about the nature of the patient's distress can best be obtained by careful

---TABLE 2–3---
Findings Best Defined by Physical Examination

Vital signs (temperature, pulse rate, respiratory rate, blood pressure)
Evidence of severity of illness
General appearance (including mental status)
Visible lesions (including integument, eyes and fundi, ears, nose, throat, joints)
Palpable lesions (including masses, local tenderness, deformities, pulsations or their absence, genitalia)
Respiratory difficulty (including signs of obstruction, weakness, splinting, cyanosis)
Murmurs, bruits, friction rubs, and bowel sounds
Neurologic signs

┌───┐
TABLE 2-5
Common Signs of Severe Illness

Excessively high or low temperature
Excessively high or low pulse rate
Excessively high or low respiratory rate
Excessively high or low blood pressure
Altered state of consciousness (anxiety, lethargy,
  confusion, delirium, coma)
Respiratory distress (noisy, labored, or ineffective)
Central cyanosis
Profuse sweating
Evidence of intense pain
Signs of pulmonary edema
Signs of increased intracranial pressure
Nuchal rigidity
└───┘

evaluation of his dyspnea, pain, or tenderness. For example, rapid, deep respiration suggests acidosis, while labored respiration with crowing inspiration suggests large airway obstruction as the cause of dyspnea.

General observation may cast doubt upon the history. A stoic may deny exertional dyspnea, while observation reveals that the effort of getting undressed produces panting. Conversely, claims of disability from back pain may be questioned if the patient bends to tie his shoes without difficulty.

The patient's position may be of diagnostic significance. Pericarditis is suggested if the patient finds relief of chest pain by sitting up and leaning forward; psoas irritation may be present if he lies with his hip flexed to relieve pain.

Changes in facial appearance may give early clues in the diagnosis of such diverse entities as myxedema, hyperthyroidism, parkinsonism, and depression. Furthermore, the body habitus may suggest one or another heritable disorder, such as the long limbs of S-S hemoglobinopathy or Marfan syndrome. Personal appearance may be important. For example, a slovenly appearance may indicate that the patient has had some deterioration of his intellectual faculties, or that he is too sick to care about his appearance. Similarly, general observation of the environment may be helpful. Is the room neat? Are the relatives attentive, anxious, or indifferent?

PRACTICAL CONSIDERATIONS

Thus far, attention has been directed toward the principles which should guide the physician in performing the physical examination. There are a number of practical matters which are equally important to the success of the examination.

Be Systematic

There is need to be systematic in the usual sequence of procedures performed in the routine physical examination. While there is no "best" order in which the examination is performed, an orderly sequence is essential to the prevention of inadvertent omissions. One such sequence developed by Hillman and Funk[21] is listed on pages 21–24.

For the same reasons it is essential that the physician be systematic and consistent in recording his physical findings. It is clear that the optimum order for *performing* the elements of a physical examination does not coincide with the most logical order for *recording* these findings.

Be Considerate

The physician should pay heed to the patient's modesty and need for privacy. He should make the patient as comfortable as possible; the thoughtless application of cold hands or a cold stethoscope can cool the doctor–patient relationship. Care should be taken in palpating tender areas; the rough and heavy-handed palpation of a tender abdomen may induce such guarding that important findings are missed. Thus, it is better to start palpating in a nontender area and to be as gentle as possible.

The Environment

The environment in which the patient is examined should be quiet and well lighted, preferably by daylight. The physician should neither stand in his own light, nor face the glare. The examining area should be free of distractions and interruptions. All of the patient's clothing should be removed and replaced by a drape or gown. Nothing deters thoroughness so much as attempting to examine over and around undergarments.

Observe Quantitatively

Both in observing and in recording observations, the physician should be quantitative. The descent of the liver edge should be measured in centimeters, not fingerbreadths; masses should be measured, rather than described in terms of fruit, eggs, golf balls, or baseballs.

Be Objective

It is important that the physician think of the abnormal physical finding in terms of the objective observation, not in terms of his interpretation of these observations, or in terms of the diagnosis derived therefrom. It is acceptable to think of a stuporous patient as smelling uremic if he is in fact uremic. However, if the uriniferous odor is due to incontinence and the patient is actually hypoglycemic, the physician may have started down an erroneous path through imprecise thinking.

Such imprecise thinking often leads to erroneous conclusions. For example, a 60-year-old man was seen because of progressive weakness and weight loss. The initial examiner found pallor and an enlarged spleen. After initial studies for causes of splenomegaly and anemia were unproductive, a consultant demonstrated that the upper as well as the lower border of the "spleen" could be demarcated. The initial observer had lost his objectivity; he palpated the left upper quadrant in search of splenomegaly, and found it. The consultant recognized that he was feeling a left upper quadrant mass and went on to determine whether it was spleen or not. In this case, it was found to be carcinoma of the splenic flexure of the colon.

Use Flexible Norms

A liver edge felt 5 cm below the costal margin in a patient with emphysema and low diaphragms would be regarded as normal, while the same finding in a young adult would be distinctly abnormal. Similarly, the experienced examiner realizes that lymph nodes are easily felt in thin patients and children. Thus, the physician must constantly adjust his standards to the situation at hand.

This flexibility does not imply a permissive attitude toward the significance of slight abnormalities. The small mass in the breast is not trivial; the faint, diastolic, decrescendo, blowing murmur along the left sternal border is not insignificant.

THE SEQUENTIAL LOGIC USED IN PHYSICAL EXAMINATION

Definition

The logical process which the physician follows in examining a patient involves not only performing the thorough, routine examination, but also in recognizing when and how to branch out from this routine.

Importance

Despite the recognized importance of the physical examination, the examination process is much misunderstood by students and physicians alike. Most of this misunderstanding arises from the disparity between what the physician believes he does (and seems to do) and what he does in fact. Students, for example, are puzzled that experienced physicians can discover more abnormalities than they can when both use the same techniques and apparently follow the

same format in examining a given patient. Physicians themselves are not always consciously aware of the process whereby they achieve their success. They are puzzled by the student's failure to observe the palmar erythema in the alcoholic patient or to elicit the plastic rigidity in the patient with early parkinsonism. Analysis of this process makes it apparent that the novice and the expert do *not* follow the same format in examining a patient. Appreciation of these differences is helpful in guiding the novice toward success and in encouraging the expert to improve his expertise.

Example

The basic difference between the novice and the expert is that the expert branches off from his routine, often quite unconsciously, during the course of his routine examination. When, for example, the examination has reached the point where the skin is being inspected, a specific question is asked, "Is the color normal?" If the answer is yes, the physician proceeds to the next question, "Is the skin free of lesions?" However, if the answer is no, his mental questioning follows another branch which pursues the nature of the color change (Fig. 2–1).

In this example, jaundice is the first condition considered as a cause of the yellowish-brown discoloration. If jaundice seems likely, the expert consciously or unconsciously enters his jaundice routine. The novice, on the other hand, simply proceeds to the next major question.

In his jaundice routine, the expert first verifies his observation by looking for scleral icterus. He next considers possible causes for jaundice, prompting him to look for excoriations which may indicate the itching of obstructive jaundice. He seeks evidence of cirrhosis. He may revert to the history to ask about drugs or to inquire in further detail about alcohol intake. He thinks ahead and will be certain to note a Kayser-Fleischer ring or splenomegaly, if present. He makes a mental note to determine urine bilirubin and urobilinogen upon completion of his examination.

To the bystander, the novice and the expert performed an identical physical examination. Yet, the expert would note the xanthomas about the patient's ankles which the novice might miss. The expert would then be quite certain the patient had chronic obstructive jaundice, while the novice would know only that the patient was jaundiced.

Knowledge of Special Routines

With increasing experience and increasing knowledge of medicine, the physician develops an increas-

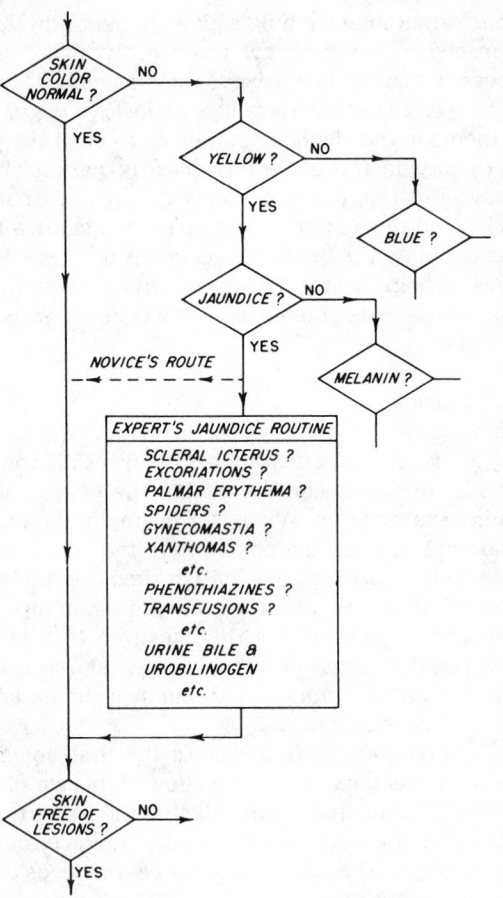

FIGURE 2–1. Schematic view of the questions asked by the experienced clinician while examining the skin. The clinician is not satisfied with merely establishing the presence of jaundice, but will probe further in order to narrow down the differential diagnosis.

ing repertoire of special routines. He comes to know what other information to seek when he encounters unequal pupils, a prominent venous pattern over the abdomen, a narrow pulse pressure, or an absent apical impulse. While the experienced physician employs these techniques unconsciously, the novice can improve his ability to examine patients by consciously considering the diagnostic implication of each abnormality which he finds in his routine examination.

From this it is clear that the novice cannot "learn" these special routines, for they encompass all of medicine. It is possible, however, to learn to be alert to the clues that are the indication for further investigation.

INDICATIONS FOR A SPECIAL ROUTINE

Jaundice has already been cited as an example of an abnormality that prompts the experienced examiner to modify his basic examination in order to insure full exploration of this finding. He should not perform his usual physical examination and *then* review the abnormal findings. He should consider the implications of any abnormalities *while* performing the examination. The perceptive examiner, then, is one who is alert to signals that suggest that he should branch off from his usual routine. These signals may arise from the history, from other physical findings, from the results of laboratory studies, from the differential diagnosis, or even from knowledge of the primary diagnosis. Illustrative examples of each will be given.

History

Clues may arise from any part of the history which alert the physician to devote extra attention to various portions of the examination. For example, a complaint of left pleuritic pain will alert the physician to palpate and compress each rib in search of a fracture, as well as to listen carefully over the spleen for a friction rub.

Physical Findings

The discovery of any abnormal finding should make the examiner ask the paired questions, "What might have caused this? What should I do to distinguish between these causes?" An early diastolic sound may represent an opening snap and should prompt an intensive search for other signs of mitral stenosis, not only at rest but also after exercise and in different positions. Similarly, vascular spiders will prompt a search for liver disease, and clubbing of the fingers suggests cyanotic heart disease, tumor of the lung or pleura, pulmonary suppuration, colitis, or enteritis.

Laboratory Results

Positive findings in the laboratory procedures should prompt the appropriate reappraisal of the physical findings, just as physical findings may suggest further laboratory studies. For example, the unexpected observation of rouleaux formation in the blood would suggest the possibility of myeloma; careful palpation in search of bony tenderness should be the response.

Whenever abnormal laboratory findings are reported, the physician should specifically consider what physical findings might be helpful in their interpretation. It must be emphasized that physical and laboratory examinations complement rather than supplant one another in the diagnostic process. This is illustrated clearly in the relationship between physical examination and x-ray examination of the pulmonary system. Physical examination may be unable to distinguish between emphysema and pneumothorax. When an emphysematous patient becomes acutely dyspneic, one should promptly obtain a chest x-ray. On the other hand, the x-ray may not be able to differentiate pleural effusion from pulmonary consolidation. These are conditions that have distinctive physical signs.

Differential Diagnosis

Indications for further or more intensive examination may arise from consideration of the differential diagnosis. In all patients with bleeding from the gastrointestinal tract, for instance, careful search should be made for physical evidence of a bleeding tendency (petechiae, ecchymoses, and positive tourniquet test) or telangiectasia. The characteristic lesions of Osler-Rendu-Weber's disease may be found in the oral mucous membranes of these patients.

It is common practice to select laboratory tests on the basis of the diagnostic possibilities under consideration. It is of equal importance to select portions of the physical examination for repeated evaluation on the same basis. For example, a common problem is distinguishing infective endocarditis from rheumatic activity in the febrile patient with rheumatic heart disease. Here, the frequent inspection of skin, mucous membranes, and fundi for emboli is as important as making frequent blood cultures. Similarly, serial examination for hot, red, swollen, or tender joints is as important as serial antistreptolysin O titers.

Another common example is the differential diagnosis of hypertension. Here the physician will look for the presence or absence of signs indicating coarctation of the aorta. Unilateral renal vascular disease will come to mind, and he will listen over the lumbar region and epigastrium for bruits which might indicate arterial stenosis.

Diagnosis

Often, the physician knows the primary diagnosis before he examines the patient. He may know the patient has diabetes mellitus or chronic myelogenous leukemia, for example. The physician's knowledge of the disease and its complications may direct him to take particular pains with certain aspects of the examination. In the instance of the diabetic in acidosis, he will look carefully at the periorbital and nasal tissues for evidence of inflammation which might indicate mucormycosis. He will also palpate the insulin injection sites to determine whether the acidosis might be due to poor insulin absorption associated with injection into an area of subcutaneous fibrosis, or whether there is evidence of cellulitis at the injec-

tion site. Thus, it is clear that the knowledge of the physician about the disease enables him to perform a better physical examination.

OUTLINE FOR PERFORMING ROUTINE PHYSICAL EXAMINATION*

In preparation for a routine physical examination, the patient is asked to remove his or her clothing, except for underpants, and put on a short paper or cloth gown which permits easy access to the chest and back. This type of gown is commonly available in most hospitals and outpatient facilities. When examining a female, it is also important to have available a half sheet to assist in the examination in the supine position.

The collection of physical examination data begins prior to the physician's examination when the nurse or physician assistant performs measurements of height, weight, blood pressure, pulse, respiration, and visual acuity using the Snellen Chart. In addition, such procedures as tonometry, dilation of pupils with neosynephrine, audiometry, and the performance of an electrocardiogram may be carried out by the nurse as a part of a systematic health profile.

Prior to the physical examination procedure, the required equipment is laid out in an organized fashion within easy reach of the examining table or bed. Depending on personal preference, instruments such as the stethoscope, pen light, tongue blades and pocket visual screener may be carried in a jacket pocket. For the routine physical examination, a full complement of equipment should include:

Stethoscope
Pen light
Tongue blades
Oto-ophthalmoscope
Reflex hammer
Sphygmomanometer
Tuning fork
Pocket visual screener
Neosynephrine
Glove and lubricating jelly
Guaiac test reagents
Pelvic speculum
Tonometer and tetracain

* Adapted from Hillman and Funk.[21] Courtesy of the Health Sciences Learning Resources Center of the University of Washington.

The examiner washes his hands and, unless contraindicated because of a physical abnormality, asks the patient to sit on the edge of the bed or the examining table. Right away considerable information may be gained from the general appearance of the patient, including impressions as to body habitus and general state of health. An almost instantaneous recognition of a distinctive body position associated with disease of the chest or spine may come from his first inspection and, with experience, a number of clues to disease, mood, or even the patient's personal image may be appreciated.

The patient is then approached and a careful inspection of his hands performed. This includes observation for the color and conformation of the nails, joint symmetry, and the status of the hand musculature. It is best done by supporting the patient's hands with your own at chest level so that each aspect of the hand may be closely scrutinized and compared to its fellow. Next, the right arm is explored by palpating the forearm and upper arm for muscle tone and tenderness, by inspecting the skin for lesions, and then by passively flexing and extending the elbow, wrist, and metacarpal joints simultaneously. The same maneuvers are repeated on the left arm.

Radial pulses are compared, checking for a major difference in amplitude. With the wristwatch, one radial pulse is counted for at least 10 seconds. During this time, the characteristics of the pulse should be further observed. The blood pressure is next taken on the right arm with a blood pressure cuff of appropriate size. Using the diaphragm of the stethoscope, good Korotkow sounds may usually be heard by placing the diaphragm over the approximate position of the brachial artery in the anticubital fossae. If, however, there is difficulty hearing these sounds, the artery should be palpated and the diaphragm should be placed over a point of strong pulsation. Additional blood pressure measurements on the left arm or the legs may be included if there is suspicion of vascular disease or hypertension.

Attention now moves to the head and proceeds in a systematic way down the body. First the face and head are inspected for overall configuration and symmetry, looking carefully for any skin lesions or tumors of the face and scalp. If the patient's visual acuity has not been evaluated using a Snellen Chart, a rapid test of near vision is carried out with a pocket visual screener or a sample of printed material. This is not a test of refractive error or distance vision and should, therefore, be performed with the patient using his glasses while the card or printed material is held at a distance of approximately 14 inches.

With a good light source, such as a pen light, the conjunctiva and sclera of the eye are inspected for changes in color or the appearance of vascular abnormalities such as petechial hemorrhages. If there is suspicion of extraocular muscle weakness, the pen light is also used as a light source to test for any displacement of the light reflex. While the patient looks directly at the light, the symmetry of the position of the reflected light image is observed. Next, direct and consensual pupillary reaction to light is tested. If it is considered important to dilate the patient's pupils prior to funduscopy, neosynephrine may be instilled at this time. A 10 percent ophthalmic neosynephrine solution will generally dilate the pupils with little if any interference with the patient's ability to focus.

The examination now focuses on the ear. The ear is first examined externally by pulling on the pinna and pushing on the tragus, looking for tenderness related to the soft tissues and cartilage of the external auditory canal. Then, with gentle traction in an upward and backward direction, the otoscope is introduced into the external auditory canal and the tympanic membrane inspected. A change in speculum size may be necessary depending on the diameter of the patient's auditory canal. Once both ears have been inspected, the otoscope light source may be used to carry out a brief inspection of the nose, specifically an observation of the lower portion of the nasal septum and turbinate.

The otoscope is now put aside, and with pen light and tongue blade the mouth is inspected. A systematic look at the buccal mucosa, teeth, gums, tongue, tonsillar fossae, and pharynx is important. In addition, the patient should be asked to phonate a vowel sound such as "ah" and the movement of the uvula and palate observed.

The final step in the examination of the head is the test of hearing using either a wristwatch, a whispered number, or, in some cases, a 256 cycles per second tuning fork. Since this is a very rough screening test, any patient suspected of a hearing deficit should be evaluated further with an audiometer.

The physician now moves behind the patient in order to carry out an examination of the neck, spine, and posterior lung fields. Neck range of motion is tested by having the patient touch his chin to his chest, to each shoulder, and then by bringing the head as far back as possible. Shoulder girdle strength and mobility are tested by first asking the patient to shrug while exerting downward pressure on both shoulders and then by asking him to extend his arms as far above his head as possible with palms together and biceps touching ears. For each of these maneuvers, the normal range of joint mobility will vary according to the patient's age.

The patient's gown is loosened and a systematic examination of the neck is performed looking for lymph node enlargement or abnormal masses. The mandibular, anterior cervical, posterior cervical, and supraclavicular areas are carefully explored. The thyroid is examined bimanually as the patient swallows.

The patient is next asked to take a deep breath while the symmetry of chest wall movement is observed. The use of accessory muscles of respiration and the length of time required for expiration is noted. The spine is percussed with the fist or by striking sharply with the fingertips on the vertebral spines looking for any tenderness. Next, percussion of the posterior lung fields is performed comparing right and left sides and noting the descent of the lung bases with a deep inspiration. This is followed by auscultation in the same position while the patient breathes through his mouth. The same procedure is followed in assessing the axillary and anterior lung fields.

The patient is next asked to lie down for the examination of anterior neck, chest, and abdomen. This begins with a systematic palpation of the breast, including each quadrant and areolar tissue. When performed on a female, care should be taken to arrange the gown or the half sheet to protect the patient's modesty. Each axillary area should also be palpated for lymph node enlargement.

Next, the pillow is removed in preparation for inspection of neck veins. While a well-filled external jugular vein is commonly seen in the fully supine position, occlusion of the vein at the angle of the jaw should result in incomplete filling from below once the vein is stripped. Rapid refilling from below with distension to the occluding finger suggests increased venous pressure. Carotid pulses are then palpated and compared.

The cardiac portion of the examination continues with inspection of the precordium for the position and character of the apex impulse and any abnormal pulsations. The apex impulse is palpated by placing the middle finger over the point of visible impulse with the index and fourth fingers in the rib spaces on either side. The force, duration, and extent of the apex impulse are noted. With the heel of the hand, the precordium is explored for any heaves, thrusts, or thrills. The heart borders are then percussed to detect gross abnormalities. Next, auscultation with the diaphragm of the stethoscope is carried out beginning at the apex and moving up the left sternal border to the pulmonic area, aortic area, and finally along the right sternal border. The timing of systole and diastole can be verified by simultaneously feeling the carotid pulse. The appreciation of any abnormality in the rhythm or quality of heart sounds should stimulate a further exploration of the precordium looking for murmur radiation and variations with phase of respiration. Then, before taking off the stethoscope, each carotid, the epigastrium, and each femoral area are listened to for bruits.

Once the examination of the chest is complete, the female patient should be assisted in replacing her gown. The abdomen is then uncovered for detailed inspection and superficial and deep palpation for any abnormalities in contour, tenderness, or palpable masses. This part of the examination should be performed gently and slowly. With one hand lifting from behind the lower ribs on the right, the liver edge is searched for as the patient takes a deep breath. If the liver is palpated, the edge is explored to define consistency, conformation, and tenderness. To confirm a suspicion of hepatic enlargement, the upper border of the liver is percussed and the overall length of the liver is estimated. Next, the spleen is palpated using the same technique of lifting the rib cage with one hand while palpating with the other. The patient is asked to take one or more deep breaths while the palpating hand is held firmly against the left upper quadrant. And finally, both femoral areas are palpated both for node enlargement and for the amplitude of femoral pulses.

Upon completing the examination of the abdomen, the legs are uncovered. Inspection of the skin, palpation of musculature and flexion of the knee and hip joints are carried out. Edema is searched for by pressing the index finger firmly against the lower tibia. The dorsalis pedis pulse is palpated and compared to its fellow. Finally, using a reflex hammer or other pointed object the plantar flexion reflex is tested bilaterally.

At this point the patient is asked to return to the sitting position. In the examination of the female, the gown is once again removed and both breasts carefully inspected for skin retraction, dimpling, or any asymmetry suggesting a tumorous growth. This examination is assisted by asking the patient to arch her back with hands first on hips then behind head. The gown is then replaced.

Next, the funduscopic examination is carried out. Initially, the red reflex is checked with plano lens in place and the ophthalmoscope held 1–2 feet from the patient's eye. A +8–12 lens is used to approach the eye and then the lens power is reduced watching for any lesions of the cornea, lens, or vitreous until the retina comes into focus. An attempt is made to view as much of the retina as possible by moving the ophthalmoscope and, with patients who have been dilated with neosynephrine, by having the patient move his eye on command in all directions. The fellow eye is examined in the same manner.

To finish neurologic testing, the patient is asked to wrinkle his forehead, show his teeth and stick out his tongue noting any muscle movement disorders. Biceps, knee, and ankle reflexes are tested and the patient is asked to extend his arms and close his eyes, looking for arm drift or tremor. Then the patient is asked to stand up and walk across the room. As he walks, the position of his feet, gait, and arm swing are observed.

The last part of any routine physical examination involves the examination of the genitalia and rectum. In the case of the male, the patient is asked to stand and remove his underpants. The penis and meatus is inspected for ulceration or discharge; the epididymis and testes are carefully palpated for tenderness, masses, or evidence of testicular atrophy. The index finger is introduced into the external inguinal canal and the patient is asked to cough or bear down while feeling for evidence of an inguinal hernia. Finally, the patient is asked to bend over the bed for inspection and palpation of the rectum. After lubricating the anus, the index finger is introduced into the rectum and careful palpation of the rectal ampulla and prostate performed. Similarly, with the examination of the female, the last step in a routine physical is the performance of the pelvic and rectal examination.

USE OF THE CLINICAL LABORATORY IN PATIENT CARE

INTRODUCTION

Ability to use laboratory data in patient care has become an essential skill required of every physician. Effective use of the laboratory should be developed as carefully as other clinical skills required in the practice of medicine.

In order to use the laboratory advantageously one must understand its functions and its limitations. Laboratory tests cannot be substituted for a careful history and examination of the patient, yet properly selected tests can give the physician information he can obtain through no other means. Thus, the function of the laboratory is to extend the physician's powers of observation. Skillful use of the laboratory requires an ability to integrate laboratory data with other clinical information, but it is a logical error to consider laboratory information as being of a different order than that obtained through the history or physical examination. All laboratory data are objective data (in contrast to the complaint of headache, for example), and they usually are expressed in quantitative terms. However, each laboratory measurement merely represents an observation of the same disordered physiology that is the object of the physician's attention during examination of the patient.

USES OF LABORATORY DATA

Screening (Detection of Disease)

Laboratory tests may be carried out on an apparently healthy individual as part of a comprehensive examination, or as part of the initial evaluation of a patient even though the history and physical examination do not suggest the need for such tests. Just as the physician measures the blood pressure in the absence of symptoms of hypertension, he may obtain a serologic test for syphilis without any clinical indication. Such screening tests usually are limited to the simpler, less expensive procedures which detect medically significant abnormalities having a high prevalence in the general population. The blood count (hemoglobin or hematocrit, white cell count, differential count, and examination of the blood film) and urinalysis (appearance, pH, specific gravity, protein, reducing substances, and microscopic examination) are done so frequently to supplement the history and physical examination that they may be considered essential components of an initial evaluation. This type of laboratory information is considered part of the "data base" in the terminology of the problem-oriented medical record.

The problems which arise when screening for disorders with a low prevalence have been discussed earlier (p. 7).

Diagnosis

During the initial evaluation of a patient, laboratory studies are usually selected on the basis of information obtained during the history and physical examination. A laboratory procedure may be used to assist the physician in establishing the presence of a suspected illness, for example, measurement of serum thyroxine to confirm a suspicion of hypothyroidism or serum creatine phosphokinase to substantiate a clinical diagnosis of myocardial infarction. In this situation, a positive laboratory result increases the probability that the clinical diagnosis is correct, and the function of the laboratory information is to enhance the reliability of that diagnosis. Conversely, laboratory tests may be used to exclude the presence of disease, for example, normal values for serum glutamic-oxaloacetic transaminase and serum glutamic-pyruvic transaminase can effectively rule out the presence of acute hepatitis. This use of laboratory data also serves to increase the reliability of the diagnostic process, since exclusion of some diagnoses increases the probability that one of the other suspected diagnoses is correct. These two applications of laboratory data are frequently used to aid the physician in selecting the most likely diagnosis from a list of several possibilities, i.e., differential diagnosis.

Following the Course of Disease

Because they are objective and quantitative, laboratory tests often provide a useful initial measure of the severity of the disease process present, and in many clinical situations they also provide the most reliable indication that therapy is having its desired effect. The erythrocyte sedimentation rate is a simple but useful indicator of improvement or exacerbation in acute rheumatic fever. Initial measurement of the reticulocyte count, and then either the hemoglobin or hematocrit, provide invaluable information regarding the effectiveness of treatment for anemia.

Selecting and Monitoring Therapy

Laboratory studies, by improving precision of diagnosis, may be of assistance in selection of appropriate therapy, for example, antimicrobial susceptibility tests in selecting the most effective antibiotic for a patient with bacterial infection. In other instances, dosage regimens of a selected therapeutic agent may be determined largely on the basis of laboratory tests; anticoagulant therapy with warfarin derivatives is hazardous without frequent measurement of the pro-

thrombin time. In circumstances where no quantitative clinical or laboratory measurements of the effects of a drug can be made, and particularly when there is reason to suspect that the dosage is too high or too low, it is often useful to measure the blood level of the agent itself. Therapeutic monitoring by measurement of blood levels of anticonvulsant drugs, cardiac glycosides, and antibiotics can indicate to the physician that the dosage schedule chosen is resulting in the desired concentration of drug in body fluids.

Other Uses

Laboratory tests are used in numerous other aspects of patient care: compatibility testing prior to blood transfusion or other types of tissue transplantation, detection of carrier states for purposes of genetic counseling, and detection of hereditary enzyme deficiencies which might be harmful under certain circumstances, for example, erythrocyte glucose-6-phosphate dehydrogenase deficiency which may result in hemolytic anemia if affected patients are administered certain drugs.

Laboratory tests are used also for such diverse purposes as environmental microbiological surveillance and provision of legal evidence in paternity litigation.

LABORATORY DATA IN THE MEDICAL DECISION-MAKING PROCESS

As explained in a previous section, medical diagnosis consists of an iterative process through which information is collected, evaluated, and utilized to determine further appropriate action.[8,20] Laboratory data are used in this process in exactly the same manner as data obtained during the history or physical examination. The iterative loop for laboratory information is more time consuming than for information collected by the physician himself, and for this reason it is usually more efficient to anticipate the possible outcomes of the iterative process and to order as promptly as possible all laboratory procedures which have a high probability of being required. Of course, the cost of the laboratory tests and any risk or inconvenience to the patient when following this practice must be balanced against prolonging the hospital stay unnecessarily, asking the patient to return repeatedly for sequential testing, and risk to the patient posed by any delay in diagnosis.

COMMON ERRORS IN LABORATORY TESTING

Serious pitfalls in the use of the clinical laboratory can occur at three points: first, with the choice of which test to perform; second, during the collection of the specimen and actual performance of the determination; and finally, in interpreting the result.

Failure to select the appropriate laboratory test usually stems from a lack of understanding of specific analytical methods used and how they relate to the patient's functional abnormality. Laboratory techniques are rapidly evolving, and tests are often methodologically complex. Lack of appreciation of the inherent limitations of a test method may mean that misleading or diagnostically valueless information will be obtained from the laboratory procedure requested. The former use of the red blood cell count as a test for anemia resulted in frequent misdiagnoses in those cases of anemia accompanied by normal red cell counts. The use of the T-3 resin uptake test as the sole means of assessing thyrometabolic status of a pregnant patient may result in an erroneous diagnosis of hypothyroidism. An understanding of the basic principles of test methodologies is critical, and appropriate consultation should be sought from the laboratory whenever there is concern that test limitations may preclude a satisfactory answer to the diagnostic question at hand.

The second point where pitfalls occur in laboratory testing is during the collection of the specimen and the actual performance of the test in the laboratory. Incorrect choice or handling of the specimen submitted frequently causes erroneous and misleading results, with the cause often not apparent to either the physician or the laboratory staff. The wrong choice of a bacterial transport medium for fastidious pathogens, or exposure of strict anaerobic organisms to the atmosphere may prevent their recovery in the laboratory, with a "negative" result then reported to the physician. Incorrect anticoagulants in tubes for blood specimens may render coagulation tests and chemical determinations grossly in error. Improper or inadequate specimens constitute a major technical problem in laboratory testing; hence, as much care should be given to collection of the specimen as to each of the other steps in the entire process.

Technical and clerical steps within the laboratory may be an additional source of errors in performance of laboratory tests. This possibility has resulted in the development of comprehensive specimen accessioning and quality control procedures which are now used almost universally in the clinical laboratory. It should be emphasized, however, that most of these quality control procedures are designed to detect systematic rather than random errors, and they are usually incapable of identifying improperly handled or deteriorated specimens. Although technical and clerical mistakes still occur, caution should be used in

summarily attributing all unanticipated results to "lab error." The unexpected test result, if valid, may contain important diagnostic information, and it should be viewed no differently than the unexpected physical finding which was not suggested by history. In both instances the finding should be pursued in depth if it could be of potential importance.

Interferences with test methodologies by medications, the nonfasting state, recumbency, or exercise, etc. is a type of technical "error" which deserves special mention. Numerous chemical interferences by medications have been documented for a variety of laboratory tests, and there is increasing awareness of the effects of both exercise and the post-absorptive state upon the results obtained with some laboratory determinations. The laboratory staff, having no information regarding the patient's drug therapy, cannot detect or circumvent these chemical interferences which may cause significant quantitative differences in the results obtained. Misleading results caused by drug interferences hopefully will diminish as new analytical methodologies are developed which are more specific for the substances in question, and as computer systems allow detection of potential interferences by automatic review of patients' therapeutic regimens.

The final point at which pitfalls can occur is in the physician's interpretation of the laboratory test results. Problems frequently arise from use of incorrect normal ranges or from overestimating the precision of the result which is reported. Differences in the technical methods of performing a test can have a profound effect upon the normal range for that test. The various methods of performing an erythrocyte sedimentation rate yield substantially different values in health and disease, and the use of the wrong range for the test may result in an erroneous diagnostic impression. Normal ranges are too often taken from the literature with the assumption that they apply to all test methodologies with that name. Age, race, and sex variations in values for tests such as blood counts and immunoglobulin concentrations may result in diagnostic errors if a single normal range is assumed. The statistical precision of the test methodology provides a second potential pitfall in interpretation of laboratory results. For example, the inherent error in the usual 100 cell WBC differential count limits the significance of changes in proportions of the various cell types on repeated determinations on the same patient. Because of the statistical sampling error a patient with a "true" value of 50 percent neutrophils may have percentages ranging from 40 to 60 on repeated determinations; hence, little significance can be attached to an apparent "increase" of this magnitude on successive determinations.

The ultimate value of a laboratory result is determined entirely by the use the physician makes of it. This, in turn, is dependent upon the physician's appreciation of the limits and capabilities of the clinical laboratory in identifying the abnormality responsible for the patient's disease.

DIAGNOSTIC ROENTGENOLOGY, ULTRASOUND, AND NUCLEAR MEDICINE

Diagnostic procedures based upon images and measurements of x-ray, ultrasound, and radioactive isotopes have proliferated rapidly in recent years. Some of these have enjoyed brief popularity and then have faded into oblivion or have been supplanted by an improved procedure or technique. Still others have proven themselves and have become a standard part of our diagnostic armamentarium.

These diagnostic methods are contributory or irrelevant depending upon the problem at hand. Accordingly, most of the consideration of indications and contraindications of these studies are discussed throughout the book in the context of the various diagnostic problems. This section focuses upon the fundamentals of these procedures, and the ways in which they differ from other sources of clinical information. Specific procedures will be discussed in connection with the clinical problem which they address.

DIAGNOSTIC ROENTGENOLOGY[29]

Diagnostic roentgenology is, in essence, a method of physical diagnosis. It provides information which cannot be obtained by classical methods of physical diagnosis, e.g., the detection of a coin lesion in the lung; or information of greater precision, e.g., the size and shape of the heart. Diagnostic roentgenology does not supplant the classical techniques, but supplements them. X-rays cannot disclose the wheeze of airway obstruction or the murmur of a diseased heart valve.

The roentgenographic examination should be conducted with the simplest technique, the minimum number of roentgenographic films, and the lowest possible radiation exposure. Static radiographic films requiring less radiation should be obtained whenever fluoroscopy is unlikely to provide additional information. Plain roentgenograms should precede examinations employing contrast substance.

Basic Considerations

NATURE AND PRODUCTION OF X-RAYS. Roentgen rays are part of the spectrum of electromagnetic radiation. They travel at the speed of light, but their wavelength is considerably shorter than that of light or radio waves. This distinctive property enables radiation to penetrate tissues and organs according to their density and thickness.

X-rays are produced in a vacuum tube, to which a potential of many thousand volts is applied between two electrodes. An increase in tube voltage will accelerate the electron stream across the tube, and will result in shorter wavelength and more penetrating (harder) radiation. Low voltage x-rays have a longer wavelength, are soft, and are more easily absorbed by the tissues than hard radiation.

ABSORPTION OF X-RAYS. It is the differential absorption of x-rays by the various tissues or by special contrast media which provides the diagnostic usefulness of the roentgenogram. The absorption increases as the *atomic number* of the material increases (lead is more absorptive than carbon), as the *density* increases (water is more absorptive than air), and as *thickness* increases (the thigh is more absorptive than the calf). The x-rays which are not absorbed pass through the tissue to form an image on the photographic film or fluorescent screen.

Most body tissues and fluids are composed of elements with low atomic numbers (hydrogen–1, carbon–6, nitrogen–7, and oxygen–8). Consequently, they have a relatively uniform absorption of x-rays and have an intermediate, homogeneous density termed "soft tissue density." Only the lesser density of fat can sometimes be delineated (retroperitoneal fat, perirenal fat, lipomas) by conventional radiography.

Bones (calcium, atomic number–20; phosphorous–15) will permit fewer x-rays to pass through the film and will appear as light areas surrounded by the darker soft tissues (Fig. 2–2).

A roentgenogram of the chest in a patient with pneumonic infiltration shows an increased tissue density because air-containing lung parenchyma has been replaced by exudate having the density of soft tissue. On an x-ray film, the infiltrate will appear lighter than uninvolved lung (or darker when viewed with the fluoroscopic screen).

CONTRAST RADIOGRAPHY. Contrasts in density may occur naturally as between the air-containing lung fields and the blood-filled cardiovascular structures. Unfortunately, these contrasts do not prevail in the abdomen or between the soft tissue structures of the extremities, and the difference in contrast shown

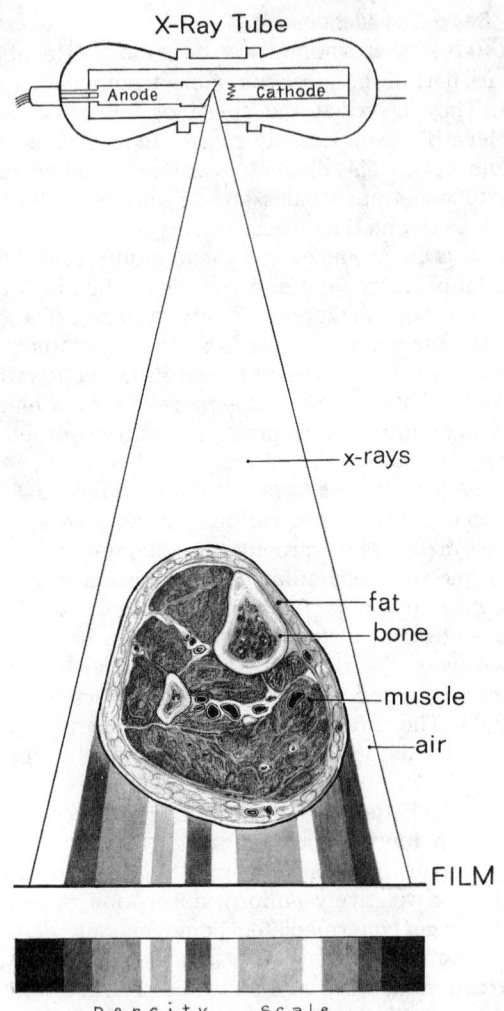

X-Ray Tube

Anode   Cathode

x-rays

fat
bone

muscle

air

FILM

Density   Scale

FIGURE 2–2. Diagram illustrating the differential absorption of x-rays by the various tissues of a leg. Note the resulting variation in contrast produced by the image-forming radiation on x-ray film (density scale) as well as the magnification of the image.

on roentgenograms is usually not sufficient for delineation. Therefore, contrast must be produced by means of solid, liquid, or gaseous substances introduced as part of the examination. These substances must either absorb more or fewer x-rays than the surrounding tissues. The contrast agents which are compounds of iodine or barium have high atomic numbers and absorb more roentgen rays than soft tissues. Other contrast agents, such as air and carbon dioxide, have approximately the same effective atomic number as soft tissues, but considerably less density and, therefore, absorb fewer x-rays.

The contrast agents can be introduced into the gastrointestinal tract, the cardiovascular system, the bronchial tree, the spinal canal, or the genitourinary system. The contrast material provides a means whereby the inside of a hollow viscus can be visualized. When it mixes with the natural contents of the system, as angiographic media mix with blood, flow patterns, and function can be observed.

COMPUTERIZED AXIAL TOMOGRAPHY.[30] In this technique a planar slice of the body is subjected to sequential sweeps, or scans of a narrow beam of x-ray. The unabsorbed emergent beam is measured by a radiation detector or an array of detectors. These data are stored in a mini-computer which also reconstructs the two-dimensional image. This image, or tomogram, is the computed distribution of radiodensity which gave the observed pattern of x-ray transmission.

Although computerized axial tomography does not have the spatial resolution of conventional roentgenograms, it has the unique capability of distinguishing the minor differences in the radiodensity of soft tissues. Thus, for example, it can reveal differences between liver and tumor, brain and hematoma, and pancreas and cyst. It is this capability and its noninvasive nature which have caused this technique to supplant older, more invasive, less revealing diagnostic imaging methods.

Its use will be discussed in connection with the clinical problems in which it is particularly helpful.

Communication with the Radiologist

The request for a radiographic study should always be accompanied by a brief clinical history and should supply pertinent data of the physical examination, and, if helpful, the result of laboratory findings. In addition, it is essential that the radiologist know the specific reason for the requested radiographic procedure. This information may determine the type and number of radiographic projections necessary to visualize the structure or anatomic part under investigation.

In certain situations, personal conversation between the clinician and radiologist is essential if maximum information is to be obtained with minimal radiation exposure to the patient. The radiologist should be consulted prior to extensive or repeated radiologic examinations of young individuals, and only absolutely essential studies should be carried out during pregnancy.

Radiographic examinations which are likely to fail in providing the necessary information should be avoided. Thus, about half intravenous urographs will be unsuccessful if the serum creatinine exceeds

8 mg/dl, and biliary ducts will not be seen during intravenous cholangiography when the serum bilirubin concentration has reached 5 mg/dl.

Consultation with the radiologist, furthermore, is important when the clinical problem calls for radiographic studies beyond the scope of routine examinations. Special views and techniques may be helpful, or films of the abdomen in studies of the small intestine may have to be adapted to the patient's special condition. For example, because of a rapid intestinal transit time, films may have to be taken at closer intervals than are called for in routine procedures. A study may have to be supplemented by compression spot films in order to detect disease of a localized area usually not examined in this fashion. Consultation in such a case may prove extremely valuable. The patient may be spared additional radiation and repeat studies.

To examine the patient with the least harmful means suited to provide all necessary information should be the aim of radiologists and referring physicians alike.

DIAGNOSTIC ULTRASOUND[19,23]

Diagnostic ultrasound provides another method of physical diagnosis. It is a purely anatomical technique except in the field of cardiology, where physiologic information about the movement of the heart wall and valves is obtainable.

Ultrasound is a noninvasive technique and has no known harmful effects. The patient lies on a stretcher during the examination; after the liberal application of mineral oil to provide satisfactory physical contact a transducer is moved around the body surface. Echos are recorded and displayed. The examination is painless and rarely takes longer than half an hour.

Nature and Production of Diagnostic Ultrasound

Diagnostic ultrasound uses sound waves with a frequency of 1 to 20 million hertz (cycles per second) which is well above the upper limit of human hearing, 20,000 hertz. At these high frequencies ultrasound is reflected and refracted from acoustic interfaces in the body in a fashion analogous to light passing through a partially transparent substance. In diagnostic ultrasound, a pulse of sound is emitted from the transducer for a few microseconds. Many sound waves are scattered or transmitted rather than being reflected back to the same transducer. The transducer thus acts both as an emitter and a receiver. Echos are only received from interfaces at right angles to the probe (see Fig. 2–3). These echos, or reflections can be translated electronically into a display on a cathode ray oscilloscope.

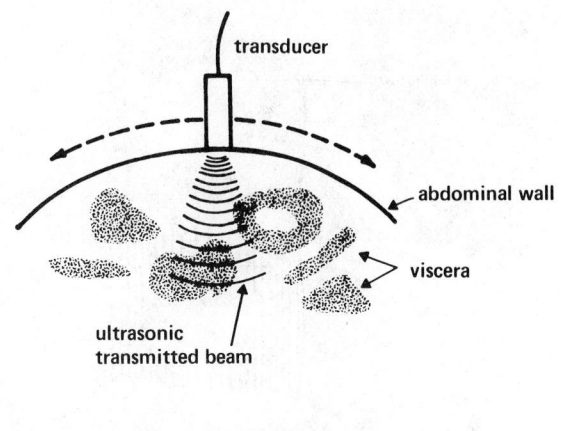

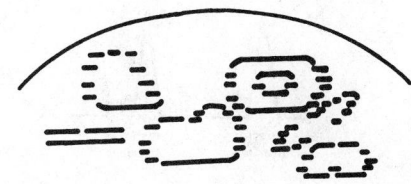

FIGURE 2–3. Diagrammatically shown are the echos produced when a transducer is moved around the wall of a structure containing a number of objects with varying shapes. Notice that only surfaces directly at right angles to the transducer produce echos.

Acoustic interfaces occur whenever a substance changes in acoustic density; thus, a reflection from an acoustic interface will occur when a sound passes from muscle to fibrous tissue. Larger reflections occur when the acoustic density difference is greater; sound is well transmitted through fluid, so a large reflection will occur when sound passes from fluid to enter soft tissues (see Fig. 2–4). Sound is very poorly conducted by gases and is reflected unduly well by bone. Thus, structures containing air such as the lung or surrounded by bone such as the pelvis are difficult to examine with ultrasound.

There are three common ways of displaying the ultrasonic reflections for observation and photographic recording. These are illustrated and described in Figure 2–5. The A-mode (amplitude *versus* depth) is especially useful in echoencephalography where the skull reflects so much of the ultrasound that it is difficult to discriminate the amplitude of the ventricles and midline structures from noise and artifacts. The B-mode (brightness *versus* depth) can be used to build up a composite two-dimensional section as the transducer is scanned across the subject. This is called echography or sonography. Such a view differs from the usual radiography in being a cross-sectional

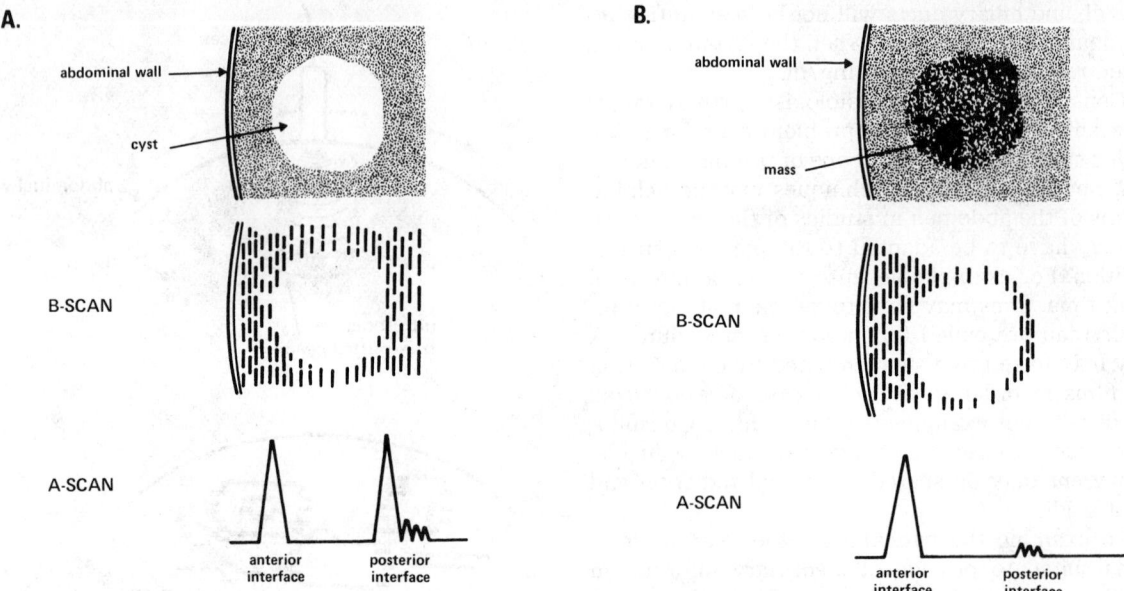

FIGURE 2-4. Diagram **A** shows the typical B-scan and A-scan appearances of a cyst. Notice that the posterior echos behind the cyst are large. Diagram **B** is the B-scan and the A-scan characteristics of a solid homogeneous mass. The posterior echos are of low amplitude.

anatomic view—each transverse section appears as if someone has taken a bandsaw and cut through the body at a vertebral level. Ultrasound therefore allows one to know the depth of a structure below the skin and to find out the anteroposterior dimension of masses. The B-mode is also used to generate a time-motion display in which the movement of a structure such as the anterior leaflet of the mitral valve can be displayed as depth *versus* time.

Some idea of the pathologic nature of a mass may be obtained from ultrasound. Whatever the acoustic density of a substance, if it is acoustically

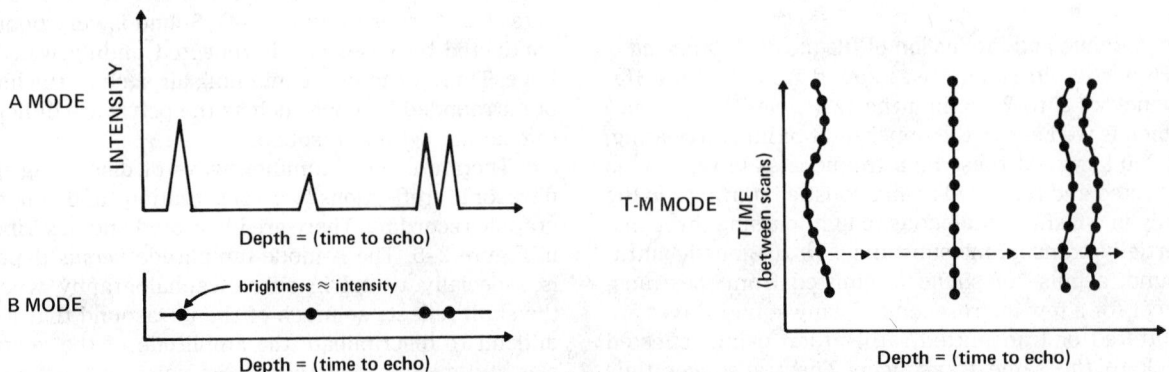

FIGURE 2-5. In A-mode the amplitude of individual echos is shown. In B-mode individual echos are shown only as dots. In TM or M-mode, individual echos are shown as dots but are placed on a moving time base so that motion can be recorded. In practice the individual dots show up as a continuous line.

homogeneous no echos will arise from it. In homogeneous tumors which contain areas of necrosis, fibrous tissue or hemorrhage will be filled with echos. Distinction of acoustically homogeneous tumors from cysts containing fluid can be made from the more prominent posterior wall echo in a cyst (Fig. 2–4).

The usefulness of ultrasound in cardiology is discussed in Chapter 17 and in neurology in Chapter 111.

NUCLEAR MEDICINE[13,15,30,31]

The instruments and radioactive tracers used in nuclear medicine have improved greatly in recent years, but the fundamental principles remain the same. One of the most fundamental is that of the dynamic state of body constituents. This principle states that the apparent constancy of body constituents, such as the level of the blood glucose or electrolytes, is the result of a delicate balance among the rates of production and breakdown of biochemical substances and cellular elements that are in a continual state of flux. Both stable and radioactive tracers played important roles in elucidating the dynamic turnover of chemical substances and body cells that formerly seemed to be quite static.

Areas of greatest use of procedures in diagnostic medicine include the thyroid, heart, brain, lung, liver, spleen, bone marrow, bone, and kidneys. These will be discussed in appropriate places in the text.

Measurements of Radioactivity

TIME DOMAIN MEASUREMENTS. Measurements at various times after administration of a radioactive tracer are characteristic of radioactive tracer studies, and are a hallmark of nuclear medicine, permitting estimation of the rate of important biochemical and physiologic processes within the intact patient. In this type of study, the survival of the patient's red cells is measured by withdrawing blood samples at various times after the injection of the labeled cells. Both stable and radioactive tracers have been used to measure rates of production and destruction of a whole host of substances, such as cellular elements of the blood and metabolic pathways of all types. These determinations of the rates of body processes involve measurements in the temporal domain.

SPATIAL DOMAIN MEASUREMENTS. Prior to the development of radiation detection devices that could localize the spatial distribution of radioactive tracers within the body, measurements were restricted to the concentrations of tracers in blood, urine, or other biologic materials that could be separated from the body at various times after administration of a tracer substance. Measurement of the spatial location of these

life processes within the human body became possible through the development of scintillation crystals which greatly increased sensitivity and spatial resolution. A scintillation crystal suitably mounted could be driven back and forth over a portion of the body, advancing a bit with each traverse. This rectilinear scanning over a patient's neck can, for example, determine whether or not a thyroid nodule accumulated radioiodine.

This scanning technique can be used to reveal brain tumors when used in conjunction with suitable radioactive materials. Radioiodinated albumin was the first successful radiopharmaceutical used for brain scanning, but has been replaced by technetium-99m pertechnetate, which is the most widely used agent at present. The latter improved greatly the image quality and reduced the radiation dose to the patient.

The subsequent invention of the scintillation camera by Anger greatly facilitated rapid dynamic studies of the time course of tracer through the brain, as well as other parts of the body. This device has a single large crystal, 11 to 15 inches in diameter, which is viewed by an array of from 19 to 37 photomultiplier tubes. Spatial localization is achieved by computer analysis of the pattern of activation of the phototube array, rather than by moving the detector back and forth as in the case of the rectilinear scanner.

The important property that radioactive tracers possess that makes possible study in the spatial as well as the temporal domain is the emission of gamma rays by many of them in the process of radioactive decay. When appropriately energetic, such gamma rays can penetrate the tissues of the body and be measured by externally placed radiation detectors. We can determine their location within the body as well as quantify the amount present. The degree of spatial resolution that can be achieved depends on the design of the radiation detector, the location of the tracer within the body, and the physical and biochemical characteristics of the radioactive tracer. For example, the "whole body counter" measures the total body content of one or more radioactive tracers within the body. It is used to study metabolic processes of the body as a whole, for example, the rate of absorption of iron in patients with nutritional anemias. The modern scintillation camera and the design of the most rectilinear scanners permit a spatial resolution of about 1 to 2 cm.

FUNCTIONAL DOMAIN MEASUREMENTS. By measuring the spatial distribution of radioactive tracers at various times we can determine *where* a physiologic or biochemical process is occurring, as well as *how fast*. The use of multiple tracers, each measuring a specific body function, adds a third domain, the *functional* domain.

We look at a diagnostic problem that a patient presents, or a question that a scientist asks, in terms of the degree of functional, spatial, and temporal resolution required for its solution or answer. For example, a single tracer that measures the phagocytic function of the liver can detect the presence of a 2½ cm lesion within the liver, provided the spatial resolution of the radiation detector is adequate. A single image can be obtained over a wide span of time after the administration of the dose, so that the temporal resolution requirement is not great. (For studies of the circulatory system, on the other hand, we have much greater need for temporal resolution; in some studies measurements must be made as frequently as every 0.1 or 0.2 seconds.) If, however, we wish to have a better idea of the nature of the lesion, it is necessary to use multiple radiopharmaceuticals to increase the diagnostic specificity. For example, we can use a radiopharmaceutical that remains in the vascular space to determine the vascular volume of the lesion, or a radiopharmaceutical that is excreted via the biliary tract, or one that has a relatively high avidity for neoplasms to elucidate further the nature of the lesion.

CHAPTER 3
The Analysis and Synthesis of Clinical Information
RICHARD J. JOHNS

Clinical information is collected and manipulated in order to solve a patient's clinical problem. Usually the problem is solved through diagnosis and therapeutic management. Sometimes the problem disappears during the procedure, and sometimes the diagnosis is not amenable to treatment. Nevertheless, the initial objective of the analysis and synthesis of clinical information is to arrive at a diagnosis.

In recent years this clinical diagnostic process has come under investigation.[4,36,39,40] While these studies do not provide clear insight into the inner workings of the diagnostic process of experienced physicians, they have been valuable in demonstrating what the process is *not*. First, it has been shown that the physician does not separate or compartmentalize the collection of information from the analysis of information—the two processes are intermingled. Second, the diagnostic process is more akin to progressing down a logical decision tree then it is to a pattern-matching *Gestalt*.

INITIAL INFORMATION ANALYSIS

In Chapter 2 it was emphasized that each piece of information should be analyzed as it is received: What does it mean? What diagnostic possibilities (hypothesis) does it suggest? What further information will be helpful in sorting out these hypotheses. This initial analysis serves two important functions. First, it guides the course of further information gathering in a rational way. Second, it permits the physician to organize, store, recall, and manipulate the clinical information. It would be impossible to deal with the informational content of the history of a present illness and the abnormal physical findings if they were treated as a list of unrelated facts. Consciously or unconsciously, physicians aggregate the facts in a meaningful way. For example, the history of chills and fever, the history of dysuria, the finding of a temperature of 39°C, and the finding of right costovertebral angle tenderness become organized by the hypothesis that the patient may have an upper urinary tract infection. Four separate pieces of information have been compressed into one concept. The importance of this aspect can be seen in the novice's difficulty in "remembering" the clinical information about a patient or in the experienced physician's difficulty in dealing with the information concerning a patient in which the manifestations "do not make sense." In both examples, there is a lack of organizing and unifying concepts.

Thus, the initial analysis of clinical information has a beneficial effect on the information-gathering process, and it is essential to the mental processing of the information.

FURTHER ANALYSIS

While the initial analysis is necessary, it is not sufficient. To rely exclusively on the analysis carried out during the information-gathering phase can lead to two possible errors.

First, if you only obtain information to test your current hypotheses you may miss important pieces of information. This is the basic reason that one performs a system review, a routine physical examination, and obtains screening laboratory studies. You seek certain basic items of information whether or not your concurrent analysis suggests that it might be worthwhile.

Second, the initial analysis is of necessity a serial process. Various hypotheses are considered and then are either abandoned or explored further. In the light of subsequent information, some of these hypotheses may have been abandoned prematurely. Furthermore, in the review of all the information, additional hypotheses must be considered. For example, if the patient described above also had cough with purulent sputum, one must also give consideration to the possibility that the problem is pneumonia at the right lung base.

This chapter is devoted to discussing this second step, the further analysis that is performed when the initial information has been collected. It also addresses the synthesis of this information with knowledge of disease. It addresses the questions of which disease best explains the patient's problems, and does one disease explain all the problems.

ANALYZE THE FACTS

The steps in the further analysis of a clinical problem can be illustrated by applying them to a specific case.

ILLUSTRATIVE EXAMPLE

A 51-year-old executive was hospitalized because of jaundice.

The past history was unrevealing. He had been advised a year previously to lose weight, and his weight had dropped from 230 to 203 pounds as the result of dieting. During that year, he had experienced occasional episodes of vague epigastric pain unrelated to food or activity. For this he had been given elixir of phenobarbital and some tablets, with questionable relief of symptoms.

Three weeks prior to admission he developed nausea and vomiting. This would occur two to three times a week, was unrelated to meals, but was accompanied by anorexia. Ten days prior to admission he noted dark urine. He noted that his eyes were yellow two days before admission.

His stools were light, but not acholic. He had no itching, no exposure to needles, blood, or jaundiced persons. He drank three to five cocktails a week.

On examination the vital signs were: temperature 99°F, pulse 96 per minute, respiration 16 per minute, blood pressure 130/70 mm Hg. The patient was mildly obese and jaundiced, but did not appear acutely ill. There were no spider angiomas, palmar erythema, or excoriations. The liver edge was smooth, slightly tender, and palpable 5 cm below the costal margin. The remainder of the examination was normal except for hemorrhoids and hypoactive tendon reflexes.

Initial laboratory examinations revealed: hematocrit 46 percent, white blood count 8000 per mm³ with a normal differential. The urine was brown, contained protein 1+, bile, and urobilinogen in a 1:4 dilution. The stool was tan and contained no occult blood.

Total serum bilirubin was 5.0 mg/dl with 3.6 mg/dl direct. The serum alkaline phosphatase was 38 Bodansky units, and the transaminases were each 320 units (normal up to 50). The serum proteins and prothrombin time were normal.

LIST THE FACTS

Chronologic List

The first step in the analysis is to list the facts in chronologic order. In this example the list would include:

Vague upper abdominal pain for 1 year
History of drug treatment
Nausea and vomiting
Anorexia
Jaundice for 10 days
Tachycardia
Hepatomegaly
Hemorrhoids
Hypoactive tendon reflexes
Proteinuria, slight
Bilirubinuria
Hyperbilirubinemia (mostly direct reacting)
Increased serum transaminase concentration
Increased serum alkaline phosphatase
concentration

RANK IN ORDER OF IMPORTANCE

Before one can arrange these findings in the order of their importance, each must be evaluated as to its possible significance. For example, the unknown medication might be a mild sedative with no adverse reactions, in which case it would be put low on the list. In this case, however, a call to the druggist revealed that it was a phenothiazine preparation capable of producing jaundice. Naturally, this would be a high priority finding. This also serves to illustrate the important point that analysis often prompts the physician to seek further information.

Findings such as hypoactive knee jerks and hemorrhoids are found in many otherwise normal individuals and, thus, would not be given a prominent place in the initial listing. Likewise, tachycardia and mild proteinuria are nonspecific findings in many types of illness and would be placed low on the list unless there were special reasons for putting them higher. Some of the items assigned lower priority might assume greater importance at a later stage in the analysis, e.g., hemorrhoids might be proven to be associated with portal hypertension.

After careful examination of the findings they can be rearranged in the order of their apparent importance as follows:

Hepatomegaly
Jaundice
Hyperbilirubinemia (mostly direct reacting)
Bilirubinuria
Increased serum transaminase concentration
Increased serum alkaline phosphatase concentration
Vague upper abdominal pain

Nausea and vomiting
Anorexia
Phenothiazine ingestion
Hemorrhoids
Proteinuria, slight
Hypoactive tendon reflexes
Tachycardia

Note the Items Which Must Be Explained

The findings italicized in the above list are those which appear to be so intimately associated with the illness that the final diagnosis should account for them. Later in the analysis it is important to verify that the diagnosis selected does explain these findings.

After the facts have been critically evaluated and listed according to their apparent importance, one may find in the list a disease manifestation that unequivocally provides a diagnosis. Such a finding would be the Kayser-Fleischer ring which is pathognomonic evidence of Wilson's disease. If the remaining findings on the list were adequately explained by a diagnosis of Wilson's disease, the analysis would not need to proceed further. However, as in the case example given above, one usually finds that the accumulated facts are common to several diseases.

SELECT A CENTRAL FEATURE

The next step is to select some outstanding feature of the illness about which one can orient the diagnostic analysis. Examples of such orienting, or central, features are fever, jaundice, hepatomegaly, ascites, renal failure, and heart failure, among others. It is preferable that the feature selected be an objective finding and, if possible, one that can be at least roughly quantified. However, in some cases, the major complaint is subjective, such as pain in a particular area, and is the only feature that can serve as the basis for the systematic analysis of the problem. The selection of a feature as the focal point about which the differential diagnosis will be centered requires practice and a wide knowledge of the important hallmarks and of the natural course of the various diseases. As one reads through this text, many examples illustrating this type of analysis will be found in the discussions of the clinical problems presented.

When the case presents two or more features that appear to have the same potential value, one should not be content to have this analysis based on only one of them. Two or more analyses should be made, each based on one of the features. By pursuing this course one may find two or more avenues which lead to the same diagnosis, thus reinforcing one's confidence in its validity.

In the example under consideration, *jaundice* was selected as the central feature. Other possibilities, such as abdominal pain or nausea and vomiting, are not as specific and would, therefore, lead to a more cumbersome list of diagnostic possibilities.

LIST THE DIAGNOSTIC POSSIBILITIES

In this example, the laboratory findings suggested that the jaundice was due to intrahepatic or extrahepatic obstruction. The list of diagnostic possibilities would include:

Intrahepatic obstruction
    Cholestatic jaundice from phenothiazine drug
    Obstructive phase of hepatitis
Extrahepatic obstruction
    Stone
    Carcinoma of pancreas, bile duct, or ampulla of Vater
    Mass in porta hepatis
    Duodenal diverticulum

In listing the diagnostic possibilities an effort should be made to be comprehensive. In this example, the uncommon possibility of duodenal diverticulum should not be overlooked. Even more important, from the standpoint of judicious management, is the recognition that hepatitis can occasionally manifest a prolonged obstructive phase. In general, readily treatable causes should always merit particular attention, even when rare.

DISTINGUISH BETWEEN THESE POSSIBILITIES

At this point in the diagnostic procedure, it is a common error to pick the most likely possibility and proceed accordingly without considering the alternatives. In this example, the past history of episodes of epigastric pain make extrahepatic obstruction a reasonable possibility. It would be tempting to proceed directly to surgical exploration. If the jaundice were caused by a drug, however, the operation would be unnecessary; if caused by hepatitis, surgery and anesthesia might prove disastrous. Thus, the prudent physician first asks, "Will further observation or examination help to distinguish between the diagnostic possibilities under consideration?"

This patient's upper gastrointestinal x-ray studies failed to reveal any abnormalities suggesting an obstructive lesion. The liver function tests remained unchanged. In order to avoid the hazard of exploratory surgery in the presence of hepatitis, a needle biopsy

of the liver was performed first. Histologic examination revealed the findings associated with posthepatic obstruction, but the diagnosis of phenothiazine-induced liver disease could not be entirely ruled out. Since the findings were inconsistent with viral hepatitis, surgical exploration was planned.

SYNTHESIS

Before the exploration was carried out, the facts were reviewed. The tentative diagnosis of extrahepatic obstruction was judged capable of explaining all of the italicized findings listed above. At operation, carcinoma of the head of the pancreas was found.

If the presumptive diagnosis does not explain all of the findings, the physician must decide whether the findings are significant, or if they may be discounted as normal variations. If the findings are significant, he must then decide whether it is necessary to make a second diagnosis to account for them.

At this stage of the analysis, attention must also be given to negative findings. For example, does a normal electrocardiogram exclude a myocardial infarction? What value may be attached to a negative serologic test for syphilis when the other findings point to a diagnosis of syphilitic aortitis?

CHAPTER 4

Issues in Diagnostic and Therapeutic Management

RICHARD J. JOHNS

Patient management involves far more than treatment. Indeed, it involves more than managing the patient's illness. *Treatment* implies the application of one or several therapeutic measures. *Management* is directed toward designing and implementing the most effective program of care for the particular patient's total problem. Management encompasses an orderly analysis of the patient's problems (including those which may or may not relate to his illness), the thoughtful planning of a solution or an approach to these problems, and an effective implementation of these plans.

Pneumococcal lobar pneumonia, for example, is adequately treated by administering penicillin. Management, however, includes investigation of alternative diagnostic possibilities (tumor, klebsiella pneumonia, and the like), assessment of possible complications (meningitis, septicemia, pericarditis), treatment of hypoxia, fluid deficit, or paralytic ileus, as well as the treatment of the infection. Management

also takes cognizance of personal and social factors, such as the role of the patient's chronic alcoholism or the impact of hospitalization on his employment. Furthermore, management includes recognition of a home situation which may preclude effective implementation of a therapeutic plan outside the hospital.

The scope of management is illustrated in Figure 4-1. Physicians commonly focus their attention on management of the patient's illness (A). As was discussed in Chapter 2, these interactions have in addition a profound direct effect on the patient (B). Nurses, other physicians, and other health professionals have an important role in management of the patient and his illness (C). This is particularly true in hospitals where many aspects of management must be shared and delegated. Under such circumstances the responsible physician must be ever mindful of the example he sets and of the need for clear and effective communication (D). Management includes attention to other problems and concerns of the patient

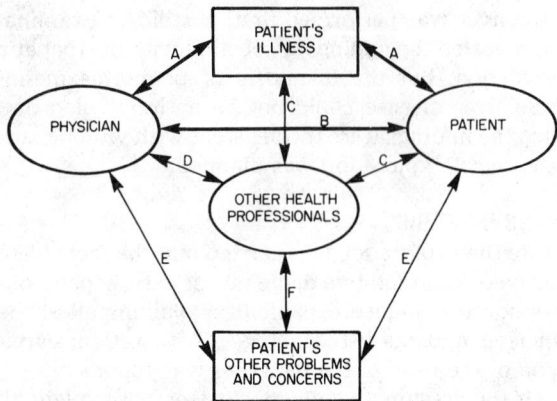

FIGURE 4–1. This illustrates the multiple interactions which occur between the various people (ellipses) and problems (rectangles). There is a tendency to focus on the interactions shown by the bold arrows. Good management, as indicated in the text, requires attention to all of the interactions.

(E). Here, too, the physician should not overlook the role of other health professionals, e.g., social workers, in discovering problems and in contributing to their solution (F and C).

This chapter will focus on the principles of good management. It will also discuss common management problems which are not related to specific disease entities, for example, the management of the dying patient. This chapter assumes that the physician has collected and analyzed the clinical information as described in the preceding chapters.

Organize and Record the Facts

Ideally, all the facts should be organized in the form of etiologic diagnoses, e.g., 1) diabetes mellitus, 2) pyelonephritis caused by *E. coli,* 3) atherosclerotic heart disease, with congestive failure, etc. As Weed points out, since this is rarely possible, it is better to start with a complete list of problems.[33] Some of these may be diagnoses while others are signs or symptoms. For example, the list for the above might initially be: 1) diabetes mellitus, 2) dysuria, 3) pyuria, 4) proteinuria, 5) exertional dyspnea, and 6) edema. This provides a list of problems which must be investigated, explained (diagnosed), and treated.

This approach has several advantages. First, it provides a framework upon which to organize laboratory studies, progress notes, and therapeutic measures, each of which should be directed toward one or another of the specific problems. Second, it avoids the pitfall of "ruling out" a given condition. For example, one might have assumed problems 2) through 5) were manifestations of the nephrotic syndrome. A diagnostic program designed to "rule out the ne-

phrotic syndrome" would not be as productive as one which investigates each problem. Third, it provides an effective means of communicating with others (nurses, consultants, house staff) involved in the patient's management. Fourth, it serves to remind the physician of problems which are unexplained or untreated which may require attention.

Have a Plan

After the physician has constructed his problem list he should list in detail all of the tests and consultative opinions considered necessary to achieve a final diagnosis. Such a work sheet should outline all, not just some, of the necessary diagnostic and therapeutic steps. Some will require immediate completion, while others may be delayed pending the results of other initial studies.

In planning studies, set a pace which is compatible with the patient's physical and emotional state. Patients are sometimes made seriously ill by poorly conceived diagnostic programs. Thus, an elderly individual with advanced arteriosclerosis may have a vascular accident when injudiciously given a series of enemas and cathartics, or when fasted and dehydrated for lengthy periods. Set the pace to fit the particular patient.

In planning the diagnostic and therapeutic program, pay particular attention to treatable possibilities. Thus, if an elderly patient is believed to have either miliary tuberculosis or a disseminated tumor, the major effort should be aimed at establishing or eliminating the diagnosis of tuberculosis which can be cured with effective treatment.

Communicate with the Patient

One of the most important skills of a physician is the ability to communicate effectively with the patient and his family. The communication of information from patient to physician should not stop with the taking of the history, nor is communication between physician and patient limited to discussion of tests, diagnoses, and drugs. The patient and his family should have the opportunity to ask any questions—both reasonable and unreasonable—which they may have, and to express any doubts, fears, or confusions which may have arisen. The patient is often troubled by an aspect of his illness which does not concern the physician. For example, an ulcer patient may be concerned because his near vision is blurred (from the parasympatholytic drug) and because he is constipated (from the antacid). The physician, in his concern that the patient is still passing occult blood, may be unaware of the patient's symptoms.

During the course of diagnostic studies the plan

of management should be explained to the patient in understandable terms. This should be done without creating anxiety, but in a way that will generate confidence and a feeling of security. It is a mistake to surprise a patient with any test or consultation. Thus, it is inconsiderate to have the patient learn from the nurse that he is on the way to have a bronchoscopic examination, nor should the patient learn only when he arrives at the consultant's office that he is being seen by a psychiatrist. The physician must lay the groundwork in such a way that understanding will be achieved, cooperation won, and anxieties dissipated.

When a patient's investigations have been completed and the physician has reached a conclusion regarding the optimum method of management, he should hold a summarizing conference with the patient and, if indicated, a relative. Such a conference is one of the most significant and important relationships of the physician to the patient, as it will almost surely determine the degree of effectiveness of the physician's advice and guidance. During this conference, the physician has several responsibilities. First, he should review each of the studies, explaining in meaningful terms why the test was done and what it indicates. The drawing of a few simple diagrams may be most helpful in explaining to the patient the nature of his illness. Next, he should outline what needs to be done in order to take care of the problem in the most effective way. Adequate time must be afforded to answer questions, as well as to prepare and explain prescriptions. The therapeutic program must be a practical one which the patient can follow without unreasonable effort or sacrifice. Throughout this discussion the physician should anticipate the probable fears and anxieties of the patient, and his conversation should be directed toward eliminating these.

The physician should take nothing for granted in making certain that the patient or his relatives understand precisely what drug and other forms of treatment are to be administered. He should not simply hand the patient several prescriptions with the instruction that, "The directions will be on the bottle." The knowledgeable physician will list on a piece of paper in brief outline the treatment to be followed, stating specific dosages and directions. Such specificity does away with confusion in the patient's mind. To be certain that the patient understands fully, he should be asked to reiterate the directions given him. On subsequent visits the patient or his relatives should be asked to repeat the program being followed. It is frequently surprising to see how grossly distorted a carefully presented therapeutic plan has become. Only repetition of directions brings ultimate understanding.

Be sure to explain to the patient the significance of important side effects a given drug may induce, and how to proceed should these develop. If serious effects are at all likely, the patient should be told to stop the drug immediately upon their appearance, and to call the physician. In thus indoctrinating the patient regarding potential side effects of various drugs, one must be circumspect and not generate needless fears or actually produce the very reactions warned against. If, in giving a patient iron, the physician says, "This may upset your stomach," there is an excellent likelihood that the prediction will come true.

Certain drugs have acquired public notoriety and, although the patient may not voice his anxieties to the physician, he may view with inward alarm the physician's admonition that such an agent is essential for his well-being. He will be torn by ambivalence, believing that he must take the medicine, and at the same time being frightened to do so. He may conjure up in his mind all sorts of bizarre notions about the drug, which are quite real to him. An example of such a drug would be prednisone: "Is it true it grows hair on your face, causes diabetes, and all your bones collapse?" Others may feel that sex hormones "make you feel queer." Such misconceptions must be anticipated, inquired about, and eradicated with a few simple words of explanation.

The Physician Must Decide

Because patients lack theoretical and technical knowledge, it is unfair for the physician to expect or to ask the patient to decide important clinical issues. On the other hand when a diagnostic or therapeutic procedure involves a risk to health or life, e.g., coronary arteriography or extensive surgery, the patient's consent must be informed consent.

In such instances the physician must weigh the risks and benefits and then advocate a course of action based upon his best judgment. In presenting the plan to the patient and his family it is important that the matter be explained clearly, honestly, and in a well-balanced fashion. He should provide ample opportunity for both questions and comments.

When advocating a course of action which involves risk, it may be difficult to avoid an overly optimistic view to protect the patient from anxiety or an overly pessimistic view to protect one's own position. A balance must be achieved between fully informing the patient without terrifying him with a recitation of every possible misadventure which can occur. This balance is especially difficult when both alternatives (action or inaction) may be associated with a grave risk, as for example the decision to explore a patient with massive gastrointestinal bleeding.

The physician should not defer the decision-making to the patient or his family, but he should present the plan fairly and openly in soliciting consent.

COMMON MANAGEMENT PROBLEMS

The foregoing general considerations apply to many clinical situations. There are, however, specific management problems which pertain to specific clinical situations. For example, a few of the diagnostic and therapeutic management problems associated with pneumococcal pneumonia have been mentioned. These are specific problems, and are quite different from the set of problems encountered in managing a patient with myocardial infarction. Indeed, one of the primary goals of this book is to describe the diagnostic and therapeutic management of common clinical conditions.

There are additional management problems which are not limited to any particular disease entity, but which are, nonetheless, quite specific. These problems include managing the uncooperative patient or the dying patient, and deciding when to embark upon a therapeutic trial or exploratory surgery. Problems of this type will be discussed in this section.

USE OF DRUGS

Indications

The physician must always have a reasonably clearcut indication for the administration of any drug. This implies that he knows what is wrong with the patient and which drug is the most effective. There is little room in therapeutic technique for the shotgun approach to drug administration. The haphazard administration of a large number of drugs is more likely to harm the patient than to benefit him. If the physician does not know what is going on, he is better advised to follow a course of watchful waiting. There are certain exceptions, usually related to life-threatening diseases, which do not permit sufficient time to reach a final diagnosis. For example, the patient with findings suggesting septic meningitis is treated with several antibiotics while awaiting bacteriologic confirmation of the presumptive diagnosis.

Contraindications

No drug should ever be given until the physician has determined whether or not the patient is sensitive to it. If a drug sensitivity exists, the fact should be noted prominently. If a patient develops a drug hypersensitivity while under treatment, this fact should be clearly explained to him, and he should be encouraged to carry on his person a notation to this effect.

Other contraindications must be carefully weighed. This implies that the physician knows both the general contraindications of the drug, and the specific drug–drug and drug–disease contraindications which may affect his patient. Barbiturates, for example, may precipitate a fatal attack in a patient with acute porphyria. The drug-drug interaction can be avoided only if the prescribing physician knows what medicines the patient is taking. When a patient is being seen by a number of physicians simultaneously, errors of this sort may easily occur.

The careful physician also avoids drugs that might further complicate his patient's problem. Thus, if a patient with viral hepatitis is nauseated, it may only complicate the illness to order a phenothiazine for nausea, since, if the jaundice becomes worse, it may be difficult to tell whether the hepatitis or a drug reaction is responsible. One must know when *not* to give drugs, as well as when to use them.

Choice of Drug

There are several important principles in the selection of drugs. First, the physician should employ drugs with which he is familiar, both in terms of beneficial effects and possible side effects or reactions. A physician should select a small number of agents to handle the various therapeutic problems, read about them, and then use them primarily. Over a period of time, he can develop a broad background of experience with a small number of drugs, rather than a fragmentary knowledge of many drugs.

Dosage and Administration

Drugs should be given on the basis of sound physiologic and pharmacologic principles, but this rule is easily broken. Thus, one finds L-thyroxin being given three times a day instead of once, or corticosteroids being administered over long periods without the use of antacids to prevent peptic ulceration; a very ill patient may awaken repeatedly during the night to void because a diuretic was given late in the evening. The physician must understand the actions of the drugs being employed, and use them to the best advantage of each particular patient.

Once a given drug is chosen, it is important to be flexible in regard to dosage. There is really no average dose of a drug; one must tailor the dose to the individual, taking into account his general health, age, size, and clinical response. At times one may need to halve or double the dose originally tried, in order to produce the desired effects.

Selecting the route of administration is as important as choosing the drug itself. For example, the patient with nausea, vomiting, or distension may not absorb oral drugs effectively. The patient with congestive failure who has hepatomegaly and nausea should receive digitalis parenterally. Patients in shock will not dependably absorb drugs injected intramuscularly. Thus, the patient with pneumococcal pneumonia who is in shock should receive penicillin intravenously. Finally, some oral medications should be given well before a meal while others should be given after meals.

New Drugs

If a new preparation clearly provides a therapeutic effect which has not been obtainable with drugs already available, its use is indicated at an early date. On the other hand, if the drug appears to do no more than older medications, it is good judgment to use the older preparations, which are likely to be both cheaper and safer. With most drugs, as experience accumulates, the therapeutic claims become more modest, and various kinds of toxicity, previously unsuspected, become manifest. One legitimate situation for using a new drug, however, is when older preparations have failed to produce the desired results in a given patient.

The physician must satisfy himself that a drug's claims of superiority to others already available are justified by the evidence at hand. In evaluating reports on the efficacy of new drugs, the physician will find these questions helpful.[45]

1. Has the agent or technique been compared against a placebo or standard therapy?
2. How has the author randomly allocated patients to the treatments under comparison?
3. How has the author controlled bias in the evaluation of results?
4. Have dose–response relationships been studied, or does the article deal only with single dose levels?
5. Is there information on the relative efficacy of different routes of administration?
6. Is there information on efficacy and toxicity of the agent when it is given chronically?
7. Is the experimental population studied of sufficient size to justify either favorable or unfavorable statements about the drug?
8. Is this patient comparable to the experimental population in which efficacy was demonstrated?

Noncompliance[43,46]

The most carefully planned therapeutic regimen will be of no benefit if the patient fails to comply with it. Noncompliance is obviously an important complication in management, and it is far more common than most physicians realize. Furthermore, physicians often do not recognize the patients who are likely candidates for noncompliance. Finally, the common reaction to noncompliance once it is discovered is to tell the patient that he is wasting the physician's time and the patient's money.

The factors contributing to noncompliance can be grouped according to those related to 1) the psychologic status of the patient, 2) his social and familial environment, 3) characteristics of the illness, 4) the therapeutic regimen, and 5) the doctor–patient relationship.

PATIENT'S PSYCHOLOGIC STATUS. The patient who is skeptical about the seriousness of his illness may be too unconcerned to follow the prescribed treatment. Such a patient is also likely to have little confidence in the general efficacy of modern medicine which further supports his noncompliance. On the other hand, the illness may evoke such intense anxiety that the patient resorts to denial of his problems and, indeed, may not have been able to pay adequate attention to the doctor's instructions; in this situation, intense anxiety may be obscured by a defensive attitude of coldness, hostility, or aggressiveness.

Therefore, lack of concern on the one hand and cold, critical, or aggressive behavior on the other, should arouse suspicion of impending noncompliance. In the former instance, the problem may be essentially an educational one and be remedied by clear, factual communication with the patient using terms understandable to him. If the patient's behavior suggests, however, a negativistic rejection of medical advice (serving to allay anxiety), the physician's task is much more difficult. He should encourage the patient to discuss his feelings about the illness and treatment and occasionally it may be necessary to modify the treatment plan, at least temporarily, in order to secure some level of cooperation.

SOCIAL AND FAMILY BACKGROUND. The physician should always pay careful attention to the patient's family situation and socioeconomic background. Lack of money or transportation and preoccupation with pressing family or occupational demands may gravely interfere with the patient's ability and willingness to comply with the management plan. In this situation it is sometimes tempting for the physician himself to ignore these aspects and to rationalize this posture by saying that his job is to prescribe treatment, the patient's to carry it out. However, tactful but frank discussion of the home and job situation may well lead to the discovery of practical aids to facilitate participation in treatment. A skilled social worker is often invaluable in the assessment of these problems and in the mobilization of community resources in their solution.

NATURE OF ILLNESS. It is likely that when the illness produces considerable discomfort such as pain, shortness of breath, or weakness which is substantially improved by the prescribed drug and which recurs when the medicine is not taken, the patient will comply with treatment. However, if the illness is relatively "silent," such as uncomplicated essential hypertension, the likelihood of noncompliance is enhanced. In these instances noncompliance should be anticipated and counteracted by a clear explanation of the benefits of treatment.

NATURE OF THE THERAPY. More complex therapeutic regimens, especially those requiring substantial changes in daily habits, are more likely to evoke noncompliant behavior than are simple treatment plans. Here, too, it is important to encourage the patient to express his feelings, ask questions, and sometimes to "negotiate" a treatment plan which, while it may fall short of the ideal, has a better chance of being carried out.

Similarly, in programs in which the benefits of the treatment are slow to appear, the tendency to noncompliance is great. The dietary management of obesity is a common example.

THE PATIENT–PHYSICIAN RELATIONSHIP. In the last analysis, the physician–patient relationship may well be the most crucial variable in determining compliance with treatment plans. In the daily work of the busy practitioner, failure to take the time for truly adequate communication is probably the most common and damaging deficiency of modern medicine. If the doctor is to maximize his effectiveness, he must cultivate a relationship of mutual respect, offer explanations in a clear manner, invite questions, and expressions of feelings and ideas, and be sensitive to psychologic and other obstacles that may stand in the way of full patient cooperation. This topic is discussed further in Chapter 136.

THERAPEUTIC TRIAL

The physician should not prematurely discontinue his step-by-step, considered attack on the patient's problem until a reasonable diagnosis is obtained. Nevertheless, it is sometimes necessary to begin specific therapy without knowing the actual cause of the patient's illness. There are other instances where a therapeutic trial must be embarked upon, based on the most probable diagnosis.

Although the nature of the illness is still obscure, if the patient is seriously ill or if essential organ function seems threatened, a program of therapy should be chosen which will cover all of the reasonable therapeutic possibilities. Even in these circumstances, however, one should try to avoid a shotgun approach. If the condition of the patient seems to warrant it, a progressive type of therapeutic trial may be begun in which first one, and then another, agent is added to the treatment program in an effort to determine its effect upon the patient's course. Drugs should be chosen that are safe, specific in action, and unlikely to cause further complications.

Once it is decided that a therapeutic trial is the wisest course of action, the treatment should be maintained long enough to test its effectiveness. In this regard, it is advisable to select criteria of improvement which can be subjected to objective analysis, e.g., fever and spleen size. The indecisive approach, where regimens are started and then abandoned, too often leads to dangerous confusion.

EXPLORATORY SURGERY

Surgical procedures are sometimes necessary to provide a diagnosis. Laparotomy and thoracotomy are major procedures requiring careful consideration. These are discussed in this section. In contrast, skin, muscle, and lymph node biopsies are considered simple procedures, involving little risk, if any. Intermediate, in terms of risk, is a group of procedures which are discussed elsewhere. These include pleural biopsy, scalene node biopsy, and mediastinoscopy (Chap. 32), liver biopsy (Chap. 62), and renal biopsy (Chap. 10).

Laparotomy

Since exploratory laparotomy is of value in determining the cause of illness in some instances, it is important to consider when such a procedure is indicated. If the clinical evidence clearly points to a localized intra-abdominal disorder, laparotomy is obviously in order. Considerable judgment is required when there is little or no evidence pointing to intra-abdominal disease. On the one hand, all operations carry some risk, especially in a seriously ill patient; on the other, surgical exploration may reveal the cause of disease even in the absence of local symptoms and signs.

Exploratory laparotomy should not be pursued until all indirect methods which afford a reasonable chance of establishing the etiology of the disease have been exhausted. Included in this category are not only history and physical examination, laboratory, x-ray, endoscopy, and other special procedures, but also, and especially, a period of searching clinical observation, during which the patient is thoughtfully requestioned and reexamined. Such a period must not become one in which the patient is allowed to drift, or in which confusing forms of therapy are added.

In deciding when to terminate such an observation period, one should neither be premature nor delay too long. One must assay the degree to which the disease has already importantly affected the patient, or is likely to do so in the near future. Such an inventory must encompass not only the physical effects of the illness, but also the personal ones. Not being able to work, periodically being forced to suspend normal living, the psychologic effects of being considered ill, the financial drain of chronic or recurrent illness, are all factors which must be weighed. From the physical standpoint, evidence that any of the organ systems are being seriously affected in a deleterious manner is the most important determinant. Clearly, significant progressive alterations would call for an immediate decision. Another consideration is the likelihood that by prolonged waiting a condition that is now curable may progress to an uncontrollable stage. A decision on this point, of course, is dependent upon the diagnostic possibilities being considered.

The risks entailed in an exploratory operation will be determined not only by the patient's general physical status, but also by what may be required surgically should a suspected abnormality be discovered. It is not enough to decide that the patient can withstand an exploration. Of equal significance is a decision regarding the patient's ability to survive surgical correction of whatever may be discovered. For example, if the clinical evidence indicates that a patient has right-sided colitis, but his general condition interdicts surgical treatment of this condition, it may be inadvisable to prove the diagnosis by a laparotomy, and further medical treatment may be preferable.

Having decided upon an exploratory operation, how should this be accomplished so that the necessary information will be forthcoming? It is most unfortunate if the operation is performed in such a way that valuable information is overlooked or discarded. Two points are worthy of emphasis. First, all suspicious lesions should be biopsied. It is impossible to distinguish tumor from inflammation with certainty without histologic study. Second, biopsy material should be studied adequately and properly. For example, cultures for tubercle bacilli, fungi, and anaerobic bacteria should be made when appropriate. Similarly, a biopsy of the skin, subcutaneous tissue, and muscle can easily be accomplished while doing a laparotomy. It is regrettable if the patient must undergo a muscle biopsy at a later date to establish the diagnosis of polyarteritis.

Thoracotomy

The principles discussed for exploratory laparotomy also apply in general to exploration of the chest, mediastinum, or pericardium. There are, however, several matters deserving special note.

First, thoracotomy for a mass lesion in the lung may require a segmental resection, or even a lobectomy. Hence, if the plan is to open the chest, the physician must be certain that the patient is able to withstand whatever procedures are necessary. Also, he must ascertain that the patient and family fully understand how extensive the exploration may ultimately be.

Second, a specific diagnosis may not be made even when adequate tissue is obtained and studied thoroughly, both histologically and biologically. This is especially true of granulomatous lesions of the lung, pleura, pericardium, and mediastinum. A wide variety of infectious agents, including tuberculosis, syphilis, fungi, parasites, and certain malignant tumors, in addition to some chemical agents, may cause a granulomatous inflammatory response which is totally nonspecific and which may become so widespread as to obscure the parent process.

Exploratory laparotomy may occasionally be undertaken on the basis of symptoms alone. In contrast, thoracotomy is almost never undertaken unless there are clear signs of disease, either on physical examination, x-ray, or other diagnostic test.

MALPRACTICE

Malpractice suits and the threat of malpractice suits represent significant and difficult issues in patient management today. Legally, medical malpractice is negligence on the part of the physician or his agent that leads to injury of the patient. These problems concerning malpractice are real, and there is no reason to expect that they will diminish.

Unfortunately, malpractice does occur. The physician forgets that the patient is allergic to penicillin and administers it, or he fails to note a coin lesion on a routine chest film. This is negligence, and the patient may be injured. Physicians aim to manage their patients in a conscientious fashion, and they intend to avoid this type of negligent error.

In current medical practice, however, avoiding negligence is necessary, but it is not sufficient to guard against being sued for malpractice. It is estimated that only one-fifth of malpractice claims reflect actual negligence on the part of the physician. Why do the other four-fifths believe they have been injured through physician negligence? A clear understanding of the basis for these claims is necessary if one is to avoid them.

Societal Factors

There is a widespread belief today that if something goes wrong and you are injured that "somebody should pay." This is seen in product liability as well as in medical malpractice. The public expects to be compensated by the automobile manufacturer if injury results from a steering gear failure. The public expects to be compensated by the physician if there is residual disability after reduction of a fracture. There is no question about the injury, but the steering gear failure may not be caused by the manufacturer's negligence and the residual disability may not be related to negligence on the part of the physician. The view that the injured party is entitled to compensation whether or not there was negligence is called *strict liability in tort* by the legal profession. Although it is not accepted in many jurisdictions, it reflects a common belief, a change in belief by our society. Much of the increase in malpractice litigation is explained by this widespread belief that one is entitled to compensation for injury (whatever its cause) when combined with the factors discussed below.

Unfavorable Outcome

Almost all claims arise from patients who experience an unfavorable medical outcome. While this is a necessary condition, it, too, is usually not sufficient. There is often another factor which prompts such a patient to claim malpractice.

Unrealistic Expectations

The most common combination of factors in precipitating malpractice claims is an unfavorable outcome in a patient who had unrealistic expectations about the outcome. Some patients die despite the best possible medical management, and others make substantially less than a full recovery. Physicians have a great propensity for wanting to spare patients and their families from anxiety. They may persuade them that everything will turn out well even when it is clear that the situation is grave or the proposed course of action is risky.

Thus, the physician himself usually gives rise to unrealistic expectations on the part of patients and families. When the results fall far short of what the patient and family were led to believe, it is understandable that they conclude that something went wrong. The sequence—1) everything was supposed to be fine, 2) it was not, 3) therefore, something must have gone wrong, 4) therefore, somebody should pay for this unfavorable and unexpected outcome—accounts for many malpractice claims.

Physicians need not burden patients or their families with the most pessimistic outcome to ensure that they will be pleased with anything short of disaster. Nevertheless, the prudent physician must give the patient or at least responsible family members a realistic appraisal of the situation. Ironically, it is the physician who is the most persuasive with patients who can impart the most unrealistic expectations.

Anger

The patient who is angry for any reason may seize upon an unfavorable outcome to gain retribution. Unfortunately for the physician, the anger may be directed at the hospital billing system, the nursing service, the physician's receptionist, or even at the patient's own illness. The physician may find himself the target of this anger and frustration even when he is not directly responsible for it. There are many reasons to be alert to anger on the part of patients, and physicians should take responsibility in seeing that the vexing issues are resolved. Considerable sensitivity is required, because patients frequently have difficulty in expressing their anger to physicians, especially if the anger is directed toward the physician.

The Litigious Patient

More patients are made litigious by circumstances than are litigious by nature. There are, however, some patients who are frankly litigious. Such patients often move from physician to physician, are deprecatory and complaining of their past medical care, and are often unreasonably demanding. This behavior tends to evoke hostility, anger, and defensiveness on the part of the physician. Even when the physician does not allow these feelings to affect his management of the patient, the scene is set for contention.

Defensive Medicine

One must practice defensive medicine. This does not imply ordering unnecessary tests or obtaining unnecessary consultations. The best defense against malpractice claims is simply good management: 1) establish an attitude of mutual trust with the patient; 2) communicate realistically with the patient; 3) be sensitive to his needs, fears, concerns (whether well founded or not); 4) be aware of your own limitations; and 5) keep good records of what was done and why it was done.

NEED FOR CONSULTATION

The physician should always be willing to ask for consultative help when it is needed. To practice first-rate medicine one must always be prepared to seek the opinion and judgment of those whose experience is greater. Even if the medical necessity is nonexistent, the physician should be alert to anxiety and restiveness in the patient or in members of his family, and respond by suggesting that the fresh viewpoint of a consultant be secured. To be fully productive, the physician and the consultant should meet and discuss the problem. Consultations carried out through an exchange of notes are often of very little value.

It is important to recognize, however, that the physician in charge of a patient cannot abdicate his responsibility for management. Management by a committee of consultants never insures that the best opinion is brought to bear on a problem.

MEDICAL EMERGENCIES

The usual orderly steps in management may need to be altered in dealing with emergencies. The details of managing these problems are discussed in Section 18.

MANAGEMENT OF EMOTIONAL DISORDERS[43]

The management of emotional disorders is of considerable importance to the practicing physician, since a number of studies show that a substantial percentage of patients seen in diagnostic clinics have no demonstrable organic abnormalities which can be related to their symptomatic complaints. The large numbers of these patients would make it impractical to refer all of them to psychiatrists, even if this were considered to be desirable.

Thus, the appropriate management of emotional problems is important to all physicians. Although this subject is treated in some depth in Section 16, it is worth outlining several aspects of the management problem here.

The recognition that an emotional problem exists is the first step in management. In general, patients whose problems are exclusively of a "mental" or emotional nature will present with complaints concerned with subjective discomfort, functional disturbance, or will have exhibited aberrant behavior which has aroused concern in others. It is important to keep in mind that apparent symptoms of emotional disturbance may in fact represent an organic entity such as thyroid dysfunction. Therefore, it is also necessary in this situation to regard symptoms and behavioral disturbances as problems which, with further fact gathering and analysis, may later become grouped under a single diagnostic entity, psychiatric or other.

It is common for an emotionally disturbed patient to complain of a physical symptom such as chronic fatigue, headache, or insomnia, and often a whole host of physical complaints will be elicited in the history taking. Among the reasons for this, two may be mentioned here: 1) The patient may be focusing upon physical discomforts as a means of minimizing painful feelings which might accompany an awareness of his emotional difficulty. 2) His preconception of what the physician's interests may be lead him to use a physical complaint as an "admission ticket" to the doctor's office.

It is apparent that in this situation, as elsewhere in medicine, treatment of the symptoms, such as prescribing aspirin for headache is doomed to failure unless it is accompanied by recognition and adequate management of the total problem. This symptomatic approach often occurs, however, and contributes to the fact that such patients frequently have had disappointing experiences with prior medical contacts and may become resentful, difficult, and demanding. Occasionally, a physical symptom may be of such psychological importance that a radical approach to it alone without appropriate evaluation and management of the whole problem may precipitate rapid psychologic decompensation. On rare occasions this may result in the development of a paranoid accusation directed at the physician.

The next questions to arise following recognition is whether the physician chooses to manage the problem himself, with or without psychiatric consultation, or to refer the patient to a psychiatrist. Parallel issues are *how* to manage the problem if the physician elects to do so, and how to facilitate the patient's acceptance of psychiatric consultation or referral. On each of these questions it is often helpful for the physician to discuss the issue with a psychiatric consultant.

Both general principles of management and management of specific problems such as suicidal behavior and anxiety states are discussed in detail in Section 16.

DIAGNOSIS OF MALIGNANCY

The doctor must make it an unbroken rule never to conclude that a patient has a malignant disease without histologic proof of the diagnosis. In these matters, he should neither trust hearsay evidence nor be willing to take anything for granted. Serious mistakes may be made by assuming that the patient has a malignant disease on the basis of an exploration of the chest or abdominal cavity in the absence of objective evidence based on the histologic study of a biopsy specimen. These mistakes can take the form of irrevocable action, e.g., irradiation of a granuloma in the lung, or the form of inaction, e.g., the failure to treat ameboma of the colon.

When the diagnosis is established, the question always arises of whether the patient should be told. While it is impossible to generalize, it is safe to say that most patients realize the nature of their illness sooner or later. If the patient has been assured that his condition is benign by his physician, he may feel betrayed. More important, the physician has then lost much of his power to support and sustain the patient through a difficult situation. Often, a gentle, honest explanation (avoiding the terms "cancer" and "malignant") will convey the information. At the same time, the physician should offer hope in the form of a specific program of management.

HOPELESS ILLNESS

Much of what has been said of malignant tumor applies to hopeless illnesses as well. The physician must be certain to have excluded all treatable conditions, even if they are much less common. For example, reasonable steps must be taken to exclude frontal lobe tumor in the patient thought to have senile dementia.

Similarly, it is important that the physician remain alert to the appearance of unassociated treatable complications. There is an understandable tendency to ascribe an unfavorable clinical course to the underlying disease without adequate investigation.

The only prudent philosophy for a physician to adopt is always to support life as long as it is present. It is dangerous to do otherwise. However, if the reasoned judgment of the physician and of his colleagues is that a patient's illness is entirely hopeless and that the patient is undergoing significant mental or physical suffering, the use of extraordinary means to support life is certainly not expected, or even desired.

THE DYING PATIENT

The patient who is dying represents a special management problem. Most patients, their families, doctors, and nurses are uncomfortable in dealing with death or in discussing its prospect. Since most persons now die in a medical institution rather than at home, physicians are centrally involved. Further-

more, since death is such an emotionally charged issue for everyone involved, it is essential that the physician be able to manage the problem effectively and with understanding.

The discomfort involved in managing a dying patient leads both doctors and nurses to avoid patient contact, to be brief and cursory when in contact with the patient, and to be evasive if the patient directs the conversation toward prognosis, outcome, and the like. At the same time the family is upset and may be struggling to suppress grief or guilt. As a result the patient, in a time of great need, may find himself cut off from counsel, emotional support, and perhaps even from conversation and full attention to physical needs.

Thus, this important clinical management problem has not been handled well by physicians or health care professionals in general, and little has been taught or learned about management of the dying patient in our educational programs. In recent years, however, this problem of the dying patient has been subjected to clinical study. Kübler-Ross[44] has identified a common pattern of emotional stages through which patients pass following the recognition of the fact that they are dying. These stages are 1) shock and denial, 2) anger, 3) bargaining, 4) depression, 5) preparatory grief, and finally 6) a peaceful acceptance. These feelings occur with some overlap and some shifting back and forth, and it is a sense of hope which sustains the patient throughout.

The physician's role is to support the patient and provide understanding. Insight into these stages permits the physician to deal with the real issues better. For example, the patient's anger may appear to be directed toward some trivial aspect of his care. His need is not simply to have the triviality corrected, and it is certainly not to have the triviality of the issue emphasized. He needs an opportunity to express his anger and resentment about the outrageous situation in which he finds himself.

It is not necessary for the physician to *tell* the patient he is terminally ill. The physician should, however, be attuned to the patient's efforts to communicate his awareness to the physician. Often this is done obliquely by patient comments such as, "I don't think there is much more that you can do for me," or, "I don't really think I am going to get better." These are not cues for hearty reassurance by the physician; they are requests for discussion of the problem. Reassurance, denial, and disclaimers by the physician promptly bar further discussion of the topic, a message which the patient clearly perceives. Inquiry into areas of particular concern to the patient, on the other hand, opens the way to a meaningful conversation about issues important to the patient. These can lead to more openness between the patient and his family as well.

REFERENCES

1. Peabody, F.W. The care of the patient. JAMA, 88:877, 1927.

Clinical Information and Clinical Problem Solving

2. Dudley, H.A.F. The clinical method. Lancet, 1:35, 1971.
3. Dudley, H.A.F. The clinical task. Lancet, 2:1352, 1970.
4. Elstein, A.S., Shulman, L.S., and Sprafka, S.A. Medical Problem Solving. An Analysis of Clinical Reasoning. Cambridge, Ma., Harvard University Press, 1978.
5. Enelow, A.J. and Swisher, S.N. Interviewing and Patient Care. New York, Oxford University Press, 1972.
6. Engel, G.R. and Morgan, W.L. Jr. Interviewing the Patient. Philadelphia, Saunders, 1973.
7. Feinstein, A.R. Clinical Biostatistics, St. Louis, Mosby, 1977.
8. Feinstein, A.R. Clinical Judgment. Baltimore, Williams & Wilkins, 1967.
9. Galen, R.S. and Gambino, S.R. Beyond Normality: The Predictive Value and Efficiency of Medical Diagnoses. New York, Wiley, 1975.
10. Morgan, W.L., Jr. and Engel, G.L. The Clinical Approach to the Patient. Philadelphia, Saunders, 1969.
11. Murphy, E.A. The Logic of Medicine, Baltimore, The Johns Hopkins University Press, 1976.
12. Whitehorn, J.C. Guide to interviewing and clinical personality study. Arch. Neurol. (Chicago), 52:197, 1944.

The Collection and Evaluation of Clinical Information

13. Belcher, E.H. and Vetter, H., (eds.). Radioisotopes in Medical Diagnosis. London, Butterworths, 1971.
14. Cochrane, A.L., Chapman, P.J., and Oldham, P.D. Observers' errors in taking medical histories. Lancet, 1:1007, 1951.
15. DeLand, F.H., Wagner, H.N., Jr., and North, W.A. Atlas of Nuclear Medicine. 3 vols. Philadelphia, Saunders, 1969, 1970, 1972.
16. Elveback, L.R., Guillies, C.L., and Keating, F.R., Jr. Health, normality, and the ghost of Gauss. JAMA, 211:69, 1970.
17. Feinstein, A.R. Scientific methodology in clinical medicine, I, II, IV. Ann. Intern. Med., 61:564, 757, 1162, 1964.
18. Feinstein, A.R., The problems of the "problem-oriented medical record." Ann. Int. Med., 78:751, 1973.
19. Goldberg, B. Diagnostic Ultrasound in Clinical Medicine. New York, Medcom Press, 1973.
20. Henry, R.J. and Reed, A.H. Normal Values. In Henry, R.J., Cannon, D.C., and Winkleman, J.W. (eds.), Clinical Chemistry, Principles and Techniques. Hagerstown, Md. Harper and Row, 1974.

21. Hillman, R.S. and Funk, D.C. Routine Examination of the Adult. Seattle, Health Sciences Learning Resources Center of the University of Washington, 1973.
22. Jelliffe, R.W. Quantitative aspects of clinical judgement. Am. J. Med., 55:431, 1973.
23. King, D. Diagnostic Ultrasound. St. Louis, Mosby, 1974.
24. Koran, L.M. The reliability of clinical methods, data and judgements. New Engl. J. Med., 293:642 and 695, 1975.
25. Metropolitan Life Insurance Co. Statistical Bulletin 40, November–December, 1959 and Bulletin 41, February–March, 1960.
26. Miller, G.A. The magical number seven, plus or minus two: some limits on our capacity for processing information. Psychol. Rev., 63:81, 1956.
27. Neuhauser, D. and Lewici, A.M. What do we gain from the sixth stool guaiac? New Engl. J. Med., 293:226, 1975.
28. Sisson, J.C., Schoomaker, E.B., and Ross, J.C. Clinical decision analysis. The hazard of using additional data. JAMA, 236:1259, 1976.
29. Squire, L.F. Fundamentals of Radiology. Cambridge, Ma., Harvard University Press, 1975.
30. Ter-Pergossian, M., Phelps, M.E., Brownell, G.L., Cox, J.R., Jr., Davis, D.O., and Evens, R.G. (eds.). Reconstruction Tomography in Diagnostic Radiology and Nuclear Medicine. Baltimore, University Park Press, 1977.
31. Wagner, H.N., Jr. (ed.). Principles of Nuclear Medicine. Philadelphia, Saunders, 1968.
32. Walker, H.K., Hurst, J.W., and Woody, M.F. (eds.). Applying the Problem-Oriented System. New York, Medcom Press, 1973.
33. Weed, L.L. Medical Records, Medical Education, and Patient Care. Cleveland, Case Western Reserve University Press, 1969.
34. Werner, A.S., Cobbs, C.G., Kaye, D., and Hook, E.W. Studies on the bacteremia of bacterial endocarditis. JAMA, 202:199, 1967.
35. Vecchio, T.J. Predictive value of a single diagnostic test in unselected populations. New Engl. J. Med., 274:1171, 1966.

The Analysis and Synthesis of Clinical Information

36. Feinstein, A.R. An analysis of diagnostic reasoning. II. The strategy of intermediate decisions. Yale J. Biol. Med., 46:264, 1973.
37. Folstein, M.F., Folstein, S.E., and McHugh, P.R. "Minimental state." A practical method for grading the cognitive state of patients for the clinician. J. Psychiatr. Res., 12:189, 1975.
38. Harvey, A.M., Bordley, J., III, and Barondess, J.A. Differential Diagnosis—The Interpretation of Clinical Evidence. 3rd ed. Philadelphia, Saunders, 1979.
39. Kassirer, J.P. and Gorry, G.A. Clinical problem solving: A behavioral analysis. Ann. Intern. Med. 89:245, 1978.
40. Schwartz, W.B., Gorry, G.A., Kassirer, J.P., and Essig, A. Decision analysis and clinical judgement. Am. J. Med., 55:459, 1973.

Issues in Diagnostic and Therapeutic Management

41. Brim, O.G., Jr., Freeman, H.E., Levine, S., and Scotch, N.A. (eds.). The Dying Patient. New York, Russell Sage Foundation, 1970.

42. Gillum, R.F. and Barsky, A.J. Diagnosis and management of patient noncompliance. JAMA, 288:1563, 1974.

43. Imboden, J.B. and Urbaitis, J.C. Practical Psychiatry in Medicine. New York, Appleton-Century-Crofts, 1978.

44. Kübler-Ross, E. Questions and Answers on Death and Dying. New York, Macmillan, 1974.

45. Lasagna, L. On evaluating drug therapy: the nature of the evidence. In Talalay, P. (ed.), Drugs In Our Society. Baltimore, The Johns Hopkins Press, 1964.

46. Rosenstock, I.M. Patients' compliance with health regimens. JAMA, 234:402, 1975.

47. Tumulty, P.A. The Effective Clinician. Philadelphia, Saunders, 1973.

SECTION TWO
Disorders of Water and Electrolyte Metabolism
W. GORDON WALKER: SECTION EDITOR

Disturbances in water and electrolyte metabolism are produced by a variety of factors, some intrinsic and some extrinsic, which affect the intake, output, or distribution of water and electrolytes. They may be the primary cause of illness, but more commonly they occur as by-products of some other disorder. Their recognition in some cases depends upon the detection of such obvious manifestations as edema or dehydration, but in other cases they are brought to light only by the use of physical or chemical measurements. Alertness to the possible presence of these disorders in certain specific clinical settings may lead to the correct diagnosis. These settings are those in which either 1) the normal regulating mechanisms are upset by disease; or 2) the fluid losses or excesses are so great that even normal regulating mechanisms cannot cope with them. Successful management depends upon 1) a correct diagnosis, 2) accurate quantitative information concerning the magnitude of the deficit or surplus to be corrected, and 3) a working knowledge of the principles underlying the regulation of water and electrolytes.

In the management of these problems, it should be emphasized that fluid and electrolyte abnormalities are not diseases, but are the manifestations of disease. The diagnosis and treatment of the underlying disease is, as always, dependent upon a careful evaluation of the history, physical examination, and laboratory data.

A semiquantitative estimate of the state of over- or underhydration should be made from information obtained from the patient or other informants. This estimate can be supplemented by the physical signs of abnormal hydration. Intelligent recruitment of information from examination of blood constituents and urine should permit more accurate quantitation of water or salt disturbances.

The physician then turns his attention to correction of the specific disturbances of water and electrolyte balance. General principles in the management of water and electrolyte disturbances will be emphasized here, with presentation of specific illustrative cases in Chapter 9 accompanied by a discussion of therapeutic management.

The physician should determine to what degree the patient's regulating mechanisms can be relied upon for assistance in correcting the disturbance. In particular, he should assess the functional capacity of the *cardiovascular system,* especially to gauge how safely water and salt can be administered without provoking congestive heart failure. This estimation of function can be very simple; adequate evaluation is accomplished by a careful history, physical examination, and determination of venous pressure. This appraisal is repeated as often as necessary during the course of fluid therapy, i.e., the patient is examined several times a day for signs of early failure. The presence of pulmonary rales is an important sign since increased venous pressure, hepatomegaly, and edema may not appear until later.

The physician should also assess *renal function.* The first step is to be sure that the patient can eliminate urine. If there is no spontaneous urination, the bladder is percussed, and, if enlarged, urine should be obtained by catheterization for the determination of specific gravity and examination of the urinary sediment.

In the following chapters, disturbances of water, sodium, potassium, and pH will be considered. It is convenient to discuss each of these separately, as though there were an isolated disturbance involving only one of them. In fact, however, they are so interrelated that isolated disturbances occur rarely. It is important, therefore, to reconstruct the events that beset the patient and to disentangle from them the basic defect that sets the disturbance in motion so that one can see clearly what alteration needs most urgent correction. It is the aim of this section to guide the physician to that goal.

CHAPTER 5

Water Metabolism

W. GORDON WALKER AND ANDREW WHELTON

BASIC CONSIDERATIONS

Water is the chief constituent of the body, and disturbances in the amount and distribution of body water are both serious and common, yet frequently are unrecognized, often to the detriment of the patient. Two aspects make recognition difficult. First, these disturbances are encountered much more frequently as a complication of some underlying disease than as isolated deficits in otherwise healthy individuals. Second, reliable physical signs are encountered relatively late in the course of development of disturbances of water balance, hence major emphasis must be placed upon careful historical evaluation of the patient's intake and output. This should include assessment of the environmental circumstances under which a deficit or excess may have occurred as well as determination of the adequacy of function of the physiologic regulatory mechanisms that operate to maintain the body water constant.

In this chapter the distribution of water, the kinetics of its movement, and the regulation of osmolality will be discussed prior to consideration of the clinical problems of water deficit and water excess.

DISTRIBUTION [3,4,5,6,18]

Body water, representing 60 percent of body weight, is the aqueous medium in which the exchanges necessary to sustain metabolic processes of the body occur. Approximately two-thirds of the water is located within the cells and the remaining one-third is extracellular (Fig. 5–1). Water moves freely back and forth across the cellular membranes and across the capillaries which separate the intravascular water from that of the interstitial fluid. This unrestricted movement of water results in the maintenance of osmotic equilibrium between the interstitial compartment of body water and that fraction of the body water within cells. This freedom of movement is *not* shared by the major solutes of the body. Sodium and its anions occupy a position that is almost exclusively extracellular while potassium and its attendant anions are largely confined to the intracellular compartment. As a consequence, the distribution of water reflects the distribution of solute within and outside the cells;

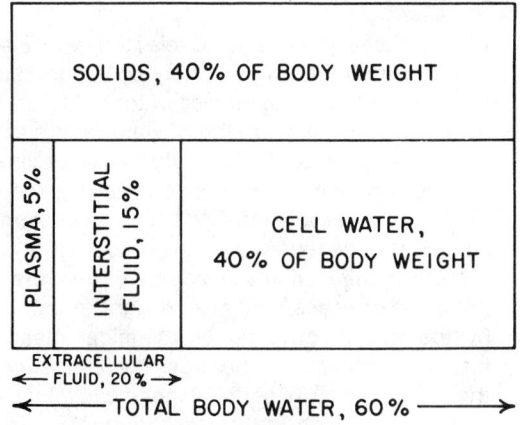

FIGURE 5–1. Distribution of body water.

there are approximately 4000 mOsm (mainly sodium chloride and sodium bicarbonate) occupying the extracellular space and approximately 8000 mOsm (potassium and anions) in the intracellular space.

Because of the marked disparity between the permeance exhibited by water and that by the major solutes of body fluid, osmotic equilibrium is achieved by water shifts between the extracellular and intracellular compartments. Thus, loss of water, as for example during prolonged sweating, represents water lost initially from the plasma and extracellular fluid. However, this water loss within the extracellular compartment results in a corresponding increase in solute concentration in this compartment. The water within the cell then exists at a higher concentration than in the extracellular fluid, and consequently a water shift from within the cell to the extracellular fluid occurs until osmotic equilibrium is reestablished and the total solute concentration is identical inside and outside the cell (Fig. 5–2). Similarly, if sodium is lost in excess of water from the extracellular compartment, the solute concentration falls in this compartment resulting in a shift of water into the cells to reestablish osmotic equilibrium; excess intracellular potassium loss results in a corresponding shift in the opposite direction. Such fluid shifts operate to maintain osmotic equilibrium across the cellular membrane in the normal state as in a wide variety of abnormal conditions.

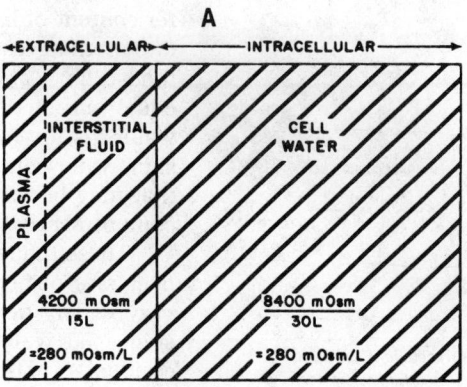

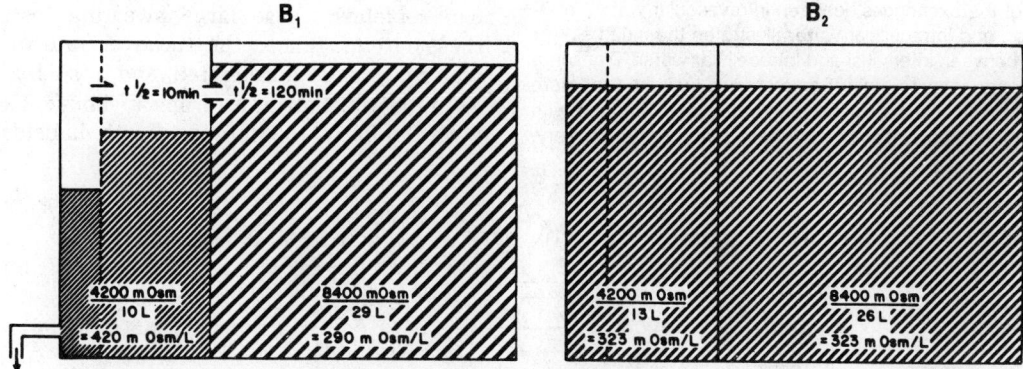

FIGURE 5-2. The compartments of body water under normal conditions are shown in diagram **A.** The extracellular fluid compartment is composed of interstitial water plus plasma water. Relative size of intracellular and extracellular compartments is determined by total solute content of each compartment.

The diagrams **B₁** and **B₂** illustrate the sequence of changes that result from water loss (6 liters) from body compartments without accompanying solute loss (as, for example, in diabetes insipidus). Initial loss in urine represents loss of fluid delivered to kidney by the blood. This loss is rapidly shared by the interstitial fluid resulting in a rapid drop in total extracellular fluid volume and corresponding increase in solute concentration in the ECF. The marked difference between intracellular and extracellular solute concentration resulting from this ECF water loss results in slower shift of water from intracellular to extracellular compartment (**B₁**). This shift continues until solute concentrations are again equal. At this point the loss is shared by both ECF and ICF (**B₂**). The distribution of the deficit is determined by the proportion of solute inside and outside the cell; a 4-liter deficit is intracellular, and a 2-liter deficit extracellular.

KINETICS[2,6]

In the steady state, the exchange of water between the plasma and extracellular fluid is extremely rapid, complete exchange occurring during the course of one circulation through the capillary bed. The exchange between the extracellular fluid and the fluid of the cells is somewhat slower and exhibits a half-time of about two hours (Fig. 5–3). These rates of movement across the barriers separating the body water compartments are the primary determinants of the rate at which osmotic equilibrium will be restored following any disturbance in solute concentration either outside or within the cell.

Excesses or deficits in body water result from disturbances in external exchanges, that is, exchanges between the total body water pool and the water of the environment. In the normal adult individual in a temperate environment the external exchange exhibits a half-time of about 10 days (Fig. 5–4). This is accomplished by a water intake that usually varies between 2500 and 3000 ml per day. The sources of this intake include ingested water, the wa-

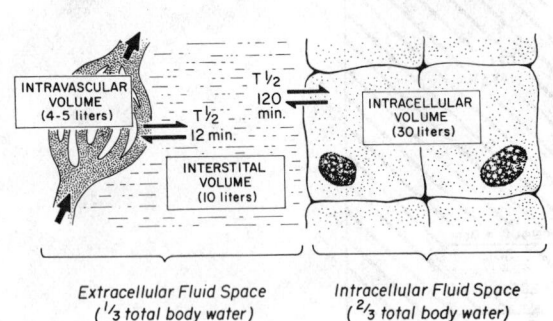

Extracellular Fluid Space
(¹/₃ total body water)

Intracellular Fluid Space
(²/₃ total body water)

FIGURE 5-3. Body water kinetics: This schematic representation of the exchanges between intravascular water, interstitial water, and intracellular water illustrates the much slower exchange between interstitial and intracellular water. Transcapillary exchange is quite rapid. Some studies indicate that more than 50 percent of the intravascular water is exchanged with that in the interstitium during each pass through the capillary.

ter content of ingested foods, as well as water of oxidation that results from the oxidation of ingested foodstuffs (Table 5–1). This intake, balanced by an equal output that includes water excreted as urine, water lost by insensible routes through the lung and skin, water content of excreted feces, as well as water that may be lost by sweating, maintains body water content nearly constant.

These figures for intake and output and the turnover rate of body water are only averages and may vary widely depending upon environmental circumstances as well as physiologic disorders. Thus, an individual sweating at a maximal rate may lose 8 to 10 liters of water per day; under circumstances where he is able to maintain an adequate oral water intake he can replenish these large sweating losses. Under these circumstances the turnover rate of the body water is greatly accelerated, and in such an extreme example the half-time drops to about 3 days (Fig. 5–5). Similarly, the individual with diabetes insipidus

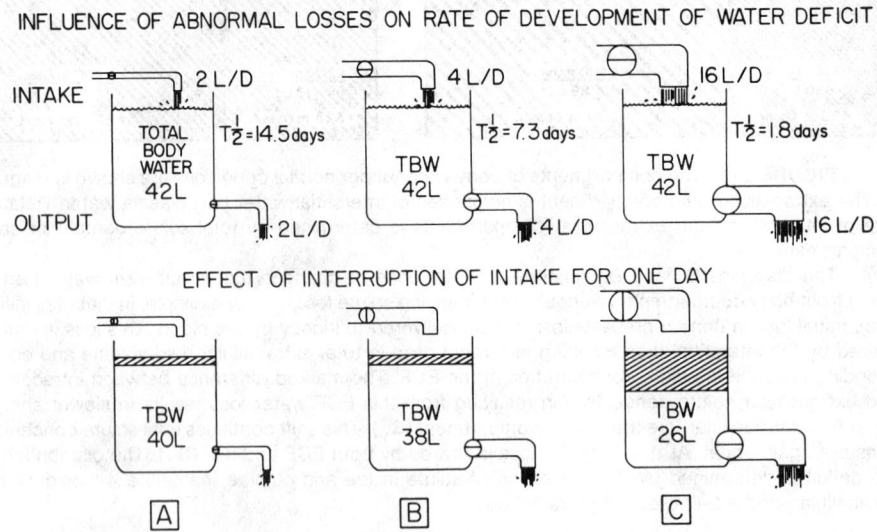

FIGURE 5-4. Schematic representation of the rate at which a deficit in body water may develop in the presence of abnormally large losses and intake. In the upper part of the illustration are shown three conditions, **A** represents normal losses and intake; **B** represents moderate increase in losses as may be encountered in sustained sweating; and **C** depicts a marked increase in water loss as for example in complete diabetes insipidus that is untreated. In each instance the individual is capable of replacing these losses and preventing development of any deficits so long as the thirst mechanism is intact and he has access to adequate water. Under these circumstances the only alteration is a considerable acceleration of water turnover rate with corresponding shortening of half-life of body water as indicated. When intake is interrupted, the rate of development of water deficit varies very greatly under these different circumstances as shown in the lower set of diagrams. After cessation of intake for any 1 day, the normal subject under usual physiologic circumstances will have lost only about 2 liters (shaded area). The individual with sustained losses through sweating may develop a deficit twice this great, and the individual with an extraordinary rate of loss, as in diabetes insipidus, may develop a life-threatening deficit in 1 day's period.

TABLE 5-1

Usual Daily Sources of Water Intake and Loss for the Average Adult

Intake	
Fluid intake	1200–1800 ml
Water content of ingested food	700–1000 ml
Water of oxidation	250–300 ml
Total	**2000–3000 ml**
Output	
Urine	1500–2000 ml
Insensible loss	
Skin	300–600 ml
Lungs	200–400 ml
Gastrointestinal loss (water content of feces)	100 ml
Total	**2000–3000 ml**

may exhibit urinary losses of water that exceed 10 to 12 liters per day. Replenishment of these losses by an increased intake will result in a comparatively rapid turnover of body water.

From both these examples, it is clear that the basis for an accelerated turnover of water is usually increased loss from some source. Only rarely is a primary increase in water intake, as in compulsive water drinking, the primary basis for an accelerated turnover of the body water. Deficits or excesses of body water arise when the homeostatic mechanisms fail to maintain equality between the intake and output. The rate at which such deficits or excesses develop is obviously determined by the magnitude of the difference between intake and output. Correction requires 1) recognition, 2) quantitative assessment of the deficit or excess, and 3) alteration of difference between intake and output in the appropriate direction to restore body water to its normal value.

REGULATION OF BODY WATER[2-5,8,10,11,16,17]

The physiologic mechanisms that control water intake and output both appear to respond primarily to serum osmolality (Fig. 5–6). Regulation of output is influenced by variation in the rate of release of the pituitary antidiuretic hormone (ADH) in response to changes in serum osmolality and intravascular volume. Osmolar changes also serve as a stimulus to modulate thirst. This mechanism is sufficiently sensitive to limit variations in osmolality in the normal individual to less than about 1 percent. The body water, through these control mechanisms, continually oscillates between a narrow range of slight excess and slight deficit as outlined in Figure 5–6.

In the presence of normal posterior pituitary function, the effectiveness of the kidney in conserving water results from its capacity to produce a urine that is hypertonic to plasma.[11] The mechanism responsible for concentrating the urine in response to the stimulus of ADH is presented in detail in Chapter 10. Since this mechanism is activated only after a modest water deficit has stimulated ADH release, it serves to retard the rate of further water loss, and concomitant stimulation of the thirst mechanism and increased water intake repairs the deficit.

The individual can tolerate disturbances in ADH release much better than disturbances in the thirst mechanism. In the absence of ADH, the kidney excretes large volumes of dilute urine, the daily urinary output often exceeding 6 to 8 liters. The resultant persistent thirst easily increases intake to equal this loss. In the absence of a normally functioning thirst mechanism, such a rate of loss can lead to development of a severe water deficit in only a few hours. Fortunately, primary disturbances of the thirst mechanism are quite rare. Any disorder that interferes with intake, such as disturbance of consciousness, etc., effectively disrupts the thirst mechanism and removes the most important defense against development of water deficit. However, disturbances of either mechanism can lead to serious, and at times life-threatening, abnormalities in water balance.

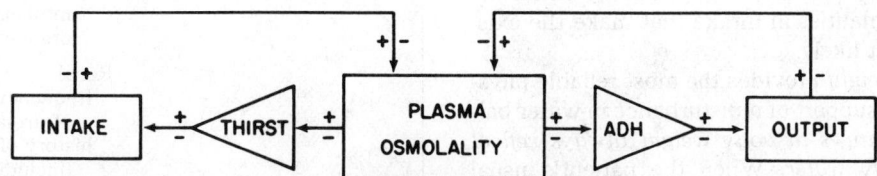

FIGURE 5-5. Control mechanisms for body water regulation. Osmolality is the parameter measured and controlled in regulating body water. Variations lead to changes in thirst stimulus and ADH release. Change in thirst stimulus results in altered water intake, and change in ADH release changes water output. Both lead to change in osmolality.

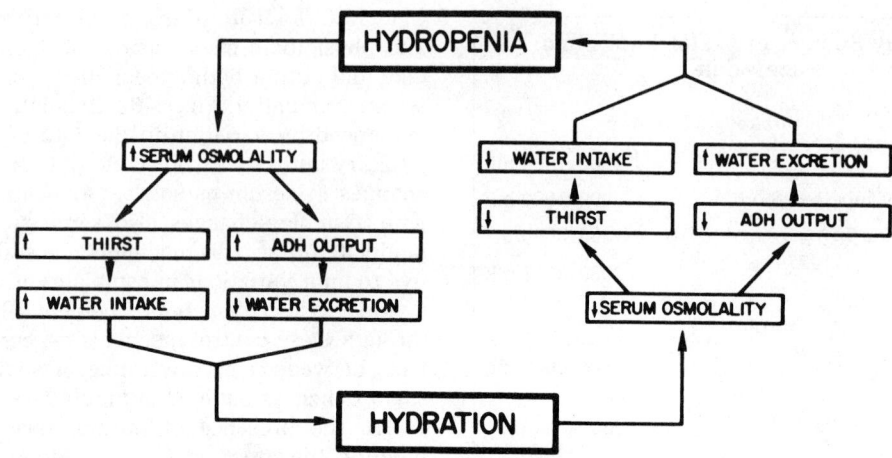

FIGURE 5-6. Regulation of water balance. This regulatory mechanism is dependent upon continuous sensing of plasma osmolality. In the normal individual it regulates the body water within such narrow limits that osmolality varies only 1 percent between hydropenia and hydration.

RECOGNITION AND MANAGEMENT OF WATER DEFICIT[12,13,14]

CLINICAL FEATURES

The clinical features of water deficit vary with the severity of the deficit. In the conscious and alert patient, loss of 1 to 2 percent of the body water leads to a severe and unrelenting thirst. Quite often, however, in the disorders where water deficit is encountered clinically, the patient is disoriented for some other reason and this important symptom may not be apparent. It is common to encounter patients who have water deficits of 5 to 7 percent who exhibit no identifiable physical signs of a deficit of this magnitude. This is particularly true in the elderly where the inelastic skin and the changes of aging make recognition of altered skin turgor difficult. With greater degrees of water loss, approaching 10 percent or more of the body water, there is regularly poor skin turgor, dry mucous membranes, stupor, and ultimately coma. Despite difficulties in diagnosis when only mild deficits exist, careful and systematic history taking as outlined in Table 5-2 will usually identify abnormal losses or abnormalities in intake that make the existence of a deficit likely.

The *body weight* provides the most reliable physical evidence in support of a disturbance in water balance. *Acute changes in body weight always reflect changes in body water.* When the patient's usual weight is accurately known, a weight at the time of the physical examination can confirm a suspected deficit of body water. Similarly, daily monitoring of body weight is the most reliable means of confirming

---TABLE 5-2---
Historical Information Sought in Assessing Water Balance

Intake	Output

Average daily intake of water and other fluids	Skin losses
	    sweating* (duration and severity)
	    abnormalities of environment leading to excessive losses

Recent alterations in intake pattern and cause (nausea or vomiting, inability to swallow, etc.)	Lungs
	    abnormal rate of breathing
	    excessively dry ambient air

Recent weight changes (acute changes in weight over period of several days are always caused by changes in body water)	Gastrointestinal
	    diarrhea or vomiting* (estimate frequency and amount)
	    fistulas, enteric or biliary* (attempt quantitative estimate)
	    gastrointestinal intubation* (quantify drainage)

	Renal
	    frequency and volume of urination
	    history of renal disease (including conditions impairing concentrating ability)

* Represent sources of loss of both water and electrolytes.

the accuracy of intake and output measurements and of identifying significant changes in body water. In the healthy adult, the daily basal weight (early morning weight after voiding and defecation and before eating or drinking) is maintained constant. Sudden deviations that exceed more than ± 1 percent represent gains or losses of body fluid, as do progressive trends upward or downward with time. Daily measurement of body weight in all patients in whom fluid balance problems are present or likely to develop provides the most reliable means of assessing day to day changes.

LABORATORY FEATURES

The most reliable laboratory evidence of a water deficit may be obtained by direct measurement of the serum osmolality, or measurement of the serum sodium concentration (Table 5–3). In the absence of renal disease, these two tests provide equivalent information. In the presence of azotemia, measurement of serum osmolality can be misleading unless "corrected" by subtracting the osmolar equivalent of urea. This is accomplished by subtracting 1 mOsm from the serum osmolality for each increment of 3 mg/dl in the serum urea nitrogen. Similarly, hyperglycemia can yield misleading results. For these reasons, measurement of the serum sodium concentration is probably the most reliable single indicator of the presence of a water deficit. It must be stressed that the serum osmolality and serum sodium provide only a relative indication of an excess or deficit of water. Thus it is possible to have a lowered serum sodium concentra-

tion indicating a relative excess of water in the presence of a deficit in total body water (see hypotonic contraction, Chap. 9).

The hematocrit *does not* provide any measure of water deficit. It shows relatively little change during the development of a pure water deficit even when the deficit is large enough to be life-threatening (Table 5–3). For example, loss of 20 percent of the body water would result in elevation of the hematocrit from 42 to 43 percent, a change of no diagnostic value. The presence of a significant elevation of the hematocrit in association with other data such as hypernatremia or hyperosmolality is strong evidence for the coexistence of a *sodium deficit.*

Table 5–3 presents data on plasma osmolality and corresponding findings in water deficits of increasing severity. Water losses that exceed 10 percent of the total body water are usually associated with a progressive disturbance in central nervous system function, and, unless the deficit is corrected, disorientation, stupor, and coma ensue. Water losses that exceed 20 percent of body weight are associated with an imminent demise.

CAUSES

Reduced Intake

Water deficits caused by a disturbance in water intake are confined to the very young, the very old, and those individuals who are too enfeebled to satisfy their own water needs. The unique features of fluid and electrolyte disorders in infancy have not been considered in this section. The subject is appropri-

---

TABLE 5–3

Clinical and Laboratory Features of Water Deficit [6,7,10,12,14]

Clinical Severity	Symptoms	Signs	Serum Na (mEq/L)	Serum Osmolality (mOsm/kg)	Hct*	Magnitude of Deficit (liters)	% Body Water Lost
Normal	—	—	144	285	42	—	—
Mild	Thirst†	None	149–151	294–298	42	1.5–2	3–4.5
Moderate	Thirst†	Dry mucous membranes	152–158	299–313	42.2	2–4	4.5–10
Severe	Thirst† Weakness	Above plus doughy skin	159–166	314–329	42.5	4–6	10–15
Very severe	Disorientation Severe weakness Fainting	Postural hypotension CNS changes Stupor Coma	>166	>330	43–44	>6	>15

*Note that these calculated changes are not clinically detectable.
†Requires that patient be alert and communicative.

ately presented in a number of pediatric treatises. Most commonly, pure water deficits are encountered in the elderly who, for a variety of reasons, may have become unable to attend to their daily needs. This is particularly likely to be encountered during hot weather when the increased rates of loss by way of the skin may lead to the rapid development of large water deficits. When the major source of water loss is perspiration, significant quantities of sodium may also be lost and a symptomatic sodium deficit that is masked by the hypernatremia resulting from water loss should always be considered in this circumstance. The demonstration of a significant rise in the hematocrit is most helpful in recognizing a coexisting sodium deficit.

Defective Thirst

Disturbances in the thirst mechanism are quite rare but may be seen following head injuries or some neurosurgical procedures. In such patients progressive hypernatremia may develop despite an ability to concentrate the urine adequately. Such individuals, who may otherwise appear to be able to function reasonably well, are totally unable to respond to a water deficit because they have no sensation of thirst. They must be placed on a regular schedule of water administration. Such a defect may persist for several years.

Excess Solute

A common disturbance of intake encountered in elderly individuals relates to excess solute intake rather than reduced water intake. The elderly victim of a cerebral vascular accident who is being fed by nasogastric tube may be given a formula whose solute load requires a greatly increased water intake. Thus, tube feeding containing 120 g of protein and 10 g of salt will result in the excretion of more than 1000 mOsm of solute. This requires the obligatory excretion of a volume of urine between 1200 and 1500 ml when the kidney is capable of concentrating normally. Since elderly individuals often have significant impairments in renal concentrating ability, water loss as urine may exceed 2000 to 2500 ml per day. Such an individual would require 3 to 4 liters of water per day simply to meet the increased demand created by this high solute intake. Failure of the physician to provide such patients with the increased water intake needed will result in a progressive water deficit that may rapidly become critical. The importance of knowing the complete composition of the tube feeding formulas used for incapacitated patients cannot be overemphasized.

---TABLE 5-4---
Possible Abnormal Daily Losses of Water

Sweat*	6000–8000 ml
Upper gastrointestinal losses† (vomiting or intubation)	2500–5000 ml
Diarrhea†	10,000+ ml
Bile	500 ml
Urine excluding diabetes insipidus*	4000–5000 ml
diabetes insipidus*	10,000+ ml

* Hypotonic losses, leading to hyperosmolality of body fluid.
† Represent isotonic losses leading to deficits of both water and electrolytes.

A water deficit may develop in a variety of other clinical situations such as severe myasthenia gravis where the patient is simply too weak to maintain an adequate water intake, extensive oral herpes where the painful condition of the mucous membranes precludes adequate fluid intake, and other disturbances leading to mechanical difficulties associated with drinking. *The physician should be alert to the possibility of inadequate water intake in any patient who is seriously ill.*

Sweating

Among the possible sources of body water loss, severe and prolonged sweating probably represents the greatest threat to maintenance of the normal body water in the healthy individual. Because the sweating rate can vary from nil to quantities in excess of 8 liters per day depending upon the environment, water loss from this source can on occasion lead to the rapid development of severe water deficits. Working in an extremely hot environment, vigorous body contact sports such as football in hot weather, and prolonged exposure to direct sunlight may all produce sweating at near maximal rates and may lead rapidly to the development of water deficits in the absence of adequate intake (Table 5-4).

Renal Loss

Renal water losses rarely contribute to the development of a water deficit in the absence of some impairment of renal function. The normal kidney under the influence of antidiuretic hormone acts promptly to retard the rate of development of water deficit when any significant loss elevates plasma osmolarity.

In the absence of the antidiuretic hormone, diabetes insipidus appears and may lead to extraordinarily large water losses from the kidneys. This condition is discussed in detail in Chapter 69.

The situation is quite different, however, when the renal concentrating ability is impaired. Such patients are more susceptible to the development of water deficits than are normal individuals. Indeed, seemingly minor reductions in water intake or increases in water loss may precipitate serious deficits. Among the disorders which impair the renal concentrating ability are the nephropathy associated with sickle cell anemia, hypercalcemia, hypokalemia, and nephrogenic diabetes insipidus (Chap. 14). With the exception of nephrogenic diabetes insipidus, all of these conditions result in only moderate increases in the daily urine volume, since the kidney is usually able to excrete a urine that is at least isotonic to plasma in these disorders. The minimum urinary volume in these patients is determined primarily by the solute output per day, a solute load of 600 mOsm requiring approximately 2 liters for its excretion. This increased obligatory water loss renders the kidney relatively ineffective at conserving water if a deficit in body water develops.

The above discussion has been concerned with the mechanisms of development of a pure water deficiency and its recognition (Table 5–5). In practice, the physician is more often faced with mixed disturbances where losses of both solute and water have occurred in varying proportions. For example, the hyperosmolar coma occasionally seen in elderly diabetics is a condition in which a water deficit predominates, but in which other disturbances including sodium and potassium deficits are also encountered. These more complicated disturbances are considered in Chapter 9.

THERAPY

The therapy of water deficit is adequate water replacement. The route and rate of this replacement depend upon the severity of the disturbance as well as upon the problems associated with the individual case.

In modest deficits, where the total water loss is less than 10 percent of the body water, oral replacement is satisfactory if the patient is capable of taking fluids orally. Should nausea be a problem, or if for any other reason oral intake is impossible, replacement must be undertaken by the intravenous route.

Solution

When the deficit is only moderate, the intravenous administration of 5 percent dextrose in distilled water may be an adequate means of achieving fluid replace-

TABLE 5–5
Clinical Conditions Leading to an Isolated Water Deficit

Type of Disturbance	Clinical Setting
Disordered Intake	
Water deprivation	Elderly feeble patients Central nervous system disorders Unavailability of water Mechanical difficulties interfering with swallowing mechanism
Absence of thirst	CNS disorders
Increased solute intake	Nasogastric tube feeding containing high protein and NaCl content
Increased Losses	
Diabetes insipidus	Pituitary or hypothalamic disorder
Nephrogenic diabetes insipidus	Hereditary renal disorder associated with marked water loss via the kidney; unresponsive to ADH
Osmotic diuresis	Diabetes mellitus Hypertonic tube feedings
Sweating	Prolonged exposure to heat—usually associated with moderate sodium deficit
Renal disease	Nephropathy of hypokalemia and hypercalcemia Nephropathy of sickle cell anemia Rarely pyelonephritis and other diffuse renal diseases after advanced renal failure supervenes

ment. The individual who can metabolize carbohydrate normally converts the dextrose in the fluids to glycogen, making solute-free water available for correcting the water deficit. This water then distributes between cells and extracellular fluid as discussed earlier. The individual who has some difficulty metabolizing dextrose (as in the diabetic) or those who also have hyperosmolarity (see Chap. 71) can be more effectively treated by giving 2.5 percent dextrose in distilled water. Similarly, in circumstances where large volumes must be administered, these more dilute solutions should be employed. The use of 2.5 percent dextrose in distilled water or 2.5 percent dextrose in a solution containing 35 mEq of sodium and chloride

TABLE 5-6
Osmolality of Commonly Employed Parenteral Fluids

Fluid	Osmolality (mOsm/kg H_2O)
2.5% Dextrose	139
2.5% Dextrose in 0.034 molar (0.2%) NaCl	209
5% Dextrose in distilled H_2O	280
5% Dextrose in 0.155 molar (0.9%) NaCl	560
Normal plasma	280
Plasma with 20% water deficit	350

per liter will provide adequate water replacement while avoiding the hemolysis which may result from the rapid administration of a more dilute solution.

While specific choice of fluid may depend very much on the individual case, as a guiding principle of therapy in the treatment of hyperosmolarity, *no fluid should be administered that exceeds the osmolality of normal plasma*. Osmolalities of some commonly used solutions of parenteral fluid are shown in Table 5-6.

Rate

Patients with severe water deficits appear to respond more satisfactorily when the therapy is planned to restore body water to normal over a period of 24 to 36 hours. For this reason when the estimated deficit exceeds 6 to 7 liters, therapy should be planned to restore about half the total deficit in the first 24-hour period.

Estimation of Deficit

An important initial aspect of planning therapy is the estimation of the initial deficit. Since, in a pure water deficit, the solute content of the body fluid compartments does not change, the change in concentration of the solute (or serum sodium concentration) can be used to estimate the deficit quantitatively. The deficit can be calculated from the expression where water deficit is given in liters and BW refers to body weight

$$H_2O \text{ deficit} = 0.6 \times BW \left(1 - \frac{144}{[Na_{obs}]}\right)$$

in kilograms. $[Na_{obs}]$ is the abnormal serum sodium concentration observed in the patient to be treated. In

practice, this calculation provides only an approximation because disturbances of consciousness or lack of knowledge by the patient concerning his usual weight introduces some uncertainty, as does lack of exact information about the percentage of the patient's body weight that is water. However, the most important objective of such a calculation is the provision of an estimate of the deficit that permits rational planning of therapy, and the results obtained are quite adequate for this purpose. Expected laboratory values and clinical data associated with deficits of increasing magnitude are shown in Table 5-3.

RECOGNITION AND MANAGEMENT OF WATER EXCESS[11,13]

CLINICAL FEATURES

Diagnostic recognition of water excess requires a careful history to identify sources and amounts of water intake and an accurate appraisal of water output. Headache, blurred vision, muscle cramps, and twitches are seen in moderate water intoxication. As the disorder progresses in severity, disorientation, stupor, and convulsions are regularly present. Although the patient who is otherwise awake and alert may experience headache and some gastrointestinal disturbance with as little as 5 to 7 percent excess body water, it is unusual to encounter significant central nervous system symptoms until much more marked degrees of the disturbance are encountered.

Physical examination is rarely helpful. *Pitting edema is virtually never seen* in the presence of pure water excess. There may, on occasion, be some scleral edema. Increased body weight provides confirmation of the suspected water excess. Table 5-7 lists the prominent clinical findings and expected laboratory data associated with water intoxication of increasing severity. The hematocrit changes represent calculated values and are included to emphasize that the hematocrit does not change significantly even in profound water intoxication unassociated with other electrolyte disturbances.

LABORATORY FEATURES

The most important single laboratory observation is measurement of the serum sodium concentration supplemented by information about change in body weight when available. Hematocrit is usually unchanged, but a low serum sodium concentration is a prerequisite to making the diagnosis of water excess. It is very rare to encounter significant symptoms until

---
TABLE 5-7
Clinical and Laboratory Features of Water Excess

Clinical Severity	Symptoms	Signs	Serum Na (mEq/L)	Serum Osmolality (mOsm/kg)	Hct	Magnitude of Excess (liters)	% Body Water Excess
Normal	—	—	144	285	42	—	—
Mild	Headache	—	139–132	275–261	41.8	1.5–4	3–8
Moderate	Headache Drowsiness Weakness	—	131–127	262–251	41.8	4–6	8–13
Severe	Above plus disorientation	Cramps Rarely seizures	126–118	250–233	41.6	6–10	13–22
Very severe	Stupor Coma	Seizures	<118	<233	41.6–41.5	>10	>22

---

the serum sodium concentration drops below 125 mEq/L. For this reason the group of disorders associated with water excess are sometimes called "asymptomatic hyponatremia."

CAUSES

Water excess also requires a persistent disparity between intake and output in a direction opposite to that leading to water deficit. The scheme depicted in Figure 5–6 is so sensitive to changes in plasma osmolality and the kidney is capable of excreting excess water at such rapid rates that *water excess is virtually never encountered as a result of increased intake* unless there is some associated disturbance in regulation of water balance. Thus, the individual who is a compulsive water drinker, the classic example of excess water intake, almost never develops water intoxication unless there is some intercurrent event that leads to increased ADH output which persists for several hours.

Nonphysiologic or inappropriate secretion of ADH may be seen in patients receiving opiate drugs for analgesic purposes, in the presence of persistent severe pain, and in several pulmonary and CNS disorders with resultant water intoxication of varying degrees of severity. Tumors producing polypeptide substances resembling ADH may also lead to inappropriate water retention. These abnormalities of ADH secretion are commonly encountered and are referred to collectively as the syndrome of inappropriate secretion of ADH (SIADH).

In summary, most cases of water excess represent 1) increased intake in circumstances associated with continued ADH output, or 2) primary renal disturbances that interfere with renal water excretion. It is rare that this latter circumstance leads to pure water excess.

Table 5–8 lists some of the conditions that may be associated with water excess, in some of which the primary disorder is associated with increased intake and in others with decreased output.

TABLE 5-8
Conditions Leading to Water Intoxication[13,16,17]

Disturbances of Intake	Clinical Setting
Compulsive water drinking	Hyponatremia likely only with associated illness, e.g., pneumonia
Iatrogenic water administration	Excess fluid administration following major surgery
Disturbances of Output	
Syndrome of inappropriate ADH secretion	Seen in carcinoma of the lung, CNS disorders, pulmonary tuberculosis, sarcoidosis
Renal impairment	Acute renal failure with oliguria Chronic renal failure
Congestive heart failure*	Seen in severe congestive failure when underperfused kidney cannot excrete water load
Cirrhosis of liver*	Occurs in presence of severe ascites

* Condition here included is dilutional hyponatremia resulting from retention of water in excess of NaCl. See Chapters 9, 10, and 11.

THERAPY

Estimation of Excess

The equation presented in the previous section, relating changes in body water to changes in sodium concentration, provides a reasonably accurate means of estimating the size of the water excess.

Fluid Restriction

The aim of therapy is a progressive reduction in body water through an appropriate reduction in fluid intake. The rate at which this is accomplished depends upon the difference between the total daily fluid intake permitted and the daily fluid losses. Assuming minimal losses (insensible losses 500 ml, urine 400 ml, and feces 100 ml; total 1000 ml), a total intake of 500 ml would result in a decrease in body water by 500 ml per day. Such a rate of loss would require a 12-day period to correct a water excess of 6 liters. Correction of water intoxication by water restriction alone is a slow process.

Water loss can be accelerated by use of osmotic agents such as urea, mannitol, or hypertonic sodium chloride, since all these agents will stimulate excretion of more water than sodium by the kidney with consequent return of the osmolality of body fluids toward normal. The hazards of overexpansion or volume overload during such treatment should be kept in mind, particularly in patients with cardiac impairment. The concomitant use of diuretics, such as furosemide and hypertonic saline replacement, provides a therapeutic approach that reduces or removes the risk of further overexpansion during therapy. It is possible that furosemide may also exert antagonistic activity to ADH and thus further enhance its usefulness in treating water intoxication. Both lithium and demeclocycline antagonize the peripheral action of ADH and thus are potentially useful in treatment of inappropriate ADH excess. The hazard of toxicity with long-term use of lithium limits its potential usefulness but demeclocycline appears promising.

Diet

It is not easy to reduce the total water intake of a patient to 500 ml per day. As can be seen from Table 5–1, the average preformed water contained in a day's intake of food usually exceeds 700 ml per day. Therefore, in order to restrict water intake to 500 ml per day, it is necessary to alter the diet so that the total daily caloric intake provides no more than 200 ml of preformed water. If this is provided as a high protein, low fat, low carbohydrate diet, the water of oxidation is kept at a minimum. Even so, this permits the patient to drink only about 150 to 200 ml of fluid per day if the total intake is to be kept at 500 ml. An additional advantage of a diet of this type results from the increased urea production and the accompanying increased minimal urine volume requirements for excreting the excess urea.

Efficacy of therapy is measured by a reduction in body weight. A successful regimen should be reflected in a weight loss of about 3/4 to 1 pound per day. If this is not achieved, extraneous water intake should be suspected and every effort made to achieve the desired limitation. The most common source of unrecognized water intake is in the daily food intake. The aid of a dietitian should be sought to insure that this source of water intake is minimal.

Hypertonic Fluids

The patient with water intoxication of sufficient severity to produce severe CNS symptoms such as stupor, coma, or convulsions requires more rapid correction of the water excess than can be achieved by fluid restriction alone. Administration of hypertonic saline, use of an additional osmotic agent such as urea or mannitol plus a diuretic such as furosemide is indicated under these circumstances.

The use of 3 percent sodium chloride solution (510 mEq/L, or about 1020 mOsm per liter) will directly elevate the osmolality of body fluids and raise the serum sodium concentration even in the absence of any excretion of the excess water. It is thus the treatment to be considered first in severe water intoxication, but only after careful evaluation of the cardiac status of the patient. Since administration of such hypertonic saline increases intracellular osmolality by osmotically drawing fluid into the extracellular space, it can rapidly produce severe overload of the cardiovascular system in individuals with significant cardiovascular disease. Because of this risk, furosemide or some other potent loop diuretic should always be used as part of the treatment regimen. The administration of 5 to 10 ml of a 3 percent NaCl solution per kg BW (2.5 to 5 mEq per kg BW) will raise the osmolality of the body fluids about 7 to 14 mOsm per liter when given slowly over a period of 2 to 4 hours and usually leads to significant improvement of the CNS disturbance. Greater quantities should be employed with great caution and only in patients with adequate renal function and a normal cardiovascular system.

The use of mannitol carries the same risks of cardiovascular overload as does hypertonic sodium chloride when given intravenously and in addition leads to further decrease in the electrolyte concentrations in the extracellular fluid as a result of fluid shifts.

When given on a daily basis to patients with the syndrome of inappropriate antidiuretic hormone secretion, it is useful in increasing renal excretion of excess water. Administration of about 0.75 g per kg BW as a 20 percent solution intravenously, given over a 6- to 8-hour period, should increase the daily urine volume by about 1 liter per day in the average sized adult.

In those individuals with seriously compromised cardiovascular function who exhibit severe CNS symptoms from water intoxication, dialysis may be necessary to remove excess water. In general, excess water may be removed either by ultrafiltration during hemodialysis or by peritoneal dialysis using a dialysate solution made hypertonic with glucose. Either method permits removal of excess water without significant expansion of the extracellular fluid volume (Chap. 11).

CHAPTER 6
Sodium Metabolism
W. GORDON WALKER AND ANDREW WHELTON

Sodium is the principal cation of the extracellular fluid of the body. The quantity of sodium determines, to a large extent, the volume of the extracellular fluid compartment. In the healthy subject this volume is maintained relatively constant by regulating the sodium content of the body. Isotope dilution studies have made data available on the quantity of sodium within the body as well as the type and magnitude of variations that are encountered in health and disease. This method identifies only about 70 percent of the total quantity of sodium within the body, the remainder being situated in poorly exchangeable portions of the skeleton. It is this exchangeable moiety of body sodium that is clinically important; Figure 6–1 (page 60) indicates the predominant extracellular location of this important fraction of the body sodium. The difference between exchangeable and nonexchangeable sodium is that the majority of sodium present in bone and cartilage is deep in the matrix of these tissues and is not readily available for equilibration with the remainder of the body sodium. Therefore, in clinical situations alteration in body sodium is synonymous with alteration in exchangeable sodium. The mean value for adult males is 41 mEq of exchangeable sodium/kg of body weight; for females, 40.

Significant symptoms are produced by either excesses or deficits in the sodium content of the body; too much sodium may lead to circulatory congestion and ultimately to pulmonary edema, while too little sodium leads to progressive circulatory collapse and shock. Either situation may be fatal if not recognized and treated. Effective treatment requires recognition of the derangement in body sodium content. Although it is widely believed that the serum sodium concentration provides the simplest and most accessible guide to recognition of these disorders, this measurement is in fact of virtually no help without a careful history and physical examination and other ancillary laboratory data. In most instances *sodium depletion of short duration is unassociated with any change in serum sodium concentration.*

All of the isotopic dilution studies of body sodium content have failed to identify any correlation between the serum sodium concentration and the total content of sodium within the body in either health or disease. In fact, the serum sodium concentration correlates most closely with serum osmolality and only provides information about the ratio of solute to water within the body fluids irrespective of whether the subject under study has an abnormally high or abnormally low body sodium content. It is thus possible for hyponatremia to be associated with excess sodium within the body and, conversely, for hypernatremia to be encountered in patients with serious sodium depletion, depending only on the relative rates of loss or gain of sodium and water by the body. For this reason the serum sodium concentration is of little value in identifying excesses or deficits of sodium. Proper recognition and treatment of these abnormalities is dependent upon a careful history and physical examination that provides information about source and quantity of possible sodium losses. A clear understanding of the homeostatic mechanisms responsible for regulating body sodium content, as well as consequences of a deficit or excess of sodium upon this regulatory system, is necessary for correctly diagnosing and treating disturbances in sodium metabolism.

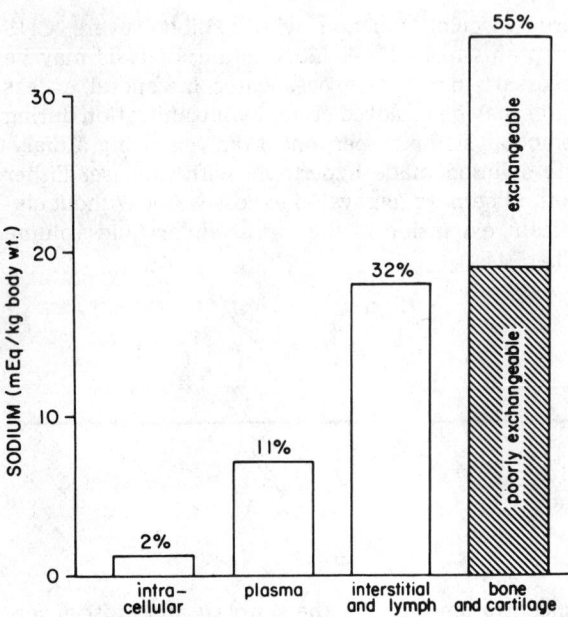

FIGURE 6-1. Distribution of exchangeable sodium within the various spaces and tissues of the body.

REGULATION OF BODY SODIUM CONTENT[1,6,22]

The sodium content of the body is closely regulated despite wide fluctuations in sodium intake. Metabolic balance studies reveal that the normal subject can tolerate a sodium intake that may vary from less than 10 mEq per day to quantities in excess of 350 mEq per day, while the total body sodium content varies by no more than 150 mEq or about 2 mEq per kg of body weight. The average intake during health usually ranges between 100 and 150 mEq per day depending upon the individual's taste and dietary habits but it has been estimated that as little as 5 mEq per day are required to sustain maximal growth during childhood. The adult human can survive without difficulty on less than 1 mEq per day for long periods of time in the absence of abnormal losses.

Sodium loss occurs in the urine, sweat, and feces (Table 6-1). In the normal individual, regulatory mechanisms operate to reduce these losses to very low levels when the intake is reduced for any reason. The kidney is capable of producing urine that contains less than 1 mEq of sodium/L when sodium conservation is required. Sodium conservation in sweat is less efficient, but in the individual acclimated to heat the sodium concentration in sweat is usually less

TABLE 6-1
Routes of Normal Sodium Loss from the Body

	Range of Loss in 24 Hours
Kidney	<1 to 150+ mEq
GI tract	<1 to 10+ mEq
Skin (sweat)	<15 to 70 mEq/L of fluid lost

than 15 mEq/L. Normally, these adjustments of sodium concentration require two to four days following change in the sodium intake, and it is during this short interval that the modest changes in the sodium content of the body occur in normal individuals when sodium intake is changed.

The renal mechanisms for regulation of sodium excretion include 1) hemodynamic alterations in response to variations in sodium intake, 2) the humorally mediated renin-angiotensin-aldosterone mechanism, and 3) a third factor that may be humorally mediated. Although the details of this last mechanism are less clearly defined, it may also have a hemodynamic component.

Increased sodium intake results in transient expansion of the plasma volume and interstitial fluid volume, and an associated increase in glomerular filtration which increases the quantity of sodium filtered. These events lead to suppression of renin release and reduction in the rate of aldosterone secretion (Fig. 6-2) and may also stimulate a third

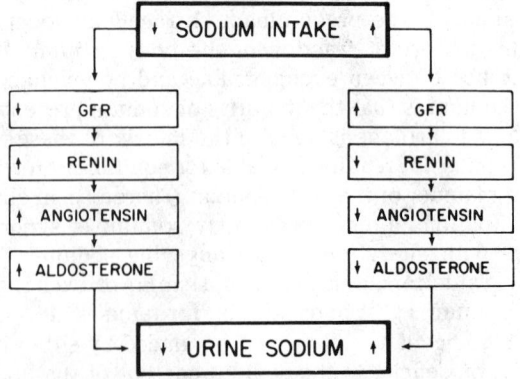

FIGURE 6-2. The role of the renin-angiotensin-aldosterone system in regulation of sodium balance. The expansion of the extracellular fluid and blood volume that results from increased intake of sodium increases glomerular filtration and reduces renin output with reduction in angiotensin production and aldosterone secretion. This reduces renal tubular reabsorption of sodium and increases urinary sodium. Reduction of salt intake reverses this sequence of events, leading to reduction in urine sodium.

factor which results in decreased tubular reabsorption of sodium. Conversely, when sodium intake is reduced, or stopped altogether, the sodium excretion which continues for a short period of time results in a decrease of extravascular volume as well as plasma volume, a reduction in the glomerular filtration rate and renal blood flow with resultant decrease in the quantity of sodium filtered at the glomerulus. This is associated with an increase in renin release and increased sodium reabsorption. When sodium intake ceases, these mechanisms are so efficient that the kidney produces urine that is virtually free of sodium.

The capacity to reduce significantly the sodium concentration of intestinal fluids is confined to the colon. Fluid entering the colon from the small bowel contains sodium at a concentration equal to plasma's. This sodium is reabsorbed in the colon. The colon, like the nephron, is capable of transporting sodium against a large gradient so that the concentration of sodium in the fecal contents can be reduced to low levels. This transport mechanism has a relatively limited capacity, however. In the presence of diarrhea, the sodium concentration in the fecal fluid rises sharply and in extreme cases approaches the concentration in plasma. Hence, sodium loss in the feces is directly related to the total quantity or volume expelled by this route. In formed stool, it rarely exceeds 10 mEq per day. In contrast, voluminous watery diarrhea may lead to losses that exceed 250 mEq per day when the fecal volume exceeds 2.5 to 3 liters per day.

In the normal individual, sweat represents the greatest potential source of sodium loss in the face of continued sodium restriction. Although the sodium concentration in the sweat varies with variation in sodium intake, the normal subject cannot elaborate sweat with a sodium concentration of less than 15 mEq/L. This small concentration may represent a significant amount of continuing sodium loss even in the normal individual when sweating continues at a significant rate and intake is inadequate.

SODIUM DEPLETION[19-21]

ROLE OF SODIUM LOSS
Serious sodium depletion is almost always the result of excessive loss, not of reduced sodium intake. As indicated in the preceding section, the body has effective mechanisms for curtailing sodium output in the face of reduced intake. For example, a stringent reduction of sodium intake produces a deficit of 90 to 150 mEq in the normal subject. An abnormal loss of sodium can, in contrast, produce deficits as large as 1000 mEq.

Rational management of sodium depletion, therefore, requires evaluation of the nature and time course of the sodium loss and an understanding of the compensatory responses to abnormal losses of sodium from the body.

EXPERIMENTAL SODIUM DEPLETION[19,20]
McCance's classical studies of sodium depletion in man demonstrated two distinct phases of sodium depletion. In these experiments normal individuals were subjected to persistent sweating and sodium restriction, but not water privation. Sweating produces a greater loss of water than sodium, since it contains less sodium than does extracellular fluid (see Fig. 6–3). However, the thirst mechanism maintains the osmolality (and sodium concentration) constant as described in Chapter 5. Thus, during the first phase there were equivalent net losses of sodium and water producing *isotonic contraction* of the extracellular fluid volume.

Only when the losses exceeded 400 mEq of sodium did the situation change. In the second phase further sodium loss evoked attempts to maintain volume by water retention. Only in this phase of *hypotonic contraction* did the serum concentration fall.

CLINICAL PHASES OF SODIUM DEPLETION
When one considers the possible sources of body sodium loss (Table 6–2, Fig. 6–3), i.e., the various sodium-containing fluids that can be lost from the body, it is evident that all their sodium concentrations are

TABLE 6-2
Routes of Abnormal Sodium Loss from the Body

Source of Na Loss	Etiology	"Effective" Osmolality of Lost Fluid
Kidney	Diuretics	Hypotonic
	Osmotic diuretics	"
	Acidosis	"
	Salt wasting nephritis	"
	Renal tubular acidosis	"
	Adrenal insufficiency	"
GI Tract	Diarrhea	Hypotonic
	Ileostomy	Isotonic
	Small bowel fistula	"
	Chronic laxative ingestion	Hypotonic
	Vomiting	"
	Nasogastric suction	"
	Villous adenoma	"
Skin	Sweating (excessive)	Hypotonic

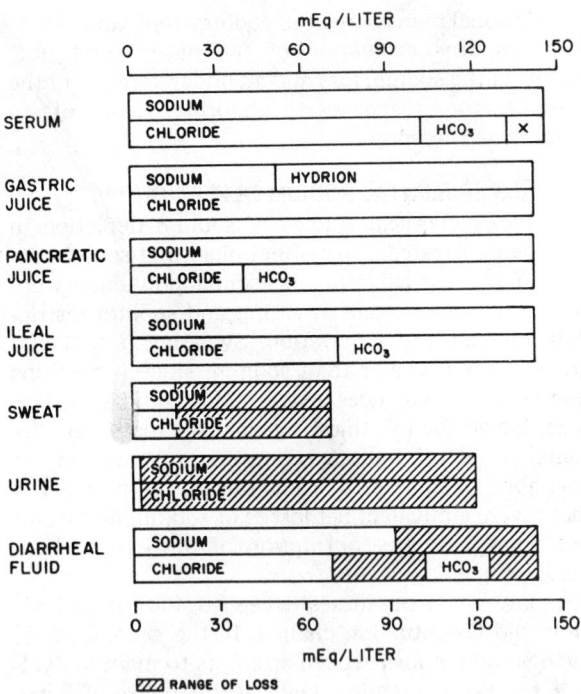

FIGURE 6-3. Sodium concentration in various body fluids and excreted fluids. The shaded areas identify the variations that may be encountered in some of these fluids.

either less than or equal to plasma sodium concentration. The most common events that lead to sodium loss from extrarenal routes (vomiting, diarrhea, and sweating) all represent fluid loss in which the sodium concentration is much less than that in plasma. Under extreme conditions, the sodium concentration in excreted fluids may approach that in the plasma. Such an occurrence is limited almost exclusively to small bowel fistulas, ileostomies, or fulminant diarrhea as in cholera. Here, in the most severe cases the sodium concentration of the fecal fluid may be virtually identical with that seen in plasma. The sequence encountered clinically in sodium depletion is in most instances similar to the experimental findings of McCance described above. Because of this, it is useful to consider these two sequential phases of isotonic and hypotonic contraction in response to sodium loss as acute and chronic stages of sodium depletion and to review the clinical findings during each phase of the disorder.

Acute Sodium Depletion (Sodium Depletion Without Hyponatremia)

Regardless of the route and rate of sodium loss, the body responds initially to restore solute concentration to normal. When intake of both salt and water are adequate, this is, of course, accomplished by retaining the quantity of salt that was lost and the corresponding amount of water. In the absence of sodium intake, however, the body adjusts the quantity of body water in a manner which returns the sodium concentration to normal. This leads to a net isotonic loss of extracellular fluid despite the fact that the initial sodium loss may have been as part of a hypotonic solution. As in the experimental example, the patient who loses a large quantity of sodium by sweating will lose much more water than sodium and the fluid loss will be hypotonic. With adequate fluid intake, however, water is retained until the sodium concentration is returned to its original normal level. Serial measurement of the body weight during an event of this sort would reveal that the net result would be significant loss of body weight with the loss representing the loss of sodium and water in isotonic proportions. At this point the serum sodium concentration is normal. Thus, isotonic contraction is the result of acute sodium depletion. This is so regardless of whether the sodium loss occurs through the kidneys, the gastrointestinal tract, or the skin.

The symptoms, physical findings, and laboratory data under these conditions all reflect a reduction in the extracellular fluid volume. The patient notes progressive weakness and lassitude followed by postural hypotension and, on occasion, syncope. Examination reveals a low blood pressure with a striking postural hypotension. This is associated with poor skin turgor; less often decreased intraocular tension, relatively dry mucous membranes, and muscular cramps are present. On occasion, particularly when the sodium loss is quite rapid, this picture may progress to that of frank shock.

An additional feature of sodium depletion that is well supported by experimental studies is a disproportionately large decrease in plasma volume. This is most easily explained by the decrease in the circulating mass of plasma proteins. This, in turn, probably represents some sequestration of protein in the interstitial space as a result of the decreased lymph flow that accompanies sodium depletion. This excessive reduction in plasma volume results in hemodynamic consequences and an increase in hematocrit beyond that to be expected from a simple isotonic contraction of the extracellular fluid volume.

The laboratory data are those to be expected whenever isotonic contraction of the extracellular fluid volume occurs. There is an elevation of the hematocrit, an increase in the serum urea nitrogen, and in serum creatinine concentrations. The *serum sodium concentration is normal*, however, in this circumstance.

Occasionally, quantities of sodium greatly in excess of 400 mEq may be lost with persistence of the picture of isotonic contraction. This is particularly true in fulminant diarrhea where several liters of fluid may be rapidly lost via the lower digestive tract during a very short period of time and unassociated with any water intake. Under such circumstances, the loss may exceed 5 liters of isotonic fluid (more than 700 mEq of sodium). In the untreated patient this leads rapidly to profound shock; death may follow shortly unless treatment is promptly implemented. Fortunately, such severe instances of diarrhea are rare in this country, but they are quite common in those areas of the world where cholera is endemic. Table 6-2 gives a partial list of the clinical disorders that may be associated with acute sodium depletion. This does not imply that these conditions may not also produce a more chronic state of sodium depletion associated with the disturbances outlined below.

Chronic Sodium Depletion (Sodium Depletion with Hyponatremia) [18-21]

In the presence of continuing net sodium loss, the homeostatic mechanisms of the body attempt to maintain the extracellular fluid volume by water retention. Figure 6-4 illustrates this phenomenon in a patient who was treated too vigorously with diuretics. He exhibits the sequence described in the preceding section; his losses were isotonic initially, resulting in no change in the serum sodium concentration. When the diuretic was stopped and rigid sodium restriction was maintained, however, he proceeded to dilute the body fluid compartments by water retention leading to hyponatremia.

For comparison, the changes produced in a normal individual in whom sodium depletion was produced by sustained sweating are also shown in Figure 6-5. The similarities are readily apparent.

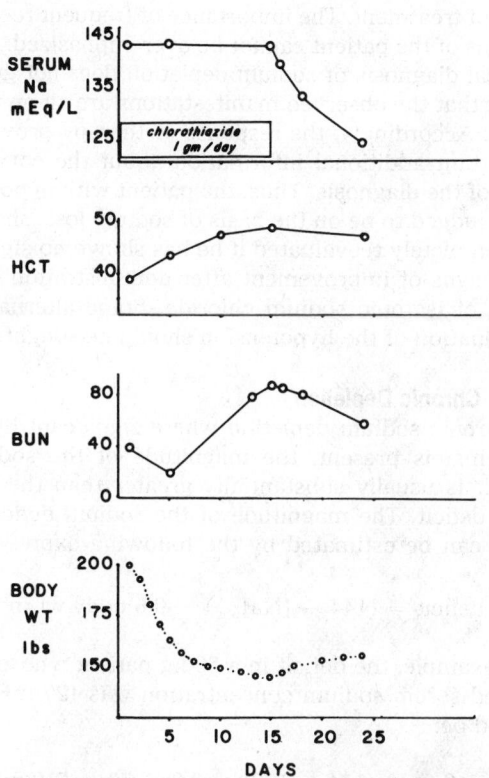

FIGURE 6-4. Sodium depletion produced by excessive diuretic therapy. Initial decline in weight was unassociated with changes in serum sodium concentration but both hematocrit and blood urea nitrogen rose. Subsequently water retention and increase in weight were associated with a decrease in serum sodium concentration.

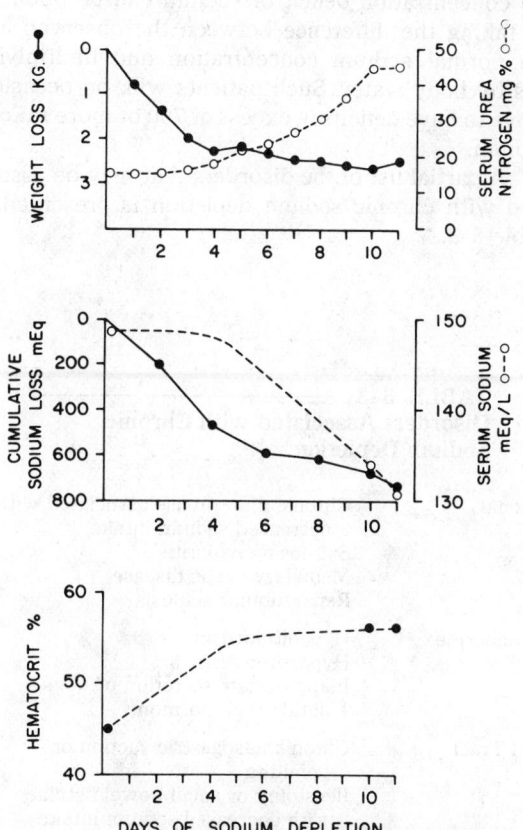

FIGURE 6-5. Experimental sodium depletion. Changes depicted in body weight, urea nitrogen, serum sodium, hematocrit, and cumulative sodium loss are drawn from data of McCance.[20] During first 3 days losses were isotonic with a 2 kg decrease in weight being associated with loss of about 300 mEq of sodium.

Patients at this stage in the evolution of sodium depletion complain of weakness, loss of appetite, giddiness, and may have experienced one or more syncopal attacks. Muscle cramps are common. If the hyponatremia becomes sufficiently severe, disorientation may develop followed by lethargy and, on occasion, convulsions. Physical findings include hypotension exaggerated by posture change. The skin turgor is poor. There may be a decrease in intraocular pressure and dry mucous membranes, but it is rare that the subjective complaint of thirst can be elicited.

The laboratory data are similar to those described above with sodium loss that develops more acutely with the exception that *the serum sodium concentration is always depressed* in the patient with chronic sodium depletion. On occasion it may be below 120 mEq/L. Loss of solute from the extracellular space results in movement of fluid into the intracellular space to readjust solute concentrations so that no osmotic gradient exists across the cell. An estimate of the concentration deficit of sodium can be obtained by taking the difference between the observed and the normal sodium concentration and multiplying this by body water. Such patients will, on occasion, prove to have deficits in excess of 700 or more mEq of sodium.

A partial list of the disorders that may be associated with chronic sodium depletion is presented in Table 6-3.

TABLE 6-3
Disorders Associated with Chronic Sodium Depletion

Renal	Chronic diuretic use associated with decreased sodium intake
	Salt-losing nephritis
	Medullary cystic disease
	Renal tubular acidosis
Endocrine	Hypopituitarism
	Hypoadrenalism
	Inappropriate secretion of antidiuretic hormone
GI Tract	Chronic nasogastric suction or vomiting
	Ileostomy or small bowel fistulae with decreased sodium intake
	Biliary fistulae
	Chronic diarrhea
	Villous adenoma
Skin	Chronic heat exposure and sweating with decreased sodium intake
	Burns with slow healing

TREATMENT OF SODIUM DEPLETION

Acute Depletion

The symptoms and findings during the acute phase of sodium depletion are caused by inadequate volume and can be rapidly corrected by administration of an isotonic (0.155 molar, 0.9 percent) sodium chloride solution. Usually, about 2000 or 2500 ml of such a solution produce marked improvement in the patient unless there is a source of continuing fluid loss or the patient is in shock when first seen. Patients who are in shock from sodium depletion, with systolic blood pressure below 90 mm Hg and tachycardia as prominent features of their clinical picture, respond more rapidly when infusions of isotonic sodium chloride are supplemented with administration of plasma.

Where continuing losses are identified, as in severe diarrhea, losses must be measured and the rate of replacement increased to provide for correction of the continuing loss as well as the initial deficit.

Careful recording of intake and output and frequent weighings of the patient should be routinely used to corroborate the clinical evaluation of the efficacy of treatment. The importance of frequent reevaluations of the patient cannot be overemphasized. The clinical diagnosis of sodium depletion does not guarantee that the observed manifestations are all on that basis. Accordingly, the response to therapy provides important additional information about the correctness of the diagnosis. Thus, the patient with hypotension, judged to be on the basis of sodium loss, should be completely reevaluated if he has shown no significant signs of improvement after administration of 3 liters of isotonic sodium chloride. Some alternative explanation of the hypotension should be sought.

Chronic Depletion

In chronic sodium depletion where significant hyponatremia is present, the magnitude of the sodium deficit is usually substantially greater than the volume deficit. The magnitude of the sodium deficit in mEq can be estimated by the following expression:

$$\text{Na deficit} = (144 - [\text{Na}]_{obs}) \times 0.6 \text{ body wt in kg}$$

For example, the deficit in a 50-kg patient whose observed serum sodium concentration was 127 mEq/L would be:

$$\text{Na deficit} = (144 - 127) \times 0.6 \times 50 = 510 \text{ mEq}$$

In an individual with normally functioning kidneys, it is preferable to replace the sodium by administration of an isotonic solution of sodium chloride. When the hyponatremia is so severe that abnormalities of central nervous system function are present, initial therapy is more effective in correcting these abnormalities if a hypertonic solution such as 0.510 molar (3 percent) sodium chloride is given. This therapy is warranted only in extreme instances of sodium depletion with hyponatremia. Even under such circumstances it is unwise to replace the entire deficit with this hypertonic solution. Replacement of one-third to one-half the estimated deficit will usually suffice to correct the central nervous system abnormalities. When the patient is sufficiently alert and able to take medication by mouth, the oral route usually suffices to achieve restoration of sodium balance, provided renal function is normal. This must be done slowly because of the marked gastric irritation produced by taking more than 1 to 1.5 g of salt orally in one dose. In general, if the deficit has developed over a protracted period and is not associated with mental aberrations, it is sufficient to plan replacement gradually over a period of several days and the oral administration of sodium chloride usually suffices.

As with acute sodium depletion, failure to achieve the expected response after an attempt has been made to correct the deficit should prompt re-evaluation of the patient. In particular, when the hyponatremia persists despite reasonable therapeutic efforts, the causes of hyponatremia discussed below should be considered (see Chap. 5).

ASYMPTOMATIC HYPONATREMIA[17]
Most instances of hyponatremia are unassociated with sodium deficit and have as their explanation a primary disturbance in water metabolism as discussed in Chapter 5. The following additional specific situations merit comment.

Hyperlipidemia may on occasion be associated with hyponatremia. This is a consequence, not of sodium deficit, but of decrease in the aqueous phase of the plasma. Because of the high lipid content of the plasma the water content is reciprocally reduced. If the correction is made for this reduction in plasma water, it is found that the sodium concentration in the serum water is normal.

Hyperproteinemia rarely is associated with hyponatremia. This may be seen in multiple myeloma but only when the total protein concentration exceeds 11 or 12 g per dl. The mechanism here is similar to the mechanism outlined above in hyperlipidemia. This change as well as the change in hyperlipidemia is not associated with symptoms and no attempt should be made to correct the hyponatremia.

Hyperglycemia, when extreme, may be associated with marked reduction in the sodium concentration. In this situation glucose accounts for a significant fraction of the total solute of plasma and

extracellular fluid. In diabetes, where it fails to enter the cells, osmotic equilibration results in a proportional lowering of the sodium concentration in the extracellular fluid. Thus, an increase in the serum glucose by 180 mg/dl will result in reduction in the serum sodium by approximately 5 mEq/L. Extreme degrees of hyperglycemia may be accompanied by severe water deficit, and under these circumstances the serum sodium concentration is unpredictable. In addition, such patients may have also developed a significant sodium deficit caused by the sustained osmotic diuresis engendered by the severe hyperglycemia.

Administration of osmotic agents such as *mannitol* may result in lowering of the plasma sodium concentration. The mechanism here is similar to that responsible for the hyponatremia associated with hyperglycemia discussed above. It may be encountered when one attempts to correct the oliguria of impending acute renal failure by mannitol administration, or when mannitol is used to sustain an osmotic diuresis during the treatment of certain instances of drug overdosage such as phenobarbital or aspirin intoxication. In these latter cases, the situation can be complicated by the coexistence of a sodium deficit, since sustained osmotic diuresis is associated with continued sodium loss in the urine. Here neither the serum sodium concentration nor the hematocrit is of any value in recognizing the development of a coexisting sodium deficit. Measurement of urinary sodium losses and replacement of these losses is the only reliable means of avoiding the development of a sodium deficit of increasing severity.

The most important distinction to be made, from the standpoint of appropriate treatment, is between the *dilutional hyponatremia* of congestive heart failure and chronic sodium depletion. The differentiation is readily made on the basis of the presence or absence of dependent edema. Although either condition may be encountered in congestive heart failure, chronic sodium depletion resulting from too vigorous use of diuretics is less common than is the hyponatremia of congestive heart failure that appears when the heart failure is so severe that the patient is unable to excrete a dilute urine in response to water ingestion. *The presence of demonstrable pitting edema excludes the diagnosis of chronic sodium depletion* in these patients. The distinction is important because of the hazard of administration of sodium to congestive heart failure patients with dilutional hyponatremia (Chap. 15).

Finally, errors can occur even in well supervised laboratories and a laboratory error should always be considered when an unexpected abnormality in the concentration of sodium is encountered. This is particularly true when there is some discrepancy between the sum of the cations measured in the plasma and the sum of the anions. The significance of the "anion gap" is discussed in Chapter 8 but a true discrepancy always occurs in an easily recognizable clinical setting such as acidosis. Historical information and physical findings are available in these situations to verify the significance of such a laboratory result.

SODIUM EXCESS

The retention of abnormal quantities of sodium occurs most commonly in renal disease, cardiovascular disturbances leading to congestive heart failure, and cirrhosis of the liver. This is discussed elsewhere in this book in the context of the specific diseases in which it is encountered.

——CHAPTER 7——
Disorders of Potassium Metabolism
W. GORDON WALKER AND DANIEL G. SAPIR

Disorders of potassium metabolism occur in a variety of clinical problems, for the mammalian organism is more vulnerable to losses or gains in body potassium (K) than to similar changes in sodium (Na). In the presence of stimuli to conserve both sodium and potassium, sodium is conserved more efficiently. In abnormal states associated with aldosterone excess, this sodium conservation may be achieved at the expense of a progressively increasing potassium deficit. The body is subject to marked disturbances in potassium metabolism not only in disease but also as a complication of some therapeutic regimens.

Severe disturbances in body content of potassium may lead to life-threatening alterations in myocardial function, skeletal muscle, and smooth muscle function leading to sudden paralysis or severe ileus. Such disturbances may also produce disorders in cell function that include cessation of growth in the young and sustained catabolic state with exaggerated nitrogen losses in the adult. Potassium disturbances often lead to changes in composition and pH of body fluids as well.

Many of the pathophysiologic effects of these disturbances in potassium content are caused by the unique distribution of potassium within the body. More than 97 percent of the total body content of potassium is located within the cells.

NORMAL DISTRIBUTION AND MOVEMENT OF POTASSIUM WITHIN THE BODY[1,6,26,27,29,30]

DISTRIBUTION
Potassium is the major intracellular cation of the body (>150 mEq/L of cell water). The total exchangeable potassium, measured by isotope dilution, differs significantly between males and females with an average value of 38 mEq per kg body weight in the female and 48 mEq/kg in the male. As shown in Figure 7–1, only about 2 percent is located in the extracellular fluid, the remainder being confined within cells. There is a significant quantity of potassium within the bone, but this is not readily exchangeable and is not reflected in the above estimates of total exchangeable potassium.

Movement
Both metabolic processes and electrical events occurring at the cell surface are associated with transmembrane movement of potassium, resulting in a continual exchange between the intracellular and extracellular potassium pools. In general, the predominant or net flux is outward into the interstitial fluid during the day. At night this trend is reversed; net movement is inward and the intracellular potassium ion concentration [K+] is restored to normal. At its peak, the resting potassium efflux from cells may add as much as 15 mEq per hour (0.5 percent of intracellular potassium per hour) to the extracellular fluid (ECF). This loss is greatly accentuated by such activities as electrical depolarization of the cell surface (muscular activity), glycogen breakdown, acidosis, and production of excess quantities of organic anions by the cell. Since this rate of accumulation in the ECF could lead to an intolerable doubling of the extracellular [K+] in only 3 to 4 hours, the importance of a renal mechanism for preventing this net rise is evident. Conversely, the importance of carefully regulating potassium intake and monitoring plasma [K+] in individuals with no renal function (anephric patients on hemodialysis or patients with acute renal failure and anuria) is critical to their survival (Fig. 7–1.).

Functions[30-34]

Potassium, as the major intracellular solute, determines the osmotic equilibrium across the cell surface and, thus, determines the volume of intracellular fluid. Potassium within the cell is usually in a constant ratio to cellular protein; the body contains 2.7 mEq of potassium for each gram of nitrogen or each 6.25 g of protein. Increase in the body store of protein (positive nitrogen balance) leads to potassium retention within the body, and conversely catabolic states (negative nitrogen balance) result in potassium loss. An adequate source of potassium is necessary for tissue growth, so potassium deficiency in the young leads to growth failure. A number of the enzymatic processes within the cell are critically dependent upon [K$^+$] and this may be the mechanism responsible for failure of anabolic processes in potassium deficient states. In addition, the electrical activity of cells is critically dependent upon the intracellular/extracellular concentration gradient, [K$_i^+$]/[K$_o^+$], of potassium across cell membranes. An increase in this ratio leads to an increase in the potential difference or hyperpolarization of the cell and a decreased concentration leads to hypopolarization. Both of these abnormal states result in disturbances of the electrical activity exhibited by cells and are primarily responsible for the adverse effects seen in cardiac and skeletal muscle function in potassium disturbances.

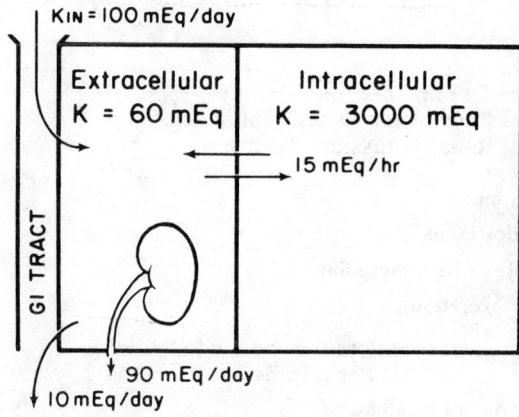

FIGURE 7-1. K$^+$ distribution and exchange in an average adult human. Total K$^+$ in the extracellular space is only about 60 mEq or approximately 2 percent of the intracellular K$^+$. The exchange between cells and the ECF is approximately 15 mEq per hour under basal conditions and can increase markedly in response to exercise, anoxia, acidosis, and other stimuli. Thus, the body is extremely susceptible to hyperkalemia when kidneys do not function adequately, since they are responsible for excretion of about 90 percent of the ingested potassium.

Disturbances in potassium content of the body may, thus, be responsible for clinical manifestations that range from diminished tendon reflexes, to muscular paralysis, pH disturbances of the body fluids, and in most extreme cases cardiac arrhythmias and cardiac standstill.

REGULATION OF BODY POTASSIUM CONTENT

Changes in the body potassium content result from a disparity between potassium intake and potassium excretion. In the normally growing child, the intake always slightly exceeds the output because of the need for progressive accumulation of potassium and protein to support growth. In adults both the concentration and amount of potassium in the body are closely regulated. Thus, intake and output are closely balanced.

Intake

Potassium is present in nearly all food. Hence decreased intake alone is probably only a factor in the development of potassium deficiency when food intake is sharply curtailed for long periods of time as in gastrointestinal disturbances, starvation, or alcoholism. The body conserves potassium, however, much less efficiently than it controls sodium and modest reductions in dietary potassium may contribute significantly to the development of a potassium deficit in many situations.

Excretion

Potassium excretion occurs by three routes: the skin, the GI tract, and the kidneys (Table 7-1). Skin losses are trivial. The concentration of potassium in sweat rarely exceeds 15 or 20 mEq/L, so that large volumes of sweat lead to only modest potassium losses by this route.

TABLE 7-1

Normal Routes of Potassium Loss from Body

Site	Average Rate of Loss
Skin	< 5 mEq/day
GI tract	5- 10 mEq/day
Kidneys	80-100 mEq/day
Total	85-110 mEq/day

GASTROINTESTINAL EXCRETION. The gastrointestinal (GI) tract is not a significant route of potassium excretion in the normal individual. Although the potassium concentration in fecal water may significantly exceed the plasma potassium concentration, the small quantity of water in feces under normal circumstances limits this source of potassium excretion to a few mEq per day.

Diarrhea can lead to significant potassium losses from the GI tract. The concentration of potassium in diarrheal fluid may rise to 20 to 25 mEq/L. When the volume of diarrheal fluid exceeds 3 to 4 liters per day, the total may be 100 mEq, a tenfold increase.

In advanced renal failure, the GI tract may function as a major route of potassium excretion with more than 60 to 80 percent of ingested potassium being excreted in the feces. Thus, these patients are particularly susceptible to potassium depletion when diarrhea occurs.

RENAL EXCRETION.[24,29] The mechanisms involved in the renal transport of potassium include filtration, reabsorption, and secretion in exchange for Na^+ (see Fig. 7-2). Potassium is freely filtered at the glomerulus and is reabsorbed passively, although active transport may also be involved to a minor degree.

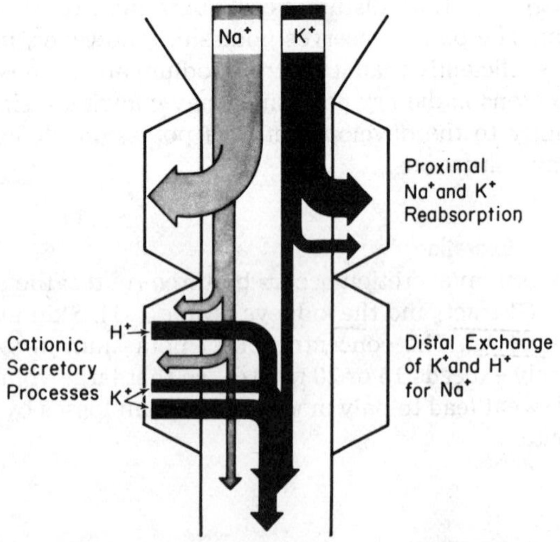

FIGURE 7-2. Schematic representation of renal K^+ transport. In the proximal tubule net K^+ transport is in the direction of reabsorption with nearly all the K^+ within the lumen being reabsorbed. Distally, the net transport is in the direction of secretion with K^+ serving as a counter ion to maintain electroneutrality as Na^+ reabsorption proceeds, although the two probably are not limited by a single coupled transport system. H^+ secretion also occurs distally, and under some conditions there is competition between K^+ and H^+ transport.

Most, if not all, the potassium that is excreted reaches the urine by a secretory process that is located in the distal tubule. Maintenance of electroneutrality within the urine requires that this potassium secretion be balanced by net movement of cation in the opposite direction. Hence, the result of this secretory process is an exchange of K for an equivalent amount of Na.

Regulatory Mechanisms

In the normal subject there is no mechanism for modulating potassium balance that operates to reduce intake or to alter GI absorption. Even though the organism responds to alteration in the intake of potassium, the kidney is the effector organ in regulating potassium balance. Table 7-2 shows the factors that modify the rate of potassium output within the distal tubule.

Generally, the potassium excretion is increased whenever the quantity of *sodium* presented to the distal tubule is increased. Conversely, potassium excretion is restricted by a reduction in the quantity of sodium presented to the distal tubule. Since sodium delivery to the distal exchange site is thought to be adequate for the potassium excretion even when the rate of urinary sodium loss is low, the variation in potassium excretion with distal tubular sodium load has been ascribed to the effects of urinary flow rate in this region.

Potassium excretion is also increased by an increased distal tubular load of poorly reabsorbed *anions*. The keto-acids that are excreted in increased

TABLE 7-2
Physiologic Stimuli Influencing Renal Potassium Transport

K^+ intake
Aldosterone
Rate of Na^+ excretion
H^+ excretion
Factors Which Lead to Increase in Renal Potassium Excretion
Increased K intake
Increased serum $[K^+]$
Increased Na^+ excretion
Increased anion excretion
Decreased H^+ excretion
Decreased NH_4^+ excretion
Increased cortisol level

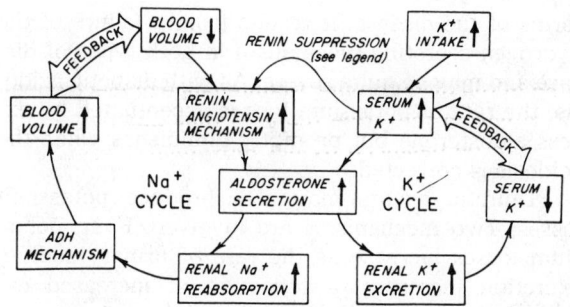

FIGURE 7-3. The relation between Na$^+$ and K$^+$ influences on aldosterone secretion. Two feedback mechanisms exist that, although independent, are capable of interaction. Plasma K$^+$ influences aldosterone secretion directly without the necessity for an intact renin-aldosterone system.[26,27] Elevated [K$^+$] in the plasma is also capable of directly suppressing renin output by the kidney. Thus, this system serves to monitor and regulate both sodium and potassium content of the body, with a capability for regulating sodium more efficiently than potassium.

quantities in diabetic acidosis thus lead to increased potassium excretion. Intake of anions such as sulfates, that are poorly reabsorbed by the kidney, may also lead to increased potassium loss (Fig. 7-2).

Distal tubular *hydrogen ion* secretion has also been shown to change the rate of potassium output. In most instances, there is a reciprocal relationship in the excretion of these two ions, so that an increased output of one will lower the excretion of the other. This reciprocal effect is thought to be responsible for the acceleration of potassium secretion observed in metabolic alkalosis.

An additional important element of control of potassium/hydrogen output is the direct effect of potassium on *renal ammonium ion production*. Production of ammonia, the major urinary buffer, is decreased by potassium loading and it is increased by potassium depletion. An increase in renal ammonia genesis will generally lead to a higher hydrogen ion output and reduced potassium excretion.

Rate of potassium output is also subject to *diurnal variation* and influenced by potassium intake and the secretory rates of the mineralocorticoid hormones (Fig. 7-3). The pattern of diurnal variation in potassium excretion coincides with the pattern of diurnal flux across cell membranes described above.

POTASSIUM DEFICITS AND HYPOKALEMIA

CAUSES

Table 7-3 lists the causes of potassium deficiency or hypokalemia. Potassium losses originate from within the GI tract or the kidneys. Many of the conditions leading to increased renal loss are primarily metabolic disorders and have been listed separately.

Deficient Intake

Potassium deficiency due exclusively to reduced intake rarely occurs except when K intake is severely restricted for prolonged periods. Since renal conservation of potassium lowers output below 10 mEq per day only with great difficulty, a chronic deficit is observed when intake is persistently nil. Alcoholism may present with this form of potassium deficiency.

Gastrointestinal Loss

Gastrointestinal losses associated with vomiting, diarrhea, or fistulae usually lead to slow development

---

TABLE 7-3
Causes of Hypokalemia

Gastrointestinal

Vomiting

Diarrhea

GI fistulae

Villous adenoma

Ureterosigmoidostomy

Ileostomy

Chronic laxative ingestion

Prolonged absence of K intake

Metabolic
Diabetic acidosis

Adrenocortical excess
  ACTH producing tumors
  Cushing syndrome
  Primary aldosteronism
    Adrenal adenomas
    Adrenal hyperplasia
  Steroid administration
  Thyrotoxicosis

Familial periodic paralysis

Renal
Renal tubular acidosis

Diuretic therapy

K-losing nephropathy

Acidosis

Alkalosis

Secondary aldosteronism
  Cirrhosis
  Nephrosis
  Bartter syndrome

of hypokalemia. The process may be hastened by the presence of conditions leading to associated increased renal losses such as aldosterone excess stimulated by associated sodium deficiency. Two conditions producing hypokalemia that are often not promptly recognized are chronic laxative abuse and villous adenoma of the colon. Patients abusing the use of laxatives are often unreliable historians, denying laxative use or liquid bowel movements. The presence of severe hypokalemia and very low concentrations of potassium in the urine should always raise suspicion of laxative abuse. Patients with villous adenoma typically give a history of frequent passage of mucoid secretions per rectum with intermittent liquid diarrhea. Since most gastrointestinal conditions leading to hypokalemia are associated with losses of rather large volumes of fluid by this route, associated sodium deficits are commonly seen.

Metabolic Disorders [28,31,32,35]

Metabolic disturbances producing increased urinary potassium losses usually result from mineralocorticoid excess or increased renal excretion of organic acids. The hypokalemia of mineralocorticoid excess may be first recognized as a result of what appears to be an inappropriate response to diuretics, with severe manifestations of hypokalemia occurring after only one or two doses of a diuretic that increases potassium excretion. This is a particularly valuable diagnostic feature in situations where overt stigmata of Cushing syndrome are not obvious on physical examination. Diabetic acidosis with progressively increasing rate of keto-acid excretion may also lead to severe and rapidly developing potassium deficits that can exceed 500 mEq after only 3 or 4 days of acidosis.

The causative factors in the loss of potassium during diabetic acidosis are similar to those producing potassium loss in other forms of acidosis. Increased excretion of acetoacetate and β-OH butyrate is not equaled by the rise in the generation and excretion of ammonium, a process that requires several days to reach maximal efficiency. The result is that potassium and sodium are excreted in excess to maintain urinary electroneutrality. Contraction of the extracellular volume incident to continued losses of sodium lead to excess mineralocorticoid hormone release and increased potassium wastage. Two of these factors, lag in ammonium production and volume stimulated aldosterone excess, are factors responsible for potassium losses in other forms of metabolic acidosis.

Renal Loss

Renal loss of potassium in renal tubular acidosis is seen in both the distal (type I) and proximal (type II)

forms of the disease. It results from a failure of the hydrogen secreting mechanism in both types of disease and may be quite severe. As with diabetic acidosis, the rate of potassium loss is accentuated by excess aldosterone but promptly diminishes when the acidosis is corrected.

Diuretic agents may also produce potassium losses. Two mechanisms are involved. First, potassium losses increase as the rate of urinary sodium excretion increases, a reflection of increased exchange of potassium for luminal sodium as increasing quantities of sodium reach the distal segments of the nephrons. This is accentuated by aldosterone excess. Second, since many diuretics produce a chloride deficiency and hypochloremic alkalosis, this increases potassium loss further. Renal potassium wastage is increased when metabolic alkalosis occurs.

Internal Shifts

The disorders covered in the preceding paragraphs are all associated with hypokalemia attributable to increased potassium losses from either the kidneys or the GI tract. There are disorders, however, in which hypokalemia occurs without either increased potassium loss or decreased intake. Familial periodic paralysis is the classic example of this type of acute hypokalemia.[32] It is associated with acute and profound decreases in plasma [K] and accompanying ascending paralyses. The episodes of hypokalemic paralysis are precipitated either by excessive exercise or ingestion of a high carbohydrate meal. In this condition the low serum potassium is a result of increased movement of this ion into the intracellular compartment, and not of external losses. Similar episodes may also occur during the course of hyperthyroidism.

CLINICAL MANIFESTATIONS OF HYPOKALEMIA

The diagnosis of potassium deficiency and hypokalemia must depend primarily upon a high index of suspicion. The disorders or conditions listed in Table 7–3 should always alert the physician to this possibility, and appropriate tests should be undertaken to diagnose or exclude potassium disturbance. Table 7–4 shows the signs and symptoms commonly associated with potassium deficits. The relation of these findings to the severity of the hypokalemia may be quite variable. Acute lowering of plasma [K] may produce profound disturbances at levels that, in chronic situations, may be associated only with weakness. Clinical manifestations are most likely to be hyperacute and catastrophic in situations where the plasma [K] is falling rapidly as in diabetic acidosis during the early stages of treatment or in familial periodic paralysis.

TABLE 7–4
Clinical Manifestations of Hypokalemia

Acute	Chronic
Weakness	Weakness
Hyporeflexia	Weight loss
Ileus	Polyuria
Flaccid paralysis	Growth retardation
Postural hypotension	Hyporeflexia
EKG abnormalities	Episodic paralysis
Respiratory distress	Postural hypotension
	EKG abnormalities
	Azotemia

Confirmation of the presence of hypokalemia rests primarily on the measurement of the serum potassium. This generally falls with losses of potassium, and is progressively depressed with larger degrees of negative potassium balance. Unfortunately, the correlation between potassium loss and depression of the serum potassium concentration is poor, so that the magnitude of deficiency cannot be accurately assessed from plasma [K]. Furthermore, the distribution of potassium between the extra- and intracellular compartments is also governed by such factors as the extracellular pH. Thus, it is not uncommon for elevations of the serum potassium to occur in the presence of total body potassium depletion when acidosis is present. Alkalosis, in contrast to acidosis, can produce a depression of the serum potassium by causing increased movement of extracellular potassium into intracellular fluid. These factors affecting the serum potassium make ancillary laboratory testing and clinical judgments important in the decision concerning the presence and magnitude of potassium deficiency. The presence of symptoms of potassium deficiency, associated with evidence of metabolic, endocrine, renal, or gastrointestinal lesions which cause potassium loss, constitutes important historical data in assessing the state of potassium stores.

The electrocardiographic changes of potassium deficiency, lowered T waves, prolongation of the QT interval (these may ultimately lead to cardiac standstill) are also helpful signs in the diagnosis of potassium deficiency (Fig. 7–4). There is not good correlation between the EKG changes and the magnitude of potassium depletion.

Irrespective of the manner in which the existence of hypokalemia is first recognized, it must be regarded as a manifestation of underlying disease. Judicious interpretation of the history, physical findings, and laboratory information is necessary to arrive at a final diagnosis. The association of hypokalemia and a history of vomiting suggests a GI disorder as the underlying cause. Hyperchloremia and decreased plasma [K] suggest renal tubular acidosis or complication of acetazolamide therapy. Metabolic alkalosis with hypokalemia in the absence of GI signs or symptoms suggests either mineralocorticoid excess or diuretic induced (chlorothiazide, furosemide, or ethacrynic acid) potassium depletion.

Alkalosis is seen in conjunction with hypokalemia when the underlying cause is persistent vomiting caused by upper GI obstruction, chronic laxative abuse, primary, secondary, or iatrogenic mineralocorticoid excess, or the administration of saliuretic diuretic agents such as chlorothiazide or furosemide.

Acidosis associated with hypokalemia is seen in the presence of severe diarrhea of relatively short duration, diabetic acidosis, renal tubular acidosis, chronic acetazolamide administration, ureterosigmoidostomy, and occasionally with diversion of the urinary stream into an ileal loop.

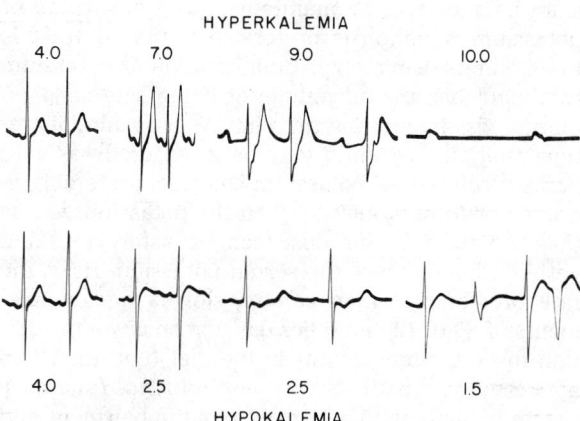

FIGURE 7–4. *Hyperkalemia.* Electrocardiographic lead V$_4$ illustrating abnormalities encountered with a progressive elevation of the serum potassium. One of the earliest changes is tall, peaked, and symmetrical T waves. As the serum potassium rises further (to 9 mEq/L) the P-R interval and the QRS duration are prolonged. Both atrial and ventricular ectopic beats may occur. At levels of serum potassium near 10 mEq/L the P waves disappear and a slow heart rate with wide QRS complexes is noted. This is followed by the development of total asystole. *Hypokalemia.* Electrocardiographic lead V$_4$ illustrating changes which may result as the serum potassium is progressively lowered. At levels below 3 mEq/L the T-wave amplitude decreases and the U wave appears or increases in magnitude. The U wave may become very prominent and the ST segment sagged or frankly depressed. Further lowering of the serum potassium may result in ectopic activity in the atria and ventricles, especially if the patient has received digitalis. Ventricular fibrillation may develop.

PATHOLOGIC CHANGES ASSOCIATED WITH POTASSIUM DEPLETION

In the presence of long-standing potassium depletion, structural changes occur in the kidney and in skeletal and cardiac muscle. Vacuolization within the renal tubular cells and peritubular scarring in the region of the distal tubules and collecting ducts represent the characteristic lesion of hypokalemic nephropathy. The scarring probably accounts for the loss of the renal-concentrating function that is seen regularly in potassium deficits of several weeks duration. Vacuolization and fragmentation of fibers may be seen in both skeletal and cardiac muscle with long-standing potassium depletion.

TREATMENT

No reliable guides are present for estimating the magnitude of the potassium deficit in a given situation. Plasma [K] below 2.5 mEq/L may be associated with deficits ranging from 400 mEq to more than 1000 mEq. The usual approach is to continue potassium administration until the plasma [K] has returned to the normal range and until an adequate oral intake of food gives additional assurance that normal potassium balance will be maintained. The oral route of potassium repletion is preferable if the GI tract is functioning adequately. Administration of potassium by mouth has the advantage of being safer and requiring less monitoring than intravenous administration. (Initially 120 mEq may be given orally as a 10 percent solution of potassium chloride, preferably in orange or tomato juice.) When the potassium is less than 2.5 mEq/L this dose can be safely repeated within 4 hours. Once the serum potassium rises, the rate of administration can be slowed and supplements of 80 to 120 mEq per day can be given in addition to potassium present in the diet (note that this applies only to patients with *normal renal function*).

In patients with advanced renal impairment and hypokalemia a much more cautious approach is mandatory. No more than 80 mEq should be given on the first day of therapy, and thereafter supplemental oral K should not exceed 30 to 40 mEq per day. Even so, careful monitoring of the serum K is essential under these circumstances (Table 7–5).

If a malfunctioning GI tract precludes oral therapy, or if the severity of the hypokalemia makes intravenous replacement desirable, no more than 30 mEq of potassium chloride should be administered hourly and this rate should not be achieved except in acute situations such as may be encountered in diabetic acidosis.

Under all other circumstances it is probably safer to keep the rate of administration at or below 10 to 15

TABLE 7–5

Some Principles of Potassium Replacement

1. Use oral route whenever possible

2. Give parenterally at less than 10 mEq/hr except in extreme emergency

3. Never exceed 30 mEq/hr intravenously

4. When parenteral K replacement exceeds 10 mEq/hr, EKG monitoring is necessary

5. Never give K parenterally to patients with renal failure (GFR <10 ml/min)

---

mEq per hour. As repletion continues and gastrointestinal motility improves, oral therapy can replace the intravenous route. Extensive drug surveillance studies in several hospitals have all shown that hyperkalemia complicating potassium administration is one of the most common and dangerous complications of hospital drug usage. It is particularly likely to occur when both oral and intravenous routes of administration are used in the same patient. *Careful monitoring of all patients receiving potassium is mandatory.*

The electrocardiogram is useful in monitoring the results of potassium administration. It should always be used to monitor the earlier therapy of severe diabetic acidosis since plasma [K] may change so rapidly that it is not practical to rely upon serum [K] measurements. As potassium balance improves U waves disappear, T-wave amplitude increases, and the QT shortens. When acidosis is present together with hypokalemia, potassium can be given with bicarbonate in order to correct both the acidosis and potassium depletion. It must be reemphasized that a severe acidosis may mask significant potassium deficits if the plasma [K] is relied upon to exclude potassium deficiency. Great caution should be exercised in the treatment of severe acidosis by bicarbonate administration even in the presence of an initially normal plasma [K]. Sudden correction of the acidosis may acutely lower plasma [K] to life-threatening levels as improvement in the acidosis results in marked shifts of potassium into the cells. When alkalosis and hypokalemia are present, there usually is an associated chloride deficit, and both potassium and chloride are necessary to completely correct the alkalosis.[30]

Adequate workup of the patient with potassium deficiency includes the identification or exclusion of sources of continuing potassium loss. In situations where potassium loss continues, as in steroid therapy, Cushing syndrome, or other disturbances associated with continuing renal or GI loss of potassium, supplemental therapy must be continued if recurrence of the hypokalemia is to be prevented.

HYPERKALEMIA

Since the total quantity of potassium present in the extracellular fluid in a 70-kg man is 80 to 90 mEq, very small increases in the extracellular fluid potassium may result in large elevations of serum potassium. Hyperkalemia may, thus, occur swiftly.[23]

CLINICAL MANIFESTATIONS

With increases in extracellular fluid potassium the resting potential of cells is lowered and results in neuromuscular irritability. Irritability of muscle may progress to a state of depolarization block resulting in paralysis if the potassium continues to rise in ECF. This occurs in both cardiac and skeletal muscle. Figure 7-4 shows sequential electrocardiographic changes that occur with increases in serum potassium. Peaking of the T waves is the most reliable measure of hyperkalemic effects upon the heart. Although it may be first seen at different [K] in different patients and in different clinical situations, it is nonetheless the earliest and most reliable indicator of cardiotoxicity caused by hyperkalemia.

CAUSES

The most common clinical settings in which hyperkalemia occurs are renal failure and acidosis (Table 7-6). Acidosis may cause hyperkalemia even when renal function is entirely normal. Hyperkalemia may be observed both early and late in the oliguric phase of acute renal failure.[32] It usually occurs late during the course of chronic renal failure when the glomerular filtration rate has fallen below 5 ml per minute. This level of renal function is usually adequate to achieve excretion of the usual daily load of ingested potassium. The imposition of an additional load, either exogenously from increased intake or endogenously from increased catabolism caused by infection, hemorrhage, tissue necrosis, or acidosis may exceed the capacity of the severely diseased kidney to excrete potassium, thereby leading to acute hyperkalemia. Use of diuretics that block potassium secretion by the renal tubule may also lead to acute hyperkalemia in renal failure. For this reason triamterene and spironolactone should never be used in the presence of renal failure.

TABLE 7-6
Causes of Hyperkalemia

Disease Related	Spurious
Renal failure	Hemolyzed blood sample
Acute	Thrombocytosis
Chronic	
	Time lapse between
Severe acidosis	drawing blood and
Addison's disease	separating cells
Hereditary episodic	
adynamia[28]	Leukocytic disintegration in
Iatrogenic	leukemia
K-retaining diuretics	
Inappropriate	
K administration	

Elevation of the serum potassium may also occur with mineralocorticoid deficiency as is seen in Addison's disease or isolated deficiency of aldosterone. This results primarily from failure of renal secretion of potassium in the absence of aldosterone.

TREATMENT

Since serious and potentially fatal elevations of the serum potassium result from small additions of this cation to the extracellular fluid in the absence of adequate renal function, successful therapy may be predicated on the removal of small amounts of potassium from this body fluid compartment (Table 7-7). A

TABLE 7-7
Treatment of Hyperkalemia

Temporary Measures

1. Ca gluconate or $CaCl_2$ intravenously 1 g given over 10–15 min period

2. Correction of acidosis (if present) with $NaHCO_3$

3. 2.5% ($\simeq$1000 mOsm/L) NaCl intravenously as slow infusion at 0.2 to 0.5 ml/min

4. Glucose and insulin intravenously 3–4 g glucose with each unit of insulin

Permanent (Corrective) Measures

1. Administration of Na polystyrene sulfonate resin, 25–75 g per day in 15–25% sorbitol orally or as retention enema. (Note: This removes K^+ and replaces an equivalent amount of Na^+.)

2. Peritoneal dialysis (do not add K^+ to first 6–8 exchanges, then use dialysate containing 1 mEq K/L).

3. Hemodialysis (use dialysate containing 2.0 mEq K/L).

---

decrease in the serum potassium may be accomplished by the transfer of this cation from the extra- to the intracellular fluids, the removal of potassium from the body, or administration of an agent which has an antagonistic effect to the action of potassium on cell membranes. In clinical situations where the serum potassium is found or suspected to be significantly increased, an EKG should be obtained immediately and treatment started immediately upon recognition of increasing amplitude of the T wave. Frequent EKG monitoring during therapy is essential. Demonstration of widening of the QRS complex is particularly ominous and requires vigorous therapy immediately if the patient's life is to be saved.

Calcium administration in the form of the chloride or gluconate salt is the most successful means of acutely counteracting the cardiac effects of hyperkalemia. This agent antagonizes the effects of potassium on all membranes. Administration of 1 to 2 g of calcium salt intravenously over 3 to 5 minutes partially reverses the characteristic EKG changes of hyperkalemia within minutes. Continuous calcium infusion at a rate of 1 g per hour may be used to control further cardiovascular toxicity of hyperkalemia. In the presence of acidosis, sodium bicarbonate can be given intravenously to increase the serum pH and transfer potassium into cells in exchange for hydrogen (Chap. 6). Insulin and glucose are also effective in transferring potassium into the cells. Generally one unit of regular insulin is given together with 3 to 4 g of glucose—the latter administered intravenously as a 10 percent glucose solution. At least 50 to 100 g of glucose may be given in this situation. All three of these forms of therapy may be given concurrently to patients with marked elevations of the serum potassium. All these measures are effective initially. Their effectiveness rapidly diminishes, however, in the presence of recurring hyperkalemia.

If hyperkalemia is refractory to the foregoing therapy, or if it occurs in the presence of poor renal function where potassium elevation may recur, dialysis is necessary. Initially peritoneal dialysis without addition of potassium to the first 6 to 8 exchanges effectively reduces plasma [K]. The other measures described above should be continued also until the serum potassium is normal. Hemodialysis is also an effective way to manage hyperkalemia, but takes more time to initiate than peritoneal dialysis.

Administration of Kayexelate, a polystyrene sulfonate resin which removes potassium from the body through exchange for sodium across the lumen of the small and large bowel, can be used to control elevations of the serum potassium. It may be given by mouth together with sorbitol (to prevent fecal impaction) or as an enema. It has a maximum binding capacity of 4 mEq K^+ per g of resin, but more than 50 percent binding is rarely achieved in practice. Although it may be used effectively for short periods of time, it suffers the disadvantage of replacing the potassium with equal quantities of sodium. Thus, in the patient with virtually absent renal function sodium overload may become a serious problem if this form of therapy is continued for long periods of time.

CHAPTER 8
Acid–Base Disturbances

DANIEL G. SAPIR AND W. GORDON WALKER

In the normal individual, the daily production of hydrogen ion exceeds 12,000 mEq. Despite this large production, the hydrogen ion concentration is maintained between 3.5×10^{-8} and 4.5×10^{-8} moles per liter in the plasma and interstitial fluid. The *buffers* in blood, interstitial and intracellular fluid, and the excretory functions of the *lungs* and *kidneys* are responsible for maintenance of the hydrogen ion concentration within these limits. Their actions, in concert, permit production and elimination of these large quantities of hydrogen ion with only very small changes in hydrogen ion concentration in body fluids. The lungs serve as the principal route of elimination of hydrogen ion when H_2CO_3 is converted to the CO_2 excreted in expired air. The kidneys provide a second route for hydrogen ion excretion that is quantitatively much smaller, but is of prime importance in restoring the buffer capacity of the body fluids (Fig. 8–1). Without the great excretory capacity of the lungs and kidneys, the buffers would be quite inadequate to regulate hydrogen ion concentration and fatal acidosis would develop in a very short time. For convenience, pH is used to represent hydrogen ion concentration, and is defined as:

$$pH = -\log [H^+] \tag{1}$$

ROUTES OF H$^+$ EXCRETION

1. LUNGS
   BASAL RATE   – 12,000 mEq/DAY AS CO_2
   MAXIMAL RATE – 30,000 mEq/DAY AS CO_2

2. KIDNEYS
   BASAL RATE   – 30 mEq/DAY AS TITRATABLE ACID
                     60 mEq/DAY AS NH_4^+
   MAXIMAL RATE –150 mEq/DAY AS TITRATABLE ACID
                    700 mEq/DAY AS NH_4^+

FIGURE 8-1. Basal and maximal rates of hydrogen excretion by the kidneys and lungs.

PHYSIOLOGY OF pH REGULATION[35-39]

SOURCES OF HYDROGEN ION PRODUCTION

The sources of hydrogen ion are shown in Figure 8–2. The major source is the production of CO_2 from metabolic processes (about 12,000 mEq per day). Metabolism of phospholipids, as well as of proteins that contain phosphate and sulfate, yields phosphoric and sulfuric acids. These latter substances account for no more than 80 to 100 mEq of hydrogen ion per day in normal individuals. Although quantitatively these sources yield only a very small fraction of the daily production, they are of special significance because the hydrogen ion thus formed is associated with non-volatile anions, phosphate and sulfate, and must be eliminated via the kidney.

ROLE OF BUFFERS

The buffers of the body fluids transport the hydrogen ion formed by all these processes from the production sources in the tissues to the lungs and kidneys for excretion.

The chemical buffering action that occurs within the body fluids is provided by mixtures of poorly dissociated weak acids and their highly ionized salts. Such buffer pairs minimize pH change by converting a strong, highly dissociated acid to a weak, poorly dissociated one, thereby reducing the concentration of hydrogen ion.

In the presence of a solution containing a buffer pair, such as carbonic acid–sodium bicarbonate, the hydrogen ion concentration of the solution is given by the relation:

$$[H^+] = K \frac{[H_2CO_3]}{[HCO_3^-]} \tag{2}$$

This can also be expressed in its logarithmic form, the Henderson-Hasselbalch equation:

$$pH = pK + \log \frac{[HCO_3^-]}{[H_2CO_3]} \tag{3}$$

The constant, pK, is related to the dissociation constant of the weak acid (K, in Eq. 2) and identifies the pH at which buffering is most effective (where pH

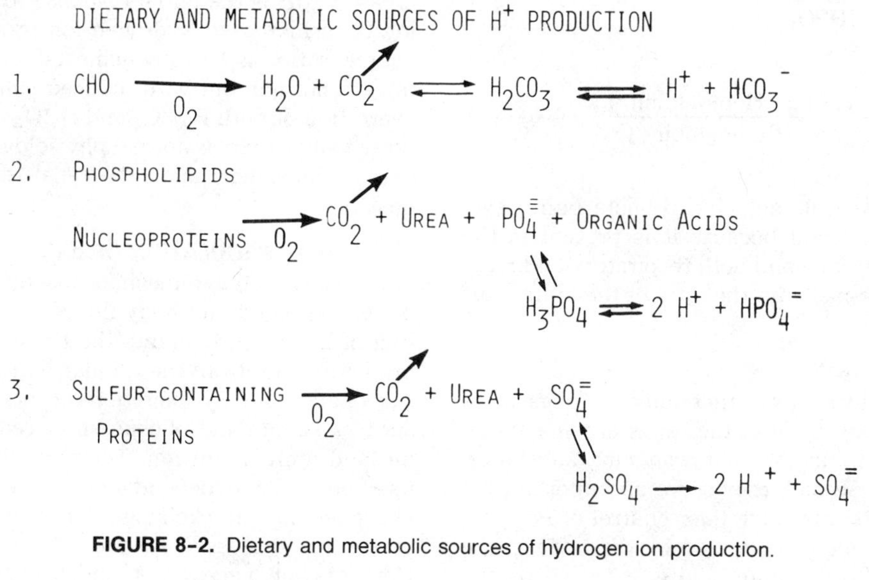

DIETARY AND METABOLIC SOURCES OF H$^+$ PRODUCTION

1. $CHO \xrightarrow{O_2} H_2O + CO_2 \rightleftharpoons H_2CO_3 \rightleftharpoons H^+ + HCO_3^-$

2. PHOSPHOLIPIDS

   NUCLEOPROTEINS $\xrightarrow{O_2} CO_2 + UREA + PO_4^= + ORGANIC\ ACIDS$

   $H_3PO_4 \rightleftharpoons 2\ H^+ + HPO_4^=$

3. SULFUR-CONTAINING $\xrightarrow{O_2} CO_2 + UREA + SO_4^=$
   PROTEINS

   $H_2SO_4 \longrightarrow 2\ H^+ + SO_4^=$

FIGURE 8-2. Dietary and metabolic sources of hydrogen ion production.

change is smallest when a given quantity of hydrogen ion is added). It is also evident from Equation (3) that it is the pH at which the concentration of the acid and its salt are equal ($\log_{10} 1 = 0$).

The concentration of CO_2 in solution is related to $[H_2CO_3]$ by the following reaction:

$$H_2CO_3 \rightleftharpoons CO_2 + H_2O$$

The concentration of CO_2 is approximately 700 times greater than the carbonic acid concentration at equilibrium. Therefore, dissolved CO_2 represents virtually all of the H_2CO_3 available, and the concentration of dissolved CO_2 can be taken as a measure of the $[H_2CO_3]$. The concentration of CO_2 is determined by its partial pressure, Pco_2, and its solubility coefficient for plasma, α. Thus, Equation (3) can be written in a more clinically useful form:

$$pH = pK' + \log \frac{[HCO_3^-]}{\alpha Pco_2} \tag{4}$$

The apparent pK' is 6.1. Since the pH of extracellular fluid is 7.4, the ratio of carbonic acid to bicarbonate can be calculated from the equation to be 1:20, a ratio quite unfavorable for optimum buffering action. However, the utility as an effective buffer depends upon the speed and facility with which the lungs and kidneys act to restore this ratio when it has been altered by addition or removal of hydrogen ion.

The principal buffer systems of the extracellular fluid and blood expressed in terms of Equation (2) are:

$$\frac{[H_2CO_3]}{[HCO_3^-]} \qquad \frac{[H_2PO_4^-]}{[HPO_4^=]}$$

$$\frac{[H^+ \, Protein^-]}{[Protein^-]} \qquad \frac{[H^+ \, Hemoglobin^-]}{[Hemoglobin^-]}$$

Of these, the carbonic acid–bicarbonate buffer system is most important because it is present in the greatest concentration and both respiratory and renal action operate to maintain the ratio of the buffer pair constant.

ROLE OF LUNGS

The lungs perform two functions in regard to acid–base regulation. First, the lungs are the *excretory route* for the major acid-producing substance, carbon dioxide. Second, they serve an important pH *regulatory function* through their control of Pco_2.

Carbon dioxide is generated by the body at the rate of 10 mEq per minute, and is excreted by the lungs at the same rate. The effect of CO_2 on $[H^+]$ is readily seen from the following reactions:

$$CO_2 + H_2O \rightleftharpoons H_2CO_3 \rightleftharpoons HCO_3^- + H^+$$

If CO_2 is permitted to accumulate, the $[H^+]$ will rise and pH will fall.

At pH 7.4, the concentration of carbonic acid is 1.3 mEq of H_2CO_3 per liter in the body fluids, representing much less than 1 percent of the total quantity of CO_2 produced per day. Thus, a large quantity of CO_2 is produced and fed into this small pool and equally rapidly removed by the respiratory system. The concentration of CO_2 (or carbonic acid) in the body fluids is determined by the balance between production of CO_2 by the tissues and excretion by the lungs. In contrast to other solutes (such as sodium, chloride, and bicarbonate ions), it is insensitive to changes in volume of body fluids and responds only to changes in respiratory rate or CO_2 production rate.

The responsiveness of the carbonic acid concentration to changes in ventilatory rate provides the respiratory system with effective control over the regulation of pH of the body fluids. For example, a drop in pH (acidosis) stimulates an increase in alveolar ventilation which increases the excretion rate of CO_2. This decrease in Pco_2, or $[H_2CO_3]$, restores the carbonic acid–bicarbonate ratio toward normal and returns pH toward normal (see Equation (4) and Fig. 8–3). It is this rapid response (half-time about 30 minutes) of $[H_2CO_3]$ to changes in respiratory rate that makes the carbonic acid–bicarbonate system an effective buffer at pH 7.4 despite the fact that this is far above this system's most effective buffering range. This increased ventilation with lowering of Pco_2 and increase in pH is the initial response to acidosis resulting from increased hydrogen ion production. Partial compensation is thereby achieved with return of pH toward normal, but with reduced values for the concentration of both H_2CO_3 and HCO_3^-. Restoration of these values to their normal physiologic ranges is ultimately dependent upon the renal responses to acidosis.

RENAL REGULATION OF pH

Three renal tubular mechanisms operate to restore pH of the blood and body fluids to normal: 1) secretion of hydrogen ions into the urine; 2) reabsorption of bicarbonate from the tubular lumen as sodium bicarbonate; and 3) excretion of nonvolatile anions such as sulfate and phosphate paired with hydrogen ion and ammonium ion. The three mechanisms are interrelated, and depend upon tubular secretion of hydrogen ion in exchange for sodium. These processes are discussed in more detail in Chapter 10. Here it is only necessary to indicate that all these pro-

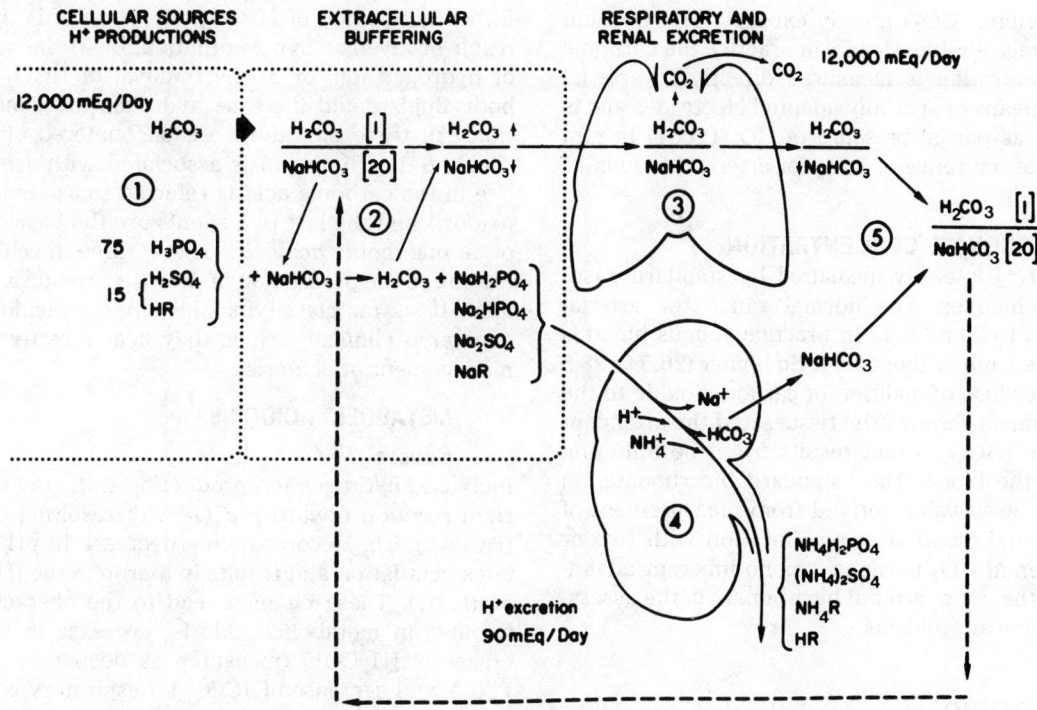

FIGURE 8–3. Buffering and excretion of daily acid production by the body. 1) Acid is produced within the cell, almost all as carbonic acid. Only about 90 mEq/day are generated as a result of production of nonvolatile acids. These strong acids cannot exist as acids at physiologic pH, hence they require immediate buffering. 2) When they enter the extracellular fluid they immediately displace or lower bicarbonate concentration with production of H_2CO_3 and sodium salts of the acids. 3) The H_2CO_3 is excreted quantitatively by the lung as CO_2 with resulting lowering of the carbonic acid concentration (P_{CO_2}). 4) The nonvolatile anions are excreted by the kidney in association with hydrogen ion and/or NH_4. The secretion of hydrogen ion is associated with reabsorption of an equimolar quantity of $NaHCO_3$. 5) This $NaHCO_3$ is returned to the blood and restores the carbonic acid–bicarbonate ratio to normal, thereby restoring the buffering capacity of the body fluids.

cesses serve to increase $NaHCO_3$ reabsorption. The exchange of hydrogen ion for sodium ion results in the return of the recovered sodium ion to the body fluids as $NaHCO_3$. The net result of this exchange is an increase in bicarbonate concentration within the body fluids and a return of the $[H_2CO_3]$ / $[HCO_3^-]$ to normal (Fig. 8–3).

The ventilatory response to acidosis, followed by the renal response, provides the body with the mechanisms for quickly restoring pH of the body fluids to normal and then regenerating the $[H_2CO_3]$ / $[HCO_3^-]$ buffering capacity of the body fluids so that subsequent pH changes, should they arise, can be effectively countered.

LABORATORY AIDS IN DIAGNOSIS OF pH DISTURBANCE

The Henderson-Hasselbalch equation (Equation 4) identifies the variables that can be measured and used to diagnose the type of acid–base disturbance present. These are: 1) direct pH measurement; 2) measurement of bicarbonate ion concentration; and 3) measurement of carbonic acid concentration.

pH MEASUREMENT

Direct measurement of the pH of arterial blood drawn anaerobically and measured immediately will identify the presence of acidosis or alkalosis, but does not provide information about the cause of the disturbance. To distinguish between metabolic and respiratory causes of the disturbance, measurement of bicarbonate and/or carbonic acid concentrations are necessary.

CARBONIC ACID CONCENTRATION (P_{CO_2})

As mentioned in the discussion of equation (4), the $[H_2CO_3]$ is determined by the partial pressure of carbon dioxide (P_{CO_2}) in the body fluids, as defined by the reaction:

$$CO_2 + H_2O \rightleftharpoons H_2CO_3$$

At equilibrium, $[CO_2]$ greatly exceeds $[H_2CO_3]$ and is readily measurable. Hence, in practice the carbonic acid concentration is measured directly in arterial blood by means of specially adapted electrodes and is expressed as partial pressure of CO_2 (Pco_2) in mm Hg. The normal range of Pco_2 for arterial blood is 37 to 42 mm Hg.

BICARBONATE CONCENTRATION

The $[HCO_3^-]$ is easily measured by standard gasometric techniques. The normal range for arterial blood is 24 to 26 mEq/L. In practice venous blood is usually used and is about 1.5 mEq higher (26.5 to 28.5 mEq/L) because of addition of carbon dioxide to the blood in transit through the tissues and the attendant increase in $[HCO_3^-]$ that results from the buffering action of the blood. The "standard bicarbonate," a commonly used value derived from measurement of pH of arterial blood after equilibration with two or more different CO_2 tensions, has no inherent advantage over the use of arterial bicarbonate in the assessment of clinical problems.

ACIDOSIS

Alterations leading to an increase in hydrogen ion concentration may be identified from inspection of the equilibrium reaction for carbonic acid, the major buffer system in the extracellular fluid, where:

$$[H^+] = K \frac{[H_2CO_3]}{[HCO_3^-]}$$

Either 1) addition of H_2CO_3 (elevation of Pco_2) as a result of alveolar hypoventilation; or 2) the addition of hydrogen ion, or 3) the removal of HCO_3^- from body fluids could increase hydrogen ion concentration. All three situations are encountered clinically (Table 8–1). The acidosis associated with a primary rise in the carbonic acid is referred to as *respiratory acidosis* and the last two events are the basic causes of a *metabolic acidosis*. These three mechanisms leading to the production of acidosis provide a convenient basis for classifying the types of acidosis encountered clinically, since they bear directly on the management of acidosis.

METABOLIC ACIDOSIS

Causes

Increased hydrogen ion production shifts the equilibrium reaction toward H_2CO_3 with resulting drop in $[HCO_3^-]$. The accompanying decrease in pH stimulates ventilation and results in a drop in the $[H_2CO_3]$ or (Pco_2). These changes lead to the characteristic findings in metabolic acidosis: decrease in pH, decrease in $[H_2CO_3]$ (measured as decreased arterial Pco_2), and decreased $[HCO_3^-]$. Respiratory compensation, the increased ventilatory response which lowers the Pco_2, moderates the decrease in pH and may, in the presence of only mild acidosis, succeed in restoring the pH to normal. In this circumstance, only a lowered $[HCO_3^-]$ and lowered Pco_2 will be observed. As the acidosis increases in severity, complete compensation cannot be achieved and the pH then falls progressively as the severity of the acidosis increases. The renal response, operating much more slowly than the ventilatory response, again tends to retard the decrease in pH by addition of HCO_3^- to the body fluids.

Metabolic acidosis may result from endogenous or exogenous sources of hydrogen ion (Table 8–1). Such metabolic derangements as overproduction of keto-acids in diabetes mellitus, excess production of lactic acid in the presence of sustained anoxia of the peripheral tissues, and drug-induced excess lactic acid production all result in addition of excess quantities of hydrogen ion to body fluids.

These acids (beta-hydroxybutyric acid, acetoacetic acid, lactic acid) react with $NaHCO_3$ to form H_2CO_3 and the sodium salt of the added organic acid. The added anion is not measured in routine clinical chemical procedures, so that the anion gap, defined as the sum of measured cations minus the sum of measured anions, ($[Na^+]$ + $[K^+]$) − ($[Cl^-]$ + $[HCO_3^-]$), is widened. This increased difference between the sums of anions and cations is a useful point in corroboration of a suspected metabolic acidosis (Fig. 8–4).

TABLE 8–1
Causes of Metabolic Acidosis

Gain of Hydrogen Ion	
Exogenous	**Endogenous**
Aspirin	Renal failure
Methanol	Renal tubular acidosis*
Ethylene glycol	
Ammonium chloride*	Diabetes
Paraldehyde	Lactic acidosis

Loss of HCO_3^-	
Exogenous	**Endogenous**
Carbonic-anhydrase-inhibiting diuretics*	Diarrhea*
	Biliary or pancreatic fistulae*
	Ureterosigmoidostomy*

* Characterized by decrease in anion gap.

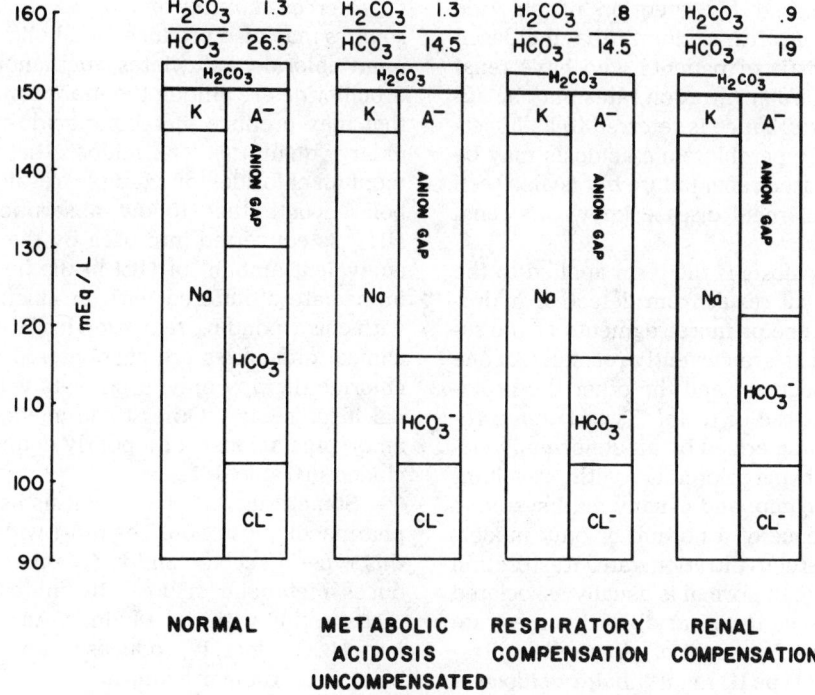

FIGURE 8-4. Recognition of unmeasured anions in metabolic acidosis. Since determination of organic anions in the blood is not a routinely available clinical procedure, the most helpful laboratory information is the difference between sum of cations and sum of anions. Shown here is the normal value for the anion gap, which is the difference between $([Na] + [K]) - ([Cl] + [HCO_3])$. Values in excess of 20 are associated with some increase in nonvolatile anion such as lactate or keto-acids. Also shown is the response to production of this unidentified anion. Initially this accumulation displaces the bicarbonate and the resultant decrease in pH stimulates respiration. The resulting drop in P_{CO_2} restores the pH partially to normal although the concentration of nonvolatile anions in the plasma remains unchanged. The renal compensation restores bicarbonate toward normal.

Decreased hydrogen ion excretion leads to the other major type of endogenous metabolic acidosis. It results from a failure of acid excretion by the kidneys. Ingestion of protein in the diet and its metabolic dissimilation and subsequent degradation as a source of energy yields urea plus phosphate and sulfate as metabolic end products (Fig. 8-2). The latter substances react with the buffer systems of the body to form H_2CO_3 and to decrease $[HCO_3^-]$ (see Fig. 8-3). These nonvolatile anions, existing as neutral salts of strong mineral acid at physiologic pH, must be excreted by the kidney and a comparable quantity of $NaHCO_3$ regenerated and returned to the blood to restore the normal pH of the body fluids. Since hydrogen ion is exchanged for sodium ion either directly (as titratable acid) or as NH_4^+, this reaction requires an intact tubular mechanism for the secretion of hydrogen ion. The rate of production of hydrogen ion

from ingested foodstuffs never exceeds the capacity of the normal kidney to secrete hydrogen ion. In chronic or acute renal failure, however, hydrogen ion secretion is limited, and a fraction of these strong mineral acids is retained instead of excreted as net acid. This daily retention produces an acidosis that is also associated with widening of the anion gap by the retained sodium sulfate and phosphate salts of the inorganic acids (Fig. 8-4).

Bicarbonate loss via the urine or other body fluids will also produce acidosis. Normally, the kidney reabsorbs all the filtered HCO_3^- plus an additional amount equal to the amount of titratable acid plus the NH_4^+ produced. This process, accomplished through hydrogen ion secretion, is deficient in some patients with renal failure, so that relatively large amounts of bicarbonate will be excreted in the urine despite systemic acidosis. When the bicarbonate wasting is accomplished by retention of chloride (through reabsorption with sodium) the increased anion gap characteristic of patients who have renal failure and low glomerular filtration rates may be absent. This type of disturbance is referred to as *hyperchloremic acidosis.* Hyperchloremic acidosis may be encountered in advanced renal failure but is also seen in a primary form of renal disease known as renal tubular acidosis.

Renal tubular acidosis is the term applied to the group of disorders that result from defective hydrogen ion transport in one or more segments of the tubule. Two basic defects are currently recognized; one involves the distal segment and the other the proximal segment. The *classic* or *distal* (Type I) *renal tubular acidosis* is characterized by an abnormally elevated urine pH, hyperchloremia with resultant decrease in the anion gap, and usually mild systemic acidosis in the presence of a normal or only moderately reduced glomerular filtration rate. Restoration of plasma bicarbonate to normal is usually associated with only mild increase in urinary bicarbonate (rate of loss rarely exceeds 2 percent of glomerular filtration rate). *Proximal* (Type II) *renal tubular acidosis* is characterized by more severe systemic acidosis (plasma HCO_3^- usually less than 15 mEq/L in untreated patients), hyperchloremia, and a urine pH usually within the normal range (<5.0) in untreated patients. Return of plasma HCO_3^- toward normal by HCO_3^- administration results in markedly alkaline urine long before systemic pH is returned to normal. Return of plasma HCO_3^- to normal by infusion of sodium bicarbonate results in profound rate of loss of urinary bicarbonate with rate of HCO_3^- excretion often exceeding 20 percent of the filtered load of bicarbonate. Incomplete or mild defects are recognized in both types and mixtures of the two defects have also been described. These disorders are considered more fully in Chapter 14.

Gastrointestinal loss of bicarbonate leading to metabolic acidosis is present in pathologic conditions involving the small and large bowel. An excellent example is the severe bicarbonate-wasting diarrhea commonly affecting children, with a less frequent incidence in adults. Other conditions of the intestine leading to bicarbonate wastage include biliary and pancreatic fistulas, ureterosigmoidostomies, and poorly functioning ileal loops used as bladder replacements. In the latter instance, bicarbonate loss results from urinary chloride exchange for bicarbonate across the ileal loop membrane. Regardless of source of bicarbonate loss, the changes in composition of body fluid are similar and hyperchloremia is usually a prominent feature of the acidosis resulting from gastrointestinal disturbances.

Increased intake of hydrogen ion from exogenous sources may also produce metabolic acidosis. Ammonium chloride, salicylates, methanol, and lysine hydrochloride are among the more common substances that may produce metabolic acidosis when ingested in large quantities. The acidosis that results from ammonium chloride, for example, results from the metabolic events that follow absorption; the ingested NH_4^+ is converted into urea by the liver, leaving an equivalent amount of HCl in the body fluids. This is immediately buffered with production of NaCl and with corresponding reduction in $[HCO_3^-]$. In general, clinical difficulties are encountered with ammonium chloride therapy only in patients with underlying renal insufficiency. Other toxic agents which produce an organic acidosis of a poorly defined nature are included in Table 8–1.

Some drugs produce acidosis as a result of their pharmacologic action. The most widely used agent of this type is acetazolamide (Diamox). This drug produces metabolic acidosis by inhibiting bicarbonate reabsorption within the kidney. As a result of the urinary HCO_3^- loss, it produces a clinical picture resembling renal tubular acidosis.

Clinical Recognition of Metabolic Acidosis

Clinical features of metabolic acidosis are similar regardless of etiology. Signs and symptoms are related to severity of the pH disturbance rather than to specific cause of the acidosis. Mild degrees of acidosis may be associated with no changes other than an increased ventilatory rate. More severe degrees of acidosis produce deep, rapid respirations (Kussmaul breathing), dryness of mucous membranes, somnolence, stupor, and coma. The specific etiology of the acidosis can only be suspected from historical data. Preexisting diabetes, renal disease, and recurrent renal stones are all conditions which should increase the index of suspicion regarding the likelihood of acidosis. In a clinical setting where there is primary liver, pulmonary, or cardiac disease, or where one of the phenformin group of hypoglycemic agents has been taken, and metabolic acidosis exists, lactic acidosis should be considered as the most probable underlying pathophysiologic event.

A clear-cut history is often difficult to obtain when a patient presents with acidosis of an unknown type which may have followed a toxic ingestion. Methanol and ethylene glycol are mistakenly taken by alcoholics, and suicide attempts or accidental poisonings in the younger age-groups often involve aspirin. A careful history of possible drug or toxin ingestions should always be obtained when acidosis is diagnosed in the absence of underlying disease.

Management of Metabolic Acidosis

In every case of acid–base disturbance, the physician's attention should be directed to the specific etiology as well as to the precise characterization of the accompanying metabolic alterations. Although the principles of therapy for the generalized electrolyte alterations occurring during metabolic acidosis are applicable in every case, knowledge of the etiology may enable the clinician to institute more effective means of treatment. The use of insulin in diabetic acidosis is an obvious example of this principle. The therapy of a case of metabolic acidosis may be illustrated by the following case presentation.

CASE PRESENTATION OF METABOLIC ACIDOSIS

An 18-year-old male with severe uremia was admitted for chronic dialysis and transplantation. After several hemodialyses, a pericardial friction rub was heard and within 24 hours he developed signs of pericardial tamponade. On examination his pulse rate was 120 per min, BP 80/50 mm Hg with marked pulsus paradoxus, respirations 20 per min and Kussmaul in character. Central and peripheral cyanosis was present and the extremities were cool. The jugular venous pressure was elevated (32 cm H_2O).

The clinical impression of an acute pericardial effusion resulting in tamponade was confirmed, and 400 ml of bloody fluid were removed by pericardiocentesis. He improved promptly and venous pressure fell to 22 cm. The systemic blood pressure rose to 110/70 mm Hg. Within a short time after the procedure the patient became semiconscious and respirations again were deep and rapid. Blood chemistries included a total CO_2 of 6 mEq/L, sodium 140, chloride 105, and K 6.6 mEq/L. The blood pH was 7.2, Pco_2 18 mm Hg, and the lactate level was 10 mM/L. A blood glucose determination was 140 per dl and there was no detectable ketonemia.

Discussion of Management

The appearance of a sudden metabolic acidosis characterized by a widened anion gap, ([140] + [6]) − ([105] + [6]) = 35 mEq/L, in a patient who exhibited signs of circulatory insufficiency strongly pointed to the diagnosis of lactic acidosis (Fig. 8–4). Confirmation was obtained by the identification of the added anion as lactate. This chemical determination is not routinely done on a clinical service so that diagnosis depends on the recognition of the clinical setting and the finding of a widened anion gap. Lactic acidosis is found in patients with circulatory insufficiency and hypoxia or in those with serious renal, hepatic, or pulmonary disease. It has also been reported in diabetic patients maintained on oral hypoglycemic agents.

An approximation of the total bicarbonate deficit in this case is obtained from the difference between a normal serum bicarbonate of 24 mEq/L and the patient's bicarbonate of 6 mEq/L and multiplying this figure by 35 percent of the patient's body weight.[37] Thus, (24 − 6) × 0.35 × 60 kg = 378 mEq of sodium bicarbonate which would theoretically be required to raise the serum bicarbonate to a normal value. In clinical practice *this calculated quantity may differ markedly from the actual amount of bicarbonate needed or that which can safely be administered* for the following reasons:

1. The production of acids may continue and increase the need for administered bicarbonate.
2. Despite the rise in serum bicarbonate and consequent rise in serum pH, alveolar hyperventilation may continue with the resulting low Pco_2 producing an alkalosis. Injudicious further bicarbonate therapy may then produce a serious alkalosis.
3. Administration of large quantities of sodium may produce extracellular volume overload resulting in congestive heart failure. The use of THAM, an organic buffer, itself an osmotic particle, does not circumvent this problem.[35]

Initially, the patient may be given one-half of the calculated deficit of sodium bicarbonate in 3 to 4 hours (in this case the administration of 200 mEq raised the CO_2 content of the serum to 17 mEq/L and the pH to 7.28) and a repeat assessment may then be made of the acid–base status. Coincident with the amelioration of the systemic acidosis the patient became fully conscious. In view of the patient's clinical improvement and the continued absence of the initial cause of the acidosis (tamponade leading to shock), no further bicarbonate was given. Within 6 hours the oxidation of the circulating lactate had increased the total serum CO_2 to 23 mEq/L.

If the initial intravenous bicarbonate administered had not resulted in a rise in the blood pH and an improvement in the patient's condition, more vigorous therapy would have been required. Bicarbonate administration could be increased by: 1) speeding the infusion rate; 2) instituting peritoneal dialysis, using a solution containing acetate which on oxidation yields an equimolar quantity of bicarbonate; and 3) employing hemodialysis which also provides acetate as a source of bicarbonate. More vigorous treatment of the acidosis by peritoneal dialysis can be effected by use of a solution made by mixing appropriate intravenous fluids containing 2 liters of water, 77 mEq/L of sodium chloride and 66 mEq/L of sodium bicarbonate, and 25 g sugar as the dialyzing fluid. Careful attention must then be directed to the maintenance of normal serum calcium, magnesium, and blood sugar concentrations. The use of some form of dialysis in the primary treatment of metabolic acidosis is indicated in patients who cannot receive added sodium.

A stable state of chronic metabolic acidosis often accompanies chronic renal failure or is seen in cases of renal tubular acidosis. This is caused either by daily retention of small quantities of hydrogen ion and/or bicarbonate-wasting. In order to compensate for this progressive acid load, body buffers (mainly from bone in the form of CO_3^-) are called upon to maintain acid–base balance. This cumulative demand upon bone buffers plays a major role in the production of renal osteodystrophy, and constitutes the major reason for therapeutic intervention, since the decline in pH is often not severe enough to produce clinical symptoms.

The oral administration of citrate, lactate, or CO_3^- as sodium or calcium salts may produce the desired rise of plasma [HCO_3^-]. Major problems with this form of therapy include: 1) gastric intolerance to these agents, 2) inherent difficulties with the cation of the administered salt, which include volume expansion with sodium or the production of hypercalcemia when calcium is given.

In the treatment of this type of acidosis, the aim of therapy should be the gradual return to normal pH over a period of several days. Acute administration of large quantities of bicarbonate often results in the creation of a metabolic alkalosis with *tetany,* and, on occasion, *seizures.* Acute hypokalemia may also be precipitated in this circumstance, since many of these patients, particularly those with renal tubular acidosis, have a latent or overt potassium deficiency.

RESPIRATORY ACIDOSIS

Cause

Respiratory acidosis is always caused by *impaired alveolar ventilation.* Failure of pulmonary ventilation results in CO_2 retention and elevation of H_2CO_3 concentration (increased arterial Pco_2). From inspection of the H_2CO_3 equilibrium reaction it is clear that CO_2 retention will produce an increased hydrogen ion and HCO_3^- concentration, but that the rise in [HCO_3^-] will be quite small. The rise in hydrogen ion concentration produces a significant fall in pH.

Any pathologic condition involving the lung, tracheobronchial tree, chest wall, or central nervous control of respiration can result in respiratory acidosis. The rise in H_2CO_3 will produce a small but definite rise in plasma bicarbonate from the action of body buffers:

$$CO_2 + H_2O \rightleftharpoons H_2CO_3 \rightleftharpoons HCO_3^- + H^+$$
$$+$$
$$Buffer^-$$
$$\Updownarrow$$
$$H\ Buffer$$

As more of the hydrogen is buffered by extra- and intracellular substances that bind hydrogen more tightly than H_2CO_3, the equilibrium is shifted to the right with resulting HCO_3^- generation. Figure 8–5 demonstrates the rise in plasma bicarbonate which occurs with acute increases in Pco_2 in the normal individual. The extra- and intracellular buffers involved in this reaction include hemoglobin and other proteins.

Manifestations of Acute Respiratory Acidosis

The clinical circumstances in which uncomplicated acute respiratory acidosis occurs are often dramatic. The presence of severe respiratory outflow obstruc-

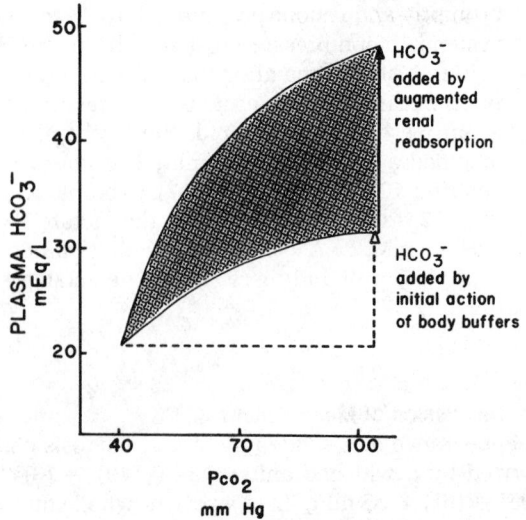

FIGURE 8–5. Relative roles of body buffers and renal response in adjusting to respiratory acidosis. The lower curve identifies the bicarbonate generated by the buffer systems in response to an elevated Pco_2 and the upper curve identifies the steady state bicarbonate concentration after renal compensation. Redrawn from Schwartz.[39]

tion should always arouse suspicion of the existence of respiratory acidosis. Only measurement of the pH and Pco_2 will adequately define the magnitude of the acid–base changes.

In general, the patient will appear acutely ill, complaining of dyspnea, and making a greater respiratory effort to increase alveolar ventilation. Hypoxemia manifested as cyanosis is a common accompanying sign of respiratory acidosis. Disorientation, stupor, and finally coma occur when the Pco_2 is markedly elevated.

Management of Acute Respiratory Acidosis

Therapy in uncomplicated acute respiratory acidosis is directed toward treatment of the underlying cause, e.g., airway obstruction, chest wall trauma, or cardiorespiratory arrest. Mechanically assisted ventilation is the treatment of choice when the initial measures do not suffice to correct the CO_2 retention. Often the severity of the patient's distress in respiratory acidosis requires treatment before the quantitative alterations in the blood pH and Pco_2 are known. These measurements may usually be obtained at a later time as a check in the adequacy of therapy.

Manifestations of Chronic Respiratory Acidosis

Long-standing obstructive and restrictive pulmonary disease results in acid–base changes that differ from those seen with acute CO_2 retention. Within several days after the elevation of Pco_2, the kidneys begin to excrete increasing amounts of net acid and to reabsorb correspondingly increased amounts of bicarbonate. Figure 8–5 shows the portion of the elevated plasma bicarbonate that is attributable to augmented renal absorption. As can be seen by analysis of the equilibrium or Henderson-Hasselbalch equations, the increased $[HCO_3^-]$ reduces hydrogen ion concentration and increases the pH.

Management of Chronic Respiratory Acidosis

The goal of therapy, namely, the relief of CO_2 retention by improvement of ventilation, is the same in chronic as in acute respiratory acidosis. However, in uncomplicated acute respiratory acidosis, removal of the underlying cause will permit the Pco_2 to return to normal, while in the patient with chronic lung disease therapeutic efforts may not overcome the underlying structural damage, so that a return to a chronic stable state of respiratory acidosis will be the therapeutic endpoint. Indeed, in many cases, the patient seen with pulmonary disease has developed a superimposed acute impairment of ventilation resulting in a combined acute and chronic respiratory acidosis. In

this instance, therapy is dictated as much by the clinical state of the patient as by the blood gas abnormalities.

CASE PRESENTATION OF CHRONIC RESPIRATORY ACIDOSIS

A 57-year-old male was admitted in a confused and somnolent state. He had smoked heavily for many years and had a chronic productive cough. For the past 2 to 3 years he had noted increasing exertional dyspnea and slight ankle edema.

On examination, his pulse was 132 per min and regular, temperature 101°F, blood pressure 105/70 mm Hg, and respiratory rate was 26 per min. There was central and peripheral cyanosis, an emphysematous configuration to the chest, and the respirations were labored with expiratory wheezing audible over the entire chest. Harsh respiratory rales and dullness to percussion were present over the whole of the left lower lobe. A forceful right ventricular impulse was present over the precordium, and there was cervical venous distension.

The hematocrit was 52 and white blood count 18,000. Electrolytes included a serum sodium of 134, potassium 5.7, HCO_3^- 39, and chloride 89 mEq/L. Measured blood gases included a Po_2 of 47 mm Hg, Pco_2 78 mm Hg, and pH 7.29. The chest film showed a left lower lobe infiltrate.

Discussion of Management

The history and physical findings were compatible with bronchitis and emphysema. A recent period of further decompensation is suggested by the patient's stupor presumably caused by a left lower lobe pneumonia. The blood gas measurements indicated the presence of hypoxemia coupled with a respiratory acidosis. Increased renal bicarbonate reabsorption accounted for the elevated $[HCO_3^-]$. Bicarbonate therapy was avoided in this situation. It would represent a large additional sodium load in the presence of right-sided heart failure. Moreover, this type of therapy might aggravate the hypoxemia by: 1) further depressing the respiratory center, which was responding to the acidosis, 2) rapidly correcting the pH by bicarbonate infusion, which would shift the oxyhemoglobin dissociation curve to the left, resulting in a decreased delivery of oxygen to the tissues.

Improvement of alveolar ventilation was therefore the primary goal of therapy in this case. This included: 1) treatment of the infection, 2) adequate tracheobronchial drainage of secretions, as well as 3) mechanical assistance to ventilation (see Chap. 31). Within 4 hours the P_{CO_2} had fallen to 65 mm Hg, pH had risen to 7.34 and the P_{O_2} increased to 60 mm Hg. After 24 hours, the clinical condition had stabilized with the patient becoming more alert so that the assisted ventilation was discontinued. At the end of 10 days in the hospital the patient felt well and repeat blood studies revealed a pH of 7.38, P_{CO_2} of 55 mm Hg, total HCO_3^- of 32 mEq/L. In view of his chronic pulmonary disease it was felt that no further improvement in alveolar ventilation was possible and the patient was discharged with stable arterial hypoxemia and chronic hypercapnia. In such cases, this is often the maximum benefit that can be achieved.

In respiratory acidosis the compensation produced by bicarbonate retention will never be sufficient to return the serum pH to completely normal levels. An apparent state of total compensation with arterial pH above 7.44 is *always* the result of a mixed pH disturbance with the secondary alteration being a metabolic alkalosis. This may be encountered, for instance, when diuretic therapy has led to superimposition of hypokalemic, hypochloremic metabolic alkalosis.

ALKALOSIS

TYPES AND CAUSES

Alkalosis results from a decrease in the hydrogen ion concentration of the extracellular fluid. The carbonic acid equilibrium reaction identifies the mechanism for production of alkalosis (see Equation 2). A decrease in the P_{CO_2} secondary to increased alveolar ventilation decreases $[H_2CO_3]$. This in turn gives rise to a decrease in hydrogen ion concentration and $[HCO_3^-]$ and is known as *respiratory alkalosis*. *Metabolic alkalosis* results from either loss of hydrogen or a gain of bicarbonate, or both. A brief outline

---

TABLE 8-2
Causes of Metabolic Alkalosis

1. Vomiting of gastric contents
2. Administration of diuretics which cause virtually equal losses of Na and Cl (thiazides, mercurials, ethacrynic acid, furosemide)
3. Hyperaldosteronism
4. Hyperadrenocorticism
5. Administration of alkali such as antacids
6. Posthypercapneic alkalosis

TABLE 8-3
Causes of Respiratory Alkalosis

1. Vigorous respirator therapy
2. Acute hyperventilation syndrome
3. Diffuse liver disease
4. Diffuse CNS disease
5. Drug induced (salicylates)

---

of the more common causes of alkalosis is shown in Tables 8-2 and 8-3. The two most common causes of metabolic alkalosis are vomiting with loss of hydrochloric acid, and diuretic therapy that produces excessive chloride and potassium loss.

RESPIRATORY RESPONSE

Respiratory compensation plays only a very minor role in compensating for metabolic alkalosis. Thus it is not unusual to find a normal or only slightly elevated P_{CO_2} in these patients. When a steady state has been achieved, metabolic alkalosis is characterized by a decrease in the hydrogen ion concentration (increased pH), an increase in the bicarbonate concentration, and a normal or slightly elevated H_2CO_3 concentration.

BUFFER RESPONSE

The immediate buffering response that acts to minimize the pH change in alkalosis is achieved by the release of hydrogen ion from intracellular and extracellular buffers. This outward shift of hydrogen from intracellular stores is accompanied by an inward movement of sodium and potassium. Although quantitatively small, this sudden shift in potassium may lead to acute lowering of plasma potassium concentration, with the resulting cardiovascular effects of hypokalemia (Chap. 7). This shift is particularly hazardous in patients with a preexisting potassium deficit from some other cause.

RENAL RESPONSE

The response of the kidneys to alkalosis does not represent simply a bicarbonate loss with concomitant retention of hydrogen. Alkalosis is usually associated with a decrease in sodium stores as, for example, in diuretic-induced alkalosis. In this situation chloride and sodium are lost from the extracellular fluid without any bicarbonate loss. There occurs a contraction of the extracellular fluid volume around the unchanged bicarbonate stores. This results in an increased bicarbonate concentration and frank alkalosis. Renal compensation with loss of bicarbonate through the urine can occur only with a significant loss of sodium. However, the stimulus to retain sodium in this situation is maximal so that virtually all filtered sodium will be reabsorbed. Since the available chloride in the glomerular filtrate is limited (decreased extracellular fluid [Cl^-]), an increased fraction of the sodium must be reabsorbed through tubular exchange mechanisms. Sodium is exchanged for hydrogen with resulting tubular reabsorption of $NaHCO_3$ and maintenance of [HCO_3^-] at an elevated level. The alkalosis is thereby maintained. Because of the increased exchange of hydrogen ion for sodium in these circumstances, a "paradoxically" acid urine is often observed in the presence of a systemic metabolic alkalosis. The hypokalemia commonly seen in alkalosis is caused by increased urinary potassium losses which result from tubular exchange of potassium for sodium and frequently to extrarenal losses, as in persistent vomiting.

CLINICAL FEATURES OF METABOLIC ALKALOSIS

The symptoms and signs of alkalosis are relatively few, and the clinical setting in which alkalosis occurs is often one in which symptoms of other electrolyte disorders predominate. Latent or overt tetany may be produced by an acute increase in the pH of the blood but few other symptoms or signs can be attributed to the alkalosis per se. Metabolic alkalosis almost always occurs in association with varying degrees of sodium and potassium depletion and often these disturbances dominate the clinical picture (Chaps. 6 and 7).

CASE PRESENTATION OF METABOLIC ALKALOSIS

A 53-year-old man was admitted to the hospital complaining of pernicious vomiting of 2 weeks' duration, weakness, and shortness of breath. He had undergone treatment for a stomach ulcer 8 years previously but developed recurrent abdominal pain 6 months before admission. Vomiting began 3 months later, and for the past 2 weeks he had had continued emesis with very poor food intake.

On examination the blood pressure was 80/40 mm Hg, pulse 140 per min and thready, respirations 30 per min, and body weight 132 pounds. The patient was cachectic with poor skin turgor. The upper abdomen was distended and a succussion splash could be elicited. La-

tent tetany in the form of a positive Trousseau and Chvostek sign were present. The reflexes were hypoactive.

Laboratory data: hematocrit 55, white count 7500, urinalysis 1+ protein, specific gravity 1.028, and pH 5.5. Serum sodium was 132, potassium 1.9, HCO_3^- 48, and chloride 75 mEq/L. Calcium was 7.8 mg/dl, SUN 40 mg/dl. Arterial blood revealed a pH of 7.62, Pco_2 48 mm Hg, and standard bicarbonate of 43 mEq/L; 24-hour urine chlorides were 33 mEq/L.

The history and physical findings together with the hypochloremic, hypokalemic alkalosis, and sodium depletion (indicated by the elevated hematocrit) were all consistent with pyloric obstruction and appropriate x-rays revealed apparently complete obstruction at the pylorus with marked gastric dilatation.

Discussion of Management

Gastric intubation with suction drainage was instituted to decompress the stomach and permit more accurate recording of intake and output. The hypotension, tachycardia, poor skin turgor, and high hematocrit represented evidence of decreased extracellular fluid volume caused by sodium depletion. The hypoactive reflexes, generalized muscle weakness, and marked hypokalemia indicated the presence of a severe potassium deficit. The latent tetany was attributed to the alkalosis. Thus, the disturbances requiring correction were sodium depletion, potassium depletion, and hypochloremic alkalosis.

As an approximation for planning therapy, the magnitude of the chloride deficit can be equated with the estimated bicarbonate excess, i.e., the quantity of chloride that was lost and replaced with bicarbonate. The chloride loss estimated in this fashion [(48 mEq/L − 25 mEq/L) × 0.35 × 60 kg] was 483 mEq. In the presence of adequate renal function, administration of chloride ion in combination with either sodium or potassium will lessen the alkalosis by the two following mechanisms: 1) Increase in serum chloride concentration increases chloride in the glomerular filtrate and permits increased renal tubular sodium chloride reabsorption. This reduces the exchange of hydrogen for sodium (which supported the increased sodium bicarbonate reabsorption and maintained the alkalotic state). As sodium retention restores a normal extracellular volume, a portion of the sodium becomes available for the urinary excretion of the excess bicarbonate. 2) Reexpansion of the extracellular volume with 0.155 molar chloride reduces the serum bicarbonate by dilution.

In this patient, 300 mEq of sodium chloride in combination with 60 mEq KCl were given intravenously during the first day of therapy. Oral replacement was impossible because of Levine tube drainage. The next morning the patient's serum bicarbonate was 44, potassium 2.2, chloride 78 mEq/L, and latent tetany was still present. A urine chloride concentration of 89 mEq/L was recorded at this time.

When chloride loss is the primary event in alkalosis, chloride repletion alone without repair of potassium deficiency will correct the alkalosis. The values at the end of the first day's therapy indicate that a very small and clinically insignificant correction occurred despite administration of 360 mEq of chloride. Alkalosis in combination with significant chloruresis suggested that severe potassium depletion with intracellular acidosis was sustaining NaHCO₃ reabsorption despite adequate chloride intake. On the second hospital day 150 mEq of sodium chloride were given together with 150 mEq of potassium chloride, and the resulting serum electrolytes included a bicarbonate of 36, potassium 2.6, chloride 83, and sodium 140 mEq/L. It was now apparent that a severe degree of potassium depletion led to the initial resistance of the alkalosis to repair with sodium chloride. Over the next several days continued potassium chloride supplementation led to full correction of the alkalosis and potassium repletion. The precise role of potassium depletion in maintenance of metabolic alkalosis remains unclear. Hypokalemia is almost always present to some degree in metabolic alkalosis. For the clinical well-being of the patient, repair of potassium deficiency should routinely be undertaken as part of the treatment for metabolic alkalosis.

One additional feature merits comment. As in this case, metabolic alkalosis usually develops over a period of several days or weeks and is relatively well tolerated by the patient. Because of this, it is satisfactory and desirable to plan repletion over a period of several days, thereby avoiding rapid administration of large quantities of sodium and potassium. In fact, the oral route for potassium repletion is preferred when this is feasible.

CLINICAL FEATURES AND MANAGEMENT OF RESPIRATORY ALKALOSIS

This form of alkalosis occurs as a result of alveolar hyperventilation which reduces the H_2CO_3 concentration (Pco_2) in the blood. Initial compensatory mechanisms include the reduction of extracellular bicarbonate by its combination with hydrogen released from extra- and intracellular buffers. A diuresis of sodium bicarbonate also serves to moderate the increase in pH, but may not be seen when a strong stimulus to conserve sodium exists. The major clinical conditions associated with respiratory alkalosis are seen in Table 8–3.

Usually only the pH disturbance occurring with artificial mechanically assisted ventilation is severe, and it requires immediate control by the reduction of the minute volume of the respirator, or increase in the dead space of the mechanical device if it is necessary to sustain the high rate to provide adequate oxygenation. The other clinical circumstance requiring treat-

---

TABLE 8–4

Clinical Findings and Expected Laboratory Values in Acid–Base Disturbances

| Condition | Clinical Findings | | Laboratory Findings (Arterial Blood) | | |
	Symptoms	Signs	pH	Pco_2 (mm Hg)	HCO_3^- (Total mEq/L CO_2)
Metabolic acidosis	Kussmaul respirations Restlessness, disorientation	Shock, coma	<7.35	15–30	2–18
Respiratory acidosis	Restlessness Disorientation Air hunger	Hypoventilation Cyanosis	<7.35	50–100	>27
Metabolic alkalosis	Weakness Paralysis Paresthesias	Latent tetany Signs of K⁺ depletion	>7.45	40–55	>27
Respiratory alkalosis	Paresthesias	Latent tetany Hyperventilation	>7.45	20–30	15–20

ment is encountered in the patient with an anxiety attack who hyperventilates and develops tetany as a consequence of the raised blood pH. Rebreathing into a paper bag or breath holding will usually suffice to increase the Pco_2 to a value sufficient to correct the disturbance. Milder forms of respiratory alkalosis are seen in hepatic and central nervous system disease and usually do not require therapeutic intervention.

The compensatory decrease of the serum bicarbonate may be misinterpreted as representing a mild metabolic acidosis in such patients if concurrent measurements of arterial pH and Pco_2 are not obtained.

A summary of the major categories of acid–base disturbances together with the major signs and symptoms and associated laboratory values are presented in Table 8–4.

CHAPTER 9
Water and Electrolyte Derangements in Practice
W. GORDON WALKER

Previous chapters have dealt almost exclusively with the clinical characteristics of isolated deficits, representing solitary discrete disturbances in body water or in the exchangeable sodium or potassium in the body. Isolated deficits are not commonly encountered in clinical practice. More often, the physician is faced with a complex situation exhibiting derangements in both body water and several of the major inorganic solutes. Because of the complexity of these disturbances, it is desirable to use an explicit diagnostic terminology that avoids such terms as dehydration and instead characterizes the abnormality in terms that describe the alterations in volume and composition of body fluids. Volume changes may be identified as representing *expansion* or *contraction* and compositional changes can be described as producing *hypotonicity, isotonicity,* or *hypertonicity.* This permits definition of six categories of disturbance in volume and composition of body fluids. These are presented in Table 9–1 with a tabulation of expected clinical and laboratory findings as well as a listing of major examples in each category. These categories, isotonic expansion or contraction, hypotonic expansion or contraction, and hypertonic expansion or contraction, cover the primary disturbances encountered in derangements of the body fluids.

Isotonic contraction represents primarily acute sodium loss accompanied by loss of water in isotonic proportions. Sodium concentration and serum osmolality are normal, but the hematocrit is elevated, reflecting isotonic loss from the extracellular fluid space. If the condition persists for several days blood urea nitrogen and creatinine are also elevated. Probably the most common cause is diarrhea that persists for a period of one or two days or more and is associated with inadequate intake. In certain situations, as

in acute severe diarrhea, acidosis may also be present because of excessive loss of bicarbonate in the fecal fluid. Other examples include moderate sodium loss from any source, but usually from the gastrointestinal tract or skin (sweating). Losses from the extracellular fluid compartment may occur without being identifiable as external losses. In severe ileus, for example, several liters of fluid may be pooled in the dilated gastrointestinal tract. A progressive increase in hematocrit may be one of the earliest signs of such fluid sequestration.

Isotonic expansion is caused by retention of sodium and water in isotonic proportions (one liter of water retained for each 145 mEq of sodium retained). It is most commonly seen in heart failure, cirrhosis, and nephrosis, but also occurs in many other situations including cases of acute glomerular nephritis, as well as toxemia of pregnancy and preeclampsia. It may also be produced iatrogenically. Characteristically, the plasma sodium concentration and osmolality are normal. Body weight is increased and the hematocrit may be decreased, depending upon the circumstances. Persistent isotonic expansion such as that encountered in heart failure and cirrhosis is usually associated with a normal hematocrit. In instances where the isotonic expansion develops more acutely, the hematocrit is reduced in proportion to the severity of the expansion.

Hypotonic contraction represents a disorder that is usually initiated by a sodium loss that exceeds 400 mEq. It is characterized by a decrease in skin turgor as well as a decrease in the serum sodium concentration and the serum osmolality. There is a variable increase in the blood urea nitrogen and hematocrit; the degree of change in these laboratory data reflect the severity of the deficits. Because of the circumstances

TABLE 9-1

Classification of Clinical Water and Electrolyte Disturbances[1,5,6,7,14,18-24]

Type of Derangement	Body Wt.	Hematocrit	Serum Sodium	Serum Osmolality	Serum* Urea Nitrogen	Urine† Sodium	Urine Osmolality	Common Clinical Examples
Isotonic contraction	↓	↑	N	N	N or ↑	± or ↓	↑	Fluid loss from diarrhea, overtreatment with diuretics, other conditions associated with acute sodium loss
Isotonic expansion	↑	N or ↓	N	N	N or ↓	±	±	Congestive heart failure, cirrhosis, nephrosis, acute glomerulonephritis, preeclampsia, iatrogenic
Hypotonic contraction	↓	↑	↓	↓	↑	↓	↑	Addison's disease, severe sodium depletion of relatively long-standing from variety of causes
Hypotonic expansion	↑	N or ↓	↓	↓	N or ↓	±	↑	Acute water intoxication, syndrome of inappropriate ADH secretion, congestive heart failure, cirrhosis
Hypertonic contraction	↓	N or ↑	↑	↑	↑	± or ↓	↑	Severe sweating, inadequate fluid intake, diabetes mellitus
Hypertonic expansion	usually ↑	↓	↑ or ↓‡	↑	± of no diagnostic value	±	±	Mannitol administration, ingestion of large quantities of NaCl

N = Normal   ↑ = increase   ↓ = decrease   ± = variable

*All these disturbances may be superimposed upon renal disease.
†Urinary sodium determination is the least helpful laboratory test for diagnostic confirmation of these disorders.
‡Depending upon whether solute responsible for expansion is NaCl or some nonelectrolyte solute.

under which such a derangement is likely to occur, potassium depletion is commonly seen, and alkalosis may be encountered. Clinical examples include chronic diarrhea, chronic adrenal insufficiency, sodium depletion resulting from sweating with inadequate salt intake, and excessive treatment with diuretics.

Hypotonic expansion is primarily the result of retention of excess water caused either by persistent antidiuretic hormone excess or some other cause of impaired water excretion as in severe congestive heart failure. In certain circumstances such as the syndrome of inappropriate ADH secretion, the resultant expansion may increase sodium excretion and lead to development of a moderate sodium deficit. In other situations such as congestive heart failure and cirrhosis there is excessive sodium retained but the water excess exceeds sodium excess and leads to hypoosmolality. The characteristic laboratory findings include lowered serum sodium concentration and lowered plasma osmolality. The clinical manifestations depend upon the severity of the hypotonicity. In edematous states such as heart failure and cirrhosis, the hypotonic expansion may be associated with other electrolyte disturbances as a result of vigorous diuretic usage. In the syndrome of inappropriate ADH secretion, the blood urea nitrogen is often quite low, frequently below 7 or 8 mg/dl.

Hypertonic contraction is produced by loss of water in excess of solute. Typically it is seen in severe and acute sweating with inadequate intake of both water and salt. It may also be seen with prolonged periods of inadequate fluid intake where sodium loss has also occurred, as for example diarrhea with poor water intake in the elderly. Laboratory findings include, most characteristically, an elevated serum sodium and serum osmolality. Where significant sodium loss is associated with the hypertonic contraction, the hematocrit will also be elevated. Since this disorder is commonly encountered in elderly individuals the hematocrit at the time the patient is initially seen may be misleading if a preexisting anemia was present.

Finally, *hypertonic expansion* is virtually always iatrogenic. The two most common circumstances leading to its development include administration of 5 percent dextrose in 0.155 molar (0.9 percent) sodium chloride in diabetics who are unable to metabolize the sugar adequately, and mannitol administration. The increasingly frequent administration of a hypertonic solution of mannitol as, for example, in an attempt to force diuresis when impending acute renal failure is suspected may lead to severe hypertonic expansion. The laboratory data that support this diagnosis depend upon the circumstances surrounding the production of the hypertonic expansion. Thus, in the former case when sodium chloride and 5 percent dextrose are given in excess, there may be only a slight reduction in the plasma sodium concentration but the osmolality of the plasma will be increased. Production of hypertonic expansion with mannitol will usually result in a much more dramatic decrease in the sodium concentration, largely because of the tendency to use solutions of mannitol that are quite hypertonic (15 to 20 percent solutions of mannitol). The hematocrit is always markedly reduced. A third condition that may lead to hypertonic expansion is ingestion of large quantities of sodium chloride or intravenous administration of a hypertonic solution of sodium chloride.

ILLUSTRATIVE CASES

As a means of further illustrating these disorders and the approach to diagnosis and therapy, illustrative cases are presented below. They have been arranged so that the reader may attempt to arrive at his own diagnosis and propose appropriate treatment. The actual treatment employed with results and pertinent comments are included in the section following the case presentations. As an exercise, the reader should attempt to arrive at an accurate diagnosis of the type of fluid and electrolyte disturbance and formulate quantitatively the appropriate treatment. The reader's diagnosis and therapy may be compared with that given for each case in the section following the case presentations.

CASE 1

A 29-year-old male was admitted to the hospital after a severe gastroenteritis of 36 hours duration. Food and fluid intake had been poor because of persistent nausea and occasional vomiting but his primary complaint was severe abdominal cramping and diarrhea with recurrent watery bowel movements. Physical examination revealed a blood pressure of 110/70, pulse of 98 per minute, and respiration of 60 per minute. The urine was unremarkable except for a specific gravity of 1.029, the hematocrit was 51, and serum electrolytes revealed a sodium concentration of 142 mEq/L, chloride 104 mEq/L, HCO_3^- 22.5 mEq/L, and a urea nitrogen of 31 mg/dl.

CASE 2

A 52-year-old male with known hypertension and a history of having had a myocardial infarction 3 years previously was seen in the out-patient department complaining of breathlessness of sudden onset that awakened him at night and swelling of the legs of 3 weeks' duration. Physical examination revealed a blood pressure of 106/100, a pulse rate of 94 per minute, respiration of 22 per minute, weight 204 pounds. The patient exhibited mild respiratory distress after walking only 20 to 30 paces. The neck veins were distended; auscultation revealed bilateral rales in lung bases, the heart was large with a protodiastolic gallop rhythm, the liver was felt 3 fingerbreadths (f.b.) below the costal margin (c.m.) and there was 3+ pitting edema extending up to the knees. Diagnosis of congestive heart failure was made and it was elected to treat the patient as an outpatient. He was given digitalis and furosemide 40 mg twice daily. He returned after 5 days complaining of weakness and giddiness on standing. He had experienced two episodes of syncope. Supine blood pressure was 105/85 and on standing dropped to 95/80. His weight was 168 pounds. There was now no evidence of venous hypertension. The lungs were clear to auscultation and percussion. The gallop rhythm was no longer heard. The liver was not palpated and there was no edema. Laboratory data revealed hematocrit 59, serum urea nitrogen 50 mg/dl, sodium concentration 145 mEq/L, chloride concentration 95 mEq/L, bicarbonate concentration 29 mEq/L, and potassium 5.1 mEq/L.

CASE 3

A 37-year-old white male with known diabetes of 22 years' duration and with a history of repeated episodes of poor control and acidosis presented at the emergency room breathing rapidly and complaining of weakness. There was a strong odor of acetone on the breath. The blood pressure was 130/70, the pulse was 112 per minute, the skin was warm and dry, and the face was flushed. The patient was breathing rapidly with increased depth of respirations and complaining of thirst. Urinalysis revealed 4+ sugar and 3+ acetone, and the hematocrit was 48. Blood chemical examinations revealed a glucose of 480 mg/dl, a serum sodium of 146 mEq/L, chlorides 102 mEq/L, bicarbonate 15 mEq/L, and serum urea nitrogen 35 mg/dl. Because the patient was alert and in no acute distress, except for the increased respiratory rate, it was elected to treat him in the emergency room with intravenous fluids. An infusion of saline was begun, and he was given 10 units of crystalline zinc insulin. During the next 12 hours he received 6 liters of 0.155 molar sodium chloride solution and a total of only 40 units of crystalline zinc insulin. At the end of this time the urine sugar remained 4+ and the acetone was persistently positive. Because of the persistent findings, he was admitted to the ward where physical examination at that time revealed some neck vein distension to the angles of the mandible with the patient sitting. There were a few moist rales in both lung bases and prominent presacral pitting edema. The hematocrit at this time was 33 and blood determinations re-

vealed a glucose of 380 mg/dl, sodium concentration of 143 mEq/L, chloride concentration of 110 mEq/L and bicarbonate of 17 mEq/L.

CASE 4

A 33-year-old truck driver with known rheumatic heart disease, aortic insufficiency, and mitral insufficiency was admitted in heart failure with marked cardiomegaly, rales at both lung bases, hepatomegaly with the liver felt 4 fingerbreadths below the costal margin, and 3+ pitting edema. He was maintained on digitalis, placed on a diet containing 2 g of salt and given 250 mg of chlorothiazide 4 times daily. On this regimen he lost 14 pounds while in the hospital, his symptoms of failure disappeared, and he felt well. He was given instruction on a 2-g salt diet and discharged on 250 mg of chlorothiazide 4 times daily and 50 mg of spironolactone twice daily. His weight at discharge was 125 pounds. His serum sodium was 143 mEq/L and his serum potassium was 4.6 mEq/L. He returned in one month complaining of marked weakness. Members of his family had noted some confusion and disorientation at times. His weight was 107 pounds. There was questionable decrease in skin turgor. The lungs were clear on auscultation and percussion. The heart had decreased markedly in size but the murmurs persisted. The liver was not felt and there was no pitting edema. Serum electrolytes revealed a sodium concentration of 111 mEq/L and potassium of 5.6 mEq/L. The marked decrease in cardiac size was confirmed by chest x-ray.

CASE 5

A 48-year-old male with remote history of three hospital admissions for tuberculosis was admitted complaining of severe back pain, occasional night sweats, and a 25-pound weight loss. Thoracic spine x-rays revealed a Pott's abscess in the region of T-10 and a surgical drainage procedure was scheduled. When induction of anesthesia was begun, he became hypotensive and the procedure was terminated. Medical consultation was obtained at that time, and evaluation revealed blood pressure of 90/60, a pulse of 120 per minute, a temperature of 99°F, and respirations of 22 and shallow. Buccal pigmentation was present and there was impressive pigmentation in both the axilla and inguinal skin folds. There was moderate evidence of muscle wasting. Laboratory data revealed a hematocrit of 38, a serum sodium concentration of 122 mEq/

L, chlorides of 88 mEqL bicarbonate 26 mEq/L, and a potassium of 5.3 mEq/L. Review of abdominal x-rays previously obtained revealed flecks of calcium situated just above the upper poles of both kidneys.

CASE 6

A 19-year-old male with a 2-year history of breathlessness on exertion and occasional hemoptysis was admitted with a diagnosis of mitral stenosis. Weight on admission was 132 pounds and he exhibited the classical physical findings of mitral stenosis. He underwent mitral commissurotomy, and postoperatively he received 2500 ml of fluid per day given intravenously as 5 percent dextrose in distilled water. On the third day following surgery, he appeared somewhat somnolent and serum electrolytes revealed sodium concentration of 130 mEq/L, and potassium 4.8 mEq/L. His urine output during this period had never exceeded 400 ml per day.

CASE 7

A 49-year-old male was admitted because of disorientation and some inappropriate behavior. He had been in an automobile accident 3 years previously and received a severe blow on the head resulting in loss of consciousness. A basilar skull fracture was diagnosed at that time, but he recovered apparently without incident. Following recovery, he was in reasonable health until the present illness. His confusion had been first noted 3 days prior to admission. On admission, his physical examination revealed a blood pressure of 125/70, pulse of 94 per minute, weight 158 pounds, temperature and respirations were normal, and the general physical examination revealed little except poor mental function. No localizing neurologic signs were identified. Laboratory data revealed a urine specific gravity of 1.022 and a hematocrit of 43. Serum electrolytes revealed sodium concentration of 112 mEq/L, chlorides of 79 mEq/L and a bicarbonate of 29 mEq/L with a potassium concentration of 4.1 mEq/L. Measurement of urinary electrolytes revealed a sodium concentration of 60 mEq/L and a total 24-hour urine volume of 550 ml. The urine osmolality was 725 mOsm/kg H_2O. The patient was given 1500 ml of 0.155 molar sodium chloride and responded with a prompt increase in urine volume. This was repeated the following day and the serum electrolytes again determined and found to be essentially unchanged, with a so-

dium concentration 114 mEq/L. Urinary electrolytes had increased markedly, however, and on the day of the second infusion the urinary sodium concentration was 110 mEq/L with a total urinary volume of 1600 ml for that day. Osmolality of this urine was 530 mOsm/kg H_2O.

CASE 8

An elderly male was brought to the emergency room in semicoma, having been found alone in his room by friends. No further history was available. On physical examination, he responded to pain but was unable to speak. The blood pressure was 120/80; the pulse was 104. Respirations were 16 per minute, and he weighed 136 pounds. The skin turgor appeared poor but this was difficult to judge because of his loose, inelastic skin. Pertinent physical findings were limited to left-sided hyperreflexia, moderate in degree. Urine specific gravity was 1.017 and the blood studies revealed a hematocrit of 55, serum sodium concentration of 163 mEq per liter, chloride concentration of 121 and bicarbonate concentration of 24 mEq/L, blood urea nitrogen 48 mg/dl, and serum osmolality of 339 mOsm/kg H_2O.

CASE 9

A 37-year-old male with long-standing history of heavy alcohol ingestion was admitted because of a severe, poorly localized pain in the upper abdomen that radiated through to the back. He had vomited once 8 hours previously at the onset of the pain without subsequent recurrence of vomiting or diarrhea. The pain had steadily increased in severity and at the time of admission he was in acute distress. His blood pressure was 110/70, pulse 115 per minute, and temperature 101°F. The skin was moist from perspiration. Remainder of the pertinent physical signs were confined to the abdomen. There was generalized abdominal tenderness with rebound tenderness present. Only an occasional bowel sound was heard. The remainder of the physical examination contributed little. Laboratory data revealed a marked leukocytosis, hematocrit of 48, serum sodium concentration of 145 mEq/L, K 3.9 mEq/L, and CO_2 of 22 mEq/L. Urinalysis revealed a specific gravity of 1.024 and a trace of protein. His condition deteriorated over the next 8 hours with increasing tachycardia and hypotension and persistence of the severe abdominal pain. The abdomen became silent. Repeat laboratory studies showed a hematocrit of 64 but the serum electrolytes remained unchanged. An amylase drawn at this time was 425 units. An upright x-ray of the abdomen showed several air-fluid levels all thought to be within the lumen of the gut.

COMMENTS ON DIAGNOSIS AND TREATMENT OF CASES

Case 1

The normal serum sodium concentration and elevated hematocrit in an individual with a history of severe diarrhea of 36 hours duration identifies the fluid disturbance as *isotonic contraction* with probable mild metabolic acidosis (HCO_3^- 22.5 mEq/L). Because of the story of continued fluid loss 2 days prior to admission, he was given 4000 ml of fluid the first day, 2000 ml of which were given as 0.155 molar (0.9 percent) sodium chloride. On the second day, he received 3500 ml of fluid, 1500 ml of which were given as 0.155 molar sodium chloride. By the third day he was able to tolerate food and fluids without difficulty. At this point, his weight had increased 2 kg over admission, his hematocrit had dropped to 41 percent, the serum sodium concentration was 146 mEq/L. The serum urea nitrogen was 19 mg/dl.

COMMENT. At presentation, the patient was thought to have both a sodium and water deficit, largely because of persistent diarrhea in the face of inadequate intake. The elevated hematocrit and urea nitrogen tended to support the diagnosis, and the presence of a normal serum sodium concentration identified this as an instance of *isotonic contraction*. During the first 2 days, the patient was given moderate excesses of both sodium and water. This represents quite acceptable therapy when renal function is adequate, since the kidneys excrete any excess sodium or water that is administered. His weight gain during this 2-day period, associated with the drop in hematocrit to 41, indicates that he retained approximately 2 liters of isotonic fluid.

Case 2

This patient developed an elevated hematocrit and blood urea nitrogen associated with a marked reduction in weight resulting from diuretic therapy. As in Case 1, the serum sodium concentration was normal, indicating *isotonic contraction*. The diagnosis of diuretic-induced sodium depletion was made. Because of the patient's cardiovascular disease, it was thought wise to treat him by an increased oral intake of salt. He was placed at bed rest and given a diet allowing an ad lib salt intake. On this regimen he gained 6

pounds in 4 days and his symptoms disappeared. Laboratory data obtained on the fifth day revealed a hematocrit of 47, serum urea nitrogen of 30 mg/dl, serum sodium concentration of 144 mEq/L, chloride of 101 mEq/L, and bicarbonate of 25 mEq/L.

COMMENT. The deficit in this case was a result of vigorous diuretic therapy. The mild elevation of bicarbonate probably represented an alkalosis that resulted from disproportionate loss of sodium and chloride. Although the deficit here was as great as that in the previous case, parenteral therapy was avoided because of the hazard of overexpansion attendant upon intravenous sodium chloride administration. On oral intake he retained sodium and water progressively and corrected the deficit. It should be emphasized that oral therapy is a perfectly appropriate, safe, and convenient means of treating sodium depletion. It should be regarded as the route of choice in all patients with cardiovascular disease unless there is some contraindication to oral administration, or unless severe signs of sodium deficit are present.

Case 3

As a result of inappropriate therapy, this patient accumulated a large excess of fluid administered as an isotonic solution of sodium chloride (*isotonic expansion*). Despite this, his diabetic acidosis remained uncontrolled. Following his admission, insulin dosage was increased on a sliding scale so that he received up to 45 units per hour depending upon the urinary glucose and the ketone concentration (see Chap. 71). On this regimen his glucosuria and ketonuria cleared during the third hour following admission to the ward. He subsequently diuresed so that his weight dropped by 4.9 kg. His hematocrit returned to normal and he felt well.

COMMENT. This case illustrates the hazards of attempting to treat diabetic acidosis under circumstances when the patient cannot be carefully watched. The hazard of overexpansion by excess sodium chloride administration is an ever present one in the management of diabetic acidosis, particularly under circumstances where the insulin dosage is inadequate and the patient is not carefully monitored. The laboratory data are all consistent with overexpansion, including the considerable drop in the hematocrit and the moderate hyperchloremia which developed. Appropriate treatment at this point depends mainly upon the condition of the patient. If he is sufficiently stable to permit such therapy, control of the acidosis and ketosis with insulin without additional fluid administration is preferable. If the patient has reasonably normal renal function, he will usually be able to excrete the excess sodium in a short period of time.

Case 4

Because of this striking improvement in his cardio-vascular status with disappearance of all manifestations of heart failure, it was thought that the hyponatremia was caused by chronic sodium depletion (*hypotonic contraction*). It was decided to attempt oral repletion and he was given 205 mEq of sodium orally on each of 2 successive days. Thereafter, he was maintained on a 25 mEq sodium diet. Throughout this period the urinary sodium did not exceed 6 mEq per day. During the 2 days of supplemental administration of sodium, his weight did not increase; in fact he lost one pound. His serum sodium concentration, however, over this 2-day period, rose from 111 to 127 mEq/L, representing an estimated increase in the sodium content of the extracellular fluid of 480 mEq. His diet plus supplemental intake during that period was estimated to be 470 mEq. Thus, he appeared to retain all of the administered sodium, a fact corroborated by measurement of urinary sodium over these 2 days which totaled 12 mEq. His mental confusion disappeared and he exhibited marked improvement over the next 7 days on increased dietary sodium alone. His sodium concentration rose further to 139 mEq/L. Throughout this period his weight changed very little, increasing only 3 pounds to 110 pounds at the end of the 10-day hospitalization period.

COMMENT. Careful questioning of this patient revealed that he had been extremely careful about his dietary intake and had probably maintained himself on as little as 2 or 3 g of salt in the diet per day. On such limited salt intake the diuretic regimen proved to be too vigorous, and he developed a severe sodium deficit. Estimation of the deficit at the time of admission (based on the initial serum sodium concentration) revealed that he had lost more than 900 mEq of sodium. Replacement of about half of this deficit, however, resulted in complete clearance of the mental symptoms and marked improvement in his general well-being. This case illustrates the hazard of producing severe sodium depletion when vigorous diuretic therapy with one of the strong nonmercurial oral agents is maintained in a patient who has also been subjected to careful sodium restriction. The necessity of following such patients closely is well illustrated. Again, as in Case 2, it is perfectly clear that oral therapy is both safe and satisfactory in treating such patients.

Case 5

A diagnosis of Addison's disease was made with associated *hypotonic contraction,* and he was given 100 mg of cortisol intravenously immediately followed by 2000 ml of isotonic sodium chloride over the next 2 hours. Continuous intravenous cortisol therapy was maintained at the rate of 100 mg intravenously every 8 hours given in 1000 ml of isotonic sodium chloride. By the following day, his blood pressure had risen to 130/85, his pulse was 100 per minute, and his temperature was 98°F. He appeared comfortable and was able to take food and fluid orally. His hematocrit measured at this time was 28, and persisted in this range for the next several days.

COMMENT. The physical findings of Addisonian pigmentation were unrecognized at the time of initial physical examination and it was only after the hypotensive episode at the time of surgery that the diagnosis became clear. Laboratory data are consistent with *hypotonic contraction;* however, his hematocrit was maintained at a level of 38, indicating that his underlying anemia had masked a significant rise in the hematocrit. This illustrates one of the difficulties associated with use of the hematocrit as a guide for sodium depletion in patients who are anemic. The hyperkalemia exhibited in this patient is modest in degree and not of a severity that warrants treatment beyond adequate hormonal replacement therapy and provision of an adequate salt intake.

Case 6

Water intoxication resulting in *hypotonic expansion* was diagnosed, and, on the basis of the lowered serum sodium concentration, it was estimated that he had accumulated an excess of 3.6 liters of water. His total fluid intake was limited to 400 ml per day. On this regimen he lost approximately 2 pounds of weight per day, and over the ensuing 4 days his serum sodium concentration returned to normal.

COMMENT. This case illustrates the hazard of continued excessive intake of water in individuals who have had extensive surgical procedures. On occasion, the antidiuretic state may persist for 2 or 3 days, particularly when the patient is experiencing a great deal of pain. More appropriate therapy should have been based on monitoring the patient's output and daily weight, and providing him with fluid adequate to cover urinary losses plus insensible losses, and to keep his weight nearly stable. In such a situation, it is desirable to avoid weight gains of more than 1 kg unless there is a specific indication for more vigorous fluid therapy as, for instance, hypotension, evidence of continued bleeding, or accumulation of fluid in the chest. In the present case, recognition of the water intoxication when the serum sodium had fallen to only 130 mEq/L warranted no more vigorous therapy than careful fluid restriction.

Case 7

On the basis of the hyponatremia, hypo-osmolality, and hypertonicity of the urine with increased urinary sodium loss, the diagnosis of inappropriate antidiuretic hormone secretion leading to *hypotonic expansion* was made. The patient was placed on a regimen of rigid fluid restriction, total intake being kept below 600 ml per day. On this regimen he lost approximately 1.5 pounds per day for the next 5 days. He cleared mentally quite well and felt well. His serum sodium concentration at this time was 125 mEq/L. Because of this improvement, his fluid intake was increased to a total of 1000 ml per day. As a result his rate of weight loss decreased to approximately 0.5 pound per day, but the plasma sodium continued to rise slowly and had returned to normal values on the 14th hospital day. Further neurologic study revealed no space-occupying lesion of the central nervous system, so he was discharged on fluid restriction to total 2000 ml per day. He was advised to maintain a daily record of his weight and to be followed regularly by a physician.

COMMENT. This patient had developed *hypotonic expansion* as a result of progressive water retention produced by the persistent elaboration of ADH. The criteria for making this diagnosis include demonstration of hypotonicity or hypo-osmolality of the plasma (as compared to normal values) and hypertonic urine. He illustrates the efficacy of fluid restriction in such patients. On occasion, such patients will excrete sufficient quantities of sodium in the urine following their hypotonic expansion to develop a serious sodium deficit. This may subsequently become symptomatic and require therapy. In the present patient, if such a deficit existed, it was sufficiently mild that it was corrected by dietary sodium intake. The failure of the hematocrit to reflect changes in body water is well illustrated in this patient.

Case 8

The diagnosis of water deficit with resulting *hypertonic contraction* was made. On the basis of the serum sodium concentration of 163 mEq/L, this deficit was estimated at 5 liters. He received half of this total replacement during the first 4 hours. Because of the elevated hematocrit and the presumption that this reflected a significant sodium deficit, the first 4 liters of fluid were given as 2.5 percent dextrose in 0.034 molar (0.20 percent) sodium chloride, thus providing him with 120 mEq of sodium during the first 6 hours. Over the next 3 days he received 3000 ml of dextrose 5 percent in water and 1000 ml of 0.155 molar sodium chloride per day. He responded slowly to this and at the end of the third day, when he had received a total

quantity of water that exceeded his deficit plus estimated continued losses, he was still somnolent. Although he could be aroused, he could not speak. He showed slow improvement during the next 5 or 6 days, became oriented and able to communicate verbally. His serum sodium concentration decreased to 145 mEq/L and his hematocrit fell to 41. His weight increased to 154 pounds.

COMMENT. This is a typical setting for the occurrence of *hypertonic contraction*. This elderly individual who lived alone probably had a mild cerebral vascular accident and became unable to maintain his fluid intake. Because of the hot environment, the most likely cause of the associated sodium depletion was persistent perspiration. Fluids chosen for replacement therapy were dictated by the need to keep the osmolality of the solution being infused well below that of his plasma osmolality. The fact that he had a significant sodium deficit is reflected in the marked decrease in his hematocrit as therapy progressed. Final hematocrit and the body weight indicate that he retained approximately 450 mEq of sodium and 8 liters of water. The difference between the estimate of the water deficit made on the basis of the elevated serum sodium concentration and the total quantity of water retained represented the water that was retained with sodium as an isotonic solution.

Case 9

The single laboratory finding in this case of pancreatitis that pointed to progressive *isotonic contraction* was the progressive rise in the hematocrit. The value of following the hematocrit closely in situations where "hidden" fluid losses develop cannot be overemphasized. Abdominal film confirmed the diagnosis of paralytic ileus with pooling of fluid in the gut. Intravenous replacement therapy was begun promptly upon recognition of the contracted state. He received 3000 ml of 0.155 molar saline and 500 ml of plasma over a period of 3 hours. His blood pressure rose to 135/75 mm Hg and his pulse dropped to 100 per minute. Peroral intubation of the duodenum with a Cantor tube with gentle suction yielded 2500 to 3000 ml per day for the succeeding 3 days. Replacement therapy consisted of giving a quantity of 0.155 molar sodium chloride solution equal to the duodenal drainage each day plus 2000 ml of 5 percent dextrose in 0.034 molar (0.20 percent) sodium chloride solution. Signs and symptoms of pancreatitis abated slowly and his hematocrit, which had returned to normal the first day, remained in the normal range.

COMMENT. This case illustrates two points. Hidden fluid losses, such as accumulation of fluid in the gastrointestinal tract, rapid development of ascites, acute swelling of an extremity as is sometimes seen with an ischemic crush injury, all can lead to severe depletion of the functional extracellular fluid volume. They are extremely difficult to recognize, and the physician must be alert to the situations where such losses are likely to occur. The hematocrit is the only useful laboratory test for confirmation of the development of isotonic contraction under these circumstances. Second, maintenance therapy is equally as important as initial replacement therapy. In the present case, continued loss of fluid via the gastrointestinal tract would have rapidly led to a return of contraction of the extracellular fluid space with hypovolemia had not the losses been quantified by measuring and replacing the Cantor tube drainage.

REFERENCES

General References

1. Brenner, B.M. and Rector, F.C., Jr. (eds.). The Kidney. Philadelphia, Saunders, 1976.
2. Elkinton, J.R. and Danowski, T.S. The Body Fluids. Basic Physiology and Practical Therapeutics. Baltimore, Williams & Wilkins Co., 1955.
   A well-referenced treatise covering clinical disorders of fluid and electrolyte content of the body.
3. Moore, F.D., Oleson, K.H., McMurrey, J.D., Parker, H.V., Ball, M.R., and Boyden, C.M. The Body Cell Mass and Its Supporting Environment. Philadelphia, Saunders, 1963.
   A compilation of data on variations in fluid and electrolyte content of the body in health and disease.
4. Orloff, J. and Berliner, R.W. Handbook of Physiology, Section 8: Renal Physiology. Baltimore, American Physiological Society, 1973.
   A comprehensive reference.
5. Schrier, R.W. (ed.). Renal and Electrolyte Disorders. Boston, Little, Brown, 1976.
6. Wesson, L.G. Physiology of the Human Kidney. New York, Grune & Stratton, 1969.
   The most complete text currently available covering renal physiology and the role of the kidney in regulating volume and electrolyte content of body fluids.

Water Metabolism

7. Austin, M.G. and Berry, J.W. Observations on 100 cases of heat stroke. JAMA, 161:1525, 1956.
8. Dunn, F.L., Brennan, T.J., Nelson, A.E., and Robertson, G.L. The role of blood osmolality and volume in regulating vasopressin secretion in the rat. J. Clin. Invest., 52:3212, 1973.
9. Miller, M. and Moses, A.M. Drug induced states of impaired water excretion. Kidney Int., 10:96, 1976.

10. Verney, E.B. Gulstonian Lectures on Polyuria. Lancet, 216:539, 645, 751, 1929.
11. ———. Croonian Lecture. The antidiuretic hormone and the factors which determine its release. Proc. R. Soc., London, Series B, 135:25, 1947.
12. Winkler, A.W., Danowski, T.S., Elkinton, J.R., and Peters, J.P. Electrolytic and fluid studies during water deprivation and starvation in human subjects and the effects of ingestion of fish of carbohydrates and of salt solutions. J. Clin. Invest., 28:807, 1944.
13. Schrier, R.W. and Berl, T. Hyponatremia and related disorders. The Kidney, 7:1, 1974.
14. Zierler, K.L. Hyperosmolarity in adults: a critical review. J. Chronic Dis., 7:1, 1958.

Sodium Metabolism

15. Bartoli, E. and Earley, L.E. Importance of ultrafiltrable plasma factors in maintaining tubular reabsorption. Kidney Int., 3:142, 1973.
16. Edelman, I.S. and Liebman, J. Anatomy of body water and electrolytes. Am. J. Med., 27:256, 1959.
17. Edelman, I.S., Leibman, J., O'Meara, M.P., and Birkenfeld, C.W. Interrelations between serum sodium concentration, serum osmolarity and total exchangeable potassium and total body water. J. Clin. Invest., 37:1236, 1958.
18. McCance, R.A. Experimental sodium chloride deficiency in man. Proc. R. Soc., Series B, 119:245, 1936.
19. ———. Medical problems in mineral metabolism. II. Sodium deficiencies in clinical medicine. Lancet, 1:704, 1936.
20. ———. Medical problems in mineral metabolism. II. Experimental human salt deficiency. Lancet, 1:823, 1936.
21. Walker, W.G. Indications and contraindications for diuretic therapy. Ann. N.Y. Acad. Sci., 139:481, 1966.
22. Wright, F.S. Intrarenal regulation of glomerular filtration rate. N. Engl. J. Med., 291:135, 1974.

Potassium Metabolism

23. Bedford, P.D. Acute potassium intoxication. Lancet, 2:268, 1954.
24. Berliner, R.W. Renal mechanisms for potassium excretion. Harvey Lect., 55:141, 1961.
25. Cheng, J.T., Sapir, D.G., Turin, M.D., and Walker, W.G. A comparison of potassium bicarbonate and potassium chloride in the repair of potassium deficiency. Johns Hopkins Med. J., 133:299, 1973.
26. Cooke, C.R., Horvath, J.S., Moore, M.A., Bledsoe, T., and Walker, W.G. Modulation of plasma aldosterone concentration by plasma potassium in anephric man in the absence of a change in potassium balance. J. Clin. Invest., 52:3028, 1973.
27. Cooke, C.R., Ruiz-Maza, F., Kowarski, A., Migeon, C.J., and Walker, W.G. Regulation of plasma aldosterone concentration in anephric man and renal transplant recipients. Kidney Int., 3:160, 1973.
28. Gamstorp, I. Adynamia episodica hereditaria. Acta Paediatr. Scand., 45:Suppl. 108, 1956.
29. Giebisch, G.H. Renal potassium excretion. In Rouiller, C. and Muller, A.F. (eds.), The Kidney, Vol. 3. New York, Academic Press, 1971, pp. 329–382.
30. Kassirir, J.P., Berkman, P.M., Lawrenz, D.R., and

Schwartz, W.B. The critical role of chloride in the correction of hypokalemic alkalosis in man. Am. J. Med., 38:172, 1965.

31. Kassirer, J.P. and Harrington, J.T. Diuretics and potassium metabolism: A reassessment of the need, effectiveness and safety of potassium therapy. Kidney Int., 11:505, 1977.

32. Shy, G.M., Wanko, T., Rowley, P.T., and Engel, A.G. Studies in familial periodic paralysis. Exp. Neurol., 3:53, 1961.

33. Steinmetz, P.R. and Kiley, J.E. Hyperkalemia in renal failure. J.A.M.A., 175:689, 1961.

34. Walker, W.G., Sapir, D.G., Turin, M., and Cheng, J.T. Potassium homeostasis and diuretic therapy. In DeWardener, H. (ed.), International Congress Series #268. Modern Diuretic Therapy in the Treatment of Cardiovascular and Renal Disease. Amsterdam, Excerpta Medica, 1973, pp. 331–342.

Acid–Base Balance

35. Kassirer, J.P. Serious acid-base disorders. N. Engl. J. Med., 291:733, 1974.

36. Orloff, J. The role of the kidney in the regulation of acid-base balance. Yale J. Biol. Med., 29:211, 1956.

37. Singer, R.B., Clark, J.K., Barker, E.S., Crosley, A.P., Jr., and Elkinton, J.R. The acute effects in man of rapid intravenous infusion of hypertonic sodium bicarbonate solution. Medicine (Baltimore), 34:51, 1955.

38. Schwartz, W.B., Van Ypersele de Strihou, C., and Kassirer, J.P. Medical progress. Role of anions in metabolic alkalosis and potassium deficiency. N. Engl. J. Med., 279:630, 1968.

39. Schwartz, W.B., Brachett, W.C., and Cohen, J.J. The response to graded degrees of chronic hypercapnia: the physiologic limits of the defense of pH. J. Clin. Invest., 44:291, 1965.

Renal Diseases and Disturbances in Renal Function
W. GORDON WALKER: SECTION EDITOR

CHAPTER 10
Renal Function and Its Clinical Evaluation
W. GORDON WALKER AND DANIEL G. SAPIR

ANATOMY

The functional unit of the kidney is the nephron, a structure composed at its proximal end of a tuft of capillaries closely invested by a covering of epithelium which is continuous with the tubule of epithelial cells.[8] This structural unit is divided into several segments that are distinctive both functionally and histologically (Fig. 10–1). In a normal man there are approximately 1 million nephrons in each kidney, and an important feature of the total renal functioning capacity is that each nephron functions separately and independently so long as its blood supply and structure are intact. Thus, destruction of the kidney and loss of renal function result from progressive loss of nephrons, while the remaining nephrons continue to function normally. Each kidney is supplied by a renal artery which divides into posterior and anterior divisions with subsequent divisions into interlobular arcuate and intralobular arteries. No anastomotic connections have been demonstrated between the major arterial networks arising from the five major branches of the renal artery, a fact of clinical importance in the development of localized areas of renal ischemia.

PHYSIOLOGIC FUNCTIONS OF THE KIDNEY

The kidneys not only excrete the end products of metabolism, such as urea, but are also responsible for regulation of body water and electrolyte concentrations. The normal physiologic function of the kidneys is best discussed in quantitative terms.

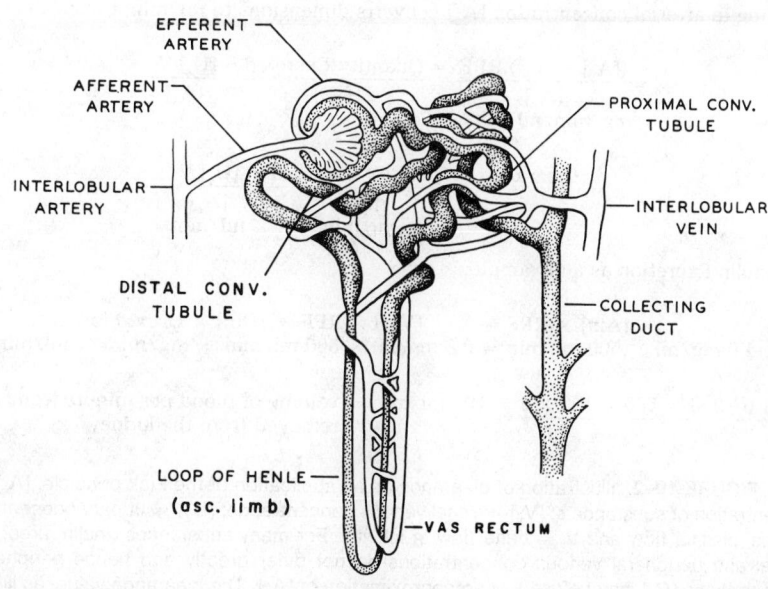

FIGURE 10–1. Schematic representation of segments of the nephron and its blood supply.

QUANTITATIVE MEASUREMENT OF RENAL FUNCTION

Renal Clearance

The principal means of studying renal function in man remains that of measuring the excretion rates of substances appearing in the urine and relating these to plasma concentrations of the substances measured. This technique, termed "clearance" by Addis, provides a valuable means for quantitative assessment of renal function.[6,8,10] For ease of understanding, it is convenient to consider calculation as a special instance of the Fick principle (Fig 10-2). For a substance which only traverses the kidney but is neither synthesized, metabolized, nor excreted, renal arterial input equals renal venous output. When a portion of the substance is excreted in the urine, arterial input

equals renal venous output plus urine output. Stated symbolically:

$$A_s \times RPF = V_s \times RPF + U_s V \qquad (1)$$

where A_s denotes arterial concentration of substance s, V_s represents renal venous concentration of the substance, RPF is renal plasma flow, U_s denotes urinary concentration of s, and V equals urine flow. Equation I may be reexpressed as the disposition of the arterial flow reaching the kidney by dividing through by A_s (Fig. 10-2). This partitioning of the arterial input of substance s into the portion leaving by way of the urine and that leaving by the renal vein expresses the urinary excretion rate as the volume of plasma *cleared* of substance s in unit time, and the expression $U_s V / A_s$ is the expression for clearance.

CLEARANCE DEFINED BY FICK PRINCIPLE

For substance remaining in plasma during transit through kidney:

$$[A_s] \times \text{Renal Plasma Flow} = [V_s] \times \text{Renal Plasma Flow}$$

For substance excreted by kidney:

$$[A_s] \times RPF = [V_s] \times RPF + \text{Quantity Excreted}$$

or:

$$([A_s] - [V_s])RPF = \text{Quantity Excreted} \quad \text{(Fick equation)}$$
$$\text{mg/min} = \text{mg/min}$$

Relating to arterial concentration $[A_s]$ converts dimensions to ml/min; thus:

$$\frac{([A_s] - [V_s]) \, RPF}{[A_s]} = \frac{\text{Quantity Excreted}}{[A_s]} = \frac{[U_s] V}{[A_s]} =$$
$$\text{mg/min/ml/min}$$

$$\text{Clearance} = \frac{\text{Quantity Excreted}}{[A_s]} = \frac{[U_s] V}{[A_s]}$$
$$\text{ml/min} \qquad \text{ml/min}$$

For Inulin Excretion as an example:

$$[Ain] \times RPF = [Vin] \times RPF + [Uin] \times \text{Urine Flow}$$
$$1.0 \text{ mg/ml} \times 500 \text{ ml/min} = 0.8 \text{ mg/ml} \times 500 \text{ ml/min} + \text{ mg/ml} \times 1 \text{ ml/min}$$

$$\frac{[1.0 - 0.8] \times 500}{1.0} = \frac{100 \times 1}{1.0} = 100 \text{ ml/min} = \text{volume of blood per minute from which inulin is removed from the kidney.}$$

FIGURE 10-2. Illustration of clearance as an application of the Fick principle. $[A_s]$ = arterial concentration of substance s; $[V_s]$ = renal venous concentration; $[U_s]$ = urinary concentration; RPF = renal plasma flow and V = urine flow in ml/min. For many substances (inulin, urea, creatinine) arterial and peripheral venous concentrations do not differ greatly and hence peripheral venous concentrations $[P_s]$ may be used as an approximation of $[A_s]$. The clearance value, as illustrated for inulin, represents a hypothetical volume of plasma from which inulin is removed each minute.

Since the concentration in renal arterial plasma (A_s) does not, in most instances, differ greatly from that in peripheral venous plasma (P_s) the latter is used and the equation

$$\text{Clearance} = \frac{U_s V}{P_s} \text{ or } \frac{UV}{P} \tag{2}$$

is the usual means of defining clearance.

The chief virtue of this concept is the ease with which it makes possible the quantitative description of renal function in the intact human. In general, it is convenient to think of renal clearances of various endogenous and exogenous substances as falling into two categories. "Fixed" clearances, such as those of inulin, urea, mannitol, creatinine, or p-aminohippurate, remain relatively constant from day to day and provide an overall measure of the functional capacity of the kidney. "Variable" clearances of such substances as sodium, potassium, water, phosphate, calcium, and others reflect the regulatory activity of the kidney and may change rapidly over a short period of time as a result of change in the individual's environment.

Glomerular Filtration Rate (GFR)

The process of urine formation begins with the production of large quantities of an ultrafiltrate of plasma at the glomerulus. Normally, approximately 19 percent of the plasma traversing the glomerulus is expressed from the blood as a protein-free ultrafiltrate in which the concentration of low molecular weight substances is equal to their concentration in plasma water. The rate at which the kidneys form this ultrafiltrate is termed the glomerular filtration rate; normally, it is about 130 ml per minute, or 180 liters per day, and can be measured by application of the clearance technique as outlined above.

Measurement of GFR as a clearance requires a substance such as inulin, which passes freely into the glomerular ultrafiltrate, but is neither removed from, nor secreted into, the urine by the renal tubule (Table 10-1).

Renal Plasma Flow (RPF)

If simultaneous measurements of arterial and renal venous blood indicate that all of a substance (such as P-aminohippurate, PAH) reaching the kidney is removed from the plasma and appears in the urine without significant storage or metabolism in the kidney, then V_s in Equation (1) becomes zero and the equation simplifies to:

$$A_s \cdot RPF = U_s V \tag{3}$$

TABLE 10-1

Measurement of Glomerular Filtration Rate by Inulin Clearance

Data

Rate of urine flow (V) = 2 ml per minute

Peripheral venous plasma inulin concentration (P_{in}) = 20 mg/dl

Urine inulin concentration (U_{in}) = 1300 mg/dl

Calculation

$$GFR = \frac{U_{in} V}{P_{in}} = \frac{\dfrac{1300\ mg}{100\ ml} \cdot \dfrac{2\ ml}{min}}{\dfrac{20\ mg}{100\ ml}}$$

GFR = 130 ml per minute

---

yielding a means of measuring renal plasma flow, thus

$$RPF = \frac{U_s V}{P_s} \tag{4}$$

PAH clearance can be used in this manner to measure renal plasma flow (Table 10-2).

TABLE 10-2

Measurement of Renal Plasma Flow by PAH Clearance

Data

Rate of urine flow (V) = 2 ml per minute

Peripheral venous plasma PAH concentration (P_{PAH}) = 1.5 mg/dl

Urine PAH concentration (U_{PAH}) = 450 mg/dl

Hematocrit (Hct) = 42%

Calculation

$$RPF = \frac{U_{PAH} \cdot V}{P_{PAH}} = \frac{\dfrac{450\ mg}{100\ ml} \cdot \dfrac{2\ ml}{minute}}{\dfrac{1.5}{100\ ml}}$$

RPF = 600 ml per minute

$$RBF = \frac{RPF}{1\text{-}Hct} = \frac{600\ ml\ per\ minute}{1\text{-}0.42}$$

RBF = 1035 ml per minute

The renal blood flow (RBF) can be estimated if the hematocrit is known:

$$RBF = \frac{RPF}{(1-Hct)} \tag{5}$$

where Hct is the hematocrit expressed as a fraction.

Clearance of Other Substances

These two substances (inulin and p-aminohippurate) can be used as references for the study of the renal mechanism involved in the excretion of other materials. Thus, a substance which has a greater clearance than inulin must be excreted, at least in part, by tubular secretion, whereas substances with clearances smaller than simultaneous inulin clearance are partially reabsorbed, following filtration. For substances partially bound to plasma proteins, correction for that fraction which is protein-bound must be taken into account, otherwise, the calculations presented above will be misleading. A more detailed treatment of this approach to quantification of renal function may be found in texts on renal physiology.[1,5,8,9]

Clinical Implications of Clearance

The clearance of a substance is thus defined as:

$$\text{Clearance of Substance X} = C_x = \frac{U_x \cdot V}{P_x}$$

To emphasize that clearance only represents the amount of plasma cleared of substance X by the kidney per unit time is to miss some of the more important clinical implications.

For example, urea is filtered just like inulin, but approximately half the urea diffuses back into plasma during passage through the tubule. The urea clearance is, thus, approximately half the inulin clearance, say 70 ml per minute. A normal subject eating 88 g of protein daily will have some 14 g of urea nitrogen to excrete per day (10 mg of urea nitrogen per minute). If he is in nitrogen balance his renal excretory rate ($U_{urea} \cdot V$) will be 10 mg per minute. From this, one can predict his plasma urea level:

$$C_{urea} = \frac{U_{urea} \cdot V}{P_{urea}}$$

$$P_{urea} = \frac{U_{urea} \cdot V}{C_{urea}} = \frac{\dfrac{10\ mg}{min}}{\dfrac{70\ ml}{min}}$$

$$P_{urea} = 0.14\ mg/ml = 14\ mg/dl$$

From such calculations, it is clear that if he doubles his protein intake he will double his plasma urea concentration.

If renal disease destroys half his nephrons, his urea clearance will be halved. Under these circumstances, also, his plasma urea concentration will be doubled:

$$P_{urea} = \frac{U_{urea} \cdot V}{C_{urea}} = \frac{\dfrac{10\ mg}{min}}{\dfrac{35\ ml}{min}}$$

$$P_{urea} = 0.28\ mg/ml = 28\ mg/dl$$

It is apparent that if he reduces his protein intake from 88 to 44 g per day, his excretory rate will be reduced from 10 to 5 mg per minute, and his plasma concentration can return to 14 mg/dl.

These important relationships between clearance, plasma concentration, and excretory rate are illustrated in Figures 10–3, 10–4, and 10–5.

REGULATION OF WATER EXCRETION

Isotonic glomerular filtrate is formed at a rate of about 125 ml per minute or 180 liters per day in the average normal adult. In contrast, urine output as the final product of this activity ranges usually between 500 ml and 2 liters per day. The kidneys must, thus, reabsorb very large quantities of both water and solute. The fraction of this large volume of filtered water and solute that finally appears as urine is determined by water and solute intake, or more precisely, the total quantity of water and solute requiring excretion. During this process, the kidney must also regulate volume and solute concentrations of the body fluids. This is achieved in such elegant fashion that the solute concentration (osmolality) varies little more than ±0.5 percent. To achieve this regulation, the kidney has the capacity to vary the rate of output of water and solute independently. Given an *excess* of body water, the kidney produces a urine that contains a much lower solute concentration than that in body fluids. Since urine formation begins as isotonic fluid, the kidney reabsorbs a hypertonic fluid in this situation. The result of this dual activity of excreting more water than solute and reabsorbing a hypertonic fluid rapidly corrects the hypotonicity (water excess) of the body fluids. Conversely, when a *deficit* of water is present in body fluids, the kidney produces a markedly hypertonic urine and reabsorbs a fluid that is hypotonic to body fluids, thus serving to correct or re-

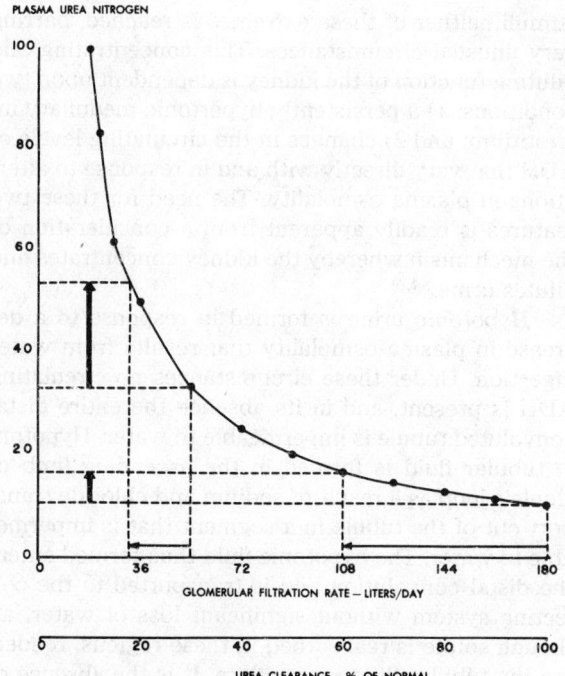

FIGURE 10-3. Relation of plasma concentration of urea to changes in glomerular filtration rate or urea clearance. In the normal subject, a 40 percent decrease in glomerular filtration rate (GFR) from 180 to 108 liters per day elevates the plasma or blood urea nitrogen only about 5 mg/dl. However, in advanced renal impairment when GFR is only about 25 percent of normal, the same percentage decrease raises the plasma concentration of urea nitrogen 20 mg/dl. Thus large changes in GFR in the presence of normal renal function may not raise plasma levels beyond those usually considered normal. This is an important fact to keep in mind when using plasma concentrations of urea as a means of monitoring changes in renal function.

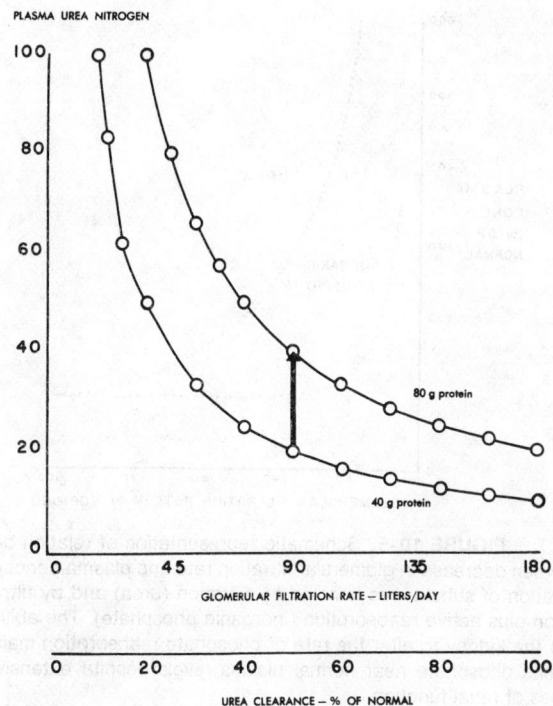

FIGURE 10-4. Variations in protein intake may produce significant changes in plasma concentration of urea in the absence of change in glomerular filtration rate. In general, when clearance is constant, the plasma or blood urea nitrogen is directly related to protein intake so that a doubling of protein intake doubles the plasma urea concentration. Conversely, halving protein intake reduces the plasma urea by half.

pair the water deficit. The mechanisms whereby the kidney achieves this remarkable regulation are dependent upon integrated behavior of the intrarenal concentrating mechanism, the modulating influence of the antidiuretic hormone, and water intake. These interrelationships are examined below.

Control of Osmolality

The osmolality of the plasma is controlled by two mechanisms: thirst and the pituitary antidiuretic hormone (ADH), vasopressin. An increase in plasma osmolality produces thirst which prompts the intake of water. This, in turn, reduces the plasma osmolality (Fig. 10-6). Increased plasma osmolality also causes ADH secretion. The ADH, through a mechanism described later, causes the kidneys to produce hyper-

tonic urine (Fig. 10-6). Thus, the urine, when compared to plasma, contains solute in excess of water; this excess solute excretion reduces the plasma osmolality.

Conversely, water intake will reduce plasma osmolality and halt ADH secretion. This leads to the production of hypotonic urine and a comparable rise in plasma osmolality. The reciprocal effect of urine osmolality on plasma osmolality can be considered as a negative feedback element in the ADH control mechanism.

The ADH mechanism responds to changes in plasma osmolality as small as 0.5 percent or less. The kidneys are the effectors in this control system. That renal disease can seriously impair the patient's ability to defend against physiologic and pathologic changes in water, and solute is, thus, a logical corollary.

Renal Concentrating and Diluting Mechanism

The kidneys' role in regulating plasma osmolality depends upon their ability to excrete, under the appro-

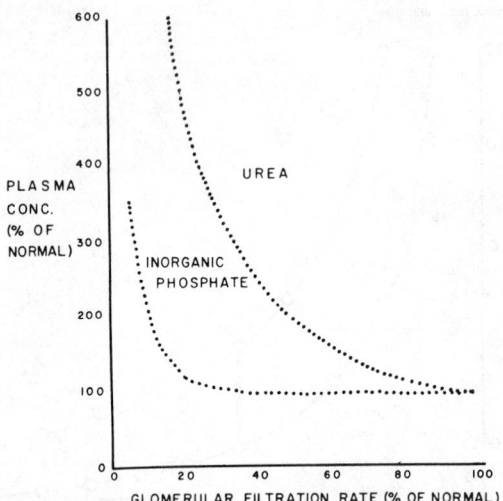

FIGURE 10-5. Schematic representation of relation between decrease in glomerular filtration rate and plasma concentration of substances handled by filtration (urea) and by filtration plus active reabsorption (inorganic phosphate). The ability of the kidney to alter the rate of phosphate reabsorption maintains phosphate near normal plasma levels despite extensive loss of renal function.

priate stimulus, urine which may be either hypertonic (up to 1200 mOsm per kg H_2O) or hypotonic (<100 mOsm per kg H_2O), with respect to an ultrafiltrate of plasma (280 mOsm per kg H_2O). As a consequence of this capacity to vary the urinary solute concentration over such a wide range, the kidney may excrete solute-free water (excess body water) at a rate that can exceed 25 liters per day under certain circumstances. Conversely, given the appropriate hydropenic conditions, the kidney can generate solute-free water and return it to body fluids at a rate that may exceed 6 to 7 liters per day. Under the usual range of physiologic

stimuli neither of these extremes is reached, barring very unusual circumstances. This concentrating and diluting function of the kidney is dependent upon two conditions: 1) a persistently hypertonic medullary interstitium; and 2) changes in the circulating levels of ADH that vary directly with and in response to alterations in plasma osmolality. The need for these two features is readily apparent from a consideration of the mechanism whereby the kidney concentrates and dilutes urine.[5,7,10]

Hypotonic urine is formed in response to a decrease in plasma osmolality that results from water ingestion. Under these circumstances no circulating ADH is present, and in its absence the entire distal convoluted tubule is impermeable to water. Hypotonic tubular fluid is formed in the ascending limb of Henle's loop as a result of sodium and chloride transport out of the tubule in a segment that is impermeable to water. The hypotonic fluid thus formed enters the distal convolution and is transported to the collecting system without significant loss of water, although solute is reabsorbed in these regions, rendering the tubular fluid more dilute. It is the absence of ADH that maintains the water-impermeable state of this segment of the nephron (Fig. 10-7).

Figure 10-7 illustrates the role of ADH in the production of *hypertonic* urine. It renders the distal convolution and collecting duct permeable to water so that the tubular fluid is permitted to come into osmotic equilibrium with the surrounding interstitial fluid as it traverses these two conduits. Thus, it becomes isotonic to plasma as it exits from the distal convolution and its surrounding isotonic interstitial fluid. In the collecting duct it equilibrates with surrounding hypertonic interstitial fluid and leaves this segment as concentrated urine. Therefore, during water deprivation the osmolality of the urine is determined by the osmolality of the medullary interstitium. The hy-

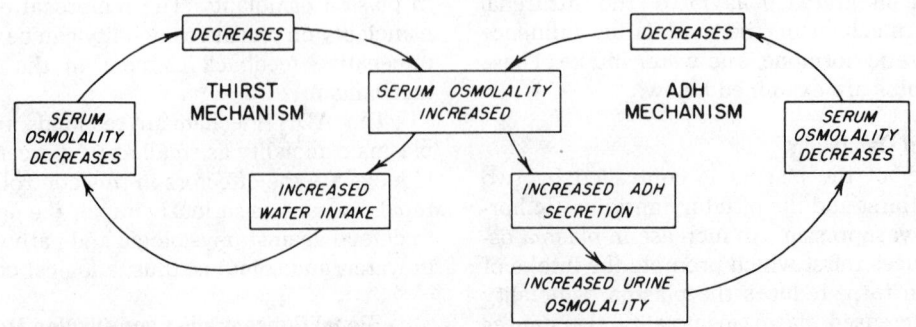

FIGURE 10-6. Sequence by which first mechanism and antidiuretic hormone output regulate serum osmolality. There is evidence that the thirst mechanism is mediated by a renin–angiotensin system, perhaps self-contained within the central nervous system.

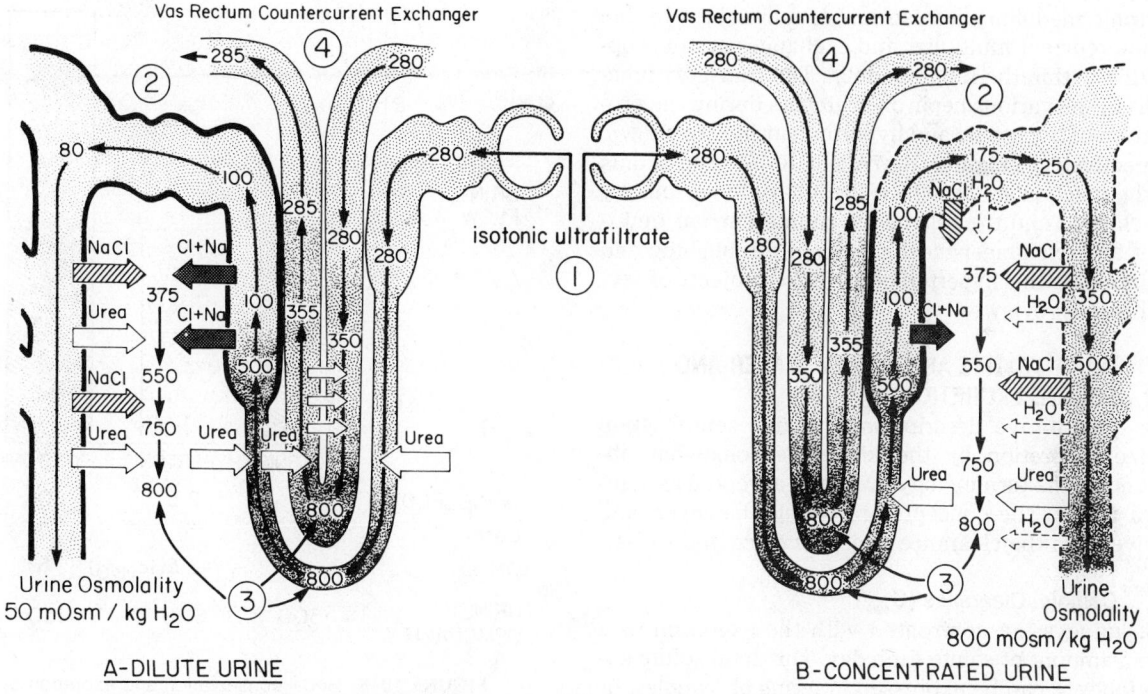

FIGURE 10-7. Formation of dilute and concentrated urine. A countercurrent multiplier and exchanger system allows the kidney to conserve water during water deficit and excrete excess water while independently regulating electrolyte excretion. During hydration and hydropenia, urine formation begins as an isosmotic plasma ultrafiltrate at the glomerulus and remains isotonic throughout the proximal convoluted tubule (1). In the loop of Henle, permeability to water and urea permits movement of water from tubular fluid into the hypertonic medullary interstitium, and urea enters the descending limb of Henle's loop from the interstitium where a high concentration of urea exists. This water removal and entry of urea raises osmolality of the tubular fluid so that it greatly exceeds the osmolality of peripheral plasma. When fluid reaches the thick ascending section of Henle's loop, this segment removes sodium chloride by active chloride transport; however, this segment is quite impermeable to water, resulting in the production of a large osmotic gradient. It is this separation of water and solute with associated increase in medullary interstitial hypertonicity which comprises the *countercurrent multiplier* segment of the system (2). Maintenance of interstitial hypertonicity thus produced depends upon the *countercurrent exchanger* system provided by the vasa rectae. These hairpin venous loops have permeability characteristics permitting rapid equilibration with the surrounding interstitium. Osmolality of entering plasma is 280 mOsm/kg H_2O but rapidly increases, often reaching or exceeding 800 mOsm/kg in the bend of the loop. In the ascending segment of the vas rectum, the process reverses itself and osmolality decreases so that exiting blood is only slightly above that entering. The multiplier and exchanger systems operating together provide a mechanism for the kidney to produce either a concentrated or a dilute urine, depending upon the presence or absence of antidiuretic hormone. Panel **7A** shows the configuration during the production of a dilute urine. The heavy lines outlining the thick ascending limb (diluting segment), the distal convolution and collecting duct signify the regions of the nephron that are impermeable to water in the absence of antidiuretic hormone. This results in further dilution of the fluid as it traverses the distal convolution and collecting duct where additional sodium chloride and other solute reabsorption occurs. The final urine may contain as few as 40–50 mOsm/kg of water during maximal water diuresis. Panel **7B** illustrates production of a concentrated urine. *The events up to and through the diluting segment are the same under both conditions.* In the presence of ADH however, water reabsorption follows the removal of sodium and chloride and urea both in the distal convolution and collecting duct. As the tubular fluid flows through the collecting duct which traverses the hypertonic medulla to reach the pelvis, it equilibrates with the interstitium. This produces urine with a solute concentration in excess of 800 to 1000 mOsm/kg. In both situations, the countercurrent multiplier and exchanger systems appear to work in approximately the same fashion and the principle difference in the two situations is contributed by antidiuretic hormone which controls the permeability of the distal nephron segments to water. For detailed reviews see references 1, 5, 19, 22.

pertonic medullary interstitium is maintained by the countercurrent multiplier and exchanger systems operating within the renal medulla. The transport functions of the various nephron segments during the production of hypotonic and hypertonic urine are shown, respectively, in Figures 10–7A and 10–7B. The details of the mechanism by which medullary hypertonicity is achieved and the role of the countercurrent multiplier and exchanger mechanisms in establishing and maintaining this hypertonicity are the subjects of several recent reviews.[5,18,19]

QUANTITATIVE ASPECTS OF WATER AND SOLUTE EXCRETION

The quantitative description of water conservation and/or excretion by the kidney is somewhat obscured by the terminology presently accepted as standard usage. The concepts are simple, however, and derive from the clearance concepts discussed earlier.

Osmolal Clearance (C_{osm})

The kidneys are confronted with the excretion of a given amount of solute each day. This total solute excretion rate can be expressed in terms of osmoles, or milliosmoles (mOsm) per minute. It can be calculated from the total solute concentration in the urine (U_{osm}) and the rate of urine excretion (V):

$$\text{Total Solute Excretion Rate} = U_{osm} \cdot V$$

The urine flow required to excrete solute at a constant rate will depend, of course, upon the solute concentration. With high urinary solute concentrations (hypertonicity), small flows will be adequate, while at low concentrations high flows will be required. In dealing with this problem it is useful to determine the urine flow required to excrete this amount of solute if the urine were *isotonic* to plasma. This is $(U_{osm} \cdot V)/P_{osm}$, where P_{osm} is the concentration of solute in plasma. This expression is also the definition of clearance:

$$\text{Osmolal Clearance} = C_{osm} = \frac{U_{osm} \cdot V}{P_{osm}}$$

When it is necessary to conserve water by excreting hypertonic urine, the observed urine flow rate (V) will be less than if isotonic urine were excreted (C_{osm}). Conversely, when it is necessary to lose water by excreting a hypotonic urine the observed flow (V) will exceed C_{osm} (Fig. 10–8). These differences between observed flows and the flows calculated for the formation of isotonic urine serve as important measures of the kidneys' ability to concentrate and dilute solute.

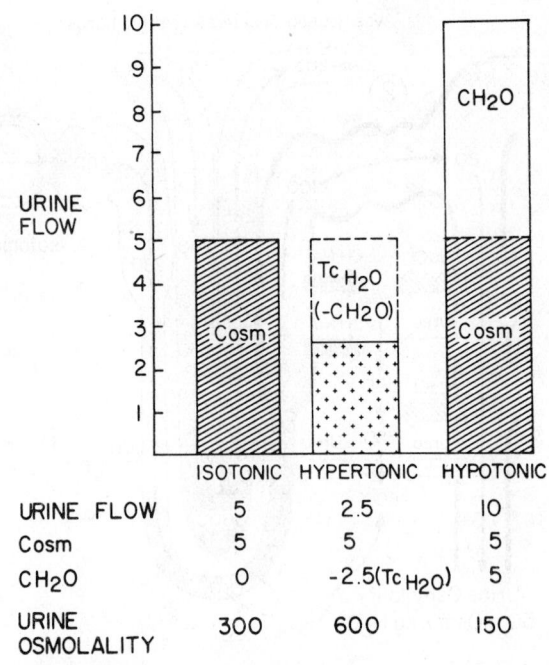

	ISOTONIC	HYPERTONIC	HYPOTONIC
URINE FLOW	5	2.5	10
Cosm	5	5	5
CH2O	0	-2.5(Tc H2O)	5
URINE OSMOLALITY	300	600	150

FIGURE 10–8. Renal conservation and excretion of water during formation of hypertonic and hypotonic urine. The relationships between urine osmolality, urine flow, osmolar clearance, and free water clearance are represented schematically. Note that when urine is hypertonic, free water clearance is negative and often designated Tc_{H_2O}.

Free Water Clearance (C_{H_2O})

This is defined as the rate at which water is excreted without solute during the production of *hypotonic* urine (Fig. 10–8):

$$C_{H_2O} = V - C_{osm}$$

Negative Free Water Clearance (Tc_{H_2O})

This is the rate at which water is reabsorbed from tubular fluid during the production of hypertonic urine (Fig. 10–8):

$$Tc_{H_2O} = C_{osm} - V$$

Limits in Normal Subjects

There are limits to the normal kidneys' ability to secrete or reabsorb water in the face of water loading or water privation. One important variable in determining these limits is the solute load.

The quantitative relationships defined above can be used to provide a quantitative description of the rate at which solute-free water is excreted from (C_{H_2O}) or added to the body (Tc_{H_2O}). Thus, free water clearance represents the amount of water that has been added to an isotonic urine (or, more precisely, the volume of urine from which all solute must be removed) in order to form a hypotonic urine with the same quantity of urinary solute. Conversely, negative-free water clearance represents the volume of water reabsorbed from an isotonic urine to produce a hypertonic urine with an identical load of solute. Normally, the rate of urine production is always less than the osmolar clearance during continued water restriction. Qualitatively, this is simply another way of saying that the final product, which begins as an isotonic ultrafiltrate of plasma, is excreted as urine that is hypertonic. Quantitatively, the difference between osmolar clearance and urine flow gives the quantity of solute-free water that is reabsorbed per unit time, i.e., it measures the rate at which pure water is being added to dilute the solute concentration of the blood and interstitial fluid. The relationship between these several parameters of the renal concentrating process is shown in Figure 10–9.

The maximal rates of free water reabsorption and excretion are determined by two factors: 1) at low rates of solute excretion, by the maximal urinary osmolal concentration which the kidney can produce; and 2) at high rates of osmolal clearance (osmotic diuresis), by the maximal rate of water diffusion. Thus, at a low rate of solute excretion the ability of the kidney to reabsorb solute-free water is limited by its capacity to increase the osmolal U:P ratio, the limit of this ratio varying between 3.5 and 4 in normal individuals. This corresponds to a maximal urinary osmolality of about 1200 mOsm per kg of water (Fig. 10–9A, hydropenia). As the solute load increases, there is a corresponding increase in reabsorption of solute-free water (Tc_{H_2O}). Solute-free water reabsorption, however, is limited by the maximal rate of water diffusion, so that Tc_{H_2O} tends to reach a maximal value at high rates of osmolar clearance (Fig. 10–9B, hydropenia). Therefore, the osmolality of the urine falls progressively toward the plasma osmolality, although the rate of free water reabsorption increases. At high values of osmolal clearance, maximal solute-free water conservation may be accompanied by a urinary osmolality of 400 mOsm per kg or less (Fig. 10–9A, hydropenia). This accounts, in part, for the large water losses during the osmotic diuresis of diabetic acidosis, for example.

Similarly, free-water excretion (C_{H_2O}) at low solute excretion rates is limited by the minimal osmolal concentration that can be produced by the kidney (Fig. 10–9A, water diuresis). With increasing solute load the rate of increase of C_{H_2O} slows remarkably and urinary osmolality approaches plasma osmolality during water diuresis just as during hydropenia.

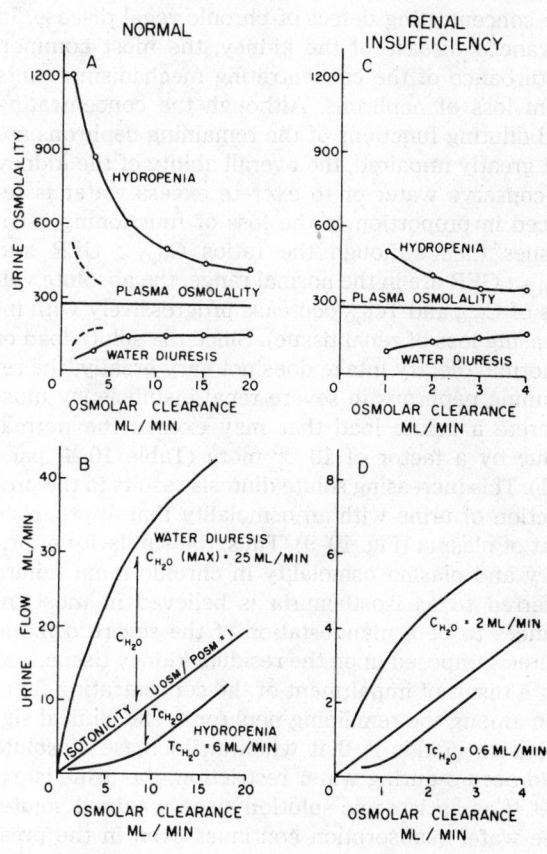

FIGURE 10–9. Relation between maximum range of renal concentrating and diluting function and urinary solute load in health and disease. The figures compare urine osmolality and solute-free water handling in the normal kidney and in the kidney in which renal function has been reduced to 10 percent of normal. **A** presents the relation between urine osmolality and osmolar clearance in the normal kidney during hydropenia and water diuresis. As solute load increases, urine osmolality approaches plasma osmolality. **B** shows the rate at which solute-free water is excreted (C_{H_2O}) or reabsorbed (Tc_{H_2O}) with increasing solute load during water excess and hydropenia. Water excretion or conservation is greatest at high solute loads despite the fact that the urine osmolality is less different from plasma than with low rates of osmolar clearance. **C** and **D** show similar relationships in the presence of severe renal impairment (GFR 10 percent of normal), assuming that the concentrating function of the remaining nephrone is unimpaired. The marked restriction of maximum values for osmolality and solute-free water transfer set narrow limits on the kidney with respect to conserving or excreting solute free water. The range of urinary osmolality in the presence of severe renal disease, as shown on the expanded scale in **C**, is also drawn in on **A** as the interrupted line.

Limits in Chronic Renal Failure

This explanation of the normal concentrating mechanism serves as a frame of reference for understanding the concentrating defect of chronic renal disease. In advanced disease of the kidney, the most common disturbance of the concentrating mechanism results from loss of nephrons. Although the concentrating and diluting functions of the remaining nephrons are not greatly impaired, the overall ability of the kidney to conserve water or to excrete excess water is reduced in proportion to the loss of functioning renal tissues (i.e., although the ratios C_{H_2O} : GFR and Tc_{H_2O} : GFR are in the normal range, the absolute values of C_{H_2O} and Tc_{H_2O} decrease progressively with increasing loss of renal tissue). Since the solute load of a normal dietary intake does not vary greatly, the remaining nephrons in severe renal insufficiency must excrete a solute load that may exceed the normal value by a factor of 10 or more (Table 10–4, page 111). This increasing solute diuresis results in the production of urine with an osmolality that approaches that of plasma (Fig. 10–9). Thus, the similarity of urinary and plasma osmolality in chronic renal failure referred to as isosthenuria is believed in most instances to be a manifestation of the severe osmotic diuresis imposed upon the residual kidney tissue, and not a result of impairment of the concentrating function among the remaining nephrons. The clinical significance of this is that when an increase in solute load occurs during water restriction, the urine is excreted as an isotonic solution since maximal solute-free water reabsorption continues even in the presence of the normal daily solute intake. With inadequate water intake, the water necessary for such an increase in solute excretion is provided at the expense of the fluid compartments of the body, a circumstance leading to rapid dehydration if uncorrected.

A comparison of limiting values for these concentrating and diluting functions in severe renal disease with those of the normal kidney is shown in Table 10–4. An average daily solute load, varying between 400 and 600 mOsm requires a minimum urinary volume of about 1200 to 1800 ml in chronic renal insufficiency. When insensible losses from all routes are added, the total daily fluid intake should be about 2.5 liters. Although this requirement can be reduced by restricting solute intake, extreme care must be employed. Conversely, caution should be used to avoid excessive water intake since these impairments also apply to the rate at which solute free water can be excreted. The maximal value for C_{H_2O} may be reduced from a normal of 25 ml per minute or greater, to less than 2 ml, depending upon the severity of the renal impairment. Under such conditions, vigorous forcing of fluids to flush out retained metabolic products can result in hyponatremia and severe water intoxication. Thus, both hypo- and hyperosmolality (Chap. 5) are presistent hazards in the presence of chronic renal failure.

DISORDERS OF RENAL FUNCTION AFFECTING THE CONCENTRATING MECHANISM DIRECTLY

There are several conditions, the most common being pyelonephritis, which result in specific disturbances of the concentrating mechanism out of proportion to the impairment of other parameters of renal function. Other conditions include hypokalemia, hypercalcemia, sickle cell disease, and less frequently, multiple myeloma and amyloidosis (Table 10–3). In these conditions, the specific derangement is loss of ability to produce a hypertonic urine. This *usually* does not result in severe degrees of water loss since production of isotonic urine under conditions of normal solute intake only obligates 1 to 2 liters of water daily. Occasionally, however, urine may be persistently hypotonic to plasma in these conditions, resulting in extreme degrees of water loss. Normally, much more water is conserved during the operation that concentrates hypotonic distal tubular fluid to isotonicity than is conserved by concentrating the isotonic fluid leaving the distal convolution. Thus, a solute output of 600 mOsm per day would require an output of 12 liters per day, if excreted at a fixed solute concentration of 50 mOsm per liter. By reducing the fluid to isotonicity, 10 of these liters of water would be conserved (only 2 liters are required to excrete 600 mOsm as an isotonic solution). Further concentration

---

TABLE 10–3
Disorders of Renal Function with Selective Disturbance of Renal Concentrating Mechanism

Systemic Diseases

Multiple myeloma
Amyloidosis
Sickle cell anemia, sickle cell trait
Hyperparathyroidism

Renal Diseases

Pyelonephritis
Hereditary nephrogenic diabetes insipidus
Renal tubular acidosis

Metabolic Disturbances

Hypercalcemia
Hypokalemia

to a value twice the solute concentration of plasma would save only an additional liter of water. Hence, a kidney limited to the production of a markedly hypotonic urine may have an obligatory water loss of several liters per day, resembling diabetes insipidus. While such extreme degrees of polyuria are uncommon, they have been observed in cases of potassium depletion and hypercalcemia. As in diabetes insipidus, the total quantity of water lost per day varies with the solute intake (Fig. 10-9) so that diets with a high solute load aggravate this defect while low solute diets diminish it.

REGULATION OF ELECTROLYTE EXCRETION AND HYDROGEN ION BALANCE

Each day the normal kidneys filter approximately 25,000 mEq of sodium, 18,000 mEq of chloride, and 4500 mEq of bicarbonate in a volume of roughly 180 liters. About 1 percent of the water and less than 1 percent of the electrolytes filtered are excreted, the remainder being absorbed by the renal tubules. The daily volume of glomerular filtrate is about 12 times as large as the extracellular fluid volume. Thus, the kidney filters and reabsorbs a volume of fluid equal to

the extracellular fluid volume every 2 hours. *By varying the composition of the reabsorbed fluids, the kidney can effectively and rapidly regulate the electrolyte composition of the interstitial fluid.* This control is impaired in severe renal disease. For instance, a kidney retaining only 10 percent of normal functional capacity would filter only 18 liters per day and reabsorb no more than 16. Thus, nearly 24 hours would be required for one cycling of the interstitial fluid, and, perhaps as long as 2 or 3 days before a new equilibrium was established. The principal mechanisms for the renal regulation of the composition of the extracellular fluid are the reabsorption of sodium, chloride, and bicarbonate in varying proportions and, in addition, the secretion of hydrogen ion and potassium. These mechanisms are schematically presented in Figure 10-10.

Sodium and Chloride

The urinary solute load is composed primarily of sodium, chloride, and urea. The daily output of sodium chloride varies normally over a wide range depending upon intake but is usually about 140 mEq (8 g). Balance studies indicate that the normal kidney responds

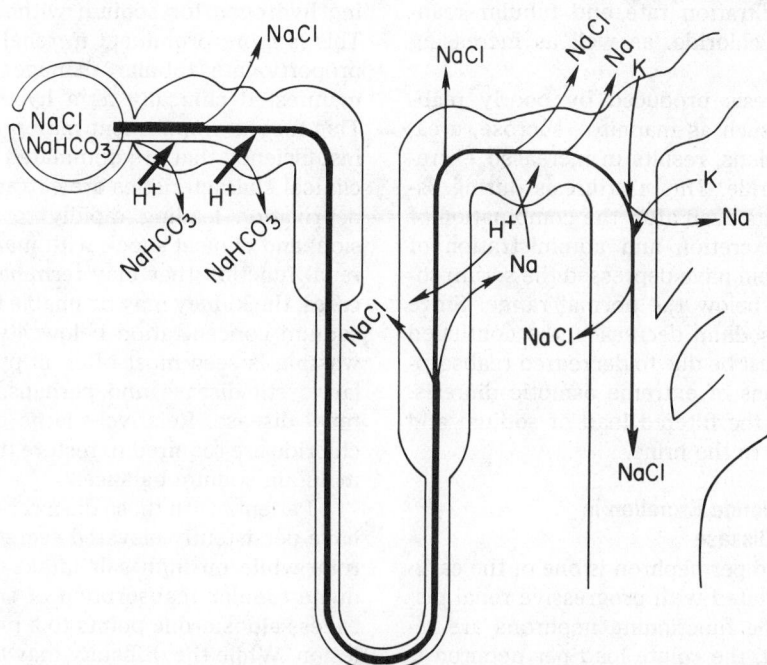

FIGURE 10-10. Mechanisms of renal sodium reabsorption. Sodium is reabsorbed in the proximal segment of the nephron as sodium chloride and, as sodium bicarbonate in exchange for hydrogen ion. In the more distal segments of the nephron, both potassium and hydrogen ions are secreted into the urine as counter ions to maintain electroneutrality as sodium is reabsorbed. These transport processes together permit the kidney to excrete urine that is virtually sodium free.

to variation in sodium intake ranging from less than 1 to more than 20 g in a manner that permits the total exchangeable sodium within the body to vary no more than 150 to 175 mEq despite these wide fluctuations in intake. The kidney is capable of producing a sodium-free (<1.0 mEq/L) urine over periods of months without any deleterious effects upon the individual so long as no extrarenal sodium losses occur. The mechanisms whereby the kidney achieves this regulation include 1) variation of filtered Na load by changes in GFR; 2) variation in renal transport of sodium by alterations in the renin-aldosterone system (Fig. 10–10); and 3) alterations in third factor (natriuretic hormone) that modulate proximal tubular reabsorption of sodium.

Relatively small increases in glomerular filtration rate may be associated with striking increases, and, conversely, virtually unmeasurable drops in glomerular filtration rate result in marked diminution in sodium excretion.

Corticosteroids increase the renal reabsorption of sodium and chloride with consequent expansion of the extracellular fluid volume, and, conversely, extracellular fluid volume decreases as a result of renal loss of sodium and chloride in the absence of corticosteroids. These hormones, especially aldosterone, increase glomerular filtration rate and tubular reabsorption of sodium chloride, as well as increasing potassium secretion.

The solute diuresis produced by poorly reabsorbed substances, such as mannitol, sucrose, urea, and a number of anions, results in increased excretion of sodium chloride. This natriuresis during osmotic diuresis persists even after the combination of increased sodium excretion and administration of large quantities of fluid have depressed the serum sodium concentration below the normal range. Since the filtered load of sodium decreases, the continued loss of this cation must be due to decreased reabsorption. Under conditions of extreme osmotic diuresis, 10 to 15 percent of the filtered load of sodium and chloride may appear in the urine.

Sodium and Chloride Excretion in Chronic Renal Disease

Change in solute load per nephron is one of the earliest alterations associated with progressive renal disease. Thus, when the functioning nephrons are reduced by 50 percent, the solute load per nephron is doubled (assuming no change in solute intake). This increase in solute excretion or osmotic diuresis impairs the ability of the kidney to conserve sodium adequately. In advanced degrees of renal insufficiency, the kidney can no longer excrete urine that is virtually sodium-free. Minimum sodium concentrations in urine after restriction of sodium intake may be no lower than 8 to 10 mEq/L (and at times higher), representing an obligatory loss of 20 to 30 mEq per day. Severe salt restriction may result in a progressive loss of sodium from extracellular fluid. This causes a decrease in the glomerular filtration rate which may result in some improvement of sodium conservation. However, when renal insufficiency is advanced, this drop in glomerular filtration rate further aggravates the uremia. Consequently, a vicious cycle is established which can, under extreme conditions, produce a pronounced sodium deficit, and may be life-threatening. In general, an intake of several grams of salt per day is adequate to avoid such sodium deficit, and significant depletion is seen only with rigid restriction of intake or extrarenal sources of sodium loss. Because it can lead to further deterioration of function, impaired sodium conservation is a very important aspect of the impairment produced by chronic renal insufficiency. In addition, the kidney's ability to excrete sodium is less easily regulated, and administration of excessive salt may result in sodium retention and edema.

Renal sodium-wasting may be further intensified by failure of the mechanism responsible for exchanging hydrogen for sodium within the tubular lumen. This is more prominent in renal diseases where disproportionate tubular damage may occur, and is manifested clinically as a hyperchloremic acidosis. This tubular impairment may produce cases of renal insufficiency that are dominated by salt-wasting. The clinical characteristics are extreme sensitivity to salt deprivation leading rapidly to weakness, hypotension, and clinical shock with marked deterioration of renal function that may terminate in death. In such cases, the kidney may be unable to reduce the urinary sodium concentration below 40 or 50 mEq/L. Salt-wasting is seen most often in pyelonephritis, medullary cystic disease, and, perhaps, other types of cystic renal disease. Relatively large quantities of sodium chloride are required to restore the sodium deficit and maintain sodium balance.

Patients with these disorders have been shown to have persistently elevated secretion rates of aldosterone while on high salt intake. This failure of adequate tubular reabsorption of sodium in the face of excess aldosterone points to a predominantly tubular lesion. While the difficulty may be aggravated by the osmotic diuresis of renal insufficiency, relative glomerular preponderance (increased rate of glomerular filtration per nephron) or a specific tubular impairment (e.g., tubular atrophy) must also be present, since the defect cannot be produced by solute-loading in patients with a comparable degree of renal insufficiency but without such marked salt-wasting tendencies.

Hydrogen Ion Regulation

The net quantity of hydrogen ions excreted by the kidney (150 to 300 mEq per day) is very small compared to that excreted by the lungs as CO_2 (15,000 mEq per day). Hence, disturbances in pulmonary function may result in acidosis within minutes, while after complete anuria several days are required for its development. The principal renal mechanism for maintenance of body pH is the regulation of bicarbonate reabsorption and, hence, control of the ratio of carbonic acid to bicarbonate.[1,10,23] This mechanism is outlined in Figure 10–11. A second renal mechanism for regulation of body pH is excretion of nonvolatile anions. The addition of an acid to the extracellular fluid provides excesses of hydrogen ion and its associated anion, both of which require excretion. Excess anions of the strong mineral acids (phosphates, sulfates, chloride) are completely excreted by the kidney, and electroneutrality demands that they be excreted with an associated cation. Since, physiologically, the lower limit of urinary pH is about 4.5, this will not permit excretion of such anions in association with hydrogen; some other cation, such as sodium, ammonium, or potassium, is required.

Since sodium is the most abundant cation available in the urine, it is the first lost in response to developing acidosis. Subsequently, a series of reactions is stimulated that results in an increase in the production of hydrogen ions and of ammonia and in the reabsorption of bicarbonate. Thus, the development of acidosis is regularly associated with a concomitantly developing sodium deficit.

The acidosis of chronic renal disease is directly related to the reduction in number of functioning nephrons. The functional impairments resulting from this reduction include inadequacy of the hydrogen ion secretory mechanism and retention of nonvolatile anions such as phosphates and sulfates. Retention of nonvolatile anions is directly related to the decreased glomerular filtration rate. The result is progressive accumulation of these nonvolatile anions in plasma (and other body fluids). This inverse relation between phosphates, sulfates, and other substances in plasma and the plasma bicarbonate concentration is the most common pattern of acidosis seen in chronic renal insufficiency, usually appearing after the glomerular filtration rate is reduced to values less than 20 percent of normal. It is aggravated by increased protein in-

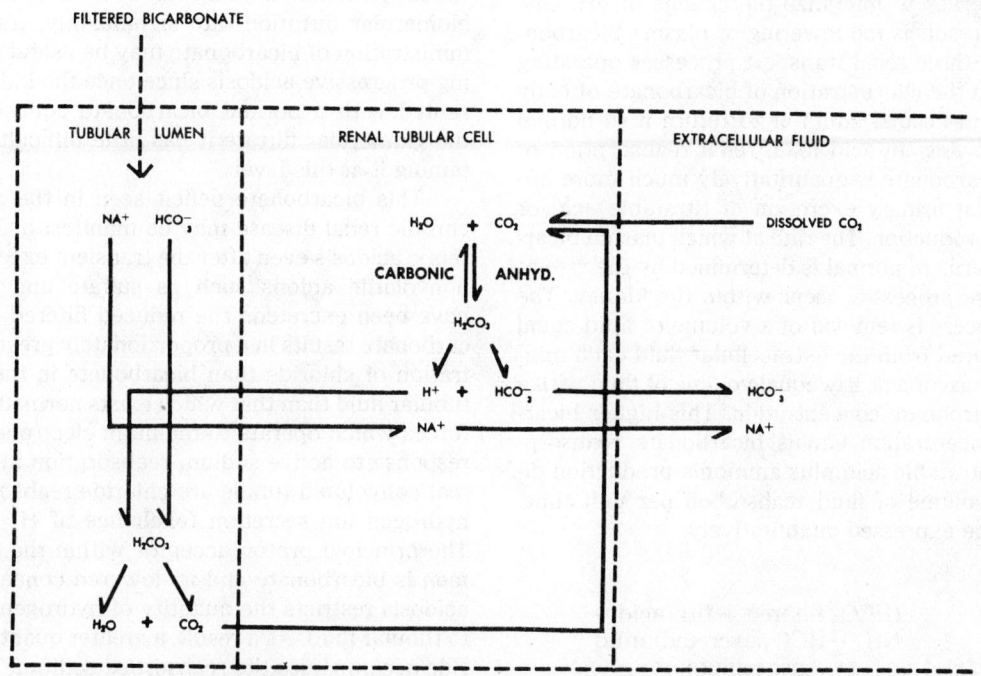

FIGURE 10–11. Proposed mechanism of exchange of hydrogen for sodium. The net effect of these reactions is reabsorption of sodium bicarbonate.

take and increased intake of substances that contain a relatively high content of chlorides or other anions in excess of cations (acid ash diet). Reduction in protein intake and substitution of carbohydrate as a food source results in improvement of this type of acidosis.

Acidosis resulting primarily from defective hydrogen ion excretion, recognized clinically as *hyperchloremic acidosis,* is seen less commonly as a pure form of acidosis in chronic renal disease. The prime example is *renal tubular acidosis* (Chap. 14), but it may be seen in a variety of renal disorders associated with renal insufficiency. Clinically, the acidosis is usually compensated but may be symptomatic with plasma chloride concentration exceeding 120 to 125 mEq/L. Plasma bicarbonate concentration is correspondingly low and plasma phosphate is usually normal. Ammonium production and titratable acidity are reduced.

Factors Regulating Bicarbonate Reabsorption

When presented with comparable loads of excess nonvolatile anions or acid loads, the major difference between the response of the normal kidney and the severely impaired kidney is in the rate at which these substances are excreted and the pH disturbance repaired. The initial systemic effect is the same in both situations; an appropriate shift in the state of the buffer pairs serves to minimize the change in pH. One important result is the lowering of plasma bicarbonate. Of the three renal transport processes operating to maintain the concentration of bicarbonate of body fluids within normal limits or to return it to normal levels following an acid load, renal reabsorption of filtered bicarbonate is quantitatively much more important than urinary excretion of titratable acid or ammonia production. The rate at which plasma bicarbonate returns to normal is determined by the rate at which these processes occur within the kidney. The overall process is removal of a volume of fluid equal to that filtered from the extracellular fluid each minute and return of a nearly equal volume of fluid with a higher bicarbonate concentration. This higher bicarbonate concentration equals bicarbonate reabsorption plus titratable acid plus ammonia production divided by volume of fluid reabsorbed per unit time. This may be expressed quantitatively:

$$[HCO_3]_{T.R.} = \frac{(HCO_3 \text{ filtered} + \text{titr. acid} + NH_4 - HCO_3 \text{ excreted}) \text{ mEq per minute}}{\text{Volume of tubular fluid reabsorbed (ml per minute)}}$$

This gives the bicarbonate concentration in mEq/L that would be found in extracellular fluid when the kidney has completely recycled the extracellular fluid. The normal kidney is capable of filtering and reabsorbing a volume of fluid equal to extracellular fluid volume in approximately 2 hours. As the glomerular filtration rate falls, however, the time required for completion of this operation varies in a reciprocal manner. Thus, the kidney with a glomerular filtration rate less than 10 percent of normal would require 20 hours. The increased time required for repair of a deficit in plasma bicarbonate concentration by the severely impaired kidney tends to make the effect of dietary ingestion of nonvolatile anions cumulative, producing progressive acidosis and other manifestations of the uremic syndrome. This decrease in plasma bicarbonate concentration results in a corresponding decrease in the amount of filtered bicarbonate which is available for reabsorption. Although the formation of titratable acid and the production of ammonia are stimulated, these increases do not offset the net effect of the diminution in the filtered load of bicarbonate as illustrated quantitatively in Table 10–2. Thus, the impaired reabsorption of bicarbonate in chronic renal disease is due to a combination of reduced glomerular filtration rate and lowered serum bicarbonate levels, both of which decrease the load of bicarbonate presented to the renal tubule. Although nothing can be done to increase the glomerular filtration rate significantly, transient administration of bicarbonate may be useful in combating progressive acidosis since once the kidney is presented with a normal bicarbonate concentration in the glomerular filtrate it has little difficulty in maintaining it at this level.

This bicarbonate deficit seen in the acidosis of chronic renal disease may be manifest as hyperchloremic acidosis even after the transient excess loads of nonvolatile anions such as sulfate and phosphate have been excreted. The reduced filtered load of bicarbonate results in a proportionately greater concentration of chloride than bicarbonate in the proximal tubular fluid than that which exists normally. The two forces which operate to maintain electroneutrality in response to active sodium reabsorption in the proximal convoluted tubule are chloride reabsorption and hydrogen ion secretion (exchange of H^+ for Na^+). The principal proton acceptor within the tubular lumen is bicarbonate and its lowered concentration in acidosis restricts the quantity of hydrogen ion added to tubular fluid. As a result, a greater quantity of chloride accompanies the reabsorbed sodium. The net effect of this disparity is an increased concentration of chloride in the fluid reabsorbed by the proximal nephron. It is likely that the increased sodium loss—a regular feature of the acidosis of chronic renal disease—stimulates aldosterone secretion, resulting in increased sodium chloride reabsorption and further accentuation of the hyperchloremia. The administration of bicarbonate elevates plasma bicarbonate concentration and corrects the acidosis. Once this is accomplished, dietary regulation may serve to prevent recurrence.

Potassium

In the normal individual, the average daily urinary excretion of potassium varies between 50 and 100 mEq per day, depending upon dietary intake. The maximum potential rate of potassium excretion is much greater, however, and under appropriate circumstances it may be twice the rate at which potassium is filtered at the glomerulus.[5,13]

The severely impaired kidney usually has more difficulty with potassium excretion than with sodium conservation. The potassium concentration in the urine becomes nearly fixed due to the limitations imposed by the tubular damage. Thus, potassium secretion must continue at a near maximal rate in order to get rid of the daily load of potassium.

In the presence of continued dietary potassium restriction, the stimulus to retain sodium, which usually persists as a consequence of the ever-present acidosis, results in increased potassium loss. Consequently, significant potassium deficits may develop in uremia. Thus, the patient with chronic renal insufficiency is prone to the development of either hyper- or hypokalemia, depending upon the intake.

CLINICAL EVALUATION OF RENAL FUNCTION

As a routine part of the examination of each patient, the physician must establish that the kidneys are free of disease and functioning normally, or alternately, establish a diagnosis of renal disease and obtain a quantitative assessment of renal function. Once renal damage appears, the resulting pathophysiologic disturbances may progress to endstage disease and terminal uremia. Quantitative appraisal of the degree of renal impairment permits the physician to anticipate these occurrences and to institute appropriate therapy. In Table 10–4 the functions of the normal kidney and the severely diseased kidney are contrasted. In the paragraphs that follow, the clinically useful facts that are employed in quantitating the severity of renal impairment are discussed.

EXAMINATION OF THE URINE

Examination of the urine constitutes the single most important test of the adequacy of renal function for clinical purposes. It should include measurement of specific gravity and of pH, testing for presence of protein, and careful examination of the urine sediment.[11,20] Examination of freshly voided concentrated urine provides more useful information than does study of a dilute specimen. Formed elements, particularly red blood cells and casts, lyse quickly in dilute urine; proteinuria may escape detection, and no information is provided about the concentrating ability of

---

TABLE 10–4

Contrasting Function of the Normal and Severely Impaired Kidney

Parameter of Renal Function	Normal	Severely Impaired GFR < 5% of normal
Glomerular filtration rate (liters per day)	180	7
Maximum urinary volume (liters per day)	25	2
Minimum urinary volume (liters per day)	0.50	1.4
Maximum solute concentration (mOsm/kg H_2O)	1200	375
Maximum free water clearance (liters per day)	24	1
Maximum free water reabsorption (liters per day)	8	0.4
Maximum total hydrogen Ion secretion (mEq per day)		
(HCO_3^- reabsorption + titratable acidity + ammonia)	5000	150
Titratable acidity (mEq per day)*	150	15
Ammonia production (mEq per day)*	350	40
Average solute excretion per day (mOsm)†	600	400
(μOsm per minute)	425	290
Average solute excretion per dl GFR		
(μOsm per dl GFR)	342	6000

* Maximum values developed in the presence of persistent systemic acidosis.
† This is determined primarily by solute intake.

the kidney. It is most desirable to use the first specimen voided in the morning, provided that it is examined *promptly*. No reliance should be placed on microscopic study of the urine sediment when more than 2 hours have elapsed between collection and examination. If the specific gravity of the urine is below 1.010, microscopic examination should be conducted immediately following collection.

Specific Gravity

Specific gravity in excess of 1.025 in otherwise normal urine usually signifies normal or adequate renal function. Specific gravity of urine is linearly related to its osmolality, but since it measures urine directly relative to the density of water, it may exhibit wide fluctuations at any given urine osmolality depending upon the nature of the major solutes in the urine. Thus glucose in the urine produces a much higher specific gravity than an equiosmolar quantity of urea. Accurate assessment of renal concentrating ability can only be provided by direct measurement of urine osmolality. The range of maximal solute concentration which the normal human kidney achieves varies between 750 and about 1100 mOsm per kg H_2O depending upon dietary intake. The urinary specific gravity provides a clinically useful estimate of this function when the urine does not contain abnormal quantities of such high density substances as glucose, phosphates, or iodine-containing compounds. Urine collected from diabetics with glycosuria, from patients following use of phosphate cathartics, or following use of intravenous radiographic contrast media will yield high values of specific gravity that do not accurately reflect the kidney's concentrating capacity.

Overnight fluid restriction usually results in urinary solute concentration that is only about 75 percent of the maximum concentration achieved after 24 hours of fluid deprivation. From a practical clinical standpoint, specific gravity measurement is of virtually no value unless carried out on the initial voiding after arising in the morning. Even then, abnormally low values do not necessarily signify impaired concentrating ability. Nevertheless, measurement of urine specific gravity on the first voided A.M. specimen is a useful screening test for evaluating renal concentrating ability. Values exceeding 1.023 to 1.025 may be regarded as signifying a normal renal concentrating mechanism and values in excess of 1.020 probably signify normal concentrating function. Protein in the urine has a relatively small effect upon urine specific gravity, each gram of protein per liter of urine raising the specific gravity by 0.00025.

Urinary pH

Measurement of pH on random urine samples has little clinical importance because of wide variation with time of day and with dietary intake. It may, however, yield valuable information in specific circumstances, as for example, renal tubular acidosis.

In the presence of systemic acidosis, a urine pH above 6.0 in the absence of urinary tract infection signifies impairment of the renal acidification mechanism and is presumptive evidence of renal tubular acidosis. Urine infected with organisms capable of splitting urea may give false high pH values.

Urinary Protein

The quantity of protein in normal urine is usually less than 50 mg per 24-hour period, representing an average concentration of less than 5 mg/dl. This concentration is too low to be detected by the usual clinical laboratory methods. The heat and acetic method, as well as the sulfosalicylic method, will regularly detect concentrations as low as 5 to 10 mg/dl. Such quantities should always be considered abnormal. Although mild degrees of proteinuria may on occasion be observed in the absence of renal disease, its detection by these methods should always be taken as presumptive evidence of renal disease.[11] The urine used in testing must have a specific gravity greater than 1.010 or cases of mild proteinuria will be overlooked.

Qualitative precipitation reactions (heat and acetic acid, and sulfosalicylic acid methods) are useful for screening purposes, but they are not satisfactory as a means of following patients with proven renal disease. The total quantity of protein excreted per 24 hours is a product of protein concentration in the urine and urine volume. Hence, wide variations in volume may produce remarkable changes in protein concentration in the presence of a constant daily protein output. For following the daily excretion of protein in renal disease, the turbidimetric sulfosalicylic method is a simple and reliable quantitative test.

Microscopic Examination of Urinary Sediment

The importance of obtaining *fresh urine* for appropriate examination of the urinary sediment has already been stressed. The significant abnormal components of urine sediment are red cells, leukocytes, epithelial cells, and casts.[20]

Red blood cells may be seen in extremely small numbers in normal urine, particularly following strenuous exercise. Centrifuged urine from normal persons rarely shows more than two to three red cells on the usual microscopic slide preparation. Red cells are present in considerable numbers, however, in almost all types of diffuse renal disease. A characteristic appearance of those associated with glomerular disease is their relatively small size and greater refractility, when compared to red cells shed from the lower urinary tract. Although it may be possible to suspect the presence of renal disease from the appearance of the red cells alone, more commonly the associated presence of red cell casts is a specific index of the presence of glomerular disease.

There are several types of casts found regularly in various sorts of renal diseases. With proper identification casts are of considerable diagnostic aid (Table 10–5).

Finally, it is frequently desirable, in caring for patients with renal disease, to obtain quantitative information about the various parameters of renal function. This is of particular value in the patient with impaired renal function in whom management will depend upon the severity of the impairment. Listed in Table 10–5 are the various routine clinical tests which provide useful quantitative information.

QUANTITATIVE ASSESSMENT OF RENAL FUNCTION

The most commonly used quantitative measures of renal function that are of clinical value are the determinations of plasma constituents that reflect changes

in clearances, or somewhat less commonly, directly measured clearances. The most valuable and most extensively used plasma constituent measurements are the blood urea nitrogen and serum creatinine concentrations. These are used almost universally to provide screening measures of the adequacy of renal function and to detect grossly impaired renal function. Although the blood urea nitrogen (BUN) is more widely used, the serum creatinine concentration provides a more precise measure of the level of glomerular function. The reasons for the uncertainty associated with interpreting the level of the BUN have been reviewed (Fig. 10–4). There are also inherent difficulties in interpreting the significance of small changes in serum creatinine values (Fig. 10–12). In the average clinical chemistry laboratory, the 95 percent confidence limits for replicate measurement of creatinine values in the normal range are greater than ± 0.35 mg/dl, thus spanning a range of 0.7 mg/dl. As is evident from Figure 10–12, it is quite difficult to be certain that a change of less than 0.4 mg/dl is significant. Since this represents a 40 percent change in GFR at a nominal creatinine value of 1.0 mg/dl, this is not a sensitive means of detecting small changes in renal function.

A more reliable means of identifying trends in directional changes in renal function in the individual

---

TABLE 10–5

Formed Elements Found in Urine in Various Renal Diseases*

	Normal	Glomerulo-nephritides	Pyelo-nephritis	Amyloid	Arteriolo-sclerosis	K-W†
Formed Elements						
RBC	rare	+	+	±	+	±
WBC	rare	+	+	±	+	±
Epi. cells	rare	+	+	±	+	+
Casts						
Hyaline	rare	+	+	+	+	+
Granular	0	+	+	+	+	+
Cellular	0	+	+	0	0	rare
WBC	0	+	+	0	0	0
Epi. Cells	0	+	rare	0	0	+
RBC	0	+	0	0	0	0
Waxy	0	+	rare	0	0	+
Fatty	0	+	0	0	0	+

* + - present; 0 - absent.
† - Kimmelstiel-Wilson syndrome.

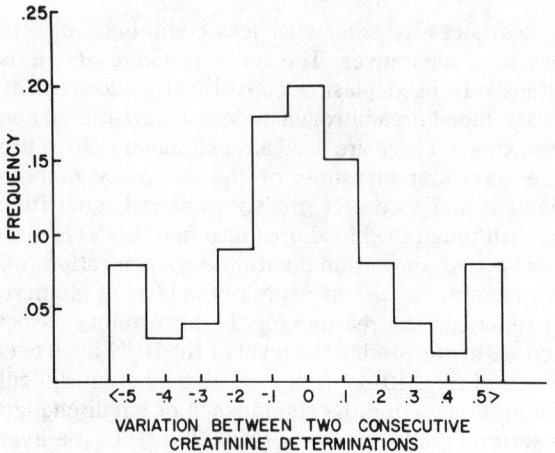

FIGURE 10–12. Distribution frequency of the difference between consecutive measurements of creatinine in 115 patients following renal transplantation (data represent 2500 creatinine measurements). The data were collected over a period of 3 years. The values included in the small peaks at the extremes are clearly significant differences and, thus, identify real changes in renal function. The larger proportion of differences appear to be normally distributed about a difference of zero with a standard deviation of 0.15 mg/dl. Thus, under the circumstances of the usual creatinine determination it is difficult to attach significance to changes in serum creatinine as great as ±0.3 mg/dl. At the normal creatinine value in the plasma of 1.0 mg/dl, this 95 percent confidence interval thus embraces a ±30 percent change in renal function. The serum creatinine is, therefore, not a particularly sensitive means of detecting small changes in renal function.

patient has been emphasized by Mitch.[21] The reciprocal of the serum creatinine value is directly related to the clearance in a constant manner. Thus, a plot of the reciprocal of the serum creatinine versus time (Fig. 10–13) identifies the direction of change in renal function and allows reasonable projection of the future appearance of renal failure. Moreover, the use of all available measurements in this type of plot greatly improves precision and enhances the utility of serum creatinine measurement.

Urea clearance has been widely used in the past as an approximate measure of glomerular filtration rate, but is unreliable for the reasons discussed on page 100. Creatinine clearance measurements yield much more reproducible results, are relatively uninfluenced by variations in urine flow rates, and are therefore preferable as a clinically useful index of glomerular filtration rate.[16] Simultaneous measurements of inulin and endogenous creatinine clearances yield values which agree comparatively well and, thus, creatinine clearance provides a practical clinical esti-

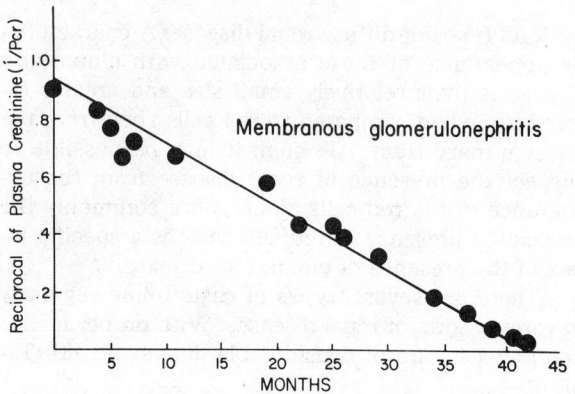

FIGURE 10–13. Monitoring change in renal function with the reciprocal of the serum creatinine. The graph of reciprocal of creatinine concentration (1/Cr) versus time in an individual with glomerulonephritis and vasculitis depicts a linear decrease with time. The slope is directly proportional to the rate of progression of disease (or rate of loss of renal function). This graphic representation of serial creatinine data permits more accurate assessment of the change in renal function than does measurement of a single value for creatinine or a small number of such measurements (Courtesy of Dr. Wm. Mitch).

mate of glomerular filtration rate. In an individual subject, replicate measurements show remarkable constancy. The 24-hour creatinine clearance is most commonly used, and consecutive measurements show a coefficient of variation of about 7 percent. In advanced renal impairment, as the plasma creatinine concentration rises, the fraction secreted by the tubules increases so that creatinine clearance exceeds the glomerular filtration rate. In spite of this fact, it remains a useful technique for following renal function quantitatively.

Quantitative aspects of renal function and the techniques used in their measurement are listed in Table 10–6, with a comparison of clinically useful tests and those useful primarily as research tools.

Other Useful Diagnostic Tests

In contrast to the tests described in the preceding section that are designed to provide quantitative or semiquantitative data on adequacy of renal function, there are a number of diagnostic tests designed to establish normalcy of structure of the genitourinary system. These include sonography and a number of radiographic procedures, both with and without the use of contrast media.

Sonography makes use of ultrasound to identify interfaces or abrupt structural changes within the body, thereby defining or delineating the structures in

---TABLE 10-6---
Quantitative Evaluation of Renal Function

Parameter of Renal Function	Precisely Defined by*	Useful Clinical Test for Evaluation
Glomerular filtration rate	Inulin clearance men—130 ml per minute women—115 ml per minute	Creatinine clearance men—95–140 ml per minute women—85–125 ml per minute Urea clearance ca. 55–80 ml per minute
Effective renal plasma flow	PAH clearance men—700 ml per minute women—600 ml per minute	PSP excretion (6 mg IV) 15 minute 30% 30 minute 45% 60 minute 60%
Tubular maxima	T_m PAH men—80 mg per minute women—70 mg per minute	PSP excretion (in advanced renal failure)
	T_m Glucose men—375 mg per minute women—300 mg per minute	
Renal concentrating ability	TC_{H_2O} determined during increasing solute load 5 to 6 ml per minute	Fishberg Conc test sp gr 1.023 or above Urine osmolality >700 mOsm/kg H_2O

* The complexity of these tests precludes their routine use in clinical evaluation of renal function.

a given two-dimensional cross-sectional plane of the body. It is of value in defining kidney size and identifying associated deformities such as cysts or masses. It is very helpful in guiding procedures such as cyst aspirations or renal biopsies. Its chief virtue is that it is completely noninvasive and without risk. Interpretation of patterns obtained by this technique is sometimes difficult because of shifting artifactual patterns created by gas bubbles in the gastrointestinal tract and the like.

Among the radiologic examinations that are used to provide information about genitourinary structure and functions, the *abdominal flat film* to identify kidneys and urinary bladder is perhaps most widely employed. With good technique, it provides useful information about *kidney size,* permits identification of radiopaque kidney stones and may, on occasion, yield information about masses in the vicinity of the kidney. It does not provide information about the urinary bladder unless there is a radiopaque structure, such as a bladder stone or foreign body, within the bladder.

The *intravenous pyelogram* (IVP) permits much clearer definition of the renal size, allows visualization of the intrarenal and extrarenal collecting system, and provides information about the adequacy of renal function. Because it requires the injection of a contrast medium, the possibility of preexisting drug sensitivity should always be carefully considered. The contrast medium yields much sharper delineation of the structures within the kidney and collecting system when administered when the patient is in the hydropenic state. The contrast media, however, have potential nephrotoxicity, and this hazard is greatest when the agents are administered in the dehydrated state. It must be stressed that use of large quantities of contrast material in ill patients is associated with a distinct risk of acute renal failure. Diabetic patients and patients with multiple myeloma and renal amyloidosis are at particularly high risk in this regard. Adequate visualization of the kidneys and collecting system by IVP requires that renal function be good. If the glomerular filtration has fallen below 25 percent of normal, the likelihood of obtaining useful information is sharply reduced, i.e., when serum creatinine is greater than 4 mg/dl or the creatinine clearance is less than 25 ml/min. In this circumstance *nephrotomography* is likely to yield better information. *Arteriography* and *computerized axial tomography* should be reserved for patients with specific indications for these procedures, such as renovascular hypertension for the former and renal masses of various sorts for the latter. These procedures are more costly, and, in the case of arteriography more risky.

RENAL BIOPSY

Specific instances where this procedure may be helpful are considered in subsequent chapters. Probably its greatest usefulness is in diagnosis and management of the nephrotic syndrome and in the diagnosis of uremia of obscure origin.[2]

Renal biopsy is technically more difficult than liver biopsy; adequate specimens are obtained with regularity only after the operator has acquired considerable experience with the procedure. It should not be undertaken casually by an inexperienced person. It is associated with a low but definite mortality, probably about 0.2 percent. Significant bleeding probably occurs in the majority of patients, and in 2 to 3 percent is of such severity as to require transfusion. Complications are minimized if: 1) all patients have been tested for bleeding, clotting, and prothrombin times prior to biopsy (abnormalities of any of these should preclude biopsy); 2) patients with a hemorrhagic diathesis are not to be biopsied, even if the above tests are normal; 3) following biopsy, the patient is watched carefully in bed for 24 hours and on limited activity for 2 weeks.

CHAPTER 11

Pathogenesis, Clinical Manifestations, and Management of Uremia

W. GORDON WALKER

CLINICAL FEATURES

Uremia is the term applied to the symptoms and signs which occur as a part of severe renal failure. These manifestations are due in part to the accompanying fluid and electrolyte disturbances. Hypo- and hyperosmolality, varying degrees of sodium depletion, potassium depletion or hyperkalemia, and acidosis may occur. The severity of each of these is variable. In addition, there are disturbances of neuromuscular, gastrointestinal, and cardiovascular function, not necessarily clearly related to any specific electrolyte abnormalities. Hypertension, anemia, and evidences of an increased bleeding tendency are also commonly observed.

Although the clinical features of the various electrolyte abnormalities are well defined, the relation between the general manifestations of uremia and a specific derangement of blood chemistry has not been established. It is clear, however, that the substances responsible can be removed by dialysis, often with spectacular improvement in the clinical condition of the patient.[1,2]

One of the earliest manifestations of uremia may be *nausea* and *vomiting* occurring upon arising in the morning or shortly thereafter. These manifestations may exist for some time without a concomitant loss of appetite, the caloric intake remaining normal despite the daily vomiting. If emesis reaches substantial proportions, however, it may lead to deficits in both potassium and sodium as well as dehydration and hypochloremic alkalosis. These extrarenal losses not only tax the limited ability of the kidneys to compensate, but may actually worsen renal function as a result of the accompanying diminution in extracellular fluid volume. Alternating constipation and diarrhea may be present. On occasion, the latter may be severe, leading to further electrolyte disturbances.

Asymptomatic pericarditis is common in uremia; associated pain is unusual. In addition, an overloaded circulation may develop as a result of too vigorous administration or ingestion of sodium chloride. Indeed, some patients with *severe hypertension* associated with uremia may exhibit a marked intolerance to salt and develop *edema* and *left ventricular failure* when the intake exceeds 30 to 40 mEq per day.

Neurologic and *neuromuscular abnormalities* may vary from mild drowsiness to lethargy and, ultimately, coma. Characteristic electroencephalographic changes have been described and are said to be promptly reversed by dialysis. Paralyses are distinctly unusual but may occur as a result of severe hypokalemia. Such occurrences are rare except in renal tubular acidosis. *Peripheral neuritis* is occasionally seen as a complication of uremia. It more often involves the lower extremities and is more common in patients with long-standing renal failure. The chief manifestations are pain, decreased sensation in the extremities, and motor involvement characterized by muscular weakness and broad-based gait. *Toxic psychoses* are occasionally seen and may include *hallucinatory experiences, manic depressive features,* or *paranoid behavior.* Most often, these behavioral disturbances are encountered under circumstances where the patient has been receiving drugs known to alter central nervous system function, such as phenothiazines, tricyclic antidepressants, and similar agents. All such drugs should be used with great caution in patients with impaired renal function. Seizures also occur frequently.

THE TREATMENT OF CHRONIC RENAL INSUFFICIENCY

The development of a successful means of prolonging life by hemodialysis or homotransplantation after all kidney function has ceased has resulted in a marked improvement in the outlook of some patients with terminal renal failure. For this reason, it is appropriate to consider first those therapeutic measures that are generally applicable to patients with uremia and to follow this with a discussion of the role of dialysis and transplantation in the treatment of terminal renal failure.

CONSERVATIVE MANAGEMENT

The therapeutic objectives of the conservative management of chronic renal failure are necessarily limited. Although the achievement of a sustained state of normal health is rarely if ever possible under these circumstances, effective management can often add many months or years of useful activity to the life of the patient with chronic renal failure. The benefits of even very difficult and restricted regimens are often so promptly evident to the patient that his cooperation is assured. The physician's general objective during this phase of management should be to make certain that the limitations of excretion and conservation placed upon the severely diseased kidney are the ones necessary to ensure adequate nutrition and fluid and electrolyte balance.

The details of management depend upon the particular physiologic disturbance responsible for the patient's discomfort (Table 11–1). Acidosis is the most common abnormality and is seen in all these patients during the later stages of their illness. The two principal contributing factors are intake of nonvolatile anion (excess protein intake) and failure of the hydrogen secretory mechanism. When acidosis first appears, the disparity between the acid load presented to the kidney and its maximal capacity for excreting

TABLE 11–1	
Principles of Management of More Common Disorders in Uremia	
Acidosis	When mild, protein restriction usually suffices for correction
	More severe degrees of acidosis may require the intermittent or continuous administration of some form of alkalinizing therapy
Water	Great care should be taken to avoid daily intake of less than 1800 ml and more than 3500 ml of fluid unless there is a well-defined reason for ignoring either of these limits
Sodium	In general, sodium intake should always exceed 25 to 35 mEq per day, unless clinical edema is present
	Even under these circumstances, greater restriction should be instituted only with great caution
Nitrogen	If acidosis is present, protein should be restricted to less than 0.5 g/kg body weight per day. Azotemia alone is not an indication for protein restriction and, in patients with severe nitrogen deficits resulting from heavy proteinuria, a high protein diet (2 g/kg per day or more) should be given as long as proteinuria persists unless acidosis supervenes

hydrogen ion is relatively small. The acidosis may be completely controlled by dietary restrictive measures; the principal source of excess nonvolatile anions is dietary protein. This is illustrated by the following.

NITROGEN RESTRICTION IN CHRONIC UREMIA

B., a 37-year-old white male with an 18-year history of chronic glomerulonephritis, was seen because of increased fatigue, irritability, anorexia, and occasional vomiting. He was hypertensive and anemic; blood urea nitrogen was 96 mg/dl, bicarbonate was 15 mEq/L, and creatinine clearance 14 ml per minute. Dietary nitrogen intake was limited to 40 g of protein per day. His bicarbonate rose to 23 mEq/L and his blood urea nitrogen fell to 42 mg/dl. He remained free of acidosis for the next 18 months with no other therapy.

As acidosis progresses in severity, dietary protein restriction alone is not sufficient to control acidosis. Failure of the hydrogen-secretory mechanism in renal insufficiency results in failure of bicarbonate reabsorption. This deficit may be offset by sodium bicarbonate administration. This may serve to combat the acidosis for long periods of time, particularly when the renal disease is not associated with hypertension. The following example illustrates this point.

BICARBONATE ADMINISTRATION IN HYPERCHLOREMIC ACIDOSIS WITHOUT HYPERTENSION

J. K., a 16-year-old boy with chronic glomerulonephritis of 7 years duration, was seen because of weakness, anorexia, and nausea. He appeared chronically ill, and respirations were increased in rate and depth. Blood pressure was 105/70 mm Hg. Blood urea nitrogen was 135 mg/dl, bicarbonate 14 mEq/L, chloride 115 mEq/L, sodium 141 mEq/L, and potassium 4.0 mEq/L. Because of hyperchloremic acidosis, he was placed on 50 mmoles of sodium bicarbonate daily. Symptoms subsided, and he returned to school. Four months later, while still receiving this dosage of bicarbonate, blood urea nitrogen was 62 mg/dl and bicarbonate 21 mEq/L. This therapy had provided the necessary bicarbonate to cover the excess anion load in his diet and had thereby relieved the acidosis.

The use of sodium bicarbonate is not without hazard in patients with a previous history of congestive heart failure or severe hypertension. In these patients such therapy should be given cautiously and only for short periods of time; the hazards of continuous administration are illustrated by the following case.

HAZARDS OF BICARBONATE THERAPY IN HYPERCHLOREMIC ACIDOSIS WITH HYPERTENSION

D. S., a 49-year-old housewife with a 12-year history of hypertension presented with muscular cramps, easy fatigability, and nocturia. She was dehydrated, chronically ill, and she breathed deeply and rapidly. The blood pressure was 190/100 and the heart was enlarged. Blood urea nitrogen was 160 mg/dl, bicarbonate 11.5 mEq/L, and chloride 111 mEq/L. The patient received sodium bicarbonate, 50 mmoles daily, and her initial response was good, with bicarbonate rising to 21 mEq/L. Appetite improved and clinical manifestation of acidosis disappeared. The initial good response was followed by the appearance of breathlessness, and 2 weeks after instituting therapy she developed acute pulmonary edema with hepato-

megaly and ankle edema. These symptoms responded to sodium restriction, but without bicarbonate supplementation she returned to her previous uremic acidotic state. Exhibition of sodium bicarbonate again corrected this state of affairs, but was followed promptly by return of symptoms of congestive heart failure.

To the extent that exchange of hydrogen for sodium is impaired, the diseased kidney sustains impairment of its sodium conserving function. Electroneutrality requires that the excess nonvolatile anions of dietary origin be excreted with a cation, and since sodium is the principal cation of the glomerular filtrate, it is the principal cation lost under these conditions. This type of salt-wasting is common in severe renal impairment, but it can nearly always be compensated for by permitting ad lib salt intake with the diet. Clinically significant salt depletion is unlikely to occur unless rigid salt restriction (intake <25 mEq per day) is instituted for relatively prolonged periods. In contrast, occasional cases exhibit remarkable salt-wasting tendencies, requiring an intake of greater than 200 mEq of sodium per day for maintenance of a normal body sodium content. Such cases are most commonly encountered with medullary cystic disease, but may on occasion be seen in advanced renal damage secondary to chronic pyelonephritis. In such cases moderate sodium restriction rapidly leads to severe sodium depletion with attendant postural hypotension and progressive uremia. Such a case is illustrated below.

SALT-WASTING RENAL DISEASE

A. R., a 29-year-old white male was admitted in uremic coma with chronic renal disease of unknown duration. He exhibited Kussmaul respiration, profound dehydration, blood pressure of 100/65, pulse 120, and a marked increase in skin pigmentation. Blood urea nitrogen was 270 mg/dl, bicarbonate 5.6 mEq/L, serum sodium 127 mEq/L, and chloride 82 mEq/L with a urinary sodium concentration of 90 mEq/L.

The poor skin turgor, hyponatremia, and large quantity of sodium in the urine supported the diagnosis of salt-wasting renal disease. Poor skin turgor was consistent with an isotonic extracellular fluid depletion of perhaps 2 liters, and the hyponatremia indicated a sodium deficit of 450 mEq. The total sodium deficit probably exceeded 600 mEq.

The patient received 450 mmoles of sodium chloride during the first day of therapy plus 250 mmoles of sodium bicarbonate in a total of 5 liters of fluid. This was followed by daily administration of 250 mmoles of sodium chloride and 140 mmoles of sodium bicarbonate daily. His coma cleared and he improved promptly as his blood urea nitrogen decreased to 65 mg/dl. He subsequently maintained stable renal function over a period of 2 years on this level of sodium intake, but on three occasions, cessation of sodium intake resulted in return of the above clinical picture. In each instance it responded dramatically to administration of large quantities of sodium chloride and sodium bicarbonate.

Protein Intake

When proteinuria is a prominent feature of renal disease, the earliest symptoms may be secondary to the progressive nitrogen deficit which results. There may be wasting of tissues as judged by loss of muscle mass, weakness, and reduced exercise tolerance. A positive nitrogen balance can usually be induced in such patients by a dietary protein intake of 2.0 to 3.0 g per kg of body weight. In general, azotemia, per se, is not a contraindication to increasing protein intake. As the severity of the renal insufficiency progresses, however, the increased acid load (associated with sulfates, phosphates, and excess chloride in the diet) leads to systemic acidosis. It then is usually necessary to curtail nitrogen intake and institute some therapy for correction, as discussed previously. Guiding principles for the management of the more common manifestations of uremia are listed in Table 11-1.

Anemia

Anemia is a regular feature of advanced renal insufficiency and may present a difficult therapeutic problem when uremia is present. The fall in hematocrit roughly parallels the diminution in renal function. The basis for this anemia is twofold. The kidney produces a hormone, erythropoietin, that stimulates red cell production; the hormone is decreased or absent in chronic renal disease. In addition, red cell survival time is shortened. These two factors may reduce the hematocrit to values less than 20 percent in severe uremia, and prominent symptoms then ensue. Chief among these is severe weakness and easy fatigability, but the high cardiac output produced by the anemia may lead to cardiac decompensation and coronary insufficiency.

Correction of the anemia is difficult and not without hazard. Although synthetic androgenic steroids have been shown to increase erythropoiesis and pro-duce modest increases in the hematocrit in uremic patients, their continued use is associated with significant hepatic toxicity. In addition to the usual hazards of transfusion, special problems are encountered in the uremic patient. The increased red cell destruction results in a relatively rapid increase in nitrogen load with its associated increased loads of phosphate and sulfate, all tending to aggravate the preexisting azotemia and acidosis. The elevated plasma potassium present in stored blood may produce acute hyperkalemia. An even more common problem is acute circulatory overload. Transfusion may precipitate acute pulmonary edema in patients who have already demonstrated a tendency to develop salt retention and congestive heart failure. Nevertheless, symptoms of anemia ultimately reach such proportions that transfusion becomes necessary. Packed cells should be used and the hematocrit should not be raised above 30 percent. On occasion the anemia may be the main precipitating factor in the development of cardiac decompensation. Such cases usually show disappointing responses to the usual therapeutic regimen for heart failure, and transfusion should be undertaken only with the greatest caution.

Excretion of Drugs

The hazards of drug overdosage are real in the uremic patient. Drugs which are excreted by the kidney are particularly likely to cause trouble. In the presence of severe renal insufficiency, streptomycin may reach toxic levels in the plasma when given in ordinary doses. For such drugs the relation between blood levels and renal clearance is similar to that for urea (Fig. 10–3). Blood levels 6 to 8 times the usual therapeutic range may develop unless dosage is adjusted appropriately.[38]

THE TREATMENT OF TERMINAL RENAL FAILURE

The anecdotal material presented in the preceding section identified the most important therapeutic approaches to alleviating or correcting the disturbances associated with chronic renal insufficiency. Inevitably, these become inadequate as the renal insufficiency progresses toward terminal renal failure. When the glomerular filtration rate (creatinine clearance) falls below 1 to 2 ml per minute, it is not usually possible to maintain life for more than a few days or weeks without some form of dialysis therapy. Judicious concern for the patient dictates that the physician anticipate this impending crisis well in advance of its occurrence, however, so that the patient and his family can be prepared emotionally to face this difficult problem.

Although it is not possible to predict accurately the subsequent course of severe renal disease from a single set of laboratory observations in a given patient, the data recently published by Maher and associates are extremely useful statistical guides in such an attempt.[30] They provide the physician with a basis for advising the patient regarding his future course after his serum creatinine reaches or surpasses 10 mg/dl. Figure 11-1 illustrates the expected progression of chronic renal insufficiency subsequent to that point in the course of the illness when the plasma creatinine level first exceeds 10 mg/dl in a group of patients with chronic renal insufficiency. It was prepared from Maher's data on patients with chronic renal failure. The group from which these data were obtained represents a mixture of the common causes of renal failure, including glomerulonephritis, vascular renal disease, pyelonephritis, obstructive uropa-thy, and polycystic kidneys. Statistically, about 20 percent show significant improvement in renal function. This improvement usually reflects response to such therapeutic efforts as relief of obstruction, treatment of infection, and correction of fluid and electrolyte disturbances. Of the remainder of patients, i.e., those failing to respond, approximately half will succumb or require dialysis within the first two months after their creatinine reaches 10 mg/dl. Nearly all the remainder will require dialysis or renal homotransplantation within five months of the time the serum creatinine reaches 10 mg/dl.

The 20 percent who showed some improvement merit further comment. This group, on the average, survived well beyond a year after the initial therapeutic effort before requiring dialysis therapy, thus underscoring the importance of attention to the conservative therapeutic maneuvers outlined in preced-

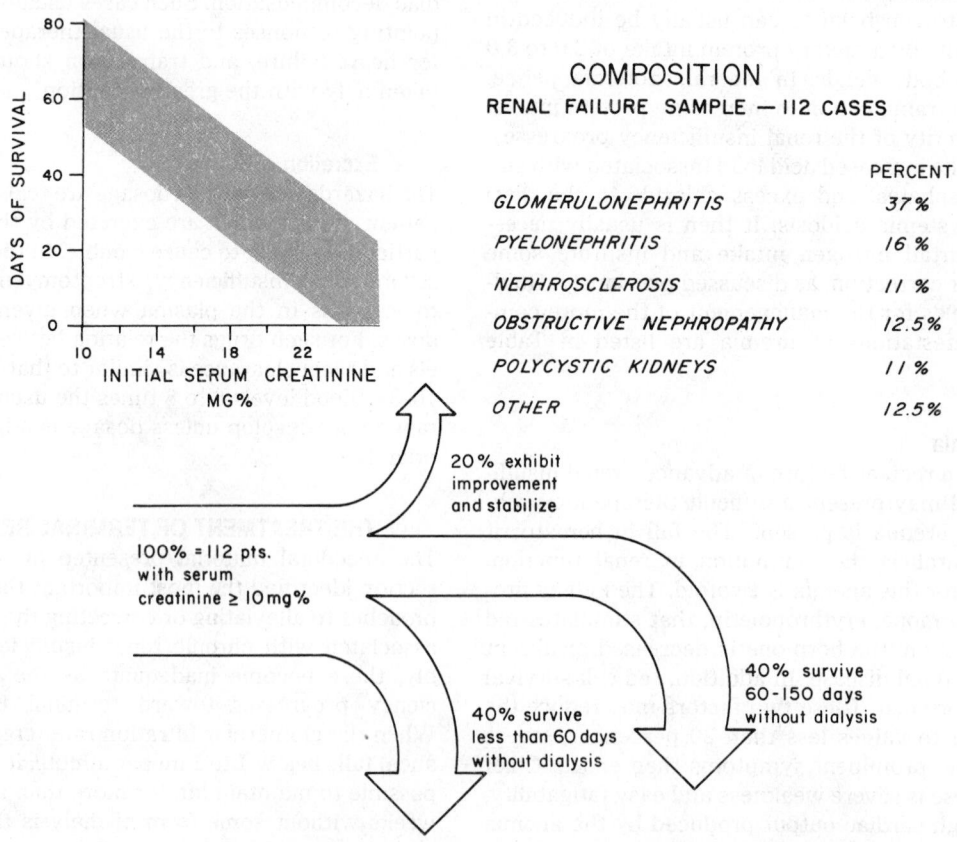

FIGURE 11-1. Expected outcome of patients with chronic renal failure who have serum creatinine values equal to or greater than 10 mg/dl when initially seen. Illustration is prepared from data of Maher et al.[30] based on study of 112 patients with chronic renal failure. Etiology varied and distribution of diseases are shown. When creatinine exceeds 10 mg/dl, prognosis is guarded and dialysis will usually be required within 2 to 4 months if patient is to survive.

ing sections of this chapter. Occasionally, when dealing with severe or acutely emergent situations in the patient with severe chronic renal disease, it may be necessary to dialyse the patient one or more times before such stability can be achieved. For those individuals showing no improvement, plans for dialysis and/or transplantation must be made with reasonable dispatch if the patient can be benefited by this form of therapy.

Not all patients reaching this advanced stage of terminal renal failure are suitable candidates for treatment by dialysis or transplantation. To cite an obvious example, the patient with diabetes mellitus and complications that include severe peripheral vascular disease with compromised circulation to his lower extremities, cerebral arteriosclerosis with deterioration of mental function, and blindness from retinopathy who has in addition terminal renal failure is not likely to be helped at all by hemodialysis or transplantation. Similarly, the patient with hypertensive disease and secondary renal failure with severe cerebral vascular disease so that he is incapable of coherent mental function should not be seriously considered a candidate for chronic dialysis. Short of these extremes, there are many patients in whom the decision regarding the reasonableness of chronic dialysis is quite difficult. While a detailed consideration of all the factors entering the decision about the appropriateness of dialysis is beyond the scope of this presentation, a useful approach may be outlined. In general, the proper orientation toward the correct decision is afforded by an attempt to answer the question, will the quality of the patient's existence be improved if he is dialysed with sufficient frequency to control his symptoms of uremia?

In the sections below are presented some of the general principles relating to peritoneal dialysis, chronic hemodialysis, and renal homotransplantation.

THE TREATMENT OF CHRONIC UREMIA BY DIALYSIS

Both peritoneal dialysis and hemodialysis provide satisfactory relief from the symptoms of uremia and either may be employed to stabilize the patient with chronic renal insufficiency. Hemodialysis is a more efficient process, but peritoneal dialysis is simple, safe, and requires little in the way of specialized equipment or specially trained personnel.

Peritoneal Dialysis

Peritoneal dialysis makes use of the peritoneal surface as a dialyzing membrane across which exchange occurs between the interstitial fluid and the dialysis fluid introduced into the peritoneum.[27] The kinetics of this exchange are illustrated in Figure 11-2.

The optimum rate of clearance obtained under ideal conditions, is about 35 ml per minute. Although less than that obtainable by the normal kidney, this is adequate to correct virtually all the manifestations of uremia within a 24-hour period. Since the peritoneum permits equilibration of both solutes and fluid in a reasonable period of time, this surface can also be used either to remove fluid from or to add fluid to the patient, depending upon the need. The rate of fluid withdrawal or addition is regulated by varying the total solute concentration of the dialysis fluid. Thus, when the quantity of glucose added to the dialyzing fluid is of the order of 5 percent, net fluid removal from the subject will usually result. The addition of a 1.5 percent glucose concentration is adequate to effect net equilibrium dialysis, that is, exchange of fluid at 30- to 45-minute intervals with the volume of fluid removed equaling that placed in the peritoneal cavity.

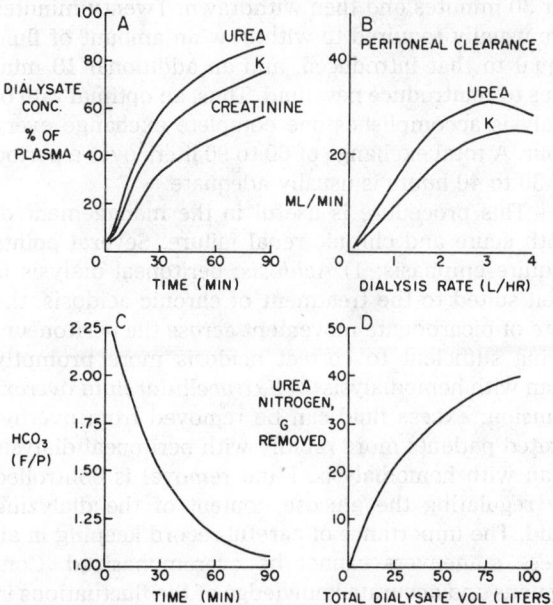

FIGURE 11-2. Kinetics of peritoneal dialysis. **A** shows the rate at which plasma urea, potassium, and creatinine equilibrate with dialyzing fluid as a function of time remaining in the abdomen. Quantitatively, the greatest net movement occurs in the first 30 minutes. **B** shows peritoneal clearance as a function of the rate of dialysis. The drop at rates for dialysis in excess of 3 liters per hour represents inadequate time for mixing and equilibration. **C** shows the relatively rapid movement of bicarbonate from the peritoneal cavity into the body fluids. F/P refers to ratio of [HCO$_3$] in dialysate to that in plasma. **D** provides an approximation of the quantity of urea removed as a function of the total volume of dialyzing fluid. This varies with the initial level of urea. (After Boen.[27])

The optimum technique for performing peritoneal dialysis on an average size adult may be summarized briefly as follows: A polyvinyl catheter with multiple perforations is inserted via a trocar and introduced through the midline into the right or left lower quadrant in such a position as to permit ready introduction or removal of dialysis fluid. Excellent positioning to ensure free flow is facilitated if insertion of the catheter is preceded by placing a liter of fluid in the peritoneum by means of a small polyethylene catheter inserted through an 18 gauge needle. The fluid should preferably be hypertonic, i.e., dialysis fluid containing 7 percent dextrose since this will continue to increase in volume during the period before insertion of the catheter. After the catheter is positioned, 2 additional liters of dialysis fluid are permitted to flow into the abdomen rapidly. To prevent chilling, the fluid should be warmed to body temperature. Introduction of the fluid is occasionally associated with some pain, but this can be controlled by analgesics. The fluid is permitted to remain in the abdomen for 30 minutes and then withdrawn. Twenty minutes are usually required to withdraw an amount of fluid equal to that introduced, and an additional 10 minutes to reintroduce new fluid. Thus, an optimal rate of dialysis accomplishes one complete exchange every hour. A total exchange of 60 to 90 liters over a period of 30 to 40 hours is usually adequate.

This procedure is useful in the management of both acute and chronic renal failure. Several points require emphasis: 1) *Acidosis:* peritoneal dialysis is well suited to the treatment of chronic acidosis, the rate of bicarbonate movement across the peritoneum being sufficient to correct acidosis more promptly than with hemodialysis; 2) *Extracellular fluid overexpansion:* excess fluid can be removed from overhydrated patients more rapidly with peritoneal dialysis than with hemodialysis. Fluid removal is controlled by regulating the glucose content of the dialyzing fluid. The importance of careful record keeping in all these maneuvers cannot be overemphasized. Continuous and accurate knowledge of the fluctuations in these data is necessary to provide adequate monitoring of the patient's extracellular fluid as the dialysis progresses. If careful attention is not paid to the cumulative fluid balance during the procedure, profound excesses or deficits may be created. Intake and output data during peritoneal dialysis should be supplemented by frequently weighing the patient; 3) *Hyperkalemia:* if potassium-free fluid is introduced, equilibration is not completed during the 30 minutes that the fluid remains in the abdomen. It will reach approximately 50 to 60 percent of the plasma concentration and may, on occasion, attain values as high as 3 to 4 mEq/L, but is usually below this. Thus, potassium removal is relatively inefficient, only 6 to 10 mEq being extracted during one exchange; during a 10-hour period, the amount removed is just equal to, or slightly in excess of, the quantity in the extracellular fluid. If the principal indication for dialysis is severe hyperkalemia of acute onset, hemodialysis may be preferable.

The two major hazards of peritoneal dialysis are infection and perforation of a hollow viscus. The risk of infection is small provided strict aseptic technique is followed. The patients should be watched very carefully, however, for the earliest sign of infection and vigorous treatment begun immediately. It is probably wiser and safer to follow this course than to maintain low concentrations of antibiotics in the dialysis fluids at all times. Perforation of a viscus is extremely rare in individuals who have not previously been operated upon, with the exception of perforation of the urinary bladder. Even this risk is only significant when the bladder is greatly distended. In general, the technique should not be used in patients who have had previous abdominal operations. If hemodialysis is not available and dialysis is imperative in such cases, the catheter may be placed under direct vision by a small surgical incision.

Peritoneal dialysis is of great value in the treatment of acute uremia both because of its simplicity and efficiency and because it can be done with virtually no highly specialized equipment. It is somewhat more difficult to use this form of dialysis to provide permanent long-range support in patients with end-stage renal disease. It has, however, been used with considerable success in such patients.[37] It is well suited as an alternate to hemodialysis in those patients in whom vascular access is difficult or impossible.

Chronic Hemodialysis

This requires a highly trained staff that includes physicians and nurses as well as dialysis technologists. For this reason, it is not feasible to maintain such a unit and its staff unless it serves a sufficiently large population to permit efficient operation. This limitation renders hemodialysis less readily available than peritoneal dialysis. The efficiency and capacity of a hemodialysis program are considerably increased by inclusion of a home-training program. The success of such a program of therapy for uremia and the potential it offers for rehabilitation are directly related to care exercised in providing the dialysis and in maintaining an appropriate regimen between dialyses. A brief consideration of the more important problems encountered in patients maintained on chronic dialysis and a review of the regimen necessary to maintain them in a reasonable state of health illustrates what may be expected of this form of therapy.

ARTERIOVENOUS SHUNTS AND FISTULAS. The continuing success of chronic dialysis depends upon the maintenance of an adequate AV communication either in the form of an external shunt or an internal AV fistula. The external silastic shunts usually provide the largest blood flows, thereby permitting the most effective dialysis. The disadvantages of external synthetic shunts are a tendency to recurrent infection around the site of entry of the shunt and some difficulty with clotting.

Daily maintenance care of the shunt, including washing of the portal of exit and entry of the shunt with hydrogen peroxide, serves to minimize infection. Careful inspection and recognition of infection at the earliest possible moment with prompt therapy usually permit adequate treatment of the infection by a combination of antibiotics and hot soaks. If treatment is instituted appropriately early, it is rare that the infection causes loss of the shunt.

Clotting of the shunt constitutes a major problem. Although it is frequently possible to declot the shunt, reestablish flow, and prevent subsequent clotting by anticoagulation, recurrent clotting always heralds the impending loss of the shunt. Declotting can be achieved much more effectively with the straight Ramirez shunt than with the Quinton-Scribner shunt. For this reason, the average shunt life is longer with the straight shunts.

For most patients an AV fistula is preferred. They provide some advantages that outweigh the major disadvantage of the lower flow rate that can be achieved during dialysis from this type of AV communication. The principal advantage lies in the convenience for the patient and the virtual absence of clotting. Indeed, if the need for hemodialysis can be anticipated sufficiently early, it is most desirable to create an AV fistula 2 to 3 months before dialysis is to start, thereby giving the fistula sufficient time to grow and mature and avoiding the necessity for inserting a shunt altogether.

MAINTENANCE REGIMEN. The maintenance in these patients is similar to that discussed below for acute renal failure. The patient with chronic renal insufficiency has no significant route of excretion for water and solutes except that provided by the intermittent dialyses. For this reason, careful regulation of fluid and food intake as well as the salts of sodium and potassium and drugs are of primary importance. In general, it is only possible to remove approximately 1.5 to 2 kg from the patient as fluid during the course of a single dialysis. This defines the quantity of ingested fluid permissible during the interval between dialyses. For routine maintenance, it is permissible to allow the patient to gain approximately 1.5 kg between dialyses and this amount can be removed relatively easily during an effective dialysis. Where the patient has already accumulated excess fluid and an attempt is being made to progressively reduce his fluid content, much more rigid restriction is necessary as outlined below.

Food intake should be arranged to provide a protein intake of approximately 40 to 50 g and a sodium intake between 1 and 2 g a day. The potassium intake should be kept as low as is compatible with palatability of the diet.

Knowledge of the behavior of drugs in the anephric state is particularly limited so that all drugs should be employed with great caution in this group of patients. For those not known to be conjugated by the liver and excreted by way of the gastrointestinal tract, substantial reduction in dosage is necessary to avoid toxicity.

COMPLICATIONS OF LONG-TERM DIALYSIS. *Anemia* is one of the most prevalent and characteristic features of chronic renal disease. It achieves its severest form in the anephric patient maintained on chronic hemodialysis for long periods. The primary cause appears to be absence of erythropoietic activity in the blood of these patients, but such things as folate deficiency, iron deficiency, and blood loss may aggravate the anemia. Folic acid administration should be maintained as long as the patient remains on chronic hemodialysis to replace the folate removed by dialysis. Blood drawn for laboratory determinations and blood remaining in the dialyser at the end of the procedure contribute to the blood loss and intermittent iron therapy should also be provided. Nevertheless, the anemia persists and the hematocrit may reach levels of 11 to 13 percent. Hematocrit values in this range are remarkably well tolerated in the absence of significant cardiovascular disease.

Frequent transfusions increase the risk of hepatitis and also increase the antibody response to foreign HLA antigens, thereby reducing the likelihood of successful tissue matching if the patient is awaiting a cadaver kidney. However, it is possible that this may improve the chances of a successful cadaver homograft if a match can be made. There is evidence which indicates that those individuals who receive a large number of transfusions and then are successfully tissue-matched and cross-matched with a cadaver kidney are more likely to have a successful result following transplantation.[39]

Hyperkalemia represents probably the most serious threat to life in the patient maintained on chronic dialysis. This may result either from dietary indiscretion or infection with increased catabolism or may be the result of inadequate dialysis. The serum potassium is probably the most important parameter to monitor in the patient who is on long-term dialysis and, if the potassium is not reduced to levels in the vicinity of 4 mEq/L at the end of dialysis, dietary readjustment is in order. If for some reason the patient does not respond to this, then the use of oral resin therapy to combat the hyperkalemia is necessary. This, of course, creates a problem with increased sodium retention if continued over long periods of time. If the hyperkalemia cannot be controlled effectively by these measures, then more frequent dialysis or more efficient dialysis is the only means of correcting this potentially life-threatening situation. It is likely that this represents the leading cause of death among patients dying while on chronic dialysis.

Fluid overload probably represents the second most hazardous problem in these patients. Since it is difficult to remove more than about 1.5 kg of fluid during dialysis, weight gain must be limited to this value or less during the interdialysis intervals. In the individual who has accumulated an excess of fluid for whatever reason, it will only be possible to remove the extra fluid provided his fluid intake between dialyses is sufficiently curtailed that he exhibits little or no weight gain during this period. This usually requires a fluid intake of 400 ml per day or less and means that the patient must be watched very carefully to be certain that this restriction is enforced. Only in this fashion is it possible to progressively remove excess fluid and reduce the weight by a corresponding amount in patients who have developed fluid overload.

Hypertension is closely related to the problem of fluid overload and in general is aggravated markedly by excess salt and water intake. It is possible at times to control the hypertension by effectively dialyzing the patients and removing sufficient fluid so that they are reduced to "dry weight." Occasionally, this is ineffective, and we have seen severe hypertension persist despite removal of more than 8 or 10 kg of fluid and no demonstrable edema. In these individuals who do not respond well to such salt and water removal, the only additional procedure available that is almost always of benefit is bilateral nephrectomy. It is the usual experience that those patients whose blood pressure does not respond well to fluid removal also show little response to antihypertensive medications until such large dosages are used that postural hypotension becomes an overwhelming problem.

Renal osteodystrophy,[28,29,31-33,35] a condition seen relatively rarely prior to the advent of chronic dialysis, has increased markedly in frequency as patients have been maintained for relatively long periods of time with inadequate renal function. These changes, characterized as a combination of osteomalacia and osteitis fibrosa, are unique to renal disease and have been attributed to relative vitamin D deficiency as well as excess parathormone production. When this condition becomes symptomatic with bone pain, gross evidence of bone resorption, and pathologic fractures, treatment may require administration of 1, 25-dihydroxycholecalciferol as the active form of vitamin D or parathyroidectomy or both. Since this condition most often appears after a relatively long period of time on dialysis and is usually preceded and likely caused by severe hyperphosphatemia, treatment in all patients with end-stage renal disease should be directed at controlling the hyperphosphatemia with a low phosphate diet, phosphate binders, such as an aluminum oxide gel (Amphogel), and adequate dialysis.[29,33,35]

PROGNOSIS. It has been estimated that the death rate among a group of patients with chronic uremia who are maintained on chronic dialysis is approximately 10 percent per year. Of those who are adequately treated by dialysis, somewhere between one-half and two-thirds are able to return to work and may be regarded as completely rehabilitated. Thus, for those patients capable of being treated by chronic dialysis, the treatment results in an average survival of about 8 to 10 years. For the most part, this represents a productive addition to the patient's life and, for those who are capable of dialyzing themselves at home at night, it may interfere relatively little with their daily activities.

Renal Transplantation

Successful renal transplantation represents the most effective means of correcting the patient's uremia. In addition to the well-established efficacy of transplants between identical twins, it is now clear that transplantation occurring between members of the same family produces superior results under certain circumstances. More recently, it has been well documented that the use of cadaver kidneys produces acceptable results.

Tissue typing based upon identification of human leukocyte antigens has greatly facilitated selection of donors among siblings within the family of the potential recipient with chronic renal failure. This technique selects siblings with apparent identity of histocompatibility antigens. When a renal transplant involving two such individuals is carried out, the 5-year survival of the renal graft exceeds 90 percent. This is substantially better than results achieved by transplantation of kidneys between siblings who share only two of the four HL-A antigens. It is very much better than the best reported results from transplants of cadaver kidneys.[36] Whether adequate histocompatibility typing between cadaver kidneys and potential recipients can improve the results with cadaver kidneys remains to be demonstrated with certainty.[34]

Continuous immunosuppression is necessary to maintain stable renal function in these patients, and this presently consists of a combination of prednisone and azathioprine. The long-term use of these drugs adds significantly to the risks incurred following transplantation. The principal hazards are persistent risk of infection, aseptic necrosis of joints (particu-

larly the hips and knees), cataracts, and an increased risk of developing malignant neoplasms. These risks mandate careful follow-up in patients who have received kidney transplants. Although bacterial infections can usually be treated successfully with antibiotics without stopping the immunosuppressive drugs, viral infections at times become life-threatening and require withdrawal of immunosuppression. This leads to prompt rejection of the graft but usually is followed by recovery from the viral illness.

Despite the risks cited above, the present results are sufficiently good to permit considerable optimism regarding the treatment of chronic uremia. Results with both chronic dialysis and transplantation continue to improve.

CHAPTER 12
Acute Suppression of Urine Formation
W. GORDON WALKER AND ANDREW WHELTON

Acute renal insufficiency associated with suppression or cessation of urine formation constitutes a most important segment of renal disease. Since the lesions responsible are usually reversible, prompt recognition and appropriate management are vital.

The minimum volume of urine necessary for adequate solute excretion on a normal intake is approximately 450 ml per day. This value varies moderately in normal individuals, depending upon the type and quantity of solute. A sustained urinary output of less than 15 ml per hour in an adult patient with previously normal renal function is evidence of significant oliguria. While this figure is arbitrary, it provides a basis for diagnosis at an early stage. A variety of abnormalities may result in the development of oliguria or anuria (Table 12–1). An orderly approach to appropriate management is facilitated by dividing these into three groups: 1) *prerenal azotemia* denotes suppression of urine formation due to inadequate perfusion of an anatomically and physiologically normal kidney and collection system; 2) *postrenal* oliguria results from obstructive lesions of the collecting system at some point below the calyceal system; and 3) *renal* disturbances are the most common causes of oliguria, since many disorders of the kidneys are associated with failure of urine formation.

PRERENAL AZOTEMIA

Prerenal azotemia results from a variety of disturbances that lead to temporary reduction or cessation of urine formation persisting long enough to permit azotemia to develop. The most common causes are prolonged dehydration and sodium depletion. A typical example of such rapid reversible azotemia is that seen in diabetic acidosis, particularly when it has persisted for several days, resulting in severe dehydration. The fluid and sodium losses produce a depletion of extracellular fluid volume with a resultant decrease in renal perfusion. This, coupled with the catabolic response to the uncontrolled diabetes, leads to rapid development of azotemia. With adequate fluid and salt replacement, the azotemia promptly disappears and no stigmata of acute renal failure develop. Similar changes occur with severe diarrhea or recurrent vomiting.

The distinctive difference between the prerenal oligurias and those associated with structural change in the kidney (acute renal failure) lies in the rapidity with which the abnormalities are reversed with appropriate therapy in prerenal azotemia. In addition to electrolyte disturbances, persistent hypotension, severe congestive heart failure, rapidly developing asci-

---TABLE 12-1---
Causes of Acute Oliguria or Anuria

Prerenal Azotemia

Shock
Acute hypovolemia
Gastrointestinal fluid loss
Severe dehydration
Addisonian crisis
?Reflex anuria
Postoperative antidiuresis
Segregated fluid accumulations

Acute Renal Failure

Nephrotoxic agents
    Heavy metals—Hg, As, Ur, Au
    Ethylene glycol
    Carbon tetrachloride
    Sulfonamides
    Kanamycin, neomycin, aminoglycoside, and
        polypeptide antibiotics
Circulatory insufficiency
    Vascular insufficiency
    Blood loss and shock
    Acute sodium depletion
        Diarrhea and vomiting
        Heat stroke
        Diabetes mellitus
    Trauma and crush injury
    Transfusion reactions
    Burns
Other disorders
    Acute glomerulonephritis
    Malignant hypertension
    Polyarteritis
    Wegener's granulomatosis
    Eclampsia
    Bilateral renal cortical necrosis
    Infections

Postrenal Obstruction

Renal calculi
Acute pyelonephritis
Cancer of pelvic organs
Irradiation, edema, and fibrosis
Prostatic obstruction
Surgical accidents

tes, and other conditions which tend to deplete plasma or extravascular fluid volume, or both, may result in prerenal azotemia. It is possible that the sequence of events may also be triggered by some reflex action. Anuria or marked oliguria may persist for relatively long periods following major surgical procedures; in some instances this occurs despite maintenance of adequate hydration at all times.

When the disturbance resulting in prerenal azotemia is correctly diagnosed and effectively treated, renal function is promptly restored to normal. Unless prompt therapy is instituted, however, protracted re-

nal ischemia may lead to necrosis of the tubules, resulting in renal failure. For this reason, prerenal causes should be sought in all cases which present initially with oliguria or anuria. As a rough diagnostic guide, oliguria associated with a urinary sodium concentration of less than 10 mEq/L or urinary osmolality of greater than 500 mOsm/kg H_2O is more likely to represent prerenal azotemia. None of the renal function tests in use for distinguishing between prerenal and renal failure is entirely satisfactory, and the final decision must be based on clinical judgment and evaluation of the patient's response to therapy designed to overcome the prerenal abnormality. The treatment of hypovolemia, sodium depletion, and other conditions leading to lowered urine output have been covered in the section on fluid and electrolyte metabolism (Section 1).

The infusion of 40 to 50 g of mannitol as a 20 percent solution when acute renal failure is suspected has gained wide acceptance. For the most part, the clinical situations in which this therapy has been used have not been clearly defined. Mannitol given early in the course of postoperative oliguria will usually be followed by an increase in urine flow simply because, in the majority of cases, oliguria is short-lived and is due to a combination of excessive ADH output and reversible reduction in renal blood flow produced by general anesthesia.

There is little evidence that mannitol can reverse the progress of acute renal failure once the oliguric phase has been firmly established; the anuria or oliguria resulting from hemolytic transfusion reactions or perhaps myoglobinuria are possible exceptions. Experimental evidence indicates that anuria associated with massive hemoglobinuria can be averted if mannitol is given within an hour after the hemolytic event occurs. There is some suggestion that the kidney undergoing osmotic diuresis is less susceptible to ischemic damage and, hence, osmotic diuresis induced by mannitol may be of some preventive value. This, however, remains to be fully evaluated. The hazards of circulatory overload and acute pulmonary edema are sufficiently great that mannitol should always be used with caution. It is questionable whether it should ever be used in the management of elderly patients with cardiovascular impairments.

POSTRENAL OBSTRUCTION

There are relatively few conditions that lead to complete cessation of urine formation as a result of urinary tract obstruction. If only one kidney or its ureter is obstructed, the remaining normal kidney is capable of performing the necessary excretory function adequately. There is no appreciable drop in urine output, and the associated symptoms are not those of renal failure, but of local obstruction. Obstruction of the lower urinary tract leading to anuria is most frequently caused by prostatic enlargement, and the discomfort resulting from overdistention of the bladder usually calls attention to this cause. Bilateral ureteral obstruction is rare and may be associated with carcinoma of the bladder, prostate, or cervix. Such obstruction may result from direct invasion by the tumor or from inflammation induced by local irradiation. Pain is variable with this type of obstruction and may even be absent. Inadvertent ureteral ligation should always be considered when postoperative anuria complicates gynecologic surgery.

Complete absence of urine formation is rare in cases of renal failure due to intrinsic renal disease, so that making a distinction between acute renal failure and postrenal obstruction is seldom difficult. Obstruction should be suspected in all patients who exhibit *complete anuria* early in their illness. Although rare, simultaneous obstruction of both ureters does occur. If complete obstruction of one ureter develops without producing symptoms, obstruction of the opposite ureter at a later date will precipitate acute anuria. Occasionally, obstruction of the ureters by uric acid crystals is encountered, particularly with the marked uricosuria which follows treatment of the lymphomas with one of the antimetabolic agents.

Diagnosis of these conditions can only be established by ureteral catheterization. This procedure is not without risk, particularly in cases with low or absent urinary output due to diffuse parenchymal damage to the kidney. Infection is more likely to be introduced in such cases since there is no mechanism for washing out the pelvis and lower collecting system with a brisk urine flow. Thus, decisions regarding ureteral catheterization must be made cautiously. If bilateral renal shadows of normal size can be identified in x-ray films, either side, but not both, may be catheterized. If there is disparity in the size of the two kidneys, the larger should always be catheterized. If the obstruction is mechanical, catheterization should result in prompt urine flow. If this does not occur, the catheter should never be permitted to remain in the ureter since the danger of introducing infection is great. Only when definite obstruction is identified should the catheters be permitted to remain in place until more definitive therapy can be instituted.

In obstruction of relatively long standing, relief may be followed by profuse diuresis; urine flow rates may approach 50 percent of the glomerular filtration rate.[41] Presumably this is attributable to tubular atrophy resulting from back pressure caused by the obstruction, and the attendant solute load (principally urea), which acts as a solute diuretic. This diuresis may lead to such profound water and sodium losses that shock supervenes within a few minutes. Appropriate fluid and sodium replacement alleviates these symptoms and the condition is usually reversible, although weeks may be required before functional restoration is complete. The management of this problem is considered in Chapter 11.

ACUTE RENAL FAILURE

The causes of acute renal failure are numerous (Table 12–1). Regardless of the condition causing the acute renal failure, only two mechanisms appear responsible for the structural changes in the kidney. Each mechanism has been demonstrated experimentally and the histologic changes classified as either *nephrotoxic* or *ischemic*. Although for many years it has been stated that the predominant lesion in both is necrosis of the tubular epithelium, it is now apparent that tubular necrosis is, indeed, the typical lesion of nephrotoxic acute renal failure but that it is an unusual histologic finding in ischemic acute renal failure.

The nephrotoxic changes are produced by specific toxic agents or chemicals (Table 12–1). The initial pathologic changes include necrosis of the epithelium lining the tubules with relatively complete preservation of the basement membrane. The glomeruli appear to be uninvolved. Regeneration of the epithelial cells can be demonstrated after about two weeks. When the tubular basement membrane is not damaged by the nephrotoxin, the epithelium grows to cover it completely, thereby reestablishing continuity of the tubule. When the basement membrane is disrupted by the necrotic process, continuity is not reestablished during regeneration and the tubule does not regain its function. In experimental studies, the length of time required for regeneration, as well as its adequacy, are directly related to the dosage of nephrotoxic substance. In general, regeneration is nearly complete by the twenty-first through the twenty-fifth day after the initial insult. In clinical situations, regeneration may take longer, and slowly increasing renal function may be demonstrated over a longer period.

It has already been indicated that in the *ischemic* form of acute renal failure the histologic findings have for many years been described as those of acute tubular necrosis. However, cellular necrosis can rarely be demonstrated in biopsy material from patients during the oliguric period of their acute renal failure. The glomeruli remain normal, and, in general, the only histologic features of note are the scattered and occasional findings of evidence of tubular epithelial cellular regeneration. This indicates that tubular cellular necrosis is of a very sporadic nature and does not readily account for the acute failure of renal function. Development of techniques which allow identification of changes in total renal and intrarenal blood flow patterns have considerably increased our understanding of the sequence of events that culminate in ischemic acute renal failure. This variety of renal failure appears better described as a *vasomotor nephropathy* rather than a syndrome of acute tubular necrosis.[42]

Studies in humans with acute oliguric renal failure from various causes reveal that total renal blood flow is decreased, usually one-half to one-third the normal flow rates. Changes in intrarenal blood flow occur with marked reduction in cortical and an increase in the inner cortical or juxtamedullary flow. There is no evidence for significant blood shunting through aglomerular sectors of the kidney. Afferent arteriole vasoconstriction develops, and net filtration pressures fall to levels commensurate with production of only minimal amounts of filtrate and clinical evidence of oliguria or anuria. Residual renal blood flow is adequate to prevent cellular necrosis.

If the initial cause of hypotension and renal ischemia is not corrected within approximately 2 to 12 hours, protracted oliguria sometimes lasting for weeks may result from the ischemia. This oliguria is associated with persistence of the pattern of decreased intrarenal blood flow over the next several days or weeks (2 to 4) despite restoration of adequate circulating volume and return of systemic blood pressure to normal levels. The humoral and local factors responsible for this persistent reduction in renal blood flow remain to be clearly identified. The renin-angiotensin system and catecholamines have been implicated in some experimental situations but their role in human disease remains to be defined.

Clinical Features of Acute Renal Failure

The clinical course of acute renal failure is characterized by three more or less distinct phases: the oligemic, the oliguric or anuric, and the diuretic.[40]

The *oligemic* phase is variable, and in a substantial number of cases is not recognizable. Clinically, this stage is characterized by hypotension and signs of shock associated with reduction or complete cessation of urine formation. Prompt recognition and treatment at this time may prevent the development of the full course of acute tubular necrosis.

The oligemic phase is followed by the *oliguric* after a variable period of time. Typically, when renal ischemia during the oligemic phase has led to tubular necrosis, urine flow increases briefly (for 12 to 20 hours) following correction of the hypovolemia and then begins to decrease. The persistence of urine flow of less than 20 ml per hour in the face of adequate hydration is strong presumptive evidence of acute renal failure. The duration of this phase is variable and depends upon the severity of kidney damage. It may last from 2 or 3 days to more than 4 weeks in patients who ultimately recover completely. If oliguria persists for 6 to 8 days, or more, signs of uremia become increasingly severe. As uremia progresses and the patient becomes obtunded, gastrointestinal disturbances including nausea and vomiting appear and there is increasing difficulty in handling respiratory secretions. The hazard of infection increases, and is a more common cause of death at this stage than the uremia per se. The principal life-threatening consequences of the uremia are hyperkalemia, acidosis, and overhydration.

The *diuretic* phase may begin from 5 to 30 days after onset, but is usually seen after 10 days to 2 weeks. In general, it is characterized by a urine output that at first increases slowly for 3 to 4 days, and which may then suddenly increase to 6 to 8 liters or more per day. During the first 3 to 4 days of this period, the signs, symptoms, and laboratory evidence of uremia may continue because the increasing urine flow indicates the function of only a small number of nephrons. As healing continues, more and more nephrons become active with a correspondingly greater increase in urine output. This urine at first has a composition which reflects the limited ability of the tubules to function. It is characterized principally by a high sodium and chloride content, the concentration of sodium frequently being greater than 50 percent of that in the plasma. There is a correspondingly low concentration of urea. This state of affairs usually persists for a week to 10 days, gradually subsiding as tubular function improves. The clinical disorders which develop at the peak of the diuretic phase are related to obligatory losses of water and solutes in the urine. Thus, severe deficits of sodium, potassium, or water may be encountered.

Management of Acute Renal Failure

The prognosis of acute renal failure depends almost entirely upon adequate management. Meticulous attention to the details of day-to-day care of the patient is essential.

If the patient is first seen at the very onset of the oliguria, attention should be directed toward the state of hydration. Since ischemic renal failure is usually due to reduction in blood and extracellular fluid volume, any deficit in either should be promptly replaced. Sources of blood loss should be identified quickly. Initially, it may be difficult to assess the state of hydration and sodium balance. If the available evidence fails to provide the needed information about fluid loss, a therapeutic trial of fluid administration may be necessary. It is most important that such treatment not be overdone. The rapid loss of more than 2 liters of extracellular fluid usually produces severe hypotension. Therefore, in the absence of continuing loss, it is unwise to give more than 1500 ml of isotonic saline intravenously. Isotonic losses (decrease in extracellular fluid volume) are most likely to lead to oliguria. Water loss alone or hypertonic dehydration, unless profound, does not produce oliguria, and under these circumstances severe hypernatremia is usually present. In managing oliguria, fluids should not be administered rapidly unless the patient is in shock. Slow administration lessens the likelihood of acute circulatory overload in the event that an error has been made in clinical evaluation of the state of hydration. If 1500 ml of fluid produces no significant change in the urinary output, one should adopt the plan of management outlined below. The role of mannitol during this phase of the disease is discussed above.

Successful management of the oliguric phase requires careful monitoring of the intake of calories, water, and salt, together with expert nursing care. Fluid (water) requirements may vary depending upon the presence or absence of sweating, the ambient air temperature, fever, or other factors which may increase insensible water loss. *A daily record should be kept of the patient's weight.* Since the catabolic response results in progressive loss of body tissue, under the regimen described above, a weight loss of approximately 0.2 to 0.3 kg per day is to be expected if proper fluid balance is being maintained. If this occurs, there should be no difficulty with circulatory overload or water intoxication. If unforeseen circumstances result in overhydration, the intake figures should be reduced to increase the rate of weight loss. It must be stressed that patients' chances for recovery are optimum when all clinical manifestations of uremia are prevented. Since in many situations, particularly in traumatic and surgical cases, other aspects of patients' illness may require acute measures that prevent the parsimonious approach to fluid therapy outlined above, *early and frequent dialysis is the hallmark of a good therapeutic regimen for acute renal failure.*

Hyperkalemia is a common problem. The rapidity with which it appears is variable and is related to the rate of catabolism. It is a special hazard in acute renal failure following hemorrhage, an enhanced catabolic response associated with extensive surgical procedures, extensive traumatic or crushing injuries, and myoglobinuria associated with oliguria. In these situations, frequent EKG monitoring for progressive T-wave elevation is desirable. The appearance of peaking of the T waves is sufficient evidence of hyperkalemia to warrant immediate therapy (Chap. 7). Both hyperkalemia and acidosis are absolute indications for dialysis. In the presence of severe and rapidly developing hyperkalemia, it may be essential to use glucose and insulin and other measures to combat the elevated potassium while preparing the patient for dialysis.

The administration of carbohydrate reduces protein catabolism; if oral intake is not possible, carbohydrate should be given intravenously. In normal individuals a maximum protein-sparing effect is probably achieved by only 100 g per day. In patients with acute renal failure, however, larger amounts are probably necessary to bring about a maximal reduction in the rate of protein breakdown. The protein-sparing effect can be enhanced by administration of anabolic steroids (testosterone and its congeners).

The two most common causes of death during oliguria are infection and gastrointestinal hemorrhage. Prophylactic antibiotic treatment is of questionable value and probably should not be used. If obvious systemic infection has developed, appropriate antibiotic therapy, based on sensitivity testing, should be instituted. Because of the impaired excretory function of the kidney careful attention to alterations in antibiotic dosage schedules is mandatory.[38] Early treatment of uremia reduces the likelihood of infection and decreases the morbidity and mortality associated with the syndrome. The decision to institute dialysis therapy should not be based solely on the blood chemistry findings but should be made in conjunction with the patient's clinical signs and symptomatology. However, acceptable guidelines for the initiation of dialysis therapy are a serum urea nitrogen of 100 to 150 mg/dl and a serum creatinine value greater than 10 to 15 mg/dl. The aim of both dialysis and the conservative techniques of patient management is to maintain the patient's health in the best state possible. Hemodialysis every 48 to 72 hours is usually effective in maintaining a patient with acute renal failure in a sufficiently stable function.

The techniques of the various modalities of dialysis are described in Chapter 11.

The *diuretic* phase appears after a variable period of time and the urinary output begins to increase slowly. Large quantities of sodium and potassium may be lost in the urine due to inadequate tubular activity during the first several days of this diuretic phase. The sodium concentration is rarely below 60 to 70 mEq/L and, since the urine output usually exceeds 2 liters, the patient may lose 120 to 140 mEq of sodium per day. Inadequate sodium replacement may lead to shock, further damage to the kidneys, and interruption of a beginning diuresis. The development of hypokalemia is less frequent. The diuretic phase, during which the kidney is unable to regulate the composition of the urine adequately, may persist for several days to 2 weeks, or longer. In severe cases, renal function does not always return completely to normal, but virtually always reaches a level that permits the kidney to regulate the volume and composition of body fluids adequately.

The prognosis in acute renal failure is influenced by the underlying cause of the renal failure. In general, those cases associated with trauma do poorly, the mortality rate in some series exceeding 60 percent. Nontraumatic cases usually exhibit a survival rate that exceeds 75 percent.[42] In general, prognosis appears best in obstetric cases.[43]

CHAPTER 13

The Proteinurias and Hematurias

W. GORDON WALKER AND KIM SOLEZ

Diffuse renal disease is most often discovered as a result of routine examination of the urine. Since it is routine practice to accept a normal urine as excluding significant diffuse renal disease, an adequate specimen must be examined (Table 13–1), and the examination must include a careful microscopic examination of the urine. The abnormality signifying the existence of diffuse renal disease may be either proteinuria, hematuria, or combinations of the two. Usually one or the other manifestation predominates.

When proteinuria exceeds 3 to 4 g per day, it produces a characteristic constellation of clinical findings irrespective of the nature of the underlying renal disease. For this reason the presentation to follow considers 1) the clinical features of the protein-losing kidney; 2) the specific diseases of the kidney which can give rise to this lesion; and 3) their management. This is followed by a similar examination of the renal disorders that may present with hematuria as the predominant initial manifestation. Although significant overlap occurs and it is rare to see hematuria as a manifestation of diffuse renal disease without some accompanying proteinuria, the division is nevertheless a useful one insofar as it facilitates the differential diagnostic process.

Presently, the differential diagnosis of many diffuse renal diseases is complicated by the lack of a single clinical entity corresponding to a unique morphologic picture and vice versa. There are a number of well-defined histopathologic entities that do not have a unique presentation but may be encountered in a variety of clinical situations. These histopathologic findings are usually based upon light microscopic, immunofluorescent, and ultrastructural changes that together present a distinctive and easily recognizable picture, but often there is no unique set of clinical findings that can be reproducibly associated with such findings. Crescentic glomerulonephritis, for example, may be seen in systemic lupus erythematosus, Schönlein-Henoch purpura, Wegener's granulomatosis, polyarteritis, and in primary renal disease without involvement of other organ systems.[60,64,67] Identical immunofluorescent staining of glomeruli may be seen in membranous glomerulonephritis with nephrotic syndrome, systemic lupus erythematosus, and in renal lesions associated with such different conditions as hepatitis and neoplasms. Con-

---

TABLE 13–1

Steps To Be Observed in Checking for Proteinuria

1. Examine first specimen voided in A.M. if possible
2. Urine should have sp gr of 1.010 or greater
3. In females, urine should be obtained as clean catch specimen
4. Testing for protein should include either heat and acetic, or sulfosalicylic acid methods
5. Patients exhibiting proteinuria should be routinely checked for postural or orthostatic proteinuria
6. *Do not rely on dye impregnated paper strips as an adequate screening procedure unless positives are confirmed by procedures under #4 above.*

versely, cases of the nephrotic syndrome with identical clinical and urinary findings may show a wide range of histopathologic findings. This overlap makes establishment of diagnosis on purely histologic or morphologic basis difficult indeed unless clinical information is available. Since clinical data must be so heavily relied upon in reaching a diagnosis, we have divided the diffuse renal diseases into those in which proteinuria predominates and those exhibiting hematuria as the principal abnormality. In considering specific diagnostic entities, we have attempted to confine our consideration of histopathologic classifications to those that have readily demonstrable clinical, prognostic, and/or therapeutic utility. More detailed histopathologic classifications without definitely established therapeutic or prognostic usefulness have usually not been included.

THE PROTEINURIAS

Minor degrees of proteinuria are readily overlooked in a very dilute specimen; a specimen is suitable for excluding proteinuria only when the specific gravity exceeds 1.010, conditions usually met by examination of the first voided A.M. specimen. Under these conditions, proteinuria is probably the most sensitive indicator of diffuse renal disease.

The list of conditions that may cause proteinuria is extensive, and benign causes should be excluded before concluding that serious renal disease is present (Table 13-2).

A routine check for postural proteinuria should be made in all patients who have proteinuria without significant changes in the urinary sediment. This is done by having the patient empty his bladder before retiring and then collecting the first specimen voided immediately upon arising in the morning. This must be compared with a specimen collected later in the day, after the patient has been up and about for several hours. When protein appears intermittently, even while the patient is upright, a possible relation to vigorous exercise should be sought.[11] Febrile proteinuria and mucus contamination from the genital tract should always be excluded as possible causes of minor degrees of proteinuria.

The practice of grading proteinuria as *trace 1+, 2+, etc.,* is inadequate. Quantitative measurement of the excretion rate is most simply accomplished by the turbidimetric method, using dilute sulfosalicylic acid,

---

TABLE 13-2
Protein Excretion Rates of Various Renal Disorders*

	Protein Excretion Rate (mg per day)			
	50–100	100–1000	1000–3000	over 3000
Exercise proteinuria	+			
Febrile proteinuria	+			
Postural proteinuria	+	+		
Arteriosclerotic renal vascular disease	+	+		
Hypertension, arterial	+	+	+ (rare)	
Congestive heart failure		+	+	+ (?)
Pyelonephritis	+	+	+ (rare)	
Polycystic renal disease	+	+		
Acute glomerulonephritis	+	+	+	+
Membranous glomerulonephritis		+	+	+
Drug-induced nephrotoxic agents (Hg, CCl_4, etc.)	+	+		
Lipoid nephrosis			+	+
Kimmelstiel-Wilson syndrome			+	+
Systemic lupus erythematosus	+	+	+	+
Polyarteritis nodosa	+	+	+ (rare)	
Multiple myeloma†	+	+	+	+
Systemic sclerosis	+	+		

* Approximate ranges of daily protein excretion in some common diseases of the kidney. Divisions should be taken as a guide, rather than absolute range of excretion in these diseases.
† Does not refer to Bence Jones proteinuria but to more general proteinuria frequently seen in multiple myeloma.

and should always be carried out. When benign causes are excluded, persistent proteinuria in excess of 0.5 g per day is unequivocal evidence of renal disease, and diagnostic renal biopsy should be considered at this point.

CAUSES OF RENAL PROTEIN LOSS

The list of diseases presented in Table 13-2 emphasizes the almost universal occurrence of proteinuria as a manifestation of diffuse renal disease. In nearly all of these entities the amount of protein lost may vary from a few hundred milligrams to over 20 g daily. Other clinical features may indicate the specific diagnosis, but the proteinuria results in the same physiologic disturbances regardless of the underlying disease. The severity of clinical manifestations secondary to proteinuria can almost always be correlated well with the severity of the protein loss. Secondary manifestations usually do not appear unless the loss exceeds 2 to 3 g daily.[49,64]

Proteinuria is nearly always caused by a disturbance in the permeability of the glomerular basement membrane. An exception is the Bence Jones proteinuria of multiple myeloma, an instance of filtration of large quantities of a protein of low molecular weight. In general, the clearance of various species of plasma proteins is inversely related to their molecular weight or molecular size, a relation which holds over a wide range of rates of protein loss. More recently the studies of Brenner and others have shown that the glomerular basement membrane is polyanionic in nature and that it is this relatively dense concentration of negative charges which tend to repel the plasma protein.[1] Glomerular injury appears to be associated with a reduction in the net negative charge on the membrane, and as a consequence the permeability of the membrane is altered, permitting larger molecular sizes to pass. By measuring the clearance of proteins of progressively higher molecular weight, an index of glomerular permeability to protein can be obtained. In this fashion it is possible to characterize the permeability of the normal glomerular membrane and to show that disease processes which lead to progressive proteinuria also produce progressive deterioration in the permeability of the basement membrane. As this permeability progressively increases, it can permit the urinary loss of quantities of protein that may exceed 100 g daily.[54]

The continuing drain upon the protein stores of the body initiates a series of changes which result in the appearance of the *nephrotic syndrome*. This may occur in any patient if the rate of protein loss is sufficiently great. Hence, the nephrotic syndrome may be a feature of a number of renal diseases of different etiology. Protein loss in the urine in excess of 3 g per day is evidence of severe glomerular disease, and recognition of its existence should not await the appearance of the nephrotic syndrome. Early diagnosis is facilitated by the daily quantitative determination of urinary protein excretion. Patients who persistently excrete 0.5 g of protein or more per day for which there is no adequate explanation should be subjected to percutaneous renal biopsy.

THE NEPHROTIC SYNDROME

The nephrotic syndrome is characterized clinically by edema of variable degree, heavy proteinuria, hypoalbuminemia, hypercholesterolemia, and hyperlipemia.

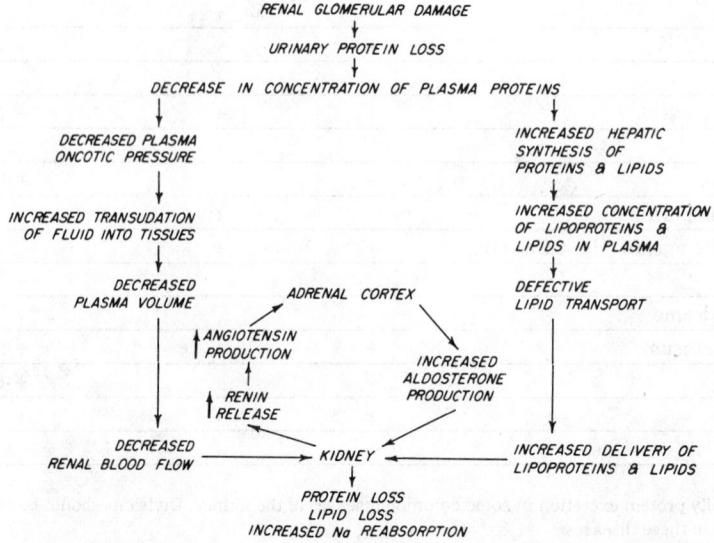

FIGURE 13-1. Sequence of events leading to the nephrotic syndrome.

Characteristically, the edema, even when severe, is associated with no complaint other than easy fatigability, unless there are large pleural effusions embarrassing respiration. A diagnosis of the nephrotic syndrome may be made in the absence of one or more of these findings, as long as heavy proteinuria is present. In general, patients who exhibit a protein loss of 3.0 g per day or greater eventually develop the clinical manifestations of this syndrome. The mechanism is shown schematically in Figure 13-1. If the proteinuria is allowed to continue it will eventually result in depletion of body nitrogen, which is, in turn, followed by an inadequate rate of synthesis of albumin by the liver, leading to a fall in the plasma albumin concentration. The two most striking consequences of this are a diminution in plasma oncotic pressure and transudation of fluid into the interstitial spaces. The net result is a tendency toward diminution of the circulating plasma volume and an increase in aldosterone production which promotes increased reabsorption of sodium and water. The mechanism for this increased aldosterone production is not completely settled, but it is likely that the primary stimulus is related to a drop in renal blood flow, consequent upon the fall in plasma volume. The kidney in turn increases renin production which stimulates liberation of angiotensin; the latter exerts a direct stimulatory effect upon the zona glomerulosa of the adrenal cortex, resulting in increased production of aldosterone. This chain of events continues until: 1) a new steady state is reached with respect to the distribution of intravascular and extravascular fluid, permitting the patient to maintain a normal plasma volume; or 2) until fluid accumulation reaches such proportions that the patient is obliged to seek medical help. Lymphatic flow is increased and, in patients with marked fluid retention, dilated lymphatics can be identified over the lateral region of the buttocks and flank.

The principal protein found in the urine is albumin, despite the fact that its concentration may be greatly reduced in the plasma. The differential permeability of the glomerular membrane results in proportionately greater losses of the plasma proteins of smaller molecular weight.[54,58] The net effect is a selective concentration of plasma proteins of larger molecular weight, such as the lipoproteins, which contribute to the lipidemia characteristic of nephrosis. Since these lipoproteins are intimately concerned with cholesterol transport, the plasma cholesterol content rises. There is also increased cholesterol synthesis by the liver. Thus, the hyperlipidemia and hypercholesterolemia result from a combination of differential retention of these substances at the glomerulus and their increased production by the liver.

Lipiduria is a regular feature of the nephrotic syndrome. It is recognized in the fatty casts present in great numbers, as well as in the cells which appear to be shed by the kidney. Occasionally, lipid is seen as free droplets or as small particles in the urine. Fat- or lipid-containing droplets can be readily identified by microscopic examination of urine under polarized light, thereby rendering them doubly refractive. It is probable that they arise as a result of increased filtration of some of the smaller lipoprotein molecules and cholesterol esters.

Although the total number of diseases that may occasionally be responsible for the protein-losing lesion associated with the nephrotic syndrome is large, over two-thirds represent primary renal diseases (Table 13-3). Differentiation between them may be impossible on clinical grounds and often can only be made histologically. This is particularly true in those individuals discovered during a routine examination to have proteinuria. The renal diseases that exhibit significant protein-losing lesions at some time during their course are: lipoid nephrosis or nil disease, membranous glomerulonephritis, mesangio proliferative

---

TABLE 13-3
Causes of the Nephrotic Syndrome[2,49,62,64]

Primary Renal Diseases

Lipoid nephrosis (minimal change or nil disease)
With glomerular mesangial hypercellularity
Membranous glomerulonephritis
Membranoproliferative glomerulonephritis
Focal sclerosing glomerulonephritis
Acute glomerulonephritis (less than 10 percent of cases)
Renal vein thrombosis
Goodpasture syndrome

Nephrotoxins and Allergens

Inorganic mercury and mercury compounds
Bismuth
Gold
Insect stings
Poison ivy
Tridione
Paradione
Snakebites

Systemic Illness

Diabetes with diabetic glomerulosclerosis
Systemic lupus erythematosus
Amyloidosis
Multiple myelosis
Syphilis
Malaria
Sickle cell anemia
Schönlein-Henoch purpura

glomerulonephritis, acute glomerulonephritis, and membranoproliferative glomerulonephritis. Less commonly, the nephrotic syndrome may be seen in: systemic lupus erythematosus, amyloidosis, multiple myeloma, renal vein thrombosis, and diabetic glomerulosclerosis, as well as in those conditions caused by an impressive list of nephrotoxins, allergenic agents, and drugs (Table 13–3).

Percutaneous renal biopsy is of great value in establishing a diagnosis. Amyloidosis, for example, is readily recognized by this means, as is diabetic glomerulosclerosis. In addition, renal biopsy permits distinction between membranous glomerulonephritis, chronic proliferative glomerulonephritis, and the other diffuse glomerulonephritides.

PRIMARY RENAL DISORDERS AND THE NEPHROTIC SYNDROME

The primary renal diseases that may present as the nephrotic syndrome can be divided into two groups on the basis of the findings obtained from the initial history and physical examination and urinalysis. The nephrotic patient with prominent hematuria and many granular and some red blood cell casts in the urine is readily placed in the group that contains chronic subacute and acute glomerulonephritis. Further justification for considering these as a group is provided by the histologic findings encountered on renal biopsy. All these patients show a picture that varies in severity but is characterized as primarily *proliferative*. These disorders are considered in more detail in the section on hematurias because they usually present in circumstances where other clinical features predominate; more often than not, the typical features of the nephrotic syndrome are absent. Hypertension of variable severity, frequently associated with evidence of circulatory overload and progressive renal failure are more common clinical presentations in this group.

The remaining group consists of those patients who present with the nephrotic syndrome and massive proteinuria but with relatively unimpressive uri-

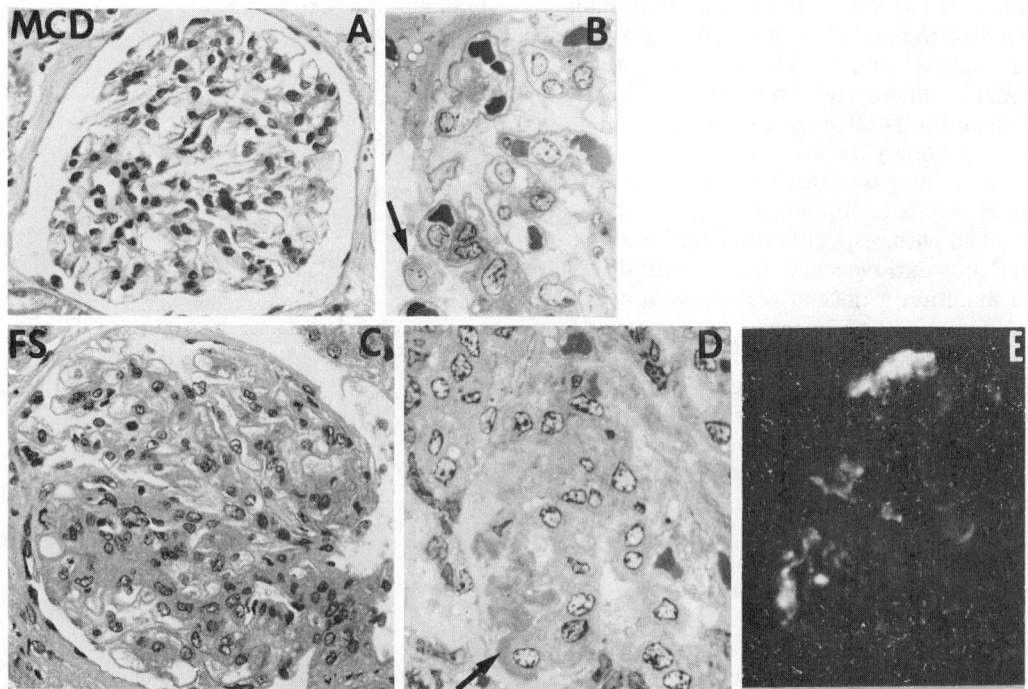

FIGURE 13–2. Characteristic glomerular changes seen in paraffin sections stained with hematoxylin and eosin (×330, left panels), plastic sections stained with toluidine blue (×750, middle panels), and frozen sections stained with fluorescein-tagged antisera (×410, right panels). In *minimal change disease* (MCD) glomeruli are essentially normal **(A)**. High power examination shows slight enlargement of epithelial cells (arrow in **B**). Immunofluorescence studies are negative. In *focal sclerosing glomerulonephritis* (FGS) portions of glomeruli are solidified (bottom of Panel **C**) with the remainder being normal. Hyaline exudative lesions may be seen in scarred regions (arrow in **D**) and these stain with IgM **(E)**.

nary sediment. Fatty casts and granular casts are almost always present but usually not in great numbers. Red cell casts are not seen and few or no erythrocytes are present. In the majority of cases, the onset of the disease is preceded by a mild upper respiratory illness but no evidence can be obtained for beta-hemolytic streptococcal infection. Renal biopsies from these patients may exhibit one of three types of changes. *Lipoid nephrosis* (nil disease) is characterized by essentially normal histologic findings on routine examination by light microscopy. *Membranous glomerulonephritis* shows marked thickening of the glomerular basement membrane including virtually all the glomeruli; there is little or no associated hypercellularity. *Focal sclerosing glomerulonephritis* is characterized by patchy involvement and does not affect all glomeruli (Fig. 13–2). Early in the course of the disease it may show abnormalities in only a very few tufts in a larger number of glomeruli. It is thus, on initial biopsy, frequently confused with lipoid nephrosis. It differs in response to therapy and, more importantly, in its clinical course.

The prognosis with this disorder is generally poor; young people particularly often progress from a state of normal renal function to end-stage renal disease in a period of less than 1 or 2 years. The pathologic changes include focal segmental sclerosis and the presence of pink-staining hyaline exudative lesions. These changes are not specific; similar lesions may be seen in diabetes, arteriosclerosis, and in the sclerosing phase of the glomerulonephritis associated with Schönlein-Henoch purpura, polyarteritis, subacute infective endocarditis, and other systemic diseases exhibiting renal involvement.

Lipoid Nephrosis (Nil Disease and Minimal Change Disease)

This disorder, thought initially to be a disease of childhood, is now recognized to occur in both adults and children but may be more common in the latter. As indicated in the preceding section, it does not exhibit any unique features that permit its recognition and separation as a distinct entity at the time of initial onset unless a renal biopsy is performed (Fig. 13–2).

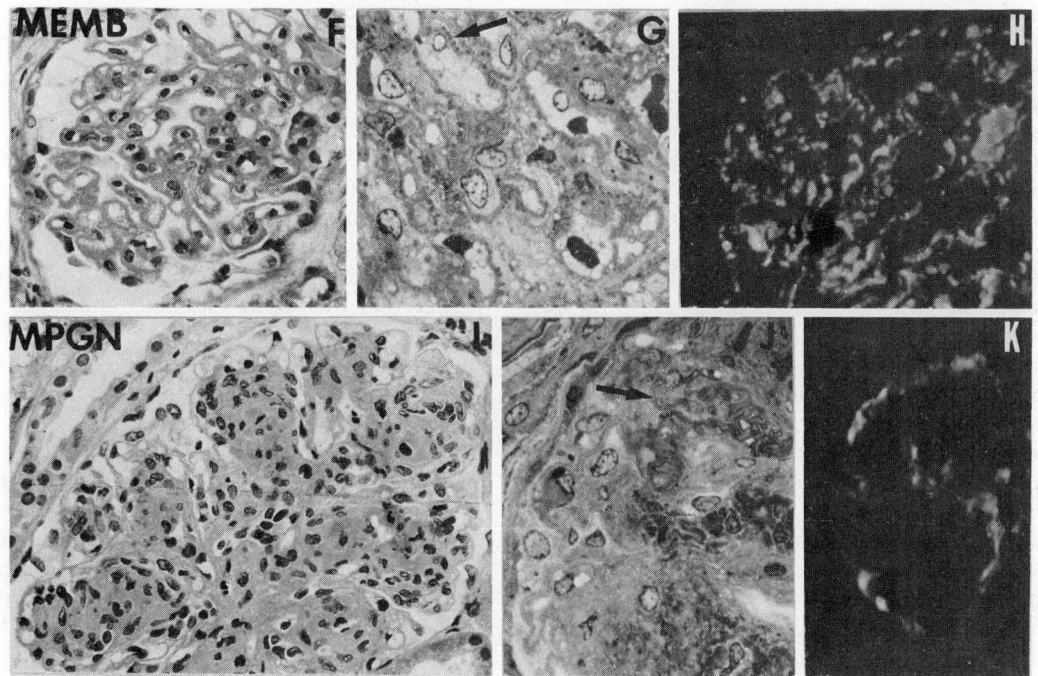

FIGURE 13–2 (cont.). In *membranous glomerulonephritis* (MEMB), capillary loops are diffusely thickened **(F)**; punctate deposits are seen on the outside of capillary loop basement membranes (arrow in **G**); and these stain with IgG **(H)**. In *membranoproliferative glomerulonephritis* (MPGN) there is increased lobulation of the glomeruli with mesangial hypercellularity and a patchy thickening of capillary loops **(I)**. "Double contours" with band-like subendothelial deposits are seen in the peripheral capillary loops (arrows in **J**); these peripheral capillaries stain with C3 **(K)**. (The differences in size of the glomeruli in the left-hand panels are due in part to variation in how near the center of the glomerulus the section was taken, and in part to glomerular enlargement in MPGN.)

A characteristic feature of the natural history of this type of nephrosis is the frequency of exacerbations and remissions and the relatively favorable long-term prognosis. There may be as many as 10 or more typical episodes of the nephrotic syndrome distributed over a 15- or 20-year period. Despite this protracted course punctuated by clinical evidence of recurrent activity, renal function may remain essentially normal. The distinguishing feature of this disorder is the completeness of the remission. Protein usually diminishes to less than 100 mg per day and often becomes undetectable during remissions. Adrenal corticosteroids are clearly of value in inducing and maintaining remissions in lipoid nephrosis (see below).

Only a small percentage of patients with lipoid nephrosis shows evidence of progression to chronic renal insufficiency. Hypertension is rarely a significant problem. Azotemia of moderate degree may be seen in association with exacerbations but appears to be due largely to the hypovolemia that accompanies the marked reduction in plasma albumin. It disappears concomitantly with reduction in proteinuria and edema.

Membranous Glomerulonephritis[44,60,67]

This descriptive term based upon histopathology identifies a subgroup of patients with the nephrotic syndrome who cannot otherwise be differentiated from lipoid nephrosis on clinical findings at the time of initial presentation. The prognosis is quite different, however, as is the response to steroid therapy. Mild hypertension and microscopic hematuria are more common in groups of patients with membranous glomerulonephritis, but these changes are not sufficiently distinctive to permit separation from patients with lipoid nephrosis without renal biopsy. About one-third of adult patients with the nephrotic syndrome fall into this group.

The histologic change, which appears as thickening of the basement membrane on H and E staining (Fig. 13–2) and a characteristic argentaffin spike and dome pattern within the basement membrane by silver stain, appears to result from deposition of immune complexes on the outer aspect of the basement membrane. Immunofluorescent studies identify gamma globulins and complement as constituents of these deposits. This is cited as evidence that this type of renal disease results from deposition of circulating immune complexes within the kidney.[47,59,63,65–67]

The clinical course of the nephrotic syndrome in these patients is different from that seen with lipoid nephrosis. In patients with membranous lesions and the nephrotic syndrome, response to steroid therapy is uniformly disappointing (see below).

The natural history is characterized by slowly progressive renal impairment with the nephrotic syndrome persisting for many years—survival for periods in excess of 10 years is not uncommon, and occasionally, spontaneous complete remission occurs. The majority, however, progress slowly to terminal or end-stage renal disease with the clinical course characterized by the nephrotic syndrome that fluctuates in severity. Hypertension appears relatively early in the course of the disease and may be quite severe. Early and effective treatment of this manifestation of the disease is important.

Nephrotic Syndrome and Glomerular Mesangial Hypercellularity

In about one-fifth of adult patients with primary renal disease presenting as the nephrotic syndrome, a distinctive histologic lesion is present characterized by hypercellularity confined exclusively to the mesangial cells. Whether this change identifies a single etiologic entity is doubtful, but the patients with this lesion do exhibit a consistent clinical pattern. They present with heavy proteinuria, normal renal function, and no blood pressure elevation. Microscopic hematuria is present in less than one-third of cases but casts are rare and there is no evidence of prior streptococcal infection. Except for the proteinuria, renal functional impairment is rare.

This disorder, like lipoid nephrosis, tends to relapse. It may exhibit spontaneous remissions, and in the majority of cases a favorable response is obtained with steroid therapy. Sustained remissions occur in more than three-fourths of these patients. Further study and long follow-up will be necessary to determine whether this is a separate and completely different entity from lipoid nephrosis.

Membranoproliferative Glomerulonephritis

A subset of the nephrotic syndrome that has a particularly bad prognosis is the group with the histologic pattern of both membranous changes and proliferative changes, termed variously membranoproliferative or mesangiocapillary glomerulonephritis. These patients tend to have somewhat more changes in the urinary sediment, particularly an increase in red cells and granular casts. The condition is much more rapidly progressive with evidence of substantial loss of renal function over a period of months. Indeed, a number of the patients have significant impairment of renal function when seen initially. Although it may be suspected from the more active urine sediment, the only means of making the diagnosis is by renal biopsy

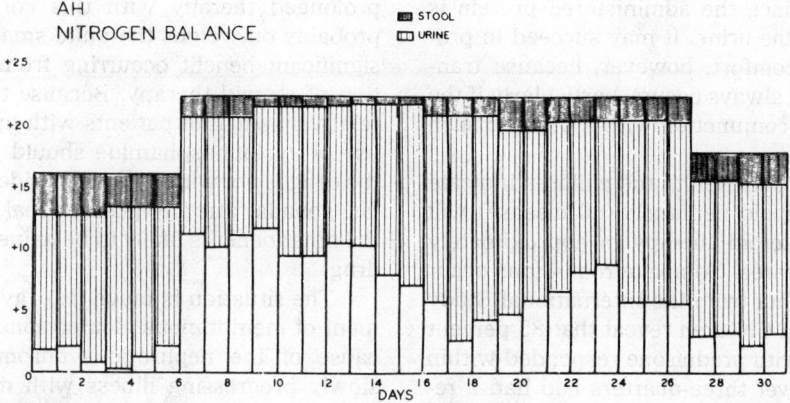

FIGURE 13-3. Nitrogen balance data on patient with lipoid nephrosis and severe proteinuria. Ordinate values are grams of nitrogen per day. Intake is plotted upward from zero and total shaded portion of each bar represents total nitrogen output for that day. Patient was studied during nitrogen intakes of 16, 23, and 18 g per day corresponding to daily protein intakes of 100, 143, and 112 g per day, respectively. White portion of each bar represents positive nitrogen balance achieved on that day. As protein intake increased, quantity of nitrogen retained each day increased. Protein loss in urine varied between 16 and 25 g per day throughout the period of study.

and appropriate immunofluorescent staining (Fig. 13-2; Table 13-5).

Focal Sclerosing Glomerulonephritis

This pathologic category is a particularly ominous one. The disease is characterized histologically by focal lesions within the glomerulus that are typically focal scars (Fig. 13-2). Because the disease is patchy in distribution, particularly early in its course, it is often misdiagnosed as nil disease, especially when only a small number of glomeruli are obtained at the time of renal biopsy. There is nothing identifiable in the urinary sediment nor in the clinical features of the disease to distinguish it from nil disease except for its markedly different clinical course. The condition responds only rarely to corticosteroids and exhibits a rapidly progressing course with deterioration of renal function that often terminates in end-stage renal disease within 12 to 18 months from the time of its initial recognition. From the standpoint of patient management, it is important to keep this entity in mind, and, in patients who have been diagnosed lipoid nephrosis or nil disease and who fail to exhibit the expected response with prednisone therapy, a repeat biopsy should be done. Immunofluorescent studies are occasionally of value in distinguishing the two since lipoid nephrosis almost never exhibits immunofluorescent staining, but this also may not be helpful if the biopsy does not succeed in obtaining glomeruli which demonstrate the lesion.

MANAGEMENT OF THE NEPHROTIC SYNDROME ASSOCIATED WITH PRIMARY RENAL DISEASES

General measures are directed toward treatment of the hypoproteinemia and the attendant edema. The persistent proteinuria characteristic of the disorder results in a marked nitrogen deficit which reduces the capacity of the liver to replace the plasma proteins lost in the urine. Positive nitrogen balance can be maintained for prolonged periods of time when protein intake is increased (Fig. 13-3). Patients can usually tolerate up to 2 or 2.5 g of protein per kg body weight per day for long periods, and the clinical features of the nephrotic syndrome can occasionally be reversed by this therapy despite continued heavy proteinuria. It is occasionally difficult to get the patient to maintain this high protein intake if sodium is rigidly restricted. When unpalatability appears to reduce protein intake, it is preferable to liberalize sodium intake to counter this. Under these circumstances diuretics may be relied upon to control edema.

On occasion, nephrotic "crises" characterized by anorexia, nausea, vomiting, and abdominal pain occur in association with profound anasarca and severe hypoalbuminemia. The cause of this clinical picture is not clear, but symptomatic improvement can on occasion be achieved by administration of intravenous albumin and the concomitant administration of diuretics. Relief often appears to be proportional to the quantity of fluid lost in response to this therapy. Its effect is transient since the administered protein is rapidly excreted in the urine. It may succeed in providing the patient comfort, however, because transient diuresis almost always occurs, particularly if the albumin is given in conjunction with a diuretic such as furosemide.

The best data in both adults and children indicate that patients with lipoid nephrosis (nil disease) will respond to corticosteroid therapy in approximately 80 to 90 percent of cases. Complete remissions occur in two-thirds. The data from the International Study of Kidney Disease in Children reveal that 85 percent of patients treated with prednisone responded within 6 weeks, of these over three-quarters had had a remission within 3 weeks of beginning therapy. Of those responding, approximately one-quarter have frequent relapses. *There is no good evidence from controlled trials to indicate that the use of maintenance corticosteroid therapy for long periods of time has any particular advantage over intermittent treatment when relapse appears.* Controlled trials have demonstrated that these results are not improved when azathioprine is added to the prednisone therapy. The use of cyclophosphamide, however, may add some advantage. This drug appears to diminish the number of patients who exhibit early relapses and, within the group of patients relapsing after cyclophosphamide therapy the frequency of relapses is reduced. These results were achieved with cyclophosphamide therapy that lasted for 2 to 3 months. Similar results, albeit with smaller numbers of subjects, have been obtained in controlled trials of these therapeutic regimens in adults. The incidence of remissions with nil disease or lipoid nephrosis is approximately the same for both adults and children. In both adults and children, the use of cyclophosphamide as adjunctive therapy in those patients with lipoid nephrosis who failed to respond to prednisone alone does not increase the number of "late" responders, i.e., those responding after 2 months. It does appear, however, that late responses are hastened somewhat when cyclophosphamide therapy is used.

The most appropriate treatment regimen for lipoid nephrosis should include a high protein (2 g/kg body weight/day), low salt (20 to 30 mEq Na/day) diet and initial treatment with prednisone (0.75 to 1 mg/kg/day) for 6 weeks. If a satisfactory response is obtained, (expected in approximately 85 percent) the prednisone should be tapered and stopped. The course should be repeated if relapse occurs. For those who fail to respond, a longer course of prednisone therapy should be given maintaining a full dosage schedule for at least 4 months. If no remission is achieved with this regimen, the added risk of more

prolonged therapy with this corticosteroid dosage probably outweighs the quite small likelihood of any significant benefit occurring from further prolongation of steroid therapy. Because the risk of death is relatively small in patients with lipoid nephrosis, the use of cyclophosphamide should be restricted since the drug is not without serious side effects. In particular, gonadal atrophy poses a real threat that offsets the other benefits likely to be gained by the use of this drug.

The situation is much less favorable in the treatment of membranous glomerulonephritis. This major cause of the nephrotic syndrome is a long-term, slowly progressing illness with mean survival time exceeding 10 years. The use of prednisone in this group provides a modest beneficial effect as judged by reduction in proteinuria in perhaps 20 to 25 percent of patients. However, in a controlled study this was offset by a slightly higher mortality rate in the treated group.[50,70] The use of agents, such as cyclophosphamide, in the treatment of membranoproliferative glomerulonephritis, focal sclerosing glomerulonephritis, and diffuse proliferative glomerulonephritis has been inadequate to make any judgment about usefulness. Although anecdotal information suggests that immunosuppressive agents may be of some benefit, the numbers included in the various controlled trials are too small to draw any conclusions.[46,50,52,53,70]

Finally, it should be stressed that in most of the results reviewed above, the use of cyclophosphamide was at a level of 5 mg/kg/day, a dose which generally induces leukopenia and thus has a significant hazard associated with it. The dosage therapy after the initial dosage was reduced to between 1 and 3 mg/kg/day and usually served to maintain the leukopenia. Therefore, great caution is necessary in the use of these drugs; the combination of cyclophosphamide and prednisone clearly increases the risk of infection and exposes the patient to hazards that may well be greater over the short-term than the hazards of the underlying disease. For this reason, caution should always be employed in reaching a decision to use such agents.

NEPHROTIC SYNDROME ASSOCIATED WITH SYSTEMIC DISEASE

Diabetic Glomerulosclerosis (Chap. 71)

The nephrotic syndrome occurs in association with diabetes mellitus in 10 to 20 percent of the reported cases. Clinically, this group can readily be distinguished from patients with membranous glomerulonephritis. In addition to evidence of preexisting diabetes which may have been present from 1 to 20 years, retinal microaneurysms are regularly found, diastolic hypertension is almost always present, and superimposed congestive heart failure is frequently noted. There is reduction in renal function with moderate to marked azotemia. Renal biopsy reveals diffuse intercapillary glomerulosclerosis, and concentric hyaline masses are frequently seen to distend capillary loops (Kimmelstiel-Wilson lesion). The diffuse intercapillary glomerulosclerosis appears to be the significant pathologic lesion since not all patients exhibit the nodular hyaline masses, and, conversely, hyaline nodules may be seen in the glomeruli of diabetics without any evidence of the nephrotic syndrome.

Treatment is disappointing. Corticosteroid therapy is contraindicated. The severity of the renal insufficiency may be such that even modest increases in protein intake produce or aggravate preexisting acidosis. Salt restriction and cautious use of diuretics may be the only therapeutic measures which can be safely used. Hypotensive therapy is advisable, but any sudden lowering of blood pressure must be avoided since it frequently worsens the renal impairment. Survival is usually measured in months.

Systemic Lupus Erythematosus

The general features of this disease and the clinical manifestations of renal involvement are discussed elsewhere (Chap. 97). Kidney disease in systemic lupus erythematosus is common, but the nephrotic syndrome occurs in less than 5 percent of these patients. Diagnosis is generally made on the basis of the systemic manifestations (fever, arthralgias, skin rash, involvement of serous surfaces, and characteristic hematologic findings). Treatment includes the therapeutic measures outlined under management of the nephrotic syndrome and the use of corticosteroid therapy.

Amyloidosis

Amyloidosis is a disorder characterized by widespread deposition or accumulation of an extracellular eosinophilic proteinaceous material in the tissues or organs of the body (Chap. 92). The symptomatology is determined by the organs predominantly involved. Renal amyloidosis may be asymptomatic throughout the course of the disease, the only manifestation being proteinuria of modest degree. On occasion, extensive accumulation of amyloid material in the kidney results in renal insufficiency leading to death in uremia. This is particularly true in the form of the disease seen in association with chronic suppuration (secondary amyloidosis). The disease presents less of-

ten as the nephrotic syndrome. The incidence in reported series varies between 5 percent and more than 40 percent of those cases of amyloidosis showing renal involvement.

In addition, renal amyloidosis with clinical features of the nephrotic syndrome may occur in association with renal vein thrombosis. This suggests that amyloid involvement of the kidney may predispose to renal vein thrombosis. Amyloidosis of the kidney is also seen in multiple myeloma presenting as the nephrotic syndrome. The diagnosis of renal amyloidosis is established by renal biopsy, this procedure appearing to be relatively safe in these cases.

Treatment should be confined to the general measures outlined for treatment of the nephrotic syndrome. Corticosteroids appear to be ineffective.

THE HEMATURIAS

Hematuria is a manifestation of many local diseases of the kidney and lower urinary tract, as well as a constant finding in a number of diffuse renal processes. The distinction between local hematuria and hematuria due to diffuse renal disease is of practical importance, and certain clinical and microscopic features serve to distinguish between the two (Table 13–5). Proteinuria may accompany the local forms of hematuria if these are severe, but it is virtually always associated with hematuria of diffuse renal disease. The excretion of protein rarely exceeds a few hundred milligrams per day when associated with local disorders of the genitourinary tract. In diffuse renal disease it varies from a few hundred milligrams to more than 10 g per day, the latter value being associated with the nephrotic syndrome. It should be stressed that both proteinuria and hematuria are usually present in diffuse renal disease, but classification into 1) those presenting with proteinuria with few or no formed elements in the urine; and 2) those presenting with hematuria with associated proteinuria is useful. The first group has been discussed in the preceding section of this chapter.

THE DIAGNOSTIC EVALUATION OF HEMATURIA

When hematuria is associated with pain and burning on micturition or suprapubic discomfort with frequency and urgency on urination, the lower urinary tract is the probable source. When the hematuria is noted only at the beginning or end of micturition, the urethra or bladder is usually the source. Hematuria associated with acute renal colic is most likely to be produced by nephrolithiasis, although clots themselves can produce renal colic on occasion when the

TABLE 13-4
Classification of Hematuria

I. Local Disorders of the Kidney and Genitourinary Tract

Disorder	Urinary Findings	Clinical Features
Exercise	Microscopic hematuria	History of vigorous exercise immediately preceding the examination
Trauma	Hematuria varying from microscopic to gross	History of trauma to region of kidney
Cystitis	WBC and clumps Proteinuria (mild) Bacteriuria No casts	Urgency, frequency, dysuria
Renal calculi	No casts or protein unless pyelonephritis present	Flank pain varying from dull ache to severe renal colic. Occasionally gross hematuria
Genitourinary tumors	Hematuria of variable severity	Local symptoms depending upon the location of the tumor
Heritable disorders Hemoglobinopathies Osler-Weber-Rendu disease Polycystic disease	Hematuria usually grossly visible No casts	Usually no symptoms Occasionally mild flank pain Rarely severe flank pain
Thrombocytopenic purpura	Only RBC in urine, no casts	No symptoms

II. Diffuse Renal Lesions [1,2,4,6,45,47,56,59,67]

Disorder	Other Urinary Findings	Clinical Features
Glomerulonephritis, acute Rapidly progressing glomerulonephritis MP glomerulonephritis	RBC casts, WBC, proteinuria, granular casts	Smoky urine Occasionally clinical features of uremia only, or heart failure and/or hypertension
Chronic	RBC casts, WBC, proteinuria, granular casts and cellular casts	Few symptoms until malignant hypertension or uremia supervene
Systemic lupus erythematosus	May resemble those in acute glomerulonephritis	Fever and joint pain are most prominent features but many systems may be involved
Polyarteritis	Telescoped urine sediment with all types of casts plus RBC and WBC	May present as acute glomerulonephritis with uremia but no hypertension; fever, anemia and nervous system involvement also common
Lung purpura with nephritis (Goodpasture syndrome)	RBC casts, gran. casts, proteinuria	Severe recurrent hemoptyses which precede onset of symptoms of uremia
Allergic nephropathies Schönlein-Henoch purpura	Urinary findings of acute glomerulonephritis with gross hematuria	Gastrointestinal and joint manifestations of this type of purpura
Thrombotic thrombocytopenic purpura	Proteinuria and RBC casts	Fever Neurologic manifestations Hemolytic anemia, jaundice
Focal embolic glomerulitis	RBC casts Mild proteinuria	Subacute bacterial endocarditis usually present; mild renal insufficiency
Malignant Hypertension	Rarely gross hematuria	Headache, decreasing vision and other manifestations of severe hypertension

---TABLE 13-4 (cont.)---

II. Diffuse Renal Lesions [1,2,4,6,45,47,56,59,67] **(cont.)**

Disorder	Other Urinary Findings	Clinical Features
Chemical or drug-induced carbon tetrachloride	RBC casts, protein	Progressive uremia, jaundice, hepatomegaly
Sulfonamides	Crystals in urine	Occasionally progressive renal insufficiency
Anticoagulants	Hematuria	Other manifestations of bleeding diathesis
Benign essential hematuria	Hematuria, often gross, RBC casts, proteinuria $<$1 g/day	Hematuria, few or no symptoms, benign course (see text)

clots form in the pelvis and are passed down the ureter.

In contrast, the hematuria of diffuse kidney disease is usually painless, is usually identifiable only by microscopic examination, and the blood is always uniformly distributed in the urine. Red blood cells which appear large and of normal morphology except for slight to moderate crenation are almost always associated with local disease somewhere in the urinary tract. When the source of the hematuria is the glomerulus or some site in the tubules, the red cells undergo considerable distortion (probably because of exposure to marked osmotic gradients in transit through the tubule). One characteristic form seen in hematuria of glomerular origin is the small, round microcyte which is one-half the size of a normal erythrocyte and exhibits increased refractility. Red cell casts, a characteristic feature of the hematuria of diffuse renal disease, unmistakably identify the nephron as the source of bleeding.

In most disorders, the severity of the hematuria varies greatly. Careful microscopic examination of freshly voided urine is necessary to establish the presence of hematuria in both local and diffuse disease and is a useful guide to further diagnostic studies. When red blood cell casts indicate that the hematuria results from diffuse parenchymal disease, renal biopsy is the procedure most likely to establish the diagnosis. Gross hematuria without casts or significant proteinuria indicates either a localized disease of the collecting system or a bleeding disturbance. Exclusion of the former requires the use of all available diagnostic aids, including a flat x-ray film of the abdomen, which may visualize radiopaque calculi; intravenous pyelography; renal arteriography; and cystoscopy with retrograde pyelography. The evaluation of hemorrhagic disorders is discussed elsewhere (Chap.

48), but it is worth noting here that several of the abnormal hemoglobins are associated with recurrent hematuria and should be excluded when painless hematuria unassociated with proteinuria or casts is encountered.

Careful studies should be made to exclude such correctable lesions as nephrolithiasis, tumors, and other surgically treatable disorders. Hematuria is frequently the last finding to disappear during the convalescent phase of acute glomerulonephritis. Patients seen initially during this stage of their illness may have little to point to a recent attack of acute glomerulonephritis. Even when the diagnosis is suspected, if no red cell casts are identified and the hematuria does not subside promptly, diagnostic evaluation as outlined above should be undertaken. After all studies are exhausted, a few instances of hematuria will remain undiagnosed, and for these the only course is continued observation.

IMMUNOLOGIC INJURY AND DIFFUSE RENAL DISEASE

In many diffuse renal diseases immunologic injury as the basis for renal damage is suggested by certain features of the clinical course of the illness plus demonstration of deposits within the kidney containing constituents of an antigen–antibody reaction. The nature of the events directly responsible for renal injury remain unknown but animal studies have defined two models of immunologic injury to the kidney that require complement fixation as the cytotoxic event. Both models, one involving production of antibodies to glomerular basement membrane and the other associated with circulating immune complexes, lead to deposition of immune globulins and complement in the kidney and result in progressive renal damage. Based upon experience with immunofluorescent his-

TABLE 13-5

Immunofluorescence in Glomerulonephritis[48,60,65,66,67,69,71]

Disease	IgG	IgA	IgM	C_3	C_4	C_{1q}	Fibrinogen
Acute glomerulonephritis	+ +	–	–	+	–	–	–
Glomerulonephritis associated with infection	+ +	–	+	+ +	+	+ +	–
Membranoproliferative glomerulonephritis Type 1	+	–	+	+ + +	+	+ +	–
Type 2 (dense deposit disease)	–	–	–	+ + +	–	–	–
Mixed cryoglobulinemia with nephritis	+ + +	–	+ + +	+ +	+	+ +	–
SLE with nephritis	+ + +	+	+	+	+ +	+ + +	–
Schönlein-Henoch*	+	+ + +	–	+	–	–	+ + +
Berger's disease*	+	+ + +	–	+	–	–	–
Malaria nephropathy	+ +	+	+				
Focal sclerosing glomerulonephritis	–	–	+ focal	+ focal	–	–	–
Goodpasture syndrome	+ + + linear	–	–	+	–	–	+
Polyarteritis nodosa	+	–	–	–	–	–	+ +

* Immunofluorescence found in mesangium.

topathology in these animals, the demonstration of gamma globulin plus one or more components of complement in any of the human glomerulonephritides have been viewed as acceptable evidence for an immunologic mechanism underlying the renal injury in these disorders. In practice, interpretation of the results of immunofluorescent studies on renal biopsies is more difficult (Table 13-5).

Identification of antigen plus antibody and complement fixation by immunofluorescent identification of the constituents of this reaction is complicated by the fact that there are two pathways for activating complement by immune reactions, and reported studies have not always been complete.[59,61,65,67,71,73] Nevertheless, such reports provide presumptive evidence for an immunologic basis for the renal diseases listed in Table 13-5.

Despite much effort directed toward associating specific patterns of immunoglobulin deposition within the glomerulus with specific disease categories, no unique associations have been observed to date (Table 13-5). Although it has been well documented that one or the other mode of complement activation may be seen most often in a particular type of renal disease, no unique clinical features or specific prognostic associations have emerged as characteristic features of a particular immunofluorescent pattern.

Acute Glomerulonephritis

CLINICAL FEATURES. The clinical features of severe acute glomerulonephritis are so striking that the disease may be recognized even before the urine is examined. The sequence of events characteristically begins with a sore throat associated with fever. This subsides in 4 to 8 days, to be followed in 2 to 3 weeks by the appearance of smoky urine, usually with reduction in urinary volume and swelling of face and ankles. The swelling is most marked in the morning and subsides during the day, only to be replaced by swelling of the ankles as evening approaches. These abnormalities are followed by progressive shortness of breath, weakness, lassitude, and anorexia. Breathlessness may be followed by acute pulmonary edema or other manifestations of circulatory congestion, particularly in older people. All the signs of uremia may soon appear and may lead to coma and convulsions. On physical examination, the facial edema is most readily apparent in the periorbital region. The dependent edema in other areas is associated with tight rubbery consistency of the overlying skin, characteristic of rapid development of edema beneath skin of normal turgor and elasticity. There is usually evidence of hyperactive circulation with full bounding pulses and variable hypertension, the diastolic blood pressure occasionally exceeding 115 to 120 mm Hg. Generalized venous hypertension may be readily apparent clinically and can be confirmed by measurement of the venous pressure. Moist rales are found in the lungs and pleural effusions may be noted; cardiomegaly and hepatomegaly may be present. Costovertebral angle tenderness is frequently noted, and, on occasion, pain in this area may be of such severity as to suggest acute renal colic.

The urine is usually turbid and has a characteristic brown or smoky color; it is rarely grossly bloody. The amount of protein in the urine usually exceeds 100 mg/dl, and microscopic examination reveals numerous red blood cells and variable numbers of casts, including red blood cell casts. Anemia is usually present, its severity varying directly with the severity of the azotemia. The blood urea nitrogen and serum creatinine are elevated, and occasionally, plasma protein concentrations are lowered with reversal of the A/G ratio. Antistreptolysin O (ASO) titer usually exhibits a rise some time during the course of the disease and may be the only evidence of antecedent beta-hemolytic streptococcal infection.

COURSE. The subsequent course is variable, but it is usually relatively short, with complete recovery in several weeks to 2 or 3 months. With appropriate treatment the symptoms of congestion subside and the fluid retention disappears after the first few days. Proteinuria may persist for several weeks and microscopic hematuria for several months, even in those cases in whom complete recovery occurs. In a small number of cases, the urinary findings show no tendency to clear. Fluid retention of variable severity persists, and the subsequent course is one of gradual deterioration—the development of progressive renal insufficiency leading to death in uremia within a few months. More often, when the urinary abnormalities fail to disappear, the acute illness is followed by a latent period of several years during which the only identifiable abnormalities are proteinuria and hematuria. This may be followed within from 1 to more than 20 years by the appearance of the nephrotic syndrome, usually refractory to therapy, which progresses slowly to uremia and death. Alternatively, the latent period may terminate in chronic renal insufficiency and uremia without appearance of the nephrotic stage. About 5 percent of patients die during the fulminant acute phase as a result of such conditions as acute pulmonary edema, acute encephalopathy, or uremia. Recovery rates appear approximately the same for adults and children.

Not infrequently, the initial episode is so mild as to go unrecognized unless the patient happens to be under medical care for his initial pharyngitis. The only manifestations may be microscopic hematuria and red cell casts in the urine. The disease may be discovered fortuitously as a result of urinalysis done as part of a routine examination. Questioning may reveal a recent history of an upper respiratory infection. However, efforts to uncover a history of an antecedent upper respiratory infection are frequently unsuccessful, and the diagnosis cannot be excluded on the basis of the absence of such a finding.

ETIOLOGY. There is no satisfactory etiologic classification of the sporadic cases of acute glomerulonephritis. The majority of cases arise as late sequelae of infections due to nephritogenic strains of beta-hemolytic streptococci. Although these infections usually involve the upper respiratory tract, they may also involve the skin or other tissues. Glomerulonephritis proven by biopsy has also been associated with pneumococcal infections with subacute infective endocarditis, usually due to the staphylococcus and sometimes viral infections.

The frequency of occurrence of acute glomerulonephritis following streptococcal epidemics is related to specific types of the Group A beta-hemolytic streptococci. Types 12, 4, 1, and Red Lake have been identified as nephritogenic strains. Epidemics due to these types are associated with a relatively high incidence of acute glomerulonephritis. Those patients who exhibit hematuria during the acute phase of the streptococcal infection appear to be more likely to develop acute glomerulonephritis subsequently than are those who do not. The importance of routine urine examination in patients with suspected streptococcal infection and the implications with respect to convalescent follow-up are self-evident.

INCIDENCE. Acute glomerulonephritis may occur at any age but is rare under the age of two. It is more common in children, but is being recognized with increasing frequency in adults. The diagnosis is probably missed more often in adults because of the greater likelihood of attributing the accompanying renal insufficiency to other diseases, such as hypertensive vascular disease with nephrosclerosis. Its occurrence in *all* age groups cannot be overemphasized, and acute glomerulonephritis should be considered as a possible cause in *any* case of undiagnosed uremia of short duration. Its higher incidence in males than in females remains unexplained.

PATHOLOGY. The commonest lesion is proliferation of cells indigenous to the glomerular tuft. The earliest change is a proliferation of the endothelial cells. When severe, it may lead to complete occlusion of the majority of the capillary lumina. A characteristic feature of the poststreptococcal variety is the involvement of almost every glomerulus. Exudation of polymorphonuclear leukocytes is frequently seen. An interstitial reaction occasionally predominates. Later, as the reaction begins to subside, the pattern of hypercellularity exhibits a focal distribution, being found mainly in the axial regions of the glomerulus. The cells involved appear to be the mesangial cells. Proliferation of epithelial cells is also noted later in the disease, but may be present within three weeks of onset. These latter changes are seen in patients who recover completely, and are not necessarily associated with a bad prognosis.

Immunofluorescent staining of the renal biopsy material obtained from patients with poststreptococcal glomerulonephritis demonstrates the presence of IgG and complement (C3) as interrupted deposits on the epithelial side of the GBM. Occasionally, only complement can be demonstrated. Electron microscopy of the GBM also confirms the presence of large subepithelial deposits ("humps"). In studies where these accumulations in the GBM have been eluted from human renal tissue, it has been possible to demonstrate the presence of antistreptococcal antibody as part of the immune complex material removed from the GBM.

In the chronic stage of the disease, glomerular destruction and fibrosis develop with varying degrees of interstitial inflammation and scarring. As progressive destruction of renal tissue occurs, the remaining tubules become dilated and hypertrophied.

TREATMENT. Because of the relation between specific types of streptococci and nephritis, it is wise to treat all cases of acute glomerulonephritis with penicillin (600,000 units per day for 8 days). Exposed members of the family should receive prophylactic penicillin therapy for a similar period.

All patients should be kept in bed during the acute phase and at rest until the urine clears. This usually requires 3 to 4 weeks. Minimal proteinuria and hematuria are not contraindications to ambulation, but should the urinary abnormalities show a persistent increase with activity, the period of bedrest must be extended. Patients with persistent heavy proteinuria and hematuria but otherwise stable urinary function should be kept at rest for 6 weeks to 2 months before ambulation is undertaken. Subsequent physical activity should be restricted as long as the urinary abnormalities persist. This advice is based upon the clear relationship which appears to exist between increasing activity and increasing urinary abnormalities.

Edema and hypertension call for rigid salt restriction. When this regimen is instituted promptly, acute hypertensive encephalopathy with convulsions can usually be avoided so that emergency measures to lower blood pressure will not be required. It is doubtful that digitalization is effective in combatting the circulatory congestion of acute nephritis. If pulmonary edema develops, some form of dialysis must be considered.

There is no need to restrict the protein intake unless there is severe oliguria, azotemia, and acidosis. The management of acute uremia in these cases does not differ from that of other forms of acute renal failure.

Rapidly Progressive Glomerulonephritis

In a small percentage of patients with acute glomerulonephritis, there is no demonstrable tendency toward improvement, but instead there is a relatively rapid deterioration with death in uremia occurring within 6 to 12 months of the initial onset of the disease. This course of glomerulonephritis, also termed "subacute" or "crescentic" glomerulonephritis, does not appear to have a unique etiology; some of the cases have been clearly identified as poststreptococcal while others have failed to yield any evidence for antecedent streptococcal infection. These patients generally do not respond to steroid or immunosuppressive therapy and when they reach end-stage renal disease the best form of management is that of chronic dialysis and renal transplantation.

Glomerulonephritis Associated with Infection

Several types of infection have an increased incidence of associated glomerulonephritis. The disturbance is seen particularly with staphylococcal sepsis of various sorts, but most commonly as a complication of staphylococcal subacute infective endocarditis. The glomerulonephritis is characterized usually by rapidly progressive renal insufficiency with all of the attendant manifestations described under acute glomerulonephritis except that hypertension is less striking. The microscopic examination of the urine shows the typical urinary sediment of acute glomerulonephritis with much hematuria, red cell casts, and numerous granular casts. This is an immune-complex type glomerulonephritis, and it tends to improve, usually reversing completely when the infection is eradicated.[3,60] It should be stressed that this entity is distinct from the focal embolic glomerulitis or glomerulonephritis that is a common accompaniment of subacute infective endocarditis regardless of the type of organism involved. The latter entity rarely is associated with any substantial degree of renal impairment and usually is characterized by the finding of microscopic hematuria and rarely red cell casts, but little in the way of clinical manifestations of the disorder.

Membranoproliferative (Hypocomplementemic) Glomerulonephritis

Membranoproliferative glomerulonephritis presents more commonly as the nephrotic syndrome (Table 13–3). In approximately one-third of cases, however, it is characterized by hematuria, azotemia, and some proteinuria without clinical manifestations of the nephrotic syndrome. It, thus, must be kept in mind when considering the patients who present with hematuria and no stigmata of the nephrotic syndrome. It occurs in both children and adults and pursues a course that is usually relentlessly progressive and terminates in renal failure within 3 to 6 years. The disease is associated with characteristic histopathologic lesions in the glomerulus, and the patients also have persistently low levels of complement. The prognosis is guarded. The course is variable but often follows an accelerated pattern. Treatment with prednisone, immunosuppressive agents, and anticoagulants has been unimpressive.

The disease has been subdivided into three types, depending upon the distribution of the deposits seen by electromicroscopy. In fact it has not been possible to associate these subtypes with clinical patterns, and the only histologic feature that permits inference regarding the clinical course is the presence or absence of crescents. In general when there is striking crescentic change seen in the glomeruli, the course is much more rapid and the prognosis particularly ominous.

There is perhaps a fourth type that should be included here. The *mixed cryoglobulinemia* associated with renal disease exhibits a pathologic picture of membranoproliferative glomerulonephritis that is indistinguishable from those above and the course and prognosis are similar.[74] Treatment including prednisone, anticoagulation, and immunosuppressive agents has been disappointing.[74]

Systemic Lupus Erythematosus

Systemic lupus erythematosus (SLE) is a disease of varied clinical manifestations which may involve—either simultaneously or at different times—the skin, joints, pleura, pericardium, spleen and lymphatic system, and kidneys (Chap. 97). Renal involvement is probably the leading cause of death, but SLE rarely presents with renal disease alone. The diagnosis is usually clinically evident before kidney involvement is identified.

Renal disease usually occurs early in this disorder and manifests itself in proteinuria and microscopic hematuria. The urinary sediment may be indistinguishable from that of acute glomerulonephritis.

The disease may present as the nephrotic syndrome with heavy proteinuria in addition to hematuria and red cell casts. The picture of acute severe glomerulonephritis with oliguria, azotemia, acidosis, and clinical manifestations of uremia may be the predominant manifestation. Although such cases are rare, early recognition is imperative since treatment of SLE differs from that of acute hemorrhagic glomerulonephritis.

PATHOLOGY. There are four histologic categories of renal involvement in systemic lupus: 1) minimal glomerular involvement with mild mesangial proliferation; 2) focal glomerulonephritis (lupus glomerulitis); 3) an extramembranous ("membranous") form of lupus nephritis with subepithelial deposits; and 4) "diffuse proliferative" lupus nephritis with subendothelial deposits. In the proliferative form, hypercellularity is seen in one or more regions of a glomerulus, together with hyaline thrombi and necrosis of portions of glomerular tufts. Very thick capillary loops ("wire loops") are seen in regions of the glomerulus that show less proliferation. The hematoxylin bodies which are generally considered to be pathognomonic of the nephritis of SLE can be demonstrated in only a small proportion of biopsies. The presence of antigen–antibody complexes in these membranous lesions has been clearly established, and such complexes have been eluted and identified as anti–DNA–DNA complexes. It appears likely that deposition of these complexes within the kidney represents one of the early initiating events in the production of lupus nephritis.[65] Electron micrographs have recently been reported to show an extraordinarily high incidence of virus-like particles in the glomeruli of patients with SLE as well as characteristic fingerprint-like whorling patterns within some of the deposits.[57,72] The etiologic significance and therapeutic implications of this finding remain to be evaluated.

TREATMENT. The general measures outlined in the section on treatment of acute glomerulonephritis also apply here. In addition, the use of corticosteroids has been shown to have a beneficial effect when given in high doses for long periods (Chap. 97).

More recent experience suggests that the combination of azotemia and nephrotic syndrome heralds a poor prognosis. Focal glomerular lesions without such severe clinical manifestations, however, carry a much more favorable prognosis. It also appears that long-term maintenance on high steroid dosage is not necessary to sustain a remission after the activity of the disease process has been arrested. The addition of azathioprine to the therapeutic regimen for lupus nephritis appears to offer some additional advantage.

Polyarteritis

Polyarteritis is a multiple system disorder exhibiting a variety of clinical manifestations which depend upon the location of the vascular lesions (Chap. 100). The symptoms and signs may be related to the joints, the gastrointestinal tract, the kidneys, and the peripheral and central nervous system, among others. This involvement of many organ systems is usually the clinical feature arousing suspicion of the disease. On occasion, however, the predominant manifestations may indicate disease of a single system.

The kidneys are involved to a variable extent in the majority of cases. The renal lesions are of two types: 1) arteritic lesions of the medium-sized renal arterioles similar to those seen elsewhere in the vascular tree; and 2) a diffuse type of glomerulonephritis. The first type may produce only microscopic hematuria without clinical evidence of renal insufficiency. In the usual case, other symptoms overshadow renal involvement, or at least are of sufficient magnitude to suggest the correct diagnosis. Less often, it presents as a primary renal disease and differentiation from acute glomerulonephritis may be difficult.[55,72] Fluid retention and signs of circulatory congestion associated with clinical manifestations of uremia of variable severity are seen, and the disease may pursue a fulminant course leading to uremia and death. Absence of hypertension in the early acute phase of polyarteritis is the most helpful characteristic serving to distinguish this illness from acute glomerulonephritis. As the disease progresses, hypertension appears and may be severe. Patients presenting with milder forms of the disease may enter a chronic phase with progressive hypertension that may ultimately become malignant and result in death.

URINARY SEDIMENT. The urinary findings are similar to those in acute glomerulonephritis. Proteinuria is variable but usually exceeds 100 mg/dl. Hematuria is almost always present and numerous red blood cell casts and cellular casts are seen. The urinary sediment has been said to represent a "telescoped" picture of all the formed elements seen in the various stages of ordinary glomerulonephritis. When the renal involvement is confined to the larger vessels in the kidney, there may be only a trace of protein and a few red cells in the urine, the latter being present only intermittently.

PATHOLOGY. The majority of the polyarteritic lesions occur in the arcuate vessels. The histologic features of the nephritis include both proliferative and destructive glomerular involvement. In the early stages, microthrombi are frequently seen, involving one or two capillary loops of the glomerulus. There may also be fibrinoid changes involving all or part of the tuft. Adhesions to Bowman's capsule are common and may be associated with epithelial proliferation and crescent formation. Hemorrhage may occasionally be seen in the capsular spaces or in the tufts, but the glomerular capillaries usually are bloodless and exhibit variable degrees of polymorphonuclear infiltration. In older lesions, complete hyalinization of glomeruli is common, and it is usual to find lesions showing virtually all stages of glomerular damage and destruction within the kidney, some glomeruli being completely spared. Immunofluorescent staining of the glomeruli and electron microscopy of the GBM indicate that the glomerular damage noted in polyarteritis is in large part caused by immune complex deposits in the GBM. In about one-third of the cases so examined, hepatitis B antigen appears to be the antigenic component in the immune complex.

TREATMENT. The administration of adrenal steroids results in suppression of the acute inflammatory and necrotic arteriolar lesions. In some patients, the evidences of renal involvement may greatly improve or disappear altogether. The prognosis appears to be determined by the extent and stage of the renal lesions before treatment is initiated (Chap. 100). Even if no new lesions develop after steroids are given, the existing renal damage may be so severe that hypertension has already appeared. Hypotensive agents may be indicated in this case. Prompt institution of steroid therapy and maintenance of full suppression as long as evidence of active arteritis exists is necessary for optimal results.

Thrombotic Thrombocytopenic Purpura

Thrombotic thrombocytopenic purpura is characterized by a decrease in the number of circulating platelets associated with purpura, hemolytic anemia, signs of central nervous system involvement, and renal disease (Chap. 48). The onset is usually acute, with malaise, headache, fatigue, and myalgia occurring frequently. Fever, nausea, vomiting, and abdominal pain are common. Mild jaundice is often seen, and hepatosplenomegaly with generalized lymph node enlargement has been observed. There may be signs of congestive heart failure. Central nervous system manifestations include confusion, delirium, psychotic behavior, and stupor, along with focal neurologic signs. The anemia is hemolytic in type, and the abnormally shaped red blood cells are called helmet cells or schizocytes; leukocytosis is common and a leukemoid reaction may be seen.

The kidneys are frequently involved, and signs of renal disease occasionally dominate the clinical picture. Examination of the urine reveals proteinuria, gross or microscopic hematuria, and frequently red blood cell, as well as granular, casts. Renal insufficiency and moderate azotemia are common and severe uremia may develop. Histologic examination reveals eosinophilic thrombi in the arterioles of the kidney and locally within segments of the glomerular capillaries. Dramatic remissions have been induced by large doses of adrenocortical steroids, but in general the prognosis is poor.

Nephritis Associated with Schönlein-Henoch Purpura

Progressive renal disease may be associated with recurrent allergic purpura, evidenced by the early appearance and persistence of microscopic hematuria. In perhaps 25 percent of the cases the hematuria persists even after the acute skin changes have cleared. There is usually an exacerbation of the urinary findings associated with recurrence of the dermal lesions. The renal disease is slowly progressive, and the associated clinical manifestations are similar to those seen in chronic glomerulonephritis. Proteinuria accompanies the hematuria and occasionally the nephrotic syndrome develops. Patients exhibiting persistent proteinuria, and hematuria when dermal manifestations are quiescent, usually develop hypertension and uremia eventually.

Renal biopsy early in the disease reveals focal nephritis with some glomeruli showing localized areas of hypercellularity—presumably due to proliferation of endothelial and mesangial cells. Adhesions and crescents are frequent. In other instances, an entire glomerulus may show these changes of hypercellularity while adjacent glomeruli appear normal. These acute lesions are replaced by generalized or focal glomerular scars, and later in the disease nearly all glomeruli are affected with changes resembling severe diffuse glomerulonephritis. Immunologic staining and electron microscopic evaluation of the glomeruli demonstrate, in particular, the presence of changes in the mesangial or stalk portions of the glomerular tuft. IgG, IgA, C3, and fibrinogen are frequently noted in the electron dense deposits in the mesangium and contiguous segments of the peripheral capillary loops.

The dermatologic manifestations of the disease usually respond promptly to treatment with corticosteroids. Such treatment also suppresses acute activity in the kidney, but it is doubtful whether the ultimate outcome of the renal disease is influenced.

Goodpasture Syndrome

The essential features of this syndrome are profuse and persistent hemoptysis, followed by the development of rapidly progressive renal insufficiency often leading to death within a few months. Hemoptysis may be the only initial manifestation, antedating all clinical evidence of renal disease by several weeks or more. Urine examination at this time usually shows albuminuria, hematuria, and red cell casts.

The glomerular lesion varies in severity, depending on the stage of the patient's clinical illness. Early lesions are of a focal nature which then become more extensive with crescent formation in the glomeruli, localized foci of necrosis in the capillary loops, and deposition of fibrin in Bowman's space. Immunofluorescent studies demonstrate the homogenous linear deposition of IgG along the basement membrane of the glomerular capillary loops.

This is the classic example of glomerular disease induced by the presence of antiglomerular basement membrane antibody. Common antigenic properties of the basement membrane of the lung and glomeruli have been identified and probably are responsible for the pulmonary involvement in the condition.[2]

Clinically, the disease usually progresses rapidly to end-stage renal disease, but high doses of corticosteroids may slow or arrest the progression of the disease in a few instances. Chronic dialysis and subsequent renal transplantation are of value. In some instances, bilateral nephrectomy after beginning dialysis has been associated with prompt cessation of hemoptysis. Recently, plasmapheresis combined with vigorous immunosuppression has been shown to be of some benefit in arresting the progress of the renal damage.

Benign Recurrent Hematuria (IgG Nephropathy)[69]

This entity is a relatively benign disease seen in childhood and early adult life which is characterized by recurrent episodes of hematuria, usually sufficiently heavy to produce gross coloration of the urine. The disturbance is more common in males. The episodes often occur following an upper respiratory infection or following strenous exercise. The attacks of gross hematuria typically are episodic, but it is usually possible to identify microscopic hematuria at intervals between the attacks. Histologic examination of the kidney usually demonstrates a focal lesion in the glomeruli, and immunofluorescent studies reveal IgA. The disease also has been called recurrent macroscopic hematuria, IgA nephropathy, Berger's disease, and IgA–IgG mesangial nephropathy.

In general, the disease is benign, and it is rare that protein loss in the urine exceeds 1 g daily. Scattered reports of renal failure and nephrotic syndrome and other more serious changes may reflect a confusion of this and other clinical entities such as Schönlein-Henoch purpura.[2,69] It is clear that IgA deposition in the kidney is seen in conditions other than the clinical entity that is termed benign essential hematuria.[69] Much of the writing on this subject has failed to make a clear distinction between whether the clinical entity of benign essential hematuria is being discussed or a collection of cases staining with IgA and in some instances other types of immunoglobulin patterns. Because of this ambiguity, it is somewhat difficult to interpret much of the published information regarding prognosis in this disorder.[48,69]

CHAPTER 14
Functional Disorders of the Renal Tubules
W. GORDON WALKER

Renal tubular dysfunction usually arises from impairment of one or more of the tubular transport mechanisms, producing specific disturbances of hydrogen ion, potassium ion, calcium and phosphorus metabolism, or loss of some particular metabolic constituent such as an amino acid. The most commonly encountered examples include renal tubular acidosis, phosphate-losing nephropathy, vitamin D-resistant rickets, and nephrogenic diabetes insipidus. In addition, a number of apparently unrelated metabolic disorders are associated with specific defects in amino acid transport by the kidney.

RENAL TUBULAR ACIDOSIS

Renal tubular acidosis (RTA) is a syndrome characterized by the presence of a variable degree of systemic metabolic acidosis that results from impairment or a failure of urinary acidification. Two distinct types are recognized. Classic or Type I RTA is caused by a defect in the distal tubule characterized by impaired hydrogen ion secretion that leads to a reduced excretion of ammonia and titratable acid. Type II, or proximal RTA, is associated with defective reabsorption of filtered bicarbonate. Both types result in systemic metabolic acidosis, but other clinical manifestations are different. Since treatment of the two types is different, distinguishing the two is of clinical importance.

Type I Distal Renal Tubular Acidosis
This disease is most commonly recognized clinically in the second and third decades of life, but may be diagnosed in virtually any age group.[76,83] Presenting symptoms may include renal stone, hematuria, periodic paralysis, or skeletal abnormalities. Presently, with the widespread use of screening laboratory determinations, the disorder is most often recognized by detection of unsuspected hyperchloremic acidosis.

The specific defect is an inability to transport hydrogen ions against a gradient comparable to that which is developed by the normal kidney in the presence of systemic acidosis (Table 14–1). This inability to lower the pH of the urine reduces both titratable acid and ammonia excretion. As a result, the kidney is forced to excrete abnormally large quantities of potassium, calcium, and sodium to maintain electroneutrality. This continuing drain of cations, particularly potassium and calcium, can lead to profound skeletal abnormalities and in some instances hypokalemia of such severity as to produce episodic paralysis. This failure of ammonia excretion and of titratable acid leads to a corresponding reduction in bicarbonate reabsorption which produces a decrease in serum bicarbonate, systemic acidosis, and hyperchloremia. The associated cation losses are responsible for the development of rickets or osteomalacia and may in some instances produce hypokalemic paralysis. Thus, hyperchloremic acidosis, hypokalemia, rickets or osteomalacia, and nephrocalcinosis usually with recurrent renal stones, represent the hallmarks of distal or type I renal tubular acidosis. When the disease presents clinically during childhood, these findings are also associated with a marked reduction in the rate of growth.

It has been demonstrated in one well-studied kindred that there was a much greater frequency of hypercalciuria than of a demonstrable acidification defect. In at least one instance a progression from hypercalciuria to nephrocalcinosis and finally renal tubular acidosis was observed in a member of the kindred who exhibited only hypercalciuria when first seen during childhood.[75] It may be that some of the clinically recognized cases of distal tubular damage and resultant renal tubular acidosis represent changes secondary to long-standing hypercalciuria and associated nephrocalcinosis. The persistent hy-

TABLE 14-1
Diagnosis of Renal Tubular Acidosis[76,77,81,85]*

	Plasma HCO₃ mEq/L	Urinary pH	Titratable Acidity μEq/min	NH₄ Production μEq/min	Total H+ Production
Normal subjects	23–25	4.8–5.2	30–40	50–60	80–100
Type I RTA (distal)	20–23	6.7–6.9	12–18	15–30	30–50
Type II RTA (proximal)	15–18	4.8–5.5	30–40	40–60	80–100

* Values represent either responses to ammonium chloride loading (0.1/kg) as described by Wrong and Davies,[85] or values obtained during untreated systemic acidosis.

percalciuria and progressive nephrocalcinosis seen in hyperparathyroidism can lead to an acidification defect and hyperchloremic acidosis.[1,2]

In general, Type I RTA is much more easily treated than is Type II. In Type I, administration of 1.5 to 2 mEq of sodium bicarbonate/kg body weight/day is usually sufficient to maintain normal arterial pH and to stop the renal losses of cations such as calcium and potassium. On occasion, however, potassium loss continues despite effective treatment with alkali.[83] Such individuals will require maintenance potassium supplements.

Type II Proximal Tubular Acidosis

Here the primary problem is failure of proximal reabsorption of filtered bicarbonate. As a consequence, the fluid reabsorbed by the kidney has a lower concentration of bicarbonate and a systemic acidosis results. However, once a steady state is reached at a lower bicarbonate level, the distal renal tubular mechanisms operate adequately. In this circumstance, the individual has a systemic metabolic acidosis characterized by a marked hyperchloremia, but with a normal urine pH. Thus, at this reduced level of bicarbonate concentration within the body fluids, the acidification mechanism within the kidney works satisfactorily, yielding normal values for titratable acid and ammonia excretion. As a result, these patients do not have a continuous drain on the cation stores of the bone, and skeletal abnormalities are not usually seen.

When treatment of Type II RTA is undertaken, two characteristic features are observed. First, large quantities of bicarbonate (up to 10 mEq/kg body weight/day) are required to return the plasma bicarbonate to normal levels and to maintain the concentration within this range. Urine pH becomes very alkaline long before the plasma bicarbonate returns to normal levels. Second, as bicarbonate administration is begun there is a marked increase in potassium loss.

Frequently, quite large quantities of supplemental potassium are required in order to maintain potassium balance and prevent severe hypokalemia.

Etiologically, a spontaneously occurring and possibly hereditary form of proximal (Type II) renal tubular acidosis has been recognized. Much more commonly, the defect is associated with Fanconi syndrome or with evidence of tubular damage secondary to various toxic agents such as heavy metals, amphotericins, and other organic compounds.[83]

Management requires large quantities of bicarbonate, frequently reaching 10 mEq/kg body weight/day. Despite this, it is more difficult to maintain the patient with a normal arterial pH, and persistent potassium loss continues which is quite marked on occasion. It is frequently necessary to provide supplements in excess of 50 to 75 mEq/day.

Phosphate-Losing Nephropathy (Vitamin D-Resistant Rickets)

Since dietary rickets is now rarely seen, phosphate-losing nephropathy is probably the leading cause of rickets in the United States.[84] Its presence is usually noted when weight bearing first begins in childhood. Tetany is uncommon, but unless the disease is treated promptly, marked rachitic deformities leading to short stature occur.

The basic defect is inability of the kidney to conserve phosphate adequately. There is an abnormally high phosphate clearance and reduced concentration of inorganic phosphorus in the blood.

It is a hereditary disorder transmitted as an X-linked dominant. Affected males have a more severe form of the disease, while females having one affected X chromosome and a normal X chromosome usually have less difficulty.

Administration of vitamin D in large doses (150,000 units or more daily) and a high phosphate intake are most successful in correcting the skeletal abnormalities. Therapy should be started as early as possible to prevent permanent skeletal deformity, but caution is necessary in order to avoid hypercalcemia with such large doses of vitamin D.

There is a nonhereditary form of the disease which has its onset between the ages of 12 and 15 years, with rapidly developing rickets and osteomalacia. There is usually severe muscular weakness.

NEPHROGENIC DIABETES INSIPIDUS

The primary lesion of nephrogenic diabetes insipidus resides in the kidney.[79] The clinical features of the disease are similar to those of diabetes insipidus associated with deficiency of the antidiuretic hormone, but the kidney fails to respond to exogenously administered vasopressin. The disease presents in infancy with signs of severe dehydration, fever, and plasma hyperosmolality, sometimes accompanied by convulsions; the dehydration may be so severe that polyuria is not recognized although the urine is hypotonic to plasma. The diagnosis is established by the failure of administered vasopressin to induce a reduction in urine flow after adequate hydration. The disease is inherited, with the greatest frequency in males of affected kindreds.

Therapy consists principally of supportive care. Solute intake should be kept low in order to reduce obligatory water loss. Restriction of protein intake in children is limited by nutritional requirements, but strict reduction in salt ingestion effectively lowers solute intake. Chlorothiazide and other diuretics will reduce urine flow by producing sodium depletion and diminishing glomerular filtration rate. This increases the proportion of filtered fluid reabsorbed in the proximal tubule, thereby reducing the rate of delivery of tubular fluid to the distal diluting segment, with a fall in total urine volume. This therapy may be hazardous since it leads to moderate sodium depletion which may be acutely aggravated by vomiting or diarrhea from any cause. Chlorothiazide induces potassium loss in the urine so that hypokalemia may develop. If such patients reach maturity, management is less difficult since they can attend to their own water requirements.

THE AMINO-ACIDURIAS[77,78,80]

The free amino acids found in the plasma appear in the glomerular ultrafiltrate and are, for the most part, nearly completely reabsorbed by the tubules. The only amino acids which appear in the urine of normal individuals in significant quantities are alanine, glycine, serine, histidine, and taurine. Excretory rates for all of these exceed 60 mg per day in the average adult. Of the other amino acids, only a few milligrams are excreted in 24 hours, despite the fact that between 1 and 5 g per day of each are filtered.

The term "amino-aciduria," as used clinically, may denote either the appearance of an abnormal quantity of a normal constituent amino acid or the appearance of an abnormal amino acid in the urine. Since renal transport involves filtration and reabsorption, it may be expected that amino-aciduria could result from filtration of increased quantities of either normal or abnormal amino acids or from impairment of the tubular reabsorptive mechanisms for the normal amino acid constituents of glomerular filtrate. In fact, examples representing each of these possibilities have been recognized. Those resulting from an increase in quantity filtered are termed "overflow amino-aciduria," and are usually, but not always, associated with elevated plasma levels of amino acids. Occasionally, the compound may have no tubular reabsorptive mechanism and, hence, filtration and excretion occur at such a rapid rate that plasma levels remain undetectable. This is so, for example, in β-amino-isobutyric aciduria and argininosuccinic aciduria.

In contrast to the overflow amino-acidurias, a few instances of specific defects in renal transport mechanisms have been recognized. The classic example is cystinuria. Lysine, ornithine, and arginine are also found in increased quantities in the urine in this disorder.

Defects in transport may be generalized or localized to the kidney. They may either reflect a hereditary disorder or be due to toxic damage to the proximal tubule. In some instances—notably the Lignac-de Toni-Fanconi type of transport defect—there is other evidence of proximal tubular damage, including defective phosphate reabsorption and defective uric acid transport.

Many of the amino-acidurias reflect a generalized metabolic disturbance and are not associated with any recognizable type of renal disorder. When amino-aciduria is associated with renal involvement, it usually is the result of either defective acidification or of stone formation. Defective acidification is usually mild and leads only to a slight compensated metabolic acidosis. It may, on occasion, be associated with rather marked calcium and potassium losses, with attendant clinical manifestations.

Renal stones are likely to occur when the amino acid appearing in the urine is relatively insoluble. Cystinuria is the most commonly encountered example of this; insolubility of cystine in acid urine leads to precipitation of cystine and the formation of radiolucent stones.

A partial listing of these syndromes is shown in Table 14–2, arranged according to the primary cause of the amino-aciduria.

---TABLE 14–2---

The Amino–Acidurias [2,77,78,80,82]

Syndrome	Amino Acids in Urine	Clinical Features	Other Disturbances of Renal Function
I. Specific Renal Tubular Transport Defects			
Cystinuria [2]	Dibasic amino acids Cystine Lysine Ornithine Arginine	Recurrent renal stone	Occasionally infection second to renal lithiasis
Hartnup disease [78]	Glutamine Asparagine Histidine Serine Threonine Phenylalanine Tryptophane Tyrosine	Pellagra-like skin rash Cerebellar ataxia Diplopia Neurologic findings intermittent	None
Glycinuria	Glycine		Renal stones
II. Amino-Aciduria Associated with Generalized Tubular Dysfunction			
Lignac-Fanconi syndrome [77]	Generalized amino-aciduria with normal plasma amino acid levels	Vomiting, poor intake, Polyuria, rickets Malnutrition Hepatosplenomegaly Cystine deposits in tissue	Glycosuria Impairment in acidification Increased uric acid and phosphate clearance
Adult Fanconi [80]	Generalized amino-aciduria	Osteomalacia most striking feature No cystine deposits in tissues	Glycosuria Increased uric acid and phosphate clearance Frequently defective acidification
Lowe syndrome [2]	Generalized amino-aciduria Increased phosphate clearance	Mental retardation, Congenital glaucoma, Nystagmus, photophobia, Hypotonia	Concentrating defect Impairment in acidification Glycosuria Keto-acids in urine
Wilson's disease [80]	Threonine Cystine, proline, Citrulline, serine Glycine, asparagine, Valine, tyrosine, Lysine	Central nervous system lesions Cirrhosis	Occasional renal stones
Heavy metal damage [2] Lead Uranium Cadmium	Reversible amino-acidurias	Variable	Variable
III. Overflow Amino-Aciduria			
Argininosuccinic aciduria [2]	Argininosuccinic acid		None
Homocystinuria [82]	Homocystine		Vascular renal disease
β-Aminoisobutyric aciduria [2]	β-Aminoisobutyric acid		None

CHAPTER 15

Renal Calculi
W. GORDON WALKER

Renal colic and hematuria are cardinal manifestations of nephrolithiasis. The hematuria is usually microscopic, but on occasion grossly bloody urine may be produced. The pain associated with renal stones is a characteristically agonizing flank pain which waxes and wanes in intensity. It may radiate along the course of the ureter to the groin and, occasionally, into the suprapubic area and urethra. Nephrolithiasis may, however, persist for years without any associated pain, and radiopaque kidney stones may be discovered incidentally as a result of abdominal x-rays made for some other purpose. Regardless of the manner in which attention is first called to the existence of renal calculi, good medical management requires that both the cause of the stone formation and the composition of the stone be identified.

COMPOSITION OF KIDNEY STONES

Almost all stones (over 95 percent) are composed of one or more of the following substances: calcium, phosphate, oxalate, uric acid, cystine, and magnesium.[2,87,88,90] The majority of these substances are normally present in urine concentrations that exceed their solubility in water, and, thus, under certain circumstances the urine may be considered to be supersaturated with respect to these constituents. Indeed, calcium oxalate, calcium phosphate, uric acid, and (under certain circumstances) cystine crystals may precipitate out of the urine on standing. Evidence indicates that there is a substance present in urine which tends to reduce the likelihood of precipitation of stone-forming components. Its nature remains to be clarified, and little can be said about its source or precise role in stone formation or stone prevention.[88,89]

The uniform staining properties and architecture of the matrix of decalcified stones suggest that the organic matrix material may be an important factor in stone formation. Finally, excretion of increased quantities of any of the above minerals in the urine may also contribute to stone formation. In most instances, stones are not pure crystals of a single substance, but are mixtures of several of those listed above. It is convenient to discuss these several substances separately, although therapy often involves attempts to lower the concentration of more than one of them in the urine in order to prevent further formation of stones or to retard the growth of those already present. Such therapy is directed toward the substance believed to play the primary role. A partial list of the causes of the common types of stones and the urinary pH usually associated with formation of specific stones is shown in Table 15–1.

CALCIUM STONES

Calcium oxalate stones may be seen in patients who persistently produce a concentrated urine, or they

TABLE 15–1
The Common Varieties of Renal Stones

Type of Stone	Urine pH	Cause(s)

Calcium oxalate	Variable	Concentrated urine
		Hypercalciuria
		  Vitamin D
		    intoxication
		  Hyperparathyroidism
		  Sarcoidosis
		Milk-alkali
		  syndrome
		Osteoporosis
		Renal tubular
		  acidosis
		Idiopathic
		  hypercalciuria
		Hyperoxaluria

Calcium phosphate	Alkaline	Renal tubular
		  acidosis
		Alkali ingestion
		Infection with urea-
		  splitters
		  (produces mixed
		  stones)

Magnesium
  ammonium
  phosphate
	Alkaline	Infection

Uric acid	Acid	Hyperuricaciduria
		  Hyperuricemia
		  Gout
		  High purine diet
		Urinary hyperacidity

Cystine stone	Acid	Cystinuria

may occur in association with an increase in urinary calcium or oxalate. These stones are endemic in certain tropical and subtropical parts of the world. It is probable that a persistently concentrated urine is the most common cause of this type of stone which is more frequently combined with calcium phosphate, uric acid, or both, than seen as a pure stone. It is doubtful whether increased oxalate consumption plays any role in their production, but a rare inborn error in metabolism, hyperoxaluria, may lead to the formation of stones, as well as to deposition of calcium oxalate crystals in soft tissue and throughout the kidneys. The latter abnormality may lead to extensive renal damage and renal insufficiency. The disease appears to be due to a defect which results in increased production of oxalate.

Hypercalciuria is frequently associated with formation of calcium stones. In the absence of ingestion of foods rich in calcium, urinary calcium should not exceed 200 mg per day. Hypercalciuria regularly accompanies hyperparathyroidism, vitamin D excess or intoxication, renal tubular acidosis, the bone resorption that follows osseous metastases of neoplasia, and very high calcium intake, as for instance ingestion of large quantities of milk. Most commonly, however, hypercalciuria is encountered unassociated with any of the above specific disturbances and has been termed *idiopathic hypercalciuria.* It is usually encountered in healthy young men who give a history of recurrent calcium stones. In these individuals the serum calcium concentration is normal and serum phosphate concentration is normal or slightly lowered despite the persistent hypercalciuria. Careful study of such individuals permits separating them into three categories: *absorptive, resorptive* and *renal hypercalciuria.*

Absorptive hypercalciuria, as implied by the name, results from increased gastrointestinal absorption of calcium. It is diagnosed by demonstrating that oral administration of calcium results in an increase in urinary excretion.[2] Serum calcium and phosphorus are normal. Calcium balance studies, if done, are virtually always positive, and dietary reduction of calcium reduces the rate of urinary calcium excretion.

Resorptive hypercalciuria represents excretion of calcium that has been resorbed from bone. Most commonly, this is caused by hyperparathyroidism, particularly when overt cases of neoplastic bony metastases are excluded. Most such patients (>75 percent) have elevated serum calciums and are, thus, easily distinguished from other forms of hypercalciuria. From the standpoint of accurate differential diagnosis, recognition of those cases of hyperparathyroidism with *normal* serum calcium values is a greater

challenge. These patients exhibit elevated levels of urinary cyclic AMP and elevations in circulating levels of parathormone. They also exhibit a persistently negative calcium balance and decreasing bone density with time, in contrast to patients with absorptive hypercalciuria who show no changes in bone density, normal or low values for parathyroid hormone, and no evidence of persistently negative calcium balance.

Surgical treatment is indicated in those cases of resorptive hypercalciuria that are due to parathyroid adenoma. In patients exhibiting hypercalcemia as well as hypercalciuria, elevated urinary cyclic AMP and renal lithiasis, diagnosis presents little difficulty and surgery is curative. In those cases with recurrent stones, elevation of urinary calcium, cyclic AMP, and elevated parathormone levels in the plasma but normal calcium values, surgical exploration is probably also the preferable therapeutic approach. It is wise, however, to see whether the elevated parathormone levels can be suppressed by calcium administration before recommending surgery.

Renal hypercalciuria represents persistent loss of calcium via the urine as a result of a renal "leak." The classical example is renal tubular acidosis. In at least one kindred with renal tubular acidosis, an increased incidence of hypercalciuria with renal stones was reported in other members of the kindred.[75] In two patients with renal hypercalciuria studied in detail, normal serum calcium, elevated parathormone levels, negative calcium balance, elevated cyclic AMP, and reduced bone density were demonstrated. The elevated parathormone levels in this condition have been suppressed by calcium administration and by thiazide administration.

Since the therapeutic regimen selected is dependent upon the distinction between these types of hypercalciuria, patients presenting with calcium stones and hypercalciuria should be studied in sufficient detail to permit categorization of the urinary calcium loss. Table 15-2 summarizes the distinguishing features of each of these types of hypercalciuria.

URIC ACID STONES

Uric acid stones develop in association with excessive excretion of uric acid or with normal excretion when the urine has a persistently acid pH (below 6.0). The principal reason for increased uric acid excretion is hyperuricemia due to a variety of causes. Less than 20 percent of uric acid stones are associated with gout. Increased intake of purines may lead to increased excretion of uric acid and predisposes to stone formation. A list of the disorders associated with formation of uric acid stones is given in Table 15-1.

CYSTINE STONES

The cystine content of urine in normal individuals is very near the limit of solubility of this amino acid. Increased excretion of cystine is seen in Wilson's disease, Fanconi syndrome, and terminal liver failure. Although crystals of cystine may be common in the urine under these circumstances, stone formation is unusual. Stones composed of cystine are almost exclusively associated with the disorder in cystine transport. In addition to cystine, arginine, ornithine, and lysine are also excreted in this metabolic defect. These substances are so soluble that they never lead to stone formation. Hence, stones are practically always composed of pure cystine. Urinary solubility of cystine varies nearly five-fold over the physiologic range of urine pH, being most insoluble in acid urine. Thus, stones are more likely to develop when the urine is persistently acid.

CLINICAL FEATURES
OF NEPHROLITHIASIS

Renal colic and hematuria are the cardinal manifestations of nephrolithiasis, but the clinical spectrum may vary from an asymptomatic opaque stone discovered incidentally on x-ray examination to a fulminant pyelonephritis. The physician's responsibility includes care of the acute attack, definition of the underlying condition leading to stone formation, and the taking of preventive measures designed to reduce the likelihood of subsequent stone formation.

Renal Colic

Typical renal colic is an excruciating, lancinating pain that begins in the flank—posteriorly or laterally—and radiates downward along the course of the ureter, and, at times, into either the testis or urethra. It is one of the more severe, frightening pains encountered in medical practice. Renal colic compares with the pain of dissecting aneurysm or angina pectoris in severity. The pain may remain unrelieved even by as much as 16 mg of morphine so that analgesic overdosage may result if vigorous therapy with opiates is used. The spectrum of pain associated with the passage of renal calculi is great. Patients with extensive nephrocalcinosis who frequently pass renal stones may have only slight to moderate discomfort for a short period.

Once the stone has entered the ureter, it must either be extruded by the peristaltic action of the ureter or extracted surgically since, if left in place, the resulting obstruction and stasis will rapidly lead to progressive loss of renal function. No invariable rules can be established for the timing of surgical intervention, but appropriate diagnostic procedures should determine promptly whether there is significant obstruction. If such obstruction is found, early surgical intervention is necessary. It is doubtful that a kidney can regain significant function if the ureter has been completely obstructed for 2 weeks or more.

Hematuria

The presence of red blood cells in the urine, in the absence of other formed elements, should always raise suspicion of renal lithiasis and should be investigated thoroughly (p. 136). Since some stones are radiolucent, contrast radiography should be employed to exclude the presence of a stone.

Obstruction

In addition to the acute obstruction produced by blockage of the ureter, intrarenal obstruction may occur due to growth of calculi and, on occasion, small stones may lodge in the ureter to produce low-grade obstruction with progressive hydronephrosis. In the latter situation, secondary infection often supervenes, producing pyonephrosis and rapid destruction of renal tissue. For this reason, periodic pyelography should be performed on patients who recurrently form stones. When the obstruction is identified, prompt surgical correction is indicated.

DIAGNOSTIC STUDY OF PATIENTS
WITH STONE FORMATION

After the indicated management of the immediate problem has been accomplished, further studies should be made to determine, if possible, the cause of the stone formation. *A complete analysis of the stone should always be done.* Usually, this analysis will shape the course of the subsequent diagnostic workup. If the stone is of calcium origin, 24-hour urinary calcium excretions followed by the studies outlined in Table 15–2 permit categorization of the type of hypercalciuria. Appropriate management depends upon the results of these studies. In similar fashion, if stone analysis results in identification of uric acid or cystine stones, subsequent efforts should be directed toward defining the conditions necessary to maintain the urine at a sufficiently high pH to prevent crystallization and stone formation by these substances. Mixed stones (containing Ca^{++}, Mg^{++}, NH_4^+, PO_4, oxalate) virtually always signify infection. Subsequent efforts should be directed toward being certain that all remaining stones are removed, if possible, and that the infection is controlled.

TABLE 15-2
Differentiation of Types of Hypercalciuria

Type	Serum Ca	Serum P	Ca Balance	Bone Density	Serum PTH	Urinary cAMP
Absorptive	NORM	NORM	POS or O	NORM	↓	↓
Resorptive	↑ or NORM	NORM or ↓	NEG	↓	↑	↑
Renal	NORM	NORM	NEG	↓	↑	↑

TREATMENT OF NEPHROLITHIASIS

Surgical treatment should be instituted if a stone in the genitourinary tract is so situated as to lend itself to removal without extensive damage to the kidney. On occasions this is not possible. Under such circumstances, the appropriate treatment outlined in Table 15–3 should be instituted and the patient watched carefully for infection. Since the presence of a stone in the upper urinary tract predisposes to infection which nearly always results in an increased rate of growth of the stone, careful management is necessary to avoid a vicious cycle leading to ultimate loss of the involved kidney. Urinary tract infection should be treated vigorously.

In addition, the specific corrective measures listed in Table 15–3 should be instituted if the composition of the stone has been established certainly enough to permit rational selection. In general, all of these therapies are designed to reduce the concentration of the offending substance in the urine and/or to maintain the pH of the urine at or near the range where solubility of the components of the stone is greatest. Once infection has become established and urinary pH has become constantly alkaline as a result of the infection, stones of any basic composition tend to grow rapidly by the accretion of calcium and magnesium ammonium phosphate in alkaline solution. For this reason, eradication of the infection is imperative whenever possible. If not, every attempt at suppression of the infection should be made by acidification of the urine. In all patients with recurrent stone formation, regular supervision and periodic urine checks are vital. The physician must be certain that the prescribed regimen is followed.

The diagnosis of hypercalciuria during the workup for calcium stone merits special attention. Absorptive hypercalciuria is most appropriately managed by reduction of calcium intake (exclusion of milk and milk products) and the use of cellulose phosphate as a calcium binding agent to further reduce calcium absorption.[1]

A diagnosis of resorptive hypercalciuria implies excess parathormone from a parathyroid adenoma or occult neoplasm. Ordinarily, surgery is indicated, but in those few cases with normal serum calcium values and little evidence of adverse effect, if the initial decision is to observe rather than carry out neck exploration, they should probably not be given orthophosphates, but watched very carefully. A propensity toward recurrent stone formation should force reconsideration of surgical exploration. Renal hypercalciuria should probably best be managed with thiazides, although the administration of neutral phosphates produces comparable results in terms of reducing the incidence of recurrence of stone formation.

Occasionally, dissolution of stones already formed may occur under appropriate therapy. When

TABLE 15-3
Therapy for Nephrolithiasis

Type of Stone	Treatment
Uric acid	Low purine diet High urine volume (>3000 ml/day) Urinary alkalinization (pH >7.4) Allopurinol
Cystine	Alkalinization (pH >7.4) High urine volume (>3000 ml/day)
Mixed stone	Most important to eradicate infection. Continuous suppression necessary if this is not achieved.
Calcium stone	
Absorptive hypercalciuria	Low calcium diet Cellulose phosphate
Resorptive hypercalciuria	Surgery
Renal hypercalciuria	Chlorothiazide 500 mg bid or Neutral phosphates (1 g of phosphorus per day as buffered neutral phosphates)

urinary pH is carefully maintained above 7.0, both uric acid and cystine stones may dissolve. Allopurinal may further facilitate dissolution of uric acid stones by reducing the quantity of uric acid in the urine bathing the stone and thereby maintaining a gradient more favorable to solution of the stone. Excretion of a dilute urine is of added benefit under these circumstances. The persistent use of neutral phosphate solution is also of value in promoting solution of small calcium oxalate stones.

REFERENCES

General References

1. Brenner, B.M. and Rector, F.C., Jr. The Kidney, Vols. I, II. Philadelphia, Saunders, 1976.
   First volume deals with physiology, second volume with pathophysiology and disease.
2. Earley, L. and Gottschalk, C. (eds.). Strauss and Welt's Diseases of the Kidney, 3rd ed. Boston, Little, Brown, 1979.
   Excellent source book for clinical renal disease.
3. Germuth, F.G., Jr. and Rodriguez, E. Immunopathology of the Renal Glomerulus. Immunocomplex Deposit and Antibasement Membrane Disease. Boston, Little, Brown, 1973.
4. Kincaid-Smith, P., Mathew, T.H., and Becker, E.L. Glomerulonephritis. New York, Wiley, 1973.
5. Orloff, J. and Berliner, R.W. Handbook of Physiology, Section 8: Renal Physiology. Baltimore, American Physiological Society, 1973.
   An excellent comprehensive reference.
6. Papper, S. Clinical Nephrology, 2nd ed. Boston, Little, Brown, 1978.
7. Schrier, R.W. (ed.). Renal and Electrolyte Disorders. Boston, Little, Brown, 1976.
8. Smith, H.W. The Kidney Structure and Function in Health and Disease. New York, Oxford University Press, 1951.
   This is an excellent source book, containing a virtually complete compilation and discussion of the physiologic studies on the kidney up to the date of its publication.
9. ———. Principles of Renal Physiology. New York, Oxford University Press, 1956.
   This monograph presents a brief and lucid account of renal physiology.
10. Valtin, H. Renal Function: Mechanisms Preserving Fluid and Solute Balance in Health. Boston, Little, Brown, 1973.
    Renal physiology lucidly presented with clinically oriented approach to the physiology of the kidney and fluid and electrolyte metabolism.

Renal Function and Its Clinical Evaluation

11. Alyea, E.P. and Parrish, A.H., Jr. Renal response to exercise. Urinary findings. JAMA, 167:807, 1958.
12. Bartoli, E. and Early, L.E. Importance of ultrafilterable plasma factors in maintaining tubular reabsorption. Kidney Int., 3:142, 1973.
13. Berliner, R.W. Renal mechanisms for potassium excretion. The Harvey Lectures 1959–1960, New York, Academic, 1961.
14. ——— and Davidson, D.G. Production of hypertonic urine in the absence of the antidiuretic hormone. J. Clin. Invest., 36:1416, 1957.
15. Bricker, N.S. Renal function in chronic renal disease. Medicine (Balt.), 44:263, 1965.
16. Doolan, P.D., Alpen, E.L., and Theil, G.B. A clinical appraisal of the plasma concentration and endogenous clearance of creatinine. Am. J. Med., 32:65, 1962.
17. Gottschalk, C.W. Osmotic concentration and dilution in the mammalian nephron. Circulation, 21:861, 1960.
18. Jamison, R.L. Countercurrent systems. In Thurau, K. (ed.), Kidney and Urinary Tract Physiology. Oxford, Medical and Technical Publishing, 1974, p. 199.
19. Kokko, J.P., Rector, F.C., Imai, M., and Rocha, A.S. Experimental and theoretical evidence for the passive equilibration model of countercurrent multiplication system. In Villareal, H. (ed.), Proceedings of the Fifth International Congress of Nephrology (Mexico, 1974), Vol. 2, 1974, p. 91.
20. Lippman, R.W. Urine and the Urinary Sediment, 2nd ed. Springfield, Ill., Thomas, 1957.
21. Mitch, W.E., Walser, M., Buffington, G.A., and Lemann, J. A simple method of estimating progression of chronic renal failure. Lancet, 2:1326, 1976.
22. Morgan, T. Movement of solute and water in the countercurrent system of the medulla. In Proceedings of the Fourth International Congress of Nephrology (Stockholm, 1969), Vol. 1, pp. 70–71.
23. Navar, L.G., Burke, T.J., Robinson, R.R., and Clapp, J.R. Distal tubular feedback in the autoregulation of single nephron glomerular filtration rate. J. Clin. Invest., 53:516, 1974.
24. Roberts, K.E., Randall, H.T., Vanamee, P., and Poppell, J.W. Renal mechanisms involved in bicarbonate reabsorption. Metabolism, 5:404, 1956.
25. Wesson, L.G., Jr. Glomerular and tubular factors in the renal excretion of sodium chloride. Medicine (Balt.), 36:281, 1957.
26. Wright, F.S. Intrarenal regulation of glomerular filtration rate. N. Engl. J. Med., 291:135, 1974.

Pathogenesis, Clinical Manifestations, and Management of Uremia

27. Boen, S.T. Kinetics of peritoneal dialysis, a comparison with the artificial kidney. Medicine (Balt.), 40:243, 1961.
28. Lemann, J., Jr., Litzow, J.R., and Lennon, E.J. Studies of the mechanism by which chronic metabolic acidosis augments urinary calcium excretion in man. J. Clin. Invest., 46:1318, 1967.
29. Litzow, J.R., Lemann, J., Jr., and Lennon, E.J. The effect of treatment of acidosis on calcium balance in patients with chronic azotemic renal disease. J. Clin. Invest., 46:280, 1967.

30. Maher, J.F., Nolph, K.D., and Bryan, C.N. Prognosis of advanced chronic renal failure. I. Unpredictability of survival and reversibility. Ann. Intern. Med., 81:43, 1974.

31. Rasmussen, H. and Bordier, P. The Physiological Basis of Metabolic Bone Disease. Baltimore, Williams & Wilkins, 1974.

32. ———, Wong, M., Bikle, D., and Goodman, D. Hormonal control of the renal conversion of 25 hydroxycholecalciferol to 1:25 dihydroxycholecalciferol. J. Clin. Invest., 51:2502, 1972.

33. Reiss, E., Canterbury, J.M., and Kanter, A. Circulating parathormone concentration in chronic renal insufficiency. Arch. Intern. Med. Symp., 3:417, 1969.

34. Seigler, H.F., Amos, D.B., Ward, F.E., Andrus, C.H., Southworth, J.G., Hattler, B.G., Jr., and Stickel, D.L. Immunogenetics of consanguineous allografts in man. I. Histocompatibility testing and skin allografts. Ann. Surg., 172:151, 1970.

35. Stanbury, S.W., Lumb, G.A., and Mawer, E.B. Osteodystrophy developing spontaneously in the course of chronic renal failure. Arch. Intern. Med. Symp., 3:274, 1969.

36. Starzl, T.E., Porter, K.A., Andres, G., Halgrimson, C.G., Hurwitz, R., Giles, G., Terasaki, P.I., Penn, I., Schroter, G.T., Lilly, J., Starkie, S.J., and Putnam, C.W. Long-term survival after renal transplantation in humans. Ann. Surg., 172:437, 1970.

37. Striber, G.E. and Tenckhoff, H.A. A transcutaneous prosthesis for prolonged access to the peritoneal cavity. Surgery, 69:70, 1971.

38. Whelton, A. Antibacterial chemotherapy in renal insufficiency: a review. Antibiot. Chemother., 18:1, 1974.

39. Opelz, G. and Terasaki, P.I. Enhancement of kidney graft survival by blood transfusions. Transplant Proc., 9:121, 1977.

Acute Suppression of Urine Formation

40. Bleumle, L.W., Webster, G.D., Jr., and Elkinton, J.R. Acute tubular necrosis: analysis of 100 cases with respect to mortality, complications and treatment with and without dialysis. Arch. Intern. Med., 194:180, 1959.

41. Bricker, N.S., Shwayri, E.R., Reardon, J.B., Kellog, D., Merrill, J.P., and Holmes, J.H. Abnormality in renal function resulting from urinary tract obstruction. Am. J. Med., 23:554, 1957.

42. Friedman, E.A. and Eliahou, H.E., (eds.). Proceedings: Conference on Acute Renal Failure, D.H.E.W. Publ. No. (NIH) 74-608. Washington, D.C., Government Printing Office, 1973.

43. Kleinknecht, D., Jungers, P., Chanard, J., Barbanel, C., Ganeval, D., and Rondon-Nucete, M. Factors influencing immediate prognosis in acute renal failure with special reference to prophylactic hemodialysis. In Hamburger, J., Crosneir, J., and Maxwell, M.H. (eds.), Advances in Nephrology, Vol. 1. Chicago, Yearbook Medical Publishers, 1971, p. 207.

The Proteinurias and Hematurias

44. Abramowicz, M., Barnett, H.L., Edelmann, C.M., Jr., Griefer, I., Kobayashi, O., Arneil, G.C., Barron, B.A., Gordillo, P.G., Hallman, N., and Triddens, H.A. Controlled trial of azathioprine in children with nephrotic syndrome. Lancet, 1:959, 1970.

45. Addis, T. Haemorrhagic Bright's disease: natural history. Johns Hopkins Med. J., 49:203, 1931.

46. Barnett, H.L. The natural and treatment history of glomerular diseases, in Children. In Giovannetti, S., Bonomini, V., and D'Amico, G. (eds.), Proceedings of the Sixth International Congress of Nephrology. Basel, Karger, 1975, pp. 470–485.

47. Bates, R.C., Jennings, R.B., and Earle, D.P. Acute nephritis unrelated to group A hemolytic streptococcus infection. Am. J. Med., 23:510, 1957.

48. Berger, J., Noel, L-H., and Yanerva, H. Complement deposition in the kidney. In Hamburger, J., Crosner, J., and Maxell, M. (eds.), Advances In Nephrology, Vol. 4. Chicago, Year Book Medical Publishers, 1974, p. 37.

49. Berman, L.B. and Schreiner, G.E. Clinical and histologic spectrum of the nephrotic syndrome. Am. J. Med., 24:249, 1958.

50. Black, D.A.K., Rose, G., and Brewer, D.B. Controlled trial of prednisone in adult patients with the nephrotic syndrome. Br. Med. J., 3:421, 1970.

51. Blainey, J.D. High protein diets in the treatment of the nephrotic syndrome. Clin. Sci., 13:567, 1954.

52. Cameron, J.S., Chantler, C., Ogg, C.S., and White, R.H.R. Long-term stability of remission in nephrotic syndrome after treatment with cyclophosphamide. Br. Med. J., 4:7, 1974.

53. Cameron, J.S., Turner, D.R., Ogg, C.S., Sharpstone, P., and Brown, C.B. The nephrotic syndrome in adults with minimal change lesions. Q. J. Med., 43:461, 1974.

54. Chinard, F.P., Lawson, H.E., Eder, H.A., Grief, R.L., and Hiller, A. A study of the mechanism of proteinuria in patients with the nephrotic syndrome. J. Clin. Invest., 33:621, 1954.

55. Davson, J., Ball, J., and Platt, R. Kidney in periarteritis nodosa. Q. J. Med., 17:175, 1948.

56. Ellis, A. Natural history of Bright's disease: clinical, histological and experimental observations. Croonian Lectures. Lancet, 1:1, 1942.

57. Grausz, H., Earley, L.E., Stephens, B.G., Lee, J.C., and Hopper, J. Virus-like particles in glomerular endothelium of patients with SLE. N. Engl. J. Med., 283:506, 1970.

58. Gregoire, F., Malmendier, C., and Lambert, P.P. The mechanism of proteinuria, and a study of the effects of hormonal therapy in the nephrotic syndrome. Am. J. Med., 25:516, 1948.

59. Habib, R., Loirat, C., Gubler, M., and Levy, M. Morphology and serum complement levels in membranoproliferative glomerulonephritis. In Hamburger, J., Crosner, J., and Maxwell, M. (eds.), Advances in Nephrology, Vol. 4. Chicago, Year Book Medical Publishers, 1974, p. 109.

60. Heptinstall, R.H. Pathology of the Kidney, 2nd ed., Vol. 1. Boston, Little, Brown, 1974, pp. 273–392.

61. Herdman, R.C., Pickering, R.J., Michael, A.F., Vernier, R.L., Fish, A.J., Gewartz, H., and Good, R.A. Chronic glomerulonephritis associated with low serum complement activity (chronic hypocomplementemic glomerulonephritis). N. Engl. J. Med., 283:506, 1970.

62. Hopper, J., Ryan, P., Lee, J.C., and Roseman, W. Lipoid nephrosis in 31 adult patients: renal biopsy study by light, electron and fluorescence microscopy with experience in treatment. Medicine, 49:321, 1970.

63. Hunsiker, L.G., Ruddy, S., Carpenter, C.B., Shur, P.H., Merrill, J.P., Muller-Eberhard, H.J., and Austen, K.F. Metabolism of third complement component (C3) in nephritis. Involvement of the classical and alternate (properdin) pathways for complement activation. N. Engl. J. Med., 287:835, 1972.

64. Kark, R.M., Pirani, C.L., Pollak, V.E., Muehrcke, R.C., and Blainey, J.D. The nephrotic syndrome in adults: a common disorder with many causes. Ann. Intern. Med., 49:751, 1958.

65. Koffler, D. and Kunkel, H.G. Mechanisms of renal injury in systemic lupus erythematosus. Am. J. Med., 45:165, 1968.

66. Michael, A.F. and McLean R.H. Evidence for activation of the alternate pathway in glomerulonephritis. In Hamburger, J., Crosner, J., and Maxwell, M. (eds.), Advances in Nephrology, Vol. 4. Chicago, Year Book Medical Publishers, 1974, p. 49.

67. Morel-Maroger, L., Leathem, A., and Richet, G. Glomerular abnormalities in non-systemic disease. Am. J. Med., 53:170, 1972.

68. Muller-Eberhard, H.J. The complement system and nephritis. In Hamburger, J., Crosner, J., and Maxwell, M. (eds.), Advances in Nephrology, Vol. 4. Chicago, Year Book Medical Publishers, 1974, p. 3.

69. Nakamoto, Y., Asano, Y., Dohi, K., Fujioka, M., Iida, H., Kida, H., Kibe, Y., Halton, N., and Takeuchi, J. Primary IgA glomerulonephritis and Schönlein-Henoch purpura nephritis. Clinicopathological and immunohistological characteristics. Q. J. Med., 47:495, 1978.

70. Report of Medical Research Council Working Party: controlled trial of azathioprine and prednisone in chronic renal disease. Br. Med. J., 2:239, 1971.

71. Ruley, E.J., Forrestal, J., Davis, N.C., Andres, C., and West, C.D. Hypocomplementemia of membranoproliferative nephritis. Dependence of nephrotic factor reaction on properdin factor. Br. J. Clin. Invest., 52:896, 1973.

72. Walker, W.G. and Solez, K. Renal involvement in disorders of connective tissue. In Strauss and Welt's Diseases of the Kidney, Earley, L.E., and Gottschalk, G.W. (eds.). Boston, Little, Brown, 1979, p. 1259.

73. Westberg, N.G., Naff, G.B., Boyer, J.T., and Michael, A.F. Glomerular deposition of properdin in acute and chronic glomerulonephritis with hypocomplementemia. J. Clin. Invest., 50:642, 1971.

74. World Health Organization Scientific Group. The role of immune complexes in disease. Geneva, World Health Organization Technical Report Series H606, 1977.

Functional Disorders of the Renal Tubules

75. Buckalew, V.M., Jr., Purvis, M.L., Shulman, M.G., Herndon, C.N., and Rudman, D. Hereditary renal tubular acidosis. Medicine (Balt.), 53:229, 1974.

76. Elkinton, J.R., Huth, E.J., Webster, G.D., Jr., and McCance, R.A. The renal excretion of hydrogen ion in renal tubular acidosis. Am. J. Med., 29:554, 1969.

77. Fanconi, G. Tubular insufficiency and renal dwarfism. Arch. Dis. Child., 29:1, 1954.

78. Jepson, J.G. and Spiro, M.J. Hartnup Disease. In Stanbury, J.B., Wyngaarden, J.B., and Frederickson, D.S. (eds.), The Metabolic Basis of Inherited Disease. New York, McGraw-Hill, 1960, Chap. 43.

79. Macdonald, W.G. Congenital pitressin resistant diabetes of renal origin. Pediatrics, 15:298, 1955.

80. Mudge, G.H. Clinical patterns of tubular dysfunction. Am. J. Med., 24:785, 1958.

81. Rodriguez-Soriano, R., Biochis, H., Stark, H., and Edelmann, C.M., Jr. Proximal renal tubular acidosis. A defect in bicarbonate reabsorption with normal urinary acidification. Pediatr. Res., 1:81, 1967.

82. Schimke, R.N., McKusick, V.A., Huang, J., and Pollack, A.D. Homocystinuria: studies of 20 families with 38 affected members. JAMA, 193:719, 1965.

83. Sebastian, A., McSherry, E., and Morris, R.C. Jr. Metabolic acidosis with special reference to the renal acidosis. In Brenner, B.M. and Rector, F.C., Jr. (eds.), The Kidney. Philadelphia, Saunders, 1976.

84. Winters, R.W., Graham, J.B., Williams, T.F., McFalls, V.W., and Burnett, C.H. A genetic study of familial hypophosphatemia with vitamin D resistant rickets with a review of the literature. Medicine (Balt.), 37:97, 1958.

85. Wrong, O. and Davies, H.E.F. The excretion of acid in renal disease. Q. J. Med., 28:259, 1959.

Renal Calculi

86. Albright, F. and Reifenstein, E.C. Parathyroid Glands and Metabolic Bone Disease. Baltimore, Williams & Wilkins, 1948.

87. Boyce, W.H. and Garvey, F.K. Incidence of urinary calculi among patients in general hospitals, 1948 to 1952. JAMA, 161:1437, 1956.

88. Howard, J.E. Urinary stone. Can. Med. Assoc. J., 86:1001, 1962.

89. Howard, J.E. Studies on urinary stone formation: a saga of clinical investigation. Johns Hopkins Med. J. 139:239, 1976.

90. Melick, R.A. and Henneman, P.H. Clinical and laboratory studies of 207 consecutive patients in a kidney stone clinic. N. Engl. J. Med., 259:307, 1958.

SECTION FOUR
Cardiovascular Disease

J. O'NEAL HUMPHRIES AND NICHOLAS J. FORTUIN: SECTION EDITORS

Patients with heart disease are discovered in many ways—from the patient with severe, unbearable chest pain indicative of life-threatening illness, to one with an asymptomatic abnormality detected on routine physical examination, chest x-ray, or electrocardiogram. In both cases, the physician must arrive at a precise etiologic, anatomic, and physiologic diagnosis, which usually requires the analysis of information from many sources. The sources of information and tools used in evaluation will be presented in the first two chapters; the problem situations or patterns of presentation occurring in practice will be discussed in the subsequent chapters.

The clinical evaluation of the cardiovascular system and the symptoms and signs of the diseases of the heart are the subjects of Chapter 16. The use of laboratory studies in the assessment of cardiovascular function is outlined in Chapter 17. Congestive heart failure is a common manifestation of disordered cardiac function, and Chapter 18 is devoted to the pathophysiology of this condition. The approach to the patient with congestive failure or an enlarged heart and the management of congestive failure are the subjects of Chapter 19. The interpretation of murmurs and the specific problems related to valvular heart disease and its surgical treatment are discussed in Chapter 20. The heart murmur may have been detected on routine physical examination or, while it may not have been the original reason to suspect cardiac disease, it may be the most reliable manifestation upon which to base a differential diagnosis. Disorders of cardiac rhythm may be responsible for the patient's seeking medical attention, as in the case of palpitation due to frequent premature contractions.

Under other circumstances, an arrhythmia may be responsible for congestive failure or circulatory collapse (Chap. 21).

Chest pain may be a symptom of potentially fatal heart disease, and the differentiation of chest pain of cardiac origin from that due to other causes is a common and important problem (Chap. 22). Myocardial and pulmonary infarction, the most common cardiovascular causes of pain in the chest and circulatory collapse, are covered in Chapters 23 and 24.

A high systemic arterial blood pressure may be detected on routine examination in the absence of symptoms, or may be the cause of congestive heart failure. In either case, it is an important finding and worthy of individual attention (Chap. 25). Another important abnormality, the cause of which must be clearly established, is pulmonary hypertension. Usually there are symptoms which, when considered with physical signs and laboratory data, lead to the recognition of the problem as one of increased pulmonary vascular resistance (Chap. 26).

Congenital heart disease is the subject of Chapter 27. Diseases of the aorta and the peripheral circulation also are discussed from the point of view of the presenting complaint (Chaps. 28 and 29). The same therapeutic agents may be used to treat a number of different cardiac disorders; in order to prevent repetition, the discussion of their mechanisms of action and uses are aggregated in Chapter 30. Acute circulatory collapse or shock often indicates serious heart disease, and prompt emergency therapy can save life. Therefore, this particular problem is discussed in the section on medical emergencies (Chaps. 144 and 145).

Clinical Evaluation of the Cardiovascular System*

RICHARD S. ROSS

Information useful in the clinical assessment of the cardiovascular system is derived from: 1) history, 2) physical examination, 3) roentgenography, 4) electrocardiography, and 5) special laboratory studies. The patient's cardiac abnormality may be detected on history, physical examination, or laboratory study, but information from all sources is often required to establish a diagnosis and to plan management. For example, the patient may present with a history of dyspnea on exertion; with the physical finding of a murmur; with the discovery of a large heart on survey x-ray; with an abnormal electrocardiogram taken as part of a screening examination; or with pulmonary hypertension discovered at the time of cardiac catheterization for investigation of a systolic murmur.

The physiologic basis for the major cardiac manifestations can be appreciated by consideration of the function of the heart as a pump interposed between two interlocking circuits. The overall function of the circulation depends upon the satisfactory performance of both cardiac muscle and heart valves. The myocardium provides energy for blood flow and the valves assure that flow is unidirectional. Dysfunction of either the myocardium or the valves leads to circulatory failure and the development of symptoms.

CARDIOVASCULAR SYMPTOMS

The major cardiovascular symptoms are described and tabulated along with the generally accepted physiologic interpretation (Table 16-1). All these symptoms and their physiologic mechanisms will be discussed in greater detail in later chapters. This and subsequent tables are concerned only with the role of heart disease in the production of a given symptom or sign and do not include all possible causes of the manifestations listed.

ELICITING THE CARDIOVASCULAR HISTORY

The general principles of history taking apply to the patient with cardiovascular disease, but certain points deserve special emphasis (Chap. 2). The patient may be short of breath (especially while talking) and, therefore, should be seated comfortably at the beginning of the interview. He should be encouraged

to discuss his present illness first, but the family and past histories must not be neglected. The past history is often important in determining whether a heart murmur represents congenital or acquired heart disease. A history of acute rheumatic fever is helpful if present but does not exclude rheumatic heart disease if it is absent. The patient may not realize that he has had rheumatic fever but may recall an illness identified as inflammatory rheumatism or St. Vitus dance. Special questioning about previous physical examinations for athletic teams, military service, or life insurance is often rewarding. The patient may remember that the auscultation of his heart received special attention on one of these occasions.

Dyspnea and chest pain may indicate major abnormalities of cardiovascular function, and the identification and quantitation of these symptoms can only be accomplished by history. The questioning of a patient with dyspnea or chest pain should be specific with regard to the relation of the symptoms to exertion. His exercise tolerance can be quantified by asking how many blocks he can walk or how many stairs he can climb without experiencing symptoms. Variability in the degree of exercise required to produce dyspnea suggests that organic valvular or myocardial disease is not responsible. Sudden isolated episodes of severe dyspnea or pulmonary edema in a patient with normal exercise tolerance indicate that the precipitating condition is inconstant as in the case of repeated episodes of pulmonary embolism or intermittent obstruction to pulmonary venous return by a left atrial thrombus or tumor.

Paroxysmal nocturnal dyspnea is an important symptom of left ventricular failure. The patient with true paroxysmal nocturnal dyspnea usually has no difficulty going to sleep but is awakened by dyspnea. The patient who reports difficulty "drawing a deep breath" when he goes to bed and, hence, has a problem getting to sleep does not have paroxysmal nocturnal dyspnea. This type of complaint is more common in anxiety. Orthopnea is shortness of breath which comes on within a few minutes after the patient lies down, and the patient learns to prevent this symptom by sleeping with his head elevated on three or more pillows. Sometimes nocturnal cough and restlessness may be early subtle signs of left ventricular failure and may be approached by asking the patient how he sleeps.

* See references 8–11.

TABLE 16-1
Major Cardiovascular Symptoms

Symptom	Description	Mechanism
Dyspnea on exertion	Difficult breathing, shortness of breath on exertion, or air hunger on exertion which is excessive relative to the patient's age, state of physical fitness, and the severity of the exercise	Pulmonary vascular congestion. Cardiac output unable to rise. Left heart unable to transfer pulmonary venous return to systemic circulation due to myocardial failure or obstruction. Congested lungs turgid, rigid, and stiff. Work of breathing increased
Orthopnea	Patient unable to lie down flat and becomes short of breath if he does	Shift of blood to heart and pulmonary circulation from veins in lower part of body
Paroxysmal nocturnal dyspnea	Patient awakens from a sound sleep with extreme shortness of breath and must stand or sit up to become comfortable	Increased plasma volume in recumbent posture, secondary to movement of fluid from extravascular to vascular space and shift of blood from peripheral veins to heart and lungs
Edema of ankles	Patient complains of swelling of the ankles, usually at the end of the day	Increased volume of extracellular fluid distributed in dependent parts, i.e., ankles
Abdominal pain	Aching pain in upper abdomen. Sometimes acute and may be confused with acute cholecystitis	Hepatic congestion and swelling with stretching of liver capsule
Palpitation	Patient aware of forceful, rapid, or irregular heartbeat	Cardiac arrhythmia, such as multiple premature systoles, tachycardia, or atrial fibrillation
Angina pectoris	Patient complains of substernal tightness or distress which comes on with exertion and disappears with rest	Relative inadequacy of myocardial blood flow, usually due to atherosclerosis of coronary arteries, but also present in aortic valve disease, hypertrophic cardiomyopathy, and pulmonary hypertension
Fatigue or decreased exertional tolerance	Patient tires easily or cannot keep up with contemporaries	Inability of cardiac output to increase in proportion to metabolic demands, or arterial oxygen unsaturation

Fatigue is a common symptom of heart failure, but it often develops gradually and the patient may be unaware of its presence. Questioning about daily habits, especially the activities after work, may be revealing. The patient may report that he goes to bed following dinner, while formerly he walked, worked in his shop, or engaged in other daily activity.

The symptoms of right heart failure are attributable to the pooling of blood in the systemic venous circulation and the extravasation of fluid into the extravascular space. These are discussed in more detail in Chapter 18. The history of ankle edema is elicited by inquiring about difficulty putting shoes back on at the end of the day after they have been removed.

CARDIAC RISK FACTORS

Special attention should be given to the presence of the major "risk factors" for coronary artery disease, which are cigarette smoking, hypertension, and elevated serum cholesterol. Numerous studies have shown that the patient who smokes more than one pack of cigarettes a day has a risk of having a heart attack that is three times that of a nonsmoker. Similar but less strong relationships exist for hypertension and elevation of serum cholesterol. If all three risk factors are present, the incidence of heart attack is approximately eight times that of subjects with none of the three.

This strong relationship between smoking and

risk makes it imperative that the patient's smoking history be recorded quantitatively in terms of pack-years of smoking. The patient who has smoked an average of two packs a day for 25 years is said to have 50 pack-years (2×25).

A history of hypertension can be obtained by asking whether blood pressure has ever been found to be elevated on physical examination or whether the patient has ever been instructed to take medicine for his blood pressure.

A history of hypercholesterolemia is usually obtained by asking the patient whether he or other members of his family have ever been told by a physician that the cholesterol was elevated. A history of premature death in male relatives is another indication that there may be an inherited defect in lipid metabolism which predisposes to premature coronary artery disease.

Other risk factors with a less strong relationship and, therefore, of less importance from the point of view of history are diabetes, gout, obesity, sedentary life, and certain personality type.

The physician should take advantage of every contact to educate his patient about the importance of risk factors. The physician's responsibility to his patient should be extended to the prevention of disease as well as to its treatment and, therefore, the patient should be persuaded to alter behavior in such a way as to minimize the risk of developing heart disease.

CARDIOVASCULAR PHYSICAL SIGNS

PHYSIOLOGIC BASIS

Cyanosis

Cyanosis is the bluish discoloration of the skin, the mucous membranes, and nail beds resulting from an increased amount of unsaturated hemoglobin in the blood and in the tissue under inspection. About 5 g of unsaturated hemoglobin per 100 ml blood is the threshold for the clinical recognition of cyanosis.

The commonest causes of cyanosis are those related to low blood flow in the peripheral vascular bed (peripheral cyanosis). The arterial oxygen saturation is normal but the flow is slow; each red cell remains in contact with the tissue for a longer period, more oxygen is lost from the cells, and more unsaturated hemoglobin is present in the venous blood. Peripheral cyanosis, due to reduced flow, will usually be more pronounced in peripheral tissues and less pronounced or even absent in central tissues, such as the mucous membranes of the mouth and the conjunctiva. The

most common cause of cyanosis of the extremities is a cold environment, but it may accompany any condition associated with reduced peripheral blood flow. Peripheral cyanosis is present in shock and heart failure because the cardiac output is decreased and, hence, the flow to the skin is slow. The impaired circulation associated with disease of the arteries and veins also results in peripheral cyanosis in the involved extremity. If cyanosis is present when the patient is warm, it is more likely to be of central origin and not the result of reduced flow. The presence of pulmonary osteoarthropathy or clubbing usually means that cyanosis is of a central type due to arterial unsaturation of long standing; its absence does not, however, guarantee that the cyanosis is peripheral.

The term "central cyanosis" has been applied to the situation in which there is arterial oxygen unsaturation. Central cyanosis occurs when blood passes from the venous circulation to the aorta without coming into contact with oxygen in the lungs. This occurs in the following situations: 1) hypoventilation, 2) right to left shunts which may be (a) intrapulmonary (ventilation–perfusion abnormality) or (b) cardiac (including the great vessels). The pulmonary conditions are described in Section 5 and the cardiac conditions in Chapter 27.

Skin Pallor and Temperature

Pallor of the skin or mucous membranes suggests anemia which may be a cause of heart failure or responsible for murmurs which are secondary to excessive blood flow. Anemia may be secondary to infective endocarditis, especially when in a patient with valvular or congenital heart disease. Skin temperature and moisture are important. Cool, damp skin in a warm environment usually indicates that the cardiac output is low and that maximum vasoconstriction is present.

Evidence of Fluid Retention

Certain aspects of the general physical examination may indicate the presence of early heart failure. Percussion of the thorax may reveal evidence of pleural effusion, and fine, moist rales in the lungs may be the earliest sign of pulmonary congestion. Hepatic enlargement and tenderness are signs of right heart failure. A careful search for edema about the ankles and over the sacrum should also be carried out.

CARDIAC SIGNS

Correct interpretation of cardiovascular signs as well as symptoms depends upon clear understanding of the physiological processes responsible. Information obtained from cardiac catheterization, angiocardiography, echocardiography, and phonocardiography has led to a better understanding of the origin of physical signs, and, therefore, the physical examination has assumed new significance. These new techniques have not replaced the old, but rather enhanced their value.

The events of the cardiac cycle are shown in relation to the common auscultatory signs in Figure 16–1. These relationships should be kept in mind during the examination of the heart. Throughout the cardiac cycle, blood returns to the right atrium from the venae cavae and to the left atrium from the pulmonary veins. When the mitral and tricuspid valves open, the blood contained in the atria flows into the ventricles, as does the blood which continues to enter from the veins. During most of diastole, ventricular filling is passive, the driving force being the venous pressure. Filling is rapid during the early part of diastole, just

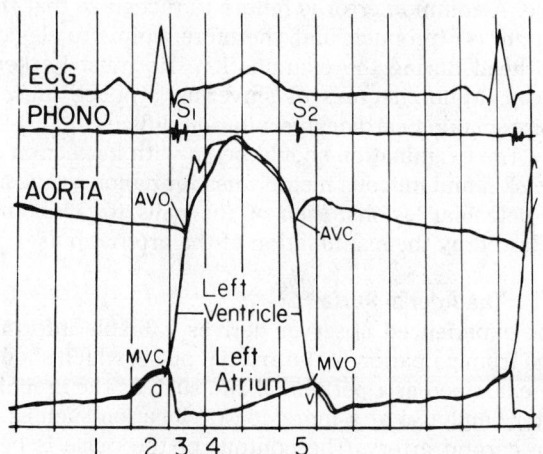

FIGURE 16–1. The hemodynamic and phonocardiographic events are related to mechanical events in the left atrium and ventricle. The temporal relation of the pressure recording to the events of the cardiac cycle is indicated by the position of the numbers. 1. Passive ventricular filling. The pressures in the left atrium and left ventricle are identical and are rising slowly. 2. Atrial systole. The atrium contracts forcing blood into the ventricle. The mitral valve approaches the closed position. The pressure in the left atrium and left ventricle rises to form the *a* wave. 3. Isometric ventricular contraction. The ventricle contracts and the mitral valve is firmly closed (MVC). The aortic valve has not opened, and pressure in the left ventricle rises. The first heart sound (S_1) is generated. 4. Rapid ventricular ejection. Ventricular contraction continues. The aortic valve opens (AVO) and aortic pressure rises. 5. Isometric ventricular relaxation. Left ventricular pressure falls, the aortic valve closes (AVC), but the mitral valve has not yet opened. The second heart sound (S_2) corresponds with the closure of the aortic valve. When the mitral valve opens (MVO), the period of rapid ventricular filling—Stage 1—begins.

after the atrioventricular valves (AV) open, and the third heart sound (S_3) is temporarily related to the culmination of this period of rapid ventricular filling. The flow of blood into the ventricle slows down later in diastole, as the ventricles become nearly full. The pressures in atria and ventricles are equal throughout diastole. Atrial systole marks the end of the period of passive filling and completes ventricular filling by the transfer of a final increment of blood from the atrium to the ventricle. The fourth heart sound (S_4) arises in the ventricle as the chamber receives the contribution of atrial systole.

Ventricular systole begins with the onset of ventricular muscle contraction and the development of pressure in the ventricle. The leaflets of the atrioventricular valves have already approached the closed position and are now firmly approximated by the rise in ventricular pressure. The first heart sound (S_1) is generated by the onset of contraction of the ventricular myocardium and the closure of the mitral and tricuspid valves. During the first part of systole, all valves are closed, and pressure develops in the ventricle without a change in volume: this is the period of isometric contraction. When the pressure in the ventricle exceeds that in the corresponding great vessels, the semilunar valves open and the period of ejection begins. The opening of the semilunar valves and the onset of ejection do not normally produce audible sound, but in the presence of disease may cause an ejection click (EC). The pressures in the ventricles and great vessels (aorta and pulmonary artery) are the same throughout ejection. The period of ejection terminates when the ventricular pressure falls below that in the great vessels and the semilunar valves close. The closure of the semilunar valves produces the second heart sound (S_2) which has two components (A_2) and (P_2) attributable to closure of the aortic and pulmonary valves respectively. A_2 normally precedes P_2. Ventricular pressure continues to fall after the semilunar valves close (period of isometric relaxation) until it falls below the pressure in the atria, at which point the AV valves open and diastole begins with the period of rapid filling. Normal AV valves open silently, but in the presence of mitral stenosis a sound known as the opening snap (OS) is generated by the opening process.

The ideal valve offers no obstruction to forward flow when it is open and prevents retrograde flow when it is closed, and the normal heart valves closely approach this ideal. Disease may impair valvular function either by preventing complete opening (stenosis) or complete closing (regurgitation). Stenosis and regurgitation may exist as separate lesions or may be present simultaneously in the same valve.

Cardiac Abbreviations

The condensation of material into tables is made possible by abbreviations commonly used in cardiologic practice.

Chambers of the Heart

SVC — Superior vena cava
IVC — Inferior vena cava
RA — Right atrium
RV — Right ventricle
PA — Pulmonary artery
PV — Pulmonary vein
LA — Left atrium
LV — Left ventricle
Ao — Aorta

Valvular Lesions

AR — Aortic regurgitation
AS — Aortic stenosis
MR — Mitral regurgitation
MS — Mitral stenosis
TR — Tricuspid regurgitation
TS — Tricuspid stenosis
PR — Pulmonary regurgitation
PS — Pulmonary stenosis

Congenital Lesions

ASD — Atrial septal defect
VSD — Ventricular septal defect
PDA — Patent ductus arteriosus
TGV — Transposition of great vessels
AVR — Anomalous venous return

Other

AF — Atrial fibrillation
PH — Pulmonary hypertension
RVH — Right ventricular hypertrophy
LVH — Left ventricular hypertrophy
LLSB — Left lower sternal border
i.s. — Interspace—between ribs
RBBB — Right bundle branch block
LBBB — Left bundle branch block

Interpretation of Cardiovascular Signs

The salient features of the cardiovascular physical examination are listed in Table 16-2. Opposite a given physical finding are listed the physiologic or pathologic mechanism and the usual interpretation. The mechanism of production of some of the physical signs remains uncertain and the explanations selected appear to be the best available.

TECHNIQUE OF CARDIOVASCULAR PHYSICAL EXAMINATION

The physical examination begins with the physician's first meeting with the patient, continues during the elicitation of the history, and ends when the patient leaves. The astute examiner also often elicits essential history while he is examining the patient, the stimulus for the additional questioning being provided by a particular physical finding. Observation of the patient's manner of moving and speaking yields information about his exercise tolerance. He may catch his breath in the midst of a long sentence or rest for a moment after entering the consultation room. In contrast, the patient whose dyspnea is due to anxiety may exhibit gasping respiration when the complaint is under discussion, but breathe quietly when attention is directed elsewhere. Counting the respirations when the patient first lies down on the examining table gives some indication of the magnitude of the circulatory load imposed by disrobing. Cyanosis or pallor may be apparent when the patient first enters the room and may disappear after he rests and becomes warm.

During the formal part of the physical examination, one must be certain that the patient is comfortable. A common error is failure to recognize that the patient is orthopneic and, therefore, failure to elevate his head during the examination. He must be kept warm. Minor degrees of shivering produce muscle noise, making cardiac auscultation difficult.

The examination should begin with inspection of the skin and mucous membranes for pallor, cyanosis, or petechial lesions, then of the nails for clubbing, followed by the examination of the arterial pulse.

The Arterial Pulse[8]

The experienced observer derives valuable information from palpation of the arterial pulse, which should be examined at a peripheral site such as the brachial artery and also at a more central location such as in the carotid artery. The contour of the pulse is best appreciated in the more central vessels. The brachial artery pulse is best examined by raising the patient's arm vertically from the examining table and compressing the brachial artery with the fingers at a point midway between the shoulder and the elbow. Attention should be directed to the rate of rise and amplitude, both of which are decreased in the patient with aortic stenosis or myocardial disease (pulsus parvus) and are greater than normal when aortic regurgitation is present (Corrigan pulse). The significance of other alterations in the arterial pulse can be determined from Table 16-2. Abnormalities of rhythm, such as atrial fibrillation and multiple premature contractions can be detected from the arterial pulse. The consulting cardiologist often stands by the patient's bedside with his hand on the patient's radial or brachial artery throughout the presentation of the history so that he samples a large number of beats and may detect short runs of arrhythmia which have not

┌───

TABLE 16-2

Cardiovascular Physical Signs

Physical Findings	Mechanism	Interpretation
Venous Pulse (JVP)		
Distention of neck veins	Elevated RA mean pressure	Right heart failure, pericardial constriction or tamponade, obstruction of superior vena cava
a wave dominant	Forceful RA systole	TS or elevated RV end-diastolic pressure as in PH or PS
v wave dominant	Transmission of RV systole to RA	TR or AF
Cannon waves—extraordinarily large waves	Simultaneous RA and RV contraction	Arrhythmia, e.g., AV dissociation
Arterial Pulse		
Quick upstroke—wide pulse pressure	Large stroke output Increased diastolic run-off Decreased peripheral resistance	AR, AV communication e.g., peripheral artery-vein fistula, patent ductus arteriosus, thyrotoxicosis, fever, anemia, etc.
Slow upstroke—narrow pulse pressure	High resistance to ejection Small stroke output	AS MS
Pulsus bisferiens—double peak pulse	Rapid left ventricular ejection	AS and AR; or hypertrophic cardiomyopathy
Pulsus alternans—alternate pulse beats less forceful	Variation in force of ventricular systole	Myocardial disease
Pulsus paradoxus—inspiratory decrease in arterial pressure >10 mm hg	Impaired filling or excessively forceful respiration	Pericardial, myocardial, or respiratory disease
Precordial Examination		
Parasternal lift (RV lift)	Right ventricular hypertrophy	PS or PH Increased pulmonary blood flow
Apical lift (LV lift)	Left ventricular hypertrophy	AS, AR, or MR Systemic hypertension, hypertrophic cardiomyopathy
Systolic bulge (adjacent to apex)	Akinetic area	Myocardial infarction and/or aneurysm
Auscultation: Sounds		
First heart sound (S$_1$)		
Normal intensity	Closure of atrioventricular (AV) valves Muscular contraction	—
Decreased intensity	Absence of pliable valve tissue Impaired myocardial contraction Mitral valve closed at onset of systole	MR or calcified mitral stenosis Myocardial infarction or cardiomyopathy Long PR—first degree heart block Severe AR—premature closure
Increased intensity	Forceful closure of stenotic valve Mitral valve wide open at onset of systole	Pliable but stenotic mitral valve Short PR interval Short RR interval, e.g., atrial fibrillation or tachycardia Ventricular premature systole
Variation in intensity	Variation in position of the mitral valve at onset of ventricular systole	AV dissociation, ventricular tachycardia, AF, ventricular premature systoles
Second heart sound (S$_2$) A$_2$		
Normal intensity	Aortic valve closure normally precedes pulmonary closure	—

(Continued)

─── **TABLE 16-2 (cont.)** ───

Physical Findings	Mechanism	Interpretation
Auscultation: Sounds (cont.)		
Second heart sound (S$_2$) (cont.)		
A$_2$ (cont.)		
Decreased intensity	Diseased aortic valve	Calcific aortic stenosis—rigid valve
	Low aortic pressure	Hypotension
Increased intensity	Forceful closure of aortic valve	Systemic hypertension
Ringing, tambour quality	Disease of aorta and valve ring	Syphilitic aortitis
P$_2$		
Normal intensity	Pulmonary valve closure normally follows aortic closure	—
Decreased intensity	Absent pulmonary valve	Destroyed by surgery or infection
	No flow through pulmonary valve	Pulmonary atresia
Increased intensity	Forceful closure of pulmonary valve	Pulmonary hypertension
Physiologic splitting (S$_2$)	Inspiratory increase in right ventricular filling	Intact atrial septum
A$_2$–P$_2$ interval increases with inspiration		
Fixed splitting	Inspiratory increase in filling of both right and left ventricles via abnormal communication	Atrial septal defect
Absence of normal inspiratory increase in A$_2$–P$_2$ interval		
Paradoxical splitting	Delayed left ventricular ejection	Left ventricular myocardial disease, aortic stenosis, systemic hypertension, LBBB
Widening of split S$_2$ with expiration	A$_2$ follows P$_2$ (Fig. 16–4)	
Variable wide splitting	Variation in ventricular activation and ejection	RBBB, PS, MR
Third heart sound (S$_3$)		
Physiologic S$_3$—no other signs of heart disease	Ventricular filling	Normal in the young (especially after exercise), pregnancy, anemia, and thyrotoxicosis
Pathologic S$_3$—other signs of heart disease	Sudden termination of filling of dilated heart	Myocardial weakness
		MR, TR
	Excessive or unusually rapid filling	VSD or PDA
Fourth heart sound (S$_4$)		
Physiologic S$_4$—no other signs of heart disease	Atrial systole	Occasionally in normal children, pregnancy, anemia, and thyrotoxicosis
		May be heard with long PR interval as only other abnormality
Pathologic S$_4$—Atrial gallop, other signs of heart disease	Atrial systole plus decreased compliance of left ventricle	Systemic hypertension
		AS or PH
		Hypertrophic cardiomyopathy
		Acute myocardial infarction
Abnormal sounds		
Opening snap (OS) of mitral valve	Sudden arrest of LA to LV flow because fusion of mitral commissures prohibits complete opening of valve	MS—pliable, movable valve tissue must be present. Absence of OS suggests valve calcified, fixed and immobile or destroyed as in MR
	Normal mitral valve opens silently	
Ejection click (EC) (early systolic)	Related to ejection of blood into great vessels and, in other situations, to the motion of valves	PS and AS
		Dilated pulmonary artery or aorta
		High pulmonary flow
		Pulmonary and systemic hypertension
Midsystolic click	Related to motion of AV valves or to extracardiac events	Abnormal chordae or prolapse of the mitral valve, old pericarditis
Friction rub	Contact between visceral and parietal pericardium. Usually three components due to atrial systole, ventricular systole, and ventricular relaxation	Pericarditis

been noted previously. At some point, the pulses in other major arteries should be examined. Coarctation of the aorta may be suspected when the femoral pulse is absent or when there is a delay in the femoral pulse wave. The significance of an absent dorsalis pedis pulse at a later examination can only be appreciated if it were known to be present initially.

The Venous System[8]

The examiner then directs his attention to the venous system with two objectives in mind: the determination of the level of venous pressure and the delineation of the character of the venous pulse wave. The venous pressure can be estimated at the bedside by adjusting the head of the patient's bed until pulsations are seen in his jugular veins. If the veins are collapsed, the head of the bed should be lowered until the veins are seen to fill, but if they are filled initially, the head of the bed should be elevated gradually to 90° to search for the point of collapse. A position will usually be found somewhere between the recumbent position and 90° (sitting up straight) at which the point of collapse lies above the clavicle but below the jaw. This is the position in which the neck veins should be examined. The height of the venous pressure can be estimated by measuring the vertical distance between the level of collapse of the veins and the second costosternal junction, and adding 5 cm to this value. The 5 cm represent a reasonably accurate measure of the distance between the surface of the chest at the level of the second rib and the center of the right atrium, which is constant in all positions. If the neck veins cannot be visualized, venous pressure can be determined by elevating the patient's arm and noting the elevation above the level of the heart at which the veins collapse.

Useful information about right heart hemodynamics can be obtained from an accurate examination of the venous pulse. The head of the patient's bed should be adjusted, the patient's head turned, and the light adjusted to provide optimal conditions for the evaluation of venous waves. Venous pulsations can be differentiated from arterial pulsations by palpation of the arterial pulse on the opposite side of the neck. Venous pulsations are visible but, usually, they cannot be felt, or are obliterated by light pressure.

The goal is to identify the *a* and *v* waves and to determine which is larger. The *a* wave is produced by atrial systole which immediately precedes ventricular systole. The venous waves are timed by the palpation of the carotid pulse on the opposite side of the neck, and the *a* wave is recognized in the neck by the fact that it appears to precede or coincide with the upstroke of the carotid pulse (Fig. 16–2). The *a* wave is a quick-up quick-down wave of very short duration. It often appears as an almost instantaneous "flicker" in the supraclavicular fossa. The *v* wave is caused by the build-up of pressure in the right atrium due to its distension by the inflow of blood from the great veins during ventricular systole while the tricuspid valve is closed. The *v* wave rises slowly and decays rapidly after the fall of the carotid pulse. It is the descent of the *v* wave which is usually noted and this is referred to as the "*y* descent." The *v* wave sometimes disappears when the patient sits up, but the *a* wave remains visible.

The *a* wave is larger than normal when the force of atrial systole is exerted against increased resistance. If the tricuspid valve has been closed prior to atrial systole by a ventricular premature contraction, the force of atrial systole cannot force blood into the ventricle and, hence, a large *a* wave appears in the jugular pulse. Similarly, the *a* wave is large in patients with tricuspid stenosis because the resistance to inflow through the tricuspid valve is increased. The *a* wave is also increased in the presence of right-ventricular hypertension due to pulmonary stenosis or increased pulmonary vascular resistance as in primary pulmonary hypertension. In this situation, there is increased resistance to atrial emptying, but it is caused by the elevated end-diastolic pressure in the right ventricle which faces atrial systole.

The *v* wave of the jugular venous pulse is increased in amplitude when the tricuspid valve is incompetent. In this situation, the force of ventricular systole is transmitted into the right atrium and, hence, into the great veins. If tricuspid regurgitation is severe, the liver may also exhibit systolic pulsation synchronous with the *v* wave in the neck vein.

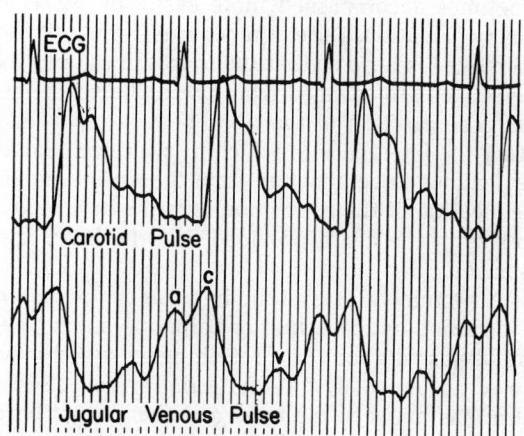

FIGURE 16–2. Venous pulse. The carotid pulse and jugular venous pulse are recorded by an external capsule on the neck of a normal subject. The *a* wave precedes and the *v* wave follows the upstroke of the carotid pulse.

An unusually rapid decay of the v wave or rapid y descent is seen in constrictive pericarditis. Filling is impaired throughout most of the cardiac cycle and is very rapid early in diastole. The veins appear to collapse during this phase of rapid filling.

It is useful to compress the liver during the examination of the neck veins. In the presence of congestive failure, a large volume of blood may be pooled in the liver, and when it is expressed into the vena cava by firm pressure on the upper abdomen, the venous pressure in the neck will rise, resulting in jugular venous distension. This response is termed "the hepatojugular reflux" and merely indicates that there is pooling of an excessive quantity of blood in the abdomen. The elevation of intrathoracic pressure by abdominal compression may also contribute to the production of this sign.

Configuration of the Chest

This is important in the interpretation of physical findings. Asymmetric enlargement of the left chest indicates that the cardiac condition developed before chest growth was complete, and may help to differentiate congenital from acquired forms of heart disease. Pectus excavatum may explain displacement of the apex beat to the left. A shallow chest resulting from a straightening of the thoracic spine may be associated with a systolic murmur in the left second interspace because of the close proximity of the pulmonary artery to the chest wall.

Inspection and Palpation of the Precordium[9]

This procedure yields information about the heart which cannot be obtained in any other way. The first step is to identify the apex impulse, which is defined as the point of maximum mechanical activity. This is sometimes accomplished more easily by inspection than by palpation. The examiner must adjust the light and move his head so that the fourth, fifth, and sixth interspaces are scanned from the axilla to the sternum. The position of the apex beat is recorded by noting the interspace in which it is located and also the distance in centimeters from the midsternal line. The location of the apex impulse is the best index of the size of the heart, provided that the heart is not displaced.

A prominent presystolic impulse can sometimes be identified by inspection or palpation and suggests careful auscultation for a fourth heart sound indicative of an unusually forceful atrial systole. Systolic pulsations between the apex and the sternal border occur when a portion of left ventricle fails to contract with systole. The extent, character, and force of the apical impulse should be noted. The left ventricle is chiefly responsible for the mechanical activity in the region of the apex beat, and with left ventricular hypertrophy, the apical impulse is sustained and forceful. In addition, left ventricular hypertrophy is sometimes associated with retraction of the precordium in the third and fourth interspaces near the sternum. This apical expansion and parasternal retraction leads to a rocking motion. It is possible to predict whether the left ventricular hypertrophy is secondary to a pressure or to a volume overload. If there is pressure overload—as in aortic stenosis or essential hypertension—the apical impulse is a sustained lift which seems to hold the examiner's hand up for a finite period of time before collapsing. In contrast, when there is a volume overload—as in aortic or mitral regurgitation—the apex impulse may have a greater amplitude, but a shorter duration.

When the right ventricle is the site of hypertrophy, the maximum activity is located in the parasternal area. The right ventricular lift is a systolic expansion in the third and fourth interspaces adjacent to the sternum. Systolic expansion in this area is sometimes associated with retraction in the area of the apex, yielding a rocking motion to the precordium which is similar but opposite in direction to that associated with left ventricular hypertrophy. Systolic expansion in the second left interspace near the sternum is indicative of enlargement of the pulmonary artery and can often be better seen than felt. Systolic expansion in the right second interspace near the sternum usually indicates that the ascending aorta is enlarged.

Systematic palpation of the precordium at the apex and along both sternal borders is indicated to detect thrills. The thrill of aortic stenosis is best felt along the right sternal border when the patient is sitting and during full expiration. The presystolic thrill of mitral stenosis is best felt with the patient in the left lateral decubitus position. Any murmur may be associated with a thrill if it is loud enough. Heart sounds can be felt, especially if they are accentuated, being referred to as "taps." The snapping first heart sound of mitral stenosis and the pulmonary valve closure sound in pulmonary hypertension are frequently palpable; a gallop is sometimes first detected by inspection and palpation and its presence confirmed by auscultation.

Percussion of the Heart

This is far less important than inspection, palpation, and auscultation, but it may be helpful in certain situations. When the apical impulse cannot be identified, the size of the heart can sometimes be determined by percussing the left border of cardiac dullness. The presence of a pericardial effusion can be confirmed by finding the apical impulse inside the left border of cardiac dullness. *A good radiologic examination of the heart provides far more accurate information about the size and shape of the heart than can be obtained by percussion.*

Auscultation [10]

Auscultation is the final step in the physical examination of the heart and must be performed in a quiet room with the patient and the physician in comfortable and relaxed circumstances. Air conditioners and fans should be turned off, and doors and windows closed to reduce background noise to a minimum. The examination usually begins with the patient in the recumbent position and always includes examination in the sitting position as well. Depending on the findings in these primary positions, the patient may also be examined in the left lateral decubitus position or after exercise. There are four prime areas for auscultation on the chest wall: apex, left lower sternal border, left second interspace, and right second interspace. It is often helpful, however, to move the stethoscope by small steps from one of these areas to the next to note changes in the amplitude and character of various auscultatory phenomena. The stethoscope should be applied over the carotid arteries in the neck, especially in the presence of a systolic murmur at the base of the heart, as murmurs generated in the great vessels may be heard over the upper chest and those of aortic valve disease may be heard in the neck. It is advisable to listen for murmurs over the back of the chest while the patient is sitting up.

At each area, attention should first be directed to the normal sounds and rhythm, then to the abnormal sounds, and lastly to the murmurs. The normal first and second sounds can usually be easily identified by their differing character, but in disease this may be difficult, and therefore, auscultation should be carried out with a finger on the carotid pulse. The first heart sound (S_1) can be identified by its occurrence coincident with the upstroke of the carotid pulse. The first sound is best heard at the apex, and the second sound (S_2) will be found to be loudest in the second interspaces both to the right and to the left of the sternum. The second heart sound consists of two parts: A_2, due to closure of the aortic valve; and P_2, due to the closure of the pulmonary valve. Both components can be heard on both sides of the sternum in the second interspace, but A_2 is the loudest component of S_2 on the right side, and P_2 is the major component of S_2 heard on the left. The two components of the second sound are identified by their temporal relationships and not by the point of maximum audibility and, therefore, it

is misleading to use the terms aortic area and pulmonic area. With inspiration, the pulmonary closure sound is delayed, the second sound splits, and P_2 can be identified as the second component. Observation of the effects of respiration on the second sound is an important part of auscultation and will be discussed in more detail later. The third and fourth heart sounds are both heard at the apex with the patient in the left lateral decubitus position.

The significance of a third heart sound depends upon the clinical setting in which it is heard. The S_3 is frequently heard in children and adolescents, in whom it is termed a "physiologic" third heart sound and has no significance. The S_3 may be heard in situations in which blood flow is increased as in anemia, thyrotoxicosis, and pregnancy. The sound is apparently generated by the termination of rapid inflow of blood into the ventricle in early diastole. The third heart sound is heard with decreasing frequency with advancing age and is a rare finding in adults who have normal hearts.

A third heart sound in a patient with heart disease has special significance. In this setting, the S_3 is termed a "pathologic" S_3 or a "ventricular gallop" and is indicative of an abnormally large diastolic inflow, as in mitral regurgitation, or of ventricular failure. The timing, character, and intensity are the same as in the case of the physiologic S_3, but in the case of myocardial failure, the generation of sound is probably related to the sudden termination of ventricular filling when the elastic limits of a dilated ventricle are reached. When the rate is rapid, as it often is in disease, the first, second, and third heart sounds are heard as a triple rhythm suggesting the sounds made by the hoofs of a galloping horse—hence the term "gallop rhythm." An S_3 gallop is usually much louder after exercise. Leg raising, which increases venous return, and hand grip exercise, which increases arterial pressure, may be used to "bring out" a gallop sound.

The fourth heart sound (S_4) is also heard occasionally in normal subjects, but this is found less commonly than the S_3. It may occur as a doubling of the first heart sound or as a sound in late diastole which suggests a presystolic murmur. The fourth sound is usually an indication of increased resistance to ventricular filling (decreased compliance) due to intrinsic myocardial disease or to an increased load as in the case of hypertension or outflow obstruction. It is generated in the ventricle in response to the thrust of forceful atrial systole. The significance again depends upon the setting. If the S_4 is heard in a patient with other manifestations of heart disease, it is known as a "pathologic" S_4 or an "atrial gallop."

After these sounds have been identified, attention is turned to a search for abnormal sounds such as clicks and friction rubs. This is best done by listening in all four areas while concentrating on systole and then on diastole. Systole and diastole are normally silent and abnormal sounds and murmurs are best identified by asking the question: Is the period between S_1 and S_2 completely silent? and then asking the same question about the period between S_2 and S_1.

CARDIAC MURMURS

Heart murmurs, which are subject to precise description with regard to timing and location of maximal audibility, frequently form a starting point in the diagnosis of cardiovascular disease. The murmur may serve as a basis for differential diagnosis in a patient ill with congestive failure, or it may be an incidental finding on routine examination.

Origin and Significance

Not all heart murmurs are indicative of organic heart disease, a fact emphasized by their classification into three groups on the basis of the mechanism of production: 1) organic murmurs due to anatomic abnormalities within the heart or central circulation, the identification of which constitutes evidence for organic heart disease; 2) physiological murmurs related to altered function within anatomically normal hearts, as with the systolic murmurs of anemia, thyrotoxicosis, and fever; and 3) innocent murmurs that cannot be related either to altered anatomy or function. The mechanisms of production of the third type are unknown, but it is known that such murmurs are not associated with organic heart disease.

The importance of distinguishing between these three types of murmurs is obvious. It is sometimes necessary to employ echocardiography, cardiac catheterization, and angiocardiography to solve the problem, but innocent murmurs can usually be differentiated from those of organic origin at the bedside.

Innocent murmurs are usually systolic. Diastolic murmurs are rarely heard in the absence of organic heart disease. The innocent systolic murmurs are usually confined either to the first or to the middle part of systole, are not loud, are rarely accompanied by a thrill, and show variability with respiration or position or both. Final judgment about the significance of a particular murmur depends on the evaluation of that finding in relation to variation within the normal population and this judgment must be based on the examiner's experience.

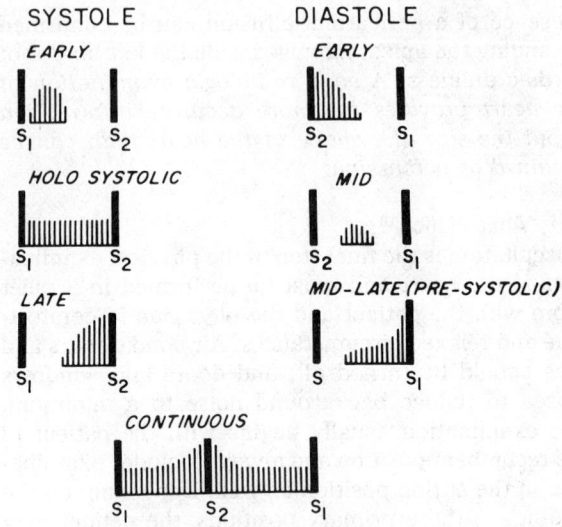

FIGURE 16–3. Timing and configuration of common murmurs in relation to the first (S_1) and second (S_2) heart sounds.

Timing and Location

Standardization of classification and description is necessary if heart murmurs are to be of maximum value in differential diagnosis, if communication between one physician and another is to be effective, and if meaningful comparison is to be made between findings recorded at different times by the same physician. Classification of murmurs on the basis of timing forms the basis for Figure 16–3. Further description with regard to intensity, character, and radiation also is possible and valuable.

The division of murmurs on the basis of timing into systolic and diastolic is indicated across the top of Figure 16–3. Each of these time periods can be subdivided into thirds and murmurs classified according to their onset as early, mid, or late. Early diastole is sometimes referred to as protodiastole and late diastole as presystole. If a murmur lasts throughout systole, it is called pansystolic or holosystolic.

Character

The character of the murmur is sometimes described as crescendo or decrescendo to indicate progressive increase or decrease in intensity. The early-diastolic murmur of aortic regurgitation is classically decrescendo and the late-diastolic murmur of mitral stenosis is crescendo. The murmur of mitral stenosis is also described as presystolic. The systolic murmur of aortic or pulmonary stenosis is best described as crescendo-decrescendo. The term "ejection systolic murmur" is applied to these and all other murmurs related to the ejection of blood into the great vessels. The terms "diamond-shaped" and "Christmas tree" are applied to the early-systolic crescendo-decrescendo murmur and refer to its phonocardiographic appearance. The quality of a murmur is described as "harsh," "blowing," or "musical." Although lacking in quantitative precision, these terms serve a useful purpose. Furthermore, the term "musical" used to describe a decrescendo diastolic murmur indicates the possibility of an unusual cause of aortic regurgitation, such as rupture of an aortic leaflet.

The radiation of a murmur is of limited help, since it is, at least in part, a function of intensity. A loud murmur may be heard all over the chest, a faint one only at one spot.

Effect of Respiration

More can be learned about the physiology of any organ system by observing its response to changing conditions or stress than by prolonged observation at rest. This general physiologic principle underlies the importance of careful observation of the effects of respiration on the heart. Normal quiet respiration results in phasic alterations in venous return, cardiac output, venous pressure, and arterial blood pressure. The response is often altered by disease.

All the hemodynamic changes depend upon the negative intrathoracic pressure which initiates inspiration. When the pressure within the chest becomes negative with respect to that in the atmosphere and in the extrathoracic airways, air flows into the chest through the respiratory tree. The veins are similar to the trachea and bronchi in that they are conduits running into the thoracic cavity from outside. The decrease in intrathoracic pressure which initiates air flow into the trachea also initiates blood flow into the thorax from the extrathoracic portions of the superior and inferior venae cavae. Venous pressure in the neck veins falls with inspiration. The return to the right atrium and right ventricle is, therefore, *increased* by the act of inspiration, and the output of the right ventricle into the lung is increased.

An important effect of respiration on physical signs is the change in the splitting of the second heart sound. Under normal circumstances, aortic valve closure precedes pulmonary valve closure, and, therefore, delay in right ventricular emptying results in the separation or splitting of the two components (P_2 and A_2) of the second sound (S_2). This normal increase in the interval between the two components of S_2 with inspiration is referred to as a physiologic splitting. If the splitting is due to left ventricular disease or aortic stenosis, left ventricular ejection is delayed, so that

aortic valve closure follows rather than precedes pulmonary closure. In this situation, inspiratory delay in pulmonary valve closure results in a narrowing of the split between the two components of the second sound, whereas the two components move apart with expiration; hence, the designation paradoxical splitting.

The effect of respiration on physical signs is also important in establishing the diagnosis of atrial septal defect. When the two atria are in free communication, the inspiratory increment in venous return is divided between the right and left ventricles; the closure of both aortic and pulmonary valves is delayed; and, hence, the interval between the two events remains relatively constant. The majority of patients with ostium secundum atrial septal defect exhibit this sign—fixed splitting of the second heart sound.

Murmurs originating on the right side of the heart are made louder by inspiration, a fact which is useful in differentiating tricuspid from mitral regurgitation. The systolic murmur of tricuspid regurgitation becomes louder and that of mitral regurgitation changes very little. This inspiratory increase is best observed in cases of minimal tricuspid regurgitation. In severe lesions, the murmur may be heard throughout both phases of the respiratory cycle.

Other Stress Maneuvers

There are several measures other than respiration which can be used to stress the heart during physical examination. Hand grip exercise is performed by asking the patient to squeeze the examiner's fingers firmly during auscultation of the heart. This maneuver increases arterial blood pressure and therefore increases the "afterload" on the left ventricle. A gallop sound of either the S_3 or S_4 type may be precipitated by this procedure. Left ventricular afterload may also be increased by asking the patient to squat down beside the examiner. This procedure increases venous return to the heart and is especially valuable in differentiating the systolic murmur of hypertrophic cardiomyopathy from that due to other abnormalities of the mitral valve. The murmur of hypertrophic cardiomyopathy decreases in intensity in this situation, while that of other forms of mitral regurgitation becomes louder or remains unchanged.

Venous return to the right heart can also be increased by raising the patient's legs and this will sometimes make it possible to hear an S_3 which is absent or only intermittently present at rest. Exercise either by passive bicycling while recumbent or hopping on one leg by the bedside is also useful as a tool for stressing the heart by increasing oxygen consumption and hence the demand for cardiac output.

CHAPTER 17

Laboratory Evaluation of the Cardiovascular System
STEPHEN C. ACHUFF AND JAMES L. WEISS

Laboratory tests supplement but never replace the history and physical examination in the evaluation of a patient with cardiac disease. No cardiovascular assessment is complete without a standard chest roentgenogram and a 12-lead electrocardiogram (12-lead ECG), but other studies are ordered only to answer specific questions. In some instances, a laboratory test will establish a diagnosis, as in the case of the electrocardiogram in the patient with atrial fibrillation. In other situations, the same test may be nonspecific, as in the case of mitral stenosis. Some tests are necessary to quantify or determine the extent of cardiac disease, as in the case of coronary arteriography.

RADIOLOGIC EXAMINATION OF THE HEART

Alterations in the cardiac silhouette seen in common forms of heart disease are presented schematically in Figure 17–1. The PA and lateral chest x-rays are the standard examinations and are used to determine overall heart size and configuration, enlargement of the aorta, pulmonary artery, and left atrium. Rib notching, characteristic of coarctation of the aorta, can also be detected on the chest roentgenogram. Intracardiac calcification can sometimes be identified on the plain roentgenogram, but image intensifier fluoroscopy is usually required for precise localization. Calcification in valves can be seen to move, while that in the pericardium and lung remains relatively motionless. Calcification of coronary arteries can sometimes be seen and when present indicates that the coronary atherosclerosis is severe. Fluoroscopic examination may also be used to evaluate mass lesions in the region of the heart. However, the distinction between a solid tumor, cyst, or aneurysm is often difficult because cardiac pulsations may be transmitted to lesions in contact with a vascular structure.

Occasionally, a routine chest roentgenogram may lead to the detection of heart disease in a totally asymptomatic patient. Pericardial cysts, benign cardiac tumors, even atrial septal defects may be discovered in this way prior to the development of symptoms.

In addition to the examination of the cardiac silhouette, evaluation of the pulmonary vasculature is equally important in a variety of cardiac disorders. Signs of pulmonary arterial and pulmonary venous hypertension and pulmonary hyperperfusion (i.e., left-to-right shunt) can be detected by careful examination of the vessels in the lung fields. The size of the central and peripheral pulmonary vessels provides information about pressure and flow in pulmonary arteries. Normally, the lower lobes receive more blood supply than the upper lobes, and the chest roentgenogram shows prominence of lower lobe vessels leading to the hilum compared to those from the upper lobes. With increased pulmonary venous pressure there is relatively less flow to the lower lobes due to regional hypoxia, and flow is shifted to the upper lobe vessels, which appear more prominent than normal. Interstitial edema may produce diffuse haziness or occasionally a reticular or nodular infiltrative appearance. Alveolar edema causes lung opacification and "fluffy" infiltrates. Kerley B lines are horizontal densities at the lung bases, best seen in the PA projection (Fig. 20–3). They are important to recognize for they reliably indicate severe pulmonary venous hypertension. In chronic states, e.g., mitral stenosis, Kerley B lines may be present without evidence of interstitial or alveolar edema.

ELECTROCARDIOGRAPHY

A resting 12-lead ECG should be obtained on every patient in whom heart disease is suspected. ECG abnormalities may accompany all types of heart disease but may also be caused by many other factors such as electrolyte disturbances or drugs. The resting ECG may be completely normal in many patients with cardiac conditions or may be abnormal in patients who have no substantiating evidence of cardiac disease. The practice of making a diagnosis of cardiac disease on the basis of minor, nonspecific ECG abnormalities has needlessly created many cardiac cripples and is to be strongly condemned. The ECG is especially valuable in the diagnosis and management of arrhythmias and conduction disturbances (Chap. 21). In addition, it provides useful information about hyper-

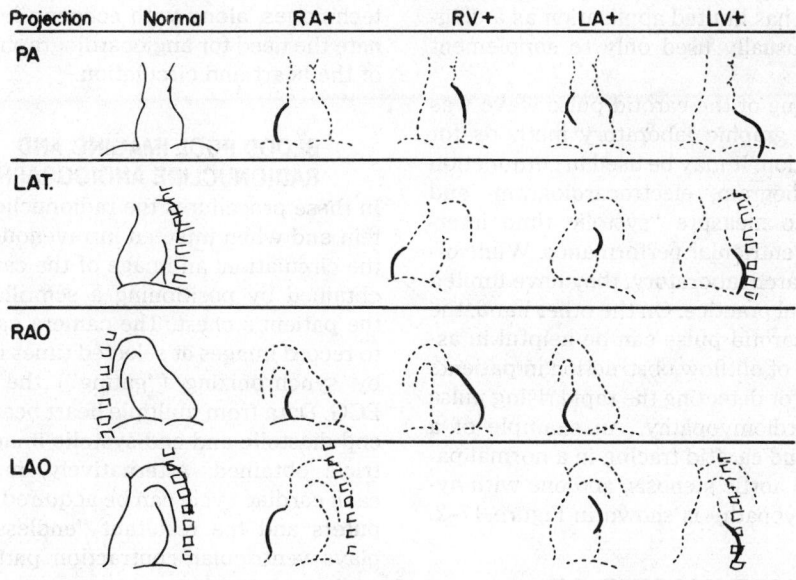

Projection	Normal	RA+	RV+	LA+	LV+
PA					
LAT.					
RAO					
LAO					

FIGURE 17-1. The usual radiographic projections of the normal heart are shown in the column labeled normal. The alterations in the silhouette produced by enlargement of specific chambers are shown in the various projections.

trophy of the right and left ventricles, especially in patients with valvular or congenital heart disease. The diagnosis of myocardial infarction can be confirmed electrocardiographically (Chap. 23), and the ECG during exercise is helpful in the differential diagnosis of chest pain (Chap. 22). Monitoring the ECG for a 12- to 24-hour period with a portable tape recorder can be of value in identifying paroxysmal arrhythmias and in further evaluation of some patients with chest pain syndromes. The reader is referred to the many excellent texts on electrocardiography for detailed descriptions of specific ECG abnormalities, as well as the indications and limitations of exercise and ambulatory ECG monitoring.[16,17,19,20]

Occasionally, the clinician is confronted with patients who have serious arrhythmias that defy interpretation by standard ECG techniques. In these circumstances, definition of the mechanism of the arrhythmias, for example ventricular versus supraventricular origin of a tachycardia, may provide important information that can direct therapeutic maneuvers. This kind of information may be obtained by recording the electrical activity of the specialized conduction system of the heart (His bundle electrocardiography), which is accomplished by selectively positioning an electrode catheter within the right heart.[18]

PHONOCARDIOGRAPHY, APEXCARDIOGRAPHY, AND INDIRECT CAROTID PULSE WAVE RECORDING

Phonocardiography is of value in certain special situations, but it has limited advantage over careful auscultation of the heart by an experienced examiner. With phonocardiography, sounds and murmurs can be timed precisely and recorded for later comparisons. For example, the exact interval between the second sound and opening snap can be determined and this measurement can be utilized to estimate the height of the left atrial pressure, which is inversely related to this interval. The phonocardiogram may be useful in discerning whether the first heart sound is preceded by a fourth sound or followed by an ejection click. The two components of the second heart sound can be identified, and variation in the interval between A_2 and P_2 in response to respiration can be studied and may be clinically useful, e.g., "fixed splitting" in patients with atrial septal defect.

Apexcardiography is a technique that records the mechanical activity of the heart on the chest wall. It is a graphic record of ultralow frequency precordial chest wall movement and may be useful as a time reference for heart sounds and for the teaching of palpation. The method has limited application as a diagnostic test and is usually used only to supplement other tests.

Indirect recording of the carotid pulse wave was one of the earliest graphic laboratory methods for study of the circulation. It may be used in conjunction with the apexcardiogram, electrocardiogram, and phonocardiogram to measure "systolic time intervals" as indices of ventricular performance. While often used in the research laboratory, they have limited application to clinical practice. On the other hand, the rate of rise of the carotid pulse can be helpful in assessing the severity of outflow obstruction in patients with aortic stenosis or detecting the rapid rising pulse of hypertrophic cardiomyopathy. An example of a phonocardiogram and carotid tracing in a normal patient, a patient with aortic stenosis, and one with hypertrophic cardiomyopathy is shown in Figure 17–2.

RADIONUCLIDE IMAGING OF THE CIRCULATION

Techniques utilizing radionuclide imaging for noninvasive evaluation of the cardiovascular system are undergoing rapid development. It is likely that these techniques, along with echocardiography, will eliminate the need for angiocardiography in many diseases of the heart and circulation.[24]

BLOOD POOL IMAGING AND RADIONUCLIDE ANGIOGRAPHY

In these procedures the radionuclide is bound to protein and when injected intravenously remains within the circulation; an image of the cardiac blood pool is obtained by positioning a scintillation camera over the patient's chest. The camera can be programmed to record images at selected times in the cardiac cycle by synchronizing ("gating") the camera with the ECG. Data from multiple heart beats are summed and end-diastolic and end-systolic images of the left ventricle obtained. Alternatively, multiple images for each cardiac cycle can be acquired with modern computers and the resultant "endless-loop" movie displays ventricular contraction patterns in a manner analogous to cineangiograms obtained in the catheterization laboratory. These techniques have proved useful in the noninvasive evaluation of cardiac performance, especially in estimating right and left ventricular size and shape, and in analyzing segmental left ventricular wall motion abnormalities such as an-

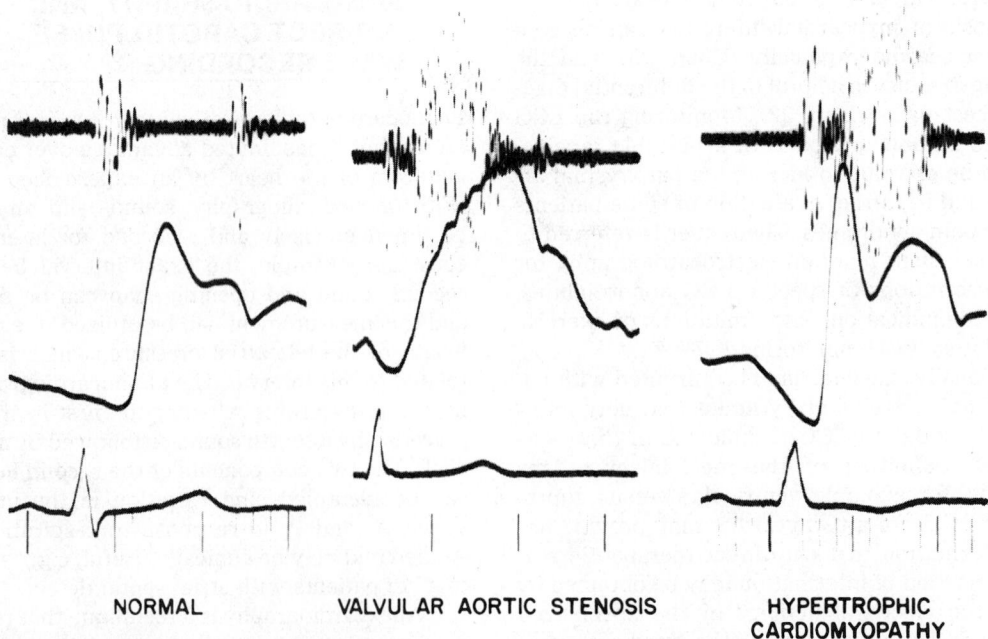

NORMAL   VALVULAR AORTIC STENOSIS   HYPERTROPHIC CARDIOMYOPATHY

FIGURE 17–2. Carotid pulse tracing and phonocardiogram comparing normal subject with patients with valvular aortic stenosis and hypertrophic cardiomyopathy (IHSS). Note that murmurs are indistinguishable but upstroke of pulse is retarded in valvular AS but rapid in hypertrophic cardiomyopathy and followed by a second late systolic peak.

eurysms. The "first pass" radionuclide angiocardio-gram, wherein an intravenously injected bolus of iso-tope is monitored during its initial passage through the central circulation, can provide information con-cerning the anatomic relationships between the var-ious cardiac chambers and the great vessels, a partic-ularly useful feature in the study of congenital cardiac lesions.[13,21]

MYOCARDIAL PERFUSION IMAGING

Radionuclides that distribute to areas of recently in-farcted myocardium, such as radio-labelled pyro-phosphate, provide so-called "hot-spot" images of the heart. This technique may be valuable in certain clini-cal situations where more conventional diagnostic tests for infarction are equivocal. Alternatively, "cold-spot" imaging utilizes potassium analogues, such as [201]thallium which are distributed to myocar-dial cells in proportion to coronary flow. Diminished radioactivity noted on these scans will represent di-minished blood flow. Defects seen on thallium scan-ning may represent ischemic or infarcted myocar-dium, the distinction often having to be made on the basis of serial scans. This technique has achieved util-ity in conjunction with stress electrocardiography, where a thallium defect appearing during exercise but resolving on the rest scan indicates viable myo-cardium that becomes ischemic with exercise. Detec-tion of significant coronary obstructive disease may thus be enhanced by combining these two techniques, especially in situations where the ECG is equivocal such as in patients with left bundle branch block or left ventricular hypertrophy.[12]

ECHOCARDIOGRAPHY[22,23]

The technique of echocardiography is based on the principle that ultrasonic waves passing through a me-dium will be reflected backward, or echoed, when they encounter a medium of different acoustic imped-ance. Blood and cardiac tissues provide such an acoustic interface causing echoes to be reflected from many intracardiac structures. Since the speed of sound in tissue is known, distance between structures can be measured accurately and specific chamber di-mensions determined. Recording the returning ech-oes as a function of time permits analysis of motion of valve leaflets or myocardium during the cardiac cycle. The echocardiographic examination is per-formed simply and painlessly by placing a transducer on the chest wall, usually in the third or fourth inter-costal space to the left of the sternum. The transducer both transmits ultrasonic waves and receives the re-

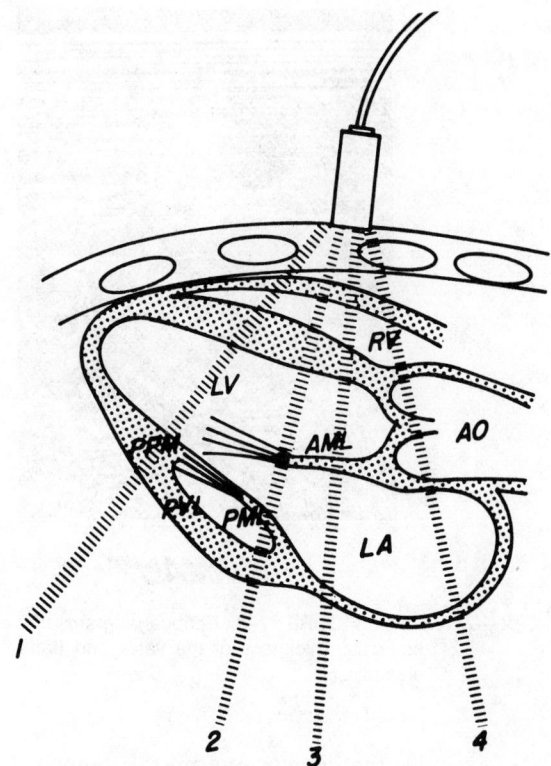

FIGURE 17-3. Sagittal section through thorax on left side of sternum to illustrate how ultrasonic beams from a single site can traverse most intracardiac structures. (Abbreviations: RV = right ventricle, LV = left ventricle, Ao = aorta, LA = left atrium, PPM = posterior papillary muscle, PML = posterior mi-tral leaflet, AML = anterior mitral leaflet.)

sultant echoes, which are displayed on a strip chart recorder along with other graphic material, i.e., ECG, heart sounds, or pulse tracings. Figure 17-3 illus-trates the direction of several ultrasonic beams through the heart and indicates that echoes can be reflected from right ventricular free wall, interven-tricular septum, left ventricular posterior wall, mitral valve, aortic valve, aortic root, and left atrial or poste-rior wall by angulation of the transducer from one position.

While the applications of echocardiography to the study of cardiac disease are numerous and ex-panding rapidly, the major diagnostic uses include:

1. Detection of mitral valve motion abnormali-ties in patients with mitral stenosis, prolapsing mitral leaflets, hypertrophic cardiomyopathy, and aortic regurgitation. An example of a nor-mal valve echogram compared with one from a patient with mitral stenosis is shown in Fig-ure 17-4. The finding of a normal mitral echo

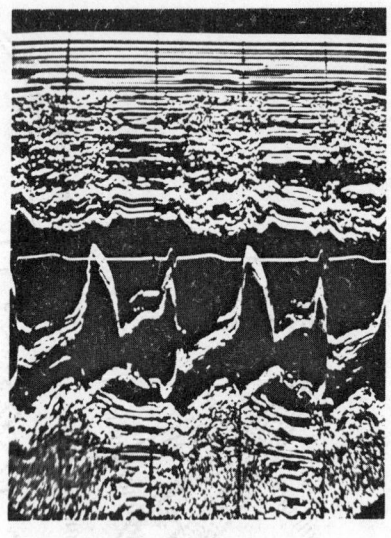
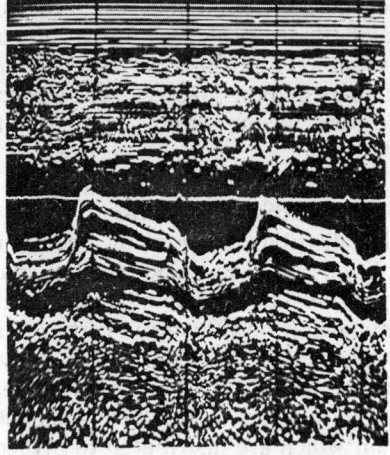

NORMAL   *MITRAL STENOSIS*

FIGURE 17–4. Echocardiograms of the mitral valve in a normal subject and patient with mitral stenosis. Thickness of the valve and flattening of the diastolic closing slope are noted in mitral stenosis.

excludes the diagnosis of mitral stenosis. Information about severity of the stenotic lesion, mobility, thickness, and degree of calcification of the valve can also be obtained by this technique

2. Determination of the presence of pericardial effusion. The echo technique can detect effusions as small as 25 ml and is the preferred method for establishing this diagnosis because of sensitivity, low cost, portability of the equipment, ease of repeatability, and absence of risk

3. Measurement of abnormal thickness of the interventricular septum in patients with hypertrophic cardiomyopathy

4. Measurement of size and function of right and left ventricular chambers

5. Detection of atrial tumors

6. Detection of abnormal motion of the interventricular septum in patients with right ventricular volume overload, e.g., ASD

7. Detailed analysis of cardiac valves, e.g., detection of bicuspid aortic valve, Ebstein's anomaly of tricuspid valve, vegetations on infected valves, etc.

Methods have been developed which permit simultaneous imaging of multiple ultrasonic beams and thereby allow visualization of multiple cardiac structures simultaneously. These new instruments are expanding the use of the technique to the study of regional left ventricular function and complex congenital lesions.

PHYSIOLOGIC AND ANGIOGRAPHIC STUDIES[15]

Most medical centers have a laboratory where the specialized techniques of cardiac catheterization and angiocardiography can be applied to the study of the physiology and anatomy of the circulation. These laboratories are essential for the solution of certain clinical problems and have contributed significantly to understanding the pathophysiology of valvular heart disease, congenital heart disease, and myocardial failure.

The basic technique utilized is cardiac catheterization. Catheters can be introduced into the peripheral veins or arteries either by surgical exposure of the vessel or by percutaneous puncture, and it is possible to position a catheter in any chamber of the heart and all the great vessels. The basic measurements are those of pressure and flow, and from these the resistance to blood flow through a vascular bed or a valvular orifice can be derived. Cardiac output or total flow can be measured by the Fick principle, which is dependent on the oxygen transport function of the circulation or by the use of the indicator dilution principle, which depends upon the injection into the circulation of a known amount of harmless dye or other marker substance. Both the Fick and the indicator dilution methods can be modified and applied to the detection of shunts in patients with congenital heart disease. Representative normal values for intracardiac pressures, cardiac output, and other derived values pertinent to the catheterization laboratory evaluation of cardiac disease are given in Table 17–1.

Anatomic information concerning the heart and great vessels is obtained by contrast radiography, which involves the injection of radiopaque material through a catheter into the heart chamber under study. The flow of this material through the chambers of the heart and great vessels is recorded radiographically. Large film roentgenograms obtained 6 to 20 times per second after injection of the contrast material provide the greatest anatomic detail. Cineangiograms recorded at 60 to 120 frames per second on movie films by coupling a motion picture camera to the fluoroscope provide more information about the dynamic aspects of the heart and normal and abnormal flow patterns.

INDICATION FOR STUDY IN A CARDIOVASCULAR DIAGNOSTIC LABORATORY

No laboratory procedure should be used indiscriminately, and this is especially true of cardiac catheterization and angiocardiography. These procedures should be undertaken only to provide an answer to a specific question formulated by the physician on the basis of clinical facts. Cardiac catheterization is seldom indicated or helpful in the patient presenting as a diagnostic problem without specific physical signs or laboratory evidence of heart disease. The techniques of the cardiovascular laboratory are best used if the physicians performing the study are thoroughly informed of the patient's problem. This is important because the same procedure is not followed with each patient, as it is in the electrocardiographic laboratory. Methods and techniques are selected to provide an answer to a specific problem in the best way possible.

INDICATIONS FOR CORONARY ARTERIOGRAPHY[14]

Coronary arteriography is usually performed to determine the location and severity of coronary atherosclerosis; and in man it is the only method that will define precisely the coronary artery anatomy. The coronary arteries are best visualized by selective

---

TABLE 17–1
Normal Values for the Cardiovascular System

Cardiac Output

Direct Fick method

$$CO = \frac{O_2 \text{ Consumption (ml/min)}}{AV\ O_2 \text{ Difference (vol \%)} \times 10}$$

Where CO = Cardiac output (L/min)
Normal = 5–6 L/min

AV O_2 difference = Difference in O_2 content of the arterial and mixed venous blood, usually expressed in volume percent (ml of oxygen/dl of blood)

Indicator dilution method

$$CO = \frac{I \times 60}{Cm \times t}$$

Where CO = Cardiac Output (L/min)

I   = Amount of the indicator injected (mg)
60 = 60 sec/min
Cm = Mean indicator concentration (mg/L)
t   = Total curve duration (sec)

Flow Resistance

$$Resistance = \frac{Mean\ driving\ pressure\ (mm\ Hg)}{Mean\ Flow\ (L/min)}$$

$$PAR = \frac{(PAm - LAm)}{CO}$$

Where PAR = Pulmonary arteriolar resistance
             Normal = < 4 units
      PAm = Mean pulmonary artery pressure
      LAm = Mean left atrial pressure
      CO = Cardiac output

$$TSR = \frac{(SAm - RAm)}{CO}$$

Where TSR = Total systemic vascular resistance
             Normal = 30 ± 5 units
      SAm = Mean systemic arterial pressure
      RAm = Mean right atrial pressure

Normal Intracardiac Pressures (mm Hg)

Right atrium mean	= 1–5
Right ventricle systolic	= 10–25
Pulmonary artery mean	= 5–15
Systolic	= 10–25
Pulmonary capillary wedge mean	= 5–13
Left atrium mean	= 2–12
Left ventricle systolic	= 85–140
End-diastolic	= 5–12
Aorta mean	= 70–100
Systolic	= 85–140
Diastolic	= 60–90

techniques whereby a catheter is positioned in the orifice of the coronary artery and an injection of contrast material is made directly into the vessel. The two most commonly used methods are 1) brachial technique (Sones), and 2) percutaneous femoral technique (Judkins). The indications for coronary arteriography (apart from the purely diagnostic study) are closely linked to the indications for myocardial revascularization surgery (Chap. 22).

The determination of left ventricular function or, more precisely, the localization and extent of left ventricular damage is an essential part of the arteriographic procedure because of the importance of ventricular function in the determination of prognosis and surgical results. This information is best obtained by careful inspection of the left ventriculogram. The vigor of left ventricular contraction, and the motion of specific portions of the ventricular wall are noted. This visual assessment of ventricular performance is usually supplemented by the measurement of end-diastolic volume, end-systolic volume, angiographic stroke volume, and ejection fraction. The level of left ventricular end-diastolic pressure is also of some value, as is the ability of the cardiac output to increase with exercise.

Evaluation of the coronary circulation is often important in patients with valvular heart disease since many patients who are undergoing evaluation for surgery are in an age group susceptible to coronary artery disease. Visualization of the coronary arteries following injection of contrast material into the aortic root may be adequate, but if satisfactory filling is not obtained selective opacification of the coronary arteries is indicated.

CHAPTER 18

Congestive Heart Failure: Pathophysiology and the Evaluation of Ventricular Function

MYRON L. WEISFELDT

The term congestive heart failure does not refer to a discrete disease entity, but rather to a functional state in which the heart is either unable to meet the needs of the peripheral organs for blood flow or is unable to meet those needs without the help of certain compensatory mechanisms. The major clinical manifestations of congestive heart failure result from fluid retention, increased pressure in the systemic and pulmonary venous system, and reduced cardiac output.

PHYSIOLOGIC CONSIDERATIONS

Cardiac output in normal man reflects the magnitude of peripheral oxygen demand. For example, during exercise[28] the increased oxygen consumption of skeletal muscle is associated with decreased vascular resistance in the arterial bed supplying the exercising muscle. Since reflex mechanisms maintain arterial pressure at or above the resting level during exercise there is increased flow to the exercising muscle (Flow = Pressure/Resistance). An increase in overall skeletal muscle flow results in increased return of venous blood to the heart.

The heart must rapidly augment its output to keep up with the venous return. If it does not, blood will rapidly accumulate in the vascular area immediately proximal to the chamber or structure unable to "keep up" and acute systemic or pulmonary venous congestion will occur. Thus, acute left ventricular failure occurs when right ventricular output is equal to systemic venous return but the left ventricle is transiently unable to eject this volume of blood. There is a sudden increase in the left atrial and pulmonary venous pressure. Pulmonary edema, as a result of this increase in pulmonary venous pressure, may appear within minutes of the onset of exercise in patients with chronic left ventricular disease or very rapidly after a decrease in left ventricular contractile function which occurs with acute myocardial infarction. It is only for a very brief period that the organism can tolerate the inability of the left ventricle to pump the volume of right ventricular output presented to it. Death due to pulmonary edema will occur unless compensatory mechanisms for augmenting cardiac function are effective.

CAUSES OF HEART FAILURE (Table 18-1)

The general causes of congestive failure are: 1) an increase in cardiac work load as a result of heightened demands for stroke volume or cardiac output or increased impedance to ejection of blood; 2) abnormalities of the contractile function of the myocardium (contractility is the functional capacity of the ventricle independent of conditions of afterload or preload. Preload is the length of cardiac muscle fibers at the onset of contraction, and afterload is the force resisting muscle shortening or ventricular ejection); or 3) restriction of the ventricular filling due to valvular obstruction or increased myocardial or pericardial stiffness. If the heart is unable to fill adequately with blood during diastole the overall pump function will be inadequate.

In a given patient there may be more than one cause of congestive failure. For example, congestive failure in the course of rheumatic heart disease with mitral regurgitation may be due to the heightened demands for stroke output as a result of valvular regurgitation as well as decreased myocardial contractile function as a result of prior rheumatic myocarditis. Likewise, in cardiac failure associated with long-standing hypertension there is an increase in work load as a result of increased impedance to ejection, restriction of ventricular filling as a result of greater stiffness of the hypertrophied ventricle and often decreased contractility as a result of associated coronary atherosclerosis. Myocardial ischemia and acute infarction likewise may result in both loss of regional myocardial contractile function and an increase in the stiffness of the ischemic or infarcted zones of myocardium.

COMPENSATORY MECHANISMS

When heart failure develops from any cause, the heart has the capacity to utilize several mechanisms which may partially or completely compensate for the alteration in cardiac performance. Some of these may be called into play immediately while others require longer periods of time to develop. In normal man there are three major physiologic mechanisms for augmenting the output of the heart under conditions of increased venous return or increased impedance to ejection. These same mechanisms are utilized to increase cardiac output during acute congestive failure, during the early stages of chronic congestive heart failure, or during acute stress in chronic heart failure states.

Heart Rate

The simplest of these mechanisms for increasing cardiac output is an increase in heart rate. If the amount of blood ejected with each beat (the stroke volume) remains unchanged, a 10 percent increase in heart rate will result in a 10 percent increase in cardiac output.

Frank-Starling Mechanism

The second mechanism available for augmenting cardiac output is the Frank-Starling mechanism which states that within limits the performance of the heart is a function of the length of the myocardial fibers at the onset of contraction. A longer initial fiber length or larger diastolic ventricular volume results in improved performance.

The performance of the heart is frequently expressed in terms of the stroke work. The stroke work, the amount of external work performed per beat, is proportional to the product of systolic pressure minus the end-diastolic pressure times the stroke volume. The left ventricular end-diastolic volume serves as a direct index of the fiber length at the onset of contraction or the preload. The relationship between stroke work and left ventricular end-diastolic volume for a heart at a given contractile state is defined by a single line: the ventricular function curve (Fig. 18-1). If there is a sudden increase in the venous return, the ventricular end-diastolic volume rises and results in augmentation of the stroke work because of the Frank-Starling relationship. In either the normal or the failing heart an increase in diastolic volume will bring the heart to a higher position on its ventricular function curve (Fig. 18-1A).

Congestive heart failure due to myocardial causes (Table 18-1) is reflected in the Starling relationship by a shift in the function curve downwards and toward the right such that a given level of stroke work can only be performed at a greater end-diastolic volume. This same principle can be stated in another manner: At the same end-diastolic volume or fiber length the failing ventricle performs less work than the normal ventricle. This shift in the ventricular function curve downward and to the right is described by many as a decrease in myocardial contractility and characterizes the change in the left ventricular function associated with left ventricular failure.

The mechanism for the shift in this curve downward and to the right in association with congestive heart failure states is often not known. Certain disorders leading to left ventricular dysfunction, such as myocardial infarction, involve the loss of contractile units of ventricular myocardium and the substitution of relatively compliant fibrous scar tissue. Such fibrotic tissue acts a "rubber band" or series compliance thus placing an additional load on the remaining muscle. In certain animal models of heart failure there are demonstrable biochemical and structural changes in the contractile proteins and in others there appear to be abnormalities of subcellular elements concerned with intracellular calcium movement. In-

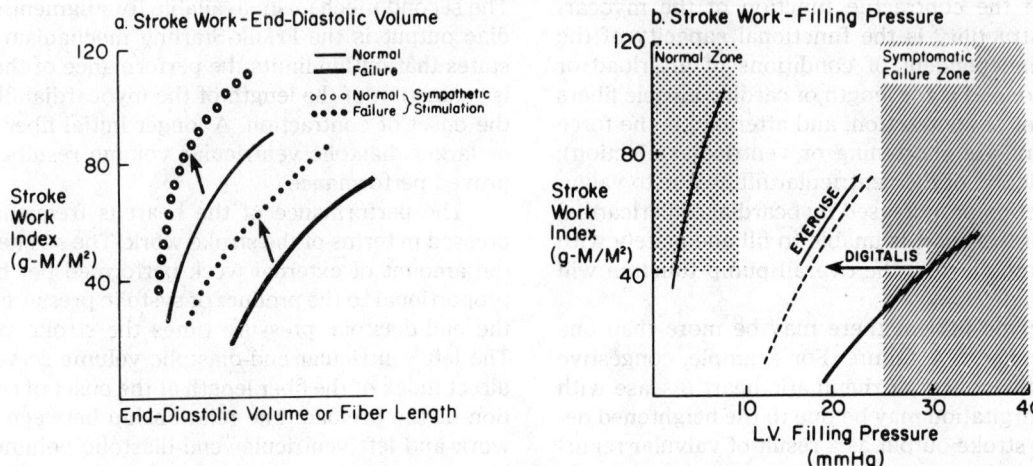

FIGURE 18-1. A. Ventricular function curves shown as the relationship between stroke work index and end-diastolic volume or fiber length. The four curves illustrate the effect of sympathetic stimulation on the ventricular function curve of the normal and failing heart. Stroke work is expressed as gram-meters per square meter of body surface (g-M/M²). **B.** Ventricular function curves depicted as the relationship between stroke work index and filling pressure. Shown are a normal curve within the normal zone and a curve for a failing heart before and after digitalis. Symptoms of dyspnea are usually encountered at filling pressures greater than 25 mm Hg.

tracellular calcium movement is the primary determinant of the intensity and duration of activation of the contractile process in cardiac muscle.

In certain heart failure states (Table 18–1) the Frank-Starling mechanism is not available as a com-

---

TABLE 18-1
Pathophysiology of Congestive Failure

A. Increased work load
   1. Increased stroke volume
      a. High output states and exercise (increased peripheral demands, e.g., hyperthyroidism and anemia)
      b. Valvular regurgitation or left-to-right shunts
      c. Severe bradycardia
   2. Increased impedance to ejection
      a. Systemic or pulmonary hypertension
      b. Pulmonic or aortic stenosis

B. Disorders of myocardial contractile function
   1. Localized—myocardial infarction (Chap. 23)
   2. Diffuse—see Table 19–5

C. Restriction of ventricular filling
   1. Mitral and tricuspid valvular stenosis
   2. Increased ventricular stiffness
      a. Ventricular hypertrophy
      b. Infiltrative myocardial diseases (e.g., sarcoid, amyloid)
      c. Myocardial ischemia and infarction
   3. Pericardial constriction

---

pensatory mechanism. In constrictive pericarditis the principal functional abnormality is the inability of the ventricles to expand their volume or fiber length during diastole. In mitral stenosis restriction of left ventricular filling is again the principal functional abnormality. With significant mitral stenosis adequate ventricular filling can only occur with a substantial increase in the left atrial pressure. If the venous return is great enough pulmonary edema results as the left atrial and thus pulmonary venous pressure rise to levels which result in transudation of fluid from the vascular space into the lung.

Sympathetic Stimulation

Sympathetic stimulation is a third means for the rapid augmentation of the left ventricular output. Under conditions of increased sympathetic stimulation, the ventricle is capable of performing more work at any given level of diastolic volume or fiber length. Such a shift in the function curve is termed an increase in contractility. A function curve which has been shifted downward and toward the right can be shifted upward and to the left and restored to the normal zone by sympathetic stimulation (Fig. 18–1A).

Heart failure is associated with a number of changes in the sympathetic nervous system.[25,37] The myocardial stores of catecholamines are depleted during heart failure. This depletion may be due to de-

TABLE 18-2
Physiologic and Pharmacologic Factors Influencing Myocardial Contractility

Increase	Decrease
Catecholamines (sympathetic tone)	Hypoxia
Digitalis glycosides	Acidosis
Angiotensin II	Hypercarbia
Heart rate	
Postextrasystolic potentiation	Sympathetic blocking agents
Certain globulins	Most antiarrhythmic and some psychopharmacologic agents and some antibiotics
	Myocardial depressant factor of intestinal origin during shock
	Antimetabolic agents

creased catecholamine synthesis but increased sympathetic stimulation may also play a role. It is not clear whether depletion under these circumstances is associated with receptor hypersensitivity. Regulation of heart rate in patients with cardiac failure is more dependent on sympathetic than parasympathetic tone when compared to normal man.

Other important physiologic and pharmacologic factors that influence left ventricular contractility in addition to sympathetic tone are listed in Table 18-2.

CHRONIC COMPENSATORY MECHANISMS

In chronic disease the heart has two important adaptive mechanisms, hypertrophy and dilatation, which allow it to maintain normal cardiac output in spite of increased demands for work. These mechanisms may allow the heart to perform almost normally for many years and keep the patient free of symptoms in spite of major increase in cardiac work. Ultimately, the compensatory mechanisms will not be adequate if the increased work demand on the heart increases progressively with time or if other disease processes affect the heart, i.e., coronary artery disease. Additionally, the compensatory mechanisms themselves may result in altered cardiac performance which may be responsible for the appearance of symptoms.

Ventricular Hypertrophy

An increase in left ventricular weight or hypertrophy occurs most commonly when the normal heart is required to generate increased wall tension for a substantial period of time. Disease states which lead to a rise in left ventricular systolic pressure and thus increased wall tension include systemic hypertension and aortic stenosis. In certain cardiomyopathic states and in ischemic heart disease, hypertrophy occurs without obvious prior hemodynamic changes. The stimulus to hypertrophy under these conditions is unknown.

There are some distinct functional advantages of left ventricular hypertrophy. The total overall pump capabilities of the hypertrophied left ventricle are greater than that of the normal ventricle. That is to say, the maximal stroke work the heart can perform at any given fiber length appears to be greater in the hypertrophied ventricle. The wall tension or systolic wall stress which must be developed by each fiber to generate a given intraventricular pressure is lower in the hypertrophied heart than in the normal heart developing the same intracavitary systolic pressure. This results from the implications of the Laplace relationship which, although derived for thin-walled spheres, appears to be applicable to the thick-walled ventricle. The Laplace relationship states that the wall stress or the grams of force for every unit cross-sectional area of ventricular muscle is equal to the pressure in the ventricle multiplied by the simultaneously determined radius of the cavity and divided by the wall thickness. Thus the hypertrophied ventricle can generate greater systolic left ventricular pressure with the *same* force per unit cross-sectional area in the ventricular myocardium than the normal ventricle because of the increase in wall thickness. Since each fiber generates less wall stress for any given level of intracavitary pressure the ventricle is able to maintain the extent of individual fiber shortening despite the increased pressure load. The oxygen demand per unit of muscle mass is reduced by hypertrophy since systolic wall stress is a major determinant of oxygen demand (see Fig. 22-1).

The disadvantages of left ventricular hypertrophy relate in part to the increase in ventricular wall stiffness associated with the hypertrophied state. At least a portion of this increase in stiffness is due to the increase in total muscle mass of the left ventricular wall. As a result of increased stiffness, atrial and ventricular filling pressures must increase in order to achieve adequate preload. Atrial systole, therefore, becomes more important in maintaining forward cardiac output. The development of atrial fibrillation with resultant loss of atrial booster function may cause marked reduction in cardiac output.

Left Ventricular Dilatation

Dilatation occurs in the failing heart as a result of a prolonged increase in diastolic pressure; also left ventricular dilatation is essential to maintenance of adequate cardiac output under conditions where an increase in stroke volume is required, for example, in high output states such as anemia, hyperthyroidism, peripheral arteriovenous shunting, valvular regurgitation, or left-to-right shunts. As long as the ventricle maintains normal contractile function, i.e., remains on the same Frank-Starling curve, increases in end-diastolic volume will result in proportional increases in stroke volume.

There are clear disadvantages of left ventricular dilatation. Based on the implications of the Laplace relationship, the wall stress necessary to generate any given intracavitary pressure is greater in the dilated heart than the normal heart in proportion to the increase in radius. Myocardial oxygen demands increase in proportion to this increase in wall stress. It is not surprising, therefore, to find that the chronically dilated heart is particularly sensitive to increases in systolic ventricular pressure and that symptomatic relief of chronic congestive failure can be obtained in the chronically dilated heart by reducing the peak pressure and thus the peak systolic wall stress of the ventricle during contraction.

Left ventricular dilatation is particularly disadvantageous in disease states where there is restriction of coronary flow or oxygen availability. Dilatation results in increased myocardial oxygen demands at a normal level of stroke work as a result of the increase in wall stress.

EVALUATION OF CARDIAC FUNCTION

LEFT VENTRICULAR FILLING PRESSURE
Ventricular function curves relating diastolic volume as an index of fiber length to stroke work are less commonly employed in clinical medicine than function curves relating left ventricular end-diastolic pressure or left ventricular filling pressure (left atrial or pulmonary capillary wedge pressure) to stroke work or cardiac output (Fig. 18–1B). The reasons for the use of end-diastolic pressure rather than end-diastolic volume include: 1) End-diastolic pressure or filling pressure is more easily measured than ventricular volume; 2) The wedge or filling pressure can be measured repeatedly in patients with unstable hemodynamics and requires only catheterization of the right heart via a peripheral vein; 3) There is great difficulty in establishing the limits of normal end-diastolic volume for patients of varying body size; and 4) The level of left ventricular end diastolic pressure or filling pressure determines the pulmonary venous pressure

(in the absence of mitral stenosis) and thus the symptoms of congestive failure: dyspnea and orthopnea. Therefore, the left ventricular filling pressure per se is of value as an indication of the probability that symptomatic dyspnea or pulmonary edema will develop.

Shown in Figure 18–1B are ventricular function curves relating filling pressure to stroke work index from a normal patient and a patient with congestive heart failure due to abnormal left ventricular myocardial contractility before and after treatment with a digitalis glycoside. Normal persons even under conditions of severe exercise stress are within the general confines of the box in the upper left hand corner of this figure. With left ventricular failure ventricular function is shifted to a curve which is downwards and to the right of normal. The left ventricular filling pressure must be very high to generate even a low-normal stroke work index (40 g-M/M²) which would be expected in the resting state. The left ventricular filling pressure is at levels greater than 25 mm Hg which is associated with pulmonary congestion. Administration of a digitalis glycoside shifts the ventricular function of the failing heart upwards and to the left to a new, more nearly normal curve, thus lowering the left ventricular filling pressure (see arrow) to a level not usually associated with congestive symptoms. If the work load is increased by exercise in this digitalized patient he moves up along the new ventricular function curve to the point at which congestive symptoms would again appear as a result of the increase in left ventricular filling pressure and pulmonary venous pressure. Dyspnea present at rest would disappear after digitalization but return with exertion.

DIASTOLIC PRESSURE–VOLUME RELATIONSHIPS
The term diastolic compliance, as used here, refers to the magnitude of the increase in ventricular diastolic pressure per unit increase in volume. In a compliant chamber the pressure rise is small for a unit increase in volume, and for a stiff or noncompliant chamber the pressure rise is great for the same unit increase in volume.

The compliance of the left ventricle is reflected in the relationship between left ventricular filling pressure or left ventricular end diastolic pressure and left ventricular volume. This relationship is exponential rather than linear as shown in Figure 18–2A. The shape of each of the two curves reflects the fact that as the diastolic volume of all ventricles is increased the myocardium becomes progressively stiffer or noncompliant and resists a further increase in volume. At normal (low) levels of end-diastolic pressure, the diastolic volume of the ventricle may increase markedly with little change in end-diastolic pressure, whereas at high levels of end-diastolic pressure (as one would encounter in severe acute congestive failure) a unit increase in end-diastolic volume would result in a substantial increase in left ventricular filling pressure. This has practical importance, for example, in treatment of acute pulmonary edema. Measures designed to reduce the level of venous return to the left ventricle, such as the application of peripheral tourniquets, may result in a small decrease in venous return and a small decrease in the end-diastolic volume of the ventricle but a substantial fall in end-diastolic pressure and pulmonary venous pressure as a result of the steep slope of the pressure–volume curve at higher pressures. Once effective treatment is initiated in acute pulmonary edema it is often surprising how rapidly the signs and symptoms of pulmonary congestion resolve. Also, severe congestive failure can be precipitated in a patient with a hemodynamic status placing him high on the diastolic pressure–volume curve by small increases in intravascular volume as might occur during transfusion or administration of intravenous fluids.

There are a number of factors which will significantly change the quantitative relationship of left ventricular end-diastolic volume to pressure. Such a change is called an alteration in left ventricular diastolic compliance or stiffness and is indicated by a shift in the pressure–volume curve. Myocardial ischemia and the early phase of acute myocardial infarction are characterized by a decrease in compliance or

increase in stiffness which is indicated by a shift in the diastolic pressure–volume relationship (Fig. 18-2A) such that there is a greater rise in diastolic pressure for any increase in volume from any initial volume. The stiffer heart has a higher filling pressure at any level of end-diastolic volume or fiber length. In terms of ventricular function curves plotted as the relationship between end-diastolic pressure (or filling pressure) and stroke work or output (Fig. 18-2B) an increase in ventricular stiffness would result in a higher end-diastolic pressure at any level of stroke work or output. A decrease in compliance would appear then as a shift in the ventricular function curve. This shift in the curve is the same as one would see as a result of a decrease in myocardial contractility. But, this is in fact not a decrease in contractility but only an alteration in left ventricular stiffness toward a stiffer ventricle. If one had plotted end-diastolic *volume* or fiber length against stroke work (Fig. 18-1A) under conditions of an alteration in left ventricular stiffness, there would be no change in the position of the ventricular function curve indicating that there is no change in contractility. From a clinical and functional point of view, however, a decrease in ventricular compliance (such as appears during myocardial ischemia or early myocardial infarction) means that symptoms of congestive heart failure will occur at a smaller ventricular volume or at a lower level of cardiac performance than under circumstances of normal left ventricular stiffness. Thus, a decrease in diastolic compliance or an increase in stiffness has the

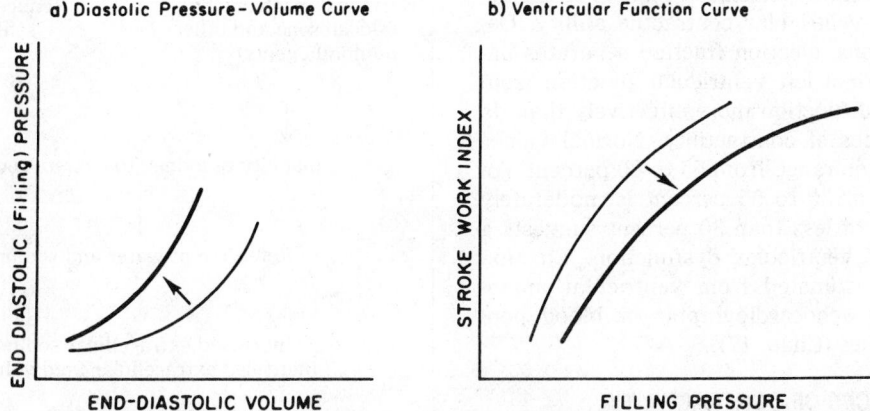

a) Diastolic Pressure-Volume Curve   b) Ventricular Function Curve

FIGURE 18-2. Effect of a decrease in left ventricular compliance on the diastolic pressure–volume curve (a) and ventricular function curve of the same heart (b). **A.** A decrease in compliance results in a higher level of end-diastolic pressure for any end-diastolic volume. The curves are steeper as volume increases. **B.** Since following a decrease in compliance the filling pressure is higher for any fiber length or volume, the ventricular-function curve using filling pressure on the abscissa is shifted downward and to the right.

same effect as a decrease in contractility: a rise in filling pressure and onset of dyspnea and pulmonary edema. A stiffer ventricle can do the same amount of work as a normal ventricle but requires a higher filling pressure.

Left ventricular hypertrophy and infiltrative cardiomyopathies (Table 18–1) also result in increased left ventricular diastolic stiffness or a shift in the end-diastolic pressure–volume relationship as shown in Figure 18–2. In disorders characterized by a stiff or noncompliant ventricle, a well-timed and forceful atrial contraction is very important in maintaining adequate forward cardiac output.

EJECTION FRACTION

At present the left ventricular "ejection fraction" is the value most frequently employed in the clinical assessment of left ventricular function and its impairment by disease. The ejection fraction is equal to the stroke volume end-diastolic volume or the end-diastolic volume minus the end-systolic volume divided by the end-diastolic volume. Since one is looking only at the percent of the total end-diastolic volume ejected, normalization of volume for body size is not necessary; this is the advantage of ejection fraction. Ejection fraction is a measure of function, not contractility. The ejection fraction (as stroke work) is sensitive to changes in end-diastolic pressure or fiber length and thus can be increased by fluid loading as with the volume of contrast material injected during angiography and decreased by fluid restriction or dehydration. An increase in systolic pressure load will decrease ejection fraction. Thus, ejection fraction may be low in severe hypertension relative to the actual level of left ventricular contractile ability. Despite the limitations, ejection fraction separates patients with abnormal left ventricular function from those with normal function more effectively than do the velocity indices of contractility. Normal values for ejection fraction range from 55 to 80 percent. An ejection fraction of 30 to 55 percent is moderately low, and a value of less than 30 percent suggests a severe degree of ventricular dysfunction. Ejection fraction can be estimated from ventricular angiograms or by the echocardiographic or blood pool scanning techniques (Chap. 17).

OTHER INDICES OF CONTRACTILITY

During recent years attempts have been made to derive other indices of overall left ventricular contractility. It would be particularly useful to have such an index which is independent of left ventricular compliance. The majority of these efforts have utilized the velocity of contractile element activity. Such indices include the maximal rate of rise of isovolumic left

ventricular pressure (dp/dt), the mean and peak velocity of circumferential fiber shortening, and the estimated theoretical velocity of circumferential fiber shortening at zero load (V_{max}). Many of these indices appear to be insensitive in separating normal from abnormal patients and are difficult to measure accurately and repeatedly.

CLINICAL MANIFESTATIONS

The major clinical manifestations of congestive failure can be divided into those due to systemic fluid retention and those due to pulmonary vascular congestion. Both are present in most patients.

FLUID RETENTION[34,35]

Cardiac output which is inadequate relative to the metabolic requirements of the body initiates the sequence of events which leads to fluid retention (Table 18–3). The renal circulation is altered by reduced total

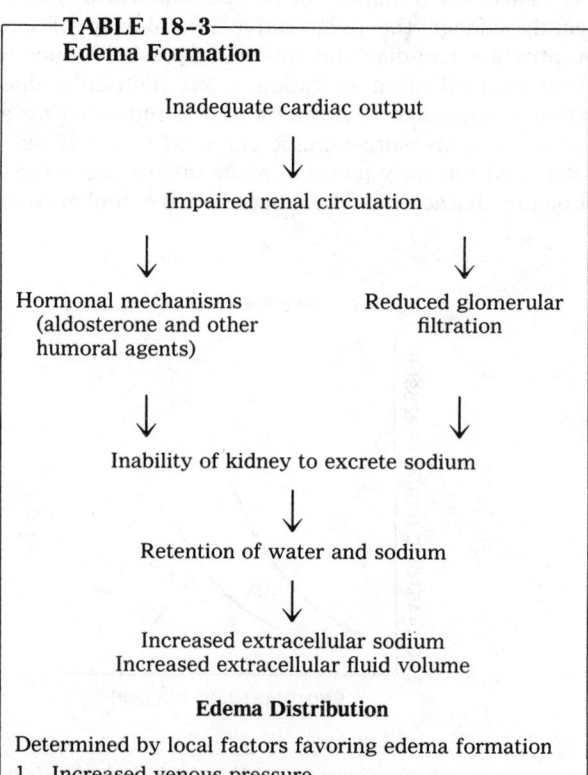

TABLE 18–3
Edema Formation

Inadequate cardiac output
↓
Impaired renal circulation
↓   ↓
Hormonal mechanisms   Reduced glomerular
(aldosterone and other   filtration
humoral agents)
↓   ↓
Inability of kidney to excrete sodium
↓
Retention of water and sodium
↓
Increased extracellular sodium
Increased extracellular fluid volume

Edema Distribution

Determined by local factors favoring edema formation
1. Increased venous pressure
2. Reduced plasma colloid osmotic pressure-low proteins
3. Decreased tissue pressure
4. Impaired lymphatic function

blood flow and redistribution of intrarenal blood flow. Glomerular filtration rate is markedly reduced. This decrease in glomerular filtration rate is accompanied by an increase in the fraction of filtered sodium which is reabsorbed. Thus, in addition to the fact that less sodium is being filtered, more of the filtered sodium is reabsorbed, and the quantity of sodium which is excreted is progressively reduced. If sodium intake is unchanged this decreased sodium excretion leads to expansion of the total body sodium content. The extracellular fluid volume expands as fluid is retained so as to maintain normal osmolality of the extracellular fluid in the face of salt retention.

Increased production of the normally occurring mineralocorticoid aldosterone has been demonstrated in a variety of conditions associated with edema formation. The administration of salt-retaining steroids to normal individuals will not produce an edematous state similar to congestive heart failure, although it does produce some increase in the total exchangeable sodium. This increase is relatively short in duration and is followed by a period of readjustment during which the output of sodium exceeds intake. Administration of aldosterone to patients with heart failure results in progressive worsening of the signs and symptoms of heart failure. Aldosterone production is increased in congestive heart failure secondary to an increase in renin release by the kidney likely in turn a result of altered renal blood flow.

Changes in the tubular reabsorption of sodium that are independent of changes in glomerular filtration rate have been identified. A receptor sensitive to changes in either vascular or total extracellular fluid volume has been postulated. Some have suggested that a hormonal "third factor" in sodium balance may be involved.

The distribution of the increased extracellular fluid resulting from increased total body sodium and water varies from patient to patient. Venous pressure is the major factor determining distribution, and its effect is emphasized by the influence of posture on the distribution of edema. An ambulatory patient will accumulate edema in the feet and ankles because gravity makes the venous capillary pressure highest in the lower extremities. If the patient is put to bed, edema appears over the sacrum. The colloid osmotic pressure of the plasma proteins tends to counteract the effects of the venous hydrostatic pressure, which favors the movement of fluid into the extravascular spaces. Edema formation, therefore, occurs more readily in the patient with low plasma proteins. Tissue pressure is important in determining the distribution of edema, which forms more readily in loose tissue, such as that around the posterior part of the ankle.

PULMONARY CONGESTION[29,30]

Pulmonary vascular congestion is the major abnormality in left ventricular failure and presents clinically as dyspnea on exertion and, in later stages, at rest. A characteristic manifestation is paroxysmal nocturnal dyspnea, in which the patient awakens from sound sleep with extreme shortness of breath. A closely related symptom is orthopnea, which requires the patient to sleep with his head and trunk elevated. On occasion, pulmonary congestion is manifest only by cough or hemoptysis.

Early in the course of left heart failure, the volume of blood contained in the pulmonary vasculature is increased and the pressure in both the arteries and veins is elevated. The turgid, congested lung becomes relatively inelastic and ventilation is impaired. The work of breathing is increased by reduced compliance of the lung, and this may be responsible in part for the symptom of dyspnea, which literally means difficult breathing. Reflex mechanisms originating in the distended vessels or compromised alveoli probably contribute to the tachypnea and sensation of air hunger (Chap. 32). If the pulmonary venous pressure is increased, the equilibrium between hydrostatic pressure and colloid osmotic pressure becomes unbalanced and fluid is extravasated into the alveolar spaces. Minor extravasation produces moist rales at the lung bases. If it is more massive and sudden in onset, pulmonary edema results.

Orthopnea and paroxysmal nocturnal dyspnea are closely related and probably depend upon the same physiologic mechanism. When the body changes from the erect to the supine position, the hydrostatic pressure in the veins of the legs falls, and that portion of the total blood volume which had been pooled there returns to the right heart to be delivered to the lungs. If the function of the left heart is inadequate, the flow of blood out of the pulmonary vascular bed is impaired, and the lungs become congested. A second, more gradual change may play a role in the development of paroxysmal nocturnal dyspnea. The reduction of venous pressure in the extremities secondary to the assumption of the supine position leads to a shift in the fluid equilibrium across the capillary membranes, and fluid enters the vascular space from the extravascular compartment. This results in an overall increase in circulatory blood volume, which acts, along with the redistribution, to produce pulmonary vascular congestion. A patient with impaired left ventricular function tends to keep his head and trunk elevated, and if he awakens from a sound sleep with severe shortness of breath, he usually seeks relief by assuming the erect posture, thereby utilizing the effect of gravity to reduce the pulmonary congestion. The congestion of the pulmonary vasculature probably initiates reflexes which result in broncho-constriction; wheezes are usually present along with moist rales.

FUNCTIONAL CAPACITY

It is useful to express the cardiac patient's functional capacity in terms of classification systems of the New York Heart Association. Such classification is valuable in transmitting information from one physician to another and also in categorizing patients with regard to their suitability for operation or to indicate the degree of improvement following therapy.

Functional Classification*

Class I Patients with cardiac disease but without resulting limitations of physical activity. Ordinary physical activity does not cause undue fatigue, palpitation, dyspnea, or anginal pain.

Class II Patients with cardiac disease resulting in slight limitation of physical activity. They are comfortable at rest. Ordinary physical activity results in fatigue, palpitation, dyspnea, or anginal pain.

Class III Patients with cardiac disease resulting in marked limitation of physical activity. They are comfortable at rest. Less than ordinary physical activity causes fatigue, palpitation, dyspnea, or anginal pain.

Class IV Patients with cardiac disease resulting in inability to carry on any physical activity without discomfort. Symptoms of cardiac insufficiency or of the anginal syndrome may be present even at rest. If any physical activity is undertaken, discomfort is increased.

* The Criteria Committee of the New York Heart Association, Inc., *Diseases of the Heart and Blood Vessels: Nomenclature and Criteria for Diagnosis*, 6th ed. Boston, Little, Brown and Company, 1964. Reprinted by permission of the publisher.

CHAPTER 19

Congestive Heart Failure and/or Enlarged Cardiac Silhouette: Approach to the Patient and Management

NICHOLAS J. FORTUIN AND RICHARD S. ROSS

CONGESTIVE FAILURE

When the patient with congestive heart failure is not in acute distress, the physician can adopt a systematic approach to diagnosis and therapy. This fact still is not universally recognized, and patients are often treated for long periods with no more specific diagnosis than congestive heart failure or myocardial insufficiency. Relief of the patient's symptoms is the ultimate goal of therapy, but the first step toward this goal is to establish the pathophysiologic mechanism and anatomic abnormality responsible for altered cardiovascular performance. Table 18–1 describes the three major mechanisms and the disease processes which are common examples of each. Careful physical examination along with an electrocardiogram and chest roentgenogram and in some cases echocardiography or radioisotope studies will define the responsible mechanism in almost all patients. When myocardial contractility is impaired, diffusely as in cardiomyopathy or regionally as in ischemic heart disease, the left ventricle must dilate in order to maintain forward cardiac output. The heart is therefore enlarged and systolic wall movement and ejection fraction are reduced. By contrast, when diastolic left ventricular function is altered and ventricular filling is impaired, the left ventricle remains normal or only slightly increased in size and wall motion or ejection fraction may be normal. Impaired diastolic filling may result from anatomic blockage of the atrioventricular valves as in mitral stenosis or atrial myxoma, from reduced compliance of the ventricle as in hypertrophy or the early phase of acute infarction or ischemia, or from pericardial or endocardial restriction. The third mechanism resulting in altered cardiac performance is excess work load. The increased work may result from excess volume work, as in congenital left to right shunts, valvular regurgitation, increased metabolic demands, or excess pressure work, as in aortic stenosis or systemic hypertension. With increased volume load the ventricle will be dilated but wall motion and ejection fraction will be normal or excessive. The pressure-loaded ventricle will show evidence of hypertrophy. In practice the patient with congestive failure may have several mechanisms working together to produce cardiac malfunction.

In addition to establishing a mechanism for heart failure, the physician must determine specific anatomic or etiologic processes underlying the pathophysiologic abnormalities. The approach to anatomic diagnosis proposed by Hamman and modified by Harvey and Bordley is useful in the solution of clinical problems (Table 19–1) and will serve as an outline for the present chapter.

Valvular heart disease, systemic hypertension, and pulmonary hypertension are discussed in more detail elsewhere (Chaps. 20, 25, and 26, respectively). Pericardial and myocardial disease receive no other discussion and, therefore, a more detailed presentation is included here.

Occasionally, patients come to medical attention because cardiac enlargement has been detected on routine screening chest roentgenograms or in the evaluation of chest pain, dyspnea, cardiac arrhythmias, or systemic embolization. Such patients usually have some form of pericardial or myocardial disease. The evaluation of the patient with cardiomegaly and the differentiation of these two conditions are considered in detail in this section.

VALVULAR HEART DISEASE AS A CAUSE OF CONGESTIVE HEART FAILURE

The diagnosis of valvular heart disease is presumed when one detects a significant heart murmur (Chap. 20). The major question posed by a patient with congestive failure and a heart murmur is: Does the murmur represent organic valvular disease? A positive answer leads to the next question: Is the valvular lesion of sufficient severity to account for the patient's symptoms? For example, the patient in congestive failure from myocardial disease may have a promi-

nent murmur of tricuspid regurgitation which disappears with improvement in cardiac function. Many patients with atherosclerotic coronary artery disease also have some degree of calcific aortic sclerosis or stenosis, which may produce loud murmurs without necessarily resulting in significant obstruction to left ventricular outflow. In such an instance, the murmur results from organic heart disease, but the valvular lesion may not be quantitatively important as a cause of the congestive heart failure. Clinical clues to the severity of individual lesions are described in Chapter 20.

Errors in the diagnosis of valvular heart disease are common in patients in whom auscultation is difficult as in the case of men with emphysematous chests or women with large breasts. Other factors which make diagnosis difficult are the presence of congestive failure with low cardiac output or pulmonary congestion with accelerated noisy breathing.

SYSTEMIC HYPERTENSION AS A CAUSE OF CONGESTIVE HEART FAILURE (Chap. 25)

Systemic hypertension is a common cause of left ventricular failure and these patients are often seen first in an attack of acute pulmonary edema. The usual presentation is with breathlessness and paroxysmal nocturnal dyspnea, but edema, elevated venous pressure, and hepatomegaly sometimes develop in the absence of pulmonary symptoms. A fourth heart sound (S_4 or presystolic gallop) commonly is heard in patients with systemic hypertension, and the left atrium may be enlarged. These findings occasionally lead to confusion with mitral stenosis.

The diagnosis of systemic hypertension is usually not difficult to establish, depending as it does on the measurement of blood pressure. Most patients will show signs of hypertension in other organs, i.e. the optic fundi, the kidneys, or the central nervous system. Diagnosis may be difficult if the patient has sustained a myocardial infarction which has caused a drop in blood pressure from hypertensive levels. The physician also must be aware that arterial blood pressure tends to be elevated in congestive failure, especially if due to myocardial disease, but in this situation, the elevation is mild and pressures in excess of 160/100 are unusual.

PULMONARY HYPERTENSION AS A CAUSE OF CONGESTIVE HEART FAILURE

Pulmonary hypertension is the most common cause of right ventricular failure. Breathlessness and fatigue are prominent, especially if the hypertension is secondary to disease of the left heart. Chest pain, similar to that of angina pectoris, may be present but

---

┌───┐
TABLE 19–1
Causes of Congestive Heart Failure

1. Valvular heart disease
2. Hypertension in the systemic circulation
3. Hypertension in the pulmonary circulation
4. Pericardial disease
5. Myocardial disease
6. Miscellaneous rare conditions including high output states, e.g., thyrotoxicosis, arterio-venous fistula, and anemia
└───┘

is rarely a primary complaint. The usual manifestations are those of right heart failure and include elevated venous pressure, hepatomegaly, ascites, and edema.

The diagnosis usually can be made by recognition of the characteristic physical findings, the most prominent of which are the cardiac signs as described in Chapter 26.

PERICARDIAL DISEASE AS A CAUSE OF CONGESTIVE HEART FAILURE[42,43,47,49]

The chronic, constrictive form of pericarditis presents as right heart failure. Recognition of this syndrome is of great importance, since it is a treatable cause of congestive failure, the discovery of which is often preceded by a prolonged period of incorrect diagnosis and unsuccessful treatment. A classification of pericardial disease is presented in Table 19-2.

In constrictive pericarditis the encompassing scar limits the inflow of blood into the right heart, resulting in a fixed restriction in the output of the heart. The problem is one of filling, whereas in myocardial failure, it is basically one of emptying. The symptoms and signs are usually those of systemic venous congestion, but if the constriction involves the

---

TABLE 19-2
Diseases of the Pericardium

I. **Acute and Subacute**

    A. Infections
        1. Bacterial
            a. Tuberculosis
            b. Purulent—pneumococcal,
                staphylococcal, etc.
        2. Protozoal—amebic
        3. Mycotic—actinomycosis,
            coccidioidomycosis
        4. Viral—Coxsackie
    B. Connective tissue and allergic disease, systemic lupus erythematosus, scleroderma, rheumatoid disease
    C. Chemical or metabolic—uremia, myxedema
    D. Neoplastic
    E. Secondary to disease of heart or great vessels. Associated with myocardial infarction, coronary embolism, dissecting aneurysm
    F. Physical injury—radiation, trauma
    G. Unknown—benign idiopathic,? viral
    H. Postmyocardial infarction, post-thoracotomy

II. **Chronic Disorders**

    A. Chronic constrictive pericarditis
    B. Chronic mediastinopericarditis
    C. Chronic pericardial effusion
        1. Myxedema
        2. Cholesterol pericarditis

TABLE 19-3
Clinical Manifestations of Constrictive Pericarditis

History	Edema, ascites
Physical examination	Elevated venous pressure
	Collapsing venous pulse
	Small, quiet heart
	Early diastolic knock
	Diastolic heartbeat
	Edema, ascites, hepatomegaly
	Paradoxical pulse
X-ray	Small or slightly enlarged heart
	Irregularly or triangularly shaped heart
	Dilated superior vena cava
	Calcium in pericardium
Electrocardiogram	Low voltage
	ST- and T-wave changes
	Atrial fibrillation
Laboratory findings	Low serum albumin, lymphopenia
Catheterization	Early diastolic dip followed by diastolic plateau in ventricular pressure
	Thickened pericardium detected by: catheter in RA, angiocardiography

---

left side—especially the left atrium—pulmonary vascular congestion may result.

The clinical features are outlined in Table 19-3. Venous congestion, hepatomegaly, ascites, and edema are the common presenting manifestations. Patients are often young people in whom heart disease is not suspected, and the protean clinical manifestations of constrictive pericarditis often lead to erroneous diagnosis. Hepatic enlargement, hypoalbuminemia, and ascites may suggest cirrhosis of the liver, or prominent albuminuria may be taken as evidence of nephrosis. Intestinal protein loss may lead to the conclusion that the patient has protein-losing enteropathy. A number of incorrect cardiac diagnoses may also arise from misinterpretation of physical findings. Probably the most common error relates to the interpretation of the pericardial knock, which may be mistaken for a gallop sound and lead to the diagnosis of cardiomyopathy or may be considered to be an opening snap leading to the incorrect diagnosis of mitral stenosis.

A high venous pressure is often the key to diagnosis, but the pressure may be abnormal only after exercise or volume loading. One feature of constric-

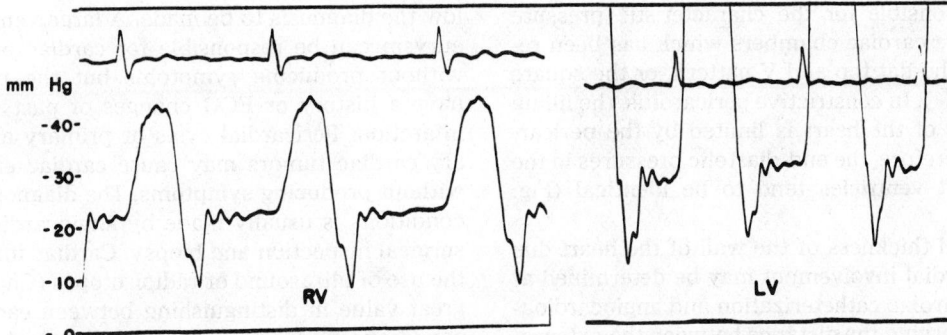

FIGURE 19-1. Intraventricular pressures from a patient with constrictive pericarditis and atrial fibrillation. The pressure does not continue to rise throughout diastole since all the filling occurs early. Right (RV) and left ventricular (LV) diastolic pressures are shown at a higher level of amplification. Note that pressures in the right and left ventricles have similar contour and reach approximately the same level at the end of diastole.

tive pericarditis is the rapid y descent of the jugular venous pulse. This finding of a collapsing pulse in the neck veins mirrors the changes in intracardiac pressure illustrated in Figure 19–1. Pulsus paradoxus is often present but is not specific for constrictive pericarditis.

In the typical case, the heart is small, and quiet. The point of maximal impulse may be difficult to localize, but finding an apex beat does not preclude the diagnosis. Murmurs and rubs are usually absent, but a characteristic early-diastolic knocking sound is sometimes heard. This sound corresponds to the period of maximal ventricular filling, and is attributed to the arrest of filling by the constricting pericardium. This early diastolic filling wave is sometimes so forceful that it can be felt on palpation or can even be seen on inspection of the precordium. Hepatomegaly, edema, and ascites may be of massive proportion.

The chest x-ray often provides the first clue to the correct diagnosis, since the heart, although sometimes small and occasionally perfectly normal in size, usually has a peculiar shape. The finding of calcific deposits in the pericardium on x-ray or fluoroscopy gives an important clue to the diagnosis (Fig. 19–2). In some cases the cardiac silhouette is enlarged, and the constricting process is due to both thickening of the pericardium and chronic pericardial effusion. The ECG usually shows low voltage, ST- and T-wave changes, and atrial fibrillation is not uncommon. A low voltage QRS complex should arouse suspicion of constrictive pericarditis or myxedema. The echocardiogram may show evidence of a small pericardial effusion, or in some cases pericardial thickening, but does not show specific signs of the constricting process. In some cases it has been normal.

The cardiovascular diagnostic laboratory may provide confirmation of the diagnosis by demonstration of a characteristic pressure tracing of arrested filling (Fig. 19–1). Ventricular filling is limited to the first part of diastole. Atrial pressure is high, and as the tricuspid valve opens blood quickly fills the ventricle to capacity. There is no further filling during the remainder of diastole and pressure and volume in the heart remain constant. The rapid inflow results in the spectacular drop in venous pressure observed in the neck veins as the collapsing pulse. The steep y de-

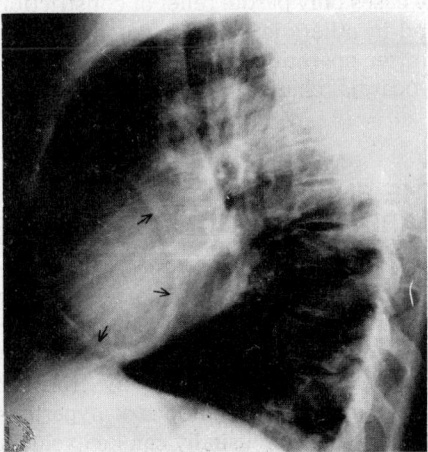

FIGURE 19-2. Lateral roentgenogram in constrictive pericarditis demonstrating pericardial calcification. The calcium is most likely to appear in the region of the atrioventricular groove and on the diaphragmatic surface of the heart. Fluoroscopy is often helpful in differentiating pericardial from pulmonary calcification.

scent is responsible for the characteristic pressure contour in the cardiac chambers which has been referred to as the flat top and V pattern, or the square root sign ($\sqrt{}$). In constrictive pericarditis, the filling of both sides of the heart is limited by the pericardium and, therefore, the end-diastolic pressures in the right and left ventricles tend to be identical (Fig. 19–1).

Abnormal thickness of the wall of the heart due to the pericardial involvement may be determined at the time of cardiac catheterization and angiocardiography by observing the distance between the external border of the heart and the cavity as indicated by the catheter or by radiopaque material. Sometimes confirmation is not possible in the laboratory, and surgical exploration is a necessary diagnostic procedure. In such a case decortication can be carried out at the same time if constriction is present. If not, a biopsy of both myocardium and pericardium can be obtained and may establish the correct diagnosis.

In most cases of constrictive pericarditis, no specific etiology can be determined and tuberculosis is no longer the most common cause of this disorder. Pericardial fibrosis and constriction can follow any injury to the pericardium, as for example, it may follow viral infection, trauma, radiation, or uremic pericarditis. If there is evidence of past tuberculous infection, antituberculosis therapy should be given. Operative removal of the constricting pericardium can be accomplished with a small risk, and in most cases this procedure will alleviate the hemodynamic abnormality and restore cardiac function to normal. In some cases only partial relief of constriction is possible and in others left ventricular dysfunction may persist after operation as a consequence of irreversible myocardial changes.

THE ENLARGED CARDIAC SILHOUETTE

Determining the cause of cardiac enlargement in patients with or without signs of congestive heart failure can be one of the most difficult differential diagnostic problems encountered by the clinician. Valvular heart disease, pulmonary hypertension, or systemic hypertension usually can be excluded in the initial evaluation. Some form of myocardial disease or pericardial effusion will be responsible for most of the remaining cases. Rarely, Ebstein's anomaly or atrial septal defect will present in adult life as unexplained asymptomatic cardiomegaly, but the other clinical features of these disorders (Chap. 27) will al-

low the diagnosis to be made. A large ventricular aneurysm can be responsible for cardiac enlargement without producing symptoms but the patient will have a history or ECG changes of past myocardial infarction. Pericardial cysts or primary and secondary cardiac tumors may cause cardiac enlargement without producing symptoms. The diagnosis of these conditions is usually made by angiocardiography or surgical inspection and biopsy. Cardiac imaging with the use of ultrasound or radioisotopes (Chap. 17) is of great value in distinguishing between each of these conditions and often obviates the need for angiographic study.

MYOCARDIAL DISEASE AND PERICARDIAL EFFUSION

The differentiation of pericardial effusion from myocardial disease may be difficult because in both situations the cardiac silhouette is enlarged and there may be dyspnea, venous hypertension, hepatomegaly, narrow pulse pressure, pulsus paradoxus, and signs of reduced cardiac output. The precordium is quiet, the heart sounds distant, and the left border of cardiac dullness displaced to the left. X-ray and ECG may be of little value. The differentiation is, however, vital since the treatment of pericardial effusion is removal of the fluid or thickened pericardium, and the prognosis is far better than in most forms of myocardial disease.

The features which may be helpful in making the distinction between pericardial and myocardial disease are listed in Table 19–4. Some features may be present in both conditions. For example, myocardial and pericardial diseases occasionally occur together, and in this situation a friction rub may be heard in a patient with myocardial disease as the primary condition. This combination may be seen as part of an acute systemic viral illness.

Pulsus paradoxus is often cited as specific for pericardial effusion, but it can also be seen in myocardial disease and is not uncommon in acute respiratory distress. The term refers to an exaggeration of the normal decrease in arterial blood pressure accompanying inspiration. Normally, this decrease may be as much as 10 mm Hg. In the presence of a pericardial effusion, however, it may reach 15 or 20 mm Hg due to the fact that inspiration increases venous return to the right heart and, since this increase in volume occurs inside the distended pericardium, it results in compression of the left heart and reduction in filling. The mechanism of pulsus paradoxus in myocardial disease, however, is less well understood. The finding of pulsus alternans or alternate weak and strong pulse wave on successive beats of the arterial pulse

TABLE 19-4

Differential Features of Myocardial and Pericardial Disease

Myocardial Disease	Pericardial Disease
History	
Family history of heart disease	Asymptomatic
Alcoholism, malnutrition, recent pregnancy	Tuberculosis, chest trauma, metastatic disease
Embolism	Chest pain relieved by leaning forward
Systemic viral illness	Systemic viral illness
Physical Exam	
Gallops, S_3 and S_4	Friction rub
Pansystolic murmur	Pulsus paradoxus
PMI at LBD	Inspiratory increase of venous pressure
Prominent v wave in JVP	Absent PMI or PMI inside LBD
Pulsus alternans	Collapsing y descent of JVP
ECG	
Abnormal QRS complexes	Normal
Atrial arrhythmias	Low voltage
ST-T changes	Atrial arrhythmias
LVH with strain	ST-T changes
Ventricular arrhythmias	

suggests left ventricular dysfunction and myocardial disease.

A specific sign of cardiac chamber enlargement (indicating myocardial disease) is the finding of a sustained cardiac impulse outside the midclavicular line which corresponds to the left border of cardiac dullness and the left heart border in the x-ray silhouette. Similarly, finding a definite impulse inside the midclavicular line and inside the left border of dullness is indicative of pericardial effusion. While the neck veins are distended in both conditions, a positive v wave reflecting tricuspid regurgitation is frequently seen in myocardial disease, whereas a collapse or exaggerated y descent is seen with pericardial effusion. The presence of a third sound or summation gallop favors the diagnosis of myocardial disease, since the filling sound typical of constrictive pericarditis is not often present in pericardial effusion.

Murmurs are relatively common in the patient with myocardial disease. The characteristic systolic murmur of tricuspid regurgitation, recognized by its inspiratory accentuation, is commonly heard in such

patients, as are murmurs due to mitral regurgitation.

The ECG usually shows nonspecific ST- and T-wave changes and low voltage of the QRS complex in both pericardial effusion and myocardiopathy. On the other hand, an entirely normal ECG is strong evidence for the diagnosis of pericardial effusion. QRS abnormalities, especially those simulating myocardial infarction and intraventricular conduction defects are more common in myocardial disease. Atrial arrhythmias are common in both conditions, but ventricular arrhythmias are more common in myocardial disease.

The standard chest x-ray is not of much help in difficult cases, but reduced pulsations on fluoroscopy and changes in shape with change in position favor pericardial disease.

Echocardiography is the simplest and most sensitive way to determine the presence of pericardial effusion (Chap. 17). The technique is also of value in describing specific chamber enlargement and alteration in ventricular wall motion and function in patients with myocardial disease and therefore allows ready differentiation of these two conditions. The diagnosis of pericardial effusion can also be established by radioisotope techniques (Chap. 17).

If the diagnosis and the etiology of pericardial effusion are established by other clinical data and cardiac function is not impaired, there is little to be gained by removing the fluid for analysis. Pericardiocentesis is a potentially dangerous procedure which should be carried out to relieve cardiac tamponade or provide fluid for diagnostic aid. In the former situation, reduction of intrapericardial pressure with removal of as little as 25 ml of pericardial fluid may dramatically restore cardiac output to normal, reduce venous pressure, and raise arterial pressure. When an infectious or malignant process in the pericardium is suspected, it is important to obtain fluid for culture and cytology. Finding bloody pericardial effusion in the absence of trauma or anticoagulation suggests malignancy or tuberculosis.

Pericardiocentesis can be performed via either the apical or the subxiphoid route. The subxiphoid is the route which should be used first, but, if fluid is not obtained, the apical route should be explored.

One hazard of pericardiocentesis is a so-called vago-vagal reaction in which profound bradycardia and even asystole may accompany puncture of the pericardium. This can be prevented by premedication with atropine. The second hazard is laceration of the myocardium or a coronary artery, but this risk is minimized by utilizing electrocardiographic or ultrasonic control.

Pericardial biopsy may be required to establish a diagnosis. Biopsy can be carried out through a small incision with low morbidity. Pericardiectomy may be necessary to prevent the recurrence of pericardial effusion. The tissue removed should be examined carefully—both histologically and bacteriologically—with special attention to the possibility of such granulomatous diseases as tuberculosis and histoplasmosis. Therapy for tuberculosis is often given even in the absence of histologic proof.

Cardiac Tamponade

Any disease process affecting the pericardium (Table 19–2) may be responsible for the development of effusion. In most cases the amount of fluid which accumulates is small and does not produce hemodynamic abnormalities. Cardiac tamponade is usually due to trauma (direct and indirect), infection, neoplastic invasion, or bleeding. Hemorrhage into the pericardium may be due to anticoagulation in the presence of active pericarditis.

Pericardial effusion, amounting to a liter or more of fluid, may be present for long periods and produce no alteration in cardiac function. The hemodynamic significance will depend on the rapidity of accumulation, the volume of fluid, and the distensibility of the pericardium. When intrapericardial pressure rises, the clinical syndrome of cardiac tamponade will ensue. Patients with tamponade are usually dyspneic and orthopneic and show signs of rising venous pressure, falling systemic arterial pressure, sinus tachycardia, and distant heart sounds. The Kussmaul sign, or paradoxic inspiratory increase in venous pressure, is usually present, as is pulsus paradoxus.

When the picture of cardiac tamponade is recognized, pericardial fluid should be removed immediately. Usually this is possible by pericardiocentesis, but occasionally surgical drainage is necessary.

In some cases cardiac tamponade may recur. Surgical creation of a pericardial window will allow drainage of fluid into the pleural spaces and prevent accumulation in the pericardium. This will rarely be effective as long-term therapy as the windows do not remain open. In most instances complete removal of the pericardium will be necessary, unless the primary disease process affecting the pericardium can be controlled.

MYOCARDIAL DISEASE [44,46]

If pericardial disease is excluded, the patient with congestive failure and an enlarged cardiac silhouette probably has a form of myocardial disease or cardiomyopathy.

Cardiomyopathy can be classified on the basis of etiology as in Table 19–5. If the heart alone is involved, the term "primary cardiomyopathy" is ap-

plied while "secondary cardiomyopathy" refers to the situation in which the heart is involved as part of a systemic disease process. The cardiomyopathies can also be classified on the basis of clinical presentation (Table 19–6). This classification into hypodynamic or congestive and hypertrophic was suggested by Goodwin for the primary cardiomyopathies.[46] Most cases secondary to the causes listed in Table 19–5 also present with hypodynamic manifestations.

Hypodynamic Cardiomyopathy

The left ventricular cavity is dilated, the wall thin, and contraction poor in this form of cardiomyopathy. The patient may first be seen because of atrial or ventricular arrhythmias, chest pain, an abnormal electrocardiogram, or vague, general complaints of fatigue and weakness. More often the clinical presentation is with congestive heart failure, which is initially of the left ventricular type with the presenting complaints being dyspnea and orthopnea. Right heart failure may follow with elevated venous pressure, hepatomegaly, and edema. The heart is enlarged, the sounds are of poor quality, and an S_3 or ventricular gallop is common. Murmurs, especially systolic murmurs of mitral or tricuspid valve insufficiency, are common and may lead to the mistaken diagnosis of primary valvular disease. These murmurs are caused by alteration in the size and shape of the ventricles, rather than by disease of the valves and may disappear with a return of compensation. The systemic arterial pressure may be elevated, especially in the presence of heart failure, and should not be taken as evidence that sys-

---

TABLE 19–5
Cardiomyopathy—Etiologic Classification

A. Ischemia: Coronary atherosclerosis (also syphilis, polyarteritis, giant cell arteritis)

B. Infectious: Bacterial, viral, rickettsial, protozoal

C. Toxic: Alcohol, emetin, sulfonamides, bacterial toxins (diphtheria), carbon tetrachloride, adriamycin

D. Metabolic or nutritional: Hyperthyroidism, hypothyroidism, beri-beri, anemia

E. Infiltrative disease: Sarcoid, amyloid, hemochromatosis

F. Collagen vascular disease: Systemic lupus erythematosus, polyarteritis, progressive systemic sclerosis

G. Neuromuscular disease: Muscular dystrophy, Friedreich's ataxia, polymyositis

H. Trauma: Mechanical, electrical, radiation

I. Postpartum

J. Idiopathic

┌─────────────────────────────────────┐
TABLE 19-6
Manifestations of Cardiomyopathy

	Hypodynamic	**Hypertrophic**
Patho-physiology	Large dilated heart, thin wall, poor contraction. Impaired emptying	Hypertrophied left ventricle. Thick wall, small cavity. Hyperdynamic contraction, impaired filling, complete ejection
History	Congestive failure	Dyspnea, angina
Physical findings	S_3 gallop. Murmur of AV valve regurgitation	LV lift. S_4 and S_3. Systolic murmur midprecordium. Quick rising, bifid pulse
Laboratory	Low output. Elevated filling pressure. Low ejection fraction	Intracavitary pressure gradient. Elevated filling pressure
Prognosis	Poor. Most dead in five years	Good. Most stable for many years
Therapy	Rest. Supportive therapy. Steroids	β-Blockade and surgery

temic hypertension is the primary cause of the congestive failure. The chest x-ray shows the heart to be diffusely enlarged and the contraction is seen to be poor on fluoroscopy; thus, the diagnosis of pericardial effusion may be suggested. The electrocardiographic changes are nonspecific ST and T wave changes, atrial or ventricular arrhythmia, and intraventricular conduction disturbances or large Q waves. The diagnosis can be established by echocardiography, which reveals the dilated ventricular cavity as well as diffusely reduced motion of the cardiac walls. Cardiac catheterization is rarely necessary, but when performed will show elevated diastolic pressures and reduced ejection fraction.

The etiology of this condition is unknown, but it is likely that a number of different insults to the myocardium may lead to the same end result. The damage may be due to a viral infection, a chemical insult such as alcohol, or be associated with the puerperium. The patient may develop severe heart failure and die in a few weeks following the initial insult or may recover from the primary illness which may be so benign that it is not recognized.

The prognosis is poor for the hypodynamic form of cardiomyopathy. The average duration of life following the onset of symptoms is 3.5 years. Death comes from congestive failure or cardiac arrest. Embolism to the systemic and pulmonary circulations and arrhythmias commonly complicate the course.

There is no specific therapy for primary hypodynamic cardiomyopathy. The possibility that the disease is a secondary cardiomyopathy must be considered as some of the systemic diseases are amenable to specific therapy. If a possible primary agent, such as excessive alcohol, can be identified, it should be removed. The negative ionotropic effects of alcohol are well established and total abstinence from alcoholic beverage is advisable in all patients with cardiomyopathy whatever the etiology may be. Rest is the keystone of management and this may need to be continued for several months to a year before maximum benefit is achieved. The patient's congestive failure should be treated by conventional means to further reduce the load on the heart. Dramatic decrease in heart size and improvement in symptoms sometimes follow the administration of adrenal steroids. Although by no means common, in certain cases it is possible to identify the effect of corticosteroids as more than that which would be expected from bed rest alone. Adrenal steroid therapy is especially effective if treatment is started at an early stage in a rapidly progressing disease.

Hypertrophic Cardiomyopathy[40,46,48,50]

This second form of primary cardiomyopathy differs with respect to presentation, natural history, and therapy from the hypodynamic form of the disease. In this condition the wall of the ventricle is thick and the cavity small. In most cases the hypertrophy is asymmetric involving the interventricular septum to a greater extent than the left ventricular free wall. The primary physiologic impairment is decreased compliance of the thickened hypertrophied ventricle, which impairs ventricular filling during diastole. This condition, which may represent a heterogeneous group of disorders, has been variously termed Idiopathic Hypertrophic Subaortic Stenosis (IHSS), Hypertrophic Obstructive Cardiomyopathy (HOCM), and Asymmetric Septal Hypertrophy (ASH).

In its early stages the clinical presentation may be with minimal symptoms, such as dyspnea on exertion or minor chest pain, but there are definite signs of left ventricular hypertrophy on physical examination, electrocardiogram, and chest x-ray. A disproportion between the minimal symptoms and the major signs of left ventricular hypertrophy should alert the clinician to this diagnosis. The physical findings include a left ventricular lift, an S_4 gallop, and a double apical impulse with a visible and palpable atrial impulse preceding the ventricular contraction. There is often a systolic murmur which may be late in onset and is heard best between the apex and the left sternal border. This murmur often leads to the mistaken diagnosis of aortic stenosis or mitral regurgitation. One of the characteristic features of the disease is the bifid upstroke of the aortic pulse wave. The first portion of ejection is unusually rapid but it is interrupted by a notch. This rapid up-stroke of the arterial pulse is useful in differentiating the disease from valvular aortic stenosis in which the up-stroke is characteristically slow (Fig. 17–2).

The electrocardiogram shows left axis deviation, left ventricular hypertrophy, widening of the QRS complex, bundle branch block, bizarre Q waves, or the pattern of Wolff-Parkinson-White syndrome. The radiologic appearance of the heart is that of left ventricular hypertrophy.

Echocardiography can be of great help in making the diagnosis. With this technique it is possible to measure the thickness of the interventricular septum and left ventricular free wall and determine the diameter of the left ventricular cavity in diastole and systole. An abnormal motion pattern of the mitral valve, present in a third to half of the cases, can also be visualized.

The diagnosis can also be established at cardiac catheterization of the left heart. The rapid up-stroke of the aortic pressure with the anacrotic notch will be demonstrated. The left ventriculogram will show the left ventricular wall to be thick, the cavity small, and the emptying of the cavity to be very rapid and unusually complete. A pressure gradient between the inflow and outflow portions of the left ventricle can be demonstrated in many patients with this disease. This pressure difference is sometimes consistently present at rest while at other times it may be seen only with the hyperdynamic beats which follow ventricular premature contractions or after the contractility of the myocardium has been enhanced by isoproterenol.

The presence or magnitude of the pressure gradient bears little relation to prognosis in this condition. It is unlikely that true anatomic obstruction to left ventricular outflow exists, since most of ventricular emptying occurs prior to the appearance of the gradient. Impaired filling rather than impaired emptying appears to be the primary problem in this disease. The thickened ventricle cannot accept diastolic inflow. The prognosis is determined by the degree of impaired filling which is reflected in the level of diastolic pressure in the ventricle.

The etiology of the condition is unknown, but there are many families in which more than one case has been reported. Echocardiographic studies of families with this disorder suggest an autosomal dominant mode of inheritance. Histologic studies of heart muscles from patients with this disorder by light and electron microscopy have shown disordered intra- and intercellular architecture in the interventricular septum, but it is not known whether these abnormalities are indicative of a primary muscle disorder or are the result of abnormal myocardial contraction.

The prognosis for hypertrophic cardiomyopathy is far better than that for the hypodynamic variety. About half the patients in most series have shown no progression of symptoms over long periods of observation. The estimated mortality in one recent series was 15 percent at 5 years and 35 percent at 10 years. Patients with milder forms of the disease discovered by more sensitive methods probably have a better prognosis. When the disease progresses the heart enlarges, atrial fibrillation appears, systemic embolism occurs and a terminal picture not unlike that of hypodynamic cardiomyopathy may result with death in congestive failure. Sudden death is the commonest terminal event and may occur at any stage of the disease.

Both medical and surgical treatments have been proposed for this disease. The surgical treatment was devised first and is based upon the belief that obstruction to left ventricular outflow is the important pathophysiologic mechanism. Myocardial tissue is resected from the outflow tract of the left ventricle and improvement in symptoms results in at least half the cases. Although designed to remove obstruction, the surgical procedure may exert its major beneficial effect by increasing compliance of the ventricle, enlarging the cavity and, hence, improving left ventricular inflow. Replacement of the mitral valve represents a second surgical approach to the treatment of this disease. This approach is based upon the observation that the aortic leaflet of the mitral valve and the hypertrophied septum come together across the outflow tract of the left ventricle late in systole.

Medical therapy with beta adrenergic blocking agents may benefit patients whose major complaints are angina or syncope. These agents may be effective in reducing the hyperkinetic character of ventricular contraction, reducing responsiveness to endogenous catecholamines during stress, and by slowing the heart rate which prolongs the diastolic filling period. As yet there is no evidence to indicate that the natural history of the disease is altered or sudden death prevented by these drugs or by surgery.

HIGH OUTPUT STATES

Congestive failure is occasionally seen in conditions characterized by an increase in cardiac output but is rare unless organic heart disease is also present. Thyrotoxicosis is associated with increased cardiac output secondary to reduced peripheral resistance and also to the direct effect of the thyroid hormone on the heart. The heart is hyperactive and the pulse pressure wide. Atrial fibrillation is common in thyrotoxicosis, but congestive failure is rarely seen in young patients. Congestive failure occurs more frequently in older patients, suggesting that thyrotoxicosis is more likely to precipitate failure when there is underlying myocardial or valvular disease.

Similar statements can be made about anemia as a cause of congestive failure. Cardiac output must increase in patients with severe anemia in order to provide for the delivery of an adequate quantity of oxygen to the tissues. The heart is hyperactive, the pulse is rapid, and there are signs of peripheral vasodilatation. Congestive failure is rare in patients with normal hearts, but anemia commonly precipitates heart failure in older individuals with underlying heart disease.

Congestive failure has been reported in patients with large arteriovenous fistulas which have usually been produced by gunshot or stab wounds. The rupture of an aneurysm of the sinus of Valsalva into the right heart produces sudden profound congestive heart failure in a patient with an otherwise normal heart. Prompt recognition and treatment of this AV communication may be life-saving. Beriberi and Paget's disease of bone are other causes of high output failure.

MANAGEMENT OF THE PATIENT WITH CONGESTIVE HEART FAILURE

The general management of the patient with congestive heart failure is outlined in Table 19–7. The first step must be to determine the pathophysiologic mechanism and anatomic abnormality responsible for altered cardiovascular function. While the general measures outlined in this chapter can be applied to most patients with congestive heart failure, definitive treatment will depend on proper diagnosis. For example, patients with valvular heart disease may improve as a result of rest, salt restriction, and digitalis, but this should not obscure the fact that mechanical problems leading to heart failure generally require mechanical solutions, i.e., valve replacement. Some patients who can be restored to Class II functional status by medical therapy may be rendered asymptomatic and prognosis improved by surgical therapy. Digitalis may not be effective when the problem is impaired left ventricular filling as in some patients with hypertensive heart disease, hypertrophic cardiomyopathy, or mitral stenosis. Patients with these and

---

TABLE 19–7
Management of Congestive Failure

I.   Establish a Diagnosis

    A. Pathophysiology
       1. Myocardial dysfunction;
       2. Excess load;
       3. Impaired filling

    B. Anatomy
       1. Localization of lesion;
       2. Severity

II. Estimate Prognosis

    A. Patient's position and rate of progession relative to the natural history of the disease

III. Identify Precipitating Factor or Factors

    A. Factors decreasing the heart's ability to meet needs of the body
       1. Discontinuation of cardiac glycoside (digitalis)
       2. Arrhythmia, e.g., onset of fibrillation, tachycardia, bradycardia, heart block
       3. Myocardial impairment
         a. Infarction
         b. Myocarditis
         c. Coronary embolism; bacterial embolism
         d. Toxic substances, e.g., alcohol
         e. Thiamine deficiency

    B. Factors increasing the load on the heart
       1. Dietary lapse: salt binge; holiday feasting
       2. Increased physical activity
       3. Infection
       4. Operation: fluid therapy; transfusions
       5. Pulmonary embolism
       6. Perforated valve or septum
       7. Anemia
       8. Thyrotoxicosis
       9. Salt and water retaining medications, e.g., corticosteroids
      10. Pulmonary infection in cor pulmonale

IV. Specific Therapy

    A. Rest
    B. Diet
    C. Cardiac glycosides
    D. Diuretics
    E. Mechanical removal of fluid
    F. Afterload reduction
    G. Surgical therapy

---

similar disorders frequently develop atrial fibrillation; the restoration and maintenance of sinus rhythm, and therefore, atrial contraction may do more to improve cardiac function than potent inotropic agents.

An important judgment concerns the patient's current position with respect to the course of his disease and its rate of progression. The patient's age and anticipated span of life also enter into this estimation. Obviously, a patient with well-compensated aortic stenosis at age 75 will be treated differently from one with increasing symptoms at age 55. The rate of progression is often best determined by making two examinations several months apart.

Social, environmental, and psychological factors deserve consideration but should never be accorded overriding emphasis. The physician's chief responsibility is to determine the best treatment for the patient's circulatory impairment and to do what he can to work this out within the social and environmental framework. Social and family factors may, for example, make it impossible for the patient to accept recommended therapy or may necessitate a delay of plans.

An estimate of the patient's prognosis without treatment must be weighed against the results of medical and surgical therapy. Failure to assess the adequacy of previous medical management accurately often leads to errors. The details of the therapeutic program must be known, and the degree of adherence to it by the patient must be evaluated. The prescription of a cardiac glycoside or a diuretic without restriction of activity and sodium intake is not an adequate trial of medical therapy. The busy physician may prescribe medication without explaining the patient's disease to him and outlining all aspects of management. A patient treated with medication alone may believe that he can be cured by a short period on the prescribed medication, and his adherence to the program is often poor. A history of the details of the patient's life covering activity, diet, symptoms, and medication must be taken before the important questions regarding the adequacy and effectiveness of medical care can be answered.

Medical therapy should be suitable for the patient at the current stage of his disease. It is as possible to overtreat patients medically as it is to undertreat them. A patient in the first episode of congestive failure need not receive all the available therapeutic measures, since such patients usually respond to salt restriction, decreased activity, and a cardiac glycoside. If, to this basic program, the physician adds powerful diuretics, the loss of fluid will be sudden and dramatic but, in some cases, deleterious. It is preferable to establish compensation slowly and to avoid sudden disastrous shifts in fluid and electrolytes. It is often best to add therapeutic measures serially, in order to assess the severity of the patient's condition. It is psychologically inadvisable to prescribe a number of medications and to impose severe restrictions on a patient who has only recently recognized that he is not totally well, unless the situation is urgent.

PRECIPITATING FACTORS

The factors responsible for precipitation of the current episode of congestive failure must be identified and removed if therapy is to be effective. These can be divided into two groups (Table 19–7). The factors in the first group operate by reducing myocardial function, those in the second group by increasing the work load placed upon the heart.

A frequent cause of reduction in the ability of the heart to function effectively is the discontinuation of cardiac glycoside medication. The sudden onset of an arrhythmia—especially atrial fibrillation in patients with mitral stenosis—is also a common precipitating factor. The onset of complete heart block or bradycardia due to another mechanism can also initiate decompensation. Myocardial function may be impaired by a number of factors, but infarction due to coronary thrombosis is one of the most common and is often the cause of sudden pulmonary edema. Coronary embolism in infective endocarditis operates in the same way. Myocardial function may be impaired by the sudden development of acute myocarditis, either the activation of long-standing rheumatic carditis, or a primary myocardial process. The sudden onset of severe and sometimes fatal congestive failure in young individuals may be due to acute infectious myocarditis following an upper respiratory infection. Alcohol is a myocardial depressant and may be an important factor in decompensation in some patients. The removal of an alcoholic intake of 60 to 120 ml a day will sometimes restore compensation.

The second major group of precipitating factors is related to an increase in the load placed upon the heart, exemplified by sudden increase in the severity of a valvular lesion due to perforation of a cusp or rupture of one of the chordae tendineae. The work of the heart is more commonly increased by the addition of an external burden, such as follows ingestion of an unusually large amount of sodium. Dietary lapses often occur at holiday seasons. Salt and water retention may also be precipitated by corticosteroid medication administered as treatment for a condition other than the heart disease. Increased physical activity is another factor of importance. A patient may feel better by virtue of good management and decide that he can resume mowing his lawn or doing heavy physical work. Infection with attendant fever and increased cardiac output is another well-known factor. Surgical operations also may be responsible, especially if excessive quantities of intravenous fluid or blood transfusions are given. The endocrine response to the surgery also contributes to the salt retention. Pulmonary embolism increases right-ventricular work and is a common precipitating factor of failure in patients with valvular heart disease. Pulmonary infection is a common precipitating cause in patients with cor pulmonale. Pregnancy places an increased load on the heart and often precipitates the first episode of failure in women with mitral valve disease.

Anemia and thyrotoxicosis, which increase the demands on the heart, are important since both can be treated effectively. The removal of the precipitating factors must accompany specific therapy for congestive failure, and the identification of these factors is important in preventing future episodes.

SPECIFIC THERAPY

The elements of the specific therapy of congestive failure are listed in Table 19–7. They are all directed at restoring the balance between the metabolic demands of the body and the heart's ability to meet those demands.

Rest

Rest is the keystone of treatment. Regardless of what has upset the balance between cardiac performance and the metabolic requirements of the body, a reduction in activity is always possible, while an increase in cardiac performance may not be. In some situations, rest may do more than just reduce the load. When failure is due to myocarditis, there is reason to believe that rest promotes healing of the myocardial process. When the patient is edematous or dyspneic, he should be placed at bedrest with the head of the bed elevated to 45°. It is also advisable to employ a cardiac bed which allows the legs to be below the pelvis while the patient is recumbent. If this is not done, fluid present in the legs may be returned to the vascular system and precipitate pulmonary edema. This shift in fluid associated with recumbency may lead to the incorrect impression that the patient is improving, since the ankle edema may decrease, but a complemental increase in sacral edema will be noted if the latter area is examined carefully.

If the patient has difficulty using the bedpan, it may be better to let him use a bedside commode twice a day. If he is properly assisted, the energy thus expended is minimal. A mild laxative or stool softener such as mineral oil, milk of magnesia, or Colace is indicated to reduce straining at stool.

Venous thrombosis and embolism are hazards of bedrest in individuals with congestive failure. The circulation to the extremities is decreased by virtue of the basic disease, and venous return is further compromised by the pressure of the edema fluid itself. For these reasons, the period of bedrest should not be longer than is necessary to initiate a good diuresis. Three measures may prevent thromboembolic complications. The first and simplest is regular leg exercise. The patient is instructed to flex his feet against a footboard. The legs may also be wrapped with elastic bandages to reduce the volume of blood pooled in the venous channels. Last, anticoagulants may be employed, but this is not without risk to a patient with hepatic congestion, a condition associated with wide spontaneous variation in prothrombin time. Low-dose heparin may effectively prevent thromboembolism without causing bleeding.

As soon as diuresis has occurred and the weight is stable, the patient should be moved to a bedside chair and encouraged to walk to the bathroom; only in the most severe situation is it necessary to maintain complete bedrest after discharge from the hospital, and a satisfactory semiambulatory regimen should be formulated whenever possible.

Diet

Diet is the second major component of therapy for congestive failure. The basic feature is restriction of salt, or, more specifically, sodium. The degree of restriction required depends upon the severity of the congestive failure. Representative dietary programs are outlined in Table 19–8. The normal hospital diet contains 10 to 15 g of sodium chloride, or 4000 to 6000 mg of sodium per day. In the treatment of heart failure we are concerned with sodium, not sodium chloride; therefore, it is preferable to designate diets by their sodium content. If the patient omits salty food and adds no salt to his food at the table, he can reduce the sodium intake to between 2000 and 4000 mg per day. If restriction to 1000 mg of sodium or below is necessary, specially prepared salt-poor milk and bread must be utilized. Restriction to 200 mg of sodium sometimes is necessary in the management of severe congestive failure. Diet of this type cannot be maintained outside the hospital without great difficulty. The patient is more likely to adhere to a low-salt diet if he is provided with a salt substitute which will make his food more palatable.

When a patient is in severe congestive heart failure, the gastrointestinal tract is edematous, and digestion and absorption are poor. Under these circumstances, the abdomen often is distended by fluid and an enlarged liver. The addition of large volumes of food makes the patient uncomfortable and may even compromise the excursion of the diaphragm. Ingestion of a large meal results in a circulatory load, diverts blood to the gastrointestinal tract, and may interfere with diuresis. It is advisable, therefore, to prescribe a liquid diet when possible and to give six small feedings daily, rather than the conventional three meals. In general, calories should be restricted,

---

TABLE 19-8
Sodium Restricted Diets

Diet Order	Sodium* (mg)	Sodium (mEq)	NaCl* (g)	General Instructions
Standard	4000–6000	170–260	10–15	
Standard without free salt	2000–4000	87–170	5–10	Standard diet without salt shaker; omit foods obviously high in salt
1000 mg sodium	800–1200	35–52	2–3	Use all salt-free foods. Limit milk to 1 to 1½ pints per day. Restrict protein to 5 ounces per day
200 mg sodium	200	9	0.5	Diet must be calculated. Use all salt-free foods. Low sodium milk is used where necessary

* 1 g NaCl = 17 mEq; Na = 395 mg Na; 23 mg Na = 1 mEq; Na = 58 mg NaCl.

---

and, if the patient is obese, more severe restriction designed to bring the patient to suitable weight is in order.

It is generally true that the patient with congestive failure cannot retain fluid without sodium and, therefore, it usually is unnecessary to control fluid intake when sodium is being restricted. If, however, the serum sodium is below the normal range, fluid restriction may be beneficial.

Cardiac Glycosides

Digitalis and the related glycosides constitute the keystone of drug therapy for congestive heart failure. Other forms of therapy are directed at the consequences of inadequate cardiac function, such as fluid retention, but the digitalis derivatives have a direct action upon the heart, increasing the force of myocardial contraction. Details regarding the pharmacology and clinical use of digitalis preparations are considered in Chapter 30.

The rapidity with which digitalization should be accomplished depends upon the severity of the patient's congestive failure and the physician's certainty about the previous state of digitalization. For example, if the physician is confident that the patient has not been receiving a cardiac glycoside, a full digitalizing dose may be given in one intravenous injection if the gravity of the failure indicates that such therapy is in order. The intravenous route is also preferable when the patient's gastrointestinal function is disordered by the congestive failure as the absorption of the drug may be slow and unpredictable and an unknown fraction of the dose may be lost by vomiting. An intravenous digitalizing dose should be administered slowly (over one minute), as rapid injection is hazardous.

Caution should be exercised when there is uncertainty about the state of digitalization. This is a circumstance in which the determination of the serum level of the cardiac glycoside may be very useful. If uncertainty remains, small divided doses should be given over several days, allowing sufficient time for the peak therapeutic effect of each dose to become manifest. The dose selected in this situation should be twice (or at the most three times) the estimated maintenance dose, e.g., 0.75 mg of digoxin daily, and should be repeated until the desired therapeutic effect or toxicity is manifest. Also, it is better in such cases to use a rapidly excreted preparation so that any toxicity which develops will be of short duration.

In outpatient treatment, it is too much to expect that patients will understand the distinctions between loading and maintenance doses. For this reason it is usually prudent to place the patient on maintenance daily dosage at the outset. This is a convenient method when digoxin is employed since full digitalization will be accomplished in approximately one week, but is not effective for longer-acting preparations, such as digitoxin, where full digitalization will require one month.

If a loading dose method is used, it is the responsibility of the physician to provide a written, *easily understood schedule,* separate from his prescription, to the patient *and* to a responsible member of the family. An explanation of the purpose of the drug also may forestall the natural inclination to "take a heart pill whenever I feel bad."

The dose of cardiac glycosides required for digitalization varies from patient to patient, and it is often difficult to recognize the level of maximum therapeutic effect without entering the toxic range. With atrial fibrillation and a rapid ventricular rate, the slowing of the ventricular rate is a useful index. In the presence of sinus rhythm, where improvement in the signs and symptoms of congestive failure may be the only evidence that a therapeutic effect has been obtained, toxic signs or symptoms may appear before therapeutic effects are clearly evident. Here again, the determination of the serum level may be helpful in defining the kinetics in a particular patient and also correlating clinical effect with serum levels.

The more dramatic toxic effects of digitalis are readily recognized and include anorexia, nausea, vomiting, diarrhea, colored and blurred vision, weakness, and abdominal pain. The appearance of multiple premature ventricular contractions is a good sign of toxicity. The serum assay is especially helpful in this clinical situation as most patients with intoxication will have serum digoxin levels above 2.0 ng/ml.

Removal of Fluid by Mechanical Means

It is occasionally necessary to remove collections of extravascular fluid by mechanical means. If large amounts are present in the serous cavities, they may retard recovery. Large pleural effusions interfere with ventilation and with venous return to the right heart. Ascites is deleterious, both because the fluid elevates the diaphragm, interfering with respiration, and because the increased intra-abdominal pressure may interfere with renal venous drainage and diuresis. When sizable accumulations are present in either chest or abdomen and a brisk diuresis does not begin within a few days, it is wise to remove the fluid by needle. It may be hazardous to remove more than 1000 ml from the pleural cavity or 2000 ml from the peritoneal cavity at one time. Premedication with atropine is advisable.

Diuretic Therapy

Since all patients with congestive heart failure retain sodium and water and develop total body sodium excess, one of the goals of therapy is to increase the excretion of sodium in the urine. There are potent diuretic agents available for this purpose, and the difficulty is not in finding an agent which can increase the loss of sodium but in selecting the appropriate regimen to accomplish this goal with a minimum of complications. The clinical pharmacology of the major diuretic agents is described in Chapter 30.

Regardless of the diuretic agent used, it is better in most instances to begin with low doses and observe the initial effect before changing the dose or adding another agent. Rapid diuresis is rarely required or even desirable, and is much more likely to produce serious complications than a slower loss of sodium which permits gradual hemodynamic adjust-

ments to the change in extracellular fluid volume. The effectiveness of diuretic therapy is best assessed by observing the patient's weight. Only in the desperately ill patient is it necessary to record precise details of fluid intake and output. The loss of 2 to 3 pounds per day is optimal. Generally, it is best to begin therapy with the milder thiazide diuretics, switching to the more potent diuretics (furosemide or ethacrynic acid) if diuresis is not accomplished. With the latter agents it is important to progressively increase the amount of drug in single doses until appropriate diuresis occurs. Sometimes substituting ethacrynic acid for furosemide will accomplish diuresis when the patient has proven refractory. The use of an aldosterone antagonist or a thiazide in combination with furosemide is often efficacious.

Almost all patients with congestive heart failure can be rendered free of excess salt and water by the use of the potent diuretic agents available today. Refractoriness to diuretic therapy is usually the result of continued high sodium intake, secondary electrolyte disturbances of hypochloremia and contraction alkalosis, or inadequate renal perfusion due to intrinsic renal disease or severe reduction in cardiac output.

Afterload Reduction[39,41]

Cardiac performance can also be improved in the patient with heart failure by reducing the impedance to left ventricular ejection and thereby reducing systolic wall stress (afterload) in the left ventricle. This permits the ventricle to empty more completely. This can be accomplished in patients with aortic stenosis by valve replacement and in patients with systemic hypertension by pharmacologic lowering of blood pressure. Recent studies have documented that reduction of peripheral resistance will benefit patients with left ventricular failure even when blood pressure is not elevated. Drugs which act as arteriolar dilators are effective in increasing cardiac output and at the same time lowering left ventricular filling pressures without reducing arterial pressure. Hydralazine and prazosin are available as oral agents for use in chronic conditions. Hydralazine acts only on arterioles, whereas prazosin has the additional advantage of causing venous dilatation. Short- and long-acting nitrates are weak arteriolar dilators but have their major effect in reducing venous tone. Reduction in venous tone may be beneficial to the patient with heart failure by reducing preload, which reduces ventricular size and systolic wall stress. A useful regimen combines the arteriolar effects of hydralazine with the venous effects of long-acting nitrates which may be administered orally in high dose, sublingually, or topically. Vasodilator therapy is generally employed when patients have proven refractory to standard treatment. The long-term efficacy of this therapy is undetermined.

Vasodilator therapy may produce dramatic effects in the patient with acute valvular regurgitation, both mitral and aortic. By lowering peripheral resistance, forward flow is promoted and regurgitant or backward flow diminished. Intravenous nitroprusside, which is a potent dilator of both arterioles and venules, is the most effective agent in this setting. This drug may also be useful in improving cardiac performance in other acute settings, such as acute myocardial infarction with pulmonary congestion or following cardiac surgery.

SURGERY IN THE PATIENT WITH HEART DISEASE[45]

The physician is often asked to aid in the management of the cardiac patient who must undergo a noncardiac surgical procedure. The physician's role in this situation will be: 1) to decide on the patient's prognosis with or without the proposed surgery; 2) to assess the risk of the operative procedure to the patient; 3) to help decide on the type of anesthetic to be employed; and 4) to aid in the perioperative and postoperative management of cardiac or other medical problems. A complete history, careful physical examination, electrocardiogram, chest x-ray, and simple blood studies will allow the physician to make proper judgment in each of these areas. It is important to carefully assess the patient's general medical status as well as his cardiac condition. Particular care is needed in searching for evidence of old or recent venous disease, pulmonary disease, urinary obstruction, or metabolic disorders such as thyroid disease, diabetes, or electrolyte disturbance, all of which may seriously alter the postoperative course.

For the purpose of determining the risk in cardiac patients, surgical procedures can be classified generally as *elective*, i.e., herniorrhaphy where there is little risk of incarceration, *necessary*, i.e., symptomatic gallbladder disease or nonobstructing carcinoma of the colon, and *emergency*, i.e., perforated viscus or leaking abdominal aneurysm. In case of advanced cardiac disease *elective* procedures should not be recommended unless the natural history of the cardiac disease itself can be improved by specific therapy. For instance, one would not recommend hernia repair for a patient with severe cardiomyopathy or aortic stenosis, because the natural history of these diseases is unfavorable for long life and the risk of surgery would be formidable. However, if the aortic stenosis

were successfully treated by valve replacement, elective surgery could be undertaken. It may be necessary to perform emergency surgery even in patients with severe cardiac disease, although the risks of surgery are great. In deciding upon the advisability of *necessary* operations, the physician must make his best judgment about the expected natural history of the cardiac disease and whether the cardiac disease or the noncardiac lesion will first cause death or further morbidity. In severe cases a period of medical treatment of the cardiac problem may lower the risk for surgery and allow necessary or elective procedures to be performed with lower risk.

Patients with cardiac disease of all types are at greater risk for death, myocardial infarction, or pulmonary thromboembolism as a result of surgery. The risk is greater with abdominal and thoracic procedures and is directly proportional to the duration of the operation. One recent study has reported the risk of perioperative myocardial infarction as 27 percent if the patient had had a previous myocardial infarction within 3 months of the procedure and 11 percent if the infarct had occurred 3 to 6 months previously. Most studies have documented that the high risk of recurrent infarction falls to four to five percent if the operative procedure is performed six months or more after infarction. The mortality of perioperative infarction is high, even when infarction is recognized early and the patient is carefully monitored. Unstable angina pectoris, severe aortic stenosis, uncompensated heart failure, and uncontrolled hypertension are also associated with a high perioperative mortality or risk of infarction. Only *emergency* procedures should be carried out in these patients. Stable angina pectoris, compensated heart failure, or abnormal electrocardiogram confer a risk which is similar to that for old myocardial infarction (four to five percent). Moderate hypertension is not a major risk factor in operative morbidity or mortality.

Table 19–9 summarizes the relative risk of several cardiac abnormalities in the patient who must face an operative procedure. In general, patients with compensated heart disease without recent acute changes withstand surgical procedures well. Cardiac arrhythmias are included in the table as a significant risk factor because recent studies have described an adverse prognosis in patients with these abnormalities who undergo surgery. This is most likely because the arrhythmias reflect underlying severe heart disease since arrhythmias themselves did not contribute to mortality. In general, patients with a major risk factor should not undergo elective or necessary operations until the cardiac condition can be properly treated.

TABLE 19-9
Relative Risk of Cardiac Disease in Noncardiac Surgery

Major	Minor
Recent MI (< 3 months)	Remote MI (> 6 months)
Unstable angina	Stable angina pectoris
Severe aortic stenosis	Abnormal ECG
Decompensated heart failure	Compensated heart failure
Severe hypertension	Compensated valvular lesions
	Cardiac arrhythmias
	Cardiac enlargement

All general anesthetic agents depress myocardial contractility, but the less potent anesthetics such as nitrous oxide have a lesser effect on the myocardium. Agents such as ether or cyclopropane also stimulate sympathetic discharge which may produce hypertension or cardiac irritability. Agents such as halothane or morphine do not have this property and may actually cause reductions in pressure through vasodilation. Spinal anesthesia does not directly affect the heart but may result in hypotension as a result of pa-ralysis of vasoconstrictor vascular reflexes. For this reason this kind of anesthesia is not preferred for patients with coronary artery disease. Spinal anesthesia may be useful for the patient with depressed myocardial function and heart failure. Most patients will do well with light, general anesthesia.

Postoperative management should include monitoring the cardiac rhythm for 12 to 24 hours and careful management of fluid balance to avoid overhydration and pulmonary congestion or underhydration and hypotension. The electrocardiogram, which may provide the only evidence of perioperative injury or infarction, should be recorded immediately after surgery and repeated 3 days later, since many cases of perioperative infarction are not detected in the initial ECG tracing. Patients who are to remain immobilized for long periods should be given low-dose heparin and those with valvular disease should receive appropriate antibiotics during and after the operative procedure. Proper case selection, anticipation of cardiac problems, and collaborative efforts between the physician and surgeon will allow most patients with cardiac disease to undergo operative procedures successfully.

CHAPTER 20
Cardiac Murmurs and Other Manifestations of Valvular Heart Disease[54,61]
J. O'NEAL HUMPHRIES AND RICHARD S. ROSS

The diagnosis of cardiovascular disease depends on the synthesis of all the available clinical information, but some objective finding must be taken as the primary point about which the differential diagnosis is developed. Heart murmurs which are subject to precise description with regard to timing and location of maximal audibility, frequently form such a starting point.

In this chapter cardiac murmurs are used as a starting point for a consideration of the physical findings and laboratory abnormalities associated with valvular lesions and acyanotic congenital abnormalities. Later sections deal with the etiology, pathophysiology, evaluation, and management of each of these lesions. Since surgical management plays such an important role in this type of cardiac disease, a portion of the chapter is devoted to general considerations of cardiac surgery and problems related to the use of prosthetic heart valves.

THE DIFFERENTIAL DIAGNOSIS OF MURMURS

The other aspects of the cardiovascular and general physical examination (Chap. 16) are essential in the differential diagnosis of murmurs. The remainder of this chapter is based upon a primary classification of murmurs by timing and point of maximum intensity as described in Figure 16–3, and is organized around a series of tables listing other physical findings and laboratory tests that are helpful in reaching a diagnosis.

Systolic Murmur—Left Second Interspace
The most common murmur is the early-systolic murmur in the left second interspace. It is usually a crescendo–decrescendo murmur of the ejection type. The six most common possibilities are listed in Table

20–1. Differentiation is difficult because all these murmurs arise in the main pulmonary artery or right ventricular outflow tract. These structures are close to the chest wall in the region of the left second interspace; the closer the apposition the more prominent the auscultatory phenomena.

The innocent murmur of a normal heart with a normal flow is usually short, not very loud, and not widely transmitted. It may be more difficult to hear during inspiration or in the sitting position. The murmur cannot be heard in the back or over the neck vessels. The absence of symptoms and other abnormal physical findings may be all that is necessary to establish this diagnosis, but if uncertainty persists, then a chest roentgenogram, an ECG, and an echocardiogram may provide support for or against this diagnosis.

The innocent murmur may be longer and louder in the presence of an abnormality of shape of the thorax, such as pectus excavatum or a small anteroposterior diameter as seen in the "straight back syndrome." Wide splitting of the second sound, palpable systolic activity parasternally, RSR′ in V_1 of the ECG, and a large cardiac silhouette on the PA chest roentgenogram are commonly seen in these patients and contribute to the suspicion of a left-to-right shunt at the atrial level. The echocardiogram shows normal right ventricular size, and right heart catheterization, if necessary, shows normal pressures and oxygen saturations.

The physiologic murmurs of high flow due to fever, thyrotoxicosis, pregnancy, and anemia are louder and longer than the innocent murmur but are still crescendo–descrescendo and end about two-thirds of the way through systole, well before the second sound. These murmurs may have a scratchy or harsh quality which may diminish when the patient sits up and takes a deep breath. The chest roentgenogram,

---

TABLE 20–1
Systolic Murmurs—Left Second Interspace

Diagnosis	Auscultation	Other Physical Examination	X-Ray	ECG	Cardio-vascular Laboratory Findings	Management
Innocent murmur	Murmur variable with respiration	Likely in normal thin chest, straight spine, or pectus excavatum	Normal or pectus deformity Straight dorsal spine	Normal	Normal	Reassurance
Physiologic murmurs	Disappears with treatment of primary condition	Signs of thyrotoxicosis, anemia, fever, pregnancy, etc.	Normal	Normal	Increased cardiac output	Treat primary condition
Atrial septal defect	S_2—wide, fixed split Middiastolic rumble LLSB	RV lift PA lift	Prominent RV Vascular lungs	Incomplete RBBB	Left-to-right shunt into RA	Surgical closure
Pulmonary stenosis	EC inspiration S_2 split, P_2 soft or absent	Thrill Venous *a* wave prominent	Prominent RV outflow Poststenotic dilatation PA	RVH—Tall RV′ RAD—Peaked P waves	Pressure gradient PA-RV	Surgery if severe
Idiopathic dilatation of pulmonary artery	EC	PA lift	Large PA	Normal	Negative except for large PA on angiography	Reassurance
Small ventricular septal defect	Pansystolic plateau murmur S_2 split	Thrill	Normal	Normal	Small left-to-right shunt into RV	If SBE or AR, surgical closure

ECG, and echocardiogram do not change unless the high flow has been present for a very long time as in a patient with sickle cell anemia where cardiac chamber enlargement develops.

Increased flow through the right ventricle and pulmonary artery is also the cause of the systolic murmur in the left second interspace of a patient with a left-to-right shunt through an atrial septal defect or anomalous pulmonary venous return to the right atrium. Other physical findings are helpful in making this diagnosis. Wide splitting of the second heart sound is usually present, and the degree of splitting does not vary or varies only slightly with respiration. Hyperactivity or even a heave may be felt in the left parasternal region. A middiastolic murmur may be heard at the lower sternal border. The simple laboratory studies provide diagnostic information; the ECG practically always shows incomplete or complete right bundle branch block, the roentgenogram cardiomegaly with prominence of the central and peripheral pulmonary vasculature, and the echocardiogram an enlarged right ventricle with paradoxical motion of the ventricular septum.

A loud and long murmur suggests pulmonary stenosis. This murmur may extend up to the aortic component of the second sound and the pulmonic component may be diminished or absent. Both the intensity and duration of the murmur are directly related to the severity of the stenosis. The murmur is widely transmitted over the precordium and is often heard in the back and even over the neck vessels. The pressure in the right ventricle is high but it is unusual to feel a parasternal heave. The ejection click may disappear during inspiration. Right ventricular hypertrophy is present on the ECG and chest roentgenogram; the latter will also show prominence of the main pulmonary artery and the proximal portion of the left pulmonary artery and normal peripheral vasculature.

Clinical evaluation is sufficient for accurate diagnosis in the vast majority of patients with a systolic murmur in the left second interspace, and cardiac catheterization and angiography are rarely necessary. Cardiac catheterization and angiography may be indicated to establish the severity and exact form of the disorder in anticipation of surgical correction in those patients determined to have organic heart disease.

Systolic Murmurs—Right Second Interspace

The ejection systolic murmurs that are loudest in the right second interspace are related to turbulence of flow in the outflow tract of the left ventricle, at the aortic valve, or in the aorta. Aortic stenosis is the most important organic lesion associated with this murmur but may be simulated by the other conditions listed in Table 20–2.

The murmur of aortic stenosis is characteristically crescendo–decrescendo or ejection in type and, if the lesion is severe, the murmur is loud and long and is associated with a systolic thrill in the right second interspace. The murmur is often well heard at the apex where it may have a musical quality. The carotid pulse is slow-rising, and the pulse pressure is small (Fig. 17–2). Although the systolic murmur is always heard, the other ausculatory signs depend on the type of lesion present. The second aortic sound is often absent when the valve is calcified and rigid, but in a young person may be loud and clear if there is congenital aortic stenosis with a flexible, mobile, diaphragm-type valve. A loud early-systolic ejection click also is heard when the valve is flexible, not when it is rigid. Mobile and flexible valves become rigid and calcified with the passage of years.

When aortic regurgitation is severe, the systolic stroke output increases and a short but very loud, early systolic murmur may be generated in the aortic root from the increased flow, even though no obstruction exists. The systolic murmur may even be associated with a thrill, but the true nature of the murmur can be recognized by the cardiac and peripheral signs of aortic regurgitation.

Murmurs of mitral regurgitation may be transmitted to the base of the heart and heard in the right second interspace. This unusual transmission is probably related to impingement of the systolic regurgitant jet on the atrial wall at its point of contact with the aorta. This murmur can be differentiated from that of aortic stenosis by its holosystolic character, the absence of peripheral signs of aortic stenosis, and the typical murmur of mitral regurgitation at the apex. Of course, aortic and mitral valve disease commonly coexist in rheumatic heart disease.

The murmur of pulmonary stenosis occasionally is heard well to the right of the sternum, but only with transposition of the great vessels is it louder on the right than on the left side. Transmission of the murmur to the neck vessels is not proof of aortic origin, since loud murmurs due to pulmonary stenosis can be heard there.

Ejection systolic murmurs in the right second interspace are often heard in elderly patients with aortic atherosclerosis. Many of these patients have sclerotic changes in the leaflets of the aortic valve, but only a few will have hemodynamically significant obstruction.

Radiologic examination of the heart is helpful (Fig. 17–1). Dilatation of the ascending aorta and enlargement of the left ventricle are seen in both aortic stenosis and regurgitation. The finding of calcification in the aortic valve area on chest roentgenogram, fluoroscopy, or echocardiography provides confirmatory

TABLE 20-2
Systolic Murmurs—Right Second Interspace

Diagnosis	Auscultation	Other Physical Examination	X-Ray	ECG	Cardiovascular Laboratory Findings
Aortic stenosis calcific (age >40 yrs)	Systolic murmur transmitted to neck and apex Diminish or absent EC and A_2 S_4 gallop	LV heave Slow-rising pulse Narrow pulse pressure Systolic thrill	Calcified aortic valve LV enlargement Dilated ascending aorta	LVH	Pressure gradient between LV and aorta
Aortic stenosis congenital (childhood and young adult)	Systolic murmur transmitted to neck and apex Loud EC and A_2 S_4 gallop	LV heave Slow-rising pulse Narrow pulse pressure Systolic thrill	LV enlargement Dilated ascending aorta	LVH	Pressure gradient between LV and aorta
Aortic regurgitation	Decrescendo diastolic murmur Early-systolic murmur Middiastolic murmur at apex (Austin Flint)	Wide pulse pressure Quick-rising pulse LV heave	Dilated aorta LV enlargement	LVH	No pressure gradient at aortic valve Aortic regurgitation on angiocardiography
Mitral regurgitation	Holosystolic murmur, not transmitted to neck, heard better at apex and axilla	LV heave	Calcium at mitral valve Big LA	LVH Broad P waves	No pressure gradient at mitral valve Mitral regurgitation on angiocardiography
Aortic sclerosis	Short systolic murmur	Age: usually over 50 Evidence of atherosclerosis	Calcium in aortic arch	Normal	No pressure gradient
Bicuspid aortic valve	Short systolic murmur Early decrescendo diastolic murmur EC	Common in youth May be associated with coarctation	Usually normal	Normal	Aortic regurgitation: none, mild, or very rarely severe
Aortic dilatation or aneurysm	Short systolic murmur Diastolic murmur may be present Tambour S_2 Lift in right second interspace	Signs of syphilis or Marfans syndrome	Dilated aorta Calcium in ascending aorta in syphilis	Normal	Dilated aorta
Hypertension	Short systolic murmur Loud A_2. S_4 may be present	Hypertension	LV enlargement	LVH	LV pressure elevated

evidence for the diagnosis of calcific aortic stenosis. The absence of aortic valve calcification in an older patient with a systolic murmur is evidence against the presence of significant aortic stenosis.

Study in the catheterization laboratory sometimes is indicated in the evaluation of systolic mur-

murs in the right second interspace. The need for study also arises in patients with aortic valve disease in order to quantitate the lesion for a decision about surgery. Patients with rheumatic heart disease frequently have findings indicating involvement of both the mitral and aortic valves, and left heart catheterization is indicated to estimate the contribution each makes to the patient's disability. Angiography also provides valuable information about coronary anatomy and left ventricular function. The principles of laboratory evaluation of the aortic and mitral valves have been outlined (Chap. 17).

Systolic Murmurs—Apex and Left Lower Sternal Border

The conditions responsible for a systolic murmur at the apex or along the lower left sternal border are listed in Table 20-3.

The organic murmurs of mitral and tricuspid re-

TABLE 20-3

Systolic Murmurs—Apex and Left Lower Sternal Border (LLSB)

Diagnosis	Auscultation	Other Physical Examination	X-Ray	ECG	Cardiovascular Laboratory Findings
Mitral Regurgitation Chronic	Holosystolic usually radiating to axilla S_1 soft S_3 common	LV heave	Big LA and LV Mitral-valve calcification	Broad, bifid P waves Atrial fibrillation common	LA pressure elevated, big v waves Mitral regurgitation by angiography
Acute	Crescendo-decrescendo murmur, holosystolic or ending before S_2, radiation to base or axilla S_4	Signs of PH	Minimal LV & LA enlargement Pulmonary congestion	Normal	Large LA v waves Mitral regurgitation by angiography
Hypertrophic Cardiomyopathy (IHSS)	Crescendo-decrescendo murmur S_4	Rapid, bifid carotid LV heave	Normal or LVH	LVH Large P wave WPW	Small LV systolic volume Gradient LV cavity to outflow tract
Ventricular septal defect (small)	Holosystolic LLSB, High-pitched, harsh	Thrill LLSB	Heart small	Normal	Left-to-right shunt Normal pressures
Tricuspid regurgitation	Holosystolic maximum toward sternum, increase with inspiration, not transmitted to axilla	v waves in JVP Pulsating liver Signs of RV hypertension and congestive failure	Big RA and VC Large heart	Right axis deviation (RAD)	Elevated v waves RA
Aortic stenosis (transmitted)	Ejection—early-systolic murmur— also heard right second interspace	Thrill—right second interspace	LV large Aortic-valve calcification	LAD and LVH	Pressure gradient aortic valve
Mitral-valve prolapse	Mid- to late-systolic murmur, may be preceded by click or clicks	Pectus excavatum	Mitral annulus calcification	Abnormal T waves	Prolapse of leaflets of mitral valve by angiography midsystole with subsequent regurgitation
Papillary muscle dysfunction	Mid, late, or pansystolic murmur S_4 gallop		Normal or mild LVH	MI or abnormal ST-T-waves	Regurgitation by angiography

gurgitation and of ventricular septal defect are heard at the apex or between the apex and the left lower sternal border and typically are holosystolic. They begin with the onset of ventricular systole, and hence S_1, and usually extend throughout systole, ending with S_2, or slightly later when the ventricular pressure falls below atrial pressure. Only the murmur of mitral regurgitation is loudest at the apex and transmitted into the axilla. That of the small ventricular septal defect, referred to as Roger's murmur, is heard best along the lower left sternal border but may be audible at the apex. The murmur of tricuspid regurgitation typically is loudest at the sternal border, or even to the right of the sternum, but frequently is loud at the apex. The increase in intensity of the murmur during inspiration, the prominent v waves in the jugular veins, and signs of right ventricular hypertension support the diagnosis of tricuspid regurgitation.

When mitral regurgitation occurs abruptly, as with rupture of chordae tendineae or severe papillary muscle dysfunction, the blowing, pansystolic murmur typical of rheumatic mitral regurgitation may not be heard. In acute mitral regurgitation the murmur may be crescendo-decrescendo in type, and harsh and rasping in character. The murmur can radiate well to the upper sternal areas. A fourth heart sound and signs of pulmonary hypertension are usually present. In this situation, the chest roentgenogram and echocardiogram will show the left atrium and ventricle to be only minimally enlarged, but there are prominent signs of pulmonary congestion.

The murmur associated with mitral valve prolapse is typically late systolic in timing and is usually introduced by one or more midsystolic clicks. The murmur and clicks may be highly variable in intensity and timing.[51,52] The late systolic timing of the murmur is explained by the fact that the mitral valve is competent early in systole, but gives way or falls back into the atrium later in systole. As the mitral regurgitation becomes more severe, it will be present throughout systole, and at this time the murmur becomes holosystolic. This change in the murmur is often associated with the onset of symptoms and enlargement of the heart. When the murmur is late in onset, it indicates that the regurgitation is not severe, and this condition is compatible with a long period of normal cardiac function. Rupture of the chordae tendineae or infective endocarditis are common explanations of the rapid progression of mild regurgitation to severe regurgitation in some of these patients.

Murmurs due to alteration in function of the papillary muscles are common in patients with ischemic heart disease. Most frequently the murmur is of low intensity, diamond-shaped, and well localized to the apex. Such murmurs and those confined to late systole do not signify hemodynamically significant mitral regurgitation. Papillary muscle dysfunction or localized rupture may cause more severe mitral regurgitation, but in this situation the murmur is usually pansystolic and the associated findings are similar to those seen in patients with acute mitral regurgitation of other etiologies. The severity of the mitral regurgitation due to papillary muscle ischemia may vary remarkably; at times the patient may be comfortable and the murmur faint and at other times the patient may be in severe respiratory distress with a loud, long apical systolic murmur.

In patients with hypertrophic cardiomyopathy (IHSS), the cardiac murmur is midsystolic and crescendo–decrescendo in shape. This murmur may simulate aortic stenosis at the left sternal edge but may sound more like mitral regurgitation at the apex. This auscultatory quandary should immediately suggest hypertrophic cardiomyopathy. A characteristic feature of the murmur of hypertrophic cardiomyopathy is modification by certain maneuvers. In most patients it will be intensified by the Valsalva maneuver and decreased by having the patient assume the squatting posture. Associated findings of a rapid, bifid carotid pulse (Fig. 17–2) and the characteristic echocardiographic findings of extreme septal hypertrophy and systolic anterior motion of the mitral valve also help to establish the diagnosis.

The murmur of a ventricular septal defect may be heard all over the precordium, including the apex, but is always loudest along the left sternal border. It is typically more harsh than that of mitral or tricuspid regurgitation. If the defect is small, the murmur may be the only abnormality detectable on physical examination. Larger defects may be associated with a middiastolic murmur at the apex caused by the increased flow across the mitral valve in diastole. Ventricular septal defects with a large left-to-right shunt are rare in adults.

Valvular aortic stenosis must be considered among the common causes of apical systolic murmurs, for the high-frequency, musical components of the aortic stenosis murmur may be transmitted down the long axis of the left ventricle to the apex. In this situation the murmur may be heard poorly in areas between the apex and the base. Its origin can be determined by the presence of other signs of aortic stenosis, such as abnormal carotid pulses and transmission of the murmur to the neck vessels, and by the absence of signs of significant mitral regurgitation such as left atrial enlargement.

Diastolic Murmurs—Apex

Diastolic murmurs at the apex are typically due to stenosis of an atrioventricular valve, but other conditions may be responsible (Table 20–4).

Mitral stenosis is the most important cause. The characteristic murmur is rumbling, low pitched, heard best at the apex, and occasionally heard only in a very small area—usually directly over the apex impulse. Exercise sometimes is necessary to bring it out, and it is also more prominent with the patient in the left lateral decubitus position. Presystolic accentuation of intensity and frequency is an important characteristic of this murmur. It may be difficult to hear, especially when there is a low cardiac output or severe congestive failure. Its presence can be suspected on the basis of other signs, such as a snapping, loud first heart sound at the apex and an opening snap of the mitral valve which gives a characteristic cadence. Silent mitral stenosis should be suspected in every patient with signs and symptoms of pulmonary hypertension with pulmonary congestion without another obvious cause, or with systemic embolization. Support for the diagnosis of mitral stenosis may be provided by the radiologic examination, which may reveal a double density along the right heart border indicating that the left atrium is enlarged (Fig. 20–1). Kerley's B lines at the lung bases are also characteristic of mitral stenosis (Fig. 20–2). Left atrial enlargement may also be detected on fluoroscopy. The ECG may show broad, notched P waves or atrial fibrillation. The echocardiogram provides the most reliable noninvasive laboratory information about the presence or absence of mitral stenosis; abnormal motion of the anterior and posterior leaflets, increased num-

TABLE 20–4
Diastolic Murmurs—Apex

Diagnosis	Auscultation	Other Physical Examination	X-Ray	ECG	Cardiovascular Laboratory Findings
Mitral stenosis	S_1 snapping OS present Mid-diastolic rumble Presystolic murmur	RV lift	Big LA Mitral-valve calcification Kerley B lines	RAD Broad notched P waves	Mitral diastolic pressure gradient
Mitral regurgitation (diastolic flow murmur)	S_1 soft or absent S_3 present Mid-diastolic murmur Systolic murmur of mitral regurgitation	LV lift	LA large LV large	LAD LVH	Gross mitral regurgitation
Flow murmur secondary to increased pulmonary blood flow, e.g., ASD, VSD, or PDA	S_1 normal S_2 fixed split in ASD Murmurs of primary lesion		Hypervascular lung fields		Proof of primary lesion
Tricuspid stenosis	Diastolic murmur heard best near sternum Increased by inspiration	Big a waves JVP	Big RA and VC		Tricuspid diastolic pressure gradient
Aortic regurgitation (transmitted)	Decrescendo diastolic murmur LLSB Onset with S_2	Signs of aortic regurgitation LV lift	Large LV	LAD LVH	Signs of aortic regurgitation
Aortic regurgitation (Austin Flint)	S_1 normal or soft OS absent Mid-diastolic rumble Presystolic rumble	Peripheral signs of aortic regurgitation LV lift	Large LV	LAD LVH	Signs of aortic regurgitation

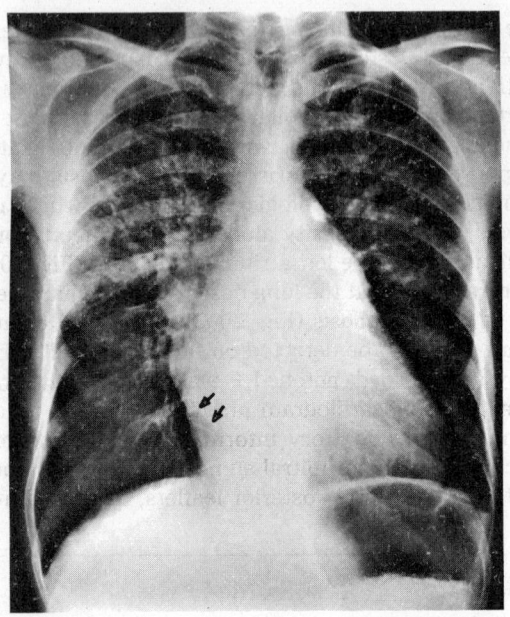

FIGURE 20-1. Chest x-ray of a patient with mitral stenosis showing double density at lower right border of the heart which represents lower border of the enlarged left atrium (arrows). The right ventricular outflow tract and the pulmonary artery are also enlarged.

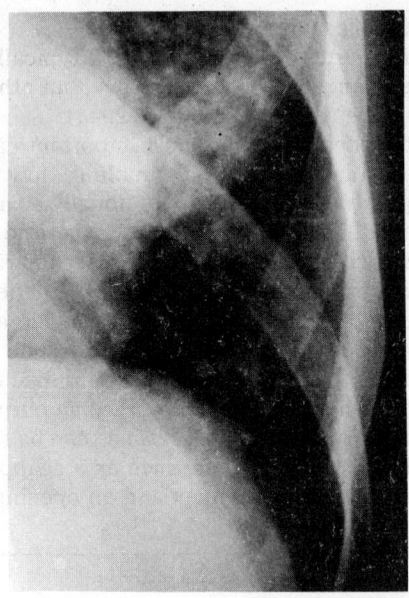

FIGURE 20-2. The left costophrenic angle from the chest x-ray of a patient with mitral stenosis showing linear streaks of increased density known as Kerley B lines.

ber of echoes from the leaflets, and enlargement of the left atrium may all be recognized.

Diastolic murmurs at the apex also may be heard in other conditions. Rarely, the tricuspid valve is involved in rheumatic heart disease and may become stenotic. The murmur usually is loudest at the lower left sternal border and may increase in intensity during inspiration. Marked distension of the jugular veins is present and the *a* wave is prominent if the patient is in sinus rhythm.

The middiastolic part of the murmur of aortic regurgitation occasionally is transmitted to the apex and may lead to the incorrect diagnosis of associated mitral stenosis. This error can be avoided by carefully tracing the transmission of the diastolic murmur from the left sternal border to the apex.

A second source of diagnostic error in the same setting is the Austin Flint murmur. This is middiastolic and/or presystolic and has the same rumbling character as the murmur of mitral stenosis. It originates at the mitral valve and is probably related to flow through the mitral valve, which is partially closed as a consequence of the regurgitant stream and rising diastolic pressures in the left ventricle.[53] The Austin Flint murmur is best differentiated from that of mitral stenosis by the absence of a snapping

first heart sound and an opening snap. If the blood pressure is elevated by a vasopressor drug the Austin Flint murmur will increase in intensity because the aortic regurgitation is increased, whereas the murmur of mitral stenosis will be unchanged. However, if the etiology is rheumatic, both valves may, of course, be involved. The echocardiogram provides valuable information to help distinguish the Austin Flint murmur from the rumble of mitral stenosis.

Increased flow through a nonstenotic atrioventricular valve can produce a diastolic murmur which simulates the murmur, but not the other auscultatory signs, of mitral stenosis. In the patient with mitral regurgitation the inflow into the left ventricle during diastole is increased and may be double or triple the normal flow. This gives rise to a diastolic murmur even in the presence of free mitral regurgitation. This murmur usually follows a very loud third heart sound gallop.

High flow through the atrioventricular valves secondary to increased pulmonary blood flow can also cause murmurs resembling those of mitral stenosis. The high flow circuit includes the tricuspid but not the mitral valve in patients with a defect in the atrial septum. In cases of ventricular septal defect and patent ductus arteriosus, the increased flow passes through the mitral but not through the tricuspid valve. Diastolic murmurs of similar character also are heard in sickle cell and other anemias and have led to the incorrect diagnosis of mitral stenosis.

Diastolic Murmurs—Second and Third Left Interspace

Diastolic murmurs at the base of the heart usually represent regurgitation at one of the semilunar valves. The lesions commonly responsible are listed in Table 20–5. These murmurs characteristically occur in early diastole and are decrescendo in type, with the maximum intensity immediately after the second heart sound. The murmurs of both aortic and pulmonary regurgitation are best heard along the left sternal border in the third and fourth interspaces, but the aortic murmur also is heard at the right of the ster-

num in the second interspace. The pulmonary diastolic murmur usually is not audible to the right of the sternum. When an aortic diastolic murmur is heard better on the right side, aortic root disease should be suspected as the cause of the aortic regurgitation. Syphilis, dissecting aneurysm, or rupture of the sinus of Valsalva must be given special consideration in these situations.

One must decide whether a decrescendo diastolic murmur at the base of the heart is due to aortic regurgitation or to pulmonary regurgitation secondary to pulmonary hypertension. This problem arises frequently in patients with mitral stenosis who might reasonably be expected to have either or both of these lesions. If the murmur is that of pulmonary regurgitation, simple mitral valvotomy is the treatment of choice, whereas if there is significant aortic regur-

TABLE 20–5
Diastolic Murmurs—Second Interspace Right and Left (Base)

Diagnosis	Auscultation	Other Physical Examination	X-Ray	ECG	Cardiovascular Laboratory Findings
Aortic regurgitation	Murmur decrescendo heard right second interspace and third left interspace S₂ may be of decreased intensity, but normal S₂ does not exclude severe AR	LV lift Peripheral signs of wide pulse pressure	Large LV	LVH LAD	Aortic regurgitation by angiocardiography
Pulmonary regurgitation	S₂ (P₂) loud if PR secondary to PH Murmur left second interspace, not to right of sternum In absence of PH P₂ normal. Murmur rough and scratchy crescendo-decrescendo	RV lift Peripheral signs of AR absent	Avascular lung fields if PH present	RAD RVH	Aortic valve competent Intracardiac phonocardiogram localizes murmur to right heart
Diastolic component of continuous murmur (transmitted)	Characteristic continuous murmur heard elsewhere, e.g., under left clavicle or over neck				

gitation, it may be an incorrect course of action. The following points may be helpful in the differentiation. Peripheral signs of aortic regurgitation—wide pulse pressures and so on—are the best evidence that the murmur arises at the aortic valve. Evidence of left ventricular hypertrophy favors an aortic origin. Finally, on statistical grounds a basilar diastolic murmur in a patient with rheumatic heart disease is most likely to be of aortic origin, even in the presence of pulmonary hypertension.

Isolated pulmonary regurgitation attributed to disease of the valve rather than to pulmonary hypertension occurs rarely. In this entity the diastolic murmur is low pitched and not of the decrescendo type.

Diastolic murmurs at the base of the heart may be transmitted from other areas. The diastolic component of the continuous murmur of a patent ductus arteriosus occasionally is heard here, but the more typical, continuous nature can be appreciated on auscultation under the left clavicle. The diastolic component of other continuous murmurs, especially that of coronary arteriovenous fistula, may be confused with the murmur of aortic insufficiency.

Continuous Murmurs

A continuous murmur is one heard throughout both phases of the cardiac cycle. The intensity may vary, but there is persistent sound throughout both parts of the cycle. It is sometimes difficult to distinguish such a murmur from prolonged systolic and diastolic murmurs of severe aortic valve disease, but there is usually an identifiable pause separating the systolic and diastolic components in the latter. The most characteristic feature of a continuous murmur is the fact that it runs over or past the second sound (S_2). The essential physiologic requirement for the generation of a continuous murmur is continuous flow through the area of murmur production throughout the cardiac cycle. Thus, there must be a pressure gradient present during both systole and diastole. These considerations lead to a physiologic classification of continuous murmurs as arising in communications between the aorta or arterial tree and any number of low-pressure chambers (Table 20–6).

The murmur of patent ductus arteriosus resembles the sound of machinery with maximum intensity in systole at or near the second sound. Both phases are best heard under the left clavicle, but sometimes one of the components will be audible in the left second interspace and will lead to the incorrect diagnosis of semilunar valve disease. Additional signs are a wide pulse pressure, evidence of left ventricular overload, and, occasionally, a middiastolic flow murmur

TABLE 20–6
Physiologic Classification of Continuous Murmurs

High Pressure	Low Pressure	Example
Aorta	Pulmonary artery	Patent ductus arteriosus
Aorta	Right heart	Ruptured sinus of Valsalva
Artery	Vein	Internal mammary artery to vein fistula
Artery	Artery (distal to stenosis)	Stenosis of artery: systemic or pulmonary
Vein	Vein (central to constriction)	Venous hum

at the apex mimicking mitral stenosis. On chest x-ray the pulmonary arteries are seen to be enlarged and the lung fields vascular. The pulmonary arteries are seen to pulsate vigorously when examined fluoroscopically.

An arteriovenous malformation of the coronary circulation is another cause of continuous murmur. The point of maximum intensity usually is over the left sternal border. Communication of a dilated coronary artery directly with one of the right heart chambers or with the coronary sinus produces a continuous murmur that may be confused with that of a patent ductus arteriosus. However, the murmur differs from that of patent ductus in usually being loudest over the lower end of the sternum or between the sternum and apex and in having a peak intensity that does not occur in association with the second heart sound.

A communication between the aorta and a chamber of the right heart may be formed by rupture of an aneurysm of the sinus of Valsalva. It is usually the right sinus of Valsalva which ruptures into either the right ventricle or the right atrium. The continuous murmur is often of grade 5 or 6 in intensity and accompanied by a thrill. The point of maximum intensity varies with the specific anatomy of an individual case but usually is best heard along the lower left sternal border. The diastolic component is louder than the systolic, which may help in its differentiation from patent ductus arteriosus. Patients with this condition usually give a history of sudden onset of congestive heart failure, sometimes associated with a feeling of tearing or breaking within the chest.

A systemic arteriovenous fistula in the chest wall may produce a continuous murmur. Such a fistulous communication most commonly develops between the internal mammary artery and vein, secondary to a penetrating wound. Pulmonary arteriovenous fistulas also must be considered and are associated with faint continuous murmurs over the part of the lung which contains them.

Other causes of continuous murmurs are congenital aortopulmonary communication, ventricular septal defect with aortic regurgitation, the surgically created subclavian artery to pulmonary artery anastomosis (Blalock-Taussig), and the aorta to pulmonary artery anastomosis (Potts procedure).

The diagnosis of the typical patent ductus arteriosus usually can be made easily without catheterization, but the differential diagnosis of the other causes of continuous murmurs requires the use of the laboratory. Right and left heart catheterization, indicator dilution studies, and contrast radiography are often necessary to locate the points of origin and termination of the shunt.

Venous hums may be confused with continuous murmurs of organic origin. If a venous hum is suspected, the diagnosis can be established by a few simple maneuvers. First, the sound is louder in the neck than over the chest. Second, it may be altered by turning the head or breathing and usually disappears entirely with pressure over the jugular vein just above the clavicle. Such a murmur is usually rough, harsh, and irregular in character. It is loudest in diastole and is diminished or absent in the recumbent position.

A stenotic area in a carotid artery or another branch of the aortic arch may be the source of a bruit heard over the chest. If the stenosis is of such degree that a pressure gradient (and, hence, flow) persists throughout diastole, the murmur will be continuous. If it arises in the innominate artery or one of its branches, it is heard better under the right clavicle and in the neck than over the heart. Abnormality of peripheral pulses or a difference between the blood pressure in the two arms may be present. A similar mechanism explains the continuous murmur heard in the presence of multiple areas of stenosis in the peripheral pulmonary arteries.

In pregnancy and the early postpartum period one may hear over the upper chest a continuous murmur that has been called a mammary souffle. This murmur may be confined to systole but may extend beyond the second sound into diastole. Characteristically, it can be obliterated by firm pressure with the bell of the stethoscope.

SPECIFIC VALVE ABNORMALITIES

Aortic Stenosis

Obstruction to left ventricular outflow can occur above (supravalvular) or below (subvalvular) the aortic valve but is most common at the aortic valve itself. Subvalvular aortic stenosis may be a congenital lesion in which a discrete fibrous membrane or tunnel causes obstruction or may result from asymmetric thickening of the interventricular septum and narrowing of the outflow tract (hypertrophic cardiomyopathy, Chap. 19). Supravalvular aortic stenosis is also a congenital lesion and practically always associated with a peculiar abnormal physiognomy; elfin facies. While rheumatic fever may damage the aortic valve and produce changes leading to aortic stenosis, isolated aortic stenosis without associated mitral involvement is rarely rheumatic in etiology but is usually due to a congenital abnormality of the aortic valve.[57]

Congenital aortic valve disease producing left ventricular outflow obstruction is seen at two different age periods. Patients with valves that are stenotic from birth usually come to the attention of the physician in childhood or early adulthood because of the presence of a heart murmur or symptoms related to left ventricular outflow obstruction. Such congenitally stenotic valves may show signs of progressive narrowing with age as a consequence of abnormal hemodynamic stress and valve calcification. A second and larger group of patients with congenitally malformed valves does not develop aortic stenosis until the sixth or seventh decade when valve calcification occurs and is responsible for progressive obstruction. These patients often have a history of a cardiac murmur from early adulthood, but signs and symptoms of left ventricular obstruction are not seen until the congenitally abnormal valve, which is usually bicuspid, becomes calcified. In elderly patients, calcification of a normal aortic valve may cause obstruction.

Patients tolerate severe degrees of aortic obstruction for long periods without symptoms. The left ventricle is able to compensate for the abnormal pressure-work which it must perform because of its ability to hypertrophy. Ultimately, however, even this compensatory mechanism proves inadequate and symptoms supervene. Thus, some patients with aortic stenosis may first present with symptoms of left ventricular failure. Angina pectoris is also a frequent symptom even in the absence of left ventricular failure or coronary atherosclerosis because left ventricular stroke work and muscle mass are increased while coronary perfusion pressure may progressively diminish with increasing valve obstruction. Coronary atherosclerosis also may be present. The third cardinal symptom of aortic stenosis is syncope, usually exertional. The mechanism underlying this symptom may be inability to augment cardiac output due to fixed outflow obstruction or even a reflex induced fall in cardiac output. In some cases cardiac arrhythmias are the cause of the syncopal episodes; heart block is especially common in patients with calcific aortic stenosis. Once any of these symptoms develop, their progression is usually rapid or the patient may die suddenly. Sudden death is unlikely to occur prior to the appearance of other symptoms, however. The appearance of any of the three cardinal symptoms in the patient suspected of having aortic stenosis demands prompt investigation.

The severity of aortic obstruction may be accurately assessed at the bedside. The key to the evaluation of the severity of aortic stenosis is the character of the arterial pulse. In severe disease the carotid pulse is retarded in upstroke and small in volume and the systolic blood pressure and the pulse pressure are reduced as seen in Figure 17–2. In older patients with coexistent sclerosis of large vessels, these arterial signs may not be present. The intensity of the systolic murmur does not necessarily correlate with the severity of the lesion, but the peak intensity will be progressively later with increasing obstruction. With severe stenosis the murmur is long and extends almost to the end of left ventricular systole, which may actually be after P_2. Left ventricular hypertrophy will usually be obvious by palpation, ECG, echocardiography, or chest roentgenogram. In older patients, significant aortic stenosis is unlikely if valve calcification is not demonstrated at fluoroscopy or echocardiography. Cardiac catheterization should be performed in preparation for surgical intervention to determine presence or absence of other valve disease, to evaluate function of the left ventricle, and to determine whether or not coronary atherosclerosis is present.

There is little justification for medical therapy in the symptomatic patient with aortic stenosis. Symptoms indicate that the left ventricular outflow obstruction is severe and that surgical therapy is indicated. In younger patients with mobile, noncalcified valves, commissurotomy may effectively relieve obstruction but this is rarely possible when the valve is calcified, and in this situation the valve must be replaced with a prosthesis. The reduction in cardiac work which occurs after successful aortic replacement will improve symptoms even in patients with coronary atherosclerosis or left ventricular dysfunction, although the immediate mortality of surgery will be higher in these patients. Bypass of significantly obstructed coronary arteries is usually performed at the time of aortic valve replacement.

Aortic Regurgitation

Aortic regurgitation may result from disease processes affecting the aortic valve leaflet (rheumatic heart disease), supporting structures in the aortic root above the valve (dissecting aneurysm), or supporting structure below the valve as in the case of a ventricular septal defect high in the septum. The most common causes of these abnormalities are listed in Table 20–7.

An understanding of the pathophysiology of aortic reflux allows an accurate assessment of the severity of the lesion at the bedside. The left ventricle dilates in order to increase stroke volume, which is necessary to maintain an adequate forward flow and accommodate the volume of blood which refluxes backward. The size of the left ventricle, determined by palpation, chest roentgenogram, or echocardiography, is a rough guide to the severity of the volume load. Systolic pressure increases because of the excess stroke volume. Aortic diastolic pressure falls in proportion to the severity of the backward diastolic leak, and the pulse pressure is therefore wide. In most cases of severe aortic regurgitation systolic pressure exceeds 140 mm Hg and diastolic pressure is less than 60 mm Hg, and in many cases accurate determi-

---

TABLE 20–7
Etiology of Aortic Regurgitation

Disease of Aortic Valve

Rheumatic
Congenital deformity
Infective endocarditis
Spontaneous rupture

Disease of Aortic Root

Syphilis
Dissecting aneurysm
Cystic medial necrosis with dilatation
Inflammatory disease
   Rheumatoid spondylitis
   Reiter syndrome
   Relapsing polychondritis
   Giant cell aortitis

Disease of Subvalvular Structure

Aneurysm of sinus of Valsalva
High ventricular septal defect
Subaortic fibrous stenosis

nation of diastolic pressure by sphygmomanometer is not possible, Korotkow sounds being heard all the way to zero pressure. Peripheral resistance decreases to promote forward blood flow; this, in conjunction with the effects of the arterial pressure, imparts the characteristic hyperkinetic circulatory signs recognized in the carotid pulse, which is quick, of full volume, and often bifid, and in peripheral arteries where palpation reveals a collapsing (waterhammer) pulse. Although the distensibility or compliance of a ventricle chronically exposed to a volume load such as aortic regurgitation increases, eventually left ventricular diastolic pressure rises as the severity of the volume load progresses; the left ventricular diastolic pressure may be very high (50 to 60 mm Hg) and may actually support the aortic diastolic pressure. A very high ventricular diastolic pressure is also likely when the aortic regurgitation develops abruptly, as seen in acute aortic dissection or acute infective endocarditis with valve rupture. In this situation the left ventricular compliance is normal and dilatation has not had a chance to develop. In addition, if the peripheral flow is reduced, reflex vasoconstriction develops. This high diastolic blood pressure in the aorta and the peripheral vasoconstriction may mask the classical peripheral signs of severe aortic regurgitation. Because the ventricular diastolic pressure rises so high and equals the aortic diastolic pressure in about middiastole the diastolic murmur may be short. Also, the high ventricular diastolic pressure closes the mitral valve in middiastole; thus, the first heart sound is absent at the onset of systole. The echocardiogram is invaluable in this setting and demonstrates fluttering of the anterior leaflet of the mitral valve and premature diastolic closure of the mitral valve.

The intensity of the aortic diastolic murmur does not correlate with the severity of reflux, but the presence of an Austin Flint murmur indicates that aortic regurgitation is severe.[53] In the patient with severe aortic regurgitation, cardiac catheterization is useful to quantitate the alteration in ventricular and aortic pressure, assess involvement of other valves, and evaluate left ventricular function. Aortic root angiography allows some degree of quantification of the severity of reflux and is helpful in describing the anatomic abnormality of the aortic root or valves.

Patients may tolerate even severe degrees of aortic regurgitation for long periods of time with preservation of excellent effort tolerance. Symptoms of congestive heart failure or angina do not occur until the left ventricle is unable to maintain an adequate forward stroke volume. In patients with chronic aortic regurgitation, this is usually due to the development of left ventricular dysfunction, possibly related to

chronic excessive stretching and tearing of sarcomeres (Chap. 18). As with aortic stenosis, once symptoms appear the progression to more severe symptoms and death is usually rapid and little affected by medical therapy. Aortic valve replacement should, therefore, be recommended for patients who are symptomatic from aortic regurgitation. Unfortunately, even successful valve replacement at this time, while important to interrupt progression of symptoms, leaves the patient with a dilated ventricle which is abnormal in its function. The dilemma of when to recommend surgery for the asymptomatic patient with evidence of severe aortic regurgitation is one of the most difficult in clinical cardiology. A prospective study of patients with rheumatic aortic regurgitation has indicated that those asymptomatic patients with any of the following had a high likelihood of developing symptoms or dying in three to six years: 1) Systolic blood pressure over 140 mm Hg and diastolic pressure less than 40 mm Hg; 2) cardiomegaly by chest roentgenogram (CT Ratio $>$ 55 percent); or 3) left ventricular hypertrophy with strain by ECG. Strong consideration should be given to surgery in this group of patients before onset of symptoms or to asymptomatic patients who show evidence of progressive cardiac enlargement.[60]

Mitral Stenosis

In the adult, mitral stenosis is almost always the result of rheumatic heart disease. In spite of this, only half the patients can recall an attack of acute rheumatic fever in childhood. Mitral obstruction occurs in the years following the initial insult to the valve sometimes as a result of continuous low-grade rheumatic activity but more commonly because of longstanding hemodynamic stress to a diseased valve. Mitral stenosis may therefore be progressive in the adult in spite of adequate prophylaxis against recurrent streptococcal infection. As the mitral orifice narrows, left atrial pressure rises in order to maintain an adequate cardiac output, and a pressure gradient is produced between left atrium and left ventricle (Chap. 17). The resultant increase in left atrial pressure is reflected backward to pulmonary veins, capillaries, and arteries and is responsible for the most common symptom of mitral stenosis—dyspnea on exertion. Patients may not notice breathlessness until unusual circulatory needs are called for, as with pregnancy or excessive physical activity or when a bout of rapid atrial fibrillation occurs. This may result in abrupt and severe elevation of left atrial pressure leading to pulmonary edema or extravasation of blood into alveoli producing hemoptysis. More commonly, the dyspnea is insidious in onset and slowly progressive.

When mitral obstruction becomes more severe, cardiac output cannot increase in response to demands, giving rise to the symptom of fatigue. This universal complaint may occur so gradually that the patient does not realize that his activities are restricted and sometimes only in retrospect, after surgical correction, does he recognize the severity of his effort incapacity. Long-standing left atrial hypertension causes enlargement of the left atrium, which is responsible for atrial arrhythmias, particularly atrial fibrillation, which produces further impairment of cardiac output. The enlarged, fibrillating atrium is a site for the formation of clot which may be dislodged as systemic emboli. In some patients marked left atrial enlargement does not occur, left atrial hypertension is more severe, and pulmonary arteries constrict to produce "reactive" pulmonary hypertension. Such patients may show predominant signs and symptoms of right heart failure early in their course. Some patients respond to elevated pulmonary venous pressure with bronchospasm so that asthmatic features may dominate the presentation. Patients with mitral stenosis are more prone to broncho-pulmonary infection. In older patients this may be responsible for the development of chronic bronchitis and emphysema. Cough, especially at night, is a frequent early symptom.

Clinical evaluation of the severity of mitral stenosis should begin with the understanding that the principal manifestations of the lesion will be predominantly in the lungs and right heart. Symptoms, generally a good guide to the severity of the valvular disease, may be misleading in mitral stenosis. Occasionally, patients with mild obstruction may develop severe pulmonary congestion during stress or a paroxysm of rapid atrial fibrillation, while some patients with severe "reactive" pulmonary hypertension may be relatively protected from pulmonary congestion and have few complaints. Signs of pulmonary hypertension on physical examination or x-ray or right ventricular hypertrophy by ECG always indicate that the mitral stenosis is severe. The chest roentgenogram is invaluable in assessing the severity of obstruction. With elevation of left atrial pressure there is a redistribution of blood flow from the lower lungs to upper lungs. This produces prominence of the vasculature in the upper lung fields and a reduction of vasculature in the lower lung fields in the upright chest roentgenogram. This finding in association with evidence of left atrial enlargement strongly suggests the diagnosis of mitral stenosis. The presence of Kerley B lines (Fig. 20–2) usually indicates that mean left atrial pressure is 25 mm Hg or higher. Lesser degrees of pulmonary congestion are seen with less severe disease. Because the mitral valve opens earlier with increasing left atrial pressure, the degree of narrowing of the A_2-opening snap interval will be a general index of the severity of obstruction.

In the young patient the diagnosis of mitral stenosis can usually be made with confidence on the basis of symptoms, physical findings, and changes on chest roentgenogram. In older patients the characteristic physical signs may be altered because of valve calcification, obesity, emphysema, pulmonary hypertension, or reduced cardiac output. However, truly "silent" mitral stenosis is distinctly uncommon. Clues to the presence of the lesion are usually apparent to the careful observer. The presence of mitral stenosis should be diligently searched for and the diagnosis suspected in any of the following clinical situations: 1) unexplained pulmonary hypertension, 2) recurrent atrial fibrillation, 3) systemic embolization, 4) asthma with atypical features, 5) chronic obstructive pulmonary disease where dyspnea is out of proportion to the objective evidence of lung disease, and 6) unexplained congestive heart failure. It is also important to recognize that the clinical findings of mitral stenosis may be mimicked closely by other conditions, for example atrial myxoma and atrial septal defect, the latter particularly in middle-aged or older patients. The diagnosis of mitral stenosis can be confirmed or established confidently in nearly all cases by echocardiography (Chap. 17). Cardiac catheterization is indicated to quantitate the severity of obstruction, (particularly when there is a disparity between clinical findings and symptoms), to determine the pliability of the valve, measure the level of pulmonary artery pressure, assess the severity of mitral regurgitation or other valvular lesions, and determine the extent of myocardial dysfunction or coronary artery disease.

There are two surgical procedures available to treat the patient with mitral stenosis: mitral commissurotomy and valve replacement with a prosthetic device. In the former operation the surgeon attempts to split the fused commissures of the mitral valve by hand or with a mechanical dilator (closed commissurotomy) or under direct inspection with a scalpel (open commissurotomy). This is a highly effective procedure in properly selected cases and may restore the mitral orifice to near normal dimensions. Many patients will continue to be free of severe mitral obstruction even 20 years after operation. The operative mortality should be 1 percent or less in well-selected patients operated upon by experienced surgeons. The disadvantages of the procedures are that 1) it cannot be performed if mitral regurgitation is present; 2) significant mitral regurgitation may be produced if the valve is very fibrotic and calcified; 3) the valve orifice may be only temporarily stretched and not actually increased in size; and 4) mitral restenosis may occur. In spite of these considerations, mitral commissurotomy should always be performed when feasible in the patient with mitral stenosis who requires surgery. Unfortunately, in not all instances is it possible to achieve successful mitral commissurotomy. With increasing thickness of the valve, fibrosis and fusion of subvalvular structures, and valve calcification, commissurotomy becomes more difficult. These factors are more likely to be found in older patients and those with a long history of symptomatic disease. These complicating factors are also more common in males. Therefore, most patients over the age of 40, particularly men, will require mitral valve replacement. The mortality of this procedure is slightly higher than that associated with commissurotomy, and the risk of subsequent embolization, although low, is significant even with anticoagulant therapy. However, valve obstruction will be effectively relieved.

The decision as to when to intervene surgically in the course of mitral stenosis will vary with the type of operative procedure anticipated. Thus, if one can confidently expect to achieve success with mitral commissurotomy, patients with early and mild (NYHA Class II) symptoms may be referred for surgery. Early operation in these patients can be expected to improve symptoms and retard the development of pulmonary vascular disease. The ideal patient will be a woman in her late 20s or 30s with modest effort intolerance and physical signs suggesting a pliable mitral valve, such as a loud and snappy S_1, loud opening snap, and prominent presystolic rumble. When mitral valve replacement is the likely procedure, operation should await the development of more severe symptomatology (Class III or IV). An exception to this general rule is the presence of pulmonary hypertension which, when confirmed by catheterization, represents an indication for commissurotomy or valve replacement even in the absence of severe symptoms.

In the past mitral surgery has been recommended for all patients with mitral stenosis who presented with systemic embolization, but this is no longer thought to be necessary. Surgery should be carried out in patients who also have moderate or severe hemodynamic abnormalities, but those with milder disease can be effectively managed with long-term anticoagulation.

Cardiac catheterization should be performed in most patients in whom surgery is considered, particularly those over the age of 40, those presenting with return of symptoms after previous mitral surgery, those with suspected pulmonary hypertension, and those with other valvular lesions. The younger patient with obvious findings of mitral stenosis and a pliable valve and who has significant symptoms can be sent to surgery without the need for catheterization.

Mitral Regurgitation [58]

Effective closure of the mitral valve requires the interaction of various components of the complex mitral apparatus consisting of valve leaflets, chordae tendineae, papillary muscles, valve annulus, and left ventricular myocardium. Disease processes affecting any of these structures may result in mitral regurgitation. The more common etiologies of mitral regurgitation are listed in Table 20–8.

The incidence of rheumatic fever is declining, but rheumatic heart disease remains the single most common cause of mitral regurgitation. Myxomatous change in the mitral valve producing valve prolapse or "floppy" valve may be a manifestation of an inherited connective tissue disorder, such as the Marfan syndrome, but occurs most commonly as an isolated abnormality.[5] The mitral regurgitation associated with this lesion is usually mild, but examples of more severe disease due to this abnormality are encountered with increasing frequency suggesting that some of these patients are prone to progression of the lesion. Rupture of chordae tendineae occurs more frequently in patients with myxomatous disease of the valve but may also occur without obvious cause or secondary to infective endocarditis or chest trauma. Dysfunction or rupture of a papillary muscle is usually a manifestation of ischemic heart disease and may occur during the evolution of acute myocardial infarction or develop insidiously in patients with chronic ischemic heart disease. Some degree of mitral regurgitation is frequent in patients with primary myocardial disease and is due to left ventricular dilatation which causes malalignment of papillary mus-

---

TABLE 20–8
Etiology of Mitral Regurgitation

Rheumatic heart disease

Congenital heart disease
  Endocardial cushion defect
  Corrected transposition of the great vessels

Mitral prolapse (myxomatous degeneration, "floppy" valves)

Ruptured chordae tendineae

Valve perforation or loss of substance (infective endocarditis)

Papillary muscle rupture or dysfunction

Calcification of the mitral annulus

Primary myocardial disease

cles or myopathic involvement of the papillary muscles themselves.

Of all valvular lesions, chronic mitral regurgitation is the best tolerated because the left ventricle ejects the extra volume load into a low-resistance chamber, the left atrium. The extra work the left ventricle must bear will be much less in this situation than when the total stroke volume must be ejected into a high resistance circuit, as in aortic regurgitation, so that excellent compensation can be maintained for many years in spite of a severe valvular leak. The left atrium enlarges gradually to accommodate the regurgitant volume; because of its distensibility, left atrial pressure may remain normal even though the volume of mitral regurgitation is severe. The posterior left atrial wall is in direct continuity with the posterior mitral valve leaflet so that progressive left atrial enlargement causes further separation of mitral leaflets and increasing incompetence of the valve. Patients with chronic mitral regurgitation pursue a slowly progressive course in which symptoms of fatigue and mild breathlessness wax and wane over many years. Signs and symptoms of severe pulmonary congestion do not appear until the regurgitant volume becomes very large and the left ventricle is unable to maintain an effective forward output. Clinical guidelines to the severity of the lesion will be best reflected in the size of the left ventricle as determined by palpation or chest roentgenogram and the severity of pulmonary venous congestion.

When mitral regurgitation occurs acutely, as with rupture of chordae tendineae or papillary muscle, the left atrium has little time to accommodate to the extra volume load, and left atrial pressure may rise precipitously to very high levels, even though the regurgitant volume may not be large. These patients will usually present with the abrupt onset of symptoms related to pulmonary congestion. The heart size may be normal or only slightly enlarged, but the lungs will show signs of pulmonary congestion. Occasionally, papillary muscle dysfunction may be responsible for intermittent acute mitral regurgitation, which may present a confusing picture of episodic pulmonary edema followed by relatively symptom-free intervals. The cardiac murmur may be absent or soft in this situation and the diagnosis of mitral valve dysfunction difficult to establish. Table 20–9 contrasts the clinical findings in acute and chronic mitral regurgitation, and Figure 20–3 shows the roentgenographic appearance associated with the two presentations. The major factor responsible for the difference in presentation is the distensibility or compliance of the left atrium.

Cardiac catheterization is indicated in the symptomatic patient with mitral regurgitation to determine the level of pulmonary artery and left atrial

---

TABLE 20–9*

Symptom	Chronic MR	Acute MR
Age at onset	Adolescence and early adulthood	>45 years
Duration of murmur	Many years	Recent onset
Natural history	CHF after many years	Sudden onset CHF
Cardiac rhythm	Atrial fibrillation	Normal sinus
Murmur	Pansystolic, blowing radiating to axilla	Pansystolic or early systolic, harsh, may radiate to base
Heart sounds	Diminished S_1	Normal or loud S_1
Gallops	S_3	S_3 and S_4
Pulmonary hypertension	Mild–moderate	Moderate–severe
Chest x-ray	Marked LV/LA enlargement. Minimal pulmonary congestion	Moderate–severe pulmonary congestion. Minimal LV/LA enlargement
Catheterization	Normal or moderate LA v waves. Marked MR	Large LA v waves. Moderate MR
Etiology	Rheumatic, congenital lesions	Ruptured chordae tendineae. Valve perforation. Papillary muscle dysfunction or rupture

* MR = Mitral regurgitation; CHF = Congestive heart failure; LV = Left ventricle; LA = Left atrium.

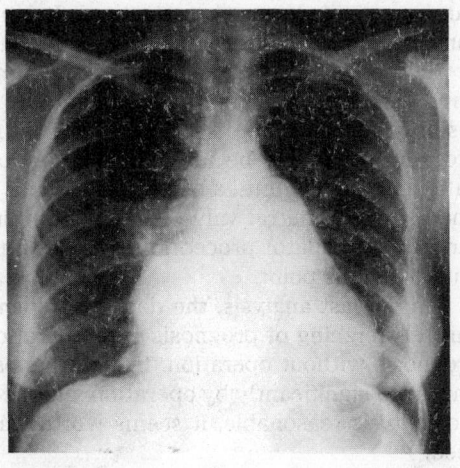
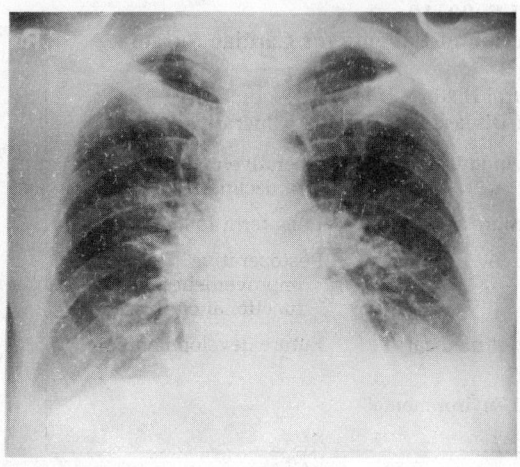

A. **B.**

FIGURE 20–3. A. Chronic rheumatic heart disease with longstanding severe mitral regurgitation. The left atrium and left ventricle are markedly enlarged but lung fields show few signs of pulmonary congestion. **B.** Acute mitral regurgitation due to ruptured chordae tendineae. Heart size is normal, but there is marked pulmonary congestion.

pressure, assess severity of the mitral leak by cineangiography, determine the presence of other significant valvular lesions, evaluate left ventricular function, and determine the presence or absence of coronary atherosclerosis. It may be difficult to distinguish between the patient with primary myocardial disease with associated mitral regurgitation and the patient with severe organic valvular disease with associated ventricular dilatation. Catheterization may be the only way to make this distinction, which is an important one, for mitral valve surgery can be of benefit in the latter situation but would be hazardous and of little help in the former.

Surgical replacement of the mitral valve with a prosthetic device should be recommended for patients severely symptomatic (Class III or IV) with mitral regurgitation. Some surgeons prefer plastic repair of the mitral valve apparatus in very selected patients with mitral regurgitation. The operative mortality of mitral valve replacement is 5 percent or less at most centers. The improvement in long-term survival and the interruption of progression of symptoms by such surgery have been amply documented. It should be recognized that delay of surgery until Class III or IV symptoms appear will leave the patient with an enlarged heart which does not function normally even after successful surgery. However, the course of mitral regurgitation may be so prolonged and benign before severe symptoms occur that it

hardly seems justifiable to recommend operation earlier.

CARDIOVASCULAR SURGERY—GENERAL PRINCIPLES

Surgical procedures will change as more forms of heart disease become amenable to definitive therapy, but certain factors will continue to be important in the selection of patients for operation. The decision depends upon the weighing of many factors, but basically it involves the comparison of the natural history of the patient's disease if he remains on medical treatment with that which can be expected if surgical treatment is provided. The elements of this decision are listed in Table 20–10. In the estimation of the prognosis without treatment it is important to remember that the physician's view is biased as his experience is greatest with those who have not done well. Rate of progression, although difficult to determine, is of great importance in selecting the appropriate time for operation and is best evaluated if the patient is seen at two points in time. The patient's age should not, per se, be a contraindication to surgery but does modify the decision. Aggressive management justified in a 40-year-old who has a life expectancy of 20 to 30 years might not be justified in an 80-

┌─ **TABLE 20-10** ─────────────────┐
Selection of Patients for Cardiac Surgery

Natural History of Disease	Operative Results
Prognosis in untreated patient	Operative mortality—rate of decline
Rate of progression	Long-term follow-up
Patient's age	Postoperative improvement in functional class
Adequacy of medical therapy	Future developments
Social and environmental factors	
└────────────────────────────────┘

year-old patient. Adequacy of medical therapy is a factor which is often neglected. Physicians are inclined to assume that they and their colleagues have provided the best possible medical therapy, and this may not be true. The doctor may not be at fault, but the patient may be unable or unwilling to follow instructions. Under ideal circumstances, social and environmental factors should not be important but in actual practice they are. It is obviously not possible for patients who are qualified by training only for manual labor to follow an ideal regime which requires extensive periods of rest. In this circumstance it is necessary to modify the decision on the basis of the patient's occupational history and capabilities.

The first item under operative results is operative mortality and the rate of decline of the mortality rate. This qualification of the operative mortality is necessary because during the early years of any operative procedure the mortality rate tends to be high as only the most severely ill patients are referred for surgery. As the surgeon gains more experience with the procedure, the physician sends him patients who constitute a lower risk. The referring physician must know the operative mortality not only in reported series but in the institution where the procedure will be done. This must be supplemented by information about the long-term efficacy and prognosis. These data must be based upon careful and complete follow-up studies which document the functional status of all patients and the incidence of complications. A procedure with a low operative mortality may eventually be discarded because of complications, such as the breakdown of prosthetic material or the development of thromboembolic complications, which appear many months after the procedure.

The amount of postoperative improvement which can be expected must be estimated. It is not necessary to require that the patient be functional Class 1 or 100 percent of normal, but if he obtains enough improvement to enable him to go back to work the result will be considered satisfactory. The anticipated procedure may not be ideal, but it may permit the patient to survive until a better operation is available. The history of mitral valve surgery from finger fracture through dilator procedures to valve replacement illustrates this point.

In the last analysis, the decision depends on the careful weighing of prognosis with operation against prognosis without operation. If the prognosis can be improved significantly by operation and the operative mortality is reasonable, it seems worthwhile to proceed.

PROSTHETIC VALVES[56]

No prosthetic valve yet designed can compare with the normal or even mildly diseased human heart valve with respect to hemodynamic design, durability, and freedom from clotting. A variety of structural modifications and materials has been utilized in the construction of prosthetic valves, aimed at improving the hemodynamic characteristics, increasing the life span, and reducing the incidence of thromboembolization. In some centers homograft human valves or heterograft porcine or bovine valves have been implanted with success.

In the majority of instances prosthetic valves function effectively for many years and the patient carries on normal activities. However, the following complications may occur:

Thromboembolism

The incidence of this complication is lower with prostheses utilized since 1970, but this complication has not been eliminated. Because of the devastating and irreversible consequences of such an event in the cerebral circulation, many centers recommend long-term anticoagulation for all patients with prosthetic valves. Early experience with the homograft and heterograft valves indicates that chronic anticoagulation is not necessary when these valves are used for replacement.

Infection

A foreign body within the circulation is a natural repository for blood-borne infection. For this reason patients should be given prophylactic antibiotics, preferably by the parenteral route, during dental or other minor surgical procedures, and at the earliest signs of any infection. Infective endocarditis on a prosthetic valve is a dread complication which carries a mortality in excess of 25 percent. More than half the patients will require valve replacement to eradicate the infection.

Prosthesis Malfunction

This may occur as a consequence of thrombus formation, alteration in the structure of the moving ball or disc by wear and tear or swelling, sticking of the ball or disc in the cage, improper seating of the prosthesis, or improper size of the prosthesis. The latter two problems will usually be evident in the early postoperative period as a refractory low-output state or intractable pulmonary congestion. The other manifestations usually develop insidiously several years after successful valve replacement. Prosthesis malfunction is notoriously difficult to detect even with the aid of catheterization and angiography. It should be suspected in the patient with a prosthetic valve who shows any of the following

1. Alteration of the timing or quality of opening and closing sounds
2. Development of a new regurgitant murmur
3. Embolization
4. Increased severity of intravascular hemolysis
5. Development of heart failure or angina after a period of improvement
6. Occurrence of syncope

Paravalvular Leak

Regurgitation of blood between the prosthetic valve ring and the heart valve annulus usually results from tearing of suture material either spontaneously or after damage of heart tissue by infection. If the regurgitation is minimal, the course is stable, but severe regurgitation requires further surgery. It has been reported that severe paravalvular leak may be present in the absence of a significant regurgitant murmur; especially around valves inserted in the mitral area.

Hemolytic Anemia

The red cell survival time is shortened in all patients with prosthetic valves, probably because of battering and destruction of cells by the intravascular foreign body. Fragments of red cells and schizocytes may be seen in the peripheral blood smear. The amount of hemolysis is usually mild and easily compensated for by increased reticulocytosis. Rarely hemolysis may be severe enough to produce anemia. This usually occurs in association with prosthesis dysfunction or a regurgitant leak. Because chronic hemolysis occurs intravascularly, iron is lost in the urine in the form of hemosiderin, and iron deficiency may be produced after several years.

CHAPTER 21
Cardiac Arrhythmias
H. LEON GREENE AND J. O'NEAL HUMPHRIES

The generation of an impulse in the sinoatrial (SA) node and the orderly spread of this impulse through the heart is essential to the efficient function of the heart. Variation in either the site or rate of impulse formation or variation in the normal sequence of spread of the impulse is termed an arrhythmia and may result in less efficient cardiac function. The severity of the dysfunction depends on both the type of arrhythmia and the associated disease of the heart. The physiology of abnormal impulse formation and transmission, recognition of the various arrhythmias, and their treatment and prevention will be the subject of this chapter. See Chapter 17 for a discussion of special techniques of evaluating and recording arrhythmias.

PHYSIOLOGY AND ANATOMY

Impulse formation can occur at many sites in the conducting system, since many cells in this specialized tissue exhibit the property of spontaneous depolarization or automaticity (Fig. 21-1). Each area of automaticity has its own intrinsic rate of impulse formation, and drugs, pH, hypoxia, and autonomic activity alter this rate. An electrical potential difference between the inside and the outside of the cell is maintained by an energy-requiring system which pumps sodium out and potassium into the cell. The potential difference (polarization) across the cell membrane may be measured by microelectrodes and recorded graphically as shown in Figure 21-1.[68]

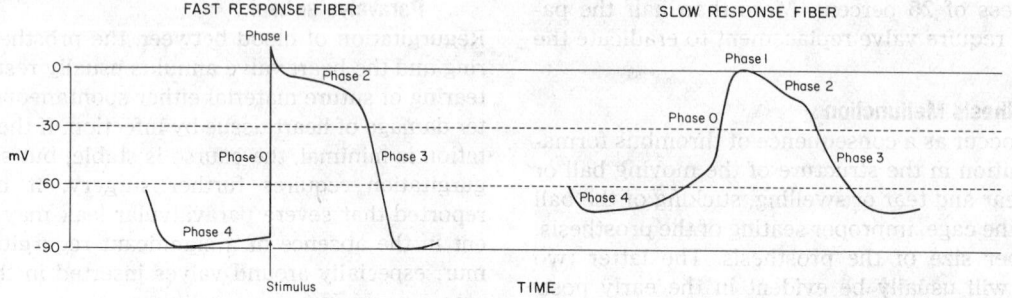

FAST RESPONSE FIBER

SLOW RESPONSE FIBER

FIGURE 21-1. Action potential of cells of the cardiac conducting system. After depolarization during Phase 0, the cell slowly recovers and is fully repolarized by the end of Phase 3. A fast response fiber is illustrated on the left, and a slow response fiber on the right. Although the fast response fiber may have some spontaneous diastolic depolarization during Phase 4, most fibers are stimulated by an outside impulse, usually by propagation of an action potential from an adjacent cell in the conducting system. The slow response fiber, on the right, has a less negative maximum diastolic potential, a slower rate of rise of Phase 0, and has distinctly separated Phases 1, 2, and 3. Working muscle cells and cells in the conducting system outside the SA and AV nodes have action potentials more similar to the fast response fibers, with even less spontaneous diastolic depolarization.

There appear to be two types of cells in the impulse formation and conduction system, one type whose action potential characteristics are dependent upon movement of sodium and potassium ions (fast response fibers), and one type whose action potential characteristics are dependent primarily upon transmembrane calcium currents (slow response fibers).[63,82] Disease processes which alter membrane properties can convert a fast response cell to a cell with properties which resemble slow response cells.

The fast-response cell in the resting state has a potential of −80 to −90 mV (the inside of the cell being negative with respect to the outside). Fast-response cells are located in working atrial and ventricular muscle and in most portions of the conducting system except SA and atrioventricular (AV) nodes. Upon stimulation from an outside impulse or an adjacent cell, membrane potential is brought to threshold, approximately −70 mV, at which time a sudden influx of sodium is accompanied by rapid loss of potential difference and is termed depolarization or phase 0 of the action potential curve. Conduction ve-

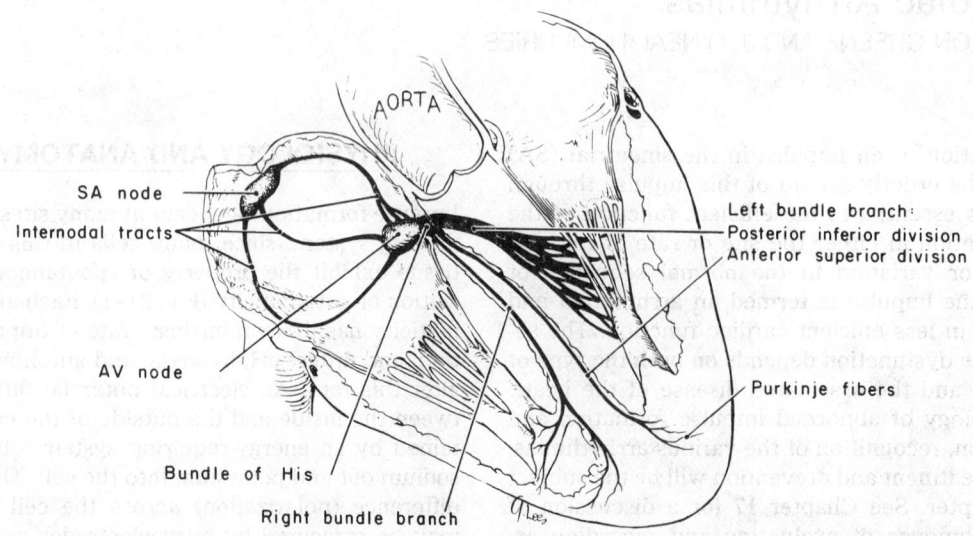

FIGURE 21-2. Anatomy of impulse conduction.

locity is directly related to the rate of rise of phase 0, and fast response cells conduct impulses rapidly (0.5 to 5.0 M per sec). Recovery of polarization occurs slowly during phases 2 and 3. Spontaneous diastolic depolarization (phase 4) occurs slowly in these cells and is caused by a gradual constant leak of sodium ions into the cell as the potassium leak out of the cell progressively diminishes.

Slow-response cells probably occur normally in the SA and AV nodes where the loss of polarization during phase 4 is thought in part to represent slow movement of calcium ions into the cell. Maximum diastolic potential is only -60 to -70 mV, and threshold potential is approximately -45 mV. When not stimulated "prematurely" by an outside impulse, continuous loss of polarization (spontaneous diastolic depolarization) will continue until threshold level is reached, at which time rapid depolarization, phase 0, occurs and an impulse is generated which can be propagated to surrounding cells and tissues. The rate of impulse formation depends on the slope of phase 4, the height of maximal polarization, and the threshold level. The conduction velocity, dependent upon the rate of rise of phase 0, is slow in these fibers (0.01 to 0.1 M per sec).

Under normal circumstances the SA node has the fastest rate of impulse formation. The impulse generated in the SA node normally spreads rapidly through the conducting system to the remainder of the heart, the lower and slower areas of automaticity being depolarized before spontaneous impulse formation occurs. The spread of the impulse in the conducting system is not recorded in the surface electrocardiogram (ECG). However, as the impulses activate the heart muscle cells, electrical forces are generated which produce the electrical forces recorded as deflections in the surface ECG. Activation of the atrial muscle results in the P wave and activation of the ventricular muscle results in the QRS complex. After activation, recovery of excitability is accompanied by the generation of other electrical forces recorded on the ECG as the T wave.

The impulse originating in the SA node (Fig. 21–2) travels rapidly to all parts of the atria and to the AV node, perhaps through specialized conducting pathways, the internodal tracts, in the atria. These pathways are easier to identify in animals than in man. Conduction of the impulse through the AV node is slow. This slow conduction through the AV node is associated with the isoelectric period between the P wave and the QRS and limits the frequency with which impulses originating in the sinus node or atrium can be conducted to the ventricles. Rapid rates of impulse formation in the atria (flutter and fibrillation) are associated with a slower ventricular rate, the exact rate depending on the conduction abil-

---

TABLE 21–1
Autonomic Nervous System

Physiological Functions	Parasympathetic		Beta Sympathetic*	
	Stimulation (Edrophonium)	Inhibition (Atropine)	Stimulation (Epinephrine, Isoproterenol)	Inhibition (Propranolol)
Rate of impulse formation				
SA node	−	+	+	−
AV junction	−	+	+	−
His bundle	0	0	+	−
Purkinje system	0	0	+	−
Conduction velocity				
Atria	+	−	+	−
AV junction	−	+	+	−
His-Purkinje system and ventricles	0	0	+	−

( ) Representative drugs
+ Increases
− Decreases
0 No change
* Alpha sympathetic receptors have no recognized influence on automaticity or conduction.

ity of the AV node. In addition to the normal slow conduction properties of this node, the number of atrial impulses which reach the ventricles may be reduced by drugs, disease, or autonomic activity which impairs conduction.

Beyond the AV node the impulse is again conducted rapidly through specialized conducting fibers. The first portion is the bundle of His which divides into three fascicles, termed the right bundle, the anterior superior fascicle of the left bundle, and the posterior inferior fascicle of the left bundle.[22] Each of these fascicles divides into the many-branched subendocardial Purkinje system. The Purkinje fibers from the anterior superior and posterior inferior fascicles meet distally in the free wall of the left ventricle.

The autonomic nervous system plays a major role in the control of the function of the conduction system, including the rate of impulse formation, rhythm, and conduction velocity (Table 21–1). Cyclic variation in autonomic activity with respiration may cause cyclic variation in the rate of impulse formation by the SA node, a condition termed sinus arrhythmia which is seen normally in children and sometimes in adults.

ARRHYTHMIAS

The significance of an arrhythmia varies not only with the specific mechanism or type of rhythm disturbance but also with the setting in which it occurs and its effect on the ability of the heart to maintain an adequate output. Premature contractions may be a completely benign finding in a healthy individual, but, when noted in a patient taking digitalis or in one with an acute myocardial infarction, may herald more serious and less well-tolerated arrhythmias. A tachycardia of any origin at a rate of 170 or 180 may be well tolerated for long periods of time by a normal heart, but in the presence of organic heart disease such a tachycardia may result in an inadequate cardiac output, severe symptoms, and even death if not quickly terminated. Likewise, the slow idioventricular rate in complete heart block may cause no trouble for decades if myocardial function is good, but results in an inadequate cardiac output and severe symptoms in the presence of a diseased myocardium or significant valvular disease.

When the primary pacemaker is suppressed or its impulse impeded in its passage through the heart, subsidiary pacemakers may take up the function of initiating the heartbeat. Cardiac arrhythmias which develop by this mechanism are termed "escape," "passive," or "default" rhythms. Since the resultant heart rate is slow, it is called bradycardia. In other circumstances the rate of spontaneous impulse formation of one of the subsidiary areas may increase and usurp the pacemaker activity of the heart. Such arrhythmias are termed "active" or "usurpation" rhythms and, because the heart rate is more rapid than normal, are called tachycardias.

The discussion of the arrhythmias is divided into three major sections; bradycardia, premature contractions, and tachycardia.

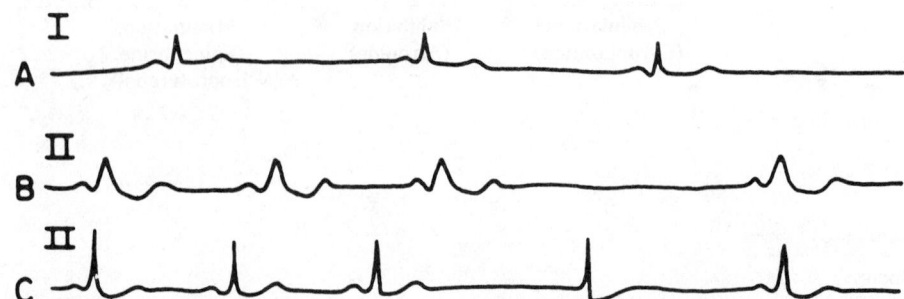

FIGURE 21–3. A. Sinus bradycardia. Atrial and ventricular rate of 37 per minute with a constant PR interval of 0.14 seconds. Chronic 2 to 1 sinoatrial block is an alternative explanation for this form of bradycardia. **B.** Sinoatrial block, 2 to 1. The interval between the third and fourth P wave is exactly twice the normal interval as seen between the first, second, and third P waves. Left bundle branch block pattern is also present. **C.** Sinus arrest. After three normal appearing P-QRS-T complexes there is no evidence of impulse formation or transmission for 1.5 seconds. At that time a QRS appears as a result of an impulse which was probably generated in the atrioventricular junction. This is an escape junctional beat. Before a second escape junctional beat is generated sequential activation of the atrium, atrioventricular node, and ventricle is resumed from the sinoatrial node.

BRADYCARDIA

The term *bradycardia* means "slow heart rate" and usually refers to the ventricular rate. The electrocardiographic features allow slow rhythms to be classified on the basis of mechanism into: (1) those due to defective impulse formation and conduction in the SA node; and (2) those due to defective impulse conduction at the AV node or in the His bundle or fascicles.

Impaired Impulse Formation

Defective impulse formation at the sinus node may be due to sinus bradycardia, sinoatrial block, or sinus standstill (Fig. 21–3).

ELECTROCARDIOGRAPHIC PATTERNS. Sinus bradycardia is recognized by normal P and QRS-T waves occurring at a slow rate. Sinoatrial block (2:1 or 3:1) is recognized electrocardiographically by a sudden decrease in atrial rate by exactly one-half or one-third (Fig. 21–3). Sinoatrial Wenckebach phenomenon is characterized by progressive decrease in P-P intervals, followed by a long P-P interval, then repeat of the cycle. Sinus arrest is characterized by the total absence of activity by the sinus node and cessation of P and QRS complexes on the ECG. Death may occur, but usually after a short preautomatic pause a lower focus initiates one or more impulses until sinus activity returns.

With extreme sinus bradycardia, high degrees of SA block or sinus arrest, the rate of impulse formation by the sinus node falls below the intrinsic rate of junctional cells in or near the AV node, 40 to 60 per minute, and the latter assumes the pacemaker function. This junctional escape rhythm continues to pace the heart until an adequate sinus mechanism returns. There are three ECG patterns associated with junctional rhythms depending upon the site of origin of the impulse which initiates atrial depolarization.[71]

Most commonly, the impulse which is formed in the junctional cells spreads to the ventricle (antegrade) and also back to the atria (retrograde). The P waves are inverted in leads II, III, and AVF and they may precede, coincide with, or follow the QRS complex, depending on the site of origin of the impulse and the comparative velocities of antegrade and retrograde conduction (Fig. 21–4A).

In the second mechanism there is no retrograde conduction of the junctional impulse. The atria are depolarized by an impulse from the very slow SA

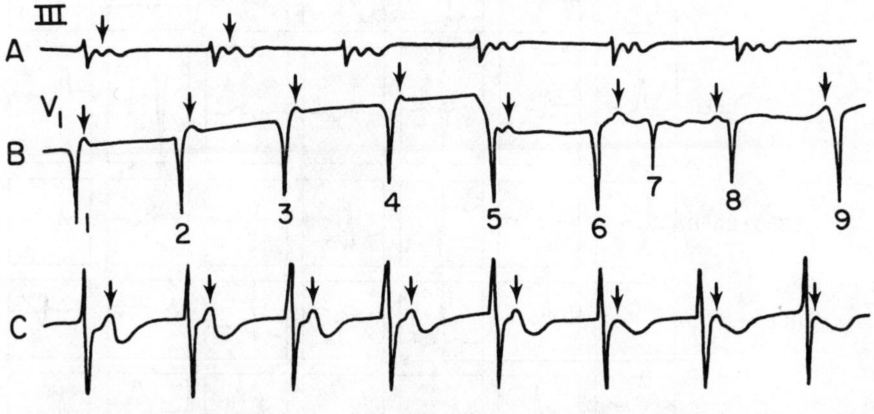

FIGURE 21–4. A. Junctional bradycardia with retrograde activation of the atrium. The P wave follows each QRS. The inverted P wave in this lead and lead II and the upright P wave in lead AVR result from the retrograde depolarization of the atrium. **B.** Junctional rhythm with capture beats also known as AV dissociation. In this strip the QRS complexes numbered 1 to 6 are the result of impulses generated in the atrioventricular junction. However, the atrium continues to be depolarized from an impulse generated in the sinoatrial node at a rate slightly slower than the rate of impulse generation in the atrioventricular junction. The fourth and fifth P waves follow the QRS complex at a time when the atrioventricular node is still totally refractory and thus are not transmitted to the ventricle. However, the sixth P wave occurs during the relative refractory period and is conducted with a prolonged PR interval. **C.** Junctional rhythm with isorhythmic dissociation. The rates of impulse formation in the sinoatrial node and atrioventricular junction are very similar, and the P waves are in close association with the QRS complexes, but sequential activation of the atrium, atrioventricular node, and ventricle is not present.

node, resulting in a normal appearing P wave, while the ventricles are under control of the faster (40 to 60 per minute) junctional cells: dissociation of atria and ventricles. Atrial impulses occurring shortly before, during, or after the QRS will find AV nodal tissue refractory and will not be conducted to the ventricle, but those occurring after the refractory period of the junctional cells will be conducted (capture beats, Fig. 21-4B). This condition has been termed "AV dissociation with capture beats" or "interference dissociation."

The third mechanism, isorhythmic dissociation, is characterized by upright P waves that closely precede, coincide with, or follow the QRS complexes (Fig. 21-4C). Although the atria and ventricles are depolarized almost simultaneously, there is no ante-

grade or retrograde conduction and the mechanism of synchronization is unknown.

ETIOLOGY. Acute stimulation of the parasympathetic fibers to the heart may result in sudden slowing of the heart rate to 40 or below, lowering of blood pressure, nausea, sweating, and weakness. Such vasovagal attacks may follow trauma to the eye, gagging, puncture of the pleura or pericardium, forceful vomiting, or noxious stimulation.

Sinus bradycardia may be normal in athletes or manual laborers. Disorders of impulse formation commonly develop in ischemic heart disease, on exposure to drugs such as digitalis, the Rauwolfia derivatives, beta adrenergic blocking agents, or with profound acidosis or hyperkalemia. Sinoatrial node disease is common in elderly persons due to degener-

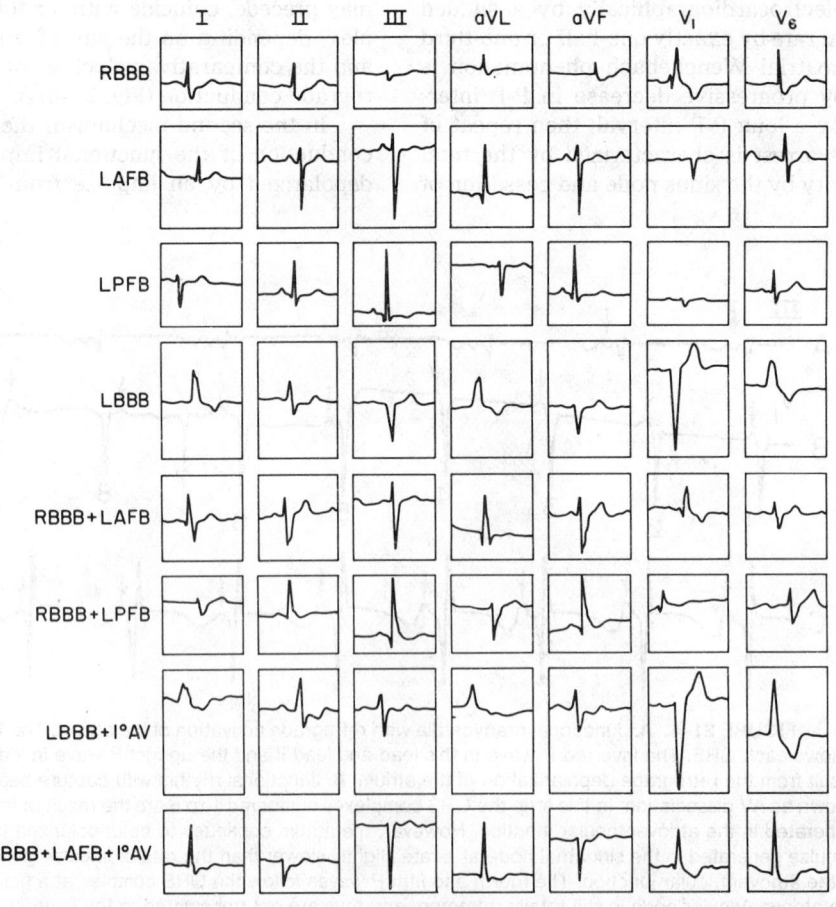

FIGURE 21-5. Electrocardiographic patterns associated with fascicular blocks. RBBB: right bundle branch block; LAFB: left anterior fascicular block; LPFB: left posterior fascicular block; LBBB: left bundle branch block; 1°AV = first degree of atrioventricular block. Upper three patterns (RBBB, LAFB, LPFB) represent unifascicular block; next three patterns (LBBB, RBBB and LAFB, RBBB and LPFB) represent bifascicular blocks; and the bottom two patterns (LBBB and 1°AV, RBBB and LAFB and 1°AV) represent two forms of trifascicular block.

ative processes or coronary atherosclerosis. Approximately one-half of the people with sinoatrial node disease also have disease of the atrioventricular node and/or His-Purkinje system.

Patients with impaired sinus node function are prone to develop premature ectopic beats and paroxysmal tachyarrhythmias, especially supraventricular. The rapid rate during the tachyarrhythmia suppresses the diseased sinus node (overdrive suppression). When the tachyarrhythmia ceases, either spontaneously or in response to therapy, sinus standstill or profound bradycardia can develop. These abrupt alterations in heart rate have been termed the "tachycardia-bradycardia syndrome."

CLINICAL MANIFESTATIONS. The patient with impairment of sinus node function, "sick sinus syndrome," may be entirely asymptomatic. However, the slow rate may lead to an inadequate cardiac output that results in congestive failure, lethargy, loss of mental agility, or azotemia. Also, transient symptoms of insufficient cerebral blood flow, such as giddiness, dizziness, or syncope, are seen. These latter symptoms often appear in patients with the "tachycardia-bradycardia syndrome" immediately following cessation of the tachyarrhythmia, although in some patients the symptoms may be due to the tachycardia itself.[74]

MANAGEMENT OF CONDITIONS CHARACTERIZED BY IMPAIRED IMPULSE FORMATION. The first principle of management is removal of the precipitating cause—e.g., discontinuing vagal stimulation, digitalis, or propranolol or correcting electrolyte imbalance.

Atropine diminishes the vagal effect on the sinus node and is especially important in the prevention and treatment of vasovagal attacks. Sympathomimetic drugs (isoproterenol and ephedrine) may be administered cautiously acutely to accelerate the sinus rate or to enhance SA node function. If the symptoms are chronic or serious and unrelated to any acute reversible process, artificial pacing may be used with success in the vast majority of patients. Atrial or ventricular pacing has been used for SA node disease. Careful search for associated AV node or His-Purkinje disease is indicated if atrial pacing is planned, since many patients will have both. Artificial pacing is discussed in more detail below.

Impaired Impulse Conduction

Conduction of an atrial impulse to the ventricles may be delayed or blocked in the AV node, the bundle of His, the fascicles, or in a combination of these areas.[62]

Delay or block of impulse conduction in one of the three ventricular conducting fascicles produces a characteristic electrocardiographic pattern (Fig. 21-5), termed right bundle branch block (RBBB), left anterior fascicular block (LAFB), or left posterior fascicular block (LPFB). These abnormalities can be caused by coronary artery disease (with or without clinical infarction), valvular heart disease, ventricular hypertrophy and fibrosis, cardiomyopathies, or degenerative processes involving the conducting bundles. Right bundle branch block produces a wide QRS complex with terminal rightward and anterior forces (deep and slurred S in V_6 and lead I, RSR′ in V_1). The QRS duration is usually $\geq$ 0.12 seconds, although RBBB can be seen with a QRS as short as 0.10 seconds. Left anterior fascicular block widens the QRS only slightly to 0.08 to 0.10 seconds, with a small Q in leads I and aVL and a leftward frontal axis deviation ($-45°$, or more characteristically $-60°$). Left posterior fascicular block produces a rightward frontal axis deviation, often $+120°$, with small Q waves in II, III, and aVF and deep S waves in lead I. The QRS duration is only slightly prolonged. Right ventricular hypertrophy, lateral myocardial infarction, and a vertical heart with chronic lung disease must be excluded clinically if a diagnosis of LPFB is entertained.

Combinations of block or delay in any two fascicles can produce additive electrocardiographic abnormalities: RBBB plus LAFB, RBBB plus LPFB, and LPFB plus LAFB which is equivalent to left bundle branch block (LBBB). Impaired conduction in all those fascicles, so-called trifascicular block, can be suspected with a combination of LBBB plus first degree AV block (see below), RBBB plus LAFB and first degree AV block, or RBBB plus LPFB and first degree AV block. However, the first degree block may be produced at the AV node with normal conduction through the third fascicle, so strict definition of the conduction abnormality is difficult or impossible from surface electrocardiography.

Impaired conduction of atrial impulses to the ventricles (AV Block) is classified as follows:

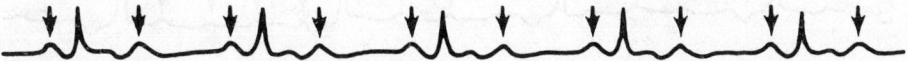

FIGURE 21-6. Incomplete heart block, 2 to 1. Every other P wave (arrows) is not followed by a QRS. The conducted P wave has a normal PR interval, but this is not true in all instances of incomplete heart block. The PP interval containing the QRS is very slightly shorter than the PP interval not containing a QRS complex. This is termed "ventriculophasic sinus arrhythmia."

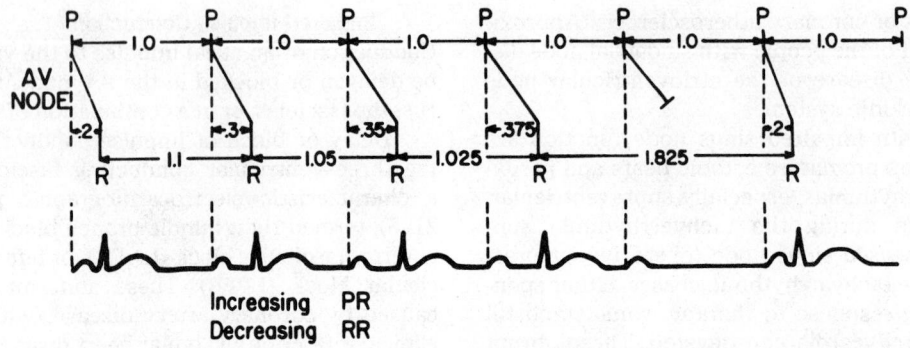

FIGURE 21-7. Schematic representation of the Wenckebach phenomenon where the PP interval remains constant but the PR becomes progressively longer while the RR interval becomes shorter. Note the fifth P wave is not conducted to the ventricle, and results in a dropped beat, which allows the atrioventricular node to rest and thus conduct the sixth P wave with a short PR interval.

First Degree—PR interval greater than 0.21 second

Second Degree (Incomplete)

1. Fixed Rate, e.g., 2:1, 3:1, etc. (Fig. 21-6)
2. Mobitz I (Wenckebach)
3. Mobitz II

Third Degree (Complete)

Various degrees of AV block may be exhibited in a single patient at different times.

Mobitz type I or Wenckebach AV block is identified by a progressive prolongation of the PR interval in each succeeding cycle until a P wave is not followed by a QRS complex (Fig. 21-7). The sequence is then repeated. Also, the R-R interval decreases in each successive cycle until an R wave is dropped, whereupon the sequence begins again. The progressively shorter R-R interval is related to a reduction in the amount of increase in the PR interval in each succeeding cycle. The ratio of P waves to QRS waves may be 2:1, 3:2, 4:3, 5:4, 6:5, and so on, and the ratio may vary from sequence to sequence. Mobitz type II

AV block is rare and characterized by a constant PR interval with an occasional P wave not followed by a QRS. The frequency of the blocked atrial impulses may be regular or varied.

Mobitz type I block (Wenckebach) is most commonly due to abnormal conduction in the AV node, whereas Mobitz type II block is usually due to abnormal conduction in the pathways below the AV node. Ratios of P waves to QRS waves of 2:1, 3:1, 4:1, etc. can represent block either at the AV node or below. Most commonly, it is AV node block, but it can be impossible to differentiate from surface ECGs.

When none of the atrial impulses is transmitted to the ventricles third degree or complete AV heart block is present. Again the block may be at the AV node, in the His bundles, in both bundle branches, or in all three fascicles. If the patient is to survive when complete heart block develops, an area of automaticity in the Purkinje system below the block must pace the ventricles. This escape Purkinje rhythm is usually regular and slow (Fig. 21-8).

The ECG in complete heart block shows a regular ventricular rhythm, with a rate of 40 or below. Occa-

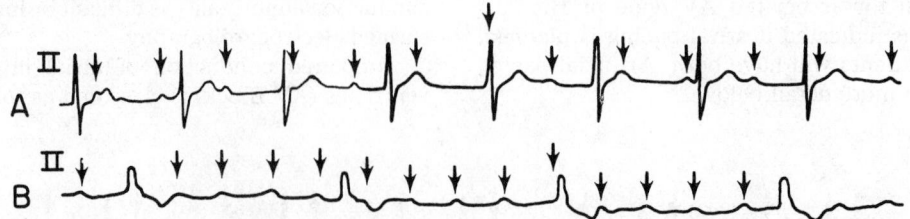

FIGURE 21-8. A. Complete heart block—junctional pacemaker. The narrow QRS complex and relatively rapid rate of 70 per minute indicate that the ventricular pacemaker is relatively high in the atrioventricular junctional tissue. P waves are indicated by the arrows. **B.** Complete heart block—idioventricular pacemaker. The wide QRS complex and very slow rate indicate that the pacemaker is located in the ventricle, usually in the distal Purkinje system.

sionally, the ventricular rate may be as high as 50 per minute, especially in congenital heart block. The atrial rhythm, whether it consists of P waves of SA origin or atrial tachycardia, flutter, or fibrillation waves, is independent of the QRS complexes; thus, the atria and ventricles are under control of different pacing centers and AV dissociation is present. The QRS complex may have a normal configuration if the idiorhythmic center distal to the site of block is located in the AV junction or the bundle of His. A variety of wide configurations resembling bundle branch block may occur if the site of origin of the impulse is in the distal Purkinje system or if intraventricular conduction defects are present. The ventricular rate varies little with the usual stimuli for tachycardia, such as exercise, emotion, and sympathomimetic drugs. An exception to this occurs when the focus of impulse formation is located in the AV junction above the His bundle because the rate may accelerate slightly with atropine or exercise. The regularity of the R-R interval may be interrupted by 1) shifting of the pacemaker to a different part of the Purkinje system; 2) premature ventricular contractions; 3) ventricular asystole or tachyarrhythmia (see below); and 4) temporary reduction in the degree of block so that some beats may be conducted and "capture" the ventricles.

ETIOLOGY. The majority of cases of heart block in the older age group result from degenerative disease in the bundle of His or proximal portion of the Purkinje system; however, all degrees of heart block may occur during an acute myocardial infarction (see Chap. 23).

First-degree and Mobitz type I block are seen frequently in acute rheumatic fever and other infectious diseases producing a myocarditis. Other causes include digitalis, gout, sarcoidosis, tumors, cardiac surgery, cardiac catheterization, and congenital anomalies.

CLINICAL MANIFESTATIONS. Isolated first-degree block is not associated with bradycardia or symptoms. Even second-degree heart block is usually not associated with serious symptoms, but the patient may be aware of slow or irregular heart action. Mobitz type II block usually implies more serious and permanent organic disease of the distal conduction tissue than does the Wenckebach (Mobitz I) type. Mobitz type II block is usually associated with a widened QRS complex.

Third-degree or complete heart block may be associated with low cardiac output and result in a variety of clinical manifestations, including congestive failure. Impaired cerebral, myocardial, or renal function and profound fatigue may result. Of greater importance are the episodic periods of totally inadequate cardiac output—the Stokes-Adams attacks.

Stokes-Adams Disease

Stokes-Adams attacks are defined as the loss of consciousness due to either 1) ventricular asystole; or 2) ventricular tachyarrhythmia in patients with complete heart block.

Transient ventricular asystole may follow the development of complete heart block in a patient with normal sinus rhythm. During sinus rhythm the ECG may be normal or more frequently may show first degree block or an intraventricular conduction defect.[18] Second-degree block is often associated with periods of complete block. Again, transient ventricular asystole may occur when all AV conduction ceases and before an idiorhythmic center below the

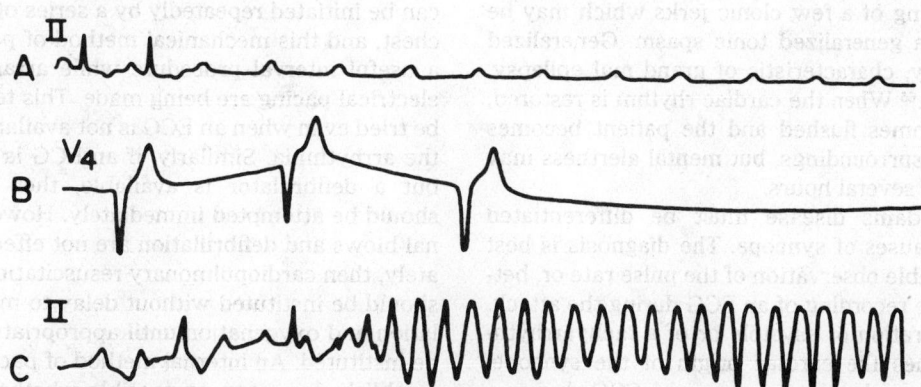

FIGURE 21–9. A. Stokes-Adams attack in a patient with sinus rhythm in whom complete heart block suddenly develops. **B.** Stokes-Adams attack in a patient with complete heart block in whom the idioventricular pacemaker suddenly ceases. **C.** Stokes-Adams attack in a patient with complete heart block in whom ventricular tachycardia suddenly develops.

block assumes the responsibility of pacing the heart (Fig. 21–9A). The complete block of AV conduction usually lasts several seconds or minutes but may persist for days or weeks. Such periods of transient complete block tend to recur, and the patient may have ventricular asystole and a Stokes-Adams attack each time the block develops.

Ventricular asystole also may occur with established complete heart block, since the idioventricular focus may suddenly stop forming impulses. Syncope and death result unless the same or another idioventricular focus begins to make impulses. This is probably the most frequent cause of Stokes-Adams attacks (Fig. 21–9B).

Ventricular tachyarrhythmia (ventricular tachycardia, flutter, and fibrillation—Fig. 21–9C) accounts for 25 to 40 percent of the Stokes-Adams attacks occurring in patients with established heart block. When the escape ventricular rate falls below a critical level in the susceptible patient a tachyarrhythmia develops (a form of the bradycardia-tachycardia syndrome). The critical level varies from patient to patient and from time to time in the same patient. If the idioventricular rate can be maintained above this critical rate, the episodes of tachyarrhythmia can be prevented.

With the typical Stokes-Adams attack the patient loses consciousness suddenly and usually without warning, although the presence of an aura cannot be used to exclude a cardiac origin for the attacks. The patient's skin is pale at first, but if the attack persists for ten seconds or more, it becomes cyanotic. Breathing is abnormally slow and deep, and Cheyne-Stokes respiration is sometimes present. If the cerebral circulation is inadequate for 20 to 30 seconds, convulsive movements may develop with incontinence of urine and feces. The convulsive activity is usually mild, consisting of a few clonic jerks which may be followed by a generalized tonic spasm. Generalized clonic activity, characteristic of grand mal epilepsy, rarely occurs.[65] When the cardiac rhythm is restored, the skin becomes flushed and the patient becomes aware of his surroundings, but mental alertness may be absent for several hours.

Stokes-Adams disease must be differentiated from other causes of syncope. The diagnosis is best made by reliable observation of the pulse rate or, better yet, by the recording of an ECG during the attack. The demonstration of asystole or of a tachyarrhythmia establishes the cardiac origin of the syncope, whereas a normal pulse or a normal ECG during a period of unconsciousness excludes Stokes-Adams disease. Frequently it is not possible to record an electrocardiogram during a time when the patient is having an attack of syncope. In this case an intracardiac electrophysiologic study may be useful to assess conduction times at various sites in the conduction system,[73,75,81] and intracardiac pacing techniques may reproduce the rhythm responsible for the patient's symptoms.[72]

TREATMENT OF HEART BLOCK. The treatment of first- and second-degree heart block consists primarily of removing any causative factor, such as digitalis. Atropine may transiently improve atrioventricular conduction if block is located at the AV node.

Complete heart block whether established and persistent or transient always requires treatment, and artificial pacing is the only acceptable form of therapy. The exception to this rule would be the survivor of certain types of myocardial infarction with transient heart block (Chap. 23) and the asymptomatic patient with congenital heart block with a regular rhythm at a rate which supports an adequate blood pressure and cardiac output.

With rare exceptions, most notably the patient with an acute inferior myocardial infarction, the patient with complete heart block is not improved by the administration of atropine. Intravenous isoproterenol will increase the rate of an idioventricular focus and improve its reliability, and therefore, may be of value in the treatment of complete block. Occasionally, it will improve AV conduction and decrease the block to second or first degree. Isoproterenol should be used only in severely symptomatic patients and only as a temporary measure until artificial pacing can be established. It is not recommended for long-term therapy. Isoproterenol may also cause ventricular irritability or worsen myocardial ischemia.

A strong blow to the precordium may terminate a Stokes-Adams attack, whether the rhythm is asystole or tachyarrhythmia. Occasionally, ventricular systole can be initiated repeatedly by a series of blows to the chest, and this mechanical method of pacing may be a useful interval procedure while arrangements for electrical pacing are being made. This technique may be tried even when an ECG is not available to confirm the arrhythmia. Similarly, if an ECG is not available but a defibrillator is available, then defibrillation should be attempted immediately. However, if external blows and defibrillation are not effective immediately, then cardiopulmonary resuscitation procedures should be instituted without delay to maintain circulation and oxygenation until appropriate therapy can be instituted. An internal method of pacing should be established as soon as possible whether the Stokes-Adams attacks are due to asystole or tachyarrhythmia. Artificial pacing practically always prevents further attacks whether the attack is due to asystole in the patient with intermittent or established complete block or to tachyarrhythmia. Suppressive antiarrhythmic agents should not be used even if the Stokes-Adams attacks are known to be due to tachyarrhythmia unless these arrhythmias persist after pacing is established.

ARTIFICIAL PACEMAKERS. [62] *External Pacemakers.* External pacers are rarely used today because of the availability and ease of insertion of internal pacemakers. External pacers are used only in an emergency situation and deliver repetitive (60 to 120 per minute), large (100 to 150 amps), very short duration (1 to 2

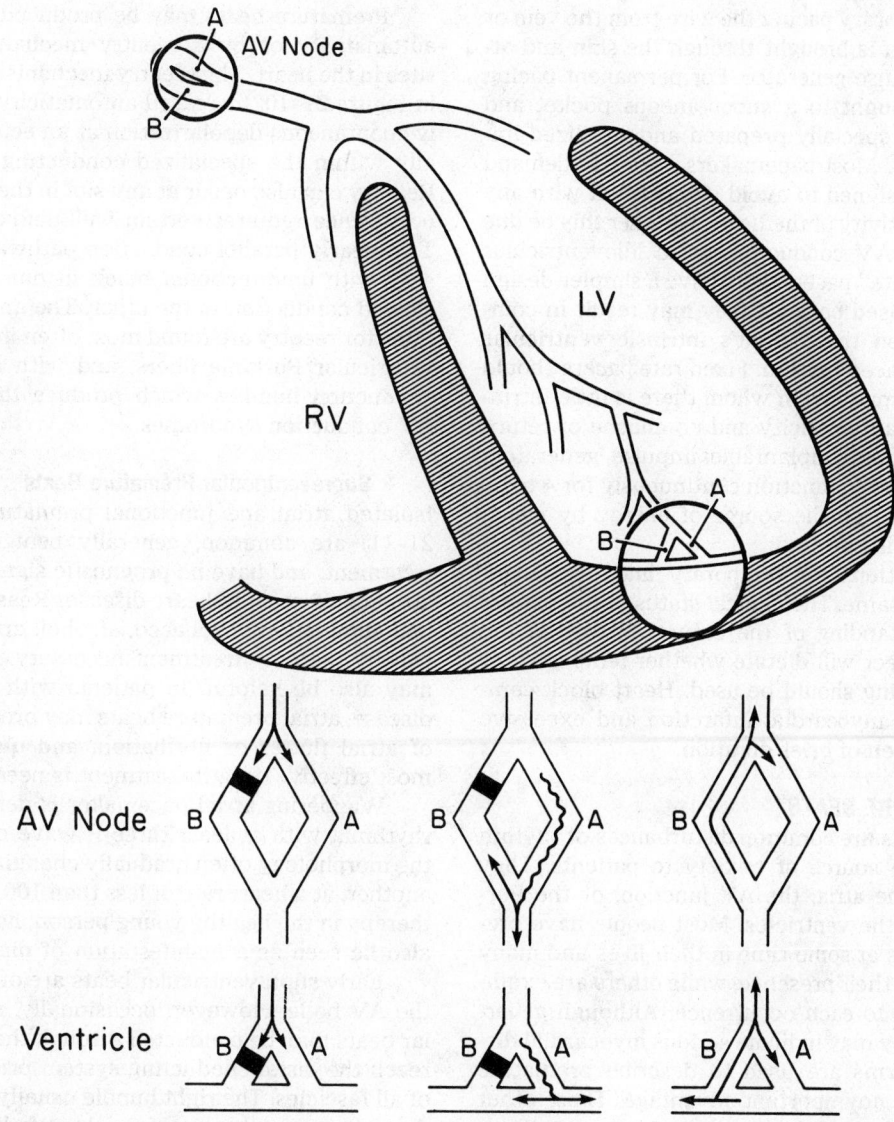

FIGURE 21-10. Reentry mechanisms diagrammed for either the AV node (upper panels) or ventricular Purkinje fibers (lower panels). An antegrade impulse encounters two separate pathways of conduction (A + B), which insert distally into other conducting tissue or myocardium (left panels). Antegrade block (stippled area) prevents conduction in Pathway B, while the impulse is conducted slowly down Pathway A (center panels). The impulse then travels to the distal end of Pathway B and finds it no longer refractory, conducting retrograde to the site of origin of the impulse and again antegrade down Pathway A (right panels). Repetitive impulses can be produced by continued circular activation of the conducting loop. RV = right ventricle; LV = left ventricle.

msec) electrical impulses with large metal paddles applied to the chest wall.

Internal Pacemakers. If the electrical impulse is delivered directly to the heart, then a small quantity of electrical energy (1 to 10 mamp) is required to pace the heart. A battery-powered impulse generator is connected by means of a wire to the endocardium (transvenous endocardial method) or to the myocardium. For temporary pacing the wire from the vein or the myocardium is brought through the skin and attached to the pulse generator. For permanent pacing the wire is brought to a subcutaneous pocket and connected to a specially prepared and sterilized impulse generator. Most pacemakers, termed "demand pacers," are designed to avoid competition with any spontaneous activity of the heart, whether this be due to a return of AV conduction or to idioventricular beats. "Fixed rate" pacemakers have a simpler design but are rarely used because they may result in competition between the patient's intrinsic ventricular beats and the paced rhythm. Fixed rate pacers should be used only in patients in whom there is little intrinsic ventricular automaticity and no chance of return of AV conduction. Implantable impulse generators are now designed to function continuously for 4 to 20 years, depending on the source of energy by which the instrument is powered.

The indications for temporary and permanent pacing are the same. The clinical status of the patient and an understanding of the natural history of the conduction defect will dictate whether temporary or permanent pacing should be used. Heart block complicating acute myocardial infarction and excessive digitalis are often of brief duration.

PREMATURE BEATS

Premature beats are common disturbances of rhythm and a frequent source of anxiety to patients. They may arise in the atria, the AV junction, or the Purkinje fibers of the ventricles. Most people have premature systoles at some time in their lives and many are unaware of their presence, while others are exquisitely sensitive to each occurrence. Although generally benign, they may indicate serious myocardial disease. Other terms are used to describe premature beats but have no important advantage. These other terms include premature contractions, premature systoles, premature complexes, and extrasystoles.

The benign types of premature beats are characteristically most noticeable at the end of the day, usually on resting after dinner or after going to bed. This occurrence at bedtime is frightening and sometimes predisposes to heart consciousness and panic. As the normal sinus mechanism slows, the premature beats may increase in frequency. Premature beats often have a cyclic pattern, appearing for days or weeks and then disappearing for long intervals.

The premature beat may cause a diminished or absent peripheral arterial pulsation. The difference between peripheral arterial and actual heart rate is called a pulse deficit. Repetitive prematures, such as bigeminy or trigeminy may cause an apparent bradycardia as detected at a peripheral artery.

Premature beats may be produced by increased automaticity or by a reentry mechanism at many sites in the heart. The reentry mechanism is described in Figure 21–10. Increased automaticity involves early spontaneous depolarization at an ectopic site, usually within the specialized conducting tissue fibers. Reentry can also occur at any site in the heart, and its occurrence requires certain well-defined conditions. Two nearly parallel conduction pathways are necessary with unidirectional block in one pathway and slowed conduction in the other. The anatomic conditions for reentry are found most often in the AV node, ventricular Purkinje fibers, and with accessory AV conduction bundles which produce the accelerated AV conduction syndromes.

Supraventricular Premature Beats

Isolated atrial and junctional premature beats (Fig. 21–11) are common, generally benign, require no treatment, and have no prognostic significance in the absence of organic heart disease. Reassurance, rest, and elimination of tobacco, alcohol, and caffeine are usually the only treatment necessary. Mild sedation may also be helpful. In patients with organic heart disease, atrial premature beats may precede the onset of atrial flutter or fibrillation, and quinidine is the most effective drug if treatment is needed.

Wandering atrial pacemaker is defined as an arrhythmia with at least three P wave configurations, the morphology often gradually changing from one to another, at a heart rate of less than 100. It requires no therapy in the healthy young person; however, it may also be seen as a manifestation of digitalis toxicity.

Early supraventricular beats are often blocked at the AV node. However, occasionally, supraventricular beats may be conducted through the AV node and reach the distal conducting system prior to recovery of all fascicles. The right bundle usually recovers conductivity after the two fascicles of the left bundle; therefore, it is possible for a conducted premature supraventricular beat to be associated with a right bundle branch block pattern. This is termed aberrant conduction. Occasionally, aberrancy occurs with other types of intraventricular conduction defects. Aberrantly conducted supraventricular beats must be distinguished from ventricular premature beats (Table 21–2) and occasionally this differentiation is impossi-

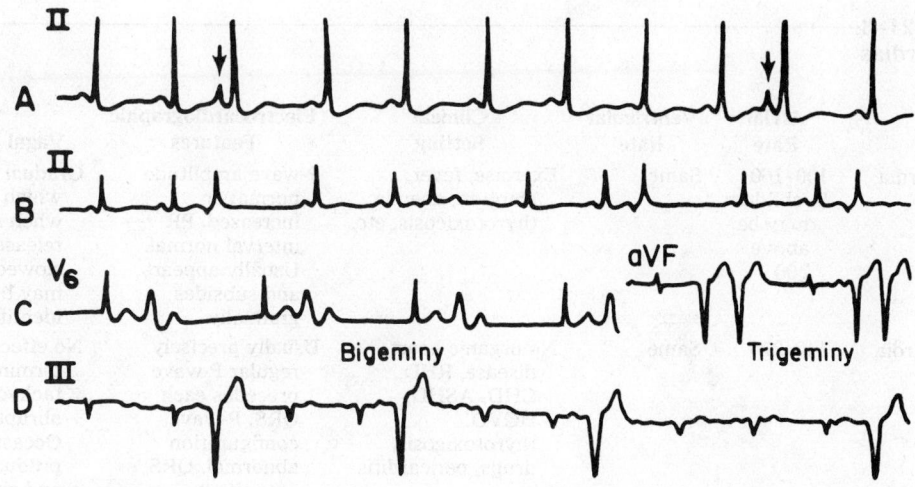

FIGURE 21–11. A. Atrial premature contraction. The P wave associated with the atrial premature contraction (third complex) appears different in configuration from the other P waves. This atrial premature beat is followed by a normal QRS pattern, but such premature beats need not be conducted to the ventricle or may be conducted in an aberrant fashion, simulating right bundle branch block. **B.** Junctional premature contraction. In this case the premature impulse was conducted not only to the ventricles but also to the atria in a retrograde fashion resulting in the inverted P wave. Retrograde conduction is not a necessary part of junctional premature contractions. **C.** Ventricular premature contraction. Lead V₆—The premature ventricular contractions are represented by the wide, bizarre QRS complexes, each of which follows a normally conducted beat. This relationship is termed "bigeminy." Lead aVF—Every normally conducted beat is followed by two premature beats of ventricular origin in this ECG demonstrating trigeminy. A less serious type of trigeminy is characterized by repetitively occurring sequences containing two normally conducted beats and a premature, ventricular beat. **D.** Ventricular premature contractions. In this patient with atrial fibrillation, the interval between the conducted beat and the premature or ectopic beat is the same on each occasion. This fixed relation of the ectopic beat to the conducted beat is termed "fixed coupling."

ble with surface electrocardiography. Intracardiac His bundle recordings may be required to clarify the mechanism of the arrhythmia.

TABLE 21-2
Differentiation of Aberrance from Ectopy

Favors Aberrance	Favors Ectopy
Variable coupling interval	Fixed coupling interval
RBBB pattern	LBBB pattern
Triphasic RSR¹ in V₁	Monophasic or biphasic QRS complex in V₁
No compensatory pause	Compensatory pause
Initial vector of QRS same as other conducted beats	Initial vector of QRS different from conducted beats
P wave preceding QRS which could have been conducted	No identifiable P wave preceding QRS

Ventricular Premature Beats

Ventricular premature beats (VPBs) are common in all age groups but increase in frequency in older patients. The presence of VPBs does not necessarily indicate organic heart disease, although in the presence of heart disease (especially ischemic) the VPB may have grave prognostic significance. The decision to treat VPB's must rest upon the clinical setting.

VENTRICULAR PREMATURE BEATS WITH NO ORGANIC HEART DISEASE. In the healthy patient without other evidence of heart disease, VPBs need not be treated. Rest, reassurance, and elimination of stimulants are the only therapies usually necessary. Occasionally, a patient may be distressed enough by symptoms of palpitations that pharmacologic antiarrhythmic therapy will be undertaken. However, risks of side effects of medications must be considered (Chap. 30). Although the presence of VPBs should stimulate further search for organic heart disease, there is no evidence to show that reduction of VPBs by therapy improves prognosis. Either VPBs at rest, or exercise-induced VPBs are seen more often in patients with occult

TABLE 21–3
Tachycardias

Diagnosis	Atrial Rate	Ventricular Rate	Clinical Setting	Electrocardiographic Features	Vagal Stimulation
Sinus tachycardia	100–160 In children may be above 200	Same	Exercise, fever, emotion, anemia, thyrotoxicosis, etc.	P-wave amplitude normal or increased. PR interval normal. Usually appears and subsides gradually	Gradual slowing which reverses when stimulation is released. When slowed, the P wave may be more easily identified
Atrial tachycardia	140–220	Same	No organic heart disease, RHD, CHD, ASHD, HCVD, thyrotoxicosis, drugs, pericarditis	Usually precisely regular P wave precedes each QRS. P-wave configuration abnormal. QRS may show aberrancy simulating ventricular tachycardia. Rhythm appears and subsides abruptly	No effect or terminates tachycardia abruptly. Occasionally may produce AV block and slow ventricular rate without altering atrial rate
Atrial tachycardia with AV block	140–220	Often a fixed fraction of the atrial rate	Digitalis, ASHD, RHD	RR interval usually two or three times atrial rate but variability may occur if degree of AV block is variable. Differs from atrial flutter by slower atrial rate and isoelectric baseline between P waves	May terminate arrhythmia abruptly, may increase degree of block, or may have no effect
Multifocal atrial tachycardia	>100	Same	Severe underlying disease, often pulmonary	Variable PP, variable PR, multiform P wave morphology	No change or transient slowing
Atrial flutter	220–320	Usually a fixed fraction of the atrial rate	RHD, ASHD, pulmonary embolus, pericarditis, thyrotoxicosis, CHD, digitalis	P or f waves occur with great regularity and result in a typical saw-tooth or picket fence undulation in leads II, III, AVF, V_1 and V_2	No effect or increases the AV block so that a 2:1 block becomes 3:1 or 4:1, etc. May rarely terminate the flutter
Atrial fibrillation		40–300	RHD, ASHD, pericarditis, thyrotoxicosis, CHD, digitalis, pulmonary embolus	Totally irregular RR interval. Baseline may have fine or coarse fibrillatory waves. In some instances no evidence of atrial activity discernible and the diagnosis rests upon the grossly irregular ventricular response	Increase the degree of AV block and a slowing of the ventricular rate

TABLE 21-3 (cont.)

Diagnosis	Atrial Rate	Ventricular Rate	Clinical Setting	Electrocardiographic Features	Vagal Stimulation
Wolff-Parkinson-White syndrome	60–100	60–100	No organic heart disease, CHD, RHD	Short PR interval due to early onset of QRS as a delta wave. Total QRS duration prolonged. P to S interval normal. May simulate posterior infarction or right-ventricular hypertrophy	May increase size of delta wave. With PAT, may terminate tachycardia abruptly or no effect.
AV junctional tachycardia	140–220	140–220	Digitalis, ASHD, RHD, CHD, no organic heart disease	Regular R-wave interval. P wave inverted in leads II, III and upright in AVR. P waves may occur before, with, or after the QRS waves. AV dissociation results in separate atrial and ventricular rates. QRS as in normal sinus rhythm	May have no effect or may terminate tachycardia abruptly
Accelerated junctional rhythm	60–130	60–130	Digitalis intoxication	Same as above except slower rate. QRS as in normal sinus rhythm	No effect or minimal slowing
Accelerated ventricular rhythm	80–130	80–130	Acute myocardial infarction	Rate often very close to sinus rate. Wide QRS complexes similar to VPBs	No effect
Ventricular tachycardia	60–140	140–280	Acute myocardial ischemia or infarction, anoxia, electric shock, digitalis, trauma, no organic heart disease	Broad, bizarre, slightly irregular QRS complexes. Independent and slower P-wave rate can sometimes be determined. Fusion beats may appear	No effect or may very rarely convert to sinus rhythm
Ventricular flutter and fibrillation		300 or greater	Acute myocardial ischemia or infarction, anoxia, electric shock, digitalis, trauma, quinidine	Disorganized, grossly irregular wave pattern	No effect

CHD = congenital heart disease
RHD = rheumatic heart disease
ASHD = arteriosclerotic heart disease
HCVD = hypertensive heart disease

coronary artery disease. However, the presence of VPBs is neither sensitive nor specific enough to be diagnostic of organic heart disease, and alteration in the frequency of VPBs with exercise can occur in either a normal or diseased heart. Another clue to the presence of underlying heart disease occasionally can be obtained by inspection of the T wave of the beat following the premature beat. Inversion of this T wave, termed "postextrasystolic T wave inversion," may be indicative of myocardial disease.

VENTRICULAR PREMATURE BEATS WITH ISCHEMIC HEART DISEASE. Ventricular premature beats in patients with angina pectoris may presage more serious arrhythmias. VPBs during the ischemia of angina pectoris induced by exercise may indicate severe coronary artery disease. Exercise-induced VPBs are more frequent in the recovery period after exercise than during exercise itself. Frequently, these VPBs are asymptomatic, but more severe arrhythmias may produce symptoms of dizziness, light headedness, or syncope. VPBs occurring on the descending limb of the T wave ("R on T phenomenon") can induce ventricular tachycardia or ventricular fibrillation especially during acute ischemia, and multiform VPBs are considered to be more serious than VPBs of a single configuration.

Symptomatic multiform VPBs, "R on T" VPBs, paired VPBs, or ventricular tachycardia should probably be treated in patients with organic heart disease. However, in patients with ischemic heart disease and VPBs, prospective trials of antiarrhythmic agents to attempt to influence mortality favorably have not shown a beneficial effect on mortality with drugs currently available in the United States. The ideal antiarrhythmic agent, which would be effective in suppressing VPBs with no adverse side effects, is not available. Digitalis may improve the arrhythmias if congestive heart failure is present, but the same arrhythmias can also be a manifestation of digitalis toxicity. Exercise conditioning can reduce the frequency of VPBs but may not prolong life.

Ventricular premature beats complicate at least 75 percent of patients with acute myocardial infarction. Sustained ventricular arrhythmias are a major cause of death, particularly in the prehospital phase of acute myocardial infarction (Chap. 23).

VENTRICULAR PREMATURE BEATS WITH OTHER ORGANIC HEART DISEASE. Valvular heart disease, cardiomyopathies, hypertensive disease, and other conditions which frequently induce hypertrophy or congestive failure may be associated with ventricular premature beats. Treatment of the underlying disorder may influence the arrhythmia, although anti-arrhythmic therapy may be necessary for symptomatic

arrhythmias. The effect of digitalis on arrhythmias in the presence of heart failure has already been mentioned, and digitalis toxicity as a cause of ventricular arrhythmias is discussed on page 242.

TACHYCARDIA

The term "tachycardia" means rapid heart rate and usually refers to the ventricular rate. However, rapid atrial arrhythmias may be associated with rapid, normal or even slow ventricular rates depending on the number of the atrial beats which are conducted from the atria to the ventricles. The most frequent cause of a rapid heart rate is an increased rate of impulse formation in the sinus node, sinus tachycardia. However, either a rapid ectopic automatic focus or a sustained reentry mechanism may usurp the pacing of the heart. The tachyarrhythmia is named according to its origin as atrial, junctional or ventricular and according to its rate as accelerated rhythm, tachycardia, flutter or fibrillation.

There are clinical features which are helpful in distinguishing one tachyarrhythmia from another, but an ECG is essential to precise diagnosis. At least one complete 12-lead ECG should be obtained, since atrial activity may be evident in only one lead. At times a recording of the electrocardiogram from the esophagus or right atrium is necessary to see the P waves and identify the tachyarrhythmia. Occasionally, recording of electrical activity from the region of the His bundle with intracardiac catheters can clarify the mechanism of difficult tachyarrhythmias. The clinical and electrocardiographic features of the more common tachycardias are presented in Table 21-3.

CLASSIFICATION AND ETIOLOGY OF THE TACHYCARDIAS

Supraventricular

SINUS TACHYCARDIA. The most common cause of a rapid heart rate is an increase in the SA rate in response to a variety of stimuli, including exercise, excitement or pain, fever, anemia, and hypovolemia. Sinus tachycardia is a compensatory mechanism and does not require treatment other than mangement of any underlying disorder.

ATRIAL TACHYCARDIA (Fig. 21-12). Atrial tachycardia may have one of two mechanisms—an ectopic automatic focus or a reentry circuit—generating impulses at a regular rate of 140 to 220 per minute;[67] the latter mechanism is by far the more common. This rhythm may complicate organic heart disease but often occurs in a patient without other evidence of heart disease, and may last from seconds to days. It has a tendency to recur after spontaneous or iatrogenic termination, and is thus frequently termed paroxysmal atrial tachycardia (PAT). In most circumstances each atrial impulse is conducted to the ventricle, but if disease or drugs impair AV conduction then only every second or more frequently a variable number of atrial impulses are conducted to the ventricle (PAT with block). In practice almost three-fourths of patients with PAT with block have digitalis intoxication.

MULTIFOCAL ATRIAL TACHYCARDIA. Multifocal atrial tachycardia is seen in patients with other severe underlying disease, often chronic lung disease.[70] It is characterized by a heart rate greater than 100, multiform (at least 3) P wave configurations, varying P-P intervals, and varying PR intervals. The high mortality of this arrhythmia is a result of a high mortality of the underlying illness. This rhythm is usually not a manifestation of digitalis toxicity, and digitalis is uniformly unsuccessful in abolishing this arrhythmia.

The only treatment is the management of the primary illness.

ATRIAL FLUTTER (Fig. 21-12). This atrial rhythm is the result of continuous activation of the atria in a circular pathway near the venae cavae (circus movement) which produces a characteristic electrocardiogram. The atrial rate is usually about 300 per minute but may be slower with enlargement of the right atrium as this elongates the circular pathway. Gross atrial enlargement may enhance the development of atrial fibrillation. In a patient with atrial flutter the ventricular rate is rarely equal to the atrial rate, and more commonly one-half, one-third, or one-fourth the atrial rate. A variation in AV conduction may result in an irregular ventricular response despite the regular atrial rhythm. Recognition of atrial flutter when every other flutter (f) wave is conducted to the ventricle may be difficult, since one f wave may be hidden in the QRS complex and the other in the T wave. Atrial flutter with 2:1 conduction should always be suspected when the ventricular rate is 140 to 160 per

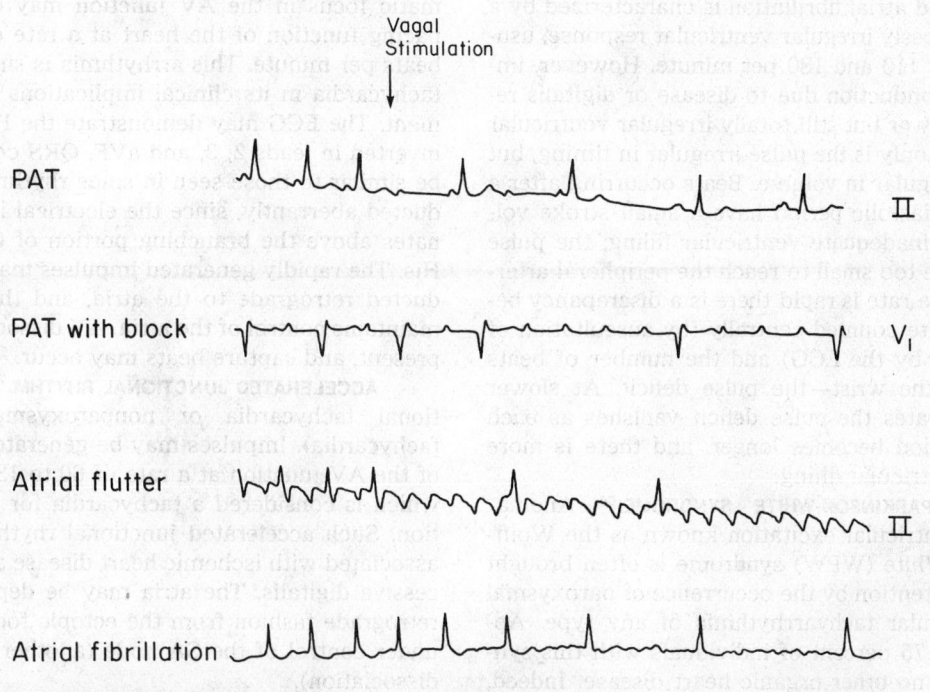

FIGURE 21-12. Common supraventricular tachycardias. The response to vagal stimulation is illustrated in the right-hand two-thirds of each tracing. Top tracing: PAT—paroxysmal atrial tachycardia. Vagal stimulation either will have little detectable effect on the rhythm or will convert it to normal sinus rhythm. Second tracing: PAT with block. Antegrade block is increased, but normal sinus rhythm rarely ensues. Third tracing: atrial flutter. AV block is increased, making flutter waves easier to identify, but conversion to normal sinus rhythm does not occur. Bottom tracing: atrial fibrillation. AV block is increased, making the atrial fibrillation waves easier to identify, but atrial fibrillation persists.

minute, especially if atrial activity is negative in leads 2, 3, and aVF and located halfway between the QRS complexes. It must be distinguished from atrial and junctional tachycardia as well as from sinus tachycardia. Vagal stimulation by retarding AV conduction may reduce the number of conducted atrial impulses and reveal easily identified flutter waves between widely spaced QRS complexes.

Atrial flutter may be impure with an irregular atrial cycle length. This type blends with coarse atrial fibrillation, and the two arrhythmias may exist at different times in the same patient. Impure flutter, coarse fibrillation, or flutter-fibrillation responds to therapy much more like atrial fibrillation than like pure atrial flutter and thus is best considered with fibrillation.

ATRIAL FIBRILLATION (Fig. 21-12).   One of the most common arrhythmias complicating organic heart disease is fibrillation of the atria. It may be seen in the absence of heart disease, terminate spontaneously, and tend to recur (paroxysmal). However, the onset of atrial fibrillation may call attention to previously unrecognized disease of the heart and it may suggest that left atrial enlargement is present.

Untreated atrial fibrillation is characterized by a rapid and grossly irregular ventricular response, usually between 110 and 180 per minute. However, impaired AV conduction due to disease or digitalis results in a slower but still totally irregular ventricular rhythm. Not only is the pulse irregular in timing, but also it is irregular in volume. Beats occurring after a very short diastolic period have a small stroke volume due to inadequate ventricular filling; the pulse wave may be too small to reach the peripheral arteries. When the rate is rapid there is a discrepancy between the rate counted centrally (by auscultation of the heart or by the ECG) and the number of beats counted at the wrist—the pulse deficit. At slower ventricular rates the pulse deficit vanishes as each diastolic period becomes longer, and there is more effective ventricular filling.

WOLFF-PARKINSON-WHITE SYNDROME.[66]   Anomalous atrioventricular excitation known as the Wolff-Parkinson-White (WPW) syndrome is often brought to clinical attention by the occurrence of paroxysmal supraventricular tachyarrhythmia of any type. Approximately 75 percent of individuals with this syndrome have no other organic heart disease. Indeed, the presence of a paroxysmal supraventricular tachyarrhythmia in a normal person should alert the examiner to the possibility of this disorder, and a careful search for the specific ECG abnormality described in Table 21-3 should be made. An ECG taken during a paroxysm of arrhythmia usually does not betray the characteristic short PR interval and delta wave. The electrocardiographic features of this syndrome are inconstant and variable, and an ECG taken during a period of sinus mechanism may not always exhibit the characteristic abnormalities. Atrial fibrillation in the WPW syndrome presents unique features mimicking ventricular tachycardia with rapid, irregular, wide, and slurred QRS complexes.

Treatment of the WPW syndrome is directed at 1) eliminating premature beats which initiate paroxysmal tachycardias; 2) equalizing refractoriness in all atrioventricular connections; 3) blocking conduction in the anomalous pathway; 4) slowing impulse conduction in portions of the reentry circuit; or 5) surgical excision of the anomalous pathway. Recent electrophysiologic techniques have allowed 1) testing to maximize efficacy of drug therapy; and 2) endocardial mapping with electrode catheters to localize the site of anomalous atrioventricular connections to guide surgical therapy.

JUNCTIONAL TACHYCARDIAS.[79]   (Rapid junctional tachycardia, paroxysmal junctional tachycardia). A reentry mechanism or more rarely an ectopic automatic focus in the AV junction may dominate the pacing function of the heart at a rate of 140 to 220 beats per minute. This arrhythmia is similar to atrial tachycardia in its clinical implications and management. The ECG may demonstrate the P waves to be inverted in leads 2, 3, and aVF. QRS complexes will be similar to those seen in sinus rhythm unless conducted aberrantly, since the electrical impulse originates above the branching portion of the bundle of His. The rapidly generated impulses may not be conducted retrograde to the atria, and the sinus node maintains control of the atria. AV dissociation is then present, and capture beats may occur.

ACCELERATED JUNCTIONAL RHYTHM.[79] (Slow junctional tachycardia or nonparoxysmal junctional tachycardia). Impulses may be generated in the area of the AV junction at a rate of 60 to 130 per minute which is considered a tachycardia for the AV junction. Such accelerated junctional rhythms are often associated with ischemic heart disease and use of excessive digitalis. The atria may be depolarized in a retrograde fashion from the ectopic focus or remain under control of the SA node (another cause of AV dissociation).

Ventricular

ACCELERATED VENTRICULAR RHYTHM.[77] (Slow ventricular tachycardia, accelerated idioventricular rhythm). A focus in the Purkinje system of either ventricle may initiate impulses only slightly faster than the sinus node, about 80 to 130 per minute, and compete for control of the heart rhythm. This rhythm is often seen in patients with acute myocardial infarction and usually generates a sufficient cardiac output and blood pressure. It does not necessarily herald ventricular fibrillation (see Chap. 23), nor does it protect against ventricular fibrillation.

VENTRICULAR TACHYCARDIA. Sudden cardiac death is the leading cause of mortality in the United States. It accounts for 400,000 to 500,000 deaths per year. It is almost always due to ventricular tachycardia that degenerates to ventricular fibrillation and is usually a complication of serious organic heart disease, particularly atherosclerotic coronary artery disease with acute ischemia or infarction. Other primary coronary causes include spasm, emboli, congenital anomalies, arteritis, or dissecting aortic aneurysm. Ventricular tachycardia and fibrillation occur frequently with cardiomyopathies. Other causes are valvular disease including mitral valve prolapse, accelerated AV conduction syndromes, long QT syndromes, hypertensive heart disease, and myocarditis and pericarditis. Most often ventricular tachycardia at a rate of 120 to 280 occurs in short paroxysms, although rarely a sustained ventricular tachycardia can continue for weeks.

Treatment of the WPW syndrome is directed at 1) eliminating premature beats which initiate paroxysmal tachycardias; 2) equalizing refractoriness in all atrioventricular connections; 3) blocking conduction in the anomalous pathway; 4) slowing impulse conduction in portions of the reentry circuit; or 5) surgical excision of the anomalous pathway. Recent electrophysiologic techniques have allowed testing to maximize efficacy of drug therapy and endocardial mapping with electrode catheters to localize the site of anomalous atrioventricular connections. Without retrograde conduction the atria remain under control of the sinus node and AV dissociation is present. Less commonly, retrograde conduction can occur. Ventricular tachycardia usually causes severe impairment of cardiac function, and efforts to terminate the rhythm should always be initiated promptly. Degeneration of the ventricular tachycardia into ventricular fibrillation is a constant and grave threat.

It is not always possible to distinguish rapid ventricular tachycardia from a supraventricular tachycardia, but a narrow or normal QRS complex favors the latter. Wide QRS complexes with no specific bundle branch block pattern favor a ventricular tachycardia, while wide QRS complexes with a typical RBBB or LBBB pattern may be seen in an atrial or nodal

tachycardia if these impulses are conducted through the Purkinje system with aberration. AV dissociation may be seen in a junctional or ventricular tachycardia but not in atrial tachycardia. Dressler beats, single narrow QRS complexes occurring earlier than the tachycardia beats, may be seen in ventricular tachycardia but not atrial or junctional tachycardia. The Dressler beat is due to a "capture" of the ventricles by the atria. In a junctional tachycardia with AV dissociation and aberrant ventricular conduction, a "capture" beat would always have a QRS at least as wide as the aberrant junctional beat itself.

VENTRICULAR FLUTTER AND FIBRILLATION. Ventricular flutter and fibrillation occur in the same setting as ventricular tachycardia and may alternate with this arrhythmia. Ventricular fibrillation always causes total collapse of the circulation. The ECG shows a totally disorganized, irregular, and impure fluctuation of the baseline.

CLINICAL MANIFESTATIONS, EVALUATION AND MANAGEMENT OF THE PATIENT WITH TACHYCARDIA

Evaluation of the history and physical findings is the first step in the management of any arrhythmia, and, although in emergencies it may be abbreviated, it must never be omitted. Information may be derived from questioning of the patient, the family, and the referring physician or by the examination of available medical records, including ECGs of previous episodes. Age, blood pressure, radial and apical pulse rates, and regularity of the pulse are data which may be obtained quickly. The physician should observe the patient's mental state and respirations and look for pallor, cyanosis, sweating, or restlessness. Valvular heart disease, shock, and signs of pulmonary congestion may be noted. The careful clinician derives significant information from inspection and palpation of the arterial and venous pulsations and by auscultation of the heart, but the precise diagnosis is most often established by electrocardiography.

A rapid ventricular rate may be due to almost any of the above mentioned arrhythmias, the nature of which may be revealed on the routine electrocardiogram, but with very rapid rhythms this may be difficult. A careful search for P waves on the routine ECG or on electrocardiograms obtained from the esophagus or the right atrium is indicated in all patients with tachycardia. Clearly seen flutter or fibrillatory waves distinguish these arrhythmias. P waves with a normal configuration before each QRS favor a sinus or atrial tachycardia; inverted P waves before or after each QRS favor a junctional tachycardia or rarely a ventricular tachycardia; and P waves independent of the QRS (AV dissociation) favor a junctional or ventricular tachycardia. One of four responses may follow vagal stimulation by the Valsalva maneuver, carotid sinus massage, gagging, intravenous infusion of pressor agents, or intravenous edrophonium (Tensilon) infusion 1) slight slowing of the atrial and ventricular rate identifying a sinus tachycardia; 2) increased AV block with no change in the atrial rate but slowing of the ventricular rate, allowing a better view of the P wave configuration of a tachycardia, flutter, or fibrillation; 3) no change, allowing no conclusion; or 4) termination of the arrhythmia. A totally irregular ventricular rhythm is strong evidence for atrial fibrillation, but slight irregularity may be seen in nodal or ventricular tachycardia due to conducted or capture beats.

Paroxysmal tachyarrhythmias may occur in patients without underlying heart disease and often exhibit a tendency to recur at irregular intervals. Paroxysmal atrial and junctional tachycardia (PAT and PJT) syndromes are the most common, paroxysmal atrial flutter and fibrillation syndromes are infrequent, and paroxysmal ventricular tachycardia and fibrillation syndromes are less common. Periods of stress, anxiety, exhaustion, excessive use of tobacco and stimulants (including coffee), and excitement enhance the possibility of precipitating one of the paroxysms of tachyarrhythmia in the susceptible individual. Any particular episode may last from seconds to days. Most end spontaneously but medical therapy may be needed. Precise diagnosis of the type of arrhythmia and the underlying heart disease is necessary because therapy must be individualized. Occasionally, intracardiac electrophysiologic studies are necessary to define the arrhythmia mechanism and dictate treatment.

Any of the arrhythmias except ventricular fibrillation may be well tolerated for a long period of time, especially in the absence of organic heart disease. However, symptoms such as palpitation, fear, breathlessness, pallor, sweating, weakness, and lightheadedness may result. Syncope or angina pectoris may develop during a supraventricular or ventricular tachyarrhythmia with relief when the rhythm is terminated spontaneously or in response to therapy. This is especially true in patients with atherosclerosis of the cerebral or coronary vessels. Syncope may also be due to total cardiac asystole or extreme bradycardia following the termination of a tachyarrhythmia. Prolonged rapid heart action may induce pulmonary edema, peripheral edema, shock, myocardial ischemic pain, or frank cerebral or myocardial infarction.

Ischemia of other organ systems is less common, but impaired renal function may result during severe attacks. On the other hand, supraventricular tachycardias can induce profound diuresis with hypotension secondary to intraventricular volume depletion.

The tachyarrhythmias which result in ventricular rates in the normal range are better tolerated and may be present for a long time without apparent change in cardiac function. These include accelerated junctional and ventricular rhythms. These rhythms are often associated with severe digitalis intoxication (page 242) or ischemic heart disease (Chap. 23). Atrial flutter may be associated with a slow ventricular rate and be well tolerated. However, maintenance of the proper ventricular rate is difficult, and it is usually advisable to eliminate atrial flutter if possible. Atrial fibrillation very commonly is associated with a normal ventricular rate, especially if an appropriate amount of digitalis is being used to slow AV conduction. Even with a normal rate cardiac function is not as good during atrial fibrillation as during sinus rhythm. This may be particularly apparent during periods of stress. Also a patient with atrial fibrillation has a greatly increased risk of systemic, and to a lesser extent pulmonary, emboli—especially in the presence of valvular heart disease.

The most critical presentation of any arrhythmia is with inadequate cardiac output and circulatory collapse. This rarely occurs in the absence of serious organic heart disease or a major cardiovascular catastrophe. Although any of the arrhythmias may produce this state if the underlying disease of the heart is advanced, the most frequent disturbance is ventricular tachycardia or ventricular fibrillation. The clinical picture is dominated by shock, left ventricular failure, severe chest pain, cyanosis, and, sooner or later, unconsciousness.

Management of Rapid Arrhythmias

The principles of management of an acute episode of a rapid arrhythmia are the same whether the specific problem is a paroxysm in the patient with a normal heart or a sustained tachycardia with circulatory embarrassment. The speed with which the physician proceeds to drug therapy or electroshock, however, varies with the severity of the clinical condition. The steps in management can be divided into four stages: 1) sedation and removal of offending stimuli, 2) vagal stimulation, 3) cardioactive drug therapy, and 4) electroshock. The physician rarely is forced to progress to the fourth stage of therapy when treating paroxysmal atrial or junctional tachycardia, but may omit stages 1 and 2 when dealing with ventricular tachycardia, and omit stages 1, 2, and 3 when dealing with circulatory collapse.

STAGE 1: SEDATION AND REMOVAL OF OFFENDING STIMULI. When there is no evidence that the circulation is compromised by the arrhythmia the physician may administer a barbiturate or diazepam which may, in conjunction with rest, allow the arrhythmia to terminate spontaneously. Any offending stimulus should be removed. If the rhythm persists for several hours or if evidence of circulatory difficulty develops, then the physician should move to stage 2.

STAGE 2: VAGAL STIMULATION AND SEDATION. Vagal stimulation is a useful diagnostic procedure as well as a form of therapy. It is important, whenever possible, to make an electrocardiographic record of the effects of vagal stimulation. The responses which may occur and their significance are tabulated in Table 21-4. It is wise to start with the Valsalva maneuver. The patient is instructed to hold his breath and strain down vigorously as if attempting to have a bowel movement. If reversion does not follow sedation and the Valsalva maneuver, carotid sinus stimulation may be tried in younger patients and in those who have no evidence of cerebral arterial disease. The patient should be in a recumbent position, and the ECG should be recorded. The bifurcation of the right carotid is located and massaged against the transverse processes of the spine. A 3-to-5 second period of gentle massage is often successful, but if not, a similar procedure may be followed on the left side. Simultaneous massage of both carotids should never be done; vigorous massage of atherosclerotic carotids should be avoided, and vagal stimulation is contraindicated with digitalis toxicity, because it may cause emergence of dangerous rhythm disturbances.

If all of these procedures fail and the arrhythmia must be terminated quickly, several choices are available. A very effective method of obtaining strong vagal activity is the intravenous administration of one or two doses of 5 mg of edrophonium. This short acting anticholinesterase may terminate the arrhythmia in one to five minutes. The Valsalva maneuver, carotid sinus massage, or the gag reflex may be again utilized at the peak of edrophonium effect. If the patient is a young, normotensive individual with an otherwise normal heart, the next step may be the use of pressor amines, which raise the blood pressure and thus stimulate the vagal pressor receptors in the aorta and carotid. Metaraminol (Aramine) is commonly administered in this situation in an intravenous infusion of 50 mg per 500 ml of 5 percent glucose. The blood pressure is monitored and the infusion continued until systolic pressures of 160 to

180 mm Hg are attained. If reversion does not occur spontaneously, carotid sinus massage should be repeated. The pressor drugs are particularly effective in patients with hypotension, but excessive elevation of the blood pressure should be avoided in the older age group. Morphine might be used at this time. Mor-

---

TABLE 21-4
Reversion of Atrial Flutter and Fibrillation

I. Purpose

1. To restore control of the heart rate to the sinus node.
2. To restore synchronous atrial and ventricular activity.
3. To reduce the incidence of systemic and pulmonary emboli.

II. Reversion Is Particularly Indicated When Atrial Flutter or Fibrillation:

1. Appears as a result of a nonrecurrent stimulus such as cardiac catheterization or surgery.
2. Is of recent onset. If cardiac surgery is anticipated, reversion may be postponed until after operation.
3. Is associated with hyperthyroidism. Reversion should follow control of metabolic state.
4. Appears following cardiac surgery. Reversion should be postponed until 6–12 weeks after operation.
5. Is symptomatic. Palpitation and easy fatigue develop after mild exercise.
6. Is associated with a history of recent embolism. Anticoagulants should usually be administered for 4–6 weeks before reversion is attempted.

III. Situations Where Reversion Is Unlikely To Be Sustained

1. Long-standing arrhythmia—especially in association with a large heart and large left atrium.
2. History of previous reversion with relapse while receiving quinidine or procainamide— not applicable in patients with paroxysmal arrhythmias.
3. Unrelieved mitral-valve disease or a dilated left atrium—occasionally reversion is worthwhile even though sinus rhythm persists for only a short period.

IV. Situations Where Reversion Is Dangerous

1. Evidence of digitalis intoxication.
2. Known left-atrial thrombus.
3. High degree AV block.
4. Sinus node disease.

phine works by potentiating the action of the vagus but also may bring about reversion by providing sedation or by producing nausea, a powerful vagotonic stimulus. Morphine can be given to patients with heart disease as well as to those with normal hearts. In older individuals or in patients with severe organic heart disease or severe lung disease, it is often wise to use cardioactive drugs before proceeding to pressors or morphine.

STAGE 3: CARDIOACTIVE DRUG THERAPY (See Chap. 30). Before using cardiac glycosides (digitalis), suppressant drugs (quinidine, procainamide, lidocaine, disopyramide, or diphenylhydantoin), or beta sympathetic blockade, the diagnostic possibilities must be reconsidered, since the order in which drugs are used varies. If the arrhythmia is supraventricular, the first step is digitalization and then beta sympathetic blockade, but if the tachycardia arises in the ventricle suppressant drugs should be used first.

Digitalization may accomplish one of two things in a supraventricular arrhythmia. The drug may cause termination of the arrhythmia, especially atrial and fast junctional tachycardias, and atrial flutter and fibrillation of recent onset. If the drug does not terminate the arrhythmia, it will reduce the number of impulses reaching the ventricle by its action on AV node conduction and result in a slowing of the ventricular rate. With the administration of the appropriate amount of digitalis the ventricular rate can be maintained between 60 and 90 per minute. This control of ventricular rate can reliably be accomplished in atrial fibrillation, only occasionally in atrial flutter, and only rarely in atrial and fast junctional tachycardia. Thus, if tachycardia or flutter persist after digitalization, other types of efforts to terminate the arrhythmia are indicated. Repetition of vagal stimulation may be successful now as a result of the vagal potentiating effects of digitalis. If repeat vagal stimulation is ineffective, then a suppressant agent, beta sympathetic blockade, or electroshock should be used. The clinical status of the patient, previous responses to therapy, and the experience of the therapist are factors which determine which of these approaches is most appropriate. Drugs should be administered as outlined in Table 30–2. Electroshock could be used at this time, but caution should be exhibited if there is the possibility of recent digitalis toxicity. The technique of overdrive pacing of the right atrium has been used to terminate supraventricular tachycardia and flutter and has proved to be especially useful if large amounts of digitalis have been recently administered and in patients with severe pulmonary disease. It is easily performed in conjunction with a diagnostic in-tracardiac electrophysiology study or routine cardiac catheterization.

If the arrhythmia is of ventricular origin, the cardiac suppressant drugs should be used before digitalis, although the cardiac glycosides are not definitely contraindicated or deleterious. Cardiac glycosides sometimes restore normal sinus rhythm in patients with ventricular tachycardia, particularly if congestive heart failure is playing a role in the arrhythmia.

Of particular importance is the recognition of the Wolff-Parkinson-White syndrome, since patients who have this syndrome may not respond to digitalization and are better managed by the suppressive drugs. In fact, the lack of response of a rapid supraventricular arrhythmia to vagal stimulation and digitalization may be a clue to the recognition of the Wolff-Parkinson-White syndrome. This is particularly true for atrial fibrillation, where large doses of digitalis may fail to slow or may actually increase the ventricular rate. Beta sympathetic blockade with propranolol also may be of use in the treatment of paroxysms of tachycardia in this syndrome.

STAGE 4: ELECTROSHOCK. Electroshock is the treatment of choice in ventricular tachycardia that has failed to respond immediately to lidocaine. Ventricular fibrillation requires the use of electroshock as promptly as possible. The patient's cardiorespiratory function should be maintained artificially until defibrillation can be accomplished. Indeed, electroshock should be employed even in supraventricular arrhythmias with circulatory embarrassment.

Management of Atrial Fibrillation

The first goal of treatment in atrial fibrillation is to gain control of the ventricular rate. Conduction at the AV node is blocked by digitalis. The net result is the passage of fewer impulses through the node, a slowing of ventricular rate, and an improvement in the cardiac efficiency. Commonly with a rapid ventricular response to atrial fibrillation, some impulses are conducted aberrantly, and these wide QRS complexes should not be confused with premature ventricular contractions. Additional digitalis is indicated in this situation but may be incorrectly withheld if the ECG is misinterpreted.

In the absence of nausea, or severe heart failure and collapse, it is preferable to administer digitalis in fractional oral doses over a period of time sufficient to observe the cumulative effects. When the situation is urgent or when the patient is vomiting, digitalis may be given intravenously in fractional doses at one to four hour intervals. Enough digitalis is generally given to slow the ventricular rate to about 70 beats per minute at rest, with reasonable rate increase under the stress of light exercise. As the ventricular rate is slowed, the pulse deficit will be eliminated. Failure of the ventricular rate to slow after digitalis administration in the patient with atrial fibrillation demands careful reappraisal with particular care taken to identify the Wolff-Parkinson-White syndrome, acute pulmonary embolism, severe lung disease with chronic cor pulmonale, hyperthyroidism, constrictive pericarditis, cardiomyopathy, or anemia.

Recently blockade of beta sympathetic activity has been introduced for the management of atrial fibrillation and a rapid ventricular response in patients with good left ventricular function. Intravenous propranolol will slow the ventricular rate in a few minutes and is preferable to digitalis when the rate must be controlled quickly. Oral propranolol may accomplish ventricular slowing effectively in some patients in whom the vigorous use of digitalis has failed.

REVERSION OF ATRIAL FIBRILLATION. Patients with atrial fibrillation of recent onset who have minimal heart disease and little evidence of decompensation may revert to normal rhythm spontaneously or within a matter of days after the institution of digitalis. For this reason aggressive measures to revert such patients are unwarranted. Patients with advanced heart disease of any type usually do not revert spontaneously. Table 21–4 lists groups of patients for whom aggressive attempts at reversion are indicated after the achievement of an optimum state of hemodynamic compensation.

Reversion can be achieved by the use of such suppressive drugs as quinidine or procainamide and by electroshock. The use of quinidine or procainamide is important to prevent relapse to atrial fibrillation.

Digitalis and quinidine (or digitalis and procainamide) are given sequentially in the pharmacologic attempt to revert atrial fibrillation, quinidine or procainamide being administered only after adequate digitalization (Table 21–5). Quinidine and procainamide slow the atrial rate and simultaneously block the vagal effect of the AV node, thereby increasing conduction. Digitalis, by its vagal effect on the AV node, will prevent the acceleration of the ventricular rate by quinidine and procainamide. Quinidine or procainamide may change atrial fibrillation to atrial flutter, and unless a high degree of block is maintained at the AV node by digitalis, atrial flutter with 1 to 1 conduction and a very rapid ventricular rate may result.

It is good practice to take an ECG before each quinidine dose to detect cardiac toxicity, manifest as

TABLE 21–5
Elective Reversion of Atrial Flutter or Fibrillation

I. **Usual Procedure**
 1. Digitalization (Table 30–3)
 2. Quinidinization—dose in grams

	Days	
	1	2
6 A.M.	0.2	0.3
9 A.M.	0.2	0.3
Noon	0.2	0.3
3 P.M.	0.2	0.3
6 P.M.	0.2	0.3
Total	1.0	1.5

 3. Omit digitalis on Days 2 and 3 (day of electroconversion)
 4. Continue quinidine 0.3 g q 6 hr evening of Day 2 and on Day 3 (Day of electroconversion)
 5. Time of electroconversion: ECG monitoring, intravenous infusion, variety of airways available
 6. Maintenance after conversion (by drug or electroshock). Quinidine 0.6 to 1.2 g daily and digitalis or procainamide 1.0 to 2.0 g daily

II. **Alternate Procedure**
 1. Digitalization
 2. Day 1: Omit digitalis. Quinidine 0.3 g q 6 hr
 3. Day 2: Omit digitalis. Quinidine 0.3 g q 6 hr and electroshock (See I-5 above)
 4. Day 3: Maintenance drugs (See I-6 above)

QRS prolongation greater than 25 percent of control QRS duration or the development of ventricular irritability. Reversion may occur after several days on a given dosage schedule; therefore, it is undesirable to increase the dose too rapidly. Immediate electrocardiographic check is desirable whenever a regular pulse is observed. Although this observation usually means that normal sinus rhythm has replaced the fibrillation, other regular rhythms may have supervened, such as atrial flutter with 3:1 or 4:1 block, or an accelerated junctional rhythm with atrial fibrillation and high-degree AV block. Institution of quinidine therapy in patients who have been digitalized can cause release of digitalis, probably from peripheral sites, causing a rise in serum digitalis levels and manifestations of digitalis toxicity.

A disadvantage of quinidine therapy is that the physician cannot select the moment of reversion. The patient may be unattended at the time of reversion, when ventricular fibrillation or asystole may occur.

With electrical cardioversion the patient is under close observation at the moment of conversion and one can deal promptly with any untoward event. These considerations have led to the current use, in many institutions, of moderate daily doses of quinidine (1.0 to 2.0 g) as preparation for electrical conversion. Thus the high, potentially toxic doses of quinidine which may be required for reversion are avoided.

One achieves successful reversion of atrial fibrillation with electroshock in about 90 percent of patients. Unfortunately, 50 to 60 percent of unselected patients successfully converted to sinus rhythm will revert to atrial fibrillation within one year's time, and greater than 90 percent will have relapsed in three years.[69] However, atrial fibrillation of short duration, atrial flutter, a small heart, and correction of the disorder precipitating the atrial fibrillation favor successful conversion and maintenance of normal sinus rhythm. The preliminary use of anticoagulants for three to four weeks will reduce the risk of embolization at the time of reversion.

One of the complications of electroshock has been the development of other rhythms suggestive of digitalis toxicity. Thus, one should omit digitalis for a day or two prior to electrical countershock, particularly in patients who have been given higher than usual dosage or who show clinical or electrocardiographic evidence of digitalis intoxication.

Prevention of Recurrence of Arrhythmias

In the paroxysmal supraventricular arrhythmias, any precipitating factors should be eliminated, such as excessive fatigue, the use of tobacco, alcohol, coffee, or tea, and stimulant drugs (such as amphetamines or ephedrine). A thorough search for such organic disease as thyrotoxicosis, pulmonary emboli, pheochromocytoma, and occult heart disease is mandatory. If attacks of paroxysmal supraventricular arrhythmias continue after the removal of precipitating factors or if there is organic heart disease with atrial flutter or fibrillation the patient should be maintained on digitalis. Maintenance doses of suppressive drugs can be used in combination with digitalis.[78] Blockade of beta sympathetic activity with propranolol may be useful to prevent recurrent attacks of supraventricular or ventricular tachycardia which recur in spite of digitalis and suppressive drug therapy. Continuous intravenous infusion of lidocaine is indicated following termination of ventricular tachycardia or fibrillation but must be replaced by oral quinidine or procainamide for long-term prophylaxis. Electrophysiologic testing with electrode catheters can detect ventricular electrical instability and can assess the effective-

TABLE 21-6		
Common Digitalis-induced Arrhythmias		
Impulse Formation	**Impulse Conduction**	**Premature Beats**
Sinus bradycardia	1° ⎫	VPBs
Sinus arrest	2° ⎬ Heart	Ventricular tachycardia
Sinus exit block	3° ⎭ block	
PAT ± AV block		Junctional premature beats
Atrial flutter		Nonparoxysmal junctional tachycardia

ness of antiarrhythmic therapy in preventing recurrences of ventricular tachycardia or fibrillation.[72]

Rarely, an arrhythmia, especially ventricular tachycardia, can be prevented by maintaining the heart rate above a critical level. This may be accomplished with an artificial pacemaker. This technique of overdrive suppression as prophylactic management of tachyarrhythmias has been particularly useful in patients with ventricular irritability complicating an acute myocardial infarction or open heart surgery. In the absence of AV heart block even atrial pacing may prevent recurrent attacks in these patients.

DIGITALIS TOXICITY

The most serious undesired effect of the cardiac glycosides is an arrhythmia (Table 21-6). Many of the arrhythmias produced by digitalis may occur spontaneously, so that when observed in digitalized patients their origin is often controversial. Serum radioimmunoassay for digoxin or digitoxin levels may be useful in evaluating patients in whom digitalis toxicity is suspected (Chap. 30). Approximately two-thirds of patients with digitalis intoxication will develop anorexia or nausea before the arrhythmia. At times this warning is not recognized as indicating an excess of digitalis. Other less common complications include bizarre neurologic disorder, personality changes and psychosis, visual disturbances, diarrhea, gynecomastia, and eosinophilia.

Treatment of Digitalis Intoxication

The method of treatment of digitalis intoxication depends on the type and severity of the adverse reaction but always includes at least temporary discontinuance of the drug (Table 21-7). The more threatening tachycardias are treated by the administration of intravenous potassium. From 40 to 100 mEq/L of 5 percent dextrose should be infused cautiously over a period of hours with electrocardiographic monitoring.

┌─────────────────────────────────────┐
│ **TABLE 21-7** │
│ **Treatment of Digitalis Intoxication** │
│ │
│ 1. Omit or reduce dose │
│ 2. Correct electrolyte or acid–base disorders │
│ 3. Suppressive drugs for ventricular │
│   tachycardia/fibrillation (procainamide, lidocaine, │
│   phenytoin) │
│ 4. Beta sympathetic blocking drugs │
│ 5. Pacemaker for severe bradycardia │
└─────────────────────────────────────┘

In most cases of digitalis intoxication characterized by a high degree of AV block, it is best not to give potassium unless the serum potassium concentration is known to be low because potassium infusion can aggravate or produce AV block.

Although caution must be exercised in the use of lidocaine and procainamide in digitalis-induced ectopic ventricular tachycardias, these drugs can be lifesaving. They must not be used when AV block is present because they may depress the only pacemaker capable of generating an impulse or increase the degree of heart block. Quinidine should not be used because of its tendency to worsen digitalis toxicity, presumably by releasing peripheral stores of digitalis. The use of electrical countershock in the treatment of digitalis-induced arrhythmias should be reserved for those resulting in circulatory collapse.

The beta-adrenergic blocking agent, propranolol, has also been used to treat digitalis-induced arrhythmias. However, it can increase the degree of AV block, and it must be used with caution in patients with congestive heart failure.

The most satisfactory approach to digitalis poisoning is to prevent it. Total elimination of digitalis intoxication seems unlikely, since the variability of dosage from patient to patient is so great. Indeed, even in the same patient there may be a change in the quantity of the drug which can be tolerated. Patients have become severely intoxicated on a maintenance dose that had been satisfactory for several years. Increased sensitivity to the drug may develop with advancing years, progression of the underlying heart disease, or progression of renal disease (the primary route of elimination of digoxin). Other situations where an increased sensitivity is noted include hypokalemia, hypercalcemia, acidosis, such infiltrative diseases of the myocardium as amyloid, sinus bradycardia, sinoatrial block, and AV block. Patients with chronic lung disease and cor pulmonale without severe hypoxia or electrolyte disturbances, thyrotoxicosis, and Wolff-Parkinson-White syndrome probably do not have increased sensitivity, but overdosage may follow an effort to slow a cardiac rate that is not responsive to digitalis. Digitalis intoxication occurs as frequently with one preparation as with another. The shorter-acting ones are more rapidly excreted, and toxic effects can be more promptly reversed.

CHAPTER 22
Thoracic Pain and Angina Pectoris
NICHOLAS J. FORTUIN AND RICHARD S. ROSS

Thoracic pain may have its origin in the various tissues of the chest wall, the neck, the intrathoracic structures, or areas below the diaphragm. When the pain arises in the skin or superficial structures it usually can be localized accurately by the patient. When it arises in deeper structures it may be diffuse and difficult to localize, or it may radiate in such a pattern as to mislead both patient and physician into believing that the abnormality lies beyond the limits of the thorax. This apparent lack of relationship between the location of the pain and the site of the lesion is explained by the fact that many thoracic structures, including the heart, the aorta, the pleura, and the esophagus, are supplied by sensory fibers from the

same segments of the spinal cord. The afferent fibers from the heart and pericardium are carried principally in the sympathetic nerves, but some reach the central nervous system by way of the vagus and phrenic nerves. The phrenic nerve also carries the pain fibers from the pericardium, diaphragm, and diaphragmatic pleura, and this pathway accounts for the referral of pericardial pain to the trapezius region and to the shoulder.

The cause of cardiac pain is not known with certainty. The myocardium and the pericardium can be the source of cardiac pain, but pain probably does not originate in the coronary arteries. Available evidence indicates that the myocardium itself gives rise to pain when coronary blood flow is inadequate. Inadequate coronary blood flow may be the consequence of obstructive disease in coronary arteries or of the imposition of an extreme demand on the myocardium in the presence of normal vessels, as in the case of aortic valve disease, hypertrophic cardiomyopathy, or systemic hypertension. Experimental observations indicate that reduced coronary blood flow can cause pain, but whether hypoxia or a buildup of some metabolite is responsible is not known.

PATHOPHYSIOLOGY OF MYOCARDIAL ISCHEMIA[85,86,91]

When the oxygen requirements of the myocardium exceed the supply of oxygen derived from coronary blood flow, the myocardium becomes hypoxic. The factors determining myocardial oxygen demand and oxygen supply are shown in Figure 22–1 and the consequences of ischemia are listed at the bottom. This diagram can be utilized to explain the way various factors precipitate angina and how various therapeutic measures bring about relief.

The major factors determining oxygen demand are heart rate, left ventricular wall tension, and the contractile state of the myocardium. Heart rate is increased in exercise, excitement, and as a response to catecholamine stimulation. Wall tension is directly proportional to ventricular volume and arterial blood pressure, and inversely proportional to the thickness of the ventricular wall. The larger the left ventricular volume the higher the oxygen cost per unit of work. Because of this, therapeutic measures which allow the ventricle to operate at a smaller volume are beneficial. The contractile state of the myocardium is most commonly altered by catecholamines or sympathetic stimulation, both of which shift the heart to a steeper function curve (Fig. 18–1), increase the rate of tension development in the myocardium, and hence, increase the oxygen cost.

The factors influencing supply are coronary blood flow and the oxygen-carrying capacity of the blood. In most situations the oxygen content is not important, and the most important factors in supply are coronary blood flow which is determined by aortic pressure and coronary vascular resistance. For this reason any disease such as atherosclerosis which alters coronary vascular resistance is important. The distribution of flow as well as total flow are of importance in providing oxygen to the myocardium. The inner subendocardial regions of the ventricle are especially liable to ischemia. Catecholamine stimulation by increasing the rate of tension development decreases the flow to the endocardium.

Pain and electrocardiographic changes are the common clinical manifestations of myocardial ischemia. The impairment of ventricular function is of importance because it initiates positive feedback loops which may tend to perpetuate the ischemic condition. The poorly functioning ventricle may dilate and this increases wall tension and oxygen consumption, which tends to aggravate the ischemic condition. The

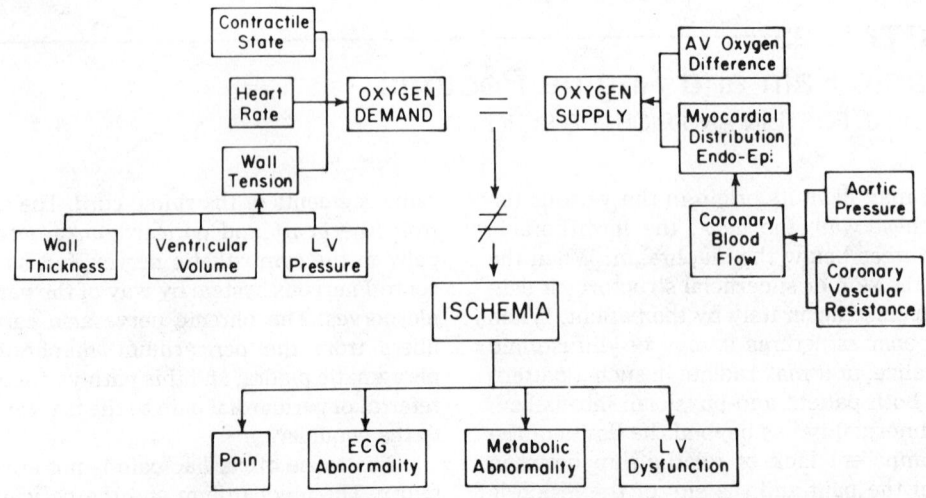

FIGURE 22–1. The pathophysiology of myocardial ischemia. The factors contributing to myocardial oxygen requirement are listed at the left. The factors regulating myocardial blood flow are listed at the right and the consequences of myocardial ischemia at the bottom of the figure.

rise in end diastolic pressure which accompanies left ventricular dysfunction is due to an acute alteration in ventricular compliance. This may also reduce subendocardial blood flow in diastole. Ventricular dysfunction may also lead to decreased arterial pressure and, hence, lower coronary perfusion pressure. The metabolic consequences of ischemia are many but the most thoroughly studied is the shift from aerobic to anaerobic metabolism which results in production of lactate by the heart. This is detected as a concentration of lactate in the coronary sinus blood which exceeds that in the arterial blood. The metabolic products of anaerobic metabolism may be important in the production of the pain of myocardial ischemia and are an important stimulus to coronary vasodilation.

Obstruction of one of the major extramural coronary arteries by an atherosclerotic plaque is responsible for myocardial ischemia in most patients with angina pectoris. Usually two or more coronary arteries are involved with significant narrowing. Proximal narrowing of a single vessel is the cause in a minority of patients, and a small percentage will show no definite evidence of atherosclerosis as detected by coronary angiography. Disease of small intramural coronary arteries may be the cause of myocardial ischemia in some of these patients. Arteriographic studies of the coronary arteries have documented the occurrence of reversible coronary artery spasm as a cause for some instances of myocardial ischemia. Spasm may occur in normal arteries or at the site of an atherosclerotic plaque. In addition to atherosclerosis, other causes of coronary artery obstruction include embolic disease, which is particularly likely in the presence of mitral valve disease, ostial obstruction from syphilitic aortitis, dissecting aortic aneurysm, Takayasu's arteritis, and other large vessel arteritides including polyarteritis and giant cell arteritis.

ANGINA PECTORIS[89,93]

Typical angina pectoris can be recognized easily. It is substernal in location and almost never inframammary or strictly precordial. Radiation into the left shoulder and down the inner aspect of the left arm into the ring and little fingers is frequent but not universally present. The character of the discomfort is often "visceral" in quality and will be described by the patient as squeezing, constrictive, oppressive, or similarly vague in nature and usually is not described as a "pain." It may also be characterized as stabbing, sharp, burning, or even tingling. "Numbness" is another word sometimes used by the patient. Sometimes the patient is not aware of discomfort but complains of dyspnea, a symptom which frequently accompanies pain. The right arm, neck, jaw, and throat may be occasional sites of radiation. Rarely, the pain is felt in these areas alone, and the chest is not involved. The discomfort usually persists for 1 to 5 minutes. Sharp, shooting pain lasting for only a few seconds or aching discomfort of several hours duration are unlikely to be due to myocardial ischemia.

The distribution and character of the pain are far less specific in establishing the diagnosis than its relationship to exertion, which is the most important feature of angina pectoris. The patient experiences pain on exertion that subsides or disappears when he rests. The amount of exertion required to produce the pain varies from day to day, but the relationship is qualitatively the same. The patient usually will say that its appearance makes him stop what he is doing. If the pain subsides while exercise continues at the same rate, it is unlikely to be angina. Distress may be provoked sooner and by less activity in cold weather or may occur more readily after eating or during emotional upset. The patient with typical angina pectoris cannot continue exertion at the same rate after the pain appears but sometimes can do more work after a brief period of rest. This so-called second-wind, or warm-up phenomenon, frequently is noted in the morning when the patient is unable to shower or shave without discomfort but within an hour is able to walk several blocks to the office.

Relief of the pain by rest is an important characteristic of angina pectoris, but the response to nitroglycerin also is important. Most patients who benefit are relieved in 3 to 4 minutes after placing the tablet under the tongue and, in many instances, after only 20 or 30 seconds. Equivocal relief or relief which comes only after ten or more minutes makes it unlikely that myocardial ischemia is responsible for the pain. The diagnosis of myocardial infarction must be considered if pain characteristic of myocardial ischemia persists for 20 minutes to an hour. The physician must remember that failure of nitroglycerin to relieve pain can be due to deterioration of the preparation as a result of age and exposure to heat, light, or moisture. This should be suspected if the patient reports that the side effects (headache, throbbing in the throat, and flushing) previously associated with the administration of the drug are now absent. The response to nitroglycerin can be helpful in establishing the diagnosis of angina pectoris, but it should never be the principal evidence on which the diagnosis is based.

STABLE AND UNSTABLE ANGINA

Patients with angina pectoris can be categorized into stable and unstable groups. Stable angina indicates that the pain has been present for some time (months to years), occurs predictably with exertion, and is alleviated rapidly by rest and nitroglycerin. In such patients there may be times when angina occurs more frequently, such as during periods of emotional stress, or periods when angina occurs infrequently. Patients with stable angina may experience pain without physical exertion, for example, after a heavy meal, during emotional upset, or when asleep during a traumatic dream experience, but there always is some event which is responsible for increasing myocardial oxygen demands.

Unstable Angina Pectoris

When ischemic cardiac pain occurs at rest without obvious provoking factors, with minimal effort, or for prolonged periods, the patient is said to suffer with *unstable angina pectoris*, a syndrome that stands in an intermediate position between stable angina pectoris and acute myocardial infarction. Other terms for this syndrome include preinfarction angina, crescendo angina, intermediate coronary syndrome, and acute coronary insufficiency. The unstable angina syndrome includes a variety of clinical presentations. Patients may experience angina for the first time with exertion and then note a crescendo pattern of increasing angina with less and less effort. Or, patients with stable angina may note an increase in the frequency of pain and a decrease in the amount of effort required to bring on pain. Angina may occur at rest or may be of increased duration and severity and require more nitroglycerin for relief. Other patients with this syndrome present with prolonged episodes of ischemic pain which resemble acute myocardial infarction but without subsequent laboratory confirmation of muscle necrosis. Such episodes may occur repeatedly. Common to each presentation is the occurrence of myocardial ischemia with minimal or no obvious increase in myocardial oxygen demands. This implies a recent change in the coronary circulation's ability to deliver oxygen, usually due to worsening or new coronary artery obstruction, although there is no clinical evidence of myocardial infarction. Thrombus formation on a preexisting area of atherosclerosis, hemorrhage into an atherosclerotic plaque, or coronary spasm all may play some role in the etiology of this syndrome.

Variant (Prinzmetal's) Angina[89]

Patients with this unusual form of unstable angina experience recurrent episodes of typical anginal pain at rest often in spite of well-preserved effort toler-

ance. The causal role of myocardial ischemia in the patient's pain may be difficult to establish unless an electrocardiogram is recorded during an episode of pain. In contrast to patients with chronic stable angina who demonstrate ST segment depression with myocardial ischemia, patients with variant angina show ST segment elevation, often of striking degree resembling acute infarction, which disappears with relief of the anginal attack. Coronary spasm may play an important role in the production of this syndrome. One-third of patients show no evidence of coronary atherosclerosis, and the remainder have major proximal obstructing lesions. Reversible spasm of both diseased and normal coronary arteries in association with the clinical manifestations of the syndrome has been observed by coronary angiography during spontaneous attacks or may be provoked by vasospastic agents such as ergot alkaloids.

Angina Decubitus

Some patients may awake with angina not associated with dreaming after they have spent several hours in the recumbent position. This is termed angina decubitus. This clinical presentation is analogous to paroxysmal nocturnal dyspnea and is due to the increased oxygen demands which occur with fluid shifts into the vascular compartment resulting in increased ventricular volume. This situation usually indicates marginal ventricular compensation and severe coronary obstruction.

DIFFERENTIAL DIAGNOSIS OF ANGINA PECTORIS

Differentiation of ischemic heart pain from other, sometimes trivial, conditions responsible for chest discomfort may present a difficult problem. The layman's knowledge that ischemic heart disease causes thoracic pain and that it may be associated with sudden death complicates the problem for the physician. Table 22–1 lists some of the more common and important causes of episodic thoracic pain that may be confused with ischemic heart pain or that may at times be present in association with it. The most common problem is the differentiation of angina pectoris from chest pain of skeletal or gastrointestinal origin. An approach to this problem is outlined in more detail in Table 22–2.

Gastrointestinal Pain

Pain arising from the esophagus, biliary tract, and less frequently the stomach or duodenum is often confused with cardiac pain because the character and location of the pain may be similar. The relation to exertion is the major differentiating feature. The pain

---

TABLE 22-1
Episodic Thoracic Pain

Presenting Condition	Symptom
Angina pectoris	Substernal visceral discomfort or distress, provoked by effort, emotion, eating, and, occasionally, by lying down. Relieved by rest and nitroglycerin
Pleural pain	Precipitated by breathing or coughing: usually described as sharp. Associated physical and radiographic findings of pleurisy
Esophageal pain	Burning and substernal, with occasional radiation to the shoulder. Nocturnal occurrence (when lying flat). Relief with food or antacids or sometimes nitroglycerin
Peptic ulcer	Nearly always infradiaphragmatic and epigastric. Nocturnal occurrence and daytime attacks relieved by food. Not worsened by activity
Biliary disease	Usually under right scapula, prolonged in duration. Biliary disease is more important as triggering mechanism for angina than as a mimic
Cervical disc	History of injury is common; may be provoked by activity. Persists after activity is discontinued. Local palpation and movement may produce pain
Arthritis-bursitis	Usually of long (hours) duration. Local tenderness or pain with movement
Neurocirculatory asthenia (vasoregulatory asthenia)	Prolonged aches in various chest locations (often with arm radiation) likely to come at the end of an active day. Lethargy and fatigue; sighing respiration
Hyperventilation	Tingling in circumoral area or hands; anxiety. Usually marked complaints of breathlessness without evidence of lung disease
Chest wall (musculoskeletal)	Provoked by movement, especially twisting, bending, etc. Usually long-lasting and often associated with local tenderness
Psychoneurosis	Virtually always after anxiety; poorly described complaints; inframammary location of pain

---

of reflux esophagitis is not usually accentuated by exertion or relieved promptly by rest. Eructation may ameliorate reflux pain but may also be beneficial to some patients with angina. Antacids may provide relief in gastrointestinal disease but do not affect cardiac pain. The response of ischemic cardiac pain to nitroglycerin is not specific since esophageal spasm which often accompanies reflux esophagitis, may be relieved by this drug. Passage of a gallstone or acute cholecystitis and esophageal spasm may produce episodic retrosternal pain which is easily confused with the acute cardiac pain of prolonged ischemia or infarction.

The differentiation of these conditions is made more difficult because ECG changes may accompany the gastrointestinal disorders and disease in the gastrointestinal tract may serve as a trigger for acute cardiac events.

Musculoskeletal Pain
The skeletal system may be the source of pain which can be mistaken for angina pectoris. Such pains may originate from arthritis or lesions in the cervical spine, or from intercostal neuritis or myositis. Skeletal pains frequently are brought on or aggravated by exertion. Walking or working with the hands, with the associated motion of the thoracic skeleton, results in pain. The hyperventilation of walking is associated with an increase in the intensity of the pain originating in the chest wall or diaphragm. In contrast to angina pectoris, skeletal pains usually are slow to subside and persist for several hours at a low level of intensity after a bout of activity. Skeletal pain may be present when the patient awakens and before he has gotten out of bed. Angina pectoris appears often while he is washing, shaving, and dressing.

A common cause of chest pain is muscle or ligament strain, frequently brought on by unaccustomed exercise and located in the costochondral or chondrosternal junction or chest wall muscles. Localized tenderness is usually present, and the pain is often clearly related to movements involving the painful site. Deep breathing, turning, or twisting, and movements of the shoulder girdle and arm often will elicit the pain. The discomfort may be brief, lasting for only a few seconds, or it may last for several hours. There-

---TABLE 22-2---
Differential Diagnosis of Angina Pectoris

General Features	Angina Pectoris	Skeletal Pain	Gastrointestinal Pain
Family history	Premature death in male relatives		
Past history	Diabetes, hypertension, obesity, and hypercholesterolemia	Trauma to neck or back	Indigestion
Onset of illness	Usually certain of month of onset, if not specific day	Uncertain of date of onset	Uncertain of date of onset
Duration of illness	Usually not more than five years without objective manifestations (i.e., ECG changes)	May have been present for many years	May have been present for many years and seasonal in occurrence
Individual Attack			
Precipitation	Effort is prime precipitator. Also may come with emotion, food, and, occasionally, on lying down	Skeletal motion or hyperventilation—associated with effort rather than work, per se	Nervous tension and food Relation to effort is vague or absent
Duration	Until effort stops. Disappears 1 to 3 minutes. Patient cannot continue. Must stop	May last many minutes to hours after rest. Patient can continue effort	Variable Up to several hours
Relief	By cessation of effort. Administration of nitroglycerin often, but not always, successful	Change in position, heat, and aspirin	Change in position, eructation, milk, or bowel movement. Nitroglycerin may be effective
Nocturnal attacks	May be awakened from sound sleep. Relief by sitting up Rare in absence of angina of effort	Trouble falling asleep	Early morning hours. Relief by antacid. May never occur in daytime or on exertion
Time of day	More likely soon after arising Shaving, washing. Effort after meals	Worse in evening, especially after day of physical exertion	Anytime. Related to food, recumbency, tension
Season and weather	Less exertion will bring on in cold weather	Worse in winter and damp weather	No relation

fore, it is often possible to distinguish it clearly from angina, which has a duration intermediate between the two extremes. Musculoskeletal pain is often sharp and sticking in the affected site but may extend upward to the shoulder and into the neck. It is aggravated by rotation of the head or forceful downward traction of the shoulder, and there may be associated circulatory disturbances in the arm.

EVALUATION OF THE PATIENT WITH CHEST PAIN
History
A careful history by an experienced physician is the most important diagnostic test for the patient with chest pain. Information about the location, character, radiation, duration, and precipitating and alleviating factors of the pain will establish the diagnosis in the

majority of patients. There is no correlation between either the duration or the severity of the complaint and the etiology of the pain. Although many physicians continue to put great emphasis on the radiation of pain into the left arm or shoulder, this is of limited value in the differential diagnosis, since conditions other than angina pectoris produce such radiation. The physician must not forget that pain provoked by activity and relieved by rest may have nothing to do with cardiac stress but rather may be caused by shoulder and neck movements during exercise.

Patients with chest pain as a manifestation of an emotional disorder are particularly difficult to evaluate. In depressive reactions and anxiety states, chest pain, which may have many features of angina may be a prominent symptom. The physician must be especially careful to establish the proper diagnosis based on objective findings in these patients because the erroneous diagnosis of cardiac disease serves to heighten anxiety creating a cycle leading to severe cardiac neurosis, worsening depression, and job disability. Early recognition of the functional nature of the pain and appropriate reassurance can alleviate the symptom and improve the emotional state. The occurrence of syndromes such as vasoregulatory asthenia or the mitral valve prolapse or Barlow syndrome in high frequency in anxious patients with cardiac complaints adds to the diagnostic difficulty since electrocardiographic changes at rest or with exercise, cardiac arrhythmias, or abnormal physical findings are frequent in these syndromes and may lend credence to the diagnosis of organic cardiac disease.

Even when ischemic heart disease is present, a second disease process often can be identified to explain certain features of the syndrome which do not fit the diagnosis of angina pectoris. Gastrointestinal disease (especially esophagitis), musculoskeletal disease, and emotional disorders frequently are present in patients who have true angina pectoris.

Physical Examination

Careful observation of the patient during the examination may provide information regarding the lability of his cardiovascular system and general emotional status. The deep breathing required for auscultation of the lungs may provoke vague chest complaints. Chest pain due to inflammation of the muscles of respiration can also be provoked by this maneuver and can be clearly differentiated from chest pain of cardiac origin. Variability in blood pressure during the examination indicates lability of cardiovascular control, as does undue cardiac acceleration with a change of position. Dermatographia, cool, moist palms, and unusual blushing may suggest the diagnosis of neurocirculatory asthenia.

Physical examination of the patient with angina pectoris is usually normal when the patient is free of pain. Hypertension, valvular disease, or obesity when present may suggest proneness to coronary artery disease. If, during examination, the patient is experiencing an attack of chest pain, cardiac auscultation should be carried out immediately. A fourth heart sound, reflecting the altered diastolic compliance of the ventricle, is invariably present. Systolic murmurs due to papillary muscle dysfunction and a precordial bulge due to localized ventricular dysfunction may appear transiently.

A most important point is the reproduction of the pain under observation. This may be accomplished by simple maneuvers during the examination, thereby satisfying both physician and patient that the cause of the pain is known and, sometimes, not serious. Manipulation of the neck and percussion of the spine may reproduce pain of skeletal origin. Palpation of the surface of the thorax also may provide evidence of arthritis or cervical disc disease, myalgia, or osteochondritis (Tietze syndrome), or, on rare occasions, may locate tenderness secondary to neoplastic disease of the ribs. When reproduction of the pain by simple means is not possible, reasonable efforts to provoke it by special procedures, such as exercise, electrocardiography, and esophageal perfusion, may be undertaken.

Special Examinations[87]

ELECTROCARDIOGRAM. An ECG taken when the patient is at rest and pain free is often normal but an ECG during an episode of spontaneous pain may provide diagnostic information. The finding of peaked or inverted T waves, ST segment depression or elevation during an episode of pain, and the disappearance of these changes after the episode is firm evidence for myocardial ischemia. Conversely, a normal or unaltered electrocardiogram during episodes of pain provides strong evidence against the cardiac origin of the pain.

EXERCISE STRESS TESTING. The goals of exercise testing are to reproduce the pain under observation, thus allowing an assessment of the electrocardiogram during pain, and to determine exercise capacity. The motor-driven treadmill is the exercise device most commonly in use in the United States, although the stationary bicycle ergometer is equally effective. Most exercise tests utilize gradual increases in work load until pain occurs or the patient's heart rate increases to 80 to 90 percent of the maximum predicted for age (submaximal test), or the patient states he can continue no longer (maximal test). While many changes may be seen in the electrocardiogram during or after exercise, only changes in the ST segment are of use in the diagnosis of myocardial ischemia. Square-wave or downsloping ST depression of 1 mm or more persisting for 0.08 seconds provides the best separation between normal subjects and those with ischemic heart disease (Fig. 22–2). When multiple electrocardiographic leads are recorded and the test is performed by an experienced physician, up to 80 percent of patients with myocardial ischemia will have abnormal tests. False positive tests reduce the utility of exercise stress testing in a variety of clinical situations. Such results are particularly prevalent in women, patients with "vasoregulatory asthenia" or the mitral prolapse syndrome, patients with preexisting ECG abnormalities, patients with other cardiac disease such as hypertension, and patients taking drugs such as digitalis, diuretics, and sedatives.

In patients with established ischemic heart disease, exercise testing can be used to define effort capacity which may be helpful in determining employment, recreational activities, response to therapeutic agents, and prognosis. ST depression of greater than 2 mm, the occurrence of complex ventricular arrhythmias, or hypotension developing during exercise suggest more severe coronary obstruction. Angina occurring at a low work load or heart rate also indicates more severe disease.

The role of exercise stress testing in the diagnosis of coronary artery disease in asymptomatic subjects remains undefined. In population groups with a low prevalence of atherosclerosis, such as healthy young men, the incidence of false positive tests may be high. Furthermore, the absence of electrocardiographic changes during exercise does not exclude the presence of major coronary obstruction. Myocardial perfusion imaging during exercise with the radioisotope [201]thallium (Chap. 17) can be of aid in the identifica-

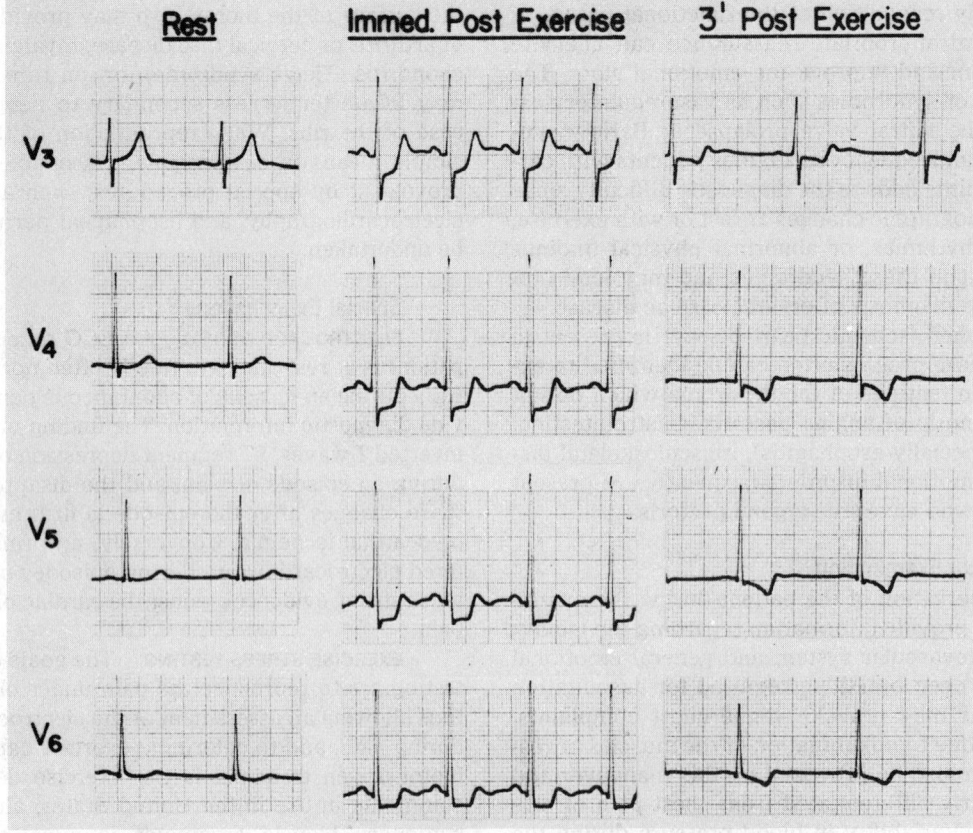

FIGURE 22–2. Exercise electrocardiogram with typical ischemic response. Resting tracing shows T wave flattening. Immediately after exercise there is 3.0 mm flat ST depression in V_5-V_6, deep junctional depression with slow rising ST segment V_3-V_4. By 3 minutes post exercise, ST depression is downsloping and T waves have become inverted.

tion of false positive responses and may improve sensitivity in the detection of myocardial ischemia.

AMBULATORY ECG MONITORING. Small, portable units capable of recording one or two electrocardiographic leads are available for continuously monitoring the ECG during daily activities. Such devices are useful in the evaluation of patients with recurrent chest pain at peculiar times during the day and for documenting arrhythmias which may occur during daily episodes of myocardial ischemia.

TESTS OF ESOPHAGEAL FUNCTION. These are described in detail in Chapter 56. Reproduction of the patient's pain by esophageal perfusion with hydrochloric acid (Bernstein test) may help to establish the gastrointestinal origin of retrosternal pain. Tests of esophageal motility or fluoroscopic visualization of the esophagus may provide evidence of esophageal spasm, but often these tests may be normal even in the patient with severe recurrent spasm.

CORONARY ARTERIOGRAPHY. Coronary arteriography is another procedure that may be valuable in the study of patients with chest pain (Chap. 17). Current techniques permit good radiologic visualization of both coronary arteries by the selective injection of radiopaque material. Atherosclerotic narrowings and obstructions can be seen and the patterns of collateral flow identified. If narrowings are seen, the diagnosis of atherosclerotic coronary artery disease is established. False positive arteriograms occur rarely, if at all. False negative arteriograms are possible, because the method either underestimates the severity of the narrowing or the lesion is located at a site which is not well visualized.

The clinical evaluation of arteriographic findings is sometimes difficult and must be based on a clear understanding that the demonstration of atherosclerotic narrowing does not prove that the patient's symptoms can be attributed to myocardial ischemia. If the arteriographic findings are clearly those of severe disease, the information is of great value. One can then be certain about the existence of ischemic heart disease and safely attribute the chest pain or electrocardiographic abnormalities to this condition. If the arteriogram fails to reveal disease, the physician must be cautious in his interpretation. Ischemic heart disease is not likely to be present if the arteriogram is normal. However, the method provides adequate visualization of only the large coronary arteries and the possibility that disease may be present in small vessels, cannot be completely excluded. Other explanations for the patient's symptoms must be sought if the arteriogram is normal. Cardiomyopathy, especially of the hypertrophic form, can be a cause of chest pain in a patient with normal coronary arteries.

It is now clear that there are patients, often females, with typical angina pectoris, an abnormal exercise test, and normal coronary arteries. This test must be evaluated along with other clinical and laboratory evidence. The clinical significance of the arteriogram that reveals only minor changes is difficult, especially when the patient is a man over 50 years of age, since atherosclerosis is common in this age group.

It is always desirable to establish the cause of the chest pain, but even negative laboratory tests can be useful in reassuring the patient. For example, a negative exercise test can be used as objective evidence that myocardial ischemia has not occurred during a given effort and demonstrates to the patient that such an effort is not harmful. In the same way, a negative coronary arteriogram can be used to assure a young man that the pains he is experiencing are not the result of life-threatening coronary artery disease.

The indications for coronary arteriography vary widely in different centers. When the diagnosis of angina pectoris is securely based on historical or electrocardiographic information and medical therapy is indicated, there is little to be gained by arteriographic definition of the arterial lesions. When the etiology of chest pain cannot be determined, arteriography may be important to exclude coronary disease in the patient who is being treated for it with insufficient evidence, or to establish the diagnosis in those with atypical angina. In some patients with established coronary artery disease, particularly those who are very young or those with demanding employment, the need for prognostic information based on arteriographic findings may be an indication for study. Arteriography will be performed in the majority of patients being evaluated for coronary bypass surgery.

AN APPROACH TO THE PATIENT WITH CHEST PAIN

On the basis of a detailed history, careful physical examination, chest x-ray, and resting ECG, the physician should categorize the patient with chest pain into one of four general diagnostic groups: 1) angina pectoris; 2) noncardiac pain; 3) cardiac pain related to other cardiac conditions, i.e., Barlow syndrome, hypertrophic cardiomyopathy, pericarditis, or pulmonary hypertension; and 4) chest pain of uncertain origin. Only a minority of patients will be classified in this last category.

If the patient has angina pectoris, and conditions such as valvular aortic stenosis or hypertrophic cardiomyopathy are excluded, medical therapy is instituted. Failure to improve with a trial of nitrates and beta-blocking drugs should prompt consideration of coronary arteriography. In some patients with angina, a stress test may be useful to determine the extent of exercise incapacity, but this information is usually obvious from the history. Major degrees of ST segment shift early in exercise, or angina occurring at a low heart rate or work load may suggest severe three-vessel disease or main left coronary obstruction and prompt earlier consideration of coronary arteriography. It should be emphasized, however, that the diagnosis of angina is made by taking a history and not by exercise electrocardiography.

If it is clear from the history that the source of pain is not myocardial ischemia, other possible causes of pain in the gastrointestinal tract or musculoskeletal system are explored. Sometimes, stress testing is performed to reassure these patients that the heart is not the cause of pain. In the patient with uncertain pain, the stress test has an important diagnostic use. Myocardial ischemia may be confirmed as the source of pain when marked ST segment shifts occur in conjunction with pain precipitated by exercise. Such patients are then managed as those with angina pectoris, and coronary arteriography is performed when there is failure to respond to medical therapy or other indication of severe coronary disease. Some patients with uncertain pain may not be able to complete an adequate stress test. In others a negative stress test may not be sufficient evidence to exclude coronary artery disease as a cause for pain particularly when no other etiology is apparent. Coronary arteriography may be the only way to establish the presence or absence of coronary artery disease in these situations.

THERAPY OF ANGINA PECTORIS[87,93]

The patient with angina pectoris needs a physician who will see him repeatedly and help him adjust to his disease. A single visit with an abbreviated diagnostic and prognostic summary is totally inadequate and may do great harm. The physician must be sure of his diagnosis and must not convey to the patient any doubts he may have. Other causes of thoracic pain must be excluded as primary or contributing causes. The patient must be taught to recognize the pains that are of cardiac origin and realize that not every chest pain he may experience is on a cardiac basis. Sometimes the majority of the pains experienced by a patient with proven angina pectoris may be on the basis of arthritis or esophagitis, and simple measures directed at these conditions may significantly reduce the number of attacks. The physician must emphasize that the prognosis is not necessarily

bad. A truthful and yet optimistic viewpoint is now possible.

General Therapeutic Measures

The ideal treatment for angina pectoris is one that brings about the regression of the atheromatous lesions. The basic cause of atherosclerosis is still unknown, but a number of factors, alone and in combination, significantly increase the risk of development of ischemic heart disease (Chap. 23). These include high concentrations of serum cholesterol, hypertension, obesity, and cigarette smoking, as well as many other less important factors. Although there is correlation between these factors and ischemic heart disease, it has not been proven that their correction will alter the basic atheromatous process. Most physicians believe that the relationship between the risk factors and disease is so strong that every effort should be made to eliminate risk factors whenever possible. Therefore correction is recommended when it can be effected by measures which are neither a hardship nor a hazard.

It is absolutely essential that patients give up cigarette smoking. Weight reduction is beneficial but often difficult to achieve in middle-aged, sedentary individuals. Weight reduction in combination with a diet appropriate for the underlying lipid disorder will help to reduce blood lipids. Control of blood pressure by weight loss, dietary sodium restriction, or drugs may reduce the frequency of anginal attacks and retard progression of atherosclerosis. Other important therapeutic measures include reduction in work involvement and avoidance of excessive fatigue, increased time for rest and relaxing activities, avoidance of chronic or acute emotional conflicts, and exercise.

The patient with angina pectoris should be encouraged to engage in moderate exercise, such as regular walking. As his tolerance increases he may be permitted to engage in a sport that does not produce pain or to pursue light jogging, swimming, or cycling. Effort capacity may improve as a result of regular exercise, and the patient's general state of well-being and confidence will also increase. Generalizations cannot be made about management, and each patient should be encouraged to establish, within his limitations, a program of activity that is as nearly normal as possible. To help the intelligent patient avoid attacks, an explanation of myocardial blood flow in terms of supply and demand will be useful; for others, simpler explanations must be provided. In any event, patients must learn that effort provokes and rest relieves the pain of angina pectoris; that effort in the cold or after eating is often less well tolerated; that more work can be tolerated if it is undertaken slowly; that he must avoid situations which require that he hurry.

Faced with a patient with recent onset angina or one who shows a changing pattern of pain, the physician should be alert to precipitating factors which may be responsible for increasing myocardial oxygen needs. Hyperthyroidism or the administration of thyroid hormone to patients with myxedema may be responsible for worsening anginal pain. In diabetic patients on insulin, hypoglycemic episodes may cause anginal attacks, particularly at night. The production of angina by paroxysmal arrhythmias may mask symptoms related to the arrhythmia itself. Worsening angina may reflect increasing left ventricular dilatation consequent to left ventricular failure, as in some cases of angina decubitus. Cardiomegaly may be a clue to such a mechanism. Such patients often improve with digitalization and diuretic therapy. It is not often appreciated that the balance between oxygen supply and demand in the myocardium may be so tenuous that a small reduction in blood hemoglobin (i.e., reduction of hematocrit by 2 or 3 points) may account for worsening angina. Such a change may be a clue to occult gastrointestinal blood loss, often from a large bowel carcinoma. Erythrocytosis, of even modest degree, also may aggravate ischemia.

Specific Therapeutic Measures

The pharmacologic therapy of angina pectoris can be appreciated by a reconsideration of Figure 22–1. The balance between myocardial oxygen demand and oxygen supply by means of coronary blood flow can be restored by either decreasing demand or increasing supply. Coronary artery bypass surgery is the only measure which acts directly to increase supply. The medications in common use act primarily by decreasing demand. Ideally, therapy should be directed at the prevention of myocardial ischemia and not just at the relief of pain. The patient may be rendered asymptomatic by any of several programs, but this does not mean that the probability of death and myocardial infarction will be reduced by the therapeutic measures.

NITROGLYCERIN.   It is probable that the most important actions of nitroglycerin are those which reduce the work of the heart by reducing wall tension. This occurs primarily by reduction in left ventricular volume as a result of peripheral venous dilatation, and to a lesser extent by reduction in arterial pressure (Chap. 30).

Patients with angina pectoris usually learn to control the number of attacks by modifying the amount and speed of physical exertion and avoiding tension-inducing experiences. When attacks cannot be avoided in this way the use of nitroglycerin is to be recommended. Patients should be encouraged to use it freely and not to try to get by without it; it does no harm to take it unnecessarily for an attack which would have passed off without it. Occasionally, mild attacks which might have been aborted by the use of nitroglycerin become severe.

Nitroglycerin taken prophylactically may permit greater effort without attacks. For example, it may be taken before facing a stressful business situation, before physical exertion, or prior to sexual intercourse.

The effective dose of nitroglycerin must be determined by experiment, since there is variability from patient to patient and in the same patient from time to time. The usual dose is 0.4 mg taken sublingually, but some physicians prefer to start with a smaller dose to avoid the unpleasant side effects at the beginning of therapy. The dose should be adjusted upward if pain is not relieved and there are no adverse effects, such as a significant drop in blood pressure or headache. It may be advisable to have the patient seated during the initial trial of the drug. The hemodynamic, and hence, the therapeutic actions of the drug are dependent on the effect of gravity and hence the medication will work less well if the patient lies down. If the initial dose (0.4 mg) results in uncomfortable headaches and flushing, it should be adjusted downward because a smaller dose may be just as effective in relieving pain. Some patients will not get relief with 0.4 mg and a regular dose of 0.6 mg may be required. Contrary to what patients often fear, it usually does not lose effectiveness with frequent use. When a dose that formerly relieved attacks suddenly becomes ineffective, it is likely that the drug has deteriorated.

Occasionally, even potent nitroglycerin in adequate amounts fails to relieve what the patient interprets as an attack of angina pectoris. He should be warned that, if chest pain is not relieved by two or three tablets within a half-hour period, his chest pain may be due to a myocardial infarction and he should seek his physician's advice before taking more medication. Rarely, the drug not only fails to relieve pain but actually seems to make it worse. This paradoxical effect is probably due to exaggerated splanchnic pooling or to an exaggerated fall in systemic blood pressure and may be circumvented by having the patient lie down before taking the medication.

LONG-ACTING NITRATES.   Nitroglycerin may be administered as a 2 percent ointment which is applied to the skin. Absorption through the skin is slower than that through the mucous membranes and the therapeutic action may persist for up to 6 hours. The dose must be determined by trial and error in each patient and is measured in inches of ointment and squeezed from a tube. Nitroglycerin ointment is especially useful in the management of nocturnal angina. An application at bedtime may make it possible for the patient to sleep throughout the night. The patient should apply the ointment gently as vigorous rubbing may lead to intense headache and a shortened duration of action.

The best effects of long-acting nitrates, such as erythrityl tetranitrate or isosorbide dinitrate, occur when the drugs are administered in chewable or sublingual form so that absorption through the buccal mucosa may occur. More prolonged action may follow oral administration of large doses of the drugs. The therapeutic effects are maximal in 20 to 30 minutes and rarely persist beyond 1.5 to 2 hours when the drug is absorbed through the mouth. While some patients may find benefit from routine administration of the drug every 4 to 6 hours, others will achieve maximal efficacy by taking the drug in anticipation of activities and repeating it every 2 hours if increased activity levels persist. In patients with unstable angina it is effective to combine two hourly administrations of a chewable or sublingual nitrate with nitroglycerin ointment.

BETA BLOCKING AGENTS. Beta blocking drugs act to reduce myocardial oxygen demands primarily by decreasing heart rate and ventricular contractility, and secondarily by decreasing blood pressure particularly during exercise (Fig. 22–1). An undesired effect is an increase in ventricular volume. Exercise performance improves after beta blocking drugs because the heart rate-contractility-systolic pressure response to any given level of exercise is reduced, which results in a delay in appearance of the critical level of oxygen demands at which angina appears.

Most patients will show dramatic improvement in angina after institution of beta blocking drug therapy, and may well be able to resume near normal activities free of pain. Most younger patients will require 160 mg or more per day to achieve effective beta blockade. If initial therapy of 20 mg four times daily is well tolerated, larger doses can be given until therapeutic effectiveness is noted or the resting pulse falls to below 60 per minute. In older patients or those with marginal ventricular function, it is advisable to begin therapy with smaller doses.

It is inadvisable to use these drugs in patients with congestive heart failure, although some such patients with severe angina may be improved by combining small doses of beta blocking drugs with digi-

TABLE 22–3

Determinants of Myocardial Oxygen Consumption	Beta Blockade	Nitro-glycerin
Wall tension		
Ventricular volume	↑	↓
Systolic pressure	↓	↓
Wall thickness		
Contractility	↓	↑ reflex
Heart rate	↓	↑ reflex

talis and diuretics. Common side effects limiting utility include lethargy, muscular weakness, mental depression, impotence, and gastrointestinal disturbance.

The beta blocking agents are usually used in combination with nitroglycerin or one of its long acting derivatives. The way in which the effects of the two drugs are complementary is shown in Table 22–3.

OTHER PHARMACOLOGIC AGENTS. Inspection of Figure 22–1 will aid in the appreciation of the mechanism of action of the cardiac glycosides and the diuretics in the treatment of angina. Left ventricular dysfunction may be improved by the cardiac glycosides and hence the ventricular volume and wall stress will be decreased. Diuretics operate by decreasing plasma volume, ventricular volume, and wall stress. Diuretics may have an additional beneficial effect by lowering elevated blood pressure and hence reducing oxygen consumption. Cardiac glycosides and diuretics are especially useful in patients with nocturnal angina. Additional measures which may be helpful in this particular type of angina are salt restriction and sleeping with the head of the bed elevated. Digitalis is also useful in slowing the ventricular rate in atrial fibrillation and preventing supraventricular tachycardia.

Surgery[83,84,90,91,92]

Bypass of obstructing lesions of the coronary arteries by connecting segments of saphenous vein removed from the legs from aorta to distal coronary artery or by implanting the internal mammary artery into the distal artery has proved highly effective in relieving anginal pain and improving functional indices of exercise capacity. Eighty to ninety percent of patients will show clinical improvement, in many associated with disappearance of objective signs of myocardial ischemia. The operative mortality is below 2 percent in centers with wide experience with the procedure. Patients with incapacitating symptoms in spite of optimal medical therapy should be considered for the bypass operation. Those with proximal vessel obstructions without severe atheromatous involvement of distal vessels and with preservation of normal ventricular function are most likely to benefit from this operation. Enhanced myocardial blood flow is the mechanism of improvement in a large proportion of patients, but other mechanisms, such as intraoperative infarction of ischemic myocardium or denervation, may be responsible or additive in some patients. There is little controversy about the utility of the bypass procedure in patients incapacitated with anginal pain. Many patients with severe symptoms have been restored to a normal life-style as a result of surgery. There is considerable uncertainty and disagreement about whether the operation can prolong life or prevent infarction in patients with coronary artery disease whether symptoms be severe, mild, or absent. To date, only patients with symptomatic left main coronary artery obstructions have shown improved survival with surgery. Whether survival can be improved by surgery in other subgroups of patients has not yet been documented. Bypass surgery has not produced improvement in ventricular function when performed on patients with chronically scarred left ventricles. The risks of surgery are greater in these patients, and the long-term benefits less good. Patients with diffuse atheromatous disease extending to the distal coronary arteries and older subjects also have poorer results. Recent studies indicate that anginal symptoms may return in 7.2 percent of patients per year following successful bypass surgery[83] indicating that for many and perhaps all, this form of therapy represents a useful but temporary palliation of myocardial ischemia in the natural history of a life-long disorder.

Management of Unstable Angina Pectoris

Patients with unstable angina should be treated in a hospital with close monitoring. In many instances hospitalization and rest alone will restore stability because the patient is removed from a stressful home or work situation. Other patients will require intensive therapy with short- and long-acting nitrates and pro-

pranolol in large doses. Nitrates are particularly important because they reduce myocardial oxygen demands and also may prevent coronary spasm which may play an important role in producing pain in this syndrome. In some patients, calcium antagonist agents which are potent vasodilators, such as Nifedipine, may be useful. Heparin may also be beneficial. In patients refractory to these measures, intra-aortic balloon counterpulsation will provide relief of pain. In almost all cases medical therapy will be effective in controlling the attacks. The short-term prognosis for such patients is excellent so that emergency arteriography or surgery are not indicated. If symptoms do not abate with medical treatment or if angina becomes incapacitating with resumption of activity, cardiac catheterization is necessary to determine if surgically bypassable coronary artery obstructions are present.

PROGNOSIS[90,93]

Many patients live long and fruitful lives after the onset of angina pectoris. The physician can be justifiably optimistic about the future, particularly if the patient adheres to a prudent program including abstinence from smoking, weight and blood pressure control, exercise, and appropriate medication. Patients with angina who have a normal electrocardiogram at rest and normal blood pressure have shown an expected yearly mortality of 1.6 percent which is only slightly different than that of healthy age-matched controls. Preservation of exercise tolerance is associated with a good prognosis. Beta adrenergic blocking drugs have resulted in improved survival in patients when administered following acute myocardial infarction and may provide similar benefit for the patient with angina. The extent of coronary arterial disease and the amount of damage to the left ventricle are the major determinants of prognosis. Patients with single vessel disease and well-preserved ventricular function have an expected 5- to 10-year survival which is similar to the normal population. One of the important outcomes of randomized clinical trials of surgery has been the realization that nonoperative treatment results in a far better course than previously suspected. In one recent study, 93 percent of patients with triple vessel disease treated medically were alive in 2 years. Severe ventricular damage is associated with a poor outlook in spite of medical or surgical treatment.

Myocardial Infarction
LEWIS C. BECKER AND JOHN T. FLAHERTY

Acute myocardial infarction occurs when the blood supply to a region of heart muscle becomes inadequate to maintain critical cell functions, and irreversible damage results. Chest pain and electrocardiographic changes characteristically accompany this process, which is followed by the release of myocardial enzymes into the circulation. The terms "coronary thrombosis" and "coronary occlusion" have been used to describe this event but are not necessarily synonymous with "myocardial infarction" since infarction may sometimes occur with normally patent coronary arteries. Conversely, complete coronary occlusion may occur without infarction if the collateral blood supply to that segment of myocardium is adequate to maintain cellular integrity.

PATHOGENESIS

The majority of myocardial infarctions are associated with severe proximal atherosclerotic narrowing of one or more of the major coronary arteries.[113] Most infarcts are thought to result from sudden thrombotic occlusion of a previously narrowed coronary artery, although there is evidence that in some instances thrombosis may occur secondarily as a result of stasis in the coronary arteries supplying the infarcted segments.

What initiates coronary artery thrombosis is unknown, but there is evidence that rupture of a complex atherosclerotic plaque occurs with the exposed ulcerated surface providing a nidus for thrombus formation. Aggregation of platelets on the intimal surface with resulting release of vasospastic substances may also be an important mechanism.

In a relatively small number of cases, infarction is caused by embolization to the distal coronary arteries from a damaged aortic valve or from an intracardiac mural thrombus. Rarely, infarction is found in young patients with normal coronary arteries. In these patients coronary artery spasm is the suspected etiology. Infarction may also occur in patients with normal or minimally diseased coronary arteries in association with episodes of hypotension during anesthesia in association with gastrointestinal bleeding or during a sustained tachycardia. Thus, infarction may be due to either a generalized or a local reduction in coronary blood flow.

PRECIPITATING FACTORS

Less than 5 percent of acute myocardial infarcts occur during unusual physical activity. In many patients one can elicit a history of recent "life crisis," such as retirement, change in job, or death of a family member. In some cases, specific precipitating factors such as anemia, hypoxemia, hypotension, or the taking of birth control pills are noted, but in the majority of patients no precipitating factors are identifiable.

RISK FACTORS

Risk factors for the atherosclerosis that underlies most myocardial infarction may be divided into major and minor groups. Analysis of populations from different countries has revealed an association between the level of serum cholesterol and the incidence of ischemic heart disease.[105] When serum cholesterol is greater than 260 mg/dl in individuals over the age of 30, the risk of clinical ischemic heart disease is increased by 100 percent. Increased fasting triglycerides and low density lipoproteins (LDL) are also associated with increased risk of ischemic heart disease, while increased high density lipoproteins (HDL) appear to be protective and are associated with lower incidence of disease. An elevated serum cholesterol, however, remains the single lipid abnormality best able to identify patients at increased risk from ischemic heart disease. Hypertension, the second major risk factor, has been shown to be important in many population studies in the United States and Europe. The third major risk factor which is independent of either serum cholesterol or hypertension is cigarette smoking. When multiple risk factors are present, their effect is more than just additive. Subjects with three major risk factors have a 16-fold increase in the incidence of ischemic heart disease over those with none. Less important risk factors include diabetes mellitus, obesity, and sedentary life-style. A familial incidence of ischemic heart disease has been recognized, but only a minority of cases involve clear-cut inheritance of known risk factors, such as lipoprotein abnormalities. More often, familial clustering appears to be related to similar lifestyles and dietary patterns in family members.

SITE OF INFARCTION

Anteroseptal myocardial infarction is due to occlusion of the left anterior descending coronary artery. The mass of infarcted myocardium and the hemodynamic disturbance resulting from occlusion of the anterior descending coronary artery is usually greater than that resulting from occlusion of the right coronary artery. Complete heart block occurring in a patient with an anterior infarction signifies extensive septal damage and suggests additional disease in the right and/or left circumflex coronary arteries.

Occlusion of the left circumflex coronary artery results in a lateral wall infarction. In the minority of individuals in whom the left circumflex coronary artery supplies a major portion of the inferior surface of the heart ("left distribution"), occlusion may result in posterior-inferior as well as lateral infarction. When the left circumflex coronary artery supplies the AV node, proximal occlusion may cause heart block. Likewise, proximal occlusion predisposes to atrial infarction and atrial arrhythmias in the 45 percent of patients in whom the sinus node artery originates from the circumflex artery. Infarction of the inferior wall of the heart more often results from occlusion of the right coronary artery. This vessel gives rise to the AV node artery in 90 percent of patients and the sinus node artery in 55 percent. Varying degrees of AV block and/or sinus bradycardia are, therefore, common. The mass of myocardium supplied by the right coronary artery is generally smaller than that perfused by the left anterior descending coronary artery, making the prognosis of patients with inferior infarction better than those with anterior infarction. Rarely, inferior wall infarctions may be associated with severe right ventricular infarction resulting in a clinical picture of right heart failure and low cardiac output.

CLINICAL PRESENTATION

Patients may present with chest pain, shock, pulmonary edema, or sudden death.[103] Occasionally, the patient may initially appear with one of the complications of myocardial infarction, such as systemic embolization or pericarditis. Severe prolonged chest pain of characteristic location is usually present, but sometimes the pain is relatively minor. About two-thirds of patients experiencing their first myocardial infarction will have had similar but less prolonged episodes of chest pain in the hours or days preceding the acute infarction. Most patients with a history of angina pectoris will have had some change in the pattern of pain prior to the episode of infarction. The pain of an infarct will generally be more severe, longer-lasting, and more refractory to nitroglycerin, and may also have a different quality compared to the patient's usual angina.

The pain of myocardial infarction is most often substernal in location, and is usually described as "squeezing," "crushing," "like a vise," "like a heavy weight," "like a fire," or "like a balloon" in the chest. Sometimes the pain is located principally in the subxiphoid or epigastric region, which explains the frequent misdiagnosis of acute indigestion by both the patient and his physician. The pain characteristically radiates to the left shoulder and down the left arm, most frequently the inner aspect. Radiation into the neck, the right arm, or down both arms is not rare. Occasionally, the pain will radiate to the back or the abdomen. In a few instances, the discomfort is felt only in one of the sites of radiation, e.g., jaw, either or both arms, or shoulder in the absence of substernal discomfort. Most commonly, the discomfort grows in severity over several minutes and remains severe for several hours, if not relieved by narcotics. Sometimes, it will wax and wane before reaching a steady level of severity. Profuse diaphoresis, dyspnea, nausea, and vomiting are common accompaniments to the pain and may dominate the clinical picture.

Myocardial infarction may be "painless" in some patients who present with acute pulmonary edema, shock, or cardiac arrest. Asymptomatic or unrecognized infarction—"silent myocardial infarction"—occurs in 10 to 15 percent of patients, based on annual physical and electrocardiographic examinations of employee groups.

Sudden Death

In one-fifth of the patients with ischemic heart disease, sudden death is the first and only clinical manifestation. Sixty percent of the people who die from ischemic heart disease do so within 24 hours of the onset of symptoms. Many experience instantaneous death without a forewarning episode of chest pain, although the majority have a history of angina or prior myocardial infarction. Autopsy studies have shown that nearly all of the patients with sudden cardiac death have severe diffuse coronary atherosclerosis involving at least two major coronary arteries. For those patients surviving their first infarct, subsequent sudden death is more common in those with persistent cardiac enlargement, ventricular ectopic activity, or ST segment abnormalities on the ECG.

DIFFERENTIAL DIAGNOSIS

Angina Pectoris

The character, location, radiation, and even severity of the anginal and infarction pain can be identical. If the pain lasts for more than 20 minutes after rest or nitroglycerin, infarction must be seriously considered. Typical changes on the ECG at this time or in later evolution are of major importance in distinguishing angina from an acute infarction. The diagnosis of acute myocardial infarction is more difficult in patients who have ECG changes of a previous infarction, or nonspecific ST-T wave abnormalities secondary to digitalis administration or left ventricular hypertrophy. Left bundle branch block presents special problems since it may mask both characteristic ST segment changes and Q waves. In these patients, serial ECGs may be of little help and the diagnosis will depend on clinical examinations or other supporting laboratory data, including changes in serum enzyme concentrations or the results of radioisotope imaging procedures. In some patients, the chest pain may be typical of infarction, but electrocardiographic or enzyme evidence may not be present. Such patients are best classified as having unstable angina pectoris (see Chap. 22).

Pericarditis

Pericarditis may be difficult to differentiate from acute infarction. Typically, pericardial pain is made worse by lying down and helped by sitting up and leaning forward. A history of preceding upper respiratory infection, and especially the presence of a pericardial friction rub on physical examination are points favoring a primary pericardial process. A pericardial rub secondary to transmural myocardial infarction does not usually appear until the second or third day after the onset of pain. During the first few days the electrocardiographic changes may be similar, but absence of typical evolution of an infarction pattern in serial tracings strengthens the case for pericarditis.

Slight elevations of serum enzyme concentrations may be seen in pericarditis, but a rise and fall typical of infarction is unusual. Common causes of pericarditis include viral infection (especially Coxsac-

kie B), bacterial infection, tuberculosis, pulmonary malignancy, and connective tissue disorder. Anticoagulants should not be given in cases of inflammatory pericarditis because of the increased risk of hemorrhage into the pericardium.

Pulmonary Embolism

Chest pain, dyspnea, and electrocardiographic changes may occur in acute pulmonary embolism and simulate acute myocardial infarction. Small rises in serum enzymes may also occur. The appearance of a pleural rub or a radiographic pulmonary infiltrate are helpful differentiating features. In addition, the electrocardiographic changes are nonspecific and do not include development of Q waves. Other acute chest conditions, such as pneumothorax, mediastinal emphysema, and pneumonia may also mimic myocardial infarction.

Other Conditions

About one-third of patients with dissecting aneurysm of the aorta are initially diagnosed incorrectly as having acute myocardial infarction. The pain of dissection is more likely to be localized in the posterior thorax and radiate up and down the spine. The demonstration of recent widening of the aorta by chest x-ray and the development of a murmur of aortic insufficiency support the diagnosis of a dissection.

Esophagitis or esophageal spasm may cause pain indistinguishable from that of acute infarction. A careful history often establishes the relationship between previous episodes of pain and ingestion of food or lying down after meals.

The pain of acute abdominal conditions, such as pancreatitis and acute biliary disease, may be located in the epigastrium and lower substernal area and simulate myocardial infarction. Gastrointestinal abnormalities and ischemic heart disease frequently coexist in the same patient since both are common conditions. Particularly in elderly patients, acute abdominal processes may cause acute myocardial infarction through stress or dehydration; sometimes the infarction is diagnosed while the underlying abdominal process is overlooked.

Occasionally, a myocardial infarction may be "silent" with respect to chest pain, but is brought to the physician's attention by complicating events, such as a systemic arterial embolus from a mural thrombus, or a pulmonary embolus from a peripheral site of deep venous thrombosis.

PHYSICAL EXAMINATION

The abnormalities to be found on physical examination depend upon the site and extent of the infarction and the complications which have resulted. Findings are modified by the residua of previous infarctions and by associated diseases. Since physical findings may change dramatically and rapidly during the first few hours following infarction, careful serial physical examinations are indicated.

Fever following myocardial infarction is seldom greater than 101°F. Sinus bradycardia and/or varying degrees of AV block are frequent occurrences during the first few hours in patients with inferior infarction. Sinus tachycardia of moderate degree is often present in patients with extensive anterior infarctions especially when cardiac failure is present. Hypotension may develop during the early phase of a large infarction, but more commonly patients suffering an acute infarction are hypertensive as a result of massive catecholamine release.

Palpable precordial bulges are frequent during the first several days in patients with large anterior wall infarctions. These areas of outward systolic motion usually disappear over several days, but their persistence may be the first clue to development of a ventricular aneurysm. Heart sounds are often faint and of poor quality. An atrial (S_4) gallop will be heard in virtually all patients with acute myocardial infarction and does not constitute evidence of ventricular failure. A ventricular (S_3) gallop is less frequently heard and indicates the development of a severe degree of left ventricular dysfunction.

Bibasilar rales are another sign of left ventricular dysfunction and may persist for as long as 24 hours following relief of left ventricular failure. However, since rales may also be secondary to atelectasis or preexistent chronic pulmonary disease, they may be misleading as a sign of failure.

Jugular venous distension is not expected in patients with left ventricular failure secondary to acute infarction. Distension of the jugular veins therefore suggests preexistent cardiac failure or an associated acute right ventricular infarction.

Approximately one-third of patients with acute infarction develop a transient, soft apical systolic murmur secondary to papillary muscle dysfunction. Systolic murmurs resulting from a ruptured ventricular septum or ruptured head of a papillary muscle are usually much louder and are often accompanied by signs of severe left ventricular failure or shock.

A classification system (Table 23–1), based on the degree of left ventricular dysfunction by clinical examination, has proved useful in evaluating and managing patients with acute myocardial infarction. The clinical class on admission is an important determinant of subsequent mortality.

TABLE 23–1

Hemodynamic and Therapeutic Implications of Clinical Class

Class	Clinical Findings	LVFP	SWI	Hospital Mortality	Initial Therapy
I (uncomplicated)	No evidence of congestive failure	N	N	5–7%	Antiarrhythmic therapy if indicated
II (mild to moderate congestive failure)	Bibasilar rales and/or an S_3 gallop	↑	N	10–15%	Diuretic
III (severe congestive failure or pulmonary edema)	Rales above the tip of the scapula, S_3 gallop, tachycardia, and/or frank pulmonary edema	↑	↓	30–40%	Routine therapy for pulmonary edema; if poor response, diuretic followed by a vasodilator
IV (cardiogenic shock)	Systolic blood pressure 80 mm Hg or less (or a drop of 80 mm Hg from previous hypertensive levels) associated with signs of circulatory insufficiency; cold clammy skin; mental confusion; oliguria	↑↓	↓	80–90%	See Table 23–2

N = normal.
LVFP = Left ventricular filling pressure equivalent to pulmonary capillary wedge pressure.
SWI = Stoke work index (g-meter/M²).

LABORATORY FINDINGS

Serum Enzymes

Serum enzyme measurements are especially important in establishing a diagnosis of acute myocardial infarction.[117] Necrosis is signaled by release of creatine kinase (CK), lactic dehydrogenase (LDH), and glutamic oxaloacetic transaminase (SGOT) into the serum, with a characteristic time course (Fig. 23–1). Serum CK typically beings to rise 4 to 6 hours after the onset of infarction, peaks within 24 hours, and returns to normal within 3 days. SGOT has a longer time course, beginning to rise 6 to 8 hours after infarction, peaking in 24 to 48 hours, and returning to normal in 3 to 4 days. LDH has the longest time course: serum levels usually start to rise 12 hours after infarction, peak in 3 to 6 days, and return to normal within 2 weeks.

Since these enzymes are present in organs other than the heart, elevations are not specific for myocardial necrosis. In addition to the heart, CK is present in skeletal muscle and brain; LDH, in skeletal muscle, kidney, liver, lung, blood, and fat; SGOT in skeletal muscle and liver. CK may therefore be elevated due to intramuscular injections, cerebrovascular disease, hypothyroidism, or other conditions associated with muscle damage such as acute alcoholism. Aortic dissection, pulmonary embolism, pancreatitis, myopathies, hemolytic disorders, drug administration (e.g., opiates, especially in the presence of biliary disease),

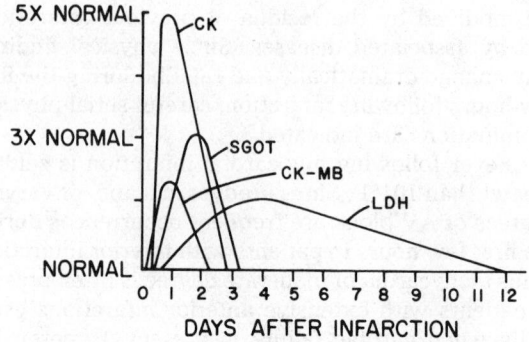

FIGURE 23–1. Time course of serum enzyme concentration following a typical myocardial infarction. CK: creatine kinase. SGOT: glutamic oxaloacetic transaminase. CK-MB: isoenzyme of CK which is found mainly in the myocardium and is, therefore, more specific for myocardial damage. LDH: lactic dehydrogenase.

and right ventricular failure with hepatic congestion are conditions which may cause a rise in serum LDH or SGOT and, therefore, confusion in diagnosis. However, attention to the time course of enzyme rise and fall may allow one to distinguish between myocardial infarction and release from other sources. In patients admitted soon after the onset of symptoms, measurement of an enzyme with a short time course, such as CK, is most useful. If the time of onset of symptoms

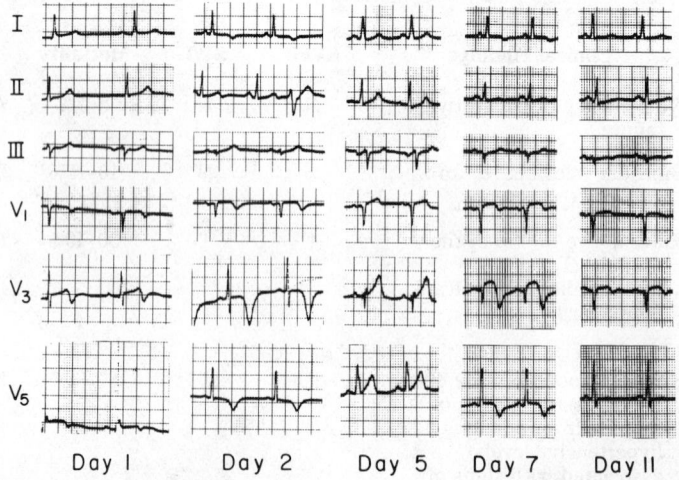

FIGURE 23–2. Serial electrocardiographic changes in a patient with acute anterior myocardial infarction. Record of Day 1 shows slight ST-segment elevation and biphasic T waves in leads V_3 and V_5. By Day 2 the T waves are deeply inverted in these leads and also inverted in lead I, suggesting nontransmural infarction. On Day 5 there is dramatic new elevation of the ST segment in V_1, V_3, and V_5 with T-wave peaking, indicating an extension of the infarction process. On Days 7 and 11, Q waves are seen in V_3, representing transmural damage. The persistence of slight ST segment elevation in V_3 may represent early aneurysm formation or coexistent pericarditis.

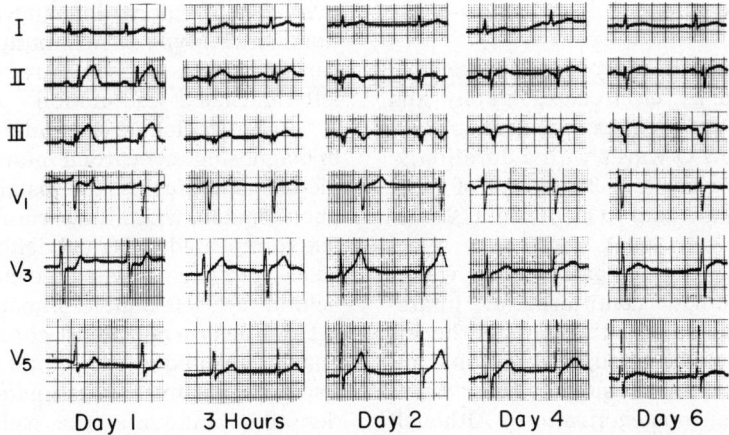

FIGURE 23-3. Typical serial electrocardiographic changes in a patient with acute inferior myocardial infarction. Initially, there is ST segment elevation and peaking of the T waves in leads II and III with reciprocal ST segment depression in V_1, V_3, and V_5. Q waves, indicating transmural infarction, are first seen at 3 hours in leads II and III. Subsequent changes include T-wave inversion in II and III with return to upright position by Day 6 and deepening of Q wave in lead III with leftward shift of electrical axis (loss of inferior forces).

is unclear, or if the patient presents to the hospital several days after a possible infarct, serial measurement of an enzyme with a longer time course, such as LDH, may be more helpful.

There has been recent emphasis on the measurement of myocardial-specific isoenzymes to reduce the incidence of false positive diagnoses of acute myocardial infarction. Measurement of the electrophoretically rapid moving isoenzyme of LDH (LDH_1) has been recommended; hepatic congestion causes a rise in the slow-moving LDH_5 fraction rather than LDH_1. However, LDH_1 may also be elevated in hemolytic anemia, hypoxia, and hypothyroidism among other conditions. More specific is the MB fraction of CK. CK-MB is found almost exclusively in myocardial tissue although it makes up only 14 percent of the total myocardial CK activity. After acute myocardial infarction, serum CK-MB begins to rise in 4 to 6 hours, like total CK, but generally peaks slightly earlier and falls slightly faster than total serum CK.

The peak serum enzyme rise appears to be related to the magnitude of the infarction. Calculation of the total amount of CK or CK-MB released into the blood and knowledge of the renal clearance of CK allows estimation of the number of grams of infarcted myocardium. Although large infarcts with high CK values are often associated with left ventricular failure and a poor prognosis, mild elevations cannot necessarily be equated with a good prognosis since pre-existing damage from prior infarctions may be present. Also, complications such as arrhythmias, systemic or pulmonary emboli, or extensions of the acute infarct may occur unpredictably.

Electrocardiogram

Electrocardiographic changes usually appear within minutes of the onset of pain and evolve in a diagnostic fashion over the next several days (Figs. 23–2 and 23–3). Occasionally, the initial electrocardiogram may be normal if the infarction is located in the lateral or direct posterior portions of the left ventricle, areas which are relatively "silent" in electrocardiography. The initial ECG may also be normal if the patient presents with unstable angina and has not actually developed an infarction yet; necrosis may begin after admission, becoming evident on later tracings. In addition, the initial tracing may be "normal" due to elevation back to baseline of previously depressed ST segments. Examination of serial tracings is important when the clinical suspicion of myocardial infarction is strong but the initial tracing is normal. Serial tracings are also of value even when the initial tracing appears to be "diagnostic" since other conditions, such as pericarditis, may closely simulate infarction on a single tracing. If reelevation of the ST segments during the first few days suggests infarct extension, this diagnosis can be confirmed by a secondary rise in serum enzymes. Persistence of ST segment elevation may indicate formation of a ventricular aneurysm and is associated with a poorer prognosis. Serial tracings are also useful to detect the development of progressive AV block or conduction disturbances of the bundle branches.

In general, the correlation between the extent of infarction as assessed by electrocardiography and that determined at postmortem examination is poor. Patients developing new Q waves with a duration $\geq$ 0.04 seconds and an amplitude $\geq$ 25 percent of the R wave in the same lead are said to have had a "transmural" infarction.

Patients who do not develop pathologic Q waves are considered to have had "nontransmural" infarctions involving less than half the thickness of the left ventricular wall. It should be noted, however, that autopsy studies do not uniformly support this "transmural"/"nontransmural" categorization. Although nontransmural infarcts are generally less extensive, there is a higher incidence of reinfarction over the next 1 to 2 years, frequently involving the segment of myocardium previously affected. The long-term prognosis does not differ for patients with transmural and nontransmural infarction, probably reflecting the fact that the extent of the underlying coronary atherosclerosis is similar.

In general, the incidence of early arrhythmias, complications, and mortality is higher with more extensive loss of myocardium. However, in some patients a very small infarction strategically located in a papillary muscle or in the septum near the His bundle may lead to serious complications by causing severe mitral regurgitation or complete heart block.

Radioisotope Studies

The diagnosis of acute myocardial infarction can also be established by scintiphotographic studies (Chap. 17). Agents such as pyrophosphate and glucoheptonate labeled with [99M]technetium have been found to localize in acutely infarcted myocardium. The appearance of radioactivity in the region of the heart on a scintiphotograph of the chest after initial clearance of the tracer from the blood suggests acute myocardial damage ("hot spot scan"). The administration of a tracer which is taken up by normal myocardial cells, such as [201]thallium, may also be of value in detecting areas of myocardial infarction and ischemia. In this instance the ischemic or infarcted area is recognized by an absence of radioactivity in an area of myocardium ("cold spot scan").

A third type of radioisotope study uses a tracer which remains in the bloodstream, such as [99M]technetium bound to albumin or red blood cells, allowing the left ventricular cavity to be imaged during the cardiac cycle (cardiac blood pool scan). The resultant picture is similar to a ventriculogram obtained at cardiac catheterization and permits assessment of both overall and regional left and right ventricular function. On this type of scan both new and remote myocardial infarcts appear as regions of absent or poor left ventricular wall motion.

These radionuclide studies are especially useful in diagnosing myocardial infarction when the clinical picture is confusing, for instance, when a history is unobtainable, when the serum enzymes are elevated due to repeated electrical defibrillations or intramuscular injections, or when the electrocardiogram is not helpful (i.e., left bundle branch block). Although not yet routinely available in coronary care units, these imaging techniques should allow more rapid diagnosis and a noninvasive estimate of the size and location of an acute infarct as well as the extent of wall motion abnormality in the majority of patients.

Other

The white blood count usually becomes elevated on the first day and returns to normal within a week. The erythrocyte sedimentation rate rises more slowly and may remain elevated for weeks even though no complications are present.

HEMODYNAMIC ASSESSMENT OF VENTRICULAR FUNCTION

The physical signs of pulmonary congestion and ventricular dysfunction are often adequate to assess prognosis as well as the need for and the effects of therapy.[98,99] However, because these signs may be inadequate or at times even misleading, hemodynamic monitoring in some cases provides objective data to assess the severity of left ventricular dysfunction and response to interventions. Hemodynamic monitoring is currently recommended for all patients in clinical Class IV, some patients in Class III, and the occasional patient in Class II who fails to respond adequately to therapy.[115] It is also used in the clinically stable patient who suddenly deteriorates after admission to the hospital. Balloon flotation catheters of the Swan-Ganz type can be passed at the bedside through a peripheral vein into the pulmonary artery for measurement of pulmonary artery and pulmonary capillary wedge pressures. Pulmonary capillary wedge pressure correlates as well with left atrial pressure and therefore can be used as an indication of left ventricular filling pressure. The pulmonary artery diastolic pressure can also be used as an estimate of left ventricular filling pressure if a satisfactory pulmonary capillary wedge pressure cannot be obtained. A thermistor located near the distal end of the balloon catheter allows intermittent determination of cardiac output by the thermodilution technique.

Insertion of a radial arterial cannula permits con-

TABLE 23-2
Hemodynamic Subsets in Cardiogenic Shock

LVFP	RVFP	SWI	Sudden Systolic Murmur	Diagnosis	Therapy
↓	↓	↓	−	Hypovolemia	Plasma volume expansion
N	↑	↓	−	Right ventricular infarction in patient with ECG diagnosis of inferior or posterior infarction	Plasma volume expansion
↑	N↑	↓	+	Ruptured intraventricular septum or papillary muscle	Vasodilator treatment followed by intra-aortic balloon augmentation and early surgery if no improvement
↑	N	↓	−	Massive left ventricular muscle loss	Dopamine, norepinephrine, intra-aortic balloon augmentation and in selected cases emergency angiography and aortic coronary bypass graft surgery

tinuous measurement of systemic arterial pressure and frequent determination of blood gases. Assessment of left ventricular filling pressure, right ventricular filling pressure, and stroke work index (SWI) reveals characteristic patterns in each of the clinical classes (Table 23–1) including those with cardiogenic shock (Table 23–2). Hemodynamic measurements in the coronary care unit have added precision to the management of critically ill patients with acute myocardial infarction. It should be emphasized that central venous pressure which reflects right ventricular filling pressure is not a valuable index of left ventricular filling pressure in patients with acute myocardial infarction. Since it is primarily the left side of the heart which is damaged, right-sided pressures are not useful for diagnosing and/or guiding therapy in patients with pulmonary congestion or systemic hypertension.

GENERAL APPROACH TO THE PATIENT

When a patient is admitted to the frightening environment of a coronary care unit, his physician must explain in detail the nature of his illness and the need for cardiac monitoring. The course of a myocardial infarction is often unpredictable, and the patient, or at least the patient's family, should, therefore, be ful-

ly informed about his prognosis and progress. In most cases, this can be done with realistic optimism and reassurance. The patient should be told how long he is expected to remain in the coronary care unit and in the hospital, and education concerning the effect of the infarct on his future employment and social life should begin after a few days. There are few clinical situations which require more individualized attention than the patient with an acute myocardial infarction.

Coronary Care Unit
The major goals in treatment of the acute stage of myocardial infarction are to relieve pain and anxiety, treat or prevent arrhythmias, minimize the size of the infarcted myocardium, and to predict, prevent, or treat any specific complications.

The coronary care unit (CCU) provides the physical facilities and trained personnel to accomplish these objectives, although in hospitals without a CCU, many of the principles of coronary care can still be utilized. The usual period for close and continuous observation is 3 to 5 days. More than 5 days may be necessary for patients with complications, such as congestive failure, ventricular arrhythmias, recurrent chest pain, or cardiogenic shock. The prophylactic aspects of the CCU rather than the potentially serious nature of the patient's illness should be emphasized to the patient and the patient's family.

Recent studies from Great Britain suggest that for uncomplicated patients, home care may be as good as or better than treatment in a hospital coronary care unit. In these low-mortality-risk patients, the proven benefits of CCU care may be canceled out by certain negative aspects, including anxiety-induced arrhythmias and iatrogenic complications. Further studies are clearly needed in this area, but physician-supervised home care may eventually be found to be suitable for selected groups of patients.

Relief of Pain

Morphine remains the drug of choice for relief of severe pain and associated apprehension. It occasionally provokes nausea and vomiting. An initial dose of 5 to 10 mg is given intravenously. Intramuscular injections should be avoided when possible since they may cause an elevation of serum enzymes. If pain persists and no untoward effects of the drug, such as hypotension, are encountered, additional doses should be given as needed. Oxygen administration is a routine measure.

A face mask provides the highest concentration of inspired oxygen but may not be tolerated well by an acutely ill patient. Nasal cannulae are usually better tolerated, maintain acceptable alveolar oxygen concentrations, and allow oral intake. Cigarette smoking is not permitted.

Preserving Ischemic Myocardium

Methods designed to minimize the size of infarcted myocardium are under active investigation in centers throughout the world.[108] Modification of infarct size is based on the concept that necrosis evolves over time and that there is initially a relatively small central area of myocardium which will inevitably undergo necrosis, surrounded by a larger area of "jeopardized" ischemic muscle. Over the next several hours increasing amounts of this jeopardized ischemic area undergo irreversible cell damage. Experimental approaches to limitation of infarct size have focused on 1) reducing myocardial oxygen requirements, for example with propranolol; 2) increasing collateral blood flow into the ischemic zone with vasodilator drugs like nitroglycerin or hyaluronidase; 3) reducing cell swelling with mannitol; and 4) promoting cellular viability by metabolic interventions like glucose–potassium–insulin.

Clinical trials are currently underway to determine which of these approaches may be used in man. It remains uncertain whether any of these agents can change the natural course of infarction when administered several hours after the onset of symptoms. However, concepts developed in the experimental laboratory have already had some impact on clinical care. Clinicians are increasingly aware of the importance of minimizing myocardial oxygen requirements and now avoid ionotropic agents, such as isoproterenol and digitalis, unless there is a specific indication.

General

During the first 24 hours the patient should be kept at bed rest. After the first 24 to 48 hours, uncomplicated patients may be allowed chair rest. Patients developing congestive heart failure or recurrent arrhythmias should be kept at bed rest for the first few days and then allowed to progress to a chair as clinical improvement is noted.

The diet should be simple and light for the first few days and contain reduced sodium content. During the early phases of infarction, gastrointestinal symptoms are common and may be controlled in part by dietary restriction. Because bed rest and opiates often cause constipation, the use of mild laxatives and stool softeners is routine. A bedside commode is preferable to a bedpan because the commode is better accepted by patients and generally requires less energy expenditure on their part.

Since the round-the-clock activity of a coronary care unit may impair a patient's ability to sleep, a point should be made to schedule periods of uninterrupted rest. Sedatives and tranquilizers may also be necessary.

Use of Anticoagulants

Asymptomatic venous thrombi of the legs have been found in up to one-third of patients with acute myocardial infarction. The incidence of pulmonary embolization is, however, much lower. Most clinical studies indicate that the incidence of thromboembolic phenomena in patients with acute infarction can be reduced by the use of anticoagulants.[97] Anticoagulants should, therefore, be used early in the course of a patient with acute myocardial infarction if there are no contraindications, and especially if the patient is in clinical Class III or IV and cannot be ambulated rapidly. Relative contraindications include bleeding diathesis, hepatic disease, chronic hypertension, suspicion of an aortic dissection, and history of a potential bleeding site in the gastrointestinal or genitourinary tracts. Anticoagulation may be accomplished with either heparin or one of the coumadin derivatives (see Chap. 30). If one of the latter is chosen, care should be taken with drugs such as barbiturates which increase the activity of the hepatic microsomal enzymes and may cause fluctuation in the effective coumadin level. In patients with a relative contraindication to anticoagulants, such as those with a history of peptic ulcer, low dose heparin has been advocated. Although in several clinical studies a low dose of heparin administered subcutaneously has reduced the incidence of thromboembolic complications, this experience has not been uniform. At present the available clinical evidence suggests that if heparin is selected and is to be optimally beneficial it should be given in full anticoagulant doses. Anticoagulant therapy is usually discontinued once the patient is ambulatory. The value of long-term anticoagulation in reducing the incidence of recurrent infarction is undetermined. Prevention of infarction by chronic administration of agents, such as aspirin or sulfinpyrazone, to reduce platelet "stickiness" is intriguing in view of the relatively minor side effects and is currently undergoing clinical trials.[95] Over the past 10 years, there has been a tendency to reduce the time of bed rest and to encourage chair rest and earlier ambulation. This probably accounts as much as anticoagulation for the declining incidence of serious thromboembolic complications.

Arrhythmia [96,104,109,114]

The CCU has reduced mortality in acute infarction by favorably influencing the detection, treatment, and prevention of arrhythmias. Any type of arrhythmia may develop in acute myocardial infarction and continuous monitoring systems have provided accurate data on their incidence (Chap. 22). If sinus tachycardia and those rhythms occurring in terminal states are excluded, over 95 percent of patients will have some arrhythmia, with atrial and ventricular ectopic beats being the most frequent. The arrhythmias which are associated with the worst prognosis, such as ventricular tachycardia, complete heart block, ventricular fibrillation, and asystole occur in at least 30 percent of cases if prophylactic antiarrhythmic agents are not aggressively employed. Ventricular fibrillation or asystole occurs in approximately 10 to 15 percent of cases and complete heart block in about 5 percent.

VENTRICULAR ARRHYTHMIAS. Ventricular premature beats (VPBs) are extremely common, occurring in at least 75 percent of patients during the first several days of acute myocardial infarction and are ordinarily treated by an intravenous lidocaine infusion. Treatment is usually begun when premature ventricular beats occur with a frequency of six or more per minute, appear early during repolarization (so-called R-on-T phenomenon), occur two or more in a row, or have multiple forms on the ECG. Ventricular beats with these characteristics frequently precede more serious arrhythmias such as ventricular tachycardia

or fibrillation. There remains controversy as to whether patients with more "stable" VPBs (unifocal, longer coupling intervals, bigeminy, etc.) or even those patients with no VPBs should also be treated. Recent evidence suggests that primary ventricular tachycardia and/or fibrillation occurs just as often in these latter patients, implying that all patients with acute myocardial infarction should be considered for prophylactic lidocaine infusion. What evidence is available suggests that prophylactic lidocaine reduces the incidence of ventricular fibrillation, but does not alter overall mortality in the setting of a well-equipped CCU.[107]

The initial dose of lidocaine is given intravenously (1 mg/kg) followed by a continuous infusion at a rate which is sufficient to suppress ectopic activity (20 to 50 μg/kg/minute) and achieve a serum level of 2 to 6 μg/ml. Above this range, side effects of hypotension and central nervous system disturbances, including tremulousness, stupor, psychotic behavior, or even seizures, may occur. Infusion rates should be kept low in older patients and patients with heart failure and/or preexisting liver disease to avoid toxicity, since clearance of lidocaine is related to hepatic blood flow. When the ventricular arrhythmias are unresponsive to lidocaine, intravenous procainamide is frequently effective. A loading dose of 500 to 1000 mg is given as 100 mg increments every 5 minutes until the arrhythmia is controlled, followed by a continuous infusion of 40 to 80 mg per hour.

Since the tendency for VPBs decreases rapidly after the first day, antiarrhythmic therapy should be discontinued after 24 to 48 hours if no VPBs are present to determine whether underlying ectopic activity still exists. If VPBs recur, it may be necessary to continue intravenous therapy longer or switch the patient to an oral agent, such as quinidine, procainamide, or disopyramide in preparation for his transfer from the CCU.

PAROXYSMAL VENTRICULAR TACHYCARDIA (PVT) AND ACCELERATED IDIOVENTRICULAR RHYTHM (AIVR). These are ventricular rhythms occurring commonly during the first several days of infarction. Ventricular tachycardia is defined as three or more consecutive ventricular ectopic beats originating from the same focus with a rate of 150 to 250 beats per minute. This rhythm may be associated with hypotension and lead to ventricular fibrillation. It is reported to occur in 15 to 40 percent of patients during the acute phase of myocardial infarction. If PVT becomes sustained and does not cease with intravenous antiarrhythmic therapy or if hemodynamic deterioration occurs, external electric shock should be employed. Accelerated idioventricular rhythm should be distinguished from PVT. It arises from a single ectopic ventricular focus, at a rate of 60 to 100 per minute and does not lead to ventricular fibrillation. Since the rate is slow and blood pressure is unaffected, no specific therapy is indicated.

Ventricular fibrillation (VF) may occur unexpectedly and without prodromal ventricular tachycardia or "malignant" VPBs during the early hours following infarction. More often, prodromal ectopic ventricular activity precedes its occurrence. When promptly detected, VF can usually be reverted easily to normal sinus rhythm by external defibrillation. An episode which occurs suddenly in an otherwise uncomplicated patient has been termed "primary ventricular fibrillation," in contrast to "complicated" fibrillation occurring in patients with evidence of left ventricular failure or shock. "Complicated" ventricular fibrillation is more often refractory to defibrillation efforts, with less than 20 percent of patients surviving to be discharged from the hospital. In contrast, more than 80 percent of patients experiencing a single episode of primary ventricular fibrillation recover to leave the hospital in good condition. After an episode of VF, an antiarrhythmic drug, such as lidocaine, is begun to prevent a recurrence.

HEART BLOCK. About 5 percent of patients with acute myocardial infarction develop complete or third degree AV block, with the incidence of heart block being higher in inferior than anterior infarction. In patients with inferior involvement, the site of heart block is usually the AV node, which is supplied by the same artery that perfuses the inferior wall. Heart block developing during an acute inferior infarction often progresses in steps from first degree, to second degree, to complete heart block. It is usually transient, lasting from a few minutes to a few days. Ordinarily, a lower junctional pacemaker takes over, and heart rate and blood pressure are well maintained. No further therapy is indicated unless hypotension and/or complex VPBs develop, in which case atropine, 0.5 to 1.0 mg intravenously, or temporary ventricular pacing may be necessary. Permanent ventricular pacing is required only rarely in patients with acute inferior infarction.

By contrast, complete heart block developing in the setting of an anterior infarction is usually caused by extensive damage to the peripheral conduction system and is, therefore, associated with infarction of a large mass of left ventricular myocardium. The mortality is much higher, approaching 80 percent. Various ventricular conduction defects, such as right or left bundle branch block or left anterior hemiblock, may precede complete heart block in an anterior in-

farction, but more often block occurs abruptly. Since the escape pacemakers are located more distally in the Purkinje fibers the rhythm is often unstable and the rate is slow (<40 per minute), with catastrophic hemodynamic consequences. A temporary pacemaker should therefore be inserted in all patients with anterior infarction who develop complete heart block and also in many who demonstrate only new conduction defects because of their high risk of progression to complete block (20 to 40 percent). Permanent demand pacing is currently recommended for patients who develop even a transient episode of complete heart block in the course of an acute anterior infarction. These patients have a high incidence of later sudden death which may be caused by recurrent heart block.

ATRIAL ARRHYTHMIAS. Sinus bradycardia is common in inferior wall infarction and should not be treated unless ventricular premature beats or significant hypotension are also present. If treatment is required, intravenous atropine may be used. An initial dose of 0.5 mg is given, followed by 1 to 3 additional 0.5 mg doses if necessary. Higher initial or total doses are more likely to produce sustained sinus tachycardia or serious ventricular arrhythmias. Transvenous pacing may be necessary in patients unresponsive to atropine.

Sinus tachycardia is commonly related to the stress of the infarction but in some patients is an indicator of congestive heart failure. Although sinus tachycardia per se does not compromise cardiac function, it does increase myocardial oxygen demands and could, in theory, lead to more extensive myocardial damage. Aside from sinus tachycardia, the most frequent supraventricular tachycardia (SVT) is atrial fibrillation, which occurs in about 10 percent of cases. It is usually transient, lasting only a few minutes to several hours, but often recurs during the first few days. Rapid ventricular rates with hemodynamic deterioration or recurrent chest pain are indications for intravenous administration of propranolol or digitalis in order to slow conduction through the AV node. Propranolol is probably preferable to digitalis if left ventricular function is adequate because of its faster action and the added benefit of reducing myocardial oxygen requirements. If slowing is not quickly accomplished, R-wave triggered DC external defibrillation may be necessary to convert the rhythm to sinus. Atrial flutter is encountered in about 5 percent of patients with acute myocardial infarction. Patients with atrial flutter require more rapid restoration of sinus rhythm because of the faster ventricular rates and the difficulty of precisely controlling the degree of AV block with drugs.

APPROACH TO THE PATIENT WITH LEFT VENTRICULAR FAILURE

The occurrence of left ventricular failure suggests the presence of either a relatively large acute infarct or a smaller acute infarct in a ventricle extensively damaged from prior infarctions. In a small subgroup of patients, left ventricular failure may develop with a small area of injury involving a critical region of the ventricle, such as the papillary muscle or the ventricular septum. The resulting acute mitral regurgitation or left to right shunt may cause decompensation of an only mildly damaged left ventricle.

The clinical classification shown in Table 23–1 is useful in planning an approach to the therapy of patients with left ventricular failure.[118]

Uncomplicated Patients: Class I

Although patients in Class I may have mild left ventricular impairment manifested by a decrease in left ventricular ejection fraction, they have no overt clinical signs of failure and specific therapy to improve function is not indicated. Therapies designed to minimize infarct size may ultimately prove to be of value in this group.[108] Mortality in this class of patients is low (3 to 5 percent) and is related to arrhythmias, ventricular rupture, and thromboembolic complications. Therapy should therefore consist of antiarrhythmic agents, treatment of hypertension, and anticoagulation.

Mild Congestive Failure: Class II

Patients with mild left ventricular failure manifested by an S_3 gallop or bibasilar rales may either improve spontaneously over 24 to 48 hours or respond to diuretic therapy and salt restriction. Pulmonary congestion in these patients may be due in part to a reduction in left ventricular compliance with a resultant elevation in left ventricular filling pressure. A small reduction in left ventricular end-diastolic volume, as a result of venous pooling and loss of plasma volume resulting from administration of a diuretic such as furosemide, often results in a decrease in left ventricular end-diastolic pressure and relief of pulmonary congestion. When furosemide is used it should be given orally or intravenously beginning with a small initial 20 mg dose. Larger doses may result in excessive diuresis and hypotension. If the initial 20 mg dose fails to induce a sufficient diuresis, larger doses (40 to 240 mg) may be given. Pulmonary congestion accompanied by small or normal heart size on chest x-ray suggests a major problem with diminished left ventricular compliance. In this setting, digitalis should not be given, since it tends to increase myocardial oxygen demands and produce cardiac arrhythmias without improving hemodynamics. However, when the heart is enlarged, digitalis is generally beneficial, since it tends to reduce heart size and thereby decrease myocardial oxygen requirements. Digitalis is ordinarily continued in patients who have been taking the drug previously for chronic congestive heart failure.

Patients in whom left ventricular failure is accompanied by hypertension may benefit by pharmacologic reduction of aortic pressure with agents such as nitroprusside or alpha-methyldopa.[100] In those with prior hypertension, reduction in systemic pressure should be carried out slowly and cautiously since a sudden or excessive reduction in aortic pressure may result in reduced coronary perfusion or in a baroreceptor mediated reflex tachycardia.

Congestive Heart Failure—Pulmonary Edema: Class III

Pulmonary edema is more likely to occur in patients with a previous history of hypertension. Pulmonary edema which is refractory to conventional therapy or appears late in the course of infarction is an ominous sign. The presence of precipitating factors, such as acute hypertension, may indicate a more favorable prognosis than would be the case if the pulmonary edema were a consequence of the extent of ventricular damage alone.

Treatment of acute pulmonary edema in the setting of an acute myocardial infarction is similar to that in the absence of infarction. Oxygen is administered by face mask or nasal cannula. The patient is placed in the sitting position, and intravenous doses of morphine are administered immediately. Aminophylline can be used to treat bronchospasm, but it should be given cautiously because of the risk of inducing excessive tachycardia and/or ventricular irritability. Intravenous diuretics, such as furosemide, are administered although their onset of action is not immediate. Digitalis should not be administered as a part of the emergency therapy unless indicated for the treatment of a specific arrhythmia such as atrial fibrillation. Rotating tourniquets are customarily applied in an attempt to reduce venous return but are of limited value.

Patients with pulmonary edema who do not respond to the initial measures outlined above or those with persistent severe pulmonary congestion may be treated by afterload reduction with vasodilators. It is generally necessary to insert a Swan-Ganz catheter into the pulmonary artery and an arterial cannula into the radial artery to allow precise regulation of vasodilator dose. By lowering the peripheral resistance the heart can generate more cardiac output with the same or lower arterial pressure and with a lower left ventricular filling pressure.[100] Since reduction of afterload also reduces myocardial oxygen consumption, it is especially beneficial for treating heart failure in patients with myocardial ischemia. The most commonly employed vasodilator is sodium nitroprusside, administered by intravenous infusion. Oral or cutaneous nitrates can also be employed either instead of, or following, initial intravenous therapy with nitroprusside.

Shock: Class IV

Hypotension is common in patients with acute myocardial infarction, especially in those with inferior infarction associated with increased vagal tone. Shock, however, is diagnosed when systolic blood pressure is < 80 mm Hg or 80 mm Hg less than a previously known control blood pressure, and when there are one or more of the following signs of insufficient organ perfusion: 1) inadequate renal blood flow, as manifested by oliguria with urine flow less than 20 ml per hour; 2) inadequate peripheral circulation with peripheral vasoconstriction, as manifested by cool, moist extremities; and 3) poor cerebral perfusion, as manifested by restlessness, confusion, or coma. Cardiogenic shock is diagnosed only when other causes of hypotension, such as hypoxia, hypovolemia, arrhythmias, or overdosage with narcotic analgesics, are excluded. Cardiogenic shock occurs in about 10 percent of patients with acute myocardial infarction and is associated with an 80 to 90 percent mortality. The most common cause is extensive damage to the left ventricle with insufficient myocardium remaining to maintain adequate cardiac function. Pathologic studies have shown infarction of more than 40 percent of the left ventricle in most patients dying of cardiogenic shock.

Although the overall mortality with cardiogenic shock is very high, certain subsets of patients can be identified in whom appropriate therapy is more successful (Table 23–2). These subsets can be recognized, or at least suspected, clinically, but definitive diagnosis and management generally requires hemodynamic evaluation with a Swan-Ganz catheter.[98,99]

The most common of the treatable subsets is characterized by a low left ventricular filling pressure and a low stroke work index, reflecting hypovolemia. In the majority of patients, this situation is the result of overzealous diuretic therapy and is easily corrected by plasma volume expansion. The left ventricular filling pressure should be carefully monitored during volume loading until a filling pressure of 15 to 18 mm Hg is reached, in order to avoid pulmonary congestion.

A second subset includes patients with extensive right ventricular infarction, but relatively limited left ventricular damage usually involving the inferior or posterior walls. These patients are characterized by an elevated central venous pressure and right ventricular filling pressure, usually in the presence of a normal or low left ventricular filling pressure. The appropriate therapy is the administration of volume, attempting to augment inadequate left ventricular filling and thereby increase cardiac output. In order to accomplish this end, right sided filling pressures may have to be forced up to levels of 25 to 30 mm Hg.

A third subset of shock patients with somewhat better prognosis are those with rupture of the interventricular septum or the head of a papillary muscle. This group constitutes only 2 percent of patients with myocardial infarction; surgical correction results in improved clinical status and prognosis.

External rupture of the heart with sudden and profound hypotension occurs most commonly during the first week following infarction. Patients with large transmural infarctions and those with hypertension are at greatest risk. Death usually occurs within minutes but occasionally, if the leakage of blood into the pericardial space is slow and the condition is recognized, there may be time to relieve the tamponade by pericardiocentesis and allow surgical correction of the defect.

Unfortunately, in the great majority of patients with cardiogenic shock, initial hemodynamic studies reveal only an elevated left ventricular filling pressure, a low cardiac output, and a low stroke work index. Therapy in this last subgroup, despite intensive research efforts and the application of new cardiac assist devices, has not significantly lowered the 90 percent mortality figure. Ionotropic agents, such as dopamine or norepinephrine, should be administered, but in most cases, the clinical improvement is only temporary. In an attempt to improve on unsatisfactory results, intra-aortic balloon counterpulsation therapy was developed.[116] The intra-aortic balloon increases coronary blood flow, improves perfusion of critical organs, and decreases left ventricular filling pressures. By appropriate timing of balloon deflation, the afterload and thereby myocardial oxygen demands can be further decreased. Diastolic augmentation begun within the first few hours of the onset of shock may increase the chance of survival. If stabilization can be accomplished and coronary angiography performed with the balloon in place, some patients may be found to have a significant component of reversible ischemic ventricular dysfunction caused by stenoses in coronary arteries remote from the infarction. Emergency aortocoronary bypass graft surgery with or without infarctectomy or aneurysmectomy can be carried out. However, since the extent of infarcted myocardium is usually great, the mortality even with surgery remains high.

COMPLICATIONS

Continuing or Recurrent Chest Pain

In most patients the pain of the acute infarction subsides within a few hours following the use of analgesics, although some patients continue to have chest pain for up to 24 hours. Recurrence of chest pain suggests a new event, such as unstable angina, infarct extension, pericarditis, pulmonary embolism, impending rupture, or expansion of the infarct with aneurysm formation. Episodic chest pain associated with reversible ST segment changes suggests unstable angina. Ischemic episodes should be treated with sublingual nitroglycerin, and like unstable angina without infarction, long-acting nitrates, propranolol, and anticoagulants may be helpful for preventing acute attacks. Reelevation of the ST segments or new ST-T wave changes associated with a rise in myocardial enzymes suggests the occurrence of additional infarction. Small infarct extensions may occur in up to 50 percent of patients during the first 10 days after an acute anterior infarction, but larger clinically evident extensions are much less common.[112] Continued episodes of ischemic pain at rest, with or without evidence of further myocardial necrosis, suggests an "incomplete" infarct in the distribution of a narrowed coronary artery. If the episodes fail to respond to intensive medical therapy, an intra-aortic balloon can be inserted and once the pain episodes are controlled, coronary angiography safely performed. Coronary bypass surgery may then be done if the coronary anatomy and left ventricular function are suitable.

Episodes of chest pain due to recurrent myocardial necrosis or ischemia must be differentiated from those due to postinfarction pericarditis. Clinically detectable pericarditis, as evidenced by precordial pain and/or a friction rub, can be found in at least 10 to 20 percent of patients with transmural myocardial infarctions. The rub appears most often between the second and fourth day. Hemodynamically significant pericardial effusions are uncommon in this situation, although atrial arrhythmias may occur from atrial inflammation. Pericarditis developing in the first 4 to 5 days after an acute infarction should be differentiated from the postmyocardial infarction syndrome.

Occurrence of a New Systolic Murmur and Congestive Heart Failure

When a patient suddenly develops a loud holosystolic murmur early in the course of a previously uncomplicated myocardial infarction, accompanied by hypotension and cardiac failure, rupture of the interventricular septum or a papillary muscle head are the most likely causes. Deciding which of these two complications is responsible may be difficult on clinical grounds and usually requires insertion of a Swan-Ganz catheter. The finding of an oxygen step-up in the right ventricle supports the diagnosis of ruptured interventricular septum, while the finding of large v waves in the pulmonary capillary wedge tracing supports the diagnosis of mitral regurgitation. When the cardiac failure developing in these situations does not improve with diuretics and digitalis, the addition of vasodilators, such as nitroprusside or nitroglycerin, may result in striking hemodynamic benefit. If the patient does not improve with this therapy, an intra-aortic balloon should be inserted and cardiac catheterization performed. If the patient can be stabilized on an intensive medical regimen including oral or cutaneous nitrates, surgery is best delayed for 2 to 3 months, since the results of more immediate surgery are disappointing. When cardiac failure is the result of a relatively small infarct causing a large shunt or gross regurgitation, the results of surgery are relatively good.[110]

Late Cardiac Failure

The development of cardiac failure during the convalescent phase of infarction should raise the suspicion of a localized left ventricular aneurysm. The patient with an aneurysm may also present with recurrent ventricular arrhythmias, systemic embolism, or chest pain. Persistent ST segment elevation may be a clue to the presence of an aneurysm, but this finding is both insensitive and nonspecific. The chest x-ray may show a localized bulge on the edge of the cardiac silhouette, but more commonly the heart is normal or shows generalized dilatation.

In the patient developing late cardiac failure, it is important to distinguish localized left ventricular aneurysm from diffuse left ventricular hypokinesis, which is not amenable to surgical therapy. These two conditions can be easily differentiated by noninvasive gated cardiac blood pool imaging. If an aneurysm is suspected, coronary angiography and left ventriculography are performed to define the coronary anatomy prior to surgery. The current indications for surgical resection of a left ventricular aneurysm include refractory congestive heart failure, uncontrolled ventricular arrhythmias, and, occasionally, unstable angina. The presence of an asymptomatic aneurysm is not an indication for surgery.

Postmyocardial Infarction Syndrome

A syndrome of fever, chest pain, and pleuritis or pericarditis develops in less than 5 percent of patients following an acute infarction. Although symptoms may appear in the first week, they are usually delayed for several weeks or even months, and recurrences are frequent. The delayed onset suggests an autoimmune process, and the course of this form of pericarditis is similar to that of the postcardotomy syndrome seen after cardiac surgery. The postmyocardial infarction syndrome may present a diagnostic problem since pneumonia, pulmonary embolism, and acute myocardial infarction must all be considered when chest pain, ST segment changes, and pleural and/or pericardial friction rubs are heard. Anticoagulants should be avoided, although the risk of pericardial hemorrhage is small. Salicylates are usually effective in controlling fever and pain. If further therapy is required, indomethacin or corticosteroids are commonly used. Steroid therapy is also indicated when there are multiple recurrences.

Shoulder-Hand Syndrome

Left shoulder pain and trophic changes of the hand occasionally occur a few weeks to months following infarction. The incidence of this complication appears to have diminished with earlier mobilization. The loss of function in the left arm and hand may be incapacitating, and physical therapy should be employed vigorously.

Chest Wall Syndrome

A significant number of patients develop complaints of chest wall discomfort, usually along the left sternal border in the weeks and months following an acute myocardial infarction. There is localized mild tenderness which may persist for several hours after exercise. Physical examination and laboratory studies are normal. Vigorous reassurance is the best therapy.

CONVALESCENCE

The duration of the hospital stay depends largely on the complications that have occurred. Convalescence for uncomplicated myocardial infarction has been

considerably shortened compared to 10 years ago. Patients are encouraged to sit up on the second, third, or fourth day and are progressively ambulated until discharge at 10 days to 2 weeks. If they have an occupation that is not physically demanding, they are encouraged to return to work in 2 to 3 months. Rehabilitation is designed to return the patient to optimal function both physically and socially and to educate him with respect to risk factors for atherosclerosis.

If the patient is overweight or has a lipid abnormality, appropriate dietary programs should be implemented. Patients with significant lipoprotein abnormalities should be encouraged to have younger family members, especially children, tested for possible lipid disturbances. Smokers should be strongly encouraged to stop. Mild physical exercise, such as walking, is encouraged. Isometric exercises are not recommended since they may cause marked increases in both blood pressure and heart rate. Later during convalescence, structured programs of graded exercise or jogging will increase exercise capacity as well as psychological well-being. Whether exercise induces growth of intercoronary collaterals remains controversial. Sexual activity is permitted, although some restraint is cautioned. The physical demands of sexual activity between married partners have been equated to "a brisk walk down the street or rapid ascent of two flights of stairs."[102] Driving an automobile is discouraged for the first several weeks. Prior to discharge from the hospital the patient's electrocardiogram should be monitored for 12 to 24 hours to detect arrhythmias. If frequent or complex premature ventricular contractions are seen, the patient is begun on antiarrhythmic therapy before discharge.

PROGNOSIS

Much attention has been directed recently to the prognostic significance of VPBs in the postinfarction period.[106] Mortality of hospital survivors of an acute myocardial infarction is approximately 10 to 15 percent in the first year and a cumulative 10 to 15 percent in the second through the fifth years. Therefore, a sizable reduction in mortality could be achieved if sudden death in the first year after myocardial infarction could be prevented. The prevalence of complex VPBs (couplets, multiform VPBs, ventricular tachycardia, R-on-T VPBs) correlated well with the incidence of sudden death, presumably from ventricular arrhythmias; therefore, many studies have attempted to influence this mortality with antiarrhythmic drugs.

Results are at best equivocal, and toxic side effects have limited long-term use of these drugs. A multicenter, double blind trial of sulfinpyrazone, an agent which decreases platelet adhesiveness, administered for 1 year after a myocardial infarction showed an improved survival of treated patients compared to placebo-treated controls.[95] The effect may have been to reduce the incidence of fatal arrhythmias, recurrent myocardial infarction, or both. Beneficial effects upon survival after myocardial infarction have been reported from Europe with the use of beta blockers which are not available in the United States.[101] A multicenter trial is currently in progress testing the effect of propranolol on survival in patients who have had a myocardial infarction.

Long-term prognosis is best in patients with normal heart size and blood pressure, and in those without symptoms, without ST segment elevations or depressions in any of the standard ECG leads, and without arrhythmias on a 24-hour ECG tape recording.[111] In these patients the 5-year survival rate is more than 80 percent. Survival is reduced by the presence of recurrent angina pectoris, congestive failure, persistent ST segment elevation, or arrhythmias on 24-hour monitoring. Patients with congestive heart failure have no more than a 20 percent chance of surviving for 5 years unless a localized left ventricular aneurysm can be detected and surgically excised.

Young individuals survive for more years after infarction than older individuals presumably because of more severe multiple vessel disease in the older patients. Most patients who sustain a myocardial infarction eventually succumb to ischemic heart disease, the majority dying from a recurrent infarction, congestive heart failure, or an arrhythmia. Sixty percent return to their former vocations and another 15 to 20 percent do less arduous work. Prognosis becomes worse with subsequent episodes of infarction.

Patient counseling is important, and patients should be appraised of their physical limitations and their life pattern discussed. Every effort should be made to return the patient to a normal social and professional life. Limitations of activity, premature retirement, and rigid dietary restriction without foundation are all too commonplace.

CHAPTER 24
Pulmonary Thromboembolism
WILLIAM R. BELL

Although pulmonary thromboembolism has been recognized for centuries, it remains one of the most common and difficult problems in the clinical practice of medicine. It is a disease that crosses all traditional compartments, specialties, and subspecialties of medical practice. There are numerous reasons why this disease is difficult to manage, but the major source of distress to the physician is the difficulty he encounters in establishing the diagnosis. Autopsy studies indicate that pulmonary thromboembolism is the most commonly missed diagnosis that is directly responsible for patient mortality. Forty to sixty percent of patients who died because of pulmonary emboli arrived for postmortem examination without correct diagnosis and treatment.[120,121]

In the United States, the annual incidence of symptomatic pulmonary emboli is estimated to be 650,000 and for approximately 38 percent of these the experience is fatal. The mortality is five- to sixfold greater in a group of patients in which the diagnosis is not established. For these reasons, it is important to emphasize early, accurate diagnosis because the majority of patients can be saved and in less than 10 percent are there associated incurable diseases.

PATHOPHYSIOLOGY
Pulmonary thromboembolism is defined as impaction of thrombus or other foreign material in the pulmonary arteries. With rare exception, the embolus originates at a distant site (distal to the right atrium) and travels to the lung via the venous circulation. The most common source of thrombi is thought to be the venous vasculature of the lower extremities. Almost all pulmonary emboli consist of thrombotic material (fibrin, red cells, white cells, and platelets) but, on rare occasions, nonthrombotic materials, such as fat, bone marrow, air, amniotic fluid ("squams"), tumor, and a wide variety of exogenous foreign bodies may embolize in the lungs.

The embolic material in the pulmonary vasculature produces complete or partial obstruction of right heart blood flow to the distal alveolar-capillary sites of gas exchange, and this initiates physiologic reactions in the heart and lungs. The hemodynamic consequences of the reduction in vascular cross-sectional area are an increase in pulmonary vascular resistance and pulmonary artery pressure and distention of the pulmonary artery. When severe, the pulmonary hypertension can result in right heart failure with reduced cardiac output. Although these hemodynamic alterations are well documented in man their precise mechanism has not been established. Theoretically, the enormous pulmonary arteriocapillary reserve capacity should provide more than adequate compensation for the areas obstructed by embolic material. In this disease, however, pulmonary hypertension has been documented when less than 50 percent of the vascular bed is obstructed. Neural reflexes or vaso-bronchoconstriction by humoral mediators, such as serotonin, bradykinin, fibrinopeptides A and B, and prostaglandin, may be responsible.

As a result of embolic obstruction, a portion of the lung may be ventilated, but not perfused with blood. This results in a respiratory microunit that is not capable of physiologic gas exchange. In response to this alteration, there is constriction of the alveolar spaces and bronchial airways to the affected area. If the vascular obstruction is complete, vessel breakdown distal to the site of obstruction may occur with hemorrhage producing damage to the ventilatory space. Portions of the lung will be without perfusion and ventilation, and when numerous alveolar units are severely damaged, focal infarction may develop. The rarity of this event is probably related to the dual blood supply of the lungs. The lungs receive blood from the bronchial arteries as well as from the pulmonary arteries and the bronchial circulation continues to function in spite of pulmonary artery obstruction. Regardless of the location and size of vessel obstructed, pulmonary infarction spreads to a pleural interlobar or visceral surface. The size of the clot(s) and vessel obstructed are not determining factors in the development of infarction. This is more likely due to the development of tissue necrosis, hemorrhage into interstitial and alveolar areas, and associated pleuritis with resultant atelectasis and hypoventilation in the adjacent pulmonary parenchyma.[122] In approximately 40 percent of patients with pulmonary infarction associated with pulmonary emboli, there is an associated effusion that may be serous, but usually is serosanguineous.

THROMBOGENESIS

The inciting event for pulmonary emboli is the formation of venous thrombosis. Although it has been known for over 100 years that damage to the vessel wall intima, stasis, and aberrations in the coagulation-fibrinolytic mechanisms are critical factors in the development of a thrombus, the precise inciting trig-

ger has not been identified. Direct damage to vessel wall intima from any cause induces thrombus formation. Stasis, the relative slowing of blood flow, facilitates interaction between coagulation factors, platelets, and vessel surface and also impedes the clearance of "activated" coagulation factors and thus provides optimal conditions for thrombus formation. Venous stasis is most commonly associated with the development of deep vein thrombosis in man. Although extensive studies have been performed on the blood coagulation system, no acceptable mechanism has been identified to explain the "hypercoagulable state." The pocket above the venous valves of the leg veins is probably the site of origin of most pulmonary emboli. The relative frequency with which pulmonary emboli originate in the leg veins, as compared with the veins of the pelvis, abdominal cavity, inferior vena cava, upper extremities, and right heart chambers, has not been established. Within the legs, the area above the knee is more frequently the source of emboli.

COEXISTING RISK FACTORS

Pulmonary thromboembolism occurs with increasing frequency in patients with certain underlying diseases.[119,124] The most common coexisting condition is immobilization resulting from a disabling illness. This is followed closely in frequency by peripheral venous disease, including thrombophlebitis, venous varicosities, with accompanying insufficiency and stasis, cardiopulmonary disease, the use of oral contraceptives, recent surgery, and obesity. Less common coexisting illnesses include endocrine and metabolic disease, pelvic disease, hypertension, the postpartum period, and malignant neoplasms. Approximately 5 percent of patients with pulmonary emboli have no recognizable concurrent or prior illness.

CLINICAL FEATURES[119]

Regardless of the clinical setting or associated symptoms or signs, pulmonary thromboembolism usually presents abruptly. Nearly all patients experience chest pain, which is more commonly pleuritic than nonpleuritic, and dyspnea. These symptoms are so common that the absence of dyspnea, chest pain, or tachypnea makes the diagnosis of pulmonary emboli unlikely. Other common symptoms include diaphoresis, cough and hemoptysis, and apprehension. In some patients, leg cramps, palpitations, syncope, nausea, vomiting, chills, and angina-like chest pain occur. Many of these symptoms are noted transiently for several days before the diagnosis is established.

Physical examination commonly reveals tachypnea, fever, and tachycardia. Hypotension leading to shock may occur in some patients and is almost always associated with massive (greater than two lobar arteries occluded) emboli. The combination of rales, rhonchi, wheezes (most likely secondary to bronchospasm), and a pleural friction rub are present in the majority of patients. Cardiac signs, which may call attention to right heart involvement, include accentuated pulmonic component of S_2, right ventricular life, S_4 gallop, ejection murmur at left sternal edge, or signs of systemic venous congestion. It is unusual to find clinically evident thrombophlebitis of the lower extremities at the time of diagnosis. More commonly observed are signs of chronic venous disease, such as tortuous varicosities, mild edema, and skin changes of stasis.

None of the above-mentioned signs or symptoms are specific for pulmonary emboli. They are present in many other diseases, including congestive heart failure, pneumonia, chronic lung disease, and myocardial infarction. It is difficult to establish the diagnosis of pulmonary emboli from clinical findings alone. The physician must first think of it when the patient presents with these nonspecific symptoms in an appropriate setting. He may then call upon laboratory aids to confirm or often deny his clinical suspicion.

LABORATORY STUDIES[124]

Electrocardiogram

In more than one-third of the patients the electrocardiogram (ECG) is normal, while in others there are nonspecific abnormalities which are not helpful in making the diagnosis. The changes observed in the ECG do not correlate with the size of the emboli, location, or hemodynamic alterations. The most frequent ECG abnormalities are changes in the ST segment and T wave in right precordial leads. The time-honored alterations of P pulmonale, peaking of P wave, right axis deviation, $S_1Q_3T_3$ pattern, atrial fibrillation, and changes of right ventricular hypertrophy are observed only occasionally. Almost all of the ECG abnormalities are transient, lasting only a few hours or days. Although the ECG may not provide specific diagnostic information, abnormalities noted here may provide a clue that an acute cardiopulmonary event has occurred. The ECG is useful in excluding myocardial infarction.

Chest Roentgenogram

Intravascular thrombi have the same radiodensity as the blood and surrounding tissues and cannot be visualized with plain x-rays. The most frequently observed abnormalities are the secondary pulmonary parenchymal changes of consolidation and atelectasis often with unilateral diaphragmatic elevation. Pleural

effusion occurs in about one-third of the patients and may be bilateral. Increase in major vessel and cardiac chamber size may occur, but is rare. Infrequently, changes compatible with pulmonary parenchymal infarction (pleural based, triangular, wedge-shaped density), abrupt vessel cut-off, and large areas of radiolucency secondary to oligemia are seen. Changes of parenchymal infarction, when present, usually occur 18 to 36 hours following the embolic event. The chest roentgenogram is normal in approximately half of the patients with documented pulmonary thromboembolic disease.

The chest x-ray is most helpful in a patient suspected of having emboli when it is normal. The combination of a normal chest x-ray and an abnormal lung isotope perfusion scan should heighten the suspicion of the diagnosis.

Hematology and Coagulation Studies

The erythrocyte sedimentation rate and white blood cell count may be minimally elevated. Infrequently, the white blood cell count (with a normal differential distribution) may increase to 15,000 to 20,000/mm³. The platelet count and the plasma fibrinogen concentration are either normal or moderately elevated. Fibrinogen–fibrin degradation products may be elevated at some time in the course of the illness, but are not elevated at the time of the acute event, and, therefore, are not helpful in making the diagnosis or making the decision to institute therapy.

Chemistry Studies

Recent studies have demonstrated that measurement of serum enzymes or isoenzymes offer little diagnostic help in patients with pulmonary emboli. Although minimal elevations in bilirubin, alkaline phosphatase, LDH, SGOT, and SGPT can be detected, they are transient and do not occur with any predictability. Presently, there is no biochemical test that has been proven to be efficacious in making or supporting the diagnosis of pulmonary thromboembolism.

Arterial Blood Gases

Although approximately 80 percent of the patients with pulmonary emboli have a reduced Pa_{O_2} on room air, this test has several limitations. At least 15 percent of the patients with even massive emboli have Pa_{O_2} levels of 90 mm Hg or greater. In diseases such as acute and chronic lung disease and cardiac disease where pulmonary embolism is common, the Pa_{O_2} level may be reduced prior to the embolic event. If a recent, normal set of arterial blood gas determinations is available for comparison, repeat study at the time of symptoms suggestive of emboli may provide evidence favoring the diagnosis.

Isotope Lung Scanning[123,125]

Pulmonary isotopic perfusion lung scanning is a valuable technique in the investigation of a patient with suspected pulmonary emboli. This technique is extremely sensitive and provides accurate information about blood flow in pulmonary vessels as small as 15 μ in diameter. It is performed by injecting isotopically labeled denatured protein particles (microspheres) into a peripheral vein. When the microspheres reach the lung, they are held up transiently in capillaries allowing external gamma detectors to image the distribution pattern of radioactivity in the lung. Currently, the detectors image six different views of the lungs: anterior, posterior, right and left lateral, and right and left oblique (Fig. 24–1). This technique can be performed easily and quickly, without discomfort or morbidity to the most seriously ill patient. The diagnostic utility of this technique is severely limited because of its lack of specificity. Anything that alters blood flow, such as infectious processes, congestive heart failure, infiltrative neoplasms, or asthma, as well as intraluminal vascular obstruction, can yield an abnormal distribution pattern of radioactivity in the lungs. If a properly performed lung scan (six views) reveals bilateral segmental defects, at best this can strongly suggest, but does not confirm the diagnosis of pulmonary emboli. The greatest utility of the lung perfusion scan is in excluding the diagnosis of pulmonary emboli. Because of its extreme sensitivity, if the perfusion scan (six views) is normal, the patient does not have emboli. An inconclusive, abnormal scan is helpful at the time of angiography, to direct the angiographer to look closely at areas suspected of having emboli.

The inhalation of radioactive gas (xenon) can be used to examine the function of the ventilatory compartments of the lung, and is often performed after the perfusion scan to determine whether ventilatory abnormalities are responsible for perfusion defects. Theoretically, if there is intraluminal obstruction due to thrombi, the perfusion scan will be abnormal, but the ventilation scan will be normal. In a patient with pulmonary emboli, the defects seen on perfusion scan will not be matched by defects on the ventilation scan. Unfortunately, this ideal situation is not always present. If the blood vessels are damaged by extensive embolic obstruction, the adjacent ventilatory compartments may be deranged. The defect seen on perfusion scan may be matched by a similar defect on ventilation scan; such a combination may be interpreted erroneously as pulmonary parenchymal disease, and not thromboembolism. Whether the combination of perfusion and ventilation lung scanning will improve the accuracy of the perfusion scan alone in supporting the diagnosis of pulmonary embolism remains to be established.

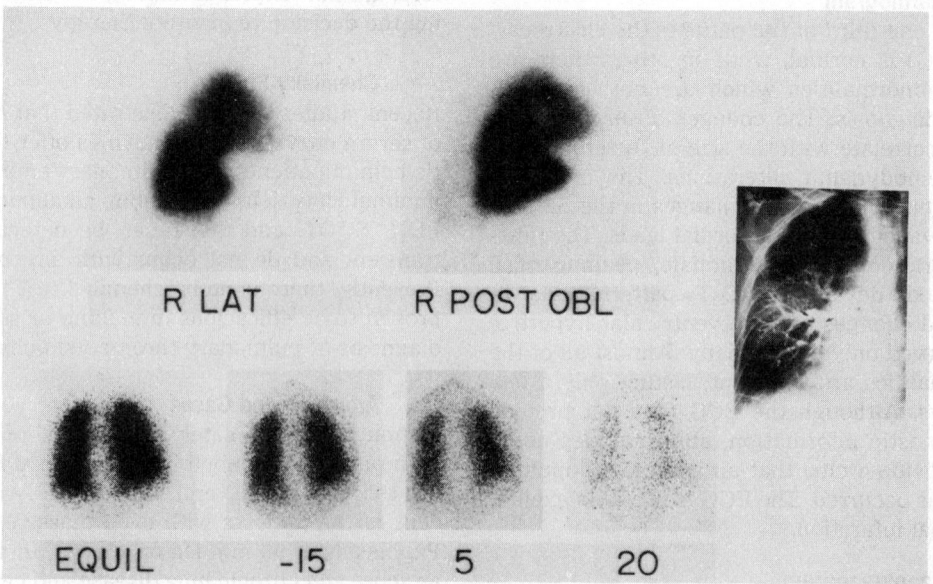

FIGURE 24-1. Ventilation and perfusion scans shown in conjunction with a selective right lower lobe pulmonary arteriogram in a patient with pulmonary embolism. There is a segmental perfusion defect in the right mid-lung field seen in the right lateral and right posterior oblique views of the perfusion scan (top). The ventilation scan (bottom) is normal. The arteriogram (right) demonstrates emboli in the artery to the right mid-lung field.

Pulmonary Angiography

The pulmonary angiogram is the best available technique to establish the presence of pulmonary emboli. Although this technique is not infallible, recent studies have demonstrated that the occurrence of false-negatives or false positives is rare. The discomfort to the patient, the personnel, expense of equipment, and time required limit the routine use of this technique but do not negate its usefulness. The morbidity and mortality are less than 1 percent.

Recent angiographic studies have documented that emboli are commonly bilateral. Infrequently (10 to 15 percent), the emboli are confined to one lung and these are usually multiple. In some patients, resolution of thrombi may occur as early as 15 to 20 days following the embolic event. The combination of angiographic and lung perfusion scanning studies has demonstrated that nearly two-thirds of the patients have residual vascular defects one year following the diagnosis.

DIAGNOSTIC APPROACH

If the history and the physical examination are suggestive of emboli, the patient should receive a lung perfusion scan directly. An arterial blood gas determination may be helpful. If the lung perfusion scan is normal, the investigations can cease; pulmonary emboli are excluded. If the lung perfusion scan is abnormal, a ventilation scan should be performed. If the ventilation scan is normal, and clinical features are appropriate, it is reasonable to accept the diagnosis of emboli and institute therapy. If the interpretation of the perfusion and ventilation scans is abnormal and compatible with emboli, but there are additional problems, such as congestive heart failure, chronic lung disease, and asthma, angiography should be performed to settle the issue.

There are other clinical situations where confirmation of the diagnosis by angiography is important. These include a past history of bleeding or untoward reaction to anticoagulants, prior to any surgical procedure, including umbrella insertion, if the patient has a past history of recurrent pulmonary emboli without angiographic documentation, or if the patient has been placed on optimal medical management without substantiating the diagnosis and his condition deteriorates.

MANAGEMENT

The most important initial step in treatment is administration of adequate fluid volume to increase the venous pressure in order to promote maximal blood return to the right heart. Anticoagulant or thrombolytic therapy should be instituted promptly, as soon as the diagnosis is made. In addition, supportive measures such as oxygen and, if indicated, minimal effective doses of analgesics, aminophyline for bronchospasm, digitalis for heart failure, and/or vasopressors for hypotension should be administered (Chap. 19). For patients with uncomplicated pulmonary emboli, the initial agent of choice is intravenous heparin, which should be administered for 10 to 14 days (Chap. 30). Before discontinuation of heparin, oral anticoagulants should be instituted and continued for 6 weeks to 6 months or longer. The duration of oral anticoagulation must be guided by the status of the patient. In those patients with risk factors such as obesity, congestive heart failure, venous disease of the lower extremities, or a history of recurrent thrombotic disease, oral anticoagulation may be continued indefinitely. In patients who are temporarily immobilized, oral anticoagulant therapy should continue until the patient is fully ambulatory.

In those patients with massive or submassive emboli who experience cardiopulmonary compromise, prompt restoration of blood flow is needed to return the cardiac index to normal. Thrombolytic agents, infused for 12 to 24 hours, can induce clot dissolution and return cardiopulmonary hemodynamics toward normal within hours, which does not occur with heparin therapy. Surgical embolectomy should be considered in the patient who is receiving optimal medical therapy but shows clinical deterioration or persisting hypotension. If anticoagulation is ineffective in preventing recurrent embolic episodes, as documented by pulmonary angiography, vena caval interruption (including umbrella insertion) may be helpful. The results of vena caval interruption have been disappointing—intraoperative mortality is high and recurrent emboli may occur because of the development of collateral vessels within 6 to 8 days. On occasion these procedures have been life saving.[126] Therefore, it is important not to wait until the situation is irreversible before obtaining surgical consultation.

In the overall management of patients with thrombotic disease, prophylaxis is important. Early ambulation after surgical procedures or parturition will help to eliminate venous stasis. In patients who must remain immobilized for long periods, such as those recovering from orthopedic procedures or when prolonged bed rest is required for treatment of heart failure or myocardial infarction, low-dose heparin or oral anticoagulation (Chap. 30) may be effective in preventing venous thrombosis. Elastic support stockings may promote venous flow in the legs as may leg muscle contraction against resistance.

CHAPTER 25

Systemic Hypertension
R. PATTERSON RUSSELL AND PAUL K. WHELTON

INTRODUCTION

An elevated blood pressure, like an elevated body temperature, may be due to any of a variety of underlying conditions. If the elevation is sustained, hypertension due to any cause will shorten life expectancy. The atherosclerotic process in all the blood vessels of the body is accelerated by hypertension, and this effect is responsible for many of the consequences of hypertension, such as cerebral infarct, coronary insufficiency, myocardial infarction, and kidney failure. In addition, microaneurysms of small cerebral vessels, first described by Charcot, are responsible for cerebral hemorrhage in association with high arterial pressures, particularly in patients over the age of 40. Hypertension also increases the work load on the left ventricle and this may lead to congestive heart failure, especially if coronary atherosclerosis coexists.

REGULATION OF BLOOD PRESSURE

Arterial blood pressure is regulated by the combined effects of cardiac output and peripheral resistance. Both are, in turn, modified by stroke volume, pulse rate, total blood volume, blood viscosity, elasticity of blood vessels, and neurogenic and humoral stimuli. While none of these modifying influences predominates throughout the entire range of blood pressure, the final integration of responses to these stimuli is chiefly attributable to two systems: the autonomic nervous system and the renin–angiotensin–aldosterone system.

The autonomic nervous system may play a primary or secondary role in hypertension. A primary role in some patients is indicated by the finding of increased cardiac output, a greater increase in systolic than in diastolic blood pressure (increased pulse pressure), and clinical signs of sympatho-adrenal hyperactivity. Eich and others have demonstrated that patients with labile or borderline hypertension frequently have increased cardiac output and normal peripheral resistance when first studied.[129] Later, cardiac output returns toward normal and peripheral resistance increases. Moreover, in subjects with volume expansion or renal ischemia as the cause of their high blood pressure, autonomic dysfunction may play a significant secondary role. The beneficial lowering of blood pressure in these instances with sympatho-

lytic and, more specifically, beta adrenergic blocking drugs tends to support this view. In essential hypertension there is little evidence to suggest that the renin–angiotensin–aldosterone system is primarily responsible for the elevated blood pressure.

EPIDEMIOLOGY

Community-based epidemiologic studies, such as the one initiated in Framingham, Massachusetts in 1949, have been influential in confirming the importance of high blood pressure as a contributor to cardiovascular morbidity and mortality.[132] In addition, certain myths concerning hypertension have been dispelled. The first concerns the value of a single casual blood pressure determination; it was found to be strongly related to the 18-year incidence of cardiovascular disease. Secondly, it had long been held that the cardiovascular consequences of hypertension derived from the diastolic component and that the systolic elevation was innocuous. However, this was not substantiated in the Framingham study and, in fact, the systolic component exerted a greater impact for every major cardiovascular sequella of hypertension. Unfortunately, the diastolic component continues to receive an inordinate amount of attention as most of the treatment studies have failed to include the systolic pressure in the formulation of guidelines for therapeutic interventions. Of all the risk factors studied, hypertension emerged as the most common, most potent, and most universal contributor to cardiovascular mortality.

Within our society there is a tendency for the blood pressure to rise with age, and the rate of the rise appears to differ between males and females (Fig. 25–1). Interestingly, an absence of hypertension and a failure of the blood pressure to rise with age has been documented in non-Western populations from widely different parts of the world.[130] In many studies the prevalence of hypertension has been shown to be inversely correlated with the degree of salt intake. To define a universally applicable figure above which one is hypertensive is to ignore the great variation in response to physiologic, environmental, emotional, and aging factors. One must recognize the arbitrary nature of any figure selected to define hypertension and, therefore, the greater the deviation the greater the certainty that values are abnormal. Even within

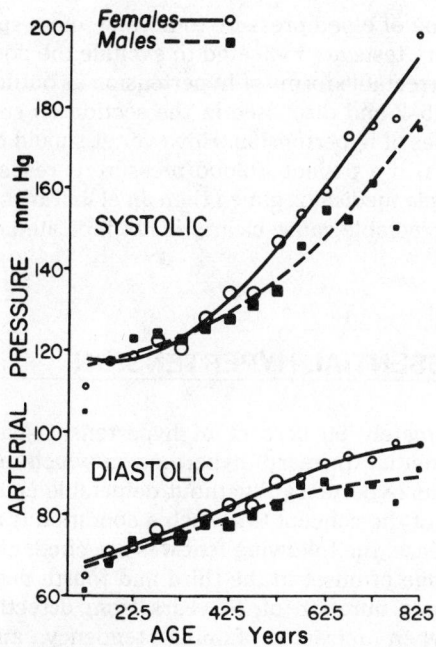

FIGURE 25-1. Systolic and diastolic pressures for females (open circles) and males (black squares) for each 5-year age group of a population sample, together with the fitted curves. The area of each circle or square is proportional to the number of subjects in that age group. (From Hamilton et al., Clin. Sci., 13:11, 1954.)

the "normal" range, subjects with higher pressure are more prone to the development of cardiovascular complications and death than are those with lower pressures.

DETECTION AND SCREENING

Is there a dividing line between normotension and hypertension? While hypertension is a diagnosis that is ultimately based on determination of the blood pressure and is said to exist when the blood pressure remains fixed above some arbitrarily defined value, it is clear that the higher the pressure the worse the prognosis. For many years systolic and diastolic pressures equal to or exceeding 160/95 mm Hg in adults were regarded as abnormal. However, the futility of selecting a precise cut-off is illustrated by current advice to treat asymptomatic, young black males with blood pressures of 140/90 mm Hg or higher. Undoubtedly these figures will change in the years ahead as more data pertaining to the natural history and benefits of therapy are applied to specific race, sex, and age groups.

Only a few years ago, fully 40 percent of hypertensive patients were unaware that their blood pressure was elevated. Today this is no longer true due to massive public education, heightened awareness of the significance of hypertension, and increased accessibility to blood pressure measurement. As a consequence, blood pressure screening is no longer considered adequate unless it is coupled with a program which facilitates referral for confirmation and, when necessary, initiation of evaluation and treatment.

Since the majority of hypertensive patients are without symptoms and are detected in the course of mass screening programs, annual checkups, or routine employment or insurance physical examinations, it is imperative to first confirm the presence of an elevated blood pressure. In this regard, specific criteria have been developed by the Joint National Committee on Detection, Evaluation and Treatment of High Blood Pressure.[138] Generally the higher the initial elevation the easier it is to confirm the deviation. However, with an isolated blood pressure reading of 140 to 159 mm Hg systolic over 90 to 104 mm Hg diastolic it is often necessary to obtain repeated measurements in both the standing and recumbent positions and under a variety of circumstances, such as at work and at home, and at different times throughout the day before a diagnosis of hypertension is confirmed.

A note of caution is indicated with regard to the use of blood pressure equipment for home determination and the increased accessibility of coin-operated automatic blood pressure measuring devices. While the former provides important information to the physician, patients must be properly instructed in the use of home blood pressure kits, and the equipment periodically evaluated for accuracy. Automated devices should provide a definition of normal, borderline, and high readings, caution consumers about the need for confirmation of elevated reading, and urge patients on treatment to share the results with their physicians and to consult them prior to changing doses or discontinuing therapy.

CLASSIFICATION OF HYPERTENSION

In this chapter the following classification of hypertension is utilized:

1. Esssential or primary
2. Secondary
   a. Amenable to correction
   b. Amenable to medical therapy

Essential or primary hypertension (Group 1) is the most common cause of high blood pressure. All other forms of hypertension are considered to be secondary to a recognizable disease process—for example, renal, adrenal, vascular, or central nervous system disease—and are separated into two groups on the basis of therapeutic response. The secondary conditions amenable to correction (Group 2a) are curable by surgical or other interventions and must be carefully considered in every patient with hypertension. Although not curable, hypertension in the remaining secondary conditions is amenable to medical therapy (Group 2b).

PATIENT EVALUATION

Figure 25-2 depicts a flow diagram for evaluating a hypertensive patient. Once it is established that the blood pressure is elevated significantly for a patient's age, race, and sex, the next step is to establish whether the elevation is primary or secondary and to ascertain the degree of involvement of such target organs as the central nervous system, eyes, heart, and kidneys. A complete history and physical examination supplemented by selective laboratory studies will provide this information. In the history taking, inquiry should be made regarding the family history of hypertension and cardiovascular complications, the presence or absence of central nervous system, cardiac, and genitourinary symptoms, dietary indiscretions, i.e., excessive consumption of salt or licorice, and, in women, any history of menstrual irregularity, previous hypertension associated with pregnancies, or use of oral contraceptives or conjugated estrogens. The physical examination enables the physician to assess the degree of target organ involvement through careful evaluation of the fundi, heart, and central nervous system. In addition, signs of specific correctable conditions such as coarctation of the aorta, Cushing syndrome, and renovascular hypertension may be detected on physical examination. Initial laboratory studies should include:

1. Urinalysis/serum creatinine
2. Serum potassium and uric acid
3. Fasting blood sugar and lipid profile
4. Electrocardiogram/chest x-ray (optional)

Additional studies may be desirable depending on the particular drug or drugs selected for therapy (see section on antihypertensive therapy). If at any time the patient does not respond as anticipated with a lowering of blood pressure to normal, more specific laboratory tests are indicated to exclude the possibility of correctable forms of hypertension as outlined in Figure 25-2 and discussed in the section on secondary causes of hypertension. However, it should be obvious that if a patient's blood pressure is responsive to a simple medical regimen then an elaborate search for a correctable cause clearly is not indicated or desirable.

ESSENTIAL HYPERTENSION

Approximately 90 percent of hypertensive patients have essential (primary) hypertension which may be defined as hypertension without detectable cause. In support of the concept that such a condition is a specific disease, the following features are cited: characteristic age of onset in the third and fourth decades, an average duration of 20 years from detection to death when untreated, familial tendency, and increased incidence in obese females and blacks. With respect to this last feature, recent studies have confirmed that in the United States hypertension is more prevalent and more severe in blacks than in whites. The National Health Survey found a blood pressure equal to or greater than either 160 mm Hg systolic or 90 mm Hg diastolic in 27 percent of black adults as compared with 14 percent of white adults and the excess prevalence was approximately the same for every age group.[139] However, the diversity of these features is more compatible with a graded characteristic like height and weight than with a specific disease.[141]

CLINICAL PRESENTATION

The four common clinical presentations of patients with hypertension are outlined in Table 25-1. In the earliest stage the patient is symptomless and hypertension is detected only during a routine physical examination. The patient is otherwise normal and there are no laboratory abnormalities. The second stage of the disease is characterized by a higher arterial pressure and mild symptoms, but major complications are absent. These early symptoms include headache, lightheadedness, vertigo, tinnitus, fatigue, nervousness, and flushing sensations of the head. Nosebleeds may occur and usually indicate that the diastolic pressure is persistently at or above 100 mm Hg. The fundi show minimal or no change. A slight left ventricular heave may be noted, but the heart is not enlarged. Symptoms at this stage may be due in part to fear and to misunderstanding of the natural history of the condition. The physician must reassure the pa-

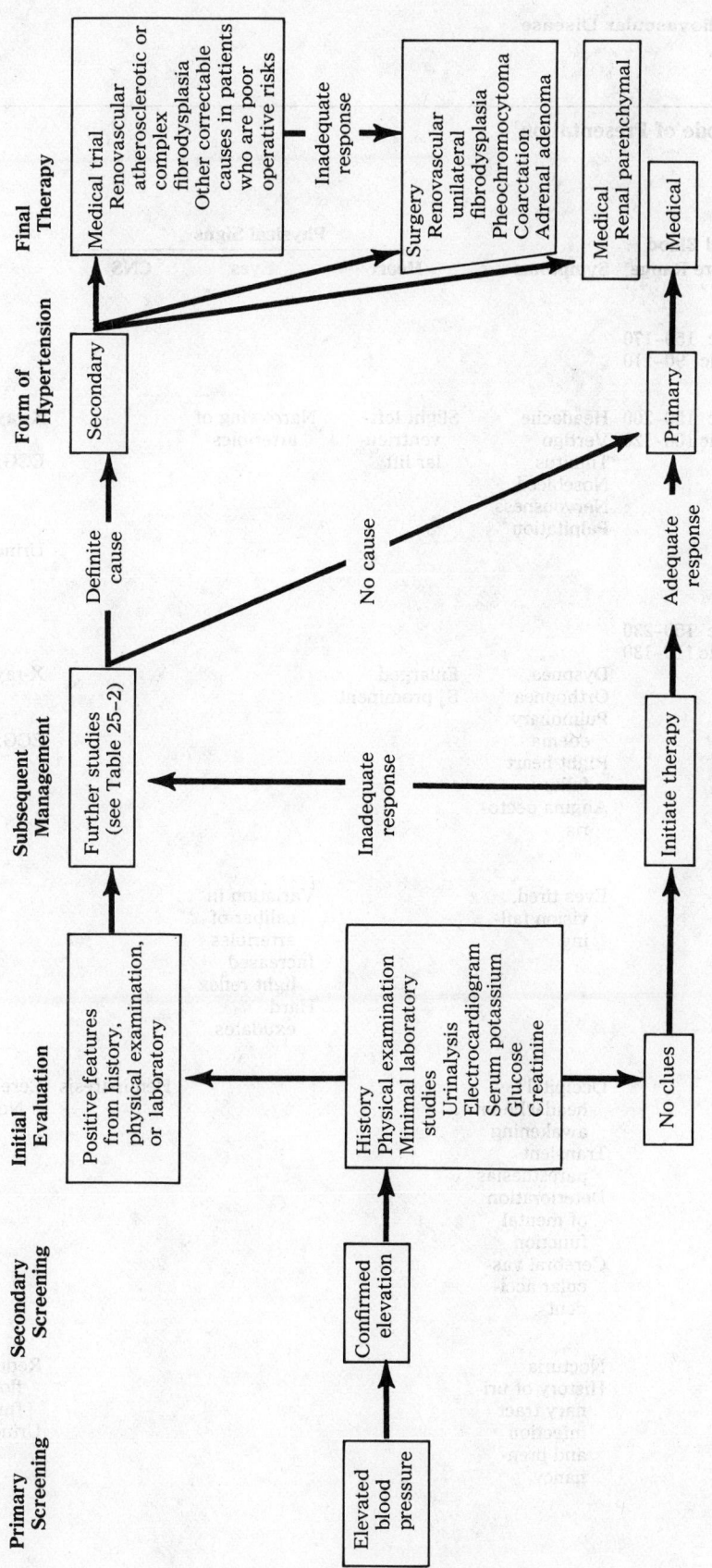

FIGURE 25-2. Flow diagram depicting the sequential evaluation of a hypertensive patient from first detection to final therapy.

TABLE 25-1
Hypertension—Mode of Presentation

Presentation	Usual Blood Pressure Range	Symptoms	Physical Signs			Laboratory
			Heart	Eyes	CNS	
Symptomless	Systolic 150–170 Diastolic 90–110					
Symptoms, no complications	Systolic 150–200 Diastolic 100–120	Headache Vertigo Tinnitus Nosebleed Nervousness Palpitation	Slight left-ventricular lift	Narrowing of arterioles		X-ray: Normal size heart ECG: Normal or minor ST-T wave abnormalities Urine: ± Trace of protein
Symptoms and complications Heart	Systolic 150–230 Diastolic 110–130	Dyspnea, Orthopnea Pulmonary edema Right heart failure Angina pectoris	Enlarged S_4 prominent			X-ray: Left ventricular hypertrophy ECG: Normal or minor ST-T wave abnormalities Left ventricular hypertrophy
Eyes		Eyes tired, vision failing		Variation in caliber of arterioles Increased light reflex Hard exudates		
Central nervous system		Occipital headache on awakening Transient paresthesias Deterioration of mental function Cerebral vascular accident			Hemiparesis	Cerebrospinal fluid: Normal or bloody
Kidney		Nocturia History of urinary tract infection and pregnancy				Reduced renal blood flow and tubular function Urine: 1–2 + protein Decreased specific gravity

TABLE 25-1 (cont.)

Presentation	Usual Blood Pressure Range	Symptoms	Physical Signs			Laboratory
			Heart	**Eyes**	**CNS**	
Malignant phase	Systolic 200–300 Diastolic 130+	Violent headaches Visual impairment Weight loss Vomiting, Drowsiness Hypertensive encephalopathy	Enlarged Left ventricular failure	Papilledema Fresh hemorrhages and soft exudates	Focal transient neurologic features	X-ray: Left ventricular hypertrophy ECG: Normal or minor ST-T wave abnormalities Left ventricular hypertrophy Urine: 2–4+ protein, microscopic and gross hematuria Serum: Urea nitrogen elevated

tient that the level of the blood pressure may be very high during examination but only moderately elevated at other times. Understanding that blood pressure is not a fixed quantity, that it varies enormously through the day, and that, in selected instances, the measurement itself causes higher readings may help to dispel much of the fear and anxiety associated with the diagnosis.

The third stage is characterized by the appearance of complications attributable to the effects of sustained high blood pressure on the heart, the eyes, the cerebral circulation, and the kidneys. Three-quarters of all patients with an elevated blood pressure develop cardiac hypertrophy, and the degree of hypertrophy is more closely related to the severity than to the duration of the hypertension. Left ventricular hypertrophy is manifested clinically by the appearance of a left ventricular heave and a prominent fourth heart sound (S_4). Electrocardiographic evidence of left ventricular hypertrophy or other less specific signs of cardiac damage are present in two-thirds of these patients. Cardiac dysfunction culminates in congestive heart failure. Right heart failure as characterized by venous distention, edema, and enlargement of the liver usually occurs only after symptoms of left heart failure have been well established. But occasionally patients with essential hypertension come to medical attention for the first time with an attack of acute pulmonary edema. Hypertension accelerates the atherosclerotic process, and, therefore, angina pectoris and myocardial infarction

may occur at an earlier age in the hypertensive patient.

The most common symptom attributable to the effects of hypertension on the cerebral circulation is headache. The typical headache of hypertension is a throbbing, occipital type of pain which is worse on awakening but gradually clears after several hours of activity. In general, the higher the pressure the more severe the headache. However, in many instances, hypertensive patients complain of headaches that are less specific and not as clearly defined. These headaches are unrelated to the level of blood pressure and frequently are dispelled by firm reassurance. Transient episodes of weakness, numbness, and tingling of the hands and feet may come and go spontaneously or proceed to a more serious complication. Both cerebral thrombosis and cerebral hemorrhage tend to occur at an earlier age in the hypertensive patient. Nonspecific disturbances of vision, such as tiredness and undue fatigability, may be early symptoms, while more specific complaints due to retinal vascular changes or to cerebral lesions may occur later on. The importance of performing an adequate funduscopic examination cannot be overemphasized because the fundi are unique in providing information about the effects of hypertension. Variations in caliber and increase in the light reflex of arteries are the earliest manifestations of hypertensive vascular damage in the retinae. Arteriovenous compression and small, sharply defined exudates, occasionally accompanied by an isolated hemorrhage, are often seen at a later stage of the disease. Hemorrhages and soft, ill-defined exudates often presage an abrupt increase in the severity of the hypertension, and the occurrence of papilledema indicates the onset of the last and most severe stage of the malignant phase.

Hypertensive encephalopathy is a term used to denote acute cerebral episodes occurring in hypertensive patients whose pressure has recently risen above previous levels, as in acute nephritis, toxemia of pregnancy, or the malignant phase. These episodes, characterized by violent headaches, vomiting, visual impairment, drowsiness, and focal, transient neurologic features, usually precede renal insufficiency. When present, these attacks represent the most positive indication for immediate reduction in blood pressure. The term "hypertensive encephalopathy" is often applied incorrectly to cerebral vascular accidents occurring in hypertensive patients. Such patients, who may have cerebral thrombosis or hemorrhage, frequently are subjected to potentially hazardous therapy with hypotensive drugs. It is usually possible to differentiate cerebral thrombosis from hypertensive encephalopathy because of the predominance of transient focal paralysis in the latter. Cerebral hemorrhage may present a more difficult problem, and a lumbar puncture may be required. In the event that cerebral hemorrhage cannot be differentiated from hypertensive encephalopathy, it is advisable to proceed with immediate blood pressure reduction.

Renal blood flow and tubular function are reduced in the early stages of essential hypertension, and mild renal insufficiency is a common late occurrence. Impairment of renal function and proteinuria develop usually in association with hypertensive vascular changes. This is demonstrated in long-standing hypertension, the malignant phase, or underlying renal parenchymal disease, such as glomerulonephritis or pyelonephritis. The hypertensive patient who suddenly develops renal insufficiency must be carefully evaluated to exclude the possibility of urinary tract infection, obstructive uropathy, sodium deficiency, or dehydration.

CLINICAL COURSE

Patients with blood pressures ranging from 140 to 159/90 to 94 mm Hg are considered to have borderline essential hypertension. Approximately half of these patients will be found on follow-up to have a higher blood pressure that warrants additional follow-up and treatment. At the other extreme is a small group of patients with accelerated or malignant hypertension in whom the diastolic blood pressure is usually greater than 130 mm Hg but of more importance than the actual level of blood pressure are the

associated signs of significant target organ damage. In between are the majority of patients with elevated blood pressure of varying degrees of severity who in the past were referred to as having "benign" essential hypertension. Unfortunately, this term has served only to confuse and in many instances belittle the seriousness of the underlying condition. Thus, in describing the clinical course of hypertension it is proposed that the term "insidious"—acting by imperceptible degrees—be substituted for the term "benign."

Patients with essential hypertension may follow an insidious or malignant course depending on the rate of progression. While this distinction is discussed here in the context of essential hypertension, it is important to emphasize that it can be applied to the other forms of hypertension as well. Figure 25–3 outlines the malignant and insidious courses (upper two panels) of untreated in contrast to treated essential hypertension (lowest panel). The differences between these courses are clearly seen in the more rapid development of complications in patients following the malignant and insidious courses. There are also differences in the causes of death in each group, with combined renal insufficiency and cardiac disease being more common in those with malignant hypertension while cardiac disease predominates in those with the insidious form.

The malignant course of essential hypertension, or malignant hypertension, is characterized by a rapidly rising or sustained diastolic blood pressure, usually in excess of 130 mm Hg, and severe progressive changes involving the brain, the eyes, and the kidneys. The earliest manifestations can often be detected on funduscopic examination. Hemorrhages, soft exudates, and papilledema are always present in the fully developed condition. Significant weight loss is often present and bespeaks the systemic nature of the syndrome. Hematuria, proteinuria, and azotemia constitute major renal manifestations. The most severe and life-threatening manifestations of malignant hypertension are renal failure and hypertensive encephalopathy. If untreated, the condition usually results in death in less than a year.[134] The malignant course may arise de novo, but is usually preceded by a period of known high blood pressure. Due to the widespread use of antihypertensive drug therapy, malignant hypertension is rarely encountered today and when it is, the patient is most likely to have a secondary form of hypertension.

With regard to the insidious course, it should be remembered that a male between the ages of 45 and 64 years with a systolic blood pressure over 150 mm Hg has more than twice the risk of heart attack and

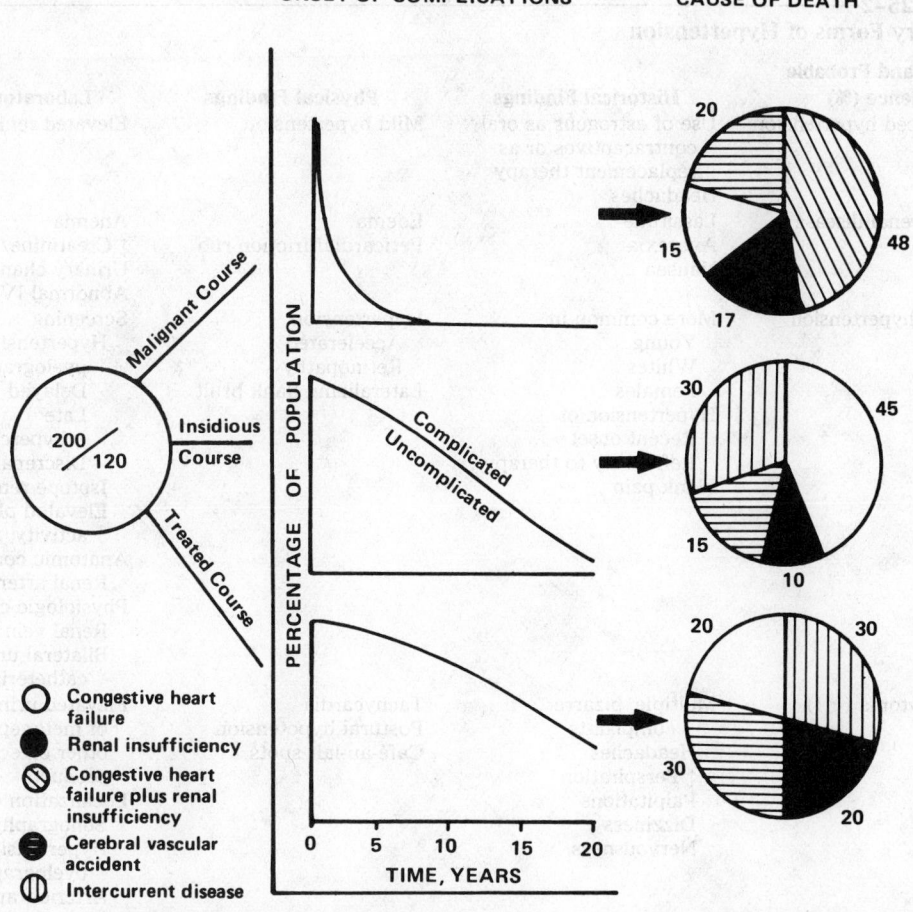

ONSET OF COMPLICATIONS

CAUSE OF DEATH

Congestive heart failure

Renal insufficiency

Congestive heart failure plus renal insufficiency

Cerebral vascular accident

Intercurrent disease

FIGURE 25–3. The natural history of the malignant, insidious, and treated courses of hypertension. The three graphs are designed to indicate the rate of development of complications in patients with untreated (malignant and insidious courses) and treated essential hypertension. This rate is most rapid in the group following the malignant course in which approximately 50 percent have developed complications within 1 year. The causes of death for each course are shown in the diagram at the right.

nearly four times the risk of stroke than a man with a systolic blood pressure under 120 mm Hg. As previously noted, the characteristic age of onset of essential hypertension is early in the fourth decade. Often the patient remains free of symptoms for 10 to 15 years, and the complications that develop are largely manifestations of atherosclerosis. Approximately 50 percent die from congestive failure, 20 percent from cerebral vascular accidents, and 30 percent from other causes, one of the most important being myocardial infarction. Benefits derived from the reduction of blood pressure in patients with malignant hypertension have been demonstrated repeatedly. Life expectancy has been increased from months to years, and if

patients are treated prior to developing significant renal insufficiency, 7- to 10-year survivals are possible. Beneficial results also have been documented for patients with less severe forms of essential hypertension. The course of such a treated population is depicted in the lowest panel of Figure 25–3.

SECONDARY CAUSES OF HYPERTENSION

Although hypertension may be associated with a wide variety of disease processes, most of the secondary causes are associated with either renal or endo-

┌─TABLE 25–2───

Secondary Forms of Hypertension

Condition and Probable Prevalence (%)	Historical Findings	Physical Findings	Laboratory Studies
Estrogen induced hypertension (?)	Use of estrogens as oral contraceptives or as replacement therapy Headaches	Mild hypertension	Elevated renin substrate
Parenchymal renal disease (<5)	Lassitude Anorexia Nausea	Edema Pericardial friction rub	Anemia ↑ Creatinine/BUN Urinary changes Abnormal IVP

Renovascular hypertension (<5)	More common in
	  Young
	  Whites
	  Females
	Hypertension of
	  Recent onset
	  Refractory to therapy
	Flank pain
		Hypertension
		  Accelerated
		  Retinopathy
		Lateralizing flank bruit
			Screening
			  Hypertensive
			    pyelography
			    Delayed visualization
			    Late
			      hyperconcentration
			    Discrepancy in size
			  Isotope renography
			  Elevated plasma renin
			    activity
			Anatomic confirmation
			  Renal arteriography
			Physiologic confirmation
			  Renal vein renin studies
			  Bilateral ureteral
			    catheterization

Pheochromocytoma (<1)	Multiple, bizarre
	  complaints
	Headaches
	↑ Perspiration
	Palpitations
	Dizziness
	Nervousness
		Tachycardia
		Postural hypotension
		Café-au-lait spots
			Elevated urinary excretion
			  of metanephrine or
			  other catecholamine by-
			  products
			Localization of tumor(s)
			  Sonography
			  Hypertensive
			    pyelography
			  Arteriography
			  Venous catheterization
			    and determination of
			    plasma
			    catecholamines

Primary aldosteronism (<1)	Weakness
	Polyuria/polydipsia
	Paresthesias
	Tetany
		Mild hypertension
		Chvostek's or Trousseau's
		  sign
			Peripheral hormonal
			  studies
			  ↓ Plasma renin activity
			    on low sodium
			    intake
			  ↑ Plasma aldosterone on
			    high sodium intake
			Localization studies
			  Sonography
			  Venography
			  Adrenal vein steroid
			    determinations

Cushing syndrome (<1)	Sexual dysfunction
	Weakness
	Backache
		Plethora
		Central obesity
		Hirsutism
		Purple striae
		Ecchymoses
			Polycythemia
			Hyperglycemia
			Osteoporosis
			Increased urinary
			  17-ketosteroids and 11-
			  oxysteroids

Coarctation of the aorta (<1)	Asymptomatic
	Hypertension in childhood
	Intermittent claudication
		Changes in legs *vs.* arms
		  Lower blood pressure
		  Diminished and/or
		    delayed pulses
		Precordial murmur
		Intercostal pulsations
			Chest x-ray changes
			  Rib notching
			  "3" sign
			Left ventricular
			  hypertrophy

crine disorders. With the advent of effective pharmacotherapy, the search for secondary causes has become more dependent on the lack of response to therapy. Indeed, in recent years it has been repeatedly demonstrated that a thorough evaluation of all patients is economically unsupportable. However, a brief evaluation which includes a thorough history and physical examination is mandatory in every patient, since even by the most conservative estimates, almost 1.5 million hypertensives in the United States have potentially correctable forms of the disease.

RENAL PARENCHYMAL DISEASE

Hypertension is one of the most frequent complications of renal failure. It is usually no more than a transient phenomenon in acute renal failure but constitutes a more serious complication in patients with chronic renal failure, since the majority of these patients ultimately die from vascular complications. It should be stressed that in the latter setting treatment of hypertension, more than any other medical intervention, provides an effective way of delaying the inevitable progression to end-stage renal disease. Generally, the hypertension appears to result from excessive salt and water retention but in 5 to 10 percent of patients it is primarily renin–angiotensin mediated. Nephrectomy, although effective in lowering blood pressure in this latter group of patients, is best reserved for those who are functionally anephric.

RENOVASCULAR HYPERTENSION

Although the exact prevalence of renovascular hypertension is uncertain, hypertension probably results from underlying renal ischemia in approximately 5 percent of hypertensive patients. The specific types of vascular, parenchymal, and capsular involvement which may induce renal ischemia include:

    I. Large vessel disease
      A. Arteriosclerotic vascular disease
      B. Fibrous displasia or fibromuscular disease
      C. Arteritis
      D. Other
   II. Parenchymal lesions
      A. Unilateral pyelonephritis
      B. Juxtaglomerular cell tumors
      C. Wilms' tumors
 III. Capsular lesions
      A. Hematoma

In certain instances surgical intervention will result in a return of blood pressure to normal, but there is never a guarantee of such an outcome. Since only a small percentage of the hypertensive population has underlying renal ischemia, it is unreasonable to embark upon an expensive and time-consuming search for renovascular disease in all patients. The pertinent clinical features that should lead one to suspect renovascular hypertension are noted in Table 25–2, and steps in the evaluation of a patient are graphically outlined in Figure 25–4. Clearly, if a patient is not a suitable candidate for surgical intervention, it is unnecessary and unwarranted to carry out any investigational procedures.

History and Physical Examination

The age, race, and sex distribution of renovascular disease suggests that the disease, especially in its correctable form, is most common in young white females, and is extremely rare in black males. Furthermore, the disease is more common in those with severe hypertension and in patients whose blood pressure is difficult to manage or abruptly rises following previously satisfactory control. The presence or absence of an abdominal bruit must be routinely documented in all hypertensive patients. Midline bruits are not uncommon in thin young females and in elderly arteriosclerotic patients, but a bruit which lateralizes to the left or right side of the midupper abdomen is strongly suggestive of renal artery stenosis. Careful abdominal auscultation in a quiet room and with application of firm pressure on the bowl of the stethoscope will facilitate detection of the distinctive high-pitched, usually continuous, bruit in 30 to 40 percent of patients with renovascular hypertension.

Although the importance of a good history and physical examination cannot be overemphasized, in many patients the decision to perform renal arteriography is strongly influenced by the results of ancillary laboratory studies. In general, the screening laboratory studies should be obtained in all patients who are under the age of 50, have untreated diastolic blood pressures >110 mm Hg, or are management problems.

Screening Laboratory Studies

Of the various screening procedures, hypertensive pyelography remains the simplest and most accurate test available in most hospitals. In addition to being a good screening test for renovascular disease, it may also reveal the presence of renal parenchymal diseases. Early films from the "rapid sequence" hypertensive pyelogram provide the most sensitive indication of renal vascular disease, namely a discrepancy in appearance time of contrast in either kidney at one minute or more. Other findings which suggest the presence of renal vascular disease are hyperconcentration of dye in the late films and a difference in renal size of at least 1.5 cm. Isotope renography is a benign procedure which supplements the information

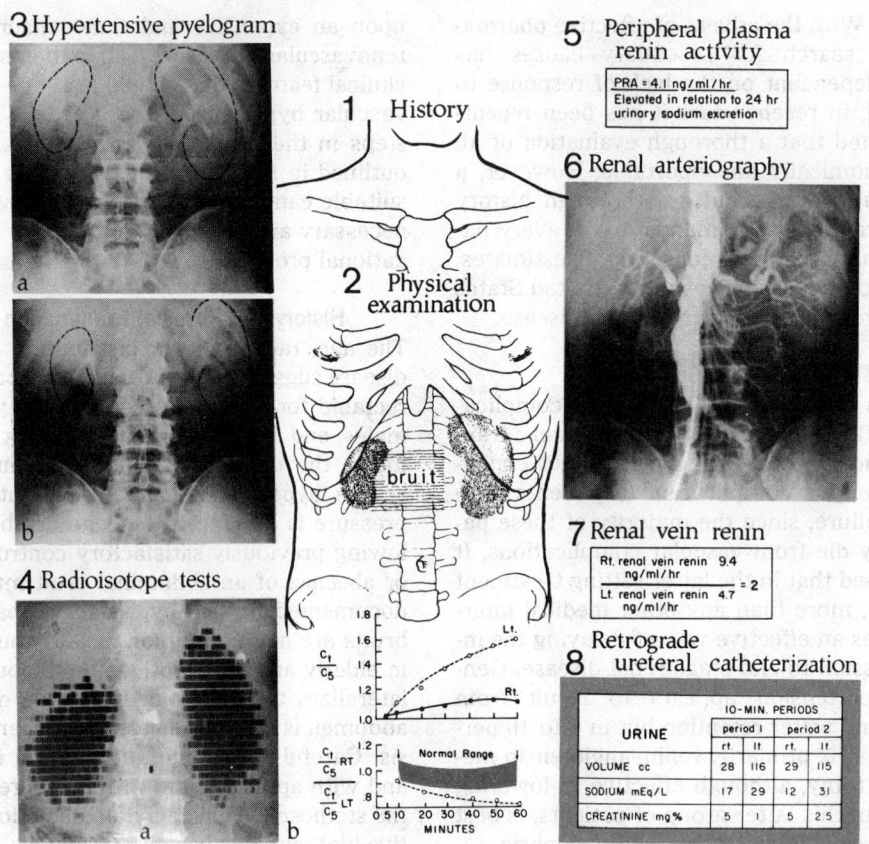

FIGURE 25–4. Hypertension secondary to unilateral renal ischemia associated with stenosis of the right renal artery in a 58-year-old white male with the following findings: 1) History of recent failure to control blood pressure adequately with treatment led to reevaluation; 2) Physical examination revealed a soft, high-pitched bruit most intense above and to the right of the umbilicus; 3) Rapid sequence "hypertensive" pyelogram revealed (a) on the 1 minute film a right kidney 3.6 cm smaller than the left and a delay in the appearance of the dye on the right, and (b) on the 30-minute film an increased concentration of dye on the right; 4) Isotope renography revealed a reduction in the (a) size, and (b) function of the right kidney; 5) Peripheral venous blood plasma renin activity elevated in relation to 24-hour urinary sodium excretion; 6) Renal arteriography demonstrated a segmental narrowing of the right renal artery—in addition, the right kidney was atrophic, the cortex thin, and the vessels crowded; 7) Comparison of renal vein renin activity levels obtained from the affected and contralateral kidneys revealed a ratio of 2.0 and a difference of 4.3 ng/ml/hr; 8) Bilateral retrograde ureteral catheterization revealed a 75 percent reduction in urine volume, a 50 percent reduction in urinary sodium excretion, and an increased urinary creatinine concentration from the right kidney in two consecutive collection periods.

obtained on pyelography and may be used as an initial screening test in patients who are allergic to pyelographic dye. However, it is less accurate than hypertensive pyelography and tends to overestimate the incidence of renovascular disease. An additional procedure which may indicate the presence of renal ischemia is the finding of elevated levels of peripheral plasma renin activity (PRA) in relation to the pa-

tient's posture and 24-hour urinary sodium excretion.[140] Again, although this finding is helpful when present, many patients with renal ischemia have levels of peripheral PRA within normal limits. The value of agents which inhibit angiotensin II and converting enzyme in diagnosing renovascular hypertension is as yet unsettled, and for the present time they are best regarded as research tools.

Renal Arteriography

In general, renal arteriography should be performed in the following groups of patients:

1. White females $<$50 years old with untreated diastolic blood pressures $>$110 mm Hg
2. Those with lateralizing upper abdominal bruits
3. Patients with positive laboratory screening procedures
4. Patients who are management problems

Renal arteriography provides accurate information in regard to the location, extent, and severity of lesions in the larger renal arteries. Indeed, angiography not only allows one to assess the technical feasibility of surgery, but when combined with the available clinical information, usually allows one to accurately predict the underlying vascular pathology, e.g., arteriosclerotic vascular disease or fibrous dysplasia.

Physiologic Studies

The mere demonstration of an arteriographic or pyelographic abnormality in a hypertensive patient is not sufficient indication for surgical intervention. It must be reasonably certain that the demonstrated lesion is responsible for the hypertension and that its surgical repair will be followed by a return of blood pressure toward, if not to, normal. To this end, there are two procedures which allow one to evaluate whether there is a physiologic alteration indicative of renal ischemia: renal vein renin activity, and retrograde ureteral catheterization.

In the presence of a lesion which reduces blood flow and/or pressure to one kidney, increased amounts of renin are released by that kidney, and consequently increased amounts of angiotensin I, angiotensin II, and aldosterone are produced. Blood for renal vein renin activity (RVRA) may be accurately obtained by sequential renal venous sampling with a single catheter after the demonstration of identifiable vascular lesions.[144] Although there are no set criteria for the diagnosis of renal ischemia, many studies have demonstrated the usefulness of comparing RVRA from both renal veins. Most often this comparison is expressed as a ratio of involved over uninvolved RVRA and ischemia is diagnosed when the ratio is 1.5 or greater. However, a ratio $\geq$ 1.5 alone does not always indicate the presence of renovascular hypertension. Additional criteria which take into consideration the absolute values for RVRA and peripheral PRA, contralateral suppression, and the absolute difference in RVRA between the two renal veins permit more accurate diagnosis.[143,144]

The other procedure which aids in the prediction of a successful outcome from surgical intervention is the retrograde catheterization of both ureters. In the presence of renal ischemia the affected kidney excretes a smaller urine volume with a lower concentration of sodium but a higher concentration of creatinine. Provided the technical aspects are well executed, bilateral retrograde ureteral catheterization permits one to predict with reasonable assurance whether a unilateral renal lesion is responsible for the patient's hypertension. However, because the technical problems and morbidity associated with the procedure are greater than with renal vein renin sampling, most investigators rely solely on the latter procedure.

Treatment

Once a presumptive diagnosis of renovascular hypertension has been established, the next question facing the physician is whether to attempt surgical revascularization of the ischemic kidney(s) or to manage the patient with a medical regimen. On the basis of the results of the cooperative study it would seem prudent, when feasible, to undertake surgery in all patients with unilateral fibrous dysplasia lesions, but initially, to manage with a medical regimen those with arteriosclerosis or more complex fibrous dysplasia lesions. Clearly with the latter approach one must ascertain that the patient's blood pressure is indeed controllable and that kidney function and size remain stable, particularly in the initial phases of follow-up. If blood pressure is not successfully controlled, or renal function begins to deteriorate, the need for surgical intervention should be carefully reconsidered. When surgery is undertaken, all possible efforts should be made to preserve renal mass, although the final decision as to whether a revascularization procedure, segmental resection, or nephrectomy is performed can only be made at the operation.

ENDOCRINE SYNDROMES

Pheochromocytoma

Pheochromocytoma, which results from excessive catecholamine production, is a rare but well-characterized and interesting form of hypertension.[133] Important end products of catecholamine biosynthesis are normally found in the brain (dopamine), autonomic nervous system (norepinephrine), and adrenal medulla (norepinephrine and epinephrine). Following release from the autonomic nervous system and adrenal medulla 90 percent of epinephrine and norepinephrine is reabsorbed unchanged. The remaining 10 percent is metabolized by catechol-o-methyl transferase (COMT) to metanephrine/normetanephrine and by monoaminoxidase to vanillymandelic acid (VMA).

Thus, the diagnosis of pheochromocytoma may be accurately confirmed by biochemical analysis of the urinary catecholamines, epinephrine and norepinephrine, or the metabolites, metanephrine, normetanephrine, and VMA. Depending on the test used, there are a number of reasons why one might obtain a "false positive" or "false negative" result, and some of these are outlined in Table 25-3. With the development of more sensitive and accurate biochemical tests, pharmacologic interventions such as histamine stimulation and phentolamine blockade have come to play a very limited role in the diagnosis of pheochromocytoma. Patients may be asymptomatic and normotensive at the time of presentation to the physician but more frequently complain of headaches, excessive perspiration, palpitation, nervousness, nausea, vomiting, and weight loss. Their hypertension is often severe and is frequently accompanied by evidence of left ventricular hypertrophy, retinopathy, and proteinuria. In addition, tachycardia is common and hyperglycemia is seen in approximately 60 percent of patients. As with renovascular hypertension, it is not reasonable to screen the entire hypertensive population for the possibility of pheochromocytoma. However, any patient with severe hypertension, paroxysmal symptoms, excessive headaches, or sweating, tachycardia, hyperglycemia, hypermetabolism without hyperthyroidism, or a paradoxical response to hypotensive or anesthetic agents should be evaluated carefully.

More than 90 percent of patients have solitary benign adenomas but the tumors can, on occasion, be multiple, ectopic, or malignant. This occurs with greater frequency in younger patients and those with familial tumors. Some of the latter will have medullary carcinoma of the thyroid and parathyroid tumors (multiple endocrine adenomatosis, Type II—Sipple syndrome). In addition, a wide variety of disease entities have been associated with pheochromocytomas including cholelithiasis, neurofibromatosis, congenital cyanotic heart disease, polycythemia, and renovascular hypertension.

Tumors can often be localized by abdominal CAT scan, sonography, or intravenous pyelography. More invasive tests, such as abdominal/thoracic arteriography and vena caval catecholamine sampling, are best reserved for patients in whom recurrent, ectopic, or multiple tumors are thought likely. These invasive tests should be performed only under carefully monitored conditions as contrast administration and catheter manipulation almost invariably activate the tu-

---

TABLE 25-3
Biochemical Diagnosis of Pheochromocytoma

Urinary Test	Accuracy (%)	False Positive Common Causes	False Negative Common Causes
Metanephrines and normeta-nephrines	95	MAO inhibitors, chlorproma-zine, severe stress, α-methyl-dopa	Contrast material
VMA	95	Naladixic acid, anileridine	MAO inhibitors, clofibrate
Catechol-amines	90	α-methyldopa, theophylline, tetracycline, quinidine, chloral hydrate	—
All of the above	99	Sympathomimetic childhood amines	Intermittent secretion; incomplete or incorrect collection

---

mor. Once the diagnosis is established, patients can be treated either medically or surgically. Since the perioperative mortality is generally less than 3 percent and the postoperative results are usually excellent, surgery is indicated in most patients. Medical therapy is usually reserved for short-term preoperative management, poor surgical candidates, and those with malignant tumors. It includes hydration, the use of alpha and/or beta receptor blockers, and on occasion, the tyrosine hydroxylase inhibitor, alpha methylparatyrosine.

Primary Aldosteronism

Primary aldosteronism is present in less than 1 percent of the hypertensive population. Although malignant hypertension is unusual, there are no other historical or physical features which help to identify these patients. The cardinal manifestations of the disease are hypertension, kaliuresis in the setting of hypokalemia, and a deranged pattern of renin–angiotensin–aldosterone secretion. In the absence of vomiting, diarrhea, excessive licorice intake, or the use of diuretics or laxatives, hypokalemia in a hypertensive patient should be carefully evaluated. Patients who develop hypokalemia after the use of thiazide diuretics deserve evaluation only if their hypokalemia cannot be easily corrected after the discontinuation of the diuretic agent. Urinary potassium excretion is best quantitated by obtaining a 24-hour urine specimen while the patient is still hypokalemic and on a liberal salt intake. In this setting, most patients with hyperaldosteronism excrete more than 30 mEq of potassium a day. The diagnosis can be subsequently confirmed by the demonstration of suppressed plasma renin activity unresponsive to restricted sodium intake and elevated plasma aldosterone concentration not suppressed by increased sodium intake. Since hypokalemia, occurring for any reason, may influence renin activity and aldosterone production, blood samples for these assays should be obtained following potassium repletion.

Although the diagnosis of primary hyperaldosteronism can usually be established with some certainty, it is more difficult to determine whether the disease results from a unilateral adrenal adenoma or from bilateral adrenal hyperplasia.[131] Since only the former is surgically correctable, the distinction is extremely important. The two conditions may be distinguished by abdominal computerized axial tomography, adrenal venography, and hormonal sampling from adrenal veins. Additional information is provided by the hormonal response to postural changes and the patient's response to short courses of spironolactone and dexamethasone. In general, patients with unilateral adenomas are best managed surgically. This is particularly true in those patients who are young, severely hypokalemic or hypertensive, and who fail to tolerate spironolactone therapy. Patients with bilateral hyperplasia usually respond well to a sodium restricted diet and low dose spironolactone therapy (less than 200 mg per day).

Idiopathic Cushing Syndrome

Idiopathic Cushing syndrome is an unusual cause of hypertension, even though most patients who have the disease are hypertensive.[133] It must be emphasized that many obese subjects exhibit hypertension and an increased excretion of urinary 17-hydroxycorticosteroids. The latter does not constitute evidence of Cushing syndrome, since this diagnosis can be made only when hyperadrenocorticalism is autonomous and nonsuppressible. The most useful clinical features in the recognition of Cushing syndrome are weakness, plethora, ecchymoses, central obesity, and osteoporosis. The evaluation and management of patients with Cushing syndrome is described in more detail in Chapter 70.

Congenital Adrenal Hyperplasia

Hypertension occasionally results from the syndrome of congenital adrenal hyperplasia, in which there is 11-hydroxylase or 17-hydroxylase deficiency. It should be suspected in hypertensive, hypokalemic children, especially when they become viralized in infancy (11-hydroxylase deficiency) or fail to develop secondary sexual characteristics at puberty (17-hydroxylase deficiency).[136] Replacement therapy with cortisol and estrogen when indicated is usually effective.

Hypertension During Estrogen Therapy

An association between oral contraceptive use and hypertension was first suggested in 1967, and it is now abdundantly clear that most patients on estrogen therapy elevate their systolic blood pressure by about 5 to 6 mm Hg and their diastolic blood pressure by about 1 to 3 mm Hg. Although severe hypertension is a rare occurrence, the rise in blood pressure is sometimes most impressive, and in this situation underlying renovascular disease has occasionally been reported. Blood pressure usually reverts back to its previous level following cessation of therapy, although this may take as long as 3 months to occur. Several investigators have reported estrogen effects on the renin–angiotensin system, but while renin substrate is increased the precise mechanisms of this form of hypertension are as yet unclear. It is important that the blood pressure of all women receiving estrogen therapy both during their reproductive years and postmenopausally be carefully monitored. Furthermore, since most women receiving estrogen therapy experience a rise in blood pressure, the criteria for selection of patients and need for subsequent close observation are most critical in those who have other cardiovascular risk factors.

COARCTATION OF THE AORTA

Coarctation must be considered in all patients with elevated blood pressure, but particularly in young patients with long-standing mild hypertension. Commonly, these patients are asymptomatic but some complain of headaches or experience intermittent claudication. Physical examination reveals arterial hypertension in the upper extremities with the pressure in the right arm often exceeding that in the left arm. Demonstration of a palpable pulse in the femoral artery does not exclude the diagnosis of coarctation, but the femoral pulse is reduced in amplitude, delayed in onset, and the pressure in the legs is less than that in the arms. There may be a systolic murmur over the precordium and sometimes over the back in the region of the narrowed aortic segment. Radiographic clues include rib notching, characteristically seen at the lower border of the outer third of the ribs, and the "3" sign contour of the left upper heart border. Angiocardiography may be desirable to define the length of the narrowed segment. The complications of untreated coarctation include aortic rupture, subacute infective endocarditis, subarachnoid hemorrhage, and congestive heart failure. Surgical results are excellent and the perioperative mortality is low if surgery is performed early in life.

MISCELLANEOUS

In many diseases hypertension is an important if not a primary manifestation. This is especially the case in arteriosclerosis, hyperthyroidism, toxemia of pregnancy, and acute disorders of the central nervous system. Arteriosclerotic hypertension is usually seen in elderly patients and results from sclerosis of the large vessels rather than from vasoconstriction of peripheral arterioles. Systolic blood pressure is often significantly elevated but the diastolic component tends to be minimally affected and is usually in the range of 90 to 100 mm Hg. Whether a reduction in systolic blood pressure alone in the elderly arteriosclerotic patient is indicated remains unsupported by present studies. Indeed, even when treatment seems appropriate, it must be instituted with great care and caution, since adverse reactions to antihypertensive therapy may be potentially more harmful in the elderly.

Systolic hypertension is often noted in patients with thyrotoxicosis, but lid lag, hand tremor, tachycardia, and thyroid enlargement or nodularity should suggest the appropriate diagnosis. Blood pressure returns to its previous level once the patient is made euthyroid and rarely requires more specific therapy.

Hypertension is also a prominent feature of toxemia of pregnancy. The disease may be mild and present no immediate problem, but can progress to a malignant phase in which convulsions and permanent renal damage may result. Toxemia presents a greater threat to the fetus than to the mother since premature birth and neonatal death are common consequences. Levels of blood pressure which would not merit treatment under ordinary circumstances should be carefully evaluated if they develop during the first trimester of pregnancy.

Hypertension may occur in patients with tumors of the brain, infections of the brain stem, and lesions of the autonomic nervous system such as spinal cord injury or acute porphyria. While these disorders of the central nervous system frequently produce striking hypertension, the blood pressure usually reverts toward normal after the acute episode has subsided.

MANAGEMENT[135]

In a chronic condition, such as essential hypertension, which extends over a 10-, 20-, or even 30-year period, the physician must concern himself with more than the mere dispensing of medications. During the period in which the patient is asymptomatic and without complications the physician occupies a unique position. He must not insist upon unnecessary restriction, petty diets, or frequent office visits, lest the patient become disillusioned, noncompliant, or semi-invalid. Yet he must be certain the patient understands the rationale for instituting therapy and that it will have to be carried out for an indefinite period. In addition to the patient's hypertension, other cardiovascular risk factors, such as obesity, cigarette smoking, and hyperlipidemia, deserve careful attention. When tension and anxiety require treatment, tranquilizers and behavioral modification should complement but never replace the more conventional forms of antihypertensive drug therapy. The value and importance of dietary sodium restriction have been recognized for many years, and this should be instituted in all patients prior to drug therapy. With the advent of more effective and acceptable forms of drug therapy, it has become customary to recommend a no-added-salt diet rather than the more restrictive diets of the past.

Both animal and human studies document the value and importance of antihypertensive drug therapy in those who remain hypertensive on a sodium restricted diet. This was first demonstrated in the late 1950s when it was shown that antihypertensive drugs could dramatically alter the course of malignant hypertension. In view of the uniformly short course and fatal outcome of patients with malignant hypertension, this was not a difficult task.[137] However, in less dramatic forms of hypertension it proved more difficult to establish unequivocally a role for antihypertensive therapy. Indeed, it was not until the Veterans Administration Cooperative Study of Antihypertensive Agents was published in 1967 that the value of therapy in nonmalignant hypertension was clearly proven (diastolic blood pressure greater than 114 mm Hg).[127] A subsequent study published in 1970 confirmed the value of therapy in patients with moderate to severe hypertension (diastolic blood pressure greater than 104 mm Hg) and suggested a role for therapy in patients with milder forms of the disease (diastolic blood pressure 90 to 104 mm Hg).[128] The beneficial effects of antihypertensive therapy as documented by these studies were dramatically manifested by a reduction in those complications directly associated with an increased level of blood pressure, such as congestive heart failure, cerebral vascular accident, and worsening renal insufficiency. More recent studies have attributed the decline in morbidity due to myocardial infarction to the greater percentage of hypertensive patients who are being treated and whose blood pressures are well controlled.

While the evidence suggests that all patients with malignant or accelerated hypertension and those with diastolic blood pressure of 105 mm Hg or greater should receive antihypertensive drug therapy, treatment of patients with diastolic blood pressure from 90 to 104 mm Hg should be individualized. In this latter group careful consideration must be given to the patient's age, race, sex, hypertensive end organ complications, family history of hypertension, and presence or absence of other cardiovascular risk factors. Patients with labile and borderline hypertension (140 to 159/90 to 94 mm Hg) should be periodically reevaluated before being subjected to the discomfort, expense, and potential hazards of lifetime drug therapy. The dilemma of managing patients with systolic hypertension was outlined previously in the section dealing with arteriosclerotic hypertension.

ANTIHYPERTENSIVE DRUGS

The primary goal of treatment is to achieve and maintain a diastolic blood pressure under 90 mm Hg with minimal side effects. This is possible in the vast majority of patients, but unfortunately it is being achieved in less than 50 percent. Many schemes for antihypertensive drug therapy have been proposed over the past 20 years, but while each has its merits, none is perfect. Obviously, therapy must be tailored to meet the needs of the individual patient. The choice of drugs will be influenced not only by the severity of the patient's hypertension and the presence or absence of hypertensive complications, but also by such widely diverse factors as the patient's financial resources and the familiarity of the physician with the drug and its side effects.

In most patients drug therapy can be initiated on an outpatient basis. Initially, patients should be seen at 2- to 4-week intervals, but once their blood pressure is well controlled, they need return no more often than every 3 to 4 months. Rarely, more frequent visits may be required in the symptomatic patient with complications secondary to therapy and/or hypertensive end organ damage. Between office visits, blood pressure control may be monitored by means of home blood pressure recordings. The patient must be able at all times to contact his physician or paramedical associate to obtain advice and encourage-

ment. Only with an open, stable, and understanding relationship is long-term benefit likely to accrue from treatment. Complicated regimens should always be avoided, and combinations of drugs with different sites of action are preferred to combinations of several drugs with similar sites of action.

Based upon their predominant site of action and certain physiologic principles, antihypertensive drugs may be conveniently divided into three categories: diuretics, sympatholytics, and vasodilators. The hemodynamic and hormonal effects of specific drugs are depicted in Table 25–4. Diuretics such as the thiazide derivatives, furosemide, and spironolactone facilitate sodium excretion by the kidney, which initially causes reductions in plasma volume, extracellular fluid volume, and cardiac output. However, with continued use these parameters return toward normal but peripheral resistance falls, and this is the major factor responsible for their long-term antihypertensive effects. Some sympatholytics, such as propranolol and trimethaphan camsylate, appear to lower blood pressure by effecting a reduction in cardiac output. Others, such as methyldopa, clonidine, prazosin, and reserpine, appear to work primarily by decreasing peripheral vascular resistance while guanethidine lowers both cardiac output and peripheral resistance. All vasodilators, such as hydralazine, minoxidil, and the more acutely acting compounds diazoxide and sodium nitroprusside, lower blood pressure as a result of direct-acting vasodilation. Fluid retention and an increase in plasma volume may limit the antihypertensive efficacy of vasodilators and sympatholytics when they are used as single agents. Table 25-4 also groups antihypertensive drugs by the frequency of their use from the most to the least. Thus, Group I is composed of diuretics; Group II, sympatholytics; Group III, direct-acting vasodilators; Group IV, guanethidine; and Group V, the rapidly acting, intravenously administered, antihypertensive drugs.

Most authorities recommend a stepped care approach to drug administration using the agents described in Table 25–4. In this scheme drug treatment is initiated with diuretics (Step 1; Group I) to which are subsequently added sympatholytic agents such as methyldopa, propranolol, prazosin, clonidine, or reserpine (Step 2; Groups I and II). If this proves ineffective, triple therapy with a combination of a diuretic, a sympatholytic, and a direct vasodilator may be instituted (Step 3; Groups I, II, and III). If a patient continues to be hypertensive on triple therapy, careful consideration should be given to the possibility of dietary or drug noncompliance or an underlying correctable cause for the hypertension. If these possibilities can be excluded, guanethidine may be added to the regi-

TABLE 25–4*
Antihypertensive Agents in Common Use

Drug Groups	Usual Dose (in mg) Initial	Usual Dose (in mg) Maximum	Cardiac Output	Peripheral Resistance	Plasma Renin Activity	Major Contraindications	Major Untoward Effects (5% or More)
Group I							
Chlorothiazide (Diuril)	500	1000	←→	↓	↑	Anuria Sulphonamide hypersensitivity	Hypokalemia Hyperuricemia
Furosemide (Lasix)	20	320	←→	↓	↑	Anuria Furosemide hypersensitivity	Volume depletion Hypokalemia Metabolic alkalosis
Spironolactone (Aldactone)	50	100	←→	↓	↑	Anuria Impaired renal function Hyperkalemia	Gastrointestinal irritation Fatigue Hyperkalemia
Group II							
Methyldopa (Aldomet)	500	2000	←→ ↓	↓	↓	Active hepatic disease Methyldopa hypersensitivity	Sedation Postural dizziness Dry mouth Headache
Propranolol (Inderal)	80	480	↓	↑ ←→	↓	Bronchial asthma AV block Congestive heart failure Labile diabetes mellitus	Nausea Anorexia Dizziness Asymptomatic bradycardia
Clonidine (Catapres)	.2	2.4	←→ ↓	↓	↓		Sedation Dry mouth Dizziness
Reserpine (Serpasil)	.75†	.5	↓	↓	↓	Mental depression Active peptic ulcer Ulcerative colitis	Nasal congestion Depression Lethargy Increased appetite Weight gain
Prazosin (Minipress)	2	20	←→	↓	←→ ↓		Postural dizziness Headaches Drowsiness
Group III							
Hydralazine (Apresoline)	50	300	↑	↓	↑	Hydralazine hypersensitivity Coronary artery disease Mitral valvular rheumatic heart disease	Headaches Nausea and vomiting Tachycardia Postural hypotension Late toxicity—lupus erythematosus-like syndrome
Minoxidil (Loniten)	2	40	↑	↓	↑		Weight gain Hypertrichosis Edema Tachycardia

* Adapted, in part, from McMahon's Management of Essential Hypertension.[137]
† Initial dose may exceed maintenance to facilitate catecholamine depletion during first 3 weeks.

┌─ **TABLE 25-4 (cont.)** ─────────────────────────

Drug Groups	Usual Dose (in mg)		Hemodynamic and Hormonal Effects			Major Contraindications	Major Untoward Effects (5% or More)
	Initial	Maximum	Cardiac Output	Peripheral Resistance	Plasma Renin Activity		
Group IV							
Guanethidine (Ismelin)	10	No limit	↓	↓	↓	Pheochromocytoma Hypersensitivity Nonhypertensive congestive heart failure Use of monoamine-oxidase inhibitors	Postural and exertional hypotension Retrograde ejaculation Impotence Diarrhea Weakness Fatigue
Group V							
Diazoxide (Hyperstat)	150–300/injection		↑	↓	↑	Compensatory hypertension Acute pulmonary edema Intracerebral hemorrhage Pheochromocytoma	Hyperglycemia Hyperuricemia Sodium and water retention Tachycardia
Sodium nitroprusside (Nipride)	.0005–.01 kg/min		↓	↓	↑	Compensatory hypertension	Nausea Abdominal cramps Sweating Vomiting
Trimethaphan camsylate (Arfonad)	3–4/min		↓	↓	↑	Uncorrected respiratory insufficiency	Mydriasis Adynamic ileus Urinary retention Nausea Vomiting Anorexia

men as a Step 4 agent (Groups I, II, III, and IV), or the Group II and III drugs may be carefully tapered and the patient treated with a combination of a diuretic and guanethidine alone. Alternatively, consideration may be given to the use of minoxidil, a potent vasodilator currently under investigation by the FDA as the Group III agent.

Of all drugs, diuretics are the most frequently used and form the basis of virtually all treatment regimens. They are effective as sole agents in the treatment of mild hypertension, and in this setting will decrease systolic blood pressure by approximately 10 to 20 mm Hg and diastolic blood pressure by 5 to 10 mm Hg. In more severe hypertension they potentiate and complement the action of sympatholytic and vasodilator agents. Of the many diuretics available, the thiazide and thiazide-like agents are the most useful and should constitute initial therapy in virtually every hypertensive patient. Chlorothiazide and hydrochlorothiazide should be given on a twice daily schedule, whereas the longer acting derivatives such as chlorthalidone and metolazone may be given once daily. Furosemide is the preferred diuretic in patients with evidence of renal insufficiency. All thiazide and thiazide-like agents may induce hypokalemia, hyperglycemia, and hyperuricemia. Hyperlipidemia, especially hypertriglyceridemia, has also been reported, but the exact importance of this finding is not yet clear. The physician should measure serum potassium, glucose, cholesterol, triglycerides, and uric acid levels prior to initiating therapy and monitor them carefully as long as diuretics are used. In addition, patients should be questioned carefully for symptoms of hypokalemia, such as muscle weakness, fatigue, and cardiac irregularities, and have a repeat serum potassium determination 6 weeks after initiation of therapy. Thereafter, potassium should be checked at 6- to 12-month intervals. Hypokalemia need only be treated when it is severe (<3 mEq/L), symptomatic, or when seen in patients with diabetes mellitus or heart disease requiring digitalis therapy. This can be accomplished in one of three ways. Restricting dietary salt intake may decrease renal potassium wasting and often corrects milder forms of hypokalemia. Supplemental potassium may be provided by dietary changes or in the form of potassium chloride tablets or elixirs. Of these, the latter is best, since dietary changes are often unreliable and potassium chloride tablets occasionally lead to small bowel ulceration or obstruction. However, in many patients the substitution or addition of a potassium sparing agent, such as spironolactone or triamterene, constitutes the most acceptable and effective form of therapy. Spironolactone is the best of these agents since in addition to its potassium sparing effects it has the most consistent antihypertensive effect. Hyperkalemia, the most dangerous side effect of spironolactone, is principally noted in patients with renal insufficiency or those in whom the agent is used in conjunction with potassium supplementation. The latter is never indicated as it is unnecessary and potentially hazardous.

Methyldopa, propranolol, clonidine, reserpine, prazosin, and guanethidine are all effective sympatholytics. Propranolol should be avoided in patients with a history of bronchospasm, asthma, congestive heart failure, cardiac conduction defects, insulin dependent and labile diabetes mellitus, and peripheral vascular disease, but in most other patients it is well tolerated and generally effective. It is particularly useful in patients with hyperdynamic circulatory states, renin–angiotensin dependent hypertension, such as renovascular hypertension, coronary insufficiency, arrhythmias, or those who are at high risk of developing acute myocardial infarction. It is worth emphasizing that the dose requirement for propranolol in the treatment of hypertension is often much higher than that used in patients with angina or cardiac arrhythmias. Methyldopa, reserpine, and clonidine have certain similarities, both in their mode of action and in the type of side effects noted with their use. All three appear to act primarily on the central nervous system even though each has additional effects on the peripheral autonomic system. Sedation, dry mouth, and dizziness are common with methyldopa and clonidine, whereas nasal congestion, lethargy, and increased appetite are associated with reserpine. Each of the three may on occasion induce

more serious side effects that are peculiar to that drug alone, such as hepatitis and hemolytic anemia with methyldopa, depression and aggravation of peptic ulcer disease with reserpine, and rebound hypertension following abrupt withdrawal with clonidine. Liver function tests and complete blood count should be periodically monitored in patients receiving methyldopa. Prazosin differs from all other sympatholytic agents in that it appears to work primarily as an alpha-receptor blocker. The most significant side effect seen with this agent is that of hypotension following initiation of therapy (first dose phenomenon). This is fairly uncommon if therapy is initiated at a dose of 1 mg twice daily and the patient is instructed to take the first capsule at bed time while supine. However, patients should be warned of the possibility of initial dizziness, and the drug is best avoided in elderly arteriosclerotic patients with impaired autonomic responses.

Guanethidine is a long-acting and very potent peripherally active sympatholytic which does not cross the blood–brain barrier in contrast to the centrally active sympatholytics discussed above. It need be taken only once a day, does not have sedative side effects, and is often effective when other agents are not. It depletes norepinephrine stores and inhibits norepinephrine release from the sympathetic neuron. This results in a modest reduction in peripheral resistance but a more striking decrease in cardiac output, since blood is pooled in the large veins. Patients should be warned about the possibility of symptomatic hypotension, and dosage should be adjusted only on the basis of postexercise blood pressures such as climbing up and down a foot stool ten times. While guanethidine has been shown to be an effective antihypertensive agent in mild to moderate hypertension, because of its side effects, including postural and exertional hypotension, retrograde ejaculation in males, impotence, and diarrhea, it is usually reserved for those patients with resistant hypertension and should be used with caution in patients with coronary, cerebral, and renal insufficiency. Guanethidine should be combined with a diuretic rather than used alone since this affords control of blood pressure with a smaller dose and with fewer side effects.

Since increased peripheral vascular resistance appears to be the primary physiologic defect in most patients with established essential hypertension, the use of direct vasodilators has for many years generated a great deal of interest. Orthostatic hypotension is uncommon during chronic vasodilator therapy, and blood flow to the brain, heart, and kidneys is unchanged or increased as these agents do not influence the sympathetic system and generally affect only arteriolar rather than venous tone. Sodium nitroprusside and diazoxide are reserved for use in hypertensive emergencies and minoxidil remains an investigational drug. Thus hydralazine is the only direct vasodilator currently approved for outpatient management of hypertension. Sodium retention and reflex tachycardia always occur with hydralazine. The resultant volume expansion and increase in cardiac output significantly decrease hydralazine's effectiveness when used as a primary agent and mandate the concomitant use of a diuretic and a sympatholytic agent whenever this drug is being administered. Although all sympatholytics improve the effectiveness of hydralazine, propranolol works best in this combination. Hydralazine is best avoided in patients with preexistent coronary artery disease, since angina may be precipitated. Hydralazine may, in addition, induce a peripheral neuropathy and a reversible lupus erythematosus-like syndrome, especially when it is used in doses greater than 300 to 400 mg per day. For this reason antinuclear antibody titers should be monitored every 6 months.

Minoxidil, while still under investigation, is important to mention since it is such a potent antihypertensive. This drug is often effective when conventional agents have failed. Its use, however, is uniformly associated with the occurrence of resting tachycardia, increased cardiac output, weight gain, and edema. In addition, hypertrichosis is common, and peculiar right atrial lesions of the heart have been reported during high-dose administration in beagle dogs. It should be considered only when conventional therapy has failed in a compliant patient. However, in this setting, when minoxidil is administered in combination with beta blockers and furosemide, normalization of blood pressure is usually possible.

Diazoxide, sodium nitroprusside, and trimethaphan camsylate are potent intravenously administered antihypertensive agents which need to be monitored carefully. They are usually reserved for the treatment of patients with hypertensive encephalopathy, malignant hypertension, and hypertension associated with acute myocardial decompensation (Group V). Usually, diazoxide is administered rapidly in a dose of 5 mg/kg, although recent studies have confirmed a beneficial effect from smaller doses which decrease the likelihood of complicating hypotension and angina.[142] The drug's hypotensive effect is potentiated by furosemide and sympatholytic agents which prevent the occurrence of reflex tachycardia. Since diazoxide is a sulphonamide derivative, its use is occasionally complicated by hyperglycemia and hyperuricemia. When administered intravenously, sodium nitroprusside lowers blood pressure within seconds. It dilates venous as well as arterial smooth muscle and often decreases cardiac output even though reflex tachycardia is a uniform occurrence. Although sodium nitroprusside can be metabolized to hydrocyanic acid on contact with the tissues, this occurs very slowly and does not constitute a problem unless the drug is used in high dosage for prolonged periods. However, since nitroprusside is unstable when it is stored in a weak solution, it must be freshly prepared prior to use and care should be taken to prevent its exposure to light. Effective in most forms of hypertensive emergencies, it is particularly useful in hypertensive patients with acute pulmonary edema where it is the treatment of choice. Trimethaphan camsylate is a short-acting ganglion-blocking drug that is especially effective in the treatment of dissecting aortic aneurysm. Like sodium nitroprusside, trimethaphan camsylate lowers the blood pressure within seconds and its administration must be supervised carefully. While elevation of the head of the bed will potentiate the hypotensive effect, when used for more than 24 hours all side effects attendant upon the use of ganglion-blocking drugs must be anticipated.

It is apparent from reviewing Table 25-4 that no single Group II, III, or IV drug possesses a unique advantage over another. In most instances between 5 and 10 percent of patients are unable to tolerate a given drug, and the physician must be prepared to recognize specific adverse effects and to recommend alternative therapy. With regard to frequency of dosage administration, while there may be therapeutic reasons to prescribe a specific drug three or four times a day when therapy is initiated, once blood pressure has come under control Group I and IV drugs may be administered once daily and Group II and III drugs twice daily.

CHAPTER 26

Pulmonary Hypertension

BERNADINE H. BULKLEY

INTRODUCTION

Not unlike its counterpart on the systemic side of the circulation, pulmonary hypertension describes a state of elevation of pulmonary artery pressure above a recognized normal range ($>$ 30/15 mm Hg), and this elevation is a reflection of some underlying disease process. Hypertension is a sign of disease, and the disease entities that may be responsible are numerous and varied. Again, not unlike its systemic counterpart, pulmonary hypertension when long-standing ceases to be only a sign of an underlying disease process and becomes additionally a cause of cardiac and of vascular pathology. Thus, an approach to a patient with pulmonary hypertension includes a documentation of the pulmonary hypertensive state, an investigation of the causes responsible for pulmonary hypertension, and a consideration of the damage to the cardiopulmonary system that has been created by the chronic elevated pulmonary pressures.

CLINICAL PRESENTATION

When the patient with pulmonary hypertension becomes symptomatic it is usually with vague complaints of fatigue, dyspnea, and weakness. As right sided heart failure develops, peripheral edema and tender liver enlargement appear, typically without signs or symptoms of left sided heart failure or pulmonary congestion. In its more advanced and severe stage, pulmonary hypertension may be associated with profound fatigue, chest pain, and syncope.

The patient with pulmonary hypertension severe enough to restrict cardiac output usually appears pale and shows signs of peripheral vasoconstriction. Cyanosis may also develop on the basis of low cardiac output and decreased cutaneous blood flow, if a foramen ovale or other congenital communication is present from a right to left shunt, or if there is associated pulmonary parenchymal disease.

Abnormalities noted by physical examination reflect the elevated pulmonary pressures and right ventricular overload. A visible and palpable parasternal lift is usually evident, and a systolic pulsation of the pulmonary artery followed by a tap of the increased second sound may be palpated over the pulmonic area. These precordial abnormalities may not be observed in the severely emphysematous patient with an enlarged AP thoracic diameter. A prominent a wave in the jugular venous pulse reflects the forceful right atrial systole due to an elevated right ventricular end-diastolic pressure, a physical finding which may antecede frank right sided failure. The prominent a wave is usually best appreciated as a quick, jerky pulsation in the suprasternal notch or above the medial end of the clavicle, which can be seen to precede the peak of the carotid pulse. If tricuspid regurgitation, which may accompany right ventricular failure, is present, the jugular venous pulse should show a prominent v wave, which often obscures the a wave but coincides with or follows the decay of the carotid pulse.

By auscultation, the pulmonary valve closure sound is accentuated and can often be detected over the entire precordium and not just in the pulmonic area. Multiple murmurs may be present. A short systolic ejection murmur is often audible in the left second interspace, presumably arising from the dilated pulmonary artery. If pulmonary insufficiency is present, a decrescendo diastolic murmur may develop along the left sternal border. One can usually readily distinguish pulmonic from aortic insufficiency both by the different location of their respective murmurs and also by the absence of peripheral signs of aortic insufficiency. Tricuspid valve regurgitation will lead to a holosystolic murmur which typically increases in intensity with inspiration and is associated with a pulsatile liver and the characteristic jugular venous pulsation. When the tricuspid regurgitation is very severe, the murmur is not influenced by respiration; in some cases no murmurs are audible. In the presence of severe right ventricular hypertrophy the murmur of tricuspid regurgitation may be best audible near the apex and may be mistaken for mitral insufficiency.

CAUSES OF PULMONARY HYPERTENSION
(Table 26-1)

The causes of increased pulmonary vascular resistance are multiple and can reflect alterations at different sites within the vascular circuit, namely increases in pulmonary arterial resistance, pulmonary venous resistance, and a combination of both. Knowledge of the specific site of resistance to flow generally leads one to the diagnosis of the underlying cause of a given patient's pulmonary hypertension.

Increased pulmonary resistance may result from vasospasm, mechanical arterial or venous obstruction, or pulmonary venous hypertension due to left heart disease. Vasoconstriction is probably a compo-

---

TABLE 26-1
Causes of Pulmonary Hypertension

I. Pulmonary Arterial Disease

A. Peripheral pulmonic stenosis
B. Massive pulmonary artery embolism or thrombosis
C. Pulmonary arteriolar disease
   1. Primary pulmonary hypertension
   2. Multiple pulmonary emboli
   3. In situ thrombosis
   4. Pulmonary hypertension, secondary to congenital heart disease
   5. Pulmonary hypertension, secondary to hypoxia, e.g., high altitude

II. Pulmonary Venous Disease

A. Left ventricular failure
B. Mitral valve disease
C. Left atrial disease
   1. Tumor—thrombus
   2. Cor triatriatum
D. Pulmonary venous obstruction
   1. Mediastinal collagenosis
   2. Veno-occlusive disease

III. Combined Pulmonary Venous and Arterial Disease

A. Parenchymal lung disease
   1. Chronic obstructive pulmonary disease (emphysema and bronchitis)
   2. Diffuse infiltration and fibrosis
   2. Sarcoidosis, collagen vascular disease
B. Extrapulmonary disease: kyphoscoliosis

---

nent of almost all forms of pulmonary hypertension. The most common stimulus for pulmonary vasoconstriction is hypoxia, which may account for the pulmonary arterial hypertension of high altitude dwellers[147] and patients with pulmonary parenchymal disease (Chap. 36). Pulmonary arterial pressure elevation resulting from hypoxia is believed to result primarily from increased pulmonary arteriolar resistance and appears to be local, a phenomenon that is aggravated by low pH.

Primary pulmonary hypertension is a form of pulmonary arterial hypertension in which spasm of the pulmonary vasculature of unknown etiology is apparently playing a role.[145] The association of Raynaud's phenomena in a significant number of patients with primary pulmonary hypertension suggests that a generalized vasospastic phenomenon may be occurring. This entity of primary pulmonary hypertension may occur as an isolated disease or in association with systemic disease such as scleroderma or collagen vascular disease. It is yet unresolved whether primary pulmonary hypertension represents a single entity or has multiple causes, and the latter appears to

most likely. Evidence for vasospasm in primary pulmonary hypertension has been derived from studies showing that exposure to oxygen or infusions of acetylcholine, tolalazine, or reserpine may cause vasodilation with lowering of pulmonary arterial pressure. Why or how the vasoconstriction occurs in primary pulmonary hypertension, however, is unknown.

Mechanical obstructions may lead to pulmonary arterial resistance changes. The most important clinical example of this in the adult is pulmonary embolism. Because of the compliant vasculature, sustained pulmonary hypertension due to emboli is unusual unless well over half of the vascular bed is obstructed.[145] The distinction between primary pulmonary hypertension and that due to multiple pulmonary emboli may be difficult to make clinically and on occasion morphologically since both conditions may be associated with histologic evidence of occluded and recanalized pulmonary vessels.

Another cause of pulmonary arterial obstruction is the vascular disease that develops in response to sustained pulmonary hypertension. Regardless of cause, if severe enough and long-standing enough, anatomic changes occur within the arterial tree and result in more rigid, less compliant vessels. Medial hypertrophy and intimal proliferation of the small pulmonary arteries and arterioles narrow and at times may lead to complete obliteration of the vascular lumen. In the most severe forms of long-term pulmonary hypertension, mostly due to congenital heart disease, extensive vascular alterations occur which include the development of vascular communications called plexiform lesions and on occasion necrotizing arteritis with thrombosis.[146]

These secondary vascular obstructive changes account for the progressive increase in pulmonary vascular resistance seen in the Eisenmenger syndrome or Eisenmenger reaction, which was originally described as an accompaniment of ventricular septal defects but can occur with any large intracardiac shunt, be it atrial, ventricular or aortopulmonary. The pulmonary vascular resistance in the Eisenmenger syndrome becomes equal to systemic vascular resistance and a bidirectional or reversed right to left shunt results. This occurs only when large defects are present from birth and pulmonary vascular resistance remains elevated from infancy, increasing as the anatomic obstructive lesions within the atrial tree develop and progress. As pulmonary vascular resistance rises and finally becomes equal to systemic, right to left shunt occurs and cyanosis results. In this setting, the volume and direction of blood flow shunting across the defect on a beat to beat basis reflects primarily the resistance in both the systemic and pulmonary circuit. Severe changes in the pulmonary vasculature accompany the Eisenmenger syndrome and account for the fixed and irreversible elevations in pulmonary vascular resistance.

In the adult population, a more common cause of pulmonary arterial hypertension is elevation in pulmonary venous pressure, which is almost always due to left heart disease. Elevation in pulmonary arterial pressure is usually a passive transmission of pressure across the capillary bed reflecting left atrial pressures and, consequently, rarely reaches systemic levels. Not uncommonly, however, in patients with mitral stenosis in particular, severe pulmonary arterial hypertension with pulmonary systolic pressure of 80 to 100 mm Hg may be present with a pulmonary venous or left atrial pressure of only 20 mm Hg. Elevated arterial or arteriolar resistance is responsible for this type of pulmonary hypertension, which is termed "reactive." Its physiologic basis is poorly understood, but it must be at least in part a consequence of reversible changes in the pulmonary circulation. In support of vasoconstriction as an important factor is the decrease in resistance which occurs after mitral valve replacement; a drop of 5 to 10 mm Hg in left atrial pressure following operation may be associated with a drop of 50 mm Hg in the pulmonary artery pressure. Other factors which may account for this pulmonary arterial versus venous pressure difference are reduced pulmonary compliance, hypoxia, and, in some instances, vascular obstruction due to thrombi or emboli.

An unusual cause of pulmonary venous hypertension is pulmonary veno-occlusive disease, a rare condition of unknown etiology seen in young men and associated with pulmonary venous intimal thickening and fibrosis of the small pulmonary veins and venules. These are generally attributed to venous thrombus but the etiology is unknown. This condition is difficult to distinguish clinically from primary pulmonary hypertension.

Diseases of the pulmonary parenchyma, such as emphysema, sarcoidosis, and interstitial fibrosis, may be associated with pulmonary hypertension. In this setting, parenchymal lesions which may destroy or alter the distensibility of vascular beds cause pulmonary pressure elevations through increased resistance to flow in the small arterial or venous pulmonary vessels. Hypoxia itself leads to increased pulmonary vascular resistance perpetuating the pulmonary hypertension due to parenchymal disease. Pulmonary hypertension due to parenchymal lung disease is usually associated with obvious signs of the parenchymal disease on physical examination and/or chest radiograph. The one possible exception would be patients with chronic bronchitis, and in this situation the his-

tory usually suggests the diagnosis. Kyphoscoliosis is another extravascular condition which may lead to alterations in the resistance of the pulmonary vascular bed and cause pulmonary hypertension without intrinsic or coexistent disease of the pulmonary parenchyma, vasculature, or heart.

APPROACH TO THE PATIENT

After the history and physical examination, the main value of further tests is to document or confirm the presence and severity of the pulmonary hypertension and in particular to look for treatable causes of the condition such as left heart lesions or pulmonary emboli. The ECG, aside from confirming right ventricular hypertrophy with peaked P waves (P pulmonale), delayed precordial transition, and increased right precordial voltage, might also suggest congenital malformations or left ventricular disease. Similarly, the chest radiograph, which usually shows a prominent pulmonary artery and central pulmonary vessels but relatively avascular lung fields in primary pulmonary hypertension (Fig. 26–1), will also be of value in detecting parenchymal lung disease or in demonstrating the typical features of an intracardiac shunt or mitral valve disease. Echocardiography may be useful for evaluating cardiac causes of pulmonary hypertension, and is especially useful for identifying otherwise silent mitral stenosis or an atrial myxoma. Pulmonary function studies with arterial blood gases are central in evaluation of any pulmonary process and in defining the extent and severity of pulmonary parenchymal disease.

Cardiac catheterization is rarely required for the diagnosis or assessment of severity of pulmonary hypertension. It is usually performed because of a suspicion of a secondary cause of pulmonary pressure elevation such as recurrent pulmonary emboli, a congenital malformation, or severe valvular abnormality. On assessing pulmonary emboli in particular, pulmonary angiography is usually necessary since clinical findings are nonspecific and currently available noninvasive tests including ventilation perfusion lung scans are so often equivocal. When entirely normal, however, a perfusion lung scan excludes the diagnosis of embolism.

Patients with severe pulmonary hypertension, and particularly those with the primary form, tolerate procedures poorly. Cardiac catheterization, angiocardiography, pulmonary scanning, anesthesia, surgery, and even venipuncture have, on occasion, been associated with death. Vasovagal reactions are common and may result in bradycardia, hypotension, and sometimes asystole. In some patients there appears to be a sudden rise in pulmonary vascular resistance,

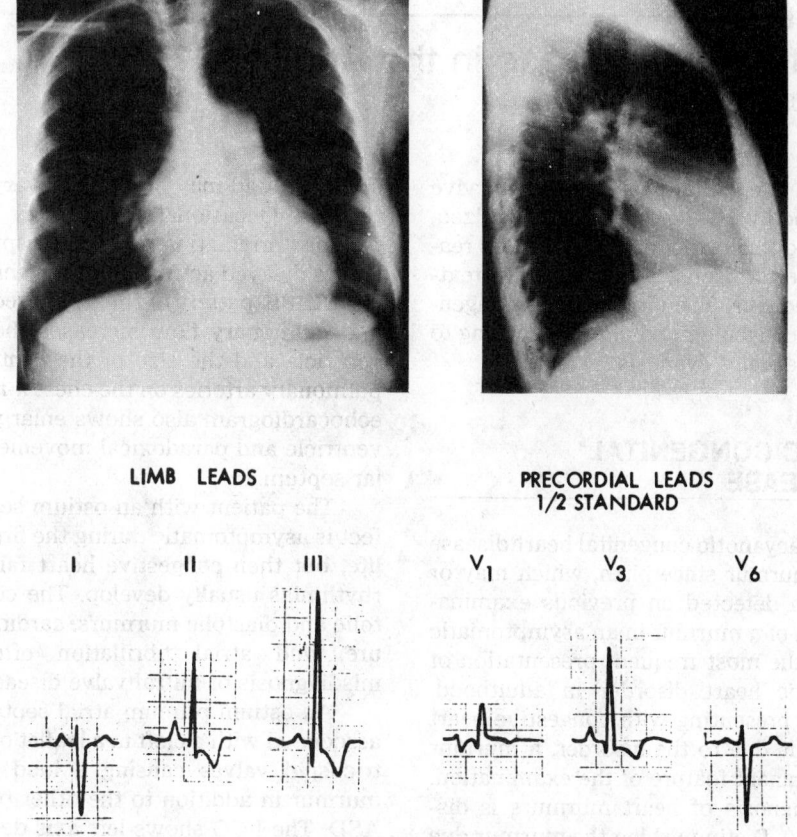

FIGURE 26–1. Chest x-ray: shows right ventricular and right atrial enlargement, enlargement of the central pulmonary vessels near the hilum, and relatively avascular peripheral lung fields. ECG: shows right axis deviation, right atrial enlargement, and right ventricular hypertrophy.

probably on a neurogenic basis, with concomitant drop in cardiac output and systemic blood pressure, failure of coronary perfusion, anoxia, and death. Premedication with atropine is mandatory, and if bradycardia develops during the procedure, additional atropine should be administered. It may be advisable to perform angiography in one lung at a time to minimize the consequences of the injection of contrast material into the pulmonary circulation.

MANAGEMENT
Management of pulmonary hypertension is predominantly management of the underlying disease process with appropriate medical and surgical therapy. Addi-

tionally, the consequences of pulmonary hypertension must be dealt with. Digitalis and diuretics have been found effective in patients with right-sided heart failure, although some argue that digitalis has no beneficial effect when the right ventricle fails. Activity which requires an increase in cardiac output should be restricted. In patients with documented pulmonary emboli, anticoagulation should be used. In some instances, the use of the vasodilating agent, such as tolalazine and nitroglycerin, have been demonstrated to be effective in lowering the pulmonary vascular resistance. A favorable effect of these agents on the natural history of the disease has not been demonstrated.

CHAPTER 27

Congenital Heart Disease in the Adult[148-151]

J. O'NEAL HUMPHRIES

Many patients with congenital heart disease survive infancy and childhood with the defect unrecognized, partially corrected, or uncorrectable, and for this reason it is appropriate to discuss this entity in a textbook of internal medicine. The discussion of congenital heart disease is conveniently divided according to the presence or absence of cyanosis.

ACYANOTIC CONGENITAL HEART DISEASE

Most patients with acyanotic congenital heart disease have had a heart murmur since birth, which may or may not have been detected on previous examinations. The detection of a murmur in an asymptomatic patient is actually the most frequent presentation of congenital acyanotic heart disorder in adulthood. Even in the patient presenting with congestive heart failure or arrhythmia due to the disorder, a murmur continues as a prominent feature of the examination. The differential diagnosis of heart murmurs is discussed in Chapter 20. Distinguishing the murmur due to a congenital defect from an innocent or physiologic murmur is at times difficult, but obviously of great importance. Evaluation of the history, physical examination, electrocardiogram (ECG), chest x-ray, and echocardiogram is usually sufficient to establish the diagnosis. Cardiac catheterization and angiography are sometimes necessary to prove the diagnosis, quantitate the severity of the defect, and exclude associated defects.

ATRIAL SEPTAL DEFECT

A defect in the lower portion of the atrial septum in the area of the foramen ovale is termed an ostium secundum atrial septal defect (ASD). The higher impedance to flow of the left ventricle as compared to the right ventricle results in shunting of blood from the left heart to the right heart through the defect and increased flow through the right ventricle and pulmonary circulation. The size of the shunt and increased right heart flow are determined by the size of the defect and the relative impedances to flow of the two ventricles.

The increased flow through the right heart causes a harsh, scratchy systolic murmur which stops before a widely split second heart sound. The splitting of the

second sound may be fixed or vary slightly with respiration. Occasionally there may be a mid-diastolic murmur originating at the tricuspid valve. The ECG shows delayed activation of the enlarged right ventricle (RBBB pattern). The increased right ventricular and pulmonary flow increases the size of the right ventricle and the size of the central and peripheral pulmonary arteries on the chest x-ray (Fig. 27–1). The echocardiogram also shows enlargement of the right ventricle and paradoxical movement of the ventricular septum.

The patient with an ostium secundum septal defect is asymptomatic during the first 40 or 50 years of life, but then congestive heart failure and atrial arrhythmias usually develop. The combination of systolic and diastolic murmurs, cardiomegaly, heart failure, and atrial fibrillation often leads to the misdiagnosis of mitral valve disease.

An ostium primum atrial septal defect usually is associated with a cleft in a leaflet of the mitral and/or tricuspid valves causing a loud apical pansystolic murmur in addition to the other physical findings of ASD. The ECG shows left axis deviation and RBBB.

Surgical closure is indicated in most patients with an ASD since the operative risk is low and the long-term results are excellent. After symptoms develop, the operative risk is higher and results not as good. Patients with isolated ASD are not at increased risk to develop infective endocarditis.

One or more pulmonary veins may drain anomalously into the right atrium either with or without an accompanying ASD. The clinical and laboratory findings and the management are very similar to those for the patient with an isolated ASD.

An occasional patient with an ASD will develop profound elevation of pulmonary vascular resistance during childhood or adolescence and present with fatigue and cyanosis due to a right-to-left shunt. These patients do not benefit from surgical closure of the defect and surgery is extremely hazardous.

VENTRICULAR SEPTAL DEFECT

A loud, harsh pansystolic murmur along the upper sternal border without other physical abnormalities and with a normal ECG, chest x-ray, and echocardiogram suggests a small ventricular septal defect (VSD). The small VSD with a very small left-to-right shunt is termed a Roger VSD and does not cause an

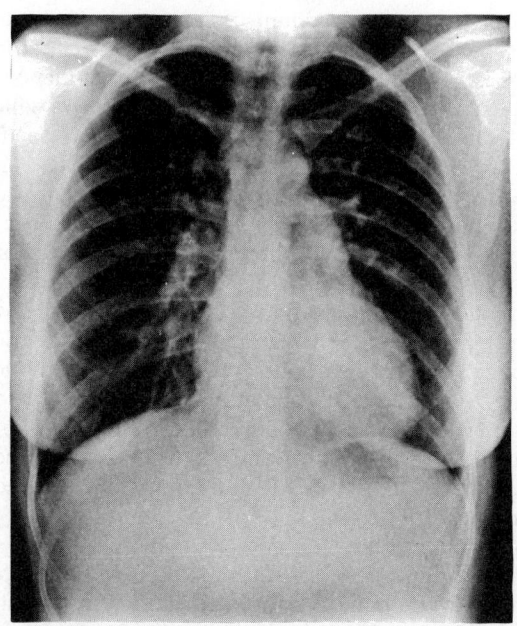

FIGURE 27-1. A 26-year-old housewife found to have ostium secundum atrial septal defect with pulmonary blood flow twice systemic blood flow. Note enlarged right ventricular outflow tract and increased vascularity of lung fields.

increase in pulmonary artery pressure or pulmonary vascular resistance. Surgical closure is necessary only if the patient has experienced one or more episodes of infective endocarditis; the risk of surgery is less than the risk of recurrent endocarditis. The patient with a Roger VSD should use prophylactic antibiotics before and after dental and operative procedures in an effort to reduce the risk of bacterial endocarditis. Occasionally, aortic regurgitation may develop since the noncoronary cusp of the aortic valve may sag into the VSD. Aortic regurgitation may be progressive in this setting; therefore, it is wise to close the VSD before severe aortic regurgitation appears.

A large congenital VSD results in either death during infancy or the development of increasing pulmonary vascular resistance which equals or exceeds the systemic vascular resistance within 2 years (Eisenmenger complex). When these patients reach adolescence or adulthood, they do not have a systolic murmur but do have a loud pulmonic second sound and a right-to-left shunt and may have a diastolic murmur of pulmonary regurgitation. This complex is discussed in the following section on cyanotic congenital heart disease.

A middle-sized VSD is very rare and presents with a loud systolic murmur, cardiac enlargement,

and prominent pulmonary arteries on chest roentgenogram. Surgical closure is indicated.

PULMONIC STENOSIS

A systolic murmur during the first half or two-thirds of systole may represent an innocent or physiologic murmur, an ASD, or a mild or moderate pulmonic stenosis (PS).

Severe pulmonic stenosis is associated with a loud systolic murmur which extends all the way to the aortic second sound; the pulmonic second sound is usually absent in severe PS. An ejection click may introduce the murmur on expiration and disappear on inspiration. The ECG shows right ventricular hypertrophy and the chest x-ray a prominent main and left pulmonary artery (due to poststenotic dilatation) and normal peripheral pulmonary arteries.

Cardiac catheterization is indicated in most patients thought to have PS in order to establish the diagnosis and its severity and to exclude associated congenital defects. Surgery is usually indicated when the gradient between the right ventricle and pulmonary artery is 40 mm HG or greater. Without surgery, patients with severe PS will develop heart failure; after the development of failure the danger of surgery is considerably increased. Patients with mild PS (gradients less than 40 mm Hg) have a normal life expectancy; the severity of PS does not increase with time. It is exceedingly rare for a patient with isolated valvular PS to develop infective endocarditis.

EBSTEIN'S ANOMALY OF THE TRICUSPID VALVE

A systolic murmur along the lower sternal border may be present in a patient with Ebstein's anomaly. Many patients with Ebstein's anomaly will present during infancy or childhood with cyanosis and severe disability. However, the severity of the anomaly of the tricuspid valve is tremendously variable; some patients may lead entirely normal lives.

Associated auscultatory features include wide splitting of both the first and second heart sounds and sometimes a mid-diastolic murmur. The systolic and diastolic murmurs may increase in intensity or change in quality with inspiration. The second component of the split first sound, which is often loud and snappy in quality and termed a "sail sound," is felt to be due to the delayed closure of the excessively large and malpositioned tricuspid valve leaflets.

There may or may not be signs of increased right atrial pressure depending on the degree of impairment to right ventricular inflow caused by the abnormal valve.

The ECG records a peculiar low-voltage RBBB pattern, prominent P waves, and atrial arrhythmias.

The chest roentgenogram shows a very large heart with normal pulmonary vasculature. The echocardiogram may show a large, easily recorded tricuspid valve.

Management includes control of atrial arrhythmias, treatment of systemic congestion, if present, and, very rarely, tricuspid valve replacement.

CONGENITAL AORTIC STENOSIS

This finding is discussed in Chapter 20.

PATENT DUCTUS ARTERIOSUS

Patency of the ductus arteriosus (PDA) produces a continuous murmur just below the left clavicle. This disorder must be distinguished from other causes of continuous murmurs described in Chapter 20.

The size of the ductus is quite variable; some are so small and the flow through them so little that there are no associated physical or laboratory abnormalities and others are very large with a sizable left-to-right shunt. With a large ductus, the systemic pulse pressure is wide, the left ventricular impulse is vigorous but not sustained, and an apical diastolic murmur may be present. The chest x-ray will show cardiac enlargement with prominence of the pulmonary vasculature. The ECG is usually normal, but tall R waves in the lateral chest leads may be present. Congestive heart failure may develop at any age.

Surgical closure is indicated in all patients with a left-to-right shunt through the PDA. This will reduce the risk of infective endocarditis on a ductus of any size and reduce the risk of heart failure and/or pulmonary vascular damage in patients with a large ductus. The operative risk is very small.

Rarely, with a very large PDA, the pulmonary vascular resistance will increase during infancy or childhood to equal or exceed systemic resistance. In this setting, surgical closure of the PDA is not helpful and the surgery is hazardous. This presentation is discussed in the following section on cyanotic congenital heart disease.

CYANOTIC CONGENITAL HEART DISEASE

As discussed in Chapter 16, cyanosis may develop from the shunting of venous blood to the systemic circulation (central cyanosis) or by the excessive extraction of oxygen from arterial blood during profoundly reduced flow in the skin and mucous membranes (peripheral cyanosis). Central cyanosis may be due to abnormal vascular or cardiac connections or to intrapulmonary shunt of venous blood through underventilated areas of lung. In the latter situation, there is usually clear clinical and x-ray evidence of significant pulmonary disease. This discussion will be limited to central cyanosis due to abnormal vascular or cardiac connections, which may be divided into three categories according to the physiologic and anatomic mechanisms which cause the cyanosis: 1) pulmonary vascular resistance equal to or greater than systemic vascular resistance and an abnormal communication between the two circulations (Eisenmenger complex); 2) anatomic obstruction to flow through the right heart and an abnormal communication between the two circulations proximal to the obstruction, such as pulmonic stenosis and a VSD, or tricuspid atresia and an ASD; and 3) abnormal vascular connections, such as the inferior vena cava connecting directly to the left atrium or a pulmonary arteriovenous fistula.

The low oxygen saturation in the arterial blood stimulates the bone marrow to increase the number of circulating red blood cells in an effort to maintain a normal delivery of total oxygen to the tissues; the level of the hemoglobin or hematocrit serves as an indirect guide to the severity of the resultant hypoxemia.

It is essential that the cause of the cyanosis be established in every patient, whether he is symptomatic or asymptomatic. The proper management is different for the different conditions; surgery may greatly improve the symptoms and/or the long-term prognosis in some patients with cyanosis, but in others surgery is hazardous and of no benefit. The most important issue is the pulmonary vascular resistance; this must be established in every cyanotic patient. If the pulmonary vascular resistance is low, then surgery can be potentially beneficial. If the pulmonary vascular resistance is elevated and equal to or greater than systemic resistance, then surgical treatment will not be helpful.

The history, physical examination, chest x-ray, ECG, and echocardiogram may be helpful in distinguishing one cyanotic condition from the other but are not absolutely reliable; therefore, it is necessary to perform cardiac catheterization and angiography in essentially all patients with central cyanosis. Many adults with cyanotic heart disease have had previous investigations and have been labeled as having a "certain congenital disorder." The physician must review these previous studies and ensure that the proper procedures were done to establish the diagnosis. It is not uncommon for a "diagnostic label" to be attached to a patient based on incomplete studies and for this "label" to be passed on from physician to physician. If the diagnosis is not firmly established, it may be necessary to repeat certain parts of the study; diagnostic procedures are far better now than they were only 10 years ago.

ELEVATED PULMONARY VASCULAR RESISTANCE AND ABNORMAL COMMUNICATION (Eisenmenger Physiology)

Eisenmenger described pulmonary hypertension and fixed elevated pulmonary vascular resistance in patients with VSDs (see Chap. 26). Subsequently, Dr. Paul Wood classified patients with any congenital defect complicated by elevated pulmonary vascular resistance as having an Eisenmenger-like complex. Thus, patients with large PDAs, single ventricle, truncus arteriosus, transposition of the great arteries with VSD or single ventricle, and a rare patient with an ASD could be part of the Eisenmenger complex if the pulmonary vascular resistance were elevated to or beyond systemic vascular resistance.

These patients present with increasing cyanosis and fatigue during adolescence and young adulthood. Hemoptysis due to intravascular thrombosis may be severe in some patients, especially those with very high hematocrits. Arrhythmias may seriously complicate the late course of this disorder and may be the cause of death in some. Syncope due to arrhythmias or low cardiac output may occur, and anginal-like chest pain can be disabling. Eventually, ventricular failure occurs and the patient develops systemic congestion with ankle edema, hepatic congestion, and ascites. Gout is not uncommon in patients with high hematocrits.

The physical examination reveals cyanosis which may or may not be difficult to detect; exercise increases the cyanosis. Prominent *a* waves are usually seen in the jugular veins and later in the course, when right heart failure and tricuspid regurgitation develop, prominent *v* waves are seen. The left precordium may actually be bowed outward if the heart has been greatly enlarged since infancy, as seen in some patients with single ventricle or truncus arteriosus. Parasternal heaves are usually present, apical heaves are not uncommon, and heaves to the right of the sternum should be sought since many of these patients will have various degrees of dextroposition of the heart.

Auscultation is not very rewarding; the second sound is loud and usually single or very narrowly split. Pulmonary and tricuspid regurgitation murmurs may develop as well as gallop rhythm.

The electrocardiogram shows signs of right or combined ventricular hypertrophy. Prominence of central pulmonary arteries, diminished peripheral pulmonary arteries, and a relatively small heart shadow are typical of Eisenmenger VSD (Fig. 27–2A), while an enlarged, elongated heart shadow and prominence of the central and peripheral pulmonary vessel are seen in patients with the more complex disorders with Eisenmenger complex (Fig. 27–2B). Echocardiography may help define the anatomic situation and give some clues as to pulmonary pressure and flow.

However, it is important to measure the pulmonary artery pressure by catheterization. If the pulmonary artery pressure is elevated, then it is necessary to measure pulmonary blood flow; this is usually done by the determination of oxygen content of blood samples obtained from the great vessels and heart chambers, applying a modification of the Fick principle, and calculating a ratio of pulmonary blood flow to systemic blood flow. The ratio of pulmonary vascular resistance to systemic vascular resistance can also be calculated. If the pulmonary flow greatly exceeds systemic flow, then the patient is usually not cyanotic and surgical correction of the defect should be considered. If the pulmonary blood flow is equal to or less than systemic flow in the presence of marked pulmonary hypertension, then the pulmonary resistance is equal to or greater than systemic resistance and operative correction of the defect is not appropriate.

The medical management of these patients is gratifying for many years, but increasing symptoms and limitations develop during the third decade, and it is most unusual for the patient to survive the fourth decade, death being due to heart failure (especially low output), cardiac arrhythmias, or thromboembolic disease. Medical management includes restriction of activities and digitalis, diuretics, and antiarrhythmic agents as indicated. The value of anticoagulation therapy is unproven but is often used because of the high risk for the development of intrapulmonary thrombosis. Pulmonary arterial dilators, such as tolazoline, have not been shown to affect the course favorably. If the hematocrit rises to very high levels, above 65, the patient may experience increased exercise tolerance after phlebotomy. Phlebotomy may also reduce, terminate, or prevent pulmonary hemorrhage. Phlebotomy should be performed cautiously; initial phlebotomies should be small and accompanied by replacement of an equal fluid volume through another intravenous route. If the initial sessions are tolerated, subsequent phlebotomies can be larger and fluid replacement need not be done. Many patients feel better with the hematocrit below 60 percent, but care should be taken to avoid reducing the hematocrit

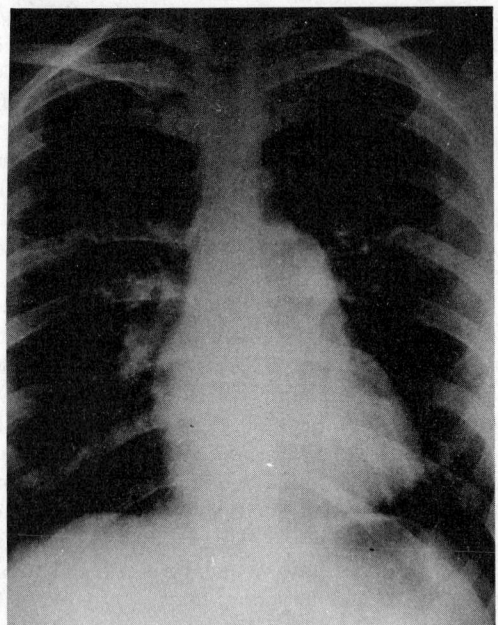 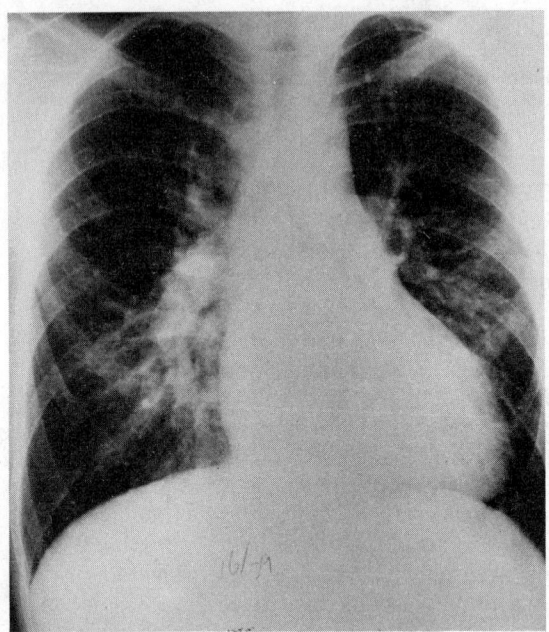

FIGURE 27-2. **Left:** Chest x-ray of a young woman with an isolated VSD and Eisenmenger syndrome showing cardiomegaly, prominent central pulmonary arteries, and a decrease in the peripheral lung vascularity (pruning effect). **Right:** Chest x-ray of a young man with transposition of the great vessels, a large VSD, and markedly elevated pulmonary vascular resistance. Note the prominent central and pulmonary vasculature. [Part B from Brest, A. (ed.), *Congenital Heart Disease in Adults*. Philadelphia, Cardiovascular Clinics, F. A. Davis Co.; reprinted by permission.]

below 50 or 55 percent because this represents an anemia for these patients. This should also be remembered if spontaneous blood loss occurs.

ANATOMIC OBSTRUCTION AND ABNORMAL COMMUNICATION (Tetralogy of Fallot Physiology)

When the obstruction to pulmonary blood flow is not at the pulmonary arterioles but rather a mechanical obstruction somewhere in the right heart, the pulmonary vascular resistance will be normal and the pulmonary artery pressure low. By far the most common abnormality of this type is Tetralogy of Fallot where there is obstruction in the outflow tract of the right ventricle and a large VSD. The resistance of the systemic arterial bed is less than the resistance of the mechanical blockage in the right ventricle, thus blood shunts from right to left through the VSD and cyanosis is present. Other examples include tricuspid atresia and ASD, Ebstein's anomaly of the tricuspid valve and ASD, transposition of the great arteries with PS and VSD, etc.

The ECG and chest roentgenogram are highly variable according to the type of disorder present. The ECG of Tetralogy of Fallot shows right ventricular hypertrophy; the ECG of tricuspid atresia and ASD shows left ventricular hypertrophy, etc. There is reduced or normal pulmonary vasculature on chest x-ray in all varieties. Echocardiogram may be helpful in establishing the relationship of the great vessels and heart chambers. Again cardiac catheterization and angiography are necessary to establish the low pulmonary artery resistance and the exact anatomic locations of the obstructions, heart chambers, and great vessels.

The management is surgical; these patients need more pulmonary blood flow. In most instances it is possible for the surgeon to relieve the obstruction and close the abnormal communication between the two circulations—so-called total correction. Even very complex combinations can now be operated on successfully because of the availability of intracardiac and extracardiac conduits. When "total correction" is not practical, these patients can be remarkably improved for many years by the surgical creation of a connection between the aorta and pulmonary artery (Blalock-Taussig, Potts, or other anastomoses).

Patients who have had surgery for cyanotic heart disease during infancy and childhood are surviving to adult life in large numbers. They may present with many new and complicated management problems, such as degeneration or infection of conduit material; serious atrial and ventricular arrhythmias and various degrees of heart block are not uncommon.

ABNORMAL VASCULAR CONNECTIONS

An anomalous vascular connection may be suspected in a cyanotic individual with a normal cardiac examination and normal ECG and chest x-ray. In patients with pulmonary arteriovenous fistulas, there may be a faint continuous murmur heard over the lung fields and there may be a cluster of peculiar shadows on the chest x-ray. The precise location of the anomalous veins can usually be determined by careful selection of sites for blood oxygen saturation determinations, indicator dilution studies, and angiographic pictures. Pulmonary arteriovenous fistulas are often multiple, and it may be very difficult to obtain complete resection without loss of unacceptably large amounts of lung. Abnormally draining systemic veins can either be ligated or transposed to the systemic venous system.

Brain abscess formation and paradoxical emboli are the most serious complications encountered in these patients.

CHAPTER 28

Diseases of the Aorta
LAWRENCE S. C. GRIFFITH

The term "aneurysm" is derived from the Greek word *aneurysma* meaning a "widening." Two types of widenings are recognized. One type is termed a saccular aneurysm and can be considered as an outpouching of a segment of aortic wall. Only a portion of the aortic circumference is involved and the opening between the aneurysm and "true" aortic lumen is often narrow. A fusiform aneurysm is more globular or cylindrical in shape and involves the entire circumference of the aorta. In this situation, there is a generalized dilatation of the aortic wall and no opening, per se, exists between the aneurysmal segment and the aortic lumen.

CLINICAL PRESENTATION

Thoracic Aneurysm Without Dissection
The clinical presentation of a patient with aneurysmal dilatation of the thoracic aorta without dissection can be misleadingly benign. Often the patient is without any symptoms and the diagnosis is suspected because an enlarged or calcified aorta is noted on routine chest roentgenogram (Fig. 28–1). If symptoms are present, the complaint is usually that of a constant substernal or interscapular aching. Occasionally, the patient will have symptoms that are secondary to compression of structures adjacent to the aorta. These symptoms include cough (bronchus), dysphagia (esophagus), hoarseness (recurrent laryn-geal nerve), or edema of the head and upper thorax (superior vena cava) (Fig. 28–2). Very occasionally, the patient will present with pain secondary to erosion of a vertebral body, rib, or the sternum. If the aneurysmal dilatation involves the aortic ring, appreciable valvular regurgitation may be present and the patient will present with symptoms of congestive failure. If a branch of the thoracic aorta becomes narrowed or occluded, the patient may present with angina pectoris if the coronary arteries are involved or transient hemiparesis or paraplegia if the cerebral or spinal circulation is compromised.

Acute Dissection of the Thoracic Aorta
The patient with an acute dissecting hematoma of the aorta will abruptly develop severe persistent precordial, interscapular, lumbar, or epigastric pain. Characteristically, the pain is described as sharp, ripping, or tearing and is often accompanied by dyspnea. Because a dissection commonly extends into one or more major branches of the aorta, migration of the pain or the occurrence of syncope, hemiplagia, paraplegia, hematuria, or myocardial infarction identifies the location or extent of this process. Often one carotid, brachial, or femoral pulse is diminished. Aortic valvular regurgitation is indicative of ascending aorta involvement. Occasionally the patient will present in shock.[159]

Aortic dissection occurs when there is a separation or "splitting" of the aortic media by extravasated

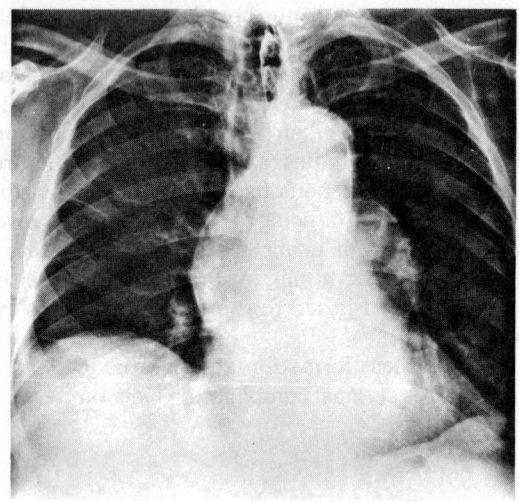

FIGURE 28-1. Thoracic aneurysm presenting as prominence of the right heart border. Note calcium in the ascending aorta. This patient had syphilis of the aorta.

blood from either the aortic lumen or the vasa vasorum. Most commonly the initial event is a tear of the aortic intima. While the dissecting hemotoma may not encircle the aorta, often the entire length of this vessel is involved. DeBakey has suggested classifying aortic dissections based on the location of the intimal tear and the extent of dissection (Fig. 28-3).[154] In Type I dissection (60 to 70 percent of cases), the intimal tear is just above the aortic valve and dissection extends around the arch into the descending and abdominal aorta. In Type II dissection (5 percent of cases), the intimal tear and dissection are limited to the ascending aorta. This is most commonly seen in patients where the underlying process is cystic medial necrosis. In Type III dissection (20 to 30 percent of cases), the intimal tear occurs in the descending aorta just distal to the arch vessels and dissection involves the descending and abdominal aorta.

In assessing the patient with suspected thoracic aortic dissection, the most important differential diagnosis is acute myocardial infarction. The patient

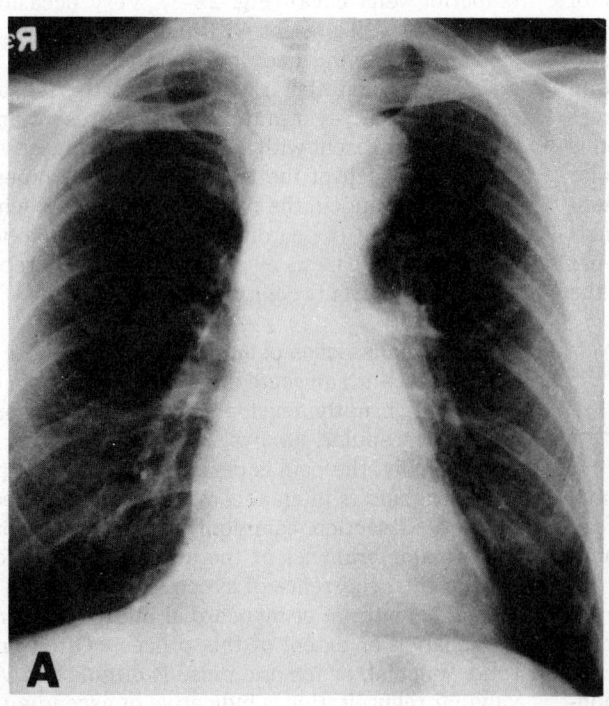
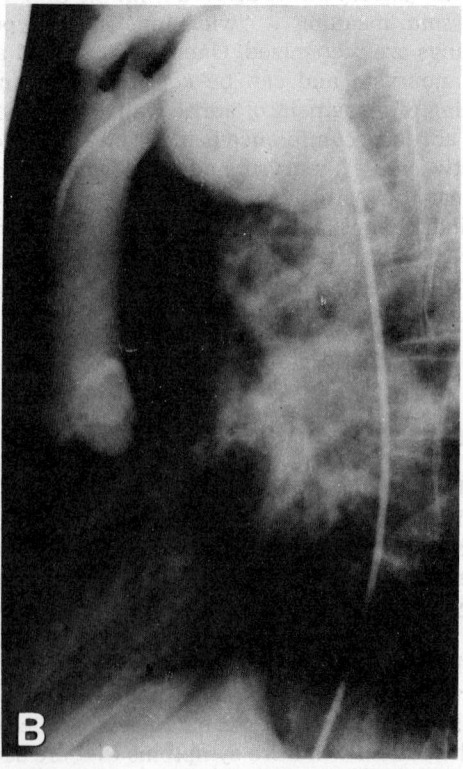

FIGURE 28-2. Mediastinal widening due to aortic aneurysm. **A.** Chest film demonstrating mediastinal widening in a patient with hoarseness. **B.** Selective aortogram demonstrating a localized saccular aortic aneurysm.

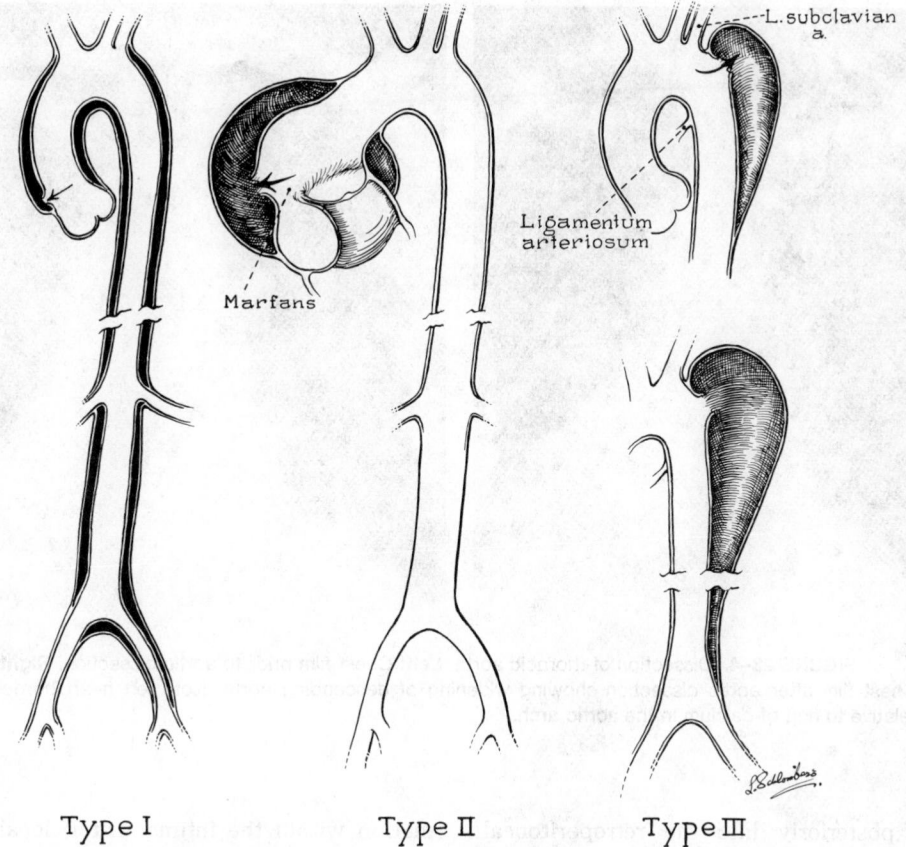

FIGURE 28–3. Types of dissection of the aorta. In Type I, the dissection begins in the ascending aorta and extends distally often into the abdominal aorta. In Type II, the dissection is limited to the ascending aorta. This most commonly occurs in Marfan syndrome. Type III dissections arise in the descending aorta at or just distal to the origin of the left subclavian artery and extend distally, often into the abdominal aorta. This classification does not include the small group (approximately 10 percent) in whom no intimal tear is found.

with acute infarction will more often have an antecedent history of angina pectoris. The pain of infarction builds more slowly and often radiates into the arms or neck. With aortic dissection, pain begins abruptly and quickly migrates to the interscapular, lumbar, or epigastric region. Physical findings such as a difference in the cuff blood pressure of each arm, a diminished carotid pulse, or findings of impaired cerebral or spinal blood flow suggest aortic dissection. A widened mediastinum on chest x-ray, especially if it represents a change, is very suggestive of dissection (Figs. 28–4, 28–5).

Abdominal Aneurysm Without Dissection
Most aneurysms of the abdominal aorta are asymptomatic and are identified as a mass on a routine examination or as an incidental finding on a roentgenogram. The patient will often be the first to identify this mass. Approximately 30 percent of these patients

will present with mild abdominal or lumbar pain that radiates to either the flank or inguinal region. The discomfort may be similar to ureteral colic or nerve root irritation secondary to herniation of an intervertebral disk. Occasionally, the patient will complain of postprandial fullness or early satiety. Some aneurysms are first recognized during the evaluation of arterial ischemia involving the legs. On physical examination, a pulsatile periumbilical mass is palpable in virtually every patient. The transverse diameter of the aneurysm can be estimated by palpation with surprising accuracy in most patients. Systolic bruits over the aneurysm may be present and pulses in the legs may be diminished or absent.

Acute Rupture of the Abdominal Aorta
In contrast to the thoracic aneurysms which dissect but do not rupture, most abdominal aneurysms rupture at the time of acute dissection. Because this most

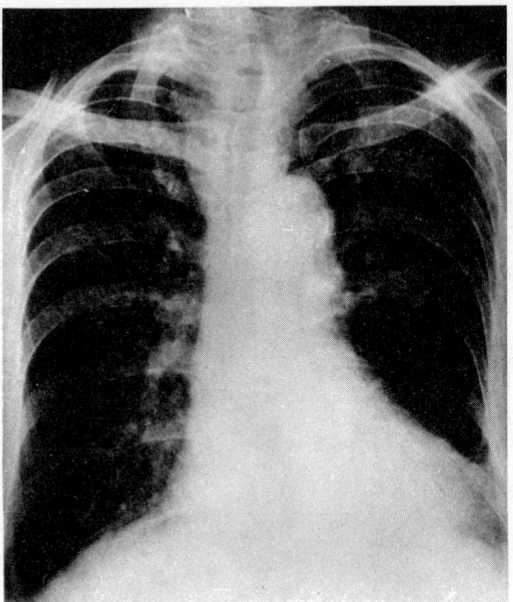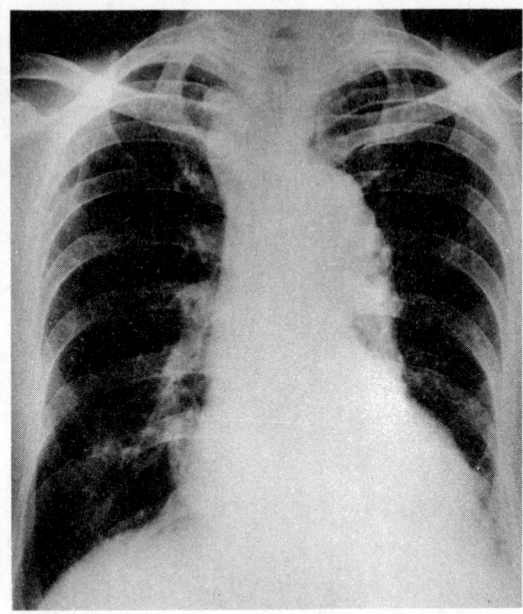

FIGURE 28–4. Dissection of thoracic aorta. **Left:** Chest film prior to aortic dissection. **Right:** Chest film after aortic dissection showing widening of descending aorta. Note left heart border relative to ring of calcium in the aortic arch.

commonly is posteriorly into the retroperitoneal space rather than anteriorly into the free peritoneal cavity, patients do not exsanguinate immediately and time is available to establish this diagnosis. The patient will present with the onset of severe and persistent boring lumbar, pelvic, or umbilical pain that will radiate to the flank or inguinal regions. Weakness, nausea, and diaphoresis are usually present. Occasionally, rupture will occur into the vena cava or the common iliac veins. Here, the presenting symptoms may be congestive heart failure or angina caused by the increased volume load on the heart. Abdominal auscultation will often reveal a continuous murmur or a loud systolic bruit. The diagnosis of acute rupture can be made by the findings of hypotension, a large often tender abdominal mass, and severe pain. All of these patients should be considered for immediate surgery.

ETIOLOGIC DISEASES

Atherosclerosis

The most common etiology of aneurysmal dilatation of both the thoracic and abdominal aorta is atherosclerosis. The initial process involves plaque for-

mation within the intima. Later, local hemorrhage, ulceration, overlying thrombus formation, and calcification follow. While it is not clear whether atherosclerosis causes degeneration of the aortic media, this process does weaken the aortic wall and aneurysmal dilatation develops. In the abdomen, atherosclerotic aneurysms most commonly involve the aorta below the renal arteries. In the thorax, the process is primarily limited to the arch and descending aorta. It is unlikely that atherosclerosis is a cause of thoracic aortic dissection. Nevertheless, this process may have an important, but yet unclear contributory role in the development of a thoracic dissection.

Cystic Medial Necrosis[157]

Cystic medial necrosis of the aorta may occur as an isolated entity (Erdheim syndrome) or as part of a congenital disorder of connective tissue (Marfan syndrome). The ascending aorta is by far the most common site involved. In both conditions, initial accumulation of a mucoid substance within the media is noted. Later, there is loss of continuity, fragmentation, and retraction of the elastic fibers. Finally, foci of medial infarction are found with associated giant cell reaction. Aortic valvular regurgitation is a common complication of this disorder. Medial degeneration of the aorta is almost a requisite for thoracic dissection.

Hypertension

Because hypertension is present in more than 80 percent of patients that develop a dissection of the thoracic aorta, it must be considered at least a contributing factor, if not a separate etiology. While hypertension probably does not cause medial degeneration, its presence may enhance development of this process. The hypertensive variables that are important include the pulse pressure and the rate of rise of the pulse wave as well as the absolute level of pressure.

Inflammatory Diseases

With the decline of syphilitic aortitis over the past three decades, inflammatory lesions of the aorta have become increasingly rare. Prior to the widespread use of early serologic detection and penicillin therapy, syphilitic aortitis was the most common etiology of a thoracic aneurysm. Between 1920 and 1940, 5 to 7 percent of all autopsied patients had evidence of syphilitic aortitis. Recent autopsy studies since 1950 place the prevalence of this disorder at approximately 0.7 percent.[156] In this condition, the *Treponema pallidum* invades the aortic wall and a low-grade inflammatory reaction may smolder for many years before necrosis and fragmentation of the elastic tissue of the media occur. This process primarily involves the ascending aorta and eventually results in a weakness of the aortic wall with aneurysm formation. A thin eggshell-like line of calcium is sometimes seen in the ascending aorta and is highly specific for syphilis (Fig. 28–1).

Mycotic aneurysms result from destruction of the aortic wall by either bacterial or granulomatous infection. These infections most commonly occur at abnormal sites such as atherosclerotic lesions, coarctation, or cystic medial necrosis. The source of infection may be intravascular (e.g., endocarditis), a remote site with hematogenous spread, or by direct erosion from the mediastinum or retroperitoneal space (e.g., tuberculosis). The clinical manifestations are frequently insidious and may not be recognized until aortic rupture has occurred.

Aortitis is an unusual manifestation of ankylosing spondylitis, Reiter syndrome, giant cell arteritis, or relapsing polychondritis. In these conditions, the inflammatory reaction results in dilatation of the ascending aorta, occasionally aneurysm formation, and aortic valvular insufficiency. Takayasu's arteritis is a rare inflammatory disorder of the aorta, its major branches, and the pulmonary artery. The origins of the branchiocephalic vessels are typically involved and result in the loss of radial or carotid pulses. This is the basis for labeling this process as "pulseless disease" or aortic arch syndrome.

Trauma

Blunt deceleration injury to the aorta is a rare but recognized cause of aneurysmal dilatation. The characteristic location of this injury is in the descending thoracic aorta just distal to the subclavian artery at the level of the ligamentum arteriosum. A false aneurysm or fistulous connection between the aorta and the vena cava or pulmonary artery can occur as the result of a penetrating injury resulting from a missle or stab wound.

DIAGNOSIS, TREATMENT, AND PROGNOSIS OF AORTIC ANEURYSMS

Thoracic Aneurysm Without Dissection

Because aortic rupture can occur abruptly and unexpectedly, consideration should be given for elective aortography of all patients with suspected thoracic aneurysms. Operative mortality for elective resection of a thoracic aneurysm varies from 20 to 40 percent. Resection should be performed on most aneurysms limited to the ascending aorta if the diameter is greater than 8 cm if symptoms secondary to the aneurysm are present or if there is moderate or severe aortic regurgitation. Sizable aneurysms involving the aortic arch and branchiocephalic vessels should also be considered for resection, but the mortality and morbidity are higher in this patient group. Aneurysms of the descending or thoracoabdominal aorta have the additional difficulty that the lower intercostal arteries which perfuse the spinal cord are commonly involved, and paraplegia is reported in 20 to 30 percent of patients surviving descending thoracic aneurysm resection. Adverse factors relating to surgery in all patients include coexisting coronary heart disease, diastolic hypertension, or age in excess of 50 years. When elective resection is not done, propranolol therapy may be beneficial in reducing both the mean arterial pressure and the rate in rise of systolic pressure.

Thoracic Aortic Dissection[158]

The catastrophic consequences of aortic dissection require immediate recognition and medical or surgical intervention. The patient should be promptly transferred to a cardiovascular center so that diagno-

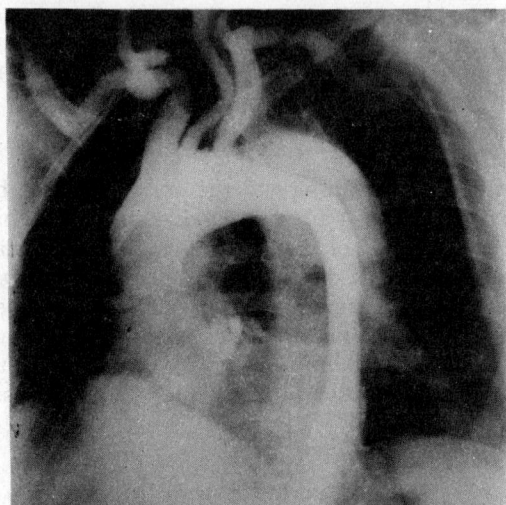

FIGURE 28-5. Aortogram of a patient with a dissection of the aorta showing a double lumen.

┌───┐
TABLE 28-1
Indication for Initial Surgical Therapy of Dissecting Aortic Aneurysm

1. Significant aortic regurgitation
2. Congestive heart failure
3. Leakage from the aneurysm with imminent rupture or pericardial tamponade
4. Occlusion of a major branch of the aorta
5. Neurologic signs suggesting cerebral ischemia
6. Intractable chest pain
7. Recurrent ventricular arrhythmias
8. Persistent oliguria
9. Failure to stop progression of the dissection by drug therapy
10. Onset of right bundle branch block
└───┘

sis can be established and surgical resection proceed if indicated (Fig. 28-5). Death is due either to occlusion of a major branch of the aorta (coronary, carotid, mesenteric, or renal) or rupture of the aorta, most commonly into the pericardium or left pleural cavity. While the risk of immediate death is approximately 3 percent, 21 percent of the patients die within 1 day, 60 percent within 2 weeks, and 90 percent within 3 months without treatment. Aortography is done to define the location of the intimal tear, extent of dissection, whether a "false" channel is present, and degree of aortic regurgitation. On the basis of this study, prognosis without surgery and expected operative risk can be defined. A Type III dissection limited to the descending and abdominal aorta has the most favorable prognosis while a Type I dissection involving all segments of the thoracic aorta including the arch has the worst prognosis. Significant aortic regurgitation and demonstration of a "false" channel are two findings associated with a more grave prognosis.

Medical therapy is started on every patient and includes relief of pain, treatment of congestive heart failure, and transfusion for blood loss. Pharmacologic efforts to limit or stop dissection include decreasing mean arterial pressure and the force of pulsatile aortic flow. Wheat and his colleagues[161] advocate the use of trimethaphan (Arfonad), guanethidine, reserpine, and propranolol to reduce systolic pressure to the 100 to 120 mm Hg range. Others are inclined to recommend surgery more quickly.[153]

Indications for immediate surgical therapy or for abandoning "medical" therapy are listed in Table 28-1. Even with current techniques, the operative risk of thoracic aortic resection for acute dissection remains formidable. Operative procedures include resection of the entire dissection, resection of the intimal tear with oversewing of the false channel, or a fenestration procedure whereby a distal reentry channel is created between the "false" lumen into the "true" lumen.

Abdominal Aortic Aneurysm

The presence and size of an abdominal aneurysm can be established by abdominal sonography or roentgenograms (anteroposterior, lateral, and oblique) of the abdomen which reveal "egg-shell" calcification within the aneurysmal wall. The size of the aneurysm is an important determinant of prognosis without operation and is the most important criterion for surgical selection of the asymptomatic patient. An abdominal aortogram is usually not done unless surgery is contemplated. This examination will determine whether important arterial branches come off the aneurysmal segment (e.g., the renal arteries) and will define the extent of atherosclerosis that will be encountered in the ileofemoral arteries at the distal end of resection. The size of the aneurysm on aortography may be misleadingly small because the dilated segment is often filled with laminated thrombus.

The prognosis of patients with an abdominal aneurysm larger than 6 cm is poor without surgical resection. Estes has reported the follow-up of 102 patients with an aneurysm seen at the Mayo Clinic prior to 1949.[155] The underlying etiology in virtually all of these patients was atherosclerosis. Survival 3 and 5 years after diagnosis was 49 percent and 19 percent. In those patients where the cause of death could be ascertained, 63 percent died from rupture of the aneurysm and 37 percent from other causes. In an autopsy study, 82 percent of aneurysms larger than 7 cm demonstrated rupture, while smaller aneurysms had a 4 percent incidence of rupture.[152] Szilagyi and his colleagues[160] have reported survival without surgery 3 and 5 years after diagnosis in patients with an aneurysm larger than 6 cm (12 and 6 percent) and for patients with an aneurysm smaller than 6 cm (68 and 48 percent). These authors have shown that survival with surgical resection is considerably better in both patient groups.

In the absence of rupture, the operative mortality for elective resection of an abdominal aneurysm has progressively declined over the past 25 years and is now under 3 percent in most major institutions. Surgical mortality for a ruptured abdominal aneurysm remains at least 35 to 45 percent. Despite improving surgical results, death due to other vascular disease (primarily cerebral and cardiac) remains an important factor in subsequent survival.

All patients with a suspected abdominal aneurysm should have either sonography or abdominal roentgenograms to confirm the measurements made by direct palpation. Surgical resection is likely indicated for any abdominal aneurysm that causes symptoms or is larger than 6 cm in diameter. Further evaluation should be done to exclude other life-threatening circumstances before a final therapeutic decision is made.

CHAPTER 29

Peripheral Vascular Disease[160,162-165]

G. MELVILLE WILLIAMS

Vascular abnormalities involving the extremities increase in frequency with age and are a major cause of disability in the United States. The challenge in managing patients with "peripheral vascular disorders" comes from the realization that peripheral manifestations are frequently symptoms of a generalized, systemic disease, yet the peripheral problem itself demands solution for the well-being of the patient. Reconstructing an occluded femoral artery will not cure atherosclerosis but it may palliate a major problem for the patient. The specificity of symptoms and the availability of extremities for examination enable the physician to make a diagnosis of the extent and severity of the disease reliably and to plan therapy rationally.

PATHOPHYSIOLOGIC CONSIDERATIONS

Blood flow to an extremity is determined by the difference between the arterial and venous pressure divided by a complex set of resistances and capacitances. Figure 29-1 illustrates these relationships. Extremity circulation is depicted as an arterial segment composed of relatively noncompliant (low capacitance) vessels and a distal or arteriolar resistance. The venous side is more complicated and is shown as a group of vessels with a large capacitance and a proximal resistance. This resistance is caused by constrictions at joints and at the diaphragm. Flow in the all important capillary bed is increased by an increase in arterial pressure, and it is diminished by an increase in resistance proximal to the capillary bed. The effects of pressure changes on the veins are far more complex because of the very large capacitance of the veins. Thus, the increase in venous pressure at the ankle produced by taking a sudden upright posture is not reflected immediately by diminished capillary flow, for blood fills the compliant veins (Fig. 29-2). The capacitance of the veins is 18 times greater than that of the arteries, permitting blood to flow prograde through capillaries during intermittent periods of high venous pressure.

An atherosclerotic plaque occluding the lumen of an artery 70 percent or less is frequently unaccompanied by reduced flow and pressure under resting conditions. However, when the distal resistance is reduced by exercise, the plaque becomes significant and restricts flow resulting in muscle ischemia which is appreciated as a crampy pain. Sclerotic plaques reducing the lumen 90 percent or more will reduce flow and pressure at rest and cause much more dramatic ischemia and pain during exercise (Fig. 29-3). Very large aneurysms increase the compliance of the arte-

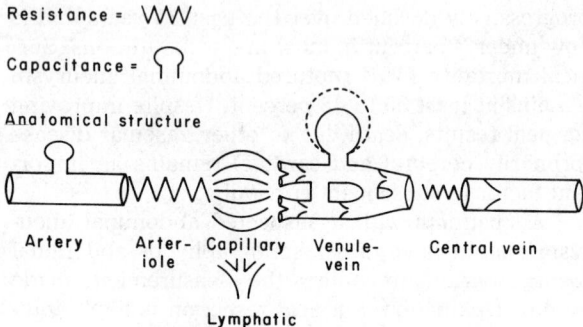

FIGURE 29-1. Diagram of the peripheral circulation.

rial tree diminishing peak systolic pressure and flow through the capillary bed. However, this rarely leads to symptoms.

The pathogenesis of venous insufficiency is far more complex and requires greater elaboration. The venous system has been likened to a ladder. The saphenous veins constitute one vertical strut while the deep veins situated between muscles represent the

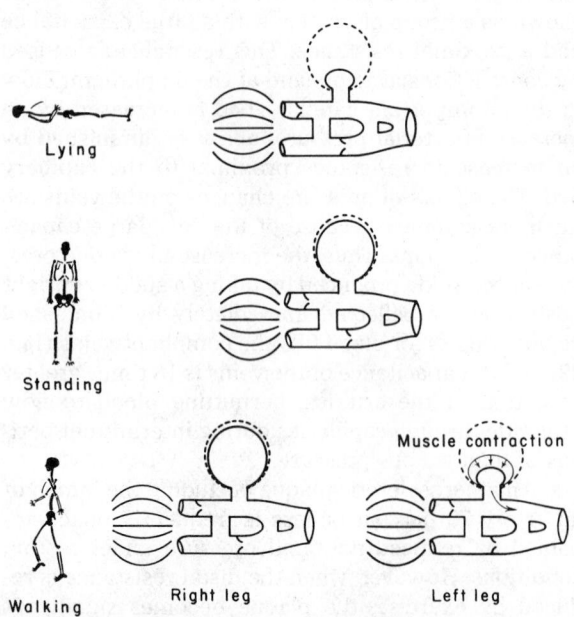

FIGURE 29-2. Diagrammatic schema illustrating the value of the venous capacitance. On standing, the effect of gravitation pressure is to cause pooling of blood in the capacitance veins. However, there will be no increase in pressure in the capillary bed until the capacitance is full. On walking or running, the capacitance modulates venous return; as one leg fills on relaxation, the other empties on pushing off.

other. The rungs of the ladder are made of multiple "perforating" veins, so called because they penetrate the fascia to drain blood from the superficial extrafascial veins to those within the muscle compartment. All major veins possess valves which permit centripetal flow only. When muscle contraction occurs the veins are compressed and blood, prevented from flowing distally by valves, is propelled up the leg. When relaxation occurs, the pressure in the deep venous system becomes lower than that in the superficial system and flow is established from superficial to deep veins through the perforating veins or rungs of the ladder.

Impaired venous return in the upright position occurs when there has been destruction of deep venous valves following thrombosis and recanalization. Patients with paralysis, severe arthritis, or other pain syndromes also develop postural venous insufficiency because muscle contraction is essential for prograde venous flow against gravity.

DIAGNOSTIC SYMPTOMS AND SIGNS

Arterial Insufficiency

The signs and symptoms of peripheral arterial disease are determined by the location and degree of vascular obstruction, the rapidity with which this obstruction develops, and the presence or absence of collateral channels. The initial symptom of arterial disease is the pain of muscle ischemia or claudication. Characteristically, this is a sensation of fatigue, dull aching, or crampiness felt in the muscle which is induced by

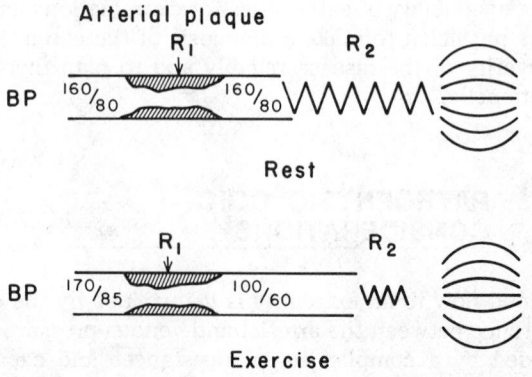

FIGURE 29-3. Illustration of the mechanism of pressure reduction distal to a partial occlusion produced by exercise. When the vascular resistance falls in the exercising muscle, the plaque becomes significant, and it is detected by measuring the pressure before and after exercise.

a constant degree of exercise and completely relieved by 5 to 10 minutes of rest. Patients with musculoskeletal disease or venous insufficiency also commonly complain of pain produced by exercise and relieved by rest. However, careful questioning of the patient will disclose clear-cut differences in most cases. The patient with arterial insufficiency acquires pain during exercise; his exercise tolerance is reasonably stable, dependent only upon the rapidity and duration of exercise; and the relief of pain occurs rapidly. By contrast, the pain associated with musculoskeletal disorders as well as those with venous insufficiency may begin during exercise or may come on several hours after a period of exercise: there are fluctuations in exercise tolerance, and the pain is relieved by rest but it may take several hours or days (Table 29-1).

The location of ischemic pain is determined by the sites of arterial obstruction. If pain is felt in the calf muscles, the major obstruction is probably in the superficial femoral artery. Pain in the thigh occurs with common femoral or external iliac disease. If pain is experienced in the buttock, there is obstruction in either the common iliac artery or distal aorta. Impotence is another sign that may reflect distal aortic disease and together with bilateral buttock and thigh claudication constitutes the Leriche syndrome.

Constant pain in a resting extremity should raise the possibility of acute arterial occlusion. Patients without any preceding history of claudication and presenting with a painful extremity most likely have had an arterial embolus. Excruciating pain is a prominent feature early after the complete occlusion of a large, normal artery. However, with the passage of time, severe pain is frequently replaced by paresthesias providing the patient with false optimism. The physician examining such a patient will find the extremity pale and pulseless below the site of occlusion. Thus, there are four adjectives all starting with "P" that describe the signs and symptoms of acute arterial occlusion—painful, paresthetic, pale, and pulseless. The site of the occlusion can frequently be deduced from the level of change of skin temperature; ankle and foot, popliteal occlusion; lower leg, superficial femoral occlusion; midthigh, iliac artery occlusion; inguinal ligament, aortic occlusion.

The patient with the preceding history of claudication who presents with chronic rest pain and/or ulceration will most often have multiple and extensive arterial stenoses or occlusions. Palpation of brachial, radial, carotid, aortic, femoral, popliteal, and pedal pulses provides important information. These pulses are graded 0 to 4+, and considerable time is required even by experienced examiners to decide if a pulse is absent. If the examiner cannot feel a pulse well enough to count it, the score is 0. Equivocation is a poor practice.

An especially valuable sign of chronic arterial ischemia is extreme pallor of the forefoot on elevation and rubor on dependency. The test is performed by elevating the extremity with the patient lying supine. The degree of blanching is noted. The extremity is then lowered by having the patient sit on the edge of the bed or examining table, and the time required for maximal "blushing" to occur is recorded. In the normal or hyperemic individual, the foot becomes only slightly pale on elevation and maximal color is present as soon as the leg is made dependent. In patients with ischemia, there is a delay of at least 20 seconds and sometimes as much as 2 minutes before the capillary blush becomes maximal. If a patient has severe rubor only on dependency, this provides a strong indication that a skin lesion or even a clean incision carried through this area of rubor will not heal. Evaluation in patients with dark skin is more difficult, but it can still be done by noting the color of the plantar surface of the foot and ankle. Dependent rubor indicates maximal small vessel vasodilatation caused by tissue ischemia.

Trophic changes in the skin are less reliable indi-

TABLE 29-1

Differential Diagnosis of Leg Pain: Signs and Symptoms

Disease Entity	Exercise-Related	Site	Pulses	Other Findings
Ischemia	4+	Muscle	↓↓ to 0	Pallor → rubor
Compression of cauda equina	3+	Sacral nerve roots	±	↓ Reflexes
Arteritis	2+	Joints, lateral thigh, shin	±	Joint effusions
Venous insufficiency	2+	Calf, foot	±	Edema, stasis dermatitis
Neuropathy	0	Glove, stocking	±	↓ Sensation

ces of ischemia. It is not uncommon to find patients with advanced ischemia, particularly if acute, with normal nail and hair growth, while abnormal skin appendages and skin texture are seen in a variety of nonvascular disorders.

Venous Insufficiency

The symptoms and signs of venous insufficiency depend in large measure upon whether the processes are acute or chronic, localized or generalized. Acute venous insufficiency may be caused by thrombophlebitis, trauma, or external venous compression. Steady pain, swelling, superficial venous distention, muscle compartment tenderness, and a dusky cyanotic skin color are the major signs and symptoms. Extreme degrees of acute venous obstruction induce arterial vasoconstriction which reduces further capillary flow. Gangrene may result. Such extremities will be massively swollen and cyanotic, giving rise to the term *phlegmasia cerulea dolens.*

Patients with chronic venous insufficiency will present with complaints of aching pain in the lower leg after periods of standing or sitting. As insufficiency progresses, the skin becomes thickened and brown colored. Secondary varicosities, pruritis, and ulceration are late manifestations. While patients frequently attribute an ulcer to trauma, ulcers caused by venous hypertension occur in predictable locations. The area of skin anterior and superior to the medial malleolus is drained by branches of the long saphenous vein and is the most common site of ulceration probably because the greatest focus of high venous pressure will occur when valves are disrupted in this system. It has been stated that the malleoli divide arterial and venous ulcerations with the former occurring inferior and the latter superior to the malleoli.

The patient with chronic venous disease should be examined in the standing and supine positions. Edema is the primary finding in most patients. Standing may disclose the presence of dilated superficial veins. The pressure in these veins is generally high when the legs are dependent. Simple palpation before and after the patient stands on his toes ten times rapidly differentiates patients with trivial varicosities from those whose varicosities are secondary to deep venous pathology. In the presence of a competent deep system, the pressure falls quite appreciably with exercise. In the presence of an incompetent deep system, the pressure will remain high despite exercise.

An attempt should be made to determine the presence and magnitude of venous valvular insufficiency. This is done by placing the patient supine, elevating the extremity to empty the veins, and applying a rubber tourniquet above the knee. When the patient

stands, the presence or absence of filling of the dilated superficial veins is noted with the tourniquet in place and immediately after it is removed. If very marked increase in filling occurs with removal of the tourniquet, the major source of filling of these superficial veins is reflux down an incompetent saphenous vein. If the veins dilate very rapidly with the tourniquet in place, they are clearly filling by means of incompetent perforators situated below the tourniquet. It is frequently possible to palpate dilated perforator veins by feeling "holes" or defects 0.5 to 1 cm in size in the fascia of the lower leg. Thus, on physical examination alone, it is possible to judge the extensiveness of the venous problem and to determine whether or not surgical resection of a few or many incompetent, valveless veins is likely to aid the patient.

LABORATORY AIDS IN THE DIAGNOSIS OF VASCULAR DISEASE

Doppler

Of the special diagnostic aids, the Doppler flow probe has assumed the most important role in the evaluation of patients. The available models are all extraordinarily sensitive detectors of flow. Thus, flow may be detected by the Doppler in pedal vessels even in cases of severe ischemia. To avoid overestimating circulatory adequacy, pressure measurements are mandatory.

The measurement of segmental limb pressures is easily done with the Doppler. Pressure in the thigh can be determined by applying a large cuff to the thigh and determining the pressure at which flow is extinguished in the popliteal or tibial artery as monitored by the Doppler probe. By placing the cuff around the calf, measurements of calf pressures can be obtained as the examiner determines what pressure is associated with the loss of pedal flow. Calf and thigh pressures are compared with each other and with the brachial artery pressure to provide an objective assessment of the degree of arterial disease. If resting calf pressures are one-fifth of those recorded in the brachial artery, severe ischemia is present and limb loss is imminent. If calf pressure is one-half the brachial artery pressure, claudication is the expected symptom. If the pressure is 80 percent or greater of the brachial artery pressure, some explanation other than arterial insufficiency must be found for the patient's symptoms, particularly if the pressure is sustained after exercise. If thigh pressure is normal and calf pressure low, the occlusion is in the distal femoral or popliteal system. If thigh pressures are also low, significant iliac or aortic disease is present. Occasionally, flow cannot be eliminated by cuff pressures greater than 200 mm. This finding suggests the presence of extensively calcified vessels and invalidates the test.

Plethysmography

A number of sensitive instruments are available which measure changes in the volume of a part. Some of these record the changes in volume associated with cardiac ejection, i.e., pulse volume recorders. Others make use of the normal compliant venous system to measure inflow. In these tests, a tourniquet is inflated to 60 mm Hg pressure to occlude venous return, and the change in volume with time during the first 10 to 20 seconds is recorded as flow. For example, the flow to a finger can be estimated by suddenly inflating a proximal tourniquet and measuring the acute increase in volume of the finger.

Deductions can also be made about the presence or absence of venous obstruction using the principles of plethysmography. If a tourniquet applied to the thigh is inflated to occlude venous return, the volume in the calf increases. However, if an occlusion is present, the increase in volume is less than expected because the capacitance is full. Further, release of the tourniquet is followed by a slower than normal return of blood volume to resting levels. Sufficient data have been generated using these principles of diminished filled volume and delayed emptying to state that plethysmography will detect significant thrombi in the femoral and iliac venous systems. Below the knee where the veins form a parallel rather than a series circuit and thrombi are far less apt to cause physiologic obstruction, plethysmographic techniques are much less accurate.

Angiography

Angiography remains the reference method for assessing the cause and severity of peripheral vascular disease. However, a better understanding of the natural history of vascular disease and the application of noninvasive techniques have changed the indications for arteriography. Seldom is arteriography required to make practical decisions in the management of patients. Rather, its major application is in those individuals who require surgery for the relief of intractable symptoms. Properly performed, it provides the surgeon with the information he needs to make judgments about the type of surgery to be performed and the likelihood of success.

Venography is indisputably the most accurate method for the detection of venous thrombi. The procedure must be carried out by skilled personnel in order to avoid problems associated with extravasation of contrast material and to be certain that the deep veins are adequately filled. Concern is still expressed about the toxicity of contrast material. However, the incidence of important complications clinically is extremely low, and venography is indicated to establish the diagnosis of phlebitis in most patients.

ISCHEMIC PERIPHERAL VASCULAR DISEASE ENTITIES

RHEOLOGIC ABNORMALITIES

Ischemia may be caused by rheologic problems as well as by structural narrowing of the blood vessel wall. Therefore, every patient presenting with ischemic manifestations should be evaluated with this thought in mind, particularly if the symptoms involve the digits and if multiple extremities are affected. The most common rheologic disorders are sickle-cell anemia, polycythemia vera, macroglobulinemia, and the presence of cold agglutinins. The effect of these various disorders is to render the blood more viscous, thereby deterring flow through the capillary bed. Raynaud's disease, which is an unusually severe vasoconstrictive response to cold, may well be a rheologic problem in some patients, for it has recently been reported that periodic plasmapheresis successfully ameliorates symptoms.

ARTERIAL EMBOLISM

An arterial embolus should be suspected in any individual who experiences the sudden loss of circulation to an extremity. While most emboli can be removed simply by modern surgical techniques, the mortality remains high and surprisingly constant at 15 to 30 percent. Thus, the problem in a significant number of patients is not so much the ischemic limb but the underlying problem such as heart failure or an unresolved nidus of thrombus providing the source for secondary emboli to important visceral and cerebral arteries.

Formerly, we believed that 90 percent of arterial emboli originated from the heart. Recent evidence suggests that 90 percent of patients with arterial emboli have heart disease, but the heart may not be the source in all. Emboli may originate from the left atrial appendage in patients with atrial fibrillation. Others originate in the left ventricle when the endocardium is damaged and the left ventricle contracts poorly. An intracardiac tumor may be the source of emboli. Emboli may come from the venous side of the circulation passing through a patent foramen ovale. Finally, thrombus may form in the aorta itself and be shed distally. Of these various sources, recent evidence suggests that paradoxic emboli originating from the venous circulation and mural aortic thrombus are more frequent causes of acute circulatory failure than previously suspected.

To reduce mortality and morbidity, it is obvious that the physician must search for the source and cause of an embolus and correct the primary cause whenever possible. The successful management of patients with arterial emboli depends upon the collaboration of physician, surgeon, and diagnostic laboratories. The first practical decision to be made is whether or not the patient can withstand angiography and general anesthesia. If the patient has had a recent myocardial infarction and is in congestive heart failure, the heart failure assumes priority and must be treated aggressively. Complicated angiographic techniques are not indicated. Rather, the patient should be transported expeditiously to the operating room, where monitoring and active treatment directed toward optimizing the cardiac function are continued. The surgical extraction of the embolus under local anesthesia is a change of scene but not of doctors. The need for prompt surgery even under these desperate circumstances must be emphasized, for the restoration of circulation to an acutely ischemic limb is likely to improve cardiac function by diminishing pain, anxiety, afterload, and the toxic products of ischemic tissue. Waiting for cardiac stability may result in such severe ischemia that myoglobin and other toxic substances are released from necrotic muscle tissue, all of which compound the patient's problems. Thus, optimal management in the very sick patient utilizes embolectomy as just one of several avenues of therapy, all of which are directed toward restoring adequate circulation to all parts of the body.

A second category of patients having arterial emboli is represented by the otherwise well patient who suddenly experiences the loss of circulation to an extremity. Under these circumstances, much is to be gained by an urgent but thorough evaluation of the patient. In the absence of bleeding or stroke, blood is drawn for coagulation studies and the patient is fully heparinized. In taking the history, special attention is directed to symptoms of preceding ischemia of the involved limb or of cardiac arrhythmias. An ECG and an echocardiogram should be carried out. Noninvasive tests of venous patency of the legs should be done. Once these tests are completed and the patient is hydrated intravenously, angiography should be performed. In cases of upper extremity emboli, the aortic arch and the origin of the involved vessel must be visualized. In the case of lower extremity embolization, biplane views of the abdominal aorta are indicated along with a demonstration of the site of occlusion. The surgical procedure is directed toward the removal of the embolus and its source whenever possible.

There is also an intermediate category of patients: those who have had a recent myocardial infarction but are stable at the time of the embolic event. More experience is needed to document the relative frequency of embolic sources in this group of patients before one can proceed with rational therapy. However, in our recent experience, the extraction of one embolus is quite likely to be followed by a second unless the cause is eradicated. Thus, we currently favor an aggressive approach in evaluating these patients as outlined above. Alternatively, the aggressive approach may be reserved for those patients who experience recurrent emboli.

ARTERIOSCLEROSIS

In actual practice, it is quite surprising to note how focal occlusive arteriosclerosis may be. Only a minority of patients have coexisting symptomatic carotid, coronary, aortic, iliac, and femoral artery occlusive disease. In terms of the practical management of the patient, more is to be gained by considering the process localized and amenable to treatment than is to be gained by an overly pessimistic view of the intractable nature of this disease.

Abundant evidence supports the concept that much more is to be gained by the medical as opposed to surgical management of patients with nondisabling claudication. Medical management consists of the following: 1) the cessation of all smoking, 2) the control of hypertension, 3) weight reduction, 4) dietary management of hyperlipidemia, 5) exercise (principally walking to the point of claudication three times a day), and 6) the proper care of the feet to prevent infection and cold exposure. The physician may expect the development of collateral circulation to take 6 months. This process can be followed by noting changes in work tolerance and in segmental limb pressures. As a general rule, surgery for the relief of claudication alone should not be undertaken when this symptom has been present for less than 6 months unless the work tolerance is clearly lessening rapidly. Vasodilator drugs have not proven effective, but there may be a role for agents which inhibit platelet aggregation such as aspirin or dipyridamole.

It is ironic that the larger the artery that is occluded the greater the chance of success achieved by surgical correction. The patient with bilateral hip and thigh claudication who has absent femoral pulses has a 90 percent chance of complete symptomatic relief by surgery. A patient with significant calf claudication and/or rest pain in the foot, who has femoral but no popliteal pulses, has a 70 percent chance of complete symptomatic relief by surgery. A patient with calf claudication and rest pain in the foot but with a popliteal pulse has a 55 percent chance of long-term symptomatic relief. In every instance of lower extremity occlusive disease, the chances for successful surgery outweigh those of failure.

Surgical reconstruction should be considered in all patients with intractable claudication, rest pain, and/or ulceration of the extremity. Intractability is a judgment based on the individual's need to perform a certain amount of work with his legs taken in the context of his overall health and of objective measurements of segmental pressures which have failed to improve or have worsened. Patients should be informed and willing to accept a surgical procedure that has a 5 to 10 percent chance of making his circulation acutely worse necessitating amputation.

Diabetic patients have four discrete problems leading to difficulties with their extremities. First, they have an increased frequency of arteriosclerosis, which also occurs at an earlier age. Second, they have arteriolar disease. Third, they have a high frequency of neuropathy, which results in anesthetic joint disease, particularly of the tarsal areas of the feet. Fourth, they have an increased susceptibility to infection. These problems render the management of the diabetic patient with a foot lesion a most complicated problem.

The so-called "trophic foot ulcer" of the diabetic is characterized by its location on the plantar aspect of the foot directly beneath a joint, most commonly the metatarsophalangeal joint. Callus surrounds the ulcer which is rarely, if ever, painful. The pathogenesis is best explained by chronic, unappreciated trauma causing deterioration and rupture of the capsule of the anesthetic joint. Fragments of the cartilage are extruded eventually eroding the skin from within out. Proper management depends upon the reduction of trauma to the joint involved, and to this end there is no substitute for special shoes. At times surgery is indicated, but the procedure should never be less than the excision of the involved joint.

THROMBOANGIITIS OBLITERANS

This disease entity initially described by Buerger was thought to be extremely rare 10 years ago, but at present virtually all physicians caring for patients with vascular disease agree that this is a distinct and not infrequent pathophysiologic entity. It is characterized by 1) necrosis of the digits of both hands and feet; 2) occurrence before the age of 40 in patients who are predominantly male, Jewish, and heavy cigarette smokers; 3) occlusion of small- and medium-sized arteries below the elbow and below the knee; and 4) the frequent coexistence of thrombophlebitis which may be either superficial or deep (Table 29–2).

Patients with Buerger's disease generally present with pain of severe nature occurring in one or more digits. A few present with claudication in the hand while writing or in the sole of the foot while walking. Virtually no other disease entity produces this type of claudication. If the physical examination demonstrates the loss of one or more tibial arteries or either the radial or ulnar artery, the diagnosis is virtually established.

Allen's sign is a useful test for demonstrating oc-

TABLE 29–2

Manifestations of Atherosclerosis, Thromboangiitis Obliterans, and Raynaud's Disease

	Atherosclerosis	Thromboangiitis Obliterans	Raynaud's Disease
Age of onset	> 40	< 40	< 40
Intermittent digital pallor	Absent	Absent	Hallmark
Persistent pain, cyanosis, and necrosis of fingers	Absent	Present	Rare and late in course
Cold sensitivity	Present	Present	Extreme
Claudication in palms and soles	Absent	May be present	Absent
Claudication in calves and thighs	Present	Late in course	Absent
Occlusion of arteries distal to the elbow and knee	Rare	Present	Absent
Occlusion of arteries above the elbow and knee	Present	Rare and late in course	Absent
History of phlebitis	Rare	Frequent	Rare

clusion of the ulnar or radial artery or of the palmar arch vessels which connect the two. The test is performed by elevating the hand and closing the fist while the examiner compresses both radial and ulnar arteries. The hand is then opened and closed until pallor is noted. After a minute, pressure on the ulnar artery is released while the examiner notes the color of the hand and fingers while maintaining pressure on the radial artery. If the ulnar artery and palmar arch are patent, the hand will assume a normal pink color immediately. If the ulnar artery is occluded, the hand will remain blanched. If the palmar arch is incomplete, the fifth or fourth fingers will assume a normal color while the first three fingers will remain blanched. Patency of the radial artery can be demonstrated in the same way by compressing the ulnar instead of the radial artery. Similar information can be obtained by use of the Doppler flow probe.

Treatment should be directed to the withdrawal from tobacco. This is easier said than done, for the extent of addiction is severe in the majority of these patients. The value of platelet antagonists, anticoagulation with warfarin, and steroids remains unproven. Some patients benefit from sympathectomy.

VASOCONSTRICTIVE DISORDERS

Vasoconstriction of the hands and feet is a normal sympathetic response to cold to preserve core body temperature. This reflex is exaggerated in a variety of systemic diseases causing patients to complain of pain and pallor in one or more fingers or toes following exposure to cold or even during emotional upsets (Table 29–2). When this symptom complex exists singly, it is called Raynaud's disease; when it exists as one manifestation of collagen vascular disorders or rheologic disorders, it is termed Raynaud's phenomenon. The work-up of patients presenting with exaggerated cold pressor responses includes assays of complement levels, rheumatoid factor, antinuclear factor, and sedimentation rate. In addition, patients with structural occlusion have increased cold sensitivity, and thorough vascular examination should be done.

In the case of Raynaud's disease, where no structural changes exist early in the course, treatment is predicated by common sense. These patients are reassured if a thorough examination demonstrates the absence of structural damage to important arteries of the involved extremities. Simple measures, such as wearing gloves inside of mittens in the wintertime and using the elbow to test for the temperature of water, should be pointed out by the physician. If symptoms persist or get worse despite common sense measures, a trial of agents blocking alpha-adrenergic

responses may be undertaken. Dibenzyline has the greatest potency and a long duration of action and should be recommended to individuals whose employment depends upon cold exposure of their extremities. Surgery, consisting of sympathectomy, is reserved for patients who have tissue loss. While early results are generally good, recurrent symptoms develop in the upper extremities in most patients after 5 years. Therefore, it must be stressed that the foremost aim of the physician in treating patients with Raynaud's disease or phenomenon is to alter habits of cold exposure, just as his aim in the patient with Buerger's disease is to have this patient eliminate smoking.

ANEURYSMS OF THE ILIAC, FEMORAL, AND POPLITEAL ARTERIES

Many instances of rupture of iliac artery aneurysms have been reported. However, iliac aneurysms are not detected on physical examination or routine x-rays, and the incidence of rupture remains unknown. In the otherwise healthy patient, surgery is the preferred method of treatment, but one could not argue with the approach of observing these by sonography or by CAT scanning in patients with cardiopulmonary disease.

Arteriosclerotic aneurysms of the femoral and popliteal arteries are likely to shed emboli and finally thrombose rather than rupture. The typical history is one of recurrent episodes of pain, principally in the foot but at times in the calf musculature. Examination at this stage of the disease will disclose the presence of the pulsating mass in the groin or behind the knee and irregular red-blue patches of skin on the foot. Continued embolization, thrombosis, and loss of the extremity are almost inevitable in untreated patients. Reconstruction of arterial circulation after thrombosis of a popliteal aneurysm is not nearly as successful as primary resection before thrombosis. Thus, all patients with extremity aneurysms should undergo resection and graft replacement when the aneurysm is found.

DISORDERS OF THE VENOUS SYSTEM

ACUTE THROMBOPHLEBITIS

The principal signs and symptoms of acute thrombophlebitis are calf pain and aching, edema, and muscle tenderness (see section on chronic venous insufficiency). However, the majority of hospitalized patients with deep venous thrombosis will have no symptoms, and only 50 percent of those thought to have phlebitis clinically have such on venography. Thus, it is hard to escape the view that reliance must be placed on the laboratory for the diagnosis of thrombophlebitis.

Venous stasis and hypercoagulability are the two major causes of thrombophlebitis. Superficial phlebitis may be a manifestation of an underlying malignancy, but may also occur in venous varicosities or for no known reason. Of itself, the process has little risk of embolizing or contributing to venous stasis. It is appropriate to treat the isolated superficial phlebitis symptomatically with heat and rest. Should other superficial veins become involved, the process must be taken more seriously and consideration be given to systemic anticoagulation. Such patients should be hospitalized and undergo venography and other tests searching for an occult malignancy.

The patient presenting with calf pain and ankle edema of acute onset should undergo an initial noninvasive assessment of venous patency. If the test is positive, heparin is begun immediately. It is still wise to confirm the diagnosis by venography, which can be done several hours or even a day later. In cases where the noninvasive test discloses no venous obstruction, heparinization may be safely deferred until a venogram can be performed. Note that irrespective of the results of the noninvasive test, venography is recommended, for neither the disease process nor the means of treatment are trivial, and it is essential to apply the reference method, i.e., venography, to establish this diagnosis. The management of patients with deep venous thrombosis may vary in its details, but there is general agreement that patients should be anticoagulated with intravenous heparin and switched to long-term therapy with warfarin after 5 to 7 days.

CHRONIC VENOUS INSUFFICIENCY

The management of a patient with chronic venous insufficiency and a stasis ulcer may be quite gratifying, for all ulcers can be healed. One needs only to put the extremity higher than the heart to correct the underlying cause of venous hypertension and treat secondary problems of infection and skin loss appropriately. Patients with large infected ulcers should be admitted to the hospital and placed on bed rest, antibiotics, and topical care of the ulcer. In a matter of 3 to 5 days, the ulcer will improve to such a degree that patients may be discharged in Unna boots or undergo skin grafts if the ulcer is greater than 3 cm in diameter. Unna boots are the best way of achieving compression of the incompetent veins allowing healing to progress while the patient is ambulatory.

Once the ulcer has healed, the patient must wear custom-made, elastic stockings to limit the increase in venous pressure which caused the problem. Surgery is reserved for those who cannot or will not wear these stockings and have recurrent ulcers. The very elderly patient may not be capable of putting these stockings on and may have to wear Unna boots permanently.

CHAPTER 30
Cardiovascular Therapeutics[166]
PHILIP R. REID, WILLIAM E. MITCH, AND WILLIAM R. BELL

The physician caring for patients with cardiovascular disease has a large array of therapeutic agents and procedures at his disposal for the management of clinical problems. Indications for drug therapy in specific disease states are considered in the preceding chapters of this section. This chapter describes the relevant clinical pharmacology for the most frequently used cardioactive drugs.

ANTIARRHYTHMIC DRUGS

An understanding of the pathophysiology of the arrhythmias (Chap. 21) is essential to the rational selection of antiarrhythmic agents. These agents are classified in Table 30–1 on the basis of electrophysiologic effects, which provide a basis for clinical application. Each of these agents has some effect in all portions of the conducting system, but some are much more potent in one area than are others. For example, since Group A or C drugs significantly prolong conduction time and effective refractory periods in atrial tissue, drugs from these groups are most useful in the treatment of atrial arrhythmias. The selection of a particular drug within a group is based upon clinical effectiveness for a specific arrhythmia and the general pharmacology of the drugs (Table 30–2). For example, both quinidine and procainamide are effective in the management of atrial flutter; procainamide would be selected for short-term control (e.g., postoper-

TABLE 30-1
Antiarrhythmic Agent Classifications

	GROUP A (Quinidine, Procainamide, Disopyramide)	GROUP B (Lidocaine, Phenytoin)	GROUP C (Propranolol)	GROUP D (Digitalis)
Atrial				
CT	↑	→	→↑	↓
ERP	↑	→	→↑	↓
AVN				
CT	↑→↓	→↓	↑	↑
ERP	↑→↑	→	↑	↑
H-P-VM				
CT	↑	→	→	→
ERP	→	→	→	→
Automaticity	↓	↓	↓	→↓

CT: Conduction Time; ERP: Effective Refractory Period; AVN: AV Node; H-P-VM: His-Purkinje-Ventricular Muscle; ↑: Increase; →: No Change; ↓: Decrease

ative) since it can be given safely as a continuous intravenous infusion whereas parenteral quinidine may produce hypotension. Alternatively, if chronic oral therapy were indicated, quinidine would be preferable because of the longer half-life and the need for fewer daily doses. Nearly all the drugs listed in Table 30-1 have allergic side effects in addition to toxic effects. These side effects are unique for each preparation so that another drug in the same group can be substituted in a patient who becomes allergic to one drug. Table 30-2 also provides information on average loading doses which should be used when it is necessary to attain a therapeutic blood level rapidly. Ideally, the use of loading doses should be reserved for patients in a hospital where appropriate monitoring is available.

QUINIDINE, PROCAINAMIDE, AND DISOPYRAMIDE

Quinidine, procainamide, and disopyramide are classified as Type A drugs because they produce a prolongation of conduction time and increased duration of the refractory period in virtually all cardiac tissue. The one exception appears to be the AV node where lower doses of these drugs may have no effect on conduction time or even enhance conduction through the AV node. In the case of quinidine, enhanced AV conduction appears to be due to an (indirect) antivagal

action. Higher doses permit domination by the direct effect which slows AV conduction. The enhancement of AV node impulse transmission by Type A drugs may become clinically important in treatment of atrial arrhythmias, such as atrial fibrillation, where this effect may "paradoxically" increase the ventricular response before the atrial arrhythmia is terminated. Therefore, in the treatment of atrial tachyarrhythmias, digitalis or propranolol is usually used to slow AV conduction and avoid the potential of a paradoxical response. Group A drugs also exert effects on ventricular tissue where they tend to slow conduction and increase refractoriness. These effects, combined with depression of phase 4 depolarization, make them effective in management of arrhythmias which result from reentry or increased automaticity.

While Type A drugs can be used for ventricular arrhythmias associated with most disease states, they should generally be avoided if ventricular arrhythmias are associated with digitalis toxicity where enhancement of impaired conduction may be an unwanted consequence. Group A drugs should also be avoided in patients with the rare syndrome of ventricular arrhythmias associated with prolonged QT interval. These patients may have ventricular repolarization slowed further by Group A drugs which may result in an increased tendency of ventricular arrhythmias due to reentry (Chap. 21). Since the Group A drugs may also slow conduction in the His-Purkinje syndrome, they should be used with caution in patients with preexisting bundle branch block.

While these drugs have similar electrophysiologic effects, their side effects are different. For example, nausea, vomiting, and diarrhea may develop in 20 to 30 percent of patients who take quinidine sulfate. Quinidine therapy may sometimes be continued if quinidine gluconate, which is better tolerated by the gastrointestinal tract, is substituted. However, the gluconate salt has approximately 20 percent less quinidine than the sulfate salt on a weight basis and, therefore, the gluconate dose must be appropriately increased. Procainamide is usually well tolerated by the gastrointestinal system but therapy may be limited by allergic side effects such as the lupus erythematous syndrome, which develops in up to 40 percent of patients who take the drug in large doses for one year. In most cases, the lupus syndrome is mild and benign and the syndrome can be suppressed by anti-inflammatory agents if continued use of procainamide is clinically necessary. The syndrome usually goes away promptly when the drug is discontinued. Disopyramide has had a shorter clinical experience; it may produce urinary retention and constipation which may limit use of the drug particularly in older

TABLE 30-2
Features of Commonly Used Antiarrhythmic Agents

	Route	Total Daily Dose	Dose Interval	Peak Levels	Elimin./Metab.	t½ ± SD	Therapeutic Serum Level	Active Metabolite	Side Effects	Indications
Quinidine sulfate	PO	800–3000 mg	4–6 hr	1–2 hr	> 90% liver	7 ± 3 hr	2–5 µg/ml	No	GI (20–30%) Cinchonism Thrombocytopenia Hemolytic anemia Skin rash Fever	Atrial fibrillation Atrial tachycardia or flutter Accelerated AV conduction syndromes PVCs
	IM	800–3000 mg	4–6 hr	½ hr						
Procainamide	PO	1000–4000 mg	3–4 hr	1–1½ hr	50% liver 50% kidney	3–4 hr	4–8 µg/ml	No	Hypotension (IV) Skin rash Fever Lupus syndrome (40%)	See quinidine
	IM	1000–4000 mg	3–4 hr	½ hr						
	IV	Bolus: 100–200 mg q̄ 5 min Infusion: 20–50 µg/kg/min		immed.						
Disopyramide	PO	400–800 mg	6 hr	1½ hr	50% liver 50% kidney	7 ± 4 hr	2–5 µg/ml	No	Blurry vision Dry mouth Constipation Urinary retention	See quinidine
Phenytoin	PO	200–600 mg	12 hr	2–6 hr	> 90% liver	22 ± 10 hr	10–20 µg/ml	No	Ataxia Nystagmus Gingival hyperplasia Fever Hepatitis Skin rash Macrocytic anemia	PVCs (digitalis toxicity)
	IV	Load: 700–1000 mg Maint.: 200–600 mg	12 hr	immed.						
Lidocaine	IV	Bolus: 0.5–2.0 mg/kg Infusion: 10–50 µg/kg/min	—	—	> 95% liver	1–2 hr	2–6 µg/ml plasma		Seizures Apnea Hallucinations	PVCs
Propranolol	PO	40–1000 mg	4–6 hr	1–2 hr	> 95% liver	3–9 hr	50–150 ng/ml		Excessive bradycardia Heart block (AV node) CHF Asthma Masked insulin hypoglycemia Mental depression Fatigue Nightmares	See quinidine
	IV	Test: 0.5 mg Load: 1–10 mg Maint.: 5–20 mg	4–6 hr	immed.						
Bretylium	IV	1000 5–10 mg/kg Infusion 1–2 mg/min (up to 30 mg/kg/day)	—	immed.*	renal	6–8 hr	?	No	Hyper/hypotension Tachycardia Nausea/vomiting	Refractory VT or VF
	IM									

* Onset of action may require several minutes.

patients. This drug also has negative inotropic effects like other Group A drugs, but in some cases this side effect appears to be more severe with disopyramide.

Toxic doses of these drugs will tend to cause loss of resting membrane potential with progressive slowing of impulse transmission. While lowering the drug dose or discontinuation may help within a few hours, immediate improvements can often be obtained by use of alkaline solutions (e.g., lactate or bicarbonate), which tend to force potassium into the cells. Since potassium is the major determinant of resting membrane potential, reestablishment of this electrical gradient may improve conduction within seconds.

Some patients show an enhanced tendency to ventricular arrhythmias after starting quinidine (quinidine syncope). There are several mechanisms for this including impaired distal conduction resulting in heart block, prolongation of the QT interval, and interaction with other drugs (e.g., phenothiazines or other Group A drugs), which may also produce slowing of conduction. More recently, it has been recognized that quinidine produces a rise in the digoxin level, sometimes to toxic levels. Thus, some of the arrhythmias observed may actually represent digitalis toxic rhythms when quinidine is added to the therapy of patients who already take digoxin.

LIDOCAINE AND PHENYTOIN

Lidocaine and phenytoin are considered together as Group B antiarrhythmic agents because they produce little effect on atrial or AV nodal conduction time or effective refractory periods of normal tissue but tend to suppress automaticity of ventricular pacemakers and may produce slowing of conduction or complete block in abnormal ventricular fibers. This last feature helps explain how a Type B antiarrhythmic agent may be effective in the treatment of ventricular arrhythmias which appear to be reentrant in nature, e.g., ventricular tachycardia following acute myocardial infarction.

Lidocaine is the primary antiarrhythmic agent for parenteral therapy of ventricular arrhythmias. It has been shown to decrease the incidence of ventricular fibrillation when used prophylactically following acute myocardial infarction. Lidocaine is always used parenterally and usually employed as an intravenous bolus and constant infusion as described in Table 30–2. Less commonly it is given intramuscularly. Lidocaine is a drug with hepatic-blood-flow-dependent elimination:[189] the lidocaine elimination rate is directly related to the hepatic blood flow and conditions such as congestive heart failure, which reduce hepatic blood flow, may therefore reduce lidocaine clearance and necessitate reduced dosage require-

ments. The wide range of doses provided in Table 30–2 reflects this blood-flow-dependent elimination. Lidocaine also has active metabolites which can occasionally contribute to toxicity, although these metabolites (monoethylglycinexylidide and glycinexylidide) are usually present in small concentrations.

Phenytoin (formerly known as diphenylhydantoin) has electrophysiologic characteristics similar to lidocaine with the advantage of a longer half-life and oral bioavailability. However, its overall effectiveness in management of ventricular arrhythmias has been generally disappointing when compared to other agents listed in Table 30–1. The one exception may be in management of ventricular arrhythmias associated with digitalis toxicity. In this situation, either lidocaine or phenytoin may be useful. When phenytoin is used intravenously, it must be infused slowly (≤ 50 mg/min) to avoid acute cardiac and central nervous system toxicity.

PROPRANOLOL

Propranolol is classified as a Group C drug because its mechanism of action appears to be through beta adrenergic blockade and possibly some effects similar to those described for quinidine. It is a nonspecific, competitive beta antagonist and, therefore, has effects related to its competitive beta antagonism in many organ systems. This nonspecificity of beta blockade gives rise to the long list of potential side effects described in Table 30–2. However, this drug is generally well tolerated and has been found useful in a variety of disease states including atrial and ventricular arrhythmias, angina pectoris, hypertrophic cardiomyopathy, and hypertension.

Propranolol is well absorbed after oral ingestion but also has hepatic-blood-flow-dependent elimination, which accounts for the difference in doses between oral and intravenous routes as noted in Table 30–2. Underlying diseases, such as sinus node dysfunction, asthma, or heart failure, may also require the use of lower doses. For example, a patient in congestive heart failure whose compensation is maintained with a high sympathetic background may require relatively little beta blockade to produce profound changes in heart rate, cardiac output, and blood pressure. A patient with mild heart failure may not be able to tolerate more than 40 mg/day, while some patients with hypertension may require 400 to 1000 mg/day.

In a few patients with angina pectoris, abrupt removal of this drug may produce the propranolol-withdrawal syndrome, which will usually occur in the first few days after propranolol discontinuation. It is manifest as a sudden exacerbation of anginal symptoms, acute myocardial infarction, ventricular arrhythmias, or sudden death. The mechanism is unclear, but the clinical appearance is that of a catecholamine hyperreactivity. The syndrome is uncommon and can be avoided by tapering the propranolol dose over several days. If recognized, propranolol therapy should be quickly restarted.

More recently, metoprolol, one of the cardioselective (β_1) beta blockers has been released for general use. At the present time, it is approved only for therapy of hypertension but probably will become available for treatment of arrhythmias in the future. The cardioselectivity of this agent permits use in patients who have relative contraindications to the nonspecific beta blockade (β_1 and β_2) produced by propranolol. However, as the dose is raised, an increasing amount of β_2 action becomes evident. Therefore, one must consider these drugs cardioselective and not cardiospecific.

BRETYLIUM TOSYLATE

Bretylium represents a recently approved antiarrhythmic for the management of ventricular arrhythmias. This drug is a quaternary ammonium which works as a ganglionic blocking agent inhibiting norepinephrine release from the adrenergic nerve terminal. The ganglionic blocking properties do not explain its antiarrhythmic effects since other ganglionic blocking agents have not been found to possess significant antiarrhythmic properties. Bretylium produces a prolongation of the action potential duration and, thus, an increase in the effective refractory period but without an increase in the conduction time. This feature distinguishes it from Group A drugs. In certain experimental conditions, such as ischemia, bretylium may increase the resting membrane potential and thereby improve impulse transmission within the distal conduction system and ventricular muscle. In some instances it has produced a pharmacologic defibrillation, which is a feature rarely seen with other drugs listed in Table 30-1. With the production of ganglionic blockade, hypotension is a regular feature; therefore, blood pressure must be closely monitored and the patient usually kept supine. In addition, the drug may initially cause transient hypertension and tachycardia, probably due to release of nerve terminal stores of norepinephrine prior to inhibition. Since catecholamines may be released, bretylium should not be used to treat the ventricular arrhythmias associated with digitalis toxicity where catecholamines regularly enhance ventricular arrhythmias. The other side effects noted in Table 30-2 may appear after prolonged use. At the present time, this drug is available only for parenteral use.

COMBINED ANTIARRHYTHMIC THERAPY

Combination therapy of antiarrhythmic agents is often considered if one agent is unsuccessful. Prior to attempting this, the physician should carefully review the adequacy of single drug therapy. Table 30-2 provides recommended drug doses, but the physician must assess each patient individually with respect to the antiarrhythmic response, side effects, and serum levels. Some patients may have an unsatisfactory response, for example, to a quinidine level of 2 μg/ml but a very good response at 4 μg/ml despite the fact that both serum levels are considered to be within the therapeutic range. Thus, higher doses of the same agent may provide all that is required, thereby avoiding the use of combined therapy with the attendent increased risks of side effects. When combined antiarrhythmic therapy is necessary, Table 30-1 may provide a rationale for choosing a drug from another group rather than use of two drugs with similar electrophysiologic effects. It is important to remember that if two drugs from the same group are used, the serum levels will reflect only the individual drug under measurement but the electropharmacologic effects will be additive. Thus, even therapeutic levels of two drugs could result in marked toxicity.

ORGANIC NITRATES[177]

The term "organic nitrate" refers to a class of compounds in which nitrate groups are substituted on a sugar moiety. Trinitroglycerin, the prototype, is trinitrated glycerol. The organic nitrates are well absorbed from the gastrointestinal tract, buccal mucosa, and skin. Together with propranolol, the organic nitrates form the therapeutic backbone in the medical management of angina pectoris. More recently, organic nitrates have been used in the therapy of congestive heart failure because of their beneficial effects on preload and afterload (Chap. 19).

The organic nitrates produce smooth muscle relaxation and thus vasodilatation, which results in an increase in venous capacitance. The increased venous capacitance produces a fall in left ventricular end-diastolic volume (an estimate of preload). The magnitude of the effect on the venous bed is usually greater than that seen on the arteriolar resistance vessels, but the route of administration may influence these results. For example, inhalation of a drug like amyl nitrite produces relatively greater effects in peripheral arterial resistance than organic nitrates administered sublingually or orally. In patients without cardiac failure there is usually a fall in the systemic blood pressure producing a reflex tachycarida with a variable decrease in cardiac output. The magnitude of this effect is dependent upon position and is greater in the upright posture. In patients with congestive heart failure, nitroglycerin may produce no change in heart rate and cardiac output may acutly increase. The different results observed in patients with or without heart failure may reflect improvement of left ventricular function in those patients with cardiac failure. The extracardiac actions described above are thought to account for the beneficial effects of nitrates in patients with angina pectoris, but the agents also produce coronary vasodilatation. This direct vasodilatation may be particularly important in patients with coronary spasm.

The major site of organic nitrate metabolism is the liver. Elimination is dependent upon hepatic blood flow as previously described for drugs such as propranolol and lidocaine. Thus, orally administered organic nitrates undergo a high hepatic clearance which reduces bioavailability. Earlier studies on the efficacy of oral organic nitrates used doses which were largely devoid of systemic effects due to high hepatic clearance. This created much controversy as to whether or not organic nitrates could ever be effective when administered orally. More recent studies, using much higher oral doses, have demonstrated hemodynamic responses which last from 2 to 6 hours. Use of the organic nitrates by sublingual administration, by chewing (without swallowing), or transcutaneously, avoids the initial portohepatic circulation and therapeutically effective doses are therefore lower. Comparative efficacy studies are not available to permit a clear choice of different preparations administered by the same route. With the recent availability of serum levels to measure organic nitrates, these important questions may soon be answered.

Side effects from different organic nitrates are similar and include extensions of their therapeutic actions: palpitations, dizziness, and headache. Occasionally, patients may complain of nausea after oral administration and usually patients note a burning sensation with sublingual trinitroglycerin. With prolonged high exposure, as has been seen in industrial nitrate workers, methemoglobinemia may appear; however, this has not been manifest in the doses of organic nitrates used clinically. Patients usually become somewhat tolerant to the headache side effect over a period of days to weeks. There is, however, no evidence of the development of tolerance to the therapeutic effects with intermittent therapy. Tolerance can be produced experimentally and perhaps with the use of higher nitrate doses for prolonged periods of time, tolerance may become a more impor-

tant question. There have been some early studies which show a reduced response of blood pressure in patients continuously treated with high dose, orally administered nitrates.

CARDIAC GLYCOSIDES[182,183]

The purpose of this section is to review the relevant pharmacology pertaining to use of cardiac glycosides in patients. The reader is also referred to Chapters 18 and 19 for discussions of the treatment of congestive heart failure and digitalis toxicity.

The cardiac glycosides are composed of a group of steroidal compounds which have structural differences that alter half-life, protein binding, extent of hepatic metabolism, or renal elimination (Table 30–3). Despite these differences, it appears that all cardiac glycosides exert their *inotropic* effect by inhibition of myocardial sarcolemmal Na-K ATPase, which results in accumulation of intracellular sodium. This produces an apparent Na^+-Ca^{++} exchange, permitting more ionized calcium interaction with the contractile proteins (myofilaments). Another major effect of cardiac glycosides is to slow AV nodal conduction (negative *dromotropic* effect) and increase the effective refractory period of the AV node. This is produced primarily by an (indirect) enhancement of vagal tone on the AV node and to some extent by a direct effect of digitalis on nodal tissue. Thus, the inotropic effect of cardiac glycosides is produced by a direct effect on the myocardium while the dromotropic effect is at least partially mediated by the central nervous system. Recent evidence also supports the role of the central nervous system in mediating many of the effects encountered during digitalis toxicity (Chaps. 19 and 21). Digitalis preparations also produce vasoconstriction of both arterioles and veins. If the glycosides are injected rapidly (less than 1 minute) intravenously, this can lead to transient hypertension.

While the actions of glycosides described above are observed in both normal subjects and patients with heart failure, the net effects observed are dependent on a combination of direct and reflex responses. For example, in patients with congestive heart failure, cardiac glycosides exert an inotropic effect which may lead to an increase in cardiac output and a subsequent withdrawal of sympathetic tone producing a net decrease in peripheral vascular resistance. If used in normal patients whose autonomic tone is normal, the inotropic effect is exerted but no increase in cardiac output is observed due to changes in other

TABLE 30-3
Cardiac Glycosides

Glycoside Preparation	Loading Dose Oral	Loading Dose IV	Daily Maintenance Dose Oral	Oral Bioavailability (%)	Half-Life	Major Elimination	IV Action Onset	IV Action Maximal Effect	Oral Action Onset	Oral Action Maximal Effect	Potentially Toxic Level (ng/ml)
Digoxin	1.5 to 4.0 mg	0.75 to 2.0 mg	0.125 to 0.75 mg	70	36 hr	Kidney (85%)	15 min	3 hr	45 min	3 hr	≥ 2.0
Digitoxin	1.0 to 1.5 mg	1.0 to 1.5 mg	0.05 to 0.2 mg	100	4–6 days	Liver (85%)	1 hr	8 hr	90 min	8 hr	≥ 35
Digitalis leaf	1.0 to 1.8 g	—	0.5 to 0.2 g	—	4–6 days	Liver	—	—	90 min	8 hr	—
Delanoside	—	1.2 to 1.6 mg	—	—	33 hr	Kidney	15 min	2 hr	45 min	4 hr	—
Ouabain	—	0.125 to 0.5 mg	—	—	21 hr	Kidney	5 min	30–60 min	—	—	—

responses, which include an increase in peripheral vascular resistance.

Digoxin and digitoxin are the most widely used cardiac glycosides in clinical medicine. Either drug may offer an advantage under certain clinical conditions. For example, digitoxin offers nearly complete oral absorption with predominantly hepatic metabolism and a half-life of 4 to 6 days. In patients with renal failure or changing renal function, digitoxin may provide more stable serum and tissue levels, permitting easier transfer from parenteral to oral therapy. However, if toxicity occurs, it may require many days to a few weeks for resolution. Digoxin, by contrast, is absorbed about 70 percent after oral administration and eliminated predominantly by glomerular filtration and, to a small extent, by renal tubular secretion. Thus, switching from parenteral to oral therapy requires dose adjustment. However, the half-life is much shorter than that of digitoxin, and if toxicity is experienced, the patient is placed at risk for a relatively shorter period of time. In choosing a glycoside preparation, the physician should consider the factors mentioned above but, perhaps more importantly, familiarity with either of these preparations.

When using the cardiac glycosides for either the inotropic or dromotropic effect (or both), the physician must be aware that the dose–response relationship for these actions is different. Experimentally, it has been demonstrated that the inotropic response increases linearly so that doubling of the dose will nearly double the inotropic response. However, the dromotropic responses appear to change less rapidly for a given dose and relatively more glycoside is required to produce a twofold prolongation of AV conduction time. It has been recognized by clinicians for many years that near toxic doses of digitalis may be required to slow the ventricular response to artial flutter. Since the effects of cardiac glycosides on conduction are largely indirect, and therefore reflect the net balance of adrenergic tone at the AV node, it is not surprising that the dose requirement may be different in clinical conditions with various degrees of sympathetic activity. For example, the postoperative patient with atrial fibrillation may require much more digitalis to slow the ventricular rate in the immediate postoperative period when sympathetic tone is high than later when sympathetic tone is reduced. The differences between the dose–response relationships for the inotropic and dromotropic effect must therefore be considered when using these drugs clinically. While the electrocardiogram may show an increase in the PR interval and ST and T wave changes as a result of digitalis administration, these effects cannot be used to gauge a therapeutic effect.

CLINICAL USE OF CARDIAC GLYCOSIDES

Most cardiovascular drugs, including the cardiac glycosides, obey what has been termed first order kinetics. This means that a constant percent of the total body stores (TBS) is excreted per unit time rather than a constant mass. Figure 30–1 demonstrates this principle for digoxin, which has a half-life of approximately 36 hours in patients with normal renal function. In 24 hours, 35 percent of TBS will be eliminated. Continued daily administration of the same dose results in an accumulation of digoxin until 35 percent of the TBS eliminated each day becomes equal to what is given each day (in Figure 30–1 this is 0.25 mg); at this point a steady-state is attained. For practical purposes, five half-lives provides a good approximation (97 percent) of the time required to reach steady-state; for digoxin this is 7.5 days (with normal renal function), and for digitoxin it is 16 to 24 days. From this discussion and use of Figure 30–1, it should be apparent that if twice the dose of digoxin were given, it would still require 5 half-lives (7.5 days) to reach steady-state but TBS would then become twice as much. The therapeutic TBS for digoxin ranges from 0.7 to 1.4 mg. In Figure 30–1, the steady-state TBS of 0.7 mg was achieved by administering 0.25 mg of the drug daily. Use of the lower end of this therapeutic range is often chosen to avoid toxicity in patients with changing renal function or altered electrolyte status. In the latter case, cardiac effects of the glycosides may be influenced by electrolyte changes

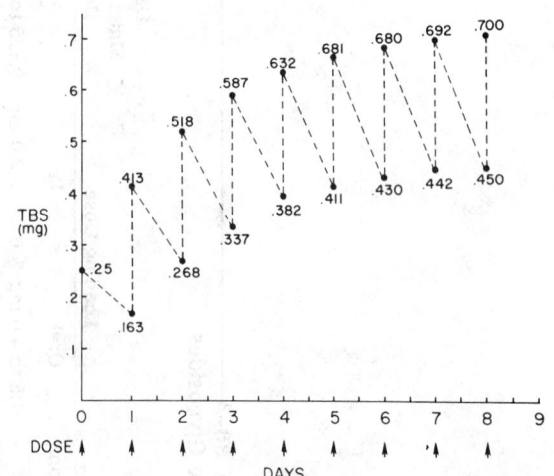

FIGURE 30–1. Example of digoxin accumulation during intravenous administration of single doses of 0.25 mg of digoxin daily in a patient with normal renal function. Steady-state is achieved by Day 8. Note the wide swings in total body stores (TBS) between doses.

(especially hypokalemia) which do not alter TBS (Table 30–4).

Clinical studies have shown that digoxin elimination is directly related to the creatinine clearance (C_{cr}) and this can be expressed as: percent TBS eliminated each day = 15 percent + $C_{cr}/5$. The 15 percent in this expression represents nonrenal digoxin elimination. In a patient with C_{cr} of 100 ml/min, 35 percent of TBS is eliminated each day, 15 percent by nonrenal mechanisms and 20 percent by the kidney. This formula can also be used to predict the TBS which will be present at steady-state for any given maintenance dose. For example, if the C_{cr} were reduced to 50 ml/min, 25 percent of TBS would be eliminated daily. A maintenance dose of 0.25 mg would result in TBS of 1.0 mg (0.25 mg/25 percent). In these examples, absorption was assumed to be 100 percent which is true if digoxin is given intravenously but only 70 percent is absorbed when the drug is administered orally. The appropriate oral dose can be determined by dividing by the bioavailability factor (0.7).

The desired therapeutic level of TBS can be achieved more rapidly by administering a loading dose. In the example shown in Figure 30–1, the loading dose would have been 0.7 mg (or 1.0 mg if given orally) followed by a maintenance dose of 0.25 mg (0.35 mg orally) per day. In actual practice the loading dose chosen is usually divided over short intervals of time to reduce the risk of unexpected toxicity. The decision as to whether a loading dose is required should be based on the clinical picture, the drug preparation used, and how rapidly the inotropic or dromotropic effect is desired. With *emergency* digitalization a loading dose may be given intravenously over a few hours. For *rapid* digitalization an oral loading dose would be used over 24 hours and the therapy continued with the selected maintenance dose. For elective digitalization only a maintenance dose would be employed. The latter approach is preferred because it reduced the risk of acute toxicity.

THE DIGITALIS RADIOIMMUNOASSAY

The use of glycoside-specific antibody has provided the required technical ease and sensitivity to permit rapid and reproducible assays for use in clinical practice. However, there is considerable overlap between the normal range and the toxic range as shown in Table 30–3. When digoxin levels exceed 2.0 ng/ml, approximately 87 percent of patients will have clinical manifestations of digitalis toxicity, but many patients may experience severe toxicity with serum levels less than 2.0 ng/ml. Table 30–4 presents factors which may alter the serum levels to produce toxicity or alter sensitivity without a change in serum levels. The latter explains part of the observed overlap between therapeutic and toxic serum levels. For digoxin, the most common reasons for toxicity are increased serum levels due to unappreciated changes in renal function and increased sensitivity (without a change in serum level) due to hypokalemia.

The timing of the blood sample for radioimmunoassay is important. Following oral administration, the glycoside requires several hours to distribute and reach an equilibrium between the tissue and the source of sampling (intravascular volume). At least 12 hours should be permitted after an oral dose to assure adequate glycoside distribution or falsely high values may be observed. If repeat serum determinations are to be made, then the sample should be obtained at the same time following the dose. Most patients take their glycoside in the morning and this becomes a convenient time for monitoring predose levels.

The digitalis radioimmunoassay may be useful under certain circumstances: 1) assessment of patient compliance; 2) uncertainty as to whether or not the patient is taking digitalis or the type of digitalis preparation being used; 3) evaluation of an unexpected response to cardiac glycosides or overdose; 4) evaluation of possible digitalis toxicity in conjunction with clinical assessment. The routine determination of the digitalis concentration without one of the above indications is unlikely to provide useful clinical information.

TABLE 30–4
Factors Altering Digitalis Effect

No Change in Serum Levels	Sensitivity
Hypokalemia	↑
Hypomagnesemia	↑
Hypercalcemia	↑
Hypothyroidism	↑
Hyperthyroidism	↓
Change in inotropic state	
e.g., propranolol or procainamide	↓

Change in Serum Level

Renal disease (digoxin), decreased elimination
Tablet bioavailibility
Gastrointestinal motility
 Increased transit time, ↑ absorption, e.g., probanthine
 Decreased transit time, ↓ absorption, e.g., malabsorption
Quinidine

DIURETICS

Diuretics are the principal therapeutic agents used in the management of edematous states whether due to cardiac or renal causes (Chaps. 11 and 19). These agents are also employed in the management of hypertension (Chap. 25). Diuretics achieve their effect by inhibiting sodium reabsorption at a particular place in the nephron, and they may be classified on the basis of the site of action (Table 30–5). This classification leads to more rational drug usage, and to an understanding of the etiology of electrolyte disorders occurring during diuretic therapy.[167,180]

CARBONIC ANHYDRASE INHIBITORS
(Acetazolamide)

These drugs inhibit carbonic anhydrase, an enzyme located in the brush border of proximal tubular cells and within cells of the distal tubule. Inhibition of carbonic anhydrase prevents reabsorption of filtered bicarbonate. Decreasing bicarbonate reabsorption has two effects: first, it produces a bicarbonate-rich, alkaline urine, and second, it depletes the body of bicarbonate, creating a metabolic acidosis.

In order to be effective, the drug must inhibit at least 99 percent of carbonic anhydrase activity, and thus urine volume does not markedly increase until a "threshold dose" is reached. The drug becomes progressively less effective with chronic administration because the concentration of bicarbonate in the serum is reduced, hence the quantity of filtered bicarbonate is decreased; the diuretic response is diminished because it depends upon the amount of filtered bicarbonate. These drugs also increase potassium losses by increasing delivery of sodium to the distal tubule and collecting duct, providing a stimulus for potassium secretion. Therefore, patients who are also receiving digitalis may be more likely to develop digitalis-induced arrhythmias. Two further complications of the drug are depression of glomerular filtration rate due to intrarenal vasoconstriction and increased respiratory rate due to production of metabolic acidosis. Although furosemide and thiazides have limited ability to inhibit carbonic anhydrase, this does not play a major role in their diuretic effect.

Because of the above complications, a drug such as acetazolamide is not used as primary therapy in the treatment of congestive heart failure. Theoretically, the drug could be used in conjunction with other drugs to increase total sodium excreted. Such usage is rarely justified because of the previously stated side effects.

ORGANIC MERCURIALS (Mercaptomerin)

Organic mercurial diuretic molecules are cleaved to liberate inorganic mercury, which binds sulfhydryl groups in the ascending limb of the loop of Henle. This binding inhibits active chloride (and hence passive sodium) reabsorption. Three factors limit the use of the drug: First, it is poorly absorbed in the gastrointestinal tract and must be given by injection; second, an acid urine is necessary for the mercurial ion

---

TABLE 30–5
Classification of Diuretics by Primary Site of Action

Primary Site of Action	Mechanism of Action	Drugs	Daily Dose	Associated Electrolyte Abnormalities
Proximal tubule	Inhibition of carbonic anhydrase; decreased reabsorption of sodium and bicarbonate	Acetazolamide	500 mg	Hyperchloremic acidosis
Ascending limb of Henle's loop	Inhibition of active chloride transport; decreased reabsorption of sodium and chloride	Furosemide Ethacrynic acid Mercaptomerin	40–80 mg 50–100 mg 1–2 ml	Hypokalemic, hypochloremic alkalosis
Distal tubule	Inhibition of active sodium transport; decreased reabsorption of sodium and chloride	Hydrochlorthiazide Metolazone Chlorthalidone	50–100 mg 5–10 mg 50–100 mg	Hypokalemic, hypochloremic alkalosis
Collecting duct	Inhibition of active transport of sodium; decreased passive secretion of potassium	Spironolactone Triamterene	100–150 mg 100–200 mg	Hyperkalemia

to be liberated, and since the drug causes metabolic alkalosis, its effectiveness is self-limited; and finally, mercury is nephrotoxic and therefore cannot be used either for long-term management or in patients with renal insufficiency.

Mercurial diuretics produce a brisk diuresis within one hour of injection. The loss of sodium chloride with little or no bicarbonate causes a contraction of body water around the same quantity of bicarbonate, creating a "contraction alkalosis." The resulting alkaline pH decreases the effectiveness of the drug. In spite of increased delivery of sodium to the distal nephron, exaggerated urinary losses of potassium are not seen because mercurials directly inhibit distal tubular potassium secretion.

The local irritation of intramuscular injection, the possibility of systemic reactions, and nephrotoxicity as well as the development of equally potent but less toxic drugs have limited the use of mercurial diuretics.

FUROSEMIDE AND ETHACRYNIC ACID

These two drugs, although structurally dissimilar, have similar pharmacologic properties. They produce a large diuresis by inhibiting active chloride and passive sodium transport in the ascending limb of Henle's loop, where 25 percent of filtered sodium chloride is reabsorbed. Both drugs are well absorbed from the gastrointestinal tract, and largely bound to plasma proteins, which prevents their filtration. Thus, they mainly reach their site of action following proximal tubular secretion into the proximal tubular lumen. When organic ions accumulate in body fluids, as in uremia, they compete with these drugs for tubular secretion, thus limiting the intratubular quantity of diuretic. Because this quantity determines diuretic effectiveness, larger doses are necessary for patients with renal insufficiency.

Furosemide and ethacrynic acid are rapid acting, with diuresis beginning within 30 to 60 minutes after oral administration, and reaching a maximum effect after 2 hours. The duration of diuretic effect is 4 to 6 hours. Both drugs have a "threshold effect," that is, diuresis does not begin until a sufficient quantity of drug has been given, and larger doses produce only a small increment in urine flow. For this reason, when the dose required for diuresis has been established, it will generally remain constant, and dividing the dose will cause the drug to appear ineffective, i.e., a patient responding to 120 mg of furosemide will have only a limited response to 40 mg given three times daily. In a rare patient, edema of the intestinal mucosal wall may falsely raise the apparent threshold dose by decreasing absorption of the drug. As extracellular vol-

ume is lowered and edema decreases, a marked increase in diuretic effectiveness may be seen.

As with mercurials, the urinary sodium and chloride loss seen with these drugs is far in excess of the bicarbonate loss, leading to a metabolic alkalosis because serum bicarbonate is proportionally increased. Enhanced delivery of sodium to the distal nephron increases the driving force for potassium secretion, and potassium depletion can also occur.

Both furosemide and ethacrynic acid result in urine with a ratio of water to sodium greater than that of extracellular fluid. Therefore, they may have an additional benefit for patients with hyponatremia. Water intake must also be restricted to take full advantage of this effect. In addition, these drugs have been shown to either maintain or increase renal blood flow (as long as marked extracellular volume depletion does not occur) and can be used safely in patients with renal insufficiency.

Furosemide and ethacrynic acid should be administered cautiously to patients with congestive heart failure because of their potent ability to deplete extracellular fluid volume. Rapid fluid shifts may interfere with the physiologic compensation of the failing heart and diminished perfusion of vital organs may result. In patients with pulmonary edema treated with furosemide, a fall in left ventricular filling pressure with improvement in pulmonary congestion occasionally occurs before diuresis. Presumably, furosemide causes venodilatation, decreasing cardiac preload to achieve this effect. Clearly, the combination of venodilatation and a major diuresis could greatly compromise cardiac output.

The side effects of these drugs include hyperuricemia, which is primarily due to competitive inhibition of proximal tubular uric acid secretion, and hyperglycemia, presumably due to potassium depletion. Impaired glucose tolerance occurs because potassium is required for insulin secretion. These side effects are rarely sufficiently severe to cause clinical problems. Both drugs can cause gastric distress, nausea, and vomiting, although ethacrynic acid is more frequently associated with such symptoms. In addition, both transient and permanent deafness have been observed following large doses of either drug, but again, this effect is more common with ethacrynic acid.

THIAZIDES

Thiazide diuretics increase urinary sodium and chloride excretion by inhibiting early distal tubular sodium reabsorption. Two structurally different drugs, metolazone and chlorthalidone, have very similar clincial effects. These latter drugs and the various thiazides differ little except in their duration of action and price.

Orally administered thiazides are well absorbed and reach their site of action primarily by proximal tubular secretion. Because these drugs increase sodium delivery to the potassium secretory site, there is an increase in urinary potassium as during treatment with furosemide or ethacrynic acid. Another common side effect of these diuretics is contraction alkalosis. Less frequent side effects, also with pathophysiologic mechanisms similar to those of furosemide and ethacrynic acid, are hyperuricemia and glucose intolerance.

Thiazides are ineffective in patients with glomerular filtration rates of less than 20 ml per minute. More importantly, they may worsen renal insufficiency by decreasing GFR, presumably by causing intrarenal vasoconstriction. Therefore, it is inadvisable to administer thiazides to patients with renal insufficiency. A possible exception is metolazone; however, clinical experience with metolazone is insufficient to recommend its use in chronic renal failure. In a few reports, both the thiazides and furosemide appear to have caused an allergic interstitial nephritis. Rarely, thiazides have been associated with the development of pancreatitis or thrombocytopenia.

SPIRONOLACTONE AND TRIAMTERENE

Spironolactone is a structural analogue of aldosterone and a specific anatagonist of its action at the renal tubule. Therefore, spironolactone inhibits aldosterone-mediated sodium reabsorption and potassium secretion, but is ineffective in the absence of aldosterone. The drug is well absorbed and has a duration of 2 to 3 days, which is clinically important because the effects of altering the dose or discontinuing the drug are not apparent for 2 to 3 days. Because sodium excretion is only minimally increased during spironolactone therapy, the main use of the drug is to diminish potassium losses occurring with thiazide, furosemide, or ethacrynic acid therapy. However, impairment of potassium excretion may cause dangerous hyperkalemia, especially when renal insufficiency is present.[171] Potassium salts are extremely dangerous when given with spironolactone, especially to patients with renal insufficiency. In addition to inhibiting potassium secretion, spironolactone may also impair renal tubular acid secretion, although this rarely presents a clinical problem. Another troublesome side effect is the development of gynecomastia, which occurs because the metabolic clearance of testosterone increases.

Triamterene acts on the same segment of the nephron as spironolactone, but does not require the presence of aldosterone. Like spironolactone, triamterene is only weakly natriuretic, and impairs secretion of both acid and potassium. Decreased potassium excretion induced by these drugs can be additive, so they should never be given concurrently. Triamterene may also induce nitrogen retention and therefore should not be used in patients with chronic renal failure.

COMPLICATIONS OF DIURETIC THERAPY

Diuretic-Induced Changes in Serum Electrolytes

Altered electrolyte concentrations are probably the most frequent complications of diuretic therapy.[187] They are usually accompanied by nonspecific symptoms such as weakness or lassitude, symptoms that are also common in patients with congestive heart failure. Evaluation of such symptoms should include measurement of serum electrolytes, in order to correctly diagnose diuretic-induced electrolyte abnormalities (Table 30–6). The pathophysiology of some of these abnormalities has been described in the discussion of individual diuretics. The following topics will emphasize the clinical setting of these problems.

Acute Sodium Depletion

Acute sodium depletion can be seen in patients with mild congestive heart failure after treatment with thiazides, furosemide, or ethacrynic acid. This complication may also be seen in patients hospitalized for ineffective diuretic response and treated with rigid dietary salt restriction for the first time. Extracellular volume depletion is recognized by a decrease in weight, orthostatic hypotension, dizziness, and tachycardia. Acute sodium depletion may also cause an increase in both hematocrit and serum urea nitrogen concentration. The syndrome can be readily treated by increasing dietary salt intake and discontinuing the diuretic.

Chronic Sodium Depletion

Chronic sodium depletion is unusual in patients with congestive heart failure. In contrast to patients with acute sodium depletion, these patients have few symptoms suggestive of hypovolemia. Serum sodium concentration is low in this condition for the same reason that symptomatic hypovolemia is unusual: the physiologic response to chronic sodium depletion is renal water retention mediated by increased release of antidiuretic hormone. The result of water retention is to minimize extracellular fluid volume loss, even though serum osmolality may become subnormal.

The symptoms of chronic sodium depletion are nonspecific, and because sodium depletion may im-

TABLE 30-7

Anticoagulants: Representative Agents

Class	Generic Name	Chemical	Trade Name	Routes of Administration	Usual Dose in Adults (units) Initial	Maintenance (mg/24 hr)	Usual Onset of Peak Activity	Dosage Monitored by Measurement of	Antidote
Heparin	Heparin sodium*	Sulfate containing mucopolysaccharide	Heparin sodium, Liquaemin sodium, Lipohepin, Panheprin	Intravenous continuous intermittent	400–700/kg/24 hr, 100–175/kg/q 4 hr		1–2 hr, <30 min	Whole blood clotting time	Protamine sulfate
Coumarin	Bishydroxycoumarin	3,3'-methylene-bis-(4-hydroxy-coumarin)	Dicumarol	Oral	200–400	25–100	1.5–3 days	One-stage prothrombin time	2-methyl-3-phytyl-1,4-napthoquinone (vitamin K_1) and/or Transfusion of blood, plasma, or plasma fractions containing the vitamin-K-dependent clotting factors
	Warfarin sodium	3-(α-phenyl-β-acetyl-ethyl)-4-hydroxy-coumarin, sodium	Coumadin, Panwarfin, Athrombin	Oral or intravenous	25–50	2.5–10	1–2 days		
Indanedione	Phenindione	2-phenyl-1,3 indanedione	Hedulin, Damlone, Indon	Oral	200–400	50–100	1–2 days		

*1.0 mg of crystalline standard heparin sodium is equivalent to 100 USP units or 130 International Units of heparin.

interrelationships.[172] Whenever heparin is employed, a flow sheet should be used to follow, on a daily basis, the patient's weight, date, hour of administration, agent (name, source, and type), dosage per 24 hours, whole blood clotting time or partial thromboplastin time (PTT), urine, and stool (for occult blood).

Administration

Aqueous heparin must be given parenterally. This agent is best administered via the intravenous route and may be given continuously or intermittently. Evenly sustained prolongation of the clotting time is most readily achieved by continuous intravenous infusion of heparin by a constant infusion pump and is the preferred manner of administration. The subcutaneous administration may cause erratic absorption, vessel puncture, bleeding, and discomfort, and is therefore a less desirable route of administration. The subcutaneous route can be used if careful monitoring of intravenous infusions is not available or if intravenous infusions interfere with ambulation. Because of the increased incidence of hemorrhage and erratic absorption, heparin should not be given intramuscularly.

INTRAVENOUS ROUTE—CONTINUOUS CONSTANT INFUSION. A loading dose of 5000 units, given slowly in 10 to 20 ml dilutent, over 10 to 15 minutes, should be administered intravenously and, immediately following this, the constant infusion (200 to 350 units heparin/kg in 250 to 500 ml of 5 percent dextrose to run 12 hours, or 400 to 700 units heparin/kg in 1000 ml of 5 percent dextrose to run 24 hours) should be started. A whole blood clotting time should be checked 6 hours later. Depending on the whole blood clotting time at 6 hours, the dose, concentration of heparin, and rate of infusion should be adjusted and the whole blood clotting time rechecked *6 hours later.* This should be done until a satisfactory whole blood clotting time is obtained, at which time the appropriate dose of heparin should be continued via constant infusion and the whole blood clotting time determined every 12 hours for the duration of therapy.

INTRAVENOUS ROUTE—INTERMITTENT INFUSION. The loading dose is given as in the case of continuous intravenous infusion. Following this, a dose of 100 to 175 units of heparin/kg body weight should be given in 10 to 20 ml of 5 percent dextrose intravenously during a 10-minute period every 4 hours. During the first 24 hours of therapy, immediately prior to each 4-hour dose, the whole blood clotting time should be determined and recorded, and the dose appropriately adjusted. Once the correct prolongation of the whole blood coagulation time is obtained, that dose of heparin should be given intravenously every 4 hours, with the whole blood clotting time checked before the second and fourth dose each day for the duration of therapy.

SUBCUTANEOUS ROUTE. When the subcutaneous route is used the approximate dosage schedule is 10,000 to 25,000 units every 6 to 12 hours. The clotting time should be measured 3 to 4 hours after the first dose and subsequent dosage adjusted to provide the desired prolongation. Therafter, the clotting time should be measured every 12 hours or just prior to administration of the heparin to determine a possible cumulative effect. Heparin has been combined with agents such as gelatin, Pitkin menstruum, peanut oil, and beeswax, in an attempt to delay absorption and produce a more sustained effect. These preparations are not recommended because of varying rates of absorption, high frequency of local reactions, other undesirable side effects, and the difficulty of reversing the anticoagulant effect with specific antidotes.

The use of low-dose (5000 units subcutaneously every 8 hours) heparin for prophylactic therapy is under investigation in several clinical areas.[168] Many studies employing low-dose heparin in prophylaxis of venous thrombosis have shown a reduction in the incidence of thrombosis. The low-dose heparin regimen has not been effective in major joint surgery, biliary tract surgery, and myocardial infarction. Because of a cumulative effect, some patients receiving low-dose heparin may become fully anticoagulated.

Toxicity

The most common untoward reaction to heparin is bleeding and, although the true incidence is difficult to quantify, it may be as high as 25 to 35 percent, when all types of bleeding are considered. The problems of maintaining a constant rate of infusion during the administration of heparin are self-evident. Reactions to heparin, other than hemorrhage, are rare and the major ones are listed in Table 30–8. Hypersensitivity and anaphylactoid reactions have ranged from mild fever, urticaria, rhinitis, and conjunctivitis, to sudden, severe hypertension, respiratory distress, and chest pain. Thrombocytopenia and transient alopecia may occur. Osteoporosis has been reported in some patients who received heparin for prolonged periods (more than one year).

Antidotes

There are several antidotes which reverse the anticoagulant effect of heparin. These include protamine sulfate, hexadimethine bromide (polybrene), clupein, polylysine, lysozyme, toluidine blue, fuchsin, and tryptophan.

The antidote which is recommended and most

TABLE 30-8
Heparin—Untoward Reactions

Hemorrhage
Allergic reactions:
    Urticaria, fever
    Asthma
    Rhinitis, conjunctivitis
Thrombocytopenia
Alopecia
Osteoporosis
Arterial thrombosis
Respiratory distress
Hypotension
Chest pain
Dysesthesia pedis
Hyponatremia
Resistance

commonly employed is protamine sulfate. The dose of protamine sulfate to be administered depends on the amount of heparin present. The amount of heparin present is dependent on the amount, the time, and route of the last dose of heparin given. The recommended dose is 1.0 mg for every 100 units (USP) heparin present in the body. It should be administered slowly, intravenously, and at a rate not greater than 5 mg per minute. No single injection of protamine sulfate should exceed 50 mg. The antiheparin effect lasts for approximately 2 hours. A clotting time should be checked approximately 15 minutes after the administration of protamine sulfate before an additional dose should be given. Some heparin effect may reappear after a single dose of protamine sulfate, especially if a large dose of heparin had been administered subcutaneously shortly before the injection of protamine.

Transfusions of blood, plasma, or other blood products are not antidotes against heparin, although they are of value in replacement therapy following hemorrhage.

COUMARIN-INDANEDIONE ANTICOAGULANTS

A large variety of coumarin-indanedione derivatives are commonly employed as anticoagulants.[169,181,186] These agents do not inhibit the rate of clotting when added to blood in vitro. When administered in vivo, they impair coagulation by altering the biologic function (clotting activity) of the end product of the vitamin K-mediated hepatic synthesis of Factors II, VII, IX, and X. Normal levels (measured by immunologic techniques) of these factors are present during the administration of the coumarin-indanedione agents. Although the synthesis of Factors II, VII, IX, and X is

not depressed by these vitamin K antagonists, their functional properties are altered. The defect has been identified and is due to the absence of the second carboxyl group on the Y carbon of glutamic acid.[173]

The coumarin-indanedione anticoagulants have certain pharmacologic actions other than those related to coagulation. These include enhancement of uric acid excretion in the urine and a rise in serum transaminase and lactic dehydrogenase activity. Some patients who receive coumarin derivatives may excrete orange or reddish-colored urine, due to a metabolic breakdown product that gives this color in alkaline medium. This is not of clinical significance.

Control of Dosage

The one-stage prothrombin time test, devised by Quick, or one of its modifications is the most widely used test to monitor the effect of the coumarin anticoagulants. Following the administration of these agents, the coagulant activity of the vitamin K-dependent factors decreases in the following sequence: VII, IX, X, and II. The order in which these disappear corresponds to the intravascular biologic half-life of these factors. The one-stage prothrombin time is influenced by changes in three of these factors (Factors II, VII, and X), but there is close parallelism in the levels of Factors VII and IX during therapy with the coumarin derivatives.[174] Thus, the one-stage prothrombin time is considered to be a reliable method for use in monitoring the effect and guiding the dosage of the coumarin anticoagulants.[169,174,181,186]

Since heparin can significantly affect the one-stage prothrombin time, the control prothrombin time should be obtained prior to the institution of heparin. It is desirable to adjust the coumarin anticoagulants to maintain the prothrombin time at a level of 15 to 25 percent of normal. This corresponds to a prolongation of the prothrombin time (in seconds) between 2 and 2.5 times the normal control.

Administration

The coumarin-indanedione derivatives are attractive because they can be administered orally. Some of these agents, e.g., warfarin (Coumadin), can also be administered intravenously. The coumarin derivatives are preferred to the chemically similar indanedione derivatives since, in clinical practice, they produce fewer adverse side effects.[169,181] The approximate dosage schedules for bishydroxycoumarin, warfarin, and one of the indanedione derivatives are shown in Table 30-7.

There are two methods commonly utilized in the initiation of therapy with the oral anticoagulants. The older technique employs a "loading dose" of one of the coumarin derivatives (e.g., warfarin, 25 to 35 mg), after obtaining a control prothrombin time. Approximately 36 hours later, the prothrombin time is determined and a daily maintenance, usually 5 to 10 mg, is selected. The final single daily dose of anticoagulant is determined on the basis of daily measurement of the prothrombin time. The direction of change, as well as the absolute value of the prothrombin time, must be known in deciding the daily dosage.

The alternative technique is based on the observation that a "loading dose" produces a rapid fall in Factor VII activity before other factor activities are depressed. Some investigators point out that even though there is prolongation of the prothrombin time, antithrombotic protection is not present until Factor X activity is also reduced. Therefore, the recommendation has been made that smaller daily doses (warfarin, 10 to 15 mg) be given when therapy is initiated. The final daily dose is determined by observing the effect on the prothrombin time. Several days are often required to reach the desired therapeutic prolongation of the prothrombin time when the second method is employed. Regardless of which induction method of coumarin administration is selected, a reasonably stable maintenance dose can be achieved within 7 to 15 days. Once this has been achieved for several consecutive days, the prothrombin time can be checked at progressively longer intervals, from daily to twice weekly, then weekly while hospitalized. After discharge from the hospital, provided the patient's condition is stable and that a stable maintenance dose has been established, the prothrombin time determinations could be done at 2- to 3-week intervals. Clinical experience suggests that no longer than 3 weeks should pass without a prothrombin time check for the duration of therapy. If at any time during therapy with these agents the dose required increases to >10 to 15 mg daily (warfarin), consultation with a coagulation specialist should be obtained.

Frequently, the oral anticoagulants are instituted near the end of a course of heparin therapy. Occasionally, therapy with the two agents may be initiated simultaneously. Because heparin can severely alter the prothrombin time, it is difficult to know when the coumarin-indanedione agents become effective. In most patients receiving continuous intravenous heparin, the prothrombin time can be reliably used as a measure of coumarin effect. In patients in whom heparin alters the prothrombin time it is possible to determine coumarin effect by using intermittent intravenous heparin therapy and determining the prothrombin time just prior to the administration of the next dose of heparin. In this way, the prothrombin time will be determined without significant influence by the presence of heparin.

A "rebound phenomenon" has been reported to occasionally follow the cessation of oral anticoagulant therapy. The precise nature of the rebound has not been defined. Some physicians feel that further thromboembolic episodes are more likely to occur at this time and recommend a gradual reduction in dosage over several days, rather than abrupt discontinuation. However, the biologic half-life of these agents varies from 40 to 75 hours and, with such a gradual disappearance from the body, additional efforts to taper the dose are unnecessary.

Factors Influencing Dosage[176,178]

A genetically determined hereditary (autosomal dominant) resistance to the anticoagulant effects of the coumarin-indanedione derivatives has been reported. To date, no heritable conditions associated with an increased sensitivity to these agents has been reported. Increased sensitivity to coumarin-indanedione derivatives may be produced by preexisting congenital or acquired hypoprothrombinemia, by disorders that interfere with the availability, absorption, or utilization of vitamin K, such as malnutrition, gastrointestinal disorders with decreased absorption of vitamin K (e.g., sprue, cystic fibrosis), oral antibiotics that alter intestinal bacterial flora, biliary obstruction, and liver disease. Hypermetabolic states, excessive intake of alcohol, and congestive heart failure may increase susceptibility of these anticoagulants. Females are more sensitive than males and dose requirements decrease with advancing age. Concomitant administration of many other drugs may either potentiate or decrease the response to the anticoagulant effects of these agents. A partial list is presented in Table 30–9. The prothrombin time of patients receiving the oral anticoagulants and any of these drugs must be monitored frequently, with great caution. The simultaneous administration of other drugs may necessitate frequent alteration in the dose of the anticoagulant, either to maintain therapeutic effectiveness or prevent potential disasters.

Toxicity of the Oral Anticoagulants

The most common untoward reaction to the coumarin-indanedione anticoagulants is hemorrhage;[186] other reactions, listed in Table 30–10 are rare.[175]

Antidotes

The anticoagulant effects of the coumarin-indanedione anticoagulants can be reversed by administration of vitamin K_1, which is a naturally occurring, oil-soluble, 3-phytyl derivative of 2-methyl-1, 4-

┌───┐
TABLE 30-9
Some Drugs That Affect the Response to
Coumarin–Indanedione Anticoagulants

I.   Anticoagulant Effects May Be Potentiated by:

Pyrazol compounds
    Phenylbutazone (Butazolidin)
    Oxyphenbutazone (Tandearil)
Antihyperlipidemic agents
    Clofibrate (Atromid-s)
    Dextrothyroxine (Choloxin)
Anabolic steroids
    Methandrostenolene (Dianabol)
    Norethandrolene (Nilevar)
    Oxymetholone (Adroyd)
    Nandrolone (Deca-Durabolin)
Muscle relaxants
    Phenyramidol (Analexin)
Salicylates—in large doses
Quinine, Quinidine
Sulfonamides and antibiotics
Disulfiram (Antabuse), mineral oil, glucagon

II.   Anticoagulant Effects May Be Decreased by:

Sedatives and hypnotics
    Barbiturates
    Glutethimide (Doriden)
    Ethchlorvynol (Placidyl)
Griseofulvin (Fulvicin, Grifulvin, Grisactin)
Rifampin (Rimactane)
Mercurial diuretics and some thiazides
Multivitamins containing vitamin K
Tranquilizers ??
    Meprobamate (Miltown, Equanil)
    Haloperidol (Haldol)

III.   Anticoagulant Effects Are Not Altered by:

    Diazepam (Valium)
    Chlordiazepoxide (Librium)
    Chlorothiazide (Diuril) in standard doses
    Flurazepam (Dalmane)
└───┘

┌───┐
TABLE 30-10
Coumarin–Indanedione Anticoagulants:
Untoward Reactions

Hemorrhage
Skin lesions—rashes, necrosis,
    petechiae, purpura, exfoliation
Syndrome of purple toes
Nausea, vomiting, diarrhea
Leukopenia
Thrombocytopenia
Agranulocytosis
Eosinophilia
Pyrexia
Hepatic damage, hepatitis, jaundice
Stomatitis, sore throat
Nephropathy
Alopecia
Resistance
└───┘

napthoquinone (vitamin K). Certain synthetic water-soluble vitamin K preparations, such as menadione and Hykinone, which are not 3-phytyl derivatives, are much less effective and should not be relied on as antagonists. The oil-soluble preparation of vitamin K_1 (Mephyton) should be administered intravenously at a rate not faster than 5 mg per minute. The water-soluble analogue of vitamin K_1 (Aqua Mephyton) is an effective antagonist and can be administered intravenously or orally, depending on the rapidity of effect that is desired. The subcutaneous and intramuscular routes can also be used, but are less desirable because of variable absorption and local hematomas.

The dose of vitamin K_1 depends on the amount and time of the last dose of anticoagulant and the urgency of the situation. In patients with life-threatening hemorrhage, where the dose of anticoagulant was not excessively large, 50 to 100 mg of vitamin K_1, given intravenously, usually will produce a therapeutic effect within 4 hours and, within 12 to 24 hours, the prothrombin time will have returned to control values. Such large doses of vitamin K_1 may make the patient resistant to subsequent doses of anticoagulants for several days. Smaller doses (5 to 10 mg) of vitamin K_1 are given if the indications for its use are less urgent. The rise in serum transaminase and lactic dehydrogenase activity and the antithyroid activity produced by these agents are not reversed by any vitamin K preparation.

The clotting factors that are functionally altered by these anticoagulants are stable on storage and are present in acid-citrate-dextrose or citrate-phosphate-dextrose bank blood and fresh frozen plasma. Transfusions of blood or plasma can act as antagonists to the coumarin-indanedione anticoagulants. A plasma fraction concentrate containing Factors II, VII, IX, and X (Konyne, Proplex) is an effective antagonist. However, because of the significant recognized risk of hepatitis transmitted by these concentrates, their use is not recommended unless a life-threatening emergency is present.

HEMORRHAGE

Hemorrhage is the most commonly encountered complication of treatment with any of the anticoagulants. The incidence of serious hemorrhage is low and it is proportional to the intensity of the regimen employed. Fatalities have been reported, and moderate hemorrhage (that does not require transfusion), such as hematuria, ecchymosis, hematomas, epistaxis, and melena, occurs in 10 to 35 percent of patients. Bleeding may involve any organ system, but certain types of hemorrhage deserve special mention. Hemopericardium occurs in some patients with myocardial infarction, and anticoagulant therapy may increase this tendency. Bleeding from the gastrointestinal tract may develop, and the term "anticoagulant ileus" has been used to describe obstructions of the small or large bowel due to hemorrhages into the abdominal wall, peritoneal cavity, mesentery, or wall of the bowel. Bleeding from the gastrointestinal, genitourinary, or respiratory tracts during anticoagulant therapy may indicate the presence of previously unrecognized lesions. Physicians should be especially alert to the possible development of subdural hematoma following head injury in patients receiving anticoagulants. Adrenal cortical insufficiency, due to bilateral adrenal hemorrhage, has been described. The occurrence of bleeding at the sites of intramuscular or subcutaneous injections of heparin has been mentioned. Patients receiving heparin should have daily physical examinations to detect abnormal bleeding and tests of urine and stool for occult blood. Unusual care is required in performance of venapunctures and prolonged pressure should be applied to venapuncture sites. Invasive procedures should be avoided and, particularly in areas in which bleeding may be especially dangerous, are contraindicated. The introduction of needles or catheters into neck and subclavian veins must be avoided. Arterial punctures, lumbar punctures, thoracentesis, paracentesis, subcutaneous, and intramuscular injections should not be performed on patients receiving anticoagulants. In general, the use of needles, cutting instruments of all varieties, and performance of invasive procedures should be avoided during therapy with anticoagulants. An exception is the use of invasive procedures required for the management of the patient on anticoagulation, such as catheterization in pulmonary embolism, acute myocardial infarction (Swan-Ganz catheter), and unstable angina.

CONTRAINDICATIONS

Anticoagulants are contraindicated in patients with an active hemorrhagic diathesis and those who are allergic to these agents. Although heparin has been reported to be of possible benefit in patients with disseminated intravascular coagulopathy, a control study has not been performed, and the role of heparin in these clinical situations remains uncertain. Relative contraindications include intestinal ulceration, surgery of the central nervous system or eye, severe hypertension (diastolic over 130 mm Hg), a past history of cerebral hemorrhage, inadequate cooperation of the patient or the absence of laboratory facilities. Anticoagulants must be used with utmost caution in pericarditis, diabetes mellitus, bacterial endocarditis, liver disease, steatorrhea, and malnutrition. Because they cross the placenta, the use of the coumarin-indanedione agents during pregnancy, and particularly at time of delivery, is felt by some to be contraindicated. These oral agents are secreted in breast milk and should not be given to nursing mothers.

THROMBOLYTIC AGENTS

Recently, two thrombolytic agents, streptokinase (SK) and urokinase (UK), have become available for the treatment of thromboembolic disease.[184] Indications for their use include massive and submassive emboli that have induced cardiopulmonary compromise, and deep vein thrombosis, particularly when it extends into the thigh veins and inferior vena cava. Both agents must be given by continuous intravenous infusion. Their mechanism of action is to convert the inert proenzyme, plasminogen, to the potent proteolytic enzyme, plasmin. The latter exerts its therapeutic effect by attacking arginyl–lysyl bonds digesting fibrin clots. The biologic half-life of these agents in the blood is short, being minutes in duration. The usual dose of SK is 250,000 IU initially, given over 20 minutes, and 100,000 IU/hour for 24 to 72 hours. UK is given in a dose of 4000 IU/kg initially over 20 minutes, followed by 4000 IU/kg/hour for 12 or 24 hours. Both agents can be administered in solutions of dextrose (5 percent), saline, or various combinations of these two excipients. The thrombin time is used to monitor therapy to ensure adequate, but not excessive, therapeutic activity of the fibrinolytic system. This test should be made initially at 4 hours to identify that activation of the fibrinolytic system has been achieved, and then following at 12 hourly intervals for the duration of therapy. For therapeutic efficacy during infusion of the thrombolytic agents, the thrombin time should be two to five times prolonged over the preinfusion value. At the termination of thrombolytic therapy, the patient should be switched over to heparin and later to coumadin. In this situation, heparin should be instituted when the thrombin time has returned to less than twice the preinfusion value, usually about a 4-hour interval. During infusion with these thrombolytic agents, absolutely no invasive procedures of any type (save careful venapuncture) should be performed. Drugs which alter the coagulation system or interfere with platelet function are contraindicated. In the recommended therapeutic doses, both SK and UK are excreted in the form of inactive metabolites in the urine.

ANTIPLATELET AGENTS

Recent studies[170,185,188] have indicated possible efficacy of agents that inhibit platelet aggregation and release in the prophylactic treatment of thrombotic disease. The three agents that have been studied in large numbers of patients are aspirin (1.2 g), dipyridamole (200 to 400 mg), and sulfinpyrazone (600 to 800 mg). All of these agents are given orally, in divided doses over 24 hours. The clinical indications for the use of these agents are different for each drug. At present, the evidence suggests that aspirin may be helpful in prophylaxis against transient cerebral ischemic attacks; the other antiplatelet agents are not useful. Although some preliminary studies suggest that antiplatelet agents may be useful in ischemic heart disease and myocardial infarction, their long-term value in reducing incidence or mortality rate remains unproved. Sulfinpyrazone may be useful in reducing the incidence of thrombotic occlusions in arteriovenous communications. Prevention of thromboembolism in patients with prosthetic devices, particularly heart valves, may be possible by combining one or more of the three antiplatelet agents with an oral anticoagulant. However, the problems with drug interaction require thoughtful consideration and careful monitoring. The value of the antiplatelet agents in the prevention of venous thrombosis is controversial. Both positive and negative results with aspirin have been reported.

The beneficial effect of aspirin, in both transient ischemic attacks and reduction in venous thrombosis following hip surgery, was demonstrated in males but not in females.

Although some studies have demonstrated a favorable effect of the antiplatelet agents in some diseases, it is clear that additional studies are needed.

REFERENCES

General References

1. Edwards, J.E. An Atlas of Acquired Diseases of the Heart and Great Vessels, Vols. 1, 2, and 3. Philadelphia, Saunders, 1961.
2. Fowler, N.O. (ed.). Cardiac Diagnosis and Treatment, 2nd ed. Hagerstown, Md., Harper & Row, 1976.
3. Hurst, J.W. (ed.). The Heart, 4th ed. New York, McGraw-Hill, 1978.
4. Julian, D.G. Cardiology, 2nd ed. London, Baillière-Tindall, 1973.
5. Willerson, J.R. and Saunders, C.A. (eds.). Clinical Cardiology. New York, Grune & Stratton, 1977.
6. Willius, F.A. and Keys, T.E. Cardiac Classics. St. Louis, Mosby, 1941.
7. Sokolow, M. and McIlroy, M.B. Clinical Cardiology. Los Altos, Calif., Lange Medical Publications, 1977.

Clinical Evaluation of the Cardiovascular System

8. Fowler, N.O. Examination of the Heart. Part II. Inspection and palpation of venous and arterial pulses. Dallas, American Heart Assoc., 1972.
9. Hurst, J.W. and Schlant, R.C. Examination of the Heart. Part Three. Precordial Pulsations. Dallas, American Heart Assoc., 1972.
10. Leonard, J.J., Kroetz, F.W., Leon, D.F., and Shaver, J.A. Examination of the Heart. Part Four. Auscultation. Dallas, American Heart Assoc., 1974.
11. Silverman, M.E. Examination of the Heart. Part I: The clinical history. Dallas, American Heart Assoc., 1975.

Laboratory Evaluation of the Cardiovascular System

12. Botvinick, E.H., Taradash, M.R., Shames, D.M., and Parmley, W.W. Thallium-201 myocardial perfusion scintigraphy for the clinical clarification of normal, abnormal, and equivocal electrocardiographic stress tests. Am. J. Cardiol, 41:43, 1978.
13. Burow, R.D., Strauss, H.W., Singleton, R., Pond, M., Rehn, T., Bailey, I.K., Griffith, L.S.C., Nickoloff, E., and Pitt, B. Analysis of left ventricular function from multiple gated acquisition cardiac blood pool imaging. Circulation, 56:1024, 1977.
14. Conti, C.R. Coronary arteriography. Circulation, 55:227, 1977.
15. Criley, J.M. and Ross, R.S. Cardiovascular Physiology. Oldsmar, Fla., Tampa Tracings, 1971.
16. Fortuin, N.J. and Weiss, J.L. Exercise stress testing. Circulation, 56:699, 1977.
17. Goldschlager, N., Selzer, A., and Cohn, K. Treadmill stress tests as indicators of presence and severity of coronary artery disease. Ann. Intern. Med., 85:277, 1976.
18. Greene, H.L. Clinical applications of His bundle electrocardiography. JAMA, 240:258, 1978.
19. Lipski, J., Cohen, L., Espinoza, J., Motro, M., Dack, S., and Donoso, E. Value of Holter monitoring in assessing cardiac arrhythmias in symptomatic patients. Am. J. Cardiol., 37:102, 1976.
20. McNeer, J.F., Margolis, J.R., Lee, K.L., Kisslo, J.A., Peter, R.H., Kong, Y., Behar, V.S., Wallace, A.G., McCants, C.B., and Rosati, R.A. The role of the exercise test in the evaluation of patients for ischemic heart disease. Circulation, 57:64, 1978.
21. Pitt, B. and Strauss, H.W. Evaluation of ventricular function by radioisotopic techniques. N. Engl. J. Med., 296:1097, 1977.
22. Popp, R.L. Echocardiographic assessment of cardiac disease. Circulation, 54:538, 1976.
23. Shah, P.M. Echocardiography of the aortic and pulmonary valves. Prog. Cardiovasc. Dis., 20:451, 1978.
24. Zaret, B.L. and Cohen, L.S. Cardiovascular nuclear medicine: (1) Evaluation of cardiac performance, (2)

Evaluation of perfusion and viability. Mod. Concepts Cardiovasc. Dis., 46:33, 1977.

Congestive Heart Failure: Pathophysiology

25. Braunwald, E. The control of ventricular function in man. Br. Heart J., 27:1, 1965.
26. ———, Ross, J., and Sonnenblick, E.H. Mechanisms of Contraction of the Normal and Failing Heart, 2nd ed. Boston, Little, Brown, 1976.
27. Covell, J.W. and Ross, J., Jr. Nature and significance of alterations in myocardial compliance. Am. J. Cardiol., 32:449, 1973.
28. Donald, K.W., Bishop, J.M., Cumming, G., and Wade, O.L. The effect of exercise on the cardiac output and circulatory dynamics of normal subjects. Clin. Sci. Mol. Med., 14:37, 1955.
29. Eichna, L.W. Circulatory congestion and heart failure. Circulation, 22:864, 1960.
30. Friedberg, C.K. Edema and pulmonary edema: pathologic physiology and differential diagnosis. Prog. Cardiovasc. Dis., 13:546, 1971.
31. Gunning, J.F., Cooper, G. IV, Harrison, C.E., and Coleman, H.N. III. Myocardial oxygen consumption in experimental hypertrophy and congestive failure due to pressure overload. Am. J. Cardiol., 32:427, 1973.
32. Laks, M.M., Morady, F., Garner, D., and Swan, H.J.C. Temporal changes in canine right ventricular volume, mass, cell size, and sarcomere length after banding the pulmonary artery. Cardiovasc. Res., 8:106, 1974.
33. Langer, G.A. Ion Movements and the Control of Contraction. In Langer, G.A. and Brady, A.J. (eds.), Mammalian Myocardium. New York, Wiley, 1974.
34. Laragh, J.H. Diuretics in the management of congestive heart failure. Hosp. Pract., 5:43, 1970.
35. ———, Cannon, P.J., Stason, W.B., and Heinemann, H.O. Physiologic and clinical observations of furosemide and ethacrynic acid. Ann. N.Y. Acad. Sci., 139:453, 1966.
36. Mason, D.T. Regulation of cardiac performance in clinical heart disease. Am. J. Cardiol., 32:437, 1973.
37. Rutenberg, H.L. and Spann, J.F. Alterations of cardiac sympathetic neurotransmitter activity in congestive heart failure. Am. J. Cardiol., 32:472, 1973.
38. Sonnenblick, E.H. Myocardial ultrastructure in the normal and failing heart. Hosp. Pract., 5:35, 1970.

Congestive Heart Failure and/or Enlarged Cardiac Silhouette: Approach to the Patient and Management

39. Braunwald, E. Vasodilator therapy: a physiologic approach to the treatment of heart failure. N. Engl. J. Med., 297:331, 1977.
40. Criley, J.M. "The bottom line syndrome." Hypertrophic cardiomyopathy revisited. West. J. Med., 130:350, 1979.
41. Editorial. Vasodilators in heart failure. Lancet, 1:972, 1978.
42. Fowler, N.O. Physiology of cardiac tamponade and pulsus paradoxus. Mod. Concepts Cardiovasc. Dis., 47:109, 1978.
43. ———. Diseases of the pericardium. Curr. Probl. Cardiol., 2:3, 1978.

44. Friedberg, C.K. (ed.). Symposium. Cardiomyopathy. Circulation, 44:935, 1971.
45. Goldman, L., Caldera, D.L., Southwick, F.S., et al. Cardiac risk factors and complications in non-cardiac surgery. Medicine, 57:345, 1978.
46. Goodwin, J.F. and Oakley, C.M. The cardiomyopathies. Br. Heart J., 34:545, 1972.
47. Hancock, E.W. Management of pericardial disease. Mod. Concepts Cardiovasc. Dis., 48:1, 1979.
48. Hardarson, T., de la Calzada, C.S., Curiel, R., and Goodwin, J.F. Prognosis and mortality of hypertrophic obstructive cardiomyopathy. Lancet, 2:1462, 1973.
49. Shabetai, R. Symposium. Pericardial disease. Am. J. Cardiol., 26:445, 1970.
50. Shah, P. IHSS-HOCM-MSS-ASH? Circulation, 51:577, 1975.

Cardiac Murmurs and Other Manifestations of Valvular Heart Disease

51. Criley, J.M., Lewis, K.B., Humphries, J.O., and Ross, R.S. Prolapse of the mitral valve: clinical and cineangiocardiographic findings. Br. Heart J., 28:488, 1966.
52. Devereaux, R.B., Perloff, J.K., Reichek, N., and Josephson, M.E. Mitral valve prolapse. Circulation, 54:3, 1976.
53. Fortuin, N.J. and Craige, E. On the mechanism of the Austin Flint murmur. Circulation, 45:558, 1972.
54. Leatham, A. Auscultation of the Heart and Phonocardiography. Edinburgh, London, New York, Churchill Livingstone, 1975.
55. Morganroth, J., Perloff, J.K., Zeldis, S.M., and Dunkman, W.B. Acute severe aortic regurgitation. Ann. Intern. Med., 87:223, 1977.
56. Murphy, E.S. and Kloster, F.E. Late results of valve replacement surgery. Mod. Concepts Cardiovasc. Dis., 48:30, 1979.
57. Roberts, W.C. Anatomically isolated aortic valve disease: a case against its being of rheumatic etiology. Am. J. Med., 49:151, 1970.
58. ——— and Perloff, J.K. Mitral valvular disease. A clinicopathologic survey of the conditions causing the mitral valve to function abnormally. Ann. Intern. Med., 77:939, 1972.
59. Ross, J., Jr. and Braunwald, E. Aortic stenosis. Circulation, 37 (Suppl. V):61, 1968.
60. Spagnuolo, M., Kloth, H., Taranta, A., Doyle, E., and Pasternack, B. Natural history of rheumatic aortic regurgitation. Criteria predictive of death, congestive heart failure, and angina in young patients. Circulation, 44:368, 1971.
61. Tavel, M. Clinical Phonocardiography and External Pulse Recordings, 3rd ed. Chicago, Year Book Medical Publishers, 1978.

Cardiac Arrhythmias

62. Cosby, R.S. and Bilitch, M. Heart Block. New York, McGraw-Hill, 1972.
63. Cranefield, P.F. The Conduction of the Cardiac Impulse: The Slow Response and Cardiac Arrhythmias. Mt. Kisco, N.Y., Futura Publishing, 1975.
64. Fisch, C. and Knoebel, S.B. Recognition and therapy of digitalis toxicity. Prog. Cardiovasc. Dis., 12:71, 1970.

65. Friedberg, C.K. Syncope: pathological physiology: differential diagnosis and treatment. Mod. Concepts Cardiovasc. Dis., 40:55, 61, 1971.

66. Gallagher, J.J., Gilbert, M., Svenson, R.H., Sealy, W.C., Kasell, J., and Wallace, A.G. Wolff-Parkinson-White syndrome. The problem, evaluation, and surgical correction. Circulation, 51:767, 1975.

67. Goldreyer, B.N. and Damato, A.N. The essential role of atrioventricular conduction delay in the initiation of paroxysmal supraventricular tachycardia. Circulation, 43:679, 1971.

68. Hoffman, B.F. and Cranefield, P.F. Electrophysiology of the Heart. New York, McGraw-Hill, 1962.

69. Jensen, J.B., Humphries, J.O., Kouwenhoven, W.B., and Jude, J.R. Electroshock for atrial flutter and atrial fibrillation: follow-up studies on 50 patients. JAMA, 194:1181, 1965.

70. Lipson, M.J. and Naimi, S. Multifocal atrial tachycardia (chaotic atrial tachycardia): clinical associations and significance. Circulation, 42:397, 1970.

71. Marriott, H.J.L. and Menendez, M.M. AV dissociation revisited. Prog. Cardiovasc. Dis., 8:522, 1966.

72. Mason, J.W. and Winkle, R.A. Electrode-catheter arrhythmia induction in the selection and assessment of antiarrhythmic drug therapy for recurrent ventricular tachycardia. Circulation, 58:971, 1978.

73. McAnulty, J.H., Rahimtoola, S.H., Murphy, E.S., Kauffman, S., Ritzmann, L.W., Kanarek, P., and DeMots, H. A prospective study of sudden death in "high-risk" bundle-branch block. N. Engl. J. Med., 299:209, 1978.

74. Moss, A.J. and Davis, R.J. Brady-tachy syndrome. Prog. Cardiovasc. Dis., 16:439, 1974.

75. Narula, O.S. (ed.). His Bundle Electrocardiography and Clinical Electrophysiology. Philadelphia, F.A. Davis, 1975.

76. ———, Scherlag, B.J., Samet, P., and Javier, R.P. Atrioventricular block. Localization and classification by His bundle recordings. Am. J. Med., 50:146, 1971.

77. Norris, R.M. and Mercer, C.J. Significance of idioventricular rhythms in acute myocardial infarction. Prog. Cardiovasc. Dis., 16:455, 1974.

78. Resnekov, L. Drug therapy before and after the electroversion of cardiac dysrhythmias. Prog. Cardiovasc. Dis., 16:531, 1974.

79. Rosen, K.M. Junctional tachycardia. Circulation, 47:654, 1973.

80. Rosenbaum, M.D. The hemiblocks: diagnostic criteria and clinical significance. Mod. Concepts Cardiovasc. Dis., 39:141, 1970.

81. Scheinman, M., Weiss, A., and Kunkel, F. His bundle recordings in patients with bundle branch block and transient neurologic symptoms. Circulation, 48:322, 1973.

82. Wit, A.L., Rosen, M.R., and Hoffman, B.F. Electrophysiology and pharmacology of cardiac arrhythmias. II. Relationships of normal and abnormal electrical activity of cardiac fibers to the genesis of arrhythmias. A. Automaticity. Am. Heart J., 88:515, 1974.

Thoracic Pain and Angina Pectoris

83. Campeau, L., Hermann, J., Lesperance, J., Grondin, C.M., and Bourassa, M.G. Loss of improvement of angina between 1 and 6 years after aortocoronary bypass surgery: correlations with changes in vein grafts and in coronary arteries. Circulation, 57 (Suppl. II):52, 1978.

84. Griffith, L.S.C., Achuff, S.C., Conti, C.R., Humphries, J.O., Brawley, R.K., Gott, V.L., and Ross, R.S. Changes in intrinsic coronary circulation and segmental ventricular motion after saphenous-vein coronary bypass graft surgery. N. Engl. J. Med., 288:589, 1973.

85. Hillis, L. D. and Braunwald, E. Coronary artery spasm. N. Engl. J. Med., 299:695, 1978.

86. ——— and Braunwald, E. Myocardial ischemia. N. Engl. J. Med., 296:971, 1034, 1093, 1977.

87. Julian, D.G. (ed.). Angina Pectoris. New York, Churchill Livingstone, 1977.

88. Kloster, F.E., Kremkau, E.L., Ritzmann, L.W., Rahimtoola, S.H., Rosch, J., and Kanarek, P.H. Coronary bypass for stable angina. N. Engl. J. Med., 300:149, 1979.

89. Maseri, A., L'Abbate, A., Pesola, A., Ballestra, A.M., Marzilli, M., Maltinti, G., Severi, S., DeNes, D.M., Parodi, O., and Biagini, A. Coronary vasospasm in angina pectoris. Lancet, 1:713, 1977.

90. Murphy, M.L., Hultgren, H.N., Detre, K., Thomsen, J., Takaro, T., and Participants of the Veterans Administration Cooperative Study. Treatment of chronic stable angina. A preliminary report of survival data of the randomized Veterans Administration cooperative study. N. Engl. J. Med., 297:621, 1977.

91. Ross, R.S. Pathophysiology of the coronary circulation. The Sir Thomas Lewis lecture. Br. Heart J., 33:173, 1971.

92. Seides, S.F., Borer, J.F., Kent, K.M., Rosing, D.R., McIntosh, C.E., and Epstein, S.E. Long-term anatomic fate of coronary artery bypass grafts and functional status of patients five years after operation. N. Engl. J. Med., 298:1213, 1978.

93. Symposium: angina pectoris. Circulation, 46:1037, 1972.

94. Weinblatt, E., Frank, C.W., Shapiro, S., and Sager, R.V. Prognostic factors in angina pectoris. J. Chronic Dis., 21:231, 1968.

Myocardial Infarction

95. The Anturane Reinfarction Trial Research Group. Sulfinpyrazone in the prevention of cardiac death after myocardial infarction. The Auturane Reinfarction Trial. N. Engl. J. Med., 298:289, 1978.

96. DeSanctis, R.W., Block, P., and Hutter, A.M., Jr. Tachyarrhythmias in myocardial infarction. Circulation, 45:681, 1972.

97. Ebert, R.V. Use of anticoagulants in acute myocardial infarction. Circulation, 45:903, 1972.

98. Forrester, J.S., Diamond, G., Chatterjee, K., and Swan, H.J.C. Medical therapy of acute myocardial infarction by application of hemodynamic subsets. Part 1. N. Engl. J. Med., 295:1356, 1976.

99. Forrester, J.S., Diamond, G., Chatterjee, K., and Swan, H.J.C. Medical therapy of acute myocardial infarction by application of hemodynamic subsets. Part 2. N. Engl. J. Med., 295:1404, 1976.

100. Franciosa, J.A., Guiha, N.H., Limas, C.J., Rodriguera, E., and Cohn, J.N. Improved left ventricular function

during nitroprusside infusion in acute myocardial infarction. Lancet, 1:650, 1972.

101. Green, K.G. Improvement in prognosis of myocardial infarction by long term beta adrenoreceptor blockade using practolol. Br. Med. J., 3:735, 1975.

102. Hellerstein, H.K. and Friedman, E.H. Sexual activity and the post-coronary patient. Ann. Intern. Med., 125:987, 1970.

103. Herrick, J.B. Clinical features of sudden obstruction of the coronary arteries. JAMA, 59:2015, 1912.

104. Julian, D.G., Valentine, P.A., and Miller, G.G. Disturbances of rate, rhythm, and conduction in acute myocardial infarction: a prospective study of 100 consecutive unselected patients with the aid of electrocardiographic monitoring. Am. J. Med., 37:915, 1964.

105. Kannel, W.B., Castelli, W.P., Gordon, T., and McNamara, P.M. Serum cholesterol, lipoproteins, and the risk of coronary heart disease: the Framingham Study. Ann. Intern. Med., 74:1, 1971.

106. Kotler, M.N., Tabatznik, B., Mower, M.M., and Tominaga, S. Prognostic significance of ventricular ectopic beats with respect to sudden death in the late postinfarction period. Circulation, 47:959, 1973.

107. Lie, K.O., Wellens, H.J., vanCapelle, F.J., and Durrer, D. Lidocaine in the prevention of primary ventricular fibrillation. N. Engl. J. Med., 291:1324, 1974.

108. Maroko, P.R. and Braunwald, E. Modification of myocardial infarction size after coronary occlusion. Ann. Intern. Med., 79:720, 1973.

109. Mason, D.T., Spann, J.F., Jr., Zelis, R., and Amsterdam, E.A. The clinical pharmacology and therapeutic applications of the antiarrhythmic drugs. Clin. Pharmacol. Ther., 11(4):460, 1970.

110. Mundth, E.D., Buckley, M.J., Daggett, W.M., Sanders, C.A., and Austen, W.G. Surgery for complications of acute myocardial infarction. Circulation, 45:1279, 1972.

111. Norris. R.M., Caughey, D.E., Mercer, C.J., and Scott, P.J. Prognosis after myocardial infarction. Six-year follow-up. Br. Heart J., 36:786, 1974.

112. Reid, P.R., Taylor, D.R., Kelly, D.T., Weisfeldt, M.L., Humphries, J.O. Ross, R.S., and Pitt, B. Myocardial-infarct extension detected by precordial ST-segment mapping. N. Engl. J. Med., 290:123, 1974.

113. Roberts, W.C. Coronary arteries in fatal acute myocardial infarction. Circulation, 45:215, 1972.

114. Rotman, M., Wagner, G.S., and Wallace, A.G. Bradyarrhythmias in acute myocardial infarction. Circulation, 45:703, 1972.

115. Russell, R.O., Jr. and Rackley, C.E. Hemodynamic Monitoring in a Coronary Intensive Care Unit. New York, Futura Publishing, 1972.

116. Sanders, C.A., Buckley, M.J., Leinbach, R.C., Mundth, E.D., and Austen, W.G. Mechanical circulatory assistance: current status and experience with combining circulatory assistance, emergency coronary angiography, and acute myocardial revascularization. Circulation, 45:1292, 1972.

117. Sobel, B.E. and Shell, W.E. Serum enzyme determination in the diagnosis and assessment of myocardial infarction. Circulation, 45:471, 1972.

118. Wolk, M.J., Sheidt, S., and Killip, T. Heart failure complicating acute myocardial infarction. Circulation, 45:1125, 1972.

Pulmonary Thromboembolism

119. Bell, W.R., Simon, T.L., and DeMets, D.L. The clinical features of submassive and massive pulmonary emboli. Am. J. Med., 62:355, 1977.

120. Freiman, D.G., Suyemoto, J., and Wessler, S. Frequency of pulmonary thromboembolism in man. N. Engl. J. Med., 272:1278, 1965.

121. Gorham, L.W. A study of pulmonary embolism. Arch. Intern. Med., 108:8, 418, 1961.

122. Moser, K.M. and Stein, M. (eds.). Pulmonary Thromboembolism. Chicago, Year Book Medical Publishers, 1973.

123. A National Cooperative Study: the urokinase-streptokinase pulmonary embolism trial. JAMA, 229:1606, 1974.

124. A National Cooperative Study: the urokinase pulmonary embolism trial. Circulation, 47(Suppl. 11):1, 1973.

125. Robin, E.D. Overdiagnosis and overtreatment of pulmonary embolism. Ann. Intern. Med., 87:775, 1977.

126. Silver, D. and Sabiston, D.C. The role of vena caval interruption in the management of pulmonary embolism. Surgery, 7:1, 1975.

Systemic Hypertension

127. Effects of treatment on morbidity in hypertension: results in patients with diastolic blood pressure averaging 115 through 129 mm Hg. Veterans Administration Cooperative Study Group on Antihypertensive Agents. JAMA, 202:1028, 1967.

128. Effects of treatment on morbidity in hypertension II: results in patients with diastolic blood pressure averaging 90 through 114 mm Hg. Veterans Administration Cooperative Study Group on Antihypertensive Agents. JAMA, 213:1143, 1970.

129. Eich, R.H., Cuddy, R.P., Smulyan, H., and Lyons, R.H. Hemodynamics in labile hypertension: a follow-up study. Circulation, 34:299, 1966.

130. Freis, E. Salt, volume, and the prevention of hypertension. Circulation, 53:589, 1976.

131. Ganguly, A., Melada, J.A., Luetscher, J.A., and Dowdy, A.J. Control of plasma aldosterone in primary aldosteronism: distinction between adenoma and hyperplasia. J. Clin. Endocrinol. Metab., 37:765, 1973.

132. Kannel, W.B. Role of blood pressure in cardiovascular morbidity and mortality. Prog. Cardiovasc. Dis., 17:5, 1974.

133. Kaplan, N.M. Adrenal causes of hypertension. Arch. Intern. Med., 133:1001, 1974.

134. Kincaid-Smith, P., McMichael, J., and Murphy, E.A. The clinical course and pathology of hypertension with papilledema (malignant hypertension). Q. J. Med. N.S., 27:117, 1958.

135. Leishman, A.W.D. Hypertension, treated and untreated: a study of 400 cases. Br. Med. J., 1:1361, 1959.

136. Mallin, S.R. Congenital adrenal hyperplasia secondary to 17-hydroxylase deficiency. Ann. Intern. Med., 70:69, 1969.

137. McMahon, F.G. Management of Essential Hypertension. Mount Kisko, N.Y., Futura Publishing, 1978.
138. Moser, M. Report of the joint national committee on detection, evaluation and treatment of high blood pressure. JAMA, 237:255, 1977.
139. National health survey: hypertension and hypertensive heart disease in adults, U.S. 1960–62. Washington, D.C., U.S. Department of Health, Education, and Welfare, Vital and Health Statistic Series 11, No. 13, U.S. Government Printing Office, 1966.
140. Oparil, S. and Haber, E. The renin angiotensin system. N. Engl. J. Med., 291:389, 446, 1974.
141. Pickering, G.W. High Blood Pressure, 2nd ed. New York, Grune & Stratton, 1968.
142. Ram, C.U.S. and Kaplan, N.W. Low dose diazoxide therapy in severe hypertension. Clinical Research, 26:368A, 1978.
143. Vaughan, E.D., Buhler, F.R., Laragh, J.H., Sealey, J.E., Baer, L., and Bard, R.H. Renovascular hypertension. Renin measurements to indicate renal plasma flow and score for surgical curability. Am. J. Med., 55:402, 1973.
144. Whelton, P.K., Harrington, C.P., Russell, R.P., White, R.I., and Walker, W.G. Renal vein renin activity: a prospective study of sampling techniques and methods of interpretation. Johns Hopkins Med. J., 141:112, 1977.

Pulmonary Hypertension

145. Brown, A.L., Jr. Primary pulmonary hypertension. Am. J. Med., 49:70, 1970.
146. Edwards, W.D. and Edwards, J.E. Clinical primary pulmonary hypertension. Three pathologic types. Circulation, 56:884, 1977.
147. Hultgren, H.N., Grover, R.F., and Hartley, L.H. Abnormal circulatory responses to high altitude in subjects with a previous history of high-altitude pulmonary edema. Circulation, 44:759, 1971.

Congenital Heart Disease in the Adult

148. Keith, J.D., Rowe, R.D., and Vlad, P. Heart Disease in Infancy and Childhood, 3rd ed. New York, Macmillan, 1978.
149. Kidd, B.S.L. and Humphries, J.O. Transposition of the great arteries in adults. In Brest, A.N. (ed.), Congenital Heart Disease in Adults. Philadelphia, F.A. Davis, 1979.
150. Nadas, A.S. and Fyler, D.C. Pediatric Cardiology, 3rd ed. Philadelphia, Saunders, 1972.
151. Perloff, J.K. The Clinical Recognition of Congenital Heart Disease, 2nd ed. Philadelphia, Saunders, 1978.

Diseases of the Aorta

152. Crane, C. Arteriosclerotic aneurysms of the abdominal aorta. N. Engl. J. Med., 253:954, 1955.
153. Daily, P.O., Trueblood, H.W., Stinson, E.D., Wuerflein, R.D., and Shumway, N.E. Management of acute aortic dissections. Ann. Thorac. Surg., 10:237, 1970.
154. DeBakey, M.D., Beall, A.C., Cooley, D.A., Crawford, E.S., Morris, G.C., Garrett, H.E., and Howell, J.E. Dissecting aneurysms of the aorta. Surg. Clin. North Am., 46:1045, 1966.
155. Estes, J.E. Abdominal aortic aneurysms: a study of one hundred and two cases. Circulation, 2:258, 1950.
156. Heggtveit, H.A. Syphilitis aortitis: a clinicopathologic autopsy of 100 cases: 1950–1960. Circulation, 29:346, 1964.
157. Hirst, A.E. and Gore, I. Marfan's syndrome: a review. Prog. Cardiovasc. Dis., 16:187, 1973.
158. ———, Johns, V.J., and Kime, S.W. Dissecting aneurysm of the aorta. A review of 505 cases. Medicine, 37:217, 1958.
159. Slater, E.E. and DeSanctis, R.W. The clinical recognition of dissecting aortic aneurysm. Am. J. Med., 60:625, 1976.
160. Szilagyl, D.E., Smith, R.F., DeRusso, F.J., Elliott, J.P., and Sherrin, F.W. Contribution of abdominal aortic aneurysmectomy to prolongation of life. Ann. Surg., 164:678, 1966.
161. Wheat, M.W. Treatment of dissecting aneurysms of the aorta: current status. Prog. Cardiovasc. Dis., 16:87, 1963.

Peripheral Vascular Disease

162. Imparato, A.M., Kim, G., Davidson, T., and Crowley, J.G. Intermittent claudication: its natural course. Surgery, 78:795, 1975.
163. Karayannacos, P.E., Yagson, D., and Vasko, J.S. Narrow lumbar spinal canal with "vascular" syndromes. Arch. Surg., 111:803, 1976.
164. Lindon, R.R. The post-thrombotic ulceration of the lower extremity: its etiology and surgical treatment. Ann. Surg., 138:415, 1953.
165. Rutherford, R.B. (ed.). Vascular Surgery. Philadelphia, Saunders, 1977.

Cardiovascular Therapeutics

166. Antonaccio, M.J. (ed.). Cardiovascular Pharmacology. New York, Raven Press, 1977.
167. Cannon, P.J. The kidney in heart failure. N. Engl. J. Med., 296:26, 1977.
168. Clagett, G.P. and Salzman, E.W. Prevention of thromboembolism in surgical patients. N. Engl. J. Med., 290:93, 1974.
169. Douglas, A.S. Anticoagulant Therapy. Oxford, Blackwell and Philadelphia, F.A. Davis, 1962.
170. Genton, E., Gent, M., Hirsh, J., and Harker, L.A. Platelet-inhibiting drugs in the prevention of clinical thrombotic disease. N. Engl. J. Med., 293:1174, 1236, 1296, 1975.
171. Greenblatt, D.J. and Koch-Weser, J. Adverse reactions to spironolactone. JAMA, 225:40, 1973.
172. Hansten, P.D. Drug Interactions. Philadelphia, Lea & Febiger, 1973, pp. 141, 230.
173. Jackson, C.M. and Suttie, J.W. Recent developments in understanding the mechanism of Vitamin K and Vitamin K-antagonist drug action and the consequences of Vitamin K action in blood coagulation. In Brown, E.G. (ed.), Progress in Hematology, Vol. 10. New York, Grune & Stratton, 1977, pp. 333–359.
174. Kazmier, F.J., Spittell, J.A., Jr., Thompson, J.J., Jr., and Owen, C.A., Jr. Effect of oral anticoagulants on Factors VII, IX, X, and II. Arch. Intern. Med., 115:667, 1965.

175. Koch-Weser, J. Coumarin necrosis. Ann. Intern. Med., 68:1365, 1968.

176. ——— and Sellers, E.M. Drug interactions with coumarin anticoagulants. N. Engl. J. Med., 285:487, 547, 1971.

177. Needleman, P. (ed.). Organic Nitrates. Heidelberg, West Germany, Springer-Verlag, 1975.

178. O'Rielly, R.A. and Aggeler, P.M. Determinants of the response to oral anticoagulant drugs in man. Pharmacol. Rev., 22:35, 1970.

179. Rosenberg, R.D. Heparin action. Circulation, 49:603, 1974.

180. Seely, J.F., and Dirks, J.H. Site of action of diuretic drugs. Kidney Int., 11:1, 1977.

181. Sherry, S. (ed.). Symposium: thrombosis and anticoagulation. Am. J. Med., 33:619, 1962.

182. Smith, T.W. and Haber, E. Digitalis. N. Engl. J. Med., 289:945, 1010, 1063, 1125, 1973.

183. ——— and Haber, E. Digoxin intoxication: the relationship of clinical presentation to serum digoxin concentration. J. Clin. Invest., 49:2377, 1970.

184. Verstraete, M. Biochemical and clinical aspects of thrombolysis. Semin. Hematol., 15:35, 1978.

185. ———. Are agents affecting platelet functions clinically useful? Am. J. Med., 61:897, 1976.

186. Vigran, I.M. Clinical Anticoagulant Therapy. Philadelphia, Lea & Febiger, 1965.

187. Walker, W.G. Indications and contraindications for diuretic therapy. Ann. N.Y. Acad. Sci., 139:481, 1966.

188. Weiss, H.J. Antiplatelet therapy. N. Engl. J. Med., 298:1344, 1403, 1978.

189. Zito, R.A. and Reid, P.R. Lidocaine kinetics predicted by indocyanine green clearance. N. Engl. J. Med., 298:1160, 1978.

SECTION FIVE
Pulmonary Disease
GARETH M. GREEN: SECTION EDITOR

CHAPTER 31
Respiratory and Nonrespiratory Functions of the Lung
GARETH M. GREEN, WILMOT C. BALL, Jr., AND HAROLD H. NEWBALL

Diseases of the respiratory tract are characterized by disorders of both respiratory and nonrespiratory functions. Abnormalities of respiratory functions account for the debilitating symptoms of dyspnea, shortness of breath, wheezing, and cyanosis. Abnormalities of nonrespiratory functions cause symptoms of sputum production and cough, cause susceptibility to infectious and other agents, and mediate tissue-damaging processes in the bronchi and pulmonary parenchyma. It may be instructive to begin this section with an overview of the functions and abnormalities that characterize both respiratory and nonrespiratory functions of the lung.

RESPIRATORY FUNCTIONS OF THE LUNG[9,26]

Respiration comprises pulmonary ventilation, alveolar gas exchange, and oxygen transport. Abnormalities in any of the components, whatever the cause, can give rise to shortness of breath, dyspnea, hypoxemia, hyper- or hypoventilation, and cyanosis. Secondary effects on the cardiovascular, hematopoietic, and central nervous system may result in cardiac arrhythmias or failure, polycythemia, and agitation or mental obtundation. A systematic assessment of the components of respiratory function is mandatory in any patient who manifests these symptoms or signs.

ABNORMALITIES OF PULMONARY MECHANICS
Disease of the lung may interfere mechanically with the process of ventilation through a variety of mechanisms, which may be conveniently divided into restrictive and obstructive types. Restrictive ventilatory defect refers to a reduction in total lung capacity. The principal mechanisms responsible for a restrictive ventilatory defect are shown in Table 31-1 with examples of each. The clinical consequences of a re-

strictive ventilatory defect depend on its severity and on the mechanism of its production. Since only a small fraction of the vital capacity is normally utilized in ventilation, even a moderately severe restrictive ventilatory defect may interfere with ventilation to a negligible degree and be unaccompanied by symptoms, even during exercise. In many instances, however, when there is reduction in the distensibility of the lung or chest wall, an abnormal degree of muscular effort will be required to exchange even a normal tidal volume. Under these circumstances, dyspnea may be present, and the patient may attempt to minimize the work of breathing by selecting a small tidal volume and rapid respiratory rate. Loss of chest bellows action resulting from muscle weakness or immobilization of the chest may result in atelectasis because of ineffective cough or inability to inflate the lungs fully. In the absence of airway obstruction only the most extreme degree of restriction will lead to overall alveolar hypoventilation and carbon dioxide retention.

With obstructive ventilatory defect, the lungs empty at a decreased rate. This can most readily be detected during a forced expiratory maneuver. Airway obstruction is the characteristic physiologic abnormality in asthma, chronic bronchitis, and emphysema and is commonly associated with respiratory failure. The mechanisms and clinical manifestations of airway obstruction are discussed in Chapter 34.

ABNORMALITIES OF GAS EXCHANGE
While physical examination and simple tests of pulmonary function will permit recognition of mechanical abnormalities of ventilation, failure of the gas-exchange function of the lung may produce less readily recognized clinical signs. In addition, hypoxemia may occur in patients with lung disease through a number of different mechanisms, the understanding of which is essential for rational management.

Figure 31-1 shows schematically the basic gas-

TABLE 31-1
Causes of Restrictive Ventilatory Defect

Mechanism	Examples
Reduction in distensibility of the lung (stiff lung)	Diffuse pulmonary infiltration, fibrosing alveolitis, pulmonary congestion
Replacement of pulmonary parenchyma by nonventilating tissue	Pneumonia, atelectasis
Compression of lung by space-occupying intrathoracic lesions	Large tumor, pleural effusion, pneumothorax, cardiomegaly
Weakness or paralysis of muscles of respiration	Poliomyelitis, phrenic nerve paralysis, muscular dystrophy
Immobilization of pleura or chest wall	Extensive pleural fibrosis, trauma, extreme obesity, thoracic deformity

TABLE 31-2
Glossary

ARDS	Adult respiratory distress syndrome
ARF	Acute respiratory failure
Barotrauma	Pneumatic injury to the lung due to elevated pressure across the lung
COLD	Chronic obstructive lung disease
CPAP	Continuous positive airway pressure
CPPV	Continuous positive pressure ventilation
FEV_1	Denotes the volume of gas which is exhaled in a given time interval during the execution of a forced vital capacity
FI_{O_2}	Fractional concentration of inspired oxygen
FRC	Functional residual capacity
FVC	Forced vital capacity: The volume of gas expired from total lung capacity and with expiration performed as rapidly and completely as possible
Pa_{O_2}	Arterial tension of oxygen
PA_{O_2}	Alveolar tension of oxygen
Pa_{CO_2}	Arterial tension of carbon dioxide
PA_{CO_2}	Alveolar tension of carbon dioxide
Pc'_{O_2}	End-capillary tension of oxygen
Pc'_{CO_2}	End-capillary tension of carbon dioxide
PEEP	Positive end-expiratory pressure
PI_{O_2}	Tension of oxygen in inspired air
$P\bar{v}_{O_2}$	Tension of oxygen in mixed venous blood
$P\bar{v}_{CO_2}$	Tension of carbon dioxide in mixed venous blood
$\dot{Q}$	Perfusion (volume flow of blood)
$\dot{V}$	Ventilation (volume flow of air)
$\dot{V}A$	Alveolar ventilation
$\dot{V}{CO_2}$	Carbon dioxide production per minute (STPD)

exchange unit of the lung, and gives typically normal values for alveolar, mixed venous, end-capillary, and arterial gas tensions in the resting adult. Reference to this diagram is made throughout the discussion which follows. A glossary of terms and symbols is found in Table 31-2.

Carbon Dioxide Transport

The partial pressure of carbon dioxide in arterial blood (Pa_{CO_2}), which does not differ substantially from the partial pressure of carbon dioxide in alveolar gas (PA_{CO_2}), is determined by the balance between delivery of carbon dioxide to the alveoli and its removal by ventilation. Maintenance of a normal arterial carbon dioxide tension requires that alveolar ventilation be kept proportional to metabolic carbon dioxide production and indicates the effect on alveolar and hence arterial P_{CO_2} of inadequate or excessive alveolar ventilation. A sustained arterial P_{CO_2} of 80 mm Hg, for example, indicates that the level of alveolar ventilation is half of normal, i.e., half that which would be appropriate for the existing rate of metabolic carbon dioxide production.

Hypercapnia is thus the result of inadequate alveolar ventilation, and may be observed in patients whose control of breathing is impaired (sedative or narcotic overdose, CNS lesion, primary hypoventilation syndrome) or who are unable to meet ventilatory

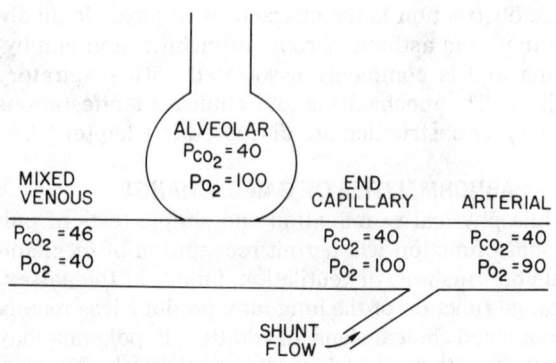

FIGURE 31-1. Scheme of the alveolar-capillary unit showing values for blood and alveolar gas partial pressures of CO_2 and O_2 in the normal subject at rest.

demands because of respiratory muscle paralysis. Chronic CO_2 retention is most common in patients with severe obstructive pulmonary disease, especially chronic bronchitis, and usually when the 1-second forced expiratory volume has fallen to 1.0 liter or less. A normal or slightly low arterial Pco_2 is maintained in most patients with a restrictive ventilatory abnormality. However, Pa_{CO_2} may rise acutely in patients very severely ill with pneumonia, pulmonary edema, or even extensive fibrosing alveolitis. Since the presence of an increased dead space may cause a marked discrepancy between alveolar ventilation and minute ventilation, the adequacy of alveolar ventilation cannot always be predicted by bedside observation. Sampling of arterial blood for measurement of Pa_{CO_2} is therefore indicated whenever alveolar hypoventilation is suspected.

An acute increase in arterial CO_2 tension is accompanied by a fall in pH of approximately 0.006 units for each mm Hg change in Pa_{CO_2}. The acidosis caused by CO_2 retention stimulates ammonia formation and acid excretion by the kidney, and after hours or days the pH rises toward normal as the plasma bicarbonate increases. During recovery, lowering of the Pa_{CO_2} may result in a pH shift to 7.45 or higher. This "metabolic alkalosis" persists until renal bicarbonate excretion restores normal acid–base balance. This process may require several days in patients with sodium retention and is often prolonged by the hypokalemic alkalosis induced by the use of diuretics.

The elevation of arterial carbon dioxide tension has important physiologic effects, although these are generally reversible. These effects are often difficult to separate from those of hypoxemia in respiratory failure. Minor degrees of carbon dioxide retention may produce an increase in systemic blood pressure, drowsiness, irritability, and headache. More marked elevation of Pa_{CO_2} results in further deterioration of mental function which can progress to coma. High levels of Pa_{CO_2} have also been shown to have an unfavorable effect on cardiac function and on renal blood flow. The cerebral effects of hypercapnea depend to some extent on the acuteness of change, so that in some instances a patient with chronic carbon dioxide retention at a level of 80 mm Hg may be fully conscious while another patient with acute elevation of the Pa_{CO_2} to 80 may be stuporous.

Hypocapnia of mild degree is common in dyspneic patients who hyperventilate because of chronic hypoxemia, or stiff lungs. An arterial Pco_2 of 30 to 35 mm Hg is often seen in diffuse pulmonary infiltration, pulmonary congestion, pulmonary embolism, and early during an attack of asthma. More marked respiratory alkalosis may be accompanied by manifestations of tetany, but is seen more frequently in anxiety than in structural lung disease.

Oxygen Transport

The O_2 tension of pulmonary capillary blood rises to reach equilibrium with alveolar gas as blood traverses the capillary. The oxygen tension of alveolar gas may be estimated from a simplification of the alveolar air equation:*

$$PA_{O_2} = PI_{O_2} - \frac{PA_{CO_2}}{R}$$

where PA_{O_2} = alveolar O_2 tension, PI_{O_2} = inspired O_2 tension (150 mm Hg for room air), Pa_{CO_2} = arterial Pco_2, which is assumed to equal alveolar Pco_2, and R = respiratory exchange ratio. The respiratory exchange ratio, defined as ratio of CO_2 output to O_2 uptake by the lungs, is equal to the respiratory quotient in the steady state, and has a numeral value of about 0.8. R may be measured by analysis of expired air, or may be estimated under nonsteady state conditions. Although the simplified equation presented here is inaccurate when inspired O_2 is above 50 percent, it provides a convenient clinical method for predicting arterial Po_2 in a patient receiving supplemental oxygen.

Arterial Po_2 is normally slightly less than end-capillary Po_2 (see Fig. 31–1) because of the admixture of venous blood. Part of this admixture is due to direct shunt through Thebesian and bronchial veins, and part is due to the effect of uneven ventilation to perfusion ($\dot{V}/\dot{Q}$) ratios in the normal lung, which results in overperfusion of portions of lung relative to their ventilation. The total shunt effect in a young normal individual is less than 6 percent of cardiac output, and results in an O_2 tension difference between alveolar gas and arterial blood (A-a O_2 difference) of about 15 mm Hg.

Oxygen content of arterial blood, which is an important factor in delivery of oxygen to peripheral tissues, also depends on the position of the oxyhemoglobin dissociation curve, which is shifted to the right by reduction in pH or elevation of body temperature, and on the concentration of normal hemoglobin in the blood. Even when arterial oxygen tension is not seriously reduced, oxygen content may be low in clinical conditions accompanied by acidosis, fever, or anemia or when an abnormal hemoglobin, i.e., sulfhemoglobin, methemoglobin, is present.

Hypoxemia may result from three separate mechanisms (see Fig 31–1):

---

* For a derivation of the alveolar air equation, see reference 9.

1. Low alveolar oxygen tension (hypoventilation, breathing low-oxygen mixtures, high altitude)
2. Failure to achieve equilibrium between alveolar and capillary oxygen tensions (diffusion defect)
3. Effective shunting of blood from the venous to the arterial side (direct anatomic shunt, perfusion of poorly ventilated alveoli)

The oxygen tension (Po_2) of alveolar gas will be reduced as a result of low inspired Po_2. In the patient breathing air at sea level it depends primarily on the alveolar ventilation. As ventilation decreases and alveolar carbon dioxide tension rises, there is a corresponding decrease in alveolar oxygen tension as predicted from the alveolar air equation. Because of the form of the oxyhemoglobin dissociation curve, however, oxygen *saturation* does not fall sharply until the oxygen tension drops below 60 mm Hg. Therefore, hypoventilation which results in elevation of the Pa_{CO_2} to 80 mm Hg and decrease in Pa_{O_2} to 50 to 60 mm Hg may be associated with impaired delivery of oxygen to the tissues.

The clinical importance of these considerations lies in the fact that a serious degree of alveolar hypoventilation invariably leads to hypoxemia in the patient who is breathing room air. When arterial Pco_2 reaches levels of 70 or 80 mm Hg, arterial oxygen saturation is nearly always sufficiently reduced so that oxygen administration is required.

When the alveolocapillary membrane has been extensively altered by disease, or when the total effective surface for gas exchange has been markedly reduced by destruction of lung parenchyma, blood leaving the pulmonary capillaries may have a significantly lower oxygen tension than alveolar air. Hypoxemia may therefore be seen in patients with marked reduction in diffusing capacity. Characteristically, O_2 unsaturation in such patients is brought on or accentuated by exercise.

Hypoxemia may also result from shunting of poorly oxygenated blood (venous admixture) through pulmonary arteriovenous communications, such as those commonly demonstrable in bronchiectasis or in chronic pulmonary hypertension of any cause. The effect is identical to that of an intracardiac right-to-left shunt or a pulmonary arteriovenous fistula. Since a mixture of well-oxygenated and poorly-oxygenated blood is always less than normally saturated, blood reaching the left heart under these circumstances will have an abnormally low oxygen tension.

An effect entirely analogous to that produced by anatomic right-to-left shunt occurs when the distribution of ventilation and blood flow is disproportionate in different areas of the lung (abnormal $\dot{V}/\dot{Q}$ ratios).

Alveolocapillary units that are underventilated with respect to their blood flow contribute unsaturated blood to the pulmonary venous circulation. Although blood from other units that are relatively overventilated will have a higher than normal oxygen tension, the oxygen saturation and content of this blood will not be significantly increased, and the mixture will remain below normal saturation. This is sometimes called venous admixture like effect. In the absence of overall hypoventilation, which can readily be identified by elevation of the arterial Pco_2, this is the mechanism most commonly responsible for cyanosis at rest in patients with diffuse pulmonary disease. Uneven distribution may also result in overventilation of some alveolocapillary units with little or no blood flow. This defect has a negligible direct effect on the composition of arterial blood but renders a portion of the ventilation ineffective in gas exchange, so that a larger minute ventilation is required to keep alveolar ventilation normal.

Hypoxemia produces important physiologic changes, especially in cerebral and cardiac function. Chronic mild hypoxemia may result only in a sense of fatigue, a subtle impairment of judgment, and a slight tachycardia with increase in cardiac output. A more abrupt and severe reduction in arterial oxygen tension may produce gross disturbances in behavior or loss of consciousness and may give rise to a fatal cardiac arrhythmia. Although disturbances of consciousness resulting from carbon dioxide retention are generally promptly and fully reversible, even a brief period of severe cerebral hypoxia may result in irreversible damage to the brain or may produce an altered state of consciousness from which recovery requires hours or days.

In the evaluation of cyanosis, which results from the presence of unsaturated hemoglobin in the tissue capillaries, factors other than reduction of arterial oxygen saturation must be considered. Severe reduction in cardiac output accompanied by a slowing of the blood flow through the peripheral tissues, seen commonly in heart disease, may produce peripheral cyanosis in the presence of normal arterial oxygen saturation.

NONRESPIRATORY FUNCTIONS OF THE LUNG

Most bronchopulmonary diseases are induced by the deposition or absorption of inhaled particulate or gaseous matter, such as silica, asbestos fibers, nitrogen dioxide, viruses or pathogenic bacteria, or immunologically reactive particles in the lung. Disease also occurs when the effectiveness of the defensive systems is diminished by genetic constitution, nutritional or immunologic deficiency, metabolic abnormalities, or by cigarette smoking, air pollutants, and occupational exposures.[8,12]

RESPIRATORY AIR CONDITIONING

In the upper respiratory tract, inspired air is drawn over a moist mucous membrane with highly reactive vascular and secretory mechanisms which warm the airstream to body temperature and saturate it with water vapor. Soluble gases, such as sulfur dioxide, are totally absorbed, and a portion of insoluble gases may be adsorbed to protein or mucopolysaccharide secretions on the surface. The nasal cavity narrows sharply in the region of the turbinates, so that the airstream is greatly accelerated in velocity and subjected to substantial turbulence. This change in velocity and turbulence exerts intense inertial forces on suspended particulates so that most particles above 10μ in aerodynamic diameter deposit on the nasal mucous membrane.[13] This air conditioned stream then resumes laminar flow in the nasal pharynx and proceeds into the trachea, bronchi, and alveoli at body temperature and vapor pressure where particles continue to be removed by inertial impaction induced where the airstream changes direction rapidly at bronchial bifurcations.

Fine particles of respirable size (0.5 to 3μ) remain suspended until they reach the terminal and respiratory bronchioles, where the airstream slows markedly as the total cross-sectional diameter of the bronchiolar passages becomes very large. Gravity exerts its effect on these small particles, and they deposit on the surfaces of the respiratory membrane. The character of respiratory tract secretions becomes more lipophilic in nature, and gases that are insoluble in the upper respiratory tract may combine with the lipid-based secretions of the respiratory membrane, oftentimes altering the chemical characteristics of the secretion as by the lipoperoxidation induced by oxidant gases.[14] Particles smaller than 0.5μ are impelled against the respiratory membrane surface by Brownian movement, but the bulk of these are expired.[13]

Exercise has a pronounced effect on respiratory air conditioning. Because of the requirement for high-volume air flow, the nasal cavity is bypassed and mouth breathing is employed. There is thus a greater burden placed on the posterior pharynx, the trachea, and the upper bronchi for temperature and humidity control of the inspired air, and the particle burden on the lower respiratory tract is far greater. Similarly, soluble gases, ordinarily removed in the nasal passages, may penetrate into the lower respiratory tract and have a greater effect on secretory responses and bronchospastic reactions of the bronchial tree. The pollutant burden of the cigarette smoker bypasses the nose during inhalation. Similarly, hard work performed in a dusty environment will place a greater burden of both particles and harmful gases on the lower respiratory tract; for this reason, an occupational history should elicit the level of physical exertion required on the job to gain some estimate of the potential exposure of the lower respiratory tract through occupational dusts and vapors. Similarly, diseases or conditions which alter the physiology of the nasal mucosa by altering the vascular hyperreactivity and secretory status or by obstructing airflow through the cavity, have a significant impact on the air conditioning physiology of the upper respiratory tract and alter substantially the air pollutant burden on the lower respiratory tract.

The aerodynamic behavior of particles of different size in the respiratory tract may be used therapeutically and prophylactically to design aerosols, such as water vapor, steroids or bronchodilators, or immunogens that have a predilection for depositing at the appropriate level in the respiratory tract. Thus, agents such as bronchodilators, to be effective in the bronchial tree, should have a size range between 3 and 10μ. Agents such as corticosteroids, for treating parenchymal disease, should have a smaller particle size, in the 0.5 to 3μ range. The local immune response of the respiratory tract reflects the site of deposition of the immunogenic particles so that secretory antibody may be localized to the nose, the bronchial mucosa, or the alveoli through an appropriate design of immunizing aerosols administered by the airborne route. Control of the spread of infectious disease in hospitals requires sound management of therapeutic nebulizers and humidifiers utilized in respiratory therapy which, without proper care, can be colonized by staphylococci and gram negative organisms and spread these nosocomial organisms widely throughout intensive care units, recovery rooms, and hospital wards. Effective control of hospital infections is critically dependent on the control of the generation and spread of small particle infectious aerosols, and is vital to the control of nosocomial pneumonias, skin infections, and other hazards of the hospital environment.

BRONCHOALVEOLAR SECRETIONS

The presence of respiratory tract fluid on the airways is critical to the function of the mucociliary escalator. The secretion on the epithelial cells has a deeper sol layer through which the cilia can freely move as they propel the overlying gel layer in a cephalad direction. Transport mechanisms in the tracheobronchial tree are influenced by the secretory activity of mucous glands and epithelial goblet cells, and on the activity of the ciliary system.[19] The mucus-producing goblet cells are affected by local irritants, such as cigarette smoke, and their numbers greatly increase in subjects with chronic bronchitis. Mucus-secreting glands and goblet cells in normal lungs do not extend to the smaller airways. On chronic exposure to irritants, such as cigarette smoke, however, the epithelium of the small airways is altered morphologically with the appearance of increasing numbers of mucus-secreting goblet cells and gland cells, which crowd the ciliated epithelial cells from the surface layer, resulting in fewer cilia to propel mucus. While the gland cells are responsive to local irritants, they also respond to parasympathetic nerve impulses. Very little is known of the biochemical composition of normal mucus (and even less of abnormal mucus); however, glycoproteins are a usual constituent.

Because mucus in the tracheobronchial tree is discontinuous, its role as a physical barrier in the airway defense mechanisms is probably limited, and emphasis is now being placed on alternative defense mechanisms such as secretory proteins. The protein composition of alveolar fluids is seemingly less complex than that of plasma.[17,21,22] Only a few major proteins are consistently found in alveolar fluids of normal subjects. IgA is found principally as 11S secretory immunoglobulin, but some IgA is in monomeric form. The following are consistently found in human alveolar lavages: transferrin, α_1-antitrypsin, 11S secretory IgA, IgG, and C3. Other proteins that are inconsistently found include: α_2-macroglobulin, IgE, IgM, unbound secretory component of IgA, C4, and C6. In addition to proteins, lipids (or lipoproteins), such as pulmonary surfactant, are also present in alveolar fluids. Of potential interest is the observation that the IgG content of alveolar fluid from smokers is twice as high as that from nonsmokers, and that even a brief history of cigarette smoking is sufficient to induce IgG changes seen in chronic smokers.

TRANSPORT MECHANISMS

In the nasal cavity and along the bronchi, transport of respiratory tract secretions is achieved by the propelling force of ciliary activity and is assisted substantially by cough. Effective propulsion of secretions by cilia requires hydrated nonviscid secretions and an intact ciliated epithelium. Exposure to oxidant air pollution and to dehydration increases viscid mucous secretion, decreases ciliary motility, and aggravates cough. Infectious agents, particularly viruses, may cause the ciliated epithelium to desquamate and may activate hypersecretion of mucous glands. Allergic

agents alter vascular permeability of submucosal blood vessels producing edema, hypersecretion, and abnormalities of respiratory tract secretions and transport. Prolonged exposure to air pollutants, particularly cigarette smoke, induces a decrease in ciliated cells and an increase in the number of mucus-secreting goblet cells with such secretory cells migrating into the smaller bronchioles where normally they are not present. The changes in respiratory tract fluid thus induced have significant effects on the characteristics of airway diameter and airflow in the distal bronchiolar tree. Two curious genetic deficiencies of ciliary motility in which chronic sinopulmonary infection is prominent attest to the importance of the ciliary mechanism:[2] Kartagener syndrome[23] and "immotile cilia syndrome."[10] These diseases are also marked by male sterility due to immobile spermatozoa. Fortunately, the bronchopulmonary tree has redundant defenses that prevent overwhelming infection in the lung in this condition despite impaired mucociliary transport.

Distal to the ciliated epithelium of the bronchioles, transport mechanisms are less well defined, as no cilia exist at that level. On the surface of the respiratory membrane, surfactant, cells, and deposited particles move from the periphery of the pulmonary lobules via the alveoli and pores of Kohn to the respiratory and terminal bronchioles at the center of the lobule. Movement may be both by the effects of expansion and contraction of the air spaces and by gradients in surface tension from the low surface activity of surfactant to the much higher surface activity of bronchiolar secretions. Transport may also occur along interstitial pathways between alveoli by forces that depend upon gradients of pressure induced by the curved surfaces of the alveoli and by the elastic tension of respiratory tissue generated by the expansion of inspiration.[24]

Immobilization is the enemy of bronchopulmonary transport. Restriction of lung expansion by positioning, by bandaging, by coma or obtundation, or by local or generalized hypoventilation of any cause, impairs fluid transport mechanisms of the pulmonary parenchyma and predisposes to fluid accumulation and pulmonary infection. Mobilization and adequate ventilation, even hyperventilation, are critical to the function of pulmonary transport defense mechanisms at all times in ill or hospitalized patients. Interference with this mechanism is an important reason for the high incidence of pneumonias in ill and hospitalized patients. Adequate ventilation of the lungs may be as important as antibiotics in maintaining pulmonary function and avoiding the complications of nosocomial pneumonias.

PHAGOCYTOSIS

Infectious, physical, or chemical particles deposited on the respiratory membrane are rapidly subjected to the phagocytic activity of the resident alveolar macrophage population or of polymorphonuclear leukocytes, monocytes, and tissue histiocytes attracted into the site of inflammatory reaction by chemotactic substances acting directly or generated by the alveolar macrophage. Alveolar macrophages develop in the bone marrow and migrate into the lungs, where there may be additional local replication. They then migrate onto the surface of the alveolus, where they differentiate into highly specialized oxygen-dependent cells that phagocytose and digest all manner of inhaled and deposited particulate material. Increased particle burden increases the number of cells in the lungs. Immunization activates the macrophages, both specifically against the immunogen and nonspecifically against other particulate substances. Phagocytic activity is accelerated by humoral antibody and digestive effectiveness by cell-mediated immune mechanisms present in the activated cell.

The alveolar macrophage is especially important in the pathogenesis of pulmonary infection because its activity is suppressed by a variety of environmental pollutants, endogenous toxicants and metabolic alterations, and by other infectious processes in the lung, specifically virus infections.[11] The alveolar macrophage is a key cell in modulating inflammation through its release of chemotactic agents, proteolytic enzymes, and lymphotactic agents. Macrophages are the principal cells to interact with organic antigens and mineral dusts to produce, along with the immune mechanisms, hypersensitivity pneumonitis and the pneumoconioses. They are active in the granuloma formation of such diverse diseases as tuberculosis, silicosis, berylliosis, and sarcoidosis, and are key cells in the transport and storage of inert and fibrogenic dusts, such as coal dust, asbestos fibers, and hematite. Some of these mineral dusts, such as silica, disable the macrophage in its bactericidal function against tubercle bacilli and other infectious organisms.[18]

PROTEASES AND ANTIPROTEASES

The role of proteolytic enzymes in the pathogenesis of lung disorders is poorly understood. Animal models suggest that granulocyte or macrophage elastase is capable of destroying the integrity of the lung parenchyma, resulting in the appearance of pathologic changes indistinguishable from human pulmonary emphysema. An example of human pulmonary emphysema resulting from proteolytic destruction of the lung is that seen in patients with severe α_1-antitrypsin deficiency, most of whom develop panlobular emphysema. In the homozygous state (phenotype Pi ZZ), patients have only 10 to 15 percent of the normal amount of α_1-antitrypsin in their serum, and the presumptive diagnosis is simply made by observing the absence of the α_1-globulin peak on a serum protein electrophoretic study. Definitive diagnosis must be made by specific phenotyping studies. In the heterozygous state (i.e., Pi MZ), the serum protein electrophoretic pattern and serum α_1-antitrypsin (α_1-AT) level may be normal, and the diagnosis must be established by phenotyping. A variety of disease states are associated with abnormal α_1-AT levels. Increased serum levels are often seen in inflammatory disorders, during pregnancy or when taking estrogens, following surgery, and in patients with cancer.

The mechanism of action of α_1-AT appears to be through its ability to inhibit the elastase of neutrophils and macrophages. Familial emphysema associated with α_1-AT deficiency (Pi ZZ) is generally characterized by the onset of progressive chronic obstructive lung disease (panlobular emphysema) in the third or fourth decade of life. When the disease appears in infancy or childhood, there may be infantile cirrhosis and/or emphysema. Large amounts of α_1-AT are found in granules in the rough endoplasmic reticulum of the liver cell cytoplasm in Pi ZZ individuals. This abnormal α_1-AT is less able to be transported into the circulation, resulting in a severe deficiency of circulating α_1-AT. It may be of importance to identify the heterozygous subject, since, as with the homozygous deficient patients, the smoking of cigarettes appears to make heterozygous individuals more susceptible to the development of panlobular emphysema.

PULMONARY IMMUNE RESPONSE[15,21]

The lung possesses a local secretory immunologic system in which secretory IgA antibody is a defense mechanism at the mucosal surface.[7] Thus, the presence of IgA antibody in lung secretions is better correlated with resistance to pulmonary infections than is the presence of serum antibody of any class. The effectiveness of IgA antibodies in resistance to viral infections is dependent on the type of virus which is invading the host, and in immunologic terms, cells such as T lymphocytes may play an equally important role. The control of some infectious processes in the lung is mediated at least in part by cell-mediated mechanisms.[16] Other infectious processes require the participation of antibodies such that antibody coating of target cells leads to enhanced killing by lymphocytes. Thus, there is cooperation and a complex interaction of B and T lymphocytes in the immune defense of the lung.[25]

CLINICAL ASSESSMENT OF PULMONARY DEFENSES

Although tests of pulmonary defense mechanisms are not yet available for routine clinical use, laboratory studies for the clinical assessment of pulmonary immune defenses are more readily available. As in all fields of medicine, a careful history is critical in the evaluation of patients with abnormal pulmonary immune defenses. The most common clinical presentation of patients with immune deficiencies is that of increased susceptibility to infections. A careful history may reveal recurrent infections, sometimes dating back to childhood, which are often severe, persistent, caused by organisms of relatively low virulence, and not infrequently in extrapulmonary as well as pulmonary sites. While the decision to evaluate the patient with abnormal pulmonary immune defenses rests primarily on clinical criteria, the documentation and definition of the defect rests primarily on laboratory studies (see Table 31-3). The laboratory evalu-

ation of the patient is based on the fact that the immune system may be arbitrarily separated into four distinct, although interrelated, functional compartments: B lymphocytes, T lymphocytes, phagocytes, and complement. B lymphocytes mature into plasma cells, which are responsible for antibody synthesis. Antibody production is of critical importance since antibodies may function in opsonization, toxin neutralization, virus neutralization, and bacteriolysis. T lymphocytes not only initiate delayed-type hypersensitivity reactions, but they also initiate graft versus host reactions, are responsible for defenses against viruses, fungi and some intracellular bacteria, function in immune surveillance, and cooperate with B lymphocytes in antibody production. Phagocytes or macrophages are responsible not only for the ingesting and killing of microorganisms, but also for the processing and presentation of certain antigens to lymphocytes. The complement components serve many functions including opsonization, chemotaxis, cytotoxicity, and as anaphylatoxins.[20] The above functions are critical to the integrity of pulmonary immune defense system.

TABLE 31-3
Laboratory Evaluation of Pulmonary Immune Defenses*

Evaluation of "B" Cell Function	Evaluation of "T" Cell Function	Evaluation of Phagocytes	Evaluation of Complement
Initial Studies	**Initial Studies**	**Initial Studies**	**Initial Studies**
1. Serum IgG, IgA, and IgM levels	1. Lymphocyte count and morphology	1. WBC and differential count	1. CH_{50} level
2. Isoagglutinins Anti-A, B	2. Skin tests (DTH): i.e., mumps, candida, trichophyton, SK-SD, tetanus, PPD	2. WBC morphology	2. Complement components C3, C4
3. Antibodies: tetanus diphtheria, pertussis, rubella, measles, and polio ΦX174		3. Look for inclusion bodies, e.g., Howell-Jolly bodies	
Advanced Studies	**Advanced Studies**	**Advanced Studies**	**Advanced Studies**
1. Specific immunization: i.e., keyhole-limpet hemocyanin, bacteriophage	1. *In vitro* response to PHA, MLC, and antigens	1. Skin window	1. Individual complement component assays
2. IgG subclasses	2. DNCB challenge	2. Chemotaxis assay	2. Serum opsonic assay
3. "B" cell quantitation; i.e., EAC rosettes	3. "T" cell quantitation: i.e., sheep RBC rosettes	3. Intracellular killing	3. Serum chemotatic assay
4. Lymph node biopsy	4. Lymphokine production: i.e., MIF	4. NBT reduction	
5. Lateral pharyngeal x-ray (especially in children)	5. Lymph node biopsy	5. Splenic scans	

* EAC: erythrocyte antibody complement; DTH: delayed-type hypersensitivity; SK-SD: streptokinase-streptodornase; PHA: phytohemagglutinin; MLC: mixed lymphocyte culture; DNCB: dinitrochlorobenzene; MIF: migration inhibition factor; NBT: nitroblue tetrazolium; CH_{50}: 50 percent hemolytic units.

CHAPTER 32

Clinical Manifestations and Diagnosis of Pulmonary Diseases

WILMOT C. BALL, Jr. AND WARREN R. SUMMER

The cardinal manifestations of pulmonary diseases are: *symptoms* of cough, dyspnea, and chest pain; *signs* of sputum production, hemoptysis, fever, wheezing or labored breathing, rales, and cyanosis; *radiologic findings* of infiltration or mass lesion; and *respiratory functional changes* of airway obstruction, diminished volumes, hypoxemia, and hypercapnia. Whereas acute respiratory diseases are largely symptomatic and associated with physical findings, chronic respiratory diseases are more likely detected, particularly in their earliest stages, only by careful assessment of radiographs, pulmonary function tests, and special studies.

The diagnosis of pulmonary diseases rests principally on a careful history and physical examination, a meticulous examination of high-quality radiographs, simple spirometry and selected additional tests of respiratory function, and special procedures such as bronchoscopy, thoracentesis, tissue biopsy, and scintigraphy. This chapter summarizes the clinical manifestations of pulmonary disease and presents diagnostic approaches to the patient so afflicted.

EVALUATION OF COUGH AND SPUTUM

HISTORY AND DIFFERENTIAL DIAGNOSIS

Cough is part of the normal defense mechanism for cleansing the tracheobronchial tree. It is a reflex act usually arising from stimulation of the bronchial mucosa at some point between the larynx and second-order bronchi or from sources as distant as the alveoli and tympanic membranes. The stimulus may be provided by inhaled particulate matter, by mucus secreted by cells lining the tracheobronchial tree, by inflammatory exudate originating in the pulmonary parenchyma or the conducting airways, by the presence of a benign or malignant tumor within the bronchus, or by pressure on the outer wall of the bronchus. Cough may occasionally be produced by conditions involving the pleural surfaces or from stimulation of the external auditory canal, as by impacted cerumen.

Dry or nonproductive cough of acute onset is the typical response to inhalation or aspiration of a foreign body or irritant, is a common early symptom of acute bronchitis or pneumonia (especially of viral origin), and may be a prominent manifestation of pulmonary embolization. Chronic, nonproductive cough

suggests an endobronchial tumor, extrinsic pressure on the trachea or on a bronchus, one of the diffuse forms of pulmonary infiltration or fibrosis, pulmonary congestion due to early heart failure, or recurrent aspiration of food or gastric contents.

GROSS AND MICROSCOPIC SPUTUM EXAMINATION

Sputum is not produced by healthy subjects, and its presence is a sign of disease. Cough productive of purulent sputum is generally indicative of infection in the tracheobronchial tree or lung, although large numbers of eosinophils associated with an allergic condition may also produce a yellow sputum. When purulent sputum is associated with an acute illness, the gross characteristics of the sputum may be a valuable differentiating feature. A rust-colored sputum, which is produced by blood evenly dispersed in yellow pus, is most commonly seen in pneumococcal pneumonia. Sputum in klebsiella pneumonia also frequently contains blood but is often bright red and more translucent and viscid. Purulent sputum with a foul odor is usually indicative of anaerobic infection, commonly due to streptococci or bacteroides in a lung abscess. Chronic cough with a purulent sputum occurs in chronic bronchitis, bronchiectasis, and a variety of other suppurative conditions. Sputum which is mucoid in character is least helpful diagnostically and may result from any form of long-standing bronchial irritation.

For microscopic examination of sputum, a sample is collected in a glass container or petri dish to facilitate the selection of a drop-sized sample of optically dense material.[34] This is smeared on a glass slide, covered and examined immediately while still wet. Under low power the slide is scanned for alveolar macrophages, the presence of which is evidence that the material arose from deep within the lung. The presence of large squamous cells, which originate in the mouth or pharynx, is caused by contamination with saliva, and indicates an inadequate specimen. In patients with asthma, low-power examination may reveal the laminated whorls called Curschmann's spirals (Fig. 32–1A), or Charcot-Leyden crystals, which are thought to represent the coalescence of eosinophilic granules (Fig. 32–1B). Cellular detail is best appreciated by use of the oil immersion lens. The sputum in patients with asthma shows a predominance of eosinophils. In contrast,

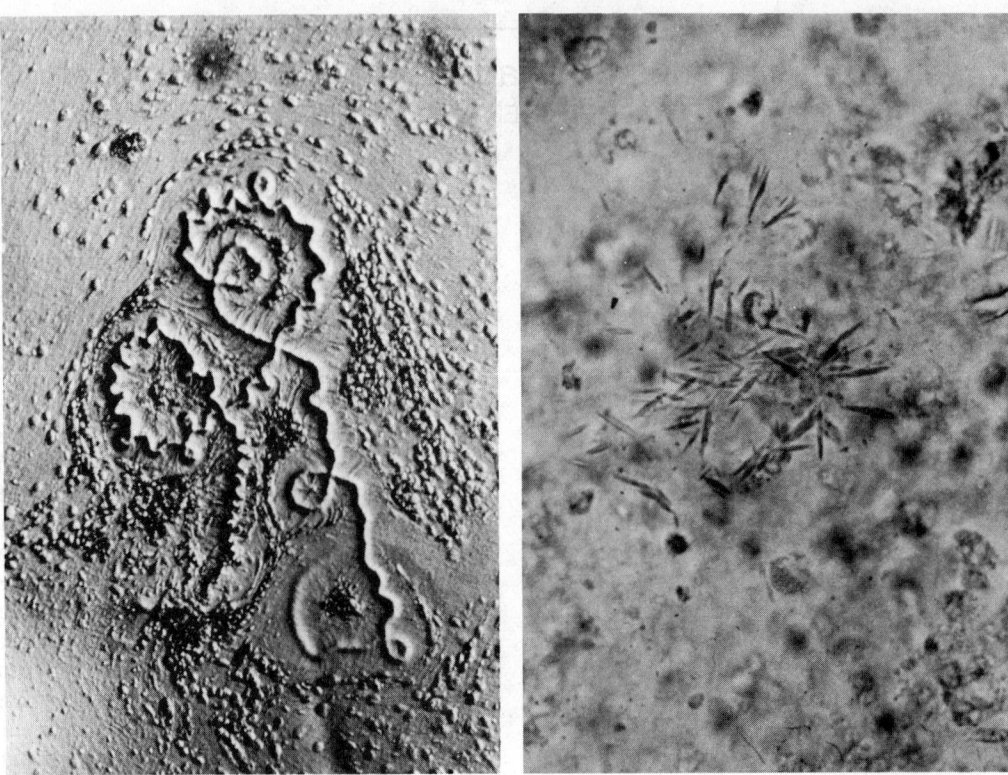

FIGURE 32–1. Left: A fully developed Curschmann spiral as seen in bronchial asthma (original magnification ×45). **Right:** Charcot-Leyden crystals. Their presence may be the only clue to the reversibility of airway obstruction (original magnification ×65). [From Epstein, R.L. Annals of Internal Medicine, 77:259, 1972, with permission.]

sputum composed predominantly of neutrophils correlates with the presence of bacterial infection, with 85 percent of such specimens showing pathogenic organisms on culture. A specimen containing a predominance of neutrophils should be gram-stained for identification of bacteria. Predominance of a specific organism, especially when bacteria are seen within polymorphonuclear leukocytes, may be used as a generally reliable guide for the selection of antibiotics in patients suspected of having pneumonia. On rare occasions the discovery of macrophages filled with large globules of fat in a patient with an unexplained infiltrate gives the only clue to the diagnosis of lipid pneumonia, and may obviate the need for thoracotomy. The presence of lipid is confirmed by Sudan III stain of the sputum. When carcinoma of the bronchus is present, cytologic study with special stains will reveal malignant cells in the majority of cases.

INTERPRETATION OF BLOOD IN THE SPUTUM

Blood-streaked sputum is an occasional occurrence in acute bronchitis, pneumonia, and other forms of bronchopulmonary suppuration. When not readily at-

tributable to one of these conditions, or when bleeding is persistent or recurrent, full investigation, including bronchoscopy, is warranted. Slight but persistent bleeding is most suggestive of bronchial carcinoma, while recurrent episodes of minor hemoptysis are more common in bronchiectasis, endobronchial tuberculosis, and mitral stenosis. Production of larger amounts of blood suggests pulmonary infarction, bleeding within a tuberculous cavity, or upper-lobe (dry) bronchiectasis. Expectoration of clots may be seen with pulmonary infarction. Care must be taken in evaluating the history of hemoptysis to be certain that the point of bleeding is not in the nose or the nasopharynx, with secondary aspiration of blood.

EVALUATION OF DYSPNEA

Shortness of breath, either during exercise or rest, is a common manifestation of many forms of pulmonary and cardiovascular disease. It denotes the patient's awareness of respiratory effort which is excessive for his level of physical activity. The neural pathways involved in the production of dyspnea are not completely understood, and no single mechanism has yet been proposed which is able to account satisfactorily for all the clinical situations in which dyspnea may be experienced.

In patients with pulmonary disease, the presence of dyspnea is closely related to abnormalities in the mechanics of breathing. There is a good correlation between the level of inspiratory work and dyspnea. Increased inspiratory work and dyspnea are found in conditions where the lungs or thorax are stiffer than normal, such as pulmonary fibrosis, because the inspiratory muscles have to develop greater tension to produce the same tidal volume. When the thoracic volume is abnormally large, as in emphysema and acute asthma, greater inspiratory muscle tension is required to produce the tidal volume. Resistance to airflow is so high at normal lung volumes that the patient breathes near his maximum inspiratory level and is using accessory inspiratory muscles. The scalenes and sternocleidomastoids do not normally participate in quiet breathing but elevate the rib cage on maximal inspiration. It has been shown that the presence of dyspnea is highly correlated with the retraction of the sternocleidomastoid muscles in the acute asthmatic attack. In emphysema, loss of elastic recoil results in a large lung volume so that accessory muscles are used during ordinary breathing at rest.

The neural pathway by which dyspnea is sensed may begin in the respiratory muscles themselves. It has been suggested that whenever the length-tension relations of the respiratory muscles are inappropriate for the task required, neural traffic reaching the central nervous system from the muscles results in the sensation of dyspnea.[32] Muscle spindles are considered the most likely site where the inappropriate length-tension is sensed.

Neural receptors within the lungs also are likely to be of great importance in dyspnea. J receptors are nonmyelinated vagal nerve endings in the interstitial space between pulmonary capillaries and alveoli.[44] When stimulated, they cause hyperpnea and a number of somatic and visceral reflex effects which decrease muscular activity during exercise. They are inactive during normal breathing, but are stimulated by pulmonary congestion and edema. It is believed that the J receptors are stimulated by the presence of pulmonary capillary hypertension and interstitial edema and that this mechanism is of paramount importance in the sensation of dyspnea associated with left ventricular failure. A similar mechanism explains orthopnea, in which these receptors are activated by increased congestion of the lungs which occurs in the supine posture. The J receptors are also stimulated by pulmonary emboli and inflammation. Some of the

dyspnea in restrictive pulmonary disease associated with stiff lungs may well be related to the excess stimulation of nerve endings within the interstitial spaces.

The level of blood gases does not appear to be directly related to the production of dyspnea. The blood gases, however, do affect the level of ventilation and are thus indirectly of great importance. The limitation of muscular exercise in the normal person at high altitude is certainly in part related to the greater ventilatory stimulus from hypoxia, for maximal exercise at any altitude is reached at an approximately equivalent level of ventilation. Muscular exercise in the patient with serious pulmonary insufficiency is likely to be limited by the sensation of dyspnea resulting from an inappropriately high degree of respiratory work. Therefore, prevention of the ventilatory stimulus from a decrease in arterial oxygen tension by increasing the level of inspired oxygen concentration allows the patient to perform a greater degree of muscular exercise at the same ventilation.

The ratio between how much a patient breathes and how much he is able to breathe is roughly related to the presence of dyspnea. When the minute ventilation becomes more than 30 percent of the maximum voluntary ventilation dyspnea is a frequent symptom. Thus, dyspnea can be viewed as an imbalance between the ventilatory stimulus and the capacity to respond to the stimulus. In the patient with pure left ventricular failure, the prime cause of the dyspnea is the increased neural stimulus from the congestion, although the congestion does cause some increase in stiffening of the lungs. The decrease in dyspnea on assuming the upright posture is probably related to the decrease in the stimulus. In the patient with asthma or emphysema, the dyspnea is primarily related to the reduced capacity to respond to the ventilatory stimulus. The dyspnea can be decreased by improving mechanical function, e.g., bronchodilators, or decreasing the ventilatory stimulus, e.g., improving the level of oxygenation.

The way in which the complaint of dyspnea is described may have diagnostic value. Most patients with obstruction of the airways recognize that their greatest difficulty consists of moving air in and out of the lungs. In contrast, patients with diffuse fibrosis or infiltrative disease complain of "breathing hard" on slight exertion and appear to experience sensations that would be normal for a much higher level of exercise. Some of these patients, however, and many patients with either pulmonary vascular disease, heart disease, or weakness of the muscles of respiration describe a sense of suffocation that appears to be qualitatively different from the sensations described above.

People frequently have considerable difficulty in describing their subjective sensations accurately and may use the term "shortness of breath" when the difficulty is actually pain on attempted deep inspiration, coughing which is triggered by attempts at hyperventilation, or even an abnormal degree of fatigue which occurs with muscular exercise. In some patients, anxiety over real or imagined disease of the heart or the lungs may result in an abnormal awareness of breathing which the patient perceives as shortness of breath. Such patients commonly manifest deep sighing respirations.

EVALUATION OF PHYSICAL SIGNS

Inspection, palpation, percussion, and auscultation are used to gain information about both anatomic and physiologic abnormalities of the lungs. Careful physical examination may provide information that could not be deduced from x-ray study. Recognition of the presence of generalized airway obstruction is a good example. Auscultation may reveal a localized rhonchus produced by a small endobronchial tumor, may identify the late inspiratory crackles of early pulmonary congestion, or may provide evidence of pleural involvement in the form of a friction rub when x-ray changes are not apparent.

PERCUSSION
Impaired resonance (dullness to percussion) results whenever something other than air-filled lung lies directly beneath the chest wall. Common causes are fluid in the pleural space, fibrous thickening of the pleura, consolidation or atelectasis of the lung, and a large peripherally located mass in the lung. A truly flat percussion note at one lung base usually signifies a large pleural effusion or elevation of the diaphragm. Increased resonance may be generalized when the lungs are hyperinflated (as in emphysema) and may be localized to one side over a pneumothorax or a large bullous lesion.

BREATH SOUNDS
Normal inspiratory breath sounds are produced by turbulent flow within airways down to the size of subsegmental bronchi, and may be heard at the open mouth as random noise which covers a wide frequency spectrum. These sounds vary in intensity with rate of airflow, and are abnormally loud when medium-sized airways are narrowed, as in asthma and bronchitis. As the sounds are transmitted through normal lung to the chest wall, most of the high frequency components are attenuated; the resulting sound heard through the stethoscope is termed *vesicular breathing*. When lung parenchyma and chest wall are normal, differences in intensity of vesicular sounds at the chest wall roughly reflect regional differences in ventilation. A local decrease in intensity may also result from impaired transmission. Pleural effusion, pleural thickening, and pneumothorax are examples of this and result in distant or absent breath sounds. An abnormal increase in intensity of breath sounds is always accompanied by a change in their character, which may range from a slight harshness of quality to fully developed bronchial breathing. These changes are due to increased transmission of the higher-frequency components of breath sounds originating in the larger airways. Bronchial breathing may be heard over consolidated, atelectatic, or compressed lung, provided the airway to this portion of the lung remains patent. Similar changes may be heard over extensively damaged lung in tuberculosis, bronchiectasis, and various forms of chronic pulmonary fibrosis.

VOICE SOUNDS
Transmission of spoken or whispered voice sounds to the chest wall may also be altered by the presence of disease. In many instances, changes in voice sounds may be more readily appreciated than the corresponding alterations in breath sounds, especially when the latter are difficult to hear because of obesity, a noisy environment, or other factors. Distant or inaudible sounds are produced by large pleural effusions, pneumothorax, and bronchial occlusion. Increased transmission of voice sounds is associated with a change in their character so that they assume a higher pitched, less muffled quality than normal and often permit distinct recognition of the words spoken. This is called bronchophony and is heard over areas of consolidation, infarction, atelectasis, or compression of lung. In its extreme form (egophony) the spoken words assume a nasal or bleating quality and the sound *ee* is heard through the stethoscope as *ay*. This sound is most common when solidified lung and pleural fluid are both present but may be heard over an uncomplicated lobar pneumonia or pulmonary infarction. Transmission of whispered voice sounds with abnormal clarity (whispered pectoriloquy) has the same significance as bronchophony.

ADVENTITIOUS SOUNDS
Much confusion in the reporting and interpretation of physical findings has resulted from the multiplicity of terms currently used to describe adventitious lung

sounds. Forgacs[36] has presented convincing arguments for referring to all the common abnormal sounds as either *crackles* or *wheezes*.

Crackles

Crackles are nonmusical individual clicking sounds often referred to as rales or crepitations. Each explosive sound is produced by the sudden equalization of pressure which follows the delayed opening of a medium or small airway in an abnormally deflated area of lung. When crackles occur only during the first half of inspiration they are generally a manifestation of severe obstructive pulmonary disease. Crackling heard entirely or predominantly during late inspiration is characteristic of fibrosing alveolitis, areas of lung contracted by fibrosis or atelectasis, and lung stiffened by pneumonia or the effects of interstitial congestion due to heart failure. In any generalized process, the less-distended dependent lung is most likely to produce crackles, which are therefore heard at the bases when the patient is erect. A few basilar end-inspiratory crackles are normally present after prolonged shallow breathing, but are abolished by a few deep breaths. A pleural friction rub, although classified as crackling, is usually recognizable as a coarse, grating or leathery sound in late inspiration and early expiration, localized low in the axilla or over the lung base posteriorly. Low-pitched discontinuous sounds may be produced by exudate within the large airways; these sounds show considerable variation from breath to breath, and are often abolished by coughing.

Wheezes

Wheezing refers to musical sounds heard either at the mouth or through the stethoscope. When low-pitched, they are sometimes called rhonchi. Studies have shown that these sounds are generated by the vibratory motion of airway closure, not by the vibration of an air column, and that there is no correlation between pitch and airway caliber. Only medium and large airways can produce these sounds. Wheezing which occurs at less than maximal expiratory flow denotes airway obstruction, and is characteristic of asthma and bronchitis.

CHEST ROENTGENOGRAPHY[39]

Posteroanterior (PA) and lateral chest roentgenograms should be obtained in any patient in whom pulmonary disease is suspected. These views constitute the basic diagnostic tool of the chest physician. The lateral projection is important because it permits visualization of lung concealed by the heart shadow and often allows precise localization of abnormal shadows seen on the PA view.

Interpretation of chest roentgenograms requires knowledge of the normal roentgen anatomy of the thorax and an ability to recognize and analyze deviations from the normal. This ability is developed through experience gained by the orderly and detailed study of many normal and abnormal films.

It is important to recognize the limitations imposed by technically suboptimal films and to repeat the examination whenever necessary. If standard views of good quality do not provide an adequate definition of the gross anatomy of an abnormal finding, additional views or special examinations may be useful.

OBLIQUE VIEWS

The oblique views are sometimes helpful in localizing a lesion and in separating a parenchymal density from overlying structures. They are also used in evaluating heart chamber size, heart valve calcification, and in separating vascular structures from mediastinal or parenchymal masses. Minimal oblique views are frequently more helpful than the standard 45° oblique films.

LATERAL DECUBITUS (RECUMBENT) VIEWS

These are used most often to demonstrate the presence of small pleural effusions and to determine if pleural fluid is loculated. On a decubitus film, free fluid runs up the dependent chest wall or layers along the mediastinum. Loculated accumulations may change shape slightly but do not change position. Free fluid in the lower hemithorax frequently shifts so that the underlying lung and pleura previously obscured by the fluid can be visualized, allowing the differentiation of effusions secondary to parenchymal infiltrates (parapneumonic effusions) from primary pleural disease. Decubitus views may aid in outlining the confines of a cavity, demonstrating air-fluid levels within cavities and differentiating pyopneumothorax from large lung abscesses.

LORDOTIC VIEW

This view projects the clavicles and first ribs above the lung, allowing the apices to be better evaluated without the clutter of overlying bony structures. The lordotic view is also extremely helpful in confirming middle lobe and lingular disease which is poorly demonstrated on routine PA and lateral views because it increases the depth of the right middle lobe and lingula projected on the film. In the lordotic position, anterior lesions are projected upward, and posterior lesions are projected downward. This effect is useful in localizing lesions seen on the PA view but inadequately identified on lateral or oblique views.

EXPIRATORY FILM

A small pneumothorax is frequently seen only on a film taken during full expiration. Superimposed inspiratory and expiratory films may be used to evaluate lack of diaphragmatic movement such as that which occurs with air trapping in empnysema or with neuromuscular disease. Unilateral hyperinflation secondary to the ball-valve effect of an endobronchial tumor or aspirated foreign body can be detected by inspiratory and expiratory films. The mediastinum shifts away from the side of the lesion because the affected lung cannot empty normally during expiration.

Compressible vascular structures such as an enlarged azygous vein and an arteriovenous malformation may be differentiated from mass lesions by a film taken during a Valsalva maneuver. The increased intrathoracic pressure causes the vascular structures to collapse.

TOMOGRAPHY

Tomography is one of the most valuable special x-ray studies available for the study of pulmonary lesions. It should be used whenever there is a question in interpretation or identification of an abnormality if the problem cannot be resolved by simpler techniques. Tomograms may demonstrate cavities masked by overlying infiltrates or bones, and allows better serial evaluation of known cavities. Fungus balls and irregularities within the walls of cavities are identified more clearly with tomograms. Calcifications within a pulmonary nodule and air bronchograms within pulmonary infiltrates frequently are defined by tomography when they are only suspected on routine views. In patients with extrapulmonary carcinoma and a pulmonary nodule, tomography may reveal multiple unsuspected metastatic lung lesions. Other key information supplied by tomography includes evaluation of normal and abnormal pulmonary vessels, detection of hilar masses and nodes, and demonstration of postintubation tracheal stenosis.

COMPUTED TOMOGRAPHY (CT)

CT examinations of the chest should not be requested indiscriminately, but should be used to resolve specific problems which are not clarified by routine examinations. Since CT can identify *pulmonary nodules* with greater sensitivity than regular tomograms, it is useful when the likelihood of small tumor metastases is high such as in the patient with melanoma or the patient with an apparently single nodule and a known primary tumor elsewhere. CT also permits quantitative measurement of the radiodensity of a small nodule, allowing very dense nodules to be recognized as granulomas even when calcification is not visible. *Mediastinal masses* can often be seen with maximum clarity in axial sections, and can readily be distinguished from vascular structures if CT examination is performed after intravenous injection of contrast material. *Pleural disease* is also more reliably distinguished from parenchymal disease by CT, which has proven useful in patients with pneumonia in whom complicating pleural effusion or empyema is suspected.

FLUOROSCOPY

Chest fluoroscopy delivers considerably more radiation than is required for exposure of films and should be used only when necessary. It is the best method for demonstrating immobility or paralysis of a diaphragm. During a rapid inspiratory sniff, the chest wall is fixed and the normal diaphragm descends; a paralyzed diaphragm will move upward because of the increased intra-abdominal pressure caused by descent of the diaphragm on the other side. Fluoroscopic examination with the application of a metallic marker is often helpful in choosing the proper location for withdrawal of fluid from a loculated pleural effusion or empyema.

BRONCHOGRAPHY AND TRACHEOGRAPHY

Bronchographic visualization of the tracheobronchial tree is less frequently used than it once was. This is partially because fiberoptic bronchoscopy has increased the area available to direct visualization and partially because the disease most definitively diagnosed by bronchography, i.e., bronchiectasis, is becoming relatively uncommon.[31] Untoward reactions to bronchographic media which contain organic iodine compounds are relatively common.

Indications for the use of bronchography are enumerated in Table 32-1.[35] The most frequent of these are hemoptysis with negative bronchoscopic studies and repeated episodes of pneumonia involving the same lobe or segments. Bronchography should be performed in a patient with suspected bronchiectasis only if surgical intervention is being seriously considered. It is not necessary to document the presence of bronchiectasis or establish its extent unless a period of conservative therapy has failed to control the clinical manifestations of the disease. However, if bronchogenic carcinoma is suspected, bronchography should be performed promptly. An area of poorly resolving pneumonia or an asymptomatic unilateral in-

TABLE 32-1
Indications for Bronchography

1. Recurrent hemoptysis of unknown cause with negative fiberoptic bronchoscopy
2. Persistent or changed pattern of cough with suspicious sputum cytology and negative bronchoscopy
3. Repeated episodes of pneumonitis involving the same lobe or segments
4. Persistent localized infiltrate of undetermined cause
5. Differential diagnosis of persistent cavity, cyst, or bronchopleural fistula

filtrate may be investigated by selective bronchography. Inflammatory disease results in dilated bronchi leading up to and entering the lesion, while carcinoma causes bronchial obstruction.[43] A characteristic bronchographic appearance may therefore allow careful observation rather than diagnostic thoracotomy. Chronically active inflammatory cavities may occasionally be better visualized after instillation of bronchographic contrast material. Although contrast material will occasionally pass from a bronchus into the pleural space and reveal the presence of a bronchopleural fistula, injection of dye into the pleural space is more likely to demonstrate such a fistula.

Bronchography for the diagnosis of bronchiectasis should not be performed for at least six weeks after recovery from an episode of pneumonia, since acute and reversible changes indistinguishable from cylindrical bronchiectasis may be seen. Markedly impaired pulmonary function and poorly compensated heart failure are contraindications to bronchographic study.

With the increased frequency of tracheal intubation and resulting tracheal stenosis, contrast visualization of the upper airway is being performed more frequently than standard bronchography.[46] Since tracheal obstruction may be dynamic and occur only on inspiration or expiration, all tracheography should be performed using the cine technique. Tantalum powder is the agent best suited for this type of study because of its ability to coat the tracheal mucosa and show fine detail without obstructing the airway. It is currently an investigational drug and is unavailable for general clinical use.

RADIOISOTOPE STUDIES

Detection of regional abnormalities in the distribution of pulmonary blood flow and ventilation can be accomplished by radioisotope scanning of the lungs.[48] Perfusion scans are made with a linear scanner or a "gamma camera" after intravenous injection of

^{99m}Tc-labeled microspheres; anterior, posterior, and both lateral views should be obtained and interpreted in conjunction with a chest radiograph taken at the same time. More recently oblique projections have been shown to increase the specificity of this test. Segmental defects unaccompanied by corresponding infiltrate on the chest film are strong evidence of pulmonary embolism.[28] If underlying pulmonary parenchymal disease, such as emphysema, is responsible for the defect, a ventilation scan using ^{133}Xe will show a filling defect in the same area. When widespread parenchymal disease is present, the absence of characteristic changes on ventilation and perfusion scans does not exclude pulmonary embolism. In addition, nonsegmental patchy filling defects may be produced by pulmonary emboli, and pulmonary arteriography may be required for confirmation of the diagnosis. Serial lung scans are useful in following the patient with pulmonary embolism. This problem is discussed further in Chapter 24.

Perfusion scans are useful in the evaluation of resectability of bronchogenic carcinoma.[29] A large area of reduced blood flow on the affected side indicates that involvement of the hilar vessels is likely, and when the entire lung is unperfused the chance of a successful resection is small.

In the patient with impaired pulmonary function who requires thoracotomy and resection of lung tissue, scans permit prediction of the effect of operation on pulmonary function, and may be critical in establishing operability.[30]

ULTRASOUND

Echo studies appear to have their greatest usefulness in localizing small areas of effusion or empyema for thoracentesis. They are not entirely reliable in distinguishing solid from liquid subpleural material, and they will not detect lesions separated from the chest wall by aerated lung.

PULMONARY FUNCTION STUDIES

Diseases that produce significant anatomic alterations in the pulmonary parenchyma or disturbances in the mechanical operation of the chest wall result in abnormalities of pulmonary function. Laboratory measurements of these derangements are clinically useful both in the diagnosis and management of chest disease.[49]

The most useful pulmonary function tests include

measurements of forced expiration (spirometry), diffusing capacity, and arterial blood gases. Measurements of alveolar ventilation, dead space, airway resistance, forced inspiratory flows, elastic recoil pressure, percent right-to-left shunt and pulmonary artery pressure may be helpful in selected cases. Exercise tolerance tests with or without supplemental oxygen are useful in the evaluation of disability and in assessing the need for ambulatory oxygen therapy. Table 32–2 shows examples of the application of physiologic testing in specific clinical problems.

SPIROMETRY

Abnormalities of pulmonary mechanics are commonly evaluated by means of spirometry, i.e., vital capacity, one or more parameters of airflow during forced expiration, and maximal voluntary ventilation. Vital capacity is defined as the largest volume of air which the patient can exhale voluntarily, beginning with the lungs fully inflated. Weakness, pain on deep breathing, poor comprehension, or lack of cooperation on the part of the patient may result in an underestimate of the vital capacity. The result is compared either with previous measurements made on the same patient or with average normal values based on sex, age, and height. Because of normal variation, an isolated measurement of vital capacity can be considered abnormal only when it is less than 85 percent of the predicted value, and then only if the patient makes an optimal effort. Reduction in vital capacity is common is association with airway obstruction of any cause. In the absence of obstruction a small vital capacity usually indicates that the total lung capacity is also reduced and that a restrictive ventilatory defect is present. The restriction may be secondary to interstitial fibrosis, pleural or parenchymal space-occupying lesions, chest wall deformities, or neuromuscular disease. Following lobectomy or pneumonectomy, the remaining lung expands, leaving the restrictive defect somewhat less than might be expected.

Spirometer tracings made during forced expiration (forced expirograms) are the most convenient indirect method of assessing the presence and severity of an obstructive ventilatory defect. A normal forced expirogram is very steep in its initial portion, is smoothly curved, and reaches a plateau in 3 to 6 seconds (Fig. 32–2). In the presence of airway obstruction, flow rates are reduced, and the tracing may continue to move slowly toward a plateau even after many seconds of expiration. No single number can characterize the contour of a forced expirogram, and a variety of parameters derived from this curve have been used to quantitate airway obstruction. The one-

---

┌─ **TABLE 32–2** ─
Examples of Application of Pulmonary Function Testing

Clinical Problem	Suggested Studies	Results and Comments
Wheezing or other clinical evidence of airway obstruction	Spirometry	Indices of expiratory flow reduced. Confirms and quantifies severity of obstruction. Immediate improvement after bronchodilator is typically seen with asthma.
	Lung volumes (He or N_2)	Increased in emphysema and asthma. May be normal in chronic bronchitis and reduced in bronchiectasis. Markedly elevated RV suggestive of pulmonary emphysema
	Diffusing capacity	Normal in asthma, normal or slightly reduced in bronchitis, low in emphysema
	Airway resistance	High in most forms of obstructive pulmonary disease, but may be normal in emphysema.
	Elastic recoil pressure	Low in uncomplicated emphysema, normal in bronchitis, asthma
Severe obstructive airway disease; suspected respiratory failure	Arterial blood	High Pco_2 indicates hypoventilation. O_2 saturation below 80 percent indicates need for oxygen therapy. Rising Pco_2 may indicate need for respirator

TABLE 32-2 (cont.)

Clinical Problem	Suggested Studies	Results and Comments
Status asthmaticus	Arterial blood	Pco_2 over 50 mm Hg usually indicates very severe impairment and need for intensive supervision
	Forced vital capacity	Excellent method for following course of attack
Evaluation of operative risk	Spirometry	Severity of obstruction related to operative risk
	Arterial blood	Elevated Pco_2 means high anesthesia risk
	Exercise ability	Inability to perform mild exercise usually correlates with high risk
Unexplained coma	Arterial blood	High Pco_2 may explain coma. Normal Pco_2 rules out hypoventilation as cause of coma
Diffuse pulmonary infiltration or fibrosis	Spirometry	Reduced vital capacity suggests stiff lung, provides baseline for evaluation of course or treatment
	Diffusing capacity	Degree of reduction indicates extent of damage to lung. Baseline for treatment
	Arterial blood	May be minimally reduced early with profound hypoxia in severe fibrosis
Pulmonary hypertension	Spirometry	Usually little loss of vital capacity in multiple emboli or primary pulmonary hypertension, marked loss in diffuse fibrosis
	Diffusing capacity	Low in diffuse fibrosis; normal or only slightly reduced value suggests pulmonary vascular disease
	Arterial blood	Recurrent small to medium sized pulmonary emboli unlikely with normal arterial oxygen tension
Polycythemia	Arterial blood	Low Po_2 and saturation suggest secondary polycythemia
Mitral stenosis	Diffusing capacity	Severe reduction suggests irreversible damage to lung
	Postexercise vital capacity	Useful in following course of disease
Suspected scleroderma with normal x-ray	Spirometry	Early restrictive ventilatory defect
	Diffusing capacity, compliance	Low values support diagnosis
High carbon dioxide combining power	Arterial blood	Normal Pco_2 with high pH and bicarbonate indicates metabolic alkalosis Pco_2 above 55 indicates compensated respiratory acidosis unless pH very high
Dyspnea without clinical signs of heart or lung disease	Spirometry and diffusing capacity	Lung disease as cause of dyspnea unlikely with normal spirograms and diffusing capacity
	Arterial blood	May be normal with significant disease. Abnormality suggests underlying pathology

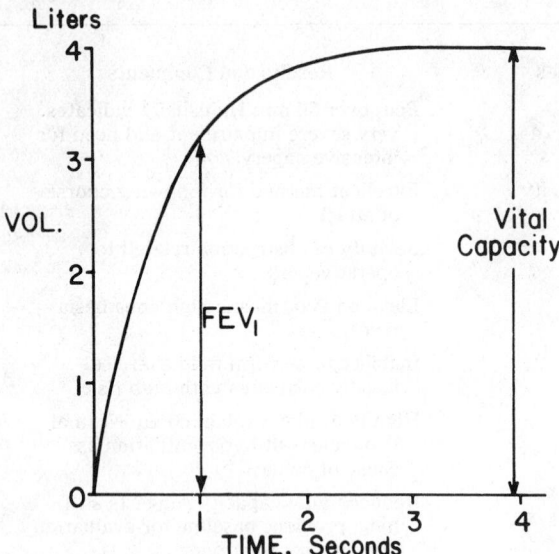

FIGURE 32–2. The normal forced expirogram. Volume in the spirometer is plotted against time. The vital capacity (VC) is represented by the total volume expired. One-second forced expiratory volume (FEV 1) is the volume expired during the first second.

second forced expiratory volume (FEV_1), expressed in liters or in percent of the measured vital capacity (FEV_1 percent) is the most convenient and useful measurement for evaluating prolonged expiration. Even in the presence of a restrictive ventilatory defect, the FEV will remain 78 to 85 percent of the vital capacity, provided the airways are not obstructed and flow is normal relative to volume.

The maximum voluntary ventilation (MVV) is the largest minute volume a patient can achieve by hyperventilation. Direct measurement of MVV is arduous for the patient, and the results are much more strongly affected by poor effort or by patient fatigue than are forced expirograms. A marked reduction in MVV is usually due to airway obstruction, but the result is also affected by a restrictive ventilatory defect. For the same degree of restriction, a neuromuscular disease will result in a greater reduction of MVV. An indirect estimate of MVV may be obtained by multiplying the FEV_1 in liters by a factor of 35.

In patients with airway obstruction, it is often of value to repeat the spirometric measurements after administration of nebulized bronchodilator since significant improvement indicates that at least part of the obstructive ventilatory defect is reversible. Serial determinations following a period of aggressive medical and physical therapy may show improvement not

seen immediately after bronchodilator administration.

COMPLIANCE AND AIRWAY RESISTANCE

More direct methods than those just discussed are available for measuring the mechanical properties of the lungs. Pulmonary compliance, defined as the number of liters change in static lung volume produced by a 1 cm H_2O change in transpulmonary (alveolar minus intrapleural) pressure, is a measure of the distensibility of the lungs. The measurement of transpulmonary (elastic recoil) pressure at functional residual capacity and at full lung inflation may be useful in the diagnosis of several diseases. For example, there is a loss of recoil in emphysema and an increase in recoil in interstitial fibrosis.

Airway resistance is the pressure difference in cm H_2O between alveoli and mouth required to produce an inspiratory or expiratory flow rate of 1 liter per second. These studies are technically much more complex than spirometry and are seldom available on a routine basis, but are valuable investigative tools and are occasionally helpful in an individual clinical problem.

LUNG VOLUMES

Functional residual capacity (FRC) may be measured by equilibration of air in the lungs with an insoluble gas such as helium, or by measuring the total amount of nitrogen washed out of the lungs during the breathing of pure oxygen. Estimates of the evenness of distribution of inspired gas may be obtained from the time it takes to achieve equilibration during lung volume measurements. Total lung capacity (TLC) is the total volume of air in the lungs at full inflation, and residual volume (RV) is the volume of air remaining in the lungs after a complete expiration. Measurements using these methods are not reliable in the presence of severe airway obstruction and abnormal distribution of inspired air since they may underestimate true lung volume. A more accurate way of determining FRC is by plethysmography.[41] An increase in RV is seen with airway obstruction of any cause, but is most marked in emphysema or during an acute attack of asthma. Reductions in TLC are seen with significant pulmonary fibrosis resulting from sarcoidosis, scleroderma or fibrosing alveolitis, neuromuscular disease, skeletal deformities, and space-occupying lesions within the chest.

DIFFUSING CAPACITY

The diffusing capacity is measured with carbon monoxide as the test gas, and is expressed in ml uptake per minute per mm Hg partial pressure difference across the alveolocapillary membrane. Various procedures have been used for determining the rate of carbon monoxide uptake and alveolar carbon monoxide concentration in order to permit calculation of the diffusing capacity. Perhaps the greatest clinical usefulness of diffusion measurements is in the group of diffuse parenchymal diseases which produce more profound abnormalities in gas exchange than in pulmonary mechanics (Chap. 34). Interstitial fibrosis even in the presence of minimal x-ray abnormality is commonly associated with a reduction in diffusing capacity. Diffusion measurements are also useful in the differentiation of emphysema from bronchitis and asthma. Pure chronic bronchitis and asthma cause little or no reduction in diffusing capacity, whereas emphysema is characterized by a significant decrease in DL_{co} (See Chap. 35). The presence of pulmonary hypertension and cor pulmonale correlates well with gross reduction in the diffusing capacity in both emphysema and in diffuse interstitial disease. The diffusing capacity for carbon monoxide may remain nearly normal in pulmonary vascular lesions, such as multiple pulmonary emboli, and may therefore occasionally be useful in differential diagnosis. In the interpretation of diffusion measurements it is important to bear in mind that a low diffusing capacity almost always results from loss of functioning alveolocapillary surface area rather than from thickening of alveolar walls.

ARTERIAL BLOOD GAS STUDIES

Measurements of oxygen tension, CO_2 tension, and pH of arterial blood have proven to be of great usefulness in the diagnosis and therapy of a wide variety of clinical conditions. From these measurements approximate values of bicarbonate and oxygen saturation can be calculated. A single arterial blood study affords a complete picture of the acid-base status of the patient and is useful in a variety of renal and metabolic problems.

The arterial Pco_2 provides the best means of determining the adequacy of alveolar ventilation. Direct measurement of a normal total minute ventilation does not mean that alveolar ventilation is adequate, since dead space ventilation may be greatly increased in patients with extensive lung disease.

When airway obstruction is severe, patients may develop acute or chronic carbon dioxide retention. This is less commonly seen with pure emphysema until the terminal phase of the disease. In the presence of ventilatory failure an elevated carbon dioxide tension should alert the clinician to the hazard of sedative or narcotic administration.

Although the oxygen saturation of arterial blood provides a useful indication of the need for therapeutic oxygen administration, the oxygen tension is a more sensitive indicator of gas transfer abnormality in the lung. Minor degrees (10 to 20 mm Hg) of reduction in oxygen tension are common in bronchitis, bronchiectasis, emphysema, atelectasis, pneumonia, the early stages of many diffuse pulmonary lesions, and a host of other conditions in which there is abnormal distribution of ventilation relative to blood flow ($\dot{V}/\dot{Q}$ abnormality). Reduction in oxygen tension may also result from overall alveolar hypoventilation or from abnormal anatomic right-to-left shunt. Rarely is it possible to draw any conclusion regarding the diffusing capacity of the lungs from a single arterial blood determination.

Single or serial arterial blood determinations have their greatest usefulness in the assessment and management of respiratory failure, in the evaluation of acid-base disorders, in the differential diagnosis of polycythemia, and as a part of more elaborate studies for the quantitation of ventilation and perfusion abnormalities.

PHYSIOLOGIC DEAD SPACE AND VENOUS ADMIXTURE-LIKE EFFECT ($\dot{V}/\dot{Q}$ Abnormalities)

When arterial blood samples are drawn in conjunction with the collection and analysis of expired air, physiologic dead space and venous-admixture-like-effect may be calculated. Physiologic dead space is the portion of each inspiration that fails to take part in gas exchange in the lung. It includes the anatomic dead space (volume of the conducting airways) and a portion of the inspired air which ventilates underperfused or nonperfused alveoli (high $\dot{V}/\dot{Q}$ ratio). Abnormally large values may be found in any disease characterized by nonuniform involvement of the lung, especially those in which vascular occlusion or obliteration is a feature. Venous-admixture-like-effect is the portion of cardiac output which is effectively shunted from right to left because of blood flow through poorly ventilated areas of lung (low $\dot{V}/\dot{Q}$ ratio). It is abnormally increased in a variety of lung diseases and, therefore, has little value in differential diagnosis.

If a patient is given 100 percent O_2 to breathe until all the nitrogen has been washed out of the lung, all alveoli will contain a high concentration of oxygen (Po_2 over 650 mm Hg), even those which are poorly ventilated. Under these circumstances, the effect on arterial blood of abnormal $\dot{V}/\dot{Q}$ ratios is abolished, and reduction in arterial Po_2 below a normal value of 600 mm Hg reflects perfusion of areas not in contact with alveolar air. Increased values of absolute shunt so calculated are commonly seen in pneumonia, severe interstitial fibrosis, pulmonary embolism, atelectasis, pulmonary AV fistula, and intracardiac right-to-left shunt.

THORACENTESIS

This technique is used in the evaluation of pleural effusion. Indications and interpretation of results are discussed in Chapter 38. It should be noted that thoracentesis involves some risk of injury to the lung and induction of pneumothorax, and they should be performed with close attention to proper technique.

BRONCHOSCOPY

The development of the flexible fiberoptic bronchoscope has greatly enhanced the capability of bronchoscopy, and has broadened the diagnostic and therapeutic indications for its use[40] (Table 32–3). The conventional rigid bronchoscope is excellent for removal of foreign bodies or tenacious secretions. The fiberoptic bronchoscope permits visualization of bronchial orifices to beyond the level of subsegmental bronchi. The optical system produces magnification of the image so that excellent detail is visible even in very small airways. The flexible shaft makes it ideally suited for patients with cervical spine abnormalities or displacement of the trachea. A number of brushes, curettes, and microbiopsy forceps devised for use with the fiberoptic bronchoscope have extended the range over which diagnostic information can be obtained. Under fluoroscopic guidance, these devices can be placed into a small lesion in the periphery of the lung.

The lowest risk is achieved when bronchoscopy is performed under topical anesthesia, which is satisfactory for most procedures. In anxious or uncooperative patients, or when a very lengthy procedure is required, general anesthesia is more satisfactory.

BIOPSY PROCEDURES

When a definitive diagnosis cannot be established by simpler means, it is often necessary to obtain tissue for microscopic examination. A wide variety of biopsy procedures are potentially useful in obtaining suitable tissue from the lung, bronchi, pleura or mediastinum, and it is important to select the procedure with the lowest risk and greatest likelihood of recovering material which will be diagnostic. Table 32–4 provides information regarding the selection of a specific biopsy procedure depending on the nature and location of the lesion.

TABLE 32–3

Indications for Bronchoscopy

Indication	Comments
Diagnostic	
Hemoptysis	Best performed when bleeding has almost stopped
Chronic unexplained cough	May be early manifestation of endobronchial tumor
Undiagnosed mass	Transbronchial biopsy may be performed
Delayed resolution of pneumonia	Excludes bronchial obstruction as cause
Localized atelectasis	Identify cause of bronchial obstruction if present
Evaluate operability in lung cancer	Extent of proximal endobronchial spread or peribronchial compression or fixation can be assessed
Positive sputum cytology with negative x-ray	Fiberoptic scope will permit localization of nearly all occult lung cancer
Lung abscess	Exclude bronchial obstruction, obtain material for culture
Tracheal extubation	Evaluate trauma to airway resulting from intubation
Therapeutic	
Control of hemorrhage	Endobronchial lesion may occasionally be cauterized
Removal of foreign body	Rigid bronchoscope preferred
Lobar atelectasis in patient on respirator	Aspiration of secretions through bronchoscope permits reexpansion
Lung abscess which drains poorly	Repeated endoscopy may promote drainage

---

BRONCHIAL BIOPSIES

During the course of diagnostic bronchoscopy with either rigid or fiberoptic instruments, any visible endobronchial lesion or abnormal-appearing area of bronchial mucosa will be biopsied. Various types of biopsy forceps are available for this purpose, and the biopsy may be performed under direct vision. Larger fragments of tissue can be obtained through the rigid bronchoscope, but various sized microforceps and curettes suitable for use with the fiberoptic instrument often yield satisfactory tissue specimens.[29] Biopsy of normal-appearing bronchial mucosa will sometimes provide histologic confirmation of the di-

TABLE 32-4
Nonthoracotomy Biopsy Techniques

Type of Lung Disease	Procedures	Indications
Diffuse parenchymal	Transcatheter bronchial brush biopsy	Most helpful in acute infections
	Bronchoscopy, open tubed or fiberoptic (FOB) with brushing, washing and biopsy	Best procedure with least risk for acute or chronic disease
	Needle biopsy (cutting)	Ability to tolerate pneumothorax. No pulmonary hypertension.
	Trephine air drill	Same as above. Bigger sample removed. Higher risk of pneumothorax.
	Mediastinoscopy	With hilar adenopathy
Localized	Pleural biopsy	With pleural effusion
Peripheral	Transcatheter bronchial brush biopsy or FOB with brushing and biopsy	Ability to visualize lesion in two planes on fluoroscopy. Excellent for cancer. Good for infectious infiltrates.
	Aspiration needle biopsy, cutting if aspiration unproductive	Obstructed bronchus preventing endoscopic diagnosis (common with larger lesions). Ability to visualize lesion in two planes. Denser lesions yield larger specimens.
Midlung	FOB with brushing, washing, and biopsy	Fluoroscope usually not necessary with FOB
	Mediastinoscopy	With lesions $\geq$ 3 cm in diameter or questionable hilar node involvement, or when tumor is known to be large cell undifferentiated carcinoma
Central	Rigid bronchoscopy, FOB on standby	Should yield diagnosis in almost all cases of epidermoid carcinoma
	Mediastinoscopy	Necessary for staging and determination of operability in all cases

agnosis in patients with pulmonary sarcoidosis. Biopsy of spurs proximal to the origin of a peripheral carcinoma is useful in establishing the presence or absence of mucosal and submucosal spread of the tumor.

BRUSH BIOPSY

This procedure, either under direct vision through the bronchoscope or under fluoroscopic guidance using a controllable catheter, is a very valuable technique because of the very low incidence of complications. Tissue fragments adhering to the stiff nylon brush may provide a specific diagnosis of infection, by smear or culture, or may permit a diagnosis of tumor on cytologic or histologic examination. If a localized lesion can be adequately seen in two projections under the fluoroscope, a brush biopsy can be obtained even when the lesion is too peripheral to be directly seen at fiberoptic bronchoscopy. The diagnostic yield from such biopsies is approximately 85 percent in bronchogenic carcinoma; a diagnosis of Hodgkin's disease,

Pneumocystis pneumonia, tuberculosis, or fungus infection can also be made by this technique.

TRANSBRONCHIAL LUNG BIOPSY

Tissue may be obtained through the bronchoscope by wedging a small biopsy forceps into the lung parenchyma.[27,38,45] In diffuse disease, lung tissue can be recovered in most instances, and is usually sufficient to provide a tissue diagnosis. In the case of a localized lesion in the periphery of the lung, fluoroscopic guidance will be required. Complications such as hemoptysis and pneumothorax are infrequent but occur more commonly with this technique than with simple bronchial brushing. The yield is substantially higher with transbronchial biopsy in most types of diffuse disease.

PLEURAL BIOPSY

Percutaneous needle biopsy of the pleura is a simple and safe procedure in the presence of pleural effusion, and is indicated whenever the etiology of an exudative effusion is not proven. This procedure is discussed further in Chapter 38. Open biopsy of the pleura by means of a limited thoracotomy will provide specimens of pleura when needle biopsy has failed and an etiologic diagnosis is mandatory.

PERCUTANEOUS LUNG BIOPSY

Biopsy through the chest wall under local anesthesia may be the procedure of choice for localized lesions near the pleural surface and in some patients with diffuse lung disease.[29] A plain needle for aspiration of tissue,[47] a cutting needle,[50] and a trephine air drill[33,37] have all been used for this purpose. In general, the aspiration technique should be tried for solid lesions, and the cutting needle used only if aspiration is not successful. The cutting needle or trephine will be necessary in patients with diffuse disease. An experienced operator may achieve a high percentage of definitive diagnoses in patients with malignancy or inflammatory disease. The chief complication is pneumothorax, which occurs in 30 percent of cases but requires insertion of a chest tube in only about 10 percent. Hemoptysis is common but is rarely serious, and intrapleural bleeding is rare.

MEDIASTINOSCOPY

Endoscopic examination of the mediastinum is performed under general anesthesia through a small skin incision at the suprasternal notch.[29] Visualization and biopsy of abnormal tissue in the area around the trachea, carina, and proximal right mainstem bronchus can be carried out. The left lower paratracheal and left mainstem bronchus area cannot be visualized by this technique. Risk of the procedure is little more than the risk associated with general anesthesia.

Mediastinoscopy is most useful in the evaluation of resectability in the patient with lung cancer. Positive nodes along the trachea or on the side opposite the primary lesion preclude resection for cure. In the case of positive lower mediastinal hilar nodes on the side of the primary, some surgeons will attempt resection if the lesion is a squamous carcinoma. Bronchogenic carcinoma presenting as a mass which is centrally located will show mediastinal node involvement in nearly half of all cases. Small cell carcinoma has an even higher rate of spread to mediastinal nodes, and mediastinoscopy is often required to establish a diagnosis. Since small cell carcinoma is not

a resectable lesion, mediastinoscopy is not indicated for staging when the cell type is already known. Peripherally located squamous and adenocarcinomas are less likely to involve mediastinal nodes than are centrally located primary tumors. Mediastinal involvement with large cell carcinoma is common regardless of the location of the primary. The routine use of mediastinoscopy prior to thoracotomy in patients with proven lung cancer which appears to be resectable will avoid unnecessary thoracotomy in almost all patients.

Mediastinoscopy is also useful in the diagnosis of sarcoidosis, tuberculosis, histoplasmosis, and Hodgkin's disease, since these conditions commonly involve mediastinal lymph nodes. This procedure has a very high yield in sarcoidosis, and should be considered when no skin lesions are present and peripheral lymph nodes appear uninvolved.[42] Mediastinoscopy has been useful in the staging of Hodgkin's disease when radiologic findings are inconclusive. Extrathoracic tumors may metastasize to the mediastinal nodes; mediastinoscopy in such cases may be the simplest procedure for demonstrating spread of the tumor.

Previous mediastinoscopy is one of the few firm contraindications to mediastinoscopy, since adhesions make an adequate dissection difficult or impossible. Superior vena cava obstruction is not a contraindication, but requires particular care in the initial incision and subcutaneous dissection. Other factors to be considered are those which increase the risk of general anesthesia, such as severe obstructive pulmonary disease or heart disease.

DIAGNOSTIC THORACOTOMY

In a significant number of patients with an undiagnosed pulmonary lesion, transbronchial or percutaneous lung biopsy may be unsuccessful or contraindicated. In this and certain other specific situations, open thoracotomy may be required for diagnosis.

The solitary peripheral nodule may be such a situation. When tumor seems likely on the basis of roentgenographic and clinical findings, excisional biopsy is usually called for. Frequently the density is too small or poorly seen for needle biopsy under fluoroscopy. A full posterolateral thoracotomy is usually performed, and the area in question examined under direct vision. Biopsies may be taken for frozen section; the extent of the disease can be accurately evaluated, and, if appropriate, definitive resection may be undertaken.

When a solitary nodule appears highly unlikely to represent a tumor, every effort should be made to establish a diagnosis short of thoracotomy. Percutaneous needle biopsy or transbronchial biopsy may succeed in proving such a lesion to be inflammatory.

Another common indication for open lung biopsy is in the patient with diffuse parenchymal lung disease which is progressive and symptomatic. Although transbronchial or percutaneous biopsies are frequently positive, they are subject to considerable sampling error, and may not provide a specimen which is fully representative of the disease process. When the process is acute and appears generalized, a lingular biopsy through a small anterior thoracotomy is a satisfactory procedure, and offers the advantages of low risk and minimal postthoracotomy discomfort. When there are multiple areas of involvement which appear by x-ray to differ in age or structure, the thoracotomy should permit inspection of a whole lung and biopsy of areas representing the most re-cently as well as the most severely involved, as well as an area of relatively normal-appearing lung.

A third situation in which open lung biopsy is preferred is in the patient with leukemia, lymphoma, or other systemic disease who develops an acute pulmonary infiltrate while on high-dose steroids and cytotoxic chemotherapeutic agents. In many of these patients it is essential that a definitive diagnosis be established without delay so that appropriate therapy may be instituted. Transbronchial or needle biopsy techniques occasionally provide too little tissue for frozen sections and may be found to be inadequate after the delay required for permanent sections. Many such patients will be found to have two or more complicating infections at the same time, and under these circumstances small biopsy samples may be seriously misleading. However, because of simplicity and low morbidity, transbronchial lung biopsy is usually attempted prior to diagnostic thoracotomy in the majority of immune compromised patients developing acute diffuse lung disease. Further discussion of this special problem will be found in Chapter 34.

CHAPTER 33
Localized Pulmonary Infiltration
E. JAMES BRITT, ROBERT A. WISE, AND JIMMIE T. SYLVESTER

INTRODUCTION

Localized pulmonary infiltrates are defined as radio-densities within the lung parenchyma which involve only a portion of the lung and which cannot be classified as mass lesions. The distinction between localized infiltrate and mass lesion is sometimes difficult and is based upon the more distinct borders and quasispherical shape of the latter. The causes of mass lesions (Chap. 37) should always be kept in mind in evaluating the etiology of an apparent localized pulmonary infiltrate. Orientation of this and many of the succeeding chapters of this section around roentgenographic findings rather than a symptom or a physical finding emphasizes the importance of the chest radiograph in the management of lung diseases. The chest radiograph may be obtained because of a symptom or physical finding or as a primary screening examination. The history and physical examination often must be interpreted in light of the chest film, rather than the other way around.

EVALUATION OF THE CHEST RADIOGRAPH

Because of the importance of the chest radiograph, physicians must learn to interpret it accurately. The following discussion describes an approach to interpretation which has proven practical. Although the discussion is oriented toward localized pulmonary infiltrates, many of the principles are generally applicable.[54]

The approach to interpretation should be systematic. First, the physician must judge the technical quality of the image; then, he must recognize the abnormality, characterize it, and search for ancillary radiographic signs.

The technically adequate chest film must be properly centered and exposed and free of motion artifact. Proper centering of the posteroanterior projection is assured by the central location of the posterior spinous processes between the heads of the clavicles. Technically similar images are essential when the chest radiograph is used to follow the course of a lung infiltrate.

Detection of subtle localized infiltrates may be accomplished by comparing the right and left intercostal spaces. This permits visualization of lung parenchyma free of overlying bone structure and also assures inspection of the entire lung from top to bottom. Close attention should be directed to the apices of the lung where the confluence of rib and clavicular shadows may obscure an infiltrate. Apical lordotic views which project the clavicles and first ribs above the lung may be necessary to elucidate further detail in this region. The retrocardiac area is difficult to evaluate due to the overlying heart shadow and the lack of contralateral symmetry. On the posteroanterior view, one should inspect this area for the presence of an *air bronchogram* (see below). In the lateral view, the lower vertebral bodies normally appear less dense than the upper vertebral bodies. Increasing density overlying the lower vertebral bodies is known as the *spine sign* and signifies the presence of an abnormally increased radiographic density in the lower lobes.

A radiodensity within the lung fields may be intrapulmonary or extrapulmonary. If the density can be seen completely surrounded by lung on both the posteroanterior and lateral views, it must be within the parenchyma. The presence of branching or linear air shadows within the density, an *air bronchogram*, is proof that the density is intrapulmonary. When the density abuts the pleural surface, the distinction between intrapulmonary and extrapulmonary location may be difficult. Specialized studies, such as ultrasonography or computerized axial tomography, may be necessary for a definitive answer.

If the abnormal density is determined to be an infiltrate within the parenchyma, precise anatomic localization within the lung may be helpful in determining the cause of the infiltrate. For example, reactivation tuberculosis commonly involves the apical and posterior segments of the upper lobes and the superior segments of the lower lobes. Localization is also valuable in directing diagnostic procedures such as bronchoscopy and therapeutic maneuvers such as postural drainage.

Aside from its location within the lung fields, the infiltrate may exhibit other features which aid in more precise localization. If an infiltrate abuts a lung fissure, it will produce a sharp border with that fissure. When it abuts a structure of similar density, the border of that structure will be obscured, producing the *silhouette sign*. Examples of these signs are shown in Figure 33–1.

Lung infiltrates may be classified as alveolar, interstitial, or cavitary. *Alveolar infiltrates* are homogeneous. Sometimes multiple rosettes several millimeters in diameter are seen at the border of these infiltrates. The presence of such rosettes, thought to represent acinar shadows, is pathognomonic for alveolar disease. Air bronchograms are frequently present. Alveolar infiltrates are found in diseases in which alveoli are filled with edema fluid, cells, blood, or other foreign material. Common causes of alveolar infiltrates are pulmonary edema, bacterial pneumonia, and pulmonary infarction.

An *interstitial infiltrate* appears as fine lines (reticular) or dots less than 3 mm in diameter (nodular) or both lines and dots (reticulonodular). This type of infiltrate is associated with diseases in which the predominant pathologic process is in the interstitium of the lung. Localized interstitial infiltrates are commonly caused by viral, mycobacterial, and fungal infections. Lymphangitic carcinomatosis, sarcoidosis, pneumoconiosis, interstitial pneumonitis, and hypersensitivity reactions usually cause diffuse interstitial infiltrates, but they may present with localized densities.

A *cavity* appears as an air density within an infiltrate. Cavitary infiltrates occur when a necrotizing process has caused sloughing of lung parenchyma which is then expectorated, leaving a hole within the lung. Incomplete drainage of such a cavity may appear as a linear air-fluid level which will change its orientation in decubitus views. Lucencies within an infiltrate do not always imply cavitation. For example, irregular resolution of a pneumonia or an infiltrate superimposed on pulmonary emphysema may produce multiple small radiolucencies which mimic a cavitary infiltrate. A list of causes of cavitary infiltrates is given in Table 33–1.

Localized infiltrates frequently produce a change in the volume of the lung previously occupied by air. A change in volume is shown by appropriate shifts of the fissures, diaphragms, mediastinum, or hila from their normal location. Decreases in volume are often seen in airway obstruction, pulmonary embolism, and in the healing stages of parenchymal inflammation. An increase in the volume of the lung associated with the infiltrate, classically seen in *Klebsiella pneumoniae* infection, is also commonly seen with the staphylococcal, mixed anaerobic, and type III *Streptococcus pneumoniae* infections. All of these infections may lead eventually to cavitation which then heals with volume loss.

Thoracic adenopathy may occur in the hilar, anterior mediastinal, paratracheal, or subcarinal re-

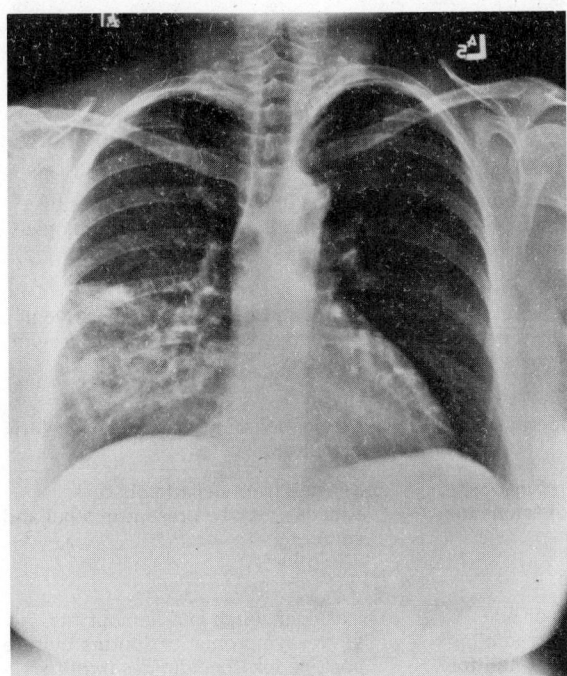
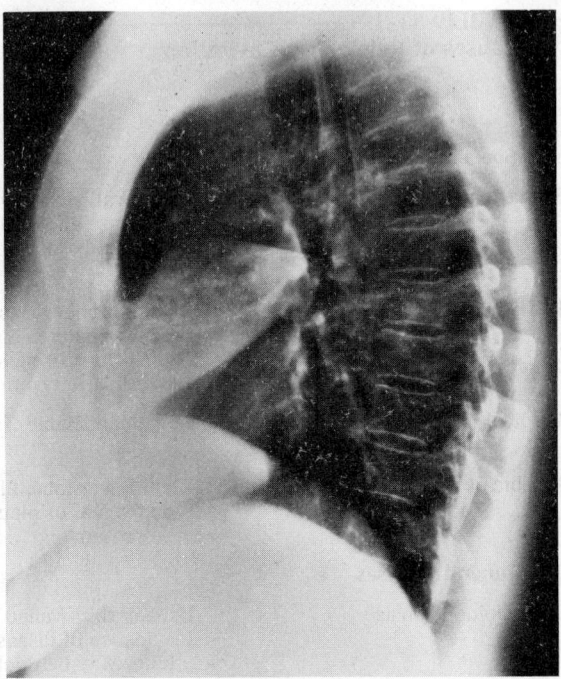

FIGURE 33–1. *The Silhouette Sign.* **Left:** Posteroanterior view of right middle lobe infiltrate. Note the blurring of the adjacent right heart border—*the silhouette sign.* **Right:** Lateral view of the same patient. In contrast, note the sharp borders of the infiltrate with the minor and major fissures. Other commonly silhouetted structures are the diaphragms by lower lobe infiltrates and the left heart border by lingular infiltrates.

gions. Causes of thoracic adenopathy are listed in Table 33–2.

The presence of a *pleural effusion* associated with a localized infiltrate is found with neoplasia, bacterial infection, or pulmonary infarction. While radiographically nonspecific, pleural fluid is an important source of diagnostic material, and therefore should carefully be sought, with additional decubitus views, if necessary.

CLINICAL EVALUATION

The clinical history should be directed toward identification of associated underlying conditions and environmental exposures and should attempt to identify the onset of the illness, its course, and the current state of the patient.

A history of associated conditions or exposures is important. Alcoholics frequently develop tuberculo-

sis, lung abscess, aspiration pneumonia, and pneumonia due to the pneumococcus or *Klebsiella pneumoniae.* Diabetics are predisposed to bacterial pneumonia, tuberculosis, and fungal infections. Immunodeficiency due to neoplasm, steroid therapy, or chemotherapy is commonly complicated by infection with opportunistic organisms such as fungi, *Pneumocystis carinii,* and viruses. The patient with a bleeding disorder may develop spontaneous pulmonary hemorrhage with localized consolidation in the face of little or no hemoptysis. Aspiration pneumonia commonly occurs after loss of consciousness or cardiac arrest. A history of travel to an endemic area may suggest a specific diagnosis such as coccidioidomycosis after travel in the southwestern United States. Exposure to parrots or parakeets may suggest psittacosis, while exposure to forest animals may suggest tularemia or pneumonic plague.

Constitutional symptoms are nonspecific, but help to date the onset and progression of the illness.

TABLE 33-1
Causes of Pulmonary Cavitation

Condition	Radiologic Appearance	Characteristic Features
I. Specific Infection		
Primary lung abscess	Thick-walled cavity with surrounding infiltrate and air fluid level; frequently located in dependent lung zones	Copious foul sputum. Predisposing conditions: alcoholism, neurologic disease, or esophageal disease
Tuberculosis	Usually upper lobes. May be multiple. Wall usually 2–5 mm thick, contour smooth or irregular. Fibrosis and calcification common	Sputum almost invariably positive in untreated cases. Positive tuberculin skin test
Atypical mycobacteriosis	Indistinguishable from tuberculosis	Identification of atypical mycobacteria on culture
Amebic abscess	Right lower lobe. Pleural effusions, empyema, or pleural adhesions may be present	Extension from hepatic abscess. Amebas may be present in stool and sputum
II. Fungus Diseases		
Coccidioidomycosis	Usually thin-walled cavity or no evidence of disease in surrounding lung. May be thick-walled, multiple, with fluid level and with extensive parenchymal disease	Occasional cough and hemoptysis, often asymptomatic. Sputum culture positive for *Coccidioides immitis*
Histoplasmosis	Simulates tuberculosis. Chronic fibrocavitary disease in apical or subapical regions	Elevated complement fixation titer. Positive sputum cultures for *Histoplasma capsulatum*
Aspergillosis	Intracavitary fungus ball (mycetoma)	Positive sputum culture for Aspergillus. Positive precipitins for Aspergillus. Secondary invasion of pre-existing cavity or cyst
Actinomycosis	Suppurative abscesses with widespread intrapulmonary consolidation. Most commonly involves lower lobes. Pleural involvement common	Chest wall sinuses, common. Cultures of sputum or sinus drainage positive. Sulfur granules in sputum
III. Cavitary Neoplasm		
Bronchogenic carcinoma	Irregular inner wall of cavity, eccentric cavitation	Cigarette smoking male over 40. Cough and hemoptysis. Sputum cytology positive
Metastatic carcinoma	Often multiple	Primary disease elsewhere may be evident. Usually squamous type
Lymphoma	Often multiple. May be associated with hilar node enlargement	Peripheral adenopathy usually present
IV. Miscellaneous		
Silicosis or pneumoconiosis	Conglomerate masses with cavitation. Associated diffuse changes	Occupational history
Pulmonary infarction	Peripheral density, often with atelectasis	Secondary infection by contamination from bronchial tree or septic pulmonary embolism
Infected bronchogenic cyst	Usually single. May be close to carina or in peripheral lung field	Asymptomatic until infected. Symptoms usually chronic

---TABLE 33-1 (cont.)----

Condition	Radiologic Appearance	Characteristic Features
IV. Miscellaneous		
Polyarteritis nodosa and Wegener's granulomatosis	Often multiple nodules which cavitate	Evidence of extrapulmonary disease
Rheumatoid lung nodules with cavitation		Associated joint manifestations. Positive serologic test for rheumatoid disease
Caplan syndrome (rheumatoid arthritis) with pneumoconiosis of coal miners	Commonly occurs in lower lobes	Occupational history. Associated joint manifestations. Positive serologic test for rheumatoid disease
Sarcoidosis	Fibrotic infiltrate and hilar adenopathy	

Fever suggests infection, but may also be seen with neoplasms, sarcoidosis, and hypersensitivity pneumonitis. An illness of acute onset suggests bacterial pneumonia or pulmonary embolism, while an insidious onset suggests malignancy or mycobacterial infection.

Cough or a change in a chronic cough pattern may also help to date the onset of the illness. The character of the sputum may suggest a diagnosis. Malodorous sputum is typical of anaerobic infection. Hemoptysis commonly accompanies bronchogenic carcinoma, tuberculosis, bronchiectasis, bacterial infections, and pulmonary infarction.

Physical examination of the chest is not as helpful as the chest radiograph in the diagnosis of localized infiltrates. There are exceptions to this rule. Crackles may be heard early in pneumonia or pulmonary edema when the chest radiograph is normal. At times, using the chest radiograph, it may be difficult to differentiate a consolidated pneumonia from a localized pleural effusion. Increased sound transmission over an area of dullness is found with consolidation of lung, while decreased sound transmission over an area of dullness is characteristic of a localized pleural effusion.

The general physical examination may prove helpful in assessing the functional status of the patient as well as the cause of the infiltrate. The presence of cyanosis and the use of accessory muscles of respiration are clues that the disease process is seriously impairing respiration. Cachexia, adenopathy, poor dental hygiene, the absence of pharyngeal reflexes, and signs of cardiac disease and venous insufficiency are helpful signs that should be sought in every patient with a localized pulmonary infiltration.

DIFFERENTIAL DIAGNOSIS

Once the roentgenographic picture, history, physical examination, and clinical setting are assessed, the differential diagnosis of the pulmonary infiltrate may be approached by routinely considering a number of etiologic possibilities (Table 33-3). The pace of the evaluation will be determined in part by the condition of the patient. Individuals who are critically ill require that a firm diagnosis be established within hours. Presumptive diagnoses may be made and treatment begun before definitive confirmation is obtained. The immunosuppressed patient represents a special class of patient in whom extensive and rapid evaluation is necessary. In the stable, less critically ill patient, there may be ample time to obtain old radiographs and to await the results of specialized laboratory testing.

INFECTION

The first consideration is whether the infiltrate is caused by infection. Productive cough, purulent sputum, fever, rales, signs of consolidation, and leukocytosis increase the likelihood of infection. The Gram stain of the sputum may provide presumptive bacteriologic information. Cultures of the sputum and blood often provide confirmatory information. Occasionally, special culture and staining techniques and serologic studies and lung biopsy may be required. The diagnosis and treatment of pneumonia is fully discussed in Chapter 84.

MALIGNANCY

Next, consider *malignancy*. Bronchogenic carcinoma (Chap. 37), the most common lung neoplasm, usually arises in the segmental bronchi. As a result, the first

TABLE 33-2
Causes of Thoracic Adenopathy

Disease	Comments
Sarcoidosis	Most common cause of bilateral hilar adenopathy. Paratracheal adenopathy common
Lymphoma	Frequently asymmetrical and involves the anterior mediastinum. One-third of cases have associated pleural effusion
Primary tuberculosis	Adenopathy is virtually always present in children and frequent in adults. When present, it is usually asymmetrical
Histoplasmosis	Commonly occurs with primary infection in children and heals with calcification. Commonly asymmetrical
Tularemia	Hilar adenopathy, usually ipsilateral, occurs in approximately one-third of pneumonic cases
Mycoplasma pneumoniae infection	Hilar adenopathy occurs in one-fourth of childhood cases and uncommonly in adults
Pneumoconiosis	Hilar adenopathy common in silicosis, and uncommon in asbestosis and simple coal workers' pneumoconiosis
Bronchogenic carcinoma	Unilateral adenopathy is the presenting radiographic finding in 12-35% of cases. Adenopathy in the radiographic absence of a primary lesion suggests small cell carcinoma
Idiopathic inflammatory lymphadenitis	Uncommon. Characteristic hilar histopathology
Infectious mononucleosis	Uncommon
Erythema nodosum	This may be a *forme fruste* of sarcoidosis
Angioimmunoblastic lymphadenopathy	Generalized lymphadenopathy. Associated interstitial pneumonitis
Cystic fibrosis	Prominent cystic bronchiectasis

radiologic manifestation of bronchogenic carcinoma may not be the mass itself, but rather obstructive pneumonitis or atelectasis. A history of weight loss, malaise, anorexia, and progressive dyspnea in a patient who smokes suggests bronchogenic carcinoma. Recurrent small amounts of hemoptysis may also be evident. With a central obstructing lesion, sputum cytology is likely to reveal malignant cells. Paraneoplastic syndromes, such as pulmonary osteoarthropathy, Cushing syndrome, and the syndrome of inappropriate ADH secretion, and hypercalcemia, also suggest carcinoma.

Bronchoalveolar cell carcinoma is a well-differentiated adenocarcinoma originating from epithelial cells in the alveoli or terminal airways.[59] It accounts for 1 to 10 percent of all primary lung cancers and presents most commonly as a persistent or poorly resolving solitary pulmonary infiltrate resembling a segmental or lobar pneumonia. It may also present as a well-circumscribed mass, single or multiple nodules, or in a diffuse form. Pleural effusion is found in 10 percent of cases. Cavitation is also described. The disease presents in middle age with no sex predominance. One half of patients are asymptomatic when the lesion is first noticed. Chest pain, cough, dyspnea, and weight loss are common complaints in the remainder. The production of mucoid sputum in quantities as great as 2 liters daily is suggestive of bronchoalveolar cell carcinoma. This symptom, however, is seen infrequently and only with extensive disease. Diffuse rales are striking on physical examination. Diagnosis, which is often delayed until other more common causes of localized infiltrates are excluded, is made by lung biopsy. Histologically, the tumor must be distinguished from metastatic adenocarcinoma. Bronchoalveolar cell carcinoma is treated surgically when the tumor is completely resectable; however, over one-half of patients selected for surgery in the past have been found to be unresectable, because the chest radiograph did not reveal the full extent of the disease. Chemotherapy and radiotherapy are unsatisfactory at this time. Prognosis is variable. When a solitary lesion has been resected, survival time can exceed 5 years. Patients with inoperable disease infrequently survive beyond 3 years.

Hodgkin's disease may present as a localized pulmonary infiltrate, although the most common roentgenographic finding is hilar and mediastinal adenopathy. Pulmonary infiltration usually occurs as a direct extension of mediastinal involvement. After radiotherapy, this lymphoma may recur as a pulmonary infiltrate in the absence of adenopathy and is usually located in areas of lung not previously irradiated. Lung parenchymal involvement by non-Hodgkin's lymphoma is present only when there is widespread

TABLE 33–3
Differential Diagnosis of a Localized Pulmonary Infiltrate

	Radiologic Appearance	Clinical	Note
Infection*			
Malignancy			
Bronchogenic carcinoma	May present as pneumonia or infiltrate distal to a proximal obstructing lesion	Weight loss, anorexia, cough, hemoptysis in a smoker, paraneoplastic syndromes may provide a clue (see text)	Sputum cytology may be positive with proximal lesions
Bronchoalveolar cell carcinoma	Indolent segmental or lobar pneumonia	Copious thin mucoid sputum	
Hodgkin's lymphoma	Parenchymal infiltrates occur only as a direct extension of mediastinal disease except in treated cases. Recurrent disease may occur as a solitary infiltrate usually outside of prior radiation fields	Painless, progressive enlargement of lymph nodes, splenomegaly, fever, weakness, pruritis	Reed-Sternberg cells have occasionally been identified in the sputum
Mechanical Obstruction			
Atelectasis	Linear or plate-like densities in dependent portions of lung	Common in postoperative and in other immobilized patients. Predisposing factors include hypoventilation, anesthesia, sedation, and analgesics	
Bronchopulmonary aspergillosis	Migratory infiltrates, evidence for mucoid impaction	Progressive or recurrent attacks of asthma in an individual with a long-standing history; fever and expectoration of brown mucus plugs	Positive skin test and precipitins against Aspergillus species. Elevated IgE level
Foreign body	Variable: hyperinflation with check valve phenomenon, atelectasis and collapse with complete obstruction	History of object in mouth, dental visit, poor dentition, etc. Right side most common because of straight right mainstem bronchus	Nonmetallic objects may not be radiopaque
Right middle lobe syndrome	Recurrent right middle lobe infiltrates	Historically, tuberculosis is most common; endobronchial tumor or foreign body must be ruled out†	Abnormal collateral ventilation may play a role (see text)
Bronchial adenoma	Localized infiltrate with atelectasis though chest film is often normal	Recurrent cough, hemoptysis, fever in a young adult	

* See Chapter 84.
† Recurrent infiltrates in the same location suggest a proximal obstructing lesion. However, recurrent pneumonia, secondary to predisposing conditions, is most common (see text).

(Continued)

TABLE 33-3 (cont.)

	Radiologic Appearance	Clinical	Note
Inhalation			
Aspiration pneumonia	Alveolar infiltrate with dependent zones or diffuse alveolar infiltrates	See text	See text
Suppurative lung abscess	Dense homogenous infiltrate progressing to cavitation with an air fluid level. Most commonly involves the superior segment of the right lower lobe	History of unconsciousness, alcoholism, seizure disorder, oropharyngeal suppuration, or copious foul sputum. Fever, weight loss and anemia	Anerobic organisms cultured from transtracheal aspirate
Lipoid pneumonia	Chronic progressive lower lobe infiltrates may simulate lung mass	History of mineral oil use	Lipid-laden macrophages in sputum
Other materials Hydrocarbons Milk Near drowning	Either localized or diffuse alveolar infiltrates	Usually acute event with specific history	
Blood	Usually lower lobe infiltrates	Epistaxis, hematemesis or hemoptysis from any cause	Clears in 3–4 days
Embolic			
Pulmonary embolism	Segmental basal homogenous infiltrate which abuts the pleural surface	Sudden onset of dyspnea and pleuritic pain in an immobilized or predisposed patient	Subtle and variable presentations make a high index of suspicion necessary
Fat embolism	Diffuse infiltrates	Skeletal trauma, petechiae, mental confusion and respiratory distress	Fat globules in the urine have been described
Septic emboli	Multiple small infiltrates which cavitate	Suspect in intravenous abuses, pelvic inflammatory diseases, and in right-sided subacute infective endocarditis	Common staphylococcal etiology
Immunologic			
Systemic lupus erythematosus	Recurrent or migratory infiltrates	Negative sputum and blood cultures; other clinical evidence for active systemic lupus erythematosus	Caution: infection is still the most common cause of infiltrates in these patients
Rheumatoid arthritis	Predominantly affects lung bases	Middle-aged men more than women; clubbing may be evident	High titer of rheumatoid factor
Dermatomyositis	Bibasilar infiltrates	Muscle weakness and skin rash	Hypoventilation and atelectasis, secondary to muscle weakness, aspiration, secondary to dysphasia and alveolitis all must be considered

---TABLE 33-3 (cont.)---

	Radiologic Appearance	Clinical	Note
Immunologic (cont.)			
Scleroderma	Bibasilar infiltrates		Aspiration must be considered because of esophageal involvement
Ankylosing spondylitis	Hyperinflation and upper lobe fibrotic and bullous disease	Clinically evident in young males more than females; chronic low back pain; spontaneous pneumothorax occurs	HLA-B27 associated
Goodpasture syndrome	Diffuse interstitial infiltrates	Dyspnea, hemoptysis, and hematuria in a young adult male	Antiglomerular basement membrane antibodies found
Idiopathic pulmonary hemosiderosis	Diffuse interstitial infiltrates	Iron deficiency, cough and dyspnea in children 10–12 years old	No renal involvement
Wegener's granulomatosis	Multiple round infiltrates with cavitation common	Sinusitis, hemoptysis, pleuritic chest pain, hematuria, and skin rash, 5th decade	A localized or limited form occurs
Other			
Radiation pneumonitis	Geometric infiltrate corresponding to radiation portal	Dry cough and dyspnea occurring days to 6 months following treatment	Diagnostic change in sputum cytopathology has been described
Congenital: Bronchopulmonary sequestration	Cystic infiltrate in posterior segment of left lower lobe more than right lower lobe	History of prior abnormal chest film helpful	
Pulmonary infiltrates with eosinophilia: Löffler syndrome	Transient migratory infiltrates		Ascariasis common, other parasites possible
Chronic eosinophilic pneumonia	Chronic peripheral infiltrates	Atopic individual: fever, malaise, cough, dyspnea for 1–2 months	
Drug allergy	Patchy infiltrates	Nitrofurantoin, para-amino salicylic acid, tricyclic antidepressants, hydrochlorothiazide	

systemic involvement. The disease is usually manifested as masses of nodules. Primary pulmonary lymphoma is uncommon.

BRONCHIAL OBSTRUCTION

Mechanical obstruction of a bronchus frequently causes loss of volume. The affected lung may appear as a localized area of increased radiodensity because of the crowding and consolidation of the normally translucent alveolar structures. Localized obstruction may result from a mucous plug, tumor, or foreign body.

Postoperative patients are subject to atelectasis secondary to mucous plugs. Impaired clearance of secretions and hypoventilation due to pain, anesthesia, and sedative and analgesic drugs are contributing factors. Dependent portions of the lung are most susceptible. Treatment of atelectasis should include suctioning, postural drainage, and encouragement to cough and inspire deeply.

Atelectasis secondary to mucous plugs may also occur in asthmatic individuals. Progressive or recurrent attacks of asthma in an individual with atopic history, accompanied by expectoration of brownish sputum and an occasional bronchial cast suggests bronchopulmonary aspergillosis. Migratory pulmonary infiltrates are common. Even the upper lobes may become atelectatic. Fever and eosinophilia are common. The diagnosis is established by the appropriate clinical picture, a positive Aspergillus skin test and serum precipitins, an elevated IgE level, and isolation of the organism from the sputum.

Bronchial adenoma is a tumor which frequently causes mechanical obstruction.[57] It is slow growing and has a low-grade malignant potential. It arises from the alveolar lining cells and is more common in women than in men and in individuals under 40 years. The majority of patients present with symptoms of cough and hemoptysis. Treatment is surgical.

Foreign body aspiration may also present as a localized infiltrate. Patients with obtundation, poor dentition, recent dental procedures, and seizure disorders are prone to aspiration. Bronchoscopy is both diagnostic and therapeutic.

Mechanical obstruction is a common cause of *recurrent infiltrates* in the same location. The "right middle lobe syndrome" is recurrent right middle lobe infiltrates and/or atelectasis, thought to result from extrinsic compression of the middle lobe bronchus by peribronchial lymph nodes. In the past, tuberculosis was a common cause. Bronchogenic carcinoma is more common today. Surprisingly, at bronchoscopy the right middle lobe bronchus is patent in many cases. Recent observations suggest that collateral ventilation to the right middle lobe is poor, rendering it more susceptible to collapse than other areas of lung.[56] Recurrent infiltrates may occur in the absence of obstruction, such as the recurrent pneumonias which occur in patients with alcoholism, diabetes, chronic sinusitis, congestive heart failure, bronchiectasis, and aspiration.[62]

EMBOLISM

Pulmonary thromboembolism may produce a pulmonary infiltrate and consolidation. The infiltrate may represent hemorrhage, edema, or tissue necrosis and is characteristically basilar and wedge-shaped, with its base against the pleural surface. *Fat embolism* must be considered in individuals suffering from skeletal trauma, who develop mental confusion, respiratory distress, severe hypoxia, and petechial hemorrhage in the skin.

ASPIRATION

Pathogenesis

Aspiration of foreign material into the lung also may cause localized pulmonary infiltrates. An example is *aspiration of gastric contents.*[51,52] The tracheal tree is

normally protected from gastric aspiration by a series of barriers. The lower esophageal sphincter prevents reflux from the stomach. The height of the esophagus in the upright position serves as a hydrostatic barrier to reflux. The coordinated swallowing mechanism closes the epiglottis while clearing the oropharynx. Laryngeal reflexes cause glottic closure following mechanical or chemical irritation. An intact cough reflex clears the material from the tracheobronchial tree.

Any disruption of these barriers favors the aspiration of gastric or oropharyngeal contents. The most common disruption is sleep. Nearly half of normal subjects have been found to aspirate pharyngeal contents during sleep. Although this aspiration is apparently of little clinical consequence in healthy persons, it may be a significant threat to persons with underlying cardiac or pulmonary disease. Risk factors which predispose to aspiration are listed in Table 33–4.

When aspiration occurs, the major deposition occurs in the dependent zones of the lungs. For example, in the supine position, the superior segments of the lower lobes and the posterior segments of the up-

---

TABLE 33–4
Risk Factors for Aspiration

Impairment of Consciousness

Anesthesia
Alcoholism
Seizure disorder
Stroke
Heroin addiction
Coma
Cardiac arrest

Impairment of Esophageal Function

Esophageal stricture, benign or malignant
Hiatus hernia, incompetent esophageal sphincter
Achalasia
Tracheoesophageal fistula
Zenker's diverticulum
Nasogastric intubation

Impairment of Swallowing Mechanism

Pseudobulbar palsy
Tracheostomy
Laryngeal carcinoma

Impairment of Cough Mechanism

Neuromuscular weakness
Local intratracheal anesthesia

Increased Bacterial Innoculum

Periodonitis
Tonsillar abscess
Dental abscess
Sinusitis

per lobes will be dependent, and in the prone position the anterior segments of the upper lobes and the middle lobes will be at risk. In general, aspirated material is more likely to be deposited on the right side than the left.

Clinical Features

The clinical episode of aspiration is frequently not observed, and the patient may present with a catastrophic illness characterized by dyspnea, hypoxemia, hypotension, and alveolar pulmonary infiltrates which may be difficult to distinguish from acute myocardial infarction, pulmonary embolism, or overwhelming sepsis. Alternatively, the patient may present with unexplained fever, an infiltrate localized to the dependent lung zones, superimposed bacterial pneumonia, or unexplained deterioration in arterial oxygenation. Silent aspiration of gastric or oropharyngeal contents may be the most common cause of hospital-acquired pneumonia.

Historical features which suggest the possibility of aspiration include a history of prolonged or violent coughing spells following a meal or an episode of vomiting, but this history is often lacking. The diagnosis can be established with confidence if particulate matter is suctioned from the tracheobronchial tree. Although gastric acid is rapidly neutralized by tracheobronchial secretions and tissue, the finding of acidic fluid in the tracheal secretions supports the diagnosis. In addition, the bronchoscopic finding of diffuse bronchial mucosal erythema and edema extending to the subsegmental bronchi is compatible with the diagnosis of aspiration of gastric contents. One should always keep in mind that illness, such as cerebrovascular insufficiency, acute myocardial infarction, and pulmonary embolism, can precede and induce aspiration of gastric contents.

Prognosis

The prognosis of aspiration pneumonia is variable. Some patients will succumb rapidly either from asphyxiation due to occlusion of the trachea or from acute overwhelming pulmonary edema, hypoxemia, and circulatory collapse. A second group of patients will develop lung infiltrates, which gradually clear over several weeks. A third group of patients show initial improvement after the acute episode, but succumb to secondary infection. The mortality of aspiration pneumonia depends upon the type and quantity of aspirated material as well as the premorbid state.

Treatment

The initial therapy of aspiration of gastric contents should be directed toward securing patency of the airway with suctioning, intubation and, if necessary, bronchoscopy. Supplemental oxygen should be administered to combat hypoxemia. If necessary, positive pressure ventilation should be applied. Positive end-expiratory pressure may be necessary to overcome hypoxemia and allow the use of nontoxic concentrations of inspired oxygen. Hemodynamic parameters should be closely monitored. Intravenous fluids should be administered to combat hypovolemia and hypotension.

Bacterial superinfection is common because of impairment of local pulmonary defense mechanisms. Infection acquired outside the hospital is commonly due to mixed aerobic and anaerobic organisms similar to those residing in the host's oropharynx. Infection acquired within the hospital frequently is caused by aerobic gram-negative bacteria as well as mixed aerobic-anaerobic infections.[58] The diagnosis of superinfection is difficult because acid aspiration per se will cause a clinical picture similar to bacterial pneumonia. Antibiotic therapy should be guided by the results of sputum smears and cultures. Transtracheal aspiration is helpful in selected cases to obtain sputum for cultures uncontaminated by oropharyngeal flora. In general, antibiotics should be reserved for patients in whom aspiration is followed by progressive lung infiltrates, purulent sputum or fever. Corticosteroids in pharmacologic doses have been long thought to be of benefit for acid aspiration, particularly if given early; however, the efficacy of such treatment is unproven.

Aspiration of gastric contents is frequently a preventable disease. Preventive measures include proper administration of tube feedings, maintenance of nasogastric tube patency, having susceptible patients sit upright during and after feeding, proper inflation of tracheostomy balloons, careful clearance of vomitus and pharyngeal secretions in patients with impaired consciousness during transport and hospitalization, positioning of unconscious or vomiting patients in the lateral decubitus or prone position, and meticulous anesthetic technique.

The lung is also vulnerable to aspiration of a variety of other foreign materials. *Lipoid pneumonia* is a chronic, slowly progressive infiltrate in the dependent lung zones caused by aspiration of mineral oil used as a stool softener or as a vehicle for nose drops. Hydrocarbon aspiration occurs commonly following ingestion of these substances and causes an acute diffuse alveolitis with pulmonary hemorrhage and edema. For this reason, hydrocarbons should not, in general, be lavaged from the stomach. Food particles when aspirated into the trachea, cause a granulomatous alveolitis with a subacute course over several days. Milk, commonly aspirated by children, causes an acute chemical bronchitis and pneumonitis. Near drowning may involve aspiration of gastric contents as well as water, and the clinical sequelae of the episode depend upon whether the water was contaminated, the duration of the submersion, and temperature of the water.

AUTOIMMUNE DISORDERS

Localized pulmonary infiltrates are seen in several so-called *autoimmune disorders*.[53,60] While infection is still the most common cause of a pulmonary infiltrate in systemic lupus erythematosus, recurrent or migratory infiltrates may represent lupus pneumonitis. Dyspnea, high fever, and nonproductive cough associated with a bilateral alveolar filling process and negative sputum and blood cultures are characteristic. Apical pleural thickening and fibrosis may mimic the early infiltrate of tuberculosis in patients with ankylosing spondylitis. Pathologically, interstitial fibrosis is found. The presence of proximal muscle weakness or tenderness and erythematous rash should suggest polymyositis or dermatomyositis as a cause of bibasilar infiltrates. These infiltrates may result from a fibrosing alveolitis or from recurrent aspiration secondary to swallowing abnormalities associated with the disorder.

Goodpasture syndrome is characterized by pulmonary hemorrhage and renal failure. It occurs most commonly in young adult males. Diffuse infiltrates are more common than localized infiltrates. Antibodies directed against glomerular basement membrane can be found. Idiopathic pulmonary hemosiderosis appears to be a separate entity, more common in children under 10 years of age. Extensive alveolar infiltration may be present on the chest radiograph, caused by alveolar hemorrhage. These pulmonary infiltrates may occur without clinically apparent hemoptysis. *Wegener's granulomatosis* is a granulomatous vasculitis which presents most commonly in the middle-aged man. The chest radiograph will reveal rounded single or multiple infiltrates, which may be cystic or cavitary, although single nodules or localized infiltrates are reported. The illness presents with malaise and weakness, sinusitis, hemoptysis and pleuritic chest pain, skin rash, and hematuria. A limited form of the illness is also described. Therapy with cyclophosphamide has resulted in an improved prognosis for these patients.

OTHER

Bronchopulmonary sequestration is a *congenital malformation* in which a portion of a lobe fails to communicate with the normal bronchial tree and receives its blood supply from a major systemic artery, usually the descending thoracic aorta. Bronchopulmonary sequestration is usually recognized as the result of pneumonia presenting radiographically, commonly as a cystic infiltrate in the posterior bronchopulmonary segment of the left lower lobe, or less often in the corresponding location on the right. The diagnosis must be confirmed by identifying the blood supply to this segment by aortography. The importance of recognizing the abnormal blood supply derives from the intraoperative hazard of surgical resection when the abnormal blood supply is not appreciated.

Localized infiltrates in patients undergoing radiation therapy suggest radiation pneumonitis.[55] The infiltrate may appear 2 to 3 months following exposure, but may occur as early as several days or as late as 6 months following treatment. The etiology is suggested by the sharp borders of the infiltrate which correspond to the outline of the radiation port. Patients have nonproductive cough and dyspnea. Lung biopsy will reveal a pneumonitis showing endothelial damage, interstitial and alveolar edema, swelling and nuclear damage in the epithelial cells, polymorphonuclear infiltration, and vascular thrombosis. Eventually, most patients will develop evidence of fibrosis in the area of pneumonitis.

The combination of *pulmonary infiltrates and peripheral blood eosinophilia* can occur in several disorders.[61] Löffler syndrome and chronic eosinophilic pneumonia are diseases of unknown etiology in which patients may be found to have nonsegmental areas of infiltration radiographically, with blood eosinophilia. In Löffler syndrome, the infiltrates are fleeting. Chronic eosinophilic pneumonia is a prolonged illness with fever, malaise, anorexia, weight loss, and dyspnea. The symptomatic and roentgenographic pictures are dramatically and promptly reversed with steroid therapy. Drugs, such as nitrofurantoin, sulphonamides, tricyclic antidepressants, and the thiazide diuretics, have been reported to produce this condition. Parasites whose life cycle involves transit through the lungs, such as ascariasis, strongyloidiasis, and ancylostomiasis, pulmonary larva migrans, and schistosomiasis, may cause the syndrome. Tropical eosinophilia is a disease seen in individuals who live or travel in the tropics in whom an asthmatic illness or an illness consisting of malaise, weight loss, fever, cough, and dyspnea develops. Roentgenographic abnormalities include a diffuse micronodular infiltrate and hilar adenopathy. High levels of antibody to filarial antigen are found and demonstrate improvement on treatment with antifilarial chemotherapy.

CHAPTER 34
Diffuse Pulmonary Infiltration and Fibrosis
CAROL J. JOHNS AND GARETH M. GREEN

This chapter is concerned with a variety of conditions that produce abnormal x-ray images widely distributed throughout both lungs. The clinical manifestations associated with this radiographic picture may be minimal or incapacitating, depending on the nature and extent of the abnormality. Some patients are asymptomatic and present because of an abnormal routine chest x-ray, while others present with cough, dyspnea, cyanosis, cor pulmonale, and heart failure resulting from impairment of lung function. Systemic manifestations of illness such as fever, anorexia, and weight loss will predominate in some disorders. In certain multisystem diseases, such as progressive systemic sclerosis (scleroderma), rheumatoid arthritis, uremia, and the lymphomas, the pulmonary manifestations may be only incidental findings. In some circumstances, diffuse disease may exist without radiographic changes.

RADIOGRAPHIC FEATURES[71]

The abnormal chest roentgenogram conveys specific information useful in guiding the clinical investigation of the patient with diffuse lung disease. The radiographic patterns can be described as alveolar, ground glass, nodular, reticular, and noduloreticular, or interstitial.

The *alveolar pattern* has a characteristic rosette pattern caused by a cluster of opacified acini, and usually has a soft, fluffy appearance. The alveolar pattern may appear and disappear rapidly as the alveoli fill and empty with edema fluid or blood, or may change more slowly when filled with granular lipid debris as in alveolar proteinosis. The process may be localized to a segment or lobe, but when it is diffuse it is most prominent in the perihilar areas with relative sparing of the peripheral portions of the lungs, forming a "butterfly" shadow as is characteristic with pulmonary edema. A so-called air bronchogram is created by the contrast between alveoli filled with dense material surrounding the less dense air-filled bronchi.

An *interstitial pattern* is produced by abnormal prominence of the connective tissue in the lung. Alveolar and interlobular septa and peribronchial and perivascular connective tissue sheaths are involved. Thickened interlobular septa are well seen in the costophrenic angles and on the diaphragmatic surface of the lung as 1- to 2-cm lines perpendicular to the pleura. These are known as Kerley B lines and become visible when they are filled with fluid, as in mitral stenosis, or when there is tumor invading the lymphatics (see Fig. 20–2).

Ground glass changes have a granular appearance with relatively homogeneous clouding or haze over the lung fields due to deposits which are too small to produce discrete shadows; *nodular* markings are discrete punctate densities and occur in miliary tuberculosis, hematogenous tumor metastases and silicosis; *reticular pattern* is a fine network of linear shadows; and *reticulonodular* changes are a combination of nodular shadows superimposed on a reticular pattern, often seen in sarcoidosis.

Radiographic changes may be evident without symptoms, and rapid change is unusual. In inflammatory disorders, cystic dilatation of distal air spaces (bronchiolectasis) may occur, producing a coarse reticular pattern with air spaces 5 to 6 mm in diameter. When extensive, this pattern is referred to a "honeycomb lung" and may be seen in any diffuse *fibrosing alveolitis*. Subpleural clusters of rounded lucencies are especially well seen at the lung bases. Proliferation of fibrous tissue may produce thick linear shadows and gross shrinkage and distortion of the lung parenchyma.

Many diseases have both alveolar and interstitial components, and it is often impossible to distinguish these pathologic processes by radiographic studies. There are serious limitations in making a diagnosis on the basis of the x-ray pattern alone, but the examination of a series of films may yield important information about the time course of a disease and therefore be of diagnostic value. Sometimes, radiographic abnormalities associated with the parenchymal densities are of great help in identifying the underlying process. Examples of this are the bilateral diaphragmatic pleural calcification, which is nearly always caused by asbestos exposure, and eggshell calcification of hilar nodes, which is rare except in patients with silicosis.

PHYSIOLOGIC ABNORMALITIES

Diseases characterized by filling of the alveoli or infiltration of the interstitial tissues of the lung usually cause abnormalities in pulmonary mechanics and gas exchange. The characteristic pattern in most of these

---
TABLE 34-1
Diagnostic Features of Diffuse Pulmonary Infiltrations

Often Asymptomatic

Sarcoidosis
Siderosis (arc welders), early pneumoconiosis
Carcinoma of thyroid with diffuse pulmonary metastases
Eosinophilic granuloma (histiocytosis X)
Löffler's pneumonia, lipoid pneumonia
Alveolar proteinosis (minimal infiltrates)

Fever

Infections, collagen diseases, leukemia, lymphoma
Extrinsic allergic alveolitis
Sarcoidosis (erythema nodosum or active hepatic disease)

Hemoptysis

Advanced fibrocystic disease with superimposed bacterial or fungal infection or mycetoma (esp. sarcoidosis)
Bronchiectasis
Idiopathic pulmonary hemosiderosis
Cavitary disease—tuberculosis, fungal disease, Wegener's granulomatosis
Vasculitis—Wegener, Goodpasture syndrome, polyarteritis
Blood dyscrasia or Coumadin overdose
Trauma—contusion

Bronchial Obstruction or Wheezing

Asthma, allergic bronchopulmonary aspergillosis
Extrinsic allergic alveolitis—infrequently
Tropical eosinophilia
Histiocytosis X (eosinophilic granuloma)

Mediastinal Adenopathy

Sarcoidosis—usually symmetrical bilateral hilar and often with right paratracheal adenopathy
Lymphoma—often asymmetrical
Granulomatous infections—tuberculosis, histoplasmosis, usually asymmetrical and often calcified when old
Fungal infections
Wegener's granulomatosis—uncommon
Silicosis—eggshell or ring calcification (seen also in sarcoidosis and postirradiation Hodgkin's)

Pleural Disease

Tuberculosis and acute pneumonias—effusion or empyema
Collagen diseases—effusion
Asbestosis—calcification, especially diaphragmatic pleura
Neoplasms, effusion, often bloody
Pulmonary emboli with or without infarction—effusion
Congestive failure—transudative effusion
Sarcoidosis—effusion rare, and usually small

---

diseases is a reduction in lung volumes (restrictive ventilatory defect) without airway obstruction, alveolar hyperventilation (low arterial Pco_2) with a reduced arterial Po_2 due largely to abnormal ventilation–perfusion ratios, and a variable but often marked reduction in diffusing capacity. The deposition of any abnormal material results in stiffening of the lungs and reduction in the volume normally occupied by air. This is manifested by a decreased compliance of the lungs and a reduction in vital capacity, total lung capacity, and residual volume.

Since the airways are only indirectly affected by processes confined to the interstitial spaces, airway obstruction is often conspicuously absent in this group of diseases. However, distortion or narrowing of airways with resulting obstruction to the flow of air may occur in complicated cases or in late stages of the chronic diffuse fibroses. A general discussion of these physiologic abnormalities and methods for the clinical evaluation of pulmonary function are discussed in Chapter 32.

APPROACH TO DIAGNOSIS

Diffuse roentgenographic abnormalities are produced by a wide variety of underlying diseases, but it is clearly important to make a definitive diagnosis whenever possible. The most practical initial approach to the problem of differential diagnosis is to narrow the range of possible causes as much as possible utilizing the appearance of the chest roentgenogram together with information from the history and physical examination. From the x-ray, one can determine the anatomic characteristics of the lesion. The history permits evaluation of the possibility of a familial disorder or a disease caused by aspiration or inhalation of a foreign substance. The importance of possible environmental and occupational exposures requires that a life time job history be taken. The duration of symptoms, together with a review of previous films if any are available, will indicate whether the process is acute, chronic, or static. The history and physical examination will provide clues to the presence of associated systemic disease. Priority in thinking should be given to any specific disorders suggested by the information so obtained, to those diseases, e.g., infections, for which specific treatment exists, and to common rather than rare diseases. A few specific clinical findings which are often helpful are shown in Table 34-1. Finally, it is useful to refer to a comprehensive list of categories (Table 34-2) to be certain that no important diagnostic possibility is being overlooked.

TABLE 34-2
Classification of Diffuse Infiltrations and Characteristic Features

Disease	Special Features
I. Familial or Congenital	
Familial fibrocystic dysplasia	Early clubbing; multiple tiny cysts
Cystic fibrosis	Children and young adults affected. Viscous tracheobronchial secretions; chronic and recurrent pyogenic infections; microabscesses; positive sweat test
Alveolar microlithiasis	Asymptomatic fine nodular alveolar calcification
Familial dysautonomia	Autonomic nervous system dysfunction; aspiration pneumonitis
II. Infections	
Bacterial	Fever, cough, sputum
Mycobacterial (tuberculosis)	Gradual onset, fever, positive PPD, cough, weight loss. Miliary disease may be indolent
Fungal	Localized or diffuse lesions. Often superimposed on underlying disease
Parasitic (schistosomiasis, ascariasis)	Bronchial asthma, eosinophilia, precipitins and complement fixing antibodies
Pneumocystic carinii	Immunosuppressed or debilitated patients
Viral	Cough, dyspnea, fever, myalgia. Patchy infiltrates or diffuse changes
III. Inhaled Irritants[93]	
Chemical fumes Nitrogen dioxide	Silo-filler's disease. Disabling dyspnea, exposure-related
Chlorine, phosgene	Exposure history. Abrupt onset of cough and dyspnea
Cadmium	Exposure history. Steroids may be lifesaving
Metal fume fever (brass and zinc)	Occupational history (galvanizing). Fever and chills on exposure

Table 34-2 (cont.)

Disease	Special Features
III. Inhaled Irritants (cont.)	
Polymerizing chemicals such as diisocyanates	Exposure to polyurethane foam, rubber, plastics, or resins. Worse beginning of work week. Minor patchy, soft opacities
Mineral dusts Asbestosis[64]	Exposure history (insulation construction, shipyard work, etc.). Long latent period. Interstitial disease progressing to diffuse coarse fibrosis, most often bibasilar. Shaggy heart border. Calcified pleural plaques, often diaphragmatic and pericardial surfaces. Associated with lung cancer and pleural mesothelioma
Berylliosis	Exposure history (aircraft manufacturing, metallurgy, rocket fuels)
Coal workers' pneumoconiosis	Coal dust exposure
Silicosis	Exposure history (sandblasting, quarrying, mining, foundry work). Associated tuberculosis. Nodular silica deposits and progressive fibrosis and retraction. Eggshell calcification of hilar nodes
Siderosis (iron oxide)	Exposure history (arc welding). No symptoms or disability. Simple nodular pattern on x-ray. Iron-laden macrophages without fibrosis
Organic dusts[63,70] Extrinsic asthma	Inhaled antigens. Mucus plugs or impactions (status asthmaticus). Eosinophilia and eosinophils in sputum
Allergic bronchopulmonary aspergillosis	Clinical asthma; eosinophilia. Multiple and varying infiltrates with rounded visible shadows of fungus plugs. Mycelia of Aspergillus cultured in sputum; Aspergillus precipitins in serum

(continued)

┌─ **Table 34–2 (cont.)** ─────────

Disease	Special Features
III. Inhaled Irritants (cont.)	
Extrinsic allergic alveolitis (Farmer's Lung)	Exposure to moldy hay. Cough and dyspnea. Granulomatous patchy pulmonary infiltrates. Remits with removal from environment. Serum precipitins for spores of *Micropolyspora faeni* and *Thermoactinomyces vulgaris*. Responds to corticosteroids
Bagassosis	Moldy sugar cane exposure. Serum precipitins for Thermoactinomyces
Byssinosis	Exposure history (raw cotton, flax, or hemp). Reversible airway obstruction. Chronic bronchitis and emphysema. X-ray changes usually minimal
IV. Neoplastic	
Bronchiolar (alveolar cell) carcinoma	Cough, sputum, weight loss. Alveolar pattern (localized or diffuse). May present as solitary nodules
Hematogenous metastases	Melanoma, breast, testis, chorioepithelioma, thyroid, pancreas, kidney
Lymphangitic carcinomatosis	Breast, stomach, pancreas, lung, biliary tract
Leukemia (lymphatic more common)	Blood and bone marrow changes. Diffuse perihilar pattern. Mediastinal nodes common
Lymphoma	Parenchymal nodules. Mediastinal nodes
V. Metabolic	
Uremia	Renal failure. Pulmonary edema pattern
VI. Aspiration	
Aspiration pneumonitis	Disturbed consciousness or disorders of swallowing. Local anesthesia of the pharynx. Drowning. Basal or posterior patchy pneumonitis
Lipoid pneumonia	Intranasal oily drops. Mineral oil laxative in elderly
Kerosene pneumonia	Kerosene ingestion

┌─ **Table 34–2 (cont.)** ─────────

Disease	Special Features
VII. Drug Reactions[90]	
Hexamethonium	Known ingestion of drugs
Hydralazine (Apresoline)	Clears with withdrawal of drugs
Busulfan (Myleran)	
Nitrofurantoin[66] (Furadantin)	
Narcotic overdose (heroin, methadone)	Known user. Transient pulmonary edema
VIII. Physical Agents	
Postirradiation fibrosis	X-ray therapy. Cough, dyspnea
Oxygen toxicity	Diffuse hemorrhagic capillary damage
IX. Circulatory	
Hemodynamic Mitral stenosis or chronic left ventricular failure	Pulmonary edema. Kerley's "B" lines. Hemosiderosis, lower lobe fibrosis.
Thromboembolic Multiple pulmonary emboli	Episodic dyspnea. Atelectatic streaks. Pulmonary hypertension. Positive lung scan
Fat embolism	Recent fracture; localized changes or diffuse pulmonary edema
Lymphangiography	Recent lymphangiogram; ground glass appearance
X. Connective Tissue Diseases	
Scleroderma	Systemic manifestations of progressive systemic sclerosis (skin changes, gastrointestinal tract and joint symptoms). Cystic changes at lung bases
Polyarteritis nodosa	Subacute febrile systemic disease. Variable manifestations of pneumonia, asthma, hemoptysis
Wegener's granulomatosis[69]	Necrotizing granulomatous lesions of upper airways, lung, and kidneys. May be limited to lungs. Multiple nodular masses which may cavitate

─Table 34-2 (cont.)─

Disease	Special Features
X. Connective Tissue Diseases (cont.)	
Systemic lupus erythematosus	Small atelectatic streaks with occasional patchy pneumonitis. Pleural effusion common. Antinuclear factor. Pulmonary disease more common in procainamide-induced disease
Rheumatoid lung disease	Rheumatoid pulmonary nodules and endarteritis. Pleural effusion common
Caplan syndrome (rheumatoid pneumoconiosis)	Coal workers' pneumoconiosis. Clinical signs of rheumatoid arthritis. Rheumatoid factor. Occasional progressive massive fibrosis
Diffuse fibrosing alveolitis[67] (synonyms—see text)	Dyspnea, clubbing. Diffuse fine fibrosis Cor pulmonale. Possible multiple agents or factors elicit this. Some respond to corticosteroids. Immunologic mechanisms possible
XI. Eosinophilic Pneumonias[81]	
Löffler syndrome	Fever, eosinophilia, asthma. Minimal or no pulmonary symptoms. Recovery usually within a month. Transitory and migratory alveolar infiltrations
Prolonged pulmonary eosinophilia	Chronic patchy infiltrations
Tropical eosinophilia	Asthmatic attacks. Biologic false positive serologic test for syphilis. Complement fixation positive for filarial antigens. May respond to diethylcarbamazine
XII. Miscellaneous	
Sarcoidosis	Granulomatous involvement of lungs, lymph nodes, eyes, skin, liver, spleen, salivary glands, muscle, etc. Variable symptoms. Hilar adenopathy frequent. Tuberculin anergy. Increase in gamma globulins. Responds to corticosteroids

─Table 34-2 (cont.)─

Disease	Special Features
XII. Miscellaneous (cont.)	
Pulmonary alveolar proteinosis	PAS-staining material occasionally in sputum. Pulmonary lavage with saline produces clearing. Chronic alveolar infiltration. Often perihilar distribution. Cellular debris fills alveoli without interstitial change
Eosinophilic granuloma (histiocytosis X)	Begins in childhood with slow progression. Airway obstruction common. May have diabetes insipidus. Pneumothorax common. Associated bone lesions common. Honeycomb cystic lung in later stages. No hilar adenopathy
Goodpasture syndrome	Hemoptysis, anemia, and renal failure. Acute hemorrhagic pneumonitis and nephritis. Patchy infiltrates. Linear irregular thickening of glomerular and alveolar basement membrane on electron microscopy. Cytotoxic specific antiglomerular basement membrane antibody
Idiopathic pulmonary hemosiderosis	Recurrent hemoptysis, anemia, hemosiderin-laden macrophages in sputum. Fine reticular shadows with interstitial fibrosis. Varying infiltrates with blood. Mechanism uncertain
Rejection phenomenon in homotransplantation	Circulating antibody against donor cells. Acute vasculitis. Destruction of grafted organ. Cytotoxic tissue-specific antibody-type II immunologic reaction
XIII. Secondary Pulmonary Fibrosis	
Bronchiectasis	Cough and purulent sputum of long standing
Bronchitis and obstructive pulmonary disease	Impaired forced expiratory flow. Hyperinflation. Increased linear markings

DIAGNOSTIC PROCEDURES

Frequently, the roentgenographic and clinical features will strongly suggest a diagnosis which can be confirmed by conventional means. For example, appropriate cultures may prove the diagnosis of infection; biopsy of a characteristic skin lesion, or a positive Kveim test for sarcoidosis may support the diagnosis of sarcoidosis; and the demonstration of a malignant tumor outside the thorax may account for diffuse metastases throughout the lungs. Seeking all readily accessible clues often will obviate the need for major invasive procedures.

SPUTUM EXAMINATION

A discussion of this subject will be found in Chapter 32. In patients with bacterial or fungal infections, appropriate smears and cultures may establish a diagnosis. Periodic acid-Schiff (PAS) stain of formalin-fixed sputum may show the characteristic alveolar material present in alveolar proteinosis. Cytologic study may reveal tumor cells. Large numbers of eosinophils in the sputum suggest a hypersensitivity disorder involving the lung. Oil droplets within macrophages support the diagnosis of lipoid pneumonia. Hemoptysis is often diagnostically helpful (see Table 34–1).

LYMPH NODE BIOPSY

Palpably enlarged cervical or supraclavicular lymph nodes may be biopsied with little discomfort and risk to the patient. Such a biopsy is often useful in the diagnosis of sarcoidosis, tuberculosis, Hodgkin's disease and other lymphomas, and metastatic carcinoma. Biopsy of clinically unimpressive nodes, or scalene fat-pad biopsy when no nodes are palpable, is likely to be unrewarding except in sarcoidosis or when large mediastinal nodes are apparent on x-ray. Scalene node biopsy has largely been replaced by mediastinoscopy, which is a safer procedure and is more likely to yield diagnostic material.

LIVER BIOPSY

Needle biopsy of the liver may be helpful in sarcoidosis, tuberculosis, lymphoma, collagen disease, and metastatic neoplasm. It will reveal tubercles in about 75 percent of patients with sarcoidosis or disseminated tuberculosis; with the latter disease tubercle bacilli can frequently be demonstrated by acid-fast tissue stains. Unless such a specific etiologic agent is demonstrated, it must always be recalled that a granulomatous reaction is nonspecific whether in the liver or a lymph node. It may occur as a response to hypersensitivity, fungus or bacterial infection, para-sitic infestation, or the deposition of foreign chemical substances, as well as in tuberculosis and sarcoidosis. Such a reaction may be seen in a node draining phospholipid-containing necrotic material from a malignant tumor or a node draining a diseased gall bladder. The histologic picture of a granulomatous reaction must thus always be interpreted in the light of the total clinical picture, but provides reasonable histologic support for sarcoidosis in the presence of highly compatible clinical findings. Careful bacterial cultures of biopsy material are always important.

LUNG BIOPSY[73,94]

Biopsy procedures are discussed in Chapter 32. The successful use of transbronchial lung biopsy in diffuse infiltrations, especially sarcoidosis, represents a significant advance. This is the procedure of choice when other features or more superficial abnormalities do not establish a diagnosis. Disorders which generally can be definitely diagnosed only by lung biopsy include bronchiolar carcinoma, pulmonary alveolar proteinosis, berylliosis, desquamative interstitial pneumonia, and idiopathic diffuse interstitial fibrosis. In patients with sarcoidosis and histiocytosis X in whom other lesions cannot be demonstrated, lung biopsy may be required. In sarcoidosis, histologic lesions are usually readily demonstrated in the lymph nodes, skin, or conjunctiva. The diagnosis of miliary tuberculosis or Farmer's Lung does not usually depend on lung biopsy.

Open lung biopsy carries a low risk, especially in young patients without complicating heart disease, and may provide more adequate tissue specimens. Percutaneous biopsies are sometimes satisfactory, but are likely to yield tissue which is not fully representative unless discrete nodular masses are present. Answers to three questions may aid in the decision regarding the need for lung biopsy: 1) Does the patient have a lesion amenable to treatment? 2) Would treatment be indicated if the suspected diagnosis proved to be correct? 3) Is it important to know of an occupational exposure or that a specific environmental agent is present in the lungs? Generally, the indications for lung biopsy are strong in young patients and in those with symptomatic and progressive disease. It is advisable to consider whether the biopsy findings are of primary importance to the patient or only to the physician. The histologic picture and the degree of fibrosis also are of prognostic value in predicting the response to corticosteroids in fibrosing alveolitis.

Lung tissue should be subjected not only to histologic study but also to a careful search for fungi and tubercle bacilli, using all appropriate staining and cultural techniques. Chemical and spectrographic analysis may be indicated to identify such substances as silicon and beryllium.

MANAGEMENT

Specific treatment obviously requires that a definitive diagnosis be established. Although many of the diseases discussed in this chapter are not responsive to therapy, it is important that all treatable possibilities be given consideration. Table 34–3 lists a number of diseases for which specific treatment is available.

ASSESSMENT OF DISEASE ACTIVITY

In considering treatment, it is clearly essential that one determine evidence of activity or progression by symptoms, previous radiographs, and measurements of pulmonary function. The degree and course of im-

---
TABLE 34–3
Therapy of Diffuse Pulmonary Lesions

A. Specific chemotherapy for infections
B. Removal from exposure for occupational pulmonary diseases
C. Corticosteroid treatment
　Sarcoidosis
　　Incapacitating or progressive disease; persistent disease, with functional impairment without evidence of spontaneous remission for more than one year
　Extrinsic allergic alveolitis if symptomatic and not responding to simple environmental removal of the offending antigen
　Pulmonary vasculitis
　　Polyarteritis nodosa, systemic lupus erythematosus
　Histiocytosis X
　　Effect uncertain
　Therapeutic trial in idiopathic fibrosing alveolitis
　　More likely helpful with more inflammatory picture and less fibrosis. "Desquamative" features, rather than "mural" changes may suggest a more favorable response or milder disease
D. Immunosuppressive or cytotoxic agents
　Neoplastic disease
　　Lymphomas, leukemia, carcinoma of breast, metastatic seminomas, etc.
　Wegener's granulomatosis (cyclophosphamide often combined with corticosteroids)
　Lupus erythematosus
　?Rheumatoid arthritis
E. Pulmonary lavage for alveolar proteinosis
F. Hormone therapy for some neoplasms, e.g., carcinoma of the breast

---

pairment will be crucial in future management decisions. The importance of diligently seeking previous radiographs cannot be overestimated. The vigor of diagnostic approach will be determined by evidences of disease activity, and similarly, biopsy studies will assist in determining activity of the process. Objective evidences of change assist in the assessment of response to treatment (radiographic changes and serial measurements of pulmonary function, as well as changes in symptoms and other clinical findings). This is particularly pertinent in patients treated with corticosteroids but applies as well to infections treated with antimicrobials (e.g., tuberculosis).

CORTICOSTEROID THERAPY

Steroid therapy appears capable of exerting a favorable effect in many patients with sarcoidosis, fibrosing alveolitis, connective tissue disease involving the lung, and certain other disorders of an immunologic type.

　Furthermore, in some instances of progressive or seriously incapacitating disease, a therapeutic trial of steroids is indicated even when a specific diagnosis has not been made. Lung biopsy may occasionally be deemed inadvisable or not likely to reveal a specific diagnostic picture. Transbronchial lung biopsy almost always can be achieved. The risks and potential value of the steroids must be weighed and the effects objectively assessed. Careful prior exclusion of infectious disease is important.

IMMUNOSUPPRESSIVE AGENTS

The role of these agents in diffuse lung disease remains relatively uncertain except in lymphomas and leukemia. Benefit from cyclophosphamide (Cytoxan) therapy has been demonstrated in Wegener's granulomatosis. These agents have an anti-inflammatory action as well as a specific inhibitory effect on immunologic reactions. Their use is indicated in patients with vasculitis, usually in combination with corticosteroids.

SUPPORTIVE TREATMENT

Supportive treatment not only is important in conjunction with specific therapy but may also be initiated when other treatment is not available or indicated. Symptomatic remedies for troublesome cough, limitation of physical activity, treatment of congestive failure, and measures to combat secondary bacterial infection may be of great therapeutic value. The relief of hypoxia by the administration of oxygen is occasionally needed. Since airway obstruction with alveolar hypoventilation is an unusual and late feature, oxygen may be administered safely with little risk of depression of respiration and carbon dioxide retention.

SPECIFIC PROBLEMS IN DIAGNOSIS AND MANAGEMENT

TUBERCULOUS AND FUNGAL INFECTIONS

The importance of identifying promptly potentially treatable infections, such as tuberculosis, cannot be overemphasized. Treatable infectious agents must always be sought, especially in patients with altered host defenses. The presence of fine miliary lesions always should suggest the possibility of *miliary tuberculosis*. The urgency of beginning appropriate chemotherapy may not be recognized. Symptoms may vary from mild illness to severe dyspnea and prostration. The presence of fever and rapidly progressive disease favors tuberculosis rather than sarcoidosis, which can produce a similar roentgenographic appearance. The tuberculin skin test is usually positive but may be negative in the presence of overwhelming disease, or in older patients whose skin reactivity is not normal. Liver biopsy is positive in over 90 percent of cases, and acid-fast tissue stains commonly show tubercle bacilli. The use of at least two to three effective antituberculous drugs is essential in tuberculosis to prevent the emergence of drug resistance. Treatment must be continued for a sufficient period of time to eradicate the disease (usually 18 to 24 months). If failure of primary treatment occurs, resistance to isoniazid may well have developed. If the patient has been treated before, it is important to include drugs to which there is reason to believe the organisms are sensitive. Rifampin is an excellent mycobactericidal drug, but neither rifampin nor any *single drug should ever be added to a failed or failing regimen.* Sensitivity studies and a careful history of previous drugs administered are essential when drug resistance is suspected. Communication with the appropriate health department is both informative and valuable in investigation of case contacts and for proper disease managment. Recognition and management of tuberculosis is outlined in Chapter 81.

Fungus infections must be differentiated from tuberculosis and appropriately treated. It is important to distinguish saprophytic fungi (i.e., *Aspergillus fumigatus* in sarcoidosis) which may not be responsible for any invasive disease.

OCCUPATIONAL DISEASES

Pneumoconiosis is a frequent cause of diffuse nodular or reticular lesions in the lung.[65] In the United States, coal workers' pneumoconiosis, silicosis, and asbestosis are the most common types seen, but a variety of metals and inorganic dusts encountered in industry can produce pulmonary injury. A careful lifelong work history and knowledge of the hazards related to specific occupations will often permit a presumptive diagnosis. The features of many of these are depicted in Table 34–2.

In addition to those diseases caused by deposition of inorganic material, numerous organic dust diseases have been described.[87] Most of these appear to represent hypersensitivity reactions and are discussed below.

IMMUNOLOGIC PULMONARY REACTIONS[74,85]

Four basic types of immunologic reaction involving the lung have been defined.

Type I is dependent on IgE and is mediated by histamine. Extrinsic asthma in response to a specific inhaled antigen is the prototype. This is not discussed in this chapter as pulmonary infiltrates are infrequent. Occasionally, eosinophilic infiltrates or mucus plugs or impactions produce radiographic shadows.

Type II reactions involve a cytotoxic tissue-specific antibody. This is observed in Goodpasture syndrome where linear, irregular thickening of glomerular and alveolar basement membrane is noted on electron microscopy. Acute hemorrhagic pneumonitis with recurrent hemoptysis and an associated nephritis is frequently rapidly progressive and fatal in spite of corticosteroid and immunosuppressive treatment.

Type III or immune-complex reactions can result in deposition of antigen-antibody complexes along alveolar-capillary membranes in response to inhalation of specific antigens. *Extrinsic allergic alveolitis* is seen in Farmer's Lung, which is caused by inhalation of spores from moldy hay. Similar reactions are seen in workers exposed to raw cotton (byssinosis) and in bird breeders exposed to pigeon or parakeet droppings. A hypersensitivity pneumonitis resulting from thermophilic actinomycetes may result from contaminated air conditioning or heating systems. Removal from the offending antigen is essential, and the process may be fully reversible if recognized early, but fibrosis will result from chronic exposure. Corticosteroid treatment may hasten regression.

Pulmonary vasculitis is another form of immune complex disease,[80] as noted in polyarteritis nodosa and Wegener's granulomatosis, where angiitis is prominent. (See Chap. 100). Response to corticosteroids and immunosuppressive treatment is often encouraging.

Type IV immune reactions are cell-mediated reactions of delayed hypersensitivity with the production of granulomatous nodules as in tuberculosis. Specific antituberculous treatment is sometimes combined with corticosteroid treatment when the degree of tissue reaction is potentially life-threatening.

SARCOIDOSIS [75-79,83,86,88]

Sarcoidosis is a granulomatous disease of unknown etiology that requires more detailed description because of its frequency as a cause of diffuse pulmonary infiltrations and its protean and variable manifestations. The most common pulmonary manifestation is hilar adenopathy, which is often associated with right paratracheal adenopathy. The pulmonary lesions vary from those which are roentgenographically invisible through small nodular lesions of 2 to 3 mm, to large confluent masses several centimeters in diameter. Soft infiltrates of an apparent "alveolar" type may also be observed. A reticulonodular pattern is frequent, with some fine interstitial infiltrates and/or fibrosis, and the disease may progress to severe diffuse fibrocystic changes. In the absence of known environmental hazardous exposure, sarcoid is the most common cause of diffuse infiltration, and it is particularly likely when symptoms and degree of illness seem mild in relation to the extent of the radiographic changes. However, the clinical presentation can vary from the incidental radiographic finding to debilitating febrile systemic illness or severe cough and dyspnea. The disease occurs most frequently in young adults and is more common and severe in black patients. Peripheral lymphadenopathy, hepatosplenomegaly, uveitis, and skin lesions are often present. Parotid and lacrimal gland enlargement and nervous system and myocardial disease with arrhythmias may be observed. Such clinical findings as depression of delayed hypersensitivity reaction (tuberculin, mumps, *Candida*), increased serum globulin, elevated alkaline phosphatase, hypercalciuria, and hypercalcemia also suggest the presence of sarcoid.

The diagnosis of sarcoidosis depends on the compatible clinical and radiologic picture and either granulomas on tissue biopsy (with reasonable exclusion of other causes of granulomatous disease) or a positive Kveim reaction. Biopsy information is sought from the most accessible tissue which seems abnormal. *Kveim reaction* is induced by the intradermal injection of a validated suspension of sarcoidal tissue (usually spleen). Any nodule appearing at the site of the injection is biopsied at 4 to 6 weeks. Although the exact nature of the reaction is poorly understood, well-formed granulomas lend support to the diagnosis. False positive reactions occur with an incidence of 5 percent and are sometimes attributable to unsatisfactory tissue suspensions. A negative reaction does not exclude the diagnosis as only about 50 to 80 percent will be positive. Satisfactorily standardized test material is of limited availability, and results must always be interpreted in the light of the clinical findings.

In sarcoidosis, many patients with mild disease will demonstrate a spontaneous remission and no treatment is required. In the absence of severe incapacitating disease, a period of observation of several months without treatment is recommended in order to assess the likelihood of a spontaneous remission. Relapses are not observed following spontaneous remissions. However, if the disease progresses, or if there is persistent significant disease in 6 to 12 months, corticosteroid treatment should be initiated. Mediastinal or hilar or peripheral lymphadenopathy alone usually is not sufficient indication for systemic treatment. With seriously ill patients, treatment should be initiated as soon as histologic support for the diagnosis is obtained, with other causes of granulomatous diseases reasonably excluded.

Corticosteroids often represent a dramatic therapeutic agent in sarcoidosis. Improvement in dyspnea, pulmonary function, and radiographs may be significant within 2 to 4 weeks, and treatment should be withdrawn if such objective improvement is not clearly documented in 2 months. Treatment is initiated with 40 mg prednisone daily for 2 weeks, 30 mg daily for 2 weeks (using divided doses for the first 4 weeks), then single daily 8 A.M. doses of 25 mg for 2 weeks, then 20 or 15 mg daily for at least 4 more months. Tapering of drugs should be gradual and cautious since relapse may occur during tapering. Monthly evaluations should be made, especially at the end of treatment and in the first 3 months thereafter. If symptoms, function tests, and chest x-rays worsen, treatment can often be reinstituted at the dose previously known to maintain stability. In some patients, lifetime low-dose maintenance therapy may be required.

Chloroquine has proven helpful in chronic indolent mucocutaneous sarcoidosis (500 mg daily for 2 weeks, then 250 mg daily for several months) but has not seemed effective in pulmonary sarcoidosis. Because of the potential of retinal and corneal damage, chloroquine is usually given no more than 6 months. Courses of treatment for skin lesions, nasal obstruction, and sinusitis can be repeated at 6-month intervals.

FIBROSING ALVEOLITIS [67,84]

A group of similar inflammatory disorders which appear to involve predominantly the alveolar walls is now commonly referred to by the term "fibrosing alveolitis."[91,92] Histologically they show varying degrees of interstitial cellular infiltration, desquamation of cells into the alveolar spaces, and deposition of fibrous tissue. The terms "interstitial pneumonitis," and "diffuse interstitial fibrosis" refer to the same group of disorders, which includes conditions referred to as "Hamman-Rich syndrome" and "muscular cirrhosis of the lung."

Liebow[82] has divided these reactions according to the predominant histologic pattern into a number of subcategories. These include usual interstitial pneumonia (UIP), an organizing form (OIP), a type with prominent desquamation (DIP), lymphocytic interstitial pneumonitis (LIP), and one in which many giant cells are evident (GIP). Although a single pattern may appear to predominate in biopsy material, many patients show features of more than one type in different areas of the lung or at different times, and no distinctly recognizable clinical or etiological counterparts have yet been identified. Many of these reactions are forms of allergic alveolitis due to specific inhaled substances or hypersensitivity reaction to a drug, but some are associated with connective tissue disorders and perhaps a majority are of unknown etiology. Even when it is anticipated that one of these reactions will be found, lung biopsy may be important, since those reactions with predominant desquamative changes are more likely to respond to steroid therapy than those showing extensive fibrosis within alveolar walls.

In fibrosing alveolitis, prednisone therapy is generally started with a dose of 60 mg per day and reduced gradually over a period of weeks until a plateau of improvement is reached, as judged by symptoms, x-ray changes, and repeated pulmonary function tests. A maintenance dose of 15 to 30 mg per day is often required to prevent relapse. In pulmonary sarcoidosis, a maintenance dose of 15 mg per day or less is sufficient to sustain remission.

PULMONARY ALVEOLAR PROTEINOSIS
Pulmonary alveolar proteinosis is a disorder of unknown etiology characterized by chronic or recurrent diffuse pulmonary consolidation of variable degree, often in a butterfly distribution, with a tendency to occur in the lower zones of the lungs.[89] Sputum examination may reveal periodic acid-Schiff-staining (PAS-staining) amorphous granular material. Pulmonary function studies reveal restriction and impairment of diffusion. Lung biopsy is generally required to establish the diagnosis. Alveoli are filled with PAS-staining material containing lipid, with varying numbers of histiocytes, but alveolar walls reveal little or no thickening. The response to steroids, enzymes, and potassium iodide has been generally unsatisfactory.

Pulmonary lavage with large volumes of saline has resulted in significant and sometimes permanent improvement in most patients in whom it has been tried.

DIFFUSE INFILTRATIVE DISEASE IN IMMUNOSUPPRESSED PATIENTS[68,72]
Patients with malignant or other serious systemic disease requiring corticosteroids or immunosuppressive treatment may present with diffuse pulmonary infiltration. This combination represents a special diagnostic and therapeutic problem. Common infections, such as tuberculosis and histoplasmosis, can produce totally uncharacteristic roentgenographic patterns in these patients, and agents which are not usually pathogenic may cause rapidly progressive infection. Table 34–4 indicates the possibilities that must be considered. The usual problem is to differentiate extension of the underlying disease, reactions to the drugs used for treatment, and superimposed infection with bacterial, viral, or parasitic microorganisms. An aggressive diagnostic approach is often justified, since many of these reactions are rapidly fatal if untreated. Needle aspiration or transbronchial biopsy of the lung may provide an answer, or open lung biopsy may be indicated.

TABLE 34–4

Diffuse Pulmonary Infiltration in the Immunosuppressed Patient with Neoplasia

Complicating Infection

Bacterial
  Gram-negative pneumonias most common
  Other bacterial pneumonias—staphylococcal
  Unusual organisms—Listeria, Herellea, Serratia
Viral
  Varicella (chicken pox, herpes zoster) pneumonia
  Measles pneumonia
  Cytomegalovirus
  Other viral agents
Parasitic—*Pneumocystis carinii*
Fungal
  Aspergillosis
  Cryptococcosis
  Candidiasis
  Histoplasmosis
  Nocardiasis
Mycobacterial—tuberculosis

Treatment Effect

Busulfan (myleran), Bleomycin, methotrexate, related drugs
Radiation pneumonitis or fibrosis

Extension of Underlying Disease

Leukemia—acute and chronic lymphatic more common
Lymphoma
Other neoplastic disease

CHAPTER 35

Obstructive Pulmonary Disease

HAROLD A. MENKES AND EUGENE R. BLEECKER

DEFINITIONS AND MECHANISMS OF AIRWAY OBSTRUCTION

Obstructive pulmonary diseases are characterized by interference with ventilation by the limitation of expiratory flow rates. They form the largest group of diseases causing cough, wheezing, and shortness of breath without radiologic shadows. They should be distinguished from airflow limitation produced by obstruction in the upper airways (e.g., larynx, trachea) caused by foreign bodies, tumors, secretions, or inflammation. In an asymptomatic individual, the diagnosis of mild airflow obstruction may depend on the use of sophisticated pulmonary function tests designed to detect early abnormalities of peripheral airways. However, the usual patient with obstructive lung disease presents with cough, sputum, wheezing, or dyspnea and has the obstruction confirmed with a simple test of forced expiration. The degree of airway obstruction is not accurately reflected by clinical manifestations, such as dyspnea and wheezing; therefore, the assessment of obstructive airway disease should include objective measures of pulmonary function.[99] Figure 35–1 illustrates the relative cross-sectional diameter of airways from trachea to alveoli (center), the relationships between supporting structures and airway caliber in the normal bronchopulmonary tree (left), and the structural abnormalities seen in chronic bronchitis, asthma, and emphysema (right). In those conditions, forced expiratory flows are limited by three factors[101]: 1) Airway resistance: In the patient with chronic bronchitis, inflammation and mucous gland hyperplasia in the bronchial mucosa reduce airway caliber. 2) Tendency for airways to collapse: In the patient with asthma, bronchial muscle spasm may narrow and collapse peripheral airways limiting airflow and trapping large volumes of air behind closed airways. 3) Elastic recoil of the lungs: At any lung volume, flows are greater in a patient with infiltrative lung disease and a stiff lung which provides the driving pressure for respiratory flows (idiopathic pulmonary fibrosis) than in a patient with obstructive lung disease and a very compliant lung which lacks recoil for expelling air during expiration (emphysema) (see Fig. 35–1).

The size of airways is determined by an interplay of 1) the pressures within and surrounding the airway, and 2) the elasticity of the airway wall or its intrinsic tendency to collapse. At high lung volumes, the pressure surrounding the airways decreases so that they tend to distend. At low lung volumes the opposite is true and airways are narrow.

Asthma, chronic bronchitis, and emphysema[105] are the three usual conditions that cause obstruction to airflow. Asthma is a clinical syndrome of varying etiology characterized by intermittent dyspnea and wheezing, which is caused by widespread narrowing of the intrapulmonary airways.[97] Unlike other causes of airflow limitation, the key feature of asthma is reversibility of airway obstruction with relatively symptom-free periods between attacks.

Chronic bronchitis refers to a clinical syndrome characterized by cough and sputum production. It may be defined[97] as a condition of chronic or excessive mucous secretion in the bronchial tree and cough on most days for at least 3 months in the year during at least 2 years. The diagnosis is made clinically when other conditions which may produce a chronic cough, such as tuberculosis, bronchiectasis, and heart disease, are not present.

Emphysema is a morphologic diagnosis made with certainty only by a pathologist. It is a condition in which there is not only dilatation of the distal air spaces of the lungs but also destructive parenchymal changes in the form of disruption of alveolar walls. Two laboratory tests which correlate best with the pathologic diagnosis of emphysema are 1) a lowered diffusing capacity which reflects loss of effective alveolar-capillary surface area, and 2) a loss of elastic recoil in the lung. The roentgenographic manifestation consistent with the presence of emphysema is hyperinflation associated with either bullous changes or loss of vascular markings characteristic of lung parenchymal destruction.

ASTHMA

CATEGORIES

Asthma can be divided into diagnostic categories based primarily on the presence or absence of allergic factors. It should be emphasized that the different categories represent a clinical spectrum and that there is overlap in the majority of patients.

Extrinsic Allergic Asthma

Asthma due to allergy commonly occurs in patients who have other atopic diseases including hay fever, eczema, and urticaria, and who have relatives with

389

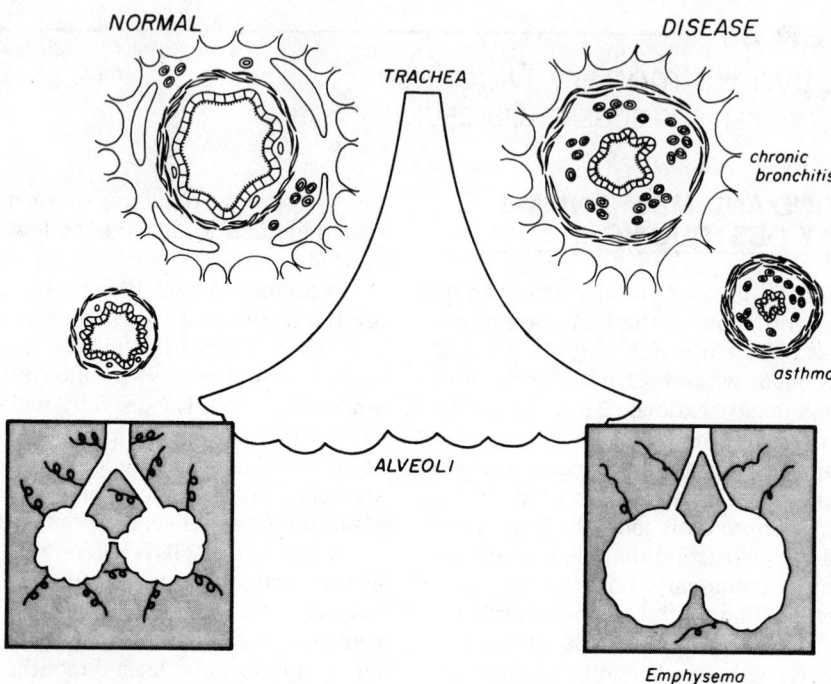

FIGURE 35-1. Airway caliber and supporting structures in asthma, chronic bronchitis, and emphysema (see text).

asthma and other atopic diseases. Allergic reactions producing acute attacks of airway obstruction are primarily of the immediate Type I immunologic reaction (Chap. 34). Specific antigen in these allergic patients will cause a wheal and flare reaction when injected intradermally and airway obstruction when inhaled. These allergic manifestations are attributable to the biologic activities of a group of chemical mediators which are immunologically released from appropriate target cells.

Exposure to an antigenic agent in susceptible individuals causes the production of specific reaginic antibody (IgE) which attaches to mast cells. Reexposure to the antigen initiates a sequence of biochemical reactions within these cells. This results in the formation, release, and/or synthesis of histamine, slow reacting substance of anaphylaxis, bradykinin, prostaglandins, platelet activating factor, and eosinophil and neutrophil chemotactic factors. These mediators contract bronchial smooth muscle, alter vascular permeability, affect pulmonary vascular muscle tone, cause platelet aggregation and degranulation, and attract inflammatory cells to the reaction site. The effects of these substances can result in all of the pathophysiologic changes characteristic of acute asthma.[95] Increases in cellular cyclic AMP inhibit mediator release while increases in cyclic GMP facilitate release. Beta adrenergic agonists increase cyclic AMP and thereby suppress mediator release while methylxanthines, such as theophylline, prevent cyclic AMP breakdown by inhibiting phosphodiesterase. On the other hand, cholinergic agents may enhance release of mediators by increasing cyclic GMP. These interactions serve as a basis for pharmacologic therapy of asthma.

Type III immunologic reactions have been implicated in the pathogenesis of reactions occurring in some allergic individuals that occur several hours after exposure to antigen. Precipitating antigen-antibody reactions can also occur in nonallergic individuals after heavy exposure to certain airborne organic dusts.

Extrinsic Nonallergic Asthma

This term refers to asthma occurring after exposure to various chemical agents which do not seem to provoke a classic IgE immunologic reaction. Many of these syndromes represent industrial diseases. For example, occupational exposure to toluene-di-isocyanate (TDI), a chemical used in the manufacture of plastics, can produce an asthmatic syndrome in some workers. Other agents, such as aspirin and nonsteroidal anti-inflammatory drugs, may also precipitate nonimmunologic asthma.[98]

Intrinsic Nonallergic Asthma

In a significant number of asthmatic subjects hypersensitivity to external allergens or chemical substances cannot explain the presence of asthma. In these patients, asthma depends on some intrinsic abnormality of the airways and has been called "nonallergic" or "intrinsic" asthma. "Intrinsic" as presently used probably encompasses a multitude of clinical syndromes which are associated with bronchial asthma.

In nonallergic asthma, although large numbers of eosinophils can be found in the blood and bronchial secretions, evidence of allergy to inhaled and ingested antigens is lacking, serum IgE levels are normal, and skin tests are negative. Symptoms of asthma in this group may begin at any age but frequently start in the second to fourth decades of life. In many of these patients the asthmatic syndrome is initiated by an upper respiratory tract infection. They improve after appropriate treatment but subsequently do not become free of asthma. The clinical manifestations are frequently severe and have a tendency to persist on a year-round basis with variations in severity rather than complete symptomatic remissions.

Mixed Allergic-Nonallergic Asthma

The asthma of many patients cannot readily be classified as allergic or nonallergic asthma. Such patients may have acute attacks that are clearly related to pollen allergy but may also have chronic symptoms that follow the pattern of nonallergic asthma. Furthermore, some patients whose asthma initially conforms perfectly to the pattern of allergic asthma may after a number of years move into a phase having all the characteristics of nonallergic asthma.

Exercise Induced Asthma

In a large percentage of subjects with asthma, exercise can produce wheezing and dyspnea a short interval after completion of the exercise. This response to exercise probably represents an example of the bronchial hyperreactivity which is characteristic of all types of asthma (see below) and is related to heat loss by the airways when cool, relatively dry air is rapidly inspired during exercise.[103] However, in some asthmatic subjects exercise induced bronchospasm is the dominant symptom.

Airway Hyperreactivity

Despite the varied etiologic factors which are responsible for asthma in these different categories, the one common feature in all asthmatic patients is an abnormal bronchial lability. Whenever a patient with asthma inhales either biochemical mediators such as histamine or prostaglandin F2α, cholinergic agents such as methacholine, or irritants such as critic acid, charcoal dust, or cigarette smoke, he responds with a degree of bronchial constriction greater than normal subjects. Inhalational challenge with either histamine or methacholine can be used to confirm the diagnosis of asthma in questionable cases, and lack of airway hyperresponsiveness to these agents casts serious doubt on the diagnosis of asthma.

CLINICAL FEATURES

In most patients with asthma, acute attacks lasting for hours or days are separated by remissions during which symptoms are reduced or absent. Even when an asthmatic is subjectively improved, there is often considerable impairment of pulmonary function which is not fully appreciated by clinical assessment.[99]

During a mild attack the patient notes wheezing and coughing but can perform ordinary tasks without dyspnea. Physical examination reveals inspiratory and expiratory rhonchi which are accentuated by a forced expiration. With increasingly severe attacks dyspnea is present with mild exertion and eventually persists even at rest. Coughing becomes more pronounced, and it is difficult for the patient to raise sputum. The chest becomes hyperinflated and breath sounds become distant with high-pitched inspiratory and expiratory wheezes. The term "status asthmaticus" connotes severe, prolonged attacks which are refractory to the usual modes of therapy. Patients in "status" are extremely dyspneic and use accessory muscles of respiration as they breathe at a high lung volume. Objective tests of lung function, such as serial spirometry and blood gases, should be employed to assess the severity of respiratory failure and to monitor therapy during status asthmaticus.

Although many cardiorespiratory diseases are characterized by wheezing, dyspnea, and cough, the differential diagnosis of an acute attack of asthma can usually be made with little difficulty on the basis of an adequate history and physical examination. The major entities that must be excluded include pulmonary embolism, acute left ventricular failure, aspirated foreign body or an endobronchial tumor, and other forms of chronic obstructive airway disease. Only occasionally is confusion between upper and lower airway obstruction likely to arise. For example, a high obstruction caused by a tracheal tumor may give rise to a clinical presentation simulating asthma. However, patients with upper airway obstruction usually present with stridor which is loudest in the region of the obstruction. In differentiating upper and lower airway obstruction, a comparison of maximum inspiratory and expiratory flow rates is useful.

PATHOPHYSIOLOGY OF THE ASTHMATIC ATTACK

Increased airway resistance alone does not explain all of the clinical and physiologic changes characteristic of asthma.[100,107] During an asthmatic attack airways tend to close at functional residual capacity, and the asthmatic must breathe at high lung volumes to keep his airways open so that gas exchange can occur. The work of breathing increases, and accessory muscles of respiration must be used to maintain this hyperinflation. In fact, sternocleidomastoid retraction correlates better than dyspnea and wheezing with severe impairment of pulmonary function during acute asthmatic episodes.[99] The severity of the asthmatic attack can be objectively measured by two simple parameters of forced expiration. The forced expiratory volume in one second (FEV_1) reflects airway obstruction while the reduction in forced vital capacity (FVC) correlates with the increased tendency for airway closure and hyperinflation of the lung. During a very severe asthmatic attack, pulmonary hypertension develops acutely. Changes in left ventricular function are clinically manifested by the development of a significant pulsus paradoxus.[102]

LABORATORY FINDINGS

Pulmonary function tests reveal the characteristic signs of bronchial obstruction including a reduction in FEV_1 and vital capacity. An FEV_1 which is less than one liter correlates with severe impairment in arterial blood gas tension. Spirometry should be used to monitor the course of the attack and the response to bronchodilator therapy. To distinguish patients with asthma from those with emphysema, measurements of diffusing capacity for CO can be made. Whereas it is typically low in emphysema, it is normal in asthmatic subjects between attacks.

Arterial hypoxemia may develop during acute attacks of asthma because of the uneven distribution of ventilation with respect to perfusion caused by bronchospasm and mucus occlusion of airways. During mild to moderately severe asthmatic attacks, there is alveolar hyperventilation and arterial CO_2 tensions are reduced. With a severe asthmatic attack, the arterial Pco_2 rises, and this should be viewed with alarm.

The characteristic radiographic abnormality during an acute attack is hyperinflation of the lungs, which is indicated by an increase in anteroposterior diameter of the chest, lowering and flattening of the diaphragm, and increased radiolucency of the lung fields. In contrast to the situation in emphysema, hyperinflation is reversed during a remission of the attack. If there is a history of nasal problems, sinus films should be obtained. The chest roentgenograms should be carefully examined for the presence of pneumonia and atelectasis secondary to mucus plugging. Sputum should be examined and cultured when indicated for the presence of infection, which may serve as a trigger of the asthmatic attack. A complete blood count with a differential white blood cell count will be useful to document the presence of eosinophilia as well as to evaluate for an infectious process.

CONTRIBUTING AND PRECIPITATING FACTORS

Regardless of whether the clinical pattern of asthma is one of allergic, nonallergic, or mixed type, a host of unrelated factors may provoke an attack. These factors include respiratory tract infections, exposure to irritating smoke, fires, dusts, emotional tension, parasympathetic activity, and allergenic agents. A comprehensive evaluation of each of these factors in the individual patient is of therapeutic importance.

MANAGEMENT OF ASTHMA

The successful management of the patient with asthma requires the simultaneous treatment of precipitating factors, clinical manifestations, and complications. Therapy will be ineffective and serious errors may result if any one of these factors is neglected. For example, proper treatment for severe wheezing due to allergy to dog dander and complicated by pneumonia must include the separation of the patient from dogs and the administration of an effective bronchodilator and an appropriate antibiotic.

General Measures

Patients with asthma should avoid exposure to irritating fumes, dusts, and aerosol sprays either occupationally or at home. No patient with asthma should smoke, and he should not be exposed to cigarette smoke in enclosed spaces such as in cars, airplanes, at home, or at work.

Excessive inhalation of nebulized bronchodilator drugs may also produce irritation of the tracheobronchial tree. The control of environmental temperature and humidity may be accomplished by the use of an air conditioner whose filter is changed regularly to avoid the accumulation of airborne molds and fungi. Use of a ventilation system will allow the asthmatic to keep pollens and pollutants out of the home environment. In exceptional circumstances removal to a more favorable climate may be indicated.

Attacks of asthma can certainly be precipitated by emotional factors, and these may present difficult therapeutic problems. Asthma can be a chronic, debilitating disease which may prove psychologically traumatic to both the patient and his family. Occasionally, in these cases, supportive psychotherapy may be very useful. In a severe attack, although hospitalization and mild sedation may be decisive factors in relieving emotional stress, the relief of anxiety resulting from the patient's confidence in his physician, nurses, and therapeutic program is often of greater importance. Oversedation, administration of morphine, and the use of drugs with undesirable cholinergic effects, drying effects, or adrenergic-blocking effects (promazine derivatives) must be avoided.

Infection

Although infection is not a part of every asthmatic attack, its presence should be looked for carefully by evaluating the clinical course, chest x-ray, and sputum. Occasionally, an asthmatic patient's sputum may appear grossly purulent because of the presence of eosinophils; therefore, microscopic sputum examination and culture are indicated before treating respiratory tract infections with the appropriate antibiotics.

Allergy to Specific Inhaled, Ingested, or Injected Substances

Allergy to specific inhaled, ingested, and injected substances may be detected by obtaining the history, by judicious skin testing, and by studying the effect of exposure and withdrawal. Attacks of asthma may be controlled in many instances by avoidance or desensitization. However, even when desensitization is performed, every attempt should be made to eliminate or decrease exposure to the offending allergens.

Pharmacologic Therapy

Five different groups of drugs are available for the treatment of asthma: 1) sympathomimetics, 2) methylxanthines, 3) anticholinergic agents, 4) drugs which prevent the release of chemical mediators such as disodium cromoglycate, and 5) corticosteroids. These drugs will now be discussed in some detail.

SYMPATHOMIMETIC AGENTS. This group of drugs includes a variety of agents which activate β_2 adrenergic receptors. Epinephrine can be administered parenterally in the management of acute asthmatic attacks and is rapidly metabolized resulting in a short duration of action. Isoproterenol is the most potent of the beta adrenergic agonists with equal β_2 and β_1 (cardiac muscle) actions. It is administered as an aerosol and metabolized by catechol-o-methyl-transferase (COMT). Its major bronchodilator effects persist for about 20 minutes and decline during the next hour. Only recommended dosage schedules should be used since commercial inhalers contain four to five times the dose necessary for bronchodilation, and overdosage may lead to tachyphylaxis, myocardial toxicity, and arrhythmias. Adrenergic agonists which have a more specific β_2 action and a longer duration of action since they are not metabolized by COMT

have recently been introduced. These agents all have some cardiac side effects and may cause skeletal muscle tremor, a β_2 side effect. They include isoetharine and metaproterenol, which are less selective β_2 agonists, and the newer agents—terbutaline, salbutamol, fenaterol, and carbuterol. Most of these drugs can be administered orally and as an aerosol. Terbutaline is also available for parenteral administration and may be preferable to subcutaneous epinephrine because of its sustained action.

METHYLXANTHINES. Theophylline derivatives are among the most useful bronchodilators and are available in a multitude of preparations. The activity of these is best compared on the basis of anhydrous theophylline equivalency. Aminophylline, the ethylenediamine salt of theophylline, is soluble and can be administered both orally and intravenously. Both absorption from the gastrointestinal tract and metabolism in the liver vary from one person to another, requiring individualization of dosage. This is best accomplished by determination of plasma theophylline levels. Plasma levels between 10 and 20 μg/ml are considered therapeutic. At higher plasma levels side effects such as nausea, vomiting, central nervous system irritability, and cardiac tachyarrhythmias are likely to occur.

Intravenous aminophylline is initially given with a loading dose of 6 mg/kg and followed by continuous infusion of 0.9 mg/kg per hour. In patients with liver disease, heart failure with chronic passive hepatic congestion, and severe obesity, the intravenous dosage should be reduced by 25 to 50 percent pending determination of blood levels. Cigarette smoking may increase metabolism, and increased doses may be required in smokers. Oral preparations are started at 200 mg four times daily, but up to three times this dose may be required in some patients.

ANTICHOLINERGIC AGENTS. These agents were used earlier in this century but have lost favor because of unwanted side effects which include drying respiratory secretions, reduced mucociliary transport, and cardiac and central nervous system stimulation. Occasionally, in refractory status asthmaticus the benefits from the use of nebulized atropine will warrant a trial of this agent.

DISODIUM CHROMOGLYCATE. This drug is not a bronchodilator, and its exact mechanism of action is not known. It may stabilize mast cell membranes, thereby suppressing immunologic and nonimmunologic release of chemical mediators. It is a dry powder which is inhaled by the patient. Because of its irritant properties, nebulized bronchodilators may have to be administered prior to its use, and it may actually worsen an acute asthmatic attack. It is best used for chronic prophylaxis and only seems to be effective in selected patients, especially young, allergic individuals and those with exercise-induced asthma. Since it is an expensive medication which is somewhat difficult to administer, it should be initially used for a 1-month trial period, and objective measurements of its therapeutic efficacy should be obtained.

CORTICOSTEROIDS. Corticosteroids are effective agents in the treatment of severe asthma and they may work synergistically with other bronchodilators. Their mechanism of action is unknown. They do not cause bronchodilation nor do they affect the release of chemical mediators in Type I immunologic reactions. They may be administered orally, intravenously, and by nebulized aerosols. Because of the serious side effects from long-term systemic steroid therapy, their use should be reserved for the moderately severe asthmatics who are not controlled with conventional therapy or for inpatients in status asthmaticus. When steroid therapy is undertaken in the ambulatory patient, pulmonary function tests should be used to judge their effectiveness, alternate day therapy should be attempted, and the lowest effective dose should be employed. Recently, inhaled steroid preparations with minimal systemic absorption have become available. Use of these agents will often permit the reduction or elimination of treatment with systemic corticosteroids. The major side effect of inhaled steroids is the development of oral candidiasis.

CHOICE OF REGIMEN. The therapeutic regimen in the treatment of asthma must be individualized for each patient. During a complete remission no medications may be required, but with incomplete remissions, airway obstruction may require chronic drug therapy. Initially, such a patient should be treated with an oral preparation of either aminophylline or a specific β_2 agonist. Nebulized bronchodilators should be used to control acute mild exacerbations, as prophylactic agents before undertaking activities which are known to cause bronchospasm, and as an adjunct to help mobilize secretions during postural drainage and respiratory therapy. When additional therapy is indicated, asthmatics should be treated with both aminophylline and β_2 agonists since these agents have different mechanisms of actions and seem to have additive effects as bronchodilators when they are used in combination.[106] Finally, prednisone should be used in the lowest effective dose as previously described. Whenever possible, nebulized steroids or sodium cromolyn should be used to reduce the dose of systemic steroids employed.

COMPLICATIONS

The course of asthma may be changed drastically by the appearance of complications, and the goal of management is their prevention if possible and treatment if necessary. Complications which should be watched for include atelectasis, pneumonia, pneumothorax, and allergic bronchopulmonary aspergillosis, a clinical syndrome characterized by febrile episodes, cough productive of brownish rubbery sputum with bronchial casts, eosinophilic pulmonary infiltrates, and proximal bronchiectasis. When this syndrome occurs, patients have serum precipitins to aspergillus antigen as well as an immediate or delayed skin reaction to this antigen.

CHRONIC BRONCHITIS AND EMPHYSEMA

DEFINITION AND ETIOLOGY

Much confusion has resulted from the indiscriminate application of the term "emphysema" to all forms of chronic lower-airway obstruction and from the failure to appreciate the potential seriousness of chronic bronchitis alone. In recognition of the fact that these conditions frequently occur together and may be difficult to differentiate clinically, terms such as "chronic obstructive pulmonary disease," "chronic obstructive lung disease," and "diffuse obstructive pulmonary syndrome" have achieved popularity. Partial clarification of this long-neglected problem has been brought about by structure-function correlation using morphologic study of diseased lungs in the inflated state, by epidemiologic studies of chronic respiratory disease, and by the extensive use of physiologic methods in the clinical evaluation of patients. Because of the close clinical relationship between these two conditions, the clinical features will be described together.

Chronic Bronchitis

Chronic bronchitis is a condition characterized by excessive secretion of mucus in the bronchi and usually by chronic or recurrent bacterial infection. Airway obstruction may be absent in some patients with chronic mucous hypersecretion, while in others it may appear transiently with superimposed acute infection or may be constant.[104] Morphologic changes are limited to the bronchial walls, which show hypertrophy of mucous glands and dilatation of their ducts. In chronic bronchitis these glands occupy a greater proportion of the bronchial mucosa and can be found in more peripheral airways than usual (Fig. 35-1).

Mutiple factors have been implicated in the etiology of chronic bronchitis. The important role played by cigarette smoking is established, and the advanced stages of clinical or morphologic bronchitis are uncommon in persons who have never smoked. Atmospheric pollution in urban areas and occupational exposure to dust are sometimes important causes of chronic bronchitis. Individual variation in susceptibility appears to be great, however, and there are undoubtedly other important factors in the pathogenesis of this disease.

Emphysema

Although emphysema is a diagnosis made on pathologic examination, an attempt should be made using clinical, physiologic, and radiologic methods to determine which patients with obstructive airway disease also have morphologic emphysema. There are two principal types of emphysema, centrilobular and panlobular, which can be recognized in fixed inflated specimens of the lung obtained at postmortem examination.

CENTRILOBULAR EMPHYSEMA. This process begins at the center of the pulmonary lobule and extends outward toward the periphery, commonly leaving alveoli at the margins of the lobule anatomically intact. The lesion is associated pathologically with the deposition of carbon pigment in the area involved, bears a well-documented relationship to antecedent chronic bronchitis, and shows a tendency to be localized more in the upper than in the lower portions of the lung.

PANLOBULAR EMPHYSEMA. This form of emphysema is characterized by uniform destruction of the pulmonary lobule in involved areas, is less clearly associated with chronic bronchitis, tends to occur in dependent regions of the lung, and is somewhat more commonly associated with the formation of bullae. In patients with advanced disease, a combination of the two types of emphysema is frequently found.

Like chronic bronchitis, emphysema is undoubtedly associated with smoking, although the factors responsible for its development in an individual are unknown. Some cases of panlobular emphysema are associated with α_1-antitrypsin deficiency, a genetically determined biochemical abnormality (see Chap. 31). This association should be suspected when emphysema develops without antecedent bronchitis, especially in patients below age 50, or when multiple members of a family are affected.

CLINICAL MANIFESTATIONS

The relation between chronic bronchitis and emphysema is such that the majority of patients with chronic lower-airway obstruction have some element of both conditions by the time serious dyspnea has developed. The usual sequence begins in a heavy smoker with chronic bronchitis, manifested by cough and sputum for a period of years before the onset of dyspnea. Dyspnea usually appears insidiously, is first noticed during exertion, and is unaccompanied by or-

thopnea. Although not episodic, as in the case of bronchial asthma, shortness of breath is frequently aggravated by dampness and cold, by exposure to dusty atmospheres, and particularly by even minor superimposed respiratory infections. It is characteristic for patients with chronic bronchitis to have frequent episodes of acute bronchitis, often attributable to *H. influenzae* or *S. pneumoniae* and they often date the onset of exertional dyspnea to such an episode. In some cases there is no history of cough preceding the onset of dyspnea.

It is common for patients to attribute their gradually decreasing exercise tolerance to age or heart disease, and many do not seek medical advice until symptoms become quite marked or until some complication has occurred. Rather severe degrees of chronic airway obstruction may thus be encountered as incidental findings in a preoperative evaluation or may first come to medical attention with the development of frank respiratory insufficiency. Gradual and progressive loss of weight may occur and is occasionally so striking as to suggest the presence of malignancy.

In early and uncomplicated chronic bronchitis the physical examination may be entirely normal, but scattered rhonchi due to the presence of mucus in the airways are commonly present. In most individuals, airway obstruction is not a problem and they seek no medical advice. Of those who eventually see a physician, evidence of airway obstruction will usually be apparent on examination. Fine wheezing of the type heard in bronchial asthma is rarely present during quiet breathing, except in the bronchitic with bronchial infection. Frequently, the recognition of airway obstruction requires that observations be made during forced expiration. It is an essential part of the physical examination to have patients exhale rapidly through the open mouth, beginning with full inflation of the lungs and continuing until no further air can be expelled. Even when this maneuver does not result in audible wheezing, prolongation of forced expiration beyond 4 or 5 seconds is indicative of airway obstruction. In patients with severe obstruction, pursed lip breathing may be observed. This probably acts to control the speed of expiration so that airway collapse is reduced.

Many physical signs once considered indicative of pulmonary emphysema actually reflect only hyperinflation of the lungs and may be seen in asthma and chronic bronchitis as well. These include an increase in the anteroposterior diameter of the chest, widened intercostal spaces, a hyperresonant percussion note, obliteration of the area of cardiac dullness, and low diaphragms. These findings should be interpreted with caution since they are subject to large observer error, correlate poorly with the severity of airway obstruction, and have little value in differentiating between asthma, bronchitis, and emphysema. The characteristic barrel chest is occasionally seen in elderly subjects without airway obstruction and is frequently absent in patients with advanced emphysema. A generalized decrease in the intensity of breath sounds is common in emphysema.

Patients having severe chronic bronchitis and little emphysema may present with repeated episodes of respiratory failure, with worsening of airway obstruction, and the development of cor pulmonale and right–sided congestive heart failure (blue bloater). The usual precipitating factor is bronchial or pulmonary infection. Here the clinical picture may be dominated by the manifestations of hypoxia and respiratory acidosis. Cyanosis and disturbances of consciousness ranging from slight drowsiness and irritability to frankly psychotic behavior or coma may be observed. Although rare, advanced degrees of carbon dioxide retention may produce a sufficient increase in intracranial pressure to cause papilledema, making differentiation from primary neurologic disease an important problem. Recovery from each episode may be accompanied by the disappearance of fluid retention and cyanosis, but some degree of hypercapnea and hypoxemia commonly persist, and secondary polycythemia may be present. Clubbing of the fingers is distinctly unusual, however, and should suggest the coexistence of bronchiectasis or carcinoma of the lung.

In contrast, the patient with severe emphysema and little bronchitis (pink puffer) usually develops carbon dioxide retention and cor pulmonale only as a terminal manifestation, when the extent of the anatomic destruction of lung is such that the maintenance of adequate alveolar ventilation is nearly a mechanical impossibility. Survival from the onset of breathlessness is likely to be shorter in these patients than in patients with predominant bronchitis.

ROENTGENOLOGIC FEATURES

Although roentgenographic assessment is important in both the diagnosis of patients with chronic obstructive airway disease and in their overall management, it may be of limited value in identifying or differentiating the common forms of obstructive pulmonary diseases. In fact, chronic bronchitis and emphysema may be present with no discernible radiologic abnormality. Increased radiolucency of the lung, increased depth of the thorax, low and flat diaphragms, a large retrosternal airspace, and a greater than 90° angle between the diaphragm and sternum on lateral films are not diagnostic of specific types of obstructive airway disease and just indicate the presence of hyperinflation. The single finding of greatest usefulness in the differentiation of emphysema from other forms of chronic obstructive airway disease is regional or generalized loss of vascularity in the peripheral lung fields with rapid tapering of the proximal branches of the pulmonary artery, although this change is often subtle and difficult to detect in the presence of congestion of the pulmonary veins or of pulmonary infiltration. Loss of vasculature may often be more readily appreciated from tomograms of both lung fields, for they give better visual separation of the vascular and other shadows. Typically, patients with α_1-antitrypsin deficiency have evidence of panlobular emphysema characterized by the loss of vascular markings predominantly in the lower two-thirds of each lung field. Plain films of the chest may reveal bullous lesions, and the presence of complicating pulmonary hypertension and right ventricular hypertrophy can sometimes be detected radiographically. Bronchograms, although definitely not recommended for the evaluation of patients with obstructive pulmonary disease, may in patients with chronic bronchitis result in the filling of markedly dilated mucous glands in the trachea and main bronchi, producing a picture suggestive of multiple diverticula. If the dilated bronchioles and emphysematous spaces in centrilobular emphysema are filled, they appear as round shadows 3 to 6 mm in diameter. A minority of patients with emphysema have chest roentgenograms which show increased vascular markings. These patients do not have hyperinflation and bullae but more frequently have evidence of pulmonary hypertension and cardiac enlargement. On the one hand, when the chest x-ray shows increased retrosternal air space, flattened or scalloped diaphragms, and loss of peripheral vascular markings, there is usually physiologic evidence of obstruction. On the other hand, there may be severe obstruction and a normal chest x-ray.

PHYSIOLOGIC CHANGES

Clinical assessment of pulmonary function in individual cases of chronic bronchitis and emphysema can be important to the physician in six ways:

1. To establish the presence and degree of airway obstruction
2. To evaluate objectively the results of treatment or the course of the disease
3. To assist in the differentiation between emphysema and other forms of airway obstruction
4. To evaluate work potential or operative risk

5. As a guide to treatment in respiratory failure
6. To serve as a basis to predict the course and prognosis of obstructive airway disease

Airway Obstruction

The characteristic functional defect occurring in chronic bronchitis and emphysema is a decrease in forced expiratory flow, which is commonly assessed by means of spirometry. Vital capacity may be normal or low, but in the presence of clinically significant emphysema the one-second forced expiratory volume (FEV_1) and the various other parameters of expiratory flow are reduced. Some estimate of the degree of limitation of exercise tolerance to be expected may be derived from the absolute value of the FEV_1. It is unusual to see patients with an FEV_1 above 2 liters who experience dyspnea during ordinary physical activity, but reduction of the FEV_1 to a value below 1 liter is usually associated with dyspnea on level walking at a normal pace or on climbing more than one flight of stairs. It is also somewhat unusual to see either carbon dioxide retention or the development of cor pulmonale when the FEV_1 exceeds 1 liter. Severe airway obstruction in which FEV_1 is less than 0.75 is associated with a significant reduction of 5-year survival to approximately one-third of normal.[96]

Serial ventilatory measurements are perhaps the most valuable objective means of determining the rate of progression of disease or of evaluating response to therapy.

Lung Volumes and Compliance

Static lung volumes are almost always abnormal in patients with airway obstruction secondary to chronic bronchitis and/or emphysema. Residual volume is elevated in both, functional residual capacity is more likely elevated with emphysema, and total lung capacity is increased with emphysema and usually normal in chronic bronchitis. With emphysema, there is typically a loss of elastic recoil.

Diffusing Capacity

Diffusing capacity is usually decreased with emphysema and correlates well with the pathologic estimation of the severity of emphysema.

Arterial Blood Studies

In the evaluation and management of patients with obstructive lung disease, arterial blood studies are necessary to determine the adequacy of alveolar ventilation and oxygenation.

MANAGEMENT OF THE AMBULATORY PATIENT

It is widely believed but has not been proven that vigorous treatment of early chronic bronchitis may help to prevent or retard the development of irreversible destructive changes in the lung. It is clear, however, that prevention or prompt treatment of complications may result in prolongation of life. Patients with predominant chronic bronchitis, especially those with a prominent asthmatic component, frequently show a dramatic response to therapy. In the patient with pure emphysema, it is sometimes impossible to achieve significant improvement in exercise tolerance. In the ambulatory patient, therapy consists primarily of measures to improve bronchial hygiene, relieve bronchospasm, improve oxygenation, and increase exercise tolerance.

The types and uses of bronchodilators are detailed in the asthma section of this chapter. There is no objective evidence to support the home use of an intermittent positive pressure ventilator to administer bronchodilators. A hand or freon-powered nebulizer is adequate for therapy with aerosolized bronchodilators. Oral beta agonists and especially aminophylline are the major therapeutic agents that are most effective in the treatment of patients with chronic obstructive airway disease.

Corticosteroids should not be used if adequate exercise tolerance can be achieved with the use of other agents. If a trial of prednisone therapy is undertaken, it should be preceded and followed by measurements of expiratory flow, and should be discontinued if no objective improvement is demonstrated.

In patients with severe hypoxemia (Pa_{O_2} less than 50 mm Hg) continuous therapy with low-flow oxygen (1 to 4 liters per minute) is indicated. This will reduce pulmonary hypertension and often improves exercise tolerance. The major complication of oxygen therapy in some patients is to depress ventilatory drive and worsen hypercapnea. Small elevations of arterial Pco_2 are tolerated by most patients. However, these patients should be monitored carefully and the lowest possible concentration of oxygen should be administered. Patients with exercise-induced dyspnea whose Pa_{O_2} is between 50 and 65 mm Hg should be evaluated with an exercise tolerance test. If Pa_{O_2} falls significantly during exercise and supplemental oxygen improves exercise tolerance, they should be treated with a portable oxygen system during routine activity. Finally, some patients, especially those who are very obese, will develop significant oxygen desaturation in the recumbent position, and they should receive supplemental oxygen during sleep.

Cessation of cigarette smoking should be considered a major therapeutic objective. Two-thirds of patients with chronic bronchitis note improvement in cough and reduction in sputum production within weeks after they stop smoking, and many report improvement in exercise tolerance. Avoidance of other irritants and conditions which cause drying of the tracheobronchial tree are also important.

Many patients with advanced bronchitis have great difficulty in mobilizing bronchial secretions; a regular program of postural drainage, breathing exercises, and assisted cough may be very helpful.

During exacerbations of chronic bronchitis, most patients will benefit from prompt antibiotic therapy which will reduce the severity and duration of these acute infections. Chronic continuous antibiotic treat-ment is usually not indicated since superinfection may develop. Mucolytic agents are occasionally useful in patients with highly viscid mucoid sputum. However, these agents may serve as irritants or cause excessive sputum production. Digitalis should only be used when there is definite evidence of left ventricular failure. In patients with severe polycythemia where the hemotocrit exceeds 65 percent, a phlebotomy is indicated to improve cardiopulmonary function and relieve a hypercoagulable state.

CHAPTER 36

Acute Respiratory Failure (ARF)
WARREN R. SUMMER

INTRODUCTION

Respiratory failure is one of the most frequent problems encountered in medicine. It represents the fifth leading cause of death in the United States. Chronic obstructive lung disease with death from respiratory failure is the only chronic disease which continues to show a yearly increase in mortality. Over 70 percent of deaths in patients with pneumonia are attributed to respiratory failure. If one considers the total number of deaths attributed to respiratory causes including the influenza-pneumonia complex, the number is slightly below 100,000 per year and is very close to that produced by accidents, which ranks fourth as a cause of death in the United States.

Respiratory failure may be divided into two main categories: that which is manifested predominantly or entirely by hypoxemia, and that which is manifested by both hypercapnia and hypoxemia.[113,115] Diseases which produce hypoxic respiratory failure are characterized by a large right-to-left intrapulmonary shunting of blood which is not corrected by high levels of supplemental oxygen. Both lungs are usually extensively involved, although the pathology may be limited to large focal areas of disease such as seen in lobar pneumonia. Total ventilation is almost always increased, and alveolar ventilation is only rarely reduced.

The combination of hypercapnic and hypoxic respiratory failure results from some insufficiency in the ventilatory apparatus. This is usually produced by marked airflow limitation as seen in chronic obstructive lung disease. However, combined hypercapnic-hypoxic respiratory failure may be produced in the presence of completely normal lungs following alterations in the control of breathing (sedative drug overdose) or inadequacies in the neuromuscular or musculoskeletal apparatus. This differentiation between hypoxic and hypercapnic-hypoxic respiratory failure, although somewhat artificial, is convenient because it allows the grouping of conditions that have either similar pathophysiologic or similar therapeutic implications (Table 36–1).

DEFINITIONS OF ACUTE RESPIRATORY FAILURE

Hypoxic respiratory failure may be defined as any condition producing severe arterial *hypoxemia* (Pa_{O_2} < 50 mm Hg) which cannot be corrected by increasing the inspired oxygen concentration to 50 percent (FI_{O_2} = 0.5). Although both Pa_{O_2} < 50 mm Hg and FI_{O_2} = 0.5 are arbitrary levels, they represent critical physiologic landmarks. At a Pa_{O_2} of 50 mm Hg, hemoglobin is approximately 80 percent saturated, and further small reductions in Pa_{O_2} produce very significant reductions in arterial oxygen content. There is little reserve under this circumstance. Although normal individuals tolerate brief reductions of arterial oxygen tension to this level, patients appear to be severely symptomatic when the Pa_{O_2} falls to 50 mm Hg or below. The symptoms, therefore, must be related to both the hypoxemia and the lung disease causing the hypoxemia. An FI_{O_2} of 0.5 is probably the highest level which can be readily achieved at a patient's airway without a closed system (intubation) or nonrebreathing mask. In addition, an FI_{O_2} of 0.5 usually corrects

┌───┐
TABLE 36-1
Pertinent Features of Hypoxic and Hypercapnic–Hypoxic Acute Respiratory Failure

	Hypoxic	Hypercapnic–Hypoxic
Age	Any	Any (bronchitis and emphysema usually > 50 years)
Previous history	Well	Chronic shortness of breath; episodic wheezing
Present illness	Acute shortness of breath temporally related to some serious event, i.e., car accident, sepsis, etc.	Recent upper respiratory infection; increase in shortness of breath, cough, sputum, and wheezing; chest pain, fever; drug overdose; muscle weakness
Physical examination	Evidence of acute illness, tachypnea (> 30), tachycardia, hypotension, lungs clear, or may have diffuse rales	Tachypnea (< 30), tachycardia, prolonged expiration, decreased breath sounds, wheezing, fever, muscle weakness, altered consciousness
Anatomy	Consolidation, atelectasis, pulmonary congestion, and edema	Mucous gland hyperplasia (bronchitis), alveolar wall destruction (emphysema); hypertrophied bronchial muscle (asthma); excess mucus; upper airway obstruction (fixed or variable); normal
Physiology	Large right-to-left intrapulmonary shunts; hyperventilation usual	Ventilation ($\dot{V}$) perfusion ($\dot{Q}$) imbalance (many low $\dot{V}/\dot{Q}$ areas); alveolar hypoventilation due to marked wasted (dead space) ventilation; hypoventilation due to reduced minute ventilation
Chest roentgenogram	Small, white lungs; patchy consolidation	Clear, prominent bronchovascular marking; hyperinflation, bullae, kyphoscoliosis; local pneumonia; hypoinflation with neuromuscular disease
Electrocardiogram	Sinus tachycardia	Normal; right ventricular hypertrophy; "p" pulmonale; low voltage; clockwise rotation
Laboratory	Nonspecific. Hematocrit low to normal; respiratory alkalosis; metabolic acidosis	Hematocrit normal to high; respiratory acidosis; mixed metabolic and respiratory acidosis
└───┘

the hypoxemia associated with hypercapnic-hypoxic respiratory failure and the vast majority of conditions in which gas exchange is not the dominant clinical problem. If hypoxemia is corrected by an FI_{O_2} of 0.5, the management of the patient is markedly simplified.

Hypercapnic-hypoxic respiratory failure may be defined as an acute, life-threatening condition in which carbon dioxide excretion by the lung is inadequate. As the carbon dioxide (CO_2) accumulates, the fractional concentration of oxygen in the alveolus decreases and hypoxemia results. Depending on the underlying physiologic condition of the lungs, hypoxemia may be substantially greater than that explained on the basis of CO_2 accumulation alone. In acute res-

piratory failure (ARF) associated with chronic obstructive lung disease, severe hypoxemia due to perfusion of poorly ventilated lung areas is also present. ARF is often defined in terms of levels of arterial CO_2 and O_2 tension. However, it is difficult to assign absolute blood gas levels because they depend on the precipitating condition and previous state of the patient. In a previously healthy individual, an arterial $Pa_{CO_2} > 45$ mm Hg constitutes ARF. This slight increase in Pa_{CO_2} has grave importance in patients suffering with acute asthma or acute neurologic weakness such as myasthenia gravis. $Pa_{CO_2} > 55$ usually indicates ARF in patients with known chronic obstructive lung disease (COLD) but previously normal carbon dioxide levels.

ACUTE HYPOXIC RESPIRATORY FAILURE

The most satisfactory designation for a variety of acute nonspecific pulmonary injuries which result in severe hypoxemia and normal Pa_{CO_2} is the "adult respiratory distress syndrome" (ARDS).[108] It usually follows a variety of seemingly unrelated systemic or pulmonary insults (see Table 36–2) and must be distinguished from acute pulmonary edema secondary to congestive heart failure (Chap. 146). The diagnosis of cardiogenic pulmonary edema is usually made eas-

ily by a history of known heart disease, the presence of heart murmurs, cardiomegaly, abnormal electrocardiogram, or elevated venous pressure.

PATHOGENESIS

The pathogenesis of the pulmonary changes in ARDS is related to the underlying etiology.[110] Table 36–3 lists some of the postulated mechanisms ultimately resulting in increased pulmonary extravascular water in acute hypoxic respiratory failure. The diagnosis of the ARDS depends on recognition of a symptom complex combined with characteristic physiologic alteration. Most patients have experienced no previous respiratory problem. Following one of the events listed in Table 36–1, there may be a period of mild to moderate respiratory embarrassment, often completely overshadowed by a variety of complex nonrespiratory problems. However, in several hours to a few days the patient begins to experience marked respiratory distress. This is associated with tachypnea (often in excess of 40 per minute) and profound cyanosis. Sputum that is pink and frothy to gross burgundy red may be expectorated. Homogeneous patchy infiltrates on the chest film quickly become diffuse, and air bronchograms are often present. A number of diseases, such as miliary tuberculosis and cardiogenic pulmonary edema, may produce similar pulmonary infiltrates. Asymmetrical or inhomogeneous infiltrates, air fluid levels, lobar atelectasis, or unexplained pleural effusions suggest etiologies other than the ARDS. These and other specific causes of diffuse pulmonary disease must be considered and

---

TABLE 36–2

Disorders Asssociated with Adult Respiratory Distress Syndrome

Aspiration
  Gastric contents
  Fresh and salt water
  Hydrocarbons

Central nervous system
  Trauma
  Anoxia
  Increased intracranial pressure

Drug overdose
  Acetylsalicylic acid
  Heroin
  Methadone
  Propoxyphene
  Barbiturate

Hematologic alterations
  Disseminated intravascular coagulation
  Massive blood transfusion
  Postcardiopulmonary bypass

Infection
  Sepsis (gram positive or negative)
  Viral pneumonia
  Tuberculosis
  Peritonitis

Inhalation of toxins
  Oxygen
  Smoke
  Corrosive chemicals (NO_2, Cl_2, NH_3, phosgene, cadmium)

Metabolic disorders
  Pancreatitis
  Uremia

Shock
  Any etiology (rare in cardiogenic)

Trauma
  Fat emboli
  Lung contusion (after cardiopulmonary resuscitation)
  Nonthoracic

TABLE 36–3

Suggested Mechanisms for Endothelial Injury and Pulmonary Edema in Adult Respiratory Distress Syndrome

1. Corrosive effects of gastric acid in aspiration pneumonia
2. Pulmonary venous hypertension following central nervous system injury or anoxia complicated by a yet unexplained persistent endothelial leak
3. Direct effect by drugs such as heroin and acetylsalicylic acid
4. Activation of alternative pathway of the complement (C)′ cascade resulting in pulmonary vascular leukostasis and release of lysozymic enzymes and superoxide radicals in hemorrhagic and septic shock and possibly many other conditions listed in Table 36-1
5. Inflammatory destruction in viral infection and pancreatitis
6. Excessive production of oxidants (H_2O_2; O_2^-) in oxygen toxicity

ruled out when clinical circumstances make their presence a reasonable possibility. However, in the majority of cases, temporal relationships alone make the precipitating events associated with the diffuse lung disease relatively obvious.

TREATMENT

Regardless of the underlying etiology, therapy is directed at relieving the patient's severe hypoxemia with oxygen while treating the underlying causes. Very high concentrations of oxygen (100 percent) cannot be continued for long periods of time because of oxidant injury to the lung parenchyma. The exact level or duration of high F_{IO_2} exposure necessary to produce pulmonary injury has not been determined. Most authorities feel that breathing greater than 90 percent oxygen for more than 24 hours should be avoided.

Increased extravascular water that produces widespread alveolar closure may be reduced by careful attention to fluid balance and careful diuresis. Left ventricular dysfunction may be assessed as a cause by measurements of pulmonary capillary pressure with a Swan-Ganz catheter. Measurements of pulmonary artery pressure and pulmonary capillary wedge pressure may also be very helpful in management of the patient's underlying fluid status during acute respiratory failure.

Lung volume can be increased by increasing transpulmonary pressure at end-expiration, i.e., a positive end-expiratory pressure (PEEP). In practice, this is accomplished by use of continuous positive airway pressure (CPAP) or continuous positive pressure ventilation (CPPV). The level of PEEP required to improve the hypoxemia varies inversely with the pulmonary compliance. Stiffer lungs require greater transpulmonary pressures for expansion. There is probably an optimal level of lung inflation to achieve the lowest rate of pulmonary extravascular water accumulation. While in normal individuals this level appears to be at the normal functional residual capacity, in the ARDS the optimum level has not been established.[114] Some experimental evidence suggests that increases in lung volume associated with a concomitant rise in pulmonary artery pressure are likely to be associated with increasing rates of extravascular fluid accumulation. Clinical or experimental evidence that PEEP *drives* extravascular water out of the lung or hastens recovery is lacking. In fact, there is some experimental evidence in simulated cases of ARDS that excessive PEEP can increase the rate of fluid accumulation within the lung.[117] Therefore, only enough PEEP should be given to allow an adequate arterial oxygen tension ($Pa_{O_2} = 60$ mm Hg which is equiv-

alent to an arterial saturation of approximately 90 percent).

Methods of instituting PEEP vary. Patients who can breathe spontaneously with adequate alveolar ventilation should be allowed to do so. Low levels of end-expiratory pressure may be delivered through a snug face mask. Levels of end-expiratory pressure above 10 cm of water require endotracheal intubation. Spontaneous ventilation lowers pleural pressure and improves venous return, thereby reducing alterations in cardiac output as a clinical problem. A rising Pa_{CO_2} or an altered level of consciousness may indicate the need for assisted ventilation, and a volume respirator is necessary to expand the very stiff lung. Overventilation which produces respiratory alkalosis must be avoided. In addition, large tidal volumes ($>$ 10 cc/kg) may overinflate the lung and produce pneumothoraces, pneumomediastinum, pneumopericardium, or subcutaneous emphysema.

Continuous positive pressure ventilation (CPPV) may increase pleural pressure, reduce the gradient for venous return, and lower cardiac output.[112] Judicious blood volume expansion can maintain cardiac output, but use of colloid is preferable to crystalloid since any reduction in intravascular osmotic pressure tends to increase the rate of extravascular pulmonary fluid accumulation.

Once an adequate Pa_{O_2} is achieved at a satisfactory F_{IO_2} ($<$ 70 percent) therapy is devoted to careful monitoring in order to avoid complications. Major complications include respiratory superinfection, gastric distension from aerophagia, upper gastrointestinal hemorrhage, fluid overload (insensible loss during artificial ventilation is usually zero), and barotrauma. General measures, such as careful aseptic suctioning, and postural drainage may help to prevent lobar atelectasis, improve Pa_{O_2}, and avoid superinfection. Intensive care unit practices that use antibiotics only when carefully documented infection requires treatment minimize the risks of superinfection with antibiotic-resistant microorganisms. A colonized tracheobronchial tree in an intubated patient is not an indication for antibiotic therapy. Probably the best prevention of superinfection, which ultimately kills 50 percent of patients suffering from ARDS, is early extubation. When the patient begins to improve, the Pa_{O_2} will begin to rise at any preestablished level of PEEP or F_{IO_2}. Slow reduction in the level of PEEP will then produce no significant hypoxemia. The rate of reduction in PEEP is therefore tailored to the change in Pa_{O_2}, and when a level of less than 5 cm maintains an adequate Pa_{O_2} on an $F_{IO_2} <$ 50 percent, the procedure may be carefully discontinued.

ACUTE HYPERCAPNIC-HYPOXIC RESPIRATORY FAILURE

Acute hypercapnic-hypoxic respiratory failure is a combination of physiologic derangements that results from one or more pathologic events. It is not a "disease," but the result of many varied insults (see Table 36–4 and Chap. 146). This form of acute respiratory failure may occur in previously healthy individuals *without* specific lung injury or in persons *with* underlying pulmonary disease.[109,111] When severe underlying chronic pulmonary disease is present, a minor precipitating event may produce severe acute respiratory decompensation. Knowledge of the pathogenesis and physiologic alterations responsible for acute respiratory failure is critical in determining a specific diagnosis and establishing appropriate therapy.

Hypercapnia may result from an increased CO_2 production (Vco_2), a decreased alveolar ventilation ($\dot{V}A$), or a combination of the two (Chap. 31). Increased Vco_2 alone (malignant hyperthermia, grand mal seizures) rarely results in increased Pa_{CO_2}. Decreased alveolar ventilation is the major cause of an elevated Pa_{CO_2}. Alveolar ventilation may be reduced by an absolute decrease in minute ventilation or when an imbalance in ventilation and perfusion causes a large percentage of dead space or wasted ventilation. In this latter case, minute ventilation may be normal or increased.

Hypoxemia may result from pure alveolar hypoventilation with the severity of the hypoxemia determined by the degree of hypoventilation as defined by the alveolar air equation (Chap. 31). Hypoxemia also results from perfusion of poorly ventilated lung units. This always occurs with lower airway disease, such as asthma and chronic obstructive pulmonary disease, and is almost always present with the obesity hypoventilation syndrome and kyphoscoliotic cardiopulmonary disease. Hypoxemia secondary to ventilation perfusion abnormalities is variable in all other causes of combined acute respiratory failure and depends on the degree of underlying or superimposed pulmonary disease.

The presentation and treatment of acute respiratory failure can be divided into those conditions in which the hypercapnia is due to decreased minute ventilation (Table 36–4, categories I–III and IVa) and those conditions in which the respiratory failure results from severe ventilation-perfusion mismatch (Table 36–4, category IVb). Categories V and VI are usually due to varying degrees of decreased minute ventilation and increased wasted ventilation. Their presentation is similar to that of category IVb. More than half of the clinical cases of hypercapnic-hypoxic respiratory failure come from category IVb. The frequency of presentation of the other multiple causes of respiratory failure depends on a particular hospital's referral base. Emergency management of acute respiratory failure is covered in Chapter 146.

ACUTE HYPERCAPNIC-HYPOXIC RESPIRATORY FAILURE SECONDARY TO DECREASED MINUTE VENTILATION

The number of diseases or conditions which may present with hypercapnic-hypoxic respiratory failure secondary to decreased minute ventilation is extensive (see Tables 146–1 and 146–3). Each entity may have characteristic signs and symptoms which initially or ultimately point to the precipitating event. Discussion of each of these conditions is beyond the scope of this chapter.

The presentation of patients with hypercapnic-hypoxic failure secondary to decreased minute ventilation varies from a sudden onset as seen in high cervical cord trauma or tetanus to the slower time

---

┌───┐

TABLE 36–4

Common Causes of Hypercapnic–Hypoxic Respiratory Failure

I. Altered Control

   a. Primary intracranial disease (tumor, vascular infection)
   b. Trauma and raised intracranial pressure
   c. Drugs, poisons, and toxins
   d. Central hypoventilation
   e. Excess oxygen administration in hypercapnic patient

II. Neuromuscular

   a. Spinal cord lesions (trauma, tumor, vascular)
   b. Acute polyneuritis
   c. Myasthenia gravis
   d. Polymyositis
   e. Parkinson's disease

III. Metabolic

   a. Severe acidosis
   b. Severe alkalosis
   c. Hypokalemia
   d. Hypophosphatemia
   e. Hypomagnesemia

IV. Lungs and Airway Disease

   a. Upper airway disease (fixed, variable, or sleep-dependent)
   b. Lower airway disease (COLD, asthma)

V. Musculoskeletal

   a. Kyphoscoliosis
   b. Ankylosing spondylitis

VI. Obesity-Hypoventilation Syndrome

└───┘

course seen in poliomyelitis, polyneuritis, or myasthenia gravis. An even slower onset is observed in hypothyroidism and muscular dystrophy. Kyphoscoliotic cardiopulmonary disease and obesity hypoventilation syndrome with decreased minute ventilation and significant ventilation perfusion imbalance have a very prolonged history of disease prior to development of acute respiratory failure. In a number of chronic neuromuscular conditions, a minor acute respiratory insult may precipitate sudden respiratory failure by worsening the underlying neuromuscular condition (myasthenia gravis) or abruptly reducing the pulmonary function (aspiration pneumonia in parkinsonism).

In conditions which alter control of respiration, the degree of respiratory failure may not correlate with the level of consciousness. This is best illustrated by barbiturate and morphine overdose, the former often resulting is coma without elevated Pa_{CO_2} and the latter showing profound hypercapnia with only moderate reductions in the level of consciousness. The degree of respiratory failure usually correlates with the loss of vital capacity in neuromuscular and metabolic conditions. The presence of respiratory failure, however, should be suspected in *all* unconscious or obtunded patients and in *all* neuromuscular patients. The diagnosis is then determined by evaluation of arterial blood gases. In addition, all patients suffering from neuromuscular disease should be followed with frequent measurements of their pulmonary vital capacity. When the vital capacity is less than 1 liter, impending respiratory failure should be anticipated and arterial blood gases closely followed.

Patients with a documented diagnosis of respiratory failure, acute coma, or severe respiratory compromise from metabolic or neuromuscular disease should be closely monitored in a respiratory intensive care unit. Monitoring should include frequent arterial blood gas analysis, serial vital capacity (in cooperative, alert patients), or serial pleural pressure measurements. Continuous pleural pressure monitoring may be of value in assessing the patient's ability to generate adequate inspiratory force. This can be accomplished by insertion of an esophageal balloon attached to a pressure transducer displayed on the bedside or central station oscilloscope.

Early intubation for this category of acute respiratory failure in potentially reversible disease is indicated. Assisted ventilation then can be easily accomplished because the underlying lung produces little resistance to adequate ventilation or gas exchange. Methods of artificial ventilatory support of these patients will be discussed later. Hypoxemia should always be corrected. High levels of inspiratory oxygen are necessary only in the presence of superimposed conditions such as atelectasis, pneumonia, or pulmonary embolism. Maintenance of good airway toilet and postural drainage usually prevents significant respiratory complications. However, minor episodes of aspiration pneumonia are frequent. Colonization of the upper respiratory tract occurs in almost all intubated or tracheostomized patients. Knowledge of the predominant flora is helpful in instituting appropriate antibiotic coverage with the onset of documented fever, leukocytosis, or pulmonary infiltration. Transient low-grade fevers or minor leukocytoses without pulmonary infiltration should be treated by increased respiratory toilet alone and a careful search for any nonpulmonary site of infection. Left lower lobe infiltrates often elude detection in patients in intensive care units because routine chest roentgenograms are usually obtained by portable anteroposterior techniques. A right lateral decubitus or left lateral film is helpful in ruling out the possibility of left lower lobe pneumonia.

Recovery from respiratory failure in hypercapnic-hypoxic patients with decreased minute ventilation depends on the nature of the underlying condition, the application of ventilatory assistance and other supportive care. Some patients with neuromuscular disease may require months or even permanent assisted ventilation. Long-term maintenance of adequate alveolar ventilation may be accomplished in some patients by the use of a rocking bed or chest plate respirator (Cuirass). These methods are primarily reserved for patients who are able to maintain borderline alveolar ventilation during the day, but show further deterioration during sleep. Electrophrenic pacing may be helpful in some central hypoventilation syndromes. A long-term commitment to respiratory support with an artificial ventilator should be avoided in patients with progressive neuromuscular disease who are not suffering from an acute reversible cause of respiratory failure.

ACUTE HYPERCAPNIC-HYPOXIC RESPIRATORY FAILURE SECONDARY TO LOWER AIRWAY DISEASE

Chronic obstructive lung disease (COLD) and asthma represent the major causes of respiratory failure. The diagnosis, detection of potentially severe attacks, and treatment of asthma are covered in Chapters 35 and 146. The majority of patients with acute respiratory failure secondary to chronic obstructive lung disease have a long background of chronic cough, sputum production, prolonged heavy cigarette consumption, wheezing, and shortness of breath. Many of these patients have been diagnosed as having "asthma," emphysema, or chronic bronchitis or have experienced multiple episodes of respiratory infection. A history of congestive heart failure or pedal edema without documented left ventricular disease is occasionally reported. A significant percentage have experienced previous or repeated episodes of respiratory failure.

The onset of respiratory failure is characterized by gradually progressive dyspnea often associated with an increase or change in chronic cough or sputum production. Impaired judgment, insomnia, agitation, and headache are not infrequent. Dyspnea eventually becomes severe over several hours, prompting medical attention. Occasionally, patients develop obtundation, twitching, asterixis, cyanosis, and coma. A recent minor respiratory infection often precedes the increasing dyspnea or cough. Sudden onset of dyspnea or chest pain occurs in the minority of patients with acute respiratory failure.

Physical examination usually reveals an anxious individual with severe respiratory distress. Breathing is often labored with some increase in respiratory rate. Accessory muscles are active. However, in the presence of severe respiratory failure, or following the use of respiratory depressant drugs (often given for agitation or insomnia), respiratory rate and depth may not appear abnormal and the patient's level of consciousness may be grossly altered. This particular clinical presentation is characteristic of patients who have received high inspiratory oxygen en route to the hospital. Examination of the chest in patients with acute respiratory failure secondary to chronic obstructive lung disease usually reveals hyperresonance, decreased breath sounds, and prolonged expiration. Wheezing or rales may or may not be present. Tachycardia is frequent and a variety of cardiac arrhythmias is common. The blood pressure may be moderately elevated, but extreme increases or decreases are occasionally seen. Signs of pulmonary hypertension or right ventricular failure are often present in acute respiratory failure, particularly in patients with a long history of severe chronic underlying lung disease. Cyanosis may be obvious, but its clinical absence does not rule out significant hypoxemia. Papilledema is occasionally seen. This is most often observed in comatose patients, but may occasionally be the only impressive finding in respiratory failure.

Abnormalities in arterial blood gases are the only definitive means of diagnosing acute respiratory failure. Therefore, a high index of suspicion is necessary in order to detect respiratory failure in some patients with COLD. Blood gas interpretation and diagnosis of acute respiratory failure in patients with established chronic respiratory insufficiency may be even more

difficult. In the pressure of an acute symptomatic respiratory, circulatory, or central nervous system alteration, a presumptive diagnosis of acute respiratory failure should be made if the arterial Pa_{CO_2} is > 55 mm Hg. There is little margin for error under these circumstances, so it is better to be cautious.

A chest film may reveal the presence of hyperinflation, obvious chronic underlying lung disease, or acute pulmonary infiltrates, but in a number of patients with severe respiratory failure, the chest roentgenogram is not helpful. The ECG may show evidence of cor pulmonale or more often simply be compatible with COLD. The hematocrit is elevated in the majority of patients with chronic hypoxemia. There may be, however, concomitant peptic ulcer disease which may be associated with low-grade gastrointestinal blood loss. Leukocytosis suggests infection, but severe leukoerythroblastic responses may follow the stress of severe hypoxemia.

MANAGEMENT OF HYPERCAPNIC–HYPOXIC RESPIRATORY FAILURE SECONDARY TO CHRONIC OBSTRUCTIVE LUNG DISEASE

Few rules are universally applicable to the treatment of acute respiratory failure even when the discussion is limited to only one of the responsible diseases. However, this chapter will offer some guidelines to management, stressing principles of patient care which apply to the majority of individual cases. These principles include: 1) application of immediate lifesaving measures; 2) determination of the precipitating factors; 3) treatment of the underlying condition; and 4) measurements.

OXYGEN

Appropriate lifesaving measures for acute respiratory failure are discussed in Chapter 146. They revolve around immediate correction of hypoxemia, need for emergency intubation or assisted ventilation, and adequate circulatory support. If, as in the majority of cases, the patient is alert or only minimally confused and has a stable cardiovascular status, low-flow controlled oxygen should be instituted ($F_{I_{O_2}}$ 0.24 via a Venturi mask). Adequate oxygenation is nearly always achieved without difficulty; however, this may take serial elevations in inspiratory $F_{I_{O_2}}$ as high as 0.4 or 0.5. The patient should be transferred to an intensive care unit or other appropriate setting for monitoring immediately after supplemental oxygen is administered. Frequent blood gas determinations, systemic arterial pressure, spirometry, and cardiac rhythm are the major parameters requiring close observation. Hemoglobin, electrolytes, and urinary output should also be monitored.

The rationale for controlled oxygen therapy is that most patients with chronic obstructive lung disease who develop acute respiratory failure have a reversible precipitating factor that has resulted in decreased alveolar ventilation. In a large number of these patients, the precipitating factor may be the reduced Po_2 itself which increases pulmonary hypertension and airway resistance, alters central nervous system function, and decreases renal function resulting in fluid accumulation. On a number of occasions the precipitating event is increased bronchospasm associated with a change in weather, minor infection, or failure to take medication. Infection may also increase bronchial secretions, replace functional pulmonary parenchyma, or increase CO_2 production, overwhelming an already limited respiratory system. Occasionally, inadvertent sedative administration or more obvious factors, such as pneumothorax, cardiac arrhythmias, left ventricular failure, or dehydration, may have developed. If adequate oxygenation can be maintained without worsening respiratory acidosis, measures can usually be applied to reverse all of these precipitating conditions.

BRONCHODILATORS

Specific measures to improve airway resistance usually include nebulized β-sympathomimetic amines, such as isoproterenol and intravenously administered aminophylline. Therapy is best monitored in cooperative patients by serial spirograms. Failure to improve air flow limitation makes the continued use of potentially dangerous bronchodilators questionable. However, many experts administer low dosages of bronchodilators even without objective airway response in the hope that unmeasurable improvements in small airways may occur. The older and more critically ill patient should receive the least amount of bronchodilators unless some evidence of improvement is associated with these drugs. It is not uncommon for the arterial oxygen tension to fall slightly during the administration of nebulized or intravenous bronchodilators.

TRACHEOBRONCHIAL SECRETIONS

Thick mucoid secretions may produce some worsening of air flow limitation. Adequate hydration is the best known expectorant since it enhances mucus flow. In the presence of purulent bronchial secretions, acute febrile bronchitis, or overt pneumonia, appropriate antibiotic therapy should be administered.

Broad spectrum coverage (ampicillin, tetracycline, or chloramphenicol) has been most successful in the absence of identification of a specific pathogen. *Streptococcus pneumoniae,* gram negative and staphylococcal species, and *H. influenzae* pneumonia are among the pathogens seen in this setting.

Postural drainage and nasal tracheal suctioning may aid expectoration in some patients. Tracheal suctioning has resulted in increased hypoxia, reflex bronchospasm, and cardiac arrhythmias. This procedure should therefore be performed with great caution.

FLUIDS AND ELECTROLYTES

Adequate hydration is also needed to maintain appropriate venous return and cardiac output in these patients. Increased filling of the right ventricle is required in the presence of pulmonary hypotension. Therefore, an increased peripheral blood volume is needed to maintain a right atrial filling pressure above the usual normal limits of 0 to 5 mm Hg. Cardiac glycosides are of questionable value in acute respiratory failure in patients with cor pulmonale and are often associated with an increased incidence of arrhythmias. The use of diuretics is indicated in patients with severe hepatic congestion and marked peripheral edema. Aggressive diuresis, however, is rarely helpful. Following institution of the above therapy, a posthypercapnic, hypochloremic, hypokalemic metabolic alkalosis often occurs. A significant metabolic alkalosis may precipitate arrhythmias and decrease respiratory drive. This metabolic derangement is especially common following induced diuresis and should be guarded against by appropriate administration of supplemental potassium.

ASSISTED AND CONTROLLED VENTILATION

Most patients hospitalized with hypercapnia and acute respiratory failure improve following conservative therapy without the need for artificial ventilatory support. Mortality has decreased significantly as the reliance on more conservative therapy has replaced early use of artificial ventilation. If a patient continues to deteriorate despite controlled supplemental oxygen, bronchodilators, antibiotics, and correction of fluid and electrolyte status, assisted or controlled ventilation may be indicated. There is no specific level of arterial Pco_2 which precludes continuation of conservative therapy. Progressive deterioration of mental status is the major indication for ventilatory support.

If inadequate alveolar ventilation is to be effectively increased by a mechanical ventilator, an endotracheal tube must be inserted. Intubation results in laryngeal and tracheal irritation and loss of effective cough, and increases the risk of infection. It is also a source of discomfort in the conscious and alert patient. For these reasons the decision to utilize artificial ventilation in a patient with acute respiratory failure should not be undertaken lightly.

Long-term intubation requires the use of nasotracheal or orotracheal tubes with a prestretched or high-compliance cuff to lessen pressure damage to the tracheal mucosa. These cuffs should be inflated to less than 25 cm of H_2O pressure or just enough to permit a small leak to occur during peak inflation. They do not have to be deflated periodically. With careful handling and frequent changes (every 3 days) endotracheal tubes may be kept in place for as long as 2 weeks. When artificial ventilation for periods longer than 2 weeks is required, a tracheostomy usually is performed. The most important indication for early tracheostomy is the presence of copious, tenacious secretions which cannot be adequately removed through the endotracheal tube. Tracheostomy is a surgical procedure which carries some risk of bleeding, pneumothorax, and production of local infection. In addition, there is an increased incidence of aspiration in the presence of a tracheostomy tube.

Once assisted ventilation is begun, the patient is usually dependent on the physician for keeping the airways clear of excessive secretions and adjusting arterial blood gas levels. Close monitoring is therefore mandatory and is best carried out in an intensive care unit or equivalent facility. If sedation is employed while attempting to control ventilation, any machine failure will almost certainly result in patient death if the problem is not immediately detected.

MECHANICAL VENTILATORS

The choice of a mechanical ventilator depends on the underlying cause of respiratory failure. Machines in common use are of two basic types: the volume, and the pressure-cycled respirator. A volume respirator may be adjusted to deliver a fixed volume during each inspiratory phase. The volume limit is determined by preselecting the inspiratory excursion of a bellows which is filled during expiration. The supply of air to the bellows may be enriched with oxygen to produce an inspired concentration of 21 to 100 percent. Peak flow rates can be adjusted with a calibrated flow control. Inspiration is begun by a timer when the respirator is used as a controller and by the inspiratory effort of the patient when the respirator is used as an assistor. To provide adequate tracheal humidity, a heated humidifier in the inspired air line saturates the delivered gas, while the temperature is monitored by a thermometer near the connection to

the patient. Most volume ventilators can generate high driving pressures, ensuring that the desired volume is delivered during each respiratory cycle.

Pressure-cycled ventilators are simpler machines which are usually driven by compressed air or oxygen. These ventilators produce inspiratory flow until a preset outflow pressure is reached. The volume delivered varies depending upon the resistance and compliance of the lungs of the patient being ventilated. If either the resistance or compliance of the lung changes, the volume delivered will also change. Most of the pressure-cycled ventilators can be used as controllers or assistors. Peak flow may or may not be adjustable, and a regulated inspired oxygen concentration is more difficult to achieve.

The major drawback to the volume-cycled ventilator is the ease with which it produces high transpulmonary pressures and large tidal volumes. These large volumes result in the production of positive pleural pressures which may significantly impair venous return and cause marked hypotension. Pressure-cycled ventilators rarely result in such high positive pleural pressures because of their mechanical inability to produce the necessary transpulmonary pressure and large tidal volumes.

Both volume- and pressure-cycled ventilators are satisfactory for controlled or assisted ventilation in patients with normal lungs. An increased alveolar ventilation in patients suffering from neuromuscular disease or barbiturate intoxication may be easily accomplished with either type of ventilator. In fact, in these patients great care must be taken to avoid production of severe hyperventilation.

Most patients with acute respiratory failure from COLD will require volume-cycled respirators to achieve adequate alveolar ventilation. These patients require large tidal volumes because of their increased dead space and severe prolongation of expiration. The latter requires long pauses between inspirations so that respiratory rates as low as 8 to 10 per minute are used. Airway resistance may change frequently due to bronchoconstriction or accumulation of secretions. Only volume-cycled ventilators can ensure adequate tidal volume in spite of these changes.

Patients with COLD and acute respiratory failure needing assisted ventilation frequently require high right ventricular filling pressures because of pulmonary hypertension. The high pleural pressure produced by artificial ventilation may reduce venous return and, hence, right ventricular filling pressure. This causes a reduction in cardiac output and systemic arterial pressure. Hypotension commonly occurs if excessive airway pressure is used, especially if diuretics have reduced systemic blood volume.

Many patients with COLD and acute respiratory failure have some degree of compensatory increase in the concentration of bicarbonate in the serum. With the institution of artificial ventilation, it is important that the arterial Pco_2 be reduced slowly so that the kidneys have an opportunity to eliminate excess bicarbonate gradually and without the development of a severe alkalosis.

Complications of assisted ventilation, in addition to the induction of hypotension and posthypercapnic metabolic alkalosis, are relatively frequent (see Table 36–5). These include complications attributable to intubation (tracheal stenosis or erosion) and ventilation (machine failure, atelectasis, gastric distension). One of the most frequent complications of assisted ventilation is hospital-acquired superinfection, which results from a variety of factors occurring in an acutely compromised host. Unnecessary use of antibiotics can contribute to the establishment of these infections. Other common complications occurring in these critically ill patients with or without assisted ventilation include cardiac arrhythmias, upper gastrointestinal bleeding, pneumothorax, pulmonary embolism, and electrolyte abnormalities.

TABLE 36–5
Complications of Artificial Ventilation

1. Machine failure (patient disconnection)
2. Airway obstruction (mucus, endotracheal tube)
3. Atelectasis
4. Arrhythmias
5. Alkalosis
6. Gastrointestinal bleeding
7. Pulmonary embolism
8. Barotrauma (pneumothorax, pneumomediastinum, pneumopericardium, subcutaneous emphysema, pneumoperitoneum, interstitial emphysema)
9. Superinfection (usually gram negative)
10. Mucosal lesions and tracheal stenosis or malacia

CHAPTER 37

Mass Lesions and Pulmonary Nodules
PETER B. TERRY AND KO-PEN WANG

A mass lesion as seen on chest x-ray may be defined as a coherent radiodensity greater than 6 cm in diameter with discrete borders, homogeneous consistency, and sphere-like or ovoid appearance. A pulmonary nodule is arbitrarily defined as a density having the roentgenographic characteristics of a mass lesion but measuring less than 6 cm in diameter and surrounded by normal lung parenchyma. Mediastinal masses and hilar nodules are distinguished by their anatomic location and suggest a specific differential diagnosis. These will be discussed first.

MEDIASTINAL MASSES

The mediastinum is the extrapleural space bounded by the sternum anteriorly, the vertebral column posteriorly, and the two pleural cavities on the left and right; it extends from the diaphragm to the thoracic inlet. The mediastinum is arbitrarily divided into four compartments (Fig. 37–1). The normal structures of the mediastinum and embryonic rests can give rise to tumors and mass lesions. Neoplasms originating outside the mediastinum, infections, and multisystem diseases such as sarcoidosis can involve the mediastinum.

CLINICAL MANIFESTATIONS
In two series, it is estimated that 35 to 44 percent of primary tumors of the mediastinum are asymptomatic when found on chest films.[118,125] In the patients who are symptomatic, the most common complaints are cough, chest pain, and dyspnea. In some instances, however, the clinical picture is dominated by extrathoracic abnormalities.

Local Effects of the Mass
Symptoms associated with mediastinal masses usually arise from the local effects of the mass and, thus, vary with the location, size, compressibility, rate of growth, and invasiveness of the lesion. Any large mass, especially a malignant tumor, may invade or erode into normal structures causing characteristic symptoms and signs.

Associated Extrathoracic Abnormalities
In some instances, the principal clinical findings are remote from the mediastinum. These may be simply the general systemic effects of infection or malig-

nancy—fever, asthenia, anorexia, weight loss, and anemia—or may be syndromes associated with a specific type of mediastinal lesion. An example is the thymoma, which may be associated with myasthenia gravis, erythroid hypoplasia, Cushing syndrome, dermatomyositis, Whipple's disease, or agammaglobulinemia. A variety of physiologic abnormalities may be seen with bronchogenic carcinoma and may be the presenting feature of the patient's illness. The most common of these are hypercalcemia, hyperadrenocorticism, hypertrophic osteoarthropathy, and certain neuromuscular syndromes.

DIAGNOSIS AND MANAGEMENT

Determination of the exact location of a mediastinal mass is of considerable value in differential diagnosis. Figure 37–1 shows the site of some of the commonly occurring lesions, and Table 37–1 indicates the divisions of the mediastinum in which each type of mass is located.[118-127]

Radiologic Studies

Posteroanterior, lateral, and oblique x-rays of the chest are essential guides to the location and character of the mass. Careful study of changes in density suggesting fat, cystic changes, calcification, or bone erosion is important. At times, overpenetrated Bucky films or tomograms will be of aid in this regard, particularly in determining the character of margins partially obscured by other mediastinal structures. Fluoroscopy permits an assessment of diaphragmatic and mediastinal mobility and will demonstrate movement of the mass in relation to swallowing, respiration, and cardiac pulsation. Movement of the vocal cords can also be observed by contrast radiography. It may

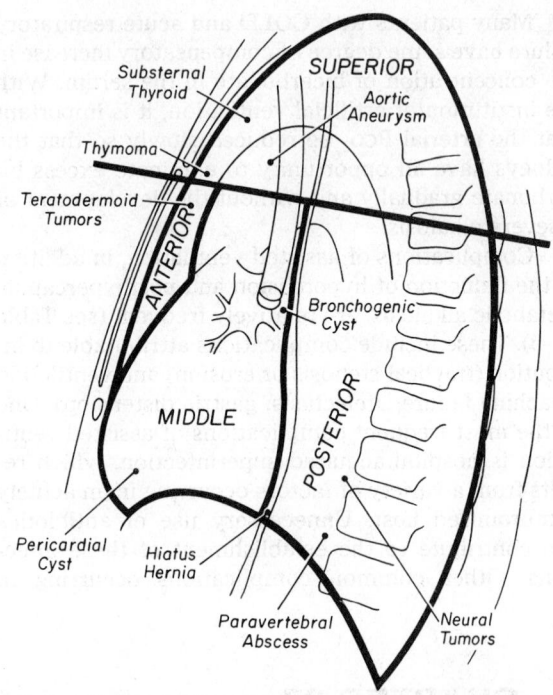

FIGURE 37–1. Diagram illustrating the mediastinum and the site of common primary lesions. The customary subdivisions are shown. Important structures in these subdivisions are: Superior mediastinum—aortic arch and major branches; superior vena cava and innominate veins; thymus; trachea, esophagus, thoracic duct; vagus, phrenic, sympathetic nerves; left recurrent laryngeal nerve; lymph nodes. Anterior mediastinum—lymph nodes, fibroareolar tissue. Middle mediastinum—heart, pericardium, ascending aorta; proximal pulmonary vessels; phrenic nerves; tracheal bifurcation; lymph nodes. Posterior mediastinum—descending aorta and branches; azygos and hemiazygos veins; esophagus, thoracic duct; vagus and sympathetic nerves; lymph nodes.

TABLE 37–1
Clinical Features of Mediastinal Masses

Mass and Incidence*	Locations	Some Clinical Manifestations	Diagnostic Aids
I. Primary Neoplasms of the Mediastinum			
Thymoma (18%) (50% are malignant)	Anterior	Associated with myasthenia gravis, erythroid hypoplasia, Cushing syndrome, or dermatomyositis	Tensilon test, bone marrow aspiration, 17-KS, 17-OHCS, plasma cortisol, antithymic, and antimuscle antibodies
Lymphoma (12%) primary in mediastinum	Anterior; may be in any part of mediastinum	Pressure on surrounding structures; lymph node enlargement elsewhere; systemic manifestations (anemia, fever, etc.)	May be lobulated, bilateral but asymmetrical; diagnosis by biopsy of other nodes

* Incidence in 1252 cases taken from 11 series, 1952 to 1972. Refers only to primary tumors of the mediastinum.[118,125]

TABLE 37–1 (cont.)

Mass and Incidence*	Locations	Some Clinical Manifestations	Diagnostic Aids
I. Primary Neoplasms of the Mediastinum (cont.)			
Teratoma (12%) (one-third are malignant)	Anterior; near base of heart	Pressure on surrounding structures; may rupture into bronchus or pleural cavity; bulging anterior chest wall; clubbing	Often very large; teeth, bone, fatty layer may be visible on x-ray, most common in young adults
Bronchogenic cyst (8%)	Anterior; often at tracheal bifurcation	Tracheal compression; secondary infection; material may be expectorated through bronchial communication	Smooth spherical mass on x-ray, may contain air-fluid level; most common in children and young adults
Substernal thyroid (6%)	Anterior Superior	Pressure on recurrent laryngeal nerve, trachea, and vessels; hyperthyroidism	May be palpable in neck; moves with swallowing; may visualize on ^{131}I scan
Pericardial cyst (6%)	Anterior	Not symptomatic	Smooth margins, shape changes with position, may pulsate; often found at right cardiophrenic angle
Enteric cyst (2%)	Anterior		
Cystic hygroma (<1%)	Anterior	Laryngeal irritation; displacement of trachea and esophagus	May be palpable in the neck; most common in infants
Mediastinal parathyroid (<1%)	Anterior	Hyperparathyroidism; seldom large enough to cause signs or symptoms of compression	X-ray findings of hyperparathyroidism; hypercalcemia, hypophosphatemia, hypercalciuria
Lipoma (<1%)	Anterior	Usually asymptomatic	Radiodensity intermediate between that of air and fluid
Neurofibroma, neurosarcoma (10%)	Posterior	Pressure on spinal cord and nerve roots	Von Recklinghausen's disease with café-au-lait spots, neurofibromata elsewhere, enlarged intervertebral foramina, erosion of vertebral pedicles; myelogram
Ganglioneuroma (5%)	Posterior	Compresses trachea, esophagus, great vessels; Horner syndrome	High urinary vanillyl-mandelic acid; gait abnormalities from extension into spinal canal; most common in young adults
Neurolemmoma (4%)	Posterior	Involves bone and encroaches on spinal canal	Myelogram
Neuroblastoma (2%)	Posterior	Nonproductive cough and wheeze; often extends into spinal canal and produces gait abnormalities	Most common in children
Pheochromocytoma (1%)	Posterior	Hypertension	Elevated urinary catecholamines; positive Regitine test

(Continued)

TABLE 37-1 (cont.)

Mass and Incidence*	Locations	Some Clinical Manifestations	Diagnostic Aids
II. Primary Neoplasms Outside the Mediastinum			
Lymphoma (25%)	Middle and anterior	Other involved nodes; systemic symptoms	Lymph node biopsy
Leukemia	Middle and anterior	Systemic signs and symptoms, anemia, thrombocytopenia, splenomegaly	Peripheral smear, bone marrow
Carcinoma of the lung, upper gastrointestinal tract, prostate, kidney	Middle	Cough, hemoptysis, dyspnea, weight loss, hematuria	Sputum cytology, bronchoscopy, mediastinoscopy, upper gastrointestinal series, increased alkaline and acid phosphatase, bone x-rays and scan, intravenous pyelogram
III. Sarcoidosis			
Mediastinal lymph nodes (common)	Middle	Often asymptomatic; other clinical evidence of sarcoidosis—erythema nodosum uveitis, parotitis, cranial nerve involvement, arthritis, and arthralgias	Commonly bilateral hilar and right paratracheal masses; hyperglobulinemia, hypercalcemia, decreased pulmonary compliance and Dl_{CO} despite clear lungs on x-ray; positive Kveim test
IV. Aortic Aneurysm			
Aortic aneurysm	Superior, middle, or posterior	Pressure on all surrounding structures including bone; may leak or rupture into adjacent viscera; Marfan syndrome; history of trauma	Mass shows expansile pulsation unless thrombosed; may have calcification in wall; tracheal tug, different B.P. in arms, evidence of arteriosclerosis or syphilis; obliteration of paraspinal shadow; arteriography
V. Infections			
Chronic tuberculosis actinomycosis brucellosis tularemia histoplasmosis	Middle or anterior	Evidence of systemic infection, symptoms of pulmonary infection, bronchial compression, erosion into a bronchus	Appropriate cultures, positive serologic titers, positive skin tests, history of exposure
Acute Infectious mononucleosis	Middle	Sore throat, rash, cervical adenopathy	Positive serologic tests
Bubonic plague (rare)	Middle	Evidence of systemic disease	History of exposure, appropriate cultures
Paravertebral abscess (acute or chronic)	Posterior	Back pain, fever, evidence of tuberculosis elsewhere	Fusiform mass, bone changes on x-ray, cultures for tuberculosis, fungi, and staphylococcus
VI. Esophageal Lesions			
Diverticulum	Posterior	Regurgitation, repeated aspiration	Barium swallow
Hiatus hernia achalasia	Posterior	Reflux symptoms; large hernias often asymptomatic	Barium swallow, mass may show air-fluid level
VII. Mediastinal Collagenosis			
Histoplasmosis Primary fibrosis (rare)	Middle	Superior or inferior vena caval obstruction, other pressure symptoms; evidence of histoplasmosis or other fibrosing lesion	Presents as mediastinal widening

also be possible to detect the expansile pulsation of an aneurysm, but errors of interpretation caused by transmitted pulsations are frequent. Examinations with radiopaque materials in the esophagus, tracheobronchial tree, or blood vessels may be definitive. Isotope scanning procedures are useful in identifying thyroid masses and in demonstrating abnormal distribution of blood flow to the lungs.

Computed tomography allows noninvasive evaluation of questionably abnormal mediastinal x-ray changes. Mediastinal fat, tortuous vessels, and questionable masses may be more clearly defined by this technique.

Ultrasound

Ultrasonic devices, which display echoes at tissue interfaces, may permit the differentiation of solid and cystic masses. Many cystic mediastinal masses are benign. A discussion of this technique will be found in Chapter 32.

Operative Procedures

Mediastinoscopy may permit a biopsy of a mass in the superior mediastinum adjacent to the trachea (Chap. 32). This simple procedure is often helpful in determining if a neoplasm is present and if it is resectable. Sometimes it can give information that makes thoracotomy unnecessary.[119,120]

Open thoracotomy is the most direct and satisfactory method of establishing an etiologic diagnosis when simpler procedures have failed. Although the risk of elective thoracotomy is low, the therapeutic implications of the anticipated findings must be weighed against the operative risk in each case.

EVALUATION OF MEDIASTINAL LYMPHADENOPATHY

Separate consideration is given to mediastinal lymphadenopathy because it is often possible to identify the lymphatic origin of a mediastinal mass even when its etiology is not known. There are many trivial causes of lymph node enlargement that would not justify thoracotomy for diagnosis. Lymph nodes are present in every division of the mediastinum, but the largest number appears in the superior and middle mediastinum in close proximity to the trachea and its bifurcation.

Enlargement of lymph nodes may be produced by infections including tuberculosis, especially the primary infection, histoplasmosis, coccidioidomycosis, actinomycosis, and other fungus diseases. Acute lymphadenopathy may be seen occasionally with pneumococcal pneumonia or lung abscess, with pertussis and tularemia, and with infectious mononucleosis. A number of cancers may present with mediastinal lymph node metastases; these are discussed in Chapter 55.

Mediastinal lymphadenopathy is best approached diagnostically by mediastinoscopy or parasternal incision.

SOLITARY PULMONARY NODULES

The solitary pulmonary nodule, often referred to as a "coin lesion," is a common abnormal roentgenographic finding. It is defined as a single rounded or oval lesion of less than 6 cm in diameter, lying within the lung parenchyma with aerated lung around it. It is a frequent incidental finding on a routine x-ray film in an asymptomatic patient. The immediate problem is to determine the likelihood of primary malignancy and the need for thoracotomy. Although most lesions are benign granulomas, as many as 40 percent of solitary nodules referred for resection are malignant tumors.[130-132] Resectability of pulmonary neoplasms is clearly related to early diagnosis, reaching 75 percent in small (less than 6 cm) asymptomatic lesions in contrast to 30 percent resectability when all types of bronchogenic carcinoma are included. Furthermore, the smaller the lesion at the time of resection, the better the survival rate.

LIKELIHOOD OF MALIGNANCY

Table 37–2 summarizes the salient features leading to a clinical diagnosis.[128] A number of clinical and radiographic features significantly alter the probability that a solitary nodule is malignant. The most important of these are age and smoking history, radiographic characteristics of the lesion (particularly the presence and type of calcification), and duration and stability as judged by serial x-ray examinations.[129] Unfortunately, very few features provide assurance that the lesion is benign. Solid or laminated calcification occurs only in granulomas. Review of prior x-rays showing either stability for at least 5 years or shrinkage characteristic of an inflammatory lesion may be accepted as evidence that the lesion is benign. In addition, an innocent-appearing lesion in a patient less than 35 years of age will almost never represent primary lung cancer.

TABLE 37-2
Differentiation of Benign and Malignant Nodules

Probably malignant
  Serial films show recent origin or rapid growth
  Umbilication or notching of the margin of the nodule
  Eccentric cavitation with irregular wall thickness
  Noncalcified fuzzy lesion in a male smoker over age 40
  Positive sputum cytology

Probably benign
  Lesion with sharp margins in patient under age 35
  X-ray stability for 2 years
  X-ray appearance characteristic of lesion associated with proven systemic disease

Almost surely benign
  Solid or laminated calcification
  X-ray stability for 5 years
  Lesion with sharp margins in patient under age 30 with positive tuberculin skin test
  Serial films show evolution characteristic of inflammatory lesion

CLINICAL FEATURES AND STUDIES

History
Symptoms related directly to the presence of the nodule are commonly absent. Suggestive points in the history include heavy smoking, hemoptysis, known previous malignancy elsewhere, and residence in endemic areas for fungi.

Physical Examination
The nodule itself can seldom be detected by examination of the chest. Careful search should be made for evidence of primary or metastatic tumor elsewhere. The presence of rheumatoid arthritis suggests the possibility of a rheumatoid nodule in the lung, especially if superficial nodules are present. Bloody nasal discharge or destructive lesions in the nasal passages suggest Wegener's granulomatosis. Cutaneous and mucosal telangiectases or a bruit over the chest wall may be present if the lesion is a pulmonary arteriovenous fistula.

Radiographic Features
Some lesions may be clearly localized and characterized from posteroanterior and lateral chest films alone, but localization is commonly aided by the use of apical lordotic or oblique views. Tomograms are usually required to obtain precise information about the character of the borders and the presence or absence of calcification and may reveal multiple nodules where only a single lesion is visible on standard radiographs. Application of a metallic marker to the nipples or cutaneous nodules removes all doubt about whether they are responsible for the roentgenographic shadow in question. Every effort must be made to obtain all previous chest films to determine the stability and duration of the lesion.

The character and location of the lesion may provide clues to its etiology. A granuloma is usually subpleural in location, has sharp margins, and is often calcified. There may be associated hilar node calcification. Primary carcinoma often shows an indistinct margin. A lesion in the anterior segment of an upper lobe strongly suggests carcinoma. Apart from the presence of solid or laminated calcification, however, no combination of radiographic features on a single examination will safely exclude malignancy.

Skin Tests
Although a positive skin test does not establish the diagnosis, negative tests with tuberculin, histoplasmin, and coccidioidin make malignancy more likely. In such instances, immediate thoracotomy generally may be indicated, even in a person under 35 years of age. A strongly positive tuberculin test does not exclude malignancy.

Sputum Studies
Sputum cytology is rarely positive with a solitary nodular malignancy. Identification of *Mycobacterium tuberculosis* in the sputum would have presumptive diagnostic value; however, sputum is seldom positive on direct smear from a tuberculoma, and resection for definitive diagnosis should not be delayed for several weeks until culture results are available.

Bronchoscopy
A fiberoptic bronchoscopic procedure is the diagnostic method of choice. When visible, biopsy of endobronchial tumor can be expected to yield a diagnosis in approximately 95 percent of cases. Nodules beyond the visual field are approached using fluoroscopic guidance. Cytologic and/or tissue samples may be obtained using a bronchial brushing technique or biopsy forceps. Malignant cells are obtained in 30 to 70 percent of malignant solitary nodules. Success varies with the expertise of the bronchoscopist and the location of the nodule.

Percutaneous Needle Biopsy

This diagnostic technique is covered thoroughly in Chapter 32. Suffice it to say that percutaneous needle biopsy is effective about 80 percent of the time in obtaining tissue sufficient for diagnosis. It is nearly always indicated to have tissue confirmation of malignancy before beginning therapy. In a patient too ill to undergo general anesthesia and thoracotomy, needle biopsy offers a simple method of obtaining a tissue diagnosis with an acceptably low morbidity and mortality rate.

Needle biopsy is a less satisfactory way of proving that a nodule is benign, since recovery of a small fragment of inflammatory tissue does not exclude tumor. The greatest value of bronchoscopic and percutaneous biopsy procedures is in proving the diagnosis of a malignant neoplasm. This information will sometimes justify thoracotomy in a poor-risk patient or will assist in persuading a patient that operation is essential.

DETECTION OF EXTRAPULMONARY DISEASE

In the absence of extrapulmonary symptoms and signs, a primary malignancy elsewhere presenting in the lungs as a solitary metastasis is most unlikely. Extensive roentgenographic surveys of the urinary tract and skeletal and digestive systems are not justified until the pulmonary lesion has been diagnosed as malignant. For a solitary nodule, the yield is small from expensive roentgenographic surveys; where multiple nodules are concerned, the yield may be higher but biopsy of the lung nodules would be necessary to confirm the presence of metastases.

DIAGNOSIS AND MANAGEMENT

Table 37–3 summarizes the clinical and radiologic features of the common and uncommon types of pulmonary nodules. Extrapulmonary lesions, such as interlobar pleural effusions, pleural plaques and tumors, chest wall tumors, and skin tumors, must be excluded by their location and appearance.

TABLE 37–3

Differential Diagnosis of Pulmonary Nodules

Type and Incidence	Radiologic Appearance	Characteristic Features
Neoplasms		
Bronchogenic carcinoma (10–25%)	Fuzzy borders, often umbilicated margin; progressive enlargement over weeks or months; calcification rare (<1%); cavitation, if present, is often eccentric	Highest incidence in cigarette smokers; often asymptomatic; occasionally hemoptysis; cytology occasionally positive; most common in men over 40
Bronchial adenoma (2% that of carcinoma)	Sharply demarcated; calcification rare; predilection for right upper lobe, middle lobe, and lingula	Cough and hemoptysis in ⅓ of cases; often visible at bronchoscopy; 10% develop distant metastases; occurs equally in men and women; younger age group than bronchogenic carcinoma
Metastatic lesions (5–15%)	Uncalcified; spherical; sharp or fuzzy margins; often multiple	Symptoms almost always absent; primary malignant tumor elsewhere; bronchoscopy and cytology usually negative
Bronchioloalveolar carcinoma (rare)	Air bronchogram; frequently slow growing	Symptoms often absent; cytology may be positive
Benign Pulmonary Tumors		
Hamartoma (5–10%)	Round or oval; majority well demarcated and lobulated; 30% calcified; very slow growth is characteristic	Symptoms usually absent

(Continued)

TABLE 37-3 (cont.)

Type and Incidence	Radiologic Appearance	Characteristic Features
Granulomas		
Tuberculosis, histoplasmosis, coccidioidomycosis, rarely brucellosis, and mineral oil aspiration (60%)	Two-thirds show calcification; laminar or solid calcification pathognomonic; sharply defined margins; occasionally linear strands to hilus or pleural surface; satellite lesions common in tuberculosis; may be multiple	Symptoms usually absent; exposure by contact or endemic area; skin tests positive; sputum cultures usually negative
Uncommon Pulmonary Nodules		
Bronchogenic cyst (2%)	Central or lower lobe location with sharp margins; occasional fluid level	Asymptomatic until communication with bronchus established
Hydatid cyst (rare)	Ovoid, sharply circumscribed; may be lobulated; fluid level may be present; meniscus of air at apex of cyst may be visible on tomogram	Association with sheepherding dogs; palpable or calcified hepatic cyst; echinococcal hooklets in sputum
Pulmonary infarct (rare as solitary nodule)	Fairly rapid resolution on serial films; small pleural effusion	Pleuritic pain and pleural rub; elevated serum lactic dehydrogenase; lung scan may show segmental defects in other areas
Rheumatoid granuloma (rare)	Well-circumscribed and uniformly dense; may be calcified; may have associated diffuse basal fibrosis; pleural effusion often present	Rheumatoid arthritis; lesion resolves rapidly oh steroid therapy; rheumatoid factor present
Pulmonary arteriovenous fistula (rare)	Spherical and usually well-circumscribed; rarely calcified; vessels leading to hilus visible on tomogram	Cutaneous and mucosal telangiectases may be present; cyanosis and polycythemia; audible bruit over lesion; angiography diagnostic
Intrapulmonary hematoma (rare)	Dense, circumscribed; progressive shrinkage on serial films	History of thoracic trauma or recent wedge resection
Chronic focal pneumonitis (rare)	Rapid resolution with antibiotics	Recent episode of pneumonia
Bronchopulmonary sequestration (uncommon)	Usually left lower lobe; may contain air-fluid level	Asymptomatic unless infected; complications rare
Hematogenous abscesses (uncommon)	Usually multiple; more numerous in lower lobes	Patient very ill; gram-negative organisms often responsible; blood cultures frequently positive
Wegener's granulomatosis (rare)	Usually multiple; nodules of varying size; cavitation frequent	Sinus, nasal, renal or other organ involvement

MULTIPLE NODULES

Multiple pulmonary nodules may represent developmental lesions, infections, neoplasms, or immunologic diseases (Table 37–4). The differential diagnosis and diagnostic approach are governed by the clinical setting and x-ray characteristics. Transthoracic needle aspiration is the diagnostic procedure of choice if there are no medical contraindications and the nodules can be seen on fluoroscopy. Diagnostic thoracotomy is rarely indicated if malignancy is suspected because curative resection is extremely rare.

TABLE 37-4
Multiple Nodules

Neoplastic	Infectious
Lymphosarcoma	Bacterial abscesses
Hematogenous metastasis	*Coccidioides immitis*
Multiple myeloma	*Paragonimus westermani*
Papilloma	
Developmental	**Immunologic**
Pulmonary arteriovenous	Wegener's granulomatosis
Fistulae	Rheumatoid necrobiotic
	nodules

MASSES

Solitary lesions larger than 6 cm in diameter are termed "masses." Virtually all the entities that may be responsible for solitary nodules may also produce larger masses. Additional diagnostic possibilities include masses resulting from conglomerate silicosis, mucoid impaction in asthmatics, and an intrapulmonary sequestration cyst.

DIAGNOSTIC THORACOTOMY

When a needle biopsy is unrewarding, thoracotomy is necessary for the proper diagnosis and management of all lesions thought to be probable or possible primary malignancies without apparent spread. Thoracotomy is required to establish a diagnosis of benign tumor as well. Thus, diagnostic thoracotomy is indicated except in those few patients showing strong evidence of a benign lesion, that is, stability of the lesion for 5 years or characteristic laminar or solid calcification. Other factors deterring one from thoracotomy include significant obstructive airway disease and serious arteriosclerotic cardiovascular disease. In uncomplicated cases the mortality and morbidity of this procedure is generally low.

BRONCHOGENIC CARCINOMA

During recent years the incidence of bronchogenic carcinoma has increased significantly. Presently, primary lung cancer is the most common cause of carcinoma related deaths in males. The incidence is far higher in smokers than nonsmokers.

Cough is the most common symptom of lung cancer. The nonspecificity and insidious onset often cause the patient to disregard this warning. Hemoptysis, wheezing, and symptoms of a postobstructive pneumonia are other common presentations. Less common but not rare symptoms are due to syndromes related to distant metastases and paraneoplastic syndromes (Table 37-5). It has been shown that symptomatic patients generally have a poorer prognosis than those asymptomatic at the time of diagnosis. Physical examination of the chest is often

TABLE 37-5
Clinical Manifestations of Bronchogenic Carcinoma

I. Syndromes Related to Primary Tumor

Endobronchial tumor may cause cough, hemoptysis, wheezing respiration, segmental emphysema, segmental atelectasis, postobstructive pneumonitis (often repeated bouts), or abscess formation

Extension to pleura and chest wall may cause chest pain, dyspnea, and serous or bloody effusion

Superior sulcus tumors may cause pain due to brachial plexus invasion, Horner syndrome due to disruption of cervical sympathetic chain, or vasomotor signs in the arm and hand

Mediastinal invasion may cause obstruction of vena cava, trachea, and esophagus, recurrent laryngeal- and phrenic-nerve palsy, chylous effusion

II. Syndromes Related to Distant Metastases

Lymphatic and vascular dissemination occur early

Palpable tumor presents in supraclavicular nodes, liver, and skin

Bone metastases may cause pain, fractures, pressure on adjacent nerves

Central nervous-system deposits may cause fits, paralysis, evidences of increased intracranial pressure

Replacement of adrenal cortex with tumor rarely causes clinical deficiency

III. Paraneoplastic Syndromes

Cutaneous abnormalities include erythema multiforme (or similar bullous lesions) and dermatomyositis

Endocrine-metabolic abnormalities include hypercalcemia, hyperadrenocorticism, carcinoid syndrome, inappropriate antidiuretic hormone secretion, gynecomastia, gonadotropin production

Connective tissue disorders include pulmonary hypertrophic osteoarthropathy and clubbing of the digits

Neuromuscular disorders include various encephalomyeloneuropathies, especially cerebellar degeneration and peripheral neuropathy, multifocal leukoencephalopathy (rarely), myopathy, and the myasthenic syndrome normal when the lesion is small or may demonstrate localized findings with airway impingement or postobstructive atelectasis.

The primary tumor is generally visible on chest x-ray at the time of diagnosis and in 95 percent of cases is present on x-ray 6 months prior to diagnosis. Specific cell types are generally correlated with typical roentgenographic appearances (e.g., small cell carcinoma presenting as a paratracheal mass).

Sputum cytology is positive in more than 80 percent of endobronchial tumors when three samples of true sputum are obtained. Peripheral coin lesions have positive sputum cytologies in only 20 percent of instances.

Fiberoptic or rigid bronchoscopy is commonly used to make the diagnosis in the presence of a lesion in the hilar areas or mid-third of the lung fields. Even in the presence of a positive sputum cytology (other than small cell carcinoma) bronchoscopy is frequently used to rule out spread to the carina, trachea, or proximal main stem bronchi, which would preclude a surgical resection. Peripheral lesions may be approached bronchoscopically under fluoroscopic guidance to allow brushings or biopsy of the suspected lesion. Transthoracic needle aspiration of malignant lesions may accurately diagnose more than 90 percent of such lesions. Mediastinal and more distant metastases are considered contraindications to surgical resection, while resection of hilar metastases may be associated with a good 5-year survival rate. Parasternal exploration of the second intercostal space is helpful in diagnosing mediastinal metastases particularly when the left upper lobe is involved with malignancy. Thoracotomy may be necessary if a coin lesion cannot be diagnosed with the previously mentioned procedures.

Prognosis is dependent upon the degree of spread. Solitary pulmonary nodules with no obvious metastatic lesions have approximately a 40 percent 5-year survival rate while carcinoma which has spread beyond the confines of curative resection is associated with a survival time of approximately 6 months.

If a workup including mediastinoscopy or parasternal incision and bronchoscopy does not suggest metastatic disease, then the patient is considered a surgical candidate. Every effort should be made to establish a diagnosis by means of tissue examination prior to surgery. Thoracotomy and pulmonary resection are not usually undertaken in any patient with the diagnosis of small cell carcinoma.

Patients with compromised pulmonary function may require careful evaluation prior to surgery. Estimates of postoperative lung function can be made from combined use of spirometric studies and ventilation perfusion scans.

Radiation therapy is the main palliative treatment modality and is helpful when a patient presents with hemoptysis, bronchial obstruction or compression of mediastinal structures, or bone pain due to metastases. Radiation has been used in conjunction with surgical resection, but its value in this situation has not been proved.[136]

Primary lung carcinomas with the exception of small cell carcinoma have not responded uniformly to antitumor drugs. Recent evidence suggests that a combination of radiation plus a cytotoxin may be helpful in extending the survival time of patients with small cell carcinoma.[135]

─────**CHAPTER 38**─────
Pleural Effusions
WILMOT C. BALL, Jr.

CLINICAL MANIFESTATIONS

SYMPTOMS

Pleural effusion is associated with symptoms which result from inflammation of the parietal pleura or compression of the lung. When the volume of fluid is small, pleural pain (pleurisy) is often present. Pleuritic pain is most commonly encountered in conditions that produce an inflammatory effusion and is often accompanied by a friction rub. The pain is commonly characterized as a sharp, stabbing sensation that is often absent or minimal during quiet respiration but that appears or is intensified abruptly during full inflation of the lungs. It must be differentiated from other types of pain that are accentuated by inspiration. These include the pain caused by rib fracture or costochondritis, compression of intercostal nerve roots, herpes zoster, acute bronchitis, and various cardiovascular and esophageal conditions. When there is direct involvement of the parietal pleura by tumor or by infection, as in empyema, constant dull aching pain independent of respiration may be seen.

The accumulation of pleural effusion, with the resulting compression of normal lung and interference with the movement of the diaphragm, may result in dyspnea, especially when the effusion is bilateral or has developed rapidly or when the amount of fluid is large. Orthopnea is uncommon in the absence of congestive heart failure. The accumulation of pleural fluid in patients with severe heart disease or with chronic obstructive pulmonary disease may result in dyspnea that seems to be out of proportion to the volume of fluid present. In this group of patients, removal by thoracentesis of even small amounts of fluid may produce marked improvement in symptoms. In many patients the accumulation of significant volumes of pleural fluid may be entirely without specific symptoms, and the presence of pleural effusion is occasionally recognized on routine radiographs of the chest or in the course of a physical examination occasioned by the appearance of other complaints.

PHYSICAL SIGNS

Accumulation of fluid usually occurs first at the bases of the lung, and the earliest physical signs are localized to this area. When the volume of pleural fluid is small, differentiation from elevation of the diaphragm, atelectasis, and consolidation may be difficult. It is usual to find a dull to flat percussion note over the area of fluid, together with reduced or absent breath sounds in this area. An area of bronchial breathing, accompanied by an alteration of the quality of voice sounds or frank egophony, is sometimes heard over the adjacent compressed lung. When the volume of fluid is large, the volume of the involved hemithorax may appear to be increased, with reduced expansion during inspiration. Unless the mediastinum has become fixed in position by invasion with tumor or portions of lung on the affected side have become completely atelectatic, the mediastinum is usually shifted away from the side of a large effusion.

RADIOGRAPHIC APPEARANCE

When there are no adhesions between the visceral and parietal pleura, the earliest sign of fluid in the pleural space which can be appreciated on plain films of the chest is blunting of the costophrenic angle and loss of sharp demarcation of the posterior portion of the diaphragm in the lateral view.[141] With the accumulation of larger volumes of fluid, the outline of the diaphragm in the lateral view is completely lost, and the posteroanterior view shows an area of opacification at the lung base, often tapering up the lateral chest wall in the form of a meniscus. When a major portion of the hemithorax is radiopaque, air-filled bronchi in the compressed and atelectatic lung may

be crowded together and displaced into the upper lung field. The heart and other mediastinal structures are characteristically shifted toward the uninvolved side.

When less than 300 ml of pleural fluid is present, the posteroanterior roentgenogram may show no abnormality. Furthermore, blunting of the costophrenic angle may be caused by old inflammatory adhesions. Lateral decubitus films may be very helpful in these situations, since as little as 15 ml of free pleural fluid may be recognized as a layer of density along the inner margin of the dependent chest wall.

In the presence of adherence of the pleural surfaces, usually resulting from inflammatory reaction, the fluid may be loculated rather than free in the pleural cavity. Under these circumstances, fluid may be confined to the region between the lower lobe and the diaphragm (infrapulmonary effusion) and may resemble an elevated diaphragm. The effusion may lie within a fissure (interlobar effusion), a situation most commonly involving the major fissure on the right in patients with congestive heart failure. The posteroanterior film in such cases may show a shadow which resembles an intrapulmonary tumor. A loculated pleural effusion may also produce a shadow which lies flat against the pleural surface and bulges into the lung field in one or more locations. The simultaneous presence of fluid and air within the pleural space produces a sharply demarcated horizontal line in an upright film and can usually be readily identified. Placement of a radiopaque marker during fluoroscopy or the use of diagnostic ultrasound may be of assistance in the more accurate localization of loculated fluid when there is difficulty in achieving complete removal by thoracentesis.

MECHANISMS OF PLEURAL EFFUSION

In health, the pleural cavity contains a small volume of thin serous fluid that acts as a lubricant during inflation and deflation of the lung. This fluid is formed for the most part by transudation from the parietal pleural surface, and water and small molecules are absorbed primarily by the capillary bed of the visceral pleura.[138] In contrast, protein, particulate matter, and cellular debris must be removed by the lymphatics of the parietal pleura and returned to the circulation via the thoracic duct, aided by the fluctuations in hydrostatic pressure which accompany normal respiration. The balance between formation and removal of this fluid may be compromised by any disorder which results in partial or complete obstruction of the lymphatic circulation, by a rise in either the pulmonary venous or the systemic venous pressures, or by a decrease in the colloid oncotic pressure of plasma. Since a significant portion of the lymphatic drainage from the abdomen passes by way of the diaphragm, especially on the right, a variety of inflammatory conditions within the abdomen or the presence of ascites may be accompanied by accumulations of pleural fluid on the right. In some cases, small perforations or defects in the diaphragm itself may result in bulk flow of ascitic fluid from the abdominal cavity into the chest. Accumulation of noninflammatory pleural fluid may therefore occur in any condition which results in ascites, in obstruction to the venous or lymphatic outflow from the thorax, or in either isolated left-sided or isolated right-sided congestive heart failure, although most commonly in the presence of combined ventricular failure. A severe reduction in the level of plasma protein concentration may contribute to the accumulation of noninflammatory pleural fluid.

Inflammatory effusions result from inflammation of the structures adjacent to the pleural space, usually just beneath the visceral pleura within the lung, but occasionally from lesions within the mediastinum, diaphragm, or chest wall. Removal of this fluid by the normal clearing mechanisms may be considerably retarded by the presence of inflammatory obstruction of the lymphatic channels draining the thorax, and secondary inflammation of larger areas of pleural surface may result in the very rapid outpouring of exudate.

The simultaneous presence of air and fluid within the pleural cavity, unless air has been introduced during thoracentesis or surgery, almost always implies the presence of a bronchopleural fistula, resulting most commonly from tuberculosis, pyogenic pneumonia, lung abscess, or malignant tumor.

When the thoracic duct is lacerated or interrupted by trauma or obstructed by tumor, lymph may accumulate in the pleural space. This condition is termed "chylothorax" and is identified by the milky appearance of the fluid, fat droplets on staining with Sudan III, and a total neutral-fat content greater than 0.5 g/dl.

DIAGNOSTIC MEASURES

Unless the etiology has been clearly established, the mere presence of fluid within the pleural cavity, identified either by physical examination or by x-ray, con-

stitutes an indication for thoracentesis. This simultaneously serves the purpose of providing fluid for examination, permitting better radiographic visualization of the lung following the removal of fluid, and relieving symptoms. The gross appearance of the fluid should be carefully noted and specimens obtained for various laboratory examinations. A minimum examination would consist of the measurement of total protein and lactic dehydrogenase (LDH) content, the determination of total and differential cell counts, and examination of the spun sediment with Wright stain. When the etiology of the effusion is not firmly established, the fluid should be subjected to appropriate bacteriologic study for pyogenic organisms, fungi, and *Mycobacterium tuberculosis* and to cytologic examination for the presence of malignant cells. Under certain circumstances (see below), it may be useful to analyze the fluid for glucose and amylase, and to determine its pH. If a milky appearance of the fluid suggests chylothorax, determination of total neutral fat should be obtained and the fluid examined for fat droplets by staining with Sudan III.

In many situations in which an inflammatory effusion is known to be present or suspected, needle biopsy of the parietal pleura with an Abrams or a Cope biopsy instrument may be performed at the time of initial thoracentesis.[142] These biopsies have shown a 60 to 75 percent positive yield in patients with tuberculous or malignant pleural effusions and may provide a diagnosis in cases where bacteriologic or cytologic examination of the fluid is unrewarding. In cases where biopsy is indicated, it is important that it be performed while free fluid is still present within the pleural cavity, since this protects the lung from injury by the biopsy instrument. In cases where ordinary measures have failed to establish a definitive diagnosis and needle biopsy of the pleura is negative, thoracotomy with exploration of the lung and biopsy of the involved areas of the pleural surface may be essential for accurate etiologic diagnosis.

DIFFERENTIAL DIAGNOSIS

In determining the etiology of a pleural effusion, it is useful to establish whether the fluid is a transudate or an exudate. Transudative effusions are caused by elevated systemic or pulmonary venous pressure or by decreased plasma oncotic pressure; the pleural surfaces are not directly involved by the primary pathologic process. In contrast, an exudative effusion results from inflammation or other disease of the pleural surface, or from lymphatic obstruction. Table 38–1 lists the principal causes of transudative and

TABLE 38–1
Causes of Pleural Effusion

Common Causes of Transudative Effusion

Congestive heart failure	Usually chronic biventricular failure Usually bilateral Pleuritic pain and friction rub uncommon
Cirrhosis	In presence of ascites Effusion usually confined to or larger on the right Serum proteins often low
Nephrotic syndrome	Associated with hypoproteinemia and generalized edema and ascites

Common Causes of Exudative Effusion

Tuberculosis	Effusion usually unilateral, may be asymptomatic Often no parenchymal lesion on x-ray
Bronchogenic carcinoma	Effusion often bloody and large, may recur rapidly after removal Parenchymal or hilar lesion usually visible on x-ray after thoracentesis
Bacterial pneumonia	Sterile effusion must be differentiated from empyema Fluid frequently becomes loculated
Viral and mycoplasma pneumonia	Pleurisy and bilateral effusion common
Pulmonary infarction	Pleural pain commonly present Effusion usually small in amount but often bloody
Lymphoma	Most common in Hodgkin's disease Often associated with mediastinal node or parenchymal involvement
Metastatic tumor	Effusion often bilateral Parenchymal lesions usually apparent
Trauma	Associated with intrapleural bleeding
Abdominal surgery	Small effusions common but usually resolve in 48 hours

Less Common Disorders in Which Effusion Occurs Frequently

Rheumatic fever	Presence of carditis usually obvious Often associated with pericardial effusion
Pleural mesothelioma (malignant)	Fluid may be high or low in protein content Effusion chronic and recurrent, may be bilateral and involve pericardium History of asbestos exposure
Asbestos pleural effusion	Recurrent exudative effusion in absence of mesothelioma
Meigs syndrome	Benign ovarian tumor with ascites and hydrothorax Fluid protein concentration usually low
Pancreatitis	Effusion more common left side Fluid may have amylase higher than in blood
Postcardiotomy syndrome	Associated with fever and pericarditis
Systemic lupus erythematosus	Usually associated with pleuritic pain, often with areas of platelike atelectasis on x-ray

Disorders Only Occasionally Accompanied by Effusion

Other collagen diseases (polyarteritis, scleroderma, Wegener's granulomatosis)	Usually associated with activity of the underlying disease
Rheumatoid arthritis	Pleural fluid glucose commonly below 12 mg/dl LDH usually very high
Fungus infections (actinomycosis, histoplasmosis, coccidioidomycosis)	Effusion or empyema occasionally complicates chronic pulmonary infection
Hypothyroidism	Low-protein effusion may occur in absence of congestive failure
Sarcoidosis	Extreme rarity of pleural effusion is useful in differentiating from tuberculosis

exudative effusions and also shows a number of less common causes of pleural effusion. Most transudative effusions contain less than 3 g of protein/dl. Exudative effusions usually contain more than 3 g of protein/dl; those due to tuberculosis or pyogenic infection frequently show a protein concentration above 5 g/dl. More reliable separation may be made from the LDH concentration of pleural fluid and by comparing pleural fluid and serum protein and LDH concentrations. An LDH concentration greater than two-thirds of the normal serum level, a pleural fluid-to-serum LDH ratio greater than 0.6, or a pleural fluid-to-serum protein ratio greater than 0.5 establishes the presence of an exudative effusion with high reliability.[139]

The presence of gross blood in the pleural fluid is most common when the effusion is due to trauma, tumor, or pulmonary infarction. It may also result from bleeding induced at the time of a previous thoracentesis and is occasionally seen in effusions due to tuberculosis and pneumonia. Blood-tinged fluid with fewer than 10,000 RBC/μl is commonly found in an inflammatory effusion of any cause and is therefore of little diagnostic aid. Noninflammatory effusions usually contain only small numbers of white blood cells, predominantly lymphocytes, but total counts above 2500 are usually seen in inflammatory exudates. The majority of these cells may be polymorphonuclear leukocytes early in the course of a bacterial or tuberculous infection or following pulmonary infarction, but later in the course of the disease mononuclear cells generally predominate. In an occasional case, the pleural fluid may contain an exceptionally high percentage of eosinophils, even in the absence of blood eosinophilia. This is a relatively nonspecific finding but may be associated with pneumothorax or may be induced by multiple thoracenteses or intrapleural bleeding. Eosinophilia is unusual in effusions due to tuberculosis and malignancy. Wright stain of the centrifuged sediment will allow identification of mesothelial cells, which are large cells with basophilic cytoplasm, a large nucleus with finely stippled chromatin, and one to three bright blue nucleoli. Tuberculous effusions very rarely show more than 1 percent of these cells, whereas most nontuberculous effusions contain over 5 percent mesothelial cells.[140]

Chemical analysis of pleural fluid may provide additional clues to diagnosis. Pleural fluid glucose is only occasionally significantly lower than serum glucose when the effusion is caused by tuberculosis or tumor, but is usually very low (0 to 16 mg/dl) in effusions due to rheumatoid arthritis. Moderate elevation of pleural fluid amylase is occasionally seen in malignant effusions, but amylase levels which are markedly elevated indicate pancreatic disease or occasionally rupture of the esophagus with leakage of salivary amylase into the pleural space. The pH of pleural fluid is usually 7.30 or greater; lower values are occasionally seen in tuberculous and malignant effusions. A value below 7.20 in a parapneumonic effusion commonly is associated with the development of an empyema.

TREATMENT

Effective management requires that the etiology of the effusion be established and that specific treatment be applied where possible. In the case of noninflammatory effusions, correction of the underlying abnormality, perhaps accompanied by thoracentesis for removal of the bulk of the fluid, will usually result in rapid clearing of the effusion. When pleural inflammation is present, reabsorption of pleural fluid may be slow, and repeated thoracentesis may be required to keep the pleural cavity dry even after institution of specific therapy. It is important in these cases that reasonable effort be made to keep the pleural cavity free of fluid, in order to prevent the development of fibrosis in the pleural space, with subsequent restriction of expansion of the lung and loss of pulmonary function. If this is not done, subsequent surgical decortication may sometimes be required. There is some evidence that in tuberculous effusions, once effective antituberculous chemotherapy has been instituted, it may be advisable to administer corticosteroids in an effort to hasten resolution of the effusion and prevent pleural fibrosis. When pleural effusion due to malignant disease recurs rapidly, requiring repeated thoracentesis, reaccumulation may be retarded by insertion of a chest tube and instillation of a sclerosing agent such as atabrine or tetracycline.

EMPYEMA

Accumulation of pus within the pleural space (empyema) is an occasional complication of bacterial pneumonia or lung abscess and should be distinguished from the more common sterile inflammatory effusion. The fluid usually is thick and has the turbid appearance of frank pus, containing over 30,000 white cells/μl and often showing the etiologic bacterial agent on Gram stain and in culture. Empyema fluid caused by anaerobic organisms, especially *Bacteroides* or anaerobic streptococci, often has a foul odor. A chronic empyema in a patient already treated with antibiotics may pose a problem in identification since the fluid may have become thinner and the culture may be sterile. The leukocyte count of the fluid under these circumstances is probably the most reliable distinguishing feature. As noted above, pleural fluid with a pH below 7.20 should strongly suggest empyema.

The presence of an empyema should be suspected whenever a patient with bacterial pneumonia shows either persistence or recurrence of fever after appropriate antibiotic treatment. Evidence of even a small amount of pleural fluid in this setting requires thoracentesis for diagnosis. Although empyemas usually arise by extension of bacterial infection through the visceral pleura from the lung, they may also result from perforation of the esophagus, subphrenic abscess, or as a complication of surgery.

Successful management of the patient with empyema requires both the administration of appropriate antibiotics *and* the maintenance of effective drainage. Prompt recognition and institution of drainage provide the greatest likelihood that the empyema space will close without becoming chronic. When a small empyema is discovered early in the course of infection, attempts to close the space by repeated thoracentesis may be justified. This is seldom successful, however, and the prompt insertion of a rubber chest tube with connection to water-seal drainage is the preferred treatment. After several days without adequate drainage, most empyemas become loculated so that a tube is no longer effective, and in this situation it is best to resect a portion of rib, open the empyema cavity widely, and allow the wound to heal from within. In neglected chronic cases, or where a bronchopleural fistula is present, decortication with or without thoracoplasty may be required.

REFERENCES

General References

1. Bates, D.V., Macklem, P.T., and Christie, R.V. Respiratory Function in Disease. Philadelphia, Saunders, 1971.
2. Baum, G.L. Textbook of Pulmonary Diseases, 2nd ed. Boston, Little, Brown, 1974.
3. Crofton, J. and Douglas, A. Respiratory Diseases. Oxford, Blackwell, 1969.
4. Felson, B. Chest Roentgenology. Philadelphia, Saunders, 1973.
5. Fraser, R.G. and Pare, J.A.P. Diagnosis of Diseases of the Chest. Philadelphia, Saunders, 1970.
6. Guenter, C.A. and Welch, M.H. Pulmonary Medicine. Philadelphia, Lippincott, 1977.

Respiratory and Nonrespiratory Functions of the Lung

7. Bienenstock, J., Clancy, R.L., and Perey, D.Y.E. Bronchus associated lymphoid tissue (BALT): its relationship to mucosal immunity. In Kirkpatrick, C.H. and Reynolds, H.Y. (eds.), Immunologic and Infectious Reactions in the Lung. New York, Marcel Dekker, 1976.
8. Brain, J.D., Proctor, D.F., and Reid, L. (eds.). Respiratory Defense Mechanisms. New York, Marcel Dekker, 1977.
9. Comroe, J.H., Jr., Forster, R.E., II, DuBois, A.B., Briscoe, W.A., and Carlsen, E. The Lung. Chicago, Year Book Medical Publications, 1962.
10. Eliasson, R., Mossberg, B., Camner, P., and Afzelius, B.A. The immotilecilia syndrome: a congenital ciliary abnormality as an etiologic factor in chronic airway infections and male sterility. N. Engl. J. Med., 297:1, 1977.
11. Green, G.M. Pulmonary clearance of infectious agents. Annu. Rev. Med., 19:315, 1968.
12. Green, G.M., Jakab, G.J., Low, R.B., and Davis, G.S. State of the Art. Defense mechanisms of the respiratory membrane. Am. Rev. Respir. Dis., 115:479, 1977.
13. Hatch, T.F. and Gross, P. Pulmonary Deposition and Retention of Inhaled Aerosols. New York, Academic Press, 1964.
14. Hueter, F.G. and Fritzhand, M. Oxidants and lung biochemistry. A brief review. Arch. Intern. Med., 128:48, 1971.
15. Kaltreider, B.H. State-of-the-Art. Expression of immune mechanisms in the lung. Am. Rev. Respir. Dis., 113:347, 1976.
16. Mackaness, G.B. The J. Burns Amberson Lecture. The induction and expression of cell-mediated hypersensitivity in the lung. Am. Rev. Respir. Dis., 104:813, 1971.
17. Newhouse, M., Sanchis, J., and Bienenstock, J. Lung defense mechanisms. N. Engl. J. Med., 295:990–998, 1045–1052, 1977.
18. Pearsall, N.N. and Weiser, R.S. The Macrophage. Philadelphia, Lea and Febiger, 1970.
19. Proctor, D.F. The upper airways. II. The larynx and trachea. Am. Rev. Respir. Dis., 115:315, 1977.
20. Reynolds, H.Y., Kazmierowski, J.A., and Newball, H.H. Specificity of opsonic antibodies to enhance phagocytosis of *pseudomonas aeruginosa* by human alveolar macrophages obtained from cigarette smokers and non-smokers. J. Clin. Invest., 56:376, 1975.
21. Reynolds, H.Y. and Newball, H.H. Analysis of proteins and respiratory cells obtained from human lungs by bronchial lavage. J. Lab. Clin. Med., 84:559, 1974.
22. Reynolds, H.Y. and Newball, H.H. Fluid and cellular milieu of the human respiratory tract. In Kirkpatrick, C.H. and Reynolds, H.Y. (eds.), Immunologic and Infectious Reactions in the Lung. New York, Marcel Dekker, 1976.
23. Sturgess, J.M., Chao, J., Wong, J., Aspin, N., and Turner, J.A.P. Cilia with defective radial spokes: a cause of human respiratory disease. N. Engl. J. Med., 300:53, 1979.
24. Tucker, A.D., Wyatt, J.H., and Undery, D. Clearance of inhaled particles from alveoli by normal interstitial drainage pathways. J. Appl. Physiol., 35:719, 1973.
25. Waldman, R.H. and Henney, C.S. Cell-mediated immu-

nity and antibody responses in the respiratory tract after local and systemic immunization. J. Exp. Med., 134:482, 1971.

26. West, J.B. Respiratory Physiology—The Essentials. Baltimore, Williams & Wilkins, 1974.

Clinical Manifestations and Diagnosis of Pulmonary Disease

27. Andersen, H. and Fontana, J.S. Transbronchoscopic lung biopsy for diffuse pulmonary diseases: technique and results in 450 cases. Chest, 62:125, 1972.
28. Ashburn, W.L. and Moser, K.M. Pulmonary ventilation and perfusion scanning in pulmonary thromboembolism. In Moser, K.M. and Stein, M. (eds.), Pulmonary Thromboembolism. Chicago, Year Book Medical Publishers, 1973.
29. Baker, R.R., Stitik, F.P., and Summer, W.R. Preoperative evaluation of patients with suspected bronchogenic carcinoma. Curr. Probl. Surg., 1–48, December 1974.
30. Boysen, P.G., Block, A.J., Olsen, G.N., Moulder, P.V., Harris, J.O., and Rawitscher, R. Prospective evaluation for pneumonectomy using the ^{99}Tc quantitative perfusion lung scan. Chest, 72:422, 1977.
31. Bronchography. A report of the committee on bronchoesophagology. Dis. Chest, 51:663, 1967.
32. Campbell, E.J.M. and Newsome, D.J. Respiratory sensation in the respiratory muscles. In Campbell, E.J.M., Agostini, E., and Newsome, D.J. (eds.), Mechanics and Neural Control. London, Lloyd-Luke, 1970,
33. Cunningham, J.H., Zavala, D.C., Corry, R.J., and Keim, L.W. Trephine air drill, bronchial brush and fiberoptic transbronchial lung biopsies in immunosuppressed patients. Am. J. Respir. Dis., 115:213, 1977.
34. Epstein, R.L. Constituents of sputum: a simple method. Ann. Intern. Med., 77:259, 1972.
35. Fennessy, J.J. Bronchographic criteria of inflammatory disease and radiologic lung biopsy techniques. Radiol. Clin. North Am., 11:371, 1973.
36. Forgacs, P. Lung Sounds. London, Baillière Tindall, 1978.
37. King, E.G., Bachynski, J.E., and Mielke, B. Percutaneous trephine lung biopsy. Chest, 70:212, 1976.
38. Levin, D.C., Wicks, A.B., and Ellis, J.H., Jr. Transbronchial lung biopsy via the fiberoptic bronchoscope. Am. Rev. Respir. Dis., 110:4, 1974.
39. Lillington, G.A. and Jamplis, R.W. A Diagnostic Approach to Chest Diseases. Differential Diagnosis Based on Roentgenographic Patterns. Baltimore, Williams & Wilkins, 1977.
40. Marici, F.N. The flexible fiberoptic bronchoscope. In Johnston, R.F. (ed.), Pulmonary Care. New York, Grune & Stratton, 1973.
41. Mead, J. Volume displacement body plethysmograph for respiratory measurements in human subjects. J. Appl. Physiol., 15:736, 1960.
42. Mitchell, D.N. and Scadding, J.G. State of the Art. Sarcoidosis. Am. Rev. Respir. Dis., 110:774, 1974.
43. Molnar, W. and Rubel, F.A. Bronchography: an aid in the diagnosis of peripheral pulmonary carcinoma. Radiol. Clin. North Am., 1:303, 1963.

44. Paintal, A.S. Vagal sensory receptors and their reflex effects. Physiol. Rev., 53:159, 1973.
45. Parks, R.D. Bronchial brushing and transbronchial biopsy. In Johnston, R.F. (ed.), Pulmonary Care. New York, Grune & Stratton, 1973.
46. Stitik, F.P., Swift, D.L., and Proctor, D.F. Bronchography with the experimental contrast agent Tantalum. In Johnston, R.F. (ed.), Pulmonary Care. New York, Grune & Stratton, 1973.
47. Turner, F.T. and Sargeant, E.N. Percutaneous pulmonary needle biopsy. An improved needle for a simple direct method of diagnosis. Am. J. Roentgenol. Radium Ther. Nucl. Med., 104:846, 1968.
48. Wagner, H.N., Jr., Sabiston, D.C., Jr., Dio, M., McAfee, J.G., Myer, J.K., and Langan, J.K. Regional pulmonary blood flow in man by radioisotope scanning. JAMA, 187:601, 1964.
49. West, J.B. Pulmonary Pathophysiology—The Essentials. Baltimore, Williams & Wilkins, 1977.
50. Zavala, D.C. and Bedell, G.N. Percutaneous lung biopsy with a cutting needle. Am. Rev. Respir. Dis., 106:186, 1972.

Localized Pulmonary Infiltration

51. Bartlett, J.G. and Gorbach, S.L. The triple threat of aspiration pneumonia. Chest, 68:560, 1975.
52. Bynum, L.J. and Pierce, A.K. Pulmonary aspiration of gastric contents. Am. Rev. Respir. Dis., 114:1129, 1976.
53. Divertie, M.D. Lung involvement in the connective tissue disorders. Med. Clin. North Am., 48:1015, 1964.
54. Felson, B. Chest Roentgenology. Philadelphia, Saunders, 1973.
55. Gross, N.J. Pulmonary effects of radiation therapy. Ann. Intern. Med., 86:81, 1977.
56. Inners, C.R., Terry, P.B., Traystman, R.J., and Menkes, H.A. Collateral ventilation and the middle lobe syndrome. Am. Rev. Respir. Dis., 118:305, 1975.
57. Lawson, R.N., Ramanathan, L., Hurley, G., Hinson, K.W., and Lennox, S.C. Bronchial adenoma: review of an 18-year experience at the Brompton Hospital. Thorax, 31:245, 1976.
58. Lorber, B. and Swenson, P. Bacteriology of aspiration pneumonia: a prospective study of community and hospital acquired cases. Ann. Intern. Med., 81:329, 1974.
59. Mario, M. and Galy, P. Bronchioalveolar cell carcinoma. Clinicopathologic relationships, natural history and prognosis in 29 cases. Am. Rev. Respir. Dis., 107:621, 1973.
60. Matthay, R.A., Schwartz, N.I., and Petty, T.Z. Pleuropulmonary manifestations of connective tissue diseases. Clin. Notes Respir. Dis., 16:2, 1977.
61. Ottesen, E.A. Eosinophilia in the lung. In Kirkpatrick, C.H. and Reynolds, H.Y. (eds.), Immunologic and Infectious Reactions in the Lung. New York, Dekker, 1976.
62. Winterbauer, R.H., Bedon, G.A., and Ball, W.C., Jr. Recurrent pneumonia, predisposing illness and clinical patterns in 158 patients. Ann. Intern. Med., 70:689, 1969.

Diffuse Pulmonary Infiltration and Fibrosis

63. Allen, D.H., Basten, A., William, G.V., and Woolcock, A.J. Familial hypersensitivity pneumonitis. Am. J. Med., 59:505, 1975.

64. Becklake, M.R. State of the Art. Asbestos related diseases of the lung and other organs: their epidemiology and implications for clinical practice. Am. Rev. Respir. Dis., 114:187, 1976.

65. Bohlig, E., Bristol, L.J., Cartier, P.H., Felson, B., Gilson, J.C., Grainger, T.R., Jacobson, G., Kiviluoto, R., Lainhart, W.S., McDonald, J.C., Pendergrass, E.P., Rossiter, C.E., Selikoff, I.J., Sluis-Cremer, G.K., and Wright, G.W. UICC/Cincinnati classification of the radiographic appearances of pneumoconioses. Chest, 58:57, 1970.

66. Bone, R.C., Wolfe, J., Sobonya, R.E., Kerby, G.R., Stechschulte, D., Ruth, W.E., and Welch, M. Desquamative interstitial pneumonia following long-term nitrofurantoin therapy. Am. J. Med., 60:697, 1976.

67. Crystal, R.G., Fulmer, J.D., Roberts, W.C., Moss, M.L., Line, B.R., and Reynolds, H.Y. NIH Conference. Idiopathic pulmonary fibrosis: clinical, histologic, radiographic, physiologic, scintigraphic, cytologic, and biochemical aspects. Ann. Intern. Med., 85:769, 1976.

68. Cunningham, J.H., Zavala, D.C., Corry, R.J., and Keim, L.W. Trephine air drill, bronchial brush, and fiberoptic transbronchial lung biopsies in immunosuppressed patients. Am. Rev. Respir. Dis., 115:213, 1977.

69. Fauci, A.S. and Wolff, S.M. Wegener's granulomatosis: studies in eighteen patients and a review of the literature. Medicine (Baltimore), 52:535, 1973.

70. Fink, J.M., Banaszak, E.F., Baroriak, J.J., Hensley, G.T, Kurup, V.R., Scanlon, G.T., Schlueter, D.P., Sosman, A.S., and Thiede, W.H. Interstitial lung disease due to contamination of forced air system. Ann. Intern. Med., 84:406, 1976.

71. Gould, D.M. and Dalrymple, G.V. A radiological analysis of disseminated lung disease. Am. J. Med. Sci., 238:621, 1959.

72. Greenman, R.L., Goodall, P.T., and King, D. Lung biopsy in immunocompromised hosts. Am. J. Med., 59:488, 1975.

73. Hanson, R.R., Zavala, D.C., Rhodes, M.L., Keim, L.W., and Smith, J.D. Transbronchial biopsy via flexible fiberoptic bronchoscope: results in 164 patients. Am. Rev. Respir. Dis., 114:67, 1976.

74. Iseman, M.D., Schwartz, M.I., and Stanford, R.E. Interstitial pneumonia in angio-immunoblastic lymphadenopathy with dysproteinemia. A case report with special histopathologic studies. Ann. Intern. Med., 85:752, 1976.

75. James, D.G., Neville, E., and Walker, A. Immunology of sarcoidosis. Am. J. Med., 59:388, 1975.

76. Johns, C.J. The prognosis and management of sarcoidois. Mt. Sinai J. Med. N.Y., 44:782, 1977.

77. Johns, C.J., Zachary, J.B., and Ball, W.C., Jr. A ten-year study of corticosteroid treatment of pulmonary sarcoidosis. Johns Hopkins Med. J., 134:271, 1974.

78. Johns, C.J., MacGregor, M.I., Zachary, J.B., and Ball, W.C., Jr. Extended experience in the long-term corticosteroid treatment of pulmonary sarcoid. Transactions of the New York Academy of Science, VII International Sarcoidosis Conference. Ann. N.Y. Acad. Sci., 278:722, 1976.

79. Koontz, C.H., Joyner, L.R., and Nelson, R.A. Transbronchial lung biopsy via the fiberoptic bronchoscope in sarcoidosis. Ann. Intern. Med., 85:64, 1976.

80. Liebow, A.A. The J. Burns Amberson Lecture. Pulmonary angiitis and granulomatosis. Am. Rev. Respir. Dis., 108:1, 1973.

81. Liebow, A.A. and Carrington, C.B. The eosinophilic pneumonias. Medicine (Baltimore), 48:251, 1969.

82. Liebow, A.A., Stear, A., and Billingsley, J.G. Desquamative interstitial pneumonia. Am. J. Med., 39:369, 1965.

83. Littner, M.R., Schachter, E.N., and Putman, C.E. The clinical assessment of roentgenographically atypical pulmonary sarcoidosis. Am. J. Med., 62:361, 1977.

84. Livingstone, J.L., Lewis, J.G., Reid, L., and Jefferson, K.E. Diffuse interstitial fibrosis: a clinical, radiological and pathological study based on 45 patients. Q. J. Med., 33:71, 1964.

85. McCombs, R.P. Diseases due to immunologic reactions in the lungs. N. Engl. J. Med., 286:1186–1194, 1245–1252, 1972.

86. Mitchell, D.N. and Scadding, J.G. State of the Art. Sarcoidosis. Am. Rev. Respir. Dis., 110:774, 1974.

87. Pepys, J. Hypersensitivity Diseases of the Lungs Due to Fungi and Organic Dusts (Monographs in Allergy, vol. 4). Basel, Karger, 1969.

88. Proceedings of the VIII International Sarcoidosis Conference, September, 1978, Cardiff, Wales. In press.

89. Rosen, S., II, Castlemen, B.J., and Leibow, A.A. Pulmonary alveolar proteinosis. N. Engl. J. Med., 258:11, 1958.

90. Rosenow, E.C., III. The spectrum of drug-induced pulmonary disease. Ann. Intern. Med., 77:977, 1972.

91. Scadding, J.G. Diffuse pulmonary alveolar fibrosis. Thorax, 29:271, 1974.

92. Scadding, J.G. and Hinsai, K.F.W. Diffuse fibrosing alveolitis (diffuse interstitial fibrosis of the lungs). Thorax, 22:291, 1967.

93. Schlueter, D.P. Response of the lungs to inhaled antigens. Am. J. Med., 57:476, 1974.

94. Zavala, D.C. Diagnostic fiberoptic bronchoscopy: techniques and results of biopsy in patients. Chest, 68:12, 1975.

Obstructive Pulmonary Disease

95. Austen, K.F. and Orange, R.P. Bronchial asthma: the possible role of the chemical mediators of immediate hypersensitivity in the pathogenesis of subacute chronic disease. Am. Rev. Respir. Dis., 112:423, 1975.

96. Burrows, B. and Earle, R.H. Course and prognosis of chronic obstructive lung disease. N. Engl. J. Med., 280:397, 1969.

97. Fletcher, C.M. (ed.). Ciba guest symposium report: terminology, definitions, and classifications of chronic pulmonary emphysema and related conditions. Symposium, September 1958. Thorax, 14:286, 1959.

98. Geraldo, D., Blumenthal, N., and Spink, W.W. Aspirin

intolerance and asthma. Ann. Intern. Med., 71:479, 1969.

99. McFadden, E.R., Kiser, R., and DeGroot, W.J. Acute bronchial asthma: relations between clinical and physiologic manifestations. N. Engl. J. Med., 288:221, 1973.

100. Permutt, S. Physiologic changes in the acute asthmatic attack. In Austen, K.F. and Lichtenstein, L.M. (eds.), Asthma Physiology, Immunopharmacology and Treatment. New York, Academic, 1973.

101. Pride, N.B., Permutt, S., Riley, R.L., and Bromberger-Barnea, B. Determinants of maximal expiratory flow from the lungs. J. Appl. Physiol., 23:646, 1967.

102. Rebuck, A.S. and Read, J. Assessment and management of severe asthma. Am. J. Med., 51:788, 1971.

103. Strauss, R.H., McFadden, E.R., Jr., Ingram, R.H., Jr., Deal, E.C., Jr., and Jaeger, J.J. Influence of heat and humidity on the airway obstruction induced by exercise in asthma. J. Clin. Invest., 61:433, 1978.

104. Thurlbeck, W.M. Aspects of chronic airflow obstruction. Chest, 72:341, 1977.

105. Thurlbeck, W.M., Henderson, J.A., Fraser, R.G., and Bates, D.V. Chronic obstructive lung disease: a comparison between clinical, roentgenologic, functional, and morphologic criteria in chronic bronchitis, emphysema, asthma, and bronchiectasis. Medicine (Baltimore), 49:81, 1970.

106. Wolfe, J.D., Tashkin, D.P., Calvarese, B., and Simmons, M. Bronchodilator effects of terbutaline and aminophylline alone and in combination in asthmatic patients. N. Engl. J. Med., 298:363, 1978.

107. Woolcock, A.J. and Read, J. Lung volumes in exacerbations of asthma. Am. J. Med., 41:259, 1966.

Acute Respiratory Failure (ARF)

108. Hopewell, P.C. and Murray, J.F. The adult respiratory distress syndrome. Annu. Rev. Med., 27:343, 1976.

109. Koerner, S.K. and Malovany, R.J. Acute repiratory insufficiency and cor pulmonale: pathophysiology, clincal features and management. Am. Heart J., 88:115, 1974.

110. Lamy, M., Fallat, R.J., Koeniger, E., and Marm-Peter, D. Pathologic features and mechanisms of hypoxemia in adult respiratory distress syndrome. Am. Rev. Respir. Dis., 114:267, 1976.

111. Malovany, R.J. and Koerner, S.K. Acute repiratory insufficiency and cor pulmonale. Am. Heart J., 88:251, 1974.

112. Scharf, S.M., Caldini, P., and Ingram, R.H. Cardiovascular effects of increasing airway pressure in the dog. Am. J. Physiol., 232(1):H35, 1977.

113. Shibel, E. and Moser, K. (eds.). Respiratory Emergencies. St. Louis, Mosby, 1977.

114. Suter, P.M., Fairley, H.B., and Isenberg, M.D. Optimum end-expiratory airway pressure in patients with acute pulmonary failure. N. Engl. J. Med., 292:284, 1975.

115. Sykes, M.K., McNichol, M.W., Campbell, E.J.M. Respiratory Failure, 2nd ed. Oxford, Blackwell, 1976.

116. Toung, T.J.K., Bordos, D., Benson, D.W., Carter, D., Zuidema, G.D., Permutt, S., and Cameron, J.L. Aspira-

tion pneumonia: experimental evaluation of albumin and steroid therapy. Ann. Surg., 183:179, 1976.

117. Toung, T.J.K., Saharia, P., Mitzner, W.A., Permutt, S., and Cameron, J.L. The beneficial and harmful effects of positive end-expiratory pressure. Surgery, 147:518, 1978.

Mass Lesions and Pulmonary Nodules

Mediastinal Masses

118. Benjamin, S.P., McCormack, L.J., Effler, D.B., and Groves, L.K. Primary tumors of the mediastinum. Chest, 62:297, 1972.

119. Doctor, A.H. Mediastinoscopy, a critical evaluation of 220 cases. Ann. Surg., 174:965, 1971.

120. Guinn, G.A., Tomm, K.E., North, L., and Mocega, E. Clinical staging of primary lung cancer. Chest, 64:51, 1973.

121. Kubic, S. Surgical Anatomy of the Thorax. Philadelphia, Saunders, 1970.

122. Leigh, T.F. and Weens, H.S. The Mediastinum. Springfield, Ill., Thomas, 1959.

123. Marshall, R.J., Edmundowicz, A.C., and Andrews, C.E. Chronic obstruction of the superior vena cava due to histoplasmosis. Circulation, 29 (Suppl.) 604, 1964.

124. Miller, R.E. and Sullivan, F.J. Superior vena cava obstruction secondary to fibrosing mediastinitis. Ann. Thorac. Surg., 15:483, 1973.

125. Rubush, J.L., Gardner, I.R., Boyd, W.C., and Ehrenhaft, J.L. Mediastinal tumors. J. Thorac. Cardiovasc. Surg., 65:216, 1973.

126. Wychulis, A.R., Payne, W.S., Clagett, O.T., and Woolner, L.B. Surgical treatment of mediastinal tumors. J. Thorac. Cardiovasc. Surg., 62:379, 1971.

127. Young, R., Pochaczevsky, R., Pollack, L., and Bryk, D. Cervico-mediastinal thymic cysts. Am. J. Roentgenol. Radium Ther. Nucl. Med., 117:855, 1973.

Solitary Pulmonary Nodules

128. Bateson, E.M. An analysis of 155 solitary lung lesions illustrating the differential diagnosis of mixed tumors of the lung. Clin. Radiol., 16:51, 1965.

129. Gracey, D.R., Byrd, R.B., and Cugell, D.B. The dilemma of the asymptomatic pulmonary nodule in the young and not-so-young adult. Chest, 60:479, 1971.

130. Katz, S., Peabody, J.W., Jr., and Davis, E.W. The solitary pulmonary nodule. Chicago, Year Book Medical Publishers, D. M., April 1961.

131. Lillington, G.A. The solitary pulmonary nodule—1974. Am. Rev. Respir. Dis., 110:699, 1974.

132. Steele, J.D. The Solitary Pulmonary Nodule. Springfield, Ill., Thomas, 1964.

Lung Cancer

133. Benfield, J.R., Juillard, G.J.F., Pilch, Y.H., Rigler, L.G., and Selecky, P. Current and future concepts of lung cancer. Ann. Intern. Med., 83:93, 1975.

134. Holland, J.F. and Frei, E.T., (eds.). Cancer Medicine. Philadelphia, Lea and Febiger, 1973.

135. Muggia, F.M., Krezoski, S.K., and Hansen, H.H. Cell kinetic studies in patients with small cell carcinoma of the lung. Cancer, 34:1683, 1974.

136. Perez, C.A. Radiation therapy for cancer of the lung. Previous experience and definition of current issues. Cancer Treat. Rep., 4:145, 1973.

137. Selawry, O.S. and Straus, M.J. Lung cancer. Semin. Oncol., 1:161, 1974.

Pleural Effusions

138. Black, L.F. The pleural space and pleural fluid. Mayo Clin. Proc., 47:493, 1972.

139. Light, R.W., MacGregor, M.I., Luchsinger, P.C., and Ball, W.C., Jr. Pleural effusions: the diagnostic separation of transudates and exudates. Ann. Intern. Med., 77:507, 1972.

140. Light, R.W., Erozan, Y.S., and Ball, W.C., Jr. Cells in pleural fluid. Their value in differential diagnosis. Arch. Intern. Med., 132:854, 1973.

141. Lowell, J.R. Pleural Effusions. A Comprehensive Review. Baltimore, University Park, 1977.

142. Salyer, W.R., Eggleston, J.C., and Erozan, Y.S. Efficacy of pleural needle biopsy and pleural fluid cytopathology in the diagnosis of malignant neoplasm involving the pleura. Chest, 67:536, 1975.

SECTION SIX
Medical Genetics
VICTOR A. McKUSICK: SECTION EDITOR

This section is concerned, not with the disorders of a particular organ system, but with an etiologic category of disease. After a discussion of general principles, each of three main categories of genetic diseases is discussed: chromosomal aberrations, mendelian disorders, and multifactorial disorders. Pharmacogenetics and immunogenetics are accorded separate chapters because, although these areas are very important to medicine, they do not primarily represent disorders, as do the other three main topics.

Of the three categories of genetic disease, mendelian disorders are discussed most extensively. Principles of diagnosis, prognosis (genetic counseling), treatment, and prevention are presented. The number of mendelian disorders is large, but they become more manageable in clinical practice when basic principles underlying all of them are familiar to the physician. Also, mendelian disorders tend to fall into one of a few major groups according to pathogenetic mechanisms. Consequently, after the discussion of principles, the major pathogenetic categories of mendelian disorders are illustrated.

CHAPTER 39
General Considerations
VICTOR A. McKUSICK

The physician who cares for adult patients, in his role as generalist and as adviser to prospective parents, must be conversant, at least in a general way, with all genetic disorders. Genetic disorders are by no means the exclusive concern of the pediatrician. Increasingly, because of improved care, patients with grave genetic disorders are surviving to adulthood, and mild forms compatible with such survival are being recognized. Cystic fibrosis of the pancreas provides an example of both features. Many diseases which were first delineated on the basis of the most severe (and, as was thought, "textbook") cases are being recognized in adult patients. Furthermore, those genetic disorders which first manifest in adolescence or later are a significant segment of medical practice. Finally, in the role that the internist often fills as family physician he has the opportunity and responsibility to observe and respond appropriately to the particular genetic characteristics of his patients and their families, and to use the information in the diagnosis and management of their health problems.

Medical genetics is concerned with genetic disorders and with the role of genetic factors in all disease. *Clinical genetics* is that part of medical genetics concerned directly with the care of patients afflicted with genetic disorders and their families.

Genetic factors play some role in most diseases and, similarly, environmental factors play a role. Most diseases can be viewed as falling somewhere on a scale or spectrum ranging from one end where genetic factors predominate in causation to the other where environmental factors predominate. For example, phenylketonuria and galactosemia are near the "genetic end" but not at the very end because diet, an environmental factor, influences these diseases. Similarly, tuberculosis is near the "environmental end," although again not at the extreme end because genetic constitution is shown by twin and ethnologic studies to play a significant role. Hypertension, peptic ulcer, diabetes, and many other disorders fall in a middle ground. Useful as this simplistic model is for conceptualizing the *relative* roles of genetic make-up and exogenous factors, few diseases can be positioned on such a scale with mathematical precision. Favism is, however, an example of a disease in which the relative roles of the two influences can be precisely stated. It would be placed in the very center of the scale; this disease has an absolute requirement for both deficiency of red cell glucose-6-phosphate dehydrogenase (an X-chromosomally determined defect) and for exposure to the fava bean (an exogenous agent). Both factors are necessary, but neither is alone sufficient in causation of favism. An exogenous factor (thiamine deficiency) and an endogenous factor (mutation in transketolase) collaborate in "causing" the Wernicke-Korsakoff syndrome.[13]

Because of the influence of environmental factors in most genetic diseases, manipulation of the environment is an approach to their treatment.

Genetic diseases tend to fall into one of three categories: 1) *Chromosomal aberrations,*[2] although usually not inherited in the usual sense of that word (they may be heritable), involve the genetic material and therefore are one form of genetic disease. 2) By typical pedigree patterns and other characteristics, many disorders reveal themselves to be the result primarily of mutation at a single genetic locus. These are called *mendelian disorders.* (See McKusick's *Mendelian Inheritance in Man*[3] for a comprehensive listing of all known mendelian disorders.) The specific chromosome or even part of the chromosome carrying the specific causative gene is becoming known for an increasing number of disorders.[31] 3) Many common disorders, such as hypertension and cardiac malformations, are termed *multifactorial* because both genetic and nongenetic factors, often multiple in each case, collaborate in causation. (*Polygenic* describes multiple genetic background.)

This three-way classification is, like many classifications, to some extent arbitrary. As indicated earlier, environmental factors influence even "single-gene" disorders, as does also the rest of the genetic make-up of the patient. Thus, all are, in this context, multifactorial. Even in multifactorial disorders the operation of individual loci has in an increasing number of instances been identified. In chromosomal aberrations many genes are present in excess or are deficient; hence, these might be termed polygenic or multifactorial. But despite its arbitrariness, the classification is useful because the approach to the three types of disease is different.

The four aspects of clinical medicine—diagnosis, prognosis, treatment and prevention (see *Foreword*)—are as significant to clinical genetics as to other aspects of medicine. Each category of genetic disease, particularly mendelian disorders, can conveniently be discussed under these four headings.

The methods of clinical genetics include pedigree construction, cytologic techniques (particularly examination for X and Y chromatin, study of the chromosomes in dividing somatic cells, mainly lymphocytes, and study of biochemical characteristics of cultured skin fibroblasts), special biochemical tests of blood and urine for the diagnosis of inborn errors of metabolism, screening of neonates or testing for heterozygous carriers of disease, amniocentesis for prenatal diagnosis and special approaches, e.g., dietary, to the treatment of inborn errors of metabolism.

CHAPTER 40
Chromosomal Aberrations
VICTOR A. McKUSICK

NORMAL MEIOSIS AND GAMETOGENESIS

The nucleus of each somatic cell of man contains 22 pairs of nonsex chromosomes (autosomes) and a pair of sex chromosomes: two X chromosomes in the female and an X and a Y in the male (Fig. 40–1). (Some cells, such as megakaryocytes, are polyploid, i.e., have chromosome counts that are multiples of the basic diploid number of 46.) In the fertilized ovum, the zygote, 23 of the chromosomes, one of each pair, are derived from the father via the sperm and 23 from the mother. In the process of mitosis, which occurs in somatic cells undergoing division, each chromosome is reduplicated so that each daughter cell receives the full complement of 46 chromosomes identical to those in the original zygote. By contrast the process of meiosis (etymologically this is the same word as *miosis,* which by usage refers exclusively to a reduction in pupil size), results in a reduction in chromosome number from the diploid number (23 pairs) found in somatic cells to the haploid number (23 unique chromosomes, one from each pair) characteristic of the gametes, eggs, and sperm.

Meiosis (Fig. 40–2) occurs during the production of gametes in the ovary or testis. The process consists of two cell divisions, with chromosome reduplication occurring only once, early in the process. In the first meiotic division the reduplicated twin-stranded pairs of homologous chromosomes (e.g., the two chromosomes come to lie side by side, attached at their cen-

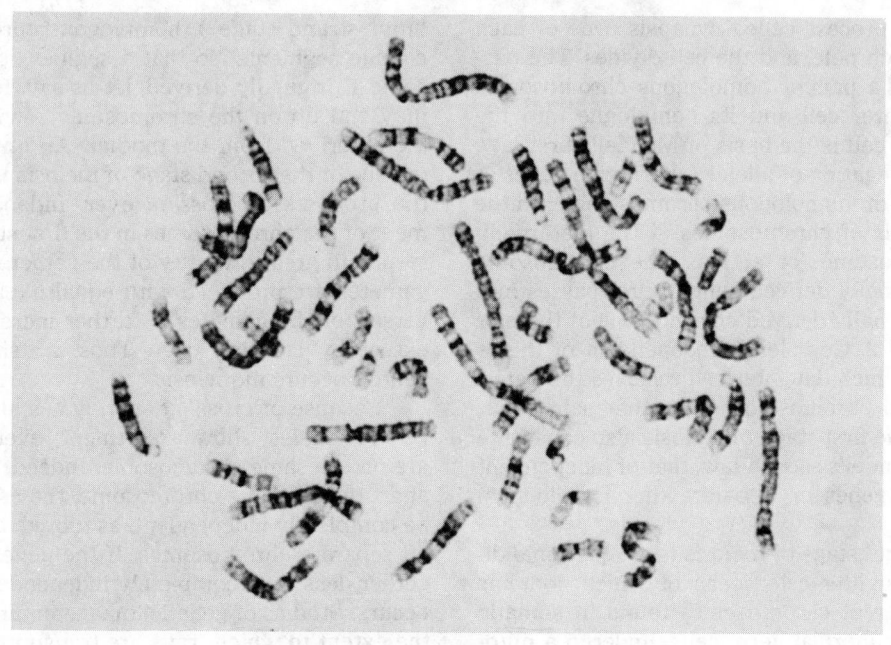

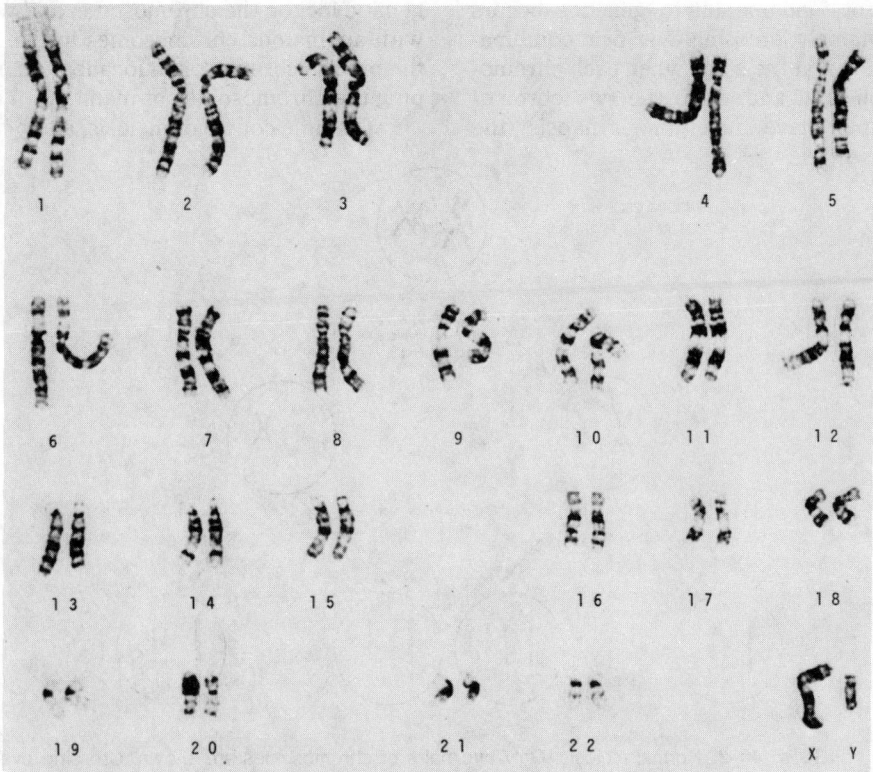

FIGURE 40–1. Top. The chromosomes (in metaphase) of a single lymphocyte from a normal male, prepared and stained by a trypsin-Giemsa banding technique.[41] Approximately 5000X magnification. **Bottom.** Same, arranged in karyotype. Courtesy of Dr. Uta Francke.

tromeres, in a process called synapsis. One of each pair goes to each pole, and the cell divides. The passage of one of a pair of homologous chromosomes into one daughter cell and its homologue into the other daughter cell is the basis of Mendel's first law, that of the segregation of alleles (alternative genes at the same locus on homologous chromosomes). In the case of one pair of chromosomes, if the maternally derived chromosome (or at least the chromosome with the maternally derived centromere) passes into cell 1, the paternally derived chromosome of the pair passes into cell 2. Completely independent of this is the matter of which daughter cell receives the paternal or maternal chromosome of another pair. Thus, the events of the first stage of meiosis also constitute the basis of Mendel's second law, that of independent assortment of genes on separate (nonhomologous) chromosomes.

In the second stage of meiosis (the equational division), the daughter cells, each of which contains half the number of chromosomes found in somatic cells and the primordial germ cells, undergo a mitosis-like division. As a result the gametes have half the somatic number of chromosomes.

Another event fundamental to genetics occurs during meiosis, namely, crossing over or recombination. Early in meiosis, at the stage when each chromosome has reduplicated and when the two chromosomes of each pair have undergone synapsis (the

"four strand stage"), homologous chromosomes exchange segments, so that a segment of the chromosome 1 originally derived, let us say, from the father may end up on the chromosome 1 with the centromere derived from the mother. An important consequence of the second stage of meiosis is separation of the products of crossing over. Independent assortment of the chromosomes in the first stage of meiosis results in great diversity of the gametes; 2^{23} different gametes are produced with equal likelihood. The diversity of the gametes is further increased to a vast extent by crossing over. Thus, a "shuffling of the genes" occurs in meiosis.

Because of crossing over, genes at different loci, i.e., nonalleles, show assortment, even though they are on the same chromosome. Indeed, if they are far apart on the same chromosome, the assortment may be completely independent, as though the genes were on separate chromosomes. If the genes are close together, less than completely independent assortment occurs. Studies of genetic linkage in families examine the extent to which traits are transmitted together in families, quantitate the degree of independence of assortment, provide a measure of the distance between genetic loci on the chromosome, and when correlated with anomalous chromosomes in the family indicate the precise chromosomal localization of genes—mapping the chromosomes of man.[31]

The time course of meiosis, and of gametogenesis

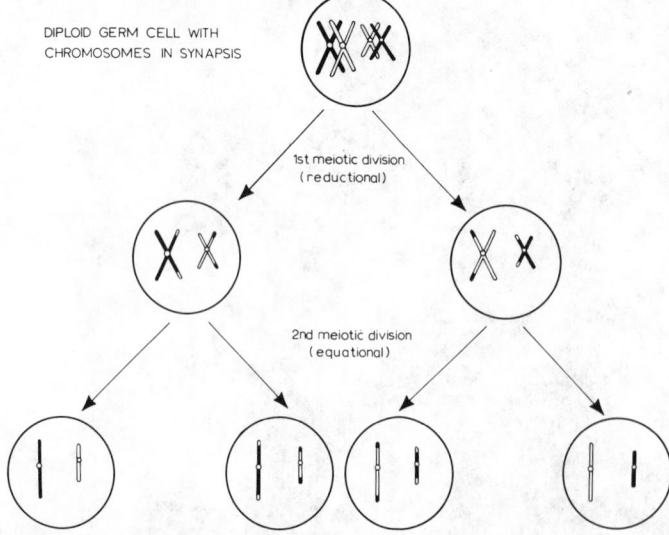

FIGURE 40-2. Normal meiosis. Only two pairs of chromosomes are shown. Crossing over, i.e., exchange of genetic information between chromosomes, of pairs occurs at the stage shown at the top. In spermatogenesis, meiosis produces four cells from each one which enters the process. In oogenesis, only one cell is produced by each primordial germ cell, since in each stage of meiosis one of the two daughter cells is cast off as a polar body.

in general, is different in males and females. In the human female, germ cells multiply rapidly during early fetal life. Oogonia (the primordial germ cells of the female) cease to propagate after the fifth or sixth month of fetal life. The female infant is born with a full stock of oocytes that must last for her entire reproductive life. Inventories of this stock have arrived at estimates of about 750,000 per individual newborn female; however, many of these oocytes degenerate at various stages of oogenesis and at various times in the life of the female.

By about the time of birth, the oocytes have completed most of the prophase of the first meiotic division and then regress into a long interphase-like dictyotene ("thick thread") stage during which the nuclear membrane remains intact and the chromosomes are visible as threadlike or netlike structures. The dictyotene stage lasts for at least 12 years and even as long as 50 years. During this stage the DNA content is tetraploid (i.e., has twice as much chromosomal material as the normal diploid body cells), since each chromosome has replicated and no cell division has taken place.

Meiosis in the oocyte is resumed about the time of ovulation, and the first meiotic, or reduction, division is completed at that time. Pituitary hormones

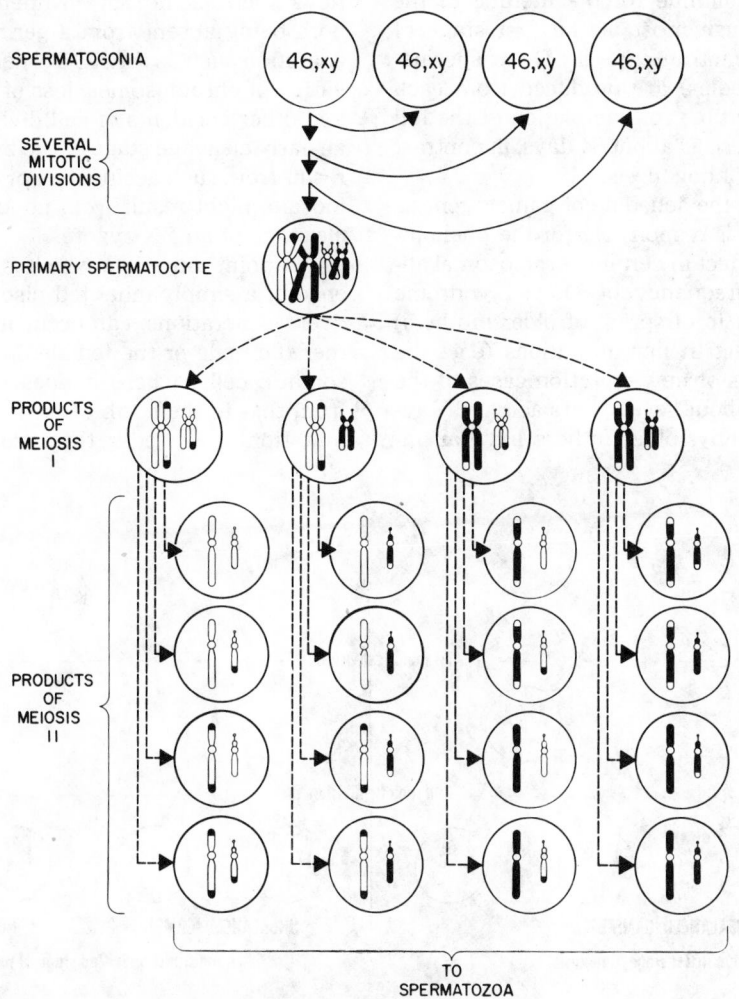

FIGURE 40-3. The basis for increasing frequency of mutations with age in the male—"paternal age effect." Opportunity for the occurrence and accumulation of mutations is illustrated. The diversifying effects of crossing over are also shown.

stimulate this resumption of meiosis. The second, or equational, division of meiosis is usually completed only after the entry of the sperm into the ovum. In the female a polar body is extruded and lost as one product of each meiotic division. When the chromosome of the male and female pronuclei come together, fertilization is complete and the cell becomes a zygote. The process of fertilization usually takes place in the ampulla of the Fallopian tube. Uterine implantation of the human embryo occurs six to seven days after ovulation.

Spermatogenesis differs from oogenesis in several important respects. The production of sperm is exceedingly abundant, and the total number produced in the lifetime of a male is astronomical. Proliferation of spermatogonia does not begin until puberty but thereafter may continue for the lifetime of the male; oogenesis through most of the first stage of meiosis is confined to intrauterine life. Four spermatids (and no polar bodies) are produced from each spermatogonium. The time for completion of the full cycle of spermatogenesis is about 64 days, in contrast to the 12 to 50 years of oogenesis.

This difference in the schedule of gametogenesis in males and females is responsible for the phenomena of maternal age effect in certain chromosomal aberrations (e.g., the frequency of Down syndrome (mongolism) is higher in offspring of older mothers) and paternal age effect in new mutations (e.g., the average age of fathers of new mutation cases of the Marfan syndrome is about seven years above the average, or said differently, older fathers have an in-creased risk of having children affected with a new mutation for some dominantly inherited disorder such as the Marfan syndrome) (Fig. 40–3).

ABNORMALITIES IN MEIOSIS AND GAMETOGENESIS

Normally, half the sperms contain 22 autosomes and a Y chromosome each. As a result, half of the fertilized eggs, or zygotes, will be XY (males) and half will be XX (females). So-called nondisjunction (Fig. 40–4) of a chromosomal pair during the process of meiosis may result in both members of a chromosomal pair being included in a germ cell, giving rise to malformations such as the XXY Klinefelter syndrome, or in both being absent from a germ cell, giving rise to a condition such as the XO Turner syndrome. Missegregation of chromosomes, loss of one member of a pair and other accidents of cell division can also occur in an early cleavage stage of the zygote. Mosaicism may result from such accidents. For example, an XXX/XO mosaic might result from nondisjunction at the first cleavage of an XX zygote.

A point mutation, which is detected by the presence of a simply inherited disorder or trait in subsequent generations, can occur in the germ cells of either the male or the female. Mutation also occurs in somatic cells, where it does not differ in principle from that in the germ cells. Theoretically, if somatic mutations occurred in the zygote or at an early post-

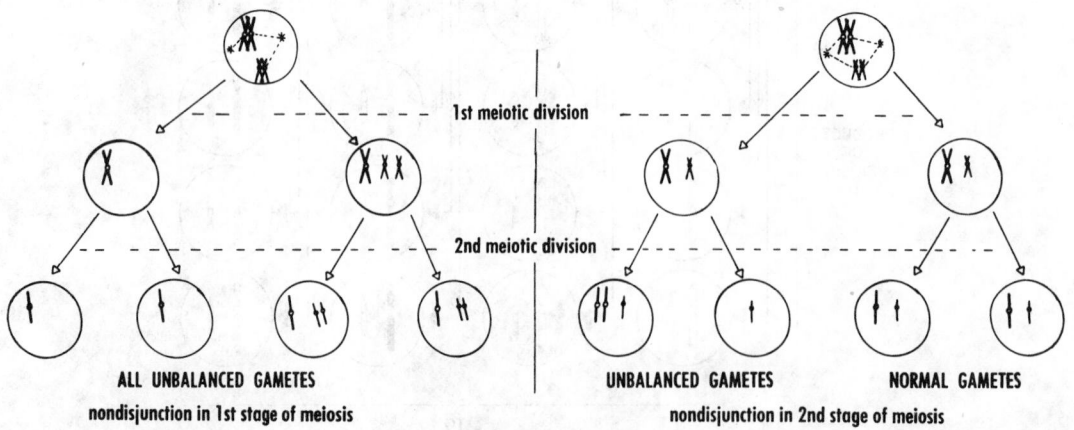

1st meiotic division

2nd meiotic division

ALL UNBALANCED GAMETES
nondisjunction in 1st stage of meiosis

UNBALANCED GAMETES   **NORMAL GAMETES**
nondisjunction in 2nd stage of meiosis

FIGURE 40–4. Abnormal meiosis, nondisjunction. Failure of the homologous chromosomes to disjoin normally in the first meiotic division (on left) and of the two chromatids to separate and pass into separate cells in the second stage of meiosis (on right) is illustrated. Nondisjunction and related accidents in the segregation of the chromosomes can also occur in mitosis, e.g., in early stages of the zygote.

zygotic stage, the individual might be affected with the given disorder. Furthermore, if a somatic mutation occurs at an appropriate postzygotic stage early in embryogenesis and if action of the mutant gene is locally manifest, a sectorial, or mosaic, situation might result. For example, if the normal allele of the gene for von Recklinghausen neurofibromatosis underwent mutation early in embryogenesis, one might observe a sector in which skin tumors and pigmented spots occur. An individual with such a condition would not transmit the disorder unless gonadal tissue was also involved. When a gonadal anlage cell suffers mutation, the situation is referred to as gonadal mosaicism. An individual with this condition, although not showing signs of the disorder and although the disorder is dominant, may have more than one affected child. (Note the difference between mosaicism and chimerism. *Mosaicism* is the presence of two (or more) classes of cells representing variations on a single genome, e.g., somatic mutation mentioned above. *Chimerism* is the mixture of cells of different genomes, e.g., sometimes a dizygotic twin is found to have a minor cell line derived from his cotwin through early crosstransfusion in utero.)

As outlined for the sex chromosomes, missegregation of autosomes can occur in meiosis or in early mitotic stages resulting in the presence of three of a particular chromosome rather than the normal two, a condition called trisomy. This is what happens with chromosome 21 to result in the Down syndrome (mongolism, or trisomy 21). Or only one of a particular autosome may end up in the zygote, a situation called monosomy. Although monosomy of the X chromosome (Turner syndrome) is relatively well tolerated, monosomy of the autosomes leads to early embryonic death as a rule; trisomy of any except chromosome 13, 18, and 21 is rarely found in liveborn infants. In rare instances patients have been found to have as many as five X chromosomes, arising, presumably, through nondisjunction in both the first and the second stages of meiosis. Such XXXXX individuals (and those who are XXXY, XXXX, and XXXXY) are severely retarded and have serious somatic malformation and abnormal sexual development. That they survive is related to the special mechanism by which X chromosomes in excess of one are rendered genetically inactive, at least in part or after a certain stage in embryogenesis. This special mechanism is responsible for normal dosage compensation in the female, in whom the excess of genetic material (two X chromosomes as compared to the one X chromosome of the normal male) would otherwise be disruptive. The one-inactive-X hypothesis (the Lyon hypothesis) concerns this mechanism of dosage compensation (Fig. 40–5).

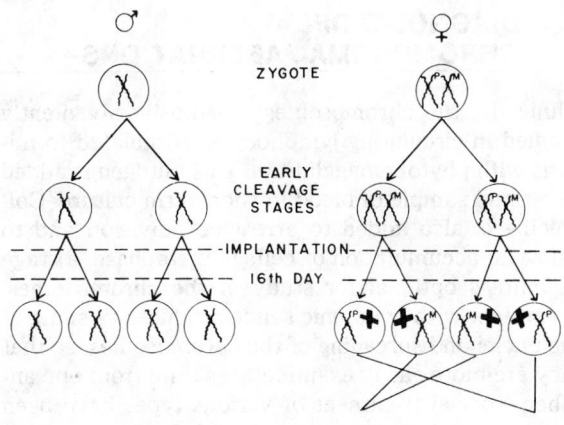

FIGURE 40–5. The Lyon principle. Sometime between implantation and the 16th day in the normal female embryo, one X chromosome in each cell becomes genetically relatively inactive and forms the Barr body, or sex chromatin. It is randomly determined whether the X chromosome contributed by the mother or the father is the inactivated one in a given cell, but once decision is made in a given cell, all descendants of that cell have the same X chromosome inactive.

Other chromosomal aberrations can occur during meiosis, not through missegregation but through chromosome breakage. A single break may lead to loss of that segment of the chromosome without a centromere. For example, the distal part of the short arm of chromosome 5 may be lost (5p-) leading to the clinical picture called the cri-du-chat syndrome. If two breaks occur in the same chromosome, an inversion may occur when the chromosome heals. If the two breaks are on the same side of the centromere, i.e., in the same chromosome arm, it is termed a paracentric inversion. If the two breaks are on opposite sides of the centromere, it is termed a pericentric inversion. If the two breaks occur in separate chromosomes, pieces may be exchanged between them, socalled reciprocal translocation. Or two breaks occurring at the end of the certain chromosome may lead to a fusion chromosome (Robertsonian translocation). The last is most frequently observed as occurring between chromosomes 21 and 14, which have their centromeres near the ends (they are so-called acrocentric chromosomes).

The individual who develops from a gamete carrying an inversion or a reciprocal translocation usually shows no abnormality but is likely to produce abnormal offspring because of the unbalanced gametes (with an excess or deficiency of genetic material, or both) that may be produced by such persons during meiosis.

DIAGNOSIS OF CHROMOSOMAL ABERRATIONS

Clinically, the chromosomes are most conveniently studied in circulating lymphocytes stimulated to mitosis with phytohemagglutinin. This mitogen is added to a small sample of blood in short-term culture. Colchicine is also added to arrest cell division and to cause an accumulation of cells in metaphase, a stage of mitosis optional for study of the chromosomes. Treatment with hypotonic saline produces swelling of the nuclei and spreading of the chromosomes, so that they are more easily examined separate from one another. Special treatment of various types have been developed, relating for example to pH, as well as special stains, to produce a banding pattern of the chromosomes. Each of the human 24 chromosomes (22 autosomes plus X and Y) has a unique and distinctive banding pattern (Fig. 40–1). After short-term culture and treatment along the lines just indicated, the cells are smeared and examined by light microscopy at high magnification. (Electron microscopy has thus far not yielded clinically useful information.)

The metaphase chromosomes of a single lymphocyte have the appearance shown in Figure 40–1A. The photographic image of each chromosome is cut out, and the chromosomes are arranged in pairs, are identified by their relative lengths, ratio of arms and specific banding patterns, and laid out in a so-called karyotype, as shown in Figure 40–1B. (The schematic representation is called an ideogram.) Each of the metaphase chromosomes is double, i.e., consists of two chromatids united at the centromere. Each chromosome has replicated in preparation for cell division, and each chromatid of a particular chromosome is destined to be that chromosome in one of the two daughter cells.

An older, and now largely screening, diagnostic technique is the test for X chromatin (sex chromatin, or Barr bodies, for Murray Barr, its discoverer). Interphase cells of females show a rounded chromatin mass subjacent to the nuclear membrane (Fig. 40–6). This mass corresponds to the single inactive X chromosome referred to earlier in connection with dosage compensation and the Lyon hypothesis. It is absent in the XY male and in the female with the XO Turner syndrome. In persons with three, four, or five X chromosomes, two, three, or four Barr bodies are present, respectively. X chromatin is easily tested for in buccal mucosal cells obtained by scraping the lining of the cheek with a tongue depressor. The scrapings are smeared on a microscope slide, fixed and stained with an agent such as Feulgen's stain or cresyl violet. In the normal female, 30 to 50 percent of cell nuclei will

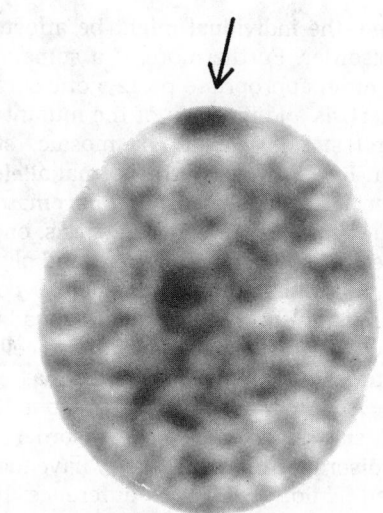

FIGURE 40–6. X chromatin (Barr body) in the nucleus of a buccal mucosal cell of a female.

show an X-chromatin mass. A routine of taking separate scrapings from each cheek is advisable in order to detect mosaicism, e.g., XX/XO karyotype.

If the buccal smear is stained with a fluorochrome and the specimen examined with a fluorescence microscope, most males (but no normal females) are found to have, in a high proportion of cells, a small fluorescent mass called the Y chromatin. This corresponds to a brightly fluorescent segment of the long arm of the Y chromosome. A few males, who are in all discernible ways normal, lack the fluorescent

---

TABLE 40–1

Phenotypes to Which Chromosomal Changes Have Been Causally Related[2,10]

1. Sex abnormalities, e.g., XO Turner syndrome, XXY Klinefelter syndrome

2. Mental retardation, e.g., trisomy-21 in Down syndrome, deleted short arm of chromosome 5 in cri-du-chat syndrome

3. Complex malformation syndrome, e.g., D_1 trisomy (trisomy-13, or Patau syndrome)

4. Behavioral abnormalities, e.g., the XYY male

5. Abortion—in one-fifth to one-third of spontaneous abortions in the first trimester, major chromosomal abnormality are demonstrable in the conceptus

6. Neoplasia, e.g., Philadelphia chromosome in chronic myeloid leukemia[20]

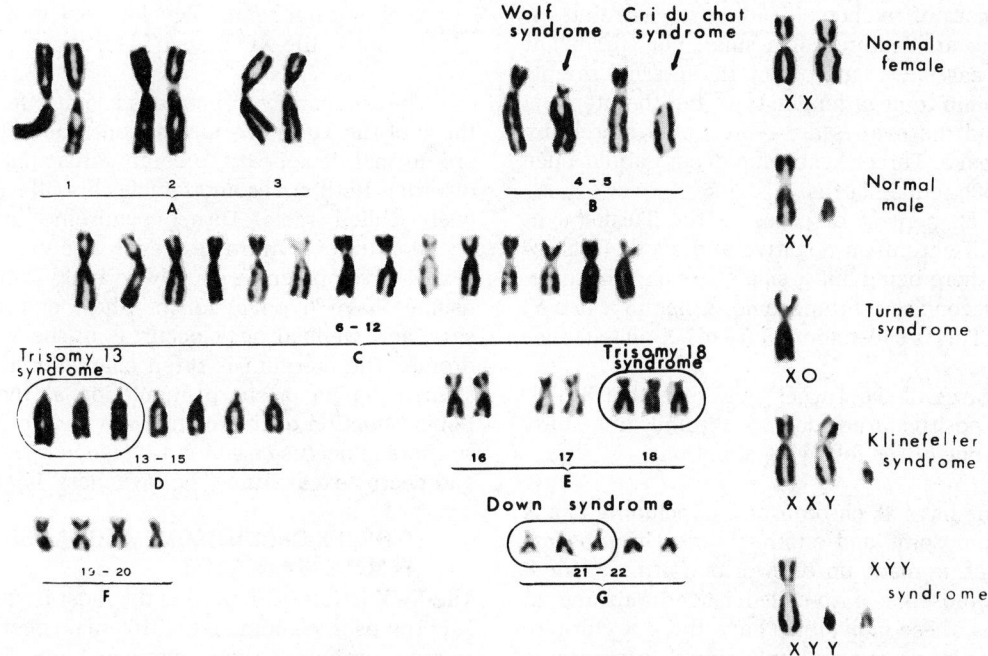

FIGURE 40-7. Composite karyotype showing selected major chromosomal aberrations. Prepared and stained by standard "prebanding" techniques.

segment of the Y chromosome and therefore are "Y-chromatin negative."

Abnormalities of the chromosomes have been related causally to disorders in six categories (Table 40-1). In addition, increased chromosomal breakage is an integral feature of some mendelian syndromes, such as Fanconi anemia. Figure 40-7 is a composite of the karyotypic findings in some leading chromosomal abnormalities.

SEX ANOMALIES RESULTING FROM ABERRATION OF THE SEX CHROMOSOMES

Primary amenorrhea and male infertility are leading presenting complaints in adults with anomalies of the sex chromosomes. In the female with primary amenorrhea, clinical features may indicate either Turner syndrome or the testicular feminization syndrome; male infertility may indicate the Klinefelter syndrome.

Buccal smear for determination of the X chromatin is a first step in the laboratory confirmation of these diagnoses (Fig. 40-6). In a majority of instances, females with Turner syndrome are X-chromatin negative, like the normal male, and males with Klinefelter syndrome are X-chromatin positive, like the normal female. Apparent females with the testicular feminization syndrome are in fact males and are X-chromatin negative. In case of uncertainty, such as those Turner syndrome patients who are chromatin positive, more direct studies of the chromosomes are indicated. In conventional cases of these three syndromes—Turner syndrome, Klinefelter syndrome, and testicular feminization—the sex-chromosome findings are, respectively, XO, XXY, and normal XY. These are described in more detail below, and some of the more complicated related conditions are discussed.

TURNER SYNDROME

Short stature, primary amenorrhea, and lack of development of secondary sex characteristics are the cardinal features of the Turner syndrome.[2] Other less consistent features are webbed neck, lowset ears, low posterior hairline, numerous pigmented nevi, broad, shield-like chest with widely spaced nipples, and brachydactyly with particular shortening of some metacarpals, especially the fourth. Coarctation of the aorta, hypertension (without coarctation and probably secondary to vascular anomaly of the kidney), and angiomata of the bowel leading to gastrointestinal bleeding are features of a small but significant number of cases. On laparotomy the internal sex organs are found to be of female type, but the uterus is infantile and the ovaries are represented merely by fibrous streaks. Turner syndrome occurs about once in every 2500 female births.

About 80 percent of cases of the Turner syndrome are X-chromatin negative and show 45 chromosomes, there being but a single sex chromosome, an X. The second sex chromosome, either an X or a Y, is missing. This is called the XO (read "X-oh") Turner syndrome.

Most cases of the Turner syndrome that are X-chromatin positive are found by chromosome study to fall into one of the following situations:

1. Some have 46 chromosomes, including one X chromosome and another large chromosome which is made up of two long arms of an X chromosome, a so-called isochromosome X. Thus, these individuals have three X-chromosome long arms and only one X-chromosome short arm. The deficiency of the short arm of the X chromosome is critical to the short stature that is part of the Turner syndrome. The Barr body and the "drumstick" of the polymorphonuclear leukocytes (which is the equivalent of the Barr body) is unusually large in these isochromosome-X cases; other evidence indicates that the Barr body in each cell of these cases is formed by the anomalous large chromosome, the isochromosome.
2. Some chromatin-positive Turner-syndrome cases are a mosaic of XO cells and other cells such as normal XX. This situation arises as a result of an accident of mitosis in the early division of the fertilized egg.
3. Other chromatin-positive Turner-syndrome cases have part of the long arm of one of the two X chromosomes deleted. In these cases the Barr body is abnormally small. Although these patients have primary amenorrhea and gonadal aplasia, as in other cases of Turner syndrome, they usually do not have short stature. Although loss of the short arm is, as was mentioned above, critical to development of short stature in Turner syndrome, factors concerned with normal sex development seem to be more generally distributed on the X chromosome. Since the germ cells do not participate in lyonization (both Xs are active in the primordial germ cells of the female), two in-

tact X chromosomes are seemingly essential to normal sexual development in man. In the mouse the XO female is fertile.

The Noonan syndrome has somatic features like those of the Turner syndrome, but the chromosomes are normal. It appears to be an autosomal dominant disorder. Both males and females are affected (previously called male Turner syndrome and female pseudo-Turner syndrome, respectively). In females sexual development is usually normal, whereas males usually have hypogonadism. Short stature, lowset ears, and webbed neck occur as in the Turner syndrome. The sternum is often characteristically misshapen, having a sharp angulation at the angle of Louis (junction of the manubrium and corpus sterni) so there is pectus carinatum ("pigeon breast") above and pectus excavatum ("hollow chest") below.

OTHER X-CHROMOSOME ANOMALIES WITH FEMALE PHENOTYPE

The XXX (triple-X) female is the most frequent of the X-chromosome anomalies with female phenotype, occurring probably about once in each 800 female births. The triple-X state is, however, less well known than many of the other X-chromosome anomalies, mainly because no characteristic disorder is produced. Although triple-X females often are mentally retarded and have a schizophrenia-like condition, somatic abnormalities do not occur consistently. Menstruation may be normal. One would expect that half the ova of such women would carry two X chromosomes rather than one and that on fertilization an XXY or another XXX individual would be formed. This is a rarity, however; most offspring have been karyotypically normal.

Quadruple-X and even penta-X cases have been identified, but these are rare.

MALE INFERTILITY AND KLINEFELTER SYNDROME

Small testes and infertility are consistent features of the Klinefelter syndrome. Gynecomastia is present in many, and the habitus is sometimes eunuchoidal, i.e., the legs are disproportionately long and the fat distribution is feminine in type, with concentration about the hips. The beard and body hair are sparse, and normal male recession of the hairline does not occur. In older cases the face tends to be unusually wrinkled. Intelligence is on the average reduced, but mental retardation is rarely severe, and some affected persons are quite intelligent. Congenital malformations are not associated with Klinefelter syndrome. About 1 in every 500 newborn males has this syndrome.

Typically, the Klinefelter patient is positive for both X and Y chromatin. High levels of pituitary gonadotropin (FSH) characterize the urinary hormone excretion. The histologic changes in the testes in postpubertal cases (ghost-like sclerosed tubules and Leydig-cell hyperplasia) are also characteristic. In the prepubertal cases these changes are not present, and the main finding is absence of germ cells. The postpubertal changes are caused by the high concentration of circulating pituitary gonadotropins.

Other sex-chromosome anomalies with male phenotype include the XXXY (triple X–Y) syndrome and the XXXXY (quadruple X–Y) syndrome. In general, the features in the genitalia, habitus, and breasts are the same as in the XXY Klinefelter syndrome. A difference is the occurrence of severe mental retardation and some congenital malformations, such as radioulnar synostosis, in the XXXY and XXXXY states.

Missegregation of the Y chromosome in the second stage of meiosis can lead to sperm carrying two Ys and an individual who is karyotypically XYY. On the average, XYY males are taller and more liable to antisocial behavior than are their XY brothers.

The study of sex chromosome anomalies has taught us much about normal sex determination. With rare exception (and these instances are themselves instructive) testes develop if a Y chromosome is present and testes do not develop if the Y chromosome is absent. To be sure, the testis may not be normally functional (e.g., in the XXY Klinefelter syndrome). Furthermore, only part of the Y chromosome near to the centromere is critical to differentiation of the indifferent embryonic gonad into a testis. Testis-determining factor (TDF) deduced from the studies of sex chromosome anomalies is probably identical with the H–Y antigen, a histocompatibility antigen coded by a Y-borne gene. Here is a clear indication of the significant role of cell-surface antigens in differentiation.[36]

MALFORMATION SYNDROMES DUE TO CHROMOSOMAL ABERRATIONS

The malformations in which microscopically identifiable chromosomal abnormality can be convincingly demonstrated are without exception complex anomalies (malformation syndromes). A prototype is the Down syndrome (mongolism). Excessive chromosome 21 material is a consistent karyotypic finding. In addition to mental retardation, leading features include round small head, typical facies (epicanthus, Brushfield spots of the iris, large furrowed tongue,

cheilosis), short stature, transverse palmar crease, brachydactyly with incurved fifth finger, alopecia areata, cardiac malformation (AV canal defect), and progressive cataract. Acute leukemia occurs in increased frequency in the Down syndrome.

Most cases of Down syndrome show three separate chromosomes 21 rather than the normal two. Meiotic nondisjunction with incorporation of both chromosomes 21 into the gamete is responsible. This accident occurs more often in older mothers. The overall frequency of the Down syndrome is about 1 in 800 live births, but the frequency becomes as high as 1 in 80 in the offspring of mothers over 40.

Some cases of the Down syndrome are found to be mosaic: Some cells are trisomy-21, whereas others are of normal karyotype. Mosaic Down syndrome originates in an accident in an early cleavage stage. It may occur at a sufficiently late stage that only a small proportion of all cells are trisomic, and the individual shows few or no stigmata. However, if the gonad participates in the trisomy, such a person can give birth to trisomic offspring. (It is biologically possible for a female with Down syndrome to be the mother of a Nobel laureate! Females with nonmosaic trisomy-21 apparently conceive trisomy-21 and normal offspring in equal proportions. Because of fetal loss of trisomy-21, karyotypically normal offspring predominate among the children of Down syndrome females.)

Other cases of Down syndrome are of one of the so-called translocation types. In many of these, a chromosomal rearrangement occurred in an earlier generation and multiple cases of mongolism occur in the family. A frequent type of translocation involves a union between a chromosome 21 and a chromosome of the 13–15 group. Carriers of a 14/21 translocation chromosome have a total of 45 separate chromosomes, but are phenotypically normal because they neither lack a significant amount of chromosomal material nor carry an excess. In such individuals, however, accidents in meiosis are likely to occur. A "balanced gamete" is formed if the translocation chromosome goes into it without any other chromosome 14 or 21. But if both the translocation chromosome and the independent chromosome 21 get into the same gamete, a state trisomic for chromosome 21 is created in the zygote (after fertilization of the anomalous gamete by a normal 21-bearing gamete). The proportions of various types of offspring—normal, balanced carriers, and Down syndrome—are not as precise as are the genetic ratios observed with "mendelizing" traits. In part, this is because many of the trisomic embryos die in utero. The proportion of children of 14/21 translocation carrier women who have Down syndrome is about 11 percent. Among the children of carrier males about 5 percent have Down syndrome.

When a parent is a translocation carrier, parental age is not a factor in the occurrence of mongolism. Translocation mongols constitute, however, less than 5 percent of all cases. Even at young maternal age, an isolated (i.e., nonfamilial) case of Down syndrome is more likely to be of conventional trisomy-21 type. For more precise prognostication, the chromosomes should be studied in any instance of more than one case of Down in a family. Even in families with two or more cases of Down, conventional trisomy-21 is frequently found. Some maintain that the karyotype should be determined in all cases of Down syndrome or suspected Down syndrome.

Two other main types of chromosomal aberrations that have been related to specific malformation syndromes are trisomy-13 and trisomy-18 (otherwise known as D_1 or Patau syndrome and E_1 or Edwards syndrome, respectively). Since chromosomes 13 and 18 are larger than chromosome 21 and, presumably, carry more genetic information, the features are more drastic in these disorders. Unlike mongolism, no instance of survival to adulthood is known.

Deletion of part of the short arm of one chromosome 5 produces a characteristic disorder called the cri-du-chat (cat cry) syndrome because of the characteristic sound made by affected infants. Patients with this disorder are rather common, especially since they survive to adulthood with microcephaly and severe mental retardation.

NEOPLASIA DUE TO CHROMOSOMAL ABERRATIONS

Since Boveri early in this century, genetic change in a clone of cells has been considered as the basis for malignancy—the "cause" of cancer. Some firmly established examples are now known in man. In cases of chronic myeloid leukemia a distal part of the long arm of one chromosome 22 is translocated to another chromosome, most often to the end of the long arm of a chromosome 9.[35] The abnormal (partially deleted) chromosome is called the Philadelphia chromosome, having been discovered by Nowell and Hungerford of that city.[20] Only blood cells show the abnormality. The chromosomal change is acquired, not congenital. Exposure to ionizing radiation is responsible in some cases for the chromosomal breakage that led to the oncogenic chromosomal rearrangement. Viral damage to the chromosomes is suspected in others.

The Philadelphia chromosome can be of diagnostic value in patients who present atypically, e.g., with the clinical picture of myelofibrosis. It also has prognostic significance. It is found in about 85 percent of chronic myelocytic leukemia (CML) cases, and cases lacking it (which can be considered a fundamentally different entity) tend to show a less chronic course and respond less favorably to therapy.

When the Philadelphia chromosome is being tested for in samples of peripheral blood, phytohemagglutinin is omitted from the preparative procedure. In CML the circulating myeloid leukocytes usually include enough mitotic cells for study; PHA stimulates the unaffected lymphocytes.

WHAT CASES SHOULD HAVE CHROMOSOME STUDIES?

A chromosome analysis is time-consuming and therefore expensive. Consequently, there must be careful selection of the cases to be studied. In X-chromosome abnormalities, buccal smear combined with informed clinical observation often suffices. For example, in a teenage boy with gynecomastia, Klinefelter syndrome can be excluded with confidence if the testes are of normal or near-normal size; normal male findings on buccal smear clinch the alternative diagnosis of adolescent gynecomastia.

Substantiation of the diagnosis of Down syndrome may be helpful in making arrangements for the care of the infant. Thus, in suspected but uncertain cases, chromosome studies are indicated. In young parents of a child with Down syndrome, chromosome analysis can improve the precision with which the risk of subsequent children's being affected is estimated. If one parent is a translocation carrier, the risk of another child's being affected is considerable.

In the differentiation of chronic myeloid leukemia from leukemoid states, such as myeloid metaplasia, finding the typical abnormal chromosome 22 is as specific as finding *Mycobacterium tuberculosis* in the sputum of a patient with a pulmonary lesion.

Cases of congenital malformations in which chromosome abnormalities might be sought are so numerous that decisions must be made as to what types of cases are likely to "pay off." Complex, multiple-system malformations are the ones in which discernible chromosomal abnormalities are most likely to be found. Malformations with mendelian patterns of inheritance, such as the Ellis-van Creveld syndrome,[26] an autosomal recessive (see Table 41–7), are not likely to show chromosomal abnormalities.

In Fanconi anemia, Bloom syndrome, and ataxia-telangiectasia (all autosomal recessive disorders) increased chromosomal breakage and other abnormali-

ties are found. The proclivity to leukemia and other malignancies shown by each of these conditions may be related to this chromosomal breakage. Study of the chromosomes can provide information corroborating the diagnosis.

CHAPTER 41
Mendelian Disorders
VICTOR A. McKUSICK

Principles of diagnosis, prognosis (genetic counseling), treatment, and prevention will be presented in this chapter. Thereafter, these principles will be illustrated with a discussion of seven special categories of mendelian disease: hemoglobinopathies; inborn errors of metabolism, including vitamin-responsive forms; lysosomal diseases; receptor disorders; defects in transmembrane transport; heritable disorders of connective tissue; and mendelian malformations. Pharmacogenetics and immunogenetics will also be discussed.

There is a large number of mendelian disorders, so that even though many of them are individually rare, in the aggregate they represent a significant aspect of clinical practice. Table 41–8 gives the numbers of firmly and provisionally identified mendelian traits, most of them "diseases," "disorders," or "defects," that have been identified in successive editions of *Mendelian Inheritance in Man.*[3] The steadily increasing numbers indicate advances in genetic nosology (classification of genetic disease). The numbers become less formidable when the information concerning all the individual conditions is systematized on the basis of advances in fundamental knowledge in the last few decades.

DIAGNOSIS

Basic to both diagnosis and prognosis is the genetic family history as incorporated in the pedigree. The mode of inheritance is an element in correct diagnosis. Three further principles of fundamental importance to the accurate diagnosis of mendelian disorders are genetic heterogeneity, pleiotropism, and variability.

THE FAMILY HISTORY
The family history carefully taken is a major tool of clinical genetics. In eliciting and recording a patient's complete history there is much to recommend obtaining the family history last. The description of the presenting problem and the past history concerning health and illness are valuable guides to the nature of the questions to be asked in taking the family history. For example, the questions to be asked of a 35-year-old man with chest pain compatible with angina pectoris are different from those to be asked of a 35-year-old man with failing vision and skin changes about the neck compatible with pseudoxanthoma elasticum.[29]

The past history and the methodical review of systems may raise suspicions of multiple-system involvement or may give evidence of long-standing minor stigmata of the disorder that brings the patient to the doctor. Thus, further background for the family history is provided. Frequently, the complaint that brings the patient to medical attention is relatively trivial. This is especially true in genetic disorders, for the patient may have become accustomed to his condition through its presence from an early age or because of its slow development. Its grave potentialities may not be known to the patient unless there are other similar cases in the family.

In obtaining the family history, there are at least four general questions to be asked:

1. Has anyone in your family had a condition similar to yours?
2. Is there any condition which seems to "run in your family?"
3. Are your parents related by blood?
4. What was the ethnic origin of your parents?

The question about consanguinity is particularly important in the case of rare recessively inherited disorders. Since it is generally held that consanguinity is "bad" and since specific regulations with regard to the marriage of relatives are laid down by some religions and by some states, patients may be embarrassed by the question, but usually the physician thinks the question will be more embarrassing than it actually proves to be.

The rarer the recessive disorder, the more frequently the parents of affected persons are found to be consanguineous. Tay-Sachs disease (infantile amaurotic idiocy) is relatively frequent in the Jews of the New York area, and the frequency of first-cousin marriages among parents of cases is relatively low, although higher than in the general population. In non-Jews the disorder is much less frequent, but a much higher proportion of the parents are first cousins or related in some other manner. In families with cystic fibrosis of the pancreas (Chap. 34), a relatively frequent disorder, little increased parental consanguinity is expected, and little or none is found. When both parents are foreign born, even if the patient does not know them to be related, the presumption of consanguinity is strong if they came from the same village. The same is true if the parents came from the same rural area of the United States, where the forebears had lived for several generations.

Ethnic background is frequently of value in the appraisal of diagnostic possibilities. Anemia in a person of Mediterranean stock brings to mind possibilities different from those suggested by anemia in one of Swedish origin. Some rare recessive diseases are much more frequent in certain ethnic groups, for example, thalassemia[37] and glucose-6-phosphate dehydrogenase (G6PD) deficiency in persons of Mediterranean origin; familial Mediterranean fever in Armenians and Sephardic Jews; acatalasia in Japanese; and so on. Other diseases are notably rare in certain groups—e.g., cystic fibrosis in blacks and phenylketonuria in Jews.

After the general questions of the family history a systematic inquiry should be made into the status, living or dead, and the state of health of all immediate relatives, particularly first-degree relatives (parents, sibs, and offspring). Whether the inquiry is carried further depends on the nature of the ailment and the results of the earlier questioning. Usually each close relative should be asked about individually, beginning with the parents. In questioning about the sibs, it is best to ask about each pregnancy of the mother in order, so that stillbirths, miscarriages, and infant deaths are not overlooked. If the patient is married and has children, the health of the spouse and all pregnancies resulting from the marital union are reviewed.

Organization of the family history is facilitated by a sketch of the family tree. The individual in a family who brings that family to study—the patient in the usual clinical situation—is referred to in pedigree studies as the proband (or as the propositus or proposita). The proband is indicated in pedigree charts by an arrow. Males and females are most often represented by squares and circles, respectively. Consanguineous matings are indicated by a double marital line. If the mating is consanguineous, it is useful to complete the pedigree sufficiently to indicate how the parents are related. Individuals affected with a given disorder can be indicated by blacked-in symbols. If several characteristics are present in the family, various special methods can be used for indicating which are present in any given individual. There are conventions for indicating twins, monozygotic and dizygotic, and for abortions. Each individual in the pedigree is indicated by a number. The generations are numbered with Roman numerals, and the persons in each generation are numbered consecutively with Arabic numerals. Thus, III-6 refers to the sixth person in the third generation of the family. These conventions are illustrated in the discussion of pedigree patterns (Figs. 41–1 to 41–6).

PEDIGREE PATTERNS OF MENDELIAN INHERITANCE

Based on the mechanics of the chromosomes in meiosis, genes are distributed in families in predictable patterns. Depending on whether the gene is located on an autosome or on an X chromosome and depending on whether the gene in single dose (heterozygous state) or only in double dose (homozygous state) results in the given phenotype, characteristic familial patterns of inheritance are demonstrated by simply inherited disorders.

When a gene in single dose causes a given effect, the phenotype is said to be dominant. When the effect is observed only in the homozygote (i.e., with the mutant gene in double dose), the phenotype is said to be recessive. In general, disorders resulting from defects in enzyme systems—e.g., all the inborn errors of metabolism—behave as recessives. Because of the margin of safety provided in most enzyme systems, phenotypic abnormality is evident only when all of a given enzyme is mutant (and deficient). On the other hand, disorders resulting from a change in a structural or other nonenzymic protein are usually dominant. Consequences of the alteration in the physical and chemical properties of the particular protein are observable in the heterozygote even though only a portion of that protein is of the mutant type. Several

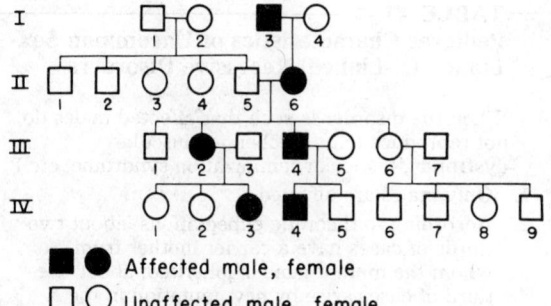

FIGURE 41-1. Autosomal dominant pedigree pattern (idealized).

of the heritable disorders of connective tissue are dominant. For example, the loose-jointedness and the cutaneous fragility, bruisability, and stretchability of the classic Ehlers-Danlos syndrome, which is inherited as a dominant, are thought to result from alteration in collagen. The differences in the nature of the defect in the dominant and recessive forms of methemoglobinemia illustrate this principle (p. 455).

Dominance and recessiveness are attributes of the phenotype, not of the gene. In population genet-

---

TABLE 41-1
Pedigree Characteristics of Uncommon Autosomal Dominant Disorders

1. Each affected individual has an affected parent, unless the condition arose by fresh mutation in the given individual (Because of wide variability in severity of dominant traits, the parent may be too mildly affected to be recognized as a case)

2. An affected individual and a normal mate will have, on the average, affected and normal children in equal proportions

3. Normal children of an affected person will have all normal offspring

4. Males and females are affected in equal proportions

5. Affected males and females are equally likely to transmit the condition to male and female offspring. Specifically, male-to-male transmission occurs

6. Homozygotes may be born if two affected persons (heterozygotes) marry. Homozygotes are usually more severely affected than heterozygotes

7. On the average, the age of fathers of sporadic (new mutation) cases is elevated

8. The more severely the disorder interferes with reproduction, the larger is the proportion of cases that are sporadic ("new mutations")

TABLE 41-2
Pedigree Characteristics of Uncommon Autosomal Recessive Disorders

1. The parents are usually clinically normal

2. The larger the family, the more often will more than one child be affected

3. The rarer the mutant gene in the population, the more often will the parents be related

4. In marriages between individuals, each with the same recessive disease, all their offspring will be affected

5. Affected individuals who marry normal individuals have only normal offspring (unless the normal spouse is a carrier)

6. The sexes are affected in equal proportions

7. If an affected individual marries a heterozygote, as is more likely to occur with consanguineous marriage, half the children would be affected, and a pedigree pattern simulating dominant inheritance would result

---

ics, for convenience, geneticists speak of dominant genes and recessive genes, but in clinical genetics confusion is avoided if the adjectives are used only in connection with specifically defined traits.

The pedigree patterns of *rare* simply inherited traits are characteristic for autosomal dominant, autosomal recessive, X-linked recessive, and X-linked dominant inheritance.

The characteristics of the pedigree of *rare autosomal dominant disorders* are outlined in Table 41-1.

The characteristics of the pedigree of *rare autosomal recessive disorders* are outlined in Table 41-2. In contrast to dominant diseases, which are transmitted to the offspring from one parent, each parent, although usually phenotypically normal, contributes a mutant gene to the affected offspring. *Recessive inheritance is inheritance from both parents.* On the average, of the children of two heterozygous parents, one-fourth (homozygotes) will be affected, one-half (heterozygotes) will carry a single mutant gene, and the remaining fourth will be normal (Fig. 41-2).

X-Linked Inheritance

Diseases or traits that result from genes located on the X chromosome are said to be *sex-linked,* or, more precisely *X-linked.* If the condition is dominant, i.e., is manifest when the gene is present in heterozygous state in the female, either sex may be affected. If the condition is recessive and rare, females will seldom be affected, since homozygosity, or a double dose of the gene, is required. In males with only one X chro-

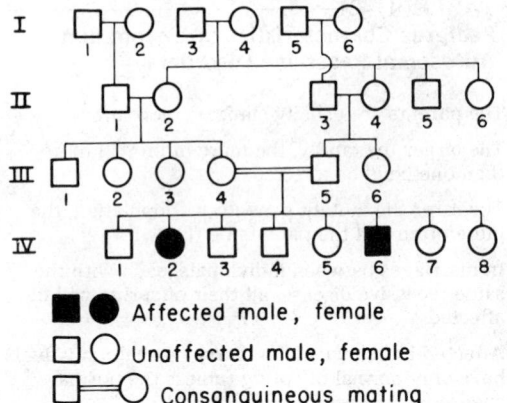

■● Affected male, female

□○ Unaffected male, female

□—○ Consanguineous mating

FIGURE 41-2. Autosomal recessive pedigree pattern. Idealized pattern. The parents are first cousins.

mosome an X-linked gene is always expressed, regardless of whether the condition is dominant or recessive in the female. Since the male cannot inherit his X chromosome from his father, male-to-male (father-to-son) inheritance rules out sex-linked inheritance. The characteristic features of *sex-linked recessive inheritance* are outlined in Table 41–3. (See Fig. 41–3.)

Some X-linked traits behave as dominants, i.e., are expressed in the heterozygous female. The features are outlined in Table 41–4. Hereditary hypophosphatemia ("vitamin-D-resistant rickets") is a good example (Figs. 41–4 and 41–5).

When an X-linked disorder is dominant but is lethal to the hemizygous affected male, a characteristic pedigree pattern, schematized in Figure 41–6 and described in Table 41–5, results. Examples are one form of incontinentia pigmenti, focal dermal hypoplasia, and orofaciodigital syndrome (OFD syndrome). The first two have, in association with congenital malformations, skin lesions whose spotty distribution may be a manifestation of the Lyon principle (Fig. 40–5). The only male cases of the OFD syndrome have been found either to have a closely simulating autosomal recessive disorder (OFD II) or to be instances of the XXY Klinefelter syndrome and are thus not true exceptions to this mode of inheritance.

In Table 41–6, disorders with dominant inheritance and those with recessive inheritance are contrasted with respect to three features. Dominant disorders tend to be more variable and also less severe than recessive ones. Because a dominant disorder may be so mild in a given individual, "skipped generations" may be observed in pedigrees. Reduced penetrance is mainly a feature of dominant traits. Re-

---

TABLE 41-3

Pedigree Characteristics of Uncommon Sex-Linked (X-Linked) Recessive Disorders

A.   When the disorder is such that affected males do not reproduce (e.g., Duchenne muscular dystrophy, testicular feminization syndrome, etc.)

1.   Only males are affected

2.   According to theoretic expectations, about two-thirds of cases have a carrier mother from whom the mutant gene is inherited; about one-third of cases arise by new mutation in the X chromosome from the mother

3.   In the inherited form, affected males may have affected brothers and affected maternal uncles. The new mutation cases are sporadic, i.e., isolated cases

4.   The sisters of inherited cases have a 50 percent chance of being carriers for the gene

5.   A carrier sister transmits the gene to half her sons, who are affected, and to half her daughters, who are carriers

6.   Unaffected males do not transmit the disorder

B.   When the disorder is such that affected males may reproduce (e.g., hemophilias A and B, G6PD deficiency, etc.)

1.   The proportion of cases that are inherited rises further above two-thirds, the less is the reduction of average number of children produced by affected males

2.   Affected males transmit the gene to *all* their daughters and to *none* of their sons

3.   All phenotypically normal daughters of affected males are carriers

4.   If married to a carrier female, affected males will have daughters, half of whom are homozygous and affected, half of whom are normal but carriers

5.   Rare heterozygous females may be affected ("manifesting heterozygotes"), because of chances of lyonization

---

duced penetrance means that the expressivity (severity) of the trait is below the level of recognition.

All simply inherited genetic disorders arose by gene mutation at some time in the past. A given case may be the result of a new dominant mutation occurring in the germ cells of one or the other of the parents. Such cases will be sporadic, and there will not be the characteristic pedigree pattern shown in Figure 41–1. If, on the average, patients with a given dominant disorder have only half as many children as do unaffected persons in the general population and one assumes genetic equilibrium, then half the probands in any large series will be new mutations. It can be shown that with an X-linked recessive condition like Duchenne muscular dystrophy, in which no

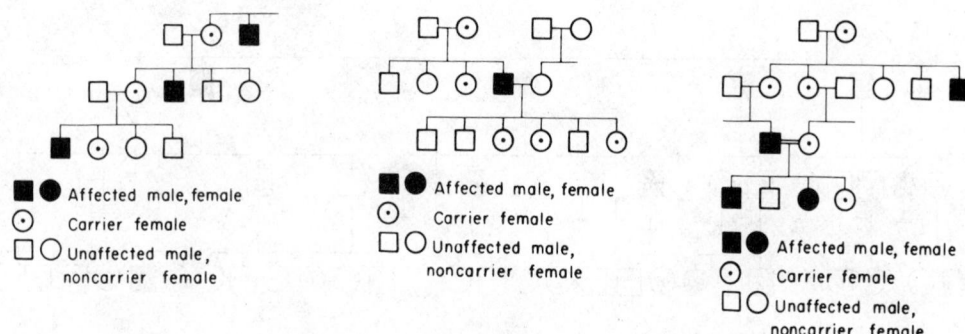

FIGURE 41–3. X-linked recessive pedigree pattern. **Left:** Oblique pattern of affected males and carrier females. **Center:** All daughters of an affected male are carriers; all sons are unaffected. **Right:** A daughter of an affected male married to a carrier female may be homozygous and affected. The fact that a son is affected is not an exception to the rule of no male-to-male transmission, since the mutant X chromosome came to the affected son from the carrier mother.

affected males reproduce, one-third of cases arise by new mutation in the X chromosome carried by the mother's ovum, and in two-thirds of cases the disorder is inherited from a carrier mother, the mutation having occurred in an earlier generation. At least such is the theoretic expectation. In fact, the mutation rate for X-linked traits may be higher in males than in females, so that fewer than one-third are new mutations.

GENETIC HETEROGENEITY[27]

It is axiomatic that the phenotype ("clinical picture") is not a necessary indication of the genotype (the genetic constitution) of the patient. This is the same as saying that any one of two or more different mutations can result in one and the same disorder. "Look-alikes" should be distinguished because the mode of inheritance may be quite different, indicating differ-

ent genetic counseling, and the clinical prognosis and appropriate management may differ. Indeed, the "look-alike" may not be mendelian, but rather environmentally produced—a so-called phenocopy.[38] (Genetic "look-alikes" are called genocopies, or genetic mimics.) A major theme of clinical genetics in the last two decades has been identification of genetic heterogeneity in conditions previously thought to be single entities. Examples are the Ehlers-Danlos syndromes, the mucopolysaccharidoses, the nonspherocytic hemolytic anemias, and the several forms of intestinal polyposis and multiple endocrine adenomatosis. As reflected by the numbers given in Table 41–7, a rapid increase in the number of known mendelian disorders

---

TABLE 41–4

Pedigree Characteristics of Uncommon X-Linked Dominant Disorders

1. Both males and females are affected, but females tend to be affected about twice as often as males

2. An affected female transmits the disorder to half her sons and half her daughters, on the average

3. An affected male transmits the disorder to *all* his daughters and to *none* of his sons

4. On the average, the heterozygous affected female tends to be less severely affected than the hemizygous male, and the disorder is more variable in heterozygous females

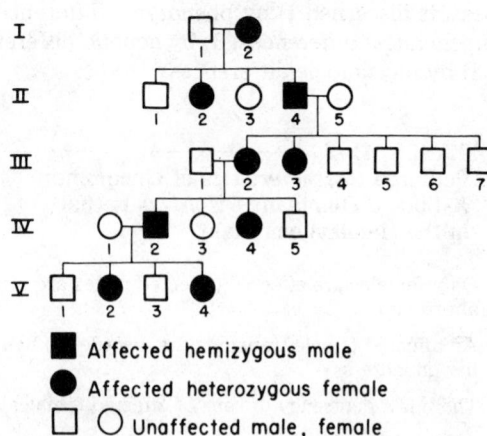

FIGURE 41–4. X-linked dominant pedigree pattern. Idealized pattern.

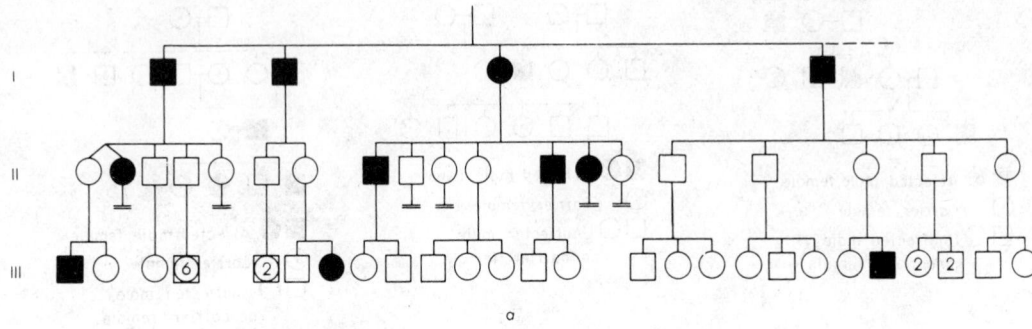

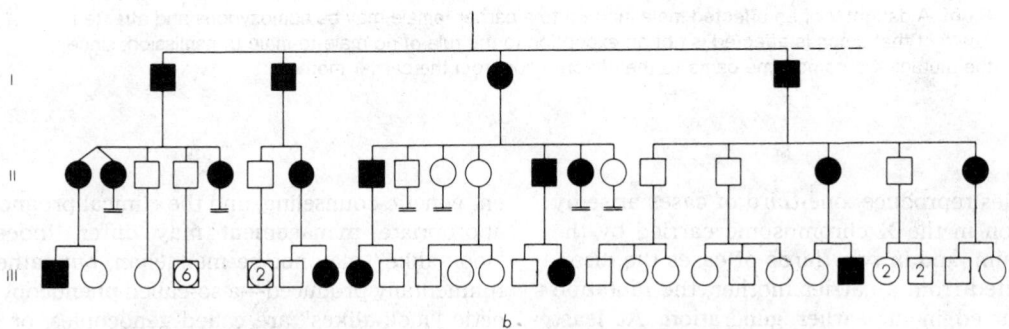

FIGURE 41–5. Hypophosphatemic (vitamin D resistant) rickets. In the pedigree in top section, skeletal signs of rickets were used as the phenotype. Some affected females were missed by this method of study. In bottom section, low serum phosphorus level was the phenotype studied. With this the pedigree pattern is completely consistent with X-linked dominant inheritance.

has occurred in the last two decades. This has resulted, not so much from identification of new phenotypes, as from discovery that one phenotype encompasses several separate genetic disorders.

Genetic heterogeneity, the existence of separate entities, is discerned 1) by phenotypic differences, 2) by biochemical differences, 3) by genetic differences, and 4) by physiologic differences.

TABLE 41–5
Pedigree Characteristics of Uncommon X-Linked Dominant Disorders Lethal in the Hemizygous Male

1. Only females are affected (affected males are lost as abortions)

2. An affected female transmits the disorder to half her daughters

3. There is a deficiency of sons of affected females

4. Affected females show an increased frequency of spontaneous abortion, these being hemizygous affected males

---

Phenotypic Differences

The presence or absence of corneal clouding is one clinical feature distinguishing two forms of mucopolysaccharidosis,[30] the autosomal recessive type de-

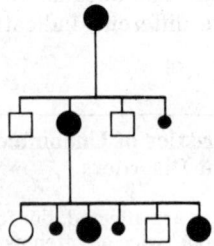

● ○ Affected and Unaffected Female

☐ Unaffected Male

• Abortion

FIGURE 41–6. Pedigree pattern of X-linked dominant lethal in hemizygous affected male.

—TABLE 41-6—
Contrasting Features of Dominant and Recessive Disorders

	Autosomal Dominant	**Autosomal Recessive**
Nature of disorder	Structural anomalies or changes in non-enzymic proteins	Enzyme defects, e.g., inborn errors of metabolism; hormone deficiencies, e.g., isolated growth hormone deficiency
Degree of variability	Large	Small
Clinical severity	Less severe	More severe

scribed by Hurler and the X-linked recessive form described by Hunter. The association of soft tissue and osseous tumors[28] distinguishes the colonic polyposis of Gardner syndrome from familial polyposis of the colon.

Biochemical Differences

The Marfan syndrome and homocystinuria, despite phenotypic overlap (subluxation of lenses and skeletal abnormalities), are distinguished by biochemical identification of homocystine in the urine. Often when a biochemical "handle" is identified phenotypic differences are then appreciated, permitting clinical differentiation. Such is, for example, now usually possible for the Marfan syndrome and homocystinuria.[29]

Genetic Differences

Differences in mode of inheritance can distinguish entities. Spastic paraplegia, retinitis pigmentosa, and Charcot-Marie-Tooth peroneal muscular atrophy are three disorders that are inherited as autosomal dominants in some families, as autosomal recessives in others, and as X-linked recessives in yet other rare instances. Usually in conditions with three different modes of inheritance, the autosomal recessive form is clinically most severe, the dominant form least severe, and the X-linked form intermediate in severity.

At least two distinct forms of elliptocytosis (ovalocytosis), both inherited as dominants, have been identified on the basis of linkage relationship, although no phenotypic differences are discernible. Linkage studies indicate that one form is determined by a gene at a locus which is close to the locus occupied by the Rh blood-group genes (now known to be chromosome No. 1), whereas a second form of elliptocytosis is determined by a gene at some locus far removed from the Rh locus.

In many instances, congenital deafness (deaf-mutism) can be shown to be inherited as a simple autosomal recessive. Assortative (i.e., nonrandom) mating is often practiced by deaf-mutes; deaf persons marry other deaf persons much more often than would occur on a random basis. All children of two deaf persons, each from a family with a recessive pattern of inheritance, are deaf if the two parents are homozygous at the same locus. Families fulfilling this expectation have been observed. In other families, however, two parents, both affected by phenotypically identical recessively inherited deafness, have children who are all normal. The explanation is that the deaf parents are homozygous at different loci and suffer from genetically distinct forms of deafness.

Somatic cell genetics provides an elegant way to identify genetic heterogeneity—fusion of cells from patients with what appear to be the same disorder (with deficiency of the same enzyme) may show complementation with restitution of normal enzyme function. The explanation may be that the enzyme in-

—TABLE 41-7—
Numbers of Loci as Identified Mainly by Mendelizing Phenotypes*

Phenotype	Verschuer 1958	McKusick's *Mendelian Inheritance in Man*[3]					October 1, 1978
		1966	1968	1971	1975	1978	
Autosomal dominant	285	269 (+568)	344 (+449)	415 (+528)	583 (+635)	736 (+753)	765 (+772)
Autosomal recessive	89	237 (+294)	280 (+349)	365 (+418)	466 (+481)	521 (+596)	533 (+620)
X-linked	38	68 (+51)	68 (+55)	86 (+64)	93 (+78)	107 (+98)	108 (+104)
Total	412	574 (+913)	692 (+853)	866 (+1010)	1142 (+1194)	1364 (+1447)	1406 (+1496)

* Numbers in parentheses refer to those not yet fully established.

TABLE 41-8

Some Hereditary Syndromes in Which External Manifestations Aid in the Diagnosis of Grave Internal Disorders*

Syndrome	External Manifestation(s) Which Is Important Clue	Internal Feature(s) of Importance	Mode of Inheritance	Basic Defect
von Hippel-Lindau syndrome	Retinal angioma(s)	Cerebellar hemangioblastoma Pheochromocytoma Hypernephroma Polycythemia	Autosomal dominant	Unknown (structural defect)
Wilson's disease (hepatolenticular degeneration)[16]	Kayser-Fleischer ring of cornea	Hepatic cirrhosis Basal ganglion degeneration	Autosomal recessive	Disorder of copper metabolism (low serum ceruloplasmin)
Pseudoxanthoma elasticum (Grönblad-Strandberg syndrome)[29]	Characteristic changes in skin of neck, axillas, and flexural areas	Gastrointestinal hemorrhage Occlusive peripheral and coronary arterial disease	Autosomal recessive	Degeneration of elastic fibers
Hereditary hemorrhagic telangiectasis (Rendu-Osler-Weber disease)	Cutaneous and mucosal telangiectases	Gastrointestinal hemorrhage Pulmonary arteriovenous fistulas Hepatic cirrhosis	Autosomal dominant	Structural anomaly of small arteries and veins
Marfan syndrome[29]	Ectopia lentis Long extremities	Aneurysm of aorta	Autosomal dominant	Connective tissue abnormality, perhaps of collagen
Holt-Oram syndrome (atriodigital dysplasia)[23]	Absent or anomalous thumbs	Atrial septal defect	Autosomal dominant	Unknown (structural defect)
von Recklinghausen neurofibromatosis	Café-au-lait spots and fibromas of skin	Pheochromocytoma Meningioma Acoustic neuroma Hypoglycemia (with intraperitoneal fibroma)	Autosomal dominant	Unknown (structural defect)
Gardner syndrome[28]	Osteomas of mandible and skull Sebaceous cysts	Premalignant polyps of colon and stomach	Autosomal dominant	Unknown (structural defect)
Peutz-Jeghers syndrome[28]	Melanin spots of the buccal mucosa, lips, and digits	Polyps of jejunum (and other portions of GI tract) producing intussusception and bleeding and rarely malignancy	Autosomal dominant	Unknown (structural defect)
Ellis-van Creveld syndrome[26]	Polydactyly and dwarfism	Single atrium	Autosomal recessive	Unknown (structural defect)
Albright hereditary osteodystrophy (pseudo and pseudo-pseudo-hypoparathyroidism)	Short metacarpals and metatarsals Round facies Subcutaneous calcification	Hypocalcemic tetany Mental retardation	Probably X-linked dominant	Unknown

* See McKusick's *Mendelian Inheritance in Man*[3] for references to specific entities.

┌─ **TABLE 41-8 (cont.)** ─────────────────────────────────────

Syndrome	External Manifestation(s) Which Is Important Clue	Internal Feature(s) of Importance	Mode of Inheritance	Basic Defect
Fabry's diffuse angiokeratoma	Characteristic angiokeratomatous lesions of skin	Episodic abdominal pain Renal failure	X-linked dominant (or intermediate, since heterozygous females are more mildly affected)	Deficiency of alpha-galactosidase (ceramide trihexosidase)
Nail-patella syndrome	Dysplastic nails, hypoplastic or absent patellas, limitation of pronation and supination of elbows	Renal failure	Autosomal dominant Linked to ABO blood group locus	Unknown (structural defect)

volved is made up of two different polypeptide chains and the cases involved have mutation in different chains. Or in one case it may be a regulator mutation, whereas the other has a structural mutation.

Physiologic Differences

This approach to identification of genetic heterogeneity is nicely demonstrated by the hemophilias. Before about 1950, all sex-linked hemophilia was assumed to be one disease, although the possibility of multiple allelism had been suggested to explain the occurrence of mild and severe forms. It was then discovered that the blood from some hemophilic subjects would correct the clotting defect in others. The explanation is that the location of the defect in the chain of clotting reactions is different, so that bloods from two hemophilic persons complement each other, each providing an essential clotting factor missing in the other. Thus, hemophilia A (classic hemophilia) and hemophilia B (Christmas disease) were distinguished. The protein clotting factors, antihemophilic globulin (Factor VIII) and PTC (Factor IX) are chemically distinct. Although both are determined by genes on the X chromosome, the genes are known to be on different parts of the chromosome; linkage studies indicate that the hemophilia A gene is fairly close to the color-blindness locus and the G6PD locus, whereas the Christmas disease gene is far removed from these loci. Thus, evidence from genetic linkage corroborates the conclusion from physiologic studies.

PLEIOTROPISM

Whereas genetic heterogeneity means that one (or almost the same) phenotype can result from any one of several genotypes, pleiotropism ("multiple effects") means that several phenotypic features can result from one gene. We have in clinical genetics many syndromes (meaning literally a "running together") based on the pleiotropism of individual genes; certain phenotypic features tend to occur together predictably. Sometimes there is an evident or at least plausible reason for the association. For example, in the Marfan syndrome, association of lens dislocation and weakness of the aortic media are explicable on the basis of a connective tissue defect, even though the precise nature of that defect is not yet known. In other cases, the reason for syndromal association is not clear. For example, why should jejunal polyps and melanin spots of the buccal mucosa, lips, and digits be associated in the Peutz-Jeghers syndrome?[28]

Syndromal association in mendelian disorders is always based on pleiotropism, not on genetic linkage.

Two genes at separate loci, even though closely situated on the same chromosome, become separated through the process of crossing-over (p. 430). The closer the genes are the longer the time (in generations) that is required for their separation. Genetic linkage does not cause a permanent association of genetic traits, does not account for mendelian syndromes. (Close linkage of loci with insufficient time for separation of specific alleles at these loci, so-called linkage disequilibrium, is probably responsible for certain HLA and disease associations [p. 467].)

The importance of pleiotropism to clinical genetics is in diagnosis. Some of the pleiotropic features are useful external clues to the presence of serious internal abnormalities. Table 41–8 lists many examples.

VARIABILITY

Not only are there many mendelian disorders, but also each may vary rather widely in affected persons, even members of the same family. This is particularly true of autosomal dominant disorders. This variability is due in part to differences in the environment, intrauterine and extrauterine, in which the individual develops and lives, and due in part to differences in the rest of the genetic make-up of the affected persons.

Variability, probably due mainly to difference in genetic background, is illustrated by two brothers with the Marfan syndrome. Both inherited the Marfan gene from their father but, whereas one had ectopia lentis, striking arachnodactyly, severe scoliosis, and marked mitral regurgitation, the second brother in his teens had no ocular or recognizable cardiac abnormality, and only rather unspecific skeletal changes which alone would not have sufficed for a firm diagnosis of the Marfan syndrome (for which there is not yet a laboratory test). That he, indeed, had the Marfan syndrome was unhappily proved by his subsequent development of dissecting aneurysm of the aorta. On the average, brothers share half their genes in common. Influence of differences in genetic background on the expression of mendelian syndromes is known in mice and other experimental animals. Usually one aspect of the syndrome, such as ectopia lentis in the example above, fails to be expressed.

Different mutations can occur in a given gene—allelic mutations—and although each may cause abnormality in a particular function controlled by that gene, the resulting abnormality may be quantitatively and even qualitatively different. Many examples are now known of allelic series as the basis of variation in genetic disease. Some enzymopathies occur in both vitamin-responsive and nonresponsive forms (see later discussion of homocystinuria), the former usually being clinically less severe. Deficiency of alpha-maltase may produce a severe form of glycogen storage disease (Pompe's disease) or a milder disorder manifest in adulthood as progressive myopathy. Cystinuria, Gaucher's disease, cystic fibrosis, glucose-6-phosphate dehydrogenase deficiency, and hemophilia are probably other examples of mendelian disorders with allelic variants.

In autosomal recessive diseases a patient may have a "double dose" of mutant genes at a given locus but they are different mutant alleles. This is called a genetic compound or compound heterozygote; "double heterozygote" is reserved for the situation of heterozygosity at two different loci. The genetic compound usually is accompanied by a phenotype intermediate in severity between that of the two homozygotes. For example, among the hemoglobinopathies SS disease (sickle cell anemia) is a severe disorder, whereas CC disease is mild; SC disease, the genetic compound, is of intermediate severity (and has some qualitative clinical differences from both sickle cell anemia and CC disease). Especially in the case of autosomal recessives, wide clinical variability in a series of cases, with little intrafamilial variation, should suggest the existence of two or more mutant alleles, resulting in different homozygous states and genetic compounds.

PROGNOSIS

In genetic disease, the question "what will be the outcome?" (see *Foreword*) has additional implications; it may apply to unborn offspring of the person seeking advice, not the person himself. Of course, prognosis in the usual sense of the implications of the disease for the length and quality of life is also important in clinical genetics. But in addition, the question often asked by patients with genetic disease or by their families is "What will be the outcome of later pregnancies?" "I have such-and such. Will I transmit it to my children?" or "My wife and I and our families do not have anything of this sort, but we have a child with such-and-such. Will our later born children have this condition also?" Providing the answers to such questions is called genetic counseling. The following principles can be given:

1. Diagnosis is of the essence. Because of genetic heterogeneity, disorders of different modes of inheritance (or not hereditary at all) may appear similar and be given the same label. Fa-

miliarity with the world's experience with the familial occurrence of a given disorder or class of disorders (as recorded in *Mendelian Inheritance in Man*[3]) is essential. A sign of the competent doctor is the ability to come to a correct diagnosis even though he has not seen the disease before. In clinical genetics the clinician is put to particular test because of the large number (Table 41–8) and individual rarity of genetic disorders.

2. In the case of autosomal dominant disorders, a sporadic case in a family may represent a new mutation. If the father is in his 40's or 50's this possibility is given increased weight. The hazard to subsequently born children is negligible, although the affected person himself can transmit the disorder to his descendants. Sporadicity may, however, be only apparent; one parent may, in fact, have the disorder in very mild form.

   In some autosomal dominant disorders, a majority of affected persons have a fresh mutation. This is the case in about 80 percent of cases of achondroplasia and an even higher proportion of cases of other conditions such as Apert syndrome (acrocephalosyndactyly). When experience teaches that the given disorder is fully penetrant (as it is in the two specific examples given), then fresh mutations can be concluded with relative confidence when both parents are unaffected. An equilibrium exists between addition of mutant genes to, and their removal from, the gene pool, i.e., the balance between new mutations on the one hand and negative selection on the other. In the Marfan syndrome, about 15 percent of cases are new mutants and reproductive fitness is reduced by about 15 percent below the population average through death of affected persons before reaching or completing the reproductive age.

3. Once a couple has given birth to a child with a well-delineated autosomal recessive disorder, such as phenylketonuria, cystic fibrosis, and many others, the risk to subsequently born children can be stated precisely as 1 in 4. Even if three, four, or any number of affected children have been born, the risk is still 1 in 4 for *each* later born child—chance has no memory. It is useful to use the coin-tossing analogy. Otherwise, parents may think that they have had their one affected child in four and can expect to have three more children who will be normal.

4. For X-linked disorders such as hemophila and Duchenne muscular dystrophy, the problems of genetic counseling are somewhat different. For example, what is the risk that a sister of the affected boy is a carrier and therefore liable to have affected sons? If the affected brother inherited his disorder from a carrier mother, the risk is very different from that if the brother's disease arose by new mutation in the X chromosome contributed to this one affected male by his mother. If there are affected maternal uncles, then the chance of the sister being a carrier is 1 in 2, the chance of her having a son (rather than a daughter) is 1 in 2, and the chance of her transmitting the hemophilia gene rather than the normal allele to said son is 1 in 2, giving a joint risk of 1 in 8 for a hemophilic son. If she already has had two normal sons the risk of her being a carrier is reduced according to Bayes principle.

5. Obviously, the ability to detect the heterozygous carrier state for recessive disorders is useful to genetic counseling. This is less the case in most rare autosomal recessives, because even if the person is a carrier (and the chances of this are 2 in 3 for the normal sib of a person with an autosomal recessive disorder), he will have affected children only if he marries another carrier. Among unrelated persons from whom he chooses his spouse, the frequency of heterozygotes is of the order of 1 in 50 to 1 in 150 for most rare recessives. The risk is, of course, much higher if he chooses a first cousin as his spouse; 1 in 4 is the chance of the first cousin being a carrier.

   On the other hand, to be able to detect female carriers of X-linked traits is of great value, because they can have affected sons regardless of the genotype of the husband. Low levels of antihemophilic globulin (or better a low ratio of Factor VIII procoagulant activity to Factor VIII antigen) is useful in detecting carriers for hemophilia A. Increased levels of creatine phosphokinase are useful in detecting females carrying the gene for Duchenne muscular dystrophy.

6. In multifactorial conditions (see p. 467), e.g., common congenital malformations such as harelip, cleft palate, and congenital heart disease, genetic risks can be estimated only in empirical terms. For example, in a collection of families with a single case of harelip, a frequency of 4 percent of harelip among offspring born subsequent to the affected child

may have been found. If one parent is also affected, the risk is increased, and so on. Empirical risk figures undoubtedly exaggerate the risk in some families and underestimate it in others. In this type of situation, as in so many others of medical genetics, the likelihood of heterogeneity must also be kept in mind. One must look for objective features which may make it possible to arrive at a more precise estimate of genetic risk. As an example, one form of cleft palate[3] is associated with a characteristic structural peculiarity of the lower lip, namely, mucous pits or mucoceles. The lip anomaly behaves as a typical autosomal dominant condition. In only a certain proportion of persons with this lip anomaly does cleft palate also occur. One can at least assure those family members without the lip anomaly that the risk of having a child with a cleft palate is not increased.

7. Prenatal diagnosis by amniocentesis[39,40] is a technique of preventive genetics. It has added a new dimension to genetic counseling.

8. In addition to a thorough knowledge of genetic principles and of the literature on the particular condition (both its genetics and its natural history), the genetic counselor should have common sense, good judgment, sense of proportion, and warmheartedness. The bald risk figures are not the whole or even the most important part of the information to be transmitted. The total "cost" must be considered. Cost can be thought of as the product of the recurrence risk and the burden (in terms of emotional and financial stress). As indicated in Table 41–9, a condition such as Duchenne muscular dystrophy, with both high recurrence risk and high burden, carries the highest cost of the examples given.

9. Genetic counseling should always be given in such a way as not to incite or aggravate anguish, although the advice should never depart from the truth. Often, genetic counseling can give great relief. The counselee frequently has an exaggerated notion of the risk involved. For example, the nonhemophilic brother of a hemophilic cannot transmit hemophilia to his descendants, but he may not know that. That the normally statured offspring of two achondroplasts cannot transmit the disorders is another example.

TREATMENT

Therapy is not the "long suit" of clinical genetics. However, mendelian disorders are not as therapeutically hopeless as they might seem. There is, of course, a difference between treatment and cure. It is true that cure is not now possible unless the surgical correction of genetically determined abnormalities can be so considered. Opportunities for treatment in genetic disease arise in part from the fact that, at least to some extent, almost all genetic diseases are the result of the action of environmental as well as genetic etiologic factors.

The following are forms of therapy in genetic disease: elimination diets, dietary supplementation, avoidance of certain drugs, elimination from the body of affected tissue or toxic material, replacement of a missing gene product, replacement of defective tissue, and other forms of surgical therapy.

Specifically Restricted Diets
In galactosemia and phenylketonuria,[3] galactose and phenylalanine, respectively, cannot be metabolized properly, and pathologic effects result from the accumulation of these substances or their metabolic products. Elimination of galactose and phenylalanine from the diet at an early stage can prevent irreversible damage. There are some indications that lifelong continuation of the elimination diet may not be necessary.

Dietary Supplementation
Avitaminosis and deficiencies of essential amino acids are not viewed as genetic disorders since, seemingly, all human beings require these dietary elements. As compared with some other mammalian species, however, man has a genetic defect in vitamin C synthesis, for example; treatment of this genetic defect is dietary consumption of vitamin C. In the

TABLE 41–9
Perspective in Genetic Counseling*

Defect	Recurrence	Burden
Anencephaly	Low	Low
Colorblindness	High	Low
Congenital heart malformation	Low	High
Duchenne muscular dystrophy	High	High

* From E. A. Murphy.

case of vitamin-dependent inborn errors of metabolism (p. 454), supplementation of the usual dietary intake with specific vitamins in pharmacologic dosage is therapeutically effective.

Avoidance of Drugs

Barbiturates and some other agents precipitate acute attacks of porphyria in the rare genetically susceptible person. Certain antimalarial and other drugs, and also the fava bean, precipitate hemolysis in persons with the X-linked genetic deficiency of erythrocyte G6PD (p. 463). Clearly, preventive treatment consists of avoiding the offending agents.

Elimination from the Body

Hemochromatosis is effectively treated by repeated venesection. The removal of the excess copper from the body in Wilson's disease (hepatolenticular degeneration) by means of penicillamine, which binds it and carries it out in the urine, is another case in point.

Replacement of a Missing Gene Product

The replacement of a missing gene product is illustrated by the administration of antihemophilic globulin in hemophilia A, of gamma globulin in agammaglobulinemia, of thyroid hormone in the several genetic defects of thyroid hormone synthesis,[3] and of cortisone in cases of genetic defects in adrenal hormone synthesis.

Enzyme Induction

At least one example of enzyme induction by pharmacologic means is known. The Arias type of hyperbilirubinemia[3] is mainly of cosmetic significance. Jaundice is lifelong. Phenobarbital in a dosage which is not objectionably sedative results in dramatic clearing of the icterus.

Cofactor (Vitamin) Administration

In the case of so-called vitamin-dependent, or better, vitamin-responsive inborn errors of metabolism, administration of the vitamin cofactor in amounts 100 times or more greater than the minimal requirement "cures" the disease. B_6-responsive homocystinuria (p. 461) is one of the best examples.

Administration of Missing Enzyme

As indicated elsewhere (Table 41-12), administration of missing enzyme is theoretically, and indeed to some extent demonstrably, effective in lysosomal diseases. Practical problems with this approach include avoidance of immunologic reactions, protection of the enzyme from enzymatic degradation until it can be taken up by cells, transport of the enzyme into cells or compartments of cells where it can act, and, of course, availability of enzyme. One example of enzyme replacement therapy is provided by the form of combined cellular and humoral immunodeficiency due to deficiency of adenosine deaminase (ADA). Accumulation of adenosine is responsible for damage to lymphocytes. Circulating red cells normally contain considerable amounts of the enzyme missing in this disease. Transfusion of normal red cells lowers levels of adenosine and effects clinical improvement. (The transfused blood must be treated in a way to remove or destroy lymphocytes, in order to avoid graft-versus-host reaction.)

Replacement of Defective Tissue

Bone marrow transplantation has been successfully accomplished in Fanconi anemia; fetal thymus has been transplanted to reconstitute the immune system in genetic immunodeficiency states; and kidney transplantation has been performed in cases of hereditary cystic disease of the kidney, cystinosis, Fabry's disease, and the amyloid kidney of familial Mediterranean fever.

Other Forms of Surgical Therapy

Removal of the spleen in hereditary spherocytosis corrects the anemia, which is the main manifestation. In the Peutz-Jeghers syndrome[3] simple removal of the polyps of the intestine (which are usually not premalignant) cures this part—the only significant one—of the syndrome. By enucleation of the affected eye, retinoblastoma, an autosomal dominant trait, is cured, if metastasis has not occurred.

PREVENTION

The most important and contributory service function of clinical genetics is preventive medicine. Primary prevention, avoidance of the occurrence of disease, is the objective of genetic counseling. Secondary prevention, avoidance or amelioration of the effects of the disease, particularly through early detection and initiation of therapy, is a significant part of clinical genetics.

Genetic preventive measures include neonatal screening for inborn errors of metabolism, family screening for disorders such as colonic polyposis and Wilson's disease, amniocentesis for prenatal diagnosis of chromosomal aberrations and inborn errors of metabolism, and population screening for heterozygous carriers of recessive disease.

---TABLE 41–10---
Practice of Preventive Medicine in the Family*

Disease	Type Inheritance	Defect	Treatment
Angioedema, hereditary	Autosomal dominant	Cl esterase inhibitor	"Impeded" androgen[11,21]
Coproporphyria	Autosomal dominant	Assay of coproporphyrinogen oxidase in white cells, fibroblasts	As for porphyria, acute intermittent (below)
Gardner syndrome[28]	Autosomal dominant	Examination for bony and soft tissue tumors, colonic polyps	Colectomy
G6PD-deficiency	X-linked recessive	RBC G6PD assay	Avoidance of hemolysis-inducing drugs
Hereditary spherocytosis	Autosomal dominant	Osmotic fragility of RBC	Splenectomy
Hemochromatosis[17]	Autosomal recessive	Measures of iron metabolism; HLA typing in families	Venosection
Homocystinuria, B_6 responsive[29]	Autosomal recessive	Homocystine in urine	Vitamin B_6
Marfan syndrome[29]	Autosomal dominant	Echography of ascending aorta	Propranolol
Malignant hyperthermia	Autosomal dominant	Blood CPK	Avoidance of anesthesia
Polyposis coli[28]	Autosomal dominant	Colonoscopy	?Colectomy
Porphyria, acute intermittent	Autosomal dominant	Uroporphyrinogen-1 synthetase in red cells	Avoidance of barbituates, etc.; hematin for acute attacks
Pseudocholinesterase deficiency (succinylcholine sensitivity)	Autosomal recessive	Assay of plasma pseudocholinesterase	Care in use of muscle relaxants in anesthesia
Porphyria cutanea tarda	Autosomal dominant	Uroporphyrinogen decarboxylase in red cells	Phlebotomy
Wilson's disease	Autosomal recessive	Ceruloplasmin, serum	Penicillamine

* This is a partial list for purposes of illustration. See McKusick's *Mendelian Inheritance in Man*[3] for additional references concerning specific disorders.

Neonatal screening becomes important for any disorder that can be treated effectively. Phenylketonuria (PKU) and galactosemia are cases in point. Early institution of therapy is essential before irreversible damage is done.

Any mendelian disorder for which there is useful therapy should be sought in other members of the family whenever an index case (proband) is detected. Examples include colonic polyposis, Wilson's disease, hemochromatosis, Marfan syndrome, the porphyrias, and G6PD deficiency (Table 41–10). In some of these conditions, such as Wilson's disease, a single testing is adequate to identify the presence of the disease. In others, such as colonic polyposis, periodic examination of persons at high risk is necessary. This is "health maintenance" practiced at the family level. The mode of inheritance is important in deciding which relatives should be screened. Ordinarily, in the case of Wilson's disease, a recessive, it is sufficient to screen sibs. In polyposis coli and acute intermittent porphyria, dominant disorders, it is essential to screen all first-degree relatives (parents, sibs, and offspring) and perhaps go further afield in the pedigree, depending on the findings in first-degree relatives.

Preclinical disease can be detected in sibs of Wilson's disease and hemochromatosis and measures to reduce body stores of copper and iron, respectively, can prevent the development of cirrhosis and other pathologic changes. In the porphyrias and in G6PD deficiency, identification of affected relatives is important so that they may be warned against agents known to precipitate abnormality.

In addition to neonates and family members, the fetus is now also subject to screening for chromosomal abnormalities and specific inborn errors of metabolism. By amniocentesis,[34,39,40] performed percutaneously in the second trimester of gestation, a sample of amniotic fluid is obtained and the fetal cells contained therein are studied after growth in culture. The chromosomes can be studied by the usual methods (p. 434). Karyotyping the fetus is the objective of amniocentesis when one of the parents carries a chromosomal rearrangement, such as fusion 14/21 chromosome, that predisposes to Down syndrome in the offspring. The fetal karyotype can also be determined in the case of older mothers, because of their relatively high risk of bearing Down syndrome offspring. It is strongly indicated in any mother over 40 and some recommend it for any mother over 35.

When parents are known to be heterozygous carriers of a particular autosomal recessive disorder (usually because of the birth of an affected child), the fetus can be tested for the disorder. Study of cultured skin fibroblasts has become a leading technique in clinical genetics. The fibroblast turns out to have, fortunate for clinical genetics, a wide enzymatic repertoire, a feature shared by amniotic cells. Theoretically any disorder for which an enzyme deficiency has been identified in skin fibroblasts—and there are over 175 such disorders, all recessive, either autosomal or X-linked—can be diagnosed antenatally by the enzymatic study of amniotic cells. (Notable exceptions to the rule that cultured skin fibroblasts can be used to diagnose enzyme deficiency states are phenylketonuria and type 1 glycogen storage disease; phenylalanine hydroxylase and glucose-6-phosphatase are not found in cultured fibroblasts.)

The objective of prenatal diagnosis[34] is to permit elective abortion of the affected fetus, and thereby help parents achieve a healthy family.[40]

Many conditions such as hemophilia cannot presently be diagnosed antenatally. The sex of the fetus can be ascertained, however, and in the case of serious X-linked recessive traits the parents may elect abortion of any male fetus when the mother is known to be a carrier.

Other methods of prenatal diagnosis[34] now under development include fetoscopy for direct observation of malformations and for fetal blood sampling.

Screening for heterozygous carriers of recessive disease at a population level is worthwhile when heterozygotes are as frequent as 1 in 30 or higher and when the information can be put to the useful service of the persons found to be heterozygous. Tay-Sachs disease is a nearly ideal example. The frequency of Tay-Sachs disease (a dreadful progressive neurologic disorder of infants, leading to death in the first decade) is about 1 in 3600 in Ashkenazi Jews. The frequency of the Tay-Sachs gene is, therefore, about 1 in 60 and the frequency of heterozygotes about 1 in 30. (These estimates follow from the Hardy-Weinberg formula, $p^2 + 2pq + q^2$, in which q is the frequency of the Tay-Sachs gene, q^2 is the frequency of Tay-Sachs homozygotes, and $2pq$ is the frequency of heterozygotes.) A test for heterozygotes—level of β-hexosaminidase A (hex A) in the blood— is available. Furthermore, the homozygous affected fetus can be identified by measurement of hex A in cultured amniotic cells. Thus, Tay-Sachs disease can, theoretically, be eliminated, if couples, both heterozygous, are identified by screening and their pregnancies are monitored by amniocentesis.

SPECIFIC CATEGORIES OF MENDELIAN DISEASE

Many of the principles outlined above, as well as special considerations, are illustrated by the seven classes of simply inherited disorders next discussed (see also Table 41-10).

THE HEMOGLOBINOPATHIES[15]
The hemoglobinopathies are prime examples of molecular disease. Indeed, the molecular abnormality of hemoglobin in sickle cell anemia, demonstrated by electrophoresis, was the original basis for Linus Pauling's seminal concept.[1] Some principles of biology and of clinical genetics learned from the study of hemoglobinopathies or illustrated by them are outlined in Table 41-11.

INBORN ERRORS OF METABOLISM[9]
In inborn errors of metabolism the mutation has occurred in a gene that codes for an enzyme controlling a step in intermediary metabolism or in a synthetic pathway. Because of deficient activity of the enzyme a block occurs in the chain of reactions, as diagrammed in Figure 41-7. Clinical abnormality results from toxic effects of metabolites that accumulate proximal to the block, or from deficiency of products of the metabolic or synthetic pathway. Alkaptonuria (p. 456) is an example of the former, and genetic defects in thyroid or adrenal hormone synthesis illustrate the latter mechanism. In some disorders, e.g., homocystinuria both pathogenetic mechanisms may be operative. In some disorders a defect in feedback inhibition occurs because of deficiency of a product of the pathway, and some of the pathologic effects are produced or aggravated through excessive production of metabolites (Fig. 41-8). This happens in the porphyrias. Administration of hematin, the deficient product of the pathway, has therapeutic value.[24] The Lesch-Nyhan syndrome[3] illustrates the same phenomenon.

┌─ **TABLE 41–11** ──────────────┐

**Some Principles Illustrated by
the Hemoglobinopathies**[15*]

I. The Genetic Code
(From the amino acid sequence of hemoglobin, normal
and variant, the triplet code of RNA and DNA in man
are deduced and checked with conclusion from
studies in bacterial systems.)

II. The Nature of Various Mutations
   a. Substitution of an amino acid (single
       nucleoside change), e.g., Hb S
   b. Deletion of one nucleoside producing frame
       shift, e.g., Hb Wayne
   c. Deletion of one codon, e.g., Hb Freiburg
   d. Deletion of several codons, e.g., Hb Gun
       Hill
   e. Deletion of a gene, e.g., α-thalassemia
   f. Deletion of 2 genes, e.g., hereditary
       persistence of fetal hemoglobin
   g. Deletion of part of 2 genes, with formation
       of fusion gene, e.g., Hb Lepore
   h. Terminator mutation, resulting in extra long
       polypeptide chain, e.g., Hb Constant Spring

**III. Two genes—One Molecule, with Following
Phenomena as a Result**
   1. Allelism (Hbs S and C) and nonallelism
       (e.g., Hb S and Hb Hopkins-2)
   2. Allelic interaction, e.g., SC diseases (a
       genetic compound)
   3. Nonallelic interaction, e.g., Hb S and Hb
       Memphis

IV. Biochemical Diversity of Man
Approximate number of single amino acid
substitutions known
   in α chains $\sim$ 100
   in β chain $\sim$ 200
   in γ chains $\sim$ 15
   in δ chain $\sim$ 10

V. Phenotypic Variability
Resulting from an allelic series, e.g., mutants in the
hemoglobin genes may produce no discernible
abnormality or one of the following

   1. Anemia
       a. Sickle cell anemia
       b. Drug-induced or aggravated hemolytic
           anemia (e.g., Hb Zurich)
       c. Chronic nonspherocytic hemolytic
           anemia (Heinz body anemia) (e.g., Hb
           Hammersmith)
   2. Methemoglobinemia (the Hbs M)
   3. Polycythemia (e.g., Hb Chesapeake)

VI. Pleiotropism
For example, the sickle cell anemia syndrome

VII. Genetic Heterogeneity
For example, the many different mutations of either
the alpha or the beta chain that lead to anemia,
methemoglobinemia, or polycythemia

* See McKusick's *Mendelian Inheritance in Man*[3] for references to specific hemoglobins.

┌─ **TABLE 41–11 (cont.)** ──────────────┐

VIII. Selection and Polymorphism
For example, malaria and the Hb S gene

**IX. Evolution Through Gene Duplication and
Divergent Mutation**
For example, the beta, gamma, and delta ("nonalpha")
globin genes

X. Pharmacogenetics
For example, Hb Zurich

└────────────────────────────────────┘

Similar pathogenetic mechanisms operate in genetic defects of cortisol and aldosterone synthesis by
the adrenal cortex. The two steroid homones are synthesized from cholesterol through intermeshed synthetic pathways. Impairment of cortisol production
results, through cybernetic mechanisms, in a compensatory increase in ACTH secretion by the anterior
pituitary. Impairment of mineralocorticoid production results in a comparable compensatory increase
in renin–angiotensin production. These compensatory
mechanisms may return cortisol or aldosterone production to normal or near normal, but at the expense
of excessive production of products and byproducts
that have undesirable hormonal effects, e.g., masculinization of the female.

Some inborn errors of metabolism are vitamin-
responsive, i.e., are alleviated by specific vitamins in
pharmacologic dosage. The vitamin in each such case
is a normal cofactor for the enzyme involved and the
mutation is of such a nature that catalytic activity of
the enzyme is defective except when it is loaded with
the vitamin-cofactor. One form of homocystinuria (p.
461) is an example.

The number of enzyme deficiencies that have
been identified is now in excess of 175. Almost all of
the resulting inborn errors of metabolism are inherited as recessives, either autosomal or X-linked. Most
enzymes are endowed with sufficient margin of safety
that the partial deficiency found in heterozygotes has
no phenotypic effects. Exceptions to this rule-of-
thumb are three enzymopathies in the hematin synthesis pathway: acute intermittent porphyria, proto-
porphyria, and coproporphyria. In part, the excessive
function of delta-amino-levulinic acid synthetase because of reduced feedback inhibition by hematin is
probably the reason for disease even in the heterozygote. Furthermore, the pathway may be stressed,
leading to intermittent attacks or clinical exacerbation. Hereditary angioedema (Table 41–10) and an-
tithrombin III deficiency ("thrombophilia") are two
other dominantly inherited enzymopathies.

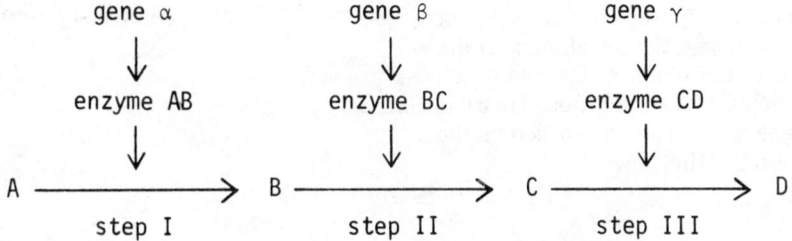

FIGURE 41-7. The genetic control of a chain of reactions in a metabolic pathway.

Dominantly inherited disorders usually involve a nonenzymic protein of structural or other function, e.g., collagen or hemoglobin. The methemoglobine-mias illustrate this principle of the basic defect of dominants *vs.* recessives. They all have the same phenotype, cyanosis (sometimes confused for congenital heart disease), but some are dominant and some recessive. Recessive methemoglobinemia is caused by deficiency of an enzyme, methemoglobin reductase. Dominant methemoglobinemia is caused by one or another of the hemoglobins M.

The principles of pathogenesis, diagnosis, and treatment of inborn errors of metabolism will be further illustrated with PKU, alkaptonuria, and the Lesch-Nyhan syndrome.

Phenylketonuria

PKU is an autosomal recessive inborn error in the metabolism of the amino acid phenylalanine. The deficiency involves the enzyme phenylalanine hydroxylase, which catalyzes the addition of a hydroxyl group to phenylalanine to make tyrosine. Phenylalanine ingested in the form of dietary protein accumulates, and the products of alternative metabolic pathways, phenylketone substances, are excreted in the urine, giving the condition its name.

Severe mental retardation is the most consistent manifestation. Patients with this disorder tend to have light complexions. Relative deficiency of tyrosine from which melanin is produced or inhibition of melanin synthesis by phenylalanine or by a metabolic product are possible mechanisms of the light coloration. The patient is often noted to have a characteristic odor, referred to as "mousy." Neurologic features and behavioral peculiarities, such as unusual posturing and spasticity, are frequently present. Chemical tests for identifying PKU in the newborn period are now available. The Guthrie test makes use of phenylalanine-requiring bacteria for a bioassay of phenylalanine in blood. A low-phenylalanine diet prevents development of retardation. If the dietary regimen is initiated early, normal development can be achieved. That restriction of phenylalanine can be safely relaxed after age 5 or 6 is hoped but not yet proved.

Like many other rare recessives, PKU varies in frequency in different ethnic groups. It is relatively frequent in persons from northern Ireland and western Scotland, less frequent in American blacks, and very infrequent in Ashkenazi Jews.

Some untreated PKU homozygous females have had children; these have all been mentally retarded, and some have shown malformations, e.g., of the heart. All of the children are heterozygotes, unless, of course, the father is a heterozygote. In utero the off-

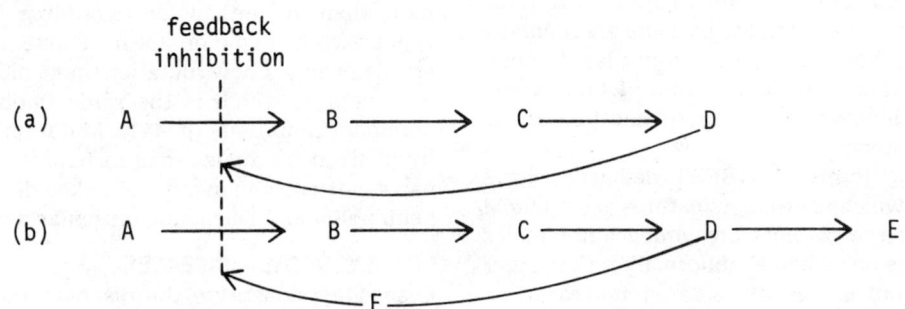

FIGURE 41-8. Control of gene action through feedback inhibition.

spring of a PKU woman is exposed to high levels of phenylalanine, which damages the developing brain. When tested after birth, the children may show no clue to the cause of the mental retardation. Theirs is an unusual form of genetic disease—one based on the genotype of the mother, not their own.[25]

Alkaptonuria

Alkaptonuria (and the abnormal phenotype that accompanies it, ochronosis) is an inborn error in the degradation of homogentisic acid, a derivative of tyrosine (that is in turn derived from phenylalanine, as noted above). Homogentisic acid oxidase is deficient. By oxidation, which is favored in alkaline urine, homogentisic acid is converted to a black alkapton. Black diapers are often the first sign of the disease.

Arthritis of the spine becomes evident in the 20s or 30s in the affected person. Calcification of the spinous ligaments or intervertebral discs produces a characteristic radiographic appearance. In vivo tanning of collagen is thought to be the mechanism of the damage to connective tissues. Sclerotic and calcific changes in the aortic valve are frequent. Black discoloration of the scleras and ear cartilages are clinically evident, and the costal cartilages are found at thoracic surgery or autopsy to be deeply pigmented. The pinnae become stiff and calcified; x-rays may even demonstrate ossification, as indicated by the presence of miniature marrow cavities. Radiopaque prostatic stones, which are black in color, are another feature of ochronosis.

The Lesch-Nyhan Syndrome

This syndrome is an X-linked recessive inborn error in purine metabolism. Hypoxanthine-guanine phosphoribosyl-transferase (HGPRT) is the enzyme deficient. This enzyme normally catalyzes the conversion of guanine to guanylic acid and of hypoxanthine to inosinic acid. Since guanylic acid no longer exercises its normal inhibitory effect on PRPP synthetase (Fig. 41–9), at the first and rate-limiting step on uric acid synthesis, hyperuricemia results. In addition to renal stones from hyperuricemia, the patients are mentally retarded, have choreoathetosis, and display compulsive self-mutilation, especially biting of fingers and lips. The pathogenesis of the neurologic features is not well understood.

Rare allelic forms of HGPRT deficiency have been found in which neurologic features are minimal or absent, and the patients are young adult males with gout as the only clinical abnormality. (Yet other patients with gout and urolithiasis are found to have a mutation of the enzyme PRPP synthetase such that it is not inhibited by guanylic acid. This disorder is also

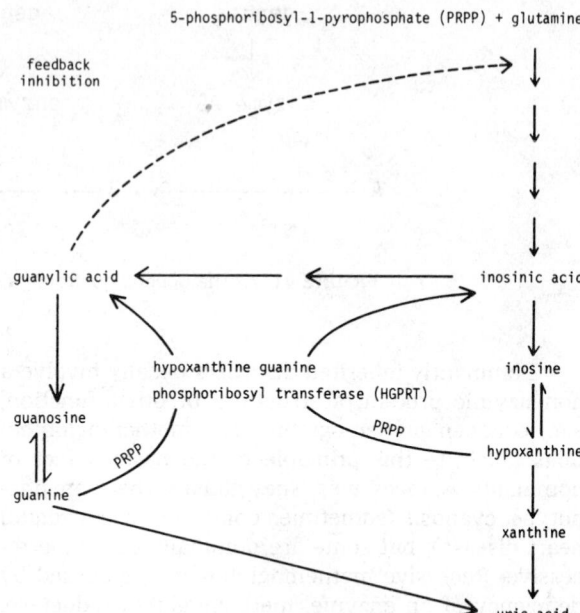

FIGURE 41–9. A schematic representation of purine metabolism with particular reference to uric acid synthesis. The basic defect in the Lesch-Nyhan syndrome is deficient activity of hypoxanthine guanine phosphoribosyl transferase (HGPRT).

X-linked recessive.) These forms of hereditary hyperuricemia constitute only a small portion of any series of gouty patients.

Among the cultured skin fibroblasts of heterozygous females, the X-linkage of the HGPRT locus is proved by demonstration of two classes of cells: one class with normal HGRPT, and one with deficient HGPRT as in affected males. This finding is predicted by the Lyon hypothesis. Studies of mouse–human somatic cell hybrids confirm the X-linkage and provide further information that the HGPRT locus is on the distal end of the long arm of the X.

Another significant genetic feature of the Lesch-Nyhan syndrome is that the great majority of mothers of cases are heterozygous carriers, which is much more than the anticipated two-thirds. Those heterozygous women who do not have heterozygous mothers, i.e., carry a new mutation, have older fathers, on the average, which is the same finding as in new dominant mutations (p. 441). Mutation may be more frequent in the males than in females, in Lesch-Nyhan syndrome and in other X-linked disorders such as hemophilia and Duchenne muscular dystrophy.

LYSOSOMAL DISEASES

Lysosomes constitute the disposal and reclamation system of the cell. They are membrane-bound sacs that maintain a low pH and contain more than 60 acid hydrolases involved in degradation of nucleic acids, proteins, lipids, mucopolysaccharides, glycogen, and other macromolecules. Deficiency of specific acid hydrolases lead to specific disorders including Fabry's angiokeratoma, Tay-Sachs disease, type II glycogen storage disease (Pompe's disease), Gaucher's disease, and at least 10 mucopolysaccharidoses (of which the Hurler syndrome, MPS I H, is the prototype). The characteristics of lysosomal diseases are listed in Table 41–12.

The mucopolysaccharidoses (Table 41–13) illustrate many of the genetic principles outlined earlier; only two will be specifically mentioned.[30]

Genetic Heterogeneity

All the mucopolysaccharidoses were confused at some stage in their history, or can be confused in some stages of the evolution of individual cases, with the Hurler syndrome. The Sanfilippo syndromes provide a particularly striking example of genetic heterogeneity. Three phenotypically identical forms of the disease (progressive mental retardation with relatively mild changes in liver, joints, and bones) show deficiency of different acid hydrolases, each responsible for cleavage of heparin sulfate at a different site in the molecule.

Allelic Variation, Including Presumed Genetic Compounds

MPS I, MPS II, MPS IV, MPS VI, and probably others have apparently allelic forms. In each case, the same enzyme is deficient, but the clinical picture, mainly in

---

TABLE 41–12
Characteristics of Lysosomal Diseases

1. Storage diseases
2. Deposits in cells are membrane-bound
3. Clinical course is progressive
4. Multiple organs and tissues are involved
5. Stored material is chemically heterogeneous
6. Treatment by providing missing enzymes potentially feasible

---

TABLE 41–13
The Mucopolysaccharidoses

Number	Eponym	Clinical	Genetics	Urinary MPS	Enzyme-Deficient
MPS I H	Hurler	Clouding of cornea, grave manifestations, death usually before age 10	Homozygous for MPS I H gene	Dermatan sulfate, heparan sulfate	α-L-iduronidase
MPS I S	Scheie	Stiff joints, cloudy cornea, aortic valve disease, normal intelligence and (?) lifespan	Homozygosity for MPS I S gene	Dermatan sulfate, heparan sulfate	α-L-iduronidase
MPS I H/S	Hurler-Scheie	Intermediate phenotype	Genetic compound of MPS I H and MPS I S genes	Dermatan sulfate, heparan sulfate	α-L-iduronidase
MPS II-XR, severe (30990)	Hunter, severe	No corneal clouding, milder course than in MPS I H, death before 15 years	Hemizygous for X-linked gene	Dermatan sulfate, heparan sulfate	Iduronate sulfatase
MPS II-XR, mild	Hunter, mild	Survival to 30s to 60s, fair intelligence	Hemizygous for X-linked allele	Dermatan sulfate, heparan sulfate	Iduronate sulfatase
?MPS II-AR (25285)	?Autosomal Hunter	Same as mild or severe MPS II-XR	Homozygous for autosomal gene	Dermatan sulfate, heparan sulfate	Iduronate sulfatase

(Continued)

TABLE 41-13 (cont.)

Number	Eponym	Clinical	Genetics	Urinary MPS	Enzyme-Deficient
MPS III A (25290)	Sanfilippo A	Indistinguishable phenotype: Mild somatic, severe central nervous system effects	Homozygous for Sanfilippo A gene	Heparan sulfate	Heparan N-sulfatase (sulfamidase)
MPS III B (25292)	Sanfilippo B		Homozygous for Sanfilippo B gene	Heparan sulfate	N-acetyl-α-D-glucosaminidase
MPS III C (25293)	Sanfilippo C		Homozygous for Sanfilippo C gene	Heparan sulfate	Acetyl-CoA:α-glucosaminide N-acetyltransferase
MPS IV A (25300)	Morquio A	Severe, distinctive bone changes, cloudy cornea, aortic regurgitation	Homozygous for Morquio A genes	Keratan sulfate	Galactosamine-6-sulfate sulfatase
MPS IV B (25301)	Morquio B	Mild bone changes, cloudy cornea, hypoplastic odontoid	Homozygous for Morquio B gene	Keratan sulfate	β-galactosidase
MPS V	—	—	—	—	—
MPS VI, severe (25320)	Maroteaux-Lamy classic severe	Severe osseous and corneal change; valvular heart disease, striking WBC inclusions; normal intellect; survival to 20s	Homozygous for Maroteaux-Lamy (M-L) gene	Dermatan sulfate	Arylsulfatase B (N-acetylgalactosamine 4-sulfatase)
MPS VI intermediate	Maroteaux-Lamy intermediate	Moderately severe changes	Homozygous for allele at M-L locus or genetic compound	Dermatan sulfate	Arylsulfatase B (N-acetylgalactosamine 4-sulfatase)
MPS VI, mild	Maroteaux-Lamy mild	Mild osseous and corneal change, normal intellect; aortic stenosis	Homozygous for allele at M-L locus	Dermatan sulfate	Arylsulfatase B (N-acetylgalactosamine 4-sulfatase)
MPS VII (25322)	Sly	Hepatosplenomegaly, dysostosis multiplex, mental retardation variable; WBC inclusions	Homozygous for mutant gene at β-glucuronidase locus	Dermatan sulfate, heparan sulfate	β-glucuronidase
MPS VIII (25323)	DiFerrante	Short stature, mild dysostosis multiplex, ring-shaped metachromasia of lymphocytes	Homozygous for MPS VIII gene	Keratan sulfate, heparan sulfate	Glucosamine-6-sulfate sulfatase

terms of severity, takes two or more different forms. The MPS I class, for example, has deficiency of α-L-iduronidase. The Hurler syndrome (MPS I H) is a severe disorder with progressive mental and somatic deterioration and death usually before age 10. The Scheie syndrome (MPS I S) is a milder disorder in which the main disability comes from corneal clouding and stiff joints of the hands, but is accompanied by normal stature and intelligence. Patients with iduronidase deficiency and an intermediate phenotype may represent the genetic compound (MPS I H/S); they are short of stature and have rather severe joint, cardiac and mental changes, but survive to their twenties. A receding chin is a feature distinct from both the Scheie and the Hurler syndrome.

DEFECTS IN RECEPTORS

Hereditary hypercholesterolemia and the testicular feminization syndrome are genetic defects in, or deficiency of, specific receptors.

The defect in *hereditary hypercholesterolemia* involves the cell membrane receptor for low-density lipoprotein (LDL). On transport into the cell, LDL normally inhibits 3-hydroxy-3-methylglutaryl coenzyme A reductase (HMG CoA reductase), the enzyme catalyzing the rate-limiting step in cholesterol synthesis. Heterozygotes for the receptor defect have levels of plasma cholesterol in the range of 300 to 500 mg per dl. They sometimes show xanthomas of tendons and have an increased risk of coronary occlusion and other complications of atherosclerosis. Homozygotes have plasma cholesterol levels in excess of 500 mg/dl, regularly have xanthomas, including a type called xanthoma plana of the palmar creases, and usually succumb to coronary occlusion before age 20.

Brown and Goldstein[14,22] discovered the defect in hereditary hypercholesterolemia by study of cultured fibroblasts from patients, particularly those homozygous for the defect. Again, heterogeneity is found. Some homozygotes have no receptor, whereas others have a functionally defective receptor. Rare homozygotes have a defective receptor which combines normally with LDL but cannot effect "internalization" of LDL. All three mutations are allelic, and genetic compounds have been observed.

Hereditary hypercholesterolemia in its heterozygous form is one of the most frequent genetic diseases, occurring in about 1 in 500 persons.

In the *testicular feminization syndrome* (androgen insensitivity), a defect occurs in a receptor which is situated in the cytoplasm and normally combines with dihydrotestosterone (DHT[13,32]). The DHT-receptor complex is translocated into the nucleus where it acts on specific chromosomal sites to induce the action of specific genes controlling male secondary sex characteristics. Again, cultured skin fibroblasts were vital in the elucidation of the defect, and again genetic heterogeneity was found. Some cases appear to have receptor but it is functionally ineffective, perhaps because that part of the molecule that interacts with DNA is defective.

Clinically, testicular feminization is a form of male pseudohermaphroditism. Patients are karyotypically normal XY males but appear to be normal females in terms of development of secondary sexual characteristics such as breasts and external genitalia. However, they have primary amenorrhea, the vagina ends blindly, and there are testes which are located in the inguinal canals and often bring the "girls" to surgical attention for presumed hernia.

Testicular feminization shows the pedigree pattern of an X-linked recessive. Since affected males are infertile, however, the pattern cannot be distinguished from that of an autosomal dominant trait that is not expressed in heterozygous females (who are, as it were, already feminized). Cloning studies of cultured skin fibroblasts from heterozygous mothers of patients with testicular feminization proved X-linked recessive inheritance by demonstrating two classes of cells: One class has deficient DHT receptor, just as in affected males, whereas the second cell line has normal DHT receptor.[32] This is the finding predicted for an X-linked trait by the Lyon hypothesis (p. 433; Fig. 40–5).

DEFECTS IN TRANSMEMBRANE TRANSPORT: CYSTINURIA

Cystinuria was one of the four disorders that Garrod spoke of as inborn errors of metabolism in his famous lectures in 1908.[4] Although the other three—alkaptonuria, albinism, and pentosuria—are indeed the result of enzyme blocks, cystinuria is a defect in an active transport mechanism in the renal tubule. Because of the mutation-determined defect, four basic amino acids—cystine, lysine, arginine, and ornithine—are imperfectly reabsorbed from the glomerular filtrate. Of these amino acids, cystine is relatively insoluble in urine, particularly acid urine, so that cystine stones form in the urinary tract. These stones are radiopaque by virtue of their high content of sulfur. The diagnosis of cystinuria is made by finding the characteristic hexagonal, platelike cystine crystals in the urine, and by a positive cyanide nitroprusside test on the urine. (Homocystine also gives a positive test; the two amino acids are distinguished by other methods such as high-voltage paper chromatography. Homocystinuria is not accompanied by urolithiasis, because homocystine is more soluble in urine than cystine and is excreted in lower amounts.) The defect in cystinuria and in some other renal tubular transport defects can be demonstrated in the intestinal mucosa as well.

Heterogeneity in cystinuria is demonstrated by the fact that in some families only homozygotes have an abnormal secretion of amino acids. In these families cystinuria is recessive. In other families, heterozygotes (e.g., both parents of affected persons as well as half the sibs and offspring) excrete cystine and lysine (but usually not the other two amino acids) in intermediate amounts, and some heterozygotes develop cystine urinary stones. Evidence indicates that the genes responsible for these two forms of cystinuria are alleles, i.e., are at the same genetic locus, and genetic compounds have been observed.

The treatment of cystine urolithiasis consists of maintenance of large urine volumes and alkaline pH. Penicillamine has also been used, on the rationale of the solubility of the mixed disulfide, cysteine-penicillamine.

Other genetic defects in transport mechanisms concern phosphate (hereditary hypophosphatemia, or vitamin-D-resistant rickets), glucose (renal glycosuria), and hydrogen ion (renal tubular acidosis).

HERITABLE DISORDERS OF CONNECTIVE TISSUE[29]

The mucopolysaccharidoses, discussed earlier as lysosomal diseases, are one class among the heritable disorders of connective tissue, since they concern one of the important elements of connective tissue, mucopolysaccharides. The fibrous elements of connective tissue—collagens and elastic fibers—are involved in the Marfan syndrome, the Ehlers-Danlos syndromes, cutis laxa, osteogenesis imperfecta, and pseudoxanthoma elasticum. Collagen is damaged by accumulating metabolites in homocystinuria (to produce a clinical picture simulating Marfan syndrome in many ways) and in alkaptonuria (to produce a characteristic arthropathy).

The Marfan Syndrome

Although the basic defect is not yet known, it is clearly a unitary one (because the Marfan syndrome is mendelian, specifically autosomal dominant) and involves the fibrous elements of connective tissue (witness the pathology of the disease). Abnormalities occur in three domains: 1) Ectopia lentis is the hallmark of ocular involvement but is found in only about three-fourths of cases. Myopia and retinal detachment are other ocular features. 2) The skeletal features include long thin limbs, giving excessive height, abnormally low ratio of upper segment to lower segment, arm span greater than height, and "spider fin-

gers" (arachnodactyly). The joints are often abnormally loose, and scoliosis is severe in many. 3) Weakness of the aortic media is the most frequent life-imperiling cardiovascular feature, but "floppy mitral valve" (the Barlow or click–murmur syndrome) is frequent, and some patients have profound mitral regurgitation.

Largely because the basic defect is not known, there is no specific laboratory test for the diagnosis of the Marfan syndrome. It remains a clinical diagnosis. Detection of ectopia lentis can help confirm the suspected diagnosis, but as noted earlier it is not always present; furthermore, ectopia lentis occurs with other conditions such as homocystinuria (see later) and the Weill-Marchesani syndrome (short stature and stiff joints with lens subluxation, an autosomal recessive). Enlargement of the aortic root by echography also supports the diagnosis of the Marfan syndrome but this finding may not be present at an early stage of the patient's disease. Family study, which should be done also for the practice of preventive medicine, can confirm the diagnosis if a history of dissecting aneurysm is obtained or if a relative is found with ectopia lentis or other clear signs of Marfan syndrome.

The aorta in the Marfan syndrome is prone to dilatation at the root and in the ascending portion, and dissection with rupture can occur. As a rule the first part to undergo progressive dilatation is that within the radiographic silhouette of the heart. Hence, because of involvement of the sinuses of Valsalva appreciable aortic regurgitation may precede aortic dilatation of a degree evident to ordinary radiographic study. Echography is a useful noninvasive means of detecting this dilatation. Dissecting aneurysm rarely, it seems, develops "out of the blue," but rather in an aorta that has already undergone dilatation. Dissections are most often of the Debakey type II (limited to the ascending aorta) but Debakey type I (extending throughout the length of the aorta) and Debakey type III (involving the aorta distal to the left subclavian) have been encountered.

Propranolol, a β-adrenergic blocker, may have usefulness in staying the progress of aortic dilatation and averting dissection. The rationale is reduction in the abruptness and force of ventricular ejection. Surgical replacement of the ascending aorta and aortic valve is performed in patients with advanced changes in the aorta.

Patients with the Marfan syndrome require lifelong periodic evaluation. In prepubertal girls induction of puberty with estrogen–progesterone to limit height and shorten the period of maximal risk of scoliosis may be indicated. The state of the aorta should be evaluated annually by echogram in patients of all ages. The ocular features require regular check.

Homocystinuria

Homocystinuria is a Garrodian inborn error of metabolism and secondarily a heritable disorder of connective tissue. The diagnosis is made by demonstration of homocystine in the urine and confirmed by demonstration of the specific enzyme deficiency in cultured skin fibroblasts. The enzyme involved is cystathionine synthase (or synthetase), which catalyzes the condensation of homocysteine and serine to form cystathionine.

As in the Marfan syndrome, ectopia lentis is a leading feature. Whereas the lenses usually are displaced upward in the Marfan syndrome, they are characteristically dislocated downward in homocystinuria. Also, whereas ectopia lentis is present at birth in the Marfan syndrome (and may progress later), the ectopia lentis of homocystinuria is acquired, usually in the first years of life, but sometimes not until the 20's or later. Myopia is an ocular feature of homocystinuria that usually develops before ectopia lentis.

Skeletal features of homocystinuria include excessive height and deformity of the anterior thorax, as in Marfan syndrome, but the joints tend to be somewhat tight rather than loose. Osteoporosis is a feature limited to homocystinuria.

The cardiovascular complications of homocystinuria are thrombotic, not aortic as in the Marfan syndrome. Occlusion of the coronary, cerebral, or renal arteries occurs with the expected clinical consequences. Venous thrombosis and pulmonary embolism are also complications.

About half the patients with homocystinuria have mental retardation, a feature not found in Marfan syndrome.

As a group homocystinurics vary widely in severity, although within one family affected persons show about the same severity. The group variation, unusual for a recessive, is due to different, presumably allelic forms of cystathionine synthase deficiency. In one form some residual activity of the enzyme is found in cultured fibroblasts and the patients respond to vitamin B_6 (or pyridoxine, a cofactor for cystathionine synthase), in dosage of 100 mg a day or more, with clearing of homocystine from the urine, cessation of thrombotic accidents, and avoidance of ectopia lentis (if it has not already developed). This category of patient tends to be at the milder end of the spectrum; intelligence is usually normal.

Patients in a second group are more severely affected, have no detectable enzyme activity in cultured fibroblasts, and do not respond to pyridoxine. Restriction of methionine intake in the diet is the mainstay of therapy, supplemented by platelet-suppressing agents to prevent thrombosis.

Homocysteine and other sulfhydryl compounds that accumulate in homocystinuria interfere with cross-linking of collagen, probably by combining with the aldols formed from lysine and hydroxylysine residues in collagen as the first step in cross-linkage. Homocysteine has a close structural similarity to penicillamine, which has a similar effect on collagen cross-linkage, witness animal experiments and observations in patients given penicillamine for Wilson's disease, cystinuria, or rheumatoid arthritis. Endothelial denudation may underlie the thrombotic propensity of the disease. The mental defect of some homocystinurics may be related to a deficiency of brain cystathionine, as well as to intracranial thromboses.

The Ehlers-Danlos Syndromes

This group of disorders once thought to be a single entity, comprises at least eight separate disorders, in several of which a basic defect in collagen formation has been identified. In each of them laxity of joints and stretchability, bruisability, and fragility of skin tend to be features, although some of these are inconspicuous in certain of the types.

Types I and II are the classic varieties, in severe and mild form, respectively. They are autosomal dominant.

Type III, also called the benign hypermobility syndrome, is characterized mainly by striking loosejointedness. Floppy mitral valve may occur in this form as in all the others. It likewise is autosomal dominant.

Type IV (ecchymotic, arterial, or Sack-Barabas type) is a grave disorder because of proneness to spontaneous rupture of the gut and large arteries. The skin is unusually thin, with readily evident subcutaneous blood vessels, and tight over the face, ears, and fingers. Its fragility is evident from frequent breaks over the shins and other areas that are subject to blunt trauma. Loosejointedness is not striking except in the fingers. Rupture of the spleen from minor impact trauma, and rupture of the gut for no apparent reason occur. Large ecchymoses or hematomas result from minor trauma or muscle tears. Rupture without dissection occurs in large arteries such as the innominate. At surgery, tissue may have the tensile characteristics of wet blotting paper. Although there is evidence of heterogeneity from both mode of inheritance and from studies of the basic defect, one form of this clinical type is inherited as an autosomal recessive and as its basic defect has deficiency in synthesis of type III collagen.

Type V is an X-linked recessive with the features of classic Ehlers-Danlos. Some affected boys have severe mitral regurgitation. The defect is thought to lie in lysyl oxidase, the enzyme that catalyzes the first step in formation of collagen cross-links.

Type VI (the ocular-scoliotic form) has the cardinal features of Type I plus more severe scoliosis than observed in the other forms and (unique to this type) marked fragility of the eye globe leading to rupture of the cornea and sclera from minor blunt trauma and retinal detachment. Dissecting aneurysm of the aorta has been observed. Collagen in this type is deficient in hydroxylysine, because of deficiency of the specific hydroxylase that converts selected lysine residues in the protocollagen chain to hydroxylysine. Defective cross-linking of collagen results because hydroxylysine is, with lysine, involved in formation of cross-links. Like almost all other enzymopathies, this is an autosomal recessive.

Type VII (arthrochalasis multiplex congenita) is characterized by profound joint laxity (leading to congenital dislocation of the hips and repeated subluxation of other joints such as the shoulders), stretchable and bruisable skin, and short stature. The basic defect in Ehlers-Danlos VII is in cleavage of the extra piece off one end of the procollagen molecule at the time it is excreted from the cell of synthesis, the fibroblast. Intermolecular cross-linking of collagen in Ehlers-Danlos VII is apparently defective because persistence of the extra long procollagen does not permit stacking of molecules in proper register.

Both Ehlers-Danlos VI and Ehlers-Danlos VII have defects in posttranslational steps in protein synthesis, that is, steps in the processing of the protein after its amino acid chain is assembled on ribosomes. Posttranslational processing occurs for many other proteins and for peptide hormones such as proinsulin and proparathormone, although genetic defect in few of these others has yet been identified.

Ehlers-Danlos VIII combines the features of Ehlers-Danlos with periodontosis, a defect in the mooring of the teeth leading to early loss. An autosomal dominant form of Ehlers-Danlos with an unusually high frequency of dissecting aneurysm of the aorta may represent yet another distinct entity.

MENDELIAN MALFORMATION SYNDROMES[8]

Although the common solitary malformations such as cleft palate, cardiac malformations, and spina bifida are multifactorial, some malformation syndromes are mendelian. Autosomal dominant examples are Apert syndrome (acrocephalosyndactyly) and the Holt-Oram syndrome (Table 41–8). Autosomal recessive examples are the Ellis-van Creveld syndrome, cartilage–hair hypoplasia, and the Kartagener syndrome. An X-linked recessive example is aquaductal stenosis (leading to hydrocephalus) with adducted thumbs.

The molecular basis of few mendelian malformation syndromes is known. In the future, study of this aspect is likely to be as contributory to normal developmental biology as study of genetic defects have been to the understanding of normal physiology and biochemistry, e.g., of coagulation, intermediary metabolism, protein synthesis, transmembrane transport, lysosomes, cell surface receptors, etc. Some mendelian defects in sexual development are now understood, e.g., 1) testicular feminization (p. 459), 2) the masculinized external genitalia of females with the several adrenal hyperplasia syndromes, and 3) the female phenotype in males with defect or absence of the H-Y gene(s), carried by the Y chromosome and normally controlling differentiation of the testes.[36]

The molecular defect in the Kartagener syndrome is likewise known. This autosomal recessive malformation syndrome comprises dextrocardia (situs inversus viscerum), bronchiectasis, sinusitis, and male infertility.[18] Bronchial cilia and sperm show, by electron microscopy, a morphologic defect in dynein, which is essential to the motor function of cilia and the sperm tail. Thus, bronchiectasis, sinusitis, and male infertility have ready explanations. Ciliated endothelium (or at least microtubules) may be involved in rotation of cardiovascular anlagen in early development. The dextrocardia may be lacking in as many as half of cases of the immobile cilia syndrome.

CHAPTER 42
Pharmacogenetics
VICTOR A. McKUSICK

Pharmacogenetics is concerned with the relationship between genetic constitution and drug effects. Particularly clear examples are the gene-determined differences[19] in the metabolism of isonicotinoyl hydrazide (isoniazid or INH), the hemolytic anemia induced by

primaquine and other drugs in persons with a defect in red cell G6PD, and hemolytic anemia induced by sulfonamides and other drugs in patients with hemoglobin Zurich.[15] The intolerance for certain substances demonstrated by patients with porphyria is another example of gene–drug interaction. Two examples from anesthesiology are succinylcholine apnea (pseudocholinesterase deficiency causing prolonged muscle paralysis) and malignant hyperpyrexia, often fatal, precipitated by any one of many anesthetic agents.

Among the examples cited, two aspects of pharmacogenetics are recognized. In connection with INH, genetic differences in the metabolism of the drug result in its having different effects in patients. In connection with primaquine sensitivity, succinylcholine sensitivity and malignant hyperpyrexia, drugs, although not metabolized in an unusual way, have abnormal effects in some persons because of their genetic peculiarity.

The pharmacogenetics of INH and primaquine sensitivity (G6PD deficiency), discussed next, is particularly instructive. They are, however, the exceptions rather than the rule. Most differences in the way drugs are handled and most differences in reactions to drugs are graded characters and probably multifactorial.

Genetic Differences in the Metabolism of INH

A number of pharmacologic agents, of which INH, a drug used in the treatment of tuberculosis, was the first to be studied from this point of view, are acetylated by a mechanism that shows genetic polymorphism.[19] About one-half of all Caucasians are rapid acetylators and one-half are slow acetylators. Slow acetylation is autosomal recessive. These phenotypes are sometimes referred to as rapid- and slow-inactivation, because the acetylated form of INH is chemotherapeutically ineffective.

Rapid acetylators get less adequate treatment of their tuberculosis from a given dosage of INH. On the other hand, slow-acetylators are more likely to develop peripheral neuropathy because of high concentration of free INH. In practice, the genetic difference in rate of INH inactivation is usually not determined in the patient who is to receive antituberculous therapy with this agent, because INH is administered in adequate dosage to treat a tuberculous infection even in a rapid-inactivator, and pyridoxine (vitamin B_6) is administered concurrently to prevent neuropathy.

Glucose 6-Phosphate Dehydrogenase (G6PD) Deficiency

A defect of G6PD is present in the erythrocytes of many Americans of African and Mediterranean origin. This disorder is inherited as an X-linked recessive, its frequency being about 10 percent in American black males and about 1 percent in black females.

The red cell enzyme defect is no apparent impediment to the patient unless some exogenous factor is superimposed. The disorder was detected in Mediterranean peoples because of the widespread consumption of fava beans and in American blacks when primaquine was given for antimalarial prophylaxis during military service. The clinical picture is that of acute hemolytic anemia following ingestion of the agent by persons with the enzyme deficiency. Hemoglobinuria, anemia, jaundice, fever, leukocytosis, and renal failure can all result, and the acute episode may be fatal.

Young erythrocytes of G6PD-deficient persons have near-normal concentrations of G6PD, but as the red cells age the enzyme decreases more rapidly than is normal and disappears relatively early in the red cell life span.

The long list of agents incriminated as factors precipitating hemolytic anemia includes such common medicaments as aspirin. Viral infections may also precipitate hemolytic crises, although the evidence is not conclusive, since antipyretic and other agents are usually administered in such cases. In the newborn infant who is G6PD-deficient, hemolysis may be induced by the administration of some vitamin K preparations, by some agent taken by the mother before delivery, or by chemicals reaching the baby through the mother's milk.

In many populations of Africa, Sardinia, Sicily, and Greece, as well as among Sephardic and Iraqi Jews, its high frequency qualifies G6PD-deficiency as a genetic polymorphism. Like the sickle gene, the G6PD-deficiency gene probably owes its high frequency to protection against malaria that it bestows on either the hemizygous male or the heterozygous female.

G6PD-deficiency provides yet another example of heterogeneity in genetic disease. The disease affecting Africans differs from that affecting Mediterranean peoples in that enzyme concentrations in the erythrocytes are not as low, and decreased G6PD activity in the leukocytes and some other tissues does not occur as it does in the Mediterranean form of the disease. Furthermore, the enzyme deficiency in blacks is accompanied by an electrophoretic peculiarity of the enzyme protein.

Some rare mutations in the G6PD molecule cause chronic nonspherocytic hemolytic anemia independent of drug exposure. About 200 mutant variants of G6PD have been identified by electrophoretic and other means. G6PD rivals hemoglobin as a demonstration of the biochemical diversity of man.

CHAPTER 43

Immunogenetics

VICTOR A. McKUSICK

BLOOD GROUPS

The blood groups (Table 43-1) share with the hemogloblins the distinction of having contributed greatly to the formulation of principles of human genetics and of genetics in general.[5] Blood groups are, furthermore, of great significance in medicine. The success of major surgery, the saving of life from exsanguinating disease or trauma, and the prevention of the congenital abnormalities or fetal loss resulting from maternofetal incompatibility illustrate their important practical role.

Most of the blood groups are genetically determined variations in certain components of the red cell membrane. However, the Lewis system antigens are adsorbed on the surface of the erythrocyte. At least 12 different blood group systems, each determined by a separate locus, have been identified.

The different antigens on the red cells are identified by means of antibodies, proteins in serum that combine with the antigens and produce such effects as agglutination of the red cells. Some of the antibodies occur "naturally"—e.g., in the ABO blood group system: group A persons have in their serum antibody against group B cells; group B persons have antibody against group A cells, and group O persons have antibody against both group A and group B cells. These "natural" antibodies are probably the result of immunization by A-like or B-like antigens that are widely distributed in nature—e.g., in foods of plant origin. Because of natural antibodies, Landsteiner in 1900 was able to demonstrate the ABO blood types simply by mixing the serum and red cells of different persons.

To demonstrate the antigens of other blood groups, it is necessary to obtain the corresponding antibody by one of two methods. In the case of MN blood groups, the antibody was produced in another species, the rabbit, by injecting human red blood cells. Rabbits injected with cells from persons of the MM genotype produced anti-M serum; cells from persons of the NN genotype stimulated production of anti-N serum. Cells from persons of the MN genotype—i.e., heterozygotes—were agglutinated by either anti-M or anti-N rabbit serum.

The other method by which antibodies demonstrating blood groups are formed is the accidental development of antibody by a pregnant woman or a transfused patient. If the mother lacks a red cell antigen that is present in the fetus (who inherited it from the father), the mother may develop antibodies against the antigen when fetal cells leak over into the mother's circulation. Most of the Rh blood groups, as well as several of the other blood group systems, were discovered in the study of cases of maternofetal incompatibility. A situation which in principle is exactly the same is that in which a patient is transfused with red cells containing an antigen he does not possess and develops a serum antibody against that antigen. The X-linked blood group Xg^a was discovered in this way.

The blood groups are inherited as codominant traits; in the heterozygote, such as the AB person, both blood types are demonstrable. In many instances—in fact, so often that it is now considered a general principle—an antibody is eventually discovered for both antigens present in the heterozygote. Thus, in the Kell system, an antiserum was first discovered that agglutinated the red cells from persons of the genotype KK or Kk but not of persons of genotype kk. Later an antiserum was found that agglutinated the red cells from persons of the genotype Kk or kk, but not KK.

The Rhesus (Rh) system is the most complex one identified in man. A transatlantic controversy has raged over whether multiple allelism or close linkage accounts for certain aspects of the diversity.[5] Specifically, Fisher and Race in England suggested that three closely linked loci are responsible for the Rh specificities that they call D, C, and E (in the order of their postulated order on the chromosome). On the other hand, Wiener in this country was of the view that a single, complex locus with many alleles is involved.[5]

The Rh blood group system has been extensively studied, mainly because the Rh_o (D) antigen is the most antigenic outside the ABO system and hence of great clinical significance.

MATERNOFETAL INCOMPATIBILITY[5]

Maternofetal incompatibility for the ABO blood groups may lead to early fetal death and abortion. It has been estimated that as many as 5 percent of con-

TABLE 43-1

Clinical Significance of Blood Group Systems in Man

System	Common Antibodies	General Type	Frequency	Transfusion Reaction	HDN*
ABO	Anti-A	Natural	Regularly	Yes	Yes
	Anti-B	Natural	Present	Yes	Yes
Rh	Anti-Rho (D)	Immune	Common	Yes	Yes
	Anti-rh'' (E)	Immune	Unusual	Yes	Yes
	Anti-rh' (C)	Immune	Unusual	Yes	Yes
Kell	Anti-Kell	Immune	Unusual	Yes	Yes
Duffy	Anti-Fy^a	Immune	Unusual	Yes	Yes
Kidd	Anti-Jk^a	Immune	Rare	Yes	Yes
Lewis	Anti-Le^a	Natural	Common	No	No
P	Anti-P$_1$	Natural	Common	No	No
Lutheran	Anti-Lu^a	Immune	Rare	No	No
MNSs	Anti-M	Natural	Rare	No	No
	Anti-S	Immune	Rare	Yes	Yes
	Anti-s	Immune	Rare	Yes	Yes

* HDN = hemolytic disease of newborn.

ceptions are lost through ABO incompatibility. This phenomenon is not surprising, since the type O mother, for example, has natural antibody against type A and B antigens of fetal red cells and other tissues, including, perhaps, the placenta, which is largely of fetal genotype.

In the Rh system, unlike the ABO bloodgroup system, the mother does not naturally carry antibodies against the Rh antigens that she does not possess. Trouble develops only if the mother becomes sensitized to what for her is a foreign antigen entering her system in the form of red cells from a fetus that contains a different Rh antigen through inheritance from the father. Sensitization of the mother is accomplished by actual bleeding from the fetus into the mother. Sensitive methods based on the demonstration of red cells containing fetal hemoglobin can detect the presence of very small amounts of fetal blood distributed in the mother's circulation. In subsequent pregnancies, if the fetus is again incompatible, the mother's titer of anti-Rh antibody may rise briskly, maternal antibody may cross the placenta to the fetus and the damaging effect on the infant may result in the characteristic clinical picture of hemolytic disease of the newborn (HDN), which can take the form of erythroblastosis fetalis, hydrops fetalis, or icterus neonatorum.

About 15 percent of Caucasians are Rh negative.

HDN would be much more frequent than it is if no other factors were involved. One factor is undoubtedly the low frequency of occurrence of sufficiently large feto-maternal bleeds; many Rh incompatible pregnancies pass without their occurrence. Another important factor protecting against Rh sensitization is accompanying ABO incompatibility. If the red blood cells that bleed from the fetus to the mother are of an ABO blood type different from the mother's, the natural antibody of the mother is likely to destroy them before they can incite sensitization.

The main offender in the Rh type of HDN has been D. It has much greater antigenic propensities than the antigens C and E and the greatest of any blood group other than the ABO groups. Furthermore, the frequencies of the different Rh groups allow greater opportunity for this strong antigen to cause clinical disease. Obviously, once HDN has occurred, the risk that future children of an Rh-negative mother and an Rh-positive father will develop erythroblastosis is 100 percent if the father is DD but is only 50 percent if he is Dd. Since in various populations some CDE combinations are more frequent than others, an estimate of whether the father is DD or Dd can be obtained from the reactions with anti-C, anti-c, anti-E, and anti-e antiserums. (Unfortunately no anti-d antiserum is available.) For example, if the father is an Englishman and reacts to anti-C, anti-D, and anti-e, but not to anti-c and anti-E, he must have CDe on one chromosome. The other chromosome may carry either CDe or Cde. Since in English populations CDe is about 41 times more common than Cde, it is likely that the man is homozygous DD (i.e., CDe/CDe).

The Rh-incompatible pregnancies most likely to lead to sensitization of the mother—those in which fetal bleeds occur into the maternal circulation—are identifiable by the demonstration of red cells containing fetal hemoglobin in the mother's blood. Such fetal bleeds are most likely to occur in late pregnancy, especially with trauma to the placenta—e.g., with forceps delivery. These observations, taken together with the natural protection afforded by ABO incompatibility, suggested that immunologic inactivation of the fetal Rh-positive red cells which leak into the mother's circulation by giving Rh antibody ("Rho-Gam") at the proper time and in the proper dosage might be a useful therapeutic approach. The approach is now fully validated and is routinely used.

HISTOCOMPATIBILITY

In addition to the ABO locus, the important histocompatibility locus in man is HLA (so-called because it is studied in human lymphocytes; A means it was the first human leukocyte locus to be designated). The HLA "locus" is in fact a region (on the short arm of chromosome 6) containing at least four separate loci, HLA-A, HLA-B, HLA-C, and HLA-D, and referred to as the Major Histocompatibility Complex (MHC). Any one person has eight HLA alleles, two at each of the four loci. The set of HLA alleles on one chromosome is referred to as a haplotype. Usually only the alleles at the two best studied loci HLA-A and HLA-B are stated. For example, HLA-Al-B8 is a frequent haplotype of Caucasians. Diversity of the HLA region is enormous. Over 30 HLA-A alleles and about 40 HLA-B alleles have been identified. Since theoretically any one of the HLA-A types may be combined with any one of the HLA-B types (or any HLA-C or -D type) the potential number of different haplotypes is enormous.

In a single family, because of the large number of different haplotypes in the population, the parents are likely to have, between them, four different ones—let us call them E, F, G and H—the father being EF and the mother GH. The offspring will be of four different types: EG, EH, FG, and FH. The chance of two sibs being of identical HLA constitution is 25 percent. The parent and child can be of identical HLA constitution only if the two parents happen to have at least one haplotype in common. For this reason, sib–sib renal transplants are more frequently successful than parent–sib transplants. (Actually more than four HLA constitutions may be found among sibs because although the HLA-A, -B, -C, and -D loci are closely linked they are still subject to low frequency recombination through crossing over during meiosis in the parents.)

HLA typing is done by serologic and cellular techniques. Antisera for identifying HLA types, especially HLA-A and HLA-B types, are derived mainly from multiparous women or multitransfused patients. Cytotoxic effects of the antiserum on lymphocytes are observed. The cellular techniques include that of mixed lymphocyte culture (MLC) and are used particularly for HLA-D types. When mixed with lymphocytes from a person of different type, lymphocytes are stimulated to mitosis in a manner similar to the effects of the nonspecific mitogen phytohemagglutinin. The reagent, or reference, cell line can be pretreated with mitomycin C to inhibit mitosis, without impairing its antigenic, i.e., mitogenic, properties toward the cell whose type is being tested. Thus, all increased mitotic activity in the mixed lymphocyte culture is attributable to the cell line under test and can be used as an index of incompatibility. Serologically determined B-lymphocyte types may actually represent the same locus as that tested by the MLC methods (HLA-D). However, until this is proved it is referred to as HLA-DR (for D-related). The D locus is of special interest because of possible homology to the immune response (Ir) locus in the H2 complex of mouse (the major histocompatibility complex equivalent to the HLA complex in man).

HLA typing is useful in kidney transplantation. Kidneys from HLA identical sibs enjoy almost 100 percent survival; kidneys from sibs that share only one haplotype fare less well; and kidneys from a sib with two different HLA haplotypes fare least well.

In the United States' experience, kidneys from HLA identical but unrelated donors fare little better than do HLA-unlike cadaver kidneys. In the experience in Europe, appropriate HLA match does correlate with survival of the transplanted kidney. The discrepancy between intrafamilial usefulness of HLA match and the populational experience may be explained by the existence of other significant histocompatibility loci in the HLA region or elsewhere in the genome. Possibly, greater homogeneity of European populations is responsible for the differences in American and European results.

The *raison d'être* of the histocompatibility antigens is not entirely clear. Possibilities are that they are structural elements of the cell membrane or receptors for specific substances and only incidentally have immunologic properties and diversity. Surveillance against cancer would be one possible biologic usefulness of this diversity. If somatic mutation or chromosomal change underlies malignancy, alteration in cell surface antigens might be expected. Recognized as nonself, such cells might be destroyed by the body's immune mechanisms. A high order of complexity in cell surface antigens, in terms of the number of loci and perhaps heterozygosity at each, would be favored in evolution by any such function.

Marker-and-Disease Association

Blood group and disease associations were identified in the 1950s. Persons of blood type O have an increased risk of peptic ulcer of the duodenum (about 1.5 times the risk of non-O persons) and persons who are also secretor-negative (do not secrete ABO blood group substance into the saliva) have a risk almost 2.5 times that of non-O, secretor persons. The basis of this (and other) blood group and disease association is not genetic linkage. The O nonsecretor association with peptic ulcer has been observed in all ethnic groups. Genetic linkage produces no permanent association of traits in a population. Genetic linkage cannot account for either syndromes or marker-disease association. Rather, blood-group-and-disease associations have their basis in the pleiotropic effect of a particular alleles.

An intimate association between a particular Duffy blood type and resistance to tertian malaria is now known. In the past when fever therapy, specifically malaria therapy, was used for central nervous system syphilis it was known that tertian malaria usually did not "take" in blacks; quartan malaria was used instead. The reason for the resistance to tertian malaria is now known to be the almost 100 percent frequency of the Duffy-null (Fy°) gene in West Africans. The Duffy a or Duffy b allele determines a cell-surface component that is essential for the *Plasmodium vivax* organism to penetrate red blood cells.[33] Duffy-null cells lack this component. The Duffy-null blood type achieved high frequency in West Africa because of the protection it afforded against vivax malaria.

Examples of association of disease with specific HLA types are now known. The most striking is that between HLA-B27 and ankylosing spondylitis. Almost all cases of ankylosing spondylitis are found to be B27; conversely any B27 male has about a 20 percent risk of developing ankylosing spondylitis of some degree. The finding suggests a central pathogenetic role of B27 in this disease; possibly the cell surface component of this specific antigenic characteristic is a specific receptor for an etiologic agent such as a virus.

Other less strong HLA–disease associations have been found. Several diseases which appear from other evidence to have important immunologic aspects to their pathogenesis, e.g., diabetes and myasthenia gravis, show strongest association with specific HLA-D alleles. In light of the suspected role of HLA-D in immune response, these findings take on special significance.

Genetic Immunodeficiencies

Another large aspect of immunogenetics concerns heritable defects in the immune mechanism: defects in immunoglobulins, cellular immunity, complement, and polymorphonuclear and macrophage function. Some of these are discussed elsewhere.

CHAPTER 44
Multifactorial Disorders
VICTOR A. McKUSICK

As indicated earlier, all disease is multifactorial. In all disorders, multiple genetic and nongenetic factors play some role even though it is a vanishing small one in some mendelian disorders. There are many common diseases, such as hypertension, atherosclerosis, cardiac malformations, emphysema, and peptic ulcer that "run in families" and in particular ethnic groups. A genetic background is indicated also by twin studies (comparisons of rate of concordance in monozygotic twins with that in like-sex dizygotic twins). Yet these conditions do not display simple mendelian pedigree patterns indicative of a monogenic basis. The genetic component of causation appears to be polygenic, i.e., there are multiple genes each contributing to the development of the disorder.

In the case of some disorders that have a quantifiable feature, such as hypertension and hypercholesterolemia, the multifactorial and possibly polygenic nature of the trait is indicated by the fact that the distribution of the variable, blood pressure and serum cholesterol, is unimodal. Measured in a population, the values show no separation into two or more classes. Where on the distribution curve for blood pressure or cholesterol an individual falls depends on the particular assortment of genes the individual inherits from his parents and the environment in which those genes function.

In connection with congenital malformations a threshold model is conceptually useful. Accumulation of a sufficient number of genetic and environmental risk factors, takes the individual above a threshold with resultant development of malformation.

Multifactorial or polygenic inheritance must not be confused with genetic heterogeneity. Diabetes, hypercholesterolemia, and hyperuricemia behave as multifactorial traits when viewed at the population level. At the family level, however, it is sometimes possible to identify a single gene locus that is mainly responsible for the disease in that family. Examples include MODY (maturity onset diabetes of the young), an autosomal dominant, hereditary hypercholesterolemia (p. 459), gout due to HGPRT deficiency (p. 456). Alpha$_1$-antitrypsin deficiency is responsible for some of the familial occurrence of emphysema. Hyperpepsinogenemic peptic ulcer is an autosomal dominant form of that disorder. Malformations of the heart and cleft lip-palate include some mendelian forms, although usually the simple inherited forms are malformation syndromes in which other pleiotropic effects of the gene reveal its unique nature. Examples are the Holt-Oram syndrome and the Ellis-van Creveld syndrome (see Table 41–8).

In due course one can anticipate that the specific biochemical function of each gene contributing to polygenic inheritance will be defined. The O-nonsecretor association with peptic ulcer indicates two loci that each make a small contribution to causation of the disease. Ankylosing spondylitis, a common disorder, is an illuminating case. It was at one time thought to be a male-influenced autosomal dominant. Then, multifactorial inheritance seemed more likely. With the discovery of the HLA-B27 association we came full circle. It can be viewed as a monogenic disease, or with equal or greater validity as a multifactorial disease. There are probably genetic factors in addition to HLA type; the reduced penetrance in female suggests this.

In genetic counseling of common disorders, recognition of a mendelian type is obviously important. Lacking that, one must rely on empirical figures for predicting risk of recurrence. To answer the question, for example, "What chance is there that our next child will have cleft palate like our first child?", it is necessary to have information on a large series of the same situation. In such a series, what is the proportion of affected children born after an index case, given that the parents and other close relatives are unaffected? For most congenital malformations, the answer to this question is a few percent (1 to 4 percent).

The empirical risk estimate is a sliding one. Whereas if three children with an autosomal recessive disorder have been born from normal parents the risk to a fourth born child is still one in four; the risk is increasingly greater for later born children in the case of more than one affected child with a common type of congenital malformation. The fact that more than one sib has been affected indicates that the parents carry particular constellations of genes that are likely to cause the malformation. For many malformations, empirical figures are now available for the recurrence risk depending on whether a single sib, a parent and child, two sibs, and so on, have been affected in the family.

REFERENCES

General References

1. Boyer, S.H. (ed.). Papers on Human Genetics. Englewood Cliffs, N.J., Prentice-Hall, 1963.
2. Grouchy, J. de and Turleau, C. Clinical Atlas of Human Chromosomes. New York, Wiley, 1977.
3. McKusick, V.A. Mendelian Inheritance in Man. Catalogs of Autosomal Dominant, Autosomal Recessive and X-linked Phenotypes, 5th ed. Baltimore, Johns Hopkins Press, 1978. (Here descriptions and bibliographic references concerning specific genetic entities can be found.)
4. McKusick, V.A. and Claiborne, R. (eds.). Medical Genetics. New York, Hospital Practice, 1973.
5. Race, R.R. and Sanger, R. Blood Groups in Man, 6th ed. London, Blackwell, 1975.
6. Riccardi, V.M. The Genetic Approach to Human Disease. New York, Oxford University Press, 1977.
7. Roberts, J.A.F. and Pembrey, M.E. An Introduction to Medical Genetics, 7th ed. New York, Oxford University Press, 1978.
8. Smith, D.W. Recognizable Patterns of Human Malformation, 2nd ed. Philadelphia, Saunders, 1976.
9. Stanbury, J.B., Wyngaarden, J.B., and Fredrickson, D.S. (eds.). The Metabolic Basis of Inherited Diseases, 4th ed. New York, McGraw-Hill, 1978.
10. Yunis, J.J. (ed.). New Chromosomal Syndromes. New York, Academic Press, 1977.

Additional References

11. Alper, C.A. The 'cure' of an inherited disease. (Editorial) J. Lab. Clin. Med., 92:497, 1978.

12. Amrhein, J.A., Meyer, W.J., III, Jones, H.W., Jr., and Migeon, C.J. Androgen insensitivity in man: evidence for genetic heterogeneity. Proc. Nat. Acad. Sci., 73:891, 1976.

13. Blass, J.P. and Gibson, G.E. Abnormality of a thiamine-requiring enzyme in patients with Wernicke-Korsakoff syndrome. N. Engl. J. Med., 297:1367, 1977.

14. Brown, M.S. and Goldstein, J.L. Familial hypercholesterolemia: genetic, biochemical, and pathophysiological considerations. Adv. Intern. Med., 20:273, 1975.

15. Bunn, H.F., Forget, B.G., and Ranney, H.M. Human Hemoglobins. Philadelphia, Saunders, 1977.

16. Cartwright, G.E. Diagnosis of treatable Wilson's disease. N. Engl. J. Med., 298:1347, 1978.

17. Edwards, C.Q., Carroll, M., Bray, P., and Cartwright, G. Hereditary hemochromatosis: diagnosis in siblings and children. N. Engl. J. Med., 297:7, 1977.

18. Eliasson, R., Mossberg, B., Conner, P., and Afzelius, B.A. The immobile-cilia syndrome: a congenital ciliary abnormality as an etiologic factor in chronic airway infections and male sterility. N. Engl. J. Med., 297:1, 1977.

19. Evans, D.A.P., McKusick, V.A., and Manley, K.A. The genetic control of isoniazid metabolism in man. Br. Med. J., 2:485, 1960.

20. Ezdinli, E.Z., Sokal, J.E., Crosswhite, L., and Sandberg, A.A. Philadelphia-chromosome-positive and -negative chronic myelocytic leukemia. Ann. Intern. Med., 72:175, 1970.

21. Gelfand, J.A., Sherins, R.J., Alling, D.W., and Frank, M.M. Treatment of hereditary angioedema with Danazol: reversal of clinical and biochemical abnormalities. N. Engl. J. Med., 295:1444, 1978.

22. Goldstein, J.L. and Brown, M.S. Familial hypercholesterolemia: pathogenesis of a receptor disease. Johns Hopkins Med. J., 143:8, 1978.

23. Holt, M. and Oram, S. Familial heart disease with skeletal malformations. Br. Heart J., 22:236, 1960.

24. Lamon, J.M., Frykholm, B.C., Bennett, M., and Tschudy, D.P. Prevention of acute porphyric attacks by intravenous haematin. Lancet, II:492, 1978.

25. Mabry, C.C., Denniston, J.C., Nelson, T.L. and Son, C.D. Maternal phenylketonuria: a cause of mental retardation in children without the metabolic defect. N. Engl. J. Med., 269:1404, 1963.

26. McKusick, V.A., Egeland, J.A., Eldridge, R., and Krusen, D. Dwarfism in the Amish. I. The Ellis-van Creveld syndrome. Bull. Johns Hopkins Hosp., 115:306, 1964.

27. ———. On lumpers and splitters, or the nosology of genetic disease. Perspect. Biol. Med., 12:298, 1969.

28. ———. Genetic factors in intestinal polyposis. JAMA, 182:271, 1962.

29. ———. Heritable Disorders of Connective Tissue, 4th ed. St. Louis, C.V. Mosby, 1972.

30. ———, Neufeld, E.F., and Kelly, T.E. The mycopolysaccharide storage diseases. Chapter 53 in Stanbury, Wyngaarden and Frederickson (9).

31. ——— and Ruddle, F.H. The status of the gene map of the human chromosomes. Science, 196:390, 1977.

32. Meyer, W., Migeon, B.R., and Migeon, C.J. A locus on the human X chromosome for dihydrotestosterone receptor and androgen insensitivity. Proc. Natl. Acad. Sci., 72:1469, 1975.

33. Miller, L.H., Mason, S.J., Clyde, D.F., and McGinnis, M.H. The resistance factor to *Plasmodium vivax* in blacks: the Duffy blood group genotype, FyFy. N. Engl. J. Med., 295:302, 1976.

34. Omenn, G.S. Prenatal diagnosis of genetic disorders. Science, 200:952, 1978.

35. Rowley, J.D. A new consistent chromosomal abnormality in chronic myelogenous leukemia identified by quinacrine fluorescence and Giemsa staining. Nature, 243:290, 1973.

36. Wachtel, S.S. H-Y antigen and genetics of sex determination. Science, 198:797, 1977.

37. Weatherall, D.J. and Clegg, G.B. The Thalassaemia Syndromes, 2nd ed. Philadelphia, F.A. Davis, 1972.

38. Winterbauer, R.H. Multiple telangiectasia, Raynaud's phenomenon, sclerodactyly, and subcutaneous calcinosis: a syndrome mimicking hereditary hemorrhagic telangiectasia. Bull. Johns Hopkins Hosp., 114:361, 1964.

39. Golbus, M.S., Loughman, W.D., Epstein, C.J., Halbasch, G., Stephens, J.D., and Hall, B.D. Prenatal genetic diagnosis in 3000 amniocenteses. N. Engl. J. Med., 300:157, 1979.

40. Powledge, T.M. and Fletcher, J. Guidelines for the ethical, social and legal issues in prenatal diagnosis. N. Engl. J. Med., 300:168, 1979.

SECTION SEVEN
Hematology
ALBERT H. OWENS, Jr.: SECTION EDITOR

INTRODUCTION

Patients with primary hemic disorders may seek medical help for a wide variety of complaints. Most common are symptoms caused by anemia (weakness, dyspnea), defective hemostasis (bleeding, bruising), abnormal cellular proliferation (lymphadenopathy, splenomegaly), or disordered immunity (infections, dysgammaglobulinemia). These clinical disorders may result from genetic or acquired abnormalities (or both acting in concert) which affect the proliferation and differentiation of the various cellular elements of the lymphoid and hematopoietic tissues, their proper functioning, or their normal survival. Since the hematopoietic and lymphoreticular cell systems are affected by alterations in vascular integrity or by the introduction of pathogens and toxins into the body, it is important that the physician distinguish between those responses which are physiologic and those disorders which reflect primary hemic abnormalities. For example, fever and lymphadenopathy are more likely the result of an infectious disease than an intrinsic lymphoreticular disorder.

Much of the nosology of contemporary hematology is based on methods for the identification and enumeration of the formed elements of the blood that were achieved some 50 to 75 years ago. In particular, several simple differential staining techniques led to a catergorization of cell types (erythrocytic, granulocytic, monocytic, megakaryocytic, etc.) in peripheral blood, bone marrow, lymphoid organs, and other tissues. Further, these techniques coupled with time-related biologic observations provided a beginning understanding of the embryologic derivation and histogenesis of these various cell types.[1]

During the past 20 years, there has been a rapid increase in knowledge related to the structure and function of the cells of the peripheral blood, the bone marrow, and the lymphoreticular system. The ontogeny of these cells and tissues is better understood. This has provided a broader appreciation of the normal functioning of mature erythrocytes, granulocytes, and megakaryocytes, as well as the various lymphoreticular cells. In addition, there is now a more specific understanding of the pathogenesis of many disease states and a more rational basis for their treatment.[10,70,72]

The continued renewal of the hemic cell systems depends on the presence of a normally responsive pool of pluripotential (uncommitted) stem cells (Fig. VII-1). These stem cells are capable of continuous and possibly unlimited self-replication. In response to specific stimuli, stem cells may differentiate along several distinctive lines. These responses are mediated by humoral stimuli and inhibitors as well as by cell–cell interactions within the tissue microenvironments of the stem cells.

Many of the hemic progenitor cells are committed to specified pathways of differentiation and maturation (e.g., erythrocytes, megakaryocytes, granulocytes) and to a restricted repertoire of physiologic functions (e.g., hemoglobin production, phagocytosis). While these progenitor cells are able to proliferate when immature, these cell lines are not capable of self-renewal per se. The several stem cell pools are the main loci of the physiologic controls of blood cell production.

Active hematopoiesis in the adult is confined to the intramedullary cavities of the centrally located bones. Thus, the bone marrow is one of the largest organs in the body. Each day it discharges around 200 billion erythrocytes, 175 billion platelets, and 105 billion granulocytes into the circulating blood. Further, the marrow serves as a storage depot for mature, functional granulocytes which are available for prompt mobilization.

Progenitor cells in the bone marrow are responsible for the production of monocytes and macrophages, also, and for the generation of uncommitted lymphocytes. In addition, the bone marrow functions as a major lymphoreticular organ and is an important site of antibody production as well as for the recognition and removal of aged, damaged, or abnormal cells.

Neither the pluripotent (uncommitted) nor the committed stem cells of the bone marrow can be distinguished by the usual morphologic methods. Indeed, they probably resemble small or medium-sized lymphocytes. However, stem cells with various biologic potentials can be separated by physical techniques and their characteristics can be appreciated by means of various in vivo "transplantation" assays or through in vitro culture techniques (Table VII–1). For example, multipotent stem cells may be identified by their ability to effect lymphohematopoietic restoration in lethally irradiated mice or by the formation of erythrocytic, granulocytic, megakaryocytic, or mixed colonies in their spleens following the intravenous infusion of small numbers of bone marrow cells. Thus, these stem cells are called colony forming units-spleen (CFU-S). Granulocyte-monocytic committed stem cells may be identified through culture on semisolid media (CFU-C). Erythrocyte committed stem cells may be identified by culture on agar or in a fibrin clot and by their responsiveness to erythropoietin (CFU-E).

The lymphoreticular system is comprised of the bone marrow, the spleen, the thymus, the lymph nodes, the tonsils, and the various aggregations of lymphocytes and macrophages which are distributed widely throughout the body mainly in subendothelial or subepithelial locations. The principal functions of these cell systems are phagocytosis (motile and fixed tissue macrophages) and humoral and cellular immunity (lymphocytes).

While lymphoreticular cells share a common ancestry with other hemic cells in the pluripotent stem cell of the bone marrow, in adult life the various cell types are likely maintained by self-replicating stem cell pools committed to restricted pathways of differentiation and maturation. Various humoral and microenvironmental factors modulate the proliferation and physiologic function of these lymphoreticular cells. For example, monocytes are produced in the bone marrow, stimulated by a macrophage-made substance (colony-stimulating activity). While relatively immature, they are released into the peripheral blood. In various tissues (microen-

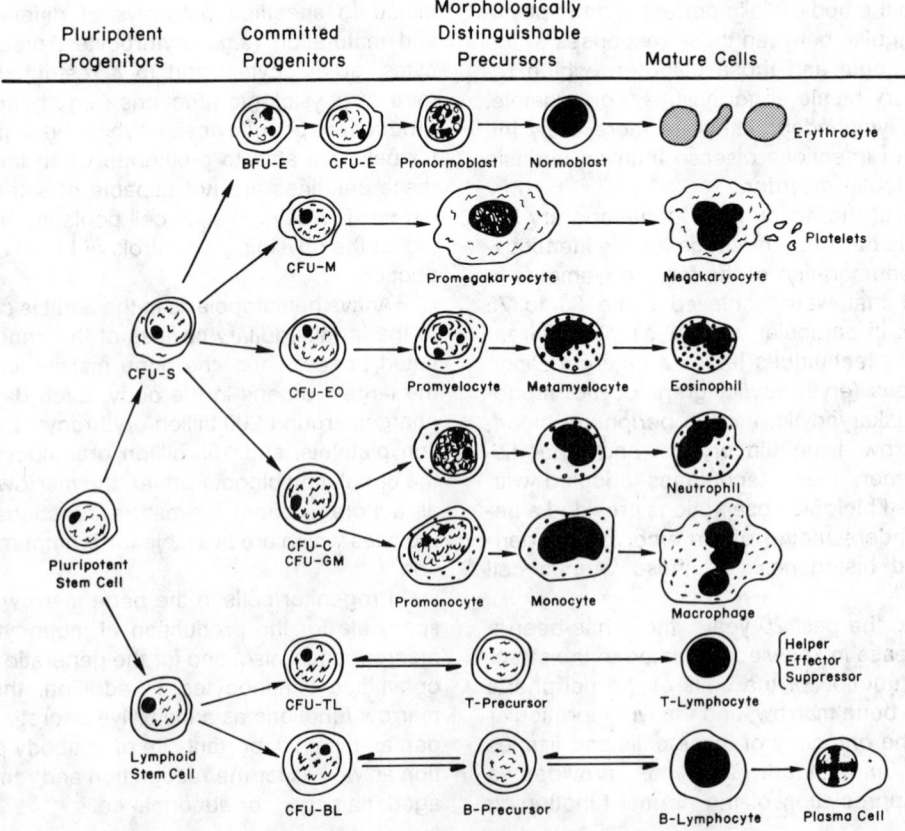

FIGURE VII-1. The cytogeneology of blood cells.

vironments), specialized "fixed" macrophages arise from these motile marrow-produced monocytes (e.g., splenic macrophages, pulmonary alveolar macrophages, and the Kupfer cells of the liver).

Normally, the peripheral blood compartment contains nearly all of the mature and functionally active erythrocytes and platelets (Table VII–2). In contrast, the granulocytes, monocyte–macrophages, and lymphocytes encountered in the peripheral blood are usually in transit to various tissue sites. The granulocytes (neutrophils, eosinophils, and basophils) are relatively mature, but perform their main functions in extravascular sites. The monocytes are relatively immature and

they undergo further cell division and maturation of function in various tissues. The lymphocytes encountered in the peripheral blood certainly are a heterogeneous population. Some are functionally undifferentiated but are able to respond to a great variety of nonself antigens. Other lymphocytes are "well differentiated," resting cells that may produce antibody or engage in various cell-mediated immune responses. (From another perspective they are "stem cells" which are responsive to specific "-poietins.") Indeed, it is likely that a small proportion of the "small lymphocytes" found in the peripheral blood are, in fact, pluripotent hematopoietic stem cells.

Cellular interactions are especially important

TABLE VII–1
Presently Defined Stages of Hematopoiesis

Stage	Characteristics	Terminology
I. Pluripotent progenitors	Unlimited self-replication Potential for differentiation along multiple cell lines Identified by bioassay	Pluripotent stem cell Colony forming unit-spleen (CFU–S)
II. Committed progenitors	Restricted self-replication Restricted differentiation Identified by bioassay	Unipotent stem cell Colony forming unit-erythroid (CFU–E) Burst forming unit-erythroid (BFU–E) Colony forming unit-megakaryocyte (CFU–M) Colony forming unit-culture (CFU–C) or Colony forming unit-granulocyte and monocyte (CFU–GM) Colony forming unit-eosinophil (CFU–Eo) Colony forming unit-T Lymphocyte (CFU–TL)

TABLE VII–1 (cont.)

Stage	Characteristics	Terminology
		Colony forming unit-B Lymphocyte (CFU–BL)
III. Morphologically distinguishable precursors	Develops into a single mature cell type Distinguishable by ordinary stains or by immuno- or histochemical techniques	Pronormoblast, normoblast Promonocyte Promyelocyte (neutrophilic, eosinophilic, basophilic) Promegakaryocyte T-lymphocyte precursor B-lymphocyte precursor
IV. Mature hemic cells	Nondividing, mature cells Performs physiologic functions according to cell type Distinguishable by ordinary stains, by immuno- or histochemical techniques, or by tests of physiologic function	Erythrocyte Monocyte; tissue macrophage Granulocyte, neutrophilic Granulocyte, eosinophilic Granulocyte, basophil; tissue mast cell Megakaryocyte; platelet T lymphocytes (helper, effector or suppressor cells) B lymphocytes (memory cells, plasma cells)

TABLE VII–2
Development and Functions of Hemic Cells

	Erythrocytes	Platelets	Granulocytes	Monocytes	Lymphocytes
Production Site	Bone marrow	Bone marrow megakaryocytes	Bone marrow production and storage	Bone marrow; multiple tissues	T cells: thymus and peripheral tissues B cells: marrow and peripheral tissues
Stimulators	Erythropoietin Thyroxin Corticosteroids Androgens Somatotropin		Colony-stimulating activity	Colony-stimulating activity	Processed antigen T-helper cells T cells: thymus hormones, thymus environment, transfer factor, somatotropin B cells: marrow environment, bursa equivalent influence
Inhibitors			Granulocytic chalone? Prostaglandin E		T cells: adrenal corticosteroids B cells: T-suppressor cell, specific antibody
Life span	120 days	3 days	Hours to days	Hours to months	Short-lived: days Long-lived B (memory) cells: months to years
Forms in blood	Reticulocyte	Platelet	Neutrophil Eosinophil Basophil Cells in transit from marrow to tissues	Immature monocytes in transit to tissues; some recirculate	Long-lived cells recirculate; most short-lived cells do not
Forms in tissues			Mature forms move through tissues Mast cells	Mature forms are motile and fixed Fixed macrophages are specialized by tissue site	
Functions	Oxygen transport Carbon dioxide transport	Hemostasis Blood clotting	Phagocytosis and lysosomal enzyme release Basophils produce heparin and histamine Eosinophils make chemotactic factor	Phagocytosis and lysosomal enzyme release Antigen processing CSA production	T-helper cells T-effector cells T-suppressor cells Transfer of cell mediated immunity B-antibody-producing cells B-memory cells Lymphokine production
Disposition	Aged and damaged cells are destroyed in spleen and tissues	Liver, spleen	Various tissues	Various tissues	Various tissues

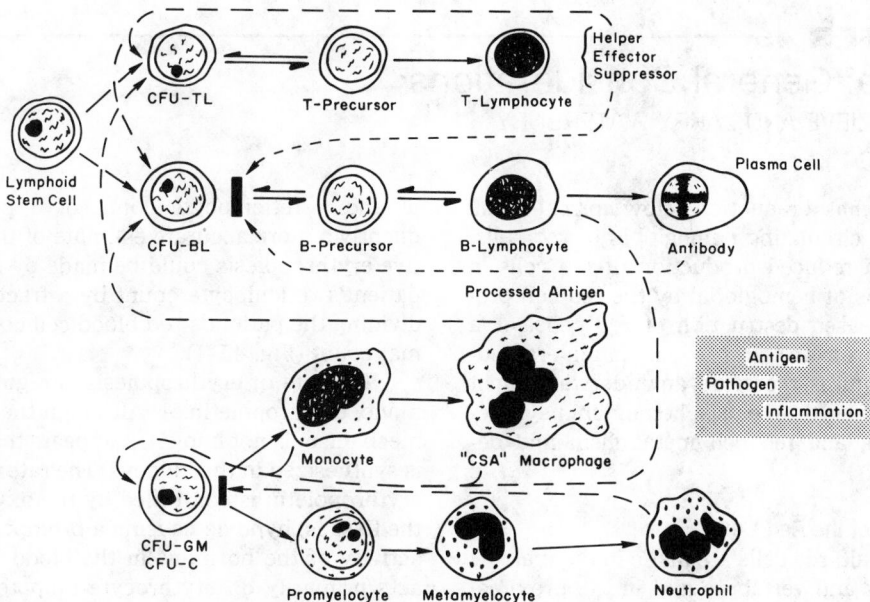

FIGURE VII-2. Controls of blood cell development.

to the physiologic integrity of the lymphoreticular cell systems. Some appreciation of these interactions may be gained by recalling a simplified version of the sequence of events which is set in motion when (wandering) neutrophils and macrophages encounter a pathogen which has penetrated a normal tissue barrier (Fig. VII-2). Likely, the macrophages will attempt to engulf the pathogen. Also, they will produce a "-poietin" (colony stimulating acitivity-CSA or CSF) which stimulates the appropriate stem cell pool to increased granulocytopoiesis and monocytopoiesis. The mature granulocytes (neutrophils) will attack the pathogen by means of phagocytosis and lysosomal enzymes. Further, they will produce a substance (chalone) which will oppose the action of CSA and exert an inhibitiory influence on granulocytopoiesis and monocytopoiesis.

Macrophages also provide a major stimulus to lymphopoiesis. By "processing antigen," they induce proliferation of T- and B-cell precursors that have been derived from uncommitted bone marrow progenitors and "influenced" by thymic or bone marrow environments.

These stimulated T cells may perform a helper function in further antigen recognition or by augmenting antibody production. T cells may also become "killer" cells capable of direct cytotoxic actions or they may produce lymphokines such as transfer factor (which recruits more un-

committed lymphocytes to the specific response) and migration inhibition factor (which causes more macrophages to localize in the pathogen-affected tissue site). T cells, in part, also perform a suppressor function by inhibiting the continuing proliferation of B cells.

While this oversimplified account does not do justice to the existing specific knowledge in this field, it is hoped that it will be indicative of the complex cellular and humoral interactions characteristic of one segment of the lymphoreticular system, and likely all of the hemic cell systems. Now one can begin to consider the complex pathogenesis of the various disorders of the blood cell systems from a newer perspective. Clearly the diagnostic tests of the future will include assessments of the functional and proliferative capabilities of the various cell lines, of the several stem cell pools, of the humoral stimulators and inhibitors, and of the appropriate cellular and microenvironmental influences. One can consider a potentially more specific rationale for therapy. The aplastic anemia that is perpetuated by a systemic inhibitor will be approached differently from an aplastic anemia due to defective stem cells. Perhaps some of the hyperproliferative disorders of the lymphoreticular system one day will be controlled more effectively by supplying a missing inhibitor or suppressor cell function or by restoring a necessary (maturing) microenvironmental influence.

CHAPTER 45

Anemia: General Considerations

PHILIP D. ZIEVE AND LARRY WATERBURY

Anemia is defined as a reduction below normal in the concentration of circulating hemoglobin or red cells. It results from a reduced production of red cells, a reduced synthesis of hemoglobin by the red cell precursors, an increased destruction of red cells, or a loss of red cells from the circulation. An understanding of anemia requires, therefore, an understanding of the physiology of erythropoiesis, hemoglobin synthesis and function, and red cell metabolism and destruction.

Production of the Red Cell[10]

In the normal adult, red cells are made in the marrow of the flat bones and vertebrae and in the proximal ends of the long bones. Pluripotential stem cells in the marrow have the capacity to differentiate into precursor cells for at least the three major cell lines: erythrocytes, granulocytes, and megakaryocytes. In addition there are unipotential stem cells which represent a functional pool of "committed" precursor cells for each of these three lines. The maturation of nucleated red cells normally takes place over 4 to 5 days. Normal maturation is dependent on the availability of two vitamins, folic acid and vitamin B_{12}, deficiency of either results in abnormal nucleic acid synthesis and the production of an abnormal erythroid precursor, the megaloblast.

Toward the end of maturation the red cell nucleus is extruded leaving a cell which is larger than the mature red cell and still contains residual RNA, stainable by supravital dyes such as new methylene blue. These *reticulocytes* remain within the sinusoids of the marrow for 1 to 2 days and then are released into the circulating blood where they are identifiable for another 24 to 30 hours. The *reticulocyte count* is one of the most useful indices of the magnitude of red cell production. Each day approximately 1 percent of the circulating red cells (about 20 ml in an adult) die and are replaced by reticulocytes. Therefore the normal reticulocyte count is approximately 1 percent of the circulating red cells. However, since this percent is influenced by the total number of mature cells, it has been suggested that it be corrected according to the concentration of red cells within the blood. For example, an anemic patient with a red cell count of 3 $\times$ 10^6 cells/μl and a reticulocyte count of 6 percent would have the same number of reticulocytes as a normal subject with a red cell count of 6 $\times$ 10^6 cells/μl and a reticulocyte count of 3 percent. Consequently a more accurate estimate of the rate of effective erythropoiesis could be made by multiplying the patient's reticulocyte count by a fraction derived by dividing the patient's red blood cell count by the normal count (Fig. 45-1).

The rate of erythropoiesis is regulated by a hormone, erythropoietin.[6,10] Although the precise site or mechanism is not known, it appears that the hormone is synthesized in the kidneys. The rate of formation of erythropoietin is controlled by the oxygen tension of the tissues, hypoxia causing a prompt increase in the activity of the hormone in the blood. Erythropoietin acts primarily on erythrocyte unipotential (committed) stem cells to increase erythroid activity in the marrow (Fig. 45-2). Its earliest measurable effect is to increase the synthesis of several classes of RNA in these cells. The maturation of developing red cells is shortened by erythropoietin; and reticulocytes, under its influence, are released earlier than usual into the circulating blood. These large grey (polychromatophilic) "shift" cells, when observed, suggest, therefore, increased erythropoietic activity.

Although in normal man erythropoietin is measurable in a concentrate of 24-hour urine, biossay, the method of measurement that is commonly used, is not sensitive enough to detect it in the blood. Radioimmunoassay, a potentially more sensitive technique, requires further development before it can be considered reliable. Erythropoietin is demonstrable, however, in the blood of hypoxic patients, including the blood of most patients with anemia. Androgens increase activity of erythropoietin in plasma and potentiate its effect on erythrocyte unipotential stem cells, in part explaining the higher red cell mass of the adult male compared to the adult female. Inappropriately increased erythropoietic activity in the blood has been observed in some patients with renal tumors or cysts, adrenal tumors, hepatomas, cerebellar hemangioblastomas, and various other neoplasms. Reduced excretion of erythropoietin in the urine has been demonstrated in patients with renal failure, in patients with reduced needs for oxygen (hypothyroidism and hypopituitarism), in hypertransfused animals, and in patients with polycythemia vera (Chap. 50).

The proportion of erythroid precursors in an aspirate of marrow provides a rough estimate of total erythropoiesis. The estimate is only valid if a cellular

CORRECTED RETICULOCYTE COUNT

1. Reported count X $\dfrac{\text{Patient's Hematocrit or RBC count}}{\text{Normal Hematocrit or RBC count}}$ = Corrected Count

2. Example: 4% (reported) X $\dfrac{22.5}{45}$ (Hct.) or $\dfrac{3 \times 10^6}{6 \times 10^6}$ (RBC Count) = 2% (Corrected)

FIGURE 45–1. Corrected reticulocyte count.

specimen has been obtained. A more accurate evaluation of the general cellularity of the bone marrow can be made by examination of a section of a clot of aspirated marrow or a biopsy of the marrow. In normal man the erythroid precursors constitute about 25 percent of the nucleated cells of the marrow.

Erythropoiesis can be increased three to five times within a week of the onset of tissue hypoxia. Patients who are chronically hypoxic (who have, for example, a chronic hemolytic anemia) may increase

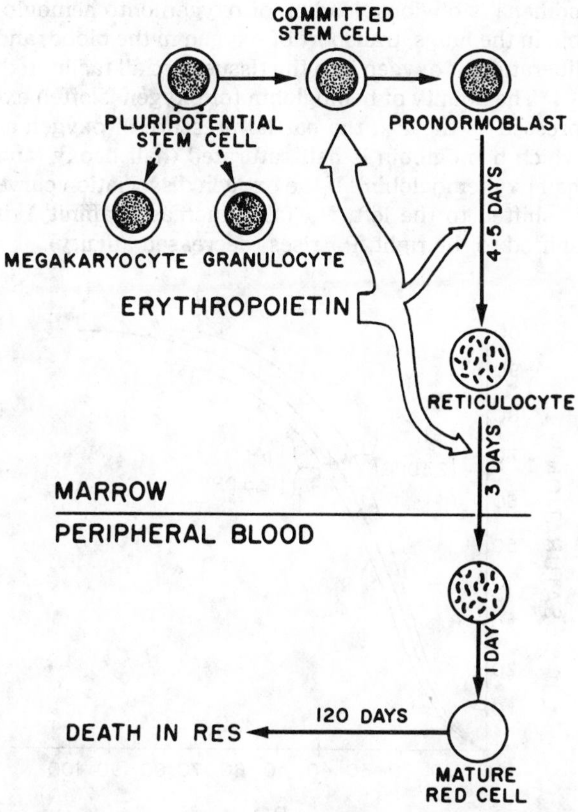

FIGURE 45–2. The effect of erythropoietin on red cell production.

erythropoiesis eight to ten times by expansion of red cell production into the fatty marrow of flat bones and into long bones.

A small but variable proportion of developing red cells die in the marrow, a process that has been called *ineffective erythropoiesis.* Ordinarily less than 10 percent of the erythroid population of the marrow are destroyed in this way but in certain disease states (megaloblastic anemia (Chap. 46), and thalassemia (Chap. 47) for example) this percentage is increased considerably. Ineffective erythropoiesis is suggested by the finding of anemia associated with a cellular erythroid marrow, and an inconsistently low corrected reticulocyte count.

The incorporation of iron into hemoglobin can be used as a measure of red cell production. By use of radioactive iron it is possible to measure the rate (and determine the sites) of erythropoiesis, but the methods are time consuming and tedious and, therefore, generally not used.[7]

The reticuloendothelial activity of the marrow can be scanned by use of radioactive colloids such as [99m]technetium sulfur colloid and [113m]Indium-ferric hydroxide which have relatively short half-lives. This activity essentially parallels the erythroid activity of the marrow and can be used as a measure of the degree and sites of hematopoiesis.

Hemoglobin Synthesis[9,13]

The synthesis of hemoglobin (Fig. 45–3) begins in the maturing erythroid precursor and ends with the loss of RNA from the reticulocyte. As in other cells, protein synthesis is directed by a genetic code contained within the DNA of the nucleus. This code transcribes information to messenger RNA which determines the sequence in which amino acids are incorporated into globin on the ribosomes in the cytoplasm of the cell.

Globin is composed of two pairs of structurally different polypeptide chains. In the normal adult, about 97 percent of globin consists of so-called α and β chains (hemoglobin A); the remainder, of α and δ chains (hemoglobin A_2, about 2 percent) and of α and γ chains (hemoglobin F, less than 1 percent).

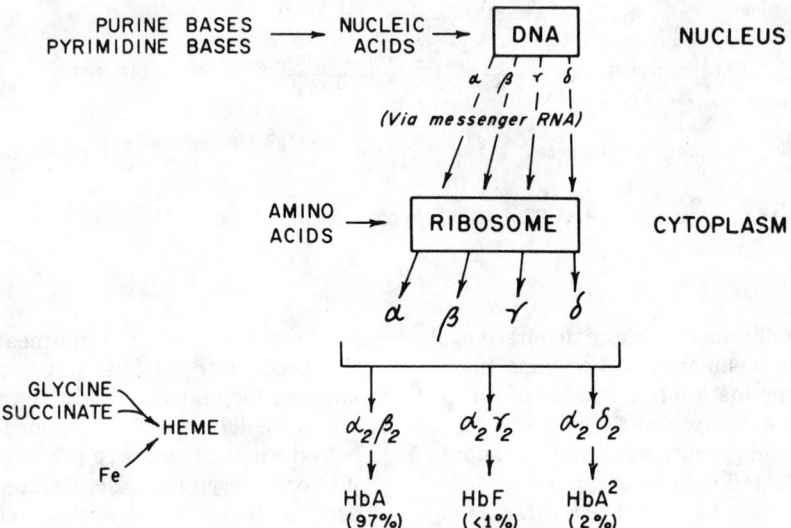

FIGURE 45-3. Synthesis of hemoglobin.

Hemoglobin results from the incorporation of the iron-protoporphyrin complex, heme, synthesized separately in mitochondria, into the globin molecule. The degree to which patients increase their rates of erythropoiesis in response to anemia is dependent primarily on the amount of iron available for heme synthesis (assuming their marrows are normal and they are able to increase appropriately the activity of circulating erythropoietin).

Any defect in the synthesis of heme or of globin results in the formation of relatively small amounts of hemoglobin within the red cell so that the mature cell appears paler than normal or *hypochromic*.

Hemoglobin Function[8,12]

The reversible binding of oxygen and carbon dioxide by hemoglobin allows the red cell to deliver oxygen from the lungs to the tissues and carbon dioxide from the tissues to the lungs (Fig. 45-4). At oxygen tensions present in the capillary beds, a small fall in the Po_2 allows a relatively large amount of oxygen to dissociate from hemoglobin and diffuse into the tissue (the steep part of the hemoglobin–oxygen dissociation curve). On the other hand, within the range of oxygen tensions likely to be present in the alveoli of the lungs or in the blood, a relatively large fall in Po_2 results in only a slight dissociation of oxygen from hemoglobin (the flat part of the curve). The shape of the curve reflects alterations in the affinity of hemoglobin for oxygen that occur as the amount of oxygen bound to hemoglobin changes. (The affinity for oxygen increases when more oxygen is bound, attribut-

able to interaction between the heme moieties of the molecule.) The physiologic advantage of these phenomena is obvious: loading of oxygen onto hemoglobin in the lungs, transport of oxygen in the blood, and liberation of oxygen into the tissues are all facilitated.

The affinity of hemoglobin for oxygen is often expressed as the P_{50}, the partial pressure of oxygen at which hemoglobin is half saturated (half deoxy- and half oxyhemoglobin). If the oxygen dissociation curve is shifted to the left, P_{50} falls (increased affinity); if shifted to the right, P_{50} rises (decreased affinity).

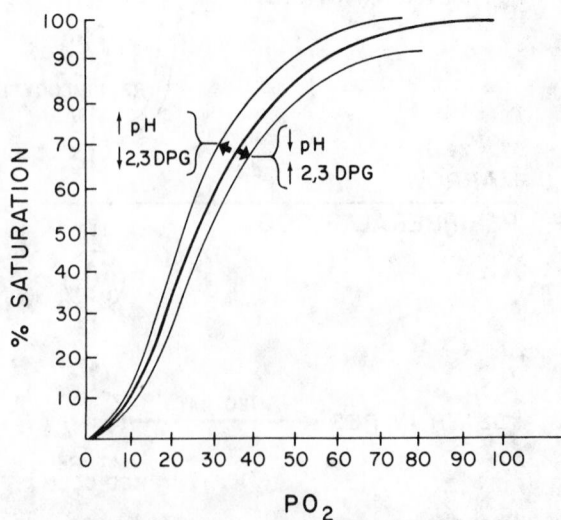

FIGURE 45-4. Hemoglobin–oxygen dissociation curve.

Several natural constituents of the red cell—hydrogen ions, carbon dioxide, ATP, and 2,3-diphosphoglycerate (2,3-DPG)—affect the binding of oxygen to hemoglobin. Increased concentrations of these substances favor oxygen dissociation. 2,3-DPG is formed by an alternate pathway of glycolysis (Fig. 45-5); its production is enhanced by hypoxia. The ability of patients to compensate for chronic anemia (Table 45-1) without an apparent alteration in cardiovascular dynamics is probably in large part attributable to an increase in the concentration of 2,3-DPG in their red cells, causing hemoglobin to liberate oxygen more readily at the oxygen tensions that prevail in the capillaries. Unlike the effect of 2,3-DPG, which is sustained, the increased oxygen dissociation that occurs in acidosis (Bohr effect) is transient since, paradoxically, increased hydrogen ion activity inhibits synthesis of 2,3-DPG.

The reversible binding of oxygen to hemoglobin is dependent upon the maintenance of reduced ionic iron (Fe^{2+}) within the molecule. The red cell is exposed continuously to conditions which favor oxidation of the iron to form methemoglobin. However, normally methemoglobin is reduced as rapidly as it is formed, primarily by the action of an enzyme, methemoglobin reductase, utilizing NADH, generated by glycolysis as a cofactor (Fig. 45-6).

Red Cell Metabolism[2,3]

The red cell normally survives in the circulation approximately 120 days. Almost 1 percent of the cells are destroyed each day, indicating that the loss of cells is by senescence rather than random destruction. The mechanisms responsible for normal death of the red cell are unknown. However, the size, shape, and plasticity of the red cell are important to its ability to withstand the continuous stress to which it is exposed in the circulation. These characteristics are dependent on the integrity of the cell membrane so

TABLE 45-1
Compensation for Anemia
Hematologic
Shift of hemoglobin–oxygen dissociation curve to right (increased synthesis of 2,3-DPG)
Increased red cell production (increased circulating erythropoietin)
Cardiovascular
Increased cardiac output (tachycardia, flow murmurs)
Altered tissue perfusion (pallor)

that any process affecting this integrity threatens the survival of the cell, especially since the mature cell is unable to synthesize protein or lipid necessary to regenerate the membrane.[5,15]

As in other cells, the membrane of the red cell is a lipoprotein barrier to the external environment. If the membrane were freely permeable to solutes, diffusion of water into the cell would produce swelling and eventually hemolysis. The internal osmotic environment is maintained by transport systems within the membrane, pumping sodium (and with it water) out of the cell and potassium into it against a gradient. These transport systems utilize energy provided by the breakdown of adenosine triphosphate (ATP) generated by glycolysis. Since there are no carbohydrate reserves in the red cell, glucose must be continuously available to it as a substrate for glycolysis. Depletion of glucose during erythrostasis, or functional deficiency of one of the glycolytic enzymes (Fig. 45-6), leads to premature death of the cell.

The membrane of the red cell contains free sulfhydryl (-SH) groups which, when oxidized, impair its function. Since the membrane, like hemoglobin, is continuously exposed to conditions which favor its oxidation, mechanisms have evolved to reduce thiol groups as they are oxidized (Fig. 45-7). Reduced glutathione (GSH), a tripeptide within the membrane, may provide hydrogen ions for this purpose. GSH is formed by the reduction of oxidized glutathione (GSSG) by glutathione reductase in a reaction utilizing nicotinamide adenine dinucleotide phosphate (NADPH) as a cofactor. NADPH is produced by the metabolism of glucose through the hexose monophosphate shunt; the rate-limiting enzyme in this reaction is glucose-6-phosphate dehydrogenase. Deficiencies of glutathione reductase or of glucose-6-phosphate dehydrogenase may lead to oxidation of sulfhydryl groups and to hemolysis (Chap. 52).

Lipids within the membrane of the red cell exchange in part with lipids in the plasma and so are to some extent sensitive to variation in plasma lipids. Patients with various diseases of the liver, especially

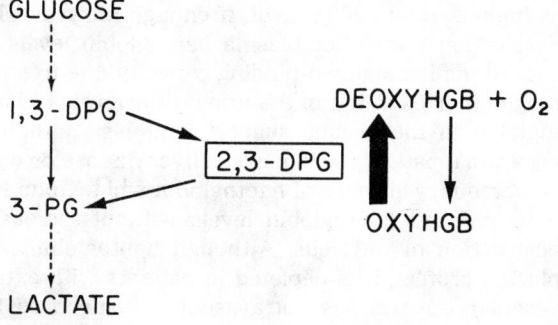

FIGURE 45-5. Metabolism of 2,3-DPG in the red cell.

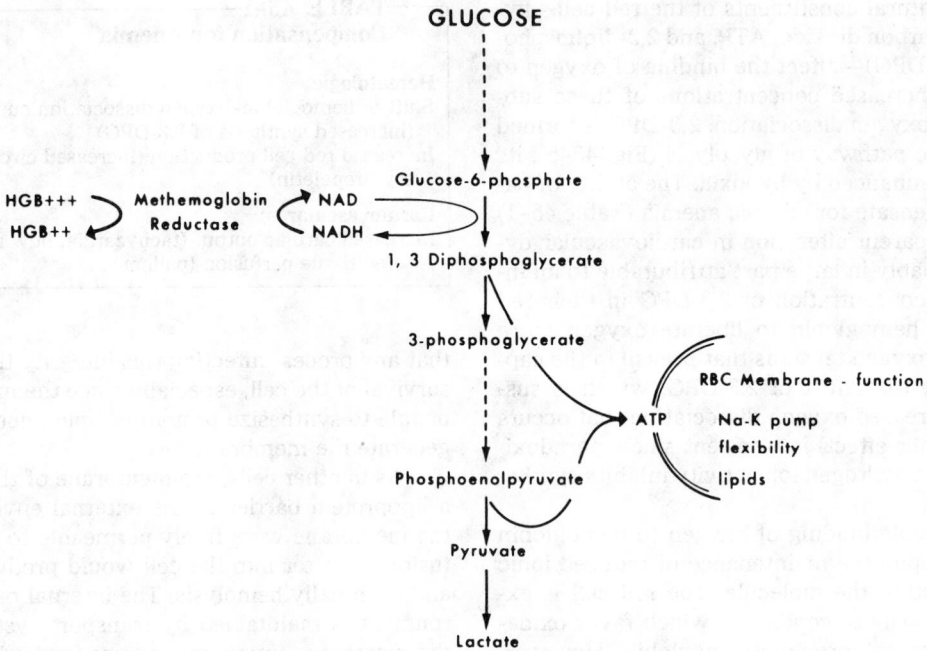

FIGURE 45-6. Schema of glycolysis in the red cell.

obstructive jaundice, have increased cholesterol (and sometimes phospholipid) within the membranes of their red cells. Increased membrane lipid causes the cells to become broader and flatter than normal; on blood smears these cells appear to have a target of hemoglobin within their central pallor and are called *target cells.* A deficiency of the enzyme which catalyzes lipid exchange between the red cell and the plasma, lecithin: cholesterol acyl transferase (LCAT), also results in increased lipid in the red cell membrane. LCAT deficiency has been reported as a rare inherited abnormality and, more often, secondary to hepatic disease. Rarely, patients with severe liver disease form *spur cells,* spiculated cells which have a marked excess of cholesterol in their membrane and whose survival is short.

A number of protein constituents of the red cell membrane have been characterized which are important in maintaining its shape and permeability. One of these, spectrin, a myosin-like protein, appears especially important in regulating the deformability and stability of the cell.[11]

Red Cell Destruction[4]
Red cell destruction normally takes place within the cells of the reticuloendothelial system. The mechanism by which the reticuloendothelial system identifies and removes the aged red cell is not known pre-

cisely. It has been suggested that an alteration in some physical property of the cell, such as "stickiness," plasticity, or the integrity of its membrane, may be the fundamental change in the aging cell. There is indirect evidence to suggest that most red cells are removed from the circulation by the reticuloendothelial system after repeated fragmentation of senescent cells. This evidence is consistent with the absence of intravascular hemolysis in normal people.

When red cell destruction occurs within the circulation rather than within the reticuloendothelial cells, hemoglobin enters the plasma (normal plasma hemoglobin is less than 0.4 mg/dl).[9] Plasma contains an α2-globulin, haptoglobin, which when present in normal amounts binds hemoglobin in concentrations as high as 150 to 200 mg/dl. If enough intravascular destruction occurs for plasma hemoglobin levels to exceed the hemoglobin-binding capacity, the free hemoglobin is excreted in the urine. Low levels of haptoglobin in the plasma suggest hemolysis although occasional patients with chronic liver disease or with an hereditary absence of haptoglobin will be found to have reduced haptoglobin levels without increased destruction of red cells. Although haptoglobin is a plasma protein, it is depleted in patients with extravascular as well as intravascular hemolysis. Increased levels of haptoglobin are found in the plasma or serum of patients with inflammatory or neoplastic

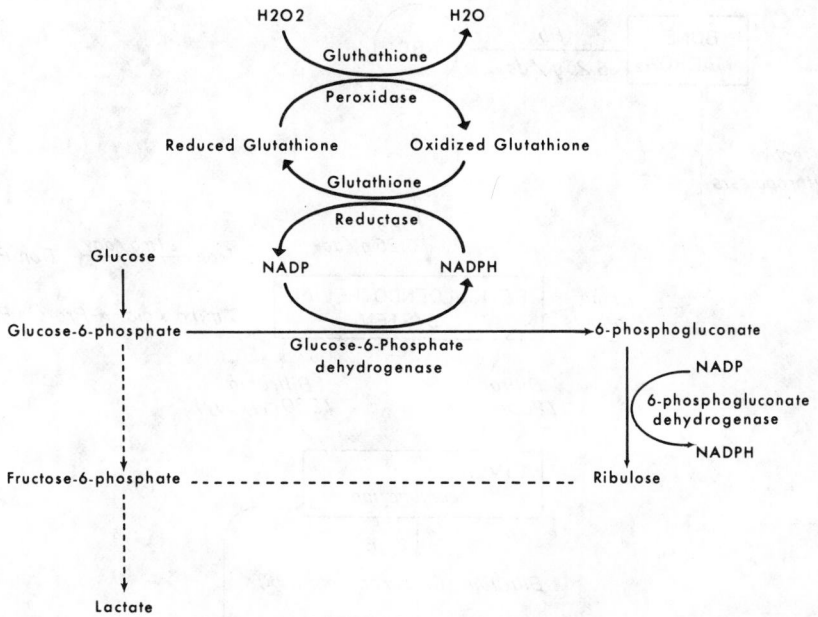

FIGURE 45–7. The hexose–monophosphate shunt.

disease. Therefore, patients who are hemolyzing and have such a disease may have haptoglobin levels that are higher than ordinarily would be expected.

Other plasma proteins also bind free hemoglobin or a portion of the hemoglobin molecule. For example, the demonstration in the plasma of methemalbumin, a complex of albumin and oxidized heme, is an indication that intravascular hemolysis has occurred. Hemopexin, a β-globulin that binds free hemin, also is depleted by hemolysis, but more slowly than haptoglobin. Unlike haptoglobin, the level of hemopexin is not increased by processes such as inflammation or neoplasia and so may be a more reliable index of the degree of hemolysis.

Red cell survival can be measured accurately by the use of radioactive compounds which are accumulated by the cell. The compound usually used in this regard is [51]Cr. The label is eluted gradually from globin, to which it is bound, so that the normal half-life of red cells by this technique is approximately 28 days. Scanning with detectors of radioactivity over the liver and spleen is used to demonstrate sequestration of the tagged cells by these organs, an indication of increased extravascular destruction.

Hemoglobin Catabolism[4,14]

The normal male has a circulating red cell mass of about 2200 ml and about 750 g of hemoglobin. Red cells containing approximately 6.25 g of hemoglobin

are removed each day by the reticuloendothelial system. The hemoglobin within these cells is catabolized by a complex series of enzymatic reactions. The amino acids and iron are reutilized, the latter primarily in the formation of new heme. The bulk of the heme of the senescent cells is converted to bilirubin. (In the process, carbon monoxide is formed by the oxidation of α-methane groups of heme so that measurement of the production of endogenous carbon monoxide is an accurate means of quantitating the catabolism of hemoglobin. The method of measurement is complicated and expensive, however, and therefore is not generally available.) The bilirubin, insoluble in water, is transported through the blood bound to albumin. It is not excreted by the kidney. In the liver it is conjugated with glucuronide and, now water soluble, excreted, for the most part, into the bile. Normally only a very small amount returns to the plasma, but that which does accounts for the "direct" reacting bilirubin measured by the van den Bergh test. In the intestinal tract bilirubin is reduced by bacteria to form urobilinogen. Some urobilinogen is absorbed from the gut and then reexcreted by the liver (the enterohepatic circulation). Small amounts (1 mg per day) are excreted in the urine (Fig. 45-8).

If the hepatobiliary system is normal, the amount of urobilinogen excreted in the feces each day is an accurate reflection of the amount of hemoglobin catabolized. The contribution of the breakdown of other

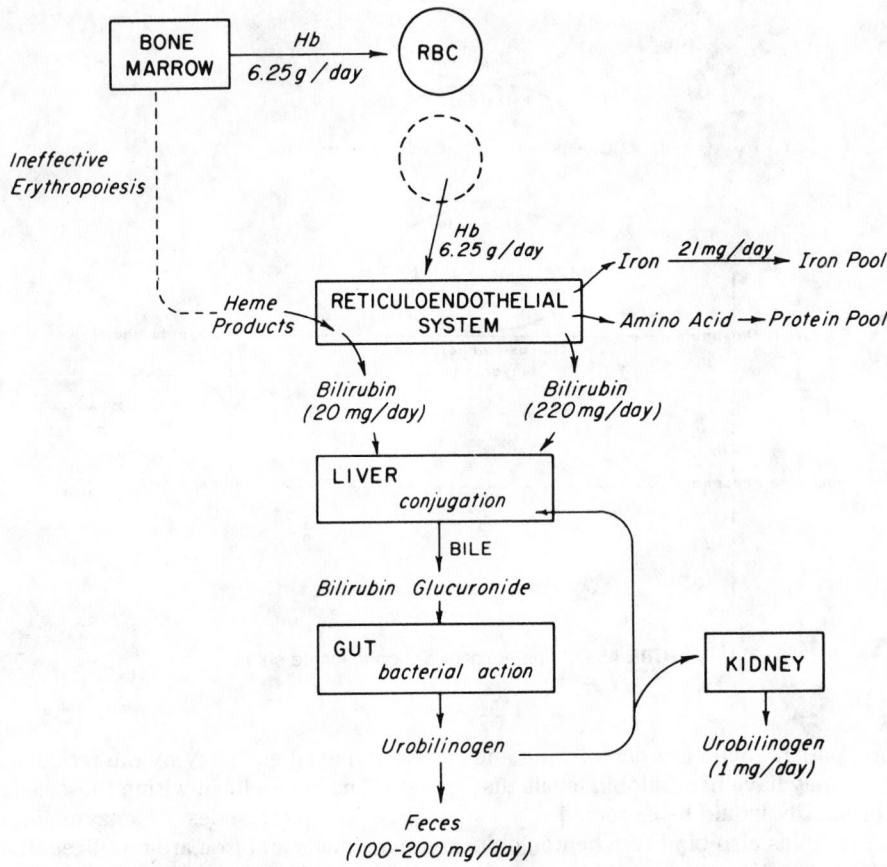

FIGURE 45–8. Hemoglobin catabolism.

heme-containing compounds (myoglobin, cytochrome, etc.) is insignificant. However, because stool cannot always be collected accurately and because the method lacks a certain esthetic appeal, measurement of fecal urobilinogen is seldom used in clinical laboratories to quantitate the extent of hemoglobin breakdown.

CLINICAL CONSIDERATIONS

The mass of hemoglobin or red cells in the circulation is almost always expressed in terms of concentration per volume of blood. Consequently the concentration of plasma (predominantly water) in the blood influences the measurement of these constituents. Therefore, a patient who has bled acutely, losing both plasma and red cells, may not appear anemic for 12 to 24 hours even though his red cell mass is considerably depleted. Obviously, dehydration also may influence the assessment of red cell or hemoglobin concentration. Furthermore, since the range of normal values is wide, a patient with a seemingly normal he-

moglobin concentration may in fact be anemic in comparison to values obtained when he was healthy.

Anemia might also be defined as a reduction in the amount of hemoglobin in the blood below that necessary to maintain, without physiologic adaptation, the normal requirements of the tissue for oxygen. By this definition a patient with reduced oxygen requirements (such as a patient with hypothyroidism) might have hemoglobin and red cell concentrations below the normal range and not be considered anemic.

Anemia is always a manifestation of an underlying disorder which must be identified before a patient can be treated optimally. Identification is made easier by recognition of the pathophysiologic process or processes that are responsible for anemia: underproduction of red cells or hemoglobin, decreased survival of circulating red cells, or bleeding. Except in the patient observed to have bled, laboratory tests are required to distinguish these processes.

It should be emphasized that there is not necessarily a correlation between the degree of anemia and the severity of the underlying disease. Bleeding hemorrhoids or benign epitaxis may produce profound anemia whereas one of the early signs of carcinoma of the colon may be a relatively slight anemia.

Symptoms and Signs[12]

In general the occurrence of symptoms attributable to anemia depends on the ability of the patient to tolerate or compensate for hypoxia (Table 45–1). Of course, if anemia is relatively mild, the reduction in delivery of oxygen to the tissues may be so slight that no physiologic compensation is necessary. More severe anemia results in an increased synthesis, by the red cells, of 2,3-DPG (Fig. 45–4), shifting the hemoglobin–oxygen dissociation curve to the right, thereby making more oxygen available to the tissues. This adaptation is in large part responsible for the observation that patients who become anemic over a period of weeks or months are less often symptomatic than those who become anemic more acutely. An alteration in cardiovascular dynamics is more likely to occur if anemia is severe, if it has developed rapidly, or if there is underlying cardiovascular disease. Increased cardiac output under such circumstances is manifested by tachycardia, especially on slight effort, and the appearance of so-called hemic murmurs, most of which are systolic flow murmurs; occasionally the murmurs sound the same as those heard typically in patients with valvular heart disease. If anemia is very severe, especially if it is chronic, even the normal myocardium may hypertrophy; and signs and symptoms of cardiac decompensation or of myocardial ischemia may appear. Patients with cardiovascular disease become symptomatic sooner. Dyspnea on exertion and orthopnea may be the first symptoms of which the patient is aware and, in fact, may be present even in the absence of other evidence of heart failure.

The shunting of blood to tissues most dependent for their viability on oxidative metabolism (brain, heart, skeletal muscle) results in decreased blood flow to the kidneys and skin and accounts in part for the pallor of anemic patients. However, the marked variation in skin color and the fact that certain disorders, such as hypopituitarism and uremia, may produce pallor out of proportion to the degree of anemia make it an unreliable sign. Pallor of the mucous membranes is more reliable, but mild, moderate, and occasionally even profound anemia may be present with little recognizable alteration in the skin or mucous membranes.

Nonspecific symptoms such as fatigue, irritability, or simply a vague feeling of loss of a sense of well-being are common complaints of anemic patients. Sometimes they are aware of these symptoms only in retrospect, after their hemoglobin concentration is raised toward normal.

Laboratory Studies[2,3,12]

Anemia can only be documented, and its pathophysiology defined by laboratory tests (Table 45–2). Because symptoms and signs of anemia may be subtle or lacking, the initial evaluation, no matter how "routine," of every patient should include an hematocrit value or measure of hemoglobin concentration and an examination of the stained blood smear. Even if anemia is not detected it is important to record baseline data so that subsequent changes (either up or down) can be appreciated. The range of normal hematocrit values or hemoglobin concentrations are so wide (Table 45–3) that a considerable loss (or increase) of red cell mass can occur without significant deviation from a statistical norm.

Microscopic examination of a stained smear of freshly shed blood (blood not mixed with an anticoagulant) is especially important if anemia has been diagnosed. The morphology of the red and white cells and a rough estimate of the number of platelets on the smear may suggest the pathophysiology of the process and occasionally may provide a specific diag-

---

TABLE 45-2
Laboratory Evaluation of Anemia

	Marrow Failure	Defect in Maturation	Defect in Hemoglobin Synthesis	Hemolysis
Peripheral RBC	No change	Normocytic	Hypochromic	Varied
Corrected reticulocyte count	Inappropriately low	Inappropriately low	Inappropriately low	High
Erythroid marrow	Reduced	Increased	Normal or increased	Increased
Morphology of erythroblasts	Normal	Megaloblastic	Reduced hemoglobin in late forms	Normal or megaloblastoid

TABLE 45–3 Normal Values		
	Males	**Females**
Hematocrit (%)	47 ± 7	42 ± 5
Hemoglobin (g/dl)	16 ± 2	14 ± 2
Red Cell Count (10^6/μl)	5.4 ± 0.8	4.8 ± 0.6
MCHC (g/dl)	33.5 ± 2	33.5 ± 2
MCV (μ^3)	90 ± 8	90 ± 8
MCH (μμg)	29 ± 2	29 ± 2

nosis (sickle cell anemia or acute leukemia, for example) (Fig. 45–9).

Some of the terms used to describe the morphology of red cells are defined in the glossary at the end of this chapter. The observer should be alert to changes in size, shape, and color of the cells and to the presence of inclusion bodies. Normal red cells appear round, have a uniform size (slightly smaller than the normal small lymphocyte), and are stained pinkish red. Since almost any abnormality can be produced artifactually in the preparation of the smear, care must be taken to use clean coverslips or slides, to use just the right amount of blood, so that the smear is neither too thick nor too thin, and to draw the blood smoothly and evenly across the glass surfaces.

An estimate of the average size and hemoglobin concentration of the red cells may be made by calculation of the so-called red cell indices (see Table 45–3 for normal values). The mean corpuscular hemoglobin concentration (MCHC) is determined by dividing the hemoglobin concentration in g per dl by the hematocrit value and multiplying by 100. A rapid estimate of the MCHC may be made by realizing that the hemoglobin concentration is normally one-third of the hematocrit value and calculating appropriately. The red cells are either normochromic or hypochromic; hyperchromia does not occur.

The mean corpuscular volume in cubic microns (MCV) is measured reliably now in most laboratories by use of an electronic counter, and is an important part of the data base used in the evaluation of anemia.

The initial evaluation of anemia also should include a reticulocyte count, appropriately corrected, as a measure of effective erythropoiesis. A low, normal, or slightly elevated corrected reticulocyte count is indicative of an inability to increase erythropoiesis appropriately in response to anemia.

A bone marrow aspirate from the patient should be examined if there is reason to suspect a disorder in the production of red cells or a disorder involving the presence of abnormal cells in the marrow (such as leukemic cells, myeloma cells, etc.). A biopsy of the marrow is more likely than an aspirate to identify tumor whose primary source is external to the marrow and provides a better estimate of cellularity.

Other studies which may be helpful in delineating the cause of anemia will be discussed in relation to specific disorders in subsequent sections.

GLOSSARY

Acanthocyte (burr cell, spur cell): A cell with spines or thorns seen primarily in a lipid disorder (abetalipoproteinemia), renal disease, and liver disease.

Anisocytosis: Variation in the size of red cells.

Antibody Screen: A series of tests (including an indirect Coombs test) used to detect the presence of anti-red cell antibodies in serum. An antibody screen is part of a routine transfusion crossmatch.

Autohemolysis Test: Screening test for hereditary hemolytic anemias due to intrinsic red cell defects. Blood is incubated under sterile conditions for 48 hours (with and without added glucose) and the degree of hemolysis determined. In hereditary spherocytosis autohemolysis is increased but corrected by adding glucose to the incubation.

Cold Agglutinins: Plasma antibodies (usually IgM) which cause direct agglutination of red cells in the cold. These antibodies commonly have anti-I specificity.

Direct Coombs Test: Used primarily to detect the presence of IgG and/or complement on the red cell surface. The patients' red cells are incubated with Coombs antiserum (antihuman gamma globulin) and observed under the microscope for agglutination.

Döhle Body: Light blue cytoplasmic inclusions in polymorphonuclear leukocytes. Associated with various infections and a congenital condition, the May-Hegglin anomaly.

Elliptocyte (ovalocyte): Oval cells seen in hereditary ovalocytosis. Macro-ovalocytes are characteristic of megaloblastic anemia.

Erythropoietin: Circulating hormonal substance elaborated by the kidney and probably other sites which stimulates bone marrow erythroid activity. Current assays for erythropoietin are still primarily research tools.

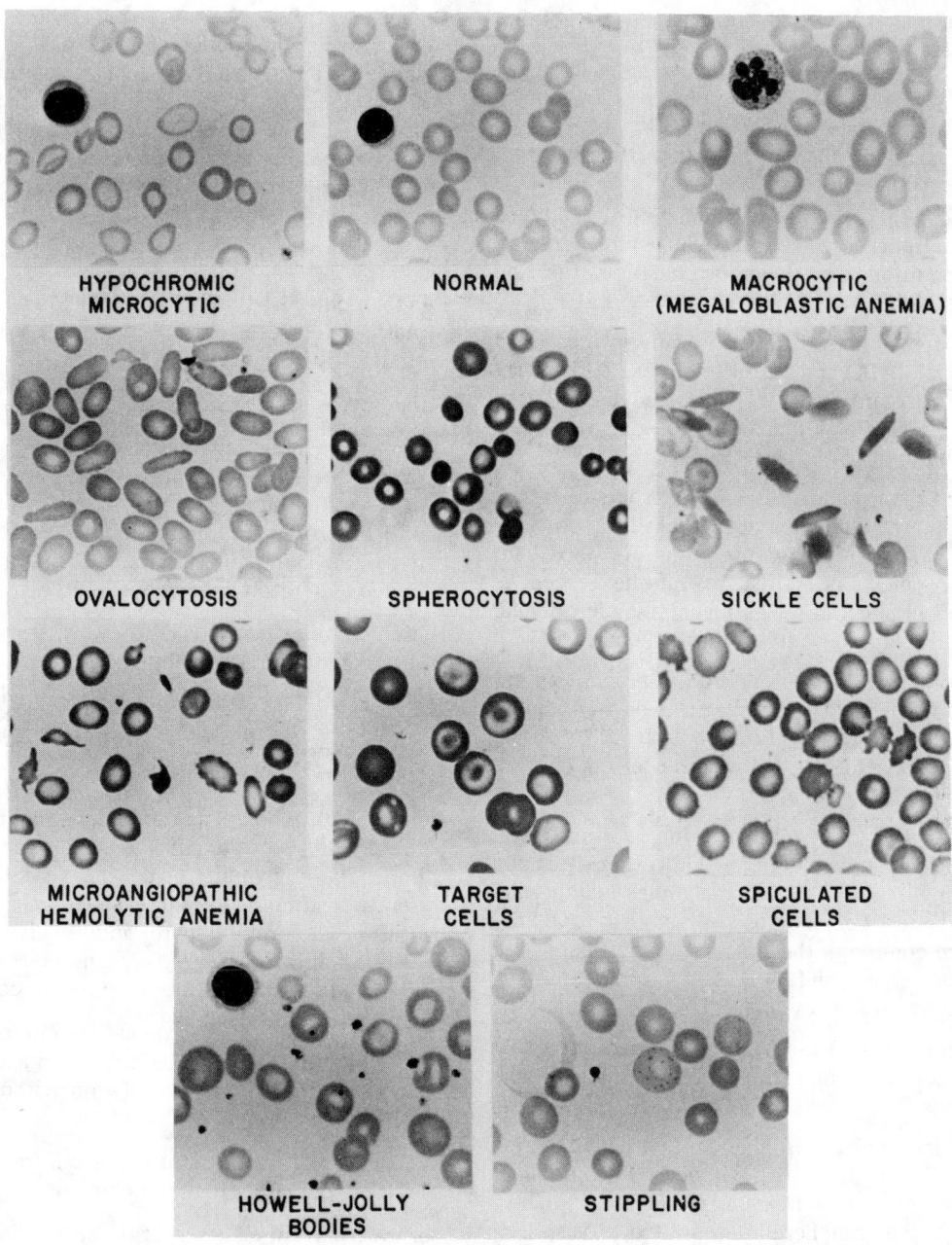

HYPOCHROMIC MICROCYTIC | NORMAL | MACROCYTIC (MEGALOBLASTIC ANEMIA)

OVALOCYTOSIS | SPHEROCYTOSIS | SICKLE CELLS

MICROANGIOPATHIC HEMOLYTIC ANEMIA | TARGET CELLS | SPICULATED CELLS

HOWELL-JOLLY BODIES | STIPPLING

FIGURE 45-9. Red cell morphology.

Ham Test (acidified-serum lysis test): A diagnostic test for paroxysmal nocturnal hemoglobinuria (PNH) based on the observation that acidified fresh normal serum (containing complement) causes lysis of red cells from patients with PNH.

Haptoglobin: A heterogenous α-2 plasma protein produced by the liver which binds free hemoglobin released during intravascular hemolysis. The hapto-globin-hemoglobin complex is rapidly removed by the reticuloendothelial system. Assay of the level of haptoglobin may therefore be useful in the diagnosis of hemolysis.

Heinz Body: An erythrocyte inclusion consisting of denatured hemoglobin and oxidized glutathione indicative of the erythrocyte's inability to handle an oxidative stress. The inclusion is seen on staining with crystal violet or other basic dyes.

Hemopexin: A β-globulin made in the liver which binds to free heme, but not hemoglobin. The heme-hemopexin complex is cleared by the reticuloendothelial system.

Howell-Jolly Bodies: Retained nuclear fragments in mature peripheral red cells. Seen after splenectomy and in conditions with defective nuclear maturation (e.g., megaloblastic anemia).

Indirect Coombs Test: Patient serum is incubated with normal ABO-compatible red cells and subsequently a Coombs test is performed using these cells. Agglutination implies the presence of free serum antibody.

Ineffective Erythropoiesis: Red cells, produced by the bone marrow, which are not released into the peripheral blood. Normally approximately 10 percent of erythropoiesis is ineffective but the percent is increased in such states as megaloblastic anemia, sideroblastic anemia and erythroleukemia.

Intrinsic Factor (IF): A glycoprotein, secreted by human gastric parietal cells, present in normal human gastric juice, which combines with B_{12}. The IF-B_{12} complex binds to receptors in the terminal ileum allowing B_{12} absorption.

Leukoerythroblastosis: Changes in the peripheral smear associated with marrow infiltration—usually tumor (myelophthisis). These changes include: anisocytosis and poikilocytosis ("tear drop" poikilocytes are common); the presence of nucleated red cells; and a "left shift" (metamyelocytes, myelocytes) in the granulocytic series.

Mean Corpuscular Hemoglobin (MCH): Hemoglobin ÷ RBC count. Normal: 29 ± 2 $\mu\mu$g. Limited clinical usefulness.

Mean Corpuscular Hemoglobin Concentration (MCHC): Hemoglobin ÷ hematocrit. Normal: 33 ± 2 g/dl red cells. Low in iron deficiency and thalassemia. Very high in hereditary spherocytosis.

Mean Corpuscular Volume (MCV): Hematocrit ÷ RBC count. Normal: 90 ± 8 μ^3. < 80 μ^3 in iron deficiency and thalassemia. Usually > 115 in megaloblastic anemias.

Megaloblast: A nucleated red cell with delayed and abnormal nuclear maturation. Seen primarily in folic acid and B_{12} deficiency.

Methemalbumin: A complex of free heme and albumin occurring after intravascular hemolysis.

Osmotic Fragility Test: Patients' red cells are incubated in varying concentrations of saline. In lower saline concentrations red cells accumulate water, swell, and lyse. By plotting the percent hemolysis at each saline concentration an osmotic fragility curve can be constructed. Increased osmotic fragility is characteristic of hereditary spherocytosis and autoimmune hemolytic anemia.

Ovalocyte: see **Elliptocyte.**

Pappenheimer Body: An iron inclusion body seen in a mature red cell in the peripheral blood when stained by Wright's or Giemsa stain.

Poikilocytosis: Variation in the shape of red cells.

Plasma Hemoglobin: Small quantities of free hemoglobin in the plasma are readily seen with the naked eye. The plasma may be pink (oxyhemoglobin) or brown (methemoglobin) at concentrations as low as 25 mg/dl. Lesser quantities may be determined accurately by various assays.

Reticulocyte: A young erythrocyte just released from the marrow identified by the presence of precipitated polyribosomes when stained using brilliant cresyl blue or similar supravital dyes. Normally reticulocytes constitute around 1 percent of the peripheral red cells.

Reticulocyte Index: The reticulocyte count corrected for the degree of anemia and the "shift" phenomenon whereby young red cells leave the marrow under the stimulus of increased erythropoietin activity. The reticulocyte index gives a better evaluation of the degree of bone marrow response to anemia than does the reticulocyte count.

Ring-Sideroblast: A sideroblast containing increased cytoplasmic iron arranged in a perinuclear distribution due to the presence of iron within mitochondria.

Schizocyte: A fragmented cell seen, for example, in microangiopathic hemolytic anemia.

Serum Iron: The concentration of iron in the serum, normally all bound to transferrin. Normal ranges from 75 to 150/dl.

"Shift" Cells: Reticulocytes released from the marrow early under the stimulus of increased erythropoietin activity secondary to anemia. When seen on routine blood smears, the cells appear as large polychromatophilic erythrocytes.

Sideroblast: A nucleated red cell containing cytoplasmic iron determined by a special stain for iron.

Spherocyte: Small, dense, round, red cell (microspherocyte). Seen in large numbers in hereditary spherocytosis, autoimmune hemolytic anemia and hemoglobin CC disease.

Stippling: Diffuse punctate basophilic deposits of RNA and sometimes iron within peripheral red cells usually denoting a young cell (reticulocyte).

Stomatocyte: Red cells containing an invaginated slitlike area of central pallor. This finding is associated with a number of heterogeneous disorders including a type of congenital hemolytic anemia and alcoholism.

Sucrose Hemolysis Test ("sugar water test"): A screening test for paroxysmal nocturnal hemoglobinuria (PNH) based on the observation that in the presence of serum and complement PNH red cells lyse in solutions of low ionic strength.

Target Cell: A cell which appears to have a target of hemoglobin in the middle of the cell's central pallor. Seen commonly in liver disease and in various hemoglobinopathies (Thalassemia, Hgb C disorders).

Total Iron Binding Capacity (TIBC): An indirect measure of transferrin in the serum. The normal TIBC is around 300 μg/dl.

Toxic Granulations: Coarse cytoplasmic granules seen in polymorphonuclear leukocytes. Although commonly associated with bacterial infections, the finding is quite nonspecific.

Transferrin: A β-globulin manufactured in the liver to which serum iron is bound. The serum transferrin concentration is around 200 mg/dl. This amount of transferrin is capable of binding around 300 μg/dl iron (total iron binding capacity).

Urine Hemoglobin, Myoglobin: The presence of free hemoglobin or myoglobin is suggested by the presence of a dark color in the supernatant of a spun urine sample which is free of red cells, documented by use of hemastix or orthotoluidine reagent test. The differentiation of hemoglobin from myoglobin may be made in a number of ways. A simple differential test is based on the observation that myoglobin is soluble in 80 percent ammonium sulfate while hemoglobin is not.

Urine Hemosiderin: Demonstrated by staining a routine urine sediment with potassium ferrocyanide. Hemosiderin is identified as blue granules within epithelial cells. A positive test indicates intravascular hemolysis. Free hemoglobin is filtered by the glomerulus and then absorbed and metabolized by renal tubular cells. The cells slough and are present in the urine several days after an intravascular hemolytic episode.

CHAPTER 46

Anemias Due to Disorders of Red Blood Cell and Hemoglobin Production

PHILIP D. ZIEVE AND LARRY WATERBURY

The bone marrow is the site of production of red cells, granulocytes, and platelets. A disruption of normal bone marrow function may result in deficient production of one or more of these formed elements of blood.

ANEMIAS DUE TO BONE MARROW FAILURE

The number of formed elements in the peripheral blood at a given time is only a static measurement of an hematopoietic system which is in a constant state of activity. Stem cells in the bone marrow are continuously differentiating into erythroid precursors that, when mature, replace erythrocytes in the peripheral circulation which are being destroyed daily. The situation is more complex in regard to granulocytes because of the large noncirculating granulocytic pool, but again net bone marrow production equals net daily loss. Platelet economy is similarly maintained by the bone marrow megakaryocytes. Whenever the bone marrow is unable to replace the normal daily loss of one or all of these formed elements of the blood, the disorder will be reflected by a diminished number of cells in the peripheral blood. By this concept, a bone marrow that is unable to increase its normal rate of erythropoiesis in response to hemolysis or blood loss is at least in a relative state of failure.

Aplastic Anemia

The term *aplastic anemia* has been used primarily to identify cases of pancytopenia associated with hypocellular or acellular bone marrow (Table 46–1). Patients with the clinical picture of aplastic anemia whose bone marrows are normocellular or even hypercellular sometimes have been called examples of refractory or aregenerative anemia rather than aplastic anemia. However, some cases once called refractory anemia have been shown subsequently to be due to a specific deficiency (such as vitamin B_{12} deficiency) or to be associated with defective heme synthesis (such as sideroblastic anemia). Also, unless a biopsy is performed, an aspirated sample may give an erroneous impression of the overall cellularity of the marrow.

About 50 percent of cases of aplastic anemia are of unknown etiology; the rest are due to a variety of physical, chemical, or pharmacologic agents or occasionally to infection (especially viral hepatitis) or neoplasia.[20,34,35] In some cases, such as those due to ionizing radiation or cytotoxic drugs, the deleterious effects of the agents that produce the disorder are generally understood and predictable. In other cases, the effects are not understood and are not, therefore, entirely predictable. Rare cases are inherited and are associated with other congenital abnormalities such as mental retardation, skeletal deformities, and patchy brown pigmentation of the skin (Fanconi's anemia). Table 46–2 lists some of the more common causes of aplastic anemia but there are a host of other agents that have been associated with it more rarely. Patients should be specifically questioned, therefore, in regard to all agents to which they have been exposed, no matter how apparently innocuous. The his-

TABLE 46–1
Aplastic Anemia

Basic mechanism	Decreased production
Peripheral smear	Red cells are normochromic, normocytic with minimal to marked anisocytosis and poikilocytosis; granulocytopenia and thrombocytopenia
Reticulocyte index	Decreased
Helpful laboratory tests	Bone marrow aspiration and biopsy

TABLE 46–2
Aplastic Anemia

Congenital—Fanconi's anemia

Acquired
1. Toxic effect, dose related
   Ionizing irradiation, cytotoxic drugs, benzene, heavy metals, etc.
2. Due to idiosyncratic reactions to drugs
   Chloramphenicol, phenylbutazone, dilantin, gold, etc.
3. Idiopathic

Other Conditions Associated with Severe Pancytopenia and Marrow Damage
1. Infection
   Hepatitis
   Miliary tuberculosis
2. Paroxysmal nocturnal hemoglobinuria
3. Preleukemia
4. Neoplastic infiltration of the marrow (myelophthisis)

tory should include details of exposure for a period of at least several months before onset since manifestations due to the noxious effects of a particular agent may be delayed. Patients should also be questioned carefully about their exposure to tuberculosis, a sometimes insidious cause of aplastic anemia.

Bone marrow failure as a cause of anemia should be suspected if there is associated granulocytopenia or thrombocytopenia or both, if the corrected reticulocyte count is low, and if, as above, there is a history of exposure to a toxic agent. The cellularity of the marrow, best assessed by examination of a section obtained by needle biopsy or perhaps by radioactive scan, is often, but not always, absent or reduced.

Uncomplicated aplastic anemia always develops gradually since, normally, slightly less than 1 percent of the circulating red cells are destroyed each day. Therefore, anemia developing within a few days is always due to bleeding or hemolysis rather than bone marrow failure. The history and physical examination usually reflect the deficiency of the various cell lines in the blood. An increased prevalence of bacterial infection and abnormal bleeding often accompanies symptoms and signs attributable to anemia. Splenomegaly or lymphadenopathy are unusual features of aplastic anemia and should suggest another diagnosis (such as leukemia).

The red cells are ordinarily normochromic and normocytic although moderate anisocytosis and poikilocytosis are sometimes seen. Nucleated red cells or young granulocytes are seldom seen in the peripheral blood and, like splenomegaly and lymphadenopathy should suggest other diagnostic possibilities (myelophthisic anemia, for example, see Chap. 50). The concentration of fetal hemoglobin in the blood is often moderately elevated.

Erythrokinetics in patients with aplastic anemia reflect bone marrow failure. The serum iron concentration is high and the percent saturation of transferrin is increased. Labeled iron is cleared from the circulating blood either very slowly, or else rapidly, but then deposited in the liver rather than the bone marrow. Red cell survival is normal or only slightly reduced.

The activity of erythropoietin in the blood and urine of these patients is high, in fact higher than observed in patients with anemia of comparable severity due to other causes.[18]

The pathogenesis of aplastic anemia is poorly understood. Because the process affects all cell lines of the marrow a defect in the pluripotential stem cell pool is suspected. The favorable response of many patients to bone marrow transplantation supports this view. There is some recent evidence to suggest a role for lymphocyte inhibition of bone marrow stem cells in the pathogenesis of aplastic anemia. There are intriguing reports of remissions following immunosuppressive therapy alone as well as in patients receiving such therapy during the course of an unsuccessful attempt at marrow engraftment.[25,34]

CHLORAMPHENICOL APLASTIC ANEMIA.[35] In the last 30 years, chloramphenicol has been the drug most often implicated in the production of aplastic anemia in this country. It has been estimated that the incidence of the disorder is approximately 1 in every 30,000 to 100,000 exposures to the drug. Actually, two types of bone marrow toxicity have been observed. One, dose related, is more common and usually is appreciated during administration of the drug. Patients with this first type develop a generally mild anemia, associated with a high serum iron, reticulocytopenia, and vacuolization of the cytoplasm of the erythroid precursors in the bone marrow. The number of circulating platelets and granulocytes are often not reduced. The toxic effects are ordinarily reversible when the drug is withdrawn. It has been reported that this more benign form of chloramphenicol toxicity is associated with inhibition of mitochondrial protein synthesis in the erythroid precursors of the bone marrow.

The other type of blood dyscrasia produced by chloramphenicol is aplastic anemia, not clearly dose related, and often diagnosed weeks to months after therapy when the antibiotic has been stopped. Pancytopenia occurs in the majority of cases. It has been said that this reaction is attributable to a different mechanism than is the more benign reversible type

but considerable overlap has been observed. There have been several reports of aplastic anemia in identical twins who had received chloramphenicol, suggesting that the predisposition to this kind of toxicity may be inherited. Clear-cut evidence of genetic influence on the development of chlorpromazine-induced granulocytopenia supports this hypothesis.

Experience with chloramphenicol has reinforced the dictum that drugs be administered only when there is a clear indication for their use. Most of the cases of aplastic anemia associated with chloramphenicol, many of them in the young, have been patients who did not require this particular antibiotic and, often, did not require an antibiotic at all.

MANAGEMENT AND PROGNOSIS OF APLASTIC ANEMIA.[3,33,34,35] Aplastic anemia is a disease with an overall mortality of 50 to 60 percent and, in severe cases, as high as 80 to 90 percent. Patients die primarily of infection and hemorrhage so that their degree of thrombocytopenia and leukopenia is of major prognostic significance, severe cases having platelet counts usually below 20 to 30,000/μl and neutrophil counts below 500/μl. Some patients do recover spontaneously after varying periods of time. Occasional patients, after prolonged periods of aplasia (months or longer), no matter what the cause, develop overt acute leukemia, usually myelomonocytic (Chap. 55); less often paroxysmal nocturnal hemoglobinuria develops (Chap. 47). These events suggest that aplastic anemia may predispose patients to somatic mutations leading to other lethal disease states.

The recommended treatment of aplastic anemia has changed significantly in the last few years. In the young patient with severe aplastic anemia, the treatment of choice is bone marrow transplantation if an HLA compatible family donor is available. Patients with potential donors should be referred after diagnosis to centers with transplantation programs before they are sensitized by random transfusions of blood components. Although the length of follow-up is still relatively short, it appears that the lives of at least two-thirds of young patients with severe aplastic anemia may be prolonged by bone marrow transplantation. Transplantation in older patients, however, is usually less successful.

In older patients and patients without HLA compatible family donors the treatment of aplastic anemia is supportive. Platelet transfusions may be life saving in the treatment of such patients with hemorrhage secondary to thrombocytopenia. It has been observed that the survival of platelets obtained from random donors becomes progressively shorter after weeks of repetitive platelet transfusions, because of the development of antiplatelet antibodies in the blood of the recipients. The use of platelets from histocompatible donors avoids this problem and maintains hemostasis for long periods of time in patients with aplastic anemia and severe thrombocytopenia.

Leukocyte transfusions are being used more and more frequently to support patients with malignancies through periods of marrow aplasia induced by cytotoxic therapy. Because of the difficulty in obtaining white cells as well as the short survival of the transfused cells, such transfusions are not yet practical in the long-term management of patients with aplastic anemia.

Corticosteroids may be of some benefit in modifying the bleeding tendency of thrombocytopenic patients but in adults rarely induce remissions. Androgenic steroids, in high doses, are often prescribed for patients with aplastic anemia. These drugs increase the activity of erythropoietin in the plasma and appear also to enhance the responsiveness to this hormone of bone marrow stem cells. The preparation presently prescribed most often is oxymetholone, 2 to 4 mg/kg per day. An increase in red cell production is more likely to occur than an increase in the production of white cells or platelets. A response is not seen ordinarily before three months of therapy. The effectiveness of androgens in the treatment of aplastic anemia is controversial, the most recent data suggesting that these drugs do not prolong survival of patients with this disease.

PURE RED CELL APLASIA.[27]   A number of patients have been observed to have failure of production of only one or two of the cell lines of the marrow (Table 46–3). Pure red cell aplasias are characterized by a selective failure of erythropoiesis with an accompanying marked reduction of erythroblasts in the bone marrow. A congenital form, the Diamond-Blackfan syndrome, responds to corticosteroid therapy. Acquired red cell aplasias have been described in association with many of the same drugs incriminated in the production of aplastic anemia. In addition there

have been a number of cases (mostly women) reported in association with thymoma and a few cases in patients with malignant disease. Many of the patients with acquired disease have been shown to have antibodies (IgG) in their serum cytotoxic to their own erythroblasts, suggesting that they have a disease of autoimmunity similar to autoimmune hemolytic anemia (Chap. 47) or autoimmune thrombocytopenia (Chap. 48). Some of these patients have been treated successfully with cytotoxic drugs, usually in combination with a corticosteroid. Splenectomy, too, occasionally has been beneficial to such patients.

The Anemia of Renal Failure[21,23]

The anemia of patients with renal failure is largely attributable to an impairment of erythropoiesis (Table 46–4). Although red cell survival is usually short, there is rarely sufficient hemolysis to account for anemia were the bone marrow able to compensate normally. The impairment in erythropoiesis apparently is due in large part to the inability of the kidneys to elaborate erythropoietin (Chap. 11). The activity of erythropoietin in the urine of such patients is extremely low. However, there seems also to be suppression of erythropoiesis by toxic factors elaborated or not excreted by the diseased kidneys. In this regard it has been observed that patients in a program of chronic dialysis occasionally increase their rate of red cell production without increasing the activity of erythropoietin in their plasma. Anephric patients, although able to maintain some degree of erythropoiesis, do, on the average, have lower hematocrit values than patients chronically dialyzed, whose kidneys have not been removed. This observation suggests that even diseased kidneys secrete some minimal erythropoietin.[18]

The hemolysis of renal failure is caused by an extracorpuscular defect; that is, transfused normal cells

---

TABLE 46–3
Pure Red Cell Aplasia

Congenital—Blackfan-Diamond Syndrome

Acquired.
1. Idiopathic
2. Secondary
   Drugs
   Thymoma
   Malignancy
   Chronic lymphocytic leukemia

TABLE 46–4
Anemia of Renal Failure

Basic mechanism	Decreased production ($\downarrow$ erythropoietin) Hemolysis (generally mild)
Peripheral smear	Red cells are normochromic, normocytic primarily. Sometimes fragmented cells and burr cells are seen
Reticulocyte index	Decreased
Helpful laboratory tests	Renal function tests

like the patients' own cells are destroyed prematurely. The shortened red cell survival is, perhaps, explained in part by a derangement of the metabolism of circulating red cells. Some patients appear to have, in addition, mechanical hemolysis attributed to narrowing of their renal blood vessels by fibrin—the so-called microangiopathic hemolytic anemia (Chap. 47).

Other mechanisms of hemolysis also are occasionally encountered. Patients dialyzed against tap water to which chloramine has been added to suppress bacterial growth may experience oxidative hemolysis. In addition some patients, frequently those multiply transfused, may develop large spleen syndromes and benefit from splenectomy.

A deficiency of essential nutrients also may contribute to the anemia of renal failure. Patients may be folate deficient because of poor diet and because folate is dialyzable, and they may be iron deficient because of the bleeding tendency associated with uremia (Chap. 48) as well as the accumulated blood loss from repeated diagnostic tests and hemodialysis.

The anemia of renal failure is characterized usually by normochromic, normocytic red cells, by a normal or slightly decreased proportion of erythroid precursors in the bone marrow, and by an inappropriately low, corrected reticulocyte count. The severity of anemia is roughly proportionate to the extent and duration of the underlying process.

If renal function is irreversibly impaired, only supportive therapy can be offered. Transfusions of packed red cells are indicated if patients are symptomatic from hypoxia but otherwise should be avoided because of the risk of iron overload, viral hepatitis, and immunization to minor blood groups. Also, potential recipients of renal allografts should, as far as possible, be spared exposure to foreign white cells and platelets, which carry histocompatibility (HLA) antigens. The use of androgens for patients in a chronic dialysis program has been shown to substantially improve the hematocrit value and eliminates transfusion requirements of some patients. Therefore, androgen therapy has become standard in many dialysis units (2 to 4 mg/kg of oxymetholone or its equivalent).

The Anemia of Hypothyroidism

Uncomplicated hypothyroidism is associated frequently with mild or moderate anemia; actually the red cell mass is considerably less than would be predicted by the hematocrit value or the hemoglobin concentration, because of a concomitant reduction in plasma volume. The red cells are characteristically

TABLE 46–5
Anemia of Hypothyroidism

Basic mechanism	Decreased production because of decreased tissue requirements. Occasionally associated with B_{12} deficiency and iron deficiency. Rarely associated with folate deficiency
Peripheral smear	Red cells are normochromic, normocytic unless associated with one of the other mechanisms for anemia mentioned above; spiculated cells are seen in the blood of some patients
Reticulocyte index	Decreased
Helpful laboratory tests	Thyroid function studies. B_{12} and folic acid assays. SI and TIBC

normochromic and normocytic; occasional spiculated cells are seen in the blood of some patients. The corrected reticulocyte count is low. Ferrokinetic studies reveal suppressed erythropoiesis although the bone marrow usually appears to contain a normal proportion of erythroid precursors. Anemia is attributed to a low activity of erythropoietin in the blood, because of the reduced needs of the tissues for oxygen. Correction of hypothyroidism results in a gradual increase in the hematocrit value over a period of 6 to 12 months, consistent with the patient's slowly increasing metabolic needs (Table 46–5).

Hypothyroid patients also are particularly prone to iron deficiency although their only consistently reported blood loss is menorrhagia. It has been shown too that malabsorption of iron is common in hypothyroidism but the contribution of that to iron deficiency in these patients is unclear. The manifestations of iron deficiency, including hypochromic, microcytic red cells, are the same in hypothyroid as in euthyroid patients.

Macrocytic anemia due to folate or vitamin B_{12} deficiency occurs occasionally in hypothyroid patients, folate deficiency because of poor diet and, perhaps, malabsorption and vitamin B_{12} deficiency because of pernicious anemia. The link between pernicious anemia and hypothyroidism is strengthened further by the finding of antibodies to gastric parietal cells in the serum of 32 percent of hypothyroid patients and of thyroid antibodies in the serum of 25 to 30 percent of patients with pernicious anemia. The significance of those antibodies is still speculative.

ANEMIAS DUE TO IMPAIRED SYNTHESIS OF NUCLEIC ACID— THE MEGALOBLASTIC ANEMIAS

The megaloblast is a relatively large erythroid precursor with delayed nuclear maturation so that, at all stages of cellular development, the nucleus appears immature relative to the apparent age of the cell. The chromatin of the megaloblast appears much more delicate than in the normoblast and does not coalesce as rapidly as the cell matures. These changes are the result of impaired DNA synthesis which affects the maturation of other cells as well, including megakaryocytes, granulocytes, and epithelial cells of the gastrointestinal and genitourinary tracts (Table 46–6).

In adults the great majority of megaloblastic anemias are due to deficiency of vitamin B_{12} or folate. Occasional cases are associated with sideroblastic anemia, acute leukemia, or the administration of various cytotoxic agents.[24,32]

Hematologic Changes

Patients with megaloblastic anemia, whether deficient in folate or vitamin B_{12}, develop symptoms gradually. Anemia is slowly progressive, and until it becomes severe, patients usually are able to compensate. Fatigue, weakness, shortness of breath, dyspepsia, and a change in bowel habits are, however, common complaints. The red cells are large, reflected in an increased MCV, and show marked variation in size and shape, especially as anemia becomes more severe. The MCV may exceed 130, values rarely seen in any other condition. An increase in the average number of lobes of the nuclei of the mature granulocytes (greater than 3.5 per cell) is an early sign of vitamin B_{12} or folate deficiency, particularly. Occasional nuclei have 5, 6, or more lobes. Leukopenia and thrombocytopenia are seen especially in patients with severe anemia. The bone marrow is markedly cellular, due primarily to an increased erythroid population. However, erythropoiesis is largely ineffective (Chap. 45) as is granulopoiesis and thrombopoiesis; and the corrected reticulocyte count is inappropriately low. The life span of the circulating red cells also is reduced considerably so that megaloblastic anemia results from a combination of hemolysis and ineffective production of red cells.

Vitamin B_{12} [24,28,31]

Vitamin B_{12} (cyanocobalamin) is a complex molecule, synthesized almost exclusively by bacteria and other microorganisms. It is found in meats, eggs, and, in smaller concentrations, in milk and cheese, but not in higher plants. The daily requirement of vitamin B_{12} is about 2 to 5 μg. It must be supplied in food, for, although bacteria in the colon synthesize the vitamin, it cannot be absorbed in the lower gut (Table 46–7).

The average dietary intake in the United States is 5 to 30 μg of vitamin B_{12} per day of which 1 to 5 μg is absorbed. Absorption requires the action of intrinsic factor, a mucoprotein which is secreted by the parietal cells of the gastric mucosa. Intrinsic factor and vitamin B_{12} form a complex which binds to receptor sites in the terminal ileum where the vitamin is absorbed.

There are several proteins in the blood that bind

TABLE 46-6
Megaloblastic Anemia

Basic mechanism	Ineffective erythropoiesis with decreased delivery of cells to the peripheral blood
Peripheral smear	Red cells are macrocytic, normochromic Macro-ovalocytes are common; marked aniso- and poikilocytosis. May see Howell-Jolly bodies and occasional megaloblastic nucleated red cells. Leukopenia with hypersegmentation of the PMNs. Thrombocytopenia
Reticulocyte index	Decreased
Helpful laboratory tests	Folate and B_{12} assay, gastric analysis, Schilling test, bone marrow

---

TABLE 46-7
Vitamin B_{12} and Folic Acid

	Vitamin B_{12}	Folate
Major dietary sources	Meat and meat products	Liver, leafy vegetables, fruits, nuts, yeast
Daily requirement	2–5 μg	50 μg
Estimated body content	2–5 mg	6–10 mg
Site of absorption	Terminal ileum (intrinsic factor necessary)	Proximal small bowel

vitamin B_{12}. The major carrier protein is transcobalamin II (TC-II), the rare deficiency of which has been associated with severe megaloblastic anemia. The vitamin is bound also to a so-called R protein(s), or cobalophilin, found also in granulocytes and in various body fluids, but the function of this factor (or factors) is unknown.

The total body content of vitamin B_{12} is estimated to be 2 to 5 mg, of which 25 percent is stored in the liver. Approximately 0.10 percent of the total is lost each day so that, if B_{12} is not ingested or if its absorption is impaired, a severe deficiency does not develop for several years.

The basic causes of vitamin B_{12} deficiency are 1) dietary inadequacy; 2) lack of intrinsic factor; 3) competition for available vitamin B_{12} by bacteria or parasites; 4) malabsorption due to intestinal abnormality; and 5) transport protein deficiency.

Folic Acid [17,28,31]

Folic acid (pteroylglutamic acid) although present in a wide variety of foods, is found in highest concentration in liver, yeast, green leafy vegetables, fruits and nuts. It exists primarily in the form of conjugates containing varying numbers of residues of glutamic acid. The daily requirement is estimated to be approximately 50 μg and the recommended dietary intake is 200 μg, easily met by the average diet in the United States (Table 46–7).

Folate is absorbed primarily as the monoglutamate so that dietary sources must be deconjugated by intestinal enzymes prior to absorption. Absorption takes place primarily in the proximal small bowel. Specific transport proteins have not been identified.

The circulating form of folate is methyltetrahydrofolate; but within cells folates exist as polyglutamates which act as coenzymes in the synthesis of DNA (see below).

Normal serum folate levels are 5 to 20 ng/ml, and the total body stores are estimated at 6 to 10 mg. The amount of folic acid stored is greater than that of vitamin B_{12}, but the daily requirement is about 100 times as large. Thus, if dietary intake ceases or absorption is impaired, the stores provide sufficient folic acid for only a few weeks, in contrast to vitamin B_{12} stores, which are sufficient for years.

The basic causes of folic acid deficiency are 1) dietary inadequacy; 2) competition for available folic acid by bacteria; 3) malabsorption due to intestinal abnormality; 4) increased requirement for folic acid, as in pregnancy and in hemolytic anemias; and 5) interference with folic-acid function by antimetabolites.

Metabolism and Interrelation of Folic Acid and Vitamin B_{12} [24,28]

The various derivatives of tetrahydrofolic acid, formed by the addition of a single carbon unit, play crucial roles in biosynthesis as one-carbon donors to other compounds. The megaloblast is the most dramatic evidence of the impairment of biosynthesis (in this case thymidylate synthesis) that is the result of folate deficiency.

The role of vitamin B_{12} in human metabolism is still unclear. Most of the B_{12} dependent systems that have been identified are bacterial. However, vitamin B_{12} clearly is essential in humans for the synthesis of DNA. The dominant hypothesis at present is that vitamin B_{12} is required for the utilization of 5-methyltetrahydrofolate, either as a cofactor in the regeneration of THFA from 5-methyl THFA and/or as a factor in the transport of 5-methyl THFA into cells.

These metabolic interrelationships may explain why greater-than-physiologic amounts of folic acid given to a patient with vitamin B_{12} deficiency correct the megaloblastic anemia. If vitamin B_{12} is not administered and folic acid is continued, anemia eventually recurs, but the marrow is hypoplastic rather than megaloblastic. Administration of vitamin B_{12} is then necessary to produce a slow return of the marrow to normal cellularity.

There is evidence that B_{12} acts by mechanisms independent of folic acid. B_{12} is needed in normal propionate metabolism as a coenzyme to methyl malonyl CoA isomerase (proprionyl CoA $\rightarrow$ methyl malonyl CoA B_{12} coenzyme $\rightarrow$ succinyl CoA). This function of B_{12} has been demonstrated in both microorganisms and mammalian tissue. The clinical significance of interference with this reaction in man is not known. It does not appear to explain the neurologic signs and symptoms associated with B_{12} deficiency even though the distribution of fatty acids (synthesized from propionate) in the myelin of patients with pernicious anemia is abnormal: Children with congential methylmalonic aciduria who lack the apoenzyme for the reaction do not have neurologic dysfunction.

VITAMIN B_{12} DEFICIENCY

Pernicious Anemia [19,24,28]

The major manifestations of pernicious anemia result from a nutritional deficiency of vitamin B_{12} conditioned by the failure of the parietal cells in the gastric mucosa to secrete intrinsic factor, thus leading to impaired absorption of vitamin B_{12} (Table 46–8). There is a relatively high prevalence of the disease in people of Northern European extraction and, in general, it is

---

TABLE 46-8
Causes of Vitamin B$_{12}$ Deficiency

1. Inadequate diet
2. Absence of intrinsic factor
   Pernicious anemia
   Gastrectomy
3. Diseases of the small intestine
   Bacterial over-growth (strictures, blind loops, etc.)
   Fish tapeworm infestation
   Resection or inflammation of the ileum
   Congenital malabsorption of B$_{12}$
4. Transcobalamin II deficiency

---

more common in whites than in other racial groups. Orientals are seldom affected. There is no predilection for the disease in people with a particular HLA genotype. The gastric abnormality may be genetically determined but is not usually expressed until after the fourth decade of life. Almost all patients exhibit achylia and achlorhydria which is refractory to stimulation by a test meal or by histamine. The gastric mucosa is atrophic. The concentration of gastrin in the serum is high, probably because of the high pH within the lumen of the stomach.

It has been suggested that pernicious anemia is an autoimmune disease.[19] The serum of most patients with pernicious anemia contains antibodies against intrinsic factor and against parietal cells. Furthermore, the prevalence of so-called autoimmune disease, such as Hashimoto's thyroiditis and hyperthyroidism, is increased in the population of patients with pernicious anemia. Some patients with pernicious anemia may have improvement of B$_{12}$ absorption following administration of corticosteroids. However, there is a poor correlation between response to steroids and fall in the titer of antibodies, and pernicious anemia has been demonstrated in a number of patients with immunologic deficiencies who have no antibodies to intrinsic factor or parietal cells.

PERNICIOUS ANEMIA IN YOUNGER PATIENTS. So-called juvenile pernicious anemia occurs rarely. One type, seen in older children, has all of the characteristics of the adult disease, including formation of antibodies to parietal cells and intrinsic factor. Some of these cases are associated with various endocrine dysfunctions. Another type, seen in younger children, results from an inability to produce intrinsic factor, even though gastric morphology and function are otherwise normal. These patients do not form antibodies to parietal cells or intrinsic factor. Two cases

of this sort have been described where intrinsic factor was present but was functionally inactive. Both groups have a high familial incidence of the disease.

Pernicious anemia, associated with immune deficiency, mentioned in the last section, also tends to occur in a younger age group (fourth decade on the average). It has many of the characteristics of the typical disease except that autoantibodies are not produced and many patients have symptoms of small bowel disease.

CLINICAL FEATURES. Pernicious anemia is for the most part a disease of middle or old age. The onset of symptoms is insidious and some time may pass, therefore, before the appropriate diagnosis is considered. As stated previously, anemia, until it is severe, is often well tolerated; but nonspecific symptoms, such as shortness of breath, anorexia, fatigue, and irritability are common. Occasional patients complain of a sore tongue, the result of a chronic glossitis, which, however, also may be a feature of folate, iron, or other nutrient deficiency. Papillary atrophy of the tongue usually accompanies this complaint. Patients frequently have prematurely gray hair and an increased proportion of them have vitiligo. Low blood pressure or, in patients with previous chronic hypertension, normal blood pressure, seems to be a characteristic of vitamin B$_{12}$ deficiency (rather than of chronic anemia per se). A distinctive lemon-yellow tint of the skin is seen occasionally, perhaps attributable to pallor in combination with slight jaundice. Low grade fever is common.

Symptoms of neurologic dysfunction when they occur are especially suggestive of Vitamin B$_{12}$ deficiency: paresthesia, weakness, incoordination, unsteady gait, and rarely (but especially if treatment is delayed), urinary and fecal incontinence and spastic paralysis (Table 46-9). An inability to perform fine movements such as typing, sewing, or buttoning clothes often occurs early in the course as does loss of vibratory sense and of two-point discrimination. Personality changes, confusion, even psychosis may also

---

TABLE 46-9
Neurologic Syndromes Seen in Pernicious Anemia

Syndrome	Prevalence
Peripheral neuropathy	Common
Dorsal column disease	Common
Corticospinal tract disease	Uncommon (late)
CNS dysfunction ("Megaloblastic madness")	Common

be present and may be mistakenly attributed to diffuse cerebral vascular disease. These neurologic abnormalities are the result of a patchy degeneration of the central and peripheral nervous systems, the precise cause of which is unknown.

The diagnosis of pernicious anemia is made on the basis of history and physical findings which suggest vitamin B_{12} deficiency and on the demonstration of megaloblastic anemia (Table 46–10). Leukopenia and thrombocytopenia are common when the anemia is severe. The bone marrow is markedly hypercellular with many megaloblasts and giant myeloid precursors. The diagnosis can be confirmed by demonstrating that the serum B_{12} level is low (< 100 $\mu\mu g/ml$), that vitamin B_{12} is poorly absorbed from the gastrointestinal tract, and that this malabsorption is corrected by intrinsic factor. Vitamin B_{12} assays presently are performed in many laboratories by a radioisotope dilution technique and are generally less reliable, because of falsely high values, than the older microbiologic assays. For reasons poorly understood, the serum B_{12} level (but not cellular stores) may be decreased in patients with folic acid deficiency and therefore a simultaneous serum folate should be obtained in the workup of any megaloblastic anemia. The Schilling test, commonly employed in the diagnosis of pernicious anemia, involves the administration of radioactive vitamin B_{12} by mouth and subsequent measurement of its excretion in the urine. If excretion is low, the test is repeated after administration of intrinsic factor to distinguish between pernicious anemia and primary disease of the bowel.

TREATMENT. The parenteral administration of vitamin B_{12} will rapidly correct all the hematologic abnormalities of pernicious anemia. There is a rise in the reticulocyte count, starting on the second or third day after therapy has been initiated and reaching a peak on the fifth or sixth day. The hematocrit or hemoglobin value starts to rise during the first week and reaches normal levels 1 to 2 months after the start of therapy. The white blood cell and platelet counts usually return to normal more rapidly. There may be transient leukocytosis or thrombocytosis. The megaloblastic bone marrow picture is altered rapidly, and within 24 hours the number of megaloblasts may be remarkably reduced.

Clinical improvement is dramatic. The low-grade fever disappears rapidly, and the soreness of the tongue is gone in 24 or 48 hours. New papillae may appear within one week. The appetite increases and a sense of well-being returns before there is striking improvement in the hematologic abnormalities.

The neurologic deficits less consistently respond to treatment. Abnormal behavior, lethargy, and confusion disappear rapidly. Evidence of spinal cord and peripheral nerve involvement may slowly improve over a matter of months, may improve rapidly, or may remain static. Occasionally there is a transient increase in neurologic complaints during the first few days of treatment. The blood pressure rises slowly to the level present before onset.

Parenteral administration of vitamin B_{12} is the treatment of choice rather than oral therapy with intrinsic factor and vitamin B_{12}. As stated above, the normal requirement for vitamin B_{12} is about 2 to 5 $\mu g/day$. Since the patient with pernicious anemia has depleted stores, the recommended dose at the onset of therapy is 100 $\mu g/day$ for 10 to 14 days. Thereafter, maintenance therapy with 100 μg per month is adequate. When larger amounts of vitamin B_{12} are administered parenterally, the excess is rapidly excreted in the urine.

If the patient fails to respond to parenteral vitamin B_{12}, two factors must be considered: 1) the diagnosis may be erroneous; this can be confirmed by appropriate absorption studies with isotopically labeled vitamin B_{12}; 2) there may be interference with the bone marrow response by infection or by medication; for example, chloramphenicol will suppress the expected response to vitamin B_{12} in a patient with pernicious anemia in relapse.

Transfusions are seldom necessary for the pa-

TABLE 46–10
Steps in the Laboratory Diagnosis of Pernicious Anemia

Problem	Interpretation
Low hematocrit value	Anemia*
Inappropriately corrected low reticulocyte count	Marrow failure†
Increased erythroid population in bone marrow	Increased ineffective erythropoiesis; decreased effective erythropoiesis
Megaloblastic marrow‡	Vitamin B_{12} or folate deficiency
Low serum vitamin B_{12} level	Vitamin B_{12} deficiency (sometimes decreased in folate deficiency)
Abnormal Schilling test	Vitamin B_{12} malabsorption
Schilling test normal with use of intrinsic factor	Pernicious anemia

* Pancytopenia common.
† Serum iron high; iron clearance low.
‡ Abnormal myeloid precursors and megakaryocytes as well.

tient in relapse because the red cell mass has diminished gradually, enabling the patient to compensate. If, however, the patient appears to have cardiac or cerebral decompensation on the basis of anoxia, packed red cells should be administered cautiously.

Pharmacologic doses of folic acid (greater than about 200 μg a day) will induce remission of the hematologic manifestations of B_{12} deficiency. Neurologic involvement is not prevented and patients treated with folic acid alone may present with primary neurologic disease without evidence of anemia or gastrointestinal involvement. Furthermore, neurologic deficits may be intensified under these circumstances (Table 46–11).

TABLE 46–11
Clinical Distinction Between Vitamin B_{12} Deficiency (Due to Pernicious Anemia) and Folate Deficiency

Feature	Pernicious Anemia	Folate Deficiency
History		
Nutrition	Usually normal	Usually poor
Age	Usually late middle-age or elderly	Any age
Race	Usually Caucasian (Northern European)	Any race
Family history	Sometimes positive	Negative
Alcoholism	No association	Strong association
Symptoms and Signs		
Neurologic (and psychiatric)	Very common	No symptoms attributable to deficiency
Loss of pigment in hair and skin	Common	No association
Laboratory		
Gastric juice	Achylia and achlorhydria (pH > 3.5)	Normal
Schilling test	Abnormal (< 7% of isotope excreted in 24 hr.)	Usually normal
Serum vitamin B_{12} level	Low (< 100 pg/ml)	Normal or low
Serum folate level	Normal or high	Low (< 4 ng/ml)

Once successful therapy has been achieved, the regular administration of vitamin B_{12} will prevent progression of neurologic disease and recurrence of anemia. If anemia recurs, it suggests not that the patient needs larger doses of vitamin B_{12} but that he has developed another type of anemia. For example, carcinoma of the stomach occurs three to ten times more often in patients with pernicious anemia than in the general population, and anemia due to chronic blood loss from this lesion may be encountered.

Other Causes of B_{12} Deficiency

Disorders other than pernicious anemia can lead to vitamin B_{12} deficiency. Whatever the pathogenesis the clinical evidence of B_{12} deficiency is the same. The diagnosis depends on evaluation of the patient's history, physical examination, and appropriate laboratory studies.

DIETARY INADEQUACY. Even with the small daily requirement and the relatively large stores of B_{12}, occasional instances of B_{12} deficiency due to dietary inadequacy are encountered in food faddists who avoid all sources of animal protein for years. Such patients, whose dietary intake of folic acid is usually high, may present with neurologic disease and little anemia. The serum level is low, but absorption of B_{12} is normal.

TOTAL GASTRECTOMY. Vitamin B_{12} deficiency inevitably will develop after total gastrectomy, but it may take as long as 10 years for signs and symptoms to appear. The absence of the stomach and, therefore, intrinsic factor results in malabsorption of B_{12} and such patients should receive, therefore, prophylactic injections of vitamin B_{12} monthly. These patients often have coexisting iron deficiency because of chronic bleeding from the esophageal-jejunal anastomosis. They may also develop folic acid deficiency because of the diarrhea and steatorrhea which often follow total gastrectomy. Rarely, vitamin B_{12} malabsorption is encountered following subtotal gastrectomy because of atrophy of the mucosa in the remaining gastric segment.

COMPETITION FOR AVAILABLE B_{12}. A number of small intestinal disorders (strictures, blind loops, jejunal diverticula) may lead to B_{12} deficiency because of an alteration in the intestinal flora allowing bacteria to compete successfully with the host for the available B_{12}. These bacteria bind, and then ingest, B_{12}, even though they do not necessarily require it for their growth. The malabsorption of vitamin B_{12} is corrected not by intrinsic factor but by administration of an appropriate antibiotic.

Patients infested with fish tapeworm also may be B_{12} deficient because of successful competition by the parasite for the vitamin. In areas where fish-tapeworm infestation is endemic, e.g., the Great Lakes area in the United States, megaloblastic anemia occurs with increased frequency in certain families despite similar degrees of infestation in other families, suggesting a genetic predisposition. The diagnosis is suspected after examining the stool for parasites and confirmed by demonstrating malabsorption of B_{12}.

INTESTINAL MALABSORPTION NOT RESULTING FROM LACK OF INTRINSIC FACTOR. Any disorder which destroys the normal absorptive sites in the terminal ileum may lead to vitamin B_{12} deficiency. Surgical resection or inflammatory diseases of the ileum (regional ileitis and celiac disease) commonly result in malabsorption of vitamin B_{12}. Some patients with pancreatic insufficiency malabsorb B_{12}, apparently because normal pancreatic secretions are necessary to degrade R protein(s) in saliva which bind B_{12} avidly and prevent its association with intrinsic factor; however, clinical B_{12} deficiency is unusual. Malabsorption of B_{12} also may be produced by certain drugs (colchicine, ethanol, and PAS, for example) but again B_{12} deficiency occurs rarely. The impaired B_{12} absorption caused by these disorders is not corrected by intrinsic factor or by the administration of antibiotics.

SELECTIVE MALABSORPTION OF VITAMIN B_{12} (IMMERSLUND-GRÄSBECK SYNDROME). A rare familial syndrome has been described in which B_{12} deficiency, usually in children, is associated with proteinuria. The malabsorption of B_{12} appears to be due to an inability of affected patients to absorb the vitamin after the intrinsic factor B_{12} complex has attached to the ileal mucosa and before B_{12} is bound to transcobalamin II.

TRANSCOBALAMIN II DEFICIENCY. A few cases of megaloblastic anemia associated with TC-II deficiency have been reported, supporting the belief that this protein is the major carrier of vitamin B_{12} in the blood.

FOLIC ACID DEFICIENCY

Nutritional Folic Acid Deficiency[17,31]

Folic acid deficiency is usually the result of an inadequate diet (Table 46–12). In the United States alcoholics in particular are prone to ingest insufficient amounts of dietary folate; these patients are especially likely to show signs and symptoms of folate deficiency because alcohol supresses the metabolic effects of folate and perhaps interferes with the release of folate from storage sites. Frequently, malnourished individuals with folate deficiency are depleted of other vitamins as well, thus complicating the presenting clinical presentation. For example, patients with combined vitamin C and folate deficiency may have the bleeding gums, hemarthroses, and perifollicular hemorrhages characteristic of scurvy as well as the signs of folate depletion. Megaloblastic anemia due to folate deficiency can develop within four months of cessation of folate intake but may occur more rapidly in patients whose requirements for folate are increased (pregnant women or patients with infection, hemolytic anemia or cancer) or in patients whose folate stores are reduced (alcoholics, for example).

SIGNS AND SYMPTOMS. Anemic patients with a history of poor diet, especially one deficient in leafy vegetables, citrus fruit, and liver should be suspected of being folate deficient. There are often associated symptoms of glossitis, anorexia, dyspepsia, flatulence, and diarrhea—similar to those elicited from patients with vitamin B_{12} deficiency.

Physical examination may show pallor, a smooth, inflamed tongue, hyperpigmentation, and signs of weight loss.

LABORATORY STUDIES. Examination of the blood and bone marrow reveals megaloblastic anemia. Serum folate, measured by a microbiologic technique utilizing *L. casei*, or in some laboratories now by radioassay, is low (less than 4 ng/ml compared to normal levels of 5 to 20 ng/ml).

The diagnosis is often confirmed by a therapeutic response to an adequate diet or to physiologic amounts of folate (50 to 100 μg per day). The megaloblastic anemia of B_{12} deficiency may respond to folic acid, but substantially larger doses are needed (200 to 1000 μg per day) (Table 46–11).

TREATMENT. Uncomplicated patients respond readily to the oral administration of 50 to 100 μg of folate a day; patients whose utilization of folate is increased or in whom erythropoiesis is suppressed by alcohol, infection, etc., may require up to 1 mg a day.

Many patients respond simply to the reinstitution of a nutritious diet. However, folate supplementation is ordinarily continued for several months to replen-

---

TABLE 46–12
Causes of Folate Deficiency

Inadequate diet
Malabsorption
Drugs
    Anticonvulsants and oral contraceptives
    Alcohol
    Antimetabolites
Increased utilization
    Pregnancy
    Chronic hemolysis
    Hemodialysis

ish body stores and then discontinued only if a proper diet has been maintained and if a state associated with increased utilization of folate is not present.

Other Causes of Folic Acid Deficiency

Tropical sprue, celiac disease, regional jejunitis, small bowel resection, and other conditions associated with the loss of the normal absorptive surface of the bowel may produce folate deficiency, sometimes associated with vitamin B_{12} deficiency. Also, bacteria in blind loops of the small intestine may utilize ingested folate and thereby diminish its absorption.

Folate depletion associated with these disorders may be treated by parenteral administration of the vitamin or, often, by administration of large amounts of oral folate (2.5 to 5 mg per day).

MEGALOBLASTIC ANEMIA OF PREGNANCY. The fetus requires large amounts of folate so that pregnant women, especially multiparous ones, are prone to folate deficiency. Consequently all pregnant women should receive dietary supplements of folate (0.5 to 1 mg per day).

FOLIC ACID ANTAGONISTS.[32] Folic acid (pteroylglutamic acid) is metabolically inactive; the enzyme, dihydrofolate reductase, is essential for the reduction of folic acid to the active compound, tetrahydrofolic acid (THFA). Certain analogues of folic acid (methotrexate is the one in general use) bind to the enzyme and prevent the formation of THFA. The use of the analogues in the treatment of patients may result in megaloblastic anemia. The hematologic effects of these folic acid antagonists can be prevented by folinic acid (citrovorum factor).

OTHER DRUGS.[32] Megaloblastic anemia due to folate deficiency has been observed in a relatively small number of patients being administered diphenylhydantoin (and even less often epileptic patients taking phenobarbital or pyrimidone), as well as in an occasional woman taking oral contraceptive medication. More often, people taking these drugs do not have megaloblastic anemia but do have low serum folate concentrations. Dilantin appears to inhibit absorption of folate, but the mechanism of action of oral contraceptive drugs in this regard is unknown. It seems unlikely that significant folate deficiency, in fact, can be attributed to oral contraceptives alone. In any case, megaloblastosis associated with the use of these drugs can be reversed by administration of folic acid by mouth.

INCREASED UTILIZATION. Chronic hemolysis with an associated increase of erythropoiesis may cause a relative deficiency of folate (for example, in patients with sickle cell anemia). Such patients develop a more profound anemia and megaloblastosis, responsive to supplementary folic acid.

SKIN DISEASE. Patients with diffuse exfoliative dermatitis lose considerable amounts of folate in their shed skin and may need folate supplementation.

INBORN ERRORS OF METABOLISM. Rare cases of congenital abnormalities of folate metabolism have been reported. Most have been associated with a megaloblastic anemia in infancy, unresponsive to physiologic doses of folic acid and most patients have had mental retardation.

MEGALOBLASTIC ANEMIAS NOT CAUSED BY VITAMIN B_{12} OR FOLIC ACID DEFICIENCY. A number of antimetabolites used in the treatment of various malignant diseases (Chap. 54) may produce megaloblastic anemia. All of these, most of them pyrimidine antagonists, interfere with the normal synthesis of DNA.

Occasionally the erythroid precursors of patients with sideroblastic anemia are megaloblastic, in the absence of folate or B_{12} deficiency. Those patients who respond to pharmacologic doses of pyridoxine resume normoblastic erythropoiesis.

Finally, commonly patients with myelomonocytic leukemia (Chap. 55), often early in their disease, develop megaloblastic anemia unresponsive to folate or vitamin B_{12}. In some of these patients, the erythroid abnormalities may be the predominant feature of the disease. When megaloblastosis is associated with marked dyserythropoiesis (bizarre cells, with fragmented or multilobed nuclei), the term erythroleukemia or Di Guglielmo's disease (Chap. 50) is often applied.

ANEMIAS DUE TO DEFECTIVE HEMOGLOBIN SYNTHESIS— THE HYPOCHROMIC ANEMIAS

Defective hemoglobin synthesis results characteristically in the appearance of hypochromic red cells. The most common cause of a hypochromic anemia is iron deficiency.

Iron Balance[22]

The bulk of dietary iron is complexed to organic foodstuffs. Therefore, of the 10 to 15 mg of iron in the average diet, only about 10 percent is normally absorbed. Certain foods, such as meat—especially veal—and wines, provide more absorbable iron than others, such as eggs and cereals. Absorption takes place all along the intestinal tract but most efficiently in the duodenum. The degree to which the mucosal cell is saturated with iron (an iron protein complex called ferritin) appears to regulate the amount of iron absorbed, but only when the intraluminal concentration of iron is low. At higher concentrations, there is no barrier to increased absorption so that iron overdose can, and does, occur. Only ferrous iron is absorbed so that ferric iron in food must be reduced prior to absorption. Gastric acid was once thought to be essential for this reduction but probably is not.

After iron is absorbed, it is transported in the blood bound to transferrin, a β-1 globulin. Only one-third of the binding sites are saturated so that, although the iron binding capacity of serum or plasma is 250 to 450 $\mu g/dl$, the normal serum or plasma iron is 80 to 150 $\mu g/dl$. The bulk of storage iron is in the form of ferritin, which is present in most cells, but in high concentrations primarily within cells of the reticuloendothelial system. In recent years, with the development of sensitive radioimmunoassays, ferritin has been found in human serum in a concentration directly proportional to the amount of reticuloendothelial iron. The measurement of serum ferritin, therefore, has become a useful clinical tool.[26,29]

Normally, iron in the blood is transported to developing erythroid cells in the bone marrow where it is incorporated into heme. About 21 mg of iron a day are required for normal erythropoiesis much of it supplied by degradation of hemoglobin that is catabolized each day in the reticuloendothelial system (Fig. 46–1). The 1 to 1.5 mg of iron absorbed daily equals the amount of endogenous iron lost in the urine, sweat, stool, and in the sloughing of skin. Iron balance in the menstruating female is made precarious by the additional loss of approximately 30 mg of iron with each menstrual period. Any further iron loss depletes stores and eventually leads to frank anemia. Table 46–13 lists average figures for iron balance in adult males and in females both before and after menopause. It can be seen that storage iron normally is sufficient to sustain hemoglobin synthesis for a relatively long period of time, if no iron is available, unless there is an increase in the daily loss of iron.

IRON DEFICIENCY ANEMIA[28]

The most obvious and dramatic result of iron deficiency, once iron stores have been depleted, is anemia (Table 46–14). In fact iron deficiency is the commonest cause of anemia in all age groups everywhere in the world. Although there is also, in iron deficiency, a reduction in the activity of at least some

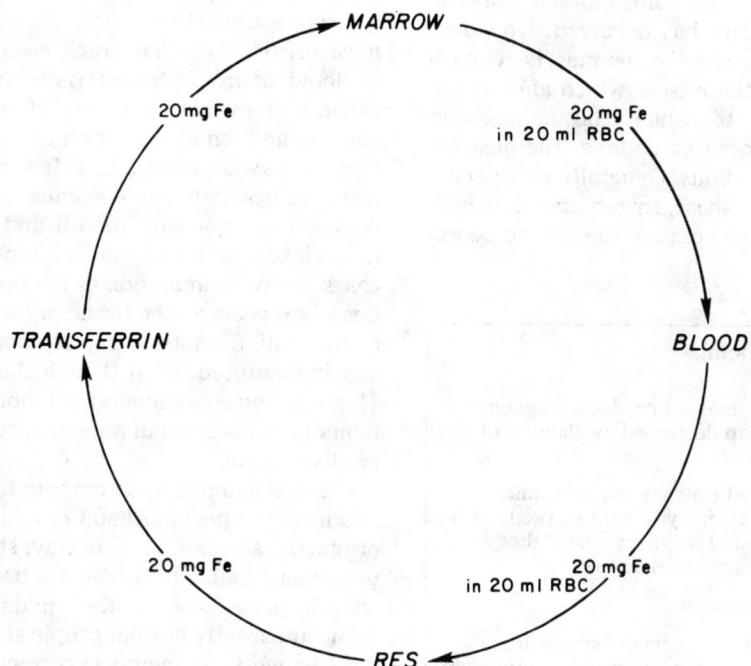

FIGURE 46–1. Schematic representation of daily exchange of iron in the adult. RES: reticuloendothelial system.

TABLE 46-13
Iron Balance

	Hemoglobin Iron (mg)	Storage Iron (mg)	Iron Intake per day (mg)	Iron Absorbed per day (mg)	Iron Loss per day (mg)
Adult Male Hemoglobin 15 g/dl	2500	1000	10–15	1–1.5	0.5–1.5
Postmenopausal Female Hemoglobin 14 g/dl	1900	500	10–15	1–1.5	0.5–1.5
Adult Female Hemoglobin 14 g/dl	1900	500	10–15	1–1.5	1–2.5* (0.5–1.5 plus 0.5–1.0 [menses])

* This apparent imbalance in menstruating females is probably corrected by increased efficiency of absorption. However, the menstruating female whose iron loss increases slightly will develop iron deficiency.

iron-containing tissue enzymes (cytochrome C, cytochrome oxidase, and succinic dehydrogenase, for example) the clinical significance of such reductions is not known.

Clinical Features

There is no convincing evidence that iron deficiency produces signs or symptoms until storage iron has been depleted and anemia has occurred. Iron deficiency anemia, like other chronic anemias, is symptomatic proportionate to the rate at which anemia develops and the depth to which the hemoglobin concentration or hematocrit value falls. The onset of symptoms is usually insidious. Generally nonspecific symptoms such as listlessness, irritability, shortness of breath, and vague weakness are the first to be expressed. Signs and symptoms of heart failure or end organ ischemia are likely to emerge relatively early or be intensified if patients have coexistent cardiovascular disease.

There are certain clinical signs which, though certainly not invariable, are particularly suggestive of iron deficiency. Most of them result from poorly understood changes in the epithelium of the skin and gastrointestinal tract. For example, patients may have brittle nails that crack easily, and, if severely depleted of iron, characteristic spoon-shaped nails, called koilonychia. A history of sore tongue may be elicited; and, on examination papillary atrophy of the tongue may be noted. In a few patients with longstanding iron deficiency anemia, glossitis may be accompanied by a sore mouth and dysphagia (Plummer-Vinson or Patterson-Kelly syndrome). In these cases, x-ray examination of the upper esophagus frequently reveals a membrane or "web" at right angles to the wall. Symptoms rapidly abate after iron therapy is instituted, even though the web may persist. This syndrome is encountered more frequently in patients of Scandinavian ancestry, suggesting a genetic predisposition.

Some patients with chronic iron deficiency anemia have the peculiar habit of eating large quantities of unnatural foods such as clay, starch, and ice. This propensity, called pica, also has been observed worldwide in patients with other kinds of severe anemia. Some apparently normal people share the same habit; but frequently, if anemia is corrected in patients with iron deficiency, pica will cease. Since some of the substances eaten have a high binding affinity for iron,

TABLE 46-14
Iron Deficiency Anemia

Basic mechanism	Decreased production secondary to decreased availability of iron
Peripheral smear	Red cells are hypochromic, microcytic with marked aniso- and poikilocytosis if the anemia is severe
Reticulocyte index	Decreased
Helpful laboratory tests	SI, TIBC, bone marrow iron stain, stool guaiac, erythrocyte protoporphyrin assay, serum ferritin

pica may contribute to the development of iron deficiency in those subjects whose intake of iron is borderline.

Laboratory Findings

The earliest sign of iron deficiency is depletion of iron stores, something that occurs, unless bleeding is acute, before the development of anemia (Fig. 46–2). Iron stores are best assessed by examination of the bone marrow for granules of hemosiderin, microscopic aggregates of ferritin, which stain bluish-green on exposure to Prussian blue. When the storage sites are exhausted, further loss of iron compromises the synthesis of heme and anemia ensues. As iron deficiency intensifies, the concentration of iron in the serum falls and the iron-binding capacity increases; the saturation of transferrin, therefore, is almost always under 15 percent and, in severe deficiency, under 10 percent. At the same time, sideroblasts, iron-containing erythroblasts in the marrow, disappear.

Patients recently depleted of iron may have a normocytic, normochromic anemia, so that the diagnosis of iron deficiency may not at first be obvious. A measurement of serum iron, iron binding capacity, serum ferritin, and an examination of the marrow iron stores may be useful, therefore, if a patient has a normochromic anemia which cannot be explained. Hypochromic, microcytic red cells are, however, characteristic of iron deficiency anemia. Usually there is moderate to marked anisocytosis and poikilocytosis as well. The degree of hypochromia is roughly proportionate to the degree of deficiency so that patients severely depleted of iron may have red cells that appear to contain virtually no hemoglobin at all. Examination of a smear of aspirated bone marrow reveals normoblastic hyperplasia; and there is decreased hemoglobin in the cytoplasm of the more mature erythroblasts, a typical finding in disorders of hemoglobin synthesis. The morphology of the marrow, in combination with a low, corrected reticulocyte count, suggests increased ineffective erythropoiesis.

Most patients with iron deficiency anemia have clearly bled; and there is no need, therefore, to measure their serum iron concentrations or to look at their bone marrows. Occasionally the diagnosis of iron deficiency is not obvious, and it is then that more extensive studies are in order. The serum ferritin assay is an extremely useful adjunct to other tests of iron deficiency. As mentioned above, the serum concentration is in direct proportion to reticuloendothelial iron stores. A reduction of serum ferritin is seen in iron deficiency. Spurious elevations of serum ferritin may be seen in inflammatory liver disease and occa-

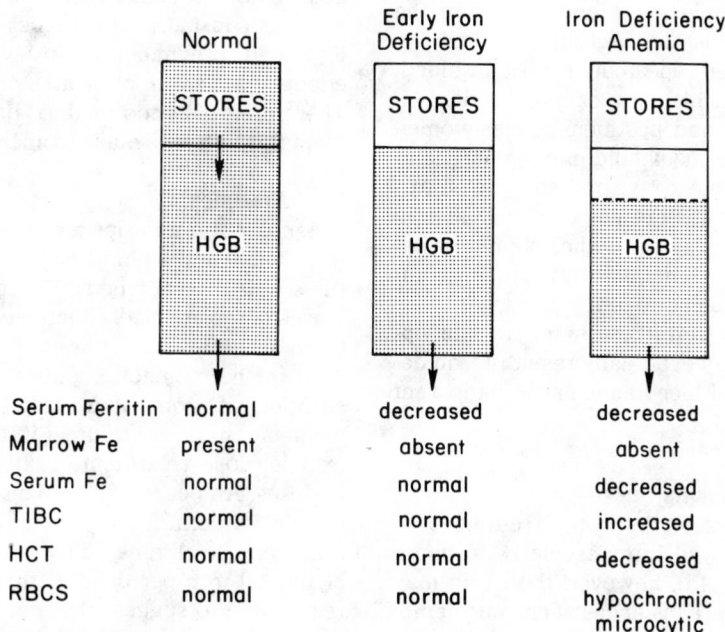

	Normal	Early Iron Deficiency	Iron Deficiency Anemia
Serum Ferritin	normal	decreased	decreased
Marrow Fe	present	absent	absent
Serum Fe	normal	normal	decreased
TIBC	normal	normal	increased
HCT	normal	normal	decreased
RBCS	normal	normal	hypochromic microcytic

FIGURE 46–2. Changes in the development of iron deficiency.

sionally in patients with various malignancies (e.g., Hodgkin's disease and acute leukemia), but for the most part it appears to be an accurate laboratory aid in the diagnosis of iron deficiency.[29] Sometimes a therapeutic trial of iron salts may establish iron deficiency as the cause of anemia when the diagnosis otherwise is not apparent.

Iron Deficiency Anemia Due to Chronic Blood Loss

The most frequent cause of iron deficiency anemia in adults is chronic blood loss, most commonly due to increased menstrual loss in females and chronic gastrointestinal bleeding in males and females.

Many women have unsuspected chronic menorrhagia. A careful history may disclose the passage of clots and heavy bleeding for seven or eight days of each cycle in a woman who believes her menses are normal. There is often an increase in menstrual bleeding just prior to the menopause. The resulting anemia may be discovered after cessation of the menses, the relation to the previous chronic blood loss being overlooked.

Chronic blood loss from the intestinal tract may be difficult to detect by history and physical findings alone. There may be a history of tarry stools, but a patient can lose as much as 50 to 75 ml of blood per day and still not have black stools. Therefore, in every patient in whom iron deficiency is diagnosed and the cause is not apparent, chronic blood loss from the gastrointestinal tract must be carefully searched for. Stools must be examined repeatedly for occult blood. Even if gastrointestinal bleeding cannot be demonstrated, however, men and postmenopausal women with iron deficiency anemia should undergo sigmoidoscopy and have complete x-rays of their gastrointestinal tract. If these studies are negative but anemia and/or bleeding continues, the studies should be repeated periodically; also many physicians recommend colonoscopy to such patients.

Chronic blood loss from the urinary tract or upper respiratory tract may eventually result in iron deficiency, but this type of bleeding is usually apparent to the patient.

Chronic Hemoglobinuria

When blood is hemolyzed, the iron is reutilized. If enough blood is destroyed intravascularly to cause hemoglobinuria (Chap. 45), however, then iron may be lost in the urine. In rare instances of chronic hemoglobinuria (paroxysmal nocturnal hemoglobinuria, post-cardiac-surgery-hemolysis) this iron loss may eventually result in iron deficiency.

It is helpful, when chronic intravascular hemolysis is suspected, to centrifuge the urine and stain the sedimented epithelial cells for hemosiderin, which accumulates there following the catabolism of excreted hemoglobin.

Other Causes of Iron Deficiency[28]

DIET. As noted in Table 46–13, the adult male loses so little iron each day that his dietary intake, at least in the United States, is more than adequate for maintenance of iron balance. It would take several years of complete lack of dietary iron, and subsequent depletion of iron stores, to produce iron deficiency in a normal adult male. The adult female is less secure but again dietary lack per se is an infrequent cause of iron deficiency. It has been emphasized, however, that the reduced contamination of food with iron, in part due to the declining use of iron cooking utensils, has resulted in a diet in this country which barely supplies sufficient iron to meet daily needs, especially in menstruating women.

MALABSORPTION. Malabsorption of iron, unless accompanied by bleeding, is an infrequent cause of iron deficiency, because the daily requirement for dietary iron is so small.

PREGNANCY. With each term birth the mother contributes 400 mg of iron to her infant. The average amount of blood lost with delivery (250 ml, containing 125 mg of iron) offsets the favorable effects of the absence of the usual menstrual iron losses. The net result is considerable iron loss with each pregnancy. Repeated pregnancies closely spaced may cause enough depletion of iron stores to cause anemia. Therefore, it is good medical practice to give supplemental iron to pregnant women.

Treatment

Diagnosis and appropriate treatment of the cause of iron deficiency anemia are the most important features of its management. The lost iron can almost always be replenished effectively with orally administered iron taken, if possible, between meals since food in the stomach significantly decreases the absorption of iron. Many different preparations are available, most containing 40 to 60 mg of elemental iron per dose; treatment usually consists of three daily doses. An occasional patient experiences gastrointestinal discomfort, e.g., cramping, diarrhea. Symptoms may be eliminated by decreasing the amount of elemental iron per dose. If that is not effective, it is reasonable to suggest that patients take the medication with meals even though absorption of iron will be decreased. The number of doses per day may be decreased as well.

The indications for parenteral administration of iron are few. Rare patients do not absorb iron adequately, cannot be relied upon to take medication, or need more rapid repletion of iron than is possible with oral administration. Severe untoward reactions can occur following intramuscular or intravenous administration, and the oral route should be used unless strong indications for parenteral administration exist.

Assuming that the underlying cause for the iron deficiency has been determined and corrected, iron therapy should be continued for some months after return of blood values to normal so that the depleted stores can be adequately replaced. Once treatment is started symptomatic improvement, including disappearance of glossitis, occurs even before there is a substantial change in the blood. The initial hematologic response to iron occurs in 4 to 5 days and is manifested by reticulocytosis and then in a gradual increase in hemoglobin concentration (about 1 g per dl per week) to normal. It is important to underscore that anemia due to long-standing blood loss may respond to iron even though there is continued occult bleeding. Thus, a satisfactory response to the administration of oral iron is no guarantee that the underlying lesion has disappeared. The cause of the blood loss must always be identified and satisfactorily treated.

OTHER CAUSES OF HYPOCHROMIC ANEMIA

Anemia Associated with Chronic Disease[36]

Anemia often complicates the course of patients with chronic disease such as malignancy, rheumatoid arthritis, and chronic infection (Table 46–15). The severity of anemia is generally proportionate to the severity of the underlying disorder. Typically the red cells are normochromic and normocytic although hypochromia is commonly seen and, less often, microcytosis. There is a slight to moderate shortening of

---

TABLE 46–15
Differential Diagnosis of Hypochromic Microcytic Erythrocytes (Common Conditions)

1. Iron deficiency anemia
2. Thalassemia
3. Sideroblastic anemia
4. Anemia of chronic disease

---

red cell survival but little or no compensatory increase in red cell production. Thus, the erythroid marrow appears normal or only slightly expanded and the corrected reticulocyte count is inappropriately low. Impaired erythropoiesis is associated in most patients with an unexplained decrease in the activity of serum erythropoietin compared to the increased activity that is expected in association with anemia. It has been reported that the serum of patients with malignancy, in contrast to the majority of patients with chronic disease, does have increased erythropoietic activity but that the marrows of these patients cannot respond normally to it.

Table 46–16 shows that iron balance is abnormal in patients with the anemia of chronic disease. The combination of a low serum iron concentration, reduced iron-binding capacity, a reduced level of serum ferritin, a decrease in the proportion of sideroblasts in the marrow, and an increase in storage iron distinguishes this anemia from other disorders of heme synthesis (Table 46–17). Abnormal iron balance results, apparently, from an impairment in the ability of these patients to mobilize iron from reticuloendothelial storage sites.

Sideroblastic Anemia[16,30]

Some anemic patients have increased serum iron, increased saturation of iron-binding capacity, and increased amounts of iron in their bone marrow (Table

---

TABLE 46–16
Iron Metabolism in Hypochromic Anemia Due to Disorders of Heme Synthesis*

	Normal	Iron Deficiency	Anemia of Chronic Disease	Sideroblastic Anemia	Thalassemia
Serum iron (μg/dl)	115 (70–180)	< 30	30 (15–65)	> 180	Elevated
Iron binding capacity (μg/dl)	340 (300–360)	> 400	200 (80–270)	250 (200–400)	250 (200–400)
Saturation of transferrin (%)	35 (25–50)	< 16	15 (10–40)	80 (60–100)	Increased
Marrow hemosiderin	2+	0	3+	4+	4+
Serum ferritin	Normal	Decreased	Slightly elevated	Elevated	Elevated

* Modified from Wintrobe, *Clinical Hematology*, 6th ed.

TABLE 46-17
Anemia Associated with Chronic Disease

Basic mechanism	Decreased production secondary to defective iron kinetics and decreased erythropoietin activity and/or erythropoietin effect on the marrow
Peripheral smear	Red cells are usually normochromic, normocytic, or slightly hypochromic
Reticulocyte index	Decreased
Helpful laboratory tests	SI, TIBC, bone marrow iron stain, serum ferritin

46-18). Transferrin levels are usually slightly decreased (Table 46-16). A Prussian blue stain of the marrow of these patients reveals an increased number of sideroblasts, and, characteristic of this disorder, in some cells the granules of iron are ringed around the nucleus—the *ring-sideroblast*. Electron microscopy has shown that the iron in the ring-sideroblast is contained in part within the mitochondria of the cell, the site of heme synthesis.

The red cells are usually dimorphic; that is, some are hypochromic and others are normochromic. Slight macrocytosis is seen occasionally; microcytosis is unusual. The corrected reticulocyte count is inappropriately low. The erythroid marrow is characteristically cellular, indicative of a degree of ineffective erythropoiesis. Sometimes the red cell precursors appear megaloblastic, even if folate deficiency (see below) cannot be demonstrated.

Sideroblastic anemia has been reported as an X-linked inherited and as an acquired disorder. Some of the acquired cases have no known cause; others occur in patients exposed to some of the drugs used in the treatment of tuberculosis—isoniazid, cycloserine, and pyrazinamide—or rarely, in patients administered chloramphenicol. One of the common causes of acquired sideroblastic anemia is acute alcoholism, almost always associated with folate deficiency. The anemia responds rapidly if ingestion of alcohol is stopped.

Lead interferes with heme synthesis at a number of points and may produce sideroblastic anemia.[16] The disease is seen most often in children who eat chips of lead paint. Adults may be poisoned by prolonged exposure to lead fumes in the course of industrial work or after ingestion of home brewed alcoholic beverages. The concentration of iron in the serum usually is not quite as high as it is in other types of sideroblastic anemia. Porphyrin metabolism is impaired resulting in an increased excretion in the urine of coproporphyrin III so that examination of the urine for coproporphyrin is a useful screening test. A definitive diagnosis is best made by measurement of the blood lead level. Anemia is usually mild in lead poisoning; encephalopathy in children and peripheral neuropathy or lead colic in adults are more troublesome complications. Basophilic stippling of the red cells is common, even in those patients who are not anemic. Chelating agents, such as British anti-Lewisite (BAL) or EDTA, are indicated only if patients are symptomatic or if the blood lead level is very high (greater than 100 μg/dl of blood).

Even when a definite etiologic agent can be identified in association with sideroblastic anemia, the precise reason that synthesis of heme is inhibited is not clear. However, it has been shown that some patients with the disorder (both inherited and acquired) respond to large doses of pyridoxine (100 to 200 mg/day). Pyridoxal phosphate is a cofactor in the synthesis of delta-amino-levulinic acid, the rate-limiting step in heme synthesis. Yet there is virtually no other evidence that responsive patients are deficient in pyridoxine. Moreover, when the anemia is corrected, red cell morphology remains abnormal, and anemia recurs if the administration of pyridoxine is stopped.

In patients who do not have sideroblastic anemia which can be attributed to an exogenous toxin and who are not pyridoxine responsive, the prognosis is dependent upon the severity of the process and the frequency at which blood transfusions are necessary.

TABLE 46-18
Sideroblastic Anemia

Basic mechanism	Decreased production secondary to defective iron metabolism
Peripheral smear	Classically a dual population of red cells is present: one normochromic, one hypochromic. Frequently aniso- and poikilocytosis is moderate to marked. Pappenheimer bodies (iron) may be seen in some cells
Reticulocyte index	Decreased
Helpful laboratory tests	SI, TIBC, bone marrow iron stain (ring-sideroblasts)

Some of these unresponsive cases eventually terminate as acute leukemia.

Thalassemia

Patients with one of the thalassemias have a hypochromic anemia due to a defect in globin synthesis. These disorders are discussed in Chapter 47.

Dyserythropoiesis[28]

Dyserythropoiesis is an imprecise term which refers to those disorders of red cell production in which there is increased ineffective erythropoiesis as well as morphologic abnormalities of the developing erythroid precursors. The abnormalities always include an alteration in nuclear structure (most often a variation in size or shape) and an unsynchronized rate of maturation of the nucleus and cytoplasm. Occasionally cells containing multiple or fragmented nuclei are seen. Increased susceptibility of red cells to immune lysis, especially by anti-I antibody, also is common, for reasons that are not yet entirely clear.

There are many acquired conditions characterized by dyserythropoiesis (megaloblastic anemia, iron deficiency, thalassemia, sideroblastic anemia, erythroleukemia, for example); but the phrase *dyserythropoietic anemia* usually is restricted to a few rare congenital disorders which overlap considerably. One of these is unique, however, in that red cells of affected patients are lysed by acidified normal serum (Ham Test—see paroxysmal nocturnal hemoglobinuria, Chap. 47) and for that reason the condition has been given the acronym, HEMPAS (hereditary erythroblastic multinuclearity with a positive acidified serum test).

The clinical manifestations of congenital dyserythropoietic anemia are variable; if anemia is intolerably severe, the only treatment is transfusion.

CHAPTER 47
Anemia Due to Hemolysis
PHILIP D. ZIEVE AND LARRY WATERBURY

The characteristic feature of hemolytic disorders is a reduction of the life span of the red cell. The occurrence of anemia or jaundice or both in association with shortened red cell survival is dependent on other factors: the ability of the bone marrow to increase red cell production and the ability of the liver to excrete biliruben pigments. Ordinarily, if there is no marrow damage and nutrients (iron, B_{12}, folate) are available, the bone marrow can compensate immediately for erythrocyte destruction rates of 2 to 3 times normal. Chronic hemolysis results in expansion of hematopoietic cells into normally fatty areas of the marrow and production of red cells may then increase up to 8 to 10 times normal.[44]

APPROACH TO DIAGNOSIS
(Table 47–1)

STEP 1: ANEMIA WITH APPROPRIATE RETICULOCYTOSIS

The observation which first leads the physician to suspect hemolysis is identification of an anemia, not explained by bleeding, associated with evidence of increased marrow production, and delivery of cells to the peripheral blood. An anemia developing acutely, with drop of the hematocrit value at a rate greater than 3 or 4 percent a week, in the absence of bleeding, also suggests hemolysis because even if erythropoiesis stops entirely, the hematocrit value does not decrease faster than that unless red cells are lost or destoyed prematurely.

In the laboratory the diagnosis of hemolysis is more easily confirmed by demonstrating increased hematopoiesis than by measuring decreased red cell survival. Thus, the corrected reticulocyte count is increased; and large polychromatophilic cells ("shift" cells) and, occasionally, nucleated red cells may be seen, reflecting increased erythropoietic activity in the plasma. The increase in hematopoiesis often is reflected also by leukocytosis and/or thrombocytosis.

Once hemolytic anemia has been diagnosed, it is important to determine, if possible, the chronicity of the process; the presence or absence of a familial pattern; whether there is a history of exposure to drugs or chemicals, and whether there is evidence of an underlying disease that is known to be associated with hemolytic anemia.

TABLE 47-1

Sequential Approach to the Diagnosis of Hemolytic Diseases

Initial Observation: Anemia associated with evidence of increased marrow production (↑ reticulocyte count, polychromatophilia, "shift" erythrocytes on smear) in the absence of clinical evidence of bleeding

Historical Data: Chronicity; familial pattern; exposure to drugs, toxins; presence of various disease states or situations associated with hemolysis

Peripheral Smear: Evaluation for morphologic features associated with specific hemolytic mechanism
a. Spherocytes, elliptocytes, spiculated cells, schizocytes, inclusions, stomatocytes, etc.
b. Morphology may be normal except for evidence of increased marrow production

Laboratory Aids (General)
a. Red urine, serum haptoglobin, urine hemosiderin, fecal urobilinogen, RBC survival

Laboratory Aids (Specific Etiology)
a. Coombs test, cold agglutinin assays, osmotic fragility, autohemolysis, enzyme screens and assays, sucrose hemolysis test, Ham test, special stains (Heinz bodies, globin inclusions, etc.), hemoglobin electrophoresis

---

STEP 2: PERIPHERAL SMEAR MORPHOLOGY

Except for evidence of increased marrow production, red cell morphology is frequently normal in patients with hemolytic anemia or at least is not specifically suggestive of hemolysis. Nevertheless, it is important to examine the peripheral blood to determine whether or not specific abnormalities are present (Table 47-2).[1]

Spherocytes are seen in many types of hemolytic disorders, but significant spherocytosis suggests hereditary spherocytosis or autoimmune hemolytic anemia. *Elliptocytes* are seen in hereditary elliptocytosis. Spiculated cells *(acanthocytes)* are seen in renal disease and hepatocellular liver disease as well as in some congenital lipid disorders. Fragmented red cells *(schizocytes)* are seen after heart valve replacement, disseminated intravascular coagulation, hemolytic uremic syndrome, vasculitis, and malignant hypertension. A number of different kinds of erythrocyte inclusions suggest hemolysis. Some may be seen on routine blood smears (such as malaria parasites, hemoglobin crystals in C hemoglobinopathies, and *stippling* in lead poisoning). Special staining methods are required to identify other types of inclusions (such as *Heinz bodies* in oxidative hemolysis, and precipitates of globin chains in the thalassemias).

TABLE 47-2

Peripheral Smear Morphology in Hemolysis

I. **Due to Increased Marrow Response to Anemia**
  A. Reticulocytosis
  B. Polychromatophilia
  C. Large "shift erythrocytes"
  D. Leukocytosis and thrombocytosis (occasionally)
  E. Nucleated red cells (usually only with severe hemolysis)

II. **Associated with Specific Hemolytic Mechanism**
  A. Congenital membrane defects
    1. Hereditary spherocytosis—spherocytes
    2. Hereditary elliptocytosis— elliptocytes/ovalocytes
    3. Hereditary stomatocytosis (increased Na/K flux)—stomatocytes
  B. Congenital hemoglobinopathies
    1. Thalassemia—hypochromia, microcytosis, target cells, inclusions
    2. SS disease—sickle cells, anisocytosis, and poikilocytosis (A & P)
    3. C Hgb.—Crystalloid inclusions, target cells, spherocytes
  C. Congenital enzyme deficiencies
    1. G6PD deficiency—nonspecific A & P during episodes of acute hemolysis. "Blister cells"
    2. Pyruvate kinase deficiency—nonspecific A & P, spiculated cells
  D. Immune hemolysis—spherocytes
  E. Associated with infection (parasites, spirochetes, nonspecific A & P)
  F. Hypersplenism—normal morphology, or minimal A & P
  G. Mechanical fragmentation (microangiopathic hemolytic anemia, intravascular coagulation, cardiac hemolysis): sharply pointed fragmented cells (schizocytes), spiculated cells
  H. Liver disease: spiculated cells, target cells
  I. Renal disease: spiculated cells, schizocytes

STEP 3: FURTHER LABORATORY EVALUATION

Following assessment of the peripheral smear one should attempt to obtain other data supportive of a diagnosis of hemolysis. *Intravascular hemolysis* is diagnosed definitively by the detection of free hemoglobin in the plasma and/or urine. At concentrations greater than 25 mg/dl the red color of free hemoglobin can be appreciated visually. Low grade intravascular hemolysis may not raise the concentration of free hemoglobin that high but will be reflected in a low serum haptoglobin concentration and, sometimes, by the appearance of abnormal cells (spherocytes, schistocytes, etc.) in the peripheral blood. Within a few days of the onset of intravascular hemolysis, hemosiderin often can be demonstrated by Prussian blue stain in renal tubular epithelial cells shed into the urine. *Extravascular hemolysis* is much more common than intravascular hemolysis but also is more difficult to diagnose, often requiring the performance of more specialized tests (red cell survival, measurement of the excretion of fecal urobilinogen or of carbon monoxide production, etc.). Serum haptoglobin is depleted whether increased destruction of red cells occurs in the circulation or in extravascular (reticuloendothelial) sites.

This stepwise assessment frequently will suggest

the presence of particular hemolytic diseases which may then be evaluated by specific tests which are described in the following sections.

CLASSIFICATION OF HEMOLYTIC ANEMIA

Hemolytic anemia may be categorized according to whether it is congenital or acquired. Congenital hemolytic diseases are due to intrinsic red cell defects whereas the majority of acquired disorders are due to "extracorpuscular" abnormalities.[44]

┌───
TABLE 47–3
Causes of Congenital Hemolytic Anemia*

A. Membrane defects
  1. Hereditary spherocytosis
  2. Hereditary elliptocytosis
  3. Hereditary stomatocytosis
  4. Associated marked abnormalities in Na and K flux
  5. Associated with abnormal membrane lipids
  6. Associated with abnormal membrane antigen composition

B. Metabolic enzyme defects
  1. Abnormalities of the hexose monophosphate shunt and related enzymes
    a. G6PD, 6-PGD
    b. GS-SG-R, GSH-Px, GSI & GSII
  2. Abnormalities of glycolysis and related enzymes
    a. HK, GPI, PFK, PGK, 2,3-DPGM, PK
    b. ATPase

C. Abnormalities in heme metabolism
  1. Erythropoietic porphyria

D. Abnormalities in globin metabolism
  1. Qualitative
    a. Sickle cell disease
    b. Other sickling disorders (Sö, SC, S-thal, etc.)
    c. Unstable hemoglobins (Köln, Zurich, etc.)
  2. Quantitative
    a. The thalassemias

* Key to abbreviations:
G6PD, glucose-6-phosphate dehydrogenase
6-PGD, 6-phosphogluconate dehydrogenase
GS-SG-R, glutathione reductase
GSH-Px, glutathione peroxidase
GSI & II, glutathione synthetase
HK, hexokinase
GSI, glucose phosphate isomerase
PFK, phosphofructokinase
TPI, triosephosphate isomerase
PGK, phosphoglycerole kinase
2,3-DPGM, 2,3-diphosphoglycerate mutase
PK, pyruvate kinase
ATPase, adenosine triphosphatase
───┘

CONGENITAL HEMOLYTIC ANEMIA (Table 47–3)

MEMBRANE DEFECTS

Hereditary Spherocytosis

In hereditary spherocytosis (HS) there is an intrinsic defect of the red cell membrane inherited as an autosomal dominant trait. The disease is more common in individuals of European ancestry. Characteristic features of the disease are: 1) microspherocytosis (small spherical erythrocytes in the peripheral blood), 2) hemolytic anemia, 3) splenomegaly, and 4) almost certain improvement following splenectomy (Table 47–4). The erythrocytes have a diminished life span both in the patient and in normal subjects. After splenectomy red cell survival is almost normal. On the other hand, normal cells survive normally when transfused into patients with hereditary spherocytosis. These observations establish that the defect in HS

┌───
TABLE 47–4
Hereditary Spherocytosis

Basic mechanism	Hemolysis due to an inherited red cell membrane defect resulting in a leaky membrane with increased sodium influx, compensating increase in activity of sodium "pump," erythrocyte damage with membrane loss in the spleen
Peripheral smear	Microspherocytes, polychromatophilia
Reticulocyte index	Increased
Helpful laboratory studies	Incubated osmotic fragility test, autohemolysis with and without added glucose
───┘

is in the red cell and that excessive destruction depends on the presence of the spleen.

PATHOGENESIS. The apparent basic defect in this disease is an abnormality in the protein structure of the red cell membrane which allows sodium to leak into the cell at an accelerated rate. Increased ATP, made available by increased glycolysis, is required to provide the energy necessary to pump sodium out of the cell. This sustained demand for energy eventually exhausts the metabolic resources of the cell, rendering it susceptible to accumulation of sodium and water and to osmotic lysis. During repeated passages through the sluggish circulation of the spleen where they are deprived of glucose and subjected to a markedly acid pH (conditions inhibitory to glycolysis), the cells lose membrane lipid, become spheroidal, lose their ability to deform, and eventually are trapped and removed from the circulation. Splenectomy does not alter the basic defect of the red cells; but in the absence of the spleen the red cell can compensate for its defect and survive almost normally.

CLINICAL FEATURES. The disease is characterized by a wide spectrum of severity ranging from abnormalities undetectible by routine clinical or laboratory studies to severe chronic hemolytic anemia. Although frequently severe enough to lead to its detection in childhood, the disease may not be diagnosed until late in adult life. There is often a family history of anemia, jaundice, and/or splenectomy. Patients usually present with anemia, jaundice, and splenomegaly. A personal and family history of gallstones and, less frequently, leg ulcers is also common. Laboratory studies reveal the characteristic findings of hemolytic anemia including microspherocytosis.

Some patients may be seen for the first time during an aplastic crisis due to a sudden diminution of red cell production often associated with infection. Severe anemia results because the increased red cell destruction continues. Jaundice may diminish as may reticulocytosis, bone marrow hyperplasia, and increased excretion of bile pigment. The diagnosis in such cases depends on recognition of spherocytes on the smear and on the previous history. A more gradual crisis has been documented in some patients as a result of relative folic acid deficiency. In these patients signs of overt hemolysis are absent and the bone marrow may be megaloblastic.

LABORATORY STUDIES. Spherocytes may consitute from 1 to 2 percent to the majority of the cells seen on peripheral smear. The cells appear hyperchromic and the MCHC is frequently increased. The presence of microspherocytes with a decreased surface/volume ratio results in an increased susceptibility to osmotic lysis by hypotonic saline (*osmotic fragility test*). The difference in susceptibility between spherocytes and normal cells to osmotic lysis by hypotonic saline can be exaggerated if the test is performed after 24 hours of sterile incubation of the cells at 37°C. Sterile incubation of the patients' blood for 48 hours (the autohemolysis test) also shows a characteristic pattern of increased hemolysis which can be prevented by added glucose.

MANAGEMENT. Splenectomy relieves the manifestations of the disease, although spherocytosis persists. Cholelithiasis and common bile duct obstruction may develop and require treatment. During an aplastic crisis transfusions may be necessary and some patients may require folic acid if they have evidence of megaloblastic anemia.

Other Membrane Defects

Although a much milder condition than hereditary spherocytosis, hereditary *elliptocytosis* is an autosomal dominant illness sometimes associated with hemolysis, splenomegaly, and increased osmotic fragility. Most of the cells appear oval in shape on peripheral smear. Hemolysis, when present, is improved by splenectomy. *Hereditary stomatocytosis* is a rare condition associated with cells which appear to have elongated slits rather than the usual central pallor. The clinical course usually is similar to that of hereditary spherocytosis, but a very severe congenital hemolytic anemia associated with marked abnormalities in membrane sodium-potassium flux also has been reported. Acquired stomatocytosis, a mild condition, may be seen in alcoholism. *Hereditary acanthocytosis* (abetalipoproteinemia) is a congenital lipid disorder associated with marked spiculation of the circulating erythrocytes due to abnormal composition of membrane lipids. The condition is not associated with hemolysis. Other rare congenital abnormalities of the red cell membrane have been reported, some of which are associated with membrane spiculation, e.g., lecithin: cholesterol acyltransferase deficiency.

ENZYME DEFECTS

Congenital nonspherocytic hemolytic anemia is an historical, descriptive phrase used to refer to inherited conditions associated with intrinsic red cell defects other than hereditary spherocytosis and the known hemoglobinopathies. The term is used less frequently as more data have accumulated regarding the pathogenesis of inherited hemolytic diseases. Many of the diseases lumped under the heading of congenital nonspherocytic hemolytic anemia have subsequently been found to be examples of inherited erythrocyte enzyme defects.

The red cell is dependent on glucose metabolism

to provide ATP for the maintenance of its shape and for the energy required to resist osmotic lysis. In addition glucose metabolism provides reduced pyridine nucleotides to maintain hemoglobin in the reduced state and combat various oxidative stresses on the cell. These metabolic requirements in the mature erythrocyte are supplied by the Embden-Meyerhof and pentose–phosphate pathways.

Abnormalities of the Hexose Monophosphate Shunt (Pentose–Phosphate Pathway)

Ordinarily about 10 percent of glucose metabolism in the red cell is by way of the hexose monophosphate shunt; however, under conditions of oxidative stress (exposure to oxidant drugs, infection) glucose metabolism through the shunt may increase markedly. Inability to increase shunt metabolism during periods of oxidative stress results in defective membrane function and the formation of intracellular precipitates of denatured hemoglobin and oxidized glutathione (Heinz bodies). These defects result ultimately in cell death.

GLUCOSE-6-PHOSPHATE DEHYDROGENASE (G6PD) DEFICIENCY.[40] G6PD deficiency is inherited as an X-linked defect (Table 47–5). The enzyme displays genetic polymorphism and more than 100 mutant enzymes associated with abnormal function and oxidative hemolysis have been described. The African variant (GdA-) is extremely common and is found in some 10 percent of black males in America. Approxi-

---

TABLE 47–6
Some Compounds Related to Hemolysis of Glucose-6-Phosphate Dehydrogenase Deficient Cells

I. **Antimalarials**
 Primaquine
 Pamaquine
 Pentaquine

II. **Antibiotics**
 Sulfonamides and sulfones
 Nitrofurantoin
 Para-aminosalicylic acid
 Chloramphenicol*

III. **Analgesics**
 Acetanilid
 Acetylsalicylic acid†
 Phenacetin
 Antipyrine

IV. **Miscellaneous**
 Naphthalene
 Vitamin K
 Dimercaprol (BAL)
 Phenylhydrazine

* Hemolytic in Caucasians, but not in blacks.
† Slightly hemolytic in very large doses.

---

mately 20 percent of black females are heterozygotes. The disease in blacks is mild with usually no evidence of hemolysis except after exposure to a variety of oxidant drugs (Table 47-6) or various infections. In hemizygous males the enzyme is present in red cells at about 10 to 15 percent of normal concentration; in heterozygous females the concentration of enzyme and consequently the propensity to hemolysis varies because of the random inactivation of one of the two X chromosomes in female cells.

In certain Mediterranean populations, Sardinians, Greeks, and Sephardic Jews, for example, a more severe deficiency of G6PD occurs in which the enzyme (Gd Mediterranean) may not be detectable in the red cells. Lower dosages of oxidant drugs cause hemolysis than in the African variant and some oxidant drugs will result in hemolysis in these patients but not in blacks. In addition, a minority of the Mediterranean group, unlike affected blacks, hemolyze after the ingestion of fava beans.

CLINICAL FEATURES. Individuals with episodes of hemolysis only following oxidant stress exhibit the features of acute intravascular hemolysis (rapid drop in hematocrit value, depletion of haptoglobin, hemoglobinemia, hemoglobinuria, reticulocytosis). On smear the erythrocytes may appear normal but are often misshaped, and peculiar cells showing eccentric

---

TABLE 47–5
Glucose-6-Phosphate Dehydrogenase Deficiency

Basic mechanism	Hemolysis due to oxidative damage to various red cell constituents (membrane, globin chains, etc.) due to the inability of the cell to adequately regenerate NADPH
Peripheral smear	Polychromotophilia, various degrees of aniso- and poikilocytosis. Occasional cells with eccentrically located hemoglobin. May be normal in the absence of oxidative stress (drugs, infection etc.)
Reticulocyte index	Increased
Helpful laboratory studies	G6PD assay or screen. Heinz body preparation at the time of hemolysis. Test for hemoglobinemia, hemoglobinuria, hemosiderinuria

concentrations of hemoglobin within the red cells may be seen ("bite" cells, "blister" cells). Wet preparations of blood stained with supravital dyes will reveal Heinz bodies which presumably damage the membrane. The concentration of G6PD within the red cell normally decreases with cell age. In the African variant young red cells have enough activity to protect the cell against oxidative stress, and it is therefore the older cells that are susceptible to hemolysis. This explains why the continuation of the administration of oxidant drugs does not result in persistent severe symptomatic hemolysis but rather a compensated hemolytic state where only cells reaching a certain age are at risk. It also explains why the diagnosis of the African variant may be difficult, especially in female heterozygotes, after a hemolytic event because an increased population of young cells is circulating. Table 47–6 lists those drugs capable of causing hemolysis in affected individuals. Infection (viral as well as bacterial) is probably a more common instigating cause of hemolysis than are drugs.

Laboratory. Although G6PD deficiency is established conclusively only by a quantitative enzyme assay, most laboratories use one of a variety of indirect screening tests to make a presumptive diagnosis. The female heterozygote is difficult to diagnose by either method especially after a hemolytic event. Differential staining techniques that can detect defective cells in a mixed population of normal and defective cells (heterozygote situation) are available primarily as research tools. It is important to identify affected individuals and counsel them about the significance of their disease and the drugs that they must avoid.

Inherited deficiencies of other enzymes of the pentose-phosphate pathway and related reactions are much less common than G6PD deficiency. The ones that have been reported are 6-phosphogluconate dehydrogenase (6-PGD), oxidized glutathione reductase (GSSG-R), glutathione peroxidase (GSH-Px) and glutathione synthetase deficiency.

Abnormalities of Glycolysis[44]

PYRUVATE KINASE DEFICIENCY. The principal source of energy for the red cell is glycolysis (Embden-Meyerhof pathway). Inherited deficiencies of most of the glycolytic enzymes have now been reported. *Pyruvate kinase* deficiency is by far the most common disorder of all the glycolytic defects (Table 47–7). Symptoms vary but most patients have mild to severe chronic hemolytic anemia with jaundice and splenomegaly. On peripheral smear there is polychromatophilia as with other hemolytic processes and there may be moderate variation in the size and

TABLE 47–7	
Pyruvate Kinase Deficiency	
Basic mechanism	Hemolysis due to defective glycolysis. Inadequate aniso- and poikilocyte production with sodium accumulation and membrane dysfunction
Peripheral smear	Polychromatophilia. Spiculated cells are common
Reticulocyte index	Increased
Helpful laboratory tests	Pyruvate kinase assay or screening test. Autohemolysis test, 2,3-DPG assay

shape of the cells; and, occasionally, large numbers of spiculated red cells are seen. In contrast to hereditary spherocytosis, osmotic fragility of the red cells is normal or decreased. Autohemolysis is increased but, unlike HS, is not lessened by glucose. ATP concentration is frequently decreased relative to cell age. In pyruvate kinase deficiency the level of 2,3-DPG is markedly elevated due to the block late in glycolysis. This elevation results in a favorable compensatory shift of the oxygen dissociation curve to the right which facilitates delivery of oxygen to the tissues (Chap. 55). Diagnosis of pyruvate kinase deficiency, as with the other glycolytic enzyme defects, may be suggested by a positive screening test (such as the cyanide-ascorbate test) but can be confirmed only by specific assay. Splenectomy seems partially to ameliorate the disease in many patients. Transfusion requirements may increase during periods of infection because of transient suppression of erythropoiesis.

ABNORMALITIES IN GLOBIN METABOLISM

General Description[46,50]

The hemoglobinopathies are inherited disorders which affect either the structure or rate of synthesis of the globin portion of the hemoglobin molecule. Normal red cells contain three distinct types of hemoglobin (A, A_2, and F), composed of four types of globin chains (Chap. 45). Mutations affecting structure have been described for each type of chain; mutations affecting rate of globin synthesis have been described for all but the gamma chain. Structural mutations produce the abnormal hemoglobins which are detected mainly by electrophoretic techniques; rate mutations produce the thalassemia syndromes.

For each type of polypeptide chain, the gene affecting the rate of synthesis appears at or very near the gene affecting the structure, so close that rate and structural mutations affecting the same chain are inherited as alleles. Therefore a person with sickle cell-thalassemia, who has one gene which directs synthesis of sickle cell hemoglobin and another gene which retards synthesis of beta chains, must pass on one or the other abnormality to each of his offspring.

The two types of mutations also interact in another fashion. In the presence of the thalassemia gene which causes impaired synthesis of globin chains, the activity of its allelic gene increases. If the allelic gene directs synthesis of an abnormal hemoglobin the effect may be striking. Persons with one gene directing synthesis of hemoglobin S and its allele directing normal (hemoglobin A) hemoglobin synthesis produce 30 to 40 percent hemoglobin S and are clinically healthy (sickle cell trait). Persons with sickle cell and beta-thalassemia genes produce 70 to 90 percent hemoglobin S and have a disease which may be severe (sickle cell-thalassemia).

Structural Mutations

With few exceptions structural mutations result from substitution of one letter in the genetic code by another. The amino acid substitutions which result produce clinical disease only if they alter the spatial or electrical configuration of the hemoglobin molecule in a critical region. In general, heterozygotes whose

red cells contain less than 50 percent of the abnormal hemoglobin have clinically significant disease when the hemoglobin is unstable (hemoglobin Zürich), have altered oxygen affinity (hemoglobin Chesapeake), or form methemoglobin of increased stability (hemoglobin M). Aberrant physical properties of the red cell may be responsible for hemolytic anemia when abnormal hemoglobins are present in high concentration (homozygous S or C hemoglobin or S or C thalassemia). Homozygosity may produce hemolytic anemia in an unknown manner (hemoglobin D_{Punjab}, E) or may be entirely benign (hemoglobin G_{Accra}). Some of the physiologically significant abnormal hemoglobins are listed in Table 47–8.

Hereditary Persistence of Fetal Hemoglobin

Another type of defect of globin synthesis is exemplified by the syndrome of hereditary persistence of fetal hemoglobin. This is a clinically benign disorder characterized by the persistence of fetal hemoglobin synthesis into adult life. The mutant gene behaves as an allele of the beta chain structural and rate-determining loci. Two forms of the disorder have been described in detail (although a number more have been recognized): in Greeks, fetal hemoblobin levels of heterozygotes range from 10 to 19 percent; and in American blacks, from 17 to 30 percent. Hemoglobin

TABLE 47–8
Some Hemoglobin Mutations of Clinical Significance

	Functional Derangement	Red Cell Morphology	Clinical Effect
Symptomatic Homozygotes			
S	Tactoid formation on deoxygenation	Sickle cells	Increased blood viscosity causing thrombosis; hemolysis
C	Reduced solubility	Target cells; microspherocytes	Hemolysis; thrombosis
Symptomatic Heterozygotes (Altered Oxygen Affinity)			
M	Stable methemoglobin formation; generally decreased O_2 affinity	Normal	Cyanosis
Kansas	Decreased O_2 affinity	Normal	Cyanosis
Chesapeake	Increased O_2 affinity	Normal	Mild erythrocytosis
Unstable			
Zürich	Unstable	Normal	Hemolysis after oxidant stress
Köln	Unstable	Heinz bodies	Hemolysis

A_2 levels are decreased, and occasional target cells are seen on blood smears. Several persons homozygous for the disorder have been described; blood smears showed many target cells and aniso- and poikilocytosis, but the patients (like the heterozygotes) were not anemic. The fundamental defect involves decreased synthesis of both beta and delta chains.

Qualitative Abnormalities

SICKLE CELL ANEMIA.[48] Sickle cell anemia is a life-long disorder that is the result of the homozygous inheritance of hemoglobin S. It is found almost exclusively in blacks (Table 47–9). About 10 percent of American blacks carry one gene and one-quarter of 1 percent have homozygous sickle cell anemia. The major clinical features are chronic hemolytic anemia; recurrent pain in the extremities, abdomen and back; and a predisposition to thrombosis.

Pathogenesis. Red cells from patients with sickle cell disease assume a peculiar sickle-like shape upon deoxygenation. The basic defect is a genetic substitution of valine for glutamic acid in position 6 of the beta chain. This substitution alters the hemoglobin molecules so that at reduced oxygen tensions they stack up into long intertwining strands which aggregate into rigid, liquid crystals called tactoids. These crystals distort the red cell and produce the characteristic sickle shape.

The sickled red cell is rigid and its mechanical fragility and permeability are increased. Hemolysis, some of it intravascular, results from these changes in the physical characteristics of the red cell. Elongated and hollyleaf-shaped cells increase blood viscosity; stagnant blood flow produces further deoxygenation, and eventually blood vessels are occluded by log-jams of sickled erythrocytes. The cells with the highest concentration of hemoglobin S irreversibly sickle when exposed to reduced oxygen tension and are the ones most responsible for these phenomena. Hemolytic anemia and vascular occlusions are hallmarks of the sickling disorders.

The degree of interaction of other hemoglobins with hemoglobin S modifies the tendency of red cells of heterozygotes to sickle and thereby determines the clinical manifestations that ensue. Patients heterozygous for hemoglobin S and D_{Punjab} are almost as sick as patients with sickle cell anemia. Persons with SC disease have some disability, and people whose red cells contain high concentrations of hemoglobin A and F as well as S, ordinarily are asymptomatic. However, sluggish capillary blood flow or hypoxia can cause patients with SA, SF, or SC hemoglobin to develop signs and symptoms characteristic of sickle cell anemia. Cyanotic heart disease, exposure to high altitudes, fever, and extreme physical exertion have precipitated thrombotic and hemolytic crises in such individuals.

Clinical Features. Most patients with sickle cell disease present with findings which immediately suggest the diagnosis. A history of chronic anemia and jaundice beginning in childhood is the rule. Recurrent severe abdominal pain and limb pain are frequently noted. Although mistaken for symptoms of acute arthritis, the limb pain is usually not in the joint. Recurrent episodes mimicking pneumonia are often the result of repeated in situ pulmonary thromboses, but bacterial pneumonia occurs with increased frequency and severity, and infection is a common cause of illness and death. There is an apparent predisposition to infection, particularly with salmonella: (especially salmonella osteomyelitis) and pneumococci. Chronic recurrent leg ulcerations occur frequently. In older patients symptoms of heart disease and cirrhosis of the liver may develop. Epistaxis and hematuria are common. Rarely patients develop a glomerulopathy. Priapism occurs occasionally, probably because of sickling in the corpus cavernosa of the penis. Most male patients show physical signs of relative androgen deficiency, with absent secondary sex characteristics, attributed to primary testicular failure. Cerebral vascular accidents, although infrequent, occur with increased prevalence due both to bleeding and thromboses.

Most patients are accustomed to chronic anemia and only complain when a complication such as thrombotic crisis, intercurrent infection, or leg ulcer develops. The frequency of painful crises is variable and may range from rare to occasional to distress-

---

TABLE 47–9
Sickle Cell Anemia

Basic mechanism	Hemolysis associated with rigid red cells of abnormal shape due to crystallization of the abnormal S hemoglobin
Peripheral smear	Polychromatophilia, sickle cells are usually seen on an untreated smear. Marked aniso- and poikilocytosis. Occasional Howell-Jolly bodies and Pappenheimer bodies may be seen in patients past age 10. Leukocytosis, thrombocytosis
Reticulocyte index	Increased
Helpful laboratory tests	Sickle cell prep. Hemoglobin electrophoresis

ingly often. The duration of crises averages several days but may last weeks.

On physical examination the patients look younger than their stated ages during childhood and late adolescence. The trunk is relatively short making the measurement from the pubic symphysis to the heel greater than that from the symphysis to the crown. The extremities are long, and the fingers are long and slender. The skull is elongated; leg ulcers may be present; and scars from previous leg ulcers may be seen. The heart is usually enlarged, and a variety of murmurs, both systolic and diastolic, may be heard, which may mimic those of valvular heart disease. The liver is usually palpable but, although the spleen is enlarged in childhood it is almost never, because of repeated infarctions, palpable in an adult. In fact, most patients, by the age of 10, are functionally asplenic; which, along with a reduction in activity of opsonins in their blood, accounts for their susceptibility to pneumococcal infections. (It is now recommended that polyvalent pneumococcal vaccine be given to all patients with sickle cell anemia.)

Laboratory Features. The laboratory findings are those of hemolytic anemia. The blood film reveals marked anisocytosis and poikilocytosis, target cells, some macrocytes, and occasional sickled erythrocytes. Nucleated red cells are frequently seen, particularly in children. The specific gravity of the urine is low, reflecting the loss of renal concentrating ability due to repeated microinfarcts in the medulla of the kidneys. There is increased unconjugated bilirubin in the plasma and increased urobilinogen excretion in the urine and feces. The bone marrow is hyperplastic; the white cell and platelet counts are usually elevated; and the numbers of reticulocytes are increased. A positive sickling test, performed by adding blood to a solution of sodium metabisulfite (a reducing agent), identifies the sickling phenomenon; and electrophoresis of the hemoglobin confirms the diagnosis by showing the typical pattern of homozygous sickle inheritance: hemoglobin S with variable amounts of hemoglobin F and no hemoglobin A.

Occasionally patients with sickle cell disease experience an aplastic crisis, usually in conjunction with an infection. There is a transient suppression of erythropoiesis during which time the severity of anemia increases and the signs of hemolysis (jaundice, reticulocytosis, erythroid hyperplasia of the marrow) disappear. During the period of aplasia, life must be maintained by transfusion, since hemolysis continues.

Management. Treatment is symptomatic. Transfusions should be avoided although they may be necessary during infection, during periods of aplastic crises, or in connection with surgical procedures. When transfusions are given electively the relationship between the viscosity of the blood and thrombosis must be kept in mind. The viscosity of the blood varies exponentially with the hematocrit and it is directly proportionate to the percent of sicklable cells. An ordinary blood transfusion which raises the hematocrit may increase the predisposition to thrombosis. A possible alternative is the use of partial exchange transfusion. This procedure results in a disproportionate reduction in percent of sicklable cells and thus decreases the predisposition to in vivo sickling and thrombosis. Partial exchange transfusions also have been employed in support of patients with chronic leg ulcers, cerebral vascular accidents, and patients to be administered anesthesia.

There is no specific curative therapy for the patient experiencing a thrombotic crisis. Treatment consists of narcotics, often in relatively high doses, for the pain, and, if bacterial infection is present, appropriate antibiotics. Oxygen, intravenous bicarbonate administration, and many different pharmacologic agents which have been advocated at different times are of no help. There is active research in the development of agents that might prevent the clinical manifestations of sickle cell anemia, but, despite transient enthusiasms, no practical therapy is yet available.

Genetic counseling should be an important feature of the care of patients who are homozygous or heterozygous for hemoglobin S.

OTHER SICKLING DISORDERS

Sickle Cell Trait[48]

Individuals with sickle cell trait (SA) are not anemic and are usually asymptomatic, but hematuria and bacteriuria occur with increased frequency. The peripheral smear is normal. In the presence of chronic hypoxia, manifestations ordinarily associated with sickle cell disease may be encountered. Splenic infarctions have occurred in individuals with sickle cell trait when they ascend to high altitudes.

Sickle Cell-Hemoglobin C Disease

The gene for hemoglobin C production is carried almost exclusively by West Africans and their descendants. The carrier rate in American blacks is about 3 percent. S and C hemoglobin genes are alleles so that a quarter of the offspring of parents, each carrying one of the two genes, will have sickle cell–hemoglobin C disease.

Mild to moderate anemia is the rule in sickle cell–hemoglobin C disease; occasional patients have normal blood values (a compensated hemolytic state). More profound anemia may be encountered during pregnancy. Painful thrombotic crises are experienced with a variable frequency, some patients being virtually asymptomatic and others severely afflicted. Complications of the disease include aseptic necrosis of the humeral and femoral heads, bone marrow infarcts, and cerebral and pulmonary infarction. Hematuria and intraocular hemorrhages have been reported. Splenomegaly is frequently encountered in the adult, and a characteristic peculiar arborization of the vessels in the periphery of the retina is seen. In the management of these patients specific attention must be paid to situations which might predispose to thrombosis.

Sickle Cell-Thalassemia

Patients with sickle cell–thalassemia have a chronic hemolytic anemia which mimics sickle cell disease but is usually less severe. Splenomegaly, hematuria, and splenic infarction at high altitudes have been described.

OTHER QUALITATIVE ABNORMALITIES. *Hemoglobin M.* Congenital methemoglobinemia is sometimes due to the inheritance of an abnormal hemoglobin in which the oxidized form of the molecule is so stable that the reducing enzyme systems are ineffective. A number of different types of hemoglobin M have been described. In several of these the distal or heme-linked histidines are replaced by tyrosine. In normal hemoglobin each globin chain contains a crevice in which the flat heme ring is anchored. The heme-linked histidine fastens the iron atom of the heme to one side of the crevice; the distal histidine, on the other side of the heme disc, participates in oxygen binding to the iron atom. If either histidine is replaced by tyrosine, trivalent iron can form a stabilizing intramolecular bond, which prevents reduction of methemoglobin by either of the erythrocytic methemoglobin reductases. Cyanosis is apparent at birth when the abnormality is in the alpha chain, for a fetal methemoglobin is then present; if the anomaly is in the beta chain, cyanosis is delayed until hemoglobin A replaces fetal hemoglobin as the major hemoglobin component. Apart from cyanosis the patients are asymptomatic.

Hemoglobins Associated with Erythrocytosis [42,50]

Over 20 hemoglobin variants have been described in which mutations occur in critical areas of the globin chains affecting the binding of oxygen to hemoglobin and resulting in erythrocytosis (Table 47–8). Many, but not all of these variants may be detected by hemoglobin electrophoresis. Oxygen-binding studies re-veal an increased affinity of the hemoglobin for oxygen, resulting in a shift of the oxygen-dissociation curve to the left. Patients may be plethoric, but are asymptomatic and the erythrocytosis is usually mild. Such an abnormal hemoglobin should be considered in the differential diagnosis of secondary erythrocytosis.

Hemoglobins with Decreased Oxygen Affinity [42,50]

Several hemoglobin variants have been described that have a decreased affinity for oxygen. (Some unstable hemoglobins associated with hemolysis also have a decreased oxygen affinity.) Because of increased oxygen delivery to the tissues there is a decreased erythropoietic response to anemia in these patients. When there is a very marked shift of the oxygen dissociation curve to the right, cyanosis may be observed (hemoglobin Kansas, Table 47–8).

Unstable Hemoglobins [46]

Unstable hemoglobins are variants which are susceptible to denaturation and precipitation within the red cell. Only heterozygotes have been described. Many different varieties have been reported associated to varying degrees, with hemolytic anemia, inclusion bodies in the red cells, splenomegaly, and dark urine (due to the increased excretion of dipyrroles). Most of these mutations involve replacement of amino acid residues in the globin molecule near the site at which it binds heme. Hemolytic anemia varies in severity from one mutation to another and for a given mutation from one patient to another. Patients with hemoglobin Zürich, for example, have not been reported to be anemic except when exposed to sulfonamides, whereas patients with hemoglobins Köln or Hammersmith are chronically anemic. The inclusion bodies are seen usually after incubation of the red cells and consist of denatured precipitated hemoglobin (Heinz bodies) which is only visible in unstained blood or in blood stained with supravital dyes. Some unstable hemoglobins are detectable by hemoglobin electrophoresis, but the best way to establish a presumptive diagnosis is to heat gently lysates of red cells from suspected patients to produce precipitated hemoglobin, a hallmark of the disease. The increased excretion of dipyrroles results apparently from the metabolism of heme liberated from precipitated hemoglobin. Hemolysis in these patients is probably a direct result of damage to the membrane of the red cells by the precipitated hemoglobin.

Quantitative Abnormalities

RETARDED GLOBIN SYNTHESIS: THE THALASSEMIAS. [37,38] The thalassemia syndromes are a heterogenous group of inherited disorders affecting the rate of synthesis of either the alpha chain (alpha-thalassemia) or beta chain (beta-thalassemia) of hemoglobin (Table 47–10). Homozygous beta-thalassemia (thalassemia major) is a life-threatening disorder associated with marked hypochromic anemia, retarded growth, hepatosplenomegaly, and severe iron overload. Hemoglobin F, unequally distributed among cells, comprises 30 to 90 percent of the circulating hemoglobin; the concentration of hemoglobin A_2 is variable. The parents of homozygotes generally have increased concentrations of hemoglobin A_2. Death in childhood or adolescence is the rule.

Heterozygous beta-thalassemia (thalassemia minor) is a benign condition, associated with no or slight anemia, slightly hypochromic red cells, increased target cell formation, and no signs or symptoms. Characteristically the MCV and MCH are extremely low. The discrepancy between the normal or almost normal hematocrit value and the markedly small cells helps to distinguish this condition from iron deficiency. Several variants exist, some with elevated concentrations of hemoglobin A_2 (about 5 percent, compared to a normal of less than 3 percent), some with elevated hemoglobin F (above 2 percent), others with elevated A_2 and F. In the United States the high A_2 variant is the most common (Table 47–10).

People heterozygous for both beta thalassemia and a gene producing a structurally abnormal beta chain mutant (such as S or C) have a disorder that is extremely variable in both its clinical and hematologic severity. These patients characteristically have a higher concentration of the abnormal hemoglobin (70 to 80 percent) than of hemoglobin A. In some patients no hemoglobin A can be detected at all. In contrast subjects who are simply heterozygous for a beta chain variant (sickle cell trait for example) consistently have a lower concentration of the abnormal hemoglobin than of hemoglobin A.

Beta thalassemia has a wide racial distribution but is found in highest incidence among people of Mediterranean ancestry and in the Indian peninsula. About 1 percent of American blacks are heterozygous for this condition.

The genetics of α chain synthesis are more complicated than those of beta chain synthesis. Alpha chain genes appear to be duplicated and thus marked variability in the clinical severity of the various thalassemia states may result depending on the number of genes affected. Deletion of only one gene results in no clinical illness, whereas deletion of three genes may be associated with a significant anemia and marked red cell abnormalities (Hemoglobin H disease). Homozygous alpha thalassemia is incompatible with life since all of the three normal human hemoglobins have alpha chains. The heterozygous state is difficult to recognize because no compensatory increase of A_2 or F is possible and because interaction with the relatively rare alpha chain structural variants is so uncommon. Heterozygous alpha thalassemia has been assumed to be present in those individuals shown to have a minor component of hemoglobin Barts (a gamma chain tetramer) in infancy or hemoglobin H (a beta chain tetramer) after infancy.

ACQUIRED HEMOLYTIC ANEMIA (Table 47–11)

INTRINSIC DEFECTS

Paroxysmal Nocturnal Hemoglobinuria (PNH)[44]
Paroxysmal nocturnal hemoglobinuria (PNH) is an acquired intrinsic erythrocyte abnormality (Table 47–12). Its cardinal features are chronic hemolytic anemia, repetitive nocturnal intravascular hemolysis with morning hemoglobinuria, and a tendency to thrombotic complications.

Although there is no evidence that the disorder is inherited it has many of the characteristics of a genetic disease. First, it is an intrinsic defect of the cell, as shown in cross transfusion experiments in which normal cells survive normally in the patient but the patient's cells are rapidly destroyed when transfused into a normal recipient. Second, there is a deficiency of an erythrocyte stromal enzyme, acetylcholinester-

---

TABLE 47–10
Heterozygous β-Thalassemia

Basic mechanism	Mild extravascular hemolysis and decreased effective production of red cells associated with decreased globin synthesis
Peripheral smear	Hypochromia, microcytosis, mild aniso- and poikilocytosis. Target cells commonly seen. Occasional inclusions. Slight polychromatophilia
Reticulocyte index	Normal or slightly increased
Helpful laboratory tests	Quantitation of hemoglobins F and A_2 (hemoglobin electrophoresis, alkali denaturation test). MCV, MCH, hematocrit.

---TABLE 47-11---
Causes of Acquired Hemolytic Anemia

Acquired Hemolytic Anemia

Intrinsic Defects

1. Paroxysmal nocturnal hemoglobinuria

Extracorpuscular (Extrinsic) Defects
1. Associated with antibodies
   a. Isoantibodies
      Transfusion reactions, hemolytic disease of the newborn
   b. Autoantibodies
      Idiopathic autoimmune hemolytic anemia ("warm" antibody)
      Idiopathic cold agglutinin disease
      Secondary immune hemolytic anemia ("warm" and "cold" antibody)
      (1) Virus infections, infectious mononucleosis, lupus erythematosus, lymphoma, drugs, paroxysmal cold hemoglobinuria
2. Associated with infection (no antibody or enzyme defect)
   a. Malaria, bartonella, bacterial infections, SBE
3. Associated with chemical agents (no antibody or enzyme defect)
   a. Dose related (lead, aniline, H_2O, snake venom, etc.)
   b. Hypersensitivity
4. Hypersplenism
5. Mechanical hemolysis
   a. Microangiopathic hemolytic anemia
   b. Exertional hemolysis
   c. Cardiac hemolysis
   d. Thrombotic thrombocytopenic purpura
6. Miscellaneous
   a. Liver disease
   b. Renal disease
   c. Inflammatory disorders

---TABLE 47-12---
Paroxysmal Nocturnal Hemoglobinuria

Basic mechanism	Intravascular erythrocyte lysis due to complement mediated erythrocyte membrane damage
Peripheral smear	Polychromatophilia
Reticulocyte index	Increased
Helpful laboratory tests	Ham test. Hypertonic sucrose hemolysis test. Bone marrow (hypoplasia sometimes seen). Serum and urine hemoglobin. Urine hemosiderin

Common presenting symptoms include weakness, jaundice, abdominal pain, the passage of dark urine upon awakening in the morning (Table 47–13) and a history of recurrent thrombosis. A history of frequent unexplained transfusion reactions also is sometimes elicited. There are, however, some patients with PNH who have few or none of these symptoms.

The red cells usually appear normal, but they may be hypochromic if sufficient hemoglobin has been lost in the urine to deplete iron stores. There is often a reticulocytosis and unlike the usual hemolytic process, leukopenia and thrombocytopenia are common. Intravascular hemolysis typically results in episodic hemoglobinemia, hemoglobinuria, methemalbuminemia, reduced serum haptoglobin, and hemosiderinuria.

The bone marrow is often hyperplastic but may be hypoplastic. In fact a number of cases of aplastic anemia due to a variety of causes have culminated eventually as PNH. Therefore, the diagnosis should be considered in every patient who presents with puzzling anemia, especially if there is unexplained hemolysis, pancytopenia, recurrent thrombosis, or a history of unexplained transfusion reactions. A num-

ase (ACE). Third, although rare remissions have been reported, the disorder is usually lifelong after onset.

A manifestation of the defect in the cell is hypersusceptibility to lysis in the presence of complement, but in the absence of demonstrable antigen-antibody reactions. Prior binding of earlier components of complement is not a prerequisite for fixation of the "third" component (C_3) to the cell, and therefore lysis occurs more efficiently in PNH than in other complement-mediated hemolytic disorders. In vitro this is expressed as enhanced hemolysis in the presence of acidified serum (Ham Test) or hypotonic sucrose (sugar water test). Platelets and granulocytes share the red cells' increased sensitivity to complement.

---TABLE 47-13---
Evaluation of Urine for Heme

	Microscopic	Benzidene	80% $(NH_4)_2SO_4$
Red cells	+	+	
Free hemoglobin	–	+	Precipitate
Myoglobin	–	+	No precipitate

ber of other illnesses affecting marrow stem cells, (leukemia and various myeloproliferative diseases), have also on occasion been associated with a PNH-like red cell lesion.

The prognosis in patients with PNH is guarded but the course is unpredictable and many patients have a relatively benign disease or long periods of relatively few symptoms. Although many patients are iron deficient, some people feel that administration of iron is contraindicated because the young cells thereby produced are more likely to be hemolyzed. Similarly, transfusion should be given cautiously because of the danger of further stimulating the hemolytic process. Occasional patients appear to decrease hemolysis in response to androgens and corticosteroids have been reported also sometimes to be effective. The major cause of death is thrombosis, perhaps attributable to thromboplastic substances liberated from red cells as they lyse. Attempts to prevent thrombosis with anticoagulants or infusion of dextran have not been impressively successful.

EXTRACORPUSCULAR DEFECTS

Associated with Antibodies[47,49]

Clinically the diagnosis of immune hemolysis mediated by antibodies rests on the demonstration of antibodies on the surface of the red cells and/or in the serum. The standard methods used for this demonstration are the Coombs test and the cold agglutinin assay.

COOMBS TEST. Antibodies coating red cells sometimes cause direct agglutination in vitro (usually IgM antibodies) and are known as "complete" antibodies. However, "incomplete" antibodies (usually IgG) coating red cells require special in vitro techniques for identification. One of these techniques utilizes an antihuman globulin reagent (Coombs antiserum) which when added to antibody-coated red cells causes their agglutination (positive direct Coombs test, Fig. 47-1). Broad spectrum Coombs' antisera identify primarily IgG and complement on red cells but also may give a weakly positive reaction with cells coated by other serum proteins such as transferrin which adsorb normally to reticulocytes. Specific Coombs antisera (anti-IgG, anti-C_3, anti-IgM, etc.) are helpful to identify specifically the coating protein. Anti-red cell antibodies when free in the serum are identified by a technique known as an antibody screen which employs among other tests the use of Coombs antiserum (indirect Coombs Test). The patient's serum is mixed with ABO and Rh compatible red cells and then the Coombs Test is carried out to identify antibody in the serum which has fixed to those red cells. Antibody specificity for various red cell antigens may be determined by using red cells of known antigenicity in the test.

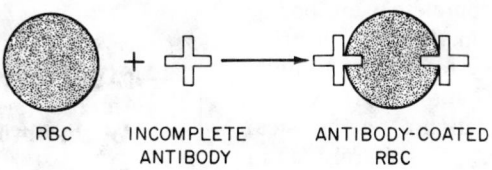

RBC   INCOMPLETE   ANTIBODY-COATED
        ANTIBODY   RBC

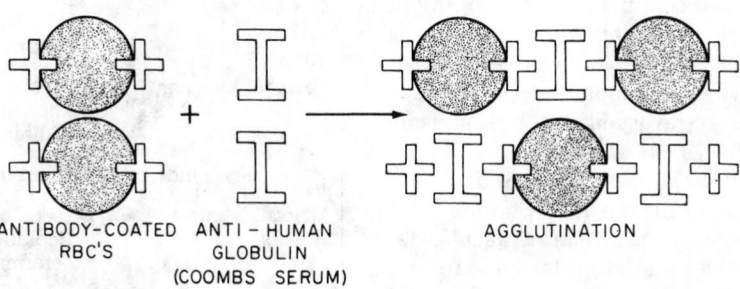

ANTIBODY-COATED   ANTI-HUMAN   AGGLUTINATION
RBC'S   GLOBULIN
                   (COOMBS SERUM)

FIGURE 47-1. Schematic representation of the Coombs test.

COLD AGGLUTININS.[45]   Some antibodies that are present in the sera of patients with immune hemolysis coat red cells and cause agglutination in vitro only when incubation is carried out in the cold (cold agglutinins). For the most part these are IgM complete antibodies which do not require a Coombs test for identification. These antibodies, however, frequently cause complement to become fixed to the red cell, resulting in a positive direct Coombs test.

OTHER LABORATORY FEATURES. In addition to evidence of increased red cell production (polychromatophilia, "shift" erythrocytes) the peripheral smear of patients with immune hemolysis frequently reveals the presence of other abnormalities. Antibody-coated cells lose membrane during their passage through the spleen resulting in microspherocytosis, a common finding in the peripheral smear in immune hemolysis. In cold agglutinin hemolysis the peripheral smear also may reveal evidence of agglutination. This agglutination also may be identified by observing a tube of the patient's anticoagulated blood placed in ice water for a few minutes.

MECHANISMS OF HEMOLYSIS. *"Warm" Antibody.* Red cells coated with IgG antibody are lysed primarily in the spleen and occasionally, when there is a very high titer of the antibody, in the liver. Coated red cells adhere to macrophages which have specific receptors for IgG. By this process the red cell loses membrane, undergoes spherocytosis and ultimately lyses.

"Cold" Antibody. Most cold antibodies, with the exception of the Donath-Landsteiner antibody, are IgM antibodies. Such "complete" antibodies cause agglutination of red cells in vivo with destruction in the reticuloendothelial system. IgM antibody (and to a lesser extent some IgG antibodies) fix complement primarily through activation of the classical complement pathway (C_1, C_4-C_2, C_3). Rarely (as in paroxysmal nocturnal hemoglobinuria, C_3 fixation and activation occurs directly. When the whole complement system is activated on the red cell surface large holes appear in the cell membrane resulting in rapid intravascular lysis of the cell. In most instances once C_3 is fixed to the red cell membrane further sequential activation of complement through C_9 does not occur and lysis is extravascular by mechanisms previously mentioned.

The extent to which the membrane is damaged when antibodies coat red cells (positive Coombs test) varies from no hemolysis to massive intravascular destruction. All the variables important for lysis are not known but include amount of antibody present, type and subclass of antibody, ability to fix complement,

antibody temperature requirements, and red cell antigen specificity of the antibody.

CLINICAL SYNDROMES[47,49]

Idiopathic Autoimmune Hemolytic Anemia, "Warm" Antibody

Approximately half the cases of Coombs-positive autoimmune hemolytic anemia are not associated with an underlying disease process (Table 47–14). Idiopathic autoimmune hemolytic anemia is seen in men and women of all ages. The onset of hemolysis is usually insidious but may be rapid and life threatening. Most of the patients have slight splenomegaly. Platelet and white cell counts are usually normal or increased but severe immune thrombocytopenia may occur in association with autoimmune hemolytic anemia (Evan Syndrome), and leukopenia is occasionally present as well. The disease is characterized by all the laboratory features indicative of an extravascular hemolytic anemia. The reticulocyte count usually is increased appropriately for the degree of anemia but rarely inappropriate reticulocytopenia is observed. The positive Coombs test is due usually to IgG binding to the red cell with little if any complement binding. The antibody frequently has specificity for one of the red cell RH antigens. A small percentage of patients with "warm" antibody autoimmune hemolysis have too few antibodies coating the red cells to be identified by the Coombs test. Antibody identification in such patients requires special techniques, not available to the routine laboratory.

TABLE 47–14
Autoimmune Hemolytic Anemia (Warm Antibody)

Basic mechanism	Immune hemolysis due to an IgG antibody causing erythrocyte adherence to phagocytic reticuloendothelial cells and extravascular destruction
Peripheral smear	Polychromatophilia. Microspherocytes are commonly seen
Reticulocyte index	Increased
Helpful laboratory tests	Direct Coombs test. Indirect Coombs test and determination of antibody specificity. Osmotic fragility test

Approximately 50 to 75 percent of patients with AIHD, whether associated with underlying diseases or with no known cause, will respond to the administration of adrenal corticosteroids. The response varies from complete control of hemolysis to minimal improvement. The effective dose of steroid varies from case to case and occasionally may be of an order that is incompatible with long-term administration. In these cases temporary administration of high doses of steroids may be of crucial value in allowing time for other therapeutic maneuvers directed at the underlying disease to be effective. The steroids may then be withdrawn or the dose reduced to an acceptable level, and the hemolytic process may remain under control. Patients with the other clinical features of autoimmune hemolysis but without a positive Coombs test also deserve a trial of steroids.

About 50 percent of patients with anemia will improve after splenectomy. This approach should be reserved for patients who do not respond to adrenal corticosteroids or to treatment of their underlying disease or in whom the continued administration of steriods is intolerable. Demonstration of excessive sequestration of chromium-labeled red cells in the spleen may be helpful in predicting the response to splenectomy. The recurrence rate of AIHD following splenectomy is substantial. Immunosuppressive agents such as azathioprine and cyclophosphamide have been used to a limited extent in these patients, and the preliminary results have been encouraging.

Secondary "Warm" Antibody Autoimmune Hemolytic Anemia

Immune hemolytic anemia may accompany, as part of the clinical spectrum, a number of diseases including chronic lymphocytic leukemia, lymphosarcoma, and collagen vascular disorders, particularly systemic lupus erythematosus (SLE). A positive Coombs test with or without hemolysis may precede the other clinical manifestations of these diseases (especially SLE) by several months or longer. The syndrome occasionally accompanies viral infections although cold hemagglutinins are more common in these patients and rarely may be seen in a large number of other disease states (such as Hodgkin's disease, teratomas, various other malignancies, tuberculosis, sarcoidosis, etc.). Patients with secondary autoimmune hemolytic anemia due to a warm antibody frequently have a milder hemolytic illness than do those who have no demonstrable underlying diseases. Their red cells are coated frequently with complement as well as IgG or with complement alone and the antibody, when present, usually has no specificity for red cell antigens.

Idiopathic Cold Agglutinin Disease

Normal persons have a low titer of a naturally occurring IgM cold reacting antibody directed against an almost universal red cell antigen designated I. Idiopathic cold agglutinin disease is a very rare disorder associated with high titers of an anti-I cold agglutinin (Table 47–15). Symptoms reflect red cell agglutination with ischemia (acrocyanosis, Raynaud's phenomenon) or hemolysis or both. Splenomegaly is unusual. Patients frequently have increased levels of a monoclonal IgM immunoglobulin which may be the cold agglutinin. These patients are generally elderly and some have a benign course requiring no other treatment than the avoidance of cold. In severe cases treatment is less than satisfactory. In general the response to steroids and splenectomy is disappointing as is therapy with agents such as penicillamine used to break up the IgM molecules. Immunosuppressant therapy may be useful in such cases. When transfusions are necessary it is wise to use red cells washed free of complement. However, shortened red cell survival occurs primarily because of agglutination of cells followed by their removal by the reticuloendothelial system rather than complement-mediated membrane disruption and intravascular hemolysis.

Secondary Cold Agglutinin Disease

ACUTE. Cold agglutinins, in high titer, are detected in the sera of some patients recovering from various viral infections and frequently in patients with mycoplasma pneumonia. Occasionally such patients may develop a hemolytic anemia which rarely

---

TABLE 47–15
Cold Agglutinin Hemolysis

Basic mechanism	Immune hemolysis due to IgM antibodies directed usually against I or i red cell antigens resulting in red cell aggregation and subsequent removal of the aggregated cell by the reticuloendothelial system
Peripheral smear	Polychromatophilia. Red cell aggregation if blood has cooled prior to the smear being made. Occasionally spherocytes are seen
Reticulocyte index	Increased
Helpful laboratory tests	Cold agglutinin titer and specificity. Direct Coombs test (Nongamma Coombs)

may be severe. These IgM antibodies usually have specificity for the I red cell antigen. Some patients with infectious mononucleosis develop an elevated cold agglutinin titer with specificity against an antigen found on newborn cells designated i. Hemolysis in these patients if present at all is usually mild and self limited and rarely necessitates treatment.

CHRONIC.   Some patients (primarily those with lymphoproliferative disorders and collagen vascular disease) have a high cold agglutinin titer with IgM antibodies directed against the I or i red cell antigen. As with secondary autoimmune disease associated with warm antibodies these patients usually have a mild hemolytic disease or no hemolysis at all. Unlike the "warm" antibody disease the response to steroids and splenectomy is poor but improvement frequently follows control of the primary disease process.

Paroxysmal Cold Hemoglobinuria

Paroxysmal cold hemoglobinuria is a very uncommon hemolytic disease associated primarily with syphilis (congenital and acquired) but occasionally seen in viral infections and other disease states. Patients exhibit severe intravascular hemolysis following exposure to cold. Hemolysis is due to the presence of an unusual IgG antibody which in vitro causes red cell agglutination in the cold and complement fixation and hemolysis upon rewarming. This "Donath-Landsteiner" cold antibody has specificity against the P red cell antigen system. The patients may demonstrate a positive direct Coombs test (nongamma Coombs) because of the presence of complement fixed to the red cell surface. Treatment is primarily directed at avoiding cold and at the underlying disease state.

Immunologic Reactions Induced by Drugs[43]

INNOCENT BYSTANDER MECHANISM.   Several drugs (quinine, quinidine, stibophen) may produce hemolysis by combining with specific antibody, adsorbing to the surface of the red cell, and activating complement. In such cases Coombs positive hemolytic anemia develops abruptly but hemolysis stops shortly after the drug is discontinued, even though the antibody can still be demonstrated in the serum. The red cell in this syndrome is an "innocent bystander." Similar reactions have been observed involving platelets and granulocytes; sometimes more than one cell is affected.

HAPTEN MECHANISM.   Hemolysis associated with penicillin is the classic example of this type of drug-induced antibody-mediated hemolysis. A covalent bond is formed between penicillin and red cells when the drug is administered in large dosages. In rare patients an antibody (7S gamma globulin) is produced which reacts with the coated cells causing hemolytic anemia. The Coombs test is positive only when performed with penicillin-coated cells. Hemolysis stops within weeks of discontinuing the drug. Many patients develop an IgM antipenicillin antibody which agglutinates in vitro red cells coated with penicillin. This antibody does not cause hemolysis.

"AUTOANTIBODY" MECHANISM.   Approximately 15 percent of patients administered alpha methyldopa (Aldomet) develop within a year a positive Coombs test; a minority of the people also develop overt hemolytic anemia. The antibody that is involved, a 7S gamma globulin, has specificity for antigens on the surface of the red cell, usually Rh antigens, and the antigen-antibody reaction does not require the presence of the drug. The mechanism whereby the drug stimulates the immune reaction is unknown. The antibody gradually disappears within months after discontinuing the drug.

NONSPECIFIC BINDING.   Cephalothin, a penicillin cogener, also may induce a positive Coombs test, apparently by binding to a serum protein which is then adsorbed on to the red cell. This reaction cannot properly be called immunologic and is not associated with hemolysis.

Other Acquired Hemolytic Anemias

INFECTION.   In the clinical course of malaria and bartonellosis, severe acute hemolytic anemia may be seen. In the United States the more common infections associated with hemolysis include *Cl. welchii,* hemolytic streptococcus, staphylococcus, and salmonella infections. The hemolysis in malaria and bartonellosis is the result of invasion of the erythrocyte by the infectious agent. The mechanism of hemolysis associated with bacterial sepsis is not completely known. In *Cl. welchii* infection, a striking spherocytosis may be noted in the peripheral blood.

CHEMICAL AGENTS.   Certain chemicals can cause hemolytic anemia that is apparently not enzyme dependent. Arsenic, lead, benzene derivatives, intravenous injections of distilled water, or the use of large volumes of water for bladder irrigation during transurethral prostatic resection can all lead to increased hemolysis. Certain drugs (such as probenecid, phenothiazines, arsphenamines) cause hemolytic anemia by some hypersensitivity phenomena in which there is no known enzyme dependency. Some biologic products, such as snake venoms are also potent hemolysins.

LIVER DISEASE.   Some patients following acute alcoholism develop transient hemolytic anemia, sometimes associated with hyperlipemia and frequently with an acute fatty tender liver (Zieve syndrome). There is characteristically little evidence of chronic alcoholic liver disease in these people. Hemolytic anemia also has been seen occasionally in patients with infectious hepatitis by mechanisms other than those associated with red cell enzyme deficiency states. In some patients with severe hepatocellular disease (both acute and chronic) hemolysis develops associated with large numbers of spiculated ("spur") cells seen on peripheral smear, a particularly ominous sign.

HYPERSPLENISM. Patients with large spleens due to a variety of causes frequently have a reduction in the number of one or more of the circulating cell lines. The spleen normally is a filter; when it is large its filtering capacity is increased. Cytopenias (especially thrombocytopenia) appear to occur primarily because cells are sequestered in a large spleen rather than because they are destroyed prematurely. The most common cause of hypersplenism in the United States is congestion due to portal hypertension in patients with cirrhosis, but in fact almost any cause of a big spleen may on occasion be associated with the syndrome of hypersplenism. Hypersplenism can be relieved by splenectomy, but prior to that operation consideration should be given to the severity of the syndrome and to the effect of the operation on the underlying disease. Therapeutic considerations should be based on the degree of clinical difficulty experienced by the patient (transfusion requirement, infection, bleeding) rather than the level of the respective blood cell counts.

Mechanical Hemolysis

Shearing stress upon the red cells, stretching them within the circulation causes them to lose membrane and eventually to be destroyed prematurely. A number of different disease states have been associated with this basic pathogenesis (Table 47–16).

CARDIAC HEMOLYTIC ANEMIA. A number of patients who have had prostheses or patches placed within their hearts have developed mild to moderate hemolytic anemia. The peripheral blood has characteristically shown spherocytes, burr cells, and schizocytes. The Coombs test is occasionally positive. Signs of intravascular hemolysis including hemosiderinuria, are present. The assumption has been that increased turbulence of flow in the vicinity of the repairs has damaged the cells. This assumption is strengthened by the observation that patients who have undergone placement of aortic valve prostheses are the group most likely to have developed hemolysis. A minority of patients exhibit overt hemolytic

---

TABLE 47–16
Mechanical Hemolysis

Basic mechanism	Hemolysis secondary to intravascular red cell injury from endothelial wall damage, turbulent flow, or partial vessel occlusion secondary to the intravascular deposition of fibrin
Peripheral smear	Polychromatophilia. Fragmented erythrocytes (schizocytes), spiculated cells
Reticulocyte index	Increased
Helpful laboratory tests	Serum hemoglobin, urine hemoglobin and hemosiderin

---

anemia but a majority of patients with aortic valve repairs have reduced serum haptoglobin and increased plasma hemoglobin indicative of compensated hemolysis. It has been observed that an increase in cardiac output, as occurs with exertion for example, may accentuate hemolysis. Reoperation is rarely necessary for treatment of hemolytic anemia and many cases have improved spontaneously with time. It has been noted that some patients with unoperated valvular disease, usually aortic but occasionally mitral disease, also show evidence of mechanical intravascular hemolysis.

EXERTIONAL HEMOGLOBINURIA. Some people, usually men after prolonged physical exertion, exhibit hemoglobinuria due to acute intravascular hemolysis. Exertion usually has involved walking or running, and it has been suggested that the red cells are damaged as they pass through the superficial vessels of the feet.

MICROANGIOPATHIC HEMOLYTIC ANEMIA. It has been postulated that the hemolytic anemia associated with a number of different disease states has been produced by fragmentation of red cells within the circulation. The hypothesis has been that these cells are damaged as they squeeze through narrowed small blood vessels occluded by fibrin or platelet plugs. Spherocytes, schizocytes, and burr cells are seen in the peripheral blood of such patients and occasionally there is detectable hemoglobinemia. The platelet count is often low, presumably because the platelets are depleted in the course of intravascular coagulation; rarely coagulation proteins are reduced as well. The disease states most often linked with microangiopathic hemolytic anemia are malignant hypertension, eclampsia and severe preeclampsia, the hemolytic-uremic syndrome in children, rejection of renal homografts, various obstetric emergencies, and sepsis.

Many of these conditions have been associated with disseminated intravascular coagulation (Chap. 48). Treatment of microangiopathic hemolytic anemia is best accomplished by treatment of the underlying disease. In selected cases, however, with progressive disease, anticoagulation with heparin has been employed with variable success.

Thrombotic Thrombocytopenic Purpura

Hemolytic anemia is also encountered in patients with thrombotic thrombocytopenic purpura. These patients usually present with an acute illness characterized by fever, bizarre neurologic and psychiatric dysfunction, hemolytic anemia, jaundice, uremia, and hemorrhagic manifestations. Occasionally the illness is more indolent, and one or several of the above fea-

tures may be absent. Splenomegaly is unusual. The peripheral blood contains bizarre erythrocytes (burr cells, schizocytes, helmet cells) and the platelet count is low. In most instances the disorder is rapidly progressive and terminates in death. Many kinds of treatments have been suggested. Corticosteroids plus splenectomy have been favored by many hematologists but are usually unsuccessful. Occasional improvements have been reported after administration of heparin, immunosuppressive drugs, and drugs that interfere with platelet plug formation. Recently, dramatic improvements have been reported after plasma exchange transfusions and even after simple transfusion of plasma. Because of the prognosis of the disease, most patients are treated with a number of these different forms of therapy.

CHAPTER 48
Bleeding Disorders
PHILIP D. ZIEVE

All animals with a circulatory system are dependent for survival on the capacity of the circulating blood to remain fluid and of the blood shed from injured vessels to clot. In man, loss of blood ordinarily is prevented by the soft tissue support to, and the integrity of, the vasculature; by certain cellular elements, the blood platelets; and by a number of plasma proteins that interact to form a clot at sites of injury.[54,69]

HEMOSTASIS

Blood Vessels

Vascular integrity is partly dependent on actively metabolizing cells of the blood vessels as well as on effective intercellular support by connective tissue. In relatively small arteries and veins vasoconstriction is an important early event in hemostasis before the formation of a clot. Bleeding can be prevented by vasoconstriction alone for several minutes, even in the face of a serious coagulation abnormality. The contraction of injured vessels is apparently a reflex, but biogenic amines released from blood platelets probably contribute to the reaction. Vasoconstriction is probably relatively unimportant in hemostasis in large blood vessels and, in fact, injury to such vessels usually requires artificial support before bleeding can be controlled. If there is major hemorrhage, the volume of blood flowing into injured vessels will decrease because of a reduction in cardiac output and a shunting of blood to vital organs.

Platelets[66]

Platelets are small, granular anucleate cells which are especially important in hemostasis in small blood vessels. They are formed in the bone marrow by megakaryocytes, large cells with multilobed nuclei from whose cytoplasm the platelets appear to demarcate. Like erythropoiesis, platelet production seems to be under hormonal control; but the characteristics of the process are much less clear than are those of red cell production.

Platelets circulate in the blood for about 10 days and then are destroyed in the reticuloendothelial system. The younger cells, those that are only a day or two old, appear larger and more dense than the rest, and are seemingly more effective in hemostasis. When platelet production is increased, the proportion of these young cells in the blood increases also. As an isolated observation, however, the size of the platelets in the blood cannot be depended upon as a reliable reflection of the rate of thrombopoiesis.

When a blood vessel is injured, platelets aggregate at the site and form a viscous plug prior to the formation of a fibrin clot (Fig. 48-1). The platelets adhere first to subendothelial collagen; and then, within seconds, a plug of aggregated cells begins to form. Aggregation is produced by small amounts of thrombin, elaborated at the site of injury, and by adenosine diphosphate released from the platelets themselves. Fusion of the aggregated platelets into an occlusive amorphous mass requires actively metabo-

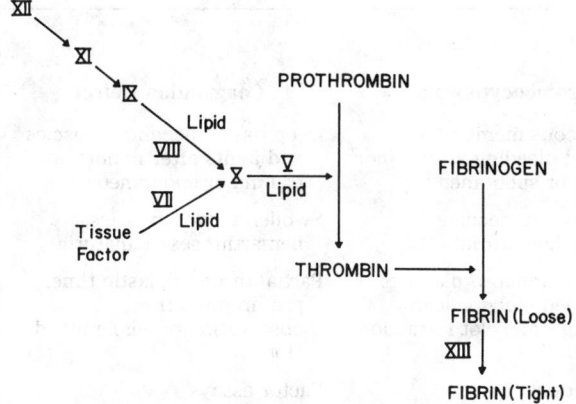

FIGURE 48-1. The coagulation mechanism.

lizing platelets and appears to involve the participation of a contractile protein, thrombosthenin, visible as microfibrils on electron micrographs of these cells.

The hemostatic plug is strengthened eventually by fibrin which within a few days replaces the platelet clot entirely. This so-called white thrombus, which consists of a head of fused platelets and a tail of fibrin within which red and white cells are trapped, is characteristic of clots that form in blood vessels in which the rate of blood flow is relatively high.

Viable platelets are also necessary to support retraction of a fibrin clot. The physiologic importance of clot retraction is unclear, although patients whose platelets are abnormal in that they do not support clot retraction have bleeding diatheses.

Coagulation[53]

Blood coagulation involves the participation of a number of plasma proteins, many of which circulate ordinarily as precursors which are activated sequentially during the course of clot formation. Two different sequences have been identified—the so-called intrinsic and extrinsic pathways (Fig. 48-1).

The intrinsic pathway is initiated by the activation of Factor XII (Hageman factor) by a negatively charged surface (for example, glass or collagen). Activated Factor XII in turn activates Factor XI. There is a complicated interrelationship between the clotting and the kinin systems which influences these early stages of intrinsic blood coagulation. Activated Factor XII catalyzes the formation of active kinins from various precursors (kininogens). Kallikrein, by positive feedback, in turn activates Factor XII and, in fact, appears responsible for most of its formation. High molecular weight (HMW) kininogen is a cofactor in the activation of prekallikrein and Factor XI by Factor XII and the activation of Factor XII by kallikrein. It has been shown, in this regard, that complexes form in plasma between kininogen and prekal-

likrein and between HMW kininogen and Factor XI (PTA, plasma thromboplastin antecedent).

Activated Factor XI activates Factor IX (Christmas factor or PTC, plasma thromboplastin component). Activated Factor IX appears to form a complex with Factor VIII (AHG, antihemophilic globulin), phospholipid, and calcium ions to activate Factor X. The phospholipid is contributed by platelet membranes, altered by exposure to thrombin. Small amounts of thrombin also modify Factor VIII so that the rate of complex formation is increased.

The extrinsic pathway is initiated by exposure of plasma to tissue factor, a lipoprotein which forms a complex with Factor VII and calcium ions to activate Factor X. Activation of Factor X through this pathway is much faster than through the intrinsic system, and it may be that trace amounts of thrombin formed in this way then feed back to accelerate clotting by modifying Factor VIII.[52]

Activated Factor X activates prothrombin (Factor II) to thrombin; the reaction is accelerated by a complex formed by Factor V, calcium ions, and platelet phospholipid. Thrombin increases the rate of this reaction also, by modifying Factor V.

In the last stage of coagulation the soluble protein fibrinogen is converted to an insoluble protein, fibrin, by the proteolytic action of thrombin. This process involves the hydrolysis of four small peptide chains (two alpha and two beta chains) from fibrinogen, and the resultant formation of fibrin monomer, the polymerization of which results in a visible clot. The clot is stabilized by transamidation catalyzed by fibrin stabilizing factor (Factor XIII).

Coagulation, once initiated, would proceed to proteolysis of all the fibrinogen within the vasculature and to permanent occlusion of blood vessels were there not circulating factors which inhibit clotting and others which dissolve the formed clot. Many of these factors are poorly characterized.

Fibrinolysis[61]

The lysis of fibrin clots is accomplished by another series of enzyme-substrate reactions, the characteristics of which are similar in many ways to those of the coagulation mechanism. The active enzyme, plasmin, is formed from an inactive precursor, plasminogen, by the action of various activators which are present in the plasma or tissues. Two of the activators, urokinase, found in human urine, and streptokinase, a bacterial enzyme, have been used therapeutically. Because there are potent inhibitors of fibrinolysis in plasma, it seems likely that significant amounts of plasminogen are formed primarily within the fibrin clot, into which the various components of the fibrinolytic system have been absorbed.

TABLE 48-1
Evaluation of the Bleeding Patient*

	Vascular Defect	Thrombocytopenia	Coagulation Defect
Symptoms	Skin, mucous membrane bleeding after minor trauma	Skin, mucous membrane, cerebral bleeding after minor trauma or spontaneously	Deep tissue bleeding (muscles and joints after minor trauma or spontaneously)
Signs	Ecchymoses, petechiae, melena	Ecchymoses, petechiae, melena, hematuria	Swollen tender muscles, hemarthroses, hematuria
Screening tests	Bleeding time	Evaluate number of platelets on stained blood smear; bleeding time; clot retraction	Partial thromboplastin time; prothrombin time; observation of whole blood clot
Specific tests		Platelet count	Factor assays

* Family and personal histories are extremely important and are discussed in the text.

APPROACH TO THE DIAGNOSIS OF HEMORRHAGIC DISORDERS

A clinical history is extremely important in evaluating the likelihood that a patient has a bleeding tendency. The duration of symptoms, the involvement of other members of the family, the factors which precipitate bleeding, and the sites of bleeding are critical points. Knowledge of the effects of minor surgery such as circumcision, tooth extraction, or tonsillectomy may be helpful in developing the story of a lifelong hemorrhagic diathesis or in identifying the point at which hemostasis became impaired (Table 48-1).

Although the various bleeding disorders produce a variety of hemorrhagic manifestations with a great deal of overlap, certain findings may suggest a particular disease process. Patients whose blood vessels are impaired bleed primarily into their skin and mucous membranes, either spontaneously or excessively after minor trauma. Petechial lesions, pinpoint hemorrhages into the skin, are characteristic of thrombocytopenia; they are most likely to be found in regions of localized high pressure, that is, dependent areas of the body and areas where clothing might be constrictive. Intracranial bleeding is a particular hazard of thrombocytopenia and, in the absence of trauma, less common in coagulation disorders. On the other hand, spontaneous soft tissue or joint bleeding occurs almost exclusively in patients deficient in either Factor VIII or IX.

It must be appreciated that bleeding from a single site (gastrointestinal tract, genitourinary tract, etc.) probably reflects an organic lesion at that site rather than a generalized defect in hemostasis. In fact, even in a patient with a proved hemorrhagic diathesis, one must be certain that visceral bleeding does not originate from such a lesion.

The similarity in the presentation of many bleeding disorders forces the physician to depend on the results of laboratory studies to make a precise diagnosis upon which appropriate therapy depends (Table 48-2). The best screening tests, because they detect an abnormality in most patients with a hemorrhagic tendency, are the platelet count, the one-stage prothrombin time (testing the extrinsic and common pathway), and the partial thromboplastin time (testing the intrinsic and common pathway). The bleeding time is an inexact test but still remains the best screening procedure in patients suspected to have a qualitative defect of their platelets. The once popular clotting time, because it is relatively insensitive, should not be used as a screening test.

VASCULAR DISEASE

Primary vascular abnormalities are not often identified as causes of a hemorrhagic diathesis, perhaps because of the lack of a good test of vascular function (Table 48-3). The bleeding time and tourniquet test are virtually the only tests used to assess the integrity of blood vessels but neither is specific or sensitive enough to be very helpful. A bleeding tendency due to vascular disease is most often expressed as purpura, a purplish discoloration of the skin caused by cutaneous hemorrhage.[63,67]

Simple Purpura

Idiopathic simple purpura is a reasonably common disorder usually mild in its manifestations and consisting primarily of easy bruising, sometimes apparently spontaneous. These lesions on the thighs and

TABLE 48-2
Screening Tests of Hemostatic Function

Bleeding Time

A gross evaluation of vascular integrity. The bleeding time is prolonged in thrombocytopenia, in most qualitative disorders of platelets, and in certain rare disorders of blood vessels. The forearm (Ivy) technique is preferred; the normal range is 2–7 minutes.

Platelet Count

Several methods for direct enumeration are available. The normal range is 150,000 to 400,000/μl. An estimate of the platelet count can be made by careful examination of the stained blood film.

Clot Retraction

In the presence of normal fibrinogen and a near normal hematocrit, clot retraction depends on the number and quality of the platelets. A qualitative estimate of clot retraction can be made at the bedside.

Whole Blood Clotting Time (Glass)

A gross evaluation of the early "stages" of clotting, specifically the formation of intrinsic thromboplastin. The results are expressed in minutes and will vary with the temperature of the reaction, the number of test tubes, the diameter of the tubes, and the size of the needle used for the venipuncture. Capillary blood clotting times are unreliable. Using an #18 needle, clean dry syringe, and 3 tubes of 13 mm in diameter, the normal range is 10 to 20 minutes.

Partial Thromboplastin Time

An evaluation of the formation of intrinsic thromboplastin. The test measures the clotting time of citrated plasma after the addition of cephalin and calcium chloride.

One-Stage Prothrombin Time

An evaluation of the extrinsic pathway of coagulation. An exogenous source of thromboplastin is added to the test plasma and calcium is introduced. The results are expressed in number of seconds required for a clot to form and converted to percent of normal. Serial dilutions of normal plasma are used to construct a curve relating 1-stage prothrombin time to prothrombin content. From this curve the prothrombin content of the test plasma may be estimated as percent of normal. Since the shape of the curve will vary with the type of thromboplastin used, estimates of prothrombin content will vary from one laboratory to another.

Thrombin Time

An evaluation of the concentration of fibrinogen. A solution of thrombin is added to plasma and the clotting time is recorded. A prolonged time indicates a low concentration of fibrinogen, the presence of an inhibitor, or a structurally abnormal fibrinogen molecule.

TABLE 48-3
Bleeding Due to Vascular Damage

Simple purpura
Senile purpura
Allergic purpura
Vitamin C deficiency
Primary amyloidosis
Dysproteinemia
Hyperglobulinemic purpura
Autoerythrocyte sensitization
Hereditary connective tissue disorders
Hereditary hemorrhagic telangiectasia

hips of women sometimes are called "devil's pinches." No generalized hemorrhagic diathesis accompanies these bruises and patients with them withstand surgical procedures normally.

Senile Purpura

Senile purpura is not clinically significant, but it is sometimes confused with other causes of abnormal bleeding. Characteristically, it takes the form of recurrent bleeding on the dorsal surface of the hand and the extensor surfaces of the forearms. The hemorrhage is intracutaneous, usually in parchment-like skin, and can be moved back and forth with the skin over the subcutaneous tissue. The hemorrhage tends to recur and thus often leaves a permanent residuum of dark brown pigmentation. There is no generalized hemorrhagic diathesis and no predisposition to bleeding following surgical procedures. Similar lesions are observed in patients with Cushing syndrome or in those who have had corticosteroid therapy for long periods of time. These latter patients occasionally may have more serious hemorrhagic diatheses.

Allergic Purpura (Schönlein-Henoch)[55]

Purpura in this disorder is part of a widespread disease whose manifestations may include malaise, fever, joint pains and swellings, and abdominal pain. The characteristic clinical presentation is a symmetrical petechial rash, the lesions occurring in clusters, in which there is often both an urticarial and an erythematous component. The limbs and trunk are more frequently involved than the chest, neck, and face. In children, gastrointestinal bleeding and/or intussusception may occur. Some patients develop an acute or subacute glomerulonephritis.

The disorder appears to represent a hypersensitivity reaction, with an accompanying vasculitis, to one of a large number of possible antigenic stimuli. In adults recognized sensitizing agents are most often drugs such as thiazide diuretics, antibiotics, and sedatives. There is no associated abnormality of platelets or coagulation. In many cases no cause is identified.

Treatment is largely supportive. Possible sensitizing agents should be withdrawn. Corticosteroids are of little help. Most patients recover spontaneously in 3 or 4 weeks but some remain symptomatic for a year or more and occasional patients develop chronic renal failure.

Vitamin C Deficiency

In the United States, vitamin C deficiency is primarily a disease of alcoholics although other malnourished people and food faddists are also susceptible. Vitamin C is essential to the formation of normal collagen so that scorbutic patients have defective blood vessels and poor intervascular support. The lesions that result from these defects include large ecchymoses around joints, particularly the knees and ankles, and perifollicular hemorrhages, petechiae which surround hair follicles, primarily of the lower extremities and anterior trunk. The follicles themselves are hyperkeratotic and the hairs protruding from them are often short and broken ("corkscrew hair"). Bleeding gums are common in patients who still have teeth. All of these manifestations disappear within a few days of administration of vitamin C.

Primary Amyloidosis

Cutaneous and, occasionally, gastrointestinal bleeding may complicate the course of patients with primary amyloidosis. Symptoms are due to impairment in vascular integrity as a result of the deposition of amyloid within the walls of blood vessels. Periorbital bleeding and bleeding in skin folds are particularly common. Sometimes amyloid plaques can be seen within the areas of hemorrhage. Rarely, patients with amyloidosis have an unexplained acquired deficiency of Factor X that contributes to their tendency to bleed.

Dysproteinemia

Patients who have myeloma or macroglobulinemia may have a hemorrhagic diathesis, either because of increased blood viscosity (producing anoxic damage to blood vessels) or because the abnormal protein is adsorbed to platelets and coagulation factors and thereby interferes with hemostatic function. Purpura also may be a sign of *cryoglobulinemia,* sometimes associated with myeloma or macroglobulinemia, sometimes present as a benign primary abnormality, and sometimes a feature of a type of immune complex disease in which the cryoprotein is a mixture of IgG and IgM immunoglobulins. In the latter condition, immune complexes also are deposited in the joints and the kidneys, with subsequent arthralgia and progressive renal failure.

Plasmapheresis usually improves hemostasis in patients with hyperviscosity of the blood due to macroglobulinemia (Chap. 92). Patients with myeloma or with mixed cryoimmunoglobulinemia respond unpredictably to cytotoxic therapy.

Hyperglobulinemic Purpura

Hyperglobulinemic purpura of Waldenström is a rare condition characterized by purpura, primarily of the lower extremities; mild anemia; an elevated erythrocyte sedimentation rate; and a polyclonal increase, in the blood, of a mixture of IgG and anti-IgG immunoglobulins. The disorder is much more common in women than men. Sometimes it is associated with an underlying collagen vascular disease. The primary disease begins usually before the age of 40 and, although there is no specific treatment for it, usually has a benign course. The secondary disease begins usually later in life, and the prognosis of affected patients depends on the severity of the underlying disorder.

Autoerythrocyte Sensitization

This disorder is characterized by recurrent, painful, apparently spontaneous ecchymoses of the extremities and anterior trunk. In many patients the lesions have been reproduced following the intradermal injection of the patient's own red cells or red cell stroma. However, virtually all affected patients, most of whom are women, are psychoneurotic; and it now seems likely that the lesions are self-inflicted.

Hereditary Connective Tissue Disorders [63]

In certain of the hereditary disorders of connective tissue, abnormal bleeding into the skin and mucous membranes occurs commonly. Pseudoxanthoma elasticum and, less often, the Ehlers-Danlos syndrome are, in addition, sometimes complicated by arterial hemorrhage.

Hereditary Hemorrhagic Telangiectasia [67]

Hereditary hemorrhagic telangiectasia is an autosomal dominant disorder which results in widespread dilatations of abnormally thin walled venules and capillaries. The characteristic lesions are 1 to 3 mm, flat, round, reddish telangiectases which blanch on pressure. They are most obvious on the lips, tongue, nasal mucous membranes, and hands but presumably occur throughout the body.

Epistaxis is the most common symptom, but gastrointestinal bleeding also occurs and may be particularly difficult to treat. Adults are much more likely than children to be symptomatic; and, in fact, the lesions may not be apparent until the patients reach early adulthood or even middle age.

Larger vascular lesions occur occasionally in the viscera of patients with this disease, especially pulmonary arteriovenous fistulas which develop in approximately one-third of the population at risk and may cause high output heart failure.

The course of hereditary telangiectasia is extremely variable. Some patients suffer enough recurrent loss of blood to become profoundly anemic. Others bleed infrequently. There is no definitive therapy. Bleeding of accessible lesions can be controlled usually by compression or cautery. Gastrointestinal hemorrhage sometimes necessitates surgery but only if all other hemostatic measures have failed.

PLATELET ABNORMALITIES

THROMBOCYTOPENIA [54,69]

The normal platelet count is 150,000 to 400,000 platelets/μl of blood. There is unlikely to be significantly defective hemostasis after trauma, due to thrombocytopenia, unless the platelet count is less than 50,000 to 60,000/μl (Table 48-4). Thrombocytopenic patients who are infected, who have multiple defects in hemostasis, or who have qualitatively abnormal platelets are particularly likely to bleed. If there is bleeding from a single site, such as the gastrointestinal tract, consideration must be given to the possible existence of a visceral lesion (carcinoma of the colon, for example) which has bled under the stress of thrombocytopenia.

The possible causes of thrombocytopenia are listed in Table 48-5.

Decreased Production of Platelets

A variety of primary and secondary disorders of the bone marrow cause thrombocytopenia. Megakaryocytes, in such conditions, usually are markedly reduced. In some cases, the marrow is generally af-

---

TABLE 48-4
Bleeding Due to Thrombocytopenia

Disorder	Thrombocytopenia
Pathophysiology	Defective hemostatic plug formation
Symptoms	Petechiae, mucous membrane bleeding
Screening test	Inspection of smear of peripheral blood
Other useful tests	Platelet count, bone marrow examination

TABLE 48-5
Thrombocytopenia

Megakaryocytes↑↑	Megakaryocytes↓↓
Immune thrombocytopenia	Aplasia
Big spleen syndrome	Leukemia
Ineffective thrombopoiesis (Folate↓, B$_{12}$↓, alcohol)	Marrow infiltration
Thrombotic thrombocytopenic purpura	Congenital*
Disseminated intravascular coagulation	

* Some cases of congenital thrombocytopenia may be associated with normal or increased numbers of megakaryocytes.

---

fected; and the production of red and/or white cells also is compromised. In other cases a disease process primarily affects megakaryocytes so that thrombopoiesis is decreased, but production of other cells remains normal. Generally, diffuse disorders of the marrow such as aplastic anemia (Chap. 46) and acute leukemia cause anemia and granulocytopenia as well as thrombocytopenia. It is useful to examine a smear of the marrow of thrombocytopenic patients to establish that thrombopoiesis is decreased and to diagnose, if possible, the underlying process. Frequently, a specimen obtained by needle biopsy is more representative than an aspirate of the total population of cells.

DRUGS [64] Cytotoxic drugs (cyclophosphamide, vinca alkaloids, and cytosine arabinoside, for example) affect production of all cell lines; the degree of suppression of the marrow depends on the dose. Often thrombocytopenia is less a clinical problem than is anemia or granulocytopenia, but there is considerable variation in response.

Chloramphenicol, a rare, unpredictable cause of aplastic anemia (Chap. 46), will, if the total dose is large enough, predictably suppress hematopoiesis. Reversible thrombocytopenia sometimes ensues, usually accompanied by a reduction in one or both of the other cell lines. A large number of other drugs have been reported occasionally to cause thrombocytopenia (especially thiazide diuretics) but in most cases the association has been only presumptive.

INFECTIONS. Both bacterial and viral infections may be associated with thrombocytopenia. The platelet count often falls slowly, and sometimes morphologic abnormalities of megakaryocytes are observed, suggesting that thrombopoiesis is impaired. It seems likely that decreased survival of circulating platelets contributes to thrombocytopenia in many cases.

CONGENITAL DISORDERS. Congenital thrombocytopenia is rare; when it does occur, it is often associated with other abnormalities. Sometimes the disease is inherited; at other times intrauterine infection (rubella, for example) may be responsible. There is one convincing report of a patient who was born thrombocytopenic because she apparently lacked a factor in her plasma necessary for platelet production; her platelet count rose when she was transfused with normal plasma.

Some patients with congenital thrombocytopenia have a normal number of megakaryocytes in the marrow even though platelet production apparently is reduced. In some of these cases, defective platelets are made which have a shortened survival. Many times, in such conditions, the platelets that do circulate appear abnormal, either large or small, or else bizarre.

MANAGEMENT OF THROMBOCYTOPENIA DUE TO DECREASED PRODUCTION OF PLATELETS. Therapy is dependent on the chronicity and severity of the process. Thrombocytopenia that is expected to be relatively transient (a month or less) may be treated with transfusion of platelet concentrates. It is possible by daily transfusions to maintain platelet counts above a dangerously low level. Patients in an aplastic phase following cytotoxic treatment for acute leukemia are treated in this way with good results. It has been noted that the survival of transfused platelets from histoincompatible donors generally diminishes after multiple transfusions. Platelets (obtained by plateletpheresis) from histocompatible donors appear to survive better, even after repeated administration. In fact, with the use of histocompatible platelets, patients with aplastic anemia have been given transfusions for months in a generally successful attempt to prevent hemorrhage. It should be noted that infection, even in these patients, diminishes survival of the transfused cells. If platelet transfusions are not feasible and if worrisome bleeding occurs, corticosteroids are often prescribed because they appear to improve hemostasis, perhaps by inhibiting the sequestration of young active platelets by the spleen. They have no effect on platelet production.

Increased Destruction of Platelets

Thrombocytopenia due to decreased survival of platelets ordinarily is associated with adequate or increased numbers of megakaryocytes in the bone marrow. The proportion of large, presumably young, platelets in the peripheral blood is usually increased.

IMMUNOLOGIC. *Autoimmune.* [56,62,65] Many patients with thrombocytopenia due to increased destruction of platelets have been said to have had idiopathic thrombocytopenic purpura (ITP). The term has been used to describe a characteristic disorder, rather than all cases of thrombocytopenia in which the cause has not been known, and therefore has never been ideal. Now, however, it seems likely that most cases of so-called ITP have an immunologic cause. In this discussion, therefore, ITP will be used to designate either established or presumptive (auto) immune disease.

Plasma from a patient with ITP transfused to a normal recipient causes thrombocytopenia within a few hours; normal platelets transfused into patients with ITP are destroyed rapidly; and infants born to mothers with ITP are frequently thrombocytopenic. The factor responsible is a 7S gamma globulin adsorbed specifically by human platelets, and, therefore, almost certainly is an antibody. The factor has been titered by measuring its effect, after transfusion, on the survival of normal platelets. If the titer is relatively high, platelets are likely to be sequestered primarily in the liver; otherwise the spleen is the major site of platelet destruction.

Conventional immunologic techniques do not detect the antibody in the serum of patients with ITP; and since transfusion of plasma of affected patients is not ethically permissible as a diagnostic procedure, the diagnosis is usually made by excluding other causes of destructive thrombocytopenia. Recently a number of new in vitro tests for antibody have been reported but none is yet generally applicable. The most specific of these is a technique that has demonstrated directly increased amounts of antibody (IgG) on the surface of platelets from patients with ITP.

Two clinical types of ITP have been described: an acute disease lasting less than 6 months and a chronic disorder lasting longer. Both are assumed to be antibody mediated. In both varieties, the number of megakaryocytes in the bone marrow is normal or increased, and platelet survival is markedly reduced. Neither variety is associated with distinctive physical signs; splenomegaly, in particular, is unusual enough to raise the suspicion of another diagnosis.

Acute ITP is much more common in children. Since it often follows viral illness, it has been postulated that the infection triggers an immune response. In such cases the disease is usually benign; but since a few deaths from severe hemorrhage have been reported, most symptomatic patients are treated with corticosteroids even though it is not proven that therapy influences the course of the disease.

Chronic ITP is more common in adults, particularly women of childbearing age. Occasionally an underlying disorder associated with altered immune reactivity, such as systemic lupus erythematosus or lymphoma, is present but frequently no other process can be identified. There is no association between this disease and a preceding viral infection.

Management. Since thrombocytopenia is a manfestation of a disease rather than a primary disorder, an attempt always should be made to identify and treat an underlying process. However, at times the accompanying hemorrhagic diathesis is so severe or the threat of major bleeding is so great that immediate therapy must be instituted even if a specific diagnosis has not been made. If thrombocytopenia due to increased destruction of platelets is thought to be antibody induced, the use of adrenal corticosteroids should be considered. The decision to treat is dependent on the severity of symptoms and on the degree of risk of a major bleed. Even if the platelet count does not rise, corticosteroids reduce the threat of hemorrhage, perhaps by inhibiting the sequestration of young active platelets by the spleen. The usual initial dose in adults is 60 mg of prednisone a day or its equivalent. The platelet count rises in 50 percent or more of the patients following administration of the drug. Response, if it occurs, may begin within hours, but often takes several days, and may take longer. If there has been no rise in the platelet count after 3 weeks of treatment with a full dose of corticosteroids, it is reasonable gradually to discontinue them. If the platelet count has risen to normal or near normal, the dose of corticosteroid is slowly tapered over a period of months. In some cases the drug may be discontinued in this way with maintenance of normal platelet counts. In others, the platelet counts fall again, sometimes to very low levels, as the dose of steroids is reduced or stopped. Frequently, a dose is reached below which severe thrombocytopenia recurs but above which platelet counts are adequate for normal hemostasis. The manifestation or serious risk of major complications of long-term steroid therapy dictate whether a given dose of drug can be given indefinitely. If not, or if steroids are ineffective, splenectomy should be considered.

Splenectomy, performed early in the course of patients with ITP, is associated with a high rate of cure (75 to 90 percent), partly due to the fact that some patients are treated who would have had spontaneous remissions in any case. If splenectomy is reserved for those patients unresponsive to or unable to tolerate steroids, the response rate is much less (about 50 percent).

There have now been several series of patients, unresponsive to steroids or splenectomy, who have been treated with immunosuppressive drugs (azathioprine, cyclophosphamide, or vinca alkaloids) with a reported high rate of remission. Vinca alkaloids may be particularly useful because long remissions after just a few weeks of therapy have been observed. Recently a regimen has been described whereby platelets are incubated with a vinca alkaloid and then infused into the blood of patients with ITP. In the reported series, remissions were produced in a high proportion of patients refractory to all other forms of therapy, allegedly because of enhanced delivery of the drug to macrophages. To date no properly controlled studies have been done to establish the precise value of any of these drugs in the treatment in ITP.[51]

Drug-Induced Immune Thrombocytopenia.[64] Rarely, patients are administered a drug (quinine and quinidine are the ones most often reported) to which they form an antibody, the immune complex then being adsorbed to platelets, which are "innocent bystanders" in the reaction. The adsorbed complex activates complement which causes premature destruction of the cell, either in the circulation or in the reticuloendothelial system. A similar process has been observed in some of the drug-induced hemolytic anemias (Chap. 47). Thrombocytopenia is characteristically abrupt and severe when the drug is administered but abates within a few days when the drug is stopped.

Isoimmune Thrombocytopenia. Rarely, in newborn infants or in patients recently transfused, transient thrombocytopenia develops, mediated by antibodies against platelet isoantigens. Thrombocytopenia is transient but occasionally severe. In the newborn, the antibody, which is of maternal origin, persists for 3 or 4 weeks, after which the infant's platelet count rises rapidly to normal. If thrombocytopenia is severe, the preferred treatment is transfusion to the child of the mother's washed platelets. Alternatively, transfusion of random platelets, to adsorb circulating antibody, or exchange transfusion is sometimes helpful. The antibodies in the transfused patients, although stimulated by foreign antigens, cause increased destruction of the transfused as well as the patient's own platelets. If bleeding is severe, exchange transfusion may be beneficial

THROMBOCYTOPENIA IN ALCOHOLICS. Chronic alcoholics without splenomegaly, after a bout of drinking, often develop moderate thrombocytopenia. The precise mechanism by which thrombocytopenia is produced is unknown. Alcohol apparently damages platelets so that their survival is short and inhibits the compensatory increase in platelet production that might otherwise prevent thrombocytopenia. Platelet counts rise, within a week, after alcohol is withdrawn, often to levels that are transiently higher than normal.

Hypersplenism or Big Spleen Syndrome

Patients who have large spleens from almost any cause, but most commonly because of congestion, may have thrombocytopenia. It is now believed that platelets in this disorder do not often have decreased survival and that thrombocytopenia merely reflects a redistribution of platelets within a large splenic pool. The degree of thrombocytopenia depends in part on the size of the spleen and in part on the ability of megakaryocytes in the bone marrow to increase the rate of thrombopoiesis. A decision to remove the spleen must be influenced by the severity of the process and by the nature of the underlying disease.

Mechanical Injury

It has been reported that platelet survival is short in patients with prosthetic heart valves and, occasionally, in patients with severe aortic stenosis. Thrombocytopenia is uncommon in this population because of a compensatory increase in the rate of platelet production.

Platelets are damaged also in patients with *thrombotic thrombocytopenic purpura* (TTP), a syndrome characterized by thrombocytopenia, hemolytic anemia, fluctuating neurologic dysfunction, renal failure, and fever. Presumably all of these phenomena are attributable to the widespread deposition of hyaline thrombi in small blood vessels throughout the body. Most reported patients have died. Early splenectomy, in combination with high dose corticosteroid therapy (60 mg of prednisone per day), is said to have cured a few patients. Heparin, aspirin, and dipyridamole (the latter are drugs that inhibit platelet plug formation) also have been advocated and more recently exchange transfusion or infusion of plasma has been said to be effective therapy. Because of the poor prognosis, most patients are treated aggressively by use of at least several, if not all, of these approaches.

DILUTION OF PLATELETS (See Chap. 52) AND INCREASED UTILIZATION OF PLATELETS (Disseminated Intravascular Coagulation)

THROMBOCYTOSIS[2,3]

The clinical disorders in which thrombocytosis is likely to be encountered are shown in Table 48-6. Patients with one of the so-called myeloproliferative diseases (polycythemia vera, myelofibrosis, and chronic granulocytic leukemia) frequently have high platelet counts, with an increased tendency both to bleed and to thrombose. Platelet counts may be higher than one million/μl and bizarre large platelets,

---

TABLE 48-6
Conditions Associated with Thrombocytosis

Myeloproliferative disorders

Malignancy

Inflammatory disease

Postsplenectomy

Acute bleeding

Hemolysis

Hodgkin's disease

---

even fragments of megakaryocytes, are seen in the stained blood smear. A spurious hyperkalemia is sometimes seen, attributable to the loss of potassium from these large cells as the blood clots in the test tube. The cause of the hemorrhagic diathesis is not known although it has been claimed that the platelets are functionally abnormal. Occasionally isolated thrombocythemia (sometimes with splenomegaly) without other evidence of myeloproliferation, is observed. In cases where bleeding cannot be controlled, cytotoxic agents have been administered to lower the platelet count.

Some other causes of thrombocytosis are carcinoma, inflammatory disease (probably the most common), splenectomy, acute bleeding or hemolysis, and Hodgkin's disease. The platelet counts in these conditions usually range between 400,000 and 800,000/μl; the platelets are morphologically normal, and bleeding attributable to thrombocytosis does not occur.

QUALITATIVE ABNORMALITIES

A number of different functional abnormalities of platelets, all associated with a hemorrhagic diathesis, have been described, some of them apparently primary and others associated with an underlying systemic disease (Tables 48-7, 48-8). In general the tendency to bleed is less pronounced in patients with these conditions than in patients with thrombocytopenia. Treatment is ordinarily not needed or possible, but, if bleeding is unusually severe, platelet transfusions should be considered.

Congenital Thrombasthenia

This is a rare autosomal recessive inherited disorder characterized by an inability of the platelets to aggregate or to support clot retraction despite usually normal platelet counts. It has been shown recently that the glycoprotein content of the platelet membrane is abnormal in these patients. Bleeding is ordinarily limited to the skin and mucous membranes.

---TABLE 48-7---
Bleeding Due to Qualitative Platelet Disorders

Disorder	Qualitative disorders of platelets
Pathophysiology	Defective hemostatic plug formation
Symptoms	Petechiae, mucous membrane bleeding
Screening test	Bleeding time
Other useful tests	Aggregation, clot retraction

Thrombocytopathy

This term has been applied to a heterogeneous group of disorders, characterized by defective platelet release reactions. The platelets are either lacking a storage pool of adenine nucleotides (so-called storage pool disease) or are unable to release that pool in response to appropriate stimuli. Platelet coagulant activity also is defective. The bleeding time usually is prolonged, and aggregation of platelets by collagen or thrombin is abnormal. Unlike the situation in thrombasthenia, clot retraction is normal. Symptoms are usually minor.

von Willebrand Syndrome (See p. 534)

Other Congenital Disorders

A number of other congenital disorders, including von Willebrand syndrome, have been described in which platelet function is abnormal but which do not fit precisely into any of the categories that have been described. In most of these conditions the bleeding time is prolonged and aggregation is abnormal, but clot retraction and platelet release reactions are normal.

---TABLE 48-8---
Qualitative Disorders of Platelets

Congenital
  a. Thrombasthenia
  b. Thrombocytopathy
  c. von Willebrand syndrome
  d. Other
Acquired
  a. Uremia
  b. Aspirin
  c. Other

Acquired Disorders

Platelet dysfunction has been reported in association with a number of acquired diseases and with the administration of a large number of drugs. Two situations which are common and well-identified are described.

UREMIA. Bleeding, especially oozing from the gastrointestinal tract and superficial cutaneous hemorrhage, is common in uremic patients. Release reactions are defective and platelets appear to adhere poorly to surfaces. Moderate thrombocytopenia also frequently is observed. Improvement has been described after hemodialysis or renal transplantation, and it has been claimed that a dialyzable inhibitor of platelet function, guanidinosuccinic acid, is responsible for the abnormalities that have been observed. Other retained metabolic products also may be involved.

ASPIRIN. This drug is now recognized to prolong the bleeding time of patients taking it, to interfere with platelet aggregation, and to interfere with the normal release of certain platelet constituents during aggregation. The abnormalities are detectable after patients have ingested as little as one 300 mg tablet of aspirin a day and persist for 24 to 48 hours. Clinical bleeding is unusual in normal people but aspirin may intensify a preexisting hemorrhagic diathesis.

COAGULATION DEFECTS

Patients with a coagulation defect have a hemorrhagic diathesis because of a deficiency of a plasma protein necessary for normal blood coagulation (Table 48-9). In general, the greater the deficiency, the more likely the tendency to bleed. For example, a patient with classical hemophilia (Factor VIII deficiency) who has 15 to 25 percent of normal Factor VIII levels usually has a milder disease than a hemophiliac whose Factor VIII levels are 1 percent of normal. On the other hand, patients with hemophilia whose clotting is delayed but ultimately occurs usually have more severe disorders than do patients with congenital afibrinogenemia whose blood never clots. Furthermore, patients with deficiencies of Hageman Factor (Factor XII) usually have no hemorrhagic diathesis even though their clotting time (in glass) may be prolonged to the same degree as that seen in severe hemophilia. Similarly, patients with prekallikrein or heavy molecular weight kininogen deficiency, whose partial thromboplastic times are prolonged, do not have defective hemostasis. Although such regi-

---

TABLE 48-9
Factors Involved in Blood Coagulation

Factor	Synonym	Site of Synthesis	In Vivo Half-Life
I	Fibrinogen	Liver	3–4.5 days
II	Prothrombin	Liver	2–5 days
V	Proaccelerin	Liver	15–36 hours
VII	Proconvertin	Liver	2–6 hours
VIII	Antihemophilic globulin (AHG)	? Endothelial cells	9–18 hours
IX	Christmas factor or plasma thromboplastic component (PTC)	Liver	20–24 hours
X	Stuart-Prower factor	Liver	32–48 hours
XI	Plasma thromboplastin antecedent (PTA)	Unknown	40–48 hours
XII	Hageman factor	Unknown	48–52 hours
XIII	Fibrin stabilizing factor (FSF)	Unknown	5–12 days

---

mens are effective, the amount of plasma that would be needed to provide concentrates prophylactically to the entire population of severe hemophiliacs in this country is far beyond that which could conceivably be made available. These observations emphasize that our knowledge of the coagulation mechanism is still incomplete.

INHERITED DISORDERS

There are a number of hemorrhagic disorders that are due to an inherited deficiency of a plasma coagulation protein. Since there is considerable similarity in these syndromes, their differentiation depends on appropriate laboratory studies.

Classical Hemophilia [52,68]

Classical hemophilia (Factor VIII or AHG deficiency) will be discussed as a prototype of inherited coagulation disorders (Table 48–10). It is an X-linked disorder that, although rare, is nevertheless the most commonly encountered inherited abnormality of clotting. Most people have believed until recently that the manifestations of the disease result from a deficiency of Factor VIII. It now appears that affected patients have in their plasma a protein structurally similar to Factor VIII which is functionally inactive.

The symptoms of the disease are lifelong. Bleeding often is noted first when an infant is circumcized. As the child grows older, hemarthroses frequently occur, ultimately leading to ankylosis of the involved joints. Hemorrhage into soft tissue, either spontaneously or following trauma, is common. Hematuria may persist for weeks or months. Intracranial bleeding seldom occurs, but occasionally an epidural or subdural hematoma presents a difficult therapeutic problem.

TABLE 48-10
Bleeding Due to Hemophilia

Disorder	Hemophilia (Factor VIII or IX deficiency)
Pathophysiology	Delayed formation of clot
Symptoms	Spontaneous soft tissue or visceral bleeding, hemarthrosis
Screening test	Partial thromboplastin time
Other useful tests	Specific factor assay

The course of the disease seems to cycle between long, symptom-free periods and periods when one catastrophic hemorrhage occurs after another. There is a tendency for the clinical manifestations to become milder as the patient grows older, either because he becomes more cautious or because the disease alters. The psychiatric implications of the disease are important. Many hemophiliacs are overprotected and lead passive, unproductive lives; others are aggressive and self-destructive.

The most precise way of diagnosing hemophilia is by means of a direct assay of the patient's plasma for AHG. Patients with severe disease almost always have levels of AHG that are less than 5 percent of normal. Table 48–2 lists four other clotting tests that are frequently performed. The most sensitive screening test is the partial thromboplastin time, usually prolonged if AHG levels are less than 20 percent of normal. As many as one-third of patients with classical hemophilia have levels of Factor VIII greater than 5 percent of normal and have normal clotting times.

MANAGEMENT. The bleeding hemophiliac is a difficult therapeutic problem and should be managed, if possible, by physicians experienced in treating patients with bleeding diatheses. Superficial wounds, including those inflicted by tooth extractions, may often be treated by pressure and local application of hemostatic solutions (such as topical thrombin). Manipulation of injured tissue should be minimal. The patient should be hospitalized if he has wounds so large that they would ordinarily be sutured or if extensive bleeding into soft tissue, into joints, or into the gastrointestinal tract occurs. Bleeding into a closed space such as a joint cavity is less dangerous than bleeding into an open space such as a muscle or the gastrointestinal tract where there are no physical barriers to limit hemorrhage.

Treatment of the bleeding hemophiliac has been revolutionized in recent years by the development of concentrates of Factor VIII, permitting optimum replacement therapy without danger of circulatory overload. These concentrates are available commercially, but many blood banks prepare their own, less potent, concentrates as cryoprecipitates (Chap. 52) from normal plasma. Factor VIII has a biologic half-life of 8 to 12 hours so that replacement must be given at 8-hour intervals when the hemophiliac is bleeding. Calculation of dosage is beyond the scope of this discussion, but is an important aspect of therapy.

Relatively minor bleeding into the soft tissues or joints usually can be controlled if Factor VIII levels are raised to approximately 10 percent of normal.

That level is attained easily by transfusion of fresh frozen plasma or cryoprecipitate. Hemarthroses, in addition, should be treated by immobilization of the joint in a position of function, followed by gradual exercise once bleeding has stopped. Aspiration of the joint to relieve symptoms is hazardous unless done by highly experienced personnel.

Patients who have sustained major soft tissue hemorrhage require levels of AHG of 20 to 40 percent of normal. Since such levels cannot be reached by transfusion with fresh frozen plasma, cryoprecipitate or commercial concentrates must be employed. Levels of AHG of 50 percent of normal or greater, achievable only by the use of commercial concentrates, may be required to control internal bleeding, a particularly dangerous complication of hemophilia.

Hemophiliacs should not receive intramuscular injections. Venipunctures are safe if properly compressed subsequently for a full 30 minutes. Tetanus immunization can, and should, be safely accomplished with intradermal injections.

Some centers have experimented with intermittent infusions of concentrates as prophylaxis against bleeding in hemophiliacs. Although such regimens are effective, the amount of plasma that would be needed to provide concentrates prophylactically to the entire population of severe hemophiliacs in this country is far beyond that which could conceivably be made available.

Genetic counseling is important for families of hemophiliacs. Carriers (heterozygotes) are usually not detectable by Factor VIII coagulant assay unless levels are below 50 percent of normal (the case in only a minority). If the techniques are available, the carrier state can be diagnosed, in about 90 percent of cases, by comparing the concentration in plasma of antigenic to functional AHG. At the present time, however, only a few laboratories are capable of the appropriate measurements.

Approximately 6 percent of hemophiliacs at some time in their lives develop a circulating anticoagulant which is an inhibitor of AHG. The inhibitor, a 7S gamma globulin, is apparently an antibody. The development of a circulating anticoagulant should be suspected if a previously stable partial thromboplastin time is observed to have become gradually more prolonged, or if seemingly adequate therapy fails to affect the AHG concentration. Unless the inhibitor is present in very low titer, it is difficult and sometimes impossible to raise the patient's Factor VIII levels by transfusion. It is, therefore, worthwhile to test the patient's blood for an inhibitor of Factor VIII after each new episode of bleeding. This test is based on the ability of the plasma containing the anticoagulant to prolong the partial thromboplastin time of normal plasma. It should be mentioned that rarely some patients who do not have hemophilia develop inhibitors against Factor VIII; their clinical presentation is identical to that of hemophiliacs except that they may be of either sex and the onset of the disease is much later in life. Patients who are symptomatic because of a circulating anticoagulant to AHG are at particular risk because of their resistance to factor replacement. Immunosuppression, either with corticosteroids or cytotoxic drugs, has proved largely ineffective. Recently, however, a number of cases have been reported in which infusion of activated prothrombin complex concentrates has been remarkably successful in terminating bleeding in patients with AHG anticoagulants; this approach is likely therefore to become more popular.

von Willebrand Syndrome[52,59]

Von Willebrand syndrome is an inherited (autosomal dominant) bleeding disorder in which there is a reduction in Factor VIII (AHG) as well as a prolonged bleeding time and decreased platelet adhesiveness (Table 48–11). Also, the platelets of patients with von Willebrand syndrome do not aggregate normally in vitro in response to the antibiotic ristocetin. There is, however, considerable variation in these laboratory tests as well as in the clinical presentation of patients with this disorder. In contrast to classical hemophilia, the antigenic and coagulant activity of Factor VIII is reduced proportionately in this syndrome. The hemorrhagic diathesis is similar to that seen in classical hemophilia but is usually milder. The major disability of patients with von Willebrand syndrome is recurrent gastrointestinal hemorrhage. The rise in Factor VIII in these patients following transfusion is often greater, more gradual, and more sustained than would be anticipated on the basis of the amount of

---

┌─ **TABLE 48–11** ─────────────────────
Bleeding Due to von Willebrand Syndrome

Disorder	von Willebrand syndrome
Pathophysiology	Delayed clot formation, defective hemostatic plug formation
Symptoms	Spontaneous mucous membrane bleeding
Screening tests	Bleeding time, partial thromboplastin time
Other useful tests	Factor VIII assay, response to infusion of plasma

---

Factor VIII infused. In fact some of these patients have shown Factor VIII elevations after transfusion with plasma from a true hemophiliac. Hemostasis in bleeding patients often can be effected by a single transfusion of three units of fresh frozen plasma a day. Transfusion may or may not shorten the bleeding time of these patients or increase platelet adhesiveness.

Other Inherited Coagulation Defects

The management of other inherited deficiencies of coagulation proteins is similar to that of classical hemophilia. The diagnosis is established by appropriate laboratory studies. In considering transfusion therapy for these disorders, it is essential to consider the biologic half-life and stability of the clotting factor in question (Table 48–9). However, because of the prolonged half-life of most of these proteins, therapy is usually simpler than it is for patients deficient in Factor VIII. Transfusion of plasma ordinarily is sufficient to control bleeding when it occurs.

Some cases of deficiencies of Factors II, VII, IX, X, and all cases of Factor XIII deficiency have, like hemophilia, been shown to be due to the synthesis of a defective coagulation protein.

ACQUIRED COAGULATION DISORDERS[54,69]

Whereas inherited disorders of coagulation almost always involve the deficiency of only one clotting factor, acquired disorders of coagulation usually involve the deficiency of several factors. Among the commonly encountered disorders are those secondary to vitamin K deficiency, those secondary to anticoagulant therapy, those associated with severe liver disease, and those due to excessive consumption of coagulation proteins in the course of intravascular clotting (defibrination syndromes). Knowledge of the underlying cause of the hemorrhagic diathesis obviously influences the therapeutic approach.

Disorders Due to a Deficiency of Vitamin K Dependent Coagulation Factors[60]

Vitamin K is the name given to several derivatives of Naphthoquinone which are essential in the synthesis of Factors II (prothrombin), VII, IX, and X in the liver. The activation of precursors of these factors requires the carboxylation of specific glutamyl residues, a process somehow dependent on vitamin K. The carboxylated residues increase considerably the affinity of the factors for divalent calcium, an essential cofactor in the reactions in which these factors participate. Vitamin K is a fat-soluble substance (or substances) and so is dependent on bile salts for its absorption in the gastrointestinal tract. The amount of vitamin K in the diet probably does not limit its availability, since it is synthesized by intestinal bacteria.

A hemorrhagic diathesis secondary to a deficiency of vitamin K dependent coagulation proteins may be due to one of a number of causes (Table 48–12):

1. A poor diet in combination with the long-term use of antibiotics that suppress bacterial growth in the intestine. Treatment with oral vitamin K corrects the deficiency. Hemorrhagic disease of the newborn is a condition due to vitamin K deficiency that presumably results from the lack of bacteria which normally synthesize vitamin K in the gastrointestinal tract.
2. Malabsorption of fat-soluble substances secondary either to biliary obstruction or to primary bowel disease (sprue, regional enteritis, ulcerative colitis). Treatment with parenteral vitamin K corrects the deficiency.
3. Severe hepatocellular disease associated with a reduction in synthesis of vitamin K dependent proteins as well as of Factor V and, occasionally, fibrinogen. Treatment with vitamin K does not correct the deficiency. Transfusions to control bleeding should employ fresh blood or plasma, since Factor V is labile on storage.
4. Administration of bishydroxycoumarin or one of its analogues. These drugs are inhibitors of vitamin K and, therefore, impair the synthesis of the vitamin K dependent clotting factors. Because of the wide use of anticoagulants in clinical medicine in the treatment and prevention of intravascular thromboses, a hemorrhagic diathesis secondary to the overuse of coumarin drugs is seen fairly frequently. Treatment with vitamin K_1 (phytonadione) is much more effective therapy than treatment with vitamin K_3 (menadione) or its water-soluble derivative. Vitamin K_1, administered intravenously in a dosage of 50 mg, ordinarily corrects the coagulation defect within 24 to 36 hours (an initial response is observed usually in 4 to 6 hours). If hemorrhage is life-threatening, transfusion with stored blood or plasma should be given prior to the onset of action of vitamin K.

Disseminated Intravascular Coagulation[58]

Isolated deficiency of fibrinogen occurs only as a rare inherited abnormality. The vast majority of fibrinogen deficiencies are acquired and are associated with reduction of a number of coagulation factors (Table 48–13). The occasional hypofibrinogenemia seen in severe hepatocellular disease already has been mentioned. However, by far the most common cause of fibrinogen deficiency in clinical medicine is a result of so-called defibrination or intravascular coagulation (also called consumption coagulopathy). It has long been known that an experimental animal can be depleted of multiple clotting factors by the intravenous infusion of tissue thromboplastin or of thrombin. In addition to hypofibrinogenemia these animals regularly develop deficiencies of other clotting factors and of platelets. In a number of disease states, deficiency of fibrinogen and, more variably, other clotting factors in combination with thrombocytopenia, has been incriminated in the production of a bleeding diathesis. All these diseases are ones in which it is postulated that the coagulation mechanism has been activated causing intravascular consumption of clotting factors. Although obviously thrombosed vessels are not often apparent, microscopic examination of the tissue of patients who have died frequently shows fibrin deposits in small blood vessels. If defibrination is

---

TABLE 48–12
Bleeding Due to Vitamin K Deficiency

Disorder	Impaired synthesis of vitamin K dependent clotting factors
Pathophysiology	Delayed clot formation due to decreased levels of Factors II, VII, IX, and X
Symptoms	Mucous membrane bleeding, excessive bleeding after trauma, ecchymoses
Screening test	Prothrombin time
Other useful tests	Liver function studies

TABLE 48–13
Bleeding Due to Intravascular Coagulation

Disorder	Disseminated intravascular coagulation
Pathophysiology	Activation of the coagulation mechanism
Symptoms	Ecchymoses, petechiae, mucous membrane bleeding, occasionally thromboses
Screening tests	Observation of whole blood clot, partial thromboplastin time, prothrombin time, thrombin time, inspection of smear of peripheral blood
Other useful tests	Specific factor assays, platelet count, measurement of fibrinogen–fibrin degradation products

gradual, partially polymerized fibrin monomer conceivably may be cleared by the reticuloendothelial system without a clot ever having been formed.

Disseminated intravascular coagulation has been described in a number of complications of pregnancy, including amniotic fluid embolism, retained dead fetus, and abruptio placenta. It is seen in patients with disseminated cancer, especially of the prostate, the stomach, and the pancreas, and in patients with acute leukemia, particularly of the promyelocytic type. The syndrome is seen also occasionally in patients with septicemia (bacterial, viral, and malarial); following hemolytic transfusion reactions; following lung surgery; after heat stroke; and in patients who are or who have been in shock. Purpura fulminans, an often fatal condition characterized by extensive gangrene of the extremities and marked prostration, which may follow an apparently benign infection, is also associated with intravascular coagulation.

Although there was at one time some question about the role of fibrinolysis in the production of this syndrome, it is now generally accepted that the increased fibrinolytic activity that is seen in this condition is a secondary manifestation. Primary fibrinolysis has been convincingly demonstrated in only a few cases.

The diagnosis of disseminated intravascular coagulation is suggested by the demonstration of thrombocytopenia, a prolonged prothrombin time, a prolonged partial thromboplastin time, and hypofibrinogenemia in a patient who is bleeding. Fibrinogen deficiency may be suspected after observation of the whole blood clot; when the level of fibrinogen is low, the retracted clot is small and is unable to retain many of the red blood cells, so that the clot appears to lyse. This phenomenon of red cell fallout is more often an indication of fibrinogen deficiency than of fibrinolysis.

One of the hallmarks of the disease is the presence of fibrinogen-fibrin degradation products (split products) in the plasma or serum of affected patients. These are intermediate products which form subsequent to the initial fibrinolysis of fibrin by plasmin. They bind to fibrin monomer and prevent its polymerization and, perhaps more importantly, they interfere in some way with the normal aggregation of platelets. Split products may be demonstrated definitively by immunoassay or presumptively by screening tests (cryoprecipitation, thrombin time inhibition, protamine sulfate precipitation) which depend on the physical properties of the soluble complexes of derivatives of fibrin in the serum.

Therapy of disseminated intravascular coagulation is not often successful unless the underlying disease can be treated. If the disease state is transient (such as an obstetrical complication), usually no therapy is necessary for the hemorrhagic diathesis since depleted factors are rapidly replenished. When bleeding is life-threatening in such cases, replacement with fresh plasma and/or platelet transfusions may be helpful. In recent years a number of patients have been treated with heparin in an attempt to retard intravascular consumption of clotting factors and thereby paradoxically relieve the hemorrhagic diathesis. Some of these patients have improved after such therapy, but it must be remembered that administration of heparin is hazardous in any patient with a preexisting coagulation abnormality, and the drug should be given cautiously. There is no universal agreement about the conditions that dictate the use of heparin in this syndrome.

Anticoagulant Therapy

The bleeding diathesis secondary to an excessive dose of one of the coumarin derivatives or of heparin already has been discussed (Chap. 30).

CHAPTER 49
Disorders of White Cells
ALBERT H. OWENS, Jr.

Current diagnostic classifications of white blood cell disorders are based primarily on the enumeration of the formed elements of the blood and the differential staining of leukocytes in the peripheral blood, bone marrow, lymphoid organs, and other tissues. It is important that physicians remain familiar with the advantages and limitations of these simple morphologic

techniques since they provide information vital to the solution of a wide variety of clinical problems.[1,2,3]

During recent times the characterization of white cells has been amplified by increasingly sophisticated technology. Electron microscopy has provided new insights into the ultrastructure of white cells and the nature of their surfaces. Tissue transplantation studies and the use of various specific biomarkers have provided evidence for the existence of a pluripotential hematopoietic stem cell which is capable of self-maintenance and differentiation along erythrocytic, granulocytic, megakaryocytic, and lymphoreticular lines. Modern marker techniques have permitted in vivo kinetic studies of the production, maturation, and tissue migration of leukocytes and a beginning appreciation of the factors which control and modulate these processes. Improved cell separation techniques together with sensitive and specific biochemical and histochemical methodology have increased our understanding of leukocyte composition, and the mechanisms involved in motility, chemotaxis, phagocytosis, and lysosomal digestion. Some of this newer physiologic and biochemical knowledge has impacted on clinical practice. For example, various qualitative defects in leukocyte phagocytosis and lysosomal digestion have been observed to be responsible for inadequate host defenses against invading microorganisms and simple studies can be performed on peripheral blood leukocytes which will lead to their correct recognition.[71]

In these chapters the white blood cells are identified briefly and their normal physiology and function outlined. The congenital and acquired qualitative defects of leukocyte function are considered together with the clinical syndromes they cause. Since the most common abnormalities in the number and tissue distribution of leukocytes are due to nonhematopoietic diseases, these several derangements are considered as diagnostic problems and the many potential underlying causes related to them. The primary proliferative abnormalities of white blood cells are considered in sequence also. Related accounts of the leukemias and plasma cell dyscrasias are contained in Chapters 55 and 92. Bone marrow failure is discussed in Chapter 46.

GENERAL CONSIDERATIONS

The total leukocyte count in the peripheral blood of normal adults ranges from 5000 to 10,000/μl. Of these, 55 to 65 percent are neutrophils, 1 to 3 percent eosinophils, 0 to 0.75 percent basophils, 25 to 35 percent lymphocytes, and 3 to 7 percent monocytes. In infants, especially in the newborn, white cell counts may be higher, even greater than 20,000/μl and over 50 percent of the cells are lymphocytes.

In adults, significant fluctuations in the total leukocyte count can be seen in a short time interval (minutes to hours) associated with a rapid redistribution of granulocytes between the marginal and circulating pools in peripheral vessels and the ready reserve in the bone marrow. For example, strenuous exercise, pregnancy and labor, convulsions, paroxysmal tachycardia, and emotional panic frequently are accompanied by a neutrophilic leukocytosis on this basis. A different type of variation in total granulocyte counts has been identified also. Cyclic changes with an amplitude of 2000 to 3000 granulocytes/μl and a periodicity of about 20 days have been observed in normal individuals and attributed to variations in the rate of production of granulocytes mediated by humoral substances.

THE GRANULOCYTIC SERIES

Origin[70,72]

The juvenile (band) and mature polymorphonuclear leukocytes (segmented cells) found in the peripheral blood are derived from granulocytic precursors located in the bone marrow. The myeloblast is the least differentiated identifiable form. As the cells mature they become smaller and their cytoplasm is less basophilic. In mature cells the nucleus is segmented and occupies proportionately less of the cell. Mature cells are described further as neutrophils, eosinophils, or basophils according to the staining characteristics of their prominent cytoplasmic granules (Table 49-1). Much evidence points to the existence of a stem cell population which remains largely in a nonproliferative state but is capable of differentiation into erythrocytic, megakaryocytic, and granulocytic cell types.

When considered in toto, the granulocytic cells compose a tissue of impressive size approximating that of the liver (1300 to 1500 g). At a given time, less than 1 percent of the cells are circulating in the peripheral blood. The remainder are located, as developing and mature cells, in the marrow (about 800 to 900 g), in marginal intravascular (capillary) compartments, and in extravascular locations in all tissues, especially the lungs, liver, and spleen (about 500 to 600 g). The relatively large pools of mature granulocytes in the bone marrow and aggregated along capillary walls serve as a ready reserve of motile phagocytic cells.

Life Span

The life span of the normal neutrophil is estimated to be between 10 and 15 days. Approximately 4 to 5 days are spent in the precursor pool in the marrow and an equal time in the marrow reserve. The time spent in the peripheral blood is less than 24 hours.

TABLE 49-1
The Granulocytic Series

Cell	Morphologic Features	Physiologic Function	Location
Myeloblast (15–20 μm)	Large nucleus, fine chromatin, usually two or more nucleoli Clear scant cytoplasm	Proliferation Marked DNA, RNA, protein synthesis	Confined to marrow except in disease
Myelocyte	Nuclear chromatin coarsens; nucleoli disappear Cytoplasm less basophilic, more abundant Prominent cytoplasmic granules develop	Progressive differentiation DNA, RNA, protein synthesis still prominent	Confined to marrow except in disease
Segmented cell (12–15 μm)	Band-shaped to multilobed nucleus; coarse chromatin Nuclear "drum stick" (Barr body) in 3% normal female cells Neutrophilic, eosinophilic, or basophilic cytoplasmic granules	Motility, chemotaxis, immune adherence, phagocytosis, and lysosomal digestion Glycolysis provides energy for phagocytosis Protein synthesis continues	Bone marrow Peripheral blood Tissues

---

The tissues in which most neutrophils are removed from the circulation are the lungs, liver, spleen, gastrointestinal tract, bone marrow, striated muscle, and kidney. Some granulocytes will survive an additional 4 to 5 days in extravascular sites.

Several factors are known to affect the concentration of circulating granulocytes (the size of the circulating pool). Rapid mobilization of granulocytes from noncirculating pools in the bone marrow and along the margins of blood vessels can result from acute physiologic events such as violent exercise and emotional events or the administration of pharmacologic agents such as endotoxin, adrenal corticosteroids, adrenalin, heparin, and etiocholanolone. The circulating leukocyte count may increase by a factor of 2 or 3, with children tending to be more reactive than adults.

While there is much to suggest a positive feedback control of granulocyte production which operates on a stem cell precursor in a manner analogous to erythropoietin in erythropoiesis, the existence of "granulopoietin" has not been proven conclusively. There are substances in the serum of humans and other species which appear to stimulate and inhibit granulocyte proliferation. A glycoprotein "colony stimulating factor" has been identified which appears to stimulate the proliferation of "committed" granulocyte precursors. The existence of "chalone" and "antichalone" has been claimed by several workers which inhibit the myelocyte (not the stem cell) or stimulate it to further proliferative activity (antichalone). Further work is needed to clarify these issues.

Function[71]

The mature granulocytes are concerned primarily with defending the body against invading microorganisms and other injurious agents. In order to achieve this purpose the granulocytes are motile, responsive to chemotactic stimuli, able to migrate through tissues, capable of recognizing foreign objects, phagocytizing them, and digesting them.

Chemotactic factors cause the active, directional migration of granulocytes to involved tissue sites by an ill understood series of events. Chemotactic factors are contained in necrotic tissue, bacterial lipopolysaccharides, complement components, and granulocytes themselves. Certain complement dependent antigen–antibody interactions (opsonins) also stimulate the directional migration of granulocytes. Neutrophils and eosinophils are more responsive to these stimuli than are basophils.

The mechanisms by which granulocytes recognize and bind to a foreign object are largely unknown. The energy required for phagocytosis is derived mainly from glycolysis. Phagocytic activity seems to be increased in anemic individuals and those with fever. Phagocytosis is impaired in malnourished individuals and in the presence of high glucose concentrations. Many bacteria produce substances which inhibit phagocytosis—for example, somatic O antigens, capsular polysaccharides, exotoxins, leukocidins.

Mature granulocytes contain two types of granules called by some "azurophilic" and "specific." The azurophilic granules (lysosomes) contain a large complement of hydrolytic enzymes that are capable of digesting phagocytized material. There are enzymes capable of degrading nucleic acids, proteins, carbohydrates, and lipids. These granules also contain enzymes which attack collagen, glucuronides, and cell membranes (hemolysins). Other granule-associated materials are pyrogenic, thromboplastin-like, phagocytin, hyaluronic acid, and several mucopolysaccharides. The "specific" granules in mature cells contain alkaline phosphatase. During early stages of development the alkaline phosphatase activity is low or absent and myeloperoxidase, acid phosphatase, and arylsulfatase activity predominate.

Granulocytes make a minor contribution to the body defense mechanisms other than phagocytosis. In individuals with agranulocytosis, antibody production and the expression of immediate and delayed hypersensitivity are unimpaired. However, the mononuclear cell response to skin inflammation is delayed, suggesting that neutrophils enhance their migration to the injured site.

Metabolism

Myeloblasts and myelocytes are capable of purine and pyrimidine biosynthesis and DNA and RNA synthesis, as well. As granulocytes mature, their DNA and RNA content declines proportionally and their nucleic acid synthetic capabilities are lost. Similarly, the tricarboxylic acid pathway enzymes decline in activity as the cells mature. Thus, glycolysis is the main energy-producing process in mature granulocytes and it is important to the completion of locomotion

and phagocytosis. Phagocytizing neutrophils are capable of converting oxygen to a series of compounds (including hydrogen peroxide) that have potent antimicrobial activity.

Granulocytes have a higher level of peroxidase, alkaline phosphatase, arginase, and arylsulfatase enzymes than do lymphocytes or other mononuclear cells found in hematopoietic tissue. Similarly, granulocytes contain more glycogen and vitamin B_{12} binding sites and their rates of glycolysis and respiration are greater. Eosinophils have higher levels of catalase and arylsulfatase activity than neutrophils. Basophils are rich in acid mucopolysaccharides, heparin, histamine, and histidine decarboxylase. The full significance of all of those observations is unknown. However, simple histochemical stains for myeloperoxidase aid in the clinical identification of myeloblasts and stains for alkaline phosphatase help distinguish normal mature neutrophils.[1]

THE LYMPHOCYTIC-PLASMA CELL SERIES

Although lymphocytes are usually classified as small, medium, or large, it is more accurate to regard them as having a continuous spectrum of sizes which change back and forth in relation to their biologic function. Small lymphocytes (4 to 10 μm) are the most numerous of these motile cells. The nucleus is large and stains a deep purple-blue, while the cytoplasm is scant and stains pale blue (Wright's stain). Rarely a few azurophilic granules may be present in the cytoplasm. Large lymphocytes (10 to 20 μm) contain larger nuclei, nucleoli, more abundant cytoplasm, and more ribosomes (Table 49-2).

TABLE 49-2
The Lymphocytic-Plasma Cell Series

Cell	Morphologic Features	Physiologic Function	Location
Lymphoblast	Large nucleus, fine chromatin, usually a single nucleolus Clear cytoplasm	Proliferation	Germinal centers of lymph nodes, spleen, tonsils, gut, and other sites Not in blood
Lymphocyte	Small: 4–10 μm Rounded, deeply staining nucleus, masses of chromatin, no nucleoli	Transformation to immunoblasts, plasma cells Cell-mediated immune responses	Lymphoid tissues Peripheral blood Bone marrow Tissues
	Large: 10–20 μm Cytoplasm clear, deeply basophilic to light	Antibody synthesis	
Plasma cell	Large: 10–20 μm Eccentric oval nucleus Dense, coarse chromatin Basophilic cytoplasm, often vacuolated; perinuclear clear zone	Antibody synthesis	Lymph nodes Bone marrow Tissues Not in blood

Lymphocytes have been divided into long-lived and short-lived subpopulations based on the results of kinetic studies employing chemically labeled cells or cells containing x-ray induced chromosomal abnormalities. The longer-lived cells are more plentiful (70 to 80 percent of the total) and have an estimated life expectancy greater than 100 to 200 days. The shorter-lived cells may exist for only 2 to 3 days. These subpopulations cannot be distinguished accurately on morphologic grounds.

Further subsets of lymphocytes have been distinguished on the basis of the molecular configuration of their surface membranes. Bone marrow derived lymphocytes (B lymphocytes, bursa-equivalent lymphocytes) contain various immunoglobulins or immunoglobulin fragments on their surface. These cells are located primarily in germinal centers and medullary cords of lymphoid organs and they are concerned mainly with humoral immune responses. Thymic lymphocytes (T lymphocytes) contain "theta-antigen" on their surfaces. They are found mostly around the germinal centers and in the deep subcortical areas. T lymphocytes are concerned more with cellular immunity.

The morphologic designation, "small lymphocyte" is rather ambiguous. Small lymphocytes may be quiescent for long periods of time, but they are not fully matured or end-stage cells. When stimulated, they may "transform" into blast-like cells, initiate DNA, RNA, and protein synthesis, and divide or further differentiate. Lymphocytes also contain triglycerides, phospholipids, and lecithin. Further, they contain small amounts of glycogen and carry on both aerobic and anaerobic carbohydrate metabolism.[73]

Origin [70,72,73]

Transplantation studies indicate that the marrow contains pluripotential stem cells fully capable of reconstituting the hematopoietic and lymphoreticular tissues. Labeling techniques show that lymphopoiesis in the marrow and thymus procedes continuously at a rapid rate. Marrow-derived cells migrate into the thymus and all other tissues. Thymus-derived cells enter the circulation, also, and the thymus seems to be the main source of the long-lived lymphocytes which recirculate continuously throughout the body. The germinal centers of the various lymphoid organs are the principal sites of production of short-lived lymphocytes in response to antigenic stimulation.

Little is known of the physiologic factors regulating the basal production and circulating levels of lymphocytes, although antigenic stimulation is involved. The administration of ACTH and cortisone is followed by a transient lymphopenia and later lympho-

cytosis. Thyroid hormone stimulates lymphopoiesis. Growth hormone enhances the development of lymphoid tissues. In contrast, testosterone in large doses seems to prevent their full development.

Function

Lymphocytes are concerned primarily with responding to antigenic substances. During the early stages of a primary response, macrophages "process" antigen and interact with lymphocytes in a stimulatory fashion. The resulting immune responses are of two major types, cellular and humoral (antibody), and lymphocytes participate in both (Chap. 91).

The Plasma Cell

Plasma cells develop from lymphoid precursors in germinal centers following antigenic stimulation. In addition, there is evidence which indicates that plasma cells may be derived from lymphoid precursors in the bone marrow. The earliest recognized plasma cell form is a large cell (20 to 30 μm) which may be difficult to distinguish from a blast cell. Mature plasma cells range in size from 4 to 20 μm. Their cytoplasm is basophilic and usually appears mottled. The nucleus contains dense clumps of chromatin (similar to a lymphocyte nucleus) which may be arranged to resemble the spokes of a wheel.

Normally plasma cells are seen in lymph nodes, bone marrow, and other tissues. They are not seen in the peripheral blood except in disease. The maturation time of plasma cells is probably less than 12 hours, and their life span ranges from 2 to 4 days after the last mitosis. Rarely, plasma cells have been reported to be phagocytic; their chief function appears to be antibody synthesis.

The plasmablast is seen in the peripheral blood and bone marrow only in multiple myeloma. It differs from the more mature plasma cell in having a large, eccentric nucleus with fine chromatin and one or more nucleoli. The cytoplasm is basophilic.

THE MONOCYTIC SERIES

Monocytes in the peripheral blood are motile, phagocytic cells of varying size (16 to 30 μm). Large monocytes have a voluminous, kidney-shaped or rounded nucleus containing a fine chromatin network with small chromatin aggregates along the nuclear membrane. Their cytoplasm is abundant and stains gray-blue (Wright's stain). It contains azurophilic granules. Small monocytes are often difficult to distinguish from large lymphocytes (15 to 20 μm). Their nucleus is usually oval or rounded. The cytoplasm stains blue and contains few azurophilic granules. Monocytes give strong histochemical reactions for lysosomal enzymes (muramidase) and nonspecific esterases.

Origin

Monocytes and macrophages constitute a family of related phagocytic cells which are found in the blood, bone marrow, lymph nodes, spleen, liver, lungs, and a wide variety of tissues and body fluids. Monocytes and granulocytes develop from the same immediate precursor. Blood monocytes arise from precursors in the marrow. They are not fully mature cells, and they will divide and differentiate further in lymphoreticular tissues throughout the body. "Promonocytes" and "monoblasts" are difficult to distinguish with light microscopy. The kinetics of monocyte production as studied by current labeling techniques are similar to granulocytes.

Function

Monocytes are often found along the margins of small blood vessels. The ingestion of India ink particles and their propensity to adhere to surfaces has been used as an aid to the identification of monocytes.

Monocytes respond to chemotactic stimuli and foreign substances as do granulocytes. As they leave their marginal locations along small vessel walls and enter tissues, monocytes may be converted into large macrophages with increased phagocytic and digestive capacities. The life span of these macrophages may be prolonged in healthy tissue for many months. When monocytes and macrophages are mobilized to inflamed tissues they function in several ways. They produce a glycoprotein (colony-stimulating activity) that stimulates granulopoiesis and monocytopoiesis. They "process" antigen and induce lymphocytes into "blastic transformation." They interact with lymphocytes to produce "monocyte migration inhibition factor" which aids in the localization of more monocytes in antigen-containing areas. Further, monocytes and macrophages interact with antigen–antibody–complement complexes and elaborate chemotactic and opsonizing factors which promote phagocytosis. In the presence of *M. tuberculosis* and similar materials, monocytes behave in a characteristic fashion by forming into epithelioid and multinucleated giant cells. They also ingest microorganisms and related particles.

Fixed-tissue macrophages, reticulum cells, or "histiocytes" have been thought to arise from the vascular endothelium, hence the term reticuloendothelial system. However, it appears that the stem cell for fixed-tissue macrophages as well as motile monocytes is in the bone marrow. The main function of the mature reticuloendothelial cells (fixed-tissue macrophages), especially those located in the lungs, liver, spleen, and bone marrow, appears to be the trapping and cleaning of particulate matter from the blood stream by phagocytosis.

WHITE CELL DERANGEMENTS IN DISEASE

A frequently encountered clinical problem concerns the evaluation of abnormalities of the leukocytes in the peripheral blood. Such derangements may be reflected in the total white cell count, the proportion of the various (expected) cell types present, or the appearance of grossly abnormal (unexpected) morphologic forms. The following text and tables consider the more commonly encountered derangements and their causes.

THE GRANULOCYTIC SERIES

Granulocytes[2,3,71]

At times, it is possible to detect enzyme defects in genetic disorders by examining the metabolic pathways, enzymatic reactions, or chemical constituents of circulating granulocytes. Among these are glycogen-storage disease, galactosemia, maple-syrup-urine disease, orotic aciduria, acatalasia, and hypophosphatasia. There need not be obvious associated abnormalities of white cell number or morphology.

There are several distinctive morphologic abnormalities which can be encountered in circulating granulocytes and which provide important clues to the diagnosis of inherited or acquired systemic disorders (Table 49-3). Several distinctive heritable functional abnormalities of granulocytes have been discovered in children and adults who were troubled by serious and repeated infections with a variety of microorganisms. These include defects in granulocyte mobility and chemotaxis (lazy-leukocyte syndrome). Chronic granulomatous disease (chronic and recurrent infections) was described initially as a sex-linked disorder affecting male offspring of asymptomatic female carriers. The granulocytes of these patients are capable of phagocytosis, but cannot digest certain microorganisms. Similar cases have been reported in females and appear to be inherited as an autosomal recessive defect. Affected individuals usually have repeated severe infections of the skin, mucous membranes, and airways with eventual systemic dissemination. Sporadic cases of similar granulocyte disorders have been reported as "variants" of chronic

TABLE 49–3
Clinically Significant Morphologic Abnormalities of Granulocytes

Abnormality	Significance
Döhle bodies Cyst-like cytoplasmic inclusions	Acquired: Infections, trauma, cancer, pregnancy, after cytotoxic drugs Inherited: May-Hegglin anomaly, with leukopenia, thrombocytopenia, giant platelets
Macropolycyte Large size (15–25 μm) with nuclear hypersegmenta-tion	Acquired: Chronic infection, granulocytic leukemia after antimetabolites, folate, or B_{12} deficiency Inherited: Autosomal dominant
Failure of nuclear lobe development (1–2 lobes only)	Acquired: Infections, leukemia, metastatic cancer, after drugs such as colchicine Inherited: Pelger-Huet anomaly autosomal dominant
Toxic granulations, vacuolization	Acquired: Infections (bacteremia)
Auer rods (malformed granules containing lysosomal enzymes)	Acquired: Acute granulocytic leukemia
Giant granules	Inherited: Disorders of polysaccharide metabolism, Alder-Reilly anomaly, with gargoylism
Large amorphous granulations, and inclusions	Inherited: Chediak-Higashi syndrome (infections, albinism, neurologic defects, lymphoma) autosomal recessive

granulomatous disease. One autosomal recessive defect has been shown to result in myeloperoxidase deficiency and consequently clinical infections due to impaired granulocyte digestion of microorganisms.

It is a common event to be called upon to evaluate reports from routine peripheral blood examinations which indicate an abnormally high or low circulating white blood cell (granulocyte) count. It is critical to determine whether the circulating elements are the normal, mature cell types expected in the peripheral blood or not. Primary proliferative disorders of the hematopoietic system are usually identified by the preponderance of an abnormal cell type and evidences of organ enlargement and tissue infiltration.

Diurnal variations are observed regularly in the granulocyte count, but the range is seldom greater than 2000 to 8000/μl. A neutrophil count as high as 15,000 to 20,000 may be encountered after strenuous exercise, maternal labor, or convulsions, and is often seen following acute hemorrhage or in the immediate postoperative period. A similar neutrophilia is noted following a transient granulocytopenia.

NEUTROPHILIA. Table 49–4 lists several common causes of significant neutrophilia. It can be seen that a frequent common denominator in these conditions is tissue inflammation, necrosis, or destruction. This neutrophilic leukocytosis is usually accompanied by an increase in the younger band or juvenile forms, and its magnitude is roughly proportional to the extent of the inflammatory or destructive process present. An orderly progression of younger and more mature morphologic forms is to be expected.

LEUKEMOID REACTIONS. A peripheral leukocyte count exceeding 50,000/μl may result from a variety of infections. Its occurrence usually raises the fear of leukemia. For example, bacterial infections, such as pneumonia and meningococcal meningitis, may produce white cell aberrations mistaken for granulocytic leukemia. Similarly, pertussis and infectious mononucleosis may induce an abnormal lymphocytosis sometimes confused with lymphocytic leukemia. Disseminated tuberculosis can cause leukocyte changes that suggest the existence of all forms of lymphocytic, granulocytic, or monocytic leukemia. The fever, lymphadenopathy, and splenomegaly that attend some of these infections may further heighten the suspicion of leukemia.

Leukemoid reactions have been reported in asso-

TABLE 49–4
Causes of Neutrophilia

Infections	Due to bacteria (especially pyogenic), mycobacteria, fungi, spirochetes, parasites May be localized or generalized
Metabolic disorders	Due to diverse causes resulting in uremia, diabetes, acidosis, gout, eclampsia
Neoplasms	Usually widely disseminated myeloproliferative disorders, lymphoma, metastatic carcinoma
Conditions causing cell necrosis or destruction	Infarction due to vascular disease (including polyarteritis) Intoxication due to drugs, especially nephrotoxins and hepatotoxins Acute hemolysis, especially intravascular

ciation with various neoplastic diseases, particularly those involving the bone marrow. Other reports have related these white cell changes to drug reactions, hemorrhage, hemolysis, eclampsia, and severe burns. At times, a number of nucleated red cells and immature white cells appear in the peripheral blood in leukemoid reactions. Their clinical significance is discussed further in the section on leukoerythroblastosis.

When granulocyte constituents are released into tissues in large amounts due to cell breakdown, untoward consequences can result. Proteolytic enzymes can damage vascular membranes, glomeruli, collagen, elastic tissue, etc. Thromboplastin can lead to fibrin formation and eventual collagen deposition and scarring as in polyarteritis, glomerulitis, or arthritis. Other substances released from neutrophils can cause problems such as slow-reacting substance which causes smooth muscle contraction and increased vascular permeability (anaphylaxis), small cationic proteins which are vasoactive, and pyrogens. Leukocytes that bind IgE, especially basophils, will release histamine on contact with antigen and initiate allergic reactions.

EOSINOPHILIA. The more common causes of a significant eosinophilia are listed in Table 49–5. Allergic disorders and hypersensitivity states associated with parasitic infestation or drug administration are the most frequently encountered etiologic entities. On occasion, eosinophilia has been reported as a familial anomaly, but in many such instances parasitic disease is responsible.

BASOPHILIA. Basophilia is encountered infrequently. When noted, it is associated most often with myeloproliferative disorders. At times it has been related to Hodgkin's disease, chronic hemolytic anemia, varicella infection, nephrosis, myxedema, and a foreign protein reaction.

NEUTROPENIA. Neutropenia results from diverse causes. Although present knowledge of granulocyte kinetics in disease states is limited, it appears that a number of conditions produce neutropenia by virtue of impaired granulocyte formation. For example, neutropenia may result from bone marrow damage due to chemical or physical agents and from maturation arrest related to dietary deficiencies or infectious diseases. Neutropenia thought to be a result of an increased rate of destruction of granulocytes has tentatively been related to several disorders resulting in splenomegaly. The precise role of leukoagglutinins is not fully understood. In one instance, that of the neutropenia induced by amidopyrine, the presence of leukoagglutinins has been demonstrated, and

---

TABLE 49–5
Causes of Eosinophilia

Allergic states	Hay fever
	Asthma
	Exfoliative dermatitis
	Erythema multiforme
	Drug reactions
Parasitic diseases	Intestinal forms (hookworm, round worm)
	Tissue forms (toxicara, trichina, strongyloides, echinococcus)
Skin disorders	Pemphigus
	Dermatitis herpetiformis
Neoplasms	Myeloproliferative disorders
	Hodgkin's disease
	Metastatic carcinomas
Other disorders	Scarlet fever
	Polyarteritis
	Eosinophilic granuloma
	Tropical eosinophilia
	Pernicious anemia

TABLE 49–6
Causes of Neutropenia

Infections	Acute viral (rubeola, hepatitis), rickettsial, bacterial (typhoid, brucella), or protozoan (malaria)
	All grave infections (bacteremia, miliary tuberculosis)
Marrow aplasia	Due to chemical or physical agents which regularly produce aplasia (e.g., antimetabolites, alkylating agents, benzol, ionizing radiation) or rarely produce aplasia (e.g., chloramphenicol, sulfonamides, thiouracil, amidopyrine)
	Due to unknown cause or related to myelophthisis (e.g., leukemia, neoplasia)
Nutritional deficits	Folic acid
	Vitamin B_{12}
Splenomegaly	Due to diverse causes (e.g., congestive, infiltrative)
Other disorders	Systemic lupus erythematosus
	Anaphylaxis, antileukocyte antibodies, immunodeficiencies, pancreatic exocrine deficiency, cyclic neutropenia (familial and sporadic)

they seem to be responsible for the agglutination of leukocytes and their rapid removal from the circulation. Another mechanism responsible for neutropenia is exemplified by the sequestration of granulocytes in the tissues, especially the gut, liver, spleen, and lungs, following anaphylactic shock.

The more common causes of neutropenia are listed in Table 49–6. A more comprehensive discussion of agranulocytosis and related abnormalities may be found in Chapter 46.

THE LYMPHORETICULAR SERIES

The lymphoreticular cell system includes monocytes, fixed and mobile macrophages, as well as the lymphocytic cell types. The monocyte-macrophage cell line shares an immediate progenitor with granulocytic cells. The lymphoreticular system responds to various stimuli in a cooperative manner. The clinical and morphologic characteristics of this response vary according to the nature of the stimulus and the overall status of the host.

Lymphocytosis

Acute viral infections and chronic granulomatous disorders are among the most frequent causes of lymphocytosis, being responsible for more than 35 percent of the cases (Table 49–7). A relative lymphocytosis is present in most cases of neutropenia. The lymphocytosis associated with hyperthyroidism is also usually relative.

Plasmacytosis

Plasma cells are not normally seen in the peripheral blood. Rarely, minimal peripheral plasmacytosis has been noted in association with the disorders listed in

---

TABLE 49–7
Causes of Lymphocytosis

Acute infections	Infectious mononucleosis
	Infectious lymphocytosis
	Pertussis
	Mumps
	Rubella
	Infectious hepatitis
	Convalescent stage of many acute infections
Chronic infections	Tuberculosis, syphilis, brucellosis
Metabolic disorders	Thyrotoxicosis
	Adrenal cortical insufficiency
Neoplasms	Chronic lymphatic leukemia
	Lymphomas

TABLE 49–8
Causes of Bone Marrow Plasmacytosis

Acute infections	Rubella
	Rubeola
	Varicella
	Infectious hepatitis
	Infectious mononucleosis
	Scarlet fever
Chronic infections	Tuberculosis
	Syphilis
	Fungus
Allergic states	Serum sickness
	Drug reactions
Collagen-vascular disorders	Acute rheumatic fever
	Rheumatoid arthritis
	Systemic lupus erythematosus
Neoplasms	Disseminated carcinoma
	Hodgkin's disease
	Multiple myeloma
Other	Cirrhosis of the liver

Table 49–8. Plasmacytosis above 10 percent has been reported in serum sickness, drug reactions, measles, scarlet fever, and the other disorders listed, but usually only an occasional plasma cell is seen. A more profound plasmacytosis or the presence of abnormal plasmablasts in the peripheral blood may be equated with the diagnosis of multiple myeloma (plasma cell leukemia).

Modest plasmacytosis is encountered more commonly in the bone marrow than in the peripheral blood. Mature plasma cells composing 5 to 15 percent (or more) of the observed nucleated cells may be related to the many disorders noted in Table 49–8. It is important in each instance to seek an explanation for bone marrow plasmacytosis. Several of the causative diseases are quite responsive to specific therapy. Others clearly carry grave prognoses.

Lymphopenia

Severe depletion or near absence of lymphocytes and plasma cells has been reported in adults in connection with hypogammaglobulinemia and thymoma. In children a variable atrophy or virtual absence of these cells has been noted in several instances of congenital immunodeficiency syndromes (Chap. 93).

Monocytosis

The most frequent causes of monocytosis are listed in Table 49–9. Monocytosis may be observed in relation to the increased myeloid activity induced by such common bacterial infections as pneumococcal pneu-

TABLE 49-9
Causes of Monocytosis

Infections	Bacterial: brucellosis, tuberculosis, subacute infective endocarditis, rarely typhoid fever
	Rickettsial: Rocky Mountain spotted fever, typhus
	Protozoan: malaria
Neoplasms	Monocytic leukemia
	Hodgkin's disease and other lymphomas
	Myeloproliferative disorders
	Multiple myeloma
	Carcinomatosis
Connective tissue diseases	Rheumatoid arthritis
	Systemic lupus erythematosus
Other disorders	Chronic ulcerative colitis
	Regional enteritis
	Sarcoidosis
	Lipid-storage diseases
	Hemolytic anemia
	Hypochromic anemia
	Recovery from agranulocytosis

monia. It is seen frequently during the period of convalescence from such sepsis and also occurs during the recovery phase of marked neutropenia.

The special relationship of the monocyte to tuberculosis and tubercle formation has been cited. In disseminated tuberculosis, less mature monocytes (promonocytes) may be encountered in the peripheral blood. On occasion, failure to pursue a complete diagnostic evaluation has led to a mistaken diagnosis of leukemia.

The proliferative activity associated with responses of the lymphoreticular system may produce distressing results. Cell breakdown products may cause fever, tissue damage (proteolytic enzymes), gout (uric acid), and so forth. Organ enlargement and tissue destruction may result from "benign" disorders. For example, the continual proliferation of macrophages in Gaucher's disease leads to destruction of liver, spleen, marrow, and bone and was once thought to be a malignant, neoplastic process. Impairments of hematopoietic function and immunoresponsiveness can be encountered during reactions of the lymphoreticular system also, as can autoimmune hemolytic anemia and heightened reactivity to insect venoms and poison ivy.

CHAPTER 50

The Myeloproliferative Disorders

ALBERT H. OWENS, Jr.

Excessive proliferation of one or more of the normal bone marrow elements is a commonly encountered clinical phenomenon.[76] These proliferative abnormalities may be categorized further with respect to their neoplastic or non-neoplastic nature (self-perpetuating or self-limiting), their rate of progress (acute or chronic), and the cell type(s) involved.

Nonneoplastic Proliferation

Most frequently, bone marrow hyperplasia occurs in response to recognizable stimuli, is rapid in onset, and resolves completely and promptly following removal of the causal agent. This type of proliferative response may be confined to one cell line or may involve all marrow elements. For example, a self-limited granulocyte response usually attends a pyogenic infection (a selective hyperplasia of the granulocytic series). In contrast, a transient increased proliferation of the erythrocytic, granulocytic, and megakaryocytic

cell lines may follow an acute hemorrhage or hemolytic episode (a self-limited response of all marrow elements).

Neoplastic Proliferation

There are several, often overlapping, clinical disorders that may be grouped together because they share the common feature of self-perpetuating proliferation of bone marrow elements and are associated often with myeloid metaplasia in extramedullary sites. Some of these disorders may run a relatively rapid course, and others may progress more slowly over a period of years (Table 50-1).

ACUTE NEOPLASTIC DISORDERS. Di Guglielmo has called attention to a rare acute myeloproliferative syndrome which is defined by anemia, increased numbers of markedly abnormal erythroblasts in the peripheral blood, and marked erythroblastic over-

TABLE 50-1

Cellular Proliferation in Myeloproliferative Disorders*

Disorder	Erythrocytic	Granulocytic	Megakaryocytic	Fibroblasts Reticulum Cells	Myeloid Metaplasia
Erythroleukemia	3+	1-3+	+/−	−	+/−
Acute granulocytic leukemia	−	3+	−	−	+/−
Thrombocythemia	+/−	+/−	3+	+/−	+/−
Chronic granulocytic leukemia	+/−	3+	1-2+	+	+
Myeloid metaplasia with myelofibrosis	+/−	1-3+	1-3+	3+	3+
Polycythemia vera	3+	1-2+	2-3+	+	+

* Modified from Gunz and Baikie (*Leukemia,* 3rd ed. New York, Grune & Stratton, 1974.

growth of the bone marrow. Individuals with this illness run a course similar to that of acute leukemia. This syndrome might more accurately be considered a "panmyelosis," since during successive periods of its evolution its erythroblastic character may blend into a myeloblastic stage indistinguishable from acute granulocytic leukemia. More frequently, there is a mixed morphologic picture, leading to the use of such terms as "erythroleukemia." Usually, increased numbers of platelets and megakaryocytes are present. Current modes of therapy are usually ineffective, although some cases respond to combination chemotherapy as for acute granulocytic leukemia. Death usually ensues in a matter of months.

Acute granulocytic leukemia may also be considered as a rapidly progressive myeloproliferative disorder with its major expression confined to one cell type. Its clinical features are described in Chapter 55.

CHRONIC NEOPLASTIC DISORDERS. In contrast to acute neoplastic disorders are polycythemia vera, myeloid metaplasia with myelofibrosis, and chronic granulocytic leukemia, which may be considered chronic myeloproliferative syndromes. Some would add thrombocythemia to this group of disorders. Chronic granulocytic leukemia is described further in Chapter 55. Brief characterizations of polycythemia vera and myeloid metaplasia with myelofibrosis follow here. These disorders are not always encountered in pure form, and may share many overlapping clinical features.

Polycythemia Vera[77]

Polycythemia vera is a chronic, self-perpetuating proliferative disorder involving all bone marrow elements and is characterized chiefly by a plethoric, cyanotic appearance, splenomegaly, and an increased red cell mass. In Vasquez's original description in 1892, he considered polycythemia to be a "special form of cyanosis" because there was no discernible cardiac or pulmonary disease. The etiology remains obscure. Polycythemia vera occurs principally during the middle and later years of life. It is more common in men than in women and more frequent in Caucasians than in blacks.

CLINICAL PRESENTATION. Individuals with polycythemia vera may experience varying degrees of general debility and symptoms referable to multiple-organ systems. Many of the clinical manifestations may be related to the increased blood volume (increased red cell mass), increased blood viscosity, tendency to hemorrhagic and thromboembolic events, as well as to the underlying vascular disease (atherosclerosis and arteriosclerosis) commonly present in individuals of this age group.

The initial manifestations are variable. At times the diagnosis is made in asymptomatic individuals. Rarely, a massive gastrointestinal hemorrhage or thrombosis of a coronary or cerebral artery may be the first recognized sign of illness. More commonly, a variety of complaints, such as irritability, easy fatigability, headache, visual disturbances, tinnitus, abdominal fullness, and aching of the lower extremities, is noted. A peculiar pruritus is experienced by approximately half the patients, and it is often particularly severe after bathing. Other common presenting symptoms include dyspnea, angina, intermittent claudication, and dependent edema. Less commonly, gout is the initial clinical problem. Infrequently, patients are mistakenly treated for conjunctivitis, allergy, or arthritis before the true nature of their illness is appreciated.

The major physical findings include a ruddy cyanosis, especially about the face and ears. The florid complexion often appears weatherworn. Ecchymoses are common. The mucous membranes are quite reddened. The retinal veins are usually engorged. Hypertension is found in about half the cases. Peptic ulcer is encountered in 10 to 20 percent of instances and gouty arthropathy in 5 percent or fewer.

Splenomegaly is a cardinal feature of polycythemia vera being present in 75 to 80 percent of cases on presentation. Early in the course of the disease the spleen may not have enlarged to palpable proportions. Later, a progressive increase in spleen size may herald increasing myeloid metaplasia with myelofibrosis or the onset of acute leukemia. Abdominal discomfort results from massive splenic enlargement, and this is periodically intensified by the occurrence of splenic infarcts. Modest hepatomegaly is observed in 30 to 50 percent of patients.

Before treatment, hematocrit values range between 55 and 80. The white cell and platelet counts are elevated; the former usually ranging from 10,000 to 50,000 and the latter from 300,000 to 600,000/μl. The red cells and white cells appear normal. There is a shift to the left in the granulocytic forms. Nucleated red cells and immature myelocytes are encountered occasionally. The granulocyte alkaline phosphatase concentration is high.

The bone marrow is usually quite cellular and the elements present in normal relative proportions. The varying degrees of hyperplasia noted affect the granulocytic and megakaryocytic elements, as well as the erythroblastic elements, giving the impression of a panmyelopathy. During the course of the disease, areas of myelofibrosis and osteosclerosis may be seen in the marrow and small foci of extramedullary hematopoiesis encountered, particularly in the liver and spleen.

The blood volume usually is increased, at times being nearly twice normal, principally because of an increase in the circulating red cell mass. Blood viscosity is increased in proportion to the hematocrit. Ferrokinetic studies reveal an increased plasma iron turnover and erythrocyte production. Red cell life span is normal, as is arterial oxygen saturation. X-rays of the bones generally reveal no abnormalities. The blood uric acid concentration is high in a significant proportion of patients. Erythropoietin concentrations in serum or urine are usually lower than normal or undetectable. Serum vitamin B_{12} concentrations are usually increased.

DIAGNOSTIC CONSIDERATIONS. The occurrence of plethora, ruddy cyanosis, splenomegaly, and hepatomegaly, coupled with polycythemia in the absence of detectable cardiac or pulmonary disease, leads

---

TABLE 50-2

Differential Features of Polycythemic Disorders

Clinical Feature	Polycythemia Vera	Secondary Polycythemia	"Stress" Polycythemia
Red cell mass	increased	increased	normal
Arterial oxygen saturation	normal	decreased	normal
Splenomegaly	present	absent	absent
Granulocytes	increased	normal	normal
Granulocyte alkaline phosphatase	increased	normal	normal
Basophils (blood histamine)	increased	normal	normal
Platelets	increased	normal	normal
Serum vitamin B_{12}	increased	normal	normal
Serum iron	decreased	normal	normal
Erythropoietin	decreased	increased	normal

---

promptly to the correct diagnosis in the majority of cases. To establish a firm diagnosis, there must be an increased red cell mass (males > 36 ml/kg, females > 32 ml/kg), normal arterial oxygen saturation (> 92 percent), and splenomegaly. Thrombocytosis (> 400,000/μl), leukocytosis (> 12,000/μl), elevated granulocyte alkaline phosphatase activity, and increased serum vitamin B_{12} concentration are important secondary criteria (Table 50-2).

Problems arise when individuals present solely with polycythemia or when the clinical features suggest an alternative myeloproliferative syndrome or an alternative cause for the hepatic and splenic enlargement. The polycythemic states (hematocrit above 55) result from increased erythropoiesis. In many instances of secondary polycythemia this increased red cell formation is mediated by erythropoietin. The increased erythropoietin secretion, in turn, may result from hypoxia or may reflect an inappropriate overproduction of this polypeptide by neoplasms or other lesions. Increased erythropoiesis has also been reported to result from the administration of androgens and adrenal corticosteroids. Furthermore, miscellaneous chemical substances, such as cobalt and coal tar derivatives, have been related to a heightened red cell production. In pursuing a systematic diagnostic plan the physician might well search for disorders productive of hypoxia or responsible for an inappropriate overproduction of erythropoietin as well as for the other hormonal and chemical agents indicated (Table 50-3).

When polycythemia is associated with increased white cell and platelet counts, thus giving evidence of a panmyelopathy, the underlying illness is probably a myeloproliferative disorder. This probability is heightened by the coexistence of splenomegaly. The existence of an increased blood (red cell) volume and increased blood viscosity may be seen in polycythemic states irrespective of their etiology. Similarly, gouty attacks and hyperuricemia have been reported in patients with secondary as well as idiopathic polycythemia.

At times, the physician is confronted by polycythemia without other evidence of myeloproliferation or any known causal condition. Rarely, such occurrences have been described as familial. Stress erythrocytosis reported infrequently in anxious or hard-driving middle-aged individuals appears to be a relative polycythemia in that the red cell mass is normal but the plasma volume is decreased. Sometimes the basic diagnosis becomes clear only when additional findings develop.

TABLE 50-3
Causes of Secondary Polycythemia

Associated with Hypoxia
Cardiovascular disease, usually congenital, resulting in
   significant venous admixture
Pulmonary disease resulting in
     Impaired gas diffusion
     Perfusion of poorly aerated lung
     Pulmonary arteriovenous fistulas
High altitude residence
Hypoventilation associated with obesity (Pickwickian
   syndrome)
Hemoglobin variants with increased affinity for oxygen

**Associated with Inappropriate Overproduction of
Erythropoietin**
Tumors, benign and malignant, of the kidney, liver,
   central nervous system, uterus, ovary
Renal cysts, rarely hydronephrosis

Associated with Adrenocortical Steroids or Androgens
Adrenal hypercorticism, all types
Virilizing tumors
Therapeutic use of androgens (rarely corticoids)

Associated with Chronic Chemical Exposure
Nitrites, sulfonamides, coal tar derivatives, and others
   producing methemoglobin and sulfhemoglobin
Cobalt, various alcohols

CLINICAL COURSE AND MANAGEMENT. Patients with polycythemia vera may be expected to survive for 10 to 20 years. The major medical problems encountered stem from the occurrence of vascular thromboses (and emboli) and hemorrhage. A peptic ulcer, which is common in these individuals, may be the site of gastrointestinal bleeding. Epistaxes, ecchymoses, and bleeding following dental extraction are more common. Intercurrent infections, particularly pulmonary, are a significant but lesser problem.

The immediate cause of death in this group of patients is principally the associated cardiovascular disease. Cerebral hemorrhage or thrombosis, myocardial infarction, and heart failure are the most frequent terminal events. In 15 to 25 percent of the patients the disease pattern changes and assumes the characteristics of granulocytic leukemia or myeloid metaplasia with myelofibrosis. At times an acute granulocytic leukemia develops toward the end of the disease.

Management is directed toward maintaining the circulating red cell mass at a near-normal level by the use of venesection, radiation therapy, or myelosuppressive drugs. Functional deficits caused by coexisting vascular disease or other processes, for example, heart failure, angina, and peptic ulcer, require attention when present.

Venesection promptly reduces symptoms due to the increased blood volume. The repeated removal of 500 ml of whole blood every 2 to 3 days until the hematocrit approximates 55 may be followed by several months remission. Symptomatic relief (and a normal red cell mass) often may be maintained by one or two similar venesections every 3 or 4 months. Erythropoiesis will not be limited until repeated phlebotomies have induced iron deficiency. Repeated bleedings are not well tolerated by some individuals and represent a significant inconvenience to others, especially if required more frequently than every other month. Myelosuppressive therapy is required to control aggressive erythropoiesis, granulopoiesis, and thrombopoiesis.

Radioactive phosphorus, ^{32}P, has been employed in the treatment of polycythemia vera for many years. Administered orally or intravenously as dibasic sodium phosphate, it is incorporated into the proliferating hematopoietic cells, thus reducing myelopoiesis. A lowering of the hematocrit, white cell, and platelet counts occurs over the next 2 or 3 months. In about half the cases, one dose of 4 to 5 millicuries will produce a satisfactory remission lasting a year or more. In many instances, a second (and rarely a third) course is required. Satisfactory ^{32}P remissions can be induced in 70 to 80 percent of cases and will last from 6 to 24 months or longer.

Recent surveys have indicated that 10 to 15 percent of patients with polycythemia treated with ionizing radiation eventually develop acute leukemia, in contrast to an incidence of less than 1 percent in patients who received no radiation. It is not clear at present that ^{32}P therapy assures sufficiently lower morbidity to justify the increased risk of leukemia which its use entails. Myelofibrosis also occurs more frequently in ^{32}P treated patients. Alkylating agents, such as busulfan, cyclophosphamide, or chlorambucil, and other cytotoxic agents, such as 6-mercaptopurine and demecolcine, have been used to inhibit the proliferation of marrow elements with about the same degree of success as ^{32}P. It is not yet clear whether the risk of acute leukemia is less with chemotherapeutic agents.[78]

Secondary gout is common in polycythemic patients with longstanding hyperuricemia. Acute attacks are treated with colchicine or indomethacin as is primary gout. Allopurinol should be used as a preventative.

Myeloid Metaplasia with Myelofibrosis

Many descriptive terms have been applied to the group of illnesses characterized by a leukoerythroblastic anemia, enlargement of the spleen and liver as the result of myeloid metaplasia, and a patchy or generalized fibrosis of the bone marrow. The etiology of this syndrome remains obscure. There is an increased incidence of myeloid metaplasia among atom bomb survivors and others exposed to ionizing radiation. One opinion relates this disorder to a neoplasm of reticuloendothelial cells involving principally the marrow, spleen, and liver. At present, many group this condition with the myeloproliferative disorders largely because of their overlapping clinical features and because of the occasional transition from one form to another.[2,3,76]

CLINICAL PRESENTATION. Myeloid metaplasia, a rather uncommon illness, occurs in both sexes with equal frequency, generally after age 50. The primary complaints are weakness, easy fatigability, abdominal discomfort, and aching in the extremities, especially the legs. Less frequent symptoms are hemorrhage (skin and gastrointestinal tract), gout, and weight loss. Common physical abnormalities include pallor, ecchymoses or petechiae, striking splenomegaly, and more modest hepatomegaly. Icterus is present at times.

Although a few patients may have a normal or even increased red blood cell mass early in their illness, one of the most characteristic features of this disorder is the leukoerythroblastic anemia. The red cells show marked anisocytosis and poikilocytosis. Nucleated red cells are often seen. The reticulocyte count is normal or moderately elevated.

The white cell count is usually elevated, and the differential shows a shift to the left. All types of immature granulocytes may be encountered in the peripheral blood, including an occasional myeloblast. The alkaline phosphatase stain shows high or normal amounts of enzyme; rarely, low values are obtained. In most cases the platelet count is elevated, and large, odd shapes are often encountered.

Attempts to secure marrow by aspiration may be unsuccessful. Biopsy techniques provide the means of demonstrating the myelofibrosis and hypocellularity present. Osteosclerosis may be seen also. These marrow changes may be patchy early in the disorder; later they may be generalized. Indeed, it is not uncommon to encounter foci of hematopoietic-cell hyperplasia. Biopsy or aspiration preparations from the spleen, the liver, and, rarely, the lymph nodes may show extensive extramedullary hematopoiesis (myeloid metaplasia).

X-rays of the bones in 25 to 50 percent of cases show a patchy irregular osteosclerosis. The cortex of the long bones is often thickened. Osteoporosis has been noted also. The blood uric acid level is elevated in about 50 percent of instances, at times to twice normal levels.

DIAGNOSTIC CONSIDERATIONS. The hallmarks of myeloid metaplasia with myelofibrosis include a leukoerythroblastic anemia, marked splenomegaly and hepatomegaly with prominent myeloid metaplasia, and fibrosis or sclerosis of the bone marrow.

The diagnostic problems commonly confronted stem in part from the transition forms which exist between polycythemia vera, chronic granulocytic leukemia, and this disorder. In other instances, myeloid metaplasia must be distinguished from an aplastic or hypoplastic anemia. In addition, the physician must remain alert to the several possible causes of leukoerythroblastosis.

"Leukoerythroblastosis" is a term used to describe the presence of nucleated red cells and various immature myelocytic forms in the peripheral blood. When severe, this abnormality is striking, persistent, and usually accompanied by anemia. In its mildest forms there may be no anemia and only a few transiently circulating abnormal cells. Leukoerythroblastosis may result from myeloproliferation or from myelophthisic disorders (Table 50–4). Carcinomatosis and other myelophthisic processes are the most frequently encountered causes of marked leukoerythroblastosis.

TABLE 50-4
Causes of Leukoerythroblastosis

Abnormal Myeloproliferation Following
Blood loss or hemolysis
Nutritional deficiency anemias

Myelophthisic Disorders
Tuberculosis, especially disseminated
Carcinomatosis (lung, breast, prostate)
Xanthomatosis (Gaucher's disease and others)
Lymphoma
Myeloma
Myeloproliferative disorders

Severe Illness, Stress, Agonal States
Infection
Heart failure
Uremia

CLINICAL COURSE AND MANAGEMENT. The average prognosis for life ranges from 4 to 5 years, but with good supportive care many patients live much longer. The main continuing clinical problems are those stemming from the anemia, the markedly enlarged spleen, or the hemorrhagic episodes.

Symptoms resulting from severe anemia are relieved by transfusion. Androgens have improved the anemia in a few instances. Not infrequently, a hemolytic anemia develops, and rarely the Coombs test may become positive. Adrenal corticosteroids have benefited these individuals as well as a few others. Splenectomy has been performed to relieve this hemolytic problem. Thrombocytopenia with bleeding also develops on occasion and may be relieved by splenectomy. In these instances splenectomy has been performed despite the fear attending removal of large amounts of hematopoietic tissue and the difficult operative and postoperative problems. Following splenectomy, the liver enlarges progressively (myeloid metaplasia), and the general course of the disease continues.

External radiation has been directed at the spleen to relieve local symptomatology or to combat hemolytic anemia or thrombocytopenia. The potential danger of irradiating the areas of extramedullary hematopoiesis has been stressed also. Busulfan has induced a decrease in spleen size in some patients and an improvement in their hematologic status, but it may have adverse effects on the remaining hematopoietic tissue.

The immediate causes of death relate to underlying cardiovascular disease affected adversely by anemia, thromboembolic events, or hemorrhage. A transition to chronic granulocytic or acute granulocytic leukemia may take place before death.

Contrasting Clinical Features of the Chronic Myeloproliferative Disorders

Polycythemia vera, myeloid metaplasia with myelofibrosis, and chronic granulocytic leukemia are considered together primarily because they manifest a chronic uncontrolled proliferation of hematopoietic cells and because their clinical features often overlap or change in an interrelating fashion with the passage of time. Although certain basic morphologic resemblances are stressed, no implication with respect to etiology is intended. Benzene and ionizing radiations are leukemogenic and will produce marrow fibrosis. Tuberculosis has been cited as possibly responsible for the induction of myelofibrosis as well as myeloid metaplasia in the spleen, although more frequently tuberculosis seems a secondary occurrence. However, present data do not permit definite conclusions concerning these or other suggested causal agents. The common proliferative abnormality seems neoplastic in character.[75,79,80]

The contrasting clinical features of these chronic myeloproliferative disorders are presented in Tables 50-5 and 50-6. Continuing clinical experience serves to emphasize the diversity of findings manifested by different patients and by the same patient during the course of his disease. A patient with classic polycythemia vera may, after many months, develop an increasing anemia and progressive enlargement of the spleen and liver. Appropriate biopsies may reveal myelofibrosis and extramedullary hematopoiesis associated with a leukoerythroblastic anemia. Similarly, an individual with polycythemia vera may develop all the features of chronic granulocytic leukemia after the passage of months or years. The granulocyte alkaline phosphatase levels are usually elevated in these patients.

One percent or fewer of patients with polycythemia vera will develop acute granulocytic leukemia. This may evolve directly from the polycythemic status or may occur as a blast crisis in a person whose illness had previously become chronic granulocytic leukemia. The use of ^{32}P therapy or other forms of radiation therapy has been linked to a tenfold or greater increase in the incidence of acute leukemia.

Some patients with clear-cut myeloid metaplasia with myelofibrosis show transient polycythemia early in the course of their disease. The myeloid metaplasia syndrome seems unique among the myeloproliferative disorders because of the occasional associated occurrence of an autoimmune hemolytic anemia and the occasional associated development of thrombocytopenic purpura unrelated to therapy. A distinctive relationship appears to exist between the Ph' chromosome and chronic granulocytic leukemia, although exceptions have been reported.

TABLE 50-5
Contrasting Clinical Features of the Chronic Myeloproliferative Disorders

Clinical Features	Polycythemia Vera	Myeloid Metaplasia with Myelofibrosis	Chronic Granulocytic Leukemia
I. Presentation			
Pruritis	50% of cases	—	—
Skin lesions	Plethora; erythema	—	Leukemic infiltrates
Ruddy cyanosis	When reduced hemoglobin exceeds 5 g/dl	—	—
Jaundice	Rare	Occasional	Rare
Thromboses	25–50% of cases	10–20% of cases	Occasional
Hemorrhage	Epistaxes, skin, central nervous system, gastrointestinal and joint bleeding	Especially gastrointestinal and skin bleeding	
Hypertension	50% of cases	Sometimes early	Occasional
Hepatomegaly	Modest, 30–50% of cases	Most cases often large	Modest
Splenomegaly	Usual, often large May be absent early	Often huge	Large
Peptic ulcer	10–20% of cases	10–20% of cases	Occasional
Gout	Approx. 5% of cases	5–10% of cases	Rare
Bone pain	Frequent	Approx. 20% of cases	Occasional
Sternal tenderness	—	+ +	+ + +
II. Course			
Average prognosis	10–20 years	4–5 years or more	3–4 years
Incidence of acute leukemia	1–10% of cases Related to ^{32}P therapy	—	Terminal acute blastic crisis usual
Terminal events	Hemorrhage Thromboembolism Cardiovascular disorder Transition to myelofibrosis or leukemia	Hemorrhage Thromboembolism Infection	Hemorrhage Infection

TABLE 50-6
Contrasting Hematologic Features of the Chronic Myeloproliferative Disorders

Laboratory Examination	Polycythemia Vera	Myeloid Metaplasia with Myelofibrosis	Chronic Granulocytic Leukemia
Hematocrit	Increased, often > 60	Decreased May show increase early	Decreased May be near normal early
Hemolysis	Normal erythrocyte survival	Occasional, with positive Coombs test	Normal erythrocyte survival
White blood cell count	Usually 10–50,000; rarely > 100,000	Usually 20–50,000; rarely > 100,000	Generally elevated; often > 100,000
Differential	Normocytic red cells Occasional nucleated red cells Occasional myelocyte	Bizarre red cell shapes Frequent nucleated red cells Frequent myelocytes, occasional myeloblast	Normocytic red cells Occasional nucleated red cells Orderly shift to left with myelocytes, occasional myeloblast

(Continued)

TABLE 50-6 (cont.)

Laboratory Examination	Polycythemia Vera	Myeloid Metaplasia with Myelofibrosis	Chronic Granulocytic Leukemia
Platelets	Usually elevated; > 400,000 in 50% of cases	Marked elevation, often bizarre forms May develop thrombocytopenic purpura	Usually elevated
Granulocyte alkaline phosphatase	Highest values	High to normal	Low to absent
Ph' chromosome	—	—	+
Bone marrow	Cellular Hyperplasia of all elements Read as normal in 50% of cases	Fibrosis and osteosclerosis Reticulum cell increase Patchy lesions early Focal areas of increased cellularity early	Myeloid hyperplasia At times increased red cells and megakaryocytes or patches of fibrosis
Myeloid metaplasia	Rare foci in liver, spleen	Marked in spleen, liver At times in lymph nodes	(Granulocytic infiltrates)
Blood (RBC) volume	Increased	Normal (anemic)	Normal (anemic)
Blood viscosity	Increased	Normal	Normal
Uric acid	Increased	Increased in 50% of cases, at times twice normal	Increased
Immunoglobulins	Rare monoclonal gammopathy	Rare increase in IgM, rheumatoid factor	—
X-rays of bones	Usually normal	Patchy or diffuse osteosclerosis, thickened cortex, or osteoporosis in 25–50% of cases	Occasional subperiosteal new bone, osteolytic lesions, transverse lines at end of long bones

CHAPTER 51
The Lymphoreticular Proliferative Disorders
ALBERT H. OWENS, Jr.

Normally functioning lymphorecticular cells are vital to the integrity of the body's defense mechanisms. The diverse anatomic distribution of the aggregates of lymphocytes, plasma cells, monocytes, fixed tissue macrophages, and the other reticuloendothelial elements that comprise the lymphoreticular cell system is important to its biologic role.

Lymphoreticular cells react against foreign microorganisms and a wide variety of toxins. They serve as the afferent and efferent elements of the immune responses. Likely they play an important role in the defense against neoplasia. They also contribute toward the physiologic regulation of granulopoiesis and erythropoiesis.[70,72]

Cell proliferation and differentiation are integral to the physiologic responses of the lymphoreticular cell system. Clinically disorders of these processes may result in such abnormalities as lymphadenopathy and splenomegaly or be recognized by assessing specific humoral or cell-mediated immune reactions.[94] Often such nonspecific systemic manifestations as fever, malaise, anorexia, and weight loss also accompany lymphoreticular disorders.

It is convenient to categorize the clinically recognized lymphoreticular proliferative disorders according to their neoplastic or nonneoplastic nature (self-perpetuating or self-limiting). Further, these disorders may be classified according to the rapidity of their course (acute or chronic), the cell type(s) involved in the proliferative process, and the associated immune reactions.

Nonneoplastic Lymphoreticular Proliferation

Table 51-1 summarizes the variable immunoproliferative phenomena attending the majority of infectious diseases. In general, the mononuclear cell response occurs promptly after antigenic stimulation and subsides on removal of the stimulus. In acute bacterial (pyogenic) infections, lymphoreticular hyperplasia and plasmacytosis may follow the initial granulocyte response, whereas in most viral infections it is the primary event. The evidence of the associated immunologic responses (e.g., antibody titer, delayed cutaneous hypersensitivity) may persist for prolonged periods.

The degree of lymphoreticular proliferation depends on a number of factors, including the nature, virulence, and amount of the stimulus, the site of entry, and the individual's capacity to react to it. For example, inguinal adenopathy is to be expected in association with a syphilitic penile chancre. Later, during the secondary stage of syphilis, generalized lymphadenopathy and splenomegaly may be noted, as well as a mild plasmacytosis in the bone marrow.

The cellular composition and morphologic pattern of the lymphoreticular response also depend to some extent on the nature and duration of the stimulus. For example, an abrupt lymphocytosis and plasmacytosis of short duration is characteristic of rubella. A more prolonged peripheral blood monocytosis, marrow plasmacytosis, and tubercle (granuloma) formation are associated with tuberculosis.

Usually, these immunoproliferative events are bland and contribute to recovery from the infectious disease. However, this is not always so. For example, in infectious mononucleosis, a disease of viral etiology, the lymphoproliferative response is exaggerated greatly, often results in the appearance of malignant-looking cells, and constitutes a major manifestation of the illness. Furthermore, on occasion the synthesis of antibody has been related to the development of a hemolytic anemia or thrombocytopenia that adds significantly to the patient's morbidity. In contrast, the synthesis of the heterophil antibody appears to have no bearing on the course of the disease.

Hypersensitivity states induced by foreign proteins or drugs and many features of the collagen-vascular diseases are thought to be in large part the result of a persistent, heightened, and inappropriate state of immune responsiveness. These disorders are

---

TABLE 51-1

Nonneoplastic Lymphoreticular Proliferative Disorders Associated with Infectious Diseases

Disease State	Etiologic Stimulus	Manifestations	
		Proliferative	**Immunologic**
Specific infections	Bacteria (pyogenic) Viral Spirochetal Mycobacterial Fungal	Lymph nodes and spleen: lymphoreticular hyperplasia Granuloma formation, especially in chronic infections due to tuberculosis, fungus	Specific immunoglobulin synthesis Hyperglobulinemia (polyclonal), especially in chronic infections Delayed cutaneous hypersensitivity
		Blood and marrow: lymphocytosis and/or monocytosis Marrow plasmacytosis, especially in chronic infections due to tuberculosis, fungus	
Sarcoid	Uncertain	Similar to tuberculosis. No necrosis Schaumann bodies characteristic	Hyperglobulinemia (polyclonal) Kveim reaction
Infectious lymphocytosis	? Viral	Peripheral blood lymphocytosis	
Infectious mononucleosis	EBV	Lymph nodes and spleen: lymphoreticular hyperplasia, characteristic atypical lymphocytes	Heterophil agglutinin; EBV titer False positive serologic test for syphilis
		Blood and marrow: characteristic atypical lymphocytes	Rarely autoimmune hemolysis and thrombocytopenia

---

TABLE 51-2

Nonneoplastic Lymphoreticular Proliferative Disorders Associated with Diseases with Prominent Immunologic Features

Disease State	Etiologic Stimulus	Manifestations	
		Proliferative	**Immunologic**
Hypersensitivity states	Foreign protein, drugs	Generalized adenopathy, splenomegaly	Specific antibody
		Blood and marrow: abnormal lymphocytosis, monocytosis, plasmacytosis	Specific cutaneous hypersensitivity (Arthus)
Serum sickness			Occasional heterophil antibody
		Nodes: lymphoreticular hyperplasia	Hyperglobulinemia (polyclonal)
Collagen-vascular diseases		Generalized adenopathy, splenomegaly may be a prominent feature (especially SLE)	Hyperglobulinemia (polyclonal)
Systemic lupus erythematosus (SLE)			SLE: autoimmune hemolytic anemia, thrombocytopenia, antinuclear antibody, decreased complement, false positive test for syphilis, LE cell phenomenon
Polyarteritis nodosa		*Nodes:* lymphoreticular hyperplasia (may be confused with lymphoma)	RA: rheumatoid factor
Rheumatoid arthritis (RA)		*Marrow:* may show plasmacytosis, especially polyarteritis	

---

summarized in Table 51-2. All these illnesses manifest prominent immunologic abnormalities as well as somewhat less conspicuous evidence of lymphoreticular hyperplasia. The pathogenetic importance of the reaction to foreign protein (antigen–antibody complexes) is relatively well understood in serum sickness. However, one cannot assign a similar importance to the antinuclear antibody of systemic lupus erythematosus or the rheumatoid factor found in the serum of individuals with rheumatoid arthritis.

At times, the proliferative aspects of these disorders may be impressive. Patients with drug reactions or collagen-vascular diseases may present with prominent lymphadenopathy and splenomegaly, and the morphologic appearance of the bone marrow or lymph nodes may suggest the incorrect diagnosis of myeloma or lymphoma.

Generalized lymphadenopathy, splenomegaly, and a (relative) peripheral lymphocytosis are associated with hyperthyroidism. These changes revert to normal upon reestablishment of the euthyroid state. There may be an increased incidence of lymphoma in individuals with long-standing hyperthyroidism. Present data are insufficient to allow comment on the possible neoplastic potential of the other types of reactive lymphoreticular hyperplasia.

Neoplastic Lymphoreticular Proliferation
In the neoplastic lymphoreticular disorders the clinical features relating to cellular proliferation are preeminent and self-perpetuating (Table 51-3). They may be accompanied by excessive immunoglobulin

synthesis, as in myeloma or Waldenström's macroglobulinemia. In the latter syndrome the macroglobulin is responsible for increased serum viscosity and, hence, many of the major manifestations of the disease.

Immunodeficiency states are known to develop in patients with lymphoreticular neoplasms. For example, increasing hypogammaglobulinemia and unresponsiveness to bacterial antigens are common in chronic lymphocytic leukemia. Furthermore, anergy to antigens causing delayed hypersensitivity responses has been related to active Hodgkin's disease.

The generally employed classifications of neoplastic lymphoreticular disorders are based primarily on cytomorphology as appreciated by conventional light microscopy. Currently, however, alternate classifications are being suggested based on biologic and immunologic observations (Table 51-4). Some neoplasms remain circumscribed as solid tumors (malignant lymphomas), especially those composed of large, cohesive cells. Others, likely derived from cells which are normally motile and circulate freely, readily disseminate and may display prominent leukemic manifestations.

INFECTIOUS MONONUCLEOSIS
Infectious mononucleosis is a self-limited febrile illness characterized by malaise, stomatitis, pharyngitis, cervical and generalized lymphadenopathy, splenomegaly, and a characteristic abnormal lymphocytosis. The disorder is encountered most often in young people. Its true prevalence is doubtless under-

TABLE 51-3
Neoplastic Lymphoreticular Proliferative Disorders

Disease State	Manifestations	
	Proliferative	Immunologic
Leukemia	Mild generalized adenopathy Splenomegaly	
Acute lymphocytic	Infiltration of blood, marrow, nodes, tissues with lymphoblasts	
Chronic lymphocytic	Infiltration of marrow, nodes, tissues with small lymphocytes	Progressive decrease in normal immunoglobulins and antibody response Decreased response of lymphocytes to mitogens
Lymphocytic lymphoma	Prominent generalized adenopathy Splenomegaly Mass lesions Infiltration of marrow common Variable small cell lymphocytosis	Autoimmune hemolytic anemia Rare monoclonal gammopathy
Plasma cell dyscrasias	Infiltration of marrow, tissues, blood with plasma cells Osteolytic bone lesions Rare adenopathy Rare splenomegaly	Overproduction of homogeneous immunoglobulin molecule or fragment (H-chain, L-chain) Progressive decrease in antibody response Low isoagglutinin titers
Histiocytic lymphoma	Regional or generalized adenopathy Splenomegaly Mass lesions Infiltration of marrow, nodes, tissue with abnormal histiocytic cells, also occasionally seen in blood	Rare monoclonal gammopathy
Hodgkin's disease	Regional or generalized adenopathy Splenomegaly Mass lesions	Impaired cell-mediated immunity Decreased response of lymphocytes to mitogens Rare monoclonal gammopathy Autoimmune hemolytic anemia
Mycosis fungoides	Skin lesions predominate Lymph nodes, viscera are involved later Abnormal cells may be seen in blood and marrow	

estimated, since the symptoms and clinical findings are often mild, nonspecific, and of only a few days' duration. Clusters of recognizable cases commonly occur in military installations, schools, and similar settings.

A herpes virus, the Epstein-Barr virus (EBV), is the cause of infectious mononucleosis. In one study of Yale undergraduate students, none of those entering with EBV antibodies detectable in their sera developed the disease, whereas 44 percent of those who had no titer on matriculation eventually came down with mononucleosis. Further, the acute illness is characterized by a marked rise in EBV antibody titer and detectable levels persist for prolonged periods.

EBV has been recovered from the leukocytes of acutely ill patients. Studies also indicate that the virus may remain in hematopoietic cells for years (latent infection).

Epidemiologic studies indicate that infection with the EB agent commonly occurs early in life, especially among those of lower socioeconomic status. Since the EBV has been linked to Burkitt's lymphoma in Africa, nasopharyngeal cancer in the Orient, and Hodgkin's disease, much interest centers around the long-term surveillance of patients recovered from infectious mononucleosis. To date, there has been no clear indication of a higher or lower incidence of neoplasia than expected.[90]

TABLE 51-4

Immunobiologic Classification of the Neoplastic Lymphoreticular Proliferative Disorders

T-Cell Diseases
Acute lymphoblastic leukemia (25% of cases)
Lymphoblastic lymphoma
Mycosis fungoides—Sézary cells
Immunoblastic sarcoma
Hodgkin's disease?

B-Cell Diseases
Chronic lymphatic leukemia (small lymphocyte)
Well-differentiated lymphocytic lymphoma
Burkitt's lymphoma
Follicular (poorly differentiated) lymphomas
Waldenström's macroglobulinemia
Multiple myeloma (plasma cell dyscrasias)
Histiocytic (large cell) lymphoma (~50% of cases)
Hairy cell leukemia
Immunoblastic sarcoma

Undefined
Acute lymphoblastic leukemia (~75% of cases)
Histiocytic (large cell) lymphomas (~50% of cases)
Malignant histiocytosis

CLINICAL PRESENTATION. The principal clinical features of infectious mononucleosis vary greatly in intensity but may be related to: 1) the infectious agent, its presumed portal of entry (e.g., stomatitis, pharyngitis), and evidences of systemic dissemination (e.g., fever, hepatitis, meningoencephalitis); 2) reactive lymphoreticular proliferation (e.g., lymphadenopathy, splenomegaly, abnormal lymphocytosis); and 3) related immunologic abnormalities (e.g., EBV antibody, heterophil antibody, autoimmune hemolytic anemia, false positive serologic test for syphilis).

The appearance of the more characteristic manifestations of infectious mononucleosis is frequently preceded by vague complaints of chilliness, malaise, mild fever, and sore throat which last 3 to 6 days. During the second or third week of illness it is common to encounter progressive fever (101 to 103°F) and debility associated with stomatitis, pharyngitis, and prominent cervical and generalized lymph node enlargement. Splenomegaly is present in half the cases and hepatomegaly somewhat less frequently. The degree of illness is usually moderate but ranges from a nearly asymptomatic state to severe prostration. At times, infectious mononucleosis is responsible for a wide variety of symptoms reflecting the involvement of multiple organ systems.

Cutaneous eruptions have been noted in 10 to 20 percent of cases. A fine, erythematous, macular rash distributed on the trunk is the type most frequently described. It is similar to that of rubella. Rarely, lesions similar to erythema multiforme or erythema nodosum occur. Conjunctivitis is encountered at times.

Jaundice has been reported in less than 10 percent of cases. It results from a diffuse hepatitis. Subclinical hepatitis is common and results in minor abnormalities of hepatic-cell function in nearly all cases.

In fewer than 1 percent of cases, involvement of the central nervous system is manifested by stupor, headache, convulsions, stiff neck, and nerve palsies, coupled with an increased cerebrospinal fluid pressure, pleocytosis, and an elevated protein concentration. Various neurologic syndromes have been described as resulting from a meningoencephalitis or polyneuronitis.

Early in the disease a transient granulocytopenia may be encountered. During the second week, the patient usually develops an absolute lymphocytosis ranging from 10,000 to 20,000/μl. The circulating mononuclear cells are mostly of an atypical type, often with bean-shaped nuclei and foamy, vacuolated cytoplasm. Sections from the enlarged lymph nodes and spleen also show a bizarre malignant-looking hyperplasia at times, with evident invasion of the capsule. Similar cells may be encountered in the bone marrow.

Serologic abnormalities develop in nearly all patients. Increasing titers of EBV antibody and a 19S, heterophil (sheep red cell agglutinating) antibody are usually seen in association with the atypical lymphocytosis. EBV titers of 1:160 and heterophil titers of 1:56 or greater usually are considered confirmatory. These patients also may develop false positive serologic tests for syphilis. Rarely, an autoimmune (Coombs positive) hemolytic anemia occurs. Thrombocytopenic purpura, presumably immunologic in genesis, develops on occasion.

DIAGNOSTIC CONSIDERATIONS. Fever, pharyngitis, lymphadenopathy, splenomegaly, and the typically atypical lymphocytosis constitute the major manifestations of infectious mononucleosis.

A frequently employed descriptive subclassification of infectious mononucleosis divides cases into febrile, glandular, and anginose forms according to their most prominent clinical features. Such a system fails to recognize fully the varied nature and intensity of the illness. It does, however, indicate the nature of the major diagnostic considerations.

The fever, headache, and malaise of infectious mononucleosis are suggestive of the symptoms of influenza or a number of similar viral illnesses. The lymphadenopathy and morbilliform rash that may occur concurrently often simulate rubella or secondary syphilis. Serum sickness or a drug reaction is a frequently considered diagnosis, particularly since some of these patients may manifest generalized lymphadenopathy, splenomegaly, abnormal peripheral blood lymphocytosis, and a heterophil antibody that reacts with sheep red blood cells. (The heterophil antibody of infectious mononucleosis may be distinguished from that encountered in serum sickness or normal individuals since the latter are absorbed on guinea pig kidney cells.)

The prominent pharyngeal findings often suggest a bacterial infection, especially a streptococcal one. Indeed, in some cases streptococcal pharyngitis and mononucleosis coexist. The appearance of a membranous exudate leads to a consideration of diphtheria. Stomatitis, when present, may simulate that due to various other etiologic agents. In these instances, a prompt and definitive diagnosis is needed in order to provide proper therapy.

Acute leukemia and infectious mononucleosis are confused at times, particularly since patients with either disorder commonly present with fever, generalized lymphadenopathy, and splenomegaly. The presence of anemia, abnormal lymphocytosis, pharyngitis, and stomatitis may add to the physician's confusion. However, the presence of very primitive (blast) leukocytes and nucleated red cells in the peripheral blood, coupled with the characteristic marrow findings, should confirm the existence of leukemia.

Infectious hepatitis, various nervous system diseases, intra-abdominal disorders, or renal abnormalities may be considered, depending on the nature of the presenting complaints, as previously indicated.

Syndromes similar to EBV and heterophil-antibody-positive infectious mononucleosis may be caused by similar viruses, for example cytomegalovirus.

CLINICAL COURSE AND MANAGEMENT. Since there is no specific treatment for infectious mononucleosis, therapy is essentially supportive in nature. Antibiotic therapy may be required for a concurrent bacterial infection (e.g., a streptococcal infection).

Complete recovery is the rule. Although convalescence is usually rapid (2 or 3 weeks), a number of patients with infectious mononucleosis may remain symptomatic. Feelings of general debility, coupled with lymphadenopathy, may persist for several weeks or months.

The frequency of major relapse is very low. Despite the acute involvement of the lymphoreticular tissues, liver, and nervous system (and rarely the heart and kidneys), no chronic impairments have been reported.

Although the usual course of the disease is uncomplicated, a small proportion of patients develop life-threatening abnormalities. The most common events leading to fatality include hemorrhage (thrombocytopenia), rupture of the spleen, edema of the glottis, respiratory failure due to nervous-system involvement, and hepatic necrosis.

THE MALIGNANT LYMPHOMAS

The malignant lymphomas are neoplasms which arise from lymphoreticular cells. They share a common cytogeneology with the lymphocytic leukemias and with the plasma cell dyscrasias. They also share a number of prominent clinical features including lymphadenopathy, splenomegaly, and a variety of hematologic and immunologic abnormalities.[70,95]

Lymphadenopathy, splenomegaly, and other evidences of excessive lymphoreticular cell proliferation are commonly encountered clinical phenomena. Therefore, careful and systematic consideration must be given to all possible diagnoses before a disorder is labeled "malignant lymphoma" (Chap. 49).[85]

The term *malignant lymphoma* emphasizes the rather predictable patterns of tumor involvement and spread which occur in the lymphoreticular tissues. However, transition states between solid tumors (e.g., lymphocytic lymphoma) and leukemia (e.g., lymphocytic leukemia) are often seen. The characterization of surface markers on malignant lymphoma cells (e.g., T-cell or B-cell markers) has led to the conclusion that they are monoclonal neoplasms for the most part. Further, it is possible to envision the patterns of tissue involvement and spread of neoplastic lymphoma cells in light of the "migration and homing" patterns of their normal counterparts. For example, follicular or nodular, poorly differentiated lymphocytic lymphoma is a monoclonal neoplasm of B cells which very commonly (about 85 percent of cases) spreads to involve the B-cell domains of the lymphoid tissues and the bone marrow. Likely the transformed cell population arose from a migratory B cell and retained its ability to move about through the body and lodge in the usual B-cell areas.

Hodgkin's Disease[87]

In 1832, Hodgkin described the autopsy findings in seven patients who died with generalized lymph node enlargment and splenomegaly. In 1856, Wilks graphically described Hodgkin's disease as "characterized by a gradual progressive enlargement of the lymphatic glands beginning usually in the cervical region and spreading throughout lymphoid tissue of the body, forming nodular growths in the internal organs, resulting in anemia and usually a fatal cachexia." The pathologic characterization of this disorder relates mainly to the presence of a polycellular infiltrate composed of giant (Sternberg-Reed) cells, lymphocytes, plasma cells, monocytes, eosinophils, and neutrophils associated with a variable degree of fibrosis and necrosis. Immunobiologic studies suggest that Hodgkin's disease is a T-cell disorder.

Hodgkin's disease is most commonly encountered in young people of all races. There is a bimodal incidence with the first peak occurring between ages 15 and 35 and the second after age 50. Males are affected nearly twice as frequently as females.

The etiology of Hodgkin's disease remains unknown. In the past a wide variety of microorganisms or filtrable agents have been suggested as causative, but none has been generally accepted. More recently, EBV has been linked to Hodgkin's disease.

CLINICAL PRESENTATION. The manifestations of Hodgkin's disease are highly variable in nature and intensity. They may be systemic in character or may be referable primarily to one or more organ systems. It is convenient to group these features as they relate to the presence of solid tumor masses and associated hematologic, immunologic, or physiologic abnormalities.

The most common presenting complaints concern the painless, progressive, asymmetrical enlargement of cervical lymph nodes. Somewhat less frequent are the symptoms that stem from compression of various adjacent structures by expanding tumor masses. For example, cough, crowing dyspnea, dysphagia, and cervicofacial and upper-extremity edema may result from a mediastinal mass impinging on the tracheobroncial tree, superior vena cava, or esophagus. Similarly, low-back or abdominal discomfort, lower-extremity edema, or urinary or gastrointestinal dysfunction may result from retroperitoneal tumor, and left flank pain may result from an enlarged spleen.

There are nontender, rubbery, matted, or lobulated masses in the peripheral lymph node bearing areas of 70 to 80 percent of affected persons. These masses usually are not attached to the overlying skin. Occasionally their size varies spontaneously over a period of several days. Palpable splenomegaly has been reported in 50 to 70 percent of cases. X-ray examinations will identify a mass lesion in most of the patients without peripheral tumors. Some 10 to 20 percent of cases may have no easily accessible mass at the onset of symptoms.

Constitutional symptoms are encountered frequently during the course of Hodgkin's disease, but they are the initial complaints in a minority of patients. However, it is these individuals who often pose the more difficult diagnostic problems, since the fever, weakness, pruritus, or cachexia observed are relatively nonspecific findings and since they may occur in the absence of detectable lymphoid tumors. For example, a patient whose complaints are recurrent fever and increasing weakness may undergo repeated diagnostic study to no avail and eventually require laparotomy to establish the existence of retroperitoneal Hodgkin's disease.

Hematologic abnormalities are observed in the majority of patients with Hodgkin's disease and are present at the time of initial diagnosis in about 30 percent. The most frequent finding is a normochromic anemia, most often a result of decreased erythropoiesis. At times, significant hemolysis can be demonstrated. The white cell count is often moderately increased, and a granulocytosis and monocytosis may be observed. An eosinophilia, usually less than 10 percent, may be seen in 10 to 20 percent of cases. Lymphopenia is common late in the disease. Thrombocytosis (platelet counts in excess of 400,000) is encountered at times, and large bizarre forms may be observed. Sternberg-Reed cells are rarely identified in marrow aspirates but may be seen in 20 to 25 percent of patients if biopsy is employed.

A number of immunologic abnormalities have been associated with progressive Hodgkin's disease. An unusual tendency toward viral, mycobacterial, and fungal infections has been noted. For example, *Herpes zoster* is encountered in 4 to 6 percent of cases. The incidence of active tuberculosis, although it remains relatively high, is declining in patients with Hodgkin's disease, as it is in the general population. In contrast, the frequency of fungus infections, especially cryptococcosis, appears to be increasing. The susceptibility to these infections has been related to the impaired ability to manifest delayed cutaneous hypersensitivity which is seen in more than half of the patients studied. Homograft rejection and lymphocyte responsiveness to mitogens are also impaired.

Recently two antigens, called F and S for their fast and slow electrophoretic mobility, have been identified in the tissues of patients with Hodgkin's disease. They are found in some normal individuals, though in lesser concentrations. In some way, the F antigen seems related to thymus-derived lymphocytes. This is in keeping with other data which suggest a T-cell disorder in Hodgkin's disease.

Electrophoretic studies of serum proteins are often normal early in the course of the disease but may show a mild hypoalbuminemia and hyperglobulinemia (commonly $\alpha2$). Infrequently, a monoclonal gammopathy is encountered that is associated with bone marrow plasmacytosis. Antibody responsiveness generally remains unimpaired. Hypercalcemia and hyperuricemia occur occasionally. Low plasma zinc and elevated serum copper concentrations are associated with progressive Hodgkin's disease.

DIAGNOSTIC CONSIDERATIONS. Since the majority of patients with Hodgkin's disease present with readily accessible tumors, it is usually easy to establish a definitive diagnosis by the demonstration of the characteristic tissue morphology. The more common problems in diagnosis occur when 1) the patient presents with nonspecific constitutional symptoms, such as fever, in the absence of an identifiable tumor mass; 2) full consideration has not been given to the several possible causes of excessive lymphoreticular proliferation (Chap. 55); 3) the morphologic pattern in the biopsy specimen is not characteristic enough to discriminate among the malignant lymphomas; 4) the report of a "positive biopsy" is accepted uncritically (e.g., biopsies from patients with disorders such as SLE or Whipple's disease); or 5) the report of a "negative biopsy" (e.g., lymphoid hyperplasia) is accepted as eliminating the possibility of Hodgkin's disease. At times, serial biopsies are required to establish a certain diagnosis.

CLINICAL COURSE AND MANAGEMENT.[81,91,93] The course of Hodgkin's disease may vary greatly. Particularly in older patients, the illness may appear to be a rapidly progressive, multicentric systemic disorder from the outset. More commonly, especially in younger individuals, Hodgkin's disease begins as a localized disorder which spreads rather predictably to involve adjacent lymphatic tissue and which is potentially curable. Since curative therapy requires that all existing disease be addressed, careful clinical staging is the cornerstone of proper patient management (Table 51-5).

It is difficult to detect all tissues involved with Hodgkin's disease. Retroperitoneal lymphography will reveal otherwise undetected disease in an impressive number of instances. For example, Lee et al. have shown that 47 percent (23 of 49) of patients whose disease had been classified previously as localized (Stage I and II) had a generalized disorder. Laparotomy will reveal Hodgkin's disease involvement of lymph nodes, spleen, and liver not detected by other means including lymphography. In one series of patients with negative lymphograms, 25 percent of those without constitutional symptoms were found to have intra-abdominal Hodgkin's disease at laparotomy and 50 percent of those with symptoms had intra-abdominal disease. Nearly all clinically enlarged spleens prove to be involved, but 25 to 35 percent of normal sized spleens are involved, too. Further, lapa-

---

TABLE 51-5

Clinical Staging of Hodgkin's Disease (Ann Arbor Classification)*

Stage	Description
I	Involvement of a single lymph node region (I) or of a single extralymphatic organ or site (I_E)
II	Involvement of two or more lymph node regions on the same side of the diaphragm (II) or localized involvement of an extralymphatic organ or site and/or one or more lymph node regions on the same side of the diaphragm (II_E)
III	Involvement of lymph node regions on both sides of the diaphragm (III) which may also be accompanied by localized involvement of an extralymphatic organ or site (III_E) or by involvement of the spleen (III_S) or both (III_{ES})
IV	Diffuse or disseminated involvement of one or more lymphatic organs or tissues with or without associated lymph node enlargement

* Each stage is subclassified as A or B to indicate the absence (A) or presence (B) of systemic symptoms not otherwise explained: viz., weight loss greater than 10 percent, fever, and night sweats.

---

rotomy has defined a small, but definite, proportion of "false positive" lymphograms.

The currently used histologic classification of Hodgkin's disease is based primarily on the observation of Lukes and his associates (Table 51-6). The predominance of lymphocytic or histiocytic proliferation (or both) has been linked to localized disease and a better prognosis. In contrast, lymphocyte depletion is encountered more often in rapidly progressive disease and signifies a poor outlook for survival. Lukes interprets these patterns as representative of the pa-

---

TABLE 51-6

Hodgkin's Disease: Relative Frequency of Histopathologic Type and Prognosis for Survival

Frequency (%)	Type	5-Year Survival (%)
10–15	Lymphocyte predominance	50–60
30–70	Nodular sclerosis*	45–55
20–40	Mixed cellularity	5–20
5–15	Lymphocyte depletion	0–10

* More common in younger age group.

tients' (immunologic) resistance and cites this as the most important determinant of the outcome of the disease. Others have pointed out that splenic involvement and histopathologic evidence of vascular invasion carry a poorer prognosis.

The more widespread disease is associated with a poorer prognosis (Table 51–7). Further, the presence of constitutional symptoms is unfavorable. The prognosis for women seems consistently better than for men, irrespective of the stage of disease. Pregnancy has not been shown to have an adverse effect on survival, but it does present problems in the use of radiation therapy and cytotoxic drugs.

A sound treatment program for Hodgkin's disease is based on an assessment of the diagnostic data, the anatomic extent of the disease and its rate of progress, the presence or absence of constitutional symptoms, and the possible existence of major physiologic abnormalities or intercurrent disorders which require more immediate therapy (e.g., bacterial infection, thrombocytopenia with bleeding, hemolytic anemia, hypercalcemia).

Truly localized Hodgkin's disease (Stage I and II) is managed best by radiation therapy (Table 51–7). Adequate tumoricidal doses (e.g., 4000 to 4500 rads in 4 to 5 weeks) must be delivered to the obviously involved areas and to adjacent lymphoreticular tissues using extended-field techniques (e.g., mantle and para-aortic fields). Since full doses are required to achieve curative results and since these dose levels are close to the tolerance of normal tissues, careful treatment planning and precise dose delivery are es-

sential. A high proportion of Stage II patients with systemic symptoms (Stage IIB) or with mixed cellularity or lymphocyte depleted histology relapse within 3 years. This has led to the use of combination chemotherapy as an adjunct to radiation therapy in these cases. With proper management, nearly 90 percent of Stage I cases and about two-thirds of Stage II cases will be disease-free at 5 years and may be presumed to be cured.

Patients with Stage IIIA Hodgkin's disease may be treated primarily with radiation therapy in centers where proper facilities exist (Table 51–7). There is a significant relapse rate, especially among patients with unfavorable histologic types. This has encouraged the adjunctive use of multiagent chemotherapy in these situations. In many institutions, patients with Stage III disease are managed primarily by means of combination chemotherapy.

Patients with Stage IIIB and IV disease are best treated per primum with multiagent chemotherapy (Table 51–7). Similar therapy is appropriate for patients who relapse following radiation therapy. A number of chemotherapeutic agents are useful in the management of Hodgkin's disease including the alkylating agents, the vinca alkaloids, procarbazine, the nitrosoureas, bleomycin, adriamycin, and the adrenal corticosteroids (Chap. 54). A combination of antitumor agents with different mechanisms of action (e.g., mechlorethamine, vincristine, procarbazine, and prednisone) given concurrently and repeatedly over a 6-month period can induce a remission in nearly every patient treated. In fact, various complementary combinations of drugs seem to be equally effective in inducing long-term, disease-free remissions provided they are given in full doses and over a sufficiently prolonged period (6 to 12 months). Radiation therapy is employed often in an adjunctive role to eradicate bulky tumors. In many centers, the treatment of patients who appear to be in complete remission is stopped only after careful "restaging" fails to reveal evidence of persistent microscopic disease.

In general, about three-quarters of previously untreated patients with advanced disease will remain in disease-free remission for 2 years. Over half of them may be expected to remain disease-free for 5 or more years and many are cured.

It is most important to an optimal long-term outcome to achieve maximal disease regression promptly during the initial course of treatment. The overall prognosis for patients with relapsing, previously treated Hodgkin's disease is much less favorable. Since the desired outcome is achieved by applying combinations of treatments at dose levels which are near the biologic tolerance of most patients, it is important that all individuals under therapy be super-

---

TABLE 51–7
Hodgkin's Disease: Clinical Stage, Initial Therapy, and Expected Survival

Clinical Stage	Initial Therapy	Disease-Free Survival	
		2 Years (%)	5 Years (%)
I	Radiation therapy	85–90	85–90
II	Radiation therapy*	85–90	60–70†
IIIA	Radiation therapy*	70–75	60–70
B	Combination chemotherapy‡	60–80	40–45
IV	Combination chemotherapy‡	60–70	30–40

* IIB and IIIA: add combination chemotherapy for mixed cellularity or lymphocyte depletion histology.
† Relapses more frequent with IIB staging and unfavorable histology.
‡ Add radiation therapy to manage bulky tumors.

vised closely and be given appropriate supportive care.

Common management problems in late stage, relapsing Hodgkin's disease result from progressive tumor growth (eventually resistant to therapy), anemia, bleeding, and other evidences of bone marrow failure, as well as from infections. Radiation therapy may be employed with profit to relieve abnormalities that result from persistent localized tumor masses. Infrequently, irradiation of an enlarged spleen will result in the resolution of constitutional manifestations and of distant tumor masses.

Adrenal corticosteroids may cause tumor lysis and a regression in systemic symptoms in a significant proportion of cases (about 25 percent). However, they are more useful in the management of such physiologic derangements as autoimmune hemolytic anemia, thrombocytopenia with bleeding, and hypercalcemia.

Rarely, acute leukemia and primary neoplasms of various types may develop in patients with long-term Hodgkin's disease. These occurrences raise questions about the carcinogenicity of radiation therapy and chemotherapeutic agents. They also pose practical problems to physicians who manage these patients and who must remain alert to these eventualities.

Non-Hodgkin's Lymphomas

Over the years, many types of malignant lymphomas have been described, most frequently on the basis of histopathologic features. In recent times, the terms giant follicle lymphoma, lymphosarcoma, and reticu-

lum cell sarcoma have been replaced by the classification suggested by Rappaport and his co-workers (Table 51–8). In general, clinicians have come to recognize that patients who have lymphomas with a nodular or follicular architecture (about one-third of non-Hodgkin's lymphomas) have a better outlook than those with a diffuse pattern. Pathologists and clinicians have employed the Rappaport system of classification (or closely related variants) under a wide variety of circumstances and it has proven to be very useful. Thus, even though many of the presumptions regarding cytogeneology implicit in this system are likely incorrect, it must be regarded as the currently accepted standard in the United States.[74,84]

At present, clinicians tend to divide the malignant lymphomas into two groups: Hodgkin's disease and the non-Hodgkin's lymphomas. The latter is a more heterogeneous grouping that encompasses rather indolent disorders such as the nodular lymphocytic lymphomas as well as more aggressive neoplasms such as diffuse histiocytic lymphoma and Burkitt's tumor (Tables 51–8 and 51–9).[84,86]

Lukes and Collins (and others) have suggested a classification of non-Hodgkin's lymphomas that is clinically relevant and based on the accumulating newer knowledge of the morphologic transformations associated with the normal functioning of the lymphoreticular cell system (Table 51–10). Their "functional classification" relates lymphoma cell morphology to the sequential stages in the histogenesis of normal T-cell and B-cell types. Their morphologic observations are reinforced by the identification of T-cell or B-cell markers on the cell surfaces. Al-

---

TABLE 51–8
Histopathologic Types of Non-Hodgkin's Lymphomas

Older Terms	Rappaport (1966)	Dorfman (1976)

Giant follicle lymphoma	Nodular lymphomas
	  Lymphocytic, poorly differentiated
	  Mixed lymphocytic and histiocytic
	  Histiocytic
		Follicular lymphomas*
		  Small lymphoid
		  Mixed small and large lymphoid
		  Large lymphoid

Lymphosarcoma	Diffuse lymphomas
	  Lymphocytic, well differentiated
	  Lymphocytic, poorly differentiated
	
	  Mixed lymphocytic and histiocytic
		Diffuse lymphomas*
		  Small lymphocytic†
		  Atypical small lymphoid
		  Lymphoblastic-convoluted and
		    nonconvoluted
		  Mixed small and large lymphoid

Reticulum cell sarcoma	Histiocytic, well differentiated
	  Histiocytic, poorly differentiated
	  Undifferentiated, pleomorphic
		Histiocytic
		  Large lymphoid†
		  Undefined

Burkitt's tumor	Undifferentiated, Burkitt's type	Burkitt's lymphoma

* Composite lymphomas comprise two well-defined cell types.
† Lymphomas showing plasmacytoid differentiated.

TABLE 51–9
Non-Hodgkin's Lymphomas: Relative Frequency of Histopathologic Type and Prognosis for Survival

Frequency (%)	Type	Survival 2 Years (%)	Survival 5 Years (%)
Nodular Lymphomas			
3	Lymphocytic, well differentiated	100	100
39	Lymphocytic, poorly differentiated	90	72
42	Mixed lymphocytic and histiocytic	93	60
16	Histiocytic	68	
Diffuse Lymphomas			
5	Lymphocytic, well differentiated	100	
19	Lymphocytic, poorly differentiated	48	32
19	Mixed lymphocytic and histiocytic	46	26
51	Histiocytic	30	18
6	Undifferentiated	35	

though clinically less useful from a practical point of view, the immunobiologic classifications provide a better conceptual framework for considering the various lymphoreticular proliferative disorders.[88]

Immunobiologic observations indicate that the majority of non-Hodgkin's lymphomas arise from the B-cell line (Table 51–10). Chronic lymphocytic leukemia and well-differentiated lymphocytic lymphoma appear to be closely related monoclonal neoplasms of B lymphocytes. On the other hand, lymphomas previously classified as histiocytic lymphoma or reticular cell sarcoma appear to have arisen from transformed lymphocytes of either the B- or T-cell type. A true histiocytic lymphoma seems to be a rare occurrence.

Lymphocytic Lymphoma

This disorder, once commonly called lymphosarcoma, is a disease characterized primarily by a progressive generalized lymphadenopathy, splenomegaly, and involvement of one or more nonlymphoid organ systems. The morphologic pattern distinctive of this disorder may be "follicular" or nodular or consist of a diffuse infiltrate of neoplastic lymphoid cells. When large, blast-like cells predominate, the term "poorly differentiated" is used. When small, mature-appearing lymphocytes are predominant, the tumor is classed as "well differentiated." This cell pattern is

similar to that seen in patients with chronic lymphatic leukemia. At times the histopathologic pattern contains a mixture of malignant lymphocytic and "histiocytic" cells (Table 51–9).

Lymphocytic lymphoma occurs with approximately the same frequency as Hodgkin's disease. It may be seen in any age group, but the age of peak incidence is between 40 and 60 years. Males are affected nearly twice as often as females. Most lymphocytic lymphomas are B-cell neoplasms. T-cell lymphomas occur more commonly in children and young adults.

CLINICAL PRESENTATION. Constitutional symptoms are encountered rarely in the course of lymphocytic lymphoma. The usual presenting problems are connected with a painless, progressive, often symmetrical, generalized lymphadenopathy. The enlarged lymph nodes are rubbery, often discrete, and rarely adherent to the adjacent structures. Palpable splenomegaly is present in 20 to 25 percent of individuals on presentation. In 20 to 25 percent of cases, lymphoid tumor masses may present in the nasopharynx or oropharynx or tonsillar areas. Furthermore, clinically detectable gastrointestinal tract involvement occurs in about 10 percent of cases. It is important to recognize extranodal lymphomas promptly because they require specific management.

TABLE 51–10
Histopathologic Types of Non-Hodgkin's Lymphomas: Functional Classification of Lukes and Collins

Type	Frequency (%)
U-Cell (Undefined) Type	17
T-Cell Types	15
Small lymphocyte	
Convoluted lymphocyte	
Sézary cell—mycosis fungoides	
Immunoblastic sarcoma	
B-Cell Types	67
Small lymphocyte	
Plasmacytoid lymphocyte	
Follicular center cells	
Small cleaved	
Large cleaved	
Small transformed (noncleaved)	
Large transformed (noncleaved)	
Immunoblastic sarcoma	
Hairy cell leukemia	
Histiocytic Type	1

Hematologic abnormalities are infrequent early in the course of lymphocytic lymphoma. However, as the disorder progresses a normochromic anemia is commonly seen. Usually this relates to impaired erythropoiesis, but at times hemolysis is the major contributing factor. In the more severe hemolytic states, the Coombs test is often positive. The platelet count generally is normal early in the disease but may be lower later on.

The relationship between well-differentiated lymphocytic lymphoma and chronic lymphatic leukemia has been mentioned. These diagnostic entities may well represent different portions of the same basic disease spectrum, since transition states are often encountered. In one large series, lymphocytic lymphoma transformed into chronic lymphatic leukemia in nearly 13 percent of the cases. Other observers have reported an absolute lymphocytosis in 15 to 30 percent of patients at some time during their course. Terms such as "leukosarcoma" have been used to describe the poorly differentiated lymphocytic lymphoma tumor cells that may be found in the peripheral blood and bone marrow.

The immunologic abnormalities which develop relatively late in the course of lymphocytic lymphoma are distinct from those which have been reported in Hodgkin's disease. Bacterial infections are encountered with increasing frequency, and their occurrence may be correlated with a progressive decrease in gamma globulin concentration and an impairment in antibody response to specific antigenic stimulation (e.g., pneumococcal polysaccharide).

Infrequently, macroglobulinemia (and its clinical consequences) is seen in association with lymphocytic lymphoma. Other monoclonal gammopathies have also been related to this disorder from time to time. Hypercalcemia may develop, too.

DIAGNOSTIC CONSIDERATIONS. The diagnosis of lymphocytic lymphoma usually presents no particular problem when an individual with little in the way of systemic symptoms manifests a painless, generalized lymphadenopathy. Biopsy is usually confirmatory.

In those instances in which the presenting manifestations are related to the presence of a solitary tumor in the nasopharynx, tonsil, mediastinum, or abdomen, a number of diagnostic possibilities must be considered (Chap. 55). Again, biopsy is relied upon as the chief means of establishing the diagnosis.

The histologic pattern of well-differentiated lymphocytic lymphoma is identical to that of chronic lymphatic leukemia. The diagnostic criteria used to separate these overlapping entities are arbitrary and vary among institutions. For example, a total white cell count in excess of $15,000/\mu l$ with more than 50 percent lymphocytes on differential count is regarded by some as one criterion of chronic lymphatic leukemia.

A syndrome, "angioimmunoblastic lymphadenopathy with dysproteinemia," has been described recently. Patients present with severe systemic symptoms, lymphadenopathy, hepatosplenomegaly, and possibly skin lesions. In most cases, there is a polyclonal hypergammaglobulinemia. At times the disorder progresses into an undifferentiated leukemia with plasmacytoid features.

CLINICAL COURSE AND MANAGEMENT.[86,92] The course of lymphocytic lymphoma is quite variable. As in Hodgkin's disease, the extent of the disorder (clinical stage) is a major determinant of prognosis for survival (Table 51-11). Histopathologic type also relates to survival (Table 51-9). Similarly, the occurrence of systemic symptoms or the development of hematologic or immunologic abnormalities indicates a poorer prognosis. Most reports note that the survival is better in women and that pregnancy seems to have no deleterious effect.

The pretreatment evaluation of patients with lymphocytic lymphoma should include a bone scan, reticuloendothelial (liver, spleen) scan, intravenous pyelogram, retroperitoneal lymphography, and (needle) biopsies of the liver and bone marrow. Following such studies, the majority of patients will be found to have Stage III or IV disease (Table 51-11); thus, diagnostic laparotomy is not generally indicated. An important subset of patients (about 10 percent) presents with extranodal lymphoma which is confined to the site of primary occurrence, especially the gastrointestinal tract and the head and neck.

Localized lymphocytic lymphomas (Stages I, II, and extranodal) respond readily to radiation therapy; usually doses of 4000 to 4500 rads are given over 4 to 5 weeks. It is not clear that extended treatment fields

---

TABLE 51-11

Nodular Lymphocytic Lymphoma: Relationship of Clinical Stage to Survival

Frequency (%)	Clinical Stage	Survival	
		2 Years (%)	5 Years (%)
2	I	100	100
5	II	90	77
14	III	85	68
79	IV	80	70
	All cases	85	70

(including total nodal irradiation) offer a better prognosis. Perhaps this is not surprising in view of the fact that the vast majority of patients treated have widely disseminated, clinically occult disease at the time of their diagnosis. Nonetheless, between 50 and 60 percent of patients with localized lymphoma will remain disease-free for 2 years or more following radiation therapy (Table 51-12). However, the frequency of relapse has led many to explore the use of combination chemotherapy given for a prolonged period (about 6 months) after the completion of radiation therapy in an attempt to eradicate the disease.

Generalized disease (Stages III and IV) is best treated by combinations of chemotherapeutic agents, each with different mechanisms of action (e.g., cyclophosphamide, vincristine, procarbazine, and prednisone). Several multiagent combinations seem equally effective if given at full dose levels for prolonged periods (6 to 12 months). Radiation therapy is often employed in an adjunctive role to eradicate bulky tumors. Although nearly 80 percent of patients so treated may appear in complete remission after 6 months or more of therapy, systematic restaging will reveal persistent lymphoma in about 20 percent of cases, especially in the sites of previous involvement. Systematic restaging has become an important part of patient management in order to prevent premature cessation of treatment while there is persistent tumor. About 20 percent of patients treated in this fashion may be expected to remain disease-free for 5 years or more, lending some credence to the hope of cure in this type of lymphoma also (Table 51-12).

At some institutions single agent chemotherapy is still used in the treatment of lymphocytic lymphoma because drugs such as chlorambucil may control the disease for months or even years without the added risks and inconvenience of more vigorous treatment. However, this approach would seem to preclude the possibility of total tumor eradication.

The major therapeutic problems encountered late in the course of lymphocytic lymphoma are infections by bacteria, viruses or fungi; anemia, at times hemolytic; progressively severe failure of all bone marrow elements; and the effects of enlarging tumor masses, eventually resistant to treatment.

Histiocytic Lymphoma[74,86]

Histiocytic lymphoma is characterized at first by the regional enlargement of lymph nodes or the development of prominent extranodal tumors and later by the generalized involvement of many organ systems. The invasive infiltrate characteristic of this disorder is composed predominantly of large mononuclear cells (15 to 35 μm) which contain delicate-appearing nuclear chromatin and often a single, prominent, dark-staining nucleolus. Recent studies indicate that histiocytic lymphomas in truth arise from transformed B- and T-cell lines of lymphoid cells in nearly all instances (Table 51-10). Although an authentic histiocytic lymphoma is a rarity, the term continues to be used in accordance with Rappaport's designation because of its clinical utility (Table 51-8).

Histiocytic lymphoma occurs half as frequently as Hodgkin's disease or lymphocytic lymphoma. It occurs in all age groups, but its peak incidence is between 40 and 60 years. The disorder is about twice as common in males as in females.

CLINICAL PRESENTATION. It is uncommon for individuals with histiocytic lymphoma to present with constitutional symptoms. The initial manifestations of this disorder most frequently are connected with a painless, asymmetrical regional lymph node enlargement, particularly in the cervical area. About one-third of the patients may become symptomatic because of extranodal tumor masses, which are most apt to be encountered in the nasopharynx or oropharynx, tonsils, skin, gastrointestinal tract, or bones. Presenting complaints may also relate to enlarging mediastinal or retroperitoneal tumors.

On examination, the palpable peripheral masses are usually nontender, matted, and free of attachment to the overlying skin. A generalized lymphadenopathy is uncommon, and palpable splenomegaly is observed less frequently than in the other lymphomas (fewer than 20 percent of cases). Retroperitoneal lymph node involvement may be demonstrated on lymphography in a high proportion of cases.

Hematologic abnormalities are uncommon in individuals with histiocytic lymphoma, especially during the early stages of the disease. Later, a normo-

---

TABLE 51-12

Lymphocytic Lymphomas: Clinical Stage, Initial Therapy, and Expected Survival

Clinical Stage	Initial Therapy	Survival 2 Years (%)	Survival 5 Years (%)
I	Radiation	50–80	35–60
II	Radiation	50–70	35–60
III	Combination chemotherapy*	50–80	20–40
IV	Combination chemotherapy*	50–80	20–40

* Single agent chemotherapy (chlorambucil) is preferred by some; radiation therapy is used to control bulky tumors.

chromic anemia is commonly seen, and other evidences of progressive bone marrow failure may develop. On occasion, an autoimmune hemolytic process may be detected. Monocytosis has been reported with some degree of frequency.

Histiocytic lymphoma at times develops into a leukemic disorder with the appearance of malignant histiocytes or monocytes in the peripheral blood and bone marrow. This outcome occurs in 3 to 5 percent of patients.

Immunologic abnormalities occur in patients with histiocytic lymphoma, but they have not been characterized as well as those of the other lymphomas. Viral infections *(Herpes zoster)* and fungal infections (histoplasmosis, cryptococcosis) seem to occur with increased frequency in these patients. The serum concentration of gamma globulin usually is not altered. However, monoclonal gammopathies have been reported in this setting, including the occasional occurrence of macroglobulinemia.

DIAGNOSTIC CONSIDERATIONS. Most commonly, the physician must evaluate complaints referable to a mass located in one of the lymph-node-bearing areas, keeping in mind the multiple possible causes of lymph node enlargement (Chap. 55). Similarly, the pressure of an extranodal mass (e.g., in the stomach, head and neck structures, mediastinum, or bones) leads to a consideration of the multiple pertinent possible causes. Tissue biopsy usually results in the establishment of a definite diagnosis.

When patients present with fever and other constitutional symptoms or with derangements referable to one or more organ systems, the diagnostic problem is more complex. However, the majority of such individuals have accessible tumor masses suitable for biopsy.

Histiocytic lymphoma develops with unusual frequency in renal homotransplant patients who are maintained on long-term immunosuppressive therapy. Such individuals should be followed carefully with this in mind. Immunosuppressive cytotoxic agents are also being given for prolonged periods to patients with rheumatoid arthritis, systemic lupus erythematosus, and other disorders with prominent manifestations of "autoimmunity." They may well have a similar risk of developing lymphoma.

CLINICAL COURSE AND MANAGEMENT.[92] The course of patients with histiocytic lymphoma is quite varied. As in the other lymphomas, the prognosis for survival is closely related to the clinical stage of the disease (Tables 51-13 and 51-14) and its histopathologic type (Table 51-9). Similarly, at all stages, women fare better than men.

The management of individuals with histiocytic

TABLE 51-13

Diffuse Histiocytic Lymphoma: Relationship of Clinical Stage to Survival

Frequency (%)	Clinical Stage	Survival 2 Years (%)	5 Years (%)
18	I	62	53
34	II	42	35
30	III	32	—
28	IV	29	18
	All cases	40	30

lymphoma follows the same basic approach used in lymphocytic lymphoma. At times, surgical excision of an extranodal tumor (e.g., tumor confined to a portion of the stomach) is followed by a prolonged disease-free period. Usually, however, Stage I and II disease is managed by radiation therapy. The dose generally employed is from 4000 to 4500 rads given in 4 to 5 weeks. Complete resolution of the tumor is to be expected in nearly all cases; disease-free status will last for 2 or more years in half of those treated. Nearly 50 percent of patients with Stage I and II disease will be alive at 5 years (Table 51-14).

Multidrug combinations (e.g., cyclophosphamide, vincristine, procarbazine, and prednisone) are the most effective means of treating Stage III and IV cases. Several combinations of chemotherapeutic agents with complementary mechanisms of action are equally effective. Adjunctive radiation therapy may be used in the management of bulky tumor masses (Table 51-14). Nearly all patients so treated will respond and about three-quarters of them will appear disease-free at 2 years. Between 25 and 45 percent of treated individuals will remain disease-free

TABLE 51-14

Histiocytic Lymphomas: Clinical Stage, Initial Therapy, and Expected Survival

Clinical Stage	Initial Therapy	Survival 2 Years (%)	5 Years (%)
I	Radiation	40–65	30–50
II	Radiation	40–65	30–40
III	Combination chemotherapy*	30–80	25–45
IV	Combination chemotherapy*	30–80	25–45

* Radiation therapy may be used to control bulky tumors.

for 5 years or more and are apparently cured. Since the results of multiagent chemotherapy in Stage III and IV diseases are similar to those achieved by radiation therapy in localized lesions, trials are underway to evaluate the role of chemotherapy in the primary management of Stage I and II disease.

It is important to achieve a complete remission during the initial course of treatment and to continue therapy for a sufficiently prolonged period (6 to 12 months) to maximize the possibility of obtaining a curative result. As in lymphocytic lymphoma, recent experience has shown that a significant portion of patients who appear in complete clinical remission will have microscopic evidence of persistent disease if they are systematically restaged. Therefore, most centers now restage patients who are in complete remission prior to discontinuing chemotherapy in order to avoid withdrawing potentially curative therapy before a complete regression of the tumor has been achieved.

A recent histopathologic subclassification of diffuse histiocytic lymphoma appears to have great clinical relevance. One subgroup (large, cleaved cells) had an excellent prognosis; two (large, uncleaved cells and follicular-center cells) had an intermediate prognosis; and 2 (blastic and pleomorphic) had a poorer prognosis for treatment response and survival.[82]

The management problems encountered late in the course of histiocytic lymphoma are similar to those associated with lymphocytic lymphoma: infections due to a wide variety of microorganisms; anemia, at times hemolytic (Coombs positive); progressively severe bone marrow failure; and the effects of enlarging tumor masses, eventually refractory to treatment. Radiation therapy applied to troublesome tumors can usually achieve useful palliation. Adrenal corticosteroids may induce tumor regression also. They are most helpful, however, in the alleviation of autoimmune hemolytic anemia, thrombocytopenic bleeding, and hypercalcemia.

Burkitt's Lymphoma

Burkitt's tumor, which occurs most commonly in well-defined areas of tropical Africa, deserves brief mention because several of its characteristics suggest important implications for the types of lymphoma more commonly encountered in temperate climates. This lymphoma has a distinctive morphologic pattern. The neoplastic cells are rather uniform in appearance and appear to be derived from B-cell lymphoid precursors (Table 51–4). Many large macrophages interspersed among the tumor cells often create a "starry sky" histologic pattern. Burkitt's lymphoma presents primarily in children under 14 years of age with a peak incidence in the 6th and 7th year. The manifestations of lymphoreticular proliferation are prominent, but leukemic transformation is rare. Particularly striking is the tumor involvement of the jaws and facial bones (about 50 percent of cases) and the intra-abdominal viscera. The disease is rapidly progressive and most cases, if untreated, die within 1 year. Small numbers of similar cases have been reported in the United States and various other parts of the world.

In Africa, the epidemiologic characteristics of the disease are compatible with an infectious etiology and an arthropod vector. There may also be a relationship to endemic malaria. The Epstein-Barr virus or a closely related agent has been identified as the possible cause of this lymphoma and EBV antibodies have been found in the sera of all patients tested.

Burkitt's tumor is highly responsive to cyclophosphamide. Nearly all treated patients improve promptly and about half enter a prolonged complete remission. Those patients responding most favorably to treatment seem to mount an immune reaction against their tumor as judged by the development of delayed hypersensitivity to isologous tumor cell membrane antigens and perhaps by a marked rise in EBV antibody titer. Whether similar phenomena occur in other types of lymphoma awaits further study.

MYCOSIS FUNGOIDES

Mycosis fungoides is a slowly progressive lymphomatous disorder which primarily involves the skin. In its advanced stages, the disorder spreads to involve lymph nodes, spleen, bone marrow, blood, and various internal organs. The diagnosis is based on a characteristic histopathologic lesion, Pautrier abscesses, which contain a variety of normal and abnormal lymphoreticular cells infiltrating epidermal structures. In some cases, abnormal lymphoid cells with highly convoluted nucleus (Sézary cells) are found in the peripheral blood. They appear to be derived from T-cell precursors.

Men are afflicted twice as often as women. The earliest skin lesions are usually rather nonspecific in appearance. At times there is much erythema and pruritis. At this stage, a casual skin biopsy may be inconclusive, and biopsies of multiple sites may be required to establish a correct diagnosis. After several months or years, the plaque-like skin lesions may thicken into tumors. Lymph node involvement is usually manifest at this juncture and disease progression accelerates. Malignant lymphoreticular cell infiltrates next affect the liver, spleen, and a variety of internal organs. Although tumor infiltrates may compromise renal, cardiac, or central nervous system function, death usually results from overwhelming bacterial, fungal, or viral infection.

Frequently, the earliest cutaneous lesions can be managed by ultraviolet radiation. The mechanisms responsible for this outcome are little understood. The more advanced plaque-like infiltrative lesions are managed best by electron beam therapy or the widespread topical application of mechlorethamine. More bulky tumor masses usually respond to radiation therapy but the duration of these responses is quite variable. Disseminated lymph node and visceral disease is best managed by multiagent chemotherapy much like lymphocytic or histiocytic lymphoma.

CHAPTER 52
Blood Transfusion
LARRY WATERBURY AND HAYDEN G. BRAINE

Rational transfusion therapy begins with a careful evaluation of each patient. The goal is to define precisely the specific blood components that are deficient and that are to be replaced by means of transfusion. With this in mind, it is important that physicians understand the essential elements of contemporary blood component preparation and transfusion technology.[103]

Blood is universally in short supply. There is good reason to fractionate freshly drawn whole blood into various components in order that each may be used where specifically indicated. In many instances, however, whole blood is required and each blood bank must maintain an appropriate supply. It is wasteful and expensive to meet the clinical needs for whole blood by "reconstituting" a suitable transfusion substitute from concentrated red blood cells, plasma fractions, and physiologic electrolyte solutions.[99]

BLOOD COMPONENT THERAPY

Red Blood Cells

Most blood banks provide several preparations containing red blood cells. These include whole blood, concentrated red blood cells, buffy-coat-poor concentrated red cells, and frozen red cells (Table 52–1). The storage life of whole blood and concentrated red cells maintained at 1 to 6°C is 21 days when acid citrate dextrose (ACD) solution is used as the anticoagulant. Currently most blood banks use citrate phosphate dextrose (CPD) solution as the anticoagulant because its higher pH results in a slower deteriorization of stored red blood cells. The removal of plasma components and leukocytes and platelets from whole blood does not adversely affect the storage life or the clinical utility of the remaining red blood cells provided proper technique is followed.

Whole blood is used primarily to treat acute bleeding that results in a loss of blood volume as well as red blood cells (Table 52–1). Patients losing 15 to 20 percent of their total blood volume in a short span of time usually develop symptoms (e.g., postural hypotension, tachycardia). The loss of 35 to 40 percent of the total blood volume usually results in shock. On the other hand, the gradual development of severe anemia (such as pernicious anemia, iron deficiency anemia, or progressive anemia secondary to renal insufficiency) may be attended by minimal signs and symptoms and frequently requires no transfusions at all. Often patients who are chronically anemic have a normal or increased total blood volume making even careful transfusions with packed cells hazardous. Elderly patients who are chronically anemic are more prone to develop signs and symptoms of cardiac ischemia (angina pectoris, ECG changes, etc.) and are also more susceptible to fluid overload making decision as to transfusion therapy more difficult. In this situation partial exchange transfusion may be used to raise the hematocrit without increasing blood volume.

Other than in the treatment of brisk hemorrhage, whole blood is usually not indicated. Most patients requiring red cells can be treated more effectively with packed red blood cells than with whole blood (Table 52–1). There are important differences between whole blood and concentrated red cells (Table 52–2). It should be noted that the hematocrit of concentrated red cells is 70 percent, not 95 percent, so that this preparation contains appreciable osmotically active protein and may induce venous congestion.

Several leukocyte-poor red cell preparations are available for patients who develop febrile transfusion reactions because of sensitization to leukocyte antigens (Table 52–1). Buffy-coat-poor erythrocytes may

---TABLE 52-1---
Clinical Use of Red Blood Cell Components

Component	Indications
Whole blood	Acute blood loss; volume replacement
Concentrated red blood cells (CRC)	Anemia
Buffy-coat-poor CRC	Allergic, febrile transfusion reactions
Washed CRC	Severe febrile reactions following CRC Severe allergic reactions to plasma proteins Paroxysmal nocturnal hemoglobinuria
Frozen CRC	Similar to washed CRC Severe alloimmunization Emergency need for rare RBC types Autologous red cell transfusions

---TABLE 52-2---
Comparison of Whole Blood and Concentrated Red Cells

	Whole Blood	Concentrated Red Cells
Volume	517/ml	300 ml
RBC Mass	200 ml	200 ml
Hemoglobin	30 g	30 g
Hematocrit	40 %	70 %
Plasma	250 ml	78 ml
Total protein	48 g	36 g
Albumin	12 g	4 g
Citrate	67/ml	22 ml

centrates have all the other advantages of washed red cell preparations since they are thoroughly cleansed of all other blood components during their preparation.

be prepared by inverted centrifugation with removal of the buffy coat and the upper red cell layers. This maneuver must be performed on blood that is less than 24 hours old and results in the loss of about one-third of the red cells in the unit. A more efficient method of removing granulocytes requires that freshly drawn, heparinized whole blood be passed through a nylon filter. Lymphocytes are not removed by this procedure, however, and the useful storage life is shortened because heparin is used as the anticoagulant and because there is a greater risk of bacterial contamination. More often, concentrated red cells washed several times with physiologic saline are used in the management of patients who have severe febrile reactions to leukocyte antigens or allergic reactions to plasma proteins.

Many blood banks use frozen red blood cells for some of their transfusion needs (Table 52-1). When mixed with preservatives such as glycerol and maintained at $-70°C$, erythrocytes may be stored for several years. Thus, red cells of rare type may be kept readily available for prompt transfusion. Also, this technique is suitable for the autotransfusion of patients with rare blood types or with multiple red cell antibodies for whom it is virtually impossible to find compatible erythrocytes. There are additional advantages to the use of frozen red cell concentrates. Normal concentrations of erythrocyte adenosine triphosphate (ATP) and 2,3-diphosphoglycerate (2,3-DPG) are maintained and this enhances continued red cell viability and function. Further, frozen red cell con-

Platelets[100,101]

Platelet transfusion strategy depends on the underlying disease process and its prognosis. When severe thrombocytopenia results from a platelet consumption rate which greatly exceeds the maximal rate of production, usually platelet transfusions are not prescribed. Exogenous platelet support cannot add significantly to the patient's own production. Treatment must be directed toward the immediate cause of the increase platelet consumption as well as the underlying disease. Splenectomy, immunosuppression, steroid therapy, or control of infection may be indicated depending on the primary disease state (Table 52-3).

When severe thrombocytopenia results primarily from decreased platelet production, generally platelet transfusions are indicated. Thrombocytopenia less than $40,000/\mu l$ is associated with a prolongation of the bleeding time and increased risk of bleeding. Platelet counts less than $10,000/\mu l$ are associated with increased morbidity from bleeding. Petechiae, ecchymoses, epistaxes, gingival bleeding, and prolonged bleeding from venipuncture may complicate severe thrombocytopenia, but sudden intracranial hemorrhage is the most significant cause of mortality. Platelet transfusions given to maintain the circulating platelet count above $20,000/\mu l$ will prevent bleeding. This "prophylactic" use of platelet transfusions has resulted in a substantial reduction in the mortality due to thrombocytopenic bleeding during the treatment of acute leukemia and related disorders.

Three platelet products are generally available for transfusion. Platelet rich plasma (300 ml plasma/

TABLE 52–3
Clinical Evaluation of Severe Thrombocytopenia (Platelet Count <50,000/μl)

Observations	Increased Production of Platelets	Decreased Production of Platelets
History	Clues for drug hypersensitivity Prior transfusions	Clues for myelophthisic disorder, toxic exposures
Physical examination	Splenomegaly Petechiae, purpura Sites of infection	Evidences of diseases which also involve marrow Petechiae
Peripheral blood smear	Thrombocytopenia Marked anisocytosis and poikilocytosis of RBC	Isolated thrombocytopenia Decrease in all elements Leukoerythroblastosis Neoplastic cells
Bone marrow aspiration/ biopsy	Normal Megakaryocytosis	Decreased megakaryocytes Generalized hypoplasia Infiltrative disease or myelofibrosis

unit) and platelet concentrates (50 ml/unit) are prepared by processing single units of whole blood. Platelet concentrates are preferable since their volume is more convenient and since packed red cells and fresh frozen plasma may be prepared simultaneously. Platelet concentrates containing 4 to 7 units may be prepared from a single donor by using one of the commercially available blood cell separators. These units separate donor blood into components by centrifugation allowing collection of leukocyte or platelet concentrates. Generally 50 ml of blood per minute are processed using regional anticoagulation with ACD. Two to three liters of a single donor's blood may be processed over a 1- to 2-hour period. Plateletpheresis is the most practical method available to harvest HLA-matched platelets in the amounts required. However, since the donor's blood is manipulated extracorporeally and then returned, the potential for complications during plateletpheresis is increased over that expected from whole blood donation.

When short periods of severe thrombocytopenia are anticipated such as during the treatment of acute leukemia, generally platelet transfusions are given daily to maintain counts above 20,000/μl (Fig. 52–1). One unit of platelets (1×10^{11} platelets) will raise the count of a patient whose body surface area is one M^2 by 10,000 to 15,000/μl. Thus, in an adult (1.7 M^2) 5 units are needed to elevate the platelet count from 20,000/μl to 50,000/μl.

In afebrile, noninfected patients (near normal platelet survival), 5-unit transfusions must be given every other day to maintain the platelet count above 20,000/μl and to prevent significant bleeding (prophylactic transfusions).

Platelet transfusions should be given by specific ABO type. In emergency situations out-of-group platelets may be given without adversely affecting platelet function. However, since significant volumes of plasma are given with each transfusion, the direct Coombs test may become positive and red cell survival may be shortened. Unless the recipient has been transfused previously or is multiparous, rarely are preformed alloantibodies to platelets encountered. Thus, HLA-specific platelets are not used routinely. When patients are multiply transfused, however, alloimmunization usually develops in 6 to 12 weeks. For this reason, patients with mild thrombocytopenia or thrombocytopenia that is of indeterminate duration (e.g., aplastic anemia) generally are not transfused unless bleeding occurs. In those instances where support may be required over a prolonged time period, HLA-matched platelets are preferred in order to minimize the risk of alloimmunization.

Refractoriness to platelet transfusions is a commonly encountered problem, especially in patients who have been multiply transfused. When patients fail to sustain an effective platelet increment 12 hours after transfusion they should be evaluated systematically for causes of increased platelet consumption (Table 52–4). If the decreased survival of platelets is associated with fever, infection, etc., the transfusion of platelets in large amounts may minimize the risk of significant bleeding during the time necessary to bring the situation under control. If the decreased survival of platelets is due to alloimmunization, the transfusion of specific HLA-matched platelets will result in satisfactory increments in about 70 percent of instances. The transfusion of platelets from an HLA-matched family member will be effective in nearly every instance (Fig. 52–2).

Granulocytes[96,102]

Leukocyte concentrates containing 1 to 3×10^{10} polymorphonuclear leukocytes may be prepared from normal donors using either leukofiltration or centrifugation. Both methods require the extracorporeal pro-

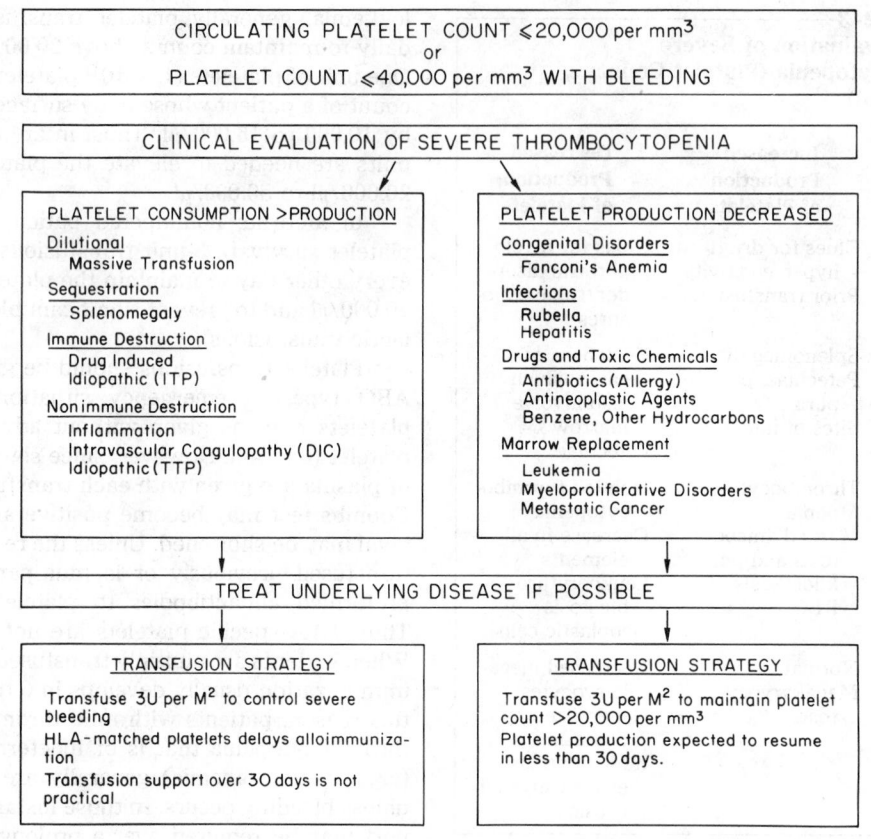

FIGURE 52–1. A clinical strategy for platelet transfusion therapy.

cessing of 3 to 5 liters of blood over a 1- to 3-hour period. Thus, the donor is exposed to more inconvenience and a greater risk of hemolysis, infection, phlebitis, hypervolemia, hypovolemia, and hypothermia than is associated with the usual blood donation. Accordingly, granulocyte donors must be selected carefully and the process supervised closely.

Filtration leukopheresis takes advantage of the fact that granulocytes adhere to nylon fibers. Thus, donors are anticoagulated with heparin and their blood is circulated through nylon "leukopacks." Subsequently, granulocytes are eluted from the nylon filters using a citrated plasma-saline solution. While clinically effective, granulocytes prepared by filtration manifest significant morphologic and physiologic abnormalities. Further, they cause more febrile transfusion reactions more frequently than granulocytes prepared by centrifugation.

The collection of granulocytes by centrifugation is inherently safer than leukofiltration since regional anticoagulation (ACD solution) is used rather than systemic heparinization. Further, it is more efficient

since plateletpheresis may be performed concurrently. However, centrifugation methods require the addition of a rouleauing agent (hydroxyethyl starch or dextran) to the blood to achieve an effective separation of granulocytes from red cells. Currently, leukopheresis methods are relatively ineffective in that at best less than 10 percent of a normal adult's daily granulocyte production can be harvested. To increase yields, donors are premedicated with etiocholanalone or adrenal corticosteroids in order to mobilize the marginating pools and bone marrow reserves of granulocytes. Further, the complete granulocyte fraction is collected and this results in substantial red cell contamination. Thus, transfused granulocyte concentrates must be ABO compatible with the recipient.

Leukocyte transfusions are used in the management of severe granulocytopenia (granulocyte count $<200/\mu l$) in order to combat infection. In patients with this degree of granulocytopenia the risk of infection is extraordinarily high, especially if effective granulocyte production remains markedly depressed longer than 5 to 7 days. In order to be effective, 1 ×

TABLE 52-4
Clinical Evaluation of Platelet Transfusion Failure

Observations	Immune Destruction of Platelets	Nonimmune Destruction of Platelets
History	Prior transfusions; often >50 units Drug hypersensitivity	None or few prior transfusions
1 hr platelet increment	<1000/μl	>3000/μl or near normal
Lymphocytotoxic antibody	Present	Absent
Clinical status		Evidences of disorders leading to increased consumption of platelets

10^{10} granulocytes (or more) must be transfused daily. Leukocyte transfusions have proven their worth in the prevention of serious infection (prophylactic transfusions) and in the successful management of a variety of established infections in granulocytopenic patients.

Unfortunately, leukocyte transfusions are not yet available widely and a variety of strategies have been developed to use them most efficiently. For example, they are often used to support patients through a self-limited period of severe bone marrow aplasia or through a course of cytotoxic, antineoplastic drug therapy which is expected to induce a disease remission (e.g., a course of remission induction chemotherapy in acute leukemia). While it is not practical to support severely granulocytopenic patients for prolonged periods, leukocyte transfusions may be helpful in the management of severe intercurrent infections. Rarely are leukocyte transfusions given to patients undergoing cytotoxic chemotherapy when the expected duration of their granulocytopenia is less than 5 to 7 days (Table 52-5, Fig. 52-3).

Leukocyte transfusion entails all the risks of blood transfusion. In addition, febrile reactions occur during 20 to 60 percent of transfusions. Transmission of graft *vs.* host disease by leukocyte concentrates has been observed and irradiation of these products to the least 1500 rad is indicated particularly if the recipient's immunity is severely compromised.

FRESH FROZEN PLASMA, CRYOPRECIPITATE, AND COMMERCIAL CONCENTRATES[99]

Plasma separated from freshly drawn blood and immediately frozen is known as fresh frozen plasma. This component maintains the functional activity of

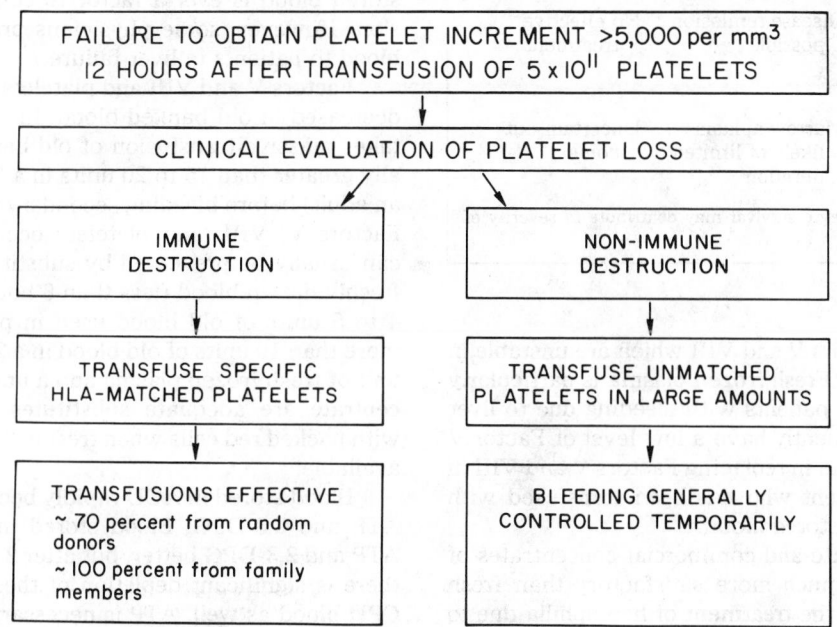

FIGURE 52-2. The management of platelet transfusion failure.

┌─────────────────────────────────────┐

TABLE 52-5

**Clinical Evaluation of Severe
Granulocytopenia (Granulocyte Count
<200/μl)***

Observations	Decreased Production (1-4 Weeks)	Decreased Production (More Than 4 Weeks)
History	Drug hypersensitivity Toxic exposure Recent infectious disease Other acquired disorder	Congenital disorders Toxic exposure Underlying acquired disease
Physical examination	Evidence of underlying disease Evidence of infection may be minimal Splenomegaly	Evidence of underlying disease Evidence of infection may be minimal Splenomegaly
Peripheral blood smear	Granulocytopenia Thrombocytopenia Evidence of leukemia or myelofibrosis	Granulocytopenia Thrombocytopenia
Bone marrow aspiration/ biopsy	Infiltrative disease Megaloblastosis Generalized hypoplasia	Generalized hypoplasia Myelofibrosis
Proposed treatment and prognosis	Disease remission possible	No effective treatment
	Marrow aplasia likely of limited duration	Uncertain outcome

* Shortened granulocyte survival may contribute to severity of granulocytopenia.

└─────────────────────────────────────┘

coagulation Factors V and VIII which are unstable in unfrozen plasma. Fresh frozen plasma is particularly useful in treating patients with bleeding due to liver disease who frequently have a low level of Factor V in their plasma and in replacing Factors V and VIII in the bleeding patient who has been transfused with multiple units of stored blood.

Cryoprecipitate and commercial concentrates of Factor VIII are much more satisfactory than fresh frozen plasma in the treatment of hemophilia due to factor VIII deficiency (Chap. 48). Cryoprecipitate is the gelatinous precipitate (approximately 3 ml from

each plasma unit) present when rapidly frozen fresh plasma is slowly rewarmed to 4C. It contains between 40 and 80 percent of the Factor VIII present in the original fresh plasma in a concentrated form. It may be stored for long periods (many months) in the frozen state. Coagulation proteins other than Factors V and VIII are stable so that stored plasma or blood may be used to correct specific deficiencies of these substances. Lyophilized concentrates of Factor VIII are commercially available as are concentrates of the "prothrombin complex." All of the commercial concentrates carry a significant hepatitis risk primarily because they are processed from large batches of plasma from muliple donors.

Fresh Blood

Table 52–6 compares the differences between freshly drawn blood (less than 8 hours old) and banked blood stored for 21 days at 4°C. The indications for the use of fresh blood hinge on these differences. As can be seen, the plasma potassium concentration increases as blood ages in vitro due to loss of erythrocyte potassium into the surrounding plasma. In actual practice, hyperkalemia is usually not a hazard in transfusion because of the large space in which the potassium is distributed in vivo. However, in patients with a high serum potassium receiving large quantities of blood and in infants undergoing exchange transfusion, fresher blood probably is indicated. There is little good evidence that the high ammonia content of stored blood is ever a factor to consider in transfusion. However, some physicians prefer giving fresh blood to patients in liver failure.

Factors V and VIII and platelets are considerably decreased in old banked blood. In actual practice, it takes massive transfusion of old banked blood (usually greater than 15 to 20 units in a 24-hour period in an adult) before bleeding secondary to deficiencies of Factors V, VIII, and platelets occurs. Hemorrhage can usually be prevented by substituting one unit of freshly drawn blood (less than 8 hours old) for every 4 to 5 units of old blood used in patients receiving more than 10 units of old blood in a 24-hour period. A unit of fresh frozen plasma and a unit of platelet concentrate are adequate substitutes when combined with packed red cells when freshly drawn blood is not available.

Blood stored in ACD rapidly becomes depleted of ATP and 2,3-DPG. Blood stored in CPD maintains ATP and 2,3-DPG better, but after 2 weeks of storage there is significant depletion of these compounds in CPD blood as well. ATP is necessary for erythrocyte viability. ATP and especially 2,3-DPG, by binding with hemoglobin, influence the blood oxygen disso-

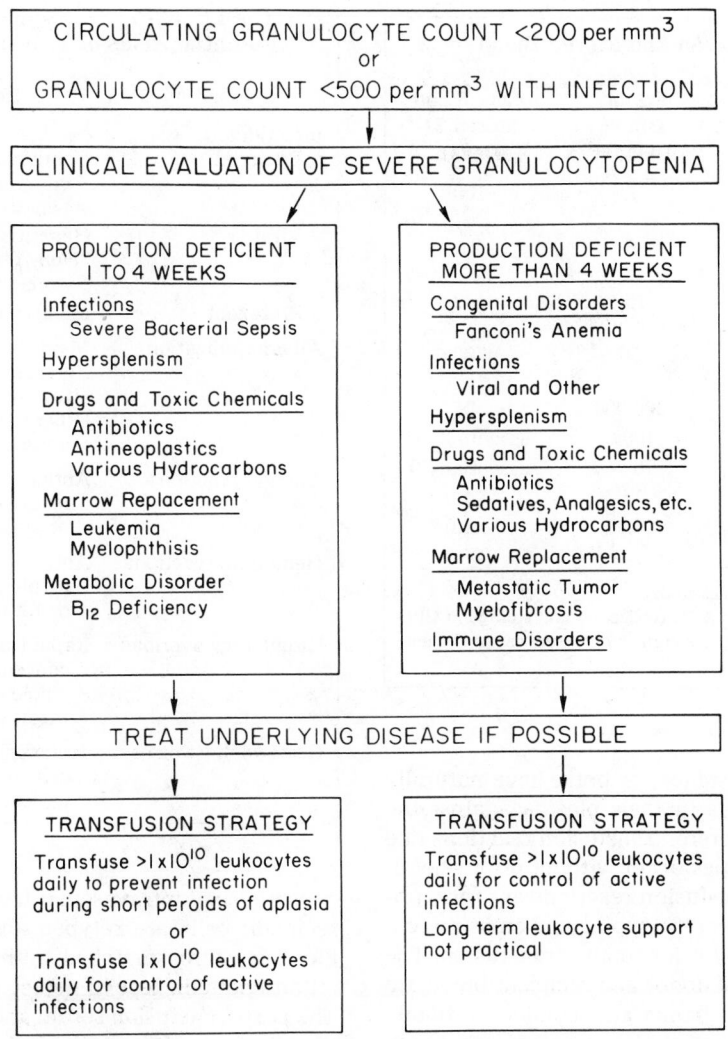

FIGURE 52-3. A clinical strategy for leukocyte transfusion therapy.

ciation curve (Chap. 45). Blood deficient in 2,3-DPG has an O_2-dissociation curve shifted to the left so that hemoglobin more strongly binds oxygen at any given Po_2, interfering with the release of oxygen to the tissues. Old banked blood probably takes several hours to regenerate 2,3-DPG post-transfusion and may be less effective as an aid to tissue oxygenation in the interim. Because of the scarcity of freshly drawn blood and the need for storage capability to meet hospital transfusion requirements, use of fresh whole blood alone is not a practical solution to these problems. Active research into methods designed to prolong the shelf life to stored blood beyond the current 21-day limit has disclosed a number of possibly useful additives. Adenine is used routinely in some European countries to prolong shelf life and may gain approval in the United States in the near future.

RISKS OF TRANSFUSION (Table 52-7)

Hemolytic Reactions[103,106]

A number of different genetically determined antigens are present on the surface of red cells. Individuals whose cells do not contain a particular blood group substance may form an antibody to it if transfused with cells that do contain the antigen. Patients may be sensitized to foreign red cell antigens by prior transfusions or pregnancy. The likelihood of eliciting an immune response is variable. Individuals whose

TABLE 52-6
Comparison of Fresh and Stored Blood

	Freshly Drawn Blood*†	Bank Blood Stored 21 Days†
Plasma Hgb mg/dl	5	100
Plasma K mEq/L	6	21
Plasma Na mEq/L	150	140
Plasma ammonia μg/dl	50	700
Viable platelets/μl	200,000	0
Factor VIII	100%	essentially 0
Factor V	100%	essentially 0
ATP μmole/ml RBCs	1.5	<1.0
2,3-DPG μmole/ml RBCs	4.5	<1.0

* Less than 8 hours postphlebotomy.
† Collection and storage in ACD (collection and storage in CPD results in lower plasma potassium, higher red cell ATP, and higher red cell 2,3-DPG).

TABLE 52-7
Potential Risks of Transfusion Therapy

Reaction	Responsible Agent
Infections	
Bacterial	Contamination of transfused components, usually by gram-negative bacteria
Viral	Hepatitis A and hepatitis B virus "Non-A, non-B" hepatitis virus Cytomegalovirus
Protozoal	Malaria, toxoplasmosis
Alloimmunization	Major blood group antigens Rh group antigens HLA antigens Other platelet and leukocyte antigens
Allergic reactions	Antigen–antibody reactions involving leukocytes, platelets, or plasma proteins
Hemolytic reactions	Antigen–antibody reactions involving major blood group or Rh antigens
Circulatory overload	Rapid transfusion of concentrated red cells or whole blood in excess of cardiovascular capacity
Graft vs. host disease	Transfusion of viable lymphoid cells to immunocompromised patients

cells lack A or B substance, or both, have naturally occurring isoantibodies in their plasma against the missing antigen. Therefore, transfusion reactions due to ABO incompatabilities occur without prior sensitization. Hemolytic transfusion reactions are rare, primarily because of the careful typing and cross-matching routines conducted prior to any transfusion. The ABO and Rh groups of donor and recipient blood are determined and blood banks also conduct antibody screening tests to detect the presence of any unexpected antibodies (e.g., anti-Kell, anti-Kidd, etc.) in donor and recipient serums. Hemolytic reactions occasionally still occur, and are associated with variable and often nonspecific signs and symptoms. Acute intravascular hemolysis following the transfusion of A or B cells into patients with anti-A or anti-B antibodies may occur within the first few minutes of beginning transfusion. On the other hand, delayed mild transfusion reactions resulting only in shortened survival of the transfused cells may go unnoticed. Pain along the transfusion vein, substernal chest pain, abdominal or back pain, extreme anxiety, chills, fever, hypotension, or dyspnea all require immediate evaluation of the possible occurrence of a hemolytic transfusion reaction. At that point, the transfusion should be stopped, and the blood remaining in the bag, a post-transfusion blood specimen, and the first voided urine specimen should be obtained to evaluate the possible presence of red cell incompatability and the occurrence of intravascular hemolysis. The donor and recipient cells are retyped and donor and recipient blood is recrossmatched by methods which include an antiglobulin test to detect incomplete antibodies. The post-transfusion serum and urine are checked for the presence of hemoglobin indicative of the occurrence of intravascular hemolysis, and a posttransfusion hematocrit is obtained to help quantitate the magnitude of red cell destruction. Acute renal failure may occur after a hemolytic reaction and there should be an early attempt to induce an osmotic diuresis. The patient should be recrossmatched immediately as he may need further transfusions. Intravascular coagulation resulting in a generalized bleeding diathesis also may occur and in the unconscious patient or the patient undergoing surgery may be the first manifestation that a hemolytic transfusion reaction has taken place.

Febrile and Allergic Reactions
Chills, fever, and urticaria during transfusion may herald a hemolytic transfusion reaction but more often are due to antigen–antibody reactions involving leukocytes, platelets, or plasma proteins. These usually occur in previously transfused patients or women

sensitized by previous pregnancies. Mild reactions frequently may be handled by symptomatic measures (such as antihistamines) if hemolysis is ruled out. Hemolytic reactions and febrile reactions may both be characterized simply by the occurrence of chills and fever. Febrile reactions involving leukocytes, platelets, or plasma proteins are common and may accompany as high as 3 percent of all transfusions. In the patient with multiple prior transfusions or the woman with multiple past pregnancies, febrile reactions are exceedingly common. Hemolytic reactions, on the other hand, are quite uncommon. However, it is safer to approach all febrile transfusion reactions as if they were hemolytic in nature. When not accompanied by other signs of a hemolytic reaction (pain, hypotension, pink serum, a drop in hematocrit) and when the reaction occurs in a multiply-transfused or multiparous patient, especially one who has experienced prior febrile reactions, the transfusion may be continued while the transfusion reaction workup is in progress. Most hemolytic reactions are due to clerical error so that one must immediately rule out the possibility that the wrong unit of blood has been administered. Severe febrile reactions may be prevented by the use of leukocyte-poor blood.

Other Reactions

The transfusion of contaminated blood, usually containing gram-negative organisms which grow in the cold (most commonly pseudomonas and coli-aerogenes groups) may result in an acute reaction characterized by shock, tachypnea, and severe abdominal pain; death may occur rapidly. In the evaluation of any transfusion reaction, a Gram stain should be made of a drop of blood from the transfusion set and appropriate cultures obtained. Circulatory overload is another important hazard of transfusions and as mentioned may occur with the use of packed cells as well as whole blood. Air embolism, another transfusion hazard, is rare with the use of collapsible plastic blood containers. Massive rapid transfusion of cold banked blood has been associated with serious cardiac arrhythmias and, in these circumstances, blood should be warmed to room temperature before administration. If blood during storage has been allowed to reach temperatures less than 0°C or greater than 10°C for extended periods, or if blood has been warmed to greater than 50°C, hemolysis will occur on transfusion.

DONOR SELECTION

One of the most important aspects of a safe transfusion service is donor selection. Strict criteria have been established to define acceptable blood donors to protect the donor and the recipient. A careful history must be taken and the following are checked: blood pressure, pulse, temperature, weight, hematocrit (or hemoglobin), and a serologic test for syphilis.

Despite improved methods of testing blood products for evidences of hepatitis A and hepatitis B virus, hepatitis remains one of the most frequent and serious complications of transfusion therapy. "Non-A, non-B hepatitis" occurs following transfusion of carefully tested components. About two-thirds of active blood donors harbor cytomegalovirus (latent infection). Presumably, their blood represents a hazard to immunocompromised recipients.[97]

HLA Matching[98,104,105]

In heavily transfused patients, alloantibodies to the HLA antigen system form rapidly. While of little consequence in red cell transfusions, antibodies against antigens of the A and B loci of the HLA system may result in absolute refractoriness to platelet and granulocyte transfusion. In such situations, platelets "matched" at the HLA-A and -B loci may be clinically effective. HLA identical siblings or unrelated donors with four antigen (A) matches may be used. However, the HLA system is highly pleomorphic and over 60 antigens have been identified making the probability of finding an A match with a random donor extremely small. Fortunately, a significant degree of antigenic similarity exists in the HLA system with substantial cross-reactivity. Matching donors with cross-reacting HLA antigens (B matches) has been shown to be nearly as effective as using A matches. This has substantially improved the outcome of platelet transfusions in alloimmunized patients. If only A matches could be used, a donor pool of 5000 would supply an average of 1.5 (0 to 21) donors per patient. Using B matches, a similar donor pool would supply 306 (7 to 1129) donors per patient. While the A and B loci of the HLA system are clearly major determinants in platelet alloimmunization, other HLA loci and platelet specific antigen systems are important also. The transfusion of platelets matched at the HLA- A and -B loci is not always successful.

Special Donors

Highly motivated, healthy donors are necessary to a successful plateletpheresis and leukopheresis support program. These donors must be willing and able to endure the inconvenience and the added risks of the cell separation procedures. Further, they must be willing to donate during the medical need since there are as yet no effective means of storing granulocytes and platelets for prolonged periods.

REFERENCES

General References

1. Hayhoe, F.G.J. and Flemans, R.J. An Atlas of Hematological Cytology. New York, Wiley, 1970.
2. Williams, W.J., Beutler, E., Erslev, A.J., and Rundles, R.W. (eds.). Hematology, 2nd ed. New York, McGraw-Hill, 1977.
3. Wintrobe, M.M., Lee, G.R., Boggs, D.R., Bithell, T.C., Athens, J.W., and Foerster, J. (eds.). Clinical Hematology, 7th ed. Philadelphia, Lea and Febiger, 1977.

Anemia: General Considerations

4. Bunn, H.F. Erythrocyte destruction and hemoglobin catabolism. Semin. Hematol., 9:3, 1972.
5. Cooper, R.A., Arner, E.C., Wiley, J.S., and Shattil, S. J. Modification of red cell membrane structure by cholesterol-rich lipid dispersions. A model for the primary spur cell defect. J. Clin. Invest., 55:115, 1975.
6. Erslev, A.J. Renal biogenesis of erythropoietin. Am. J. Med., 58:25, 1975.
7. Finch, C.A., Deubelbeiss, K., Cook, J.D., Eschbach, J.W., Harker, L.A., Funk, D.D., Marsaglia, R.G., Hillman, R.S., Slichter, S., Adamson, J.W., Ganzoni, A., and Giblett, E.R. Ferrokinetics in man. Medicine, 49:17, 1970.
8. Finch, C.A. and Lenfant, C. Oxygen transport in man. N. Engl. J. Med., 286:407, 1972.
9. Hershko, C. The fate of circulating hemoglobin. Br. J. Haematol., 29:199, 1975.
10. Izak, G. Erythroid cell differentiation and maturation. In Brown, E.B. (ed.), Progess in Hematology, Vol. 10. New York, Grune & Stratton, 1977, p. 1.
11. Kirkpatrick, F.H. Spectrin: current understanding of its physical, biochemical, and functional properties. Life Sci., 19:1, 1976.
12. Linman, J.W. Physiologic and pathophysiologic effects of anemia. N. Engl. J. Med., 279:812, 1968.
13. Nienhuis, A.W. and Benz, E.J. Regulation of hemoglobin synthesis during the development of the red cell. N. Engl. J. Med., 297:1318, 1371, 1430, 1977.
14. Schmid, R. Bilirubin metabolism in man. N. Engl. J. Med., 287:703, 1972.
15. Weed, R.I. The importance of erythrocyte deformability. Am. J. Med., 49:147, 1970.

Anemia Due to Disorders of Red Blood Cell and Hemoglobin Production

16. Cartwright, G.E. and Deiss, A. Sideroblasts, siderocytes, and sideroblastic anemia. N. Engl. J. Med., 292:185, 1975.
17. Erbe, R.W. Inborn errors of folate metabolism. N. Engl. J. Med., 293:753, 807, 1975.
18. Fried, W. Erythropoietin and the kidney. Nephron, 15:327, 1975.
19. Goldberg, L.S., Bluestone, R., Stiehm, E.R., Terasaki, P.I., and Weisbart, R.H. Human autoimmunity, with pernicious anemia as a model. Ann. Intern. Med., 81:372, 1974.
20. Hagler, L., Pastore, R.A., and Bergin, J.J. Aplastic anemia following viral hepatitis: report of 2 fatal cases and literature review. Medicine, 54:139, 1975.
21. Hendler, E.D., Goffinet, J.A., Ross, S., Longnecker, R.E., and Bakovic, V. Controlled study of androgen therapy in anemia of patients on maintenance hemodialysis. N. Engl. J. Med., 291:1046, 1974.
22. Hershko, C. Storage iron regulation. In Brown, E.B. (ed.), Progress in Hematology, Vol. 10. New York, Grune & Stratton, 1977.
23. Higgins, M.R., Grace, M., Ulan, R.A., Silverberg, D.S., Bettcher, K.B., and Dossetor, J.B. Anemia in hemodialysis patients. Changing concepts in management. Arch. Intern. Med., 137:172, 1977.
24. Hoffbrand, A.V., Ganeshaguru, K., Hooten, J.W.L., and Tripp, E. (eds.). Megaloblastic anemia. Clin. Haemotol. 5(3), 1976.
25. Hoffman, R., Zanjani, E.D., Lutton, J.D., Zalusky, R., and Wasserman, L.R. Suppression of erythroid-colony formation by lymphocytes from patients with aplastic anemia. N. Engl. J. Med., 296:10, 1977.
26. Jacobs, A. and Worwood, M. The biochemistry of ferritin and its clinical implications. In Brown, E.B. (ed.), Progess in Hematology, Vol. 9. New York, Grune & Stratton, 1975.
27. Krantz, S.B. Pure red cell aplasia. N. Engl. J. Med., 291:345, 1974.
28. Lewis, S.M. and Verwilghen, R.L. Dyserythropoiesis and dyserythropoietic anemias. In Brown, E.B. (ed.), Progress in Hematology, Vol. 8. New York, Grune & Stratton, 1973.
29. Lipschitz, D.A., Cook, J.D., and Finch, C.A. A clinical evaluation of serum ferritin as an index of iron stores. N. Engl. J. Med., 290:1213, 1974.
30. Pierce, H.I., McGuffin, R.G., and Hillman, R.S. Clinical studies in alcoholic sideroblastosis. Arch. Intern. Med., 136:283, 1976.
31. Rosenberg, I.H. Folate absorption and malabsorption. N. Engl. J. Med., 293:1303, 1975.
32. Stebbins, R., Scott, J., and Herbert, V. Drug-induced megaloblastic anemias. Semin. Hematol., 10:235, 1973.
33. Storb, R., Prentice, R.L., and Thomas, E.D. Marrow transplantation for treatment of aplastic anemia. An analysis of factors associated with graft rejection. N. Engl. J. Med., 296:61, 1977.
34. Thomas, E.D., Fefer, A., Buckner, C.D., and Storb, R. Current status of bone marrow transplantation for aplastic anemia and acute leukemia. Blood, 49:671, 1977.
35. Williams, D.M., Lynch, R.E., and Cartwright, G.E. Drug-induced aplastic anemia. Semin. Hematol., 10:195, 1973.
36. Zucker, S., Friedman, S., and Lysik, R.M. Bone marrow erythropoiesis in the anemia of infection, inflammation, and malignancy. J. Clin. Invest., 53:1132, 1974.

Anemia Due to Hemolysis

37. Bank, A. The thalassemia syndromes. Blood, 51:369, 1978.
38. Benz, E.J., Jr. and Forget, B.G. The molecular genetics of the thalassemia syndrome. In Brown, E.B. (ed.), Progress in Hematology, Vol. 9. New York, Grune & Stratton, 1975, p. 107.

39. Dean, J. and Schechter, A.W. Sickle cell anemia: molecular and cellular bases of therapeutic approaches. N. Engl. J. Med., 299:752, 804, 863, 1978.
40. Desforges, J.F. Genetic implications of G-6-PD deficiency. N. Engl. J. Med., 294:1438, 1976.
41. Frank, M.M., Schreiber, A.D., Atkinson, J.P., and Jaffe, C.J. Pathophysiology of immune hemolytic anemia. Ann. Intern. Med., 87:210, 1977.
42. Nagel, R.L. and Bookchin, R.M. Human hemoglobin mutants with abnormal oxygen binding. Semin. Hematol., 11:385, 1974.
43. Petz, L.D. and Fudenberg, H.H. Immunologic mechanisms in drug-induced cytopenias. In Brown, E.B. (ed.), Progress in Hematology, Vol. 9. New York, Grune & Stratton, 1975, p. 185.
44. Prankerd, T.A.J. and Bellingham, A.J. (eds.). Haemolytic anaemias. Clin. Haematol. 4(1), 1975.
45. Pruzanski, W. and Shumak, K.H. Biologic activity of cold-reacting autoantibodies. N. Engl. J. Med., 297:538, 1977.
46. Rieder, R.F. Human hemoglobin stability and instability: molecular mechanisms and some clinical correlations. Semin. Hematol., 11:423, 1974.
47. Rosse, W.F. Correlation of in vivo and in vitro measurements of hemolysis in hemolytic anemia due to immune reactions. In Brown, E.B. (ed.), Progess in Hematology. Vol. 8. New York, Grune & Stratton, 1973, p. 51.
48. Sears, D.A. The morbidity of sickle cell trait. A review of the literature. Am. J. Med., 64:1021, 1978.
49. Swisher, S.N. (ed.). Immune hemolytic anemias. Semin. Hematol., 13(4), 1976.
50. Weatherall, D.J. (ed.). Abnormal haemoglobins. Clin. Haematol. 3(2), 1974.

Bleeding Disorders

51. Ahn, Y.S., Byrnes, J.J., Harrington, W.J., Cayer, M.L., Smith, D.S., Brunskill, D.E., and Pall, L.M. The treatment of idiopathic thrombocytopenia with vinblastine-loaded platelets. N. Engl. J. Med., 298:1101, 1978.
52. Barrow, E.M. and Graham, J.B. Blood coagulation factor VIII (antihemophilic factor): with comments on von Willebrand's disease and Christmas disease. Physiol. Rev., 54:23, 1974.
53. Bennett, B. Coagulation pathways: interrelationships and control mechanisms. Semin. Hematol., 14:301, 1977.
54. Biggs, R. (ed.). Human Blood Coagulation, Haemostasis and Thrombosis, 2nd ed. Oxford, Blackwell, 1977.
55. Cream, J.J., Gumpel, J.M., and Peachey, R.D. Schönlein-Henoch purpura in the adult. A study of 77 adults with anaphylactoid or Schönlein-Henoch purpura. Q. J. Med., 39:461, 1970.
56. Dixon, R., Rosse, W., and Ebbert, L. Quantitative determination of antibody in idiopathic thrombocytopenic purpura. N. Engl. J. Med., 292:230, 1975.
57. Grey, H.M. and Kohler, P.F. Cryoimmunoglobulins. Semin. Hematol., 10:87, 1973.
58. Heene, D.L. Disseminated intravascular coagulation: evaluation of therapeutic approaches. Semin. Thromb. Hemostas., 3(4):291, 1977.
59. Hoyer, L.W. von Willebrand's disease. In Spaet, T.H. (ed.), Progress in Hemostasis and Thrombosis, Vol. 3. New York, Grune & Stratton, 1976, p. 231.
60. Jackson, C.M. and Suttie, J.W. Recent developments in understanding the mechanism of vitamin K and vitamin K antagonist drug action and the consequences of vitamin K action in blood coagulation. In Brown, E.B. (ed.), Progress in Hematology, Vol. 10. New York, Grune & Stratton, 1977, p. 33.
61. Kaplan, A. Initiation of the intrinsic coagulation and fibrinolytic pathways of man: The role of surfaces, Hageman factor, prekallikrein, high molecular weight kininogen, and factor XI. In Spaet, T.H. (ed.), Progess in Hemostasis and Thrombosis, Vol. 4. New York, Grune & Stratton, 1978, p. 127.
62. Mammen, E.F. (ed.) Immunoantibodies in blood coagulation. Semin. Thromb. Hemostas. 1(4):184, 1975.
63. McKusick, V.A. Heritable Disorders of Connective Tissue, 4th ed. St. Louis, Mosby, 1972.
64. Miescher, P.A. Drug-induced thrombocytopenia. Semin. Hematol., 10:311, 1973.
65. Mueller-Eckhardt, C. Idiopathic thrombocytopenic purpura (ITP): clinical and immunologic considerations. Semin. Thromb. Hemostas., 3(3):125, 1977.
66. Nurden, A.T. and Caen, J.P. Membrane glycoproteins and human platelet function. Br. J. Haematol., 38:155, 1978.
67. Osler, W. On a family form of recurring epistaxis, associated with multiple telangiectases of the skin and mucous membrane. Bull. Johns Hopkins Hosp., 12:333, 1901.
68. Ratnoff, O.D. and Jones, P.K. The laboratory diagnoses of the carrier state for classic hemophilia. Ann. Intern. Med., 86:521, 1977.
69. Zieve, P.D. and Levin, J. Disorders of Hemostasis. Philadelphia, Saunders, 1976.

Disorders of White Cells

70. Cline, M.J. and Golde, D.W. Cellular interactions in haematopoiesis. Nature, 277:177, 1978.
71. Humbert, J.R. (ed.). Neutrophil physiology and pathology. Semin. Hematol., 12:1, 1975.
72. Metcalf, D. Hematopoietic colonies. In Connors, T.T. and Roberts, J.J. (eds.), Recent Results in Cancer Research, Vol. 61. New York, Springer-Verlag, 1977.
73. Nowell, P.C. and Wilson, D.B. Lymphocytes and hemic stem cells. Am. J. Pathol., 65:641, 1971.
74. Rappaport, H. Tumors of the Hematopoietic System (Atlas of Tumor Pathology, Section 3, Fascicle 8). Washington, D.C., Armed Forces Institute of Pathology, 1966.

The Myeloproliferative Disorders

75. Canellos, G.P. The treatment of chronic granulocytic leukemia. Clin. Haematol., 6:113, 1977.
76. Clarke, W.J., Howard, E.B., and Hackett, P.L. (eds.). Myeloproliferative Disorders of Animal and Man. Oak Ridge, Tenn., U.S. Atomic Energy Commission, 1970.
77. Golde, D.W. and Cline, M.J. Pathogenesis of polycythemia vera—new concepts. Am. J. Hematol., 1:1149, 1976.

78. Landaw, S.A. Acute leukemia in polycythemia vera. Semin. Hematol., 13:33, 1976.
79. Miescher, P.A. and Farquet, J.J. Chronic myelomonocytic leukemia in adults. Semin. Hematol., 11:129, 1974.
80. Stryckmans, P.A. Current concepts in chronic myelogenous leukemia. Semin. Hematol., 11:101, 1974.

The Lymphoreticular Proliferative Disorders

81. Aisenberg, A.C. Current concepts in cancer: the staging and treatment of Hodgkin's disease. N. Engl. J. Med., 299:1228, 1978.
82. Berard, C. Clincial relevance of the histopathological subclassification of diffuse histiocytic lymphoma. N. Engl. J. Med., 299(25):1382, 1978.
83. DeVita, V.T. and Arsenan, J.C. Intensive chemotherapy for Hodgkin's disease—long term complications. Natl. Cancer Inst. Monogr., 36:447, 1973.
84. Dorfman, R.F. Pathology of the non-Hodgkin's lymphomas: new classifications. Cancer Treat. Rep., 61:45, 1977.
85. Dorfman, R.F. and Warnke, R. Lymphadenopathy simulating the malignant lymphomas. Hum. Pathol., 5:519, 1974.
86. Jones, S.E., Fuks, Z., et al. Non-Hodgkin's lymphomas. IV. Clinicopathologic correlation in 405 cases. Cancer, 31:806, 1973.
87. Kaplan, H.S. Hodgkin's Disease. Cambridge, Mass., Harvard University, 1972.
88. Lukes, R.J. and Collins, R.D. Lukes-Collins classification and its significance. Cancer Treat. Rep., 61:971, 1977.
89. Murphy, S. and Hersh, E. Immunotherapy of leukemia and lymphoma. Semin. Hematol., 15:181, 1978.
90. Niederman, J.C., Evans, A.S. Prevalence, incidence and persistence of EB virus antibody in young adults. N. Engl. J. Med., 283:361, 1970.
91. Rosenberg, S.A. The management of Hodgkin's disease. N. Engl. J. Med., 299:1246, 1978.
92. Rosenberg, S.A. Validity of the Ann Arbor staging classification for non-Hodgkin's lymphomas. Cancer Treat. Rep., 61:1023, 1977.
93. Rosenberg, S.A. and Kaplan, H.S. The management of stages I, II, and III Hodgkin's disease with combined radiotherapy and chemotherapy. Cancer, 35:55, 1975.
94. Roubinian, J.R. and Talal, N. Neoplasia, autoimmunity and the immune response. Adv. Intern. Med., 23:435, 1978.

95. Weissman, I.L., Warnke, R., et al. The lymphoid system: its normal architecture and the potential for understanding the system through the study of lymphoproliferative diseases. Hum. Pathol., 9:25, 1978.

Blood Transfusion

96. Alavi, J.B., Root, R.K, Djerassi, I., Evans, A.E., Gluckman, S.J., MacGregor, R.R., Guerry, D., Schreiber, A.D., Shaw, J.M., Koch, P., and Cooper R.A. A randomized clinical trial of granulocyte tranfusions for infection in acute leukemia. N. Engl. J. Med., 196:706, 1977.
97. Conrad, M.E., Knodell, R.G., Bradley, E.L., Flannery, E.P., and Ginsberg, A.L. Risk factors in non-A, non-B posttransfusion hepatitis. Transfusion, 17(6):579, 1977.
98. Duqesnoy, R.J., Filip, D.J., Rodey, G., and, Aster, R.H. Transfusion therapy of refractory thrombocytopenic patients with platelets from donors selectively mismatched for cross-reactive HLA antigens. Transplant Proc., 9:221, 1977.
99. Greenwalt, T.J. and Perry, S. Preservation and utlilization of the components of human blood. In Brown, E.B. and Moore, C.V. (eds.), Progress in Hematology, Vol. 6. New York, Grune & Stratton, 1969.
100. Grumet, F.C. and Yankee, R.A. Long-term platelet support to patients with aplastic anemia. Effects of splenectomy and steroid therapy. Ann. Intern. Med., 73:1, 1970.
101. Levine, A.S., Schimpff, S.C., Graw, R.G., Jr., et al. Hematologic malignancies and other marrow failure states: progress in the management of complicating infections. Semin. Hematol., 11:141, 1974.
102. Lowenthal, R.M., Goldman, J.M, Buskard, N.A., Murphy, B.C., Grossman, L., Storring, R.A., Park, D.S., Spiers, A.S.D., and Galton, D.A.G. Granulocyte transfusions in treatment of infections in patients with acute leukemia and aplastic anemia. Lancet, 1:353, 1975.
103. Mollison, P.L. Blood Transfusion in Clinical Medicine, 5th ed. Oxford, Blackwell, 1972.
104. Schiffer, C.J. (ed.). Platelet Physiology and Transfusion—A Technical Workshop. American Association of Blood Banks, 1978.
105. Yankee, R.A., Grumet, F.C., and Rogentine, G.N.: Platelet transfusion therapy. The selection of compatible platelet donors for refractory patients by lymphocyte HLA typing. N. Engl. J. Med., 281:1208, 1969.
106. Zmijewski, C.M. Immunohematology, 2nd. ed. New York, Appleton-Century-Crofts, 1972.

SECTION EIGHT
Neoplastic Diseases

ALBERT H. OWENS, Jr.: SECTION EDITOR

Neoplastic disorders are the second most common cause of death in the United States. Their frequency and the variety of their clinical manifestations have resulted in a voluminous descriptive literature. Extensive studies detail the morbid anatomy of neoplasia. A less extensive knowledge exists about the causative agencies involved. Current clinical investigation is increasingly concerned with the physiologic and biochemical abnormalities associated with tumors as well as with the proper evaluation of therapeutic results.

The physician who must base his therapeutic and preventive practices on existing knowledge is faced with a bewildering array of reported facts. The following chapters are designed to orient the student to the major concepts concerning human neoplasia and to direct him to the relevant literature.

Chapter 53 considers the salient features of the biology of human tumors—causal factors, modes of clinical presentation, and expected course and survival. These features are introduced as the physician most commonly encounters them, and then their pathogenesis is explained.

Chapter 54 deals with the principles underlying the management of patients with neoplastic disorders. A general scheme of systematic patient evaluation is suggested, and the utility and limitations of presently available therapeutic modalities are discussed. Particular attention is paid to the biologic effects of irradiation and systematic therapy, as well as to their specific indications and therapeutic results, in order to provide a logical approach to management.

In Chapter 55 the leukemias and bronchogenic and breast cancer are discussed to illustrate the several biologic and therapeutic principles previously presented.

CHAPTER 53
Biology of Human Neoplasia
ALBERT H. OWENS, Jr.

Neoplastic diseases are ubiquitous and protean in their manifestations. They are properly considered in virtually every differential diagnosis. Their prompt identification and rational treatment are derived from our current understanding of the circumstances of their origins, their anatomic extents, the associated physiologic abnormalities, and their expected clinical courses.

Fundamentally, neoplastic diseases are defined by their biologic characteristics. In general, a neoplastic disease consists of an altered cell population that has become unresponsive to normal controls and to the organizing influences of adjacent tissues. Relatively unrestrained cell proliferation and growth are common to all neoplasms. In contrast to benign tumors, malignant neoplasms exhibit the additional general properties of local tissue invasion and metastatic spread to distant anatomic sites.[2,6,10,29]

Experience in correlating the microscopic examination of tissue with the nature of clinical disease has allowed the identification of certain histologic abnormalities as being predictive of neoplastic biologic behavior. Among these histologic abnormalities are a high frequency of mitotic figures, derangements of nuclei and nucleoli, an alteration of normal tissue architecture, and evidence of the invasion of adjacent structures or distant metastatic spread. Cytogenetic studies of tumor cells have revealed various abnormalities of chromosome number and appearance, although none universally characteristic of the neoplastic state. However, the foreshortened (Philadelphia) chromosome 22 has been related closely to chronic granulocytic leukemia.

Histologic examination of tissue specimens or exfoliated cell preparations is the main clinical diagnostic method. Characteristic histologic aberrations predict neoplastic diseases with a high degree of accuracy. Hence, common clinical parlance includes the phrase "proved by biopsy." However, this predictive relationship is not infallible. Both types of interpretive errors occur. For example, lymph node abnormalities associated with insect bites, diphenylhydantoin administration, or systemic lupus erythematosus may be mistaken for malignant lymphoma. Conversely, the microscopic appearance of follicular carcinoma of the thyroid or chondrosarcoma may not reflect the malignant nature of these diseases.[1-3]

Great diversity exists among the biochemical characteristics of tumor cells and much of it correlates with growth processes. To date no single alteration has been defined which is responsible for all types of neoplastic transformation. Changes in chromosomal DNA may result in oncogenesis, but it is not clear that this is a necessary requisite in all cases. Activation of latent genes or suppression of others may occur by processes analogous to those of normal cell differentiation. Further, occasional observations suggest that the transformation of a normal cell to a cancerous one can be reversed to some extent, but the control mechanisms involved are largely unknown. Changes in the chemical architecture of the surface membrane of malignant cells are associated with their loss of contact inhibition and intercellular adhesiveness. For example, in contrast to their normal counterparts, the surfaces of malignant cells contain N-acetylglucosamine moieties which react with a glycoprotein (phytoagglutinin) obtained from wheat germ lipase causing them to clump. Cancer cells also elaborate distinctive substances which may aid in their clinical recognition. These include the "carcinoembryonic antigen" present in the blood of patients with gastrointestinal cancers, α-fetoprotein associated with hepatoma and embryonal cancers, and "gamma-protein" encountered in several tumor types, as well as a wide range of physiologically active polypeptides. The synthesis of these materials, which often occurs normally during fetal development, may well relate to derepression of gene function during oncogenesis. Knowledge in this area is rapidly expanding.[11,22,23]

CLINICALLY APPARENT CAUSAL FACTORS

Epidemiologic studies have identified environmental hazards, social practices, and heritable factors that seem responsible for variations in the incidence and clinical course of several cancers. These interrelationships are quite complex, and the discovery of the precise etiologic agents responsible for most cancers is thwarted further by the prolonged period of oncogenesis. However, certain environmental factors and host (patient) characteristics are of proven practical clinical utility.[12,17,20,26]

Heritable Human Neoplasms[14,25]

The increased incidence of neoplastic diseases within certain families has been noted frequently. However, a clearly defined pattern of inheritance has been established only rarely, and it is often difficult to assess the importance of environmental factors. Retinoblastoma, lipomatosis, colonic polyposis, and so on (Table 53–1) may present in families with a pattern of dominant inheritance. In some families the association of pheochromocytoma and medullary (amyloid-producing) carcinoma of the thyroid, cerebellocortical hemangioblastoma, or neurofibromatosis seems to be inherited as a dominant trait. More recently two other groups of tumors have been shown to follow a dominant inheritance pattern in some cases: polyendocrine adenomas (pituitary, parathyroid, pancreas) including the Zollinger-Ellison syndrome and hereditary adenocarcinomatosis (adenocarcinomas of the colon, stomach, uterus, and ovary occurring in different members of the same family). In contrast, there are several relatively rare heritable nonneoplastic disorders and hamartomatous abnormalities that have been associated with malignant tumors with great frequency (Table 53–2). For the most part, the chromosomal abnormalities and the immunodeficiency disorders are transmitted as autosomal recessive characteristics as are albinism and xeroderma pigmentosa.

The association of leukemia with abnormalities of chromosome 21 is of interest. The inheritance of mongolism and trisomy of chromosome 21 is well established, as is the increased incidence of acute granulocytic leukemia in this setting. The inheritance of a chromosome 21 from which a portion of the short arm has been deleted or translocated has been shown and cited as predisposing to the development of chronic lymphocytic leukemia. Bloom syndrome and Fanconi's anemia are heritable disorders with marked chromosomal abnormalities in which there is a high incidence of acute leukemia.

The relative incidence of various neoplastic diseases with respect to age, sex, and other constitutional factors indicates that several additional host determinants exist. Acute (lymphocytic) leukemia is essentially a disease of childhood. Malignant melanoma is essentially a postpubertal phenomenon. Testicular tumors and Hodgkin's disease are most frequently diseases of young adults. Breast cancer is far

TABLE 53-1
Heritable Neoplasms

Neoplasm	Clinical Manifestations
Skin and subcutaneous tissue	
Nevoid basal cell cancers	Dominant inheritance. Onset from childhood to middle age. Associated with multiple anomalies of skin, connective tissue and skeleton
Trichoepithelioma	Dominant inheritance. Onset usually at puberty. Basal cell cancers may be associated
Lipomatosis	Dominant inheritance. Sarcomatous change occurs rarely
Gastrointestinal tract colonic polyposis	Dominant inheritance. Malignant potential high
Nervous system retinoblastoma	Dominant inheritance; incomplete penetrance. Familial history in 5-10% of cases; bilateral tumors more likely than in sporadic cases
Chemodectoma	Dominant inheritance. Carotid-body tumors may be bilateral; may secrete catecholamines
Endocrine Medullary thyroid cancer	May be associated with pheochromocytoma, neurofibromatosis, mucosal neuromas, parathyroid hyperplasia and neoplasia. May secrete calcitonin, histaminase, catecholamines
Multiple endocrine adenomas	Onset in third to fifth decades. Associated adenomas of pituitary, parathyroid, and pancreatic islet cells. Various hormones secreted

TABLE 53-2
Heritable Disorders and Neoplasia

Non-neoplastic Disorder	Neoplasm
Chromosomal abnormalities	
Mongolism (Trisomy-21)	Acute leukemia (granulocytic)
Bloom syndrome	Acute leukemia
Fanconi's anemia	Acute leukemia (monocytic)
Immunodeficiencies	
Ataxia telangiectasia, Wiskott-Aldrich Bruton (X-linked) Late-onset deficiencies Chediak-Higashi (lysosomal)	Lymphoreticular neoplasia, possibly other tumor types
Skin and subcutaneous tissue abnormalities	
Albinism (pigmentation)	Squamous skin cancer
Xeroderma pigmentosa (DNA repair)	Squamous and basal cell skin cancers
Dyskeratosis congenita	Squamous cancer of skin and mucous membranes
Tylosis	Esophageal cancer
Café-au-lait pigmentation	Neurofibromatosis and related tumors Sarcomas occur in 10% of cases
Mucocutaneous pigmentation (Peutz-Jegher)	Intestinal polyposis (hamartomas); malignant potential low
Hamartoma syndromes	
Retinal angiomas (von Hippel-Lindau)	Multiple angiomas of cerebellum
Tuberous sclerosis	Multiple cerebral gliomas
Multiple exostoses	Chondrosarcomas develop, 5-10% of cases

Acquired Antecedent Disorders[1,7,8]

Acquired non-neoplastic clinical disorders have been associated with an increased incidence of malignant tumors. Several of these antecedent diseases are listed in Table 53-3. In general, these neoplasms have arisen from tissues undergoing prolonged regenerative activity. Perhaps the increased rate and extent of cellular proliferation enhances the development of true neoplasia. In any event, it is important that a physician observing patients with these non-neoplastic disorders be aware of their association with true neoplastic states. In some instances immediate therapy is indicated, and in others careful serial observation is required to detect evolving tumors before they become extensive.

There are additional disorders to be considered in this category because they too are significant with respect to the development of malignant neoplasms.

more common in women than in men, and its frequency declines noticeably after the menopause. In both sexes the incidence of the chronic leukemias, myeloma, and the common cancers has been observed to increase progressively with advancing age.

TABLE 53-3
Acquired Clinical Disorders and
Related Neoplasms

Acquired Disorder	Neoplasm
Skin and mucous membranes	
Actinic dermatitis, keratoses	Squamous cancer of skin
Thermal burns	Chronic sunlight (ultraviolet) exposure of farmers, sailors, etc.
Leukoplakia	Squamous cancer of mouth, vagina, bladder
	Leukoplakia is a term often loosely defined
Paget's disease of nipple	Adenocarcinoma of breast
	Associated intraductal cancer defines therapy of Paget's lesions
Bowen's disease	Cutaneous carcinoma-in-situ sometimes associated with arsenic ingestion or ionizing irradiation. Often associated with respiratory, gastrointestinal, or genitourinary cancers.
Hematopoietic tissue	
Aplastic anemia	Acute leukemia
Paroxysmal nocturnal hemoglobinuria	Acute leukemia
Gastrointestinal tract	
Sideropenic dysphagia	Squamous cancer of oropharynx and proximal esophagus (Plummer-Vinson, Patterson-Brown-Kelly syndrome)
Cirrhosis of liver	Hepatic cell adenocarcinoma with postnecrotic and alcoholic cirrhosis
	Deficient diet (protein), parasitism related in some geographic areas
Chronic ulcerative colitis	Adenocarcinoma of colon, multiple sites, developing in relation to pseudopolyp formation
Genital tract	
Chronic cervicitis	Squamous cancer of cervix, especially with multiparity, lower socioeconomic status
	Rare in Jews
Chronic balanitis	Squamous cancer of penis
	Rare in men with neonatal circumcision
Skeletal system	
Paget's disease of bone	Osteogenic sarcoma

For example, Bowen's disease of the skin, regarded as a low-grade neoplasm by some, tends to evolve into a squamous cancer. In many cases, Bowen's disease is also associated with cancers of the respiratory, gastrointestinal, or genitourinary tract.

Nonfamilial polyps (benign neoplasms) developing in the intestinal tract are regarded by many as "premalignant lesions." Colonic polyps are observed more frequently in older age groups, but there is a difference of opinion regarding the tendency of various types of polyps to develop into carcinoma. Their malignant potential is lower than that of the various familial polyposes. Similarly, chondromas of bone will occasionally develop into sacromas.

Our knowledge of clinical disorders currently recognized as "premalignant" is largely limited to those occurring in sites accessible to serial examination. Pathologic studies strongly suggest the lesions with similar clinical significance also exist in more inaccessible sites. For example, squamous metaplasia of the bronchial epithelium has been correlated with an increased incidence of squamous cancer.

Environmental Carcinogens [12,17,19,20,25]

Specific etiologic agents have been identified and associated with several clinical neoplastic diseases. These external environmental factors are primarily chemical or involve ionizing or ultraviolet radiation. Table 53–4 lists the more common carcinogens and relates them to the resulting neoplasms. Comments concerning the populations usually at risk (by occupation), the nature of the exposure, and other clinical evidences of such contact are also included. In each instance, the chemical compound (or mixtures) or physical energy has been shown to be carcinogenic in laboratory animals. Studies of atom bomb survivors have also clearly shown an increased incidence of acute and chronic granulocytic leukemia as well as myelofibrosis with myeloid metaplasia. Further, fetal x-radiation markedly increases the risk of dying from a malignant disease before 10 years of age.

In general, occupational cancers appear at the site of the most intense and prolonged exposure to the carcinogen. These sites, of course, vary with the type of exposure and the physiologic disposition of the carcinogens that are taken into the body. Usually there is a relatively long latent period (years) before the clinical emergence of the neoplasm. The characteristics of these tumors and their subsequent courses appear to differ little from their spontaneous counterparts.

Several epidemiologic surveys have linked cigarette smoking to an increased incidence of cancer, cardiovascular disease, chronic bronchitis, and pulmonary emphysema. Cigarette smokers have a sub-

TABLE 53-4

Etiologic Agents in Human Neoplasms—Environmental Carcinogens

Causal Factor	Neoplasm	Evidence of Exposure	Occupation and Type of Exposure
Chemical Agents			
Aromatic amines, especially β-naphthyl-amine	Papilloma and cancer of bladder, urinary tract	Compounds in urine	Cutaneous, respiratory exposure; chemical workers producing dye stuffs, rodenticides, laboratory reagents
Benzol	Leukemia, lymphoma	Anemia, bone marrow aplasia	Cutaneous, respiratory exposure; coal tar refiners, solvent manufacturers, painters, printers, mechanics using solvents
Coal tar, pitch, creosote, anthracene	Cancer of skin, larynx, bronchus	Chronic dermatitis, warts, photosensitivity of hands, face, exposed areas	Cutaneous, respiratory exposure; coke oven workers, coal tar distillers, lumber industry, chemical workers
Petroleum, shale and paraffin oils, waxes, tars	Cancer of skin	Chronic dermatitis, wax boils, warts in exposed areas	Cutaneous exposure; workers in oil refineries, wax and asphalt producers, mechanics
Isopropyl oil	Cancer of sinus, larynx, bronchus		Respiratory exposure; producers of isopropyl alcohol
Asbestos	Cancer of bronchus, mesothelioma	Pulmonary asbestosis, asbestos bodies in sputum, asbestos warts on fingers	Respiratory exposure generally, >2 years; asbestos miners, shippers, millers, pipe fitters, others Generalized pulmonary fibrosis (asbestosis) present
Chromium	Cancer of bronchus	Chronic dermatitis, chrome holes in skin, perforated nasal system	Respiratory (and cutaneous) exposure; workers engaged in chromate ore reduction
Nickel	Cancer of nasal cavity, sinus, bronchus	Nasal polyps, chronic bronchitis, dermatitis	Respiratory exposure; nickel miners, shippers, and refiners Nickel carbonyl responsible agent (?)
Arsenic	Cancer of skin, bronchus, bladder	Keratoses (especially palms and soles)	Smelters, pesticide manufacturers
Vinyl chloride	Hemangiosarcoma of liver		Chemical workers
Physical Agents			
Ionizing radiation	Cancer of skin, thyroid, tongue, tonsil, sinus, osteogenic sarcoma, leukemia	Radiation dermatitis	Percutaneous or systemic exposure for therapeutic purposes (e.g., treatment of spondylitis, polycythemia), or by accident (radium-dial workers)
	Cancer of bronchus		Respiratory exposure; pitch-blende miners
Ultraviolet radiation	Cancer of skin	Chronic active dermatitis, hyperkeratosis, exposed areas	Cutaneous exposure; farmers, watermen, other outdoor workers Rarely predisposing factors (e.g., xeroderma pigmentosa)

stantially greater risk than nonsmokers of developing cancer of the bronchus, larynx, oral cavity, esophagus, and urinary bladder. Further, smoking compounds the carcinogenicity of other agents such as asbestos.

Our burgeoning technology is producing potential carcinogens at an ever-increasing rate, and the population is exposed to them through air, water, and food. Mycotoxins from various molds associated with foodstuffs are among the most potent tumor inducers in laboratory animals. The relative cancer-causing risks of artificial sweeteners, other food additives, pesticides, and so on are a matter of great public concern. Physicians must remain alert to the potential long-term effects produced by hormones or other therapeutic agents. The high incidence of uterine cancer in postmenopausal women treated with estrogens and the high incidence of vaginal cancer in children born to mothers who were given stilbestrol during pregnancy are cases in point.

Viruses have been shown to be oncogenic in several animal species. At least 12 strains of human adenoviruses are capable of inducing tumors in newborn laboratory animals or causing neoplastic transformation in cells in vitro. The human wart virus is known to induce papillomas in man. The Epstein-Barr (EBV) virus, the cause of infectious mononucleosis, is linked to the occurrence of Burkitt's tumor in Africa and nasopharyngeal cancer in the Orient. Herpes simplex Type II virus has been associated with cancer of the uterine cervix. RNA viruses (B-type particles) resembling murine mammary tumor agents have been found in cultured cell lines derived from human breast cancers. C-type particles have been found in the blood of patients with acute lymphoblastic leukemia. Further, leukemic cells contain abundant RNA-dependent DNA-polymerase enzyme activity similar to that of oncogenic RNA viruses, and they contain tumorlike RNA as judged by DNA-RNA molecular hybridization studies.[16,26]

A relatively unique experience in acute leukemia patients who have undergone allogeneic bone marrow transplantation also provides a commentary on the possibility of viral etiology. In a few cases, it has been established clearly that the acute leukemia which recurred after successful marrow transplantation emerged in donor type cells (cytogenetic evidence).[52]

Serologic studies have identified tumor-related antigens in patients with osteogenic sarcoma, melanoma, and other soft tissue sarcomas. Similar antibodies have been found in family members. These observations are compatible with a virus or other infectious agent being causative in these tumors and

producing unrecognized infections in normal individuals. However, despite these and the many other provocative findings alluded to previously, no unequivocal evidence of a human cancer virus has been forthcoming.

Cancer Prevention[39]

Recognition of these oncogenic agents is of significance to the clinician in terms of preventive medicine. Identification of industrial hazards has relieved workers of the risks of exposure. More than one study has shown that a reduction in cigarette smoking has resulted in a decline in the incidence of bronchogenic cancer. Some virus-caused cancers might well be prevented by vaccination or other prophylactic measures, but more research is needed to identify the pertinent basic biologic factors.

Tumor Immunity[15,35]

In animal models, tumor specific transplantation antigens have been demonstrated clearly. Distinctive antigenicity has been shown in "spontaneous" tumors and in tumors caused by chemicals, physical agents, or various viruses. The major antigens in chemically induced tumors seem specific for each tumor. Tumors caused by the same DNA virus usually have common neoantigens but lack virion antigens. Tumors caused by the same RNA virus usually share common transplantation-type antigens and virion antigens. Certain tumor-associated antigens seem to be specified by genetic information intrinsic to the host (in contrast to the genetic material added by an oncogenic virus) and they may be expressed normally during an earlier stage of development (fetal or embryonic antigens). It is postulated that these fetal antigens reappear during oncogenesis by means of gene derepression and by mechanisms similar to those leading to ectopic hormone production.

Observations in man suggest that there are analagous tumor-related and fetal antigens associated with a variety of neoplasms. For example, distinctive antigenicity is associated with Burkitt's lymphoma, nasopharyngeal cancer, melanoma, osteogenic sarcoma, several types of soft tissue sarcoma, and neuroblastoma. Fetal antigens have been demonstrated in cancers of the large bowel, pancreas and lung (carcinoembryonic antigen), hepatoma and embryonal carcinoma (α-fetoprotein), and in a wider variety of benign and malignant tumors (γ-fetoprotein). Carcinoembryonic antigen is also present in the blood of pregnant women, heavy smokers, and some patients with hepatic cirrhosis, pulmonary emphysema, and ulcerative colitis.

Studies in animals have defined humoral and cell-mediated immune responses to tumor-related antigens. It has been shown also that sensitized lymphocytes can be prevented from acting against tumor cells by the presence of "blocking or enhancing antibodies." Immunologic responsiveness to tumor antigens may be thwarted by the presence of suppressor T cells, large amounts of tumor (immune paralysis), or tolerance due to the introduction of tumor antigen very early in life (e.g., vertical transmission of murine leukemia or mammary tumor agents). In one experimental system (the induction of squamous cell skin cancers in mice by ultraviolet light), there is a specific nonresponsiveness to the tumor in animals fully capable of expressing a wide range of other immune reactions.

Again, there is evidence for analogous situations in man, but the data are more incomplete. In general, cancer patients with a greater degree of immunoresponsiveness have a better prognosis. It also seems clear that patients are capable of responding to autochthonous tumor antigens and that a reasonable biologic basis exists for useful immunotherapy. "Spontaneous remissions" in human cancer are a rare, but well documented, phenomenon. Immune mechanisms are thought responsible in some cases, but direct and conclusive evidence is lacking.

MODES OF CLINICAL PRESENTATION

The manner in which neoplastic diseases present themselves clinically is varied and inconstant. Whereas categorization and generalization are necessary, oversimplification is unwarranted in that it frequently leads to an undesirable lessening of clinical diagnostic awareness. Our current ability to define, detect, and quantitate the neoplastic state clinically is limited, and the thoughtful clinical observer will often find himself taxed to his capacity.[6-9]

The onset of the neoplastic state is difficult to date in humans. When there has been a known carcinogenic exposure (e.g., atom bomb casualties, thymic irradiation, and chromate exposure), a prolonged latent or induction period is likely before clinically detectable disease evolves.

IN SITU LESIONS
Commonly, carcinoma in situ is cited as a premalignant lesion or as the earliest recognizable stage of clinical cancer. Although discussed most often in relation to the uterine cervix, such morphologic abnormalities have been observed at many tissue sites.

However, current knowledge of their biologic cause and consequences is imperfect. It is probable that a significant portion of such noninvasive lesions do not develop into clinical cancer. Frequently, the entire in situ abnormality is removed by the biopsy procedure. In many instances these tissue changes evolve in sites that are inaccessible to serial observation and therapeutic resection. As the diagnostic terminology implies, current therapeutic practice calls for the removal of these in situ lesions where practicable.

QUIESCENT NEOPLASMS
Malignant neoplastic diseases may exist in man for months or years and produce few symptoms. Their presence may be detected by chance during the course of a routine medical survey related to cancer detection or begun for some unrelated purpose. Although every reasonable effort should be made to treat minimal and potentially curable lesions appropriately and to treat progressive neoplasms as effectively as possible, the detection of a malignant disease does not lead to an active therapeutic program in all cases. At autopsy (after death from any cause), cancer of the prostate is found in men with an increasing frequency related to their age, such that 15 percent of men over age 40 will have this pathologic diagnosis. However, only 2 to 3 percent of men will develop clinical illnesses caused by advancing prostate cancer. Similarly, chronic lymphocytic leukemia may exist for long periods with few symptoms. Hence, in the absence of effective curative therapy, treatment is begun for palliative purposes only.[10,13,21,29]

The varied clinical abnormalities produced by advancing neoplastic diseases may be grouped into two categories based on their presumed pathogenesis. These clinical categories are 1) abnormalities that stem directly from the presence of a tumor; and 2) physiologic derangements that are produced indirectly.

MASS LESIONS AND RELATED SYNDROMES
The clinical syndromes commonly associated with progressive nonleukemic neoplasms are related primarily to the growth of tumor masses and the consequent physical alterations produced in adjacent organ systems. The findings include the presence of an obvious tumor mass; the existence of an ulcerative lesion that does not heal satisfactorily; chronic bleeding and the consequences of blood loss; bone destruction and its sequelae; involvement of the central or peripheral nervous system, with attendant seizures, paralysis, and pain; acute or chronic obstruction of a hollow viscus and related findings; obstruction of mediastinal

structures and its sequelae; and involvement of serous surfaces, with the consequent fluid accumulation. These syndromes are, of course, nonspecific and may be produced by noncarcinomatous mass lesions of other etiologies that alter the structure and function of organ systems in a similar manner.[5,7]

A commonly encountered clinical problem derives from the initial presentation of a tumor at a site distant from its origin. The more frequent sites of presentation of metastatic neoplasms are the cervical and supraclavicular lymph nodes, lungs, liver, bones, and brain. These and other sites are listed in Table 53–5, together with the most probable primary source of the tumor.[10,13]

PHYSIOLOGIC ABNORMALITIES

The study of human neoplastic diseases has been concerned largely with cell morphology, tissues of origin, tendency to metastasize, and attempts to eradicate or control the growth of the neoplasms by surgery, radi-

ation, and chemotherapy. Recently there has been an increased appreciation of the many physiologic functional abnormalities that are associated with neoplastic diseases but that are not primarily related to the physical consequences of their presence. Indeed, these functional derangements may constitute the presenting symptom complex which confronts the physician. They may determine the nature of the patient's morbidity and shape the design of his therapeutic program.[24]

Tumors may arise in organs that normally produce physiologically active substances, such as hormones. When such tumors produce excessive amounts of these substances unmodified by normal feedback control mechanisms, characteristic clinical illnesses ensue. Such are the consequences of functional adenomas of the pituitary, parathyroid, thyroid, islet cells of the pancreas, and adrenal cortex and medulla.

More commonly, tumors arise from organs that

TABLE 53–5
Common Sites of Clinical Presentation of Obscure Primary Tumors

Site	Primary Tumor	Commentary
Skin and subcutaneous tissue	Melanoma, breast, bronchus, stomach, kidney	Lesions are generally infiltrative and widespread. Stomach, colon, and ovarian cancers may present with metastatic masses in the umbilical area
Cervical lymph nodes	Nasopharynx, pharynx, oral cavity, thyroid	More distant metastases rarely seen except when progression of local disease has been curbed
Supraclavicular lymph nodes	Bronchus, breast, stomach, esophagus, pancreas, colon, testis, ovary, uterine cervix	Nonpalpable scalene lymph nodes infrequently yield the diagnosis of metastatic cancer
Inguinal lymph nodes	Genitalia, rectum	Inflammatory disease frequently encountered
Lung	Breast, colon, kidney, testis, stomach, melanoma, thyroid	Radiographic patterns may vary from a solitary lesion (rare), multiple nodules (most common) to that of lymphangitic or hematogenous spread
Liver	Colon, breast, bronchus, stomach, pancreas	Hepatomegaly, usually without hepatic insufficiency. Metastases commonly cause disproportionate elevation of alkaline phosphatase (hepatic isozyme)
Ovary	Colon, stomach	Metastases to the ovary (Krukenberg tumors) may exceed the size of the primary by several-fold
Bones	Breast, bronchus, kidney, prostate, thyroid	Marrow bearing bones involved most frequently. Lesions usually lytic; at times sclerotic
Central nervous system	Bronchus, breast, colon, kidney	Metastases usually multiple (70% of cases)
Serous cavities	Bronchus, breast, ovary, lymphoma	Cytologic studies to be interpreted with caution

do not produce physiologically active substances currently recognized under normal conditions of health. Certain of these tumors appear to elaborate polypeptides with hormonal activity. Bronchogenic neoplasms, for example, may produce an ACTH-like substance that can induce hyperadrenocorticism or a parathormone-like substance that can induce hypercalcemia. Similarly, physiologically active secretions of bronchogenic tumors may be responsible for the inappropriate secretion of antidiuretic hormone, the disproportionate anorexia and wasting, or the hypertrophic pulmonary osteoarthropathy occasionally encountered.[24]

This behavior of tumor cells is also of considerable biologic importance. It seems probable that the unnatural synthesis of physiologically active polypeptides results from a derepression or activation of a latent DNA coding function. Perhaps this further uncovering of genome is not a completely random event occurring during oncogenesis. Some morphologic tumor types seem more commonly associated with aberrant hormone production than others.[22,23]

Ectopic-hormone-producing tumors may be classified into two groups according to their embryologic origin, morphologic features, histochemical properties, and the types of hormones they secrete. One group of tumors arise from neural crest cells which migrated to the foregut and the branchial arches— small cell lung cancer, medullary cancer of the thyroid, thymoma, pancreatic islet cell tumors, carcinoid tumors. These tumor cells contain large neurosecretory granules, contain biologically active aromatic amines, and similar enzymatic activities (Pearse's APUD cells). They may secrete calcitonin, ACTH, MSH, vasopressin, insulin, gastrin, secretin, glucagon, serotonin, histamine, and other biogenic amines.[45] The second group of tumors are endodermal or mesodermal in origin—cancers of the bronchus, gastrointestinal tract and kidney, sarcomas of connective tissue and blood vessels, lymphoreticular neoplasms, non-germ-cell gonadal tumors, and adrenal cortical tumors. They may secrete parathormone, erythropoietin, gonadotrophins, prolactin, growth hormone, renin or thyrotrophin.

PARANEOPLASTIC SYNDROMES

The characteristics of the more commonly encountered physiologic derangements associated with neoplastic diseases are presented in Tables 53-6 to 53-13. These abnormalities are listed in relation to the organ systems which they primarily affect and the neoplasms with which they are associated most com-

monly. Some of these derangements may be visualized as consequent to the elaboration of excessive amounts of normal cell products, others as being caused by deficiencies. However, the pathogenesis of many of them remains ill-defined.

Skin and Mucous Membranes

The skin and mucous membranes react in various ways to the presence of a neoplasm, as is shown in Table 53-6. In a strict sense, the mucous membrane pigmentation described by Peutz and Jeghers is not caused by the presence of intestinal polyposis but, rather, represents a closely associated heritable abnormality. The pathogenesis of the acquired hyperpigmentation characteristic of acanthosis nigricans is unknown. Similarly, the generalized pruritus seen most commonly with Hodgkin's disease remains an enigma. The *Herpes zoster* infections in patients with Hodgkin's disease are probably related to deficiencies in immune responsiveness, especially since the process frequently becomes disseminated, the generalized cutaneous lesions being clinically similar to those of varicella.

Several of these clinical manifestations are related to disturbances of the cutaneous circulation. Carcinoid tumors are believed to contain an enzyme which activates a bradykinin-like polypeptide responsible for the vasodilatation and flush observed in patients having such tumors. This physiologically active polypeptide may also be responsible for the associated asthma (bronchoconstriction). After a protracted period, a thickened, violaceous change develops in the skin and over the face, neck, and upper anterior thorax of many of these patients. Over similar periods of time, clinical evidences of pulmonary hypertension and tricuspid valve deformity may evolve.

Systemic mast cell disease is characterized primarily by the presence of urticaria pigmentosa, diarrhea, hepatosplenomegaly, and sclerotic bone lesions. Abnormal proliferation of mast cells is noted in several tissues, particularly the bone marrow. These cells are responsible for the excessive production of histamine that causes at least part of the symptomatology.

The pathogenesis of Raynaud's phenomenon associated with neoplastic diseases is not known in every instance. At times the presence of cryoglobulins is responsible. Purpura may be associated with macroglobulinemia and the resultant increased serum viscosity. More commonly, it is associated with thrombocytopenia. The latter may be related to the underlying neoplasm (generally of the hematopoietic tissue) or may result from the bone-marrow-suppressant effects of chemotherapeutic agents or ionizing radiation. Care should be taken not to overlook the

---

TABLE 53–6

Physiologic Abnormalities Due to Neoplasia: Skin and Mucous Membranes

Manifestations	Mechanism	Neoplasm
Pigmentation Abnormalities		
Acanthosis nigricans		Carcinomas of gastrointestinal tract; other viscera
Diffuse hyperpigmentation	ACTH-MSH secretion	Small cell cancers of lung, thymoma, carcinoid, islet cell cancer of the pancreas
Mucocutaneous pigmentation (Peutz-Jeghers)	Autosomal dominant inheritance	Intestinal polyps (malignant potential low)
Café-au-lait pigmentation	Autosomal dominant inheritance	Neurofibromatosis
Xeroderma pigmentosa	Autosomal recessive inheritance	Squamous cancer of skin
Erythemas and Vascular Abnormalities		
Erythroderma and exfoliative dermatitis		Lymphoma, leukemia; many tumor types
Flushing, vasodilatation violaceous	Bradykinin-like polypeptide secretion	Carcinoid tumors
Superficial thrombophlebitis		Cancers of pancreas, bronchus, stomach, and other sites
Urticaria		
Urticaria pigmentosa,	Histamine secretion	Mast cell tumor
Urticaria, transient		Several tumor types
Bullous Lesions		
Erythema multiforme		Leukemia, lymphoma, other tumors
Pemphigoid		Melanoma, cancers of bronchus, stomach, other sites
Purpura and Ecchymoses	Thrombocytopenia, macroglobulinemia, cryoglobulinemia, intravascular coagulation, fibrinolysin secretion	Leukemia, lymphoma, myeloma, other tumor types
Pruritis	May be associated with urticaria, erythema	Hodgkin's disease, polycythemia vera
Benign Tumors		
Dermal inclusion cysts (Gardner)	Autosomal dominant inheritance	Colonic polyposis and brain tumors
Mucosal neuromas	Autosomal dominant inheritance pheochromocytoma	Medullary cancer of thyroid
Dyskeratosis congenita		Cancer of esophagus
Varied Pathogenesis		
Pyoderma (various microorganisms)	Depressed granulocyte function; impaired immunity	Leukemia, lymphoma, myeloma
Virus infections, often disseminated (*Herpes zoster*)	Impaired immunity	Hodgkin's disease
Dermatomyositis	Cancer-associated in 5–50% of cases > age 40.	Several tumor types
Lichen sclerosis et atrophicans		Several tumor types
Paget's disease of the nipple		Intraductal breast cancer
Hypertrichosis	Viralizing hormones, ectopic ACTH, gonadotrophin	Ovarian and adrenal tumors; lung cancer and other types

possibility that purpuric lesions are manifestations of a coexistent bacteremia.

The erythema multiforme, exfoliative dermatitis, bullous pemphigoid lesions, and dermatomyositis seen with leukemia, lymphoma, and a wide variety of cancers are spoken of as "allergic manifestations" of the underlying neoplasm or hypersensitivity states that somehow derive from the presence of the tumor. Erythema multiforme has been described, on occasion, in association with surgical manipulation of the tumor mass or with radiotherapeutic treatment. Bullous skin lesions, exfoliative dermatitis, and, probably, dermatomyositis are of diverse etiologies, but the clinician should be aware of the possible presence of an associated neoplastic disease.

Hematopoietic System[3,9]

The most commonly encountered hematologic abnormalities are presented in Table 53–7.

Polycythemia, induced by erythropoietin, is a rare manifestation of neoplastic disease that has been reported in association with hypernephromas, hepatomas, benign uterine myomas, and vascular cerebellar tumors, as well as with renal cysts. On occasion a patient's rubor and suffused conjunctivas and mucous membranes, considered together with his elevated hematocrit, and with what is taken as his palpable spleen, have led to an incorrect diagnosis of polycythemia vera, the renal tumor palpable in the left upper quadrant being mistaken for an enlarged spleen.

Anemia is one of the more frequent accompaniments of neoplastic disease. Commonly, it results from prolonged blood loss, especially from the gastrointestinal tract, which results in iron deficiency. This chronic bleeding represents a direct conse-

---

TABLE 53–7

Physiologic Abnormalities Due to Neoplasia: Hematopoietic System

Manifestation	Mechanism	Neoplasm
Abnormal Red Cell Mass		
Erythrocytosis	Erythropoietin secretion	Renal cancer, hepatoma uterine myoma, cerebellar hemangioma
Anemia Normochromic	Erythrocyte destruction by antibody	Leukemia, lymphoma, ovarian cancer
	Erythrocyte distortion and destruction due to mechanical forces (microangiopathic hemolytic anemia)	Cancers of the stomach, prostate, breast, lung, pancreas, colon
	Deficient erythrocyte production ("pure red cell aplasia") possibly caused by suppressor lymphocytes	Thymoma, chronic lymphocytic leukemia
	Decreased production and survival of erythrocytes ("anemia of cancer")	Many tumor types
Hypochromic	Blood loss, sometimes occult (gastrointestinal tract)	Tumors of GI and GU tracts, and head and neck
Abnormal Circulating White Cell Mass		
Leukemoid reactions	Marrow invasion by tumor (Granulopoietin secretion?)	Many tumor types
Leukopenia	Decreased production (marrow invasion); decreased survival (sepsis, antibody)	Leukemia, lymphoma, other tumors
Abnormal granulocyte function	Impaired chemotaxis, phagocytosis, or digestion	Acute leukemia, rarely other tumors
Abnormal Circulating Platelet Mass		
Thrombocytosis (often bizarre forms)	Marrow invasion by tumor (thrombopoietin secretion?)	Myeloproliferative disorders, lymphoma, bronchogenic cancer, other types
Thrombocytopenia	Decreased production (marrow invasion); decreased survival (sepsis, antibody)	Hematopoietic tumors, also other types
Abnormalities of Bleeding and Clotting		
Prolonged bleeding	Various clotting factor deficiencies (liver failure)	Many tumor types
	Fibrinolysin secretion	Prostate cancer
	Circulating anticoagulants (antibodies)	Plasma cell dyscrasias
Intravascular coagulation	Tumor produced "thromboplastin"	Many tumor types

quence of erosion of the tumor surface. At times a normochromic anemia results from an increased rate of erythrocyte destruction with or without demonstrable erythrocyte autoantibodies and with or without demonstrable increased splenic sequestration of red cells. In contrast to normal individuals, those with disseminated neoplasia often are unable to compensate for this increased red blood cell destruction; their maximal erythropoietic response is a fraction of that normally expected.

A depression of all formed elements of the peripheral blood is often seen in patients with disseminated neoplastic disease, particularly those with tumors of hematopoietic tissues. The older concepts of myelophthisis as a determinant of decreased bone-marrow function are being modified. Massive replacement of marrow by tumor cells is an infrequent occurrence and an insufficient explanation for the majority of the pertinent clinical abnormalities encountered. Several other factors known to depress erythropoiesis are commonly identified in this clinical setting. They include active infection, renal insufficiency, cytotoxic drugs and hormonal agents, and ionizing radiation. An additional factor, ill-understood at present, is the existence of substances produced by the tumor that depress erythropoiesis. For example, this is presumed to explain the erythroid hypoplasia seen on occasion in patients with thymic tumors.

The precise agency responsible for the leukemoid reactions and the thrombocytosis associated with neoplastic diseases is unknown. These phenomena are encountered more commonly in tumors that in-volve bone marrow. It is important to remember that leukemoid reactions are of diverse etiologies, some of which merit specific therapy—tuberculosis, for example.

Infections—Host Resistance[30,33]

Clinically significant infections with a variety of microorganisms are common accompaniments of neoplastic diseases, as indicated in Table 53-8. Infectious diseases may cause the presenting manifestations of neoplastic disorders or may complicate their course or treatment. Frequently, it is difficult to distinguish between fever related to the neoplastic process and that stemming from a coexisting infection.

Commonly, the microorganisms responsible for infectious disorders in this setting are indigenous to the patient. These infections are frequently associated with an obstructed hollow viscus, or they may be related to surface ulceration or perforation. For example, pneumonia, lung abscess, cholangitis, or pyelonephritis may result from obstruction of the bronchi or of the biliary or lower urinary tracts by tumor. Similarly, urinary tract infections may be associated with neoplastic erosion of the bladder mucosa, and abdominal abscesses or peritonitis may stem from perforation of the gastrointestinal tract.

Clinically significant characteristics of this type of infectious disease are slow resolution despite adequate antimicrobial therapy and recurrence in the same site. Hence, it is important for the physician encountering these phenomena to suspect the possibility of an underlying neoplasm.

In addition to the local tissue or structural factors

TABLE 53-8

Physiologic Abnormalities Due to Neoplasia: Infections and Host Resistance

Infection	Abnormality	Neoplasm
Localized infections due to a variety of microorganisms	Hollow viscus obstruction, surface erosion, break in physical barriers	Several tumor types
Systemic infections due to variety of microorganisms, especially gram-negative, staphylococcus, rare pathogens, fungi	Impaired granulocyte response (quantitative) and perhaps function (qualitative). Often associated with bleeding into tissues	Leukemia, lymphoma, myeloma, and a variety of tumor types
Bacterial infections especially pneumococcal and other "extracellular" microorganisms	Impaired antibody response, hypogammaglobulinemia	Myeloma, chronic lymphocytic leukemia
Salmonella bacteremia	Uncertain	Lymphoma, gastrointestinal neoplasms
Tuberculosis, fungal, and viral (*H. zoster*) infections, often disseminated	Impaired cell-mediated immune responses	Hodgkin's disease, other tumor types

that predispose patients with neoplasia to infectious diseases, factors of lessened host resistance, not fully characterized, seem operative. For example, pseudomonas bacteremia, an uncommon clinical occurrence is apt to be found in association with neoplastic diseases as well as in other debilitating states. Similarly, staphylococcal bacteremia or postoperative wound infection is commonly encountered in patients with neoplasms.

Hematopoietic or lymphoreticular neoplasms predispose patients to certain recurrent acute infections, indolent infections, or infections caused by uncommon microorganisms. Patients with acute leukemia are prone to develop staphylococcal infections as well as gram-negative bacteremias. Individuals with chronic lymphocytic leukemia and myeloma are subject to recurrent infections of the skin, lung, and urinary tract, caused by a variety of organisms, including the staphylococcus, streptococcus, pneumococcus, and gram-negative bacilli. Pneumococcal meningitis without an associated infection at the portal of entry (e.g., sinus, middle ear, or lung) is particularly likely to occur in association with multiple myeloma. Perirectal abscess is often encountered in patients with monocytic leukemia.

The increased incidence of *Herpes zoster* infections in association with Hodgkin's disease and other lymphomas is well known. This is regarded as an activation of a latent varicella infection by many although many cases occur shortly after exposure to children with chicken pox. Similarly, tuberculosis and infections due to Listeria and fungi are linked to Hodgkin's disease and other hematopoietic neoplasms. In these patients, these infections are often widespread.

Several underlying abnormalities of host defense mechanisms have been identified (Table 53–8). In acute leukemia, deficient granulocyte response to stimulation has been noted in skin window studies. Acquired hypogammaglobulinemia and impaired responsiveness to a primary antigenic stimulus have been described in patients with lymphoid neoplasms. Anergy to tuberculin despite previously established hypersensitivity has been seen to develop in relation to relapsing Hodgkin's disease. Impaired homograft rejection and other evidences of deficient cell-mediated immune responses have been noted in patients with Hodgkin's disease and several disseminated cancers.[38]

Myeloma is usually characterized by the presence of an increased serum concentration of an immunoglobulin of a single molecular species. These patients may be regarded as having a monoclonal gammopathy in that the synthesis of one type of immunoglobulin or immunoglobulin fragment increases to the virtual exclusion of all others. An impairment in normal humoral antibody responses seems to correlate most closely with the increased incidence of bacterial infections seen in these patients.

The increased frequency of infections in patients with neoplastic diseases is due to multiple factors. It seems clear that impairments of granulocyte response and function, humoral antibody responses, and cell-mediated immunity play a role. However, more needs to be learned about the importance of local tissue factors and a variety of circulating factors such as properdin, interferon, and perhaps other important determinants as yet unidentified. In addition, physicians must remain aware of the fact that antitumor treatments (irradiation, cytotoxic drugs, cortisone analogues) affect hematopoiesis, immune responsiveness, and the systemic dissemination of several microorganisms.

Endocrine[4,5,24]

The various endocrine abnormalities attributable to neoplastic diseases may be related to tumors of the endocrine organs or tissues not known to produce hormones normally. An experienced physician, when caring for a patient ill because of hormonal overproduction, will search for an underlying tumor. Also, when caring for a cancer patient, the experienced physician will remain alert to the possible ectopic secretion of hormones.

Benign or malignant tumors of the various endocrine glands at times elaborate physiologically active hormones in supranormal amounts and are unresponsive to the normal feedback control mechanisms. On occasion, further growth and infarction of such a tumor may lead to an abrupt deficiency of the related hormone. Similarly, nonsecretory tumors or metastatic deposits have been responsible for the ablation of various endocrine glands, such as the anterior pituitary ablation caused by an expanding intrasellar chromophobe adenoma or the addisonian syndrome caused by the bilateral replacement of the adrenal cortex with metastatic bronchogenic cancer.

There is a wide variety of paraneoplastic syndromes due to the ectopic secretion of hormonal substances by tumors of nonendocrine tissue (Table 53–9). These hormones may be similar to their "normal" counterparts or they may have a somewhat altered molecular configuration or metabolic effects. However, the ectopic hormone production processes are not responsive to the normal physiologic controls.[24,53]

TABLE 53–9

Physiologic Abnormalities Due to Neoplasia:
Endocrine Syndromes Due to Ectopic Hormone Secretion

Manifestation	Mechanism	Neoplasm
Hyperadrenal corticism	Ectopic ACTH secretion "corticotrophin-releasing factor" secretion	Small cell cancer of the lung, thymoma, carcinoid tumors, cancers of breast, ovary and prostate
Hyperthyroidism	Ectopic "TSH secretion" (may be due to excessive HCG)	Choriocarcinoma, placental tumors, embryonal cancer of testis
Hyperglycemia	Excessive secretion of HGH, catecholamines, glucagon, adrenal steroids estrogens; body wasting	Many tumor types
Hypoglycemia	Ectopic insulin or insulin-like hormone (somatomedin) Impaired glycogenolysis Excess tumor consumption of glucose Under alimentation	Many tumor types
Feminization—sexual precocity	Ectopic gonadotrophin secretion	Teratomas, bronchogenic cancer, esp. giant cell, breast cancer, melanoma
Virilization—sexual precocity	Ectopic gonadotrophin or ACTH secretion	Hepatoblastomia, melanoma, cancers of the lung and breast
Hypertension	Ectopic ACTH secretion Pressor amine secretion Renin secretion	Lung, thymic cancers Neurogenic tumors Renal tumors

Metabolic[24,45,53]

Tumors are known to produce several types of physiologically active substances including hormones, enzymes, immunoglobulins and immunoglobulin fragments, prostaglandins, bioactive aromatic amines, and vasoactive peptides. Since the pathogenesis of many systemic tumor-associated syndromes remains in doubt, it seems likely that additional physiologically active tumor secretions will be identified. For example, humoral substances may be responsible for the tissue wasting, certain hepatic dysfunctions, certain cerebral dysfunctions, hematopoietic disorders, coagulopathies, and neuropathies.

Hypercalcemia is a common cause of morbidity in patients with a wide variety of neoplasia (Table 53–10). The onset of symptoms is usually insidious and may occur shortly after the patient is immobilized for some reason. Somnolence, dementia, constipation, polyuria, and polydypsia are the usual mani-

TABLE 53–10

Physiologic Abnormalities Due to Neoplasia: Metabolic Disturbances

Manifestation	Mechanism	Neoplasm
Hypercalcemia	Ectopic PTH secretion Prostaglandin secretion Osteoclast activating Factor secretion	Cancer of the bronchus, breast, kidney, colon; many tumor types Myeloma, lymphoma
Hypocalcemia	Hypomagnesemia inhibits PTH secretion Hyperphosphatemia due to rapid tumor (DNA) lysis ? Blastic bone metastases ? Excessive calcitonin secretion	Several tumor types Lymphoma, Burkitt's tumor
Osteomalacia with hypophosphatemia	Tumor-derived factor, possibly a vitamin D antagonist	Mesenchymal tumors
Hyperuricemia, gout	Due to rapid tumor cell proliferation and break down	Myeloproliferative disorders, lymphomas

festations. The hypercalcemia and hypercalciuria results from the breakdown of bone. This progressive demineralization may be due to the action of parathyroid-like hormone or tumor-secreted prostaglandins.

Hyponatremia and water retention have been associated with bronchogenic cancer for many years (Table 53–11). Similar phenomena occur in association with chronic pulmonary diseases (tuberculosis, lung abscess); central nervous system trauma (skull fracture, concussion), vascular compromise (hemorrhage and thrombosis), infection (meningitis, syphilis, encephalitis); and a variety of other diseases. Inappropriate vasopressin secretion is responsible for the abnormalities of many of these cases. More recently, it has been appreciated that hyponatremia and volume expansion can result from the action of vincristine, a metabolite of cyclophosphamide and other drugs on the renal tubule.

Metabolic acidosis in cancer patients is usually due to progressive renal insufficiency. However, metabolic acidosis may result from renal tubular dysfunction caused by the excretion of immunoglobulin fragments (e.g., L-chains), or other proteins (e.g., lysozymes) in the urine of patients with leukemia, lymphoma, or myeloma. The pathogenesis of renal tubular defects in other instances is unclear. However, certain anticancer agents can cause similar renal tubular dysfunction, e.g., streptozotocin and isophosphamide.

One form of metabolic acidosis encountered in patients with acute leukemia and lymphoma is due to excessive production of lactate by tumor cells ("lactic acidosis"). Lactic acidosis is seen more often in association with the massive tissue anoxia which accompanies shock and it has been suggested that tissue anoxia caused by leukemia-cell related blood hyperviscosity and sludging is responsible for lactate overproduction in some cases (Table 53–11).

The overproduction of hypoxanthine, xanthine, and uric acid is a consequence of the excessive cellular proliferation and destruction which accompanies a variety of neoplasms. In neoplastic disorders of some chronicity, continued hyperuricemia is associated with gout in some cases (e.g., the myeloproliferative disorders). At times, drug-induced massive tumor lysis results in transient hyperuricemia and uricosuria, especially in patients with leukemia and lymphoma. Indeed, anuria may result from the precipitation of uric acid crystals in the renal tubules. This may be prevented by maintaining an alkaline urine, pH 7 or above, and a daily urine volume in excess of two liters. However, it is more effective to use allopurinol, a xanthine oxidase inhibitor, since it retards the conversion of the more soluble precursors to uric acid.

Transient hyperkalemia is another consequence of massive tumor lysis. At times this has complicated the management of patients with tumors which are very responsive to chemotherapy, e.g., leukemia and lymphoma. Proper anticipation and prompt recognition are keys to successful management with fluids, glucose, and insulin as needed (Chap. 10).

TABLE 53-11

Physiologic Abnormalities Due to Neoplasia: Water and Electrolyte Disturbances

Manifestations	Mechanism	Neoplasm
Hyponatremia (volume expansion)	Ectopic vasopression secretion	Lung cancer, lymphoma, other tumor types
Hypernatremia (volume depletion)	Hypercalciuria, hypokalemia, dysproteinemia (L-chain) or protein fragment effect on renal tubule	Many tumor types Myeloma, lymphoma
Hypokalemia	Ectopic ACTH secretion L-chain nephropathy, lysozymuria (renal tubular damage)	Lung cancer, other tumors myeloma, leukemia
Hyperkalemia	Massive tumor breakdown Lactic acidosis	Leukemia, lymphoma
Metabolic acidosis	Renal tubular defects Lactic acidosis	Hematopoietic tumors
Metabolic alkalosis	Ectopic ACTH secretion	Bronchogenic cancer, other types
Nephrotic syndrome	Amyloidosis Antigen–antibody complexes	Cancers of bronchus, kidney, ovary, lymphoma

Gastrointestinal[4,5]

A syndrome of intractable peptic ulcer, gastric hypersecretion, and diarrhea has been described in association with non-β, islet-cell tumors of the pancreas (Table 53–12). About two-thirds of the tumors are malignant and one-third are benign adenomas. In about 25 percent of cases, the functioning islet-cell tumor occurs in patients with familial polyendocrine adenomas (anterior pituitary, parathyroid, thyroid). A gastrin-like substance secreted by the islet-cell tumor seems responsible for the gastric hypersecretion. In some cases, non-β, islet-cell tumors are associated with a profound watery diarrhea and hypokalemia ("pancreatic cholera"). Achlorhydria is present, also. It has been postulated that these tumors secrete a gastrin-like substance as well as a humoral factor which stimulates the small bowel (vasoactive intestinal peptide).

Connective Tissue[4,5]

The connective tissue disorders occurring in association with neoplastic diseases are presented in Table 53–13. Critical evaluation of these associations is often difficult because of the lack of detailed clinical and pathologic study. Few fundamental observations have been made about their precise pathogenesis, particularly with respect to the articular abnormalities.

Metastatic tumor involvement of muscles, joints, or adjacent connective tissue structures is rare, although involvement of bony structures is common. At times, rheumatic or arthritic complaints are due to these underlying bony lesions and may occur before the bone has been destroyed sufficiently to permit the lesions to be detected by x-ray examination.

During the course of acute leukemia, especially in children, joint symptomatology is encountered frequently. The clinical picture may imitate that of acute rheumatic fever. Rarely, arthralgia has been reported to precede the diagnosis of leukemia by several months. Usually, however, ample evidence of the leukemic process exists in association with the arthropathy. Leukemic infiltration of the synovia and subperiosteal tissue associated with hemorrhage is responsible for the clinical manifestations.

Rheumatoid arthritis, systemic lupus erythematosus, and periarteritis nodosa have been reported in association with lymphoreticular neoplasms. These associations must be accepted cautiously, since the morphologic changes in the lymph nodes of patients with collagen-vascular disorders may mimic those of lymphoma. An unexpectedly frequent association between Sjögren syndrome and histiocytic lymphoma has been reported also.

Arthropathies resembling rheumatoid arthritis have been seen with a variety of tumors, although the pathogenesis is unclear. In a small series of cases, acute arthritis of the small joints of the hands and feet in patients with adenocarcinoma of the pancreas was related to fat necrosis of the synovium or adjacent tissue. In another small series of patients with carcinoma of the prostate and rheumatoid-like arthropathy involving the hands, feet, shoulders, and knees, significant improvement was reported 7 to 12 days after estrogen administration was begun.

Although hypertrophic pulmonary osteoarthropathy may occur in a high proportion of individuals with mesothelioma, it is most commonly encountered clinically in association with bronchogenic carcinoma. Rarely, it is seen with intrathoracic metastatic lesions. The symptomatology derives from the subperiosteal new-bone formation, which occurs more frequently along the tibiae, radii, and phalanges. The ankles, knees, wrists, and fingers are the most commonly symptomatic points. At times the periarticular swelling and the presence of a joint effusion, especially of the knees, may simulate rheumatoid arthritis. In most instances the digits are clubbed. All the factors which cause hypertrophic pulmonary osteoarthropathy are not known, but the inappropriate secretion of

---

TABLE 53–12

Physiologic Abnormalities Due to Neoplasia: Gastrointestinal Disturbances

Manifestation	Mechanism	Neoplasm
Peptic ulcer Gastric, pancreatic hypersecretion	Ectopic gastrin or secretin secretion	Pancreatic islet cell tumors, carcinoids, rarely other types
Diarrhea, abdominal cramps, asthma, flushing (carcinoid syndrome)	Secretion of serotonin, bradykinin-like peptides	Carcinoid tumors
Watery diarrhea syndrome	Secretion of "vasoactive-intestinal-peptide"	Pancreatic tumors, bronchogenic cancer, rarely other tumors

TABLE 53-13
Physiologic Abnormalities Due to Neoplasia: Connective Tissue Disorders

Clinical Manifestations	Neoplasm
Arthropathy Signs, especially in children, imitate rheumatic fever Due to subperiosteal and synovial leukemic infiltrates and hemorrhage	Acute leukemia
Arthropathy similar to rheumatoid arthritis involving small and large joints Special incidence with cancer of prostate and pancreas suggested	Lymphoma, several cancers
Hypertrophic pulmonary osteoarthropathy generally seen with digital clubbing; linked to ectopic HGH secretion Subperiosteal new bone formed, tibiae, radii, phalanges Arthropathy similar to rheumatoid arthritis	Intrathoracic tumors, especially bronchogenic cancer
Amyloidosis Rheumatic complaints frequent Arthropathy of large joints probably due to amyloid deposits in synovium Inflammatory signs rare Para-articular deposits occur; chronic tenosynovitis, carpal-tunnel syndrome	Myeloma
Gout Increased uric acid concentrations, serum and urine, and secondary gout, especially in myeloproliferative disorders and myeloma	Hematopoietic tumors, myeloma
Dermatomyositis or myopathy without skin changes with onset after 40 years of age has 5 to 50% association with neoplasia Increased incidence of scleroderma with tumors uncertain	Several cancers, hematopoietic tumors

growth hormone (HGH) is responsible for some of the manifestations.[53]

Remissions of this syndrome have been seen after resecting the underlying tumor or simply interrupting the vagus nerves above the lung root. Response to corticosteroids and salicylates is inconsistent.

Amyloidosis occurs in 5 to 15 percent of patients with myeloma and has been reported in persons with Hodgkin's disease, renal cell cancer, and several nonneoplastic disorders. Patients with amyloidosis have frequent rheumatic complaints. An arthropathy involving the larger joints has been noted and ascribed to amyloid deposits in the synovium. Signs of inflammation are uncommon. Para-articular deposits of amyloid on occasion result in a chronic tenosynovitis or pain and numbness in the hand along the distribution of the median nerve (carpal-tunnel syndrome).

The incidence of neoplasia in patients developing dermatomyositis after the age of 40 is high, ranging from 5 to 50 percent. Cancers of the bronchus and breast are most commonly associated with dermatomyositis, but many diverse tumor types have been reported. The precise pathogenesis of the dermatomyositis (which may occur without dermal lesions) is uncertain, although it is generally related to allergy or hypersensitivity to an unknown tumor component. Improvement in the dermatomyositis may take place following tumor resection.

Scleroderma has been reported in association with various tumors, but it is not clear that this association is statistically significant. In a few cases, sclerodermatous skin changes have been related to a secreting carcinoid tumor. Bronchiolar carcinoma has been reported as a terminal event in a few patients with the chronic lung disease of progressive systemic sclerosis.

Neuromuscular[4,5]

The neurologic disorders that accompany neoplastic diseases are most commonly caused by the involvement of the central nervous system by primary or metastatic tumors. On occasion, neurologic deficits are the initial clinical manifestations of illness, as, for example, in 3 or 4 percent of patients with bronchogenic carcinoma.

Metastatic deposits commonly develop within the brain and rarely develop within the spinal cord. Metastases account for approximately 20 percent of all intracranial tumors. The brain and cord may be affected indirectly by metastases developing within their bony coverings, the skull, and the spine, with a consequent extension inward through the dura or with a compromise of vascular supply. Spinal cord compression associated with tumorous destruction of the adjacent vertebral body is a not infrequent occurrence during the course of many neoplastic diseases.

Several reports note the prolonged survival of patients who have undergone resection of solitary cerebral metastases and the primary tumors, and serve to remind physicians of the practical importance attached to the clinical demonstration of the solitary deposit. However, cerebral metastases are multiple in at least 70 percent of cases, and in only a small minority of instances are the remaining organ systems free of obvious involvement.[10,29]

Diffuse metastatic involvement of the meninges, particularly about the base of the brain, occurs less frequently. In contrast to carcinomas, the leukemias and lymphomas spread to the meninges more often than to the substance of the brain. "Tumor meningitis" may present a difficult diagnostic problem, particularly when there are no other clinical manifestations of the neoplastic process. The patient may present with headache, signs of increased intracranial pressure, cranial nerve palsies, or diabetes insipidus (rarely) or as a case of aseptic meningitis.

A practical problem results from the appearance of neurologic symptoms in patients with neoplasms, particularly those as responsive to therapy as the leukemias and lymphomas. At present the nerve cell degenerations and the demyelinating disorders are unresponsive to known therapy. On the other hand, tumor cell infiltrates of the meninges or mass lesions will yield satisfactorily to treatment. The physician must also remain mindful of the not infrequent meningeal infections with cryptococcus, listeria, mycobacteria, and other microorganisms in these patients. Neurologic symptoms may also result from small vessel damage attendant on marked erythrocytosis or leukocytosis, intravascular clotting or the bleeding diatheses associated with thrombocytopenia, clotting-factor deficiencies, or the macroglobulinemic high serum viscosity state.

Certain neuromuscular disorders associated with neoplastic diseases cannot be attributed to actual involvement with tumor tissue, although their pathogenesis has not been clarified (Table 53–14). There is paucity of pathologic studies dealing with such disorders, particularly of the spinal cord and peripheral nerves. Additional interpretive problems arise because apparently identical abnormalities are seen as accompaniments of nonneoplastic disorders (sarcoid, tuberculosis, alcoholism) and because ionizing radiations can produce such a lesion as myelitis, vincristine may induce a peripheral neuropathy, and corticosteroids may cause myopathy.

TABLE 53–14

Physiologic Abnormalities Due to Neoplasia: Nonmetastatic Neuromuscular Disorders

Clinical Manifestations	Neoplasm
Encephalomyeloneuropathy Degeneration of neural cells causes psychologic disorders (dementia, depression); cerebellar disorders (dysarthria, ataxia); sensory, motor, or mixed neuropathies; mixed syndromes	Several cancers, especially bronchogenic, ovary, breast
Multifocal leukoencephalopathy Demyelinating lesions bilateral, asymmetrical especially of cerebral hemispheres causing dementia, hemiparesis, speech defects, occasional cerebellar signs	Lymphoma, leukemia
Carcinomatous myopathy Weakness and wasting especially of proximal limb and girdle muscles, with or without inflammation (polymyositis) or skin lesions (dermatomyositis)	Several cancers, especially bronchogenic
Myasthenic syndrome Weakness of proximal limb muscles, rarely cranial muscles Transient improvement with repeated contractions Poor response to neostigmin Sensitive to curare	Bronchogenic cancer, especially small cell
Myasthenia gravis Thymoma occurs in 15 to 30% of cases Improvement noted after resection	Thymoma

"Carcinomatous encephalomyeloneuropathy" is a term that encompasses the overlapping clinical syndromes resulting from neural cell degeneration in the cerebellar cortex, the dorsal spinocerebellar tracts, the posterior columns, and the corticospinal tracts. Less frequently, neuronal damage is seen in the brain stem nuclei, dorsal root ganglia, and anterior horns of the spinal cord. The corresponding clinical syndromes may be primarily disorders of mentation or cerebellar function, syndromes of sensory or motor neuropathy, or mixed polyneuropathy. Overlapping of these syndromes is common. Carcinomas of the bronchus, ovary, and breast are the most frequently associated tumors, although a few cases associated with Hodgkin's disease have been reported.

"Progressive multifocal leukoencephalopathy" is a term used for the syndromes that result from the bilateral, asymmetrical demyelinating lesions most commonly observed in the cerebral hemispheres, cerebellum, brain stem, and, rarely, spinal cord. These result in dementia, visual impairment, hemiparesis, speech abnormalities, and, rarely, cerebellar dysfunction. These disorders are related more frequently to leukemia and lymphoma, although instances have been reported in patients with carcinoma of the bronchus and breast. In general the clinical course of this demyelinating disorder is more rapid than that associated with nerve cell degeneration. There is some evidence that a slow virus infection is involved.

Slowly progressive weakness and wasting, especially of proximal limb and girdle muscles, are common presenting complaints of carcinomatous myopathy. In general the onset is insidious, although there are reports of an abrupt onset following the administration of a muscle relaxant during anesthesia. This myopathy may occur in association with clinical or pathologic evidence of inflammation (polymyositis) or skin involvement (dermatomyositis). It may also occur in association with neurologic abnormalities (neuromyopathy), making precise clinical definition difficult. Of practical importance is the association of cancers of the bronchus, breast, and other sites with myopathy of late onset unaccompanied by other systemic abnormalities. Adrenal corticosteroids may induce remissions in this syndrome, particularly in those patients with dermatomyositis.

A consistent relationship between these degenerative changes, which affect the nerve cells, myelin, or muscles, and the associated neoplasm has not been demonstrated. The demyelinating disorders have been identified relatively late in the course of the neoplastic disease, but the encephalomyeloneuropathies and myopathies may precede or develop subsequent to the initial tumor diagnosis. Remissions of the last group of disorders have been related to the resection or successful treatment of the underlying neoplasm. However, spontaneous remission and exacerbations have also been noted, making interpretation of these events difficult.

A few patients with tumors who complain of weakness exhibit additional features which suggest myasthenia. Proximal muscle weakness is common, but cranial muscle weakness is rare. Although increased fatigability follows repeated contraction of the involved muscles, a transient increase in strength is noted commonly. There is little or no increase in muscular strength after neostigmine or edrophonium administration. In some, symptoms have abated following the administration of guanidine. Thus far, the vast majority of patients with this myasthenic syndrome have had small-cell cancer of the bronchus. However, the Eaton-Lambert syndrome has also been associated with breast cancer and other tumors and has been described in otherwise normal persons.

Among individuals with typical myasthenia gravis there is a 15 to 30 percent incidence of thymoma. There is not an unusual incidence of other neoplasms among them. The precise pathophysiologic relationship between the thymoma and myasthenia is not clear. Remission of the myasthenia, however, has been noted following resection or radiation of the thymic tumor.

Another ill understood and rare clinical syndrome relates to the somatic pain induced by drinking alcohol in certain patients with Hodgkin's disease. This is also seen occasionally with other neoplasms.

EXPECTED CLINICAL COURSE AND SURVIVAL

The prognosis for patients with neoplastic diseases is based on a complex series of biologic interactions between the tumor and the host. Certain factors have been related to a desirable or undesirable outcome in groups of patients, but good judgment must be shown in applying such data directly to an individual patient. The efficacy of various types of therapeutic intervention is an important prognostic factor, also. However, even in the most "favorable" or "localized" lesions which can be "excised completely" or "ablated" by radiation therapy, it seems likely that the integrity of the patients' biologic defense mechanisms is a major determinant of the overall outcome.

TUMOR-RELATED FACTORS

In general, the major prognostic determinants that relate to the tumor are the site of origin, the histologic type and grade, and the extent of disease at diagnosis (clinical stage). In certain sites, such as the breast and prostate, hormone responsiveness is an important prognostic characteristic. In other neoplasms, the tumor cell's sensitivity to drugs or the emergence of drug resistance affect the course and survival significantly.[1-5,18]

The histologic pattern of tumors arising in the same site has been related to prognosis. Selected examples are shown in Table 53–15. The relationships between cell type and survival in breast cancer and bronchogenic cancer are shown in Chapter 55. Histologic criteria for the degree of malignancy of a tumor have been based primarily on the degree of cellular differentiation, the degree of cellular and nuclear pleomorphism, and the frequency of mitoses. For example, Broder's original studies divided squamous cell carcinomas into four grades of malignancy (Grades I to IV). In general, Grade I (differentiated) patterns were predictive of the least aggressive tumor growth and dissemination whereas Grade IV (undifferentiated) patterns were associated with the most rapid rates of tumor growth and spread and the least favorable prognosis for life (e.g., Table 53–15).

Precise cancer grading as introduced by Broder is a time-consuming procedure and is not too helpful in predicting the biologic behavior of a tumor in an individual patient. Grading is applied mainly to squamous cancers and is useful in the analysis of groups of patients. In cancers of the thyroid, ovary, testis, a clear definition of the cell type is more informative (Table 53–15).

Neoplasms arising in different sites have differing potentials for growth and spread. In this regard, cancers of the tongue, thyroid, and skin, which commonly spread to regional lymph nodes but rarely spread to distant parts of the body may be contrasted with that of bronchogenic carcinoma and malignant melanoma, where death is often related to distant metastatic deposits.

Patients who present with localized neoplasms have the best chances of survival, and their expected survival decreases in proportion to the observed ex-

TABLE 53–15
Survival with Common Neoplasms Related to Histologic Type

Site	Morphology	Survival at 5 Years (%)
Thyroid	Follicular and Papillary	80–90
	Medullary	50–60
	Undifferentiated	10–12
Testis	Seminoma	80–90
	Embryonal carcinoma	50–60
	Choriocarcinoma	5–10
Salivary glands	Acinar cell	80–85
	Low-grade mucoepidermoid	80
	High-grade mucoepidermoid	20–25
	Mixed malignant	35–40
	Squamous	15–20

tensiveness of disease (Table 53–16). Although this generalization is supported by data from many sources, there are also individuals who present with localized tumors but succumb rapidly to metastatic disease despite optimal therapy. Conversely, a few with widespread tumors survive for prolonged periods, sometimes with no treatment. The extent of a patient's neoplastic disease at a given point in time is expressed as its clinical stage. The systems employed in various institutions differ somewhat; however, Stage I usually indicates a neoplasm confined to its site of origin and Stage IV distant metastatic spread, with Stages II and III representing intermediate gradations. Similar schemes have been applied to the

TABLE 53–16
Survival with Common Neoplasms Related to Extent of Disease at Diagnosis

Neoplasm	Total Cases	Percent Relative Survival at 5 Years*			
		All Stages	Localized	Regional	Distant
Breast (female)	25,698	62	84	53	10
Bronchus	22,585	8	30	8	1
Colon	19,461	46	73	42	5
Ovary	5,240	32	72	36	8
Prostate	13,790	51	64	51	17
Rectum	11,515	40	64	31	4
Stomach	9,983	12	39	13	2
Uterus, body	7,614	72	83	50	14
Uterus, cervix	10,577	60	79	46	12

* Relative survival adjusts for mortality expected in general population with characteristics similar to cancer cases.[18]

clinical classification of Hodgkin's disease and other lymphomas. In this instance, Stages I and II designate localized and more widespread regional involvement, respectively, and Stages III and IV indicate more widespread involvement, often associated with systemic symptomatology (Chap. 50).

Another system for describing the clinical extent of neoplastic disease has been devised by the International Union Against Cancer. This TNM system is a rather straightforward description: T meaning tumor, N meaning nodes, and M meaning distant metastases. Numerical modifers (1, 2, 3) indicate the degrees of involvement. For example, a patient with a breast cancer in excess of 5 cm with axillary node involvement but no evidence of more distant spread would be classified as $T_3N_2M_0$. It seems likely that this staging system will gain wider use in clinical practice.[8,27]

HOST-RELATED FACTORS

Several host-related characteristics affect the prognosis of patients with neoplastic disease, but many are ill defined.[18,25] Overall, the survival of female patients is greater than that of males and this holds true when cancer outcomes are examined site by site. Pregnancy per se does not seem to alter the course of malignant diseases in a major way, although there are many reports which indicate that accelerated tumor growth occurred in the postpartum period. The patient's race also relates to prognosis. In most cancers, the prognosis is better for whites than blacks.

Clearly age is of major importance. Neoplasms occur more commonly in older individuals than in younger ones, as do various degenerative diseases, notably of the cardiovascular system. These nonneoplastic diseases also limit life expectancy, particularly if they are responsible for a significant functional insufficiency of one of the major organ systems, such as the heart, kidneys, or liver. The several major physiologic abnormalities produced by neoplasms themselves may also be life-limiting, and these are not necessarily expressions of extensive neoplasia. Examples are hemolytic anemia, thrombocytopenic bleeding, hypercalcemia, and infection. At least half of cancer patients die of physiologic abnormalities due to their cancers or associated degenerative disorders and not from the direct consequences of tumor

---

TABLE 53-17
Trends in Survival with Common Neoplasms

Neoplasms	(Percent Relative Survival at 3 Years)*					
	1940–1949		1950–1959		1960–1969	
	No. Cases	3-Year Survival	No. Cases	3-Year Survival	No. Cases	3-Year Survival
Breast (female)	12,184	63	22,105	71	14,911	72
Bronchus	4,772	6	16,072	10	15,941	11
Colon	7,488	36	16,153	49	10,152	50
Hodgkin's disease	1,013	35	2,008	44	1,990	61
Larynx	1,462	47	3,259	60	2,725	67
Leukemia (acute)	922	4	2,837	14	2,432	30
Leukemia (chronic)	1,599	24	3,627	35	1,587	41
Melanoma (skin)	749	49	1,982	63	1,966	74
Myeloma	391	10	1,328	13	1,116	27
Ovary	2,339	30	4,296	33	3,085	35
Pancreas	2,009	2	4,391	2	2,888	2
Prostate	6,008	49	11,647	59	7,384	66
Stomach	7,390	12	9,987	15	3,889	15
Thyroid	697	67	2,377	81	1,445	86
Uterus, body	3,509	66	6,529	74	4,400	76
Uterus, cervix	7,075	53	10,280	64	4,888	63

* Relative survival adjusts for mortality expected in general population with characteristics similar to cancer cases.[18]

mass, ulceration, or obstruction. Methods of defining host resistance to tumors are yet imperfect and this assessment in patients is complicated by the use of cytotoxic and immunosuppressive treatments. However, it seems clear that impaired functioning of the reticuloendothelial system is related to oncogenesis and that progressively more severe deficiencies of immune reactivity are associated with advancing neoplastic diseases. Defects in cell-mediated responses are particularly notable in disseminated lymphoma and many cancers.

On the other hand, it is quite clear that patients are capable of responding to (autochthonous) tumor antigens. In Burkitt's tumor, patients developing a delayed-hypersensitivity response to tumor membrane extracts during treatment have a better prognosis than those who did not. Other studies indicate that the ability to develop (non-tumor-specific) cell-mediated immune responses correlates with a better prognosis following surgical resection of a wide variety of cancers. Thus, there is a beginning appreciation of host resistance factors important to prognosis.

Clinicians often use the observed rate of tumor growth and spread as guides to management and prognosis in individual cases. In some instances where there is no potential for curative therapy, antitumor treatment may be withheld while the tumor remains indolent. A long interval between treatment of the primary tumor and recurrence usually signifies a better prognosis.

Changing Cancer Survival[1,18]

During recent years, the prognosis for survival in several types of cancer has improved significantly (Table 53–17). Among the tumor types showing improvement are: acute leukemia, chronic leukemia, Hodgkin's disease, myeloma, melanoma, and cancers of the bladder, larynx, prostate, and thyroid. The outlook for cancers of the colon, rectum, breast, uterine body and uterine cervix improved between 1940 and 1950, but during the past 20 years there has been little change. The prognosis for cancers of the bronchus, pancreas, stomach, and certain other inaccessible sites has remained poor throughout the past 30 years or more.

CHAPTER 54

Principles of Management

ALBERT H. OWENS, Jr.

Traditionally, the internist's interest in neoplastic diseases was confined largely to early and precise diagnosis. With the exception of the hematologist's continuing concern with neoplasms of hematopoietic tissue, the mangement of patients with neoplasms remained primarily the responsibility of the surgeon and radiotherapist.

Most recently the internist has assumed a major role in the management of these patients. A growing appreciation of the diverse physiologic derangements produced by tumors and the advent of effective systemic therapy for several of these diseases have stimulated the internist's interest and supplemented his characteristic evaluation of the whole patient's physiologic and psychologic status as the basis of a meaningful program of supportive care.

Prior to the formulation of a specific therapeutic program for a patient with a neoplastic disease, a thorough review must be made of his clinical status. As in most clinical situations, the overall result of treatment will be related to the interaction of the disease, the patient (host), and the therapy; the outcome can be anticipated in these terms. A general scheme of systematic patient evaluation is suggested by these factors. It would include making a precise diagnosis and delineating any associated physiologic abnormalities and additional disease processes.

A Precise Diagnosis[1,4,8,27]

A precise anatomic diagnostic formulation includes knowledge of the neoplasm's site of origin, tissue type, or both, as well as the anatomic extent of the disease process. The diagnosis is supported primarily by the microscopic examination of a tissue biopsy specimen or cell preparation considered in conjunction with the clinical disease state.

Clearly every effort should be made to avoid the inappropriate treatment of nonneoplastic disease and the failure to identify correctly a disease process (e.g., tuberculosis) with alternate (and perhaps greater) therapeutic implications. Furthermore, the location of the neoplasm and the extent to which it has spread throughout the body bear directly on the choice of a potentially curative or palliative therapeutic procedure.

The International Union Against Cancer has devised a systematic procedure for describing the extent of neoplastic disease which is being adopted widely as the basis for uniform diagnostic reporting and treatment planning (Chap. 53). This TNM classification applies to the clinical staging of patients not treated previously. The formulation describes the degree of involvement by the neoplastic process (numerals 1 to 3) as it relates to the Tumor, the regional lymph Nodes, and distant Metastases. Thus, a patient with a small epidermoid cancer of the uterine cervix confined to the primary site would be classified as T_1 N_0 M_0.[8,27]

The morphologic pattern (cell type and grade) of a tumor and its anatomic extent (clinical stage) are key data for treatment planning. All pertinent clinical data should be developed fully and all factors considered carefully when deciding on an individual program of therapy. In most cases this requires the input of several specialists.

Tumor type is of prime importance in the formulation of a program of systemic treatment which is palliative in the majority of instances. Neoplasms likely to respond to endocrine therapy are those arising from tissue that is normally responsive to hormonal stimuli. A well-differentiated follicular thyroid carcinoma containing colloid may be expected to concentrate [131]I.[^] A further consideration of tumor type in relation to the use of other chemotherapeutic agents will be presented in more detail subsequently.

The clinically apparent rate of tumor growth and spread also determines the timing of noncurative therapy. In a small proportion of patients, tumors may remain indolent for prolonged periods and demand no therapeutic intervention.

Physiologic Abnormalities

The spectrum of physiologic abnormalities that may be related to a given patient's neoplasm has been summarized previously. These functional abnormalities may be the primary determinants of the patient's prognosis and thus may demand primary therapeutic attention. Examples are massive hemorrhage from gastrointestinal tumor, a profound hemolytic process, hypercalcemia, and a major infectious process, such as pneumococcal meningitis.

The prime importance of logical physiologic therapy and thoughtful emotional support cannot be overemphasized. Often, in instances where the clinical application of potentially curative procedures is not possible or has failed, such supportive management provides far more comfort to the patient and his family than does the use of antitumor drugs.

Additional Disease Processes

Neoplastic diseases are most common in the older age groups. Therefore, patients with tumors may have coexisting disease processes, particularly of a degenerative nature. At times these nonneoplastic disorders are of prime clinical importance and determine the patient's prognosis. At other times the physiologic deficits produced by these disorders prohibit a major operative procedure or a potentially curative surgical resection. For example, a thoracotomy for the resection of a bronchogenic carcinoma would not be feasible in a patient with severe coronary artery disease, marked myocardial insufficiency, or marked respiratory insufficiency due to emphysema and bronchitis.

THERAPEUTIC MODALITIES

The optimal goal of an antitumor treatment regimen is complete eradication all manifestations of the disease. With this in mind the neoplastic cell has come to be regarded as the offending foreign organism or pathogenic parasite, and therapeutic efforts have been directed at removing or destroying the population of offensive cells.

Surgery[4,7,9]

The earliest successful treatment of neoplasms and the current main curative therapy is surgical excision. The major treatment benefits have accrued in cancers at accessible sites, where techniques of diagnostic surveillance are easily applied and excision can be carried out before the tumor has become extensive. The surgical approach is limited by the location and extent of the neoplasm rather than by the type of neoplastic cells of their metabolic characteristics. Consideration must be given, however, to the relative mortality risks of anesthesia and surgery and the functional morbidity after the procedure.

Radiation[28,37]

Ionizing radiations of varying type and energy are employed to eradicate localized populations of neoplastic cells. As with surgical therapy, these procedures are limited chiefly by the location and anatomic extent of the lesion being treated. The greatest therapeutic successes are achieved with relatively small neoplasms that are detected before they have produced major organ-system alterations or have spread beyond feasible treatment fields. Tumor cell eradication is limited by the lack of cytotoxic specificity in ionizing radiations. Thus, the tolerance of adjacent normal tissue limits the amount of radiation that can be directed at the tumor.

Additional known biologic effects of irradiation must be considered when treating patients. At times, its effects on gonadal tissue are utilized in ablative therapy, but the possible mutagenic consequences of inadvertent nonlethal germ cell irradiation or unknown exposure of an early fetus must always be borne in mind. The carcinogenic potential of ionizing radiation has been clearly demonstrated in humans. In many therapeutic situations this delayed effect is of little practical consequence, but it should strongly militate against treating relatively young individuals for benign lesions or tumors that can be easily excised. Under certain circumstances (such as Stage I cancer of the larynx), complete tumor cell ablation can be achieved by irradiation without the sacrifice of organ function (voice) that a curative surgical procedure might require.

Systemic Therapy[32,34,36,40]

There are compelling reasons to seek effective systemic treatments of neoplastic diseases. Certain of these disorders, such as leukemia and multiple myeloma, are disseminated in their earliest recognizable form. Similarly, a great many patients with solid tumors present for treatment when their diseases have progressed beyond regional confines. Furthermore, regional or distant recurrence of cancer is common in many tumor types despite the most favorable clinical presentation and treatment. The frequent recovery of apparently viable neoplastic cells from the regional venous blood and systemic circulation of these patients emphasizes some therapeutic problems which remain to be solved.

Antineoplastic chemotherapy is considered curative in certain tumor types (e.g., trophoblastic tumors, acute lymphoblastic leukemia, Burkitt's tumor, Hodgkin's disease, histiocyctic lymphoma) because of the high frequency of disease-free remissions that extend for 5 years or more. In other circumstances, complete resolution of all clinically detectable disease can be achieved, but not for an indefinite period. With many tumor types, the results are variable and less useful overall.

The determinants of the overall outcome of antineoplastic chemotherapy are complex and ill understood. Most currently available antitumor drugs appear to act on similar metabolic pathways in normal and neoplastic cells, hence a lack of tumor specificity continues to be one of the chief limitations to their use. Nonetheless, drugs with consistent and clinically useful tumor-inhibitory effects have been identified. With these, additional problems of drug resistance limit their long-term use. Only in rare circumstances (such as those involving the blood–brain barrier) is the utility of drug treatment limited by the anatomic location of the neoplasm.

The chief limitation of short-term anticancer drug therapy is toxicity to the patient's organ systems, notably the bone marrow, liver, kidneys, and nervous system. Several of these drugs have been shown to possess mutagenic, teratogenic, and carcinogenic properties that should be considered carefully, particularly when the treatment of benign conditions is contemplated.

Hormonal therapy, supplemental or ablative, is not considered potentially curative. Present evidence indicates that these treatments are effective in tumors arising from endocrine-responsive tissue whose growth remains responsive to hormonal stimuli. The limitations of this form of treatment follow from that fact.

Various forms of tumor-specific or nonspecific immunotherapy are being evaluated. The results to date are variable (some promising; many disappointing) and often matters of scientific controversy. Unfortunately, this is the status in even the most favorable clinical situations in which immunotherapy is instituted in patients with minimal tumor burdens.

Combined or Adjuvant Therapy[41,42]

Therapeutic modalities have been combined in an effort to circumvent the limitations inherent in each. Radiation therapy has been used preoperatively to reduce the mass of tumor and render it resectable and to prevent distant metastatic spread by devitalizing tumor cells prior to surgical manipulation. Preoperative radiation is clearly useful in managing cancer of the body of the uterus. There are some indications of its utility in the larger cancers of the head and neck and rectum, but this is not a matter generally agreed upon.

Postoperative radiation therapy is more widely used. Such radiation therapy can improve the result when tumors cannot be excised completely as in the case of malignant brain tumors or large soft tissue sarcomas. Postoperative radiation therapy may be used to permit a smaller surgical procedure. For example, some advocate a limited resection of primary breast cancers followed by radiation therapy in lieu of a radical mastectomy. There is of course, no general agreement on this matter. Postoperative radiation therapy is used routinely and with good effect in the management of selected tumors such as Wilms' tumor.

Chemotherapeutic agents have been used as adjuvants to radiation therapy with the thought of increasing the radioresponsiveness of the tumor and treating distant metastases that were not clinically apparent. Such a combined approach has proven advantageous in the treatment of retinoblastoma, Wilms' tumor, and possibly in the management of head and neck cancers. Sequential combinations of multiagent chemotherapy and radiation therapy may improve the outcome for patients with Hodgkin's disease and lymphoma. It appears that radiation therapy is most successful in dealing with large tumor masses whereas chemotherapeutic agents can cope more effectively with widely disseminated deposits. Whether this approach will be feasible or useful in other tumors (e.g., testicular tumors) is uncertain.

Chemotherapeutic agents have been used as adjuvants to surgery mainly to deal with clinically occult tumor dissemination. Most early trials failed to show any therapeutic advantage for this approach. However, in each instance very short periods of drug treatment were prescribed for cancers that are notably "slow growing." More recently, for example in breast cancer, it has been shown that the prolonged administration of cytotoxic drugs will delay or prevent tumor recurrence following surgery (Chap. 55).

Supportive Care

Extensive surgical procedures, intensive radiation therapy, and the vigorous use of chemotherapeutic agents have improved the results of cancer treatment. However, a favorable outcome is often dependent on sustaining patients through limited periods of major physiologic impairment and readjustment. Intensive alimentation, reconstructive surgery, various restorative devices, blood component transfusion, and the control of infections are key considerations.[31] Proper programs of rehabilitation and psychologic support should be initiated with the beginning of antitumor treatment, especially in those cases where complete functional restoration is possible. The larger treatment centers are usually better prepared to render these comprehensive services.

PALLIATIVE THERAPY— GENERAL INDICATIONS

Patients with neoplastic diseases that have progressed beyond hope of cure frequently develop symptoms which are mechanical in their genesis and are related to the presence of a tumor mass. Among these symptoms are pain due to a bony deposit or nerve root pressure, bleeding from a tumor surface, obstruction of viscera, unhealing ulceration, paralysis

due to central nervous system or peripheral nerve compression, and serous cavity or subcutaneous fluid accumulation. Such impairments, or their imminent development, constitute adequate indication for treatment, provided there is a reasonable likelihood of achieving a good result.

In general, symptoms and lesions of this type are best treated by radiotherapy. The chronic leukemias, lymphomas, Wilms' tumor, and neuroblastoma are radioresponsive tumors, whereas adenocarcinomas of the intestine, lung, kidney, and pancreas, melanoma, and osteogenic and fibrosarcomas are generally nonradioresponsive. Head and neck squamous tumors and cancers of the genitalia, bronchus, and esophagus are among those displaying an intermediate response to radiotherapy. The use of ^{131}I offers satisfactory palliation to patients with colloid-forming carcinoma of the thyroid because of the selective uptake of iodine by this tumor.

On occasion a surgical procedure is most suitable, as in the relief of intestinal obstruction or the removal of an ulcerated breast lesion. At times a surgical procedure should be followed by a course of radiotherapy, as in acute spinal cord compression or extensive head and neck tumors.

When distressing functional derangements are secondary to neoplasms which are responsive to antitumor drugs, appropriate therapy should be started. When the likelihood of a significant drug-induced remission is reasonable, it is important to support the patient in every way possible to permit completion of an adequate course of therapy. Many symptoms can be relieved by the judicious use of simple supportive measures.

BIOLOGIC EFFECTS OF ANTITUMOR THERAPY

A physician contemplating a specific therapeutic program must be thoroughly familiar with the varied biologic effects of available treatment modalities. He must appreciate the nature and basis of the effects of ionizing radiations and the chemotherapeutic agents available to prevent unintended discomfort in the individual being treated.

IONIZING RADIATION

The ionizing radiations employed therapeutically are of varying energies, but they produce qualitatively similar effects on exposed tissues. The sources of therapeutic ionizing radiations may be external to the patient, may be implanted in his tissues or body cavities, or may be given systemically in soluble chemical form such as $Na_2H^{32}P_2O_4$ and ^{131}I.[37]

Whole-body irradiation is used infrequently in clinical practice. When used, therapy may be given from external sources, usually at a relatively low dose rate, or it may be given systemically in soluble isotopic form. Animals receiving high sublethal doses of whole-body irradiation quickly become listless and anorectic and may vomit. Similar effects are produced in patients who receive whole-body irradiation, 1000 rads at a dose rate of 5 rads per minute for purposes of immunosuppression prior to bone marrow transplantation.

Animals receiving lethal doses of whole-body irradiation usually die 7 to 14 days later as a consequence of bone-marrow failure (marrow aplasia). The usual immediate causes of death are bleeding (thrombocytopenia) and infection (granulocytopenia). Animals receiving larger lethal doses die sooner because of gut damage or central nervous system derangement.

Most radiation therapy used clinically is directed toward specific anatomic sites or regions. The practical factors which limit the application of regional radiation therapy are the patient's systemic reaction and the effects produced on normal tissues within the field of treatment. Radiation sickness is characterized by general debility, anorexia, and vomiting. Symptoms that begin soon after the onset of treatment are related to dose and to volume and type of tissue treated, and subside promptly on cessation of therapy or reduction in dosage.[4,37]

The normal tissues most commonly exposed in a treatment field include skin, mucous membrane, fat, connective tissue, muscle, bone, and cartilage. The intensity of the acute reaction observed in the skin or mucosa varies with the energy of the ionizing radiation and usually defines the tolerable dose when low energy radiation is being used. In many situations the acute or delayed changes produced in such tissues as the bone marrow, central nervous system, eyes, epiphyses, gonads, kidneys, and lungs are of great importance.[4,28,43] These are summarized in Table 54–1.

In general the early tissue effects of radiation (those produced in a matter of days) result from acute cell injury and death. At times this tissue necrosis is complicated by infection. Later (after a few weeks), tissue regeneration is completed but may be impaired by scarring and fibrosis. More severe late radiation effects (after months have elapsed) stem largely from vascular damage and include tissue atrophy or necrosis and ulceration, often in the skin. Vascular damage also determines the delayed development of impairments in other exposed organs—for

example, radiation nephritis and radiation myelitis. Years later, neoplastic changes may become evident.

Ionizing radiations cause cell death, which may be defined as a loss of reproductive integrity. Exposed cells develop abnormalities of the nucleus, with

TABLE 54–1
Biologic Effects of Ionizing Radiation—External Source

Tissue Exposed	Clinical Manifestations
Skin and mucosa	Early erythema, desquamation followed by reepithelialization, fibrosis (days) Later atrophy, telangiecstasia develop Late necrosis, ulceration due to devascularization (months) Still later, neoplasia
Hair	Epilation May recover in 5 to 12 months depending on dose
Hematopoietic	Transient fall in reticulocytes, white cells, platelets, several days More marked when larger volume of marrow exposed during treatment of hematopoietic tumors May later result in marrow aplasia, fibrosis (months)
Eye	Conjunctivitis, possible ulceration Sequence similar to mucosa Late cataract formation (months to years)
Lung	Acute radiation pneumonitis (days) related to lung volume exposed, perhaps related infection Late fibrosis (months)
Heart	Acute and chronic pericarditis
Kidney	Delayed radiation nephritis (8 to 12 months) due to vascular damage
Gonad	Sterility Mutational changes
Bone	Stops growth of ununited epiphyses; skeletal distortion results Late bone necrosis due to devascularization
Central nervous system	Delayed effects (months) due to vascular damage, e.g., radiation myelitis More marked when larger volume of central nervous system exposed

visible chromosomal fragmentation and cross-link-ing. These result from the disruption of chemical bonds of the macromolecular cellular components, presumably through the intermediary of free radical formation. These changes may be modified by repara-tive mechanisms within the cell. The net damage to deoxyribonucleic acid (DNA) seems to be of critical importance in determining the biologic expression of radiation effects.

ANTITUMOR DRUGS

The antitumor drugs most commonly employed in current practice are classified as polyfunctional alkyl-ating agents or as metabolic antagonists of various sorts, according to their presumed mechanisms of ac-tion (Table 54–2). Although information is available concerning their effects on diverse biologic systems

at varying levels of physiologic organization, the pre-cise relationships of these laboratory data to the therapeutic situation in tumor-bearing man are most complex and difficult to integrate satisfactorily. Fig-ures 54–1 and 54–2 are simplified schematic represen-tations of the biochemical sites of action of cancer chemotherapeutic agents developed to depict their relationships to normal cellular metabolic processes. The goal is to provide a frame of reference, not to encourage uncritical thinking.[32,34,36]

Cell Kinetics[40]

The effects of antitumor drugs on normal and neo-plastic tissues vary according to their proliferative activity. Certain drugs, such as mechlorethamine (HN2) and 1,3 bis(2-chloroethyl)-1-nitrosourea (BCNU), as well as γ-radiation react with cellular

---

TABLE 54–2
Characteristics of Commonly Used Antitumor Drugs

Classification	Cell Cycle	Mechanism	Drug
Alkylating agent	Cell cycle nonspecific React with biologic molecules irrespective of cell proliferation Arrest cell division at G_2 Cyclophosphamide; cycle active	Alkylation of nucleic acids, proteins, electron-rich molecules Probable critical target is DNA; covalent binding to purine and pyrimidine bases Cross-linking of DNA strands	Mechlorethamine Cyclophosphamide Melphalan Chlorambucil Busulfan Carmustine Lomustine Semustine
Antimetabolites	Cell cycle specific Drug action may relate to specific phase of cell cycle S-phase most sensitive	Interfere with critical enzyme functions Drugs are usually structural analogues of normal enzyme substrates	Methatrexate 6-Mercaptopurine 6-Thioguanine 5-Fluorouracil Florafur Cytosine arabinoside 5-Azacytidine Hydroxyurea
DNA intercalators	Cell cycle specific S-phase seems most sensitive Adriamycin; cycle nonspecific	Compounds of diverse structure which intercalate in the minor groove of DNA and interfere with transcription Drugs also cause breaks in DNA strands	Adriamycin Daunorubicin Bleomycin Actinomycin-D Mithramycin Mitomycin-C "Cis-platinum"
Mitotic inhibitors	Cell cycle specific Metaphase arrest	Interactions with microtubular proteins prevent mitotic spindle formation and possible other microtubular functions	Vinblastine Vincristine Colchicine "Podophyllotoxins"
Miscellaneous	Cell cycle nonspecific	Reacts with DNA causing strand fragmentation	Procarbazine
		Impairs 17-hydroxy-corticosteroid synthesis; damages adrenal cortex	Mitotane
		Asparagine-dependent tumor cells are susceptible to deprivation	L-Asparaginase

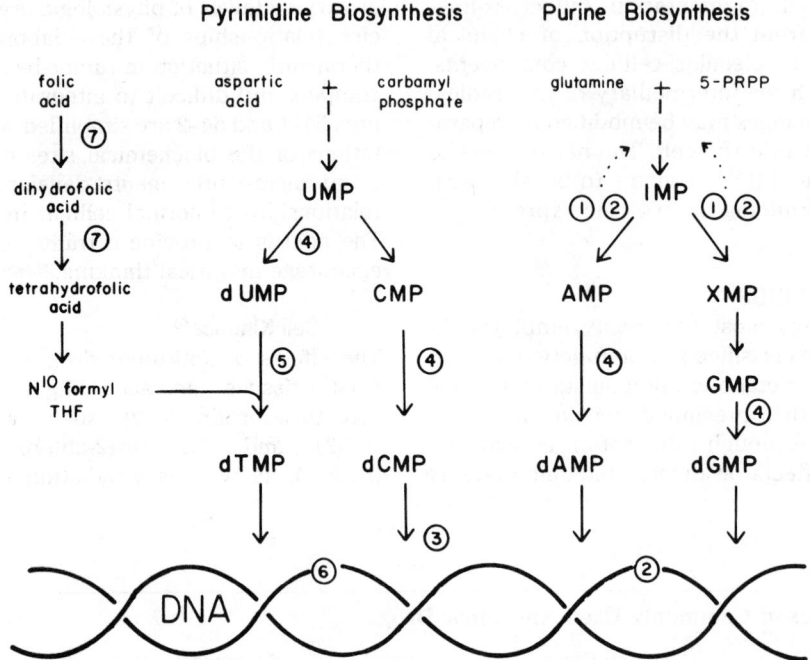

Figure 54-1. Major sites of action of antitumor drugs affecting DNA synthesis: 6-mercaptopurine ①, 6-thioguanine ②, arabinosyl cytosine ③, hydroxyurea ④, 5-fluorouracil ⑤, 5-iodo-2'-deoxyuridine ⑥, methotrexate ⑦. Steps in purine biosynthesis: 5-phosphoribosyl 1-pyrophosphate (5—PRPP), inosinic monophosphate (IMP), xanthine monophosphate (XMP), guanosine monophosphate (GMP), deoxyguanosine monophosphate (dGMP), adenosine monophosphate (AMP), deoxyadenosine monophosphate (dAMP). Steps in pyrimidine biosynthesis: cytidine monophosphate (CMP), deoxycytidine monophosphate (dCMP), uridine monophosphate (UMP), deoxyuridine monophosphate (dUMP), deoxythymidine monophosphate (dTMP).

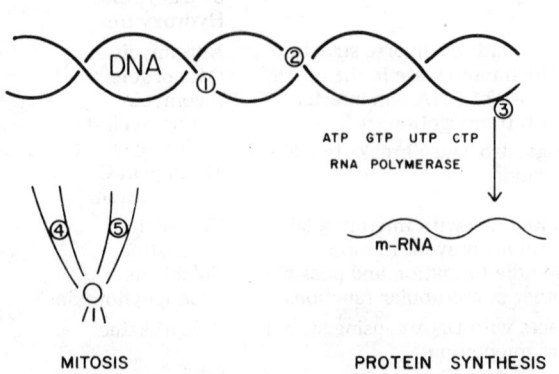

FIGURE 54-2. Major sites of action of antitumor drugs that interact with DNA or inhibit mitosis: alkylating agents ①, procarbazine ②, intercalators (dactinomycin, mithramycin, adriamycin, daunomycin) ③, colchicine ④, vinca alkaloids ⑤.

constituents irrespective of their proliferative activity (cell cycle nonspecific agents). Other drugs, such as methotrexate, arabinosyl cytosine and hydroxyurea, seem cycle-specific in their effect and indeed their actions are related to the phase of the cell cycle during which DNA is synthesized (S-phase specific).

By custom, the proliferative cycle which all types of dividing cells go through is divided into four phases—mitosis, G_1 (Gap$_1$), S (DNA synthesis), and G_2 (Gap$_2$). In most mammalian cells, S, the period of DNA synthesis, is of 6 to 8 hours duration and the G_2 phase lasts for approximately 2 hours. The G_1 phase is quite variable and it is during this period that cells perform many functions and increase their size. The G_0 phase has been added to describe cells which remain in G_1 for prolonged periods (nonproliferating). These resting cells are insensitive to the effects of most antitumor drugs.

There are several detailed descriptions of the events of the cell cycle and cell kinetic studies in normal and neoplastic tissues. In reviewing the mechanism of action of the commonly used antitumor drugs, their relationship to the phases of the cell cycle will be noted.

Alkylating Agents

The polyfunctional alkylating agents in current use are nitrogen mustards and sulfonic acid esters. These include mechlorethamine (HN2), cyclophosphamide, chlorambucil, busulfan, and melphalan. In all animal species studied, drug effect is most prominent in those tissues undergoing continual proliferative activity—hematopoietic tissue, intestinal epithelium, gonads, and hair follicles. Larger doses may cause convulsions or other evidence of central nervous system derangements. Cardiac toxicity and water retention due to renal tubular cell dysfunction has been ascribed to large doses of cyclophosphamide. Chronic administration of busulfan has been associated with pulmonary fibrosis, skin hyperpigmentation, and a "pseudo addisonian syndrome." Most of the alkylating agents except busulfan are immunosuppressants. Most alkylating agents are also mutagenic and carcinogenic.

Alkylating agents are highly reactive chemically and they combine with a wide variety of biologic materials, especially proteins and nucleic acids. In vivo and in vitro alkylating agents cause chromosomal breaks and clumping, cross-linking of DNA strands, and they arrest cell division at the premitotic interval (G_2). Alkylation at the N-7 position of the guanine moiety of DNA seems a very important determinant of cell injury and this chemical reaction can take place during all phases of the cell cycle. Alkylating agents are more efficient inhibitors of DNA viruses than RNA viruses and they inhibit mitosis much more readily than protein synthesis or enzyme actions.

Special attention should be drawn to cyclophosphamide, a polyfunctional alkylating agent widely used as an antitumor agent or as an immunosuppressant. Cyclophosphamide is metabolized, mainly by the oxidative enzymes located in the hepatic microsomes. Some of the metabolites are biologically inert and one is the "proximate alkylating agent" which interacts with nuclear DNA. The nitrosoureas (BCNU, CCNU, and methyl-CCNU) are metabolized in vivo, also. Their breakdown products appear to be involved in biologically important reactions with nucleic acids and proteins.

Antimetabolites

Most antimetabolites in current use are purine or pyrimidine analogs or folic acid antagonists. Prior to producing their biologic effects, the purine and py-

rimidine analogs must be converted in the target cell into a nucleotide. The antimetabolites block DNA synthesis or cause defects in its structural integrity, and this occurs almost exclusively during the S-phase of the mitotic cycle (phase specific). Their major toxic effects are observed in tissues with the greatest proliferative activity—hematopoietic tissue, intestinal epithelium, gonads, and hair follicles. In addition, 6-mercaptopurine and methotrexate may cause hepatic cell damage.

Three purine analogs are employed widely. The administration of 6-mercaptopurine impairs several purine interconversions and inhibits de novo purine biosynthesis. Azathioprine (Imuran), a congener designed to protect the -SH group of 6-mercaptopurine from rapid metabolic breakdown, is used primarily as an immunosuppressant. Although 6-thioguanine interferes with purine biosynthesis and metabolic interconversions as much as 6-mercaptopurine, a significant amount of the analog is incorporated into DNA. In some animal models the amount of DNA incorporation parallels therapeutic utility. In man, the overall results of 6-thioguanine therapy are similar to those of 6-mercaptopurine.

When administered, the fluorinated pyrimidine analogs 5-fluorouracil and 5-fluoro-2′-deoxyuridine undergo a series of metabolic interconversions. In part, they are converted to 5-fluorodeoxyuridine monophosphate which inhibits the normal action of thymidylate synthetase. This appears to be the most important determinant of biologic effect. Some 5-fluoruracil is also incorporated into RNA. In contrast, 5-iodo-2′-deoxyuridine is phosphorylated in mammalian cells and incorporated into DNA in place of thymidine. This compound inhibits the growth of *Herpes simplex* and vaccinia (DNA viruses) and is used clinically to treat diseases they cause.

Arabinosyl cytosine is an unnatural analog by virtue of its sugar moiety. It is converted to its nucleotide and as such exerts its main effects by inhibiting DNA polymerase (competitive inhibitor of deoxycytidine triphosphate). Arabinosyl cytosine has been used in the treatment of disseminated *Herpes simplex* infections but it seems ineffective.

Methotrexate and related compounds impair DNA synthesis by inhibiting the folic acid reductase enzymes. No congener has greater overall clinical utility than methotrexate. Citrovorum factor (tetrahydrofolic acid) administered shortly after (or before) methotrexate can prevent much of its toxicity, and the technique of "citrovorum factor rescue" has been used clinically to permit higher doses of methotrexate.

Hydroxyurea inhibits DNA synthesis without blocking RNA or protein synthesis. One of its main effects seems to be interference with the conversion of ribonucleosides to deoxyribonucleosides (inhibition of ribonucleoside diphosphate reductase).

Antibiotics

A great many antibiotics have been shown to have antitumor activity in various laboratory test systems. Of these, dactinomycin (Actinomycin-D), mithramycin, daunomycin, adriamycin, and bleomycin are in common clinical use.

Large doses of dactinomycin cause damage to proliferating tissues in the bone marrow, gastrointestinal tract, skin, and mucous membranes. These biologic effects are mainly due to the binding of dactinomycin to helical DNA and the consequent inhibition of DNA-dependent RNA synthesis. In greater concentration, the antibiotic will affect DNA synthesis and protein synthesis more directly. This selective action of dactinomycin has been used by molecular biologists as an investigative tool in clarifying many aspects of cell metabolism.

Mithramycin apparently has a very similar mechanism of action. However, the biologic effects which limit the clinical utility of the drug are dissimilar. They include bleeding (precipitous thrombocytopenia, multiple coagulation factor defects, capillary damage), hepatocellular damage, and hypocalcemia. In addition to its use as an antitumor agent, mithramycin is employed effectively to treat hypercalcemia and to control Paget's disease of bone. It appears that the effectiveness of mithramycin in hypercalcemic patients is based on the antibiotic's ability to inhibit the action of parathyroid hormone on bone.

Daunomycin and adriamycin have very similar chemical structures. However, they have a somewhat different spectrum of biologic effects and antitumor action. The usual treatment-limiting effects in man are due to damage to the proliferating cells of the bone marrow, gastrointestinal tract, and skin and mucous membranes. Both antibiotics can cause serious damage to the heart. It is of interest that these antibiotics are metabolized in vivo and that some of the metabolic products are biologically active. The mechanism of action of these compounds is thought to be similar to dactinomycin. Clearly, daunomycin and adriamycin, intercalate in the minor groove of helical DNA and interfere with the transcriptional process. There is some evidence also that higher concentrations of the drugs will inhibit DNA synthesis.

Bleomycin is a mixture of antibiotics which react with DNA causing strand fission. Bleomycin also appears to inhibit some of the enzymes involved in DNA repair. Cells in the early S-phase seem most sensitive to the action of this antibiotic and chromosomal fragmentation and mitotic arrest results. After administration of the antibiotic, high concentrations of bleomycin remain in the skin, lungs, and in responsive tumors. Damage to the skin and lungs usually limits clinical therapy.

Mitotic Inhibitors

Colchicine and the vinca alkaloids cause cells to arrest in metaphase primarily because they interfere with proper formation of spindle proteins. Colchicine affects tissues with a high degree of proliferative activity (bone marrow, intestinal epithelium, hair follicles). The continued clinical use of vinblastine is limited primarily by bone marrow depression whereas vincristine usage is limited most commonly by neurotoxicity. It is likely that these seemingly diverse biologic results are due to the effect of the alkaloids on various microtubular proteins in dividing and nondividing cells as well.

Miscellaneous Agents

Procarbazine causes a great deal of chromosomal damage. The drug reacts with DNA and causes strand fragmentation. DNA and RNA synthesis is impaired. It is an oxidant, but relatively little is known about its precise mechanisms of action. Nausea and vomiting and bone marrow depression usually limit the clinical use of procarbazine. Neurotoxicity is also encountered. Since procarbazine is an oxidant it may produce hemolytic anemia in susceptible individuals (Chap. 45). Procarbazine is also an amine oxidase inhibitor. It is of some interest that procarbazine is a potent immunosuppressant. It is also a potent carcinogen.

Cis-diaminedichloroplatinum is representative of a series of inorganic platinum coordination complexes that are chemically reminiscent of the mustard-type bifunctional alkylating agents. The general biologic effects of these compounds include antimicrobial, immunosuppressive, and mutagenic properties as well as antineoplastic. While interstrand (DNA) cross-linking has been observed, it seems more likely that the major biologic damage caused by the drug results from its intercalation with helical DNA. The continued use of "cis-platinum" clinically is limited by renal toxicity and to a lesser extent by hearing loss and myelosuppression.

Mitotane (o-p'-DDD) came into clinical use because of its selective toxicity to adrenal cortical cells. Early degenerative lesions develop in the zona reticu-

TABLE 54–3
Biologic Effects of Steroid Hormones

Effects	Androgens	Estrogens	Progestin	Adreno-Corticoids
Tissues	Stimulates growth of male sex tissues, body hair follicles, sebaceous glands, larynx, soft tissue and bones, erythropoietic tissue, closure of epiphyses	*Females:* Stimulates growth of breasts, nipples, uterus, pubic hair; proliferation of endometrium, myometrium, vaginal mucosa. *Males:* Feminization of breasts, skin, hair, fat distribution. Atrophy of genitalia	Maturation of breasts, endometrium, vaginal mucosa	Atrophy of thymus and lymphatic tissues and lympholysis. Decrease in blood lymphocytes, eosinophiles; increase in neutrophiles, platelets. Increased liver glycogen. Atrophy of muscles; osteoporosis
Metabolism	Increased RNA in target tissues. Protein, calcium, and potassium anabolism. Antagonizes estrogen action	Increased RNA in target tissues. Protein and calcium anabolism. Lowers blood lipids. Antagonizes androgen action	Inhibits anabolic effects of androgens	Protein catabolism. Enhances gluconeogenesis. Increased secretion of gastric acid and pepsinogen. Increased secretion of angiotensin, aldosterone. Antagonizes insulin and HGH. Stimulates erythropoiesis
Whole Organism	Masculinization. Growth spurt (prepubertal). Increased tissue mass. Sodium and water retention	Feminization. Loss of libido (males). Sodium and water retention Nausea	Sodium and water retention (large doses)	Sodium and water retention. Hypertension. Antiinflammatory. Immunosuppression
Antitumor Mechanisms	Directly on tumor cells; nuclear functions. Anterior pituitary suppression Antiestrogenic effect (?)	Direct effect on tumor cells; nuclear functions. Anterior pituitary suppression	Effects on tumor unclear. Anterior pituitary suppression	Effect on tumor cells. Decreased glucose uptake

laris and the zona fasiculata and are accompanied by an impairment of 17-hydroxycorticosteroid synthesis. There is some evidence that mitotane inhibits enzymes important to steroid hormone production in the adrenal gland and enzymes responsible for the transformation of steroids in tissues as well. The clinical use of mitotane is limited primarily by skin eruptions, gastrointestinal intolerance and mental derangements.

L-Asparaginase is an enzyme prepared from *E. coli* or other microorganisms. Tumor cells lacking the capacity to synthesize asparagine are uniquely susceptible to this experimental agent. However, many soon become refractory through the induction of the enzyme asparagine synthetase. The administration of L-asparaginase is limited by fever (endotoxin), chills, coagulation defects, hepatotoxicity, and pancreatitis.

STEROID HORMONES

The steroid hormones of clinical importance in the treatment of neoplastic disease are androgens, estrogens, corticosteroids, and progestational agents. A simple description of the metabolic basis of steroid-hormone-induced effects is not warranted.

There is a complex relationship between the end organs or tumors, pituitary trophic hormones, and the steroids, which is further complicated by the interconversion of steroid hormones in vivo.

The biologic effects of androgens, estrogens, progestins, and adrenal corticosteroids are summarized in Table 54–3. These hormones alter the morphology of responsive tumors, but the precise biochemical effect responsible for their tumor-controlling properties or their relatively tissue-specific action is not a matter of general agreement.

During the past four years, much has been learned about the sequence of events which relate to the binding of a steroid hormone to a target cell and the biologic effects which result. For example, there are specific estrogen-binding proteins or estrogen receptors in estrogen-responsive cells. When the combined hormone and receptor protein enter the nucleus, specific stimulation of RNA polymerase and nucleic acid synthesis results. The resulting protein synthesis, etc. enables the cell to fully "respond to estrogen." It is believed that similar mechanisms may be involved with other steroid hormones and their tissue responses.[36]

Satisfactory oral and parenteral forms of these hormonal agents exist. To a large extent they are metabolized by the liver and the breakdown products eliminated in the urine and bile. Several of the listed tissue or metabolic effects of these hormones constitute their limiting toxicity clinically. On the other hand, certain of these effects, such as those of the corticosteroids on thrombocytopenic bleeding, hemolytic anemia, and calcium metabolism, are employed to advantage in the supportive care of patients.

Nafoxidine and tamoxifen have been introduced into clinical use relatively recently because of their antiestrogenic properties. It appears that these compounds block the effects of estrogens at the cellular level. For example, studies of tamoxifen in the rat uterus indicated that the drug binds with cytoplasmic estrogen receptors and translocates into the nucleus where it seems to stimulate some "early" estrogen responses but inhibit markedly the "late" actions of estrogen. (Nafoxidine frequently induces troublesome photosensitivity and ichthyosis which will likely limit its clinical use.)

SYSTEMIC THERAPY: SPECIFIC INDICATIONS AND RESULTS

The general indications for the systemic treatment of neoplastic diseases have been discussed previously. Specific therapeutic indications are summarized here in relation to disease entities. Approximations of therapeutic usefulness are indicated by the frequency with which a neoplasm responds in relation to the cost in toxicity (Table 54–4).

A response is defined chiefly in terms of the objective clinical abnormalities that described the disease state at the beginning of therapy. For example, a (complete) response in acute leukemia implies a reversion to normal of the peripheral blood and marrow findings, as well as a resolution of all related symptomatology. In solid tumors, response implies a resolution of symptomatology and a decrease in tumor size or number by at least 50 percent without any evidence of disease progression. It must be pointed out, however, that the interpretation of clinical reports is difficult due to varied patient selection, response criteria, and other factors.

CHEMOTHERAPY

During the past few years it has become apparent that the use of cancer chemotherapeutic agents in combination may potentiate their effect on tumor cells. Drugs with differing mechanisms of action may be given simultaneously or in sequence with good effect. Combination chemotherapy is bearable because the adverse (toxic) effects of the drugs can, in some cases, be distributed over several tissues and yet not summate to severe intensity. Thus, the overall thera-

---

TABLE 54–4

Clinical Results of Systemic Chemotherapy in Common Disseminated Cancers

Potential Cure	Extended Survival	Useful Responses	Refractory
Acute lymphoblastic leukemia	Acute myeloblastic leukemia	Breast cancer	Bladder cancer
Hodgkin's disease	Chronic granulocytic leukemia	Osteogenic sarcoma	Bronchogenic cancer
Histiocytic lymphoma	Lymphocytic lymphoma	Colon cancer	Esophageal cancer
Burkitt's tumor	Plasma cell dyscrasias	Prostate cancer	Hepatic cancer
Trophoblastic tumors	Chronic lymphocytic leukemia	Endometrial cancer	Pancreatic cancer
Testis tumors	Lung: small cell cancer	Thyroid cancer	Stomach cancer
Ewing's sarcoma	Ovarian cancer	Adrenal cortical cancer	Renal cancer
Rhabdomyosarcoma	Soft tissue sarcomas	Head and neck cancer	Uterine cervix cancer
Wilm's tumor	Neuroblastoma		Melanoma
Retinoblastoma	Thyroid: follicular cancer		

peutic outcome is much improved (Tables 54–5, 54–6).

In many instances, more effective control of the tumor can be achieved by intermittent, intense courses of drug treatment spaced at intervals to permit recovery from toxicity. The success of this technique requires excellent supportive patient care.

Leukemia[9,49,50]

All types of acute leukemia are rapidly progressive and demand prompt treatment. Prolongation of useful life bears a direct relationship to the length of drug-induced disease remission (Table 54–5).

Acute lymphocytic leukemia, predominantly a disease of childhood, will respond (complete re-

---

TABLE 54–5
Expected Results of Initial Chemotherapy in Responsive Neoplasms

Neoplasm	Drugs in Combination	Expected Results	Comment
Leukemia			
Acute lymphoblastic	Prednisone Vincristine Daunorubicin	Complete remission in 90–95% of patients <age 15	"Prophylactic therapy" for meningeal leukemia "Maintenance therapy" for ~ 3 years 50% disease-free remissions >5 years
Acute myeloblastic	Daunorubicin Arabinosyl cytosine 6-Thioguanine	Complete remission in 50–60% of patients <age 65	Value of meningeal and maintenance therapy is uncertain Median disease-free remissions ~ 2 years
Chronic lymphocytic	Chlorambucil	Partial remission in 50–70% of cases	Disease often indolent Remissions maintained by continued therapy for 2–3 years
Chronic granulocytic	Busulfan	Partial remission in >95% of cases	Remissions maintained by continued therapy for 3–5 years
Lymphoma			
Hodgkin's disease (Stage III and IV)	Mechlorethamine Cyclophosphamide Vincristine Procarbazine Prednisone	Complete remission in 80% of cases	Radiation therapy to bulky tumors Continued therapy for 1 year 30–60% disease-free remissions >5 years
Lymphocytic (Stage III and IV)	As in Hodgkin's disease	Complete remission in 50–80% of cases	Radiation therapy to bulky tumors Continued therapy for 1 year 20–40% disease-free remissions >5 years Well-differentiated lymphoma often indolent
Histiocytic (Stage III and IV)	As in Hodgkin's disease	Complete remission in 30–80% of cases	Radiation therapy to bulky tumors Continued therapy for 1 year 25–45% disease-free remissions >5 years
Plasma Cell Dyscrasias			
Myeloma	Cyclophosphamide Prednisone Melphalan	Partial remission in 25–30% of cases	Remissions maintained by continued therapy for 1–2 years Radiation therapy to mass lesions

TABLE 54-6

Expected Results of Initial Chemotherapy in Responsive Neoplasms

Neoplasm	Drugs in Combination	Expected Results	Comment
Lung cancer: small cell	Cyclophosphamide Adriamycin Vincristine Nitrosourea	Complete remission in 20–30% of cases	Radiation therapy to bulky tumors Median remission duration >2 years
Breast cancer	Cyclophosphamide Methotrexate 5-Fluorouracil Adriamycin	Partial remission in 60–70% of cases	Radiation therapy to mass lesions Hormonal therapy useful in ER positive tumors ER negative tumors have higher growth fraction
Colon cancer	5-Fluorouracil Semustine Mitomycin C	Partial remission in 15–20% of cases	
Ovarian cancer	Cyclophosphamide Melphalan Adriamycin	Partial remission in 50–70% of cases	Surgery, radiotherapy for bulky tumor Some complete remission obtained with combination chemotherapy
Trophoblastic tumors	Methotrexate Dactinomycin	Complete remission in >95% of cases	Nearly all cases remain disease-free >5 years
Testis cancer	Cyclophosphamide Cis-platinum Bleomycin	Complete remission in 30–40% of cases	Remissions maintained by continued therapy for 1 to 2 years Many disease-free remissions >5 years
Wilm's tumor	Dactinomycin Vincristine	Complete remission in 80–90% of cases	Surgery, radiotherapy for bulky tumor 60–80% cases disease-free >5 years
Osteogenic sarcoma (localized)	Methotrexate Adriamycin	Surgery and chemotherapy yield ~ 50% disease-free survival >5 years	Chemotherapy maintained ~ 2 years Limb-preserving surgery possible
Ewing's sarcoma	Cyclophosphamide Adriamycin Vincristine	Radiotherapy and chemotherapy yield ~ 50% disease-free survival >5 years	Chemotherapy maintained ~ 2 years
Rhabdomyosarcoma	Adriamycin Cyclophosphamide Vincristine	Surgery, radiotherapy, chemotherapy yield ~ 50% survival at 5 years	Chemotherapy maintained 1–2 years
Neuroblastoma	Cyclophosphamide Adriamycin Vincristine	Complete remission in 30–50% of cases	Surgery, radiotherapy for bulky tumor 20–25% of cases disease-free at 5 years

sponse) to a number of drugs used singly—prednisone (55 percent), vincristine (50 percent), 6-mercaptopurine (35 percent), methotrexate (20 percent), arabinosyl cytosine (20 percent), and cyclophosphamide (20 percent). More effective remission induction (~90 percent) can be achieved by using prednisone in combination with vincristine, 6-mercaptopurine, or methotrexate.

At present, patients should be treated promptly on diagnosis with a multidrug "remission induction" regimen (e.g., vincristine and prednisone) which includes prophylactic therapy for meningeal leukemia. Once a complete remission is achieved, prolonged "remission maintenance" or "consolidation" therapy is undertaken using multiple drugs intermittently in a planned sequence. It is to be expected that 50 percent or more of individuals on maintenance therapy will be alive at 5 years and free of evident leukemia.

Acute granulocytic leukemia, encountered most frequently in adults, is more refractory to treatment. The frequency of remission induction with single drugs is low—6-mercaptopurine (20 percent), arabinosyl cytosine (20 to 30 percent), and methotrexate (10 percent). Cyclophosphamide is not effective at the usual dose levels, but can induce complete remissions when given in high doses on an intermittent schedule.

Combination chemotherapy is clearly superior in inducing complete remissions in acute granulocytic leukemia. The drugs used in the most effective combinations include daunorubicin, arabinosyl cytosine, and 6-thioguanine. Remission induction rates of 50 percent or more are to be expected in patients not previously treated. In contrast to acute lymphoblastic leukemia, median disease-free remission periods in excess of 2 years can be obtained without continued maintenance therapy.[30]

Preleukemia (Chap. 55) represents a special case in that the disease process may remain static for prolonged periods (smoldering leukemia). The decision to begin multiagent chemotherapy is usually based on evidence of progressive marrow failure (especially thrombocytopenia and granulocytopenia) and progressive leukemia cell proliferation. The chronic leukemias, especially chronic lymphocytic leukemia, may pursue an indolent course for months or years. Since there is no evidence that prompt and aggressive therapy achieves superior long-term results, treatment is initiated only when the disease is progressing.

Busulfan will induce excellent and prolonged (years) partial remissions in nearly all patients (>95 percent) with chronic myelocytic leukemia. Splenic irradiation will achieve similar results, but it is generally more difficult to maintain satisfactory remission status without rather wide swings in disease activity. Hydroxyurea and 6-mercaptopurine may be used to control disease manifestations, also.

Chlorambucil, cyclophosphamide, and other alkylating agents can bring about prolonged partial remissions in 60 to 70 percent of patients with chronic lymphatic leukemia. Prednisone is also effective and is especially helpful in the management of hemolytic anemia, thrombopenic bleeding, and hypercalcemia. Combination chemotherapy to date, has not yielded superior treatment results.

Lymphoma[9,49,50]

Advanced stage lymphoma is usually a progressive disorder at the time of diagnosis and this makes treatment mandatory. It is important to achieve the best remission status possible since patients entering complete remission early in their course have a better prognosis (Table 54–5).

Several agents given singly for 6 to 8 weeks will achieve remissions in 60 to 80 percent of patients with Hodgkin's disease (10 to 20 percent complete remissions). Among the most efficacious drugs are mechlorethamine, cyclophosphamide, vinblastine, and procarbazine. Prednisone will cause prompt tumor lysis to 25 to 30 percent of cases, and is most helpful in the management of certain systemic disorders such as hypercalcemia, thrombocytopenic bleeding, hemolytic anemia, and marked pyrexia.

Clearly, combination chemotherapy is superior and is preferred in the initial management of all patients with advanced stage lymphoma. For example, when patients with Hodgkin's disease are treated with courses of mechlorethamine, vincristine, procarbazine, and prednisone over a 6-month period, about 80 percent will enter complete remission and 60 percent will remain disease-free for 5 years or more. The results in lymphocytic lymphoma and histiocytic lymphoma are similar, but the proportion of patients apparently freed of their disease is somewhat less (Chap. 51).

The results of cyclophosphamide therapy in Burkitt's lymphoma are of great interest. Most patients enter complete remission following relatively short courses of single drug treatment. More than half of these patients can be expected to remain disease-free for prolonged periods encouraging the thought of cure. There is good evidence that heightened host immunity plays a role in this outcome.

Myeloma[7,9]

Plasma cell myeloma often pursues an indolent course and may not require treatment. Cyclophosphamide, melphalan, and prednisone given as single drugs over an 8- to 12-week period will induce disease remissions in 20 to 30 percent of patients (Table 54–5). (The serum concentrations of myeloma protein provide an excellent guide to therapy.) These remissions generally are not as satisfactory as those achieved in the chronic leukemias. The combined use of prednisone and one of the alkylating agents seems a superior treatment. Higher doses of cyclophosphamide given intermittently are also effective.

Trophoblastic and Germ Cell Tumors[4,7]

Choriocarcinoma is a rapidly progressive disease and should be treated promptly. (Chorionic gonadotropin titers are a helpful guide to treatment.) Experience has shown that 90 percent or more of patients will respond to methotrexate or dactinomycin (Table 54–6). About one-half will remain disease-free for 5 years or longer and appear cured. The use of these drugs together or in sequence has increased the cure rate to about 75 percent. Refractory choriocarcinoma will respond to combination chemotherapy (e.g., methotrexate, dactinomycin, chlorambucil) and regressions have been reported following treatment with daunomycin, adriamycin, and bleomycin. Metastatic hydatidiform mole is a less aggressive disease and nearly all patients (95 percent) can be cured with methotrexate or dactinomycin.

It is of some importance that complete disease control can be achieved without sacrificing the reproductive organs. Many post-treatment pregnancies have been carried to term successfully.

Prompt treatment of disseminated embryonal tumors of the testis with mithramycin or dactinomycin has produced remissions in one-third or more of individuals. A small fraction, perhaps 10 percent, has remained disease-free for 5 years or more. Combination chemotherapy (e.g., cyclophosphamide, vincristine, bleomycin, cis-platinum) is also effective.

Metastatic seminoma is quite responsive to alkylating agents, as are adenocarcinomas of the ovary. Meaningful remissions can be induced in 30 to 50 percent of cases with drugs such as mechlorethamine or cyclophosphamide. Vincristine has been helpful in some cases. Here again, combination chemotherapy seems more useful.

Childhood Tumors[7,8]

Acute lymphocytic leukemia and lymphocytic lymphoma are among the most common neoplasms encountered in childhood. They are best managed with combination chemotherapy and with radiation therapy (Chaps. 51 and 55). Hodgkin's disease is also managed similarly. It is important to begin treatment promptly in order to insure the best outcome. It may be expected that prolonged drug therapy will result in a retardation of linear growth.

Brain tumors in children are managed primarily by surgery and radiation therapy according to their cell type. The role of chemotherapeutic agents in their treatment is under investigation. The intrathecal installation of antimetabolites such as methotrexate and arabinosyl cytosine is useful in managing meningeal tumor and other superficial deposits. Vincristine and the nitrosoureas, given systemically, have produced regression of certain brain tumors. These leads are being explored, but it can be appreciated that the methodology for following the clinical effects of drugs on brain tumors is difficult.

Over the past several years the prognosis for Wilms' tumor has improved steadily (Table 54–6). In patients presenting with localized disease, surgical excision of the tumor should be followed by radiation therapy to the region and by prolonged, cyclic administration of dactinomycin. About 80 percent of such patients will be disease-free at 5 years. In patients presenting with metastatic disease or bilateral Wilms' tumor, surgery and radiation therapy are the best means of managing the large tumor masses, and courses of dactinomycin and vincristine are used to treat widespread disease. Complete remissions may be expected in two-thirds of the cases or more and about 40 percent will be alive and disease free 2 years later.

Neuroblastoma presents usually as a disseminated disease. Surgical excision and radiation therapy are used to manage local tumor masses. (Neuroblastoma is very radioresponsive.) Vincristine, cyclophosphamide, dactinomycin, and adriamycin when employed as single agents have induced remissions in 30 to 50 percent of patients treated for disseminated disease. There is a body of opinion which suggests that surgical excision of apparently localized neuroblastoma (Stages I, II, and III) should be followed by repeated courses of cyclophosphamide. More widely disseminated disease (Stage IV) with bony metastases seems best managed with multiagent chemotherapy and radiation therapy.

The outlook for osteogenic sarcoma has improved greatly. Amputation is usually recommended when the tumor is resectable and when there are no evident pulmonary metastases. Intermittent courses of high-dose methotrexate followed by citrovorum factor, have been given to patients following amputation. It would appear that such a combined approach has resulted in a 50 percent, 5-year, disease-free survival. High dose methotrexate-citrovorum factor and adriamycin cause regressions in some patients with metastatic osteogenic sarcoma when given as single agents. Combination chemotherapy seems more efficacious, although the outlook is poor.

Ewing's sarcoma may be difficult to distinguish from histiocytic lymphoma. It is a very radioresponsive tumor. The most successful plans of management employ radiation therapy to control the primary tumor mass and repeated courses of multiagent therapy to treat more widespread deposits (e.g., vincristine, adriamycin, and cyclophosphamide).

Similar therapeutic regimens have emerged for the soft tissue sarcomas, especially rhabdomyosarcoma. Surgical excision and radiation therapy are the best means of managing bulky tumor masses. Combination chemotherapy (e.g., vincristine, adriamycin, and cyclophosphamide) can then be given in short courses over a 1- to 2-year period. With this approach complete remissions have been achieved in 50 to 75 percent of patients who presented with metastatic disease and most patients remain disease-free for over 1 year.

Solid Tumors in Adults[4,7,8]

Although the overall results of drug treatment of the commonly occurring cancers of the breast, colon, bronchus, and other sites are not completely satisfactory, useful palliation can be obtained in selected patients (Table 54-6). The nature of the possible tumor response must be balanced carefully against potential toxicity.

In breast cancer, single agent chemotherapy seems useful when combined with surgical resection of limited stage disease (Chap. 55). Melphalan appears to reduce the risk of recurrent disease in premenopausal women who have tumor involvement of axillary nodes as does prolonged treatment with a combination of drugs. In patients with metastatic disease, multiagent chemotherapy has proven very useful, especially in managing individuals with progressive visceral organ involvement. For example, several large trials have revealed the efficacy of various drug combinations which include 5-flouroracil, methotrexate, vincristine, cyclophosphamide, and adriamycin given in short, intermittent courses over prolonged periods. Some 50 to 80 percent of cases respond with extensive tumor regression, and this status may be maintained for 8 to 10 months or more on the average. Thus, multiagent chemotherapy has replaced hormonal treatment as the initial modality in the management of rapidly progressive metastatic disease, especially in estrogen receptor negative tumors.[47]

Best results in the treatment of metastatic cancer of the rectum, colon, or stomach are achieved with 5-fluorouracil. Partial remissions of relatively short duration result in 15 to 20 percent of patients, especially those with less extensive tumor involvement of the parenchymal organs. It is curious that an S-phase specific drug (5-fluorouracil) should be the most active one against tumors with such a low proliferative (growth) fraction. Trials with combination chemotherapy in cancers of the gastrointestinal tract suggest that 5-fluorouracil, mitomycin-C, and the nitrosoureas used together in various ways do not improve clinical results very much.

Metastatic adrenal cortical cancer will respond satisfactorily to several weeks of mitotane therapy in 30 to 35 percent of cases. Gastrointestinal intolerance, muscle aches, mental derangement, skin rashes, etc., make long-term treatment difficult.

Bronchogenic cancer responds to alkylating agents with significant tumor shrinkage in only 10 to 15 percent of patients (Chap. 55). However, even minimal tumor shrinkage may be helpful in the management of airway obstruction or painful body deposits.

The results achieved in small cell cancer of the lung have improved remarkably in recent years (Chap. 55). Combination chemotherapy including such agents as adriamycin, cyclophosphamide, vincristine, a nitrosourea, and epipodophyllotoxin yields complete remissions in 20 to 30 percent of cases and partial responses in an additional 30 to 40 percent. The most successful programs employ radiation therapy in the management of bulky tumor masses. At present the median period of disease-free remission is about 2 years.[44,51]

Regional Chemotherapy

Topical applications of 5-fluorouracil or mechlorethamine have proven quite useful in the management of extensive squamous cell cancers of the skin and, in some instances, the lesions of mycosis fungoides. Alkylating agents instilled locally in high concentration are as efficacious as colloidal radioactive isotopes in the management of malignant effusions. The intrathecal administration of methotrexate or arabinosyl cytosine can control meningeal leukemia, and prophylactic injections seem to prevent the clinical emergence of this complication in children with acute lymphocytic leukemia. Regional perfusion or infusion therapy of a wide variety of tumors has been attempted with variable results. The best outcomes have followed the perfusion of extremities bearing melanomas or sarcomas.

HORMONAL THERAPY

Hormonal therapy is used primarily for metastatic tumors of the breast and prostate that retain a degree of responsiveness of endometrial cancer. Corticosteroids frequently induce remissions in acute lymphocytic leukemia and occasionally cause regressions of lymphomatous tumor masses and multiple myeloma. Thyroid hormone is used to suppress TSH secretion in patients following resection of their tumor and hence reduce the likelihood of recurrent tumor growth.[5,7,8]

The clinical usefulness of hormonal agents and endocrine ablative procedures in selected neoplastic diseases is indicated in Table 54-7. The availability of clinically useful techniques for the measurement of estrogen receptors, progesterone receptors, and receptors for other steroidal hormones has provided a reliable basis for guiding hormonal therapy. This is especially true in breast cancer where the presence or absence of estrogen receptors (ER) in each patient's

---
TABLE 54–7

Expected Results of Hormonal Therapy of Disseminated Neoplasms

Neoplasm	Therapy	Expected Result	Comment
Breast cancer (premenopausal, ER+)	Castration	Partial remission in 60–70% of cases	Estrogens will stimulate tumor growth
Breast cancer (postmenopausal, ER+)	Antiestrogen	Partial remission in 40–50% of cases	Adrenalectomy or hypophysectomy may yield a second remission in responsive patients
	Androgen	Partial remission in 30–40% of cases	
Breast cancer (ER−)		Rare response	Neither pre- nor postmenopausal patients are likely to respond
Prostate cancer	Estrogen	Symptomatic relief and some tumor regression ∼ 60% of cases	Well-differentiated tumors (acid phosphatase +) likely responsive
Endometrial cancer	Progestin	Partial remission in 25–30% of cases	
Thyroid cancer	Thyroid hormone	Suppression of recurrent tumor growth (well-differentiated tumors)	Thyroid hormone continued indefinitely after surgery to suppress TSH

---

tumor has become one of the prime determinants of the initial treatment prescribed for disseminated disease. For example, premenopausal patients with ER positive cancers are likely to be treated with ovariectomy and ER positive, postmenopausal patients with an antiestrogen unless they have rapidly progressing disease with visceral organ involvement. There seems to be no value to "prophylactic castration" for the prevention or recurrence of breast cancer following primary curative resection. Adrenalectomy and hypophysectomy are helpful in the secondary management of patients with hormone responsive breast cancers, but a precise summary statement is hard to formulate.[47]

IMMUNOTHERAPY

Clinical cancer immunotherapy is in its infancy.[15,35] Many promising leads have been developed in animal models and limited human studies. However, the controlled therapeutic trials completed to date are insufficient to define precise recommendations for clinical practice.

It would appear ideal to immunize patients against their tumor when their tumor cell population is at its lowest ebb and their capacity for immunoresponsiveness is least impaired (e.g., following a potentially curative resection of breast cancer or on induction of a complete remission in acute lymphocytic leukemia). For example, Mathé et al. have reported that remissions lasted longer in patients immunized with BCG, formalinized or irradiated "autologous" acute leukemic cells, or a mixture of both, than in those not immunized. However, a similar trial shows no advantage to immunization.

Numerous attempts have been made to heighten effective tumor immunity by means of nonspecific stimulants such as *Corynebacterium parvum*, BCG, or dinitrochlorobenzene (DNCB). Clinical results are not clear, but early experiences indicate that BCG therapy may be of some use in the management of malignant melanoma and local recurrences of breast cancer and that DNCB treatment has produced good results in squamous cell and basal cell cancers of the skin.

Studies of active, passive, adoptive, and nonspecific immunotherapy in patients doubtless will become more informative in the future. Further, laboratory studies such as those in Marek's disease (a herpes virus-caused tumor in fowl) are providing a conceptual basis for prophylactic immunization trials in man.

CHAPTER 55

Illustrative Neoplastic Diseases
ALBERT H. OWENS, Jr.

A description of the leukemias and bronchogenic and breast cancer will serve to illustrate several of the biologic phenomena and principles of therapeutic management reviewed in preceding chapters. The manner in which these disorders may come to the physician's attention will be considered, the major factors involved in the diagnostic evaluation indicated, and the expected clinical course and chief considerations in treatment presented.

These neoplasms may be contrasted with respect to known causal factors or predisposing conditions. Genetic factors are related to the development of some cases of acute leukemia (mongolism), chronic lymphocytic leukemia, and breast cancer. Ionizing radiation and chemicals which damage chromosomes have been causally related to some instances of leukemia and bronchogenic cancer. Some evidence for viral etiology has accumulated in leukemia and breast cancer.

Aside from their varying sites of origin, these neoplasms represent varying cell types. The leukemias are defined by the proliferation of mature or immature lymphoid or granulocytic cells and monocytes. One-half of bronchogenic cancers are of squamous cell type, one-third are undifferentiated, and the remainder are adenocarcinomas. Breast cancers are mostly adenocarcinomas of a reasonably differentiated type.

The leukemias present as disseminated neoplasms with principally systemic symptoms. Breast cancer frequently is confined to an area near its point of origin and becomes symptomatic because of obstruction to regional lymphatics or involvement of the overlying skin. Bronchogenic tumors are intermediate in nature in that more than two-thirds of the patients present with disease too extensive for complete surgical resection. Initial symptoms may be related to the local tumor mass, metastatic lesions, or systemic abnormalities evoked by physiologically active tumor-secreted substances.

The primary curative treatment for breast and bronchogenic cancer is surgical resection or radiation therapy. Two-thirds or more of patients with localized breast cancer are alive after 5 years, but only 20 percent of those with resectable bronchogenic cancer. Irradiation is a major palliative modality in bronchogenic cancer, breast cancer, and the chronic leukemias but is of little utility in acute leukemia.

Multiagent chemotherapy and general supportive care have improved the outlook in the leukemias and in breast cancer. The results of combination chemotherapy in bronchogenic cancer are less satisfactory.

These clinical characteristics and therapeutic considerations are summarized in Table 55–1.

THE LEUKEMIAS

The leukemias are neoplastic disorders of hematopoietic tissues which are disseminated in their earliest recognizable stages. Large numbers of abnormal leukocytes are usually present in the peripheral blood, bone marrow, and lymphoreticular tissues. Actually, as the disorders progress, leukemic infiltrates may involve every organ system or tissue in the body.

The leukemias are commonly classified according to their clinical course and the predominant abnormal cell type (Table 55–2). Acute leukemia is usually abrupt in onset, and the prognosis of untreated cases is very poor. Over 90 percent of untreated patients die within 6 months.

Acute leukemia is categorized further as lymphocytic or granulocytic. At times the predominant abnormal cell type in acute leukemia in children is so primitive in appearance that the terms stem cell or undifferentiated cell leukemia are used. However, most authorities consider the term acute lymphocytic leukemia to include these variants.

Acute granulocytic leukemia occurs more commonly in adults. Acute myelomonocytic leukemia (Naegli) is a variety of acute granulocytic leukemia in which monocytes and their precursors appear to arise from abnormal marrow myeloblasts. Acute monocytic leukemia (Schilling) is recognized also, but the frequency with which this diagnosis is made varies greatly from one institution to another.

Preleukemia is a term used to describe patients who present with indications of marrow failure, but in whom clear-cut morphologic evidence of acute leukemia may not emerge for several months or years. Erythroleukemia is a term applied to patients with acute (granulocytic) leukemia in which there is a great deal of abnormal erythroid hyperplasia (Chap. 50).

The chronic leukemias are usually more gradual

TABLE 55-1
Contrasting Clinical Characteristics of Illustrative Neoplasms

	Acute Leukemia	Chronic Granulocytic Leukemia	Chronic Lymphocytic Leukemia	Bronchogenic Carcinoma	Breast Cancer
Causal factors	Ionizing radiation Chemicals Chromosomal abnormalities Virus?	Ionizing radiation Chemicals	Genetic	Cigarette smoke Asbestos Metals Chromate Ionizing radiations	Genetic factors Virus?
Cell types	Myeloblast Lymphoblast Monoblast	Granulocytes	Lymphocytes	Squamous cell Small cell Adenocarcinoma Large cell	Adenocarcinoma
Clinical presentation	Abrupt onset Systemic disorder Multisystem findings due to cell infiltrates and marrow failure	Slow onset Systemic disorder Multisystem findings due to cell infiltrates and marrow failure	Slow onset Systemic disorder Multisystem findings due to cell infiltrates, marrow failure, and immuno-incompetence	Intermediate onset (months) Findings due to mass lesion in chest or distant spread Physiologic abnormalities due to ectopic hormonal secretion	Slow onset Findings due to mass lesion in breast or regional nodes
Expected course	Rapid progression (months)	Slow progression (years) Huge splenomegaly, later anemia and bleeding	Slow progression (years) Adenopathy, anemia, progressive immune deficiency	Rapid progression (months)	Slow progression (years)
Treatments	Drugs induce frequent complete remissions. Hemorrhage, anemia, infection main problems demanding supportive care. Drug resistance develops (months). Sites inaccessible to drugs (CNS)	Drugs and radiation therapy equally effective (years). Preterminal blastic phase	Drugs, supportive care, and radiation therapy useful (years)	Curative resection less than one-third cases; their 5-yr survival, 20%. Death due to distant spread. Radiation therapy main palliation	Curative resection possible in 50 to 60% of cases; 5-yr survival >60% Chemotherapy improves prognosis in mastectomy patients with positive nodes Radiation therapy and multiagent chemotherapy useful

TABLE 55-2
Clinical Characteristics of the Leukemias

Leukemia	Occurrence	Cell Type	Course
Acute lymphocytic	Most common in children	Lymphoblast Stem cell or undifferentiated cell	Abrupt onset Prognosis 4 to 5 months untreated
Acute granulocytic	More common in adults	Myeloblast	Abrupt onset Prognosis 3 to 4 months untreated
Myelomonocytic		Monocytes and promonocytes present with myeloblasts	
Monocytic		"Pure" monocytic infiltrates	
Erythroleukemia		Erythroblasts in blood and marrow along with myeloblasts	Eventually myeloblasts predominate. Course similar to AGL
Chronic lymphocytic	Increasing incidence after age 45 Twice as common in males	Mature lymphocyte	Insidious onset Slow, variable progression Prognosis 4 to 5 years untreated
Chronic granulocytic	Peak incidence second to fourth decades	Mature and immature granulocytes Philadelphia chromosome	Insidious onset Prognosis 2 to 4 years

in onset and the prognosis of patients who receive no specific treatment is measured in years. Chronic lymphocytic leukemia is recognized by the large number of mature lymphocytes which circulate in the blood and infiltrate the bone marrow and lymphoreticular tissues. Chronic granulocytic leukemia is recognized by the abundance of mature and immature granulocytes which are usually present in the blood and bone marrow but may occasionally accumulate in peripheral tissues (chloroma).

ACUTE LEUKEMIA

Etiology[9,26]

Genetic and environmental factors have been linked to the occurrence of acute leukemia. If one of a pair of identical twins develops acute leukemia, the risk of the other twin developing leukemia is severalfold greater than a similar sequence in fraternal twins or siblings living together in the same household. Individuals with certain chromosomal abnormalities are predisposed to acute leukemia, e.g., Down syndrome (Trisomy-21), Bloom syndrome, Fanconi's aplastic anemia, and ataxia-telangiectasis. Certain environmental factors which damage chromosomes also increase the risk of acute leukemia, e.g., ionizing radiation and chemicals such as benzene, and alkylating agents. An increased incidence of acute leukemia has been noted following whole body exposure to ionizing radiation (atomic bomb, ^{131}I, ^{32}P) and regional irradiation (ankylosing spondylitis treatment).

In several animal species, including sub-human primates, it is clear that viruses cause acute leukemia. C-type particles, morphologically similar to known RNA tumor viruses, have been found in blood and tissue specimens from patients. Further, RNA-tumor-virus-like, RNA-dependent, DNA polymerase, and genetic DNA sequences complementary to RNA tumor virus, and RNA tumor virus-related antigens have been demonstrated in leukemic cells.

A provocative series of events has been reported in patients with acute leukemia who have had their hematopoietic and immune system replaced by means of bone marrow transplantation from HL-A identical siblings of different sex. Briefly stated, acute leukemia recurred, in one case as early as 60 days following transplantation, but only in donor-type cells. This outcome is compatible with virus causation. A few clinical studies have indicated the existence in healthy family members of immunity (cellular and humoral) to leukemia-associated antigens of patients. These findings are also compatible with an infectious etiology.

Studies in animal models indicate that an interaction between genetic and environmental factors is required in the pathogenesis of acute leukemia. A similar multifactorial etiology may underly the disease in humans.

---TABLE 55-3---
Clinical Manifestations of the Leukemias

I. Findings Suggestive of Infectious Disease

The fever, headache, malaise, and increasing
prostration associated with the pharyngeal lesions or
lymphadenopathy or bone lesions suggest a variety of
infectious ills

These findings more common in acute leukemia and
occasionally confused with acute viral illnesses,
mononucleosis, tuberculosis, drug reactions, or
collagen vascular disease

II. Skin and Mucous Membrane Manifestations

These include specific leukemic skin infiltrates as well
as nonspecific erythema, exfoliation, vesicle
formation, and lesions due to pyogenic infection and
hemorrhagic diathesis

Skin infiltrates are found more frequently in chronic
lymphocytic, granulocytic, and monocytic leukemia

Petechial lesions and ecchymoses commonly seen in
mucous membranes

Sore throat, swollen, inflamed gums, and anorectal
inflammation commonly encountered in monocytic
leukemia

Pallor due to anemia common to all forms

Mild icterus seen on occasion due to increased red cell
destruction

III. Lymph Node Enlargement

Generalized lymphadenopathy is common in acute
leukemia but less conspicuous than in chronic
lymphocytic leukemia

IV. Findings Suggestive of Chest Disease

Thymic enlargement or other lymphoid tumor masses
infrequently cause presenting symptoms of acute
leukemia, more commonly in chronic lymphocytic
leukemia

Pain of bone lesions at times suggests lung or heart
disease (especially acute leukemia)

Palpitation, weakness due to anemia suggest heart
disease

V. Findings Suggestive of Abdominal Disorders

Splenomegaly prominent in the chronic leukemias;
present but less conspicuous in acute leukemia

Pain due to splenic infarction

Leukemic masses may involve all viscera,
retroperitoneal nodes, especially chronic lymphocytic
leukemia

VI. Findings Relative to Genitourinary Tract

Obstructive uropathy, flank pain, infection especially
chronic lymphocytic leukemia

Infrequent hematuria (hemorrhagic diathesis)

Kidney infiltrates common; symptoms and signs rare

Infiltrates in epididymis and seminal vesicles

VII. Findings Suggestive of Bone and Joint Disease

Bone pain and tenderness due to periosteal disease,
lytic lesions, pathologic fractures, and so forth

Rare chloroma in acute granulocytic leukemia

Acute arthritis due to periosteal disease, synovial
infiltrate or hemorrhage, especially acute leukemia

Rare secondary gout, especially chronic granulocytic
leukemia

---TABLE 55-3 (cont.)---

VIII. Findings Suggestive of Nervous System Disease

Meningeal infiltrates lead to nerve palsies, signs of
increased intracranial pressure

Diffuse central nervous system derangement due to
hemorrhagic diathesis, leukemic cell thrombi,
infiltrates, especially acute leukemia

Frequent retinal hemorrhage, infiltrate, especially acute
leukemia

Rare peripheral neuropathy

Clinical Manifestations

The symptoms of acute leukemia are generally abrupt
in onset and progressive in character. The clinical
manifestations may be related to the relentless proliferation of leukemic cells and their invasion into various tissues or to progressive failure of bone marrow
function (Table 55-3). Most frequently, these presenting complaints are associated with lymph node enlargement, marked anemia, hemorrhagic diathesis,
fever, and increasing prostration. However, it should
be remembered that leukemic infiltrates may develop
in any region of the body, and the early indications of
this illness may suggest diverse diseases of many organ systems.

The fever, prostration, anemia, and abnormal leukocytosis may mimic the symptoms of several infectious diseases, particularly mononucleosis, acute viral illnesses, disseminated tuberculosis, and fungal
diseases. They sometimes suggest the diagnosis of a
drug reaction or collagen-vascular disease. Infrequently, patients presenting with prominent joint and
bone complaints will be considered to have acute
rheumatic fever, sickle cell crisis, or even osteomyelitis. The true significance of the noninfiltrative,
nonhemorrhagic cutaneous lesions may not be
promptly appreciated.

The often protracted course of "preleukemia" deserves special comment.[9] At times the prominent feature is a refractory anemia, associated with aplasia of
the bone marrow. Recurrent skin lesions, particularly
apparent pyoderma or tinea barbae, as well as anorectal infections and inflammation of the gums and
pharynx, may precede the more characteristic leukemia stigmata. Splenomegaly or "hypersplenism" has
been a feature of preleukemia or "smoldering leukemia" in some cases. Paroxysmal nocturnal hemo-
globulinuria has been a preleukemic finding also.

Diagnosis[9]

The diagnosis of acute leukemia is substantiated
mainly by the findings of the blood and bone marrow
examinations. Among these are the characteristic im-

maturity of the leukocytes as well as their increased number, anemia with young red cells often present in the peripheral blood, and thrombocytopenia. Excessive numbers of the characteristic blast cells are found in the bone marrow. These criteria distinguish leukemia from the abnormal leukocytosis or leukemoid reactions seen with infectious diseases, drug reactions, metastatic (bone) solid tumors, diabetic coma, and eclampsia and following marked hemorrhage or hemolysis.

Course and Management

Acute leukemia is a rapidly progressive fatal illness. The chief problems in the care of these patients are hemorrhage, infection, anemia, and, less frequently, the consequences of enlarging leukemic tumor masses. Appropriate specific therapy should be instituted immediately (Chap. 54). Vigorous supportive care is also of prime importance, including red blood cell, platelet and granulocyte transfusion, antibiotic therapy, fluid and electrolyte replacement, and a protected environment (protective isolation).

ACUTE LYMPHOCYTIC LEUKEMIA.   Multiagent chemotherapy has improved the prognosis of acute lymphocytic leukemia in children dramatically. Formerly over 90 percent of (untreated) cases were dead within 6 months. Now over 90 percent of patients can be brought into complete remission with the expectation that about half of them can be kept disease-free for 5 years.[49,50]

A variety of agents employed singly are capable of inducing remissions in acute leukemia. Among them are prednisone, vincristine, daunorubricin, methotrexate, 6-mercaptopurine, arabinosyl cytosine, and cyclophosphamide. However, the therapeutic advantages of combination chemotherapy have been demonstrated clearly. Prednisone combined with vincristine will induce complete remissions in 80 to 90 percent of patients under 15 years of age. When daunorubricin, 6-mercaptopurine, or methotrexate are added to the vincristine and prednisone regimen, complete remissions can be induced regularly in over 90 percent of cases.

Continued treatment is necessary to maintain the patients' complete remission status. Various successful treatment regimens have been developed which employ several of the active antileukemic drugs in sequence at prescheduled intervals. Important too, is the prophylactic treatment for meningeal leukemia with intrathecal methotrexate or arabinosyl cytosine and radiation therapy to the skull and neuraxis. Most commonly used antileukemic drugs given systemically cannot achieve therapeutically effective concentrations in the meninges and cerebrospinal fluid.

Commonly, "maintenance treatment" regimens are continued for 3 years or more. One-half of the patients so treated may be expected to remain free of leukemia for 5 years or more.

In recent years, a subset of patients with T-cell acute lymphocytic leukemia has been identified. These patients are likely to present with mediastinal masses and high peripheral white (tumor) cell counts. Their disease is often aggressive and less responsive to combination chemotherapy.

ACUTE GRANULOCYTIC LEUKEMIA.   About one-half to two-thirds of adults with acute granulocytic leukemia can be brought into complete remission with multiagent chemotherapy.[9,31,50] Drugs are frequently combined in short intensive courses repeated at intervals sufficient to permit some recovery of normal marrow elements. The drugs used in the most effective combinations are arabinosyl cytosine, 6-thioguanine, and daunorubricin. Sequential regimens using daunorubricin and arabinosyl cytosine at intervals timed in relation to their cell-cycle specificity (Chap. 54) are equally effective.

The value of maintenance therapy in acute granulocytic leukemia has not been demonstrated clearly. Indeed, one recent report indicates that a median disease-free remission period in excess of 2 years can be achieved by a relatively short induction regimen without the need for maintenance therapy.[31] There are relatively few long-term disease-free survivors, although the number is growing.

Radiation therapy has a limited role in the management of acute leukemia. It can be used to good effect in treating meningeal leukemia and solid tumors (chloroma). Meningeal leukemia can also be managed very effectively by the intrathecal administration of methotrexate or arabinosyl cytosine.

CHRONIC GRANULOCYTIC LEUKEMIA

Etiology[9,26]

Present evidence indicates that chronic granulocytic leukemia is a monoclonal neoplastic disorder that results from an abnormality of hematopoietic stem cells. The Ph' chromosome, which is the hallmark of chronic granulocytic leukemia, has been demonstrated in granulocytes, megakaryocytes, and erythroid precursors. Further, in a few well-studied glucose-6-phosphate dehydrogenase heterozygotes with chronic granulocytic leukemia, the red cells and granulocytes contained only one enzyme type. While some studies indicate that multiple factors may cooperate in the leukemogenic process, it seems clear that ionizing irradiation and chemicals such as benzene can induce chronic granulocytic leukemia in man, probably by means of causing chromosomal damage in specific loci (chromosome 22).

Clinical Manifestations

The onset of chronic granulocytic leukemia is insidious. Patients with this disorder may remain asymptomatic for many months. Common presenting complaints are weight loss, low-grade fever, weakness, dyspnea, palpitations, pallor, splenomegaly, and evidence of a generalized bleeding tendency. These manifestations may be attributed to the continued slow proliferation of long-lived granulocytes and progressive bone marrow failure (Table 55–3). The abnormalities of granulocyte proliferation and survival often result in the accumulation of myeloid tissue 5 or 10 times larger than the normal total mass. Aside from the symptoms due to tissue infiltration and mass lesions, patients with a large number of tumor cells may show signs of hypermetabolism or develop gout due to prolonged hyperuricemia.

Diagnosis[9]

Chronic granulocytic leukemia is classified among the myeloproliferative disorders because of its clinical relationship to polycythemia vera and myeloid metaplasia. The blood picture characteristically encountered early in the illness shows an orderly shift to the left with a rare myeloblast, more numerous myelocytes and metamyelocytes, and a preponderance of segmented forms. The leukocyte count may be as high as 1,000,000/μl. Anemia is commonly absent, and the platelet count is often higher than normal. The hallmark of this disease is the foreshortened chromosome 22 (Philadelphia chromosome), most readily demonstrated in myeloid marrow cells. Marrow smears reveal excessive numbers of myeloid cells similar to those found in the blood. Their alkaline phosphatase activity is lower than normal. The serum concentrations of vitamin B_{12} and its binding protein are characteristically increased.

Chronic granulocytic leukemia must be distinguished from the other myeloproliferative disorders and the several conditions which may cause leukoerythroblastosis (Chap. 50).

Course and Management[9,49,50]

The course of chronic granulocytic leukemia is variable. Since the disease may remain relatively quiescent for prolonged periods, and since the goal of therapy is palliative, treatment is initiated when there is clear evidence of progression. The chief problems encountered in patients with progressive chronic granulocytic leukemia are related to the large spleen (and infarcts thereof), increasing anemia, hemorrhagic diathesis due to thrombocytopenia, increasing weight loss and debility, and, to a lesser extent, bone pain.

Primary therapeutic attention is directed toward reducing the mass of proliferating myeloid tissue. Busulfan can control the major manifestations of the disease in nearly all patients on initial treatment and for months or years thereafter (Chap. 54). Radiation therapy to the spleen will induce remissions similar to those caused by busulfan and may also be used to palliate the consequences of splenomegaly or the involvement of bone or other tissue. With proper management most patients will survive 5 years or more and enjoy good remission status.

The terminal events of this illness are commonly related to the evolution of an acute phase characterized by the rapid proliferation of immature aneuploid myeloid cells, progressive anemia, thrombocytopenia, and an overall picture which resembles that of acute leukemia. Hemorrhage and infection are common causes of death. The disease in this phase is resistant to therapy. Treatment with combinations of chemotherapeutic agents (e.g., prednisone, vincristine, and arabinosyl cytosine) on occassion produces a meaningful remission (Chap. 54).

CHRONIC LYMPHOCYTIC LEUKEMIA

Etiology[9,26]

There is little to suggest that ionizing radiations or chemicals which damage chromosomes result in chronic lymphocytic leukemia. More likely genetic factors play a role. Several reports of an unusually high incidence of lymphocytic leukemia and lymphoma in siblings and family members have been published. In some of these patients and families there is an apparent increased incidence of other neoplasms. In one interesting study, a distinctive chromosomal anomaly (Ch' chromosome) was noted in three siblings who developed chronic lymphocytic leukemia and other family members who did not. Recent studies characterize chronic lymphocytic leukemia as a monoclonal B-cell neoplasm.

Clinical Manifestations

As in the granulocytic form, the clinical manifestations of chronic lymphocytic leukemia evolve gradually. Since this is a disease of older age groups, it is not uncommon to observe it as an incidental illness.

In contrast to chronic granulocytic leukemia, the lymphocytic form frequently presents with painless, generalized lymphadenopathy. Splenomegaly is rarely of the magnitude encountered in the chronic granulocytic disorder. Anemia and bleeding tendencies are also seen (Table 55–3). The clinical manifestations of chronic lymphocytic leukemia may be re-

TABLE 55–4
Causes of Lymph Node Enlargement

Anatomic Site	Neoplastic	Non-Neoplastic

Generalized enlargement	Leukemia
	  Chronic lymphocytic, acute, chronic
	    granulocytic (acute phase)
	Lymphoreticular neoplasms
	  Hodgkin's disease, lymphocytic and
	    histiocytic lymphoma
		Acute infections
		  Bacterial, rickettsial, viral
		Chronic infections
		  Tuberculosis, syphilis, toxoplasmosis
		Hypersensitivity states
		  Serum sickness, drug reactions
		Collagen-vascular disorders
		  Systemic lupus erythematosus,
		    rheumatoid arthritis
		Endocrine metabolic disorders,
		  hyperthyroidism,
		    hypoadrenocorticism,
		    hypopituitarism

Cervical nodes	Lymphoreticular neoplasms
	Metastatic neoplasms
	  Nasopharynx, oral cavity, pharynx,
	    thyroid
		Acute infections (as above)
		Chronic infections
		Tuberculosis, fungus
		Sarcoid

Supraclavicular nodes	Lymphoreticular neoplasms
	Metastatic neoplasms
	  Bronchus, breast, stomach,
	    esophagus, pancreas, colon,
	    genitalia
		Acute infections (as above)
		Chronic infections
		  Greater incidence reflecting
		    intrathoracic tuberculosis, fungus
		    diseases
		Sarcoid

Axillary nodes	Lymphoreticular neoplasms
	Metastatic neoplasms
	  Breast, rarely from bronchus
		Acute infections
		  Streptococcus, staphylococcus,
		  P. tularensis, cat-scratch disease

Mediastinal nodes	Lymphoreticular neoplasms
	Metastatic neoplasms
	  Bronchus, breast, stomach, pancreas,
	    colon, genitalia
		Acute infections
		  Pneumonia, lung abscess, viscus
		    perforation
		Sporotrichosis
		Chronic infections
		  Tuberculosis, fungus
		Sarcoid
		Erythema nodosum

Retroperitoneal nodes	Lymphoreticular neoplasms
	Metastatic neoplasms
	  Stomach, pancreas, colon, genitalia
		Acute Infections
		  Salmonella (other enteric fevers),
		    viscus ulceration and/or
		    perforation, abdominal abscess
		Chronic infections
		  Tuberculosis, fungus

Inguinal nodes	Lymphoreticular neoplasms
	Metastatic neoplasms
	  Genitalia, rectum
		Acute infections
		  Streptococcus, staphylococcus
		Venereal infections
		  Syphilis, lymphopathia venereum,
		    granuloma inguinale

All sites	Congenital anomalies Lymphangioma, cystic hygroma	

lated to the proliferation and accumulation of long-lived, immunologically-inert lymphocytes, progressive bone marrow failure, and increasing immunologic unresponsiveness (humoral immunity).

The clinical phenomenon of lymph node enlargement deserves special comment. Lymphoid tissue is responsive to many stimuli and participates in many regional or systemic diseases. Infections of all types, hypersensitivity states, collagen-vascular disorders, and thyrotoxicosis can produce regional or generalized lymphadenopathy. Some of these diseases can also produce transient abnormal blood lymphocytosis. Primary and metastatic neoplastic diseases also commonly involve the lymph nodes.

Neoplastic and nonneoplastic causes of lymph node enlargement are summarized in Table 55–4. It is often difficult to establish the cause of clinically significant lymphadenopathy, particularly at one point in time. The accurate pathologic interpretation of lymph node biopsy material demands an experienced pathologist and careful correlation with all available clinical data. A nonspecific clinical syndrome with nonspecific morphologic lymph node abnormalities may resolve completely or may develop into one of the lymphomatous neoplasms. On occasion, the neoplastic nature of the lymph node abnormality is appreciated correctly, but its precise classification is not possible. A patient with an undifferentiated malignant tumor may prove to have a lymphomatous disease on further study. Similarly, an abnormal cervical lymph node initially classified as lymphoma or histiocytic lymphoma may prove to be a metastatic deposit from an occult undifferentiated nasopharyngeal or bronchogenic primary neoplasm. Or the initial impression of neoplasia may prove incorrect and the lymph node alterations found to be part of a disorder such as systemic lupus erythematosus.

Clinically significant enlargement of the spleen also merits special attention. The spleen is part of the lymphoid organ of the body, and many of the comments made concerning the causes of lymph node enlargement are pertinent to splenomegaly. In contrast to the regional lymph nodes, the spleen is rarely involved with metastatic neoplasia. Involvement with primary lymphoid neoplasms is relatively common. The most frequent causes of splenomegaly are summarized in Table 55–5.

The pathologic interpretation of altered splenic morphology may be difficult. On occasion, a spleen several times its normal size fails to yield a pathognomonic histologic abnormality on comprehensive microscopic examination. Not infrequently, patients with classic manifestations of Hodgkin's disease or lymphocytic lymphoma have had enlarged spleens re-

---

TABLE 55–5
Causes of Splenomegaly

Neoplastic

Primary lymphoreticular neoplasms
  Hodgkin's disease, lymphocytic lymphoma, histiocytic lymphoma, chronic and acute lymphocytic leukemia, monocytic leukemia
Primary hematopoietic neoplasms
  Acute granulocytic leukemia, myeloproliferative disorders (chronic granulocytic leukemia, myeloid metaplasia, polycythemia vera)
Metastatic neoplasms (rare)
  Breast, melanoma, chorionepithelioma

Non-Neoplastic

Acute infections
  Bacterial, rickettsial, viral
Chronic infections
  Bacterial (brucellosis, subacute bacterial endocarditis), tuberculosis, fungal, spirochetal, protozoan
Sarcoidosis
Hypersensitivity states
  Serum sickness, drug reaction
Collagen vascular disorders
  Systemic lupus erythematosus, rheumatoid arthritis (Still's disease, Felty's syndrome)
Endocrine-metabolic disorders
  Hyperthyroidism, lipoid storage disorders (Gaucher's disease, Niemann-Pick disease)
Hematologic disorders
  Pernicious anemia, Cooley's anemia, iron deficiency anemia, congenital and acquired hemolytic anemias, thrombocytopenic purpura
Congestive splenomegaly
  Portal or splenic vein thrombosis, cirrhosis of liver
Cystic lesions
  Lymphangioma, hemangioma, post-traumatic

---

moved earlier in their courses with inconclusive pathologic descriptions after microscopic study. The appreciation of altered splenic morphology as it relates to the clinical evaluation of lymphoid neoplasms is limited by the infrequency or impossibility of serial studies.

Diagnosis[9]

The diagnosis of chronic lymphocytic leukemia is at times somewhat arbitrary. This entity is near one end of a spectrum which includes lymphocytic lymphoma at the opposite extreme. A monotonous small cell lymphocytosis is present in the blood; counts range from near normal to 400,000 to 500,000/μl. Similar cells characteristically involve the bone marrow and lymph nodes. Anemia and thrombocytopenia develop as the disorder progresses.

Course and Management[9,50]

Chronic lymphocytic leukemia may remain indolent for months or years and require no particular therapeutic attention. When progressive, the major management problems stem from progressive increase in the size of lymph nodes and lymphoid tumor masses, a progressive anemia that may have a significant hemolytic component, a bleeding diathesis associated with thrombocytopenia, or infectious diseases attendant on hypogammaglobulinemia and other results of an acquired immunologic deficiency state. The most suitable therapeutic program will, therefore, combine pertinent elements of supportive and specific treatment.

Alkylating agents (chlorambucil, cyclophosphamide) given for 4 to 8 weeks or more will induce good partial remissions in 60 to 70 percent of the patients. Prednisone will show an antitumor effect in about 50 percent. Combination chemotherapy with drugs such as cyclophosphamide, vincristine, and prednisone have not proven superior. Adrenal corticosteroids are used frequently to suppress immune hemolysis, bleeding tendencies due to thrombocytopenia, or hypercalcemia. Ionizing radiations may induce a marked resolution of lymphoid tumor masses.

The course of chronic lymphocytic leukemia usually extends over a period of five years or longer. One-third of cases are alive at 10 years after diagnosis. It is less common to observe a preterminal acute phase of this disorder than in chronic granulocytic leukemia. Death frequently results from an infectious disease, bleeding, the sequelae of severe anemia, or an unrelated disease.

BRONCHOGENIC CARCINOMA

Bronchogenic carcinoma is a malignant neoplastic disorder which arises from bronchial epithelial structures. The majority of these cancers are squamous cell or epidermoid in type (over half), and about one-fifth are adenocarcinomas. The remaining cell types include large cell (giant cell, clear cell) cancers and small cell (oat cell, anaplastic) cancers. It seems likely that small cell cancers are distinct from the other types biologically and they appear to arise from nonepithelial cells of neuroectodermal origin (APUD cells, Chap. 53).

Bronchogenic carcinomas arise peripherally as well as centrally. Studies in humans and in animal models indicate that neoplasia is preceded by and associated with multifocal dysplastic and in situ lesions. This is especially true for squamous cell cancers. Similar pre-neoplastic changes are not usually associated with adenocarcinomas, many of which arise in peripheral locations.

Etiology[26]

Environmental agents are preeminent among the causal factors presently associated with bronchogenic cancer. These include cigarette smoke, asbestos, chemicals (chromate, coke oven gases, bis-chloromethyl ether, nickel) and ionizing irradiation (uranium ore). All are assimilated by inhalation.

Recent studies have indicated that genetic factors which relate to tissue repair or carcinogen metabolism may affect the carcinogenic process. For example, high concentrations of a carcinogen-activating enzyme (aryl hydrocarbon hydroxylase) in bronchial epithelium appears to be associated with an increased susceptibility to bronchogenic carcinoma.

During modern times the incidence of bronchogenic carcinoma has increased continuously. The incidence remains higher in men than in women, in cigarette smokers than nonsmokers, and greater in urban areas than rural settings. A few studies have shown that cessation of cigarette smoking has resulted in a decreasing incidence of cancer.

Clinical Manifestations[3,53]

Over 95 percent of patients with bronchogenic cancer are symptomatic when first seen. The modes of clinical presentation are varied and may be related to the primary tumor mass, symptomatic secondary deposits, or associated nonthoracic, nonneoplastic abnormalities. These syndromes are summarized in Table 55–6. Manifestations unrelated to the primary tumor frequently are the first to become apparent clinically. For example, approximately one-third of all bronchogenic cancers produce intracranial metastases, and 10 to 12 percent of these produce symptoms that precede those of the primary growth.

The primary tumor is generally visible on chest x-ray. It can be visualized by bronchoscopy in one half of the cases. Biopsy remains the major diagnostic method, tissue being obtained from the primary or a secondary growth. Sputum cytologic studies reveal malignant cells in about 90 percent of the cases when care is taken to obtain true sputum and minimize endobronchial infection. Technologic improvements such as the fiberoptic bronchoscope, tantalum dust bronchography, small brushes, and irrigation systems to obtain cytologic specimens from distal bronchopulmonary segments, and refinements in cytodiagno-

TABLE 55-6

Clinical Manifestations of Bronchogenic Carcinoma

I. Syndromes Related to Primary Tumor

Endobronchial tumor may cause cough, hemoptysis, wheezing respiration, segmental emphysema, segmental atelectasis, postobstructive pneumonitis (often repeated bouts), or abscess formation

Extension to pleura and chest wall may cause chest pain, dyspnea, serous or bloody effusion

Superior sulcus tumors may cause pain due to brachial plexus invasion, Horner syndrome due to disruption of cervical sympathetic chain, or vasomotor signs in the arm and hand

Mediastinal invasion may cause obstruction of vena cava, trachea and esophagus, recurrent laryngeal- and phrenic-nerve palsy, chylous effusion

II. Syndromes Related to Distant Metastases

Lymphatic and vascular dissemination occur early

Palpable tumor presents in supraclavicular nodes, liver, and skin

Bone metastases may cause pain, fractures, pressure on adjacent nerves

Central-nervous-system deposits may cause fits, paralysis, evidences of increased intracranial pressure

Replacement of adrenal cortex with tumor rarely causes clinical deficiency

III. Non-Neoplastic Syndromes

Cutaneous abnormalities include erythema multiforme (or similar bullous lesions) and dermatomyositis

Endocrine-metabolic abnormalities include hypercalcemia, hyperadrenocorticism, carcinoid syndrome, inappropriate antidiuretic hormone secretion, gynecomastia, gonadotropin production

Connective tissue disorders include pulmonary hypertrophic osteoarthropathy and clubbing of the digits

Neuromuscular disorders include various encephalomyeloneuropathies, especially cerebellar degeneration and peripheral neuropathy, multifocal leukoencephalopathy (rarely), myopathy, and the myasthenic syndrome

sis may enhance the screening of asymptomatic individuals and the pretreatment evaluation of suspected cases.

Diagnosis

There are certain practical difficulties involved in establishing the precise diagnosis of bronchogenic carcinoma because of the varied cell types involved and because some of the specimens obtained by bronchoscopy or needle aspiration are small and distorted. The recognition of the better differentiated tumors is relatively easy, but anaplastic lesions often provide difficulties which cannot be resolved even with electron microscopy. The recognition of precise cell types in sputum samples also have similar problems. Hopefully immunohistochemical techniques which identify tumor-associated cell markers may resolve some of these difficulties.

Intrathoracic tumors deserve special comment, because of their varied nature and to underscore the need for a thorough diagnostic evaluation. The varieties of tumors are summarized in Table 55–7. Each of these diagnostic possibilities carries a distinctive prognosis and often carries specific therapeutic implications. For example, tuberculous or pyogenic infection requires proper antibacterial chemotherapy and perhaps a surgical procedure. Even among the tumors, a precise knowledge of their type is needed, since thymoma, bronchogenic cancer, thyroid cancer, and lymphoma require different therapeutic approaches.

Course and Management[54]

The course of bronchogenic carcinoma is surprisingly short with the exception of well-treated small cell cancer. Although it seems to begin most commonly in a solitary site, lymphatic and blood vessel spread occurs early on. Death commonly results from the effects of distantly metastatic tumor, for example, from central nervous system involvement.

During recent years an increasing experience has been gained with the clinical staging of bronchogenic carcinoma and the TNM system is being adopted more widely. Briefly stated, the survival of patients with squamous cancer, large cell cancer, and adenocarcinoma can be related to the extent of disease at diagnosis and the number of identifiable physiologic complications. Overall, the median survival of patients with nonresectable lesions is approximately 4 months.

The major curative therapy is pulmonary resection. Unfortunately, less than one third of symptomatic cases prove resectable. Prior to thoracotomy an expeditious patient evaluation program should be completed. Every reasonable effort should be made to establish the diagnosis by means of tissue examination. Consideration should be given to the possibility that the thoracic tumor is a metastatic lesion or the major manifestation of a lymphomatous disorder. Thoracotomy and pulmonary resection are not usually undertaken in patients with small cell cancers.

Before thoracotomy careful study should be made of the clinical extent of the disease. Particular attention should be directed to possible regional lymph node involvement, mediastinal invasion (vena caval,

TABLE 55-7
Common Intrathoracic Tumors

Site	Primary Neoplasm	Metastatic Neoplasm	Non-Neoplastic Masses
Superior mediastinum	Lymphoma Thymoma Thyroid cancer Parathyroid adenoma	Bronchus Breast Gastrointestinal tract Genitalia	Lymphadenopathy Tuberculosis, fungus, sarcoid, cystic hygroma Goiter Aneurysm Bronchial and thymic cysts
Anterior mediastinum	Lymphoma Mesenchymal tumors (benign and malignant) Teratodermoid tumors	Breast Bronchus	Lymphadenopathy Tuberculosis and fungus
Middle mediastinum	Lymphoma-leukemia Plasmacytoma Atrial myxoma	Bronchus Gastrointestinal tract Genitalia	Lymphadenopathy Tuberculosis, fungus, sarcoid, pyogenic infection, abscess, mononucleosis, erythema nodosum Aneurysm Mediastinal collagenosis (histoplasmosis) Bronchial and pericardial cysts
Posterior mediastinum	Lymphoma Neural tumors (benign and malignant)	Bronchus Esophagus Stomach	Esophageal dilatation; diverticulum Diaphragmatic hernia Paravertebral abscess Aneurysm Gastroenteric cyst Meningocele
Pulmonary parenchyma	Bronchogenic cancer Bronchial adenoma, including carcinoid Alveolar cell carcinoma Lymphoma Mesodermal tumors (benign and malignant)	Wide variety of tumors presenting as single or multiple nodules Hematogenous (miliary) or lymphangitic spread of metastases	Infections: pyogenic, tuberculosis, fungus Sarcoid Pneumoconioses Vascular anomalies, infarction Foreign body Pulmonary cysts Hamartoma Peculiar edema patterns

tracheal, or esophageal obstruction, as well as recurrent laryngeal or phrenic nerve palsies), or carinal involvement (seen on biopsy), pleural or chest wall involvement, and the existence of occult distant metastases. Even after these factors have been evaluated thoroughly, about one half of all patients operated on will be found to have disease extended beyond curative resection.

An additional evaluation must be made of the patient's general suitability for undergoing anesthesia and major surgery. Furthermore, the effect of the proposed pulmonary resection on the patient's respiratory function must be estimated.

Radiation therapy is the main palliative treatment modality and is helpful in the management of hemoptysis, bronchial obstruction, compression of mediastinal structures, and pain due to bony deposits or nerve-root involvement. Radiation therapy is used also in the management of nonresectable, localized tumors and with some short-term success.

Several types of antitumor drugs can induce tumor regressions in small proportion of patients with non-small-cell bronchogenic cancer when used singly or in combination. These include alkylating agents, antimetabolites, and various antibiotics. Overall, however, these tumor types are quite refractory. Alkylating agents and radioactive colloidal isotopes are employed with some success in the management of malignant effusions.

While the general prognosis is poor, the 5-year survival rate being 5 percent or less, there are a few patients who live for long periods. Survivorship among females is somewhat better than among males.

Small Cell Cancer[44,45,51]

It is most important to identify small cell cancer promptly and to determine carefully the extent of each patient's disease. Often tumor-secreted polypeptides (some of which are physiologically active) serve as effective biomarkers for the disorder, although distinctive markers initially present may be lost as the disease recurs and progresses.

During recent times, the therapeutic outcome for this disorder has improved remarkably. The initial management of "limited disease" (confined to one hemithorax and the ipsilateral supraclavicular lymph node area) employs radiation therpy to the primary tumor-bearing area together with multiagent chemotherapy given for a period of 6 to 12 months. Nearly 40 to 60 percent of patients may be expected to enter complete remission with a median disease-free period extending for 2 years or more. In "extensive disease" (tumor involvement spread beyond the hemithorax) combination chemotherapy (adriamycin, cyclophosphamide, vincristine, nitrosourea) is the main therapeutic modality. Drugs are given in intermittent courses for 6 months or more. Radiation therapy is used for bulky tumor masses. Overall, about 25 to 30 percent of patients in this category will have a complete remission of their disease with a median duration between 1 and 2 years. More intensive chemotherapy may improve this result.

BREAST CANCER

Breast cancer is a rare occurrence in women under the age of 25, but it steadily increases in incidence throughout the years thereafter. Indeed, breast cancer is the chief cause of death in American women during their fifth decade of life, and remains among the leading causes of death in older age groups.

Etiology[3,26,46]

Genetic factors appear to affect the incidence of breast cancer. Female relatives of breast cancer patients have a risk of developing breast cancer that is 3 to 5 times greater than the general population. When daughters of patients develop breast cancer it tends to occur at an earlier age. Orientals are less susceptible to breast cancer than Caucasians. Although the incidence in Orientals increases on migrating to the Western world, it is still less than in Caucasian women.

In mice, there is clear evidence for a mammary tumor virus which causes breast cancer and which is transmitted to infants through nursing. In humans, B-type virus particles resembling mammary tumor virus have been found in milk. Further, there is evidence for an RNA-dependent DNA polymerase and chromosomal DNA sequences complementary to RNA tumor viruses. However, the evidence for a human mammary tumor virus is inconclusive to date.

In rats, hydrocarbon carcinogens can cause mammary cancer. There is no human counterpart known. It has been suggested that radiation therapy given in past years for mastitis resulted in an increased incidence of breast cancer. Women with cystic disease of the breast also have a two- to threefold increased risk of developing breast cancer.

Pathogenesis[2,46]

Pathologic studies indicate that the majority of breast cancers arise in the small mammary ducts. Several independent lesions are often found on careful examination and they may be found in the opposite breast in a small proportion of cases. A commonly used histologic classification of these neoplastic lesions recognized infiltrating ductal carcinomas, scirrhous carcinomas, adenocarcinomas, or carcinomas of other types (less than 10 percent of cases).

It appears that breast cancer is a relatively slow growing neoplastic process. Spread to the regional nodes is achieved via the draining lymphatics, and to distant sites via the bloodstream. The likelihood of regional or distant spread is greater when the primary tumor has grown to 3 to 5 cm or more.

Clinical Manifestations[29,47]

Fully 80 percent of women with breast cancer present with a painless lump which they found themselves. In 90 to 95 percent of cases, a firm breast mass is the major clinical finding. Retraction of the skin or nipple, patchy edema of the skin, or discharge from the nipple likely relate to an underlying cancer. On rare occasions, there are eczematoid changes or signs of tissue inflammation that are associated with a rapidly growing, aggressive cancer (inflammatory cancers).

It is rare for patients with breast cancer to present with systemic symptoms or with disseminated cancer. Breast cancer has been associated with various physiologic abnormalities which appear to be mediated by humoral substances (e.g., ectopic hormone secretion), but these syndromes are encountered less frequently than in other tumor types.

The extent of disease at diagnosis is an important determinant of prognosis (Table 55–8). Even in patients with distant metastases, the number of sites

TABLE 55-8
The Relationship Between Clinical Stage and Survival with Breast Cancer

Clinical Stage	Survival (%)	
	2 Years	5 Years
I. Tumor < 2 cm	95	82
II. Tumor 2–5 cm Regional nodes + or −	88	63
III. Tumor > 5 cm, or extension Regional nodes + or −	70	42
IV. Distant metastases	22	0

involved bears on longevity. The clinical staging system coming into more common use is based on the TNM system proposed by the International Union Against Cancer (Chap. 53).

The size of the primary tumor is also an important prognostic factor. It is quite unlikely that lesions 2 cm or less in size have metastasized and it is also quite unlikely that they will recur after removal. If cancer does recur, the outlook is more favorable if the interval between primary therapy and recurrence is prolonged.

Diagnosis[1]
The diagnosis of breast cancer usually is not difficult. Certain benign lesions present as painless masses. These include adenofibromas, cystosarcoma phylloides (rare cases are malignant), cystic disease, plasma cell mastitis, and fat necrosis. Intraductal papillomas may be appreciated as small masses, but there is generally a nipple discharge. Rarely soft tissue sarcomas, lipomas, and other connective tissue tumors present in the breast.

Surgical biopsy is the definitive diagnostic procedure and this should not be delayed. In premenopausal women, less than 20 percent of breast masses will be malignant; but in postmenopausal women, over 80 percent will be cancers.

Clinical Course and Management[4,47]
Breast cancer is one disease in which the utility of early detection has been demonstrated. In one well-designed study, clinical and mammographic screening detected 2.72 breast cancers per 1000 women, ages 40 to 60. In contrast, 1.44 cancers per 1000 were diagnosed in the control group who were not

screened. At operation 70 percent of screened cases had axillary nodes free of tumor, whereas tumor-free nodes were found in only 45 percent of control cases. Thus, the prognosis for the screened cases is distinctly better (Table 55–8).

A careful and expeditious clinical staging evaluation is a necessary prerequisite to the decision for primary therapy. Localized cancers (Stage I and II) can be managed with a "less than radical" mastectomy, but Stage III cases require wider excision. No trial clearly defines the optimal surgical methodology. The long continued use of melphalan alone or of cyclophosphamide, methotrexate, and 5-fluorouracil in combination following surgical excision of the primary lesion will protect against tumor recurrence in patients with tumor-involved axillary nodes. (Thus far, this advantage has been shown in the premenopausal age group.) Recent data indicates the radiation therapy is an equally effective method of managing the primary tumor. Further, one large, well-controlled trial in Sweden shows an advantage for preoperative radiation therapy in the prevention of recurrence. No advantage has been shown for performing "prophylatic oophorectomy" at the time of initial therapy.

Disseminated breast cancer is managed best with hormonal therapy or multiagent chemotherapy depending on the disease extent, the organ sites involved, and the rate of progression of the disorder (Table 55–9). The presence or absence of estrogen receptors (ER) on the tumor cells is pivotal in constructing a rational treatment plan and it is most important that proper assays be performed on freshly excised tumor tissue. In ER positive, premenopausal patients, oophorectomy will result in tumor regression in 60 to 65 percent of cases. In ER positive, postmenopausal patients, nearly half will respond to antiestrogens such as tamoxifen or to androgens. Patients whose tumors are responsive to hormonal manipulations, are likely to benefit from further endocrine therapy when their disease becomes progressive again (e.g., adrenalectomy, alternate hormone administration).

The major indication for multiagent chemotherapy is progressive, disseminated disease. Among the drugs used in current combinations are cyclophosphamide, methotrexate, 5-fluorouracil, and adriamycin. Meaningful partial remissions will be achieved in 50 to 70 percent of cases, but complete remissions are rare. The onset of antitumor action is more rapid (1 to 2 weeks) than with hormone therapy (4 to 8 weeks). Thus, chemotherapy is more effective in dealing with aggressive metastatic breast cancer. Remissions are maintained by continuing treatment over a period of several months, perhaps 12 to 24.

---TABLE 55-9---
Treatment of Disseminated Breast Cancer

Patient Status	Tumor Characteristics			Initial Treatment
	Receptor	Metastatic Sites	Progression	
Clinically Occult Metastases				
Premenopausal	+ or −	Involved regional nodes	Slow	Adjuvant chemotherapy, 6–12 months
Postmenopausal	+ or −	Involved regional nodes	Slow	Adjuvant chemotherapy under evaluation
Clinically Obvious Metastases				
Premenopausal	+	Regional, bones	Slow	Ovariectomy. Following with chemotherapy may provide greater, long-term benefit
Postmenopausal	+	Regional, bones, pleura	Slow	Antiestrogen
Premenopausal	+	Liver, lungs, "poor prognosis viscera"	Rapid	Combination chemotherapy
Postmenopausal	+			
Premenopausal	−	Any site	Slow or rapid	Combination chemotherapy
Postmenopausal	−			
		Inflammatory cancer	Rapid	Combination chemotherapy Radiation therapy to primary tumor

Radiation therapy is useful in the management of symptomatic tumor masses.

Chemotherapy is the most effective treatment for ER negative disseminated breast cancer. (The likelihood of ER negative tumors responding to hormonal manipulations is quite small.) Although there is some evidence that ER negative tumors have higher growth fractions, the clinical results to date are conflicting as to whether ER positive or negative tumors are more responsive to multiagent chemotherapy. In ER positive tumors, there are indications that a more complete and long-lasting therapeutic result is achieved if chemotherapy is prescribed after the maximal hormonal result has been achieved.

Inflammatory breast cancer represents a special case, especially in view of its very aggressive nature and its poor prognosis. Vigorous multiagent chemotherapy is used to manage the primary tumor. Antiestrogens may be an effective adjunct in the management of ER positive tumors. At times, surgical resection is helpful in the local management of refractory primary tumors.

REFERENCES

General References

1. Committee on Pathology of the National Research Council. Atlas of Tumor Pathology, 2nd ed. Washington, D.C., Armed Forces Institute of Pathology, 1967.
2. Ackerman, L.V. and Del Regato, J. H. Cancer: Diagnosis, Treatment and Prognosis, 5th ed. St. Louis, Mosby, 1977.
3. Becker, F.F. (ed.). Cancer: A Comprehensive Treatise. New York, Plenum, 1975.
4. Holland, J.F. and Frei, E.T. (eds.). Cancer Medicine. Philadelphia, Lea & Febiger, 1973.
5. Horton, J. and Hill, G.J. Clinical Oncology. Philadelphia, Saunders, 1977.
6. Pitot, H.C. Fundamentals of Oncology. New York, Dekker, 1978.
7. Rubin, P. and Bakemeier, R.F. (eds.). Clinical Oncology for Medical Students and Physicians: A Multidisciplinary Approach, 5th ed. New York, American Cancer Society, 1978.
8. Veronasi, U. (ed.). Clinical Oncology: A Manual for Students and Doctors, 2nd ed. Prepared by the Committee on Professional Education, International Union Against Cancer. New York, Springer-Verlag, 1978.
9. Williams, W.J., Beutler, E., Erslev, A.J., and Rundles, R.W. (eds.). Hematology, 2nd ed. New York, McGraw-Hill, 1979.
10. Willis, R.A. The Spread of Tumors in the Human Body, 3rd ed. London, Butterworth, 1973.

Biology of Human Neoplasia

11. Drewinko, B. and Humphrey, R.M. (eds.). Growth Kinetics and Biochemical Regulation of Normal and Malignant Cells. Baltimore, Williams & Wilkins, 1976.
12. Evans, H.J. and Lloyd, D.C. (eds.). Mutagen-Induced Chromosome Damage in Man. Edinburgh, University Press, 1978.
13. Gilbert, H.A. and Kagan, A.R. (eds.). Metastasis. Semin. Oncol., 4(1), 1977.
14. Goepp, C.E. (ed.). Heredity and cancer. Semin. Oncol., 5(1), 1978.
15. Green, I., Cohen, S., and McCluskey, R.T. (eds.). Mechanisms of Tumor Immunity. New York, Wiley, 1977.

16. Ito, Y. Viruses and Human Cancer. New York, Karger, 1978.
17. Kraybill, H.F. and Mehlman, M.A. (eds.). Environmental Cancer. New York, Halsted Press, 1977.
18. Levin, D.L., DeViesa, S.S., Godwin, D.J., Jr., and Silverman, D.T. (eds.). Cancer Rates and Risks, 2nd ed. Washington, D.C., Department of Health, Education, and Welfare Publication No. 76-691, 1974.
19. Magee, P.N. Carcinogenesis and aging. Adv. Exp. Med. Biol., 97:133, 1978.
20. Miller, E.C. Current perspectives on chemical carcinogens in humans and experimental animals. Cancer Res., 38(6):1479, 1978.
21. Nicholson, G.L. and Bronson, K.W. Specificity of arrest, survival, and growth of selected metastatic variant cell lines. Cancer Res., 38(2):4105, 1978.
22. Pierce, G.B., Shikes, R.H., and Fink, L.M. Cancer: A Problem in Developmental Biology. Englewood Cliffs, N.J., Prentice-Hall, 1978.
23. Saunders, G.F. (ed.). Cell Differentiation and Neoplasia. New York, Raven, 1978.
24. Waldenström, J. Paraneoplasia: Biologic Signals in the Diagnosis of Cancer. New York, Wiley, 1978.
25. Wellington, D.G., MacDonald, E.J., and Wolf, P.F. Cancer Mortality: Environmental and Ethnic Factors. New York, Academic, 1979.
26. Wynder, E.L. and Rauscher, F.J., Jr. (eds.). Etiology of cancer. Semin. Oncol., 3(1), 1976.

Principles of Management

27. American Joint Committee for Cancer Staging and End Results. Manual for Staging of Cancer. Chicago, American Joint Committee, 1977.
28. Andrews, J.R. The Radiobiology of Human Cancer Radiotherapy, 2nd ed. Baltimore, University Park, 1978.
29. Baldwin, R.W. Secondary Spread of Cancer. New York, Academic, 1978.
30. Burke, P.J., Karp, J.E., Braine, H.G., and Vaughan, W.P. A timed sequential therapy of human leukemia based upon the response of leukemic cells to humoral growth factors. Cancer Res., 37:2138, 1977.
31. Burke, P.J., Braine, H.G., Rathbun, H.K., and Owens, A.H., Jr. The clinical significance and management of fever in acute myelocytic leukemia. Johns Hopkins Med. J., 139:1, 1976.
32. Carter, S.K., Barkowski, M.T., and Hellman, K. Chemotherapy of Cancer. New York, Wiley, 1977.
33. Canellos, G.P. (ed.). Oncologic emergencies. Semin. Oncol., 5(2), 1978.
34. Capizzi, R.L. (ed.). Pharmacologic bases of cancer chemotherapy. Semin. Oncol., 4(2), 1977.
35. Clinical Conference on Cancer. Immunotherapy of Human Cancer. New York, Raven, 1978.

36. Goodman, L.S. and Gilman, A. The Pharmacologic Basis of Therapeutics, 5th ed. New York, Macmillan, 1975.
37. Kagan, A.R., Gilbert, H.A., and Nussbaum, H. Modern Radiation Oncology. Hagerstown, Md., Harper & Row, 1978.
38. Litwin, S.D., et al. (eds.). Clinical Evaluation of Immune Function in Man. New York, Grune & Stratton, 1976.
39. Niebergs, H.E. (ed.). Prevention and Detection of Cancer. New York, Dekker, 1977.
40. Norton, L. and Simon, R. Tumor size, sensitivity to therapy and design of treatment schedules. Cancer Treat. Rep. 61:1307, 1977.
41. Salmon, S.E. and Jones, S.E. (eds.). Adjuvant Therapy of Cancer. Amsterdam, New York, North-Holland, 1977 and 1979.
42. Schabel, F.M. Concepts for systemic treatment of micrometastases. Cancer, 35:15, 1975.
43. Vaeth, J.W. (ed.). Combined Effects of Chemotherapy and Radiotherapy on Normal Tissue Tolerance. New York, Karger, 1979.

Illustrative Neoplastic Diseases

44. Abeloff, M.D., Ettinger, D.S., and Khouri, N. Intensive induction therapy for small cell carcinoma of the lung. Cancer Treat. Rep., 63:4, 1978.
45. Baylin, S.B., Weisburger, W., Eggleston, J.C., and Mendelsohn, G. Variable content of histaminase, L-dopa decarboxylase and calcitonin in small cell carcinoma of the lung. N. Engl. J. Med., 299:105, 1978.
46. Black, M.M., Zachran, R.E., Shore, B., Moore, D.H., and Leis, H.P. Prognostically favorable immunogens of human breast cancer tissue: antigenic similarity to murine mammary tumor virus. Cancer, 35:121, 1975.
47. Bonnadonna, G. and Veronasi, U. (eds.). Breast cancer. Semin. Oncol. 5(4), 1978.
48. Fialkow, P.J., Bryant, J.I., Thomas, E.D., and Nieman, P.E. Leukemic transformation of engrafted human marrow cells in vivo. Lancet, 1:251, 1971.
49. Freireich, E.J. and Hersh, E.M. (ed.). Leukemia and lymphoma. I. Semin. Hematol. 15(2), 1978.
50. Freireich, E.J. and Hersh, E.M. (eds.). Leukemia and lymphoma. II. Treatment and diagnosis. Semin. Hematol., 15(3), 1978.
51. Greco, F.A. and Einhorn, L.H. Small cell lung cancer. Semin. Oncol., 5(3), 1978.
52. Thomas, E.D., Buckner, C.D., Fofer, A., Nieman, R.E., and Storb, R. Marrow transplantation in the treatment of acute leukemia. Adv. Cancer Res., 27:269, 1978.
53. Yesner, R. Spectrum of lung cancer and ectopic hormones. Pathol. Annu. 13:207, 1978.
54. Zubrod, C.G. and Selawry, O. The treatment of lung cancer. Arch. Intern. Med., 23:451, 1978.

SECTION NINE
Diseases of the Gastrointestinal Tract
THOMAS R. HENDRIX: SECTION EDITOR

The major symptoms of alimentary tract disease are dysphagia, heartburn, abdominal pain, bleeding, nausea and vomiting, diarrhea, and constipation. All these symptoms arise from disordered function, but their description in physiologic terms is limited because our knowledge of normal alimentary tract function is so incomplete.

The alimentary tract has many functions, but its raison d'être is absorption. To prepare ingested food and fluid for absorption and subsequent elimination of the residue, the alimentary tract is separated by sphincters into functional segments (oropharynx, esophagus, stomach, intestine, and colon), each with a characteristic motor function.[3] It is not disorders of absorption (malabsorption) that give rise to the bulk of alimentary tract symptoms but, rather, disorders of motility. With increased understanding of gastrointestinal function, and particularly of motor activity, it will be possible to describe all gastrointestinal symptoms in physiologic terms. Empiric therapy will give way to treatment directed at the correction of the primary disorder.

The diagnosis of and the therapeutic approach to gastrointestinal disorders will be discussed under the following topics: 1) dysphagia and heartburn; 2) abdominal pain; 3) peptic ulcer; 4) gastrointestinal bleeding; 5) diarrhea and constipation; and 6) malabsorption. Important clinical examples will be given in each category. Although nausea and vomiting are very common symptoms, in reaching a diagnosis it is not particularly helpful to consider them alone.

CHAPTER 56
Dysphagia and Heartburn
THOMAS R. HENDRIX AND TURNER E. BYNUM

Dysphagia, or difficulty in swallowing, is one of the most reliable of all alimentary tract symptoms. It indicates an abnormality of the swallowing mechanism, and it should never be dismissed as an emotional disorder.

The patient with dysphagia initially becomes aware of swallowing and later notes interference or discomfort during passage of the bolus. This latter sensation may be localized anywhere from the oropharynx to the epigastrium. Dysphagia occurs only during swallowing and should not be confused with the sensation of a lump or tightness in the throat or of fullness in the epigastrium. Interference with the passage of the bolus may or may not be painful.

It is useful to divide dysphagia into that of oropharyngeal and esophageal origins because the symptoms as well as the diagnostic and therapeutic approaches are different. Oropharyngeal dysphagia is frequently associated with choking caused by aspiration of a fraction of the swallowed bolus and less commonly with regurgitation into the nose. It is most frequently caused by a neuromuscular disorder and usually dysphagia is only part of the symptom complex.[29] It may, however, be the presenting or most prominent symptom in disorders such as myasthenia gravis and oculopharyngeal muscular dystrophy. Painful, ulcerative lesions of the pharynx are obvious causes of dysphagia whereas a retropharyngeal abscess may not be so apparent. The dysphagia of Plummer-Vinson (Paterson-Kelly) syndrome or sideropenic dysphagia is more difficult to classify for it is associated with atrophic changes of both the epithelium and muscle. Dysphagia in this disease is not due to the characteristic pharyngeal web because the web often persists for years after dysphagia has been relieved by iron replacement. Finally, oropharyngeal dysphagia is caused by narrowing of the lumen of the pharynx by tumor, granulomatous infiltration or extrinsic pressure from a Zenker's diverticulum, or an enlarged thyroid.

633

Esophageal dysphagia is associated with a sense of retrosternal fullness, or pain with swallowing. Often the patient's localization of the site of obstruction corresponds quite closely with the site demonstrated by x-ray examination. Esophageal dysphagia is most commonly caused by motility disorders. Narrowing of the lumen by carcinomatous or inflammatory strictures are also common causes of esophageal dysphagia. Only rarely is dysphagia produced by extrinsic pressure on the esophagus.

PHYSIOLOGY OF NORMAL SWALLOWING

Swallowing consists of elaborately coordinated contractions of the striated muscle of the pharynx and upper esophagus and of the smooth muscle of the middle and lower esophagus. In the resting state, the esophageal lumen is separated from the adjacent segments of the alimentary canal by two sphincters. A sphincter is a segment with a resting pressure greater than that of adjacent segments and which relaxes in response to the appropriate stimulus (swallowing, in this case). The upper esophageal sphincter (cricopharyngeus) prevents air from filling the esophagus during inspiration, and the lower sphincter prevents the reflux of gastric contents into the esophagus.

The first phase of swallowing, the propulsion of the bolus out of the mouth into the pharynx, is voluntary, but subsequent events are involuntary. As the tongue forces the bolus into the pharynx, the nasopharynx is closed by the soft palate and the larynx is closed to prevent the bolus from entering the trachea. The upper esophageal sphincter relaxes, and the pharynx propels the bolus into the esophagus by a broad moving ring of contraction (peristalsis). The peristaltic wave proceeds into the upper esophagus and continues to the cardia. Prior to the arrival of the bolus in the distal esophagus, the lower esophageal sphincter relaxes. This sphincter, which is the principal barrier to gastroesophageal reflux, is 2 to 4 cm in length, extending from below the diaphragm to 1 to 2 cm above it. At rest, its intraluminal pressure averages 20 mm Hg greater than intragastric pressure (Fig. 56-1).[3]

Failure of peristalsis, failure of sphincter relaxation, or disorganization of motor function of the esophagus or pharynx may produce dysphagia just as severe as that associated with a constricting lesion.

DIAGNOSTIC PROCEDURES

To establish the cause of dysphagia, radiologic studies, esophagoscopy, biopsy, exfoliative cytology, and esophageal motility recordings may be necessary.

Radiologic Studies

The most important diagnostic technique is a barium swallow, by which it is usually possible to determine whether the dysphagia is caused by a mechanical obstruction or by an abnormality of esophageal motor function. Since the action of the pharynx is so rapid, it is necessary to record the barium swallow on cine film when studying lesions of the pharynx and the upper esophagus. The film then can be run at slow speed, and abnormalities of the swallowing mechanism can be detected more easily.[33] The absence of peristalsis in the esophagus is best demonstrated by having the patient drink the barium in Trendelenberg's position (head down). If there is no esophageal peristalsis, the barium will remain in the esophagus until the patient is tilted to an upright position. Since dysphagia usually is first noted with solid food, the passage of a barium-impregnated marshmallow should be observed if routine barium swallow does not demonstrate a lesion.

Esophagoscopy, Biopsy, and Cytology

If an x-ray examination has shown either a lesion within the esophagus or a constant narrowing of the lumen, esophagoscopy is the most direct method of establishing the nature of the abnormality. By this technique, the lesion can be inspected and biopsies and specimens for cytologic examination taken, making it possible to distinguish between inflammatory and neoplastic lesions. A malignancy is not ruled out, however, if the biopsy shows only inflammatory changes, because tumors of the esophagus or tumors extending into the esophagus often spread beneath the mucosa and might not be reached by superficial biopsies. In such situations, repeat biopsies or exfoliative cytologic studies are required.

Esophageal Motility Studies[25]

Motor abnormalities may be suggested by the movement of the radiopaque bolus as seen by fluoroscopy or cineradiography. To establish these abnormalities more definitely, the motor function of the pharynx and esophagus can be recorded by the simultaneous measurement of intraluminal pressure from several points. This is accomplished usually by means of perfused, water-filled catheters connected to external pressure-recording devices. Examination of such manometric records will demonstrate whether a swallow triggers progressive peristalsis, whether the strength of the peristaltic wave is normal and sufficient to propel the bolus, whether the peristaltic wave is propagated sequentially throughout the length of

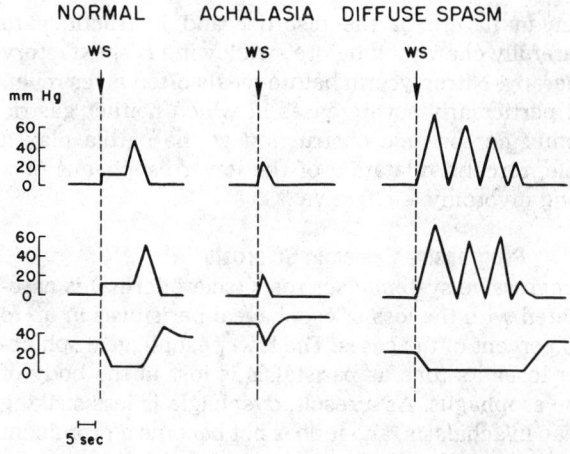

FIGURE 56-1. Esophageal manometric records from patients with normal esophageal function, achalasia, and diffuse esophageal spasm. Intraluminal pressure is recorded in the lower esophageal sphincter (lowest tracings) and 5 and 10 cm above the sphincter. In the normal, a swallow of water is followed by relaxation of the lower esophageal sphincter, then the esophagus is cleared by a peristaltic wave proceeding ab-orad, and finally the sphincter closes. In achalasia, the resting pressure in the sphincter is elevated and does not relax completely in response to a swallow. The simultaneous elevation of pressure in the esophagus is caused by the pharynx propelling the bolus into an esophagus that is closed because of incomplete relaxation of the sphincter. In diffuse spasm, a swallow triggers a series of high amplitude simultaneous repetitive esophageal contractions. In this record, sphincter pressure and relaxation are normal. Relaxation is prolonged in association with continuing motor activity in the body of the esophagus. Some patients with diffuse spasm have sphincter dysfunction with elevated pressure and intermittent incomplete relaxation.

the esophagus, and whether the sphincters open properly (Fig. 56-1). Combining manometric with cineradiographic techniques has added greatly to our knowledge of esophageal function.

CLINICAL EXAMPLES OF MOTILITY ABNORMALITIES[13,25]

Achalasia[10]

Achalasia, failure of relaxation of the lower esophageal sphincter, characteristically presents as slowly progressive dysphagia, although the dysphagia may go unrecognized and the patient comes to medical attention because of pneumonia caused by the aspiration of esophageal contents during sleep or because an unusual mediastinal shadow is seen on a chest x-ray. At the other end of the spectrum are the few patients with achalasia whose symptoms are abrupt

in onset and associated with severe pain caused by an esophageal spasm.

Barium swallow shows that the lumen of the distal esophagus tapers smoothly to a point. The body of the esophagus is dilated and, in the neglected patient, may reach enormous proportions—the so-called sigmoid esophagus. Peristalsis is absent, although striking segmental contractions are seen at times, especially in early cases. The loss of esophageal tone and peristalsis is caused by the loss of normal parasympathetic innervation of the esophagus.[30]

Although the loss of esophageal tone and peristalsis is caused by the loss of normal parasympathetic innervation of the esophagus, the etiology of this neural injury is unknown. In South and Central America, Chagas' disease, a chronic infection with *Trypanosoma cruzi*, may include achalasia in its manifestations but involvement of other organs such as the heart, colon, ureters, and intestine accompany the esophageal disorder.[11] The parasympathetic denervation of the esophagus in achalasia causes the muscle to be supersensitive to cholinergic agents, such as methacholine.[30] This sensitivity to methacholine has been used as a diagnostic test, but since a positive methacholine test is not specific for achalasia and no therapeutic decisions are based on its result, its continued use is not warranted.

Manometric studies show that the resting pressure in the lower esophageal sphincter is elevated with pressures as high as 110 mm Hg. With swallowing, the hypertensive sphincter relaxes incompletely; there is always a barrier of 10 to 30 or more mm Hg between the esophagus and stomach.[22] The sphincter in achalasia has, in addition, been shown to be supersensitive to gastrin.[21] The diagnosis of achalasia is confirmed by passage of the esophagoscope through the narrowed segment and demonstration that there is no obstructing lesion in the distal esophagus or cardia. Achalasia is the consequence of 1) aperistalsis in the body of the esophagus, 2) hypertensive sphincter (cardiospasm), and 3) incomplete sphincter relaxation (achalasia). Since peristalsis and normal sphincter function cannot be restored pharmacologically, treatment is directed at decreasing the tone in the lower sphincter so that the combined forces of pharyngeal contraction and gravity can empty the esophagus. Sphincter tone can be reduced by forceful pneumostatic dilatation of the lower esophageal sphincter or by surgical myotomy. Pneumostatic dilatation is preferable because the morbidity rate is lower than that associated with surgery and reflux esophagitis, which occasionally follows surgical treatment, does not follow dilatation.[17] If dysphagia recurs after adequate reduction of sphincter resistance, three possible explanations should be considered: 1) achalasia itself, 2) carcinoma, and 3) peptic stricture. The latter is seen almost exclusively as a complication of surgical treatment of achalasia.

Diffuse Esophageal Spasm[16,35]

Diffuse esophageal spasm in its symptomatic form produces retrosternal chest pain or dysphagia or both. These symptoms are associated with multiple segmental contractions in the lower esophagus. Peristalsis proceeds normally from the pharynx to the upper esophagus, but as the bolus enters the lower esophagus the entire segment contracts synchronously and repetitively rather than in the normal sequential pattern. One-third of symptomatic patients have elevated resting sphincter pressure and incomplete relaxation with swallowing. The abnormality in an occasional patient evolves into typical achalasia.[23] The frequency of diffuse spasm increases with age. In its mildest form it produces no symptoms but is responsible for the tertiary (nonperistaltic) contractions commonly seen on a barium swallow. The nature of the underlying neuromuscular dysfunction is unknown, but the esophagus acts as though the threshold of the stretch receptors is set too low. It is useful to consider diffuse spasm as a motility disorder caused by several unrelated conditions (Table 56–1). In patients with mild symptoms reassurance as to the benign nature of the disorder and instructions to carefully chew food before swallowing is satisfactory therapy. Nitroglycerin before meals often gives relief. In particularly severe cases in which neither gastric reflux nor organic obstruction at the cardia play a role, forceful dilatation of the lower esophagus or a long myotomy is effective.[35]

Progressive Systemic Sclerosis[11,34]

Progressive systemic sclerosis (scleroderma) is associated with the loss of esophageal peristalsis in up to 80 percent of the cases. The lower esophageal sphincter loses its tone as peristalsis is lost in the body of the esophagus. As a result, dysphagia is less striking than in achalasia, and it does not become a prominent symptom unless reflux esophagitis and stricture develop. Normally, when gastric material refluxes into the esophagus a peristaltic wave is initiated that sweeps the esophagus clean and closes the sphincter behind it. Since both peristaltic and sphincter activities are lost, patients with scleroderma are particularly prone to develop peptic esophagitis. In addition to scleroderma, esophageal aperistalsis is seen occasionally in patients with Raynaud's phenomenon without sclerodermatous skin changes and in other disorders, such as systemic lupus erythematosus (SLE) and Sjögren syndrome.

The only treatment is that designed to prevent peptic esophagitis by limiting the esophageal reflux.

CLINICAL EXAMPLES OF STENOSING LESIONS OF THE ESOPHAGUS

The pathogenesis of the dysphagia caused by stenotic lesions is obvious: The lumen is too narrow for the bolus. Since the obstruction is mechanical, excision of the narrowed segment or dilatation of the lumen by bougies is required.

Carcinoma of the Esophagus[13,31]

Carcinoma of the esophagus makes its presence known by dysphagia. At first, the difficulty is intermittent and noted only with a large bolus of solid food. Unfortunately, even at this early symptomatic stage the tumor growth is so advanced that curative surgery rarely can be accomplished. Carcinoma of the esophagus is primarily a disease of the elderly. Neoplasms of the lower two-thirds of the esophagus are five times as common in men as in women, whereas carcinoma of the upper esophagus is more common in women. The incidence of esophageal carcinoma is 3 to 4 times as great in the nonwhite as in the white population. In central Asia the incidence is 500 times that in the United States. Such differences suggest that environmental factors play an etiologic

---

TABLE 56–1
Clinical Classification of Diffuse Esophageal Spasm

1. Idiopathic symptomatic	Symptoms often severe Occasionally mimics angina pectoris
2. Irritant-induced	Gastroesophageal reflux Corrosive ingestion
3. Obstruction at cardia	Carcinoma Stricture or benign obstruction Malfunctioning lower esophageal sphincter Lower esophageal (Schatzki) ring
4. Ganglion degeneration	Achalasia Chagas' disease
5. Presbyesophagus	Increasing frequency with age Symptoms usually mild or absent
6. Neuromuscular disorders	Diabetic neuropathy Amyotropic lateral sclerosis

role. In this country heavy use of cigarettes and alcohol are associated with the occurrence of this malignancy.

The diagnosis is suggested by the finding of an irregular narrowing of the esophageal lumen on barium swallow and is confirmed by the finding of malignant cells on esophagoscopic biopsy or cytology. Surgery is generally recommended for carcinomas of the lower one-third of the esophagus and cardia, whereas radiotherapy is generally employed for the others. Five-year survival, regardless of the type of therapy, is less than 5 percent. Therefore, the aim of therapy for most patients is palliation. In many patients this is best provided by bouginage or the insertion of a silastic tube.

Inflammatory Stricture [13,27]

Reflux esophagitis is the most common cause of benign strictures. The second most common cause of benign strictures is the ingestion of corrosive materials. In children, the accidental swallowing of a cleaning material, such as lye, is the most frequent cause of chemical burns of the esophagus, whereas in adults a suicide attempt is the most common cause. [32]

Heartburn, Gastroesophageal Reflux, and its Consequences [25,27]

Heartburn is the symptom of reflux of acid gastric juice into the esophagus. Typically, heartburn is a burning sensation originating in the subxyphoid region that spreads upward into the chest, and in severe episodes into the neck, shoulders, and ulnar aspects of the arms. The symptom appears after meals, especially with overindulgence, and is accentuated by lying down or bending over. Relief is obtained by standing up and by drinking liquids, especially antacids. When the symptoms of gastroesophageal reflux are not typical, their differentiation from angina pectoris and peptic ulcer and other causes of dyspepsia may be difficult. Also, symptomatic gastroesophageal reflux may accompany angina pectoris and peptic ulcer, so its identification and adequate treatment contribute to the symptomatic relief of the patient [15,18] (Chap. 22).

The esophageal epithelium is protected from damage by reflux of gastric contents by three mechanisms: 1) the lower esophageal sphincter which acts as a barrier to reflux, 2) secondary peristalsis which sweeps refluxed material back into the stomach and closes the sphincter, and 3) antacid effect of swallowed saliva. Two components are necessary for symptomatic gastroesophageal reflux: 1) a failure of these protective mechanisms, and 2) sensitivity of the esophagus to the refluxed materials. Acid gastric

juice is the most common offending material but duodenal juice with bile acids and pancreatic juice are equally noxious to the esophageal epithelium. Gastroesophageal reflux produces a vicious cycle in that reflux of acid into the esophagus delays clearing the esophagus by peristalsis and during this delay sphincter tone is diminished, thus facilitating further reflux. This reflux leads to increased rate of loss of esophageal epithelial cells which in turn impairs the ability of the epithelium to prevent the diffusion of acid into the mucosa. If the loss of epithelial cells exceeds the ability of the germinal layer to provide replacements, esophagitis and ulceration develop. [27]

EVALUATION OF GASTROESOPHAGEAL REFLUX. [14,28] Most patients with heartburn will respond to simple antacid therapy and, hence, require no additional confirmation of the nature of the underlying disorder. However, patients with atypical symptoms, symptoms that do not respond promptly and completely, or who have other disorders such as angina pectoris will require documentation that gastroesophageal reflux is the cause of the patient's symptoms. There are three clinically important questions:

1. Is the esophagus the origin of the pain?
2. Is reflux occurring?
3. Has reflux been severe enough to lead to esophagitis (which is the precursor of the serious complications of reflux, e.g., stricture and bleeding)?

Acid Perfusion Test. The acid perfusion test provides an answer to the first question. It determines the sensitivity of the patient's esophagus to acid but does not necessarily prove that reflux is present. It is performed by perfusing the esophagus first with normal saline and then with 0.1 N HCl at 120 drops per minute. The test is positive if the patient's symptoms are induced by acid perfusion but not by saline.

Acid Reflux Test. The acid reflux test answers the second question. It is performed by measuring the pH in the distal esophagus with a pH electrode during a variety of maneuvers that increase intra-abdominal pressure. In a normal individual, the lower esophageal sphincter provides an effective barrier between stomach and esophagus, and esophageal pH remains above 5. If the pH does not fall, 300 ml of 0.1 N HCl is placed in the stomach and the maneuvers are repeated. Over 90 percent of patients judged to have clinically significant reflux by other criteria have a positive acid reflux test. Even better correlation between symptoms and esophageal pH is provided by recording intraesophageal pH for 12 hours, 6 P.M. to 6

A.M.[12] If reflux can be demonstrated radiographically the presence of reflux is established, but is found in only 40 percent of patients judged to have clinically significant reflux by other criteria.

Esophagoscopy and Biopsy.   The answer to the third question is provided by esophagoscopy and biopsy. Less than 20 percent of patients with symptomatic reflux have esophagitis, i.e., inflammation of the esophagus, demonstrated by biopsy.[25,27]

TREATMENT OF REFLUX.[11,28]   The aim of therapy is to relieve reflux symptoms and heal esophagitis, if present. The initial treatment of reflux should be intensive in order to interrupt the vicious cycle and to establish whether or not the symptoms are responsive to therapy. The patient should avoid large meals. No special diet is indicated; but since success of therapy is gauged by the extent to which symptoms have been relieved, food and beverages that the patient associates with dyspepsia should be avoided. In addition, no food should be eaten 2 to 3 hours before retiring. Antacids should be taken either in the form of 2 alginate-antacid tablets after meals and at bedtime or Mg-Al OH 2 tablespoonsful 1 and 3 hours after meals and at bedtime. The head of the bed should be elevated on 6 to 8 inch blocks. Most patients' symptoms will be controlled in 2 weeks and the intensity of the regimen can be relaxed. If the symptoms have not responded, it should be established that they are reflux in origin. If symptoms are reflux-induced, Bethanechol (25 mg), a cholinergic drug that increases sphincter tone and hastens gastric emptying, should be given before meals and at bedtime.[24] In the occasional patient who is resistant to conventional therapy, cimetidine, which blocks gastric acid production, should be given a trial before considering surgical therapy. Less than 5 percent of patients with significant reflux symptoms will require antireflux surgery.

COMPLICATIONS OF REFLUX. *Esophagitis.*   If reflux is severe or prolonged, the reparative capacity of the esophageal epithelium may be exceeded and esophagitis will follow. There is, however, no clear correlation between severity of symptoms and the presence of esophagitis; but if symptoms are persistent or recurrent, esophagoscopy with biopsy should be performed to determine if reflux has led to esophagitis. It should be noted that esophagitis, i.e., inflammation of the esophageal mucosa, is a histologic rather than a clinical diagnosis.

Reflux esophagitis will usually respond to the measures employed for simple reflux. The end point of therapy is, however, healing of the esophagitis rather than symptomatic relief. If the esophagitis does not clear or returns when the intensity of the regimen is decreased to a level acceptable for long-term management, surgical therapy with one of the antireflux procedures such as the Belsey, Nissen, or Hill should be considered.[13,25] If the patient is not a satisfactory surgical risk, esophagitis may be treated successfully by suppressing gastric acid production with cimetidine.

Occasionally esophagitis follows vomiting or prolonged intubation. Of particular note are patients with scleroderma who are particularly prone to develop severe esophagitis because they have neither a sphincter to form a barrier to reflux nor a peristaltic wave to return refluxed material to the stomach.

Barrett Syndrome.   Occasionally the squamous epithelium of the distal esophagus is destroyed by reflux and is replaced by columnar epithelium from the cardia. The new squamocolumnar junction is prone to develop peptic ulcer and stricture. Indeed, benign strictures or ulcers in midesophagus are most likely to be a manifestation of the Barrett syndrome.[26]

Esophageal Ulcer.   Severe reflux frequently leads to superficial ulceration of the esophagus. Penetrating peptic ulcers also occur in the esophagus. They may produce esophageal strictures or lead to severe hemorrhage or perforation into the mediastinum.

Esophageal Stricture.   The end stage of reflux esophagitis is stricture. Since the treatment of stricture is difficult, the major effort should be directed toward its prevention by effective management of reflux and esophagitis. Unfortunately, many patients who develop stricture do not have impressive reflux symptoms and do not seek medical aid until the stricture has progressed to the stage of dysphagia. It is as though their esophagi were insensitive so that severe inflammation and consequent scarring progress unnoticed. Temporary relief of dysphagia usually can be achieved by dilatation, but it is unlikely to be lasting unless reflux can be controlled or the irritant quality of the refluxed fluid decreased.[13] These therapeutic goals are accomplished most satisfactorily by antireflux surgery or the use of cimetidine (see Chap. 58).

Aspiration Pneumonitis.   Patients with free reflux may aspirate, especially while asleep, and occasionally this leads to pneumonitis. On the other hand, it is debatable how often chronic pulmonary disease is the result of repeated aspiration of refluxed gastric contents.

Hiatal Hernia

Hiatal hernia, the herniation of part of the stomach through the esophageal hiatus into the thorax, is frequently diagnosed on upper gastrointestinal barium studies obtained in the search for the explanation of a variety of common symptoms such as heartburn, postprandial epigastric pain, and ill-defined abdominal distress. This association of hiatal hernia and symptoms is frequently accepted as evidence that the hernia causes the symptoms. Evidence is rarely available, however, to support such a cause and effect relation.[20]

Anatomically, hiatal hernias are of three types: sliding, paraesophageal, and combined. The sliding type is characterized by the cardioesophageal junction being displaced into the chest. This displacement has been thought to put the lower esophageal sphincter at a mechanical disadvantage and provide an explanation for the reflux symptoms often associated with this type of hernia. The diagnosis of sliding hiatal hernia is based primarily on the radiographic demonstration of herniation of part of the stomach above the diaphragm; but this demonstration is not as simple as it might seem since radiologists do not agree as to the criteria on which to base the diagnosis. In fact, among patients having "routine gastrointestinal series," the incidence of hiatal hernia has been reported as low as 10 percent and as high as 90 percent.

The lower esophageal or Schatzki ring is one of the commonly accepted criteria of hiatal hernia because it has been thought to be the cardioesophageal junction. Combined radiographic, manometric biopsy studies have shown that this easily identified radiographic landmark is not located at the cardioesopha-

geal junction but at the upper margin of the lower esophageal sphincter.[19] In summary, the presence of a sliding hiatal hernia is unimportant; in fact, it has been said that reflux is no more common in patients with a hiatal hernia than in those with the cardioesophageal junction in normal position. The clinically important question is whether or not the lower esophageal sphincter is competent and not the presence of a hiatal hernia. Therefore, repair of hiatal hernia in the absence of demonstrated reflux is never indicated.

The paraesophageal type of hernia is characterized by maintenance of the cardioesophageal junction in a normal position with herniation of the fundus of the stomach through a defect in the diaphragm lateral to the esophagus. Reflux symptoms are not commonly associated with paraesophageal hernias. They may cause postprandial fullness, and occasionally bleed because of erosive gastritis. In the combined type of hernia both the cardioesophageal junction as well as the fundus of the stomach are displaced into the chest. Those latter two types of hernia may become enormous, particularly in the elderly, and at times produce a volvulus and strangulation of the stomach requiring emergency surgery.

Eventration of the diaphragm (abnormal elevation of one leaf because of aplasia, trauma, or paralysis) may produce a striking radiographic picture but rarely causes symptoms.

—CHAPTER 57—
Abdominal Pain
THOMAS R. HENDRIX AND JOHN L. CAMERON

Abdominal pain is a frequent and often baffling symptom. Many of the diseases which present with abdominal pain require prompt surgery, and therefore accurate differentiation is important.

ORIGIN OF ABDOMINAL PAIN[55,58]
A review of the origins of abdominal pain is a useful introduction to its differential diagnosis.

Pain Due to Tension
The alimentary tract from the esophagus to the anal canal is insensitive to many stimuli that produce pain in somatic structures. Mucosal biopsies produce acute ulcers but never produce pain at the time of biopsy nor during the healing phase, whereas similar lesions in the buccal or anal mucosa or in the skin are

very painful. The intestine can be cut, crushed, or burned without pain. In contrast, if distended or the muscle coat contracts with spasm, pain is felt. It appears that the primary cause of pain is tension in the muscle of the gut.

Colic, the wave-like pain associated with forceful peristaltic contractions, is the most characteristic type of pain arising from the viscera. Powerful peristalsis may be initiated by an irritant substance, such as the oxalic acid from green apples, or by an attempt to force the luminal contents through an obstruction. Other disorders, such as ulcers or ischemia, produce painful spasm that is not colicky.

Tension on the mesentery and acute stretching of the capsules of solid organs such as the liver, spleen, and kidney also produce pain. Stretch receptors similar to those in muscle presumably are the source of the impulses interpreted as pain.

Pain Due to Ischemia

Ischemia of somatic, cardiac, or visceral muscle produces pain. Visceral pain of ischemic origin is encountered when circulation is impaired. The most common cause is strangulation of the bowel due to adhesion, hernia, or volvulus. Less frequently, ischemic pain is caused by mesenteric vascular occlusion. Intermittent vascular insufficiency, so-called intestinal agina, is quite rare.

Pain Due to Peritoneal Irritation

Inflammation of the peritoneum is the third major source of abdominal pain. Localized peritonitis results from the extension of inflammation to the peritoneum from an adjacent viscus, such as an inflamed appendix or gallbladder. Generalized peritonitis may be sterile when gastric juice, pancreatic juice, or bile leaks into the peritoneal cavity, or septic when contaminated with contents of the colon or an abscess. Peritonitis causes reflex spasm of the overlying muscles, resulting in rigidity and tenderness of the abdominal wall.

LOCATION OF ABDOMINAL PAIN

Pain arising from parietal structures is usually well localized. For example, pain associated with appendicitis becomes localized in the right lower quadrant of the abdomen only when the inflammation involves the contiguous parietal peritoneum.

If the involved organ has migrated from its original embryonic position, the location of the pain will not correspond to the location of the organ. For example, diaphragmatic irritation leads to shoulder pain, and the discomfort caused by the involvement of gut is usually felt anteriorly in the midline.

The study of pain responses in human subjects has provided useful information about localization:

1. Distension of the stomach or duodenum produces pain between the xiphoid and umbilicus in the midline or slightly to the right. The nearer the stimulus is to the third portion of the duodenum, the nearer the pain is to the umbilicus.
2. Stimulation of the small intestine results in periumbilical pain, but ileal pain also may be referred to the right lower quadrant.
3. Colon pain is referred to the midline between the umbilicus and the symphysis; pain from the ascending or descending colon or from the

hepatic and splenic flexures may also be localized to the side involved presumably due to pressure on adjacent structures.

4. Rectosigmoid distension produces suprapubic pain, and distension of the rectum leads to pain in the area of the sacrum and perineum. Bladder distension also produces suprapubic pain.
5. Gallbladder distension produces midepigastric pain spreading to the right upper quadrant or to the right scapular area as the distension increases. With common bile duct distension, pain appears in the midepigastrium, and sometimes radiates to the shoulders.
6. Pancreatic pain is midepigastric. The pain spreads laterally and to the back, when the posterior parietes become involved.

ACUTE ABDOMINAL PAIN

There are few situations in clinical medicine that demand decisive action as frequently as the initial evaluation and management of acute abdominal pain. The failure to immediately recognize a "surgical abdomen" in an acutely ill patient results in a delay in operative intervention, which often means an increase in morbidity and mortality. For example, the results of prompt surgery for acute appendicitis are almost uniformly excellent with minimal morbidity and almost no mortality. In contrast, if recognition is delayed until a perforation has occurred, postoperative morbidity is frequent and the chance of death is greatly increased. Although the physician should always attempt to make a specific diagnosis at the time of initial evaluation, the main purpose of the work-up is to determine whether or not a "surgical abdomen" exists. The specific diagnosis can be made promptly at the time of laparotomy and the proper surgical treatment determined. The operative procedure should never be delayed to more accurately determine the etiology of the "surgical abdomen." Thus, the main purpose of the initial evaluation is to decide whether or not peritoneal signs are present, signifying a "surgical abdomen" and the need for prompt laparotomy.

HISTORY

Careful documentation of the onset and subsequent course is an important aid in determining the cause of acute abdominal pain.

Onset of Pain

Sudden onset is most frequently caused by the perforation of a viscus, such as the perforation of a peptic ulcer. Intestinal ischemia, such as follows a superior mesenteric artery embolus, can also present with sudden pain. In conditions causing the obstruction of a hollow viscus or an inflammation of its walls, such as volvulus, appendicitis, cholecystitis, and salpingitis, the onset of pain is more gradual, taking several hours to reach its peak.

Character of Pain

Colic is the most characteristic type of abdominal pain and usually indicates obstruction of a hollow viscus. Pleuritic pain is present when the inflammatory process involves the diaphragm or when the movement of the diaphragm brings the inflamed organ against the peritoneum. Patients may describe their abdominal pain as sharp, dull, burning, tearing, or aching, but unfortunately these terms give little insight into the nature of the underlying disorder.

Location and Radiation of Pain

Severe abdominal pain that rapidly becomes generalized is often caused by the leakage of an irritating fluid into the peritoneal cavity. The irritating material may be gastric juice, bile, blood, or pus. Pain that is more localized may give help in indicating what organ is involved in the disease process. For example, midepigastric pain is associated with structures innervated by T6 to T8, namely, the stomach, duodenum, pancreas, liver, and biliary tree. Periumbilical pain is related to innervation from T9 to T10 including such structures as small intestine, appendix, upper ureters, testes, and ovaries. Lower abdominal pain has its origin in structures innervated by T11 and T12, such as the colon, bladder, lower ureters, and uterus.

Vomiting

Vomiting is a common accompaniment of abdominal pain. It may be a manifestation of intestinal obstruction, or a visceral reflex secondary to abdominal pain. In patients with intestinal obstruction it may occur early if the obstruction is high, but late or not at all if the obstruction is low.

PHYSICAL EXAMINATION

Observation of the Patient

In performing a physical examination on an acutely ill patient there is a tendency to cut corners and to center attention on the obvious. It is important first to observe the patient carefully to evaluate the gravity of his illness. Is there evidence to suggest impending shock or vascular collapse? Is the patient restless, as is commonly seen with colic, or does he lie immobile in bed, as is commonly seen with peritonitis or ischemia of the bowel?

Signs of Impending Vascular Collapse

In many disorders associated with acute abdominal pain, such as peritonitis, acute pancreatitis, and intestinal obstruction, there is striking hypovolemia caused by the large and rapid translocation of fluid from the vascular space to the peritoneal cavity or the intestinal lumen. Rapid, weak pulse, hypotension, cold, moist skin, and restlessness are the signs of shock. Early recognition of these signs and vigorous replacement of fluid will improve the prognosis, regardless of the nature of the underlying disorder.

Examination of the Abdomen

The specific questions that should be answered by the abdominal examination are:

1. Are there signs of peritonitis? This is determined by examining for direct and referred tenderness. If peritonitis is present, is it localized or diffuse?
2. What is the character of the bowel sounds? Are they hyperactive and come in rushes, as is typical of intestinal obstruction, or are they absent, as is characteristically seen with peritonitis or ischemia and strangulation of the bowel? It is important to follow the character of the bowel sounds. They may be present early in the course of ischemia and strangulation but disappear as the process evolves.
3. Are there any masses to be seen or felt? Occasionally a dilated loop of bowel or a distended gallbladder is more clearly seen than felt. Care should be taken to exclude inguinal and femoral hernia.
4. Is there evidence of free fluid in the abdomen? If so, aspiration through a 20-gauge needle in the flank often gives definite information. For example, the presence of fat droplets or a high amylase content in the aspirate usually is indicative of pancreatitis, but also may accompany a perforation of a duodenal ulcer. Gross blood suggests a ruptured aneurysm or spleen or an ectopic pregnancy; cloudy, dirty fluid is present after a perforation of the bowel.

Pelvic and Rectal Examination

These examinations help differentiate disorders of the female reproductive tract from inflammatory diseases of the bowel. Occasionally, an abdominal examination in cases of appendicitis or diverticulitis is unremarkable, whereas a rectal examination demonstrates a tender localized mass.

Other Important Observations

A rectal temperature above 102° F is less frequently found in abdominal than in acute pulmonary and renal infections. If fever of this magnitude is associated with abdominal pain, consideration should be given to the possibility that the pain is referred from an extra-abdominal site. Pulses should be evaluated in all four extremities to avoid overlooking a dissecting aneurysm. Observation of the pupillary reactions and the deep tendon reflexes is crucial to avoid missing the diagnosis of tabes dorsalis.

LABORATORY AIDS

Blood Examination

The hematocrit provides important information in patients with acute abdominal pain. When elevated it calls attention to hemoconcentration and hypovolemia, and when low intra-abdominal hemorrhage should be considered. However, a normal hematocrit does not exclude a massive hemorrhage. Leukocytosis is indicative of inflammation and usually accompanies those disorders that may require surgery. Leukocytosis over 20,000 is particularly frequent in mesenteric vascular occlusion.

Urine Examination

In addition to providing evidence of urinary-tract infections, calculi, or acute glomerulonephritis, urinalysis may provide the first indication of diabetes mellitus, which can present with acute abdominal pain. Bilirubinuria may provide the first clue to the presence of hepatobiliary disease. Finally, examination of the urine for porphobilinogen is the simplest way to establish the diagnosis of porphyria.

Stool Examination

Blood in the stool suggests that the abdominal pain originates in the gut. Melena is usually seen with intussusception, mesenteric vascular occlusion, and obstructing neoplastic or inflammatory lesions.

Serum Determinations

Serum determinations of amylase and bilirubin should be obtained if involvement of the pancreas or biliary tract seems possible. For the interpretation of the laboratory results it is important to know when in the course of the illness the blood sample was examined.[75] The serum amylase, for example, frequently returns to normal 48 hours after the onset of pain in patients with pancreatitis even though they are still symptomatic.

Lactescent or hyperlipemic serum may be found in as many as 20 percent of patients with acute pancreatitis. Hyperlipemia may obscure the diagnosis since the serum amylase is often normal in its presence.[41] Serum electrolytes and urea nitrogen should also be determined so that imbalances can be corrected, particularly if surgery is anticipated.

X-Ray Examination

A flat and upright film of the abdomen and a chest film should always be obtained when evaluating a patient with an acute abdomen. Findings which may provide an explanation of the patient's abdominal pain include a lower lobe pneumonia, free air under the diaphragm indicating a perforated viscus, absent psoas shadows suggesting retroperitoneal bleeding or mass, displaced stomach or bowel gas shadows, small bowel air fluid levels suggesting a paralytic or mechanical ileus, large bowel gas and/or air fluid level suggesting an ileus, volvulus, or obstruction, and pancreatic, biliary, or urinary calcifications.

If an emergency barium enema is done to define the site and nature of a colonic obstruction, the full amount of barium is not necessary because the location of the obstructing lesion rather than a detailed study of the mucosa is the question. A water soluble contrast medium should be used if a perforation of the colon is considered to be a possibility. Barium should not be given by mouth if an obstruction of the colon is suspected, but its use to confirm the presence of a small bowel obstruction is perfectly safe.

CLINICAL EXAMPLES

Appendicitis[36,67]

Inflammation of the appendix is a common cause of peritonitis. The aim, however, is to perform an appendectomy before the peritonitis becomes more than a sympathetic reaction to the underlying inflamed appendix.

A consideration of the clinical course of appendicitis illustrates the importance of serial observation of the patient. The first symptom of acute appendicitis frequently is epigastric discomfort attributed to indigestion. When epigastric symptoms predominate there may be no tenderness in the right lower quadrant. In other patients the first symptom will be a colicky periumbilical pain; if the pain is associated with diarrhea the patient will conclude, and the physician will most likely agree, that gastroenteritis is the cause of the symptoms. Anorexia, nausea, and vomiting are common at this stage. In a matter of hours the pain shifts to the right lower quadrant. Frequently, but by no means invariably, tenderness on deep palpation is elicited at McBurney's point. A fever of a degree or two appears together with leukocytosis. If the patient remains untreated, a perforation occurs followed by generalized peritonitis or periappendiceal abscess. The accurate diagnosis of appendicitis would not be so difficult if it regularly followed this pattern, but probably no more than one-fifth of the patients with the disease have the characteristic course. The variable clinical picture seen in patients with acute appendicitis is caused in part by the mobility of the cecum and appendix and the consequent absence of contact between the inflamed appendix and the parietal peritoneum in the right lower quadrant. In large series of cases of acute appendicitis the most common sign was localized abdominal tenderness, which unfortunately is not very specific. The physical signs of appendicitis evolve slowly and are frequently atypical thus making early diagnosis difficult. When the cecum resides high in the midabdomen appendicitis may simulate cholecystitis or pyelonephritis. When the appendix lies deep in the right lower quadrant, appendicitis may mimic Crohn's disease, psoas abscess, ureteral calculus, or even hip disease. In the pelvis, an inflamed appendix may produce bladder symptoms or, in women, symptoms suggestive of disease of the right tube or ovary. Most of this confusion can be resolved by careful serial examinations of the patient, including rectal, pelvic, and urinary examinations.

Acute Diverticulitis[49,72]

The spectrum of diverticular disease of the colon extends from multiple asymptomatic diverticula involving the entire colon on one hand to a few diverticula in the sigmoid colon, associated x-ray evidence of spasm and irritability, and symptoms of irritable bowel syndrome. The asymptomatic diverticula are a degenerative phenomenon in which the mucosa protrudes through the muscle coats in the absence of evidence of motor abnormality. The diverticula associated with chronic or recurring symptoms can be shown to be associated with increased motor activity with striking elevation of intraluminal pressure.[69,71] Acute diverticulitis most frequently involves the sigmoid colon and may appear with no premonitory symptoms, or it may be superimposed on long-standing symptoms of irritable colon. The pathologic process is a microperforation of the mucosa of a single

diverticulum rather than diffuse inflammation of diverticula.[49] The symptoms are pain in the left lower quadrant with severe constipation, nausea, and, uncommonly, vomiting. The patient becomes febrile and has leukocytosis. It is not surprising that it has been called "left-side appendicitis." Usually the attack subsides in a few days, but unlike appendicitis rarely proceeds to free perforation or pericolic abscess.

The diagnosis is suspected with the clinical findings of left lower quadrant pain, fever, and leukocytosis. If peritoneal signs suggest a perforation or an abscess, water-soluble contrast media should be used. Care must be taken to avoid attributing narrowing of the lumen, mucosal irregularity, and blood in the stool to diverticulitis when in fact carcinoma of the colon is present. After the acute attack subsides, this difficult differentiation is made most directly by fiberoptic colonoscopy, which permits direct inspection of the lesion and mucosal biopsies.

The therapy of an acute attack is antibiotics such as ampicillin and intravenous fluids. After the attack subsides, the bulk in the diet should be increased by supplements of bran or bulk laxative so that the stools are soft and constipation is avoided. If attacks with fever and leukocytosis are recurrent or pericolic inflammation and abscess complicate the picture, resection is indicated.

Acute Cholecystitis[50,56,73,77]

Acute cholecystitis presents with pain in the epigastrium and the right upper quadrant. The pain, which is steady in nature, increases over several hours. Obstruction of the cystic duct by a stone initiates the attack. As the stone attempts to pass the cystic duct, pain is also felt at the inferior angle of the right scapula. If the attack is severe, nausea, vomiting, and a low-grade fever appear. Signs of irritation of the parietal peritoneum develop in the right upper quadrant. Leukocytosis is usual, and after 24 hours mild bilirubinemia and bilirubinuria are occasionally found. Constipation and mild paralytic ileus with an air-filled jejunal loop (sentinel loop) seen on an abdominal x-ray film usually accompany attacks of cholecystitis.

Gallstones are found in 85 to 95 percent of patients with cholecystitis, but unfortunately for diagnostic purposes less than one-fifth are radiopaque. Cholecystitis was formerly thought to be caused by an infection of the gallbladder, but present evidence indicates that synthesis of unstable bile by the liver leads to gallstone formation,[53] and then, if interference of gallbladder emptying occurs, acute cholecystitis develops as the consequence of distension and chemical irritation. Any bacterial infection is a secondary phenomenon, rarely appearing in less than 48 hours.[38]

Immediate surgery is the treatment of choice unless there are other medical problems that greatly increase the operative risks.[81] It avoids the small risk of perforation and makes a second hospitalization unnecessary. If perforation does occur, usually it is contained in a well-localized abscess, but occasionally it leads to bile peritonitis or to one of the rare complications, such as the passage of a large stone into the intestine with a subsequent obstruction at the ileocecal valve (gallstone ileus), or a permanent fistula (cholecyst-duodenal or cholecyst-colonic) with a chronic retrograde infection of the biliary tract.[54]

Acute Pancreatitis[37,41,42,46]

The clinical presentation of pancreatitis is as variable as the setting in which it occurs, ranging from a sudden acute abdominal catastrophe with shock and cyanosis to mild episodes of deep epigastric pain and vomiting. It is common in the latter situation, since it occurs so frequently in alcoholics, to attribute the episodes to "alcoholic gastritis." A patient may be carried on the emergency room records as having "gastritis" for several attacks until an elevated serum amylase is found during an acute attack.

There is no specific clinical feature that allows the clinician to make the diagnosis of pancreatitis. The measurement of amylase is the most specific aid to the diagnosis, but it is only transiently elevated and often returns to normal in 48 to 72 hours even in the presence of continuing clinical activity. In addition, as many as 20 percent of the patients with acute pancreatitis have either normal or only borderline elevation of the serum amylase. Striking elevations are almost always caused by pancreatitis if mumps can be excluded. Mild to moderate elevations are seen in a variety of situations, such as with a perforated esophagus or peptic ulcer, strangulated bowel, mesenteric thrombosis, and renal insufficiency. The administration of morphine can also produce mild elevations of the serum amylase.

Since pancreatitis is associated with an increased renal clearance of amylase, the ratio of amylase to creatinine clearance has been advocated as a useful index of pancreatitis in these borderline situations.[59] Enlargement of the pancreas detected by ultrasonography or computed axial tomography (CAT scan) increases the certainty that pancreatitis is the cause of the attack of acute abdominal pain. Unfortunately, early in the attack when help is most needed, changes in the pancreas are infrequently great enough to be diagnostic. These diagnostic procedures are ex-

tremely accurate in the diagnosis of late complications such as pseudocysts and abscesses.

Other manifestations of pancreatitis include bilirubinemia and bilirubinuria (seen in about one-fifth of patients), hyperglycemia (seen in about one-quarter of patients), and hypocalcemia. In severe cases serum calcium falls between the 3rd and 10th days, occasionally low enough to cause tetany.

The pathogenesis of pancreatitis in man is not known, and it seems unlikely that there is a single pathogenic mechanism. Pancreatitis, like pneumonia, is a clinicopathologic syndrome that may be seen in assocation with the conditions listed in Table 57–1. Recently hypertriglyceridemia has been detected in as many as 40 percent of patients presenting with acute pancreatitis. These lipid abnormalities usually persist following resolution of the inflammatory disease. In addition, estrogen administration has recently been shown to induce hyperlipemia and pancreatitis in some females.[47] These findings have suggested to some that hyperlipidemia may act as an intermediary in the pathogenesis of acute pancreatitis in many clinical settings.[42]

Regardless of antecedent factors, the final common pathway in the pathogenesis of pancreatitis is the liberation of activated pancreatic juice into the tissues of the pancreas. In its mildest form only edema develops, which clears without residual changes in the structure or function of the pancreas. In its most severe form, tissue destruction extends to the blood vessels, leading to hemorrhagic pancreatitis, a disease with a fatality rate of 50 to 85 percent. In more severe cases, and especially with repeated attacks, there is a loss of acinar tissue and islets of Lan-

---

TABLE 57–1

Factors Associated with Acute Pancreatitis

Alcohol

Gallstones

Hyperlipoproteinemia
(Types I and V)

Trauma (including surgical)

Drugs (corticosteroids, estrogens, furosemide, azothioprine, thiazides)

Carcinoma

Viral infection

Ischemia

Duodenal ulcer

Hypercalcemia

Hereditary[51]

gerhans, with the development of pancreatic insufficiency with steatorrhea or diabetes or both.

For activated pancreatic juice to gain access to the interstitial tissue of the pancreas, two events must take place: rupture of the ductules of the pancreas and activation of pancreatic enzymes. Normally, activation of proteolytic enzymes of pancreatic juice does not occur until they encounter enterokinase in the duodenum. Experimentally it can be initiated within the pancreas by the retrograde injection of a variety of agents, such as bile, bacteria, and elastase. Ischemia may also lead to the escape of activated pancreatic juice into the tissues.

The treatment of acute pancreatitis is supportive. Since hypovolemia may be severe, the restoration of the blood volume with plasma expanders is imperative. The continued secretion of pancreatic juice into the substance of the pancreas increases tissue damage; therefore an effort to suppress pancreatic secretion should be made. This includes the following: 1) the patient takes nothing by mouth (food in the duodenum stimulates the release of pancreozymin, which in turn stimulates the pancreatic acinar cells to discharge their digestive enzymes); 2) effective gastric suction is used to minimize the amount of acid reaching the duodenum (acid in the duodenum stimulates the release of the hormone secretin, which in turn causes the pancreas to secrete a large volume of watery, bicarbonate-rich juice). Cimetidine, which blocks acid secretion, may achieve the same effect without the discomfort and complications of intubation.

The complications of acute pancreatitis are pseudocyst formation, renal failure, massive pleural effusion, hypocalcemia, pancreatic abscess, and pancreatic ascites.

Perforation of Peptic Ulcer[57,68,79]

Approximately 5 to 10 percent of patients with duodenal ulcer perforate. Perforation of a gastric ulcer is much less common. Most patients (90 percent) give a history of periodic dyspepsia compatible with the diagnosis of a peptic ulcer antedating the perforation. In a few patients, however, the sudden, severe, prostrating pain of perforation is the first indication of peptic ulcer disease.

With the escape of gastric contents into the peritoneal cavity, severe pain appears first in the epigastrium and rapidly spreads over the entire abdomen. The patient appears critically ill, with shallow thoracic respirations; he has a rigid, board-like abdomen and is reluctant to move. As fluid pours out from the peritoneal surface the pain may lessen, but this should not be misinterpreted as a sign of recovery. Fluid becomes detectable in the flanks, and liver dullness may be lost if a large amount of air escapes into the peritoneal cavity (more likely with the perforation of a gastric than of a duodenal ulcer).

About 80 percent of the patients with perforations can be shown by radiography to have free air in the peritoneal cavity. An upright chest x-ray is the study most likely to detect free air under the diaphragm. If the patient cannot stand, a left lateral decubitus film of the abdomen will usually detect free air. Free air in the abdomen may come from other causes such as perforation of the bowel, either spontaneous or traumatic. It is regularly found after laparotomy, and, finally, pneumatosis cystoides intestinalis produces benign asymptomatic pneumoperitoneum.

As soon as a perforated peptic ulcer is suspected the patient should be readied for laparotomy. In the past, simple closure of the ulcer was the acceptable procedure. Studies over the past decade, however, have revealed recurrence rates as high as 60 to 70 percent following simple ulcer closure, even in the absence of a history suggesting chronic ulcer disease. Currently, most surgeons feel that unless the perforation has been present for an excessive period (greater than 12 hours) or the patient is elderly or extremely ill, definitive surgical therapy for peptic ulcer, such as a pyloroplasty and vagotomy, rather than simple closure should be carried out.

Intestinal Obstruction[70]

The hallmarks of intestinal obstruction are abdominal pain, distension, vomiting, and obstipation. All four symptoms are not necessarily present in every case, and the severity of each of these clinical manifestations varies with the level and type of obstruction. When an obstruction is high in the small intestine, vomiting appears early and may be copious and distension minimal. With low intestinal obstruction in the colon, distension may be marked and vomiting not occur at all. Obstipation may be overlooked because the patient has two or three bowel movements early in the course of intestinal obstruction until the bowel distal to the point of obstruction is evacuated. On physical examination bowel sounds typically are high-pitched and occur in rushes. The abdomen is usually distended, but in the absence of ischemic bowel should not be tender.

Intestinal obstruction is most usefully classified into small and large bowel obstruction. Within each of these two categories the obstruction may be: 1) simple obstruction, in which the lumen of the bowel is obstructed but with the blood supply intact; 2) strangulation obstruction, in which there is compromise of the blood supply to the intestine as well as blockage of the lumen; and 3) closed loop obstruction, where the blood supply may or may not be interfered with but where the egress of the intestinal contents is blocked both proximally and distally causing rapid distension of the loop with the risk of perforation.

There are many etiologic mechanisms that produce intestinal obstruction. Extrinsic lesions such as adhesions cause obstruction; lesions in the bowel wall itself such as a neoplasm cause obstruction; or an intraluminal mass such as a bezoar may produce intestinal obstruction. In years past, incarcerated inguinal hernias were the most common cause of small bowel intestinal obstruction. In recent years, however, with the ready access of hernia repair, and with the increasing amount of female pelvic surgery being done, adhesions have become the most frequent cause of small bowel obstruction. Incarcerated hernias probably remain as the second most common cause with other disorders such as regional enteritis, intussusception, volvulus, internal hernias, and small bowel neoplasms following thereafter. The predominant cause of large bowel obstruction is carcinoma. Diverticulitis is the second most common cause of obstruction with volvulus being third.

Large bowel obstruction should always be treated as an emergency because it is a closed loop obstruction when the ileocecal valve is competent. Thus surgical decompression with a colostomy is necessary to avoid cecal distension and perforation. Small bowel obstruction in the absence of signs of ischemic bowel is less of a surgical emergency and more time can be taken to prepare the patient for surgery. This includes the passage of a long intestinal tube and administration of intravenous fluids. However, if signs of intestinal ischemia develop, such as fever, leukocytosis, peritoneal signs, or the loss of bowel sounds, immediate surgery is indicated.

Differentiation of Mechanical Obstruction from Paralytic Ileus

The differentiation of a mechanical obstruction of the bowel from paralytic ileus (failure of the propulsive motor activity of the bowel) requires careful serial observations. Typically, in paralytic ileus there are no bowel sounds, but early in the course feeble sounds may be heard. The early stage of a mechanical obstruction is associated with strong, high-pitched, active bowel sounds. Later, bowel sounds may decrease or disappear as dilatation of the bowel, strangulation,

or peritonitis develops. Paralytic ileus can be found in association with any severe disease and is regularly present temporarily after anesthesia and abdominal surgery. It is frequently caused by peritonitis or by severe electrolyte disturbances, especially by potassium deficiency, and may follow the use of anticholinergic drugs or ganglion-blocking drugs. The treatment of paralytic ileus is supportive (intestinal decompression and restoration of fluid and electrolyte balance). If the primary disorder is correctable, the ileus is self-limiting.

Mesenteric Vascular Occlusion [61,64,84]

Occlusion of the mesenteric blood supply leads to infarction of the intestine. If necrosis of the intestine is to be avoided and the life of the patient saved, early diagnosis and surgical correction are vital. Miraculous recoveries are possible, and many patients who lose a large percentage of the small intestine do surprisingly well.

Infarction of the bowel may be caused by either arterial or venous occlusion. With the former, the symptoms are acute in onset. Patients with superior mesenteric artery occlusion present with the history of sudden, severe, diffuse abdominal pains. Often the pain has decreased to a dull ache by the time the patient is seen by a physician. On physical examination bowel sounds are greatly diminished or absent. There may be only mild or even no tenderness. Hemoconcentration and a striking leukocytosis are usually found. With supportive care the patient's condition may appear stable for 2 to 4 days until necrosis, perforation, and peritonitis occur. If the patient is to survive, the diagnosis must be confirmed early by superior mesenteric arteriography and surgery performed within hours of the occlusion. [85] Most superior mesenteric artery occlusions are caused by emboli in patients with atrial fibrillation or a recent myocardial infarction. If surgery is performed early, embolectomy may be possible; otherwise massive bowel resection is necessary.

The symptoms associated with venous occlusions are usually slower to evolve, symptoms often being present for days or even weeks. Because the clinical picture is less dramatic, diagnosis may be delayed and the chance of recovery after surgery decreased. The etiology of venous occlusion is not usually determined. Often the patients are polycythemic. The extent of bowel involvement is usually more limited than with arterial occlusion, but postoperative extension is frequent and anastomic disruption common (see Chap. 60).

Intestinal infarction can be shown to be produced

by obstruction of the mesenteric vessels in less than 40 percent of patients. In the remainder, an episode of hypotension produces intestinal hypoperfusion and ischemia which proceeds to enterocolitis with necrosis of the mucosa or to frank intestinal infarction.[45]

SURGERY IN ACUTE ABDOMINAL DISEASE

In some diseases presenting with acute abdominal pain the prognosis worsens if operative intervention is delayed. A perforated viscus (duodenal ulcer), bowel with compromised blood supply (strangulation obstruction), and inflammatory disease that is apt to lead to necrosis and perforation (appendicitis) are common examples. With the exception of a perforated peptic ulcer, the history is usually not of great value in making the decision that immediate surgery is necessary. The A-P chest x-ray or upright abdominal film can predict the urgency if free air is seen. Laboratory data can be confirmatory, but rarely does the decision to operate ever rest on a laboratory value. The decision in most instances rests on the physical examination. The diagnosis of a surgical abdomen depends on the presence of "peritoneal signs." Peritoneal signs are detected by rebound tenderness—pain elicited by sudden release of gentle pressure over the area of the abdomen remote from the area of pain. Markedly decreased or absent bowel sounds generally accompany peritoneal signs in a surgical abdomen. Making the exact diagnosis is secondary; what is most important is determining that a surgical abdomen is present. Often the decision cannot be made on the basis of the initial examination, and close observation with repeated examinations (every 30 minutes to one hour) by the same physician are required.

DISEASES IN WHICH LAPAROTOMY IS CONTRAINDICATED

There are a variety of diseases that can mimic an acute surgical abdomen. Unnecessary surgical intervention can be avoided only if they are considered in the differential diagnosis. These conditions are as diverse as acute pyelitis, hepatitis, acute hepatic congestion secondary to congestive failure, abdominal crisis associated with sickle cell anemia, and tabes dorsalis, diabetic ketosis, lactic acidosis, and acute porphyria.[78a]

Little can be accomplished at laparotomy for the patient with acute pancreatitis. If pancreatitis is found unexpectedly because of a mistake in the diagnosis, then the operation should be terminated promptly and certainly no attempt should be made to manipulate the pancreas or to perform a biopsy.

CHRONIC ABDOMINAL PAIN

Many patients with chronic abdominal pain are not found to have any significant organic disease, hence, they are said to have "functional" or "psychophysiologic" disorders. On the other hand, many patients with serious organic diseases, when first seen, have symptoms that are equally nonspecific. If such diseases are to be diagnosed correctly and promptly, each patient must be carefully evaluated and the diagnosis of functional disorder used only as a diagnosis of exclusion.

DIAGNOSTIC APPROACH

History

A careful history gives direction to the diagnostic work-up. As new diagnostic possibilities arise the patient should be questioned further, since decisive topics are unlikely to be pursued with sufficient tenacity if a specific diagnosis is not suspected.

ONSET. Pain whose onset can be accurately dated is significant. The explanation may be organic as in the case of pain caused by an intermittent intestinal obstruction or by porphyria, or the pain may have its origin in emotional problems precipitated by a stressful event. On the other hand, pain that has been present for years, or pain that the patient cannot remember ever being free of, is unlikely to be caused by a specific organic or psychological factor.

LOCATION OF SYMPTOMS. Radiation or spread of the pain may give diagnostic clues. For example, if the distress radiates up into the retrosternal region, it is likely that the reflux of gastric contents into the esophagus is responsible. If the pain radiates through to the back, the posterior penetration of an ulcer or a pancreatic lesion is suggested. Radiation to the right upper quadrant or through to the tip of the right scapula suggests the involvement of the gallbladder or the bile ducts.

The location of the symptoms is not an infallible guide to the location of the involved organ. For example, the initial symptoms of a carcinoma of the body and tail of the pancreas are usually indistinguishable from those of an "irritable colon."

TYPE OF PAIN. The characterization of abdominal pain other than colic gives little help in diagnosis.

TIMING OF SYMPTOMS. Several points are sufficiently helpful in differential diagnosis for their presence or absence to be specifically determined:

1. Pain that awakens a patient an hour or two after he goes to sleep is indicative of organic

disease, usually a duodenal ulcer or gastro-esophageal reflux, and should never be labeled "functional."

2. Pain relieved by eating is highly suggestive of the presence of a peptic ulcer (Chap. 58). However, if eating initiates distress, then biliary tract disease, pancreatitis, carcinoma of the stomach, or esophageal reflux should be suspected. In addition, some patients with peptic ulcers, especially gastric ulcers and ulcers causing pyloric obstruction, have pain initiated or exaggerated by eating.

3. Pain before breakfast is infrequent with a peptic ulcer and is more likely to be a manifestation of the functional gastrointestinal disorder. It is not safe, however, to ignore this symptom, since a carcinoma of the stomach may present in this way.

4. An inquiry into what type of food causes pain is rarely illuminating. Certainly, the presence of indigestion after eating fatty foods or cabbage is not specific for gallbladder dysfunction. True epigastric colic, however, appearing within half an hour after a meal, especially if the meal contained fatty foods, strongly suggests biliary-tract dysfunction.

5. Periumbilical colic appearing after meals is a characteristic sign of an obstructing lesion of the small bowel, or rarely intestinal angina. The typical history of intestinal angina is that the patient has no abdominal pain if he fasts or eats sparingly. With larger meals, colicky pain appears within a half hour of eating and lasts 1 to 2 hours. This sequence leads to diminished intake and weight loss.[39]

6. If abdominal distress or colic is relieved by defecation, the responsible lesion is likely to be in the colon or distal ileum.

Associated Findings

Heartburn indicates the reflux of gastric juice into the esophagus and it may accompany an exacerbation of a variety of gastrointestinal disorders (Chap. 56).

Aerophagia with eructation is regularly increased by indigestion from any cause; hence, it is no more characteristic of cholecystitis than of functional disorders.

ANOREXIA AND WEIGHT LOSS. Anorexia and weight loss are indicative of serious underlying disease until proven otherwise. The underlying disease need not be neoplastic, however, for many patients with benign gastric ulcers present with greater weight loss than patients with carcinomas of the stomach.

CONSTIPATION AND OBSTIPATION. A change in bowel function should receive careful attention. It may be constipation in a patient who paid no attention to bowel function in the past. It may be alternating diarrhea and constipation; or it may be such severe obstipation that the patient resorts to enemas. It is generally recognized that these symptoms suggest an obstructing lesion in the bowel, especially in the colon. It is not, however, well recognized that severe obstipation is often the initial symptom of such extracolonic disorders as carcinomas of the stomach, gallbladder, and pancreas.

Physical Examination

Physical findings, such as jaundice, a palpable gallbladder, and hepatomegaly, direct attention to the liver, bile ducts, or pancreas as a possible source of the pain. A succussion splash indicates delayed gastric emptying. An epigastric or a left upper quadrant mass suggests a tumor of the stomach or pancreas. Although the finding of an abdominal mass always brings to mind neoplastic disease, one should always rule out inflammatory diseases, which have better prognosis and may be responsive to specific therapy. For example, a rolled-up matted tuberculous omentum is sometimes mistaken for a carcinoma of the colon.

Visible peristalsis, hyperactive bowel sounds, and visible or palpable distended loops of bowel point to an obstructing lesion of the intestine.

Ascites should be carefully looked for; if present, an examination of the fluid may indicate the diagnosis and eliminate the necessity for expensive diagnostic procedures.

If fever is present it must be explained. Even though abdominal pain is the presenting symptom, if it is associated with fever, the cause may be a systematic disease. In this case the diagnosis may be established more readily by special examinations, as in the diagnosis of lymphoma by lymph node biopsy, tuberculosis by finding acid-fast organisms in the sputum, SLE by finding LE cells in the blood, polyarteritis by finding arteritic lesions in a muscle biopsy, and so on.

Laboratory Aids

The initial choice of laboratory studies will be determined by the diagnostic impression gained from the history and physical examination. Only rarely should a barium enema, gastrointestinal series, and cholecystogram be requested as the initial diagnostic study.

In addition to the routine examination of blood and urine, evidence for partial obstruction of the biliary tract should be sought by testing the urine for bilirubin and by determining the bilirubin and alkaline phosphatase levels in the serum. If the problem is one of recurrent abdominal pain, then the serum amylase, urine porphobilinogen, sickle cell preparation, and serologic tests for syphilis are important aids in the differential diagnosis. Blood in the stool indicates a mucosal lesion and should be investigated by proctoscopy and x-ray studies.

RADIOLOGIC EXAMINATION. A plain film of the abdomen, with both upright and supine views, is the first roentgen examination. The films should be reviewed for any evidence of renal, pancreatic, or biliary calculi. Dilated loops of bowel or abnormal gas shadows may indicate the site and nature of intrinsic bowel disease. Displaced gastric or colonic gas pattern may be produced by a mass. An air fluid level or lucency in the mediastinum may be indication of a large hiatus hernia. Only after the abdominal films have been carefully studied should more elaborate roentgen examinations be undertaken.

The most useful diagnostic examination for the evaluation of upper abdominal pain is the radiographic study of the upper gastrointestinal tract. The major abnormalities demonstrable by the technique, listed in the order of their frequency, are hiatus hernia, duodenal and gastric ulcers, gastric neoplasms, displacement of the duodenum by inflammatory or neoplastic involvement of the pancreas, and hypertrophic gastric rugae (hypertrophic gastritis). The second most important diagnostic aid is the cholecystogram, which will demonstrate either a normally visualized gallbladder, a nonfilling of the gallbladder, or cholelithiasis. It must be stressed, however, that the finding of an anatomic abnormality does not prove that it is the cause of the patient's symptoms. This admonition is particularly relevant to the demonstration of hiatus hernia, hypertrophic gastric rugae, nonfilling gallbladder, and cholelithiasis.

ULTRASONOGRAPHY AND COMPUTERIZED AXIAL TOMOGRAPHY (CAT SCAN).[60,78] These new but expensive procedures provide a new dimension to the diagnosis of intra-abdominal masses. Ultrasonography, which involves no x-ray exposure nor side effects, is proving to be the best method for screening for cholelithiasis. In addition, ultrasonography is ideally suited for identification of cystic lesions. CAT scanning provides extraordinary detail in a narrow cross section of the body. Because of x-ray exposure, limited area studied and expense, CAT scanning cannot be considered a screening procedure.

PROCTOSCOPY. Lower-abdominal symptoms should be investigated by proctoscopy and barium enema. Proctoscopic examination should be completed prior to the barium enema for the following reasons: 1) it is simpler to perform and more easily tolerated; 2) proctoscopy examines the segment of large bowel that is poorly visualized by barium enema; and 3) if a lesion is found by proctoscopy, biopsy can be performed and a tissue diagnosis obtained.

Patients with Normal Studies

If all studies are either normal or inconclusive in a patient with recurrent abdominal pain, an arrangement should be made for reexamination at the time of the next attack. This will allow the physician to determine whether the pain is associated with any diagnostic clues; it will also permit the physician to get a clear idea of the onset and pattern of the pain while these features are fresh in the patient's mind; and finally it will provide an opportunity to get laboratory and x-ray studies at a time when they are most likely to show an abnormality.

CLINICAL EXAMPLES OF CHRONIC AND RECURRENT ABDOMINAL PAIN

The most important causes of chronic and recurrent abdominal pain, excluding peptic ulcer (Chap. 58), are discussed here.

CHRONIC CHOLECYSTITIS AND CHOLELITHIASIS[53,56,83]

Gallstones are formed from precipitated pigment (bilirubin) or cholesterol. Pigment stones occur in patients with increased bilirubin excretion (as occurs in hemolytic disorders such as sickle cell disease). Cholesterol gallstones form from "lithogenic bile." In lithogenic bile, the concentration of bile acids and lecithin are not sufficient to maintain the cholesterol in solution, especially when the bile is concentrated in the gallbladder.[77,82] Gallstones intermittently obstruct the cystic duct, and thus produce cholecystitis.

The symptoms attributed to chronic cholecystitis and gallstones[53,56] range from recurrent attacks of biliary colic, fever, and jaundice to symptoms indistinguishable from functional dyspepsia.

Typical biliary colic appears in the epigastrium with radiation to the right upper quadrant and subscapular regions. In about one-fourth of the cases the pain also radiates to the left upper quadrant or left subscapular area, and, occasionally, left-sided discomfort may be the most prominent feature. The pain builds up to a peak intensity in 15 to 45 minutes and subsides over several hours, but the patient may be aware of residual soreness for a day or two. Since the gallbladder is stimulated to contract by humoral (cholecystokinin) and neural (vagus) stimuli released by eating, typical biliary colic appears 1 to 3 hours after a meal.

Not all clinically significant gallbladder disease is associated with recognizable biliary colic; however, if the episodes of pain are associated with a mild jaundice or with a right upper quadrant mass, the likelihood of establishing cholelithiasis as the cause is increased.

Frequently, the diagnosis of chronic cholecystitis rests on a history of pain after eating fatty food and on the absence of abnormalities in the gastrointestinal series. The impression is strengthened if the gallbladder fails to be visualized on a cholecystogram or if gallstones are found. There are, however, several flaws in this formulation.

1. Gallstones and an inflammation of the wall of the gallbladder are increasingly common with advancing age, so that as many as 50 percent of the patients at postmortem examination in the seventh decade have gallbladder disease. These pathologic changes cannot be equated with a clinical syndrome with any regularity.
2. The dyspepsia and eructation associated with the eating of fatty food, cabbage, and so on, traditionally have been considered characteristic of chronic cholecystitis. A number of investigations have shown this not to be true. In fact, if a history of intolerance of fatty food is elicited, the patient is more likely to have a functional gastrointestinal disease than gallbladder disease.
3. A distressing number of patients who have had cholecystectomies for chronic cholecystitis return with symptoms similar to the preoperative symptoms. Though often labeled "postcholecystectomy syndrome," these patients' symptoms are usually caused by one of the following conditions: (a) an unrecognized peptic or functional gastrointestinal disease, with symptoms erroneously attributed to gallbladder disease; (b) stones remaining in the common duct or cystic duct; (c) a partial obstruction of the common duct; or (d) associated pancreatitis. Before advising surgery for chronic cholecystitis, serious consideration should be given to the possibility that the patient's symptoms might be the result of one of these conditions.

Since practically all clinically significant cases of chronic cholecystitis are associated with gallstones, the presence of gallstones should be demonstrated before this diagnosis receives serious consideration. Approximately 15 to 20 percent of all gallstones can be seen on a plain x-ray film of the abdomen. If the gallbladder retains any function, the gallstones can be seen as negative shadows of the contrast medium. If the patient's gallbladder fails to be visualized by oral cholecystography, gallstones if present can be demonstrated by ultrasonography.

Confidence that gallbladder disease is the cause of the patient's symptoms is increased if there is a history of biliary colic, jaundice, fever, or an elevated alkaline phosphatase. If the patient has symptoms leading to the suspicion of gallbladder disease, if other diseases which may mimic gallbladder disease have been excluded, if evidence of gallstones is found, and if the patient does not have some underlying illness that increases the hazard of a cholecystectomy, the treatment of calculous gallbladder disease is surgical. However, the case for cholecystectomy in the treatment of asymptomatic gallstones is not clear. Although the risks of an elective cholecystectomy are small and the likelihood of the patient's developing symptomatic gallbladder disease is said to be 50 percent in the next 5 to 10 years,[63,83] the risk to life from elective surgery occurs on the day the surgery is performed, whereas the "silent" stone may not become symptomatic for another 5 to 20 years. If, however, surgery is delayed until the patient develops a complication such as common duct stones with jaundice, surgery will carry a several times greater risk than if it had been performed electively.

Much interest has been generated in the "medical treatment" of gallstones. In experimental studies it has been shown that feeding one (chemodeoxycholic acid), but not the other (cholic acid), primary bile acid, leads to the dissolution of cholesterol gallstones.[80] The role of chemodeoxycholic acid in the management of cholelithiasis, if released for general use, is unclear because of expense and necessity to continue its use for long periods of time if not indefinitely. It is interesting to note that surgical treatment (cholecystectomy) also decreases the lithogenicity of bile.

CHRONIC RELAPSING PANCREATITIS[44,46]

The most common recurrent form of pancreatitis appears as episodes of acute pancreatitis, associated with bouts of alcoholism. An elevated serum amylase may be found, especially if the blood is drawn early in the attack. With each succeeding episode, however, pancreatic exocrine function decreases and the likelihood of finding an elevated amylase diminishes. In patients not having diagnostic pancreatic calcifications seen on abdominal x-ray, several recently introduced procedures may be useful in establishing the presence of chronic pancreatic disease. Ultrasonography is a useful screening procedure for demonstrating enlargement of the pancreas, dilated ducts, pseudocysts, and small calcifications. Endoscopic pancreatography enables visualization of the characteristic abnormalities of pancreatic ducts.[74] Finally, CAT scanning gives the most detailed views of the pancreas, but since the therapeutic options are limited these procedures usually give more information than can be used clinically.[78] Although chronic pancreatitis is characterized by a triad consisting of pancreatic calcification, diabetes mellitus, and steatorrhea, no more than one-third of the cases present the complete syndrome. Pancreatic exocrine insufficiency is discussed in Chapter 61.

There is no specific medical treatment for chronic pancreatitis, but patients are usually placed on antacids and anticholinergic drugs with the aim of decreasing stimulation of pancreatic secretion. Many surgical procedures have been advocated, but most have given inconstant results. The major reason for failure is that most cases of recurrent pancreatitis are associated with alcoholism, and no operation has been devised that will permit these patients to drink with impunity. Ninety-five percent pancreatectomy leaving a rim of pancreas in the duodenal C-loop gives the greatest success with 85 percent good results, even in alcoholics.[44] This operation requires no anastomosis between ducts and intestine and hence has a low operative mortality. However, roughly one-half of the patients not diabetic before surgery, require insulin thereafter. In some patients pancreatitis is associated with cholelithiasis, peptic ulcer, hyperparathyroidism, or hyperlipidemia. The correction of these conditions is associated with an amelioration or cessation of the attacks of pancreatitis.

INTERMITTENT OR CHRONIC INTESTINAL OBSTRUCTION[70]

Postoperative adhesions are frequently blamed for chronic or recurrent abdominal pain. Before a second operation is undertaken to "lyse the adhesions," objective evidence of partial intestinal obstruction should be demonstrated. An intermittent incomplete volvulus is occasionally the cause of recurrent abdominal pain but can be diagnosed only if abdominal x-rays are taken during an attack. The most common inflammatory lesion of the bowel producing partial intestinal obstruction and chronic abdominal pain is Crohn's disease (Chap. 60).

Neoplastic lesions are a frequent cause of chronic obstructive symptoms. The most common is carcinoma of the colon, especially on the left side. Lymphoma of the small bowel also produces symptoms of progressive obstruction. Intestinal polyps, such as those found with the Peutz-Jeghers syndrome, and small intestinal carcinoid give rise to intermittent obstructive symptoms.

Vascular lesions, in addition to producing acute abdominal pain when there is an acute mesenteric vascular occlusion, may also produce symptoms of intestinal obstruction. The ischemic segment produces partial obstruction as it becomes narrowed and fibrotic.

Intestinal pseudo-obstruction is a rare intestinal motor abnormality which presents with episodic abdominal distension and vomiting.[65,76] Abdominal x-rays show dilated intestinal loops with air fluid levels which may be interpreted as indicating the presence of a mechanical obstruction, but at laparotomy no obstructing lesion is found. To avoid unnecessary operation, careful small bowel contrast studies should be done if a site of obstruction is not clear.

CHRONIC PERITONITIS

Chronic peritonitis caused by a tuberculous infection causes chronic diffuse abdominal pain, minimal tenderness, and low-grade fever.[40] It may occur with or without ascites. When associated with cirrhosis and ascites, the diagnosis of tuberculous peritonitis is difficult to establish and is frequently overlooked.

SYSTEMIC DISEASES AND INTOXICATIONS WITH RECURRENT ABDOMINAL PAIN[66]

Systemic diseases and intoxications that may present with chronic or recurrent abdominal pain are too numerous to discuss in this section. Included in this group are diseases as dissimilar as polyarteritis nodosa, systemic lupus erythematosus, lead poisoning, hypercalcemia, diabetic acidosis, ketoacidosis, porphyria, hyperlipemia, and tabes dorsalis.

CARCINOMA OF THE STOMACH[4]

Although steadily decreasing in incidence over the past several decades, gastric carcinoma is still the seventh cause of cancer deaths in the United States and remains an important cause of abdominal pain. Early detection is to be hoped for since 5-year survival after surgery is greater than 50 percent if the tumor has not extended into the submucosa, whereas only 10 percent of all patients treated surgically have 5-year cures. It appears that intestinal metaplasia of the gastric mucosa represents the precursor lesion to gastric carcinoma. This lesion also is associated with hypochlorhydria, achlorhydria, and gastric ulcer, hence it is not suprising they all are found in association with gastric cancer. Unfortunately, the clinical manifestations of gastric carcinoma can be so vague that a tumor may develop and become inoperable despite the fact that a patient is being followed closely by a physician. Weight loss, anorexia, vomiting, and pain are the most common symptoms. Weakness and dizziness secondary to chronic blood loss anemia also may be the initial symptoms. A palpable mass is present in only one-third of the patients, and usually is a sign of incurability. An upper gastrointestinal series is the first diagnostic test to be ordered in patients suspected of having a gastric malignancy and its accuracy in differentiating between benign and malignant lesions is about 90 percent. Gastroscopy with brushings for cytologic examination and biopsy will increase the accuracy to greater than 98 percent. Gastric analysis offers too little diagnostic help to make its continued use justifiable. Surgery is the therapy for gastric carcinoma, and it appears that survival can be improved somewhat by multiple chemotherapy combinations.

CARCINOMA OF THE PANCREAS[4,52]

Whereas gastric cancer is decreasing, cancer of the pancreas is increasing to the point that it is now the fourth most common cause of cancer death. To make matters worse, early diagnosis is only by accident and as a result the 5-year survival is no more than 1 percent. Even when the tumor is in the head of the pancreas and jaundice is an early symptom, the survival is less than 10 percent. Pain is the most common presenting symptom, being noted by three-fourths of the patients with carcinoma of the head of the pancreas and by practically all patients with involvement of the body and tail of the pancreas. Usually the pain is a dull ache in the epigastrium that may radiate into the right upper quadrant if the tumor is in the head and to the left if it is in the body and tail. In addition, patients frequently note sharp intermittent epigastric pain. Many have crampy lower abdominal pain, and since over three-fourths of the patients with carcinoma of the body or tail also present with severe constipation, many are initially thought to have the irritable-colon syndrome. A steady pain in the back or in the lower lumbar region is found in one-fifth of the patients as the presenting complaint or as a second pain separate from the epigastric distress.

Seventy percent of patients with carcinoma of the head of the pancreas present with jaundice, whereas fewer than 15 percent of the patients with involvement of the body of the pancreas are jaundiced. Likewise, an abdominal mass is more frequently encountered in cancer of the head than of the

body and tail of the pancreas. Not more than 50 percent of the patients show any displacement of the gastrointestinal tract by x-ray. The only two diagnostic procedures that have any promise of leading to earlier diagnosis and as a consequence increased survival are CAT scanning and endoscopic cannulation of the pancreatic duct (ERCP).[74,78] Isolated examples of early diagnosis have been reported but to date there is no evidence of improvement in the overall grim picture presented by pancreatic cancer. By the time the mass has grown large enough to show characteristic compression of the duodenum on barium studies or changes in pancreatic vessels on angiography, the chance for long-term survival is past. Most surgery ends up as a palliative effort and the tumor has not been responsive to chemotherapy nor radiation therapy.

IRRITABLE COLON[43,48,62]

Irritable colon, functional bowel disorder, and spastic colon are all terms used to designate the most common cause of chronic or recurrent abdominal pain. The pain is most frequently localized to the left lower quadrant or hypogastrium. Sometimes it is localized in the left or right upper quadrant and may be called splenic flexure or hepatic flexure syndrome. The later is confused with gallbladder dysfunction if strict criteria are not observed. The abdominal pain is likely to be associated with bloating, constipation, or diarrhea alternating with constipation. Eating often aggravates the pain; in some patients defecation or passing flatus gives relief but more often defecation seems incomplete and the patients' symptoms are aggravated. Physical examination is normal except that palpation over the colon, especially the sigmoid, may produce distress. Increased motor activity is observed at times during proctoscopy. In some patients there is increased mucus on the mucosa but there is never bleeding and mucosal biopsy is always normal. Routine diagnostic studies including x-rays are normal.

Irritable colon is more common after age 30. The patient is most often an obsessive or perfectionistic woman. An attack of diarrhea due to salmonellosis, shigellosis, or antibiotic administration may precede the appearance of irritable colon symptoms. Irritable colon symptoms occasionally are associated with active peptic ulcer, and are sometimes produced by lactose intolerance. Irritable colon can never be accepted as the cause for blood in the stool, anemia, or weight loss. The symptoms of irritable colon are attributed to spastic and incoordinated muscle contraction of the colon. If the abnormality persists it may lead to diverticulosis. Indeed, the irritable bowel symptoms are erroneously attributed to diverticulitis (Chap. 60).

Treatment consists of reassurance by explaining the nature of the symptoms in physiologic terms and use of bulk laxative to even out the swings from constipation to diarrhea.

Irritable colon should be differentiated from hysterical or conversion reactions. The pain associated with hysteria is likely to be described as unbearable but has persisted unchanged day and night for weeks, months, or even years. Mellinkoff has characterized hysterical pain colorfully and clearly: "It is as though the individual's anxieties and fears were all melted, washed from his mind, and recrystallized in the form of a painful abdomen. The pain is then guarded jealously, and he is preoccupied with his abdomen as though he dreaded losing his pain lest he bear instead the anxiety from which the pain was molded."[66] All too often these patients are treated in desperation with surgical procedures or opiates, both of which only compound the problem.

CHAPTER 58
Peptic Ulcer and Dyspepsia
THOMAS R. HENDRIX

Dyspepsia, originally meaning difficulty in digestion, now refers to a variety of symptoms associated with the ingestion of food. Such symptoms range from postprandial bloating, distension, and eructation to gnawing or burning epigastric pain. Most patients find accurate description of these symptoms difficult, and they often come to use terms learned while being questioned by physicians.

Peptic ulcer is the most common organic cause of dyspepsia. It is a generic term applied to ulcers caused directly or indirectly by active gastric juice, that is, containing acid and pepsin. These ulcers may be found in the esophagus, stomach, and duodenum; at the site of a gastroenterostomy (marginal ulcer); in the jejunum at multiple levels (as seen at times in the Zollinger-Ellison syndrome); and in ectopic gastric tissue in a Meckel's diverticulum. Of these locations, the duodenum and stomach are the most common.

There are many reasons for considering a duodenal ulcer and a simple gastric ulcer to be different diseases. They have different sex distribution; different genetic distributions as indicated by blood types; different age, social, and economic distributions; different gastric secretory responses; and differences in their responses to medical and surgical treatment. Duodenal ulcer characteristically is associated with a high rate of gastric secretion, not only after a meal but in the fasting state as well.

If gastric hypersecretion alone were the whole explanation for peptic ulcer disease, diffuse rather than localized ulceration would be expected. Additional factors are operative. One such factor is the striking tendency for peptic ulcers to occur at muco-sal junctions, for example, at the esophagogastric, fundopyloric, and pyloroduodenal junctions.[113] Another weakness in the concept that "acid hypersecretion equals ulcer" is that, although duodenal ulcer patients as a group secrete twice as much acid as do normal individuals, there is a striking overlap of the acid outputs of the two groups. In addition, patients with gastric ulcers tend to secrete less acid than normal individuals do. For these reasons, the measurement of gastric secretion has no value in the differential diagnosis of dyspepsia.[99]

Not only is the pathogenesis of peptic ulceration unresolved, but the simpler question of how peptic ulcer pain is produced is also unanswered. The two major views are: 1) pain is produced *directly* by acid irritating exposed nerve endings in the ulcer; 2) pain is produced *indirectly* by an increase in the tone of the wall of the duodenum and gastric antrum. The second view has more appeal, but it has not been proved. In addition, patients with and without demonstrable ulcers may have identical symptoms, hence the suggestion that the symptoms are not dependent on the presence of an ulcer.

EVALUATION OF DYSPEPSIA
The onset of dyspeptic symptoms in relation to food intake, as well as their duration, relief by antacids, nature, location, and radiation are helpful in suggesting the cause of the dyspepsia. However, none of these is specific and must be regarded only as a clue to the diagnosis which must be established by more definitive means. In addition to peptic disease, dyspepsia may be the presenting symptom of a variety of

disorders including gastric and pancreatic carcinoma, cholelithiasis, pancreatitis, abdominal angina, intestinal obstruction, functional disorders, and depression.

Location of Pain

The pain of a peptic ulcer is referred to the epigastrium. If it is associated with a component radiating through to the back, a posterior perforation or at least inflammation extending into the posterior parietes is strongly suggested.

Type of Pain

In its mildest form ulcer pain is best described as hunger pain. It slowly builds up, is steady for one-half to 2 hours, and then gradually subsides. As the pain becomes more severe, such adjectives as "gnawing" and "burning" are used to describe it, but the pattern of its onset and disappearance remains the same.

Time of Pain

At first the ulcer patient may note hunger distress only prior to the evening meal, but as symptoms progress in intensity he becomes aware of pain from 30 minutes to 4 hours after other meals. Pain that awakens the patient from sleep 1 to 2 hours after retiring is so characteristic of a peptic ulcer, and especially of a duodenal ulcer, that this must be considered to be the diagnosis until convincing evidence to the contrary is presented. Conversely, pain before breakfast is so infrequent that this symptom strongly suggests that the patient's dyspepsia is not caused by a peptic ulcer.

Relief of Pain

The pain of a peptic ulcer is promptly relieved by the taking of food or antacids. Traditionally, milk is thought to be most effective, but almost any food gives temporary relief. Vomiting or the removal of the gastric contents by aspiration also is followed by subsidence of the pain. Patients with gastric ulcers may not give such clear stories of prompt improvement with the taking of food or antacids. If a history is obtained of a typical food–pain relief pattern that changes so that eating can no longer be depended on to help, and may even exaggerate the pain, partial pyloric obstruction or deep penetration of the ulcer should be suspected.

Less Common Symptoms of Duodenal Ulcer Activity

Constipation is a symptom commonly associated with ulcer activity, and a small percentage (about 5 percent) of the patients with chronic duodenal ulcers have predominantly colonic symptoms.

Heartburn and eructation are also commonly associated with ulcer activity. Occasionally, heartburn is so prominent that the primary disease is thought to be esophageal.

Radiographic Studies[98]

Upper gastrointestinal barium series is the most readily available method of diagnosing peptic ulcer and should be the initial diagnostic study. However, this x-ray examination does have limitations, in that:

1. It is unable to define mucosal disease, e.g., gastritis.
2. It is not definitive in differentiating benign from malignant gastric ulcer.
3. It cannot delineate superficial, subacute gastric or duodenal erosions which have not yet developed well defined craters.
4. It is unable to define complete healing of an ulcer.

Furthermore, as an ulcer heals, the surrounding tissue, especially in the duodenum, becomes scarred and deformed and radiologic assessment of activity of the ulcer becomes more difficult.

Endoscopic Studies[111]

For the reasons listed above and because endoscopy can provide visual, cytologic, and histologic information, it is playing an increasing role in the differential diagnosis of patients with dyspepsia. In addition, endoscopy provides accurate assessment of the healing of gastric and duodenal ulcers. Endoscopy should be employed to establish benignity of any gastric ulcer with atypical radiographic features. It provides the best measure of complete healing of gastric ulcer and is the only method of establishing healing of a duodenal ulcer. Because of cost, endoscopy can be recommended only for the evaluation of atypical or complicated ulcer disease.

CONTROL OF GASTRIC SECRETION

An understanding of the physiology of gastric secretion[1,3] is valuable even though the measurement of gastric secretion provides little data of diagnostic or prognostic value in peptic disease. Since therapy for peptic ulcer is aimed, in the main, at limiting gastric secretion, understanding of the normal control of gastric secretion is useful in the design of medical and surgical therapy.

Normal Secretion

Hydrochloric acid is secreted by the parietal cells of the proximal four-fifths of the stomach by an incompletely understood mechanism that involves the active transport of H^+ and Cl^- ions into the gastric juice. The epithelium of the stomach stringently limits the diffusion of ions and is so tight that a concentration gradient of one to one million is normally achieved for H^+ between plasma and gastric juice. Parietal cells secrete acid in response to three interacting endogenous stimuli: 1) acetylcholine from postganglionic cholinergic neurons; 2) gastrin, the peptide hormone of the gastric antrum; and 3) histamine.

In man, the fasting acid secretory rate is about 15 percent of the maximal rate and shows diurnal variation with a peak in the evening (10 P.M.) and low in the morning (8 A.M.). Physiologic control of gastric secretion is divided into three interrelated phases. First is the cephalic phase, in which vagal efferent pathways, activated by the thought, smell, and taste of food, stimulate the parietal cells directly through the release of acetylcholine and indirectly by stimulating the G cells (gastrin containing) of the antrum to release gastrin. Second is the gastric phase, in which distension of the stomach leads to direct (neural) and indirect (hormonal) stimulation of acid secretion through vagovagal and intramural reflexes. In addition, contact of the epithelium with the products of protein digestion also leads to direct and indirect stimulation of the parietal cells. Calcium increases the responsiveness of the parietal cells as well as the G cells. The responsiveness of the G cells is decreased as the pH in the antrum falls, thus providing a negative feedback control of gastric secretion. Third is the intestinal phase, in which the release of duodenal gastrin as well as other intestinal hormones stimulates gastric secretion. The intestine also exercises a negative feedback control over gastric secretion. A number of duodenal and intestinal hormones released in response to acid, hyperosmolar fluid, and products of fat and protein digestion inhibit gastric secretion and emptying. The list includes secretin, cholecystokinin-pancreozymin, enteroglucagon, gastric inhibitory peptide (GIP), and vasoactive intestinal peptide (VIP). The relative importance of these hormones in normal control of gastrointestinal function remains to be determined.

The concentration of acid in the stomach is determined by three factors: 1) rate of gastric secretion; 2) buffering capacity of gastric contents; and 3) rate of gastric emptying. Although the rate of gastric secretion is the greatest in the first hour after a meal, the concentration of H^+ falls because of the buffering capacity of the food. During the second and third hour after a meal, the H^+ concentration rises in spite of decreasing acid secretion because the buffering capacity of gastric contents decreases due to saturation

of proton acceptors of the food and loss of buffer from the stomach by gastric emptying. As a consequence the highest rate of delivery of acid into the duodenum occurs in the second hour after eating; the pH of the duodenal contents is raised as a result of neutralization of acid by bicarbonate secreted by the pancreas, liver, and duodenum in response to secretin, which also limits gastric secretion and emptying. Hence the control of gastric and duodenal pH as well as gastric emptying is the result of complex series of interacting "feedback" mechanisms.

Hypersecretion[99]

Average normal basal (fasting acid) output is 2 mEq per hour with an upper range of normal about 5 mEq per hour but basal secretion as high as 10 mEq per hour is occasionally found in patients without symptoms or obvious disease. Average normal maximal acid output is 20 mEq per hour with an upper limit of 40 mEq per hour. Hypersecretion or secretion above these "normal" levels is found in:

1. 5 percent of asymptomatic individuals
2. 25 percent of patients with duodenal ulcer
3. Hypergastrinemia due to (a) gastrinoma of the pancreas (Zollinger-Ellison syndrome), duodenum, or antrum; (b) hyperplasia of G cells of antrum or pancreas; (c) retained antrum in which a portion of antrum is left with the duodenal stump at the time of surgery (partial gastrectomy with gastrojejunostomy). The retained antral G cells no longer bathed with gastric acid are removed from normal inhibition and release large amounts of gastrin
4. Portacaval shunts presumably due to failure of hepatic inactivation of histamine and other gastric secretagogues from the intestine
5. Small bowel resection possibly due to removal of gastric inhibitory factors of intestinal origin
6. Pyloric obstruction possibly stimulating acid secretion through stimuli evoked by antral distension
7. Hypercalcemia of any origin
8. Malignant carcinoid, systemic mastocytosis, and basophilic leukemia due to hyperhistaminemia
9. Severe brain damage leading to increased vagal discharge
10. Pancreatitis or pancreatic duct obstruction

Hyposecretion

Hyposecretion of gastric acid is the result of 1) decreased parietal cell secretion; 2) back diffusion of secreted acid through an abnormal mucosa; or 3) a combination of the two factors. The gastric atrophy of pernicious anemia involves the acid producing mucosa but spares the antrum. Not only is the secretion of intrinsic factor necessary for vitamin B_{12} absorption lost but also the ability to secrete acid and pepsin. The more common form of gastritis, antral gastritis, involves the antrum and, to a lesser degree, the fundus. Although there is decreased secretion of acid with antral gastritis, probably of more importance is the damage to the mucosa which allows back diffusion of acid which in turn leads to more mucosal damage. The damaged mucosa may be replaced with intestinal metaplasia, a very permeable epithelium that is unable to maintain a normal hydrogen gradient. A variety of agents lead to disruption of the gastric mucosal barrier: bile acids and lysolecithin refluxed from the duodenum, and drugs such as aspirin and alcohol.[86,96] Their role in the pathogenesis of antral gastritis is unknown. Finally, benign gastric ulcer and gastric carcinoma are usually associated with antral gastritis and gastric hyposecretion.[114]

MEDICAL THERAPY OF PEPTIC ULCER

The treatment of peptic ulcer is empiric and is based on the assumption that the mechanism of symptom relief and ulcer healing is through the neutralization of acid gastric juice.

Diet[87,106]

The patient with a peptic ulcer should take a normal diet with three meals a day and should avoid only those foods that he has found to cause dyspepsia. None of the so-called ulcer diets have been shown to hasten relief of symptoms or rate of healing. All meals stimulate gastric secretion by distension of the stomach and their protein content. Although protein stimulates acid secretion, it also buffers the pH of gastric contents.

After the symptoms have come under control the use of coffee and occasional alcohol with meals is not contraindicated unless their use results in a recurrence of symptoms.

When the patient presents with severe, constant pain or with vomiting, therapy should be initiated in the hospital by a period of 24 to 48 hours of continuous gastric suction. Then the patient may be placed on a regimen consisting of liquid or soft feedings. This needs to be maintained only for a day or so if the patient has an appetite for a regular diet.

Cimetidine[90]

Cimetidine is a potent inhibitor of gastric acid secretion. It is an H_2 receptor antagonist and as a consequence blocks histamine stimulation of the parietal cell. Histamine's action is mediated through two types of receptors, H_1 receptors blocked by traditional antihistamine drugs and H_2 receptors that are unaffected by antihistamines and are responsible for histamine stimulation of gastric secretion. Blocking the H_2 receptor on the parietal cell also blunts the response to the other physiologic stimuli, acetylcholine and gastrin. The basal and nocturnal acid secretion is reduced with 300 mg orally by 90 to 95 percent and food-stimulated acid secretion by 70 percent. Anticholingeric drugs, which have been employed extensively in the past in the treatment of peptic ulcer disease, reduce food-stimulated acid secretion by only 25 to 30 percent. In prospective double-blind randomized 4 to 6 week trials, 70 percent of duodenal ulcers in the cimetidine group were healed as compared to 40 percent in the placebo group when evaluated by duodenoscopy. Cimetidine is given as 300 mg tablets with meals and at bedtime. Since cimetidine is rapidly excreted by the kidneys, its dosage must be decreased when used in patients with renal insufficiency.

The use of cimetidine has been associated with infrequent and reversible side effects including granulocytopenia, gynecomastia, and mild elevations of serum creatinine and aminotransferases. In the elderly, especially those with renal insufficiency, reversible confusion and coma have been reported when the dose has not been scaled down.[90]

Antacids[88,92,112]

Antacids have been the cornerstone of medical therapy for the past 25 years. Their effectiveness is determined by their capacity to buffer gastric acid and the rate of gastric emptying. Recent studies have shown that an intensive antacid regimen of 210 ml per day (30 ml of antacid [aluminum-magnesium hydroxide with an in vitro buffering capacity of 123 mEq HCl per dose] 1 and 3 hours after meals and at bedtime) was as effective as cimetidine in healing duodenal ulcers. After 4 weeks of treatment, 64 percent of ulcers treated with cimetidine were healed as demonstrated by duodenoscopy as compared to 52 percent of those treated with intensive antacid regimen.[101] Although intensive antacid therapy is as effective as cimetidine and the cost is similar, in practice fewer patients complete the full course, hence fewer heal their ulcers because of the inconvenience of taking medicine seven times a day after symptoms have disappeared.

TABLE 58-1
Antacids*

	In Vitro Buffer Capacity (mEq HCl/ml antacid)	Sodium Content (mg/5 ml)
Mylanta II	4.14	8.0
Aludrox	2.81	4.5
Maalox	2.58	5.6
Mylanta	2.38	3.9
Gelusil-M	2.23	5.7
Riopan	2.23	0.7
Amphojel	1.93	8.2
Gelusil	1.33	6.5
Phosphojel	0.42	13.0

* Data from Fordtran, JS, et al.[94]

In addition, 25% of patients on an intensive antacid regimen will develop diarrhea.

In Table 58-1 are listed some of the more commonly used commercial antacid mixtures along with their buffering capacity and sodium contents.

Soluble antacids, such as sodium bicarbonate and calcium carbonate, are the most effective. However, in large doses they produce alkalosis, and with prolonged use in some individuals they lead to the milk-alkali syndrome (hypercalcemia, renal insufficiency, and alkalosis).[109] In addition, calcium-containing antacids produce acid rebound to secretory rates twice basal acid secretion.[91] For this reason, nonabsorbable antacids, such as aluminum hydroxide gel and magnesium trisilicate gel, are usually employed.

Since aluminum hydroxide is extremely constipating, most antacids containing this substance also contain varying amounts of magnesium oxide (milk of magnesia). Intensive antacid regimens based on magnesium-oxide-containing preparations cause diarrhea in 25 percent of patients. This is corrected by a change to an antacid containing less laxative.

Anticholinergics[103]

Anticholinergic drugs decrease gastric acid secretion, but the dosages required produce other undesirable effects, such as dry mouth, blurred vision, and urinary retention. At present the only role of anticholinergics in the treatment of peptic ulcer disease is to augment the antisecretory effect of cimetidine (see p. 656).[89]

Sedation

Sedatives should be given only on specific indication rather than as a routine part of the ulcer regimen.

Experimental Drugs

Several experimental drugs have been demonstrated to result in ulcer healing but their advantage over cimetidine or an "intensive antacid regimen" has not been demonstrated. Carbenoxolone, a licorice extract, has been shown to hasten the rate of healing of gastric ulcers but has an aldosterone-like action so that 50 percent of patients have sodium retention and hypertension.[116] Prostaglandin E_2 reduces gastric secretion and has been shown to enhance the rate of healing of gastric ulcers but has diarrhea as a side effect.[95] A colloidal bismuth compound, tripotassium dicitrate bismuthate has shown increased healing of both duodenal and gastric ulcer without troublesome side effects.[97]

Long-Term Management

The advent of cimetidine has simplified medical therapy of peptic ulcer. On the basis of current experience, patients with duodenal ulcer should be treated for 8 weeks with cimetidine 300 mg with meals and at bedtime (q.i.d.). Because of its convenience, more patients continue therapy to healing with cimetidine than with antacids. It is hoped that as a consequence the frequency of the complications of ulcer will decrease. If the patient has a recurrence within 6 months, a second 8-week course of cimetidine should be instituted and serum gastrin measured to exclude hypergastrinemia as the cause of the ulcer disease. With this recurrence, healing should be documented by duodenoscopy. If the ulcer is healed, maintenance therapy with 300 mg of cimetidine at bedtime may decrease the chance of recurrence.[100] If, on the other hand, the ulcer is unhealed, cimetidine therapy should be supplemented with antacid or anticholinergics.[89]

There is less agreement concerning the role of cimetidine in the treatment of gastric ulcer. Although not shown to be more effective than intensive antacids, more patients are able to comply fully with the cimetidine regimen, hence more should heal their ulcers with cimetidine than with traditional antacid therapy.[90] Healing of gastric ulcers should be documented by endoscopy before discontinuing therapy. The concern for complete healing of a gastric ulcer is prompted by the high rate of recurrence and by the complications of a chronic incompletely healed gastric ulcer.

COMPLICATIONS OF PEPTIC ULCER

In 20 percent of patients with chronic peptic ulcer, medical management fails to prevent the progression of the disease or the development of complications.

Hemorrhage

Hemorrhage complicates the course of 16 percent of duodenal ulcers and 12 percent of gastric ulcers (Chap. 59). If hemorrhage is massive and is not under control in 12 to 24 hours, surgical therapy should be considered.

Perforation

Perforation occurs in 1 percent of peptic ulcers. (Chap. 57). All such patients require surgery.

Obstruction[105]

Obstruction complicates the course of 7 percent of duodenal ulcers and less than 0.5 percent of gastric ulcers.

Minor degrees of pyloric obstruction are common in patients with duodenal ulcers; indeed, much of the intractability seen in chronic disease has been attributed to partial pyloric obstruction. In fully developed pyloric obstruction, vomiting is the most characteristic symptom. Prior to this stage, the patient notes that meals aggravate his distress rather than relieve it.

In ulcer patients presenting with these symptoms, a succussion splash or clapotage may be elicited, confirming the suspicion of gastric retention. Clapotage is a splashing sound heard in the epigastrium when the abdomen is gently rocked to and fro. This sign should not be elicitable from a normal stomach more than 1 hour after a glass of water has been drunk or 3 hours after a meal.

The differentiation between benign and malignant obstruction can best be established by endoscopy with cytology and biopsy. Rarely are symptoms of pyloric obstruction caused by adult pyloric hypertrophy.

Endoscopy to establish the cause of gastric retention should not be performed until the patient has been on gastric aspiration for 24 hours. If the obstruction is benign the patient should be started on small feedings daily (soft diet) and cimetidine.

After 3 days the adequacy of gastric emptying can be assessed by aspirating and measuring the gastric contents 4 hours after the evening meal. If gastric emptying has returned to normal, less than 200 to 300 ml of gastric juice should be recoverable. Another simple useful test is performed by instilling 750 ml saline into the stomach and withdrawing the residue after 30 minutes. Ninety percent of normal individuals have less than 200 ml remaining whereas patients with gastric retention have more than 400 ml.[115] The initial episodes of pyloric obstruction are due to edema and spasm caused by ulcer activity. They can be treated satisfactorily with an ulcer regi-

men. Recurrent episodes indicate that the ulcer is resistant to medical therapy or scarring has led to irreversible narrowing. In either case the treatment is surgical.

Intractable or Recurrent Peptic Ulcer

Most intractable or recurrent ulcers are a manifestation of the severity of the ulcer diathesis and/or the inability of the patient to follow an effective regimen. However, before this formulation is accepted, several questions should be considered:

1. Have other causes of dyspepsia been excluded?
2. Is the patient receiving optimal ulcer therapy?
3. Are the patients' symptoms truly due to the ulcer or to an associated unresolved emotional problem?
4. Are complications related to the ulcer, such as obstruction or penetration through the wall causing symptoms?
5. Have all specific causes of gastric hypersecretion been ruled out?

ZOLLINGER-ELLISON (Z-E) SYNDROME AND RELATED DISORDERS.[102,117] Originally Zollinger and Ellison called attention to a group of patients with jejunal ulcers and gastric hypersecretion associated with non-beta-cell islet tumors of the pancreas. These tumors are composed of G cells and secrete large amounts of gastrin which causes gastric hypersecretion and peptic ulcers. As experience has accumulated, it is recognized that 75 percent of ulcers caused by gastrinomas are in locations expected in uncomplicated peptic ulcer disease. Z-E syndrome should be suspected in patients with intractable ulcer disease, giant or multiple ulcers, or rapid recurrence after surgery. In addition, the following findings should lead to a consideration of Z-E in the differential diagnosis: 1) gastric hypersecretion; more than two-thirds of patients with Z-E syndrome have basal secretory rates over 10 mEq per hour and one-half are greater than 15 mEq per hour; 2) diarrhea or even steatorrhea; in more than one-third of patients diarrhea is a prominent symptom; 3) hypertrophy of gastric rugae seen with endoscopy or x-ray studies. The diagnosis is confirmed, however, by finding an elevated serum gastrin ($>$500 pg/ml). In patients with Z-E syndrome with intermediate elevation (200 to 500 pg/ml), calcium or secretin infusions lead to striking elevations of serum gastrin.[104] Ultimate proof of the diagnosis is demonstration of a non-beta-cell tumor in the pancreas at time of surgery. Since approximately two-thirds of these tumors are malignant and very few cures have been achieved by attempting to remove the tumor, total gastrectomy to remove the end-organ had been the treatment of choice until recently. Z-E syndrome has been shown to respond to cimetidine. Two-thirds of the patients are controlled on the usual dose of 1200 mg per day, but some require double the dose. In Z-E syndrome, cimetidine must be given continuously to keep the ulcer disease under control.[108]

A Z-E-like syndrome has been seen with gastrinomas of the antrum and duodenum as well as G cell hyperplasia of the antrum and pancreas. In addition, gastrinomas may be one of the abnormalities encountered in familial multiple endocrine adenomas, the Wermer syndrome.[117] Since as many as 20 percent of Z-E patients have other endocrine adenomas, it has been suggested that Z-E syndrome is really only one manifestation of the so-called Wermer syndrome.

SURGERY FOR PEPTIC ULCER

The aim of the surgical treatment of peptic ulcer is to decrease gastric secretion to a level at which healing will occur and recurrences will be eliminated while interfering as little as possible with alimentary tract function.

The four types of operation most frequently employed are 1) subtotal gastrectomy, in which the antrum and a substantial part of the body of the stomach (the acid-producing mucosa) are resected; 2) vagotomy and antrectomy, designed to remove both the neural and humoral stimuli of gastric secretion; 3) vagotomy and pyloroplasty, in which the neural stimuli are interrupted and the resulting gastric retention is minimized by pyloroplasty; and 4) parietal cell or highly selective vagotomy which denervates the acid secreting portion of the stomach and leaves the innervation and motor function of the antrum intact. In the first two procedures gastrointestinal continuity is reestablished by either gastroduodenostomy (Billroth I) or gastroenterostomy (Billroth II).[118]

In general, the greater the gastric resection, the greater is the frequency and severity of postgastrectomy dumping symptoms. Postgastrectomy malabsorption tends to be more severe after gastroenterostomy than after gastroduodenostomy. Since the incidence of recurrent ulcer is greater in patients treated with vagotomy and pyloroplasty, vagotomy with antrectomy is currently the preferred surgical treatment for duodenal ulcer.

The choice of the surgical procedure to be employed in the treatment of a peptic ulcer is based more on the experience and preference of the surgeon than on any fundamental physiologic considerations.

COMPLICATIONS OF THERAPY

Medical Therapy

The four main complications of medical therapy—diarrhea, delayed gastric emptying, hypophosphatemia, and the milk-alkali syndrome—should disappear as cimetidine becomes the preferred treatment for peptic ulcer disease.

Surgical Therapy

Surgery provides completely satisfactory relief of ulcer symptoms in 80 percent of the patients. In 4 to 10 percent of patients so treated, the results are unsatisfactory, and in a few the complications may be more severe than the original ulcer symptoms.

DUMPING SYNDROME.[107]   The dumping syndrome is experienced in mild form by many patients after a partial gastrectomy. In most, symptoms disappear within a month but in a few patients these symptoms continue to be prominent and on rare occasion disabling. Within 15 minutes of eating the patient becomes aware of an epigastric fullness at times associated with nausea. If the attack is severe, tachycardia, sweating, and weakness appear. These symptoms may be followed by abdominal cramping and a loose stool or two. The attack is aggravated by walking about and relieved by lying down.

When the stomach and duodenum are anatomically and functionally intact, gastric emptying is controlled so that the intestinal contents never become hypertonic. In the postgastrectomy dumping syndrome, this control is lost. The appearance of hypertonic fluid in the intestine calls forth a rapid secretion of fluid into the jejunum. The resulting distension of the intestine causes a sensation of epigastric fullness and stimulates intestinal motility and diarrhea. The abrupt shift of water from the blood to the intestinal lumen gives rise to symptoms of hypovolemia—that is, tachycardia, sweating, and syncope.

The dumping syndrome can be minimized by taking small, frequent feedings which are low in carbohydrates and by separating the solid and liquid portions of the meal by 1 hour. Initially it may be necessary to lie down for ½ hour after meals.

POSTPRANDIAL HYPOGLYCEMIA SYNDROME. The symptoms of the postprandial hypoglycemia syndrome are sweating, palpitations, and syncope 2 to 3 hours after meals. When the stomach empties rapidly, glucose is absorbed quickly and the blood sugar reaches hyperglycemic levels. This results in a compensatory liberation of insulin that overshoots, resulting in hypoglycemia.

AFFERENT LOOP SYNDROME.[110] The afferent loop syndrome is caused by a partial obstruction of the afferent loop of the gastroenterostomy. As a result, bile and pancreatic juice accumulate. When the loop empties, usually after the meal has passed into the efferent loop, the stomach is flooded with the retained duodenal fluid, and bilious vomiting occurs.

POSTGASTRECTOMY ANEMIA. A variety of factors contribute to postgastrectomy anemias, among them: 1) bleeding from the stomach or jejunum; 2) decreased absorption of iron; and 3) least commonly, decreased absorption of vitamin B_{12} caused by the failure of the stomach to produce intrinsic factor. Patients who have had total gastrectomies regularly develop a B_{12} deficiency.

MARGINAL ULCER. Peptic ulcers may form in the jejunum adjacent to a gastroenterostomy. They rarely occur when the surgery is performed for a gastric ulcer, but, depending on the procedure employed, they appear in about 1 to 10 percent of the patients with duodenal ulcers treated surgically. The first concern in the patient with a marginal ulcer is the adequacy of the surgical procedure. On occasion the vagotomy is incomplete or antral tissue is left in with the duodenal stump. When acid is excluded from contact with the antrum, gastrin output is increased which in turn increases gastric secretion. In these patients, as well as in others in whom ulcer disease is poorly controlled by routine treatment, unusual forms of peptic ulcer disease should be looked for (see p. 658).

POSTGASTRECTOMY MALABSORPTION (SEE P. 686)

OTHER CAUSES OF DYSPEPSIA

X-Ray Negative Dyspepsia

In patients with dyspepsia who have negative upper gastrointestinal series and no other apparent cause for their symptoms, the use of fiberoptic endoscopy has provided new insight into the causes of their symptoms. In these patients, gross endoscopic or histologic abnormalities are found in approximately 75 percent. The more common findings include: unsuspected gastric or duodenal ulcers, atrophic gastritis, antral gastritis, and duodenitis. It is not clear how these mucosal abnormalities are related to or cause dyspepsia. Nevertheless, the symptoms in these patients usually respond to the same therapy given to ulcer patients.

Chronic Cholecystitis (See Chap. 57)

Functional Dyspepsia

Patients with dyspepsia for which no organic cause is demonstrated are arbitrarily put into one of two groups. The first contains those whose symptoms simulate the symptoms associated with organic disease of the upper gastrointestinal tract such as peptic ulcer, cholecystitis, and peptic esophagitis. In this group the symptoms probably arise from a motor disturbance of the gastroduodenal segment induced by emotional turmoil and other poorly understood factors rather than by anatomic abnormalities. At present, the techniques for studying gastroduodenal motility are not refined to the point that this hypothesis can be put to a test.

Patients in the second group have symptoms that are bizarre compared with the symptoms of patients with known organic disease. It is thought that these patients are describing their emotional disturbances in somatic terms. These patients most frequently show features of hysteria, conversion reaction, or depression.

In the first group, simple symptomatic treatment, combining reassurance with an attempt to resolve the anxiety-producing situation, is usually satisfactory. The second group gets no relief from symptomatic therapy and usually needs more formal psychotherapy.

CHAPTER 59
Gastrointestinal Bleeding
THOMAS R. HENDRIX, MARVIN M. SCHUSTER, AND ROBERT I. WHITE, Jr.

Gastrointestinal bleeding may present as a life-threatening emergency with hematemesis and melena or, at the other extreme, it may be occult and chronic and only discovered in a search for the cause of anemia.

ACUTE GASTROINTESTINAL BLEEDING
Acute gastrointestinal bleeding is particularly difficult to deal with because its appearance is usually unexpected, the source of the bleeding often is uncer-

tain, and the volume of blood lost and the rate of continuing loss are difficult to determine.

The therapy of gastrointestinal bleeding is supportive and definitive. Supportive therapy aims to restore and maintain normal functioning blood volume regardless of the source of hemorrhage in order to avoid hypovolemia and its complications, such as renal shutdown, hepatic failure, myocardial ischemia, and cerebral vascular insufficiency. Definitive therapy requires that the nature and location of the bleeding lesion be identified. For example, arterial bleeding from a peptic ulcer or Mallory-Weiss tear is treated definitively by surgical closure of the bleeding point; on the other hand, surgical treatment of erosive gastritis or bleeding varices is indirect and can introduce as many problems as it attempts to correct. Finally, if the cause of the bleeding is not a local lesion but a blood dyscrasia, such as von Willebrand syndrome, surgery is contraindicated.

The successful management of a gastrointestinal hemorrhage requires the close cooperation of the physician, radiologist, and surgeon. The decisions should be based on joint medical–surgical consideration of each patient.

Hypovolemia and Rate of Bleeding

The primary reason that the mortality from gastrointestinal bleeding has not improved over the past 40 years is that there is no simple, direct measure of functional blood volume.[127] As guides to blood replacement, the clinician, at present, must rely on clinical estimates which have been validated by tedious investigative procedures.[142,143]

HEMATEMESIS.[139] The greater the rate of bleeding and the higher the lesion is in the gastrointestinal tract, the more likely it is the patient will vomit blood. The patient who has had a massive hematemesis should be considered to have lost one-third to one-half his blood volume. If blood replacement is based on this assumption, the chances of underestimating the blood loss and of suddenly finding it necessary to combat severe vascular collapse will be minimized.

MELENA. As little as 50 to 80 ml of blood introduced into the upper gastrointestinal tract will make the stools black. The appearance of more than one black stool, tarry in consistency, within a 24-hour period usually is associated with a loss of 25 percent or more of the blood volume.

BLOOD PRESSURE AND PULSE.[142] Features of shock (hypotension, tachycardia, and cold, clammy skin), if present when the patient is recumbent, are indicative of a 50 percent loss of the blood volume. If

signs of shock are present only when the patient assumes an upright position, a loss of 20 to 30 percent of the blood volume should be assumed.

The blood pressure is not a reliable indication of the extent or rate of bleeding because it may be maintained at near-normal values until vasoconstrictor capacity is exceeded; further blood loss then leads to sudden and severe vascular collapse.[120] On the other hand, a systolic blood pressure below 100 mm Hg or a pulse above 110 indicates that as much as 50 percent of the normal blood volume has been lost. Half the patients with systolic blood pressure below 100 mm Hg on admission have a massive hemorrhage requiring more than 2.5 liters blood replacement whereas only 13 percent of patients requiring less than 2.5 liters have admission blood pressure below 100 mm Hg. A rising pulse rate also is an ominous sign. A steady pulse rate, however, is not a reliable indication that the blood volume is being maintained in a safe range.[120]

Most gastrointestinal hemorrhages, and especially those of arterial or variceal origin, occur in episodes lasting about 30 minutes. After each bleeding episode the patient's blood pressure and pulse stabilize, and the physician may be lulled into a false sense of security. However, each recurrent episode of bleeding depletes the patient's vascular reserve and, if blood replacement is inadequate, further bleeding leads to vascular collapse.[128]

Skin and conjunctival pallor are poor indices of the extent of bleeding. Pallor of the palmar creases, however, suggests a loss of 50 percent of the blood volume.[138]

CENTRAL VENOUS PRESSURE.[120,138] Central venous pressure (CVP) is a useful indicator of functional blood volume but requires the insertion of a catheter into the superior vena cava. Since the largest fraction of the blood volume is in the venous compartment, one of the first indications of decompensation is a falling CVP. Rapidly falling CVP (2 mm H_2O per minute with an overall fall of 5 cm H_2O) was always found to be associated with arterial bleeding and should alert the clinician to the likelihood that emergency surgery will be required.[119] Since the range of normal CVP is wide, 5.5 to 13.5 cm, the direction and rate of change is of more significance than the initial pressure. Monitoring CVP also helps guard against overtransfusion since the CVP rises before pulmonary congestion and edema occur.

HEMATOCRIT.[119,143] The hematocrit is not a useful index of the extent of gastrointestinal bleeding. It tells only what percentage of the blood volume is composed of red cells, but provides no direct measure of blood volume. Since it takes from 6 to 24 hours or more after a hemorrhage for hemodilution to be complete, the hematocrit determined soon after a massive hemorrhage will be near normal. Hematocrit changes in gastrointestinal hemorrhage differ from those in hemorrhage elsewhere, because the gut is able to absorb up to 75 percent of the water from blood passing through. Such reabsorption helps preserve the intravascular volume, but the process is not rapid enough to protect the patient with a massive hemorrhage from hypovolemia. Nitrogenous materials are also absorbed, so the serum urea nitrogen, even in the absence of kidney disease, can rise to levels twice normal within 8 hours of the loss of one pint of blood into the gut.

Site of Bleeding[132]

As soon as measures have been instituted to correct hypovolemia, clues suggesting the location of the lesion should be sought by history and physical examination.

UPPER OR LOWER GASTROINTESTINAL TRACT. The first step is to determine whether the bleeding is from the upper or lower gastrointestinal tract so that relevant diagnostic and therapeutic procedures can be employed. If the patient vomits blood, the bleeding lesion is most certainly proximal to the ligament of Treitz. If the patient has not vomited blood, a tube should be passed into the stomach.[135] If the gastric aspirate contains blood, then the bleeding site is above the ligament of Treitz. If the stomach is free of blood, there are three possibilities: 1) the site of bleeding is below the ligament of Treitz; 2) bleeding has stopped and all the blood has passed into the intestine; and 3) the site of bleeding is distal to the pylorus and proximal to the ligament of Treitz, but at the time of intubation the bleeding is not brisk enough to cause reflux of blood into the stomach.

If a tarry stool is passed, the lesion is not lower than the ileocecal sphincter. However, red blood can be passed with a bleeding lesion as high as the esophagus. The color of the blood passed is as much a function of the rate of bleeding and passage through the gastrointestinal tract as it is the site of bleeding. In general, the larger the hemorrhage, the more rapid the passage through the gut.

HISTORY. First, are there recent or remote symptoms of peptic ulcer disease? Peptic ulcer is the most common cause of massive upper gastrointestinal hemorrhage[132,135] (Table 59–1). Statistical data, however, cannot be relied on to provide the correct diagnosis in the individual patient.

Next, is there a history of recent heavy alcoholic

TABLE 59–1

Lesions Causing Upper Gastrointestinal Hemorrhage in 827 Patients at Johns Hopkins Hospital 1972–1977

Lesion	Incidence (%)
Erosive gastritis or duodenitis	27
Duodenal ulcer	22
Esophageal varices	15
Gastric ulcer	12
Mallory-Weiss	7
Marginal ulcer	3
Carcinoma	
Gastric	2
Esophageal	1
Miscellaneous*	4
Undiagnosed	7
Total	100

* Miscellaneous group includes: bleeding disorders, benign tumors (especially leiomyoma and neurofibroma), congenital disorders such as Peutz-Jeghers syndrome, pseudoxanthoma elasticum, hereditary telangiectasia, esophageal ulcer, and rupture of an aneurysm into the duodenum or biliary tract (hemobilia).

intake or of drug ingestion, especially of aspirin, corticosteroids, phenylbutazone, or anticoagulants? The recent ingestion of any of these substances suggests the possibility of diffuse gastric erosions, an acute peptic ulcer, or an iatrogenic bleeding disorder. A history of blood appearing only after vomiting, especially after an alcoholic binge, should lead to a consideration of the Mallory-Weiss syndrome, in which retching leads to a longitudinal mucosal tear at the gastroesophageal junction.

Historical evidence of liver disease should be sought. Of course, not every alcoholic with hepatomegaly has cirrhosis, not every cirrhotic has varices, and finally, not every cirrhotic with varices bleeds from this site. Indeed, in a large series of patients with upper gastrointestinal bleeding, it was found that one-third of the patients with cirrhosis and varices were actually bleeding from other lesions.[140]

PHYSICAL EXAMINATION. Many of the rare causes of gastrointestinal hemorrhage are associated with characteristic physical findings that may be missed unless they are specifically looked for (see Section VI).[125] These include 1) melanin spots on the lips and buccal mucosa, found in the Peutz-Jeghers syndrome with bleeding from intestinal polyps; 2) telangiectatic lesions of Osler-Weber-Rendu disease (hereditary hemorrhagic telangiectasia) seen on the face, head, fingertips, and mucous membranes with bleeding from similar vascular lesions in the gastrointestinal tract; 3) characteristic skin changes of pseudoxanthoma elasticum are associated with vascular lesions, especially in the stomach, which may bleed; 4) less commonly, café-au-lait spots may be associated with bleeding neurofibromas of the intestinal tract. Cutaneous caviar vascular lesions may be found with bleeding gastrointestinal vascular anomalies. Finding the cutaneous manifestations of these rare diseases, however, cannot be taken as proof that they are the cause of gastrointestinal hemorrhage; finally, 5) purpura, ecchymoses, or bleeding gums, which can be overlooked easily if not specifically sought, are evidence of a bleeding diathesis.

UPPER GASTROINTESTINAL HEMORRHAGE. *Endoscopy.*[132,140] If the clinical evidence favors an upper gastrointestinal source of the bleeding, endoscopy should be performed as soon as hypovolemia has been corrected. Fiberoptic endoscopes make it possible to examine the esophagus, stomach, and first part of the duodenum with ease and safety. Endoscopy can be performed in the patient's room so that the patient is not removed from observation of the ward medical and nursing staff. To insure that the lesion is visualized, it is necessary to lavage the stomach with ice water through a large bore gastric tube (36 French). During lavage the patient should be positioned on his side to minimize the chances of aspiration.

Angiography.[121,122] If endoscopy has failed to identify the source of bleeding or bleeding is so rapid the stomach cannot be cleaned of blood sufficiently for endoscopy and the patient is continuing to bleed briskly, angiography should be performed. Selective visceral arteriography has become an important technique not only in the localization of the site of bleeding but in control of hemorrhage by direct infusion of vasoconstricting drugs into the bleeding vessel. A catheter is introduced percutaneously into the femoral artery and guided by fluoroscopy into the branches of the celiac, superior mesenteric, and/or inferior mesenteric arteries. Extravasation of contrast material into the bowel lumen is the roentgenographic sign of active bleeding. In order to consistently see extravasation of contrast material, the injected artery must be bleeding at a rate greater than 1.5 ml per minute (3 units per day). Since arterial bleeding is episodic and slows or ceases when the patient is hypovolemic, careful attention must be given to maintaining a normal blood volume during angiography to insure the greatest chance of identifying the site of bleeding. Angiography is the only technique available for identifying a bleeding lesion in the small intestine.[136] Occasionally a patient with recurrent gastrointestinal hemorrhage which eluded diagnosis is shown by angiography to have a vascular tumor of the intestine or a bleeding Meckel's diverticulum which can be resected.[136]

Barium Studies. Emergency barium studies are not recommended as part of the evaluation of massive gastrointestinal hemorrhage because they rarely provide a definitive diagnosis and preclude more accurate techniques of endoscopy and angiography until the barium clears the gastrointestinal tract.

LOWER INTESTINAL HEMORRHAGE. *Proctoscopy and Angiography.*[126] If the clinical findings suggest the lower bowel is the source of bleeding, proctoscopy should be the first diagnostic procedure. Proctoscopy will determine whether or not the bleeding is from the rectosigmoid, rectum, or anal canal. Bleeding lesions commonly identified by proctoscopy include diffuse mucosal lesions, such as ulcerative and ischemic colitis; local vascular lesions, such as hemorrhoids; and tumors, such as polyps or cancer. If proctoscopy fails to identify the source of bleeding and bleeding continues at a rapid rate, angiography of the superior and inferior mesenteric arteries is the most effective method of localizing the source of the bleeding. With more frequent use of angiography in patients with colonic hemorrhage, the necessity for emergency surgery has diminished since local infusion of vasopressin stops the bleeding in most patients (Fig. 59–1). Angiography has shown vascular ectasia or angiodysplasia of the colon to be a common cause of massive as well as chronic colonic bleeding.[124] Since this lesion is difficult or impossible to detect by direct inspection at operation or colonoscopy, diagnosis and successful surgical management are dependent upon angiography. In the past when barium enema was the primary diagnostic procedure, two-thirds of the cases of massive colonic bleeding were found to be associated with diverticula as the only demonstrable abnormality. Association does not, however, prove a cause-and-effect relation. With increased use of angiography only a small percentage of these patients are shown to have a bleeding diverticulum. When bleeding is demonstrated to originate from a diverticulum, it is most frequently in the ascending colon, whereas the greatest concentration of diverticula are found in the sigmoid and descending colon (Table 59–2).

If bleeding is not massive, carcinoma of the colon, polyps, and inflammatory diseases such as ulcerative colitis, Crohn's disease, amebic or ischemic colitis should be considered. Colonoscopy and barium enema examination are useful in the evaluation of these causes of less rapid colonic bleeding.[123]

Radioisotope Imaging. Radioisotope imaging

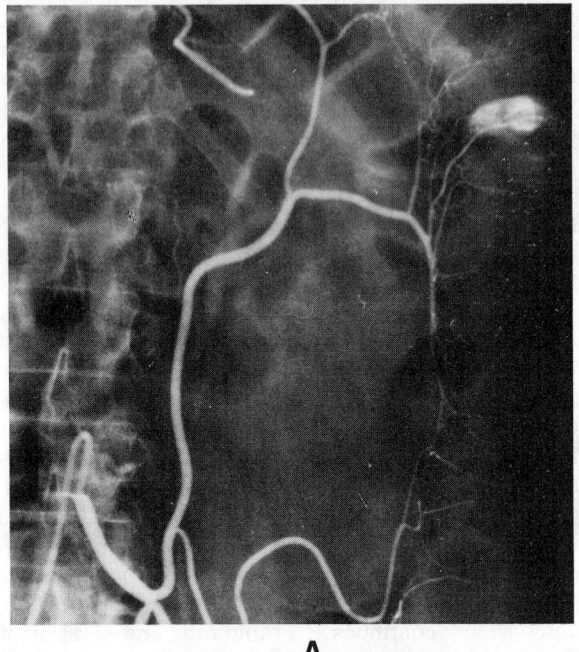

A.

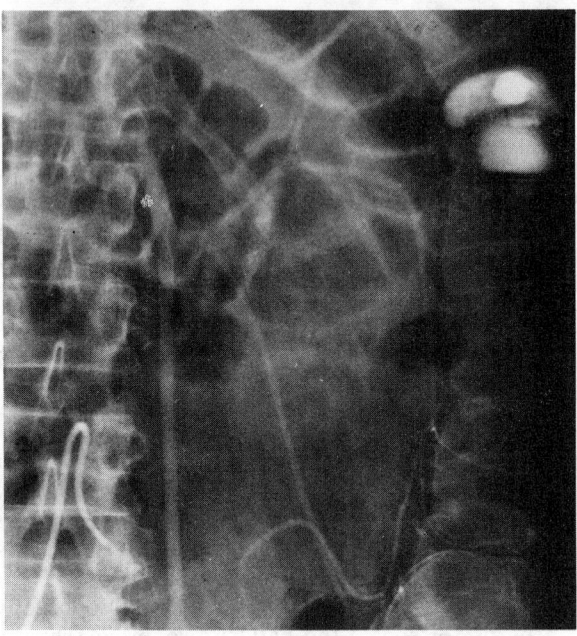

B.

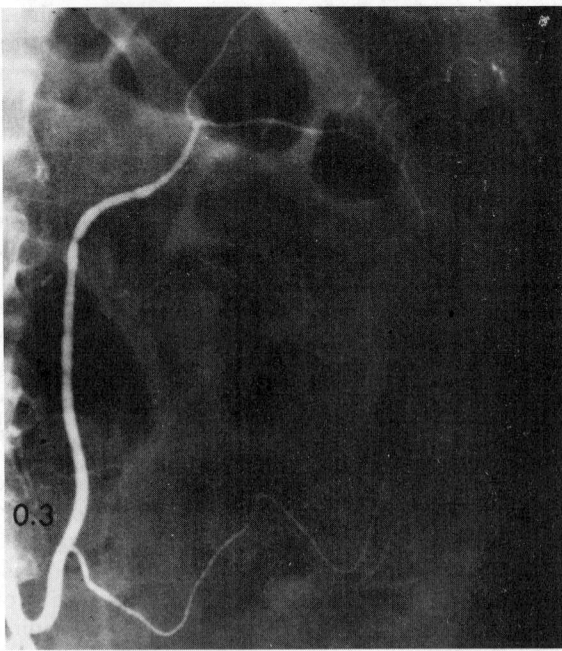

C.

FIGURE 59–1. Inferior mesenteric angiogram, arterial **(A)** and venous **(B)** phase from a patient with a bleeding diverticulum in the splenic flexure. A large area of extravasation of contrast material is seen on the arterial phase **(A)** and in the venous phase **(B)** contrast material fills up the base of the diverticulum. After 20 minutes of a selective arterial infusion of vasopressin (0.3 U/min), the bleeding is largely controlled **(C)** as evidenced by minimal extravasation of contrast material.

is helpful in the detection of Meckel's diverticulum, which is a rare cause of intermittent hemorrhage. The hemorrhage is almost always red blood and occurs in patients under the age of 25. Small bowel x-rays usually miss the diverticulum and angiography is often not available during the brief episodes of bleeding. 99Technetium pertectnitate is taken up by the ectopic gastric mucosa contained in most bleeding diverticula, thus providing a simple noninvasive technique for identifying this occult cause of bleeding.[129]

TABLE 59-2
Lesions Causing Lower Bowel Bleeding in 353 Patients at Johns Hopkins Hospital 1972-1977

Lesion	Incidence (%)
Cancer of left colon	24
Benign polyps	12
Bleeding diverticula	7
Cancer of right colon	4
Angiodysplasia	3
Inflammatory bowel disease	3
Miscellaneous*	8
Undiagnosed†	39
Total	100

* Miscellaneous group includes small bowel tumors, Meckel's diverticulum, vascular malformation, ischemic bowel disease.
† Half of the undiagnosed group had colonic diverticula which could not be demonstrated to be cause of bleeding.

Therapeutic Approach to Massive Gastrointestinal Hemorrhage

The therapy of massive gastrointestinal hemorrhage is, first, supportive, that is, restoring and maintaining the blood volume, regardless of the source of the bleeding, and second, definitive, that is, treatment designed to stop the bleeding.

SUPPORTIVE THERAPY. When a patient with a massive hemorrhage is first seen, the blood volume deficit should be estimated and replacement begun immediately; first, with whatever fluid is readily available, e.g., saline or plasminate, and shifting to whole blood as soon as possible. It is not necessary, however, to transfuse to a normal hematocrit; the goal is to prevent shock, to maintain normal vital signs, and to raise the hematocrit to a level (30 percent) which will provide a margin of safety should bleeding recur or surgery be required. Careful monitoring of central venous pressure is most useful in avoiding fluid overload as well as determining the need for further transfusions.[120,138] Rapid transfusion, which is often life saving, is performed more safely with the aid of central venous pressure measurements. As soon as hypovolemia is corrected, packed red cells may be transfused instead of whole blood, especially if blood substitutes have been used to treat shock while awaiting the arrival of blood. Packed red cells are useful also when an acute hemorrhage is superimposed upon chronic bleeding, since under these conditions compensatory mechanisms have often led to hemodilution. Slow bleeding into the gastrointestinal tract allows time for more reabsorption of fluid than rapid bleeding. Therefore, replacement with packed cells is more appropriate for slow bleeding and whole blood for rapid bleeding.

The adequacy of blood replacement is determined by regularly recording blood pressure, supine and sitting, pulse, CVP, urine output and specific gravity, hematemesis, stools, and volume of blood and fluid replacement. If there is continued rapid bleeding after the correction of hypovolemia or if bleeding recurs after an apparent arrest of 24 hours or more, definitive therapy of the bleeding lesion should be instituted.

DEFINITIVE THERAPY. The vigorous approach to the identification of the source of gastrointestinal hemorrhage is advocated so that if bleeding continues or recurs, definitive therapy can be promptly instituted. Arterial bleeding, e.g., from a peptic ulcer or a Mallory-Weiss tear is, on one hand, most treacherous because of its intermittency and the rapidity with which it can lead to shock; but on the other hand, it is most effectively treated by surgical ligation. Bleeding from a duodenal ulcer, especially in young patients, tends to stop spontaneously; but if massive, recurrent, or in a patient with a long history of ulcer disease, it is likely that a sclerotic artery in the ulcer base has been eroded. In this case, surgery with direct suture of the artery provides the most effective lasting control of the bleeding. A history of previous hemorrhages does not necessarily imply the need for surgery. Both the severity and frequency of recurrences must be taken into account. Mallory-Weiss bleeding can often be controlled by cautery applied when the lesion is identified endoscopically. In patients not considered good candidates for surgery, selective angiography can be used both to identify the bleeding artery and stop the bleeding by embolization with gelfoam or small detachable balloons.[145]

Small arterial-capillary hemorrhage from erosive gastritis is usually self-limiting if the agent causing the damage, e.g., acetylsalicylic acid, alcohol, etc., is withdrawn. If bleeding is massive and continuing, selective angiography with infusion of vasopressin into the left gastric or celiac artery should be instituted.[121] Surgery should be avoided because the diffuse distribution of the bleeding lesions requires a major gastric resection, even total gastrectomy, to remove the bleeding points.

Cimetidine is being widely used, not only for the treatment of bleeding peptic ulcers and erosive gastritis, but also in an attempt to prevent stress ulcers in seriously ill and postoperative patients. These uses are based on the belief that gastric acid production is involved in the pathogenesis of all of these bleeding lesions. It should be emphasized that at this time the efficacy of these uses of cimetidine has not been established. Peptic ulcers, however, are best treated with cimetidine regardless of whether presentation is with pain or bleeding (Chap. 58).

Bleeding from colonic diverticula and angiodysplasia can be demonstrated only by angiography. These bleeding lesions are usually located in the right colon and are visualized by superior mesenteric arteriography. When the bleeding has been demonstrated, it should be treated by intra-arterial vasopressin perfusion. If this fails, definitive surgery can be performed because the site of bleeding has been localized.

The patient bleeding from esophageal varices has two problems: the acute bleeding episode and the chance or even likelihood that liver failure will follow. If the patient's hepatic reserve is unknown or limited, the best way to increase the chance for long-term survival is to control the bleeding and postpone portal-systemic shunt surgery until hepatic function is restored to an optimal level. Since the mortality rate for bleeding varices and the incidence of rebleeding is so high, immediate control should be obtained by infusion of vasopressin.[133] Infusional therapy coupled with adequate transfusion to maintain a normal functional blood volume provides the cirrhotic the maximal chance of surviving a variceal hemorrhage. Vasopressin decreases the inflow into the engorged portal bed with a resultant fall in portal pressure and cessation of variceal bleeding, while adequate transfusion maintains normal blood pressure and hepatic artery flow which is the major source of blood supply to the liver in cirrhosis. If this form of control is unsuccessful, the Blakemore-Sengstaken tube can be utilized to tamponade the varices. Emergency portal-systemic shunting is an alternative to control variceal hemorrhage but it carries a high mortality. If tamponade is to be maintained as a therapeutic measure, a tracheostomy should be performed to minimize the chance of aspiration. Fresh whole blood is preferred for transfusion of patients with cirrhosis and bleeding because it replaces clotting factors which are often diminished in these patients. For more details of the treatment of bleeding esophageal varices, see Chapter 64.

Some patients have recurrent acute bleeding episodes that go undiagnosed in spite of complete diagnostic studies. Some of these patients have von Willebrand syndrome (see Chap. 48). Their bleeding diathesis is obscured by transfusions. In fact, they usually have no difficulty when surgery is performed after transfusion, but the AHG deficiency found in this disease can be detected only in the intervals between hemorrhages. If no bleeding disorder is detected, patients with undiagnosed, recurrent, acute gastrointestinal hemorrhages should be studied by angiography at the onset of a bleeding episode. If the bleeding site is still not localized, surgical exploration should be undertaken during active bleeding, thus giving the surgeons the best chance to identify the lesion responsible. This approach has been successful when interval exploration has not identified the source of bleeding.

CHRONIC GASTROINTESTINAL BLEEDING

Chronic blood loss can be continuous or intermittent, or an acute hemorrhage may be superimposed upon prolonged, slow bleeding. If the patient has a low hematocrit but shows only minimal symptoms of hypovolemia, the blood loss has been slow enough for compensatory adjustment to take place. The pattern of the bleeding should be established by testing daily stools for occult blood. Guaiac-positive stools indicate a blood loss of at least 10 ml per day (for comparison, 30 to 70 ml of blood are lost in a normal menstrual period).

Site of Bleeding

Endoscopic examination of the upper and lower gastrointestinal tract should be undertaken, preferably at a time that bleeding is active. If no explanation is found, then x-rays of the entire gastrointestinal tract should be taken. If still no lesion has been found, angiography should be performed to determine if a vascular malformation or tumor is present. Bleeding into the lumen will not be great enough to be seen angiographically. Therefore, an attempt should be made to establish that the abnormality demonstrated by angiography is the source of bleeding by introducing a small plastic tube weighted so that it will pass to the cecum. When blood appears in the drainage, the tube should be fastened in position and x-ray studies performed using contrast medium through the tube. The location of the tube will also give the surgeon indication of where he should begin his search for the bleeding lesion. The two most commonly encountered causes of occult chronic gastrointestinal bleeding are peptic ulcer and carcinoma. Continuous occult bleeding, demonstrated by daily stool guaiac determinations, strongly suggests malignancy as a source, whereas intermittent bleeding is more likely due to benign lesions, such as polyps, Crohn's disease, angiodysplasia, anal fissures, and hemorrhoids.

Treatment

The treatment of chronic gastrointestinal bleeding is the treatment of the primary lesion. The anemia which results from chronic blood loss can often be treated by oral administration of iron. In order to replete tissue stores, iron therapy should be continued for 3 months after the hematocrit has returned to normal levels. When the hematocrit is very low or when symptoms of anemia are prominent, especially in the elderly patient with compromised cardiovascular or cerebrovascular reserve, transfusion may be necessary. Packed red blood cells are preferred to whole blood since plasma volume is usually normal, although the percentage of red cells is low.

Carcinoma of the Colon and Rectum

Rectal bleeding, gross or occult, is the earliest sign of colorectal carcinoma. This malignancy deserves special comment because of 1) its frequency (second only to skin cancer and second to lung cancer as a cause of death); 2) its potential for cure (although the 5-year survival is only 50 to 60 percent, it approaches 100 percent in early tumors confined to the bowel wall)[144]; and 3) its precursor, the colonic polyp, which antedates the appearance of malignancy by 5 to 15 years. Unlike many other precursor lesions, polyps are easy to identify and simple to remove in toto.[130] Only half of patients with colorectal cancer reach definitive surgical therapy before the tumor has extended through the bowel wall or metastasized to regional lymph nodes. Five-year survival in those with spread beyond the bowel wall is only 14 percent. To improve these results, more effective screening for colorectal cancer is needed. Seventy-five percent of colorectal cancer occurs in patients over 55 years of age, and 95 percent after age 45. Also, other high risk groups need to be brought under surveillance, e.g., patients with ulcerative colitis, familial polyposis, Gardner syndrome, previous polyps or colorectal cancer, and a family history of colorectal cancer.

When first described, it was hoped that carcinoembryonic antigen (CEA) would provide a serologic screening test for colorectal cancer. Although positive in 90 percent of patients with metastatic colorectal cancer, it is not specific for colonic nor malignant disease; but of more practical note, it is positive in only 40 percent of early disease. The major use of CEA is to follow patients for evidence of recurrent tumor.

Patients over the age of 40 should have a series of five stool specimens examined for occult blood annually.[131] These examinations have been greatly facilitated by the development of hemoccult slides which can be collected at home and mailed to the doctor. Patients with stools positive for occult blood or who have symptoms suggesting colorectal cancer—e.g., recent change in bowel habits, either constipation or diarrhea; sense of incomplete evacuation; crampy abdominal pain; or anal pain or mass—should be evaluated for colorectal cancer.

First, these patients should be sigmoidoscoped, although somewhat less than 50 percent of colorectal cancers are within the reach of the rigid sigmoidoscope. In the past sigmoidoscopy had been advocated as the primary screening procedure for colorectal cancer, but even if used optimally it would find no more than 50 percent of the malignancies.[137] Any polyps found should be removed. If sigmoidoscopy does not identify a source of the bleeding, a barium enema, preferably air contrast examination, should be performed, even if a bleeding polyp has been identified by sigmoidoscopy, because polyps are frequently multiple. If polyps are seen, they should be removed by colonoscopy. If no lesions are seen on barium enema, colonoscopy should be performed since polyps and early cancers not visible by x-ray evaluation may be picked up by endoscopy.[141] If a carcinoma is found, the primary treatment is surgical resection. If pathologic examination of the specimen shows invasion of vessels or penetration to the serosa, it is almost certain there have been micrometastases that will not be cured by surgery. Adjuvant chemotherapy with 5-fluorouracil alone or in combination with drugs such as methyl-lomustine (methyl-CCNU), vincristine, and streptozotocin should be given in an attempt to prevent or delay metastatic recurrence.[134]

The best available evidence indicates that colorectal cancer does not arise de novo but rather passes through a stage of adenomatous growth, then epithelial atypia, and finally invasive carcinoma. It has been estimated that of 1000 colonic polyps, only 100 are neoplastic, of these 10 will be large adenomatous polyps, and only one will have become an invasive carcinoma.[130] Thus it can be seen that there should be ample opportunity to make an early diagnosis of carcinoma if the tools available are used regularly.

CHAPTER 60

Diarrhea and Constipation
THOMAS R. HENDRIX AND THEODORE M. BAYLESS

DIARRHEA

Diarrhea is caused by increased water in the stools. Normally 100 to 150 ml of water is lost in the stools daily, but when the volume increases the stools lose their form and diarrhea results. Increased fluid in stools can be caused by impaired absorption, increased secretion, or a combination of these factors. In addition, the disorder may involve the small intestine or colon singly or in combination. The alimentary tract normally is presented with a fluid load of over 10 liters per day derived from exogenous (dietary) and endogenous sources (salivary, gastric, biliary, pancreatic, and intestinal secretion). In health all but 1500 to 2000 ml are absorbed by the time the cecum is reached, and the colon then absorbs all but 100 to 150 ml of the remaining fluid. Since the colon has a limited absorptive capacity, about 2.5 liters per day, diarrhea appears if a larger volume is presented to the colon by the small intestine.[182]

The volume of fluid presented to the colon by the small intestine is increased if: 1) there is a failure of intestinal absorption, e.g., diffuse mucosal disease such as celiac disease, deficiency of a digestive enzyme such as lactase or ingestion of a nonabsorbable solute such as magnesium sulfate (epsom salts); or 2) there is increased fluid secretion, e.g., toxin-induced such as in *E. coli* or *V. cholera* diarrhea, hormone induced such as VIP (Vasoactive Intestinal Peptide) in pancreatic cholera or prostaglandin in medullary carcinoma of the thyroid. Similarly disordered colonic function may be the cause of diarrhea, for example, 1) decreased colonic absorption due to diffuse mucosal disease, such as in ulcerative colitis or shigellosis; or 2) increased colonic secretion induced by unabsorbed bile salts or fatty acids entering the colon or caused by a fluid secreting tumor, such as villous adenoma.

The contents of the intestine at each level has a characteristic composition: jejunum-Na^+148, K^+5.6, Cl^-138, HCO_3^-15; ileum-Na^+146, K^+5.7, Cl^-121, HCO_3^-42; and stool-Na^+55, K^+90, Cl^-20, HCO_3^-7.0 mEq/L.[167] The greatest change in ionic composition occurs during passage through the colon. Since the colon's absorptive capacity is limited, stool electrolyte composition approaches ileal composition as the volume of diarrhea increases.

To design definitive therapy for diarrhea, the physician must determine the site and nature of the intestinal abnormality, as well as the volume and composition of the fluid lost.

CLASSIFICATION AND CLINICAL MANIFESTATIONS

It is convenient to categorize diarrhea on the basis of the onset and duration of the illness: 1) acute diarrhea with sudden onset and short duration; and 2) chronic diarrhea, often with an insidious onset and a long duration.

Acute Diarrhea

Infectious agents (viral, bacterial, or parasitic), toxins, poisons, and drugs are the major causes of acute diarrhea. Enteric infections are discussed in Chapter 86. Enterotoxins produced by noninvasive bacteria, most often toxigenic *E. coli* (in this country), and viral enteritis are probably the most common causes of acute diarrhea. Since simple, specific diagnostic tests have not been developed for these infections, their diagnosis in clinical practice is by exclusion. Recent advances, however, provide promise that specific diagnostic procedures may become available. At times, ulcerative colitis presents as an acute, fulminant illness. Other inflammatory causes of acute diarrhea include appendicitis and diverticulitis. Causes of drug and diet related diarrhea are listed in Table 60–1. Pseudomembranous enterocolitis has been described with increasing frequency with the use of antibiotics, including lincomycin, clindomycin, and cephalin.[147] Characteristic plaques which may become confluent develop on the colonic mucosa as the disease progresses. If these lesions are not apparent at proctoscopy in a suspected case, rectal biopsies should be taken to look for microscopic pseudomembranes. This antibiotic-associated colitis is caused by an enterotoxin produced by *Clostridium difficile* which proliferates in the colon when the normal flora is eliminated by antibiotics. If unrecognized and untreated, it is associated with a high fatality rate. There are, however, two effective therapies: 1) vancomycin which eliminates the toxin-producing organism; and 2) cholestyramine, an anion-binding resin, which promptly reverses the clinical and histologic finding by binding the toxin.[153] Ischemic colitis and partial intestinal obstruction present with diarrhea. Psychogenic stress is an important cause of acute diarrhea.

---TABLE 60-1---
Drug- and Diet-Related Diarrhea

I. **Drug**

  A. Osmotic overload
    1. Magnesium-containing antacid
    2. Lactulose (in treatment of hepatic coma)
    3. Cathartics

  B. Mucosal injury
    1. Cancer chemotherapy
    2. Antibiotic associated colitis
      (pseudomembranous colitis—clindamycin,
      lincomycin, and cephalin most common)
    3. Colchicine
    4. Neomycin (causes steatorrhea)

  C. Alteration of motility
    1. Parasympathomimetic agents
    2. Thyroid
    3. Cardiovascular drugs (digitalis, quinidine,
      ganglionic blocking drugs)

II. **Diet**

  A. Osmotic overload
    1. Lactose-containing food (in lactase deficient
      patients)
    2. Dumping syndrome
    3. Elemental diets

  B. Increased secretion and/or mucosal injury
    1. Caffeine (secretion)
    2. Food poisoning
      a. Bacterial (staphylococcal, clostridia,
        salmonella, shigella, *Vibrio*
        parahemolyticus)
      b. Toxin (mushroom, staphylococcus
        enterotoxin, botulism)
    3. Fat in patients with steatorrhea
    4. Heavy metals (mercury, arsenic, cadmium,
      lead)

DIAGNOSTIC PROCEDURES. The initial diagnostic procedure should be a Wright's stain or methylene blue stain of a fecal smear to determine whether or not fecal leukocytes are present.[166] In enteric inflammatory disorders, both those caused by specific invasive organisms and idiopathic inflammatory bowel disease, the fecal leukocytes are predominantly polymorphonuclear leukocytes. In typhoid fever, mononuclear cells predominate. If no leukocytes are seen, the diarrhea is most likely viral or toxigenic. In addition, the stools should be examined for amebae and blood and they should be cultured for pathogenic bacteria. Proctoscopy should be performed, especially if there is blood in the stool to obtain mucus for direct smear for amebae and biopsy to determine the nature of the inflammatory process. Gonococci are at times found to be the cause of heavy purulent exudate.[181] If the history suggests that contaminated food might be the source of the infection, food samples should also be cultured.

THERAPY. Most acute diarrheal episodes are self-limiting and do not require specific therapy. If, on the other hand, the patient is dehydrated and especially if vomiting occurs, parenteral fluid replacement with Ringer's lactate solution should be instituted. Suppressants of intestinal transit such as deodorized tincture of opium (DTO) 5 drops after each movement (not more than 5 doses per day), paregoric 5 ml after each movement (up to 5 doses per day), or diphenoxylate hydrochloride and atropine (Lomotil) 2.5 to 5 mg or loperamide 2 mg 4 or 5 times per day may be given to patients who have neither fever nor leukocytes in their stool. Because diarrhea is a defense mechanism to wash away offending organisms, antidiarrheal agents should not be given early in the course of acute infectious bowel disease.

Chronic Diarrhea

Diarrhea that has persisted for several weeks usually requires a detailed diagnostic investigation. A classification of chronic diarrhea based on the predominant pathophysiologic mechanism is presented in Table 60–2. In some disorders, such as Crohn's disease (regional enteritis), there are a number of physiologic derangements occurring at the same time, for example, increased exudation as a result of inflammation, decreased absorption, and increased secretion and motility. In others, e.g., giardiasis and "food allergy," no satisfactory hypotheses are available. Indications of whether the lesion causing diarrhea is in the small or the large bowel are to be found in the patient's history. Crohn's disease of the small bowel and celiac disease are examples of chronic diarrhea originating in the small intestine. Although the material entering the right colon is more voluminous than normal because of impaired small intestine absorption, the reservoir and absorptive capacity of the colon is still intact, and the patient may therefore have only one or two large bowel movements a day. If abdominal discomfort occurs, it is usually worse after meals or just before a bowel movement. A barium enema with ileal reflux, a small bowel series, and screening tests for malabsorption should confirm the clinical suspicion of small bowel disease. In contrast, ulcerative colitis involving the descending colon and rectum illustrates the clinical findings of large bowel diarrhea. Inflammation of the rectum lowers the threshold for stimulation by bowel contents, and small amounts of stool produce the urge to defecate. This symptom complex of frequent small stools, urgency, and blood and mucus in the stools points toward large-bowel diarrhea.

TABLE 60-2
Pathophysiologic Classification of Chronic Diarrhea

I. **Decreased Absorption (see Chap. 61)**
   A. Small intestine
      1. Generalized malabsorption
         a. Mucosal damage (celiac disease)
         b. Impaired intraluminal digestion (pancreatic insufficiency)
         c. Bacterial overgrowth (bile salt deconjugation and mucosal injury—scleroderma
      2. Specific malabsorption
         a. Enzyme deficiency (disaccharidases)
         b. Transport defect (chloridorrhea, glucose-galactose malabsorption)
         c. Nonabsorbable solute (magnesium, lactulose)
   B. Colon
      1. Idiopathic inflammatory bowel disease
         a. Ulcerative colitis
         b. Crohn's disease
      2. Specific inflammatory bowel disease
         a. Amebiasis
         b. Ischemic colitis
         c. Radiation colitis

II. **Increased Secretion**
   A. Small intestine
      1. Dumping syndrome
      2. Gastric hypersecretion (Zollinger-Ellison syndrome)
      3. Endogenous secretogogues (vasoactive intestinal peptide, prostaglandins, serotonin, etc.)
   B. Colon
      1. Unabsorbed fatty acids[146]
      2. Bile acids (failure of ileal reabsorption)[168,177]
      3. Unabsorbed carbohydrates (lactase deficiency)
      4. Fluid secreting tumor (large villous adenoma)

III. **Motor Disturbances (Decreased Mixing Activity)**
   A. Small intestine and colon
      1. Carcinoid syndrome
      2. Postvagotomy diarrhea
      3. Hyperthyroidism
      4. Diabetic visceral neuropathy[195]
      5. Scleroderma
   B. Colon
      1. Irritable bowel syndrome

IMPORTANT ASSOCIATED FINDINGS TO BE EVALUATED IN THE PATIENT WITH CHRONIC DIARRHEA. There are other clinical features that aid in the differential diagnosis of diarrhea. At times, these other signs and symptoms may be the presenting problem, and diarrhea may not be a major complaint.

Weight Loss. Weight loss is an important symptom, indicating a serious underlying disease until proved otherwise. Diarrhea and marked weight loss may be caused by the following conditions: 1) those that cause anorexia; 2) partial intestinal obstruction with postprandial pain and a resultant decrease in food intake; 3) malabsorption; and 4) generalized diseases that affect the intestinal tract, such as hyperthyroidism, Addison's disease, diabetes with autonomic neuropathy, lymphoma, leukemia, polyarteritis, systemic lupus erythematosus, scleroderma, carcinoid syndrome, and tuberculosis. Weight loss is not part of the irritable bowel syndrome (functional bowel disease).

Malabsorption. The typical patient with intestinal malabsorption presents with weight loss and bulky, light-colored, greasy, foul-smelling stools. Secondary deficiencies due to the malabsorption of specific substances, such as calcium, iron, vitamins B, D, and K, folic acid, and proteins, and not diarrhea may dominate the clinical picture. Malabsorption should be considered in the differential diagnosis of unexplained weight loss, even though diarrhea is not a prominent symptom (Chap. 61).

Arthritis. Arthritis may occur in any patient with chronic diarrhea, but particularly in patients with Crohn's disease, ulcerative colitis, polyarteritis, systemic lupus erythematosus (SLE), and Whipple's disease.

Skin Manifestations. Skin manifestations of diagnostic significance associated with diarrheal diseases include 1) flushing, in the carcinoid syndrome; 2) hyperpigmentation sparing the mucous membranes, in Whipple's disease; 3) generalized pigmentation, in Addison's disease; 4) dermatitis, in pellagra; 5) urticaria pigmentosa, with mast cell tumors; 6) dermatitis herpetiformis, coexisting with celiac disease; 7) erythema nodosum, with Crohn's disease or ulcerative colitis; 8) pyoderma gangrenosum, with ulcerative colitis; 9) dermatomyositis. Glossitis and cheilosis occur most commonly with vitamin deficiencies and malabsorptive states. Clubbing occurs with Crohn's disease and cirrhosis. Thrombophlebitis migrans may occur with intra-abdominal malignancies, including carcinoma of the pancreas.

Fistula or Sinus Tract. A fistula or sinus tract in the lower abdomen or perianal region is a common presentation of Crohn's disease, but it may also be seen with tuberculosis and actinomycosis. Peri-intestinal abscesses caused by perforations due to foreign bodies or diverticulitis also produce fistulas on occasion.

Severe Abdominal Pain. Severe abdominal pain preceding the onset of diarrhea occurs with ischemic colitis, perforation of a gallstone into the intestine, or with a marginal or gastric ulcer forming a gastrocolic fistula. Patients with the severe ulcer diathesis of the Zollinger-Ellison syndrome frequently have diarrhea and may have steatorrhea.

Nocturnal Diarrhea. Nocturnal diarrhea usually indicates a definite organic disease. It may be associated with any severe disorder, but it is especially common in diabetic visceral neuropathy, hyperthyroidism, and ulcerative colitis. It is unusual for the patient with a functional diarrhea to be awakened at night by the urge to defecate.

DIAGNOSTIC PROCEDURES IN CHRONIC DIARRHEA.
Stool Examination. The first step in determining the cause of diarrhea is examination of the stool. Blood, gross or occult, indicates ulceration of the mucosa or a neoplasm. Fecal leukocytes (Wright strain) also indicate an inflammatory lesion in the colon. Stool examination for ova and parasites should be performed. Giardiasis is the most common parasitic cause of diarrhea in this country. If the stools contain fat as indicated by a positive test for split fats (Sudan III stain), malabsorption is the likely cause of the diarrhea (see Chap. 61).[175] Finally, if a fecal smear turns red upon alkalization, the patient has been taking phenolphthalein laxatives and the diarrhea may be factitious.

Proctosigmoidoscopy.[192] A proctosigmoidoscopic examination should be performed on every patient with chronic diarrhea before x-ray studies are done. The examination is done without an enema preparation because hypertonic cleansing solutions produce edema and an excessive secretion of mucus that may be mistaken for early ulcerative colitis. Enemas may also wash away the mucus containing amebic trophozoites and decrease the likelihood of seeing these organisms in a smear of rectal mucus or in a rectal biopsy.

The normal rectal mucosa is smooth and translucent so that the submucosal vessels are clearly visible and is covered with a thin, shiny layer of mucus. Abnormalities range in severity from hyperemia and edema which obscure the mucosal vascular pattern to friability (small bleeding points in response to minor trauma such as rubbing with a cotton swab) to frank ulceration. In addition polyps may be seen which may be adenomas (true neoplasia) or "pseudopolyps." The latter are heaped up masses of hyperplastic disordered epithelium and inflamed granulation tissue that represent an unsuccessful attempt to repair severe mucosal damage.

Rectal Biopsy.[198] Rectal biopsy is useful 1) as a diagnostic tool in the evaluation of diarrheal diseases; 2) to provide follow-up information concerning the activity of inflammatory bowel disease and response

to therapy; and 3) to detect "precancer" in patients with ulcerative colitis.

Rectal biopsy should be taken if the mucosa appears abnormal. In addition, biopsies should be taken in those patients in whom the diagnosis is in doubt because a biopsy of normal appearing rectal mucosa may provide the first objective indication of diseases such as Crohn's disease, Whipple's disease, amyloidosis, schistosomiasis, and cystic fibrosis.

Tests of Malabsorption. (See Chapter 61 for discussion of tests of malabsorption.)

Roentgenologic Examination. Roentgenologic examination of the gastrointestinal tract is often helpful in unraveling the puzzle of chronic diarrhea. First, a plain film of the abdomen without contrast media may reveal evidence of large or small bowel obstruction, pancreatic calcification, calcified tuberculous lymph nodes, or the colonic dilatation of fulminant ulcerative colitis.

In most situations it is best to proceed with a barium enema before upper gastrointestinal and small bowel studies. Severe ulcerative colitis is an exception; barium enema should not be performed until the patient improves lest toxic megacolon be induced. The barium enema, in addition to filling the entire colon, is the best method for visualizing the terminal ileum and for demonstrating a gastrocolic fistula.

An upper gastrointestinal series will show those forms of peptic ulcer disease commonly associated with diarrhea, such as the Zollinger-Ellison syndrome and pyloric stenosis. Gastrocolic fistulas or inadvertent gastroileal fistulas after partial gastrectomy may also be demonstrated.

A small bowel study normally reveals delicate intestinal folds, with continuity of the barium column and with no dilated segments. The small bowel pattern is abnormal in over 90 percent of all patients with intestinal malabsorption due to mucosal involvement as occurs in celiac disease or tropical sprue (Chap. 61). Dilution of barium in the small bowel by excessive intestinal secretion often is an important clue to the presence of chronic secretory diarrhea.

In Crohn's disease, the small bowel changes may be localized to the terminal ileum with narrowing of the lumen (string sign); may affect separate segments, including the jejunum, duodenum, and colon, with narrowing and proximal dilatation (skip areas); or may involve the entire small bowel (ileojejunitis). Prominent thickened intestinal folds can be seen if the bowel wall is infiltrated by amyloidosis, lymphoma, Whipple's disease, or intestinal lymphangiectasia.

Colonoscopy. Fiberoptic instruments have made it possible to examine visually the entire colonic mucosa and by biopsy to determine the histologic nature of any abnormalities seen. It is particularly helpful in differentiating inflammatory from neoplastic masses. Less frequently it is used to obtain histologic evidence to support the diagnosis of Crohn's disease when rectal biopsy is normal but there is inconclusive evidence of abnormality on barium enema, and to determine the extent of involvement in ulcerative colitis. The usefulness of information obtained by colonoscopy must be weighed against the increased risk in inflammatory bowel disease of perforation during colonoscopy.

Stool Volume. Measurement of daily stool volume with patient on a regular diet and during a 48-hour fast (fluid intake maintained by intravenous infusion) is helpful in distinguishing endogenous from exogenous secretory stimuli. For example, if diarrhea is caused by an endocrine-secreting tumor, such as a vasoactive intestinal peptide-secreting pancreatic adenoma, fecal volume will not fall significantly when the patient fasts. On the other hand, if diarrhea is caused by some dietary component which is not absorbed, such as lactose, fecal volume will decrease strikingly during the fast.

CLINICAL EXAMPLES

The examples of diarrheal diseases selected for presentation are ulcerative colitis, Crohn's disease, humorally-mediated diarrheal syndromes, amebiasis, and functional bowel disease (Table 60–3).

Ulcerative Colitis

Ulcerative colitis[159] is a chronic inflammatory disease of unknown etiology involving the mucosa of the colon. The typical but by no means pathognomonic lesion is the crypt abscess, in which the epithelium of the crypt breaks down and the lumen fills with purulent exudate. The lamina propria is densely infiltrated with polymorphonuclear leukocytes and round cells. As the crypts are destroyed, the normal mucosal architecture is lost and scarring eventually leads to the shortening and narrowing of the colon.

To date, the cause of this epithelial destruction is unknown. Although genetic and psychosomatic factors may play a role, identification of the sequence of events at the colonic epithelium is most likely to provide the basis for definitive therapy.[178] It is unclear whether the damage is in response to some unique agent or material from the lumen of the colon or whether the damage is the consequence of some exaggerated immunologic response of the host to a common stimulus.

CLINICAL MANIFESTATIONS. Ulcerative colitis occurs in all age groups from infancy to old age, but the majority of those affected are young adults at the time of onset.

The incidence in family members of patients with ulcerative colitis and in the Jewish population is greater than in the general population, whereas blacks are less frequently affected. In the mildest form, called ulcerative or hemorrhagic proctitis, only

---

TABLE 60–3
Differential Diagnosis of Colitis

	Ulcerative[170] Colitis	Crohn's Disease[151]	Amebic[183] Colitis	Ischemic[176] Colitis
Onset	Gradual or abrupt	Gradual	Abrupt or gradual	Abrupt
Symptoms	Rectal bleeding and diarrhea	Diarrhea with little or no bleeding	Diarrhea Streaks of blood	Sudden pain Rectal bleeding
Perianal inflammation	Occasionally	Common; at times presenting symptom	None	None
Proctoscopy	Diffuse with friability	Normal, or focal, discrete ulcers, or diffuse	Diffuse or isolated ulcers	Usually normal
X-ray distribution	Distal, continuous segmental	Right side most frequent, often discontinuous and asymmetric	Sigmoid or cecum	Segmental, splenic flexure often
Ileal involvement	Normal or dilated	Sometimes normal, often narrowed	Normal	Occasionally involved
Pathologic findings	Diffuse involvement of mucosa	Involvement of mucosa, muscularis and serosa with deep fissures	Mucosa and submucosal	Mucosa or transmural
Fistula	None	Common	None	None

the rectal mucosa is involved.[160] Often the only symptom is blood in the stool and initially is erroneously attributed to hemorrhoids. In this form, the disease inflammation almost never extends to the proximal colon and is rarely a serious threat to health. At the other extreme, the entire colon is irreparably damaged when first seen and may progress to life-threatening toxin megacolon with perforation.

The onset of ulcerative colitis may be insidious, with vague abdominal discomfort, anorexia, lassitude, and a gradual change in bowel habits. Rectal bleeding, with or without diarrhea, frequently is the first symptom that brings the patient to his doctor. The majority of patients with ulcerative colitis have frequent small bowel movements containing pus, blood, and mucus mixed with small amounts of fecal material. As rectal involvement progresses, the threshold for stimulation by fecal contents is lowered and the patient experiences urgency and tenesmus. Cramping lower-abdominal pain relieved by defecation is a common complaint. One-third of the patients have an abrupt onset with bloody diarrhea, fever, anorexia, and weakness.

In two-thirds of the patients, ulcerative colitis is intermittently symptomatic, but in the other third the disease is continuously active. In about 5 percent the disease follows an extremely rapid and progressive (fulminant) course. Acute fulminant ulcerative colitis may be the first manifestation of ulcerative colitis, or may appear in the course of established disease. Rectal discharge is almost constant and bleeding may be massive. Fever, hypovolemia, tachycardia, and hypoproteinemia are major manifestations. Toxic megacolon and colonic perforation are highly lethal complications.

DIAGNOSIS.[170] Ulcerative colitis is a diagnosis of exclusion. When the onset is acute, it is essential to exclude infective colitis caused by shigella, salmonella, gonococcus, and amebae, as well as antibiotic-associated colitis and ischemic colitis before the diagnosis of ulcerative colitis is seriously entertained. Although no single finding is pathognomic, the prime diagnostic procedure is proctoscopy. In mild active ulcerative colitis, the rectal mucosa is hyperemic, edematous, granular, and, most characteristically, friable, that is, small mucosal bleeding points appear when the mucosa is rubbed with a cotton swab. In more severe disease, purulent exucate, spontaneous bleeding, and small ulcerations are seen.

Rectal biopsy is a useful confirmatory measure.[198] The inflammation and crypt abscesses are characteristic but not specific for ulcerative colitis. Histologic features suggestive of Crohn's disease, ischemic colitis, antibiotic-induced pseudomembranous colitis, amebiasis, schistosomiasis, tuberculosis,

and lymphogranuloma venerum should be looked for, since these diseases may sometimes present as an ulcerative colitis.

A barium enema is not required to make the diagnosis of ulcerative colitis and should not be done in acutely ill patients, lest toxic megacolon be induced. It does, however, indicate the extent of the disease and hence is useful in determining the prognosis.

The barium enema will be abnormal in almost all patients with ulcerative colitis except in those with ulcerative proctitis or disease limited to the rectosigmoid. Early changes include blurring of the bowel margins in the distal colon and obliteration of haustral folds. As the disease progresses, ulcerations appear and are seen as fine serrations and irregularities along the colon wall. If destruction of the mucosa is severe, the islands of remaining mucosa appear as pseudopolyps. With scarring there is a shortening and narrowing of the bowel with the further loss of haustrations. The involvement of the colon in ulcerative colitis is continuous proximal from the rectum, whereas in Crohn's disease it may be segmental. The smooth colon without haustral folds may be simulated by the changes produced by chronic purgation with laxatives.

TREATMENT.[156,191] Medical therapy is usually effective in suppressing disease activity in ulcerative colitis, but less than 5 percent of patients are "cured" or have no recurrences. Colectomy with an ileostomy is eventually required in about 20 percent. Adrenal corticosteroids and salicylazosulfapyridine (Azulfidine) are the mainstays of medical treatment. The aim of therapy is to produce and maintain a symptomatic remission. This is best accomplished by starting the patient on full doses of steroids (60 mg prednisone per day) and tapering to a maintenance dose (15 to 30 mg on alternate days) when the desired clinical response is achieved. Salicylazosulfapyridine, a combination of sulfonamide and salicylic acid (3 g per day orally), is used as an adjunct in the treatment of active disease and for maintaining a remission. The establishment of a strong patient–physician relationship is an important part of the long-term treatment of ulcerative colitis.

In ulcerative proctitis and mild disease localized to the rectum and sigmoid colon, local administration of hydrocortisone or prednisolone (30 mg prednisolone in 100 ml of water) in the form of small retention enemas at night is often effective.

Fulminant ulcerative colitis requires intensive care in the hospital. The initial therapy is directed at correcting the large fluid and electrolyte losses that result from severe diarrhea. The replacement of the blood volume and plasma protein is essential. Some patients lose as much as 50 g of protein per day. Parenterally administered hydrocortisone (300 mg per day) or ACTH is used. If toxic dilatation of the colon appears, these same measures are used, plus parenteral feedings, antibiotics, avoidance of narcotics, and careful observation for signs of impending perforation. If the patient with severe fulminant colitis has not improved within 48 hours, total colectomy with ileostomy should be performed. The surgical mortality with an urgent operation is about 7 percent whereas it is over 20 percent if a perforation occurs.

Surgery cures ulcerative colitis.[162] In all but exceptional cases, the procedure should be total colectomy with ileostomy. When done as an elective procedure, the mortality is about 1 percent. The indications for colectomy include: 1) failure to respond to medical therapy; 2) life-threatening complications, such as toxic megacolon, impending perforation, bleeding, chronic malnutrition, and in children, growth failure; 3) severe extracolonic complications, unresponsive pyoderma gangrenosum, persistent incapacitating arthritis, progressive ocular disease, or progressive liver dysfunction; 4) strictures of the colon or extensive perirectal complications; and 5) "precancer" and carcinoma itself. The aim of therapy is to have the patient live a full and active life. If this cannot be accomplished by medical measures, then surgery should be employed. The use of well-fitted appliances and disposable bags has lessened the burden of self-care of an ileostomy.[171] Many patients have found ostomy societies helpful in their adjustment to the inconvenience and psychological problems associated with an ileostomy. "Continent ileostomies" provide an alternative to help some patients accept an indicated colectomy.[161] This procedure frees the patient of the necessity of wearing an ileostomy bag. The bowel is evacuated by inserting a catheter into the stoma periodically.

THE COMPLICATIONS OF ULCERATIVE COLITIS. The complications of ulcerative colitis may be divided into local complications related to the colonic disease and systemic or extracolonic manifestations. Anemia, rectal bleeding, and hypoproteinemia are common and frequently require transfusion. On occasion, hemorrhage is massive and may require colectomy for its control. Perianal fistulas and abscesses occur but are much less frequent than with Crohn's disease. Marked dilatation of the colon with abdominal distension and tenderness may appear in the course of an acute exacerbation. In this syndrome, known as "acute toxic dilatation" or "toxic megacolon," the colon loses all tone, becomes greatly dilated, and may perforate if effective treatment is not begun promptly. Toxic megacolon often is iatrogenic, induced in severe active colitis by anticholinergic drugs, opiates, or preparation for barium enema.[180]

Pseudopolyposis is the result of a severe disease and indicates an extensive destruction of the colonic mucosa. The polypoid lesions may be seen on proctoscopy or as multiple sessile filling defects on barium enema. They are not precancerous.

The incidence of carcinoma of the colon not only is increased in ulcerative colitis but also occurs at a lower age (average 40 years) than the general population (average 60 years).[174,197] Factors associated with a high incidence of carcinoma of the colon are: 1) involvement of the entire colon, 2) long duration, even if inactive, and 3) onset in childhood. The risk of developing a carcinoma is not significantly greater than age-matched controls in the first five years of the disease, but by the time the patient with pancolitis has had the disease for 15 years, the incidence may be as high as 1 in 25. This risk is more than ten times that of the general population. Regular follow-up rectal and colonoscopic biopsies with particular attention to "precancerous" or dysplastic changes are useful in identifying those patients destined to develop carcinoma of the colon.[148]

Carcinoembryonic antigen (CEA) is elevated in the serum of patients with advanced carcinoma of the colon. It is not a sensitive indicator of early disease, is not specific for colonic carcinoma and is elevated in as many as 27 percent of patients with ulcerative colitis without cancer.[197]

The extracolonic complications of ulcerative colitis are varied and may be severe.[164] In general, they occur when the colitis is active. Skin lesions are occasionally seen, including pustules, erythema multiforme, erythema nodosum, and pyoderma gangrenosum. Arthritis may affect either large or small joints, but it is especially likely to involve the knees and ankles. There is also an increased incidence of rheumatoid spondylitis in patients with ulcerative colitis, and the spine changes may precede the recognized onset of colonic disease. Ocular complications, such as iritis, conjunctivitis, and uveitis, infrequently appear and usually coincide with colonic, skin, or joint activity.

Liver involvement in ulcerative colitis may take several forms.[158] Mild diffuse fatty change is frequent but usually without clinical effect. Hepatitis, chronic active hepatitis, postnecrotic cirrhosis, biliary cirrhosis, sclerosing cholangitis, and bile duct cancer have been described in association with ulcerative colitis. Intermittent fever, liver tenderness, and elevation of serum alkaline phosphatase concentration have been attributed to pericholangitis possibly resulting from bacterial drainage from the colon. The hepatic disease may regress after colectomy.

PROGNOSIS.[159]   Eighty-eight percent of the patients with ulcerative colitis have at least one subsequent attack during the 5 years after the initial episode. The severity of the first attack and the extent of involvement at that time influences both the short-term and the long-term prognosis. Although patients with mild disease, distal involvement or both have the best outlook, the 20-year survival for all cases of ulcerative colitis is only 65 percent of the age- and sex-matched controls.

Crohn's Disease[149,155]

Crohn's disease (also called regional enteritis, regional ileitis, or granulomatous colitis) is an inflammatory disease of unknown etiology most commonly affecting the terminal ileum or colon, but may involve any part of the gastrointestinal tract from the stomach to the rectum. It is a chronic recurrent illness affecting adolescents and young adults with abdominal cramps, diarrhea, loss of weight, fever, anemia, right lower quadrant mass, and perianal fistulas as the most common symptoms. As with ulcerative colitis, there appears to be a high familial incidence of Crohn's disease and its occurrence in Jews is greater than expected by chance.[189]

The pathologic changes are limited to the terminal ileum in one-half of the patients. Several sharply demarcated skip areas separated by normal bowel occur in the others. Involvement of the adjacent proximal colon as well as of the terminal ileum occurs in about 25 percent of the patients. Isolated lesions of the duodenum or stomach are much less common. In addition, Crohn's disease may involve the colon without small bowel changes in 15 percent of cases. The colonic lesions are often segmental and sometimes spare the rectum. The differential diagnostic features of Crohn's disease and ulcerative colitis are listed in Table 60–3. About 20 percent of patients with chronic inflammatory bowel disease restricted to the colon cannot be clearly classified as either ulcerative colitis or Crohn's disease hence are called "indeterminate."[170]

Grossly, the involved intestine in Crohn's disease is thickened. The mesentery contains numerous hyperplastic lymph nodes and is also thickened, with mesenteric fat extending up over the bowel. The lumen is narrowed and the mucosa is ulcerated with intervening edematous areas causing a cobblestone appearance. The microscopic pathology includes focal mucosal inflammation and ulceration, with chronic inflammation, extending through all layers of the bowel. Noncaseating granulomas (hard tubercles) can be found in 30 to 50 percent of the resected specimens. Deep fissures extend into the areas of inflammation. Histologic alterations often extend into areas that appear grossly normal. In later stages, scarring leads to strictures.

Fistulas develop through fissures in the thickened bowel and usually are found to originate in the proximal portion of a stenotic area thus serving to partially decompress the obstructed bowel.

No unified hypothesis is available to explain the pathogenesis of Crohn's disease and its characteristic inflammatory pattern. It has been suggested, however, that an infectious agent from the lumen initiates the disease in individuals with an unusual inflammatory response but unexplained are the segmental distribution of the inflammatory process, its predeliction for the terminal ileum and right colon, and the frequency of perianal disease.

CLINICAL MANIFESTATIONS. The disease usually begins in the teens and twenties, with over 10 percent appearing before age 15; 50 percent beginning in the third decade; and over 90 percent before age 40.[152] An insidious onset and a long course before a specific diagnosis is made are characteristic, the average duration of symptoms before diagnosis being 2½ years.

Another feature of the disease is the variation in the clinical picture. In the early phase, patients may notice a gradual decrease in their sense of well-being and a vague, cramping abdominal pain. The discomfort may be localized to the periumbilical area or to the right lower quadrant. It often occurs one or two hours after meals, may be preceded by audible bowel sounds (borborygmi), and is relieved by defecation or vomiting. Because of anorexia, nausea, or the fear of abdominal cramps, food intake is decreased, and weight loss almost invariably results. In adolescents a decrease in growth rate may precede the appearance of intestinal symptoms by 1 to 2 years.[196] In small bowel Crohn's disease, there is usually some moderate increase in the number of bowel movements, rarely over five per day, and stools become soft and unformed. As many as one-fifth of the patients with ileal disease deny having diarrhea, and thus the intestinal origin of the disease remains obscure until other manifestations appear. An unexplained low-grade fever may be the only objective evidence of disease for many months. Some patients present with iron deficiency anemia and occult blood in the stool. Rectal bleeding and diarrhea are symptoms of Crohn's disease of the colon. Gross hemorrhage occurs but is rare. In a 20-year follow-up of patients originally evaluated because of fever of undetermined origin, Crohn's disease was the second most common final diagnosis. In children, since fever and arthralgia are often the presenting symptoms, many are initially thought to have rheumatic fever or juvenile rheumatoid arthritis.

In Crohn's disease of the colon the involvement may be segmental or diffuse and in the latter may be difficult to distinguish from ulcerative colitis. On histologic examination of rectal biopsies the involvement of the mucosa is usually focal rather than uniform as encountered in ulcerative colitis and granulomas may be found.

COMPLICATIONS OF CROHN'S DISEASE. The complications of Crohn's disease often bring the patient to medical attention. At least half the patients form fistulas—internal, perianal, vaginal, vesical, or cutaneous through an appendectomy or laparotomy scar. On the other hand, free perforation is rare. These fistulas may make their appearance as abscesses or tender masses. Toxic megacolon may complicate the course of Crohn's disease involving the colon, especially in adolescents.

Extensive ileal involvement will produce impaired vitamin B_{12} absorption and eventually megaloblastic anemia. Impaired ileal absorption of bile salts causes depletion of the bile salt pool with resultant steatorrhea which is associated with oxaluria and nephrolithasis in some patients. Malabsorption may also be produced in Crohn's disease by bacterial overgrowth, extensive mucosa involvement, or "short bowel" syndrome as a consequence of multiple intestinal resections. The frequency of oxalate renal calculi and gallstones has been found to be increased.[157] Arthritis and ankylosing spondylitis occasionally occur. Eye manifestations include iritis and scleritis. Erythema nodosum is not uncommon with colonic involvement. Patients with perianal abscesses or fistulas should always be examined for the possibility of Crohn's disease.

DIAGNOSIS. The diagnosis of Crohn's disease is made on the basis of the combination of clinical, radiologic, and pathologic finding. There are no truly pathognomic findings, rather confidence in the diagnosis of Crohn's disease is strengthened only as the patient's course is followed. In any patient suspected of Crohn's disease, proctoscopy and rectal biopsy should be performed. Often on histologic examination, suggestive abnormalities will be found even though no gross findings were encountered. Usually proctoscopic examination is followed by a barium enema because this examination demonstrates the right colon and terminal ileum, the areas most frequently involved in Crohn's disease. The loss of mucosal detail and cobblestone filling defects are seen. The ileal lumen may be narrowed by spasm or scarring, producing the classic string sign. In acutely ill patients or those suspected of having an abcess in whom preparation for a barium enema may seem unwise, a small bowel series with colon follow-through will usually provide adequate information for making diagnostic and therapeutic decisions. A small bowel series demonstrates the proximal extent of disease, skip areas,

and stenosis and dilatation indicating a partial obstruction. Other diseases having the distribution of Crohn's disease include ileal or ileocecal tuberculosis, yersinosis, lymphoma, carcinoid tumors, actinomycosis, carcinomas of the cecum, and amebic involvement of the cecum.[179,193]

In tuberculosis the cecum is usually fibrotic and narrowed. In about half of the patients, there is evidence of pulmonary tuberculosis. Typical calcified abdominal nodes are seen in a small percentage of cases with intestinal tuberculosis. Biopsy and culture studies should be performed on fistulae, if present, in order to rule out tuberculosis and actinomycosis. When a positive tuberculin skin test and other clinical features make tuberculosis a possibility, treatment with both antituberculosis drugs and steroids may be desirable. At times, a laparotomy is necessary to establish a diagnosis prior to undertaking therapy.

Rectal or fistula biopsies contain granulomas in about half the patients with Crohn's disease of the colon.

TREATMENT.[190,196] The aims of therapy should be to suppress active inflammatory disease and conserve small bowel with medical treatment, and to reserve surgery for the complications of fistulae and abscess and for a "fresh start" in obstruction.

Adrenocortical steriods alone or in combination with antibiotics produce symptomatic and x-ray improvement in the majority of patients treated during the first few years of their disease, especially in those with predominately ileal involvement. Extensive colonic disease is less responsive to steroid therapy. Fistulae proximal to an inflammatory segment will close if steroid treatment relieves the associated partial obstruction. Steroids can only suppress the inflammatory reaction. If symptoms are obstructive and caused by a fibrotic, stenotic segment, little relief can be expected from steriods. If a surgical resection is performed while the disease is clinically active, the early recurrence rate approaches 50 percent.

Initially Crohn's disease should be treated with prednisone starting with 40 to 60 mg per day and salicylazosulfapyridine 3 g per day if there is no clear evidence of an abscess. If there are deep fissures in the involved bowel, antibiotics such as tetracycline are added. Symptoms such as fever, anorexia, crampy pain, and abdominal tenderness should improve. As soon as clinical improvement is apparent the steroids are tapered over a 2-to-3 month period to a maintenance dose of 20 to 30 mg every other day. If symptoms do not respond promptly, the presence of an obstruction, abscess, or an error in diagnosis must be carefully considered. Patients requiring antiinflammatory therapy, but who cannot tolerate steroids because of side effects or have failed to respond, sometimes respond to azothiaprine 1 to 1.5 mg per kg per day.[186]

Surgery is employed for the complications of Crohn's disease in the fibrotic stage: 1) obstruction, 2) abscess, and 3) fistula. Crohn's disease tends to recur after surgery, a rate of 50 to 80 percent in some series.[151,165] Abscesses require drainage, but it is wise to delay the definitive resection of the involved bowel or of fistulous tracts until the inflammatory reaction is controlled.

Intravenous hyperalimentation has been useful in preparing seriously ill patients for surgery by improving nutrition and by putting the bowel at "rest" so the inflammatory process may subside. In some patients fistulae have closed, particularly if the bowel is not deformed by fibrosis; and in some the improvement has been so striking that surgery is postponed indefinitely.

Amebiasis[173,183]

Infestation with *Entameba histolytica* may cause an asymptomatic carrier state, chronic mild diarrhea, or acute diarrhea if the infestation is heavy or if the patient is malnourished and debilitated.

DIAGNOSIS.   The diagnosis is confirmed by identifying the trophozoites of *E. histolytica* in freshly passed diarrheal stools or in mucus or exudate scraped or aspirated from the edge of an ulceration. The examination of fecal material or rectal mucus fixed in polyvinylalcohol (PVA fixative) also is useful. Only cysts are found in the stools of patients without diarrhea.

The typical proctoscopic findings are irregular, punched-out ulcers with relatively normal mucosa between the ulcerations. Rectal involvement may not be distinguishable from ulcerative colitis, Crohn's disease, or shigellosis, but the uncertainty should be resolved by rectal biopsy. Serologic tests (hemagglutination) are usually positive in the presence of tissue invasion and approach 100 percent with extracolonic disease such as liver abscess.

Although metronidazole (750 mg three times daily for 5 to 10 days) is considered by many as the treatment of choice because of low toxicity and over 85 percent success rate, multiple drug therapy such as corbasone and diodoquin, has also provided a high cure rate with few recurrences. Relapses after a cure are rare and are probably due to reinfection.

Local complications in the colon include perforation, appendicitis, scarring, and granuloma formation with obstruction. Large amebomas in the cecum may present a difficult differential diagnostic problem with carcinoma, tuberculosis, and actinomycosis.

Amebic hepatitis and liver abscess occur in approximately 5 percent of those with amebic dysentery. Abscesses are usually in the right lobe of the liver. Liver involvement may occur without either diarrhea or a history of previous intestinal symptoms, and stool examinations may be negative for amebas but serologic tests will be positive.

Humorally Mediated Diarrheal Syndromes

An uncommon but important cause of chronic secretory diarrhea is hormone-producing tumors. The release of these secretogogues is not under normal physiologic control hence is uninfluenced by meals or fasting. In these disorders, diarrhea continues unabated when oral intake is eliminated and fluid intake is provided via the intravenous route. Except for the Zollinger-Ellison syndrome (which is characterized by peptic ulcer), there is no histologic alteration in the gastrointestinal mucosa hence no blood, leukocytes, nor fat in the stool.

GASTRIN-SECRETING ADENOMAS OF THE PANCREAS. Diarrhea or steatorrhea occurs in one-third of patients with the Zollinger-Ellison syndrome. The mechanisms for diarrhea include the cathartic effects of excessive gastric secretion, acid inactivation of pancreatic enzymes, mucosal damage, and increased fluid and electrolyte secretion by the small bowel. Patients or family members may have other endocrine adenomas. Cimetidine or gastrectomy will control the diarrhea.

NONGASTRIN-SECRETING ADENOMAS OF THE PANCREAS.[187,194]   These have been associated with massive watery diarrhea and hypokalemia. The term "pancreatic cholera" or watery diarrhea syndrome has been applied to these patients. Decreased gastric acid secretion, flushing, hypercalcemia, and hyperglycemia are encountered in some patients. The diarrhea sometimes responds to tumor excision or to administration of adrenal cortical steroid hormones. Vasoactive intestinal peptide (VIP) has been isolated from some of these tumors and is believed to account for the clinical findings by activation of intestinal adenylate cyclase. In others, prostaglandins seem to be the secretory agents and indomethacin therapy has been helpful when surgical resection was not possible.

SYMPATHETIC NERVOUS SYSTEM TUMORS.[185]   Sympathetic nervous system tumors including gangliomas, neuroblastomas, and ganglioneuroblastomas, have been associated with diarrhea which was controlled by removal or destruction of the tumors. The catecholamines secreted by these tumors do not seem to be the cause of the diarrhea. A smooth muscle active substance as well as trace amounts of bradykinin-like activity have been recovered from tumor tissue of one patient. Another patient's retroperitoneal tumor contained vasoactive intestinal peptide. It is not known if the primary gut disturbance is due to alteration of motility or secretion of fluid by the mucosa but vasoactive intestinal peptide (VIP) is found in some of these tumors.

MEDULLARY CARCINOMA OF THE THYROID.[169] Medullary carcinoma of the thyroid with metastasis is commonly associated with watery diarrhea. The diarrhea decreases with resection of large amounts of tumor tissue suggesting the presence of a humoral agent. These tumors are, at times, associated with an overproduction of prostaglandins, while others have high calcitonin or VIP content.

MALIGNANT CARCINOID SYNDROME.[163] This syndrome is associated with diarrhea. These patients have increased blood levels of serotonin as well as bradykinin. Serotonin increases smooth muscle contractions and intestinal motility, as well as stimulating intestinal secretion. The diarrhea can be controlled by serotonin antagonists.

Functional Bowel Diseases—Irritable Colon[199]

Functional bowel disease can be looked upon as an accentuation and prolongation of the normal responses of the colon to stimuli such as meals or emotional tension—for example, the diarrhea of students just before final examinations. Similar functional derangements may persist for weeks or months after an episode of gastroenteritis. Numerous other terms have been used to describe this disorder, including "spastic colon," "mucous colitis," and "adaptive colitis." It is manifested by episodes of diarrhea; diarrhea alternating with passage of small hard stools with increased mucus; or constipation with abdominal pain. Nocturnal diarrhea is unusual in functional bowel disease and would be a point against this diagnosis. Pain in the hypogastrium, left lower quadrant, splenic flexure, or hepatic flexure is common. Abdominal distension with hyperresonance to percussion is also a frequent finding. Extracolonic symptoms including anorexia, nausea, belching, aerophagia, sour taste, and sweating may be part of the clinical picture. Significant weight loss is unusual and cannot be attributed to functional bowel disease until organic disease has been excluded. Patients with hyperthyroidism may have diarrhea as the presenting symptom and as a consequence be misdiagnosed as functional bowel disease. It should be kept in mind that even organic causes of diarrhea can be aggravated by stressful situations.

The diagnosis of functional bowel disease is based on the characteristic symptom complex and on the exclusion of organic illness. Normal proctoscopy, barium enema, hematocrit, sedimentation rate, white blood count, and negative stool examination for blood, ova and parasites are necessary to make the diagnosis. In the irritable-colon syndrome, proctoscopy and barium enema may reveal spasticity of the distal colon, but this is not invariably found. This syndrome is believed to be the precursor of diverticulosis because high pressure is generated in the colon as a result of the motility disturbance (see Chap. 57).

Management includes reassurance, which is partially provided by the detailed interview under relaxed circumstances and by the diagnostic procedures. The syndrome should be described to the patient as a specific entity, emphasizing it as a variation of normal physiology. Therapy includes the use of a high fiber diet or bulk laxative, such as psyllium hydrophilic mucilloid, to interrupt the constipation-diarrhea cycle and to reestablish regular bowel habits.[154] The use of anticholinergics are, at times, tried to relieve painful spasm and antidiarrheals such as diphenoxylate HCl to control diarrhea. Dietary restriction and manipulation have been grossly overemphasized in the management of this syndrome. Lactose and milk intolerance, however, should be ruled out as a contributing factor, if bloating, flatulence, crampy pain, or diarrhea are prominent symptoms.

CONSTIPATION

Chronic constipation[188] has been called "a peculiar disorder of both the bowel and the mind." It is clinically useful, though not established on a physiologic basis, to categorize patients suffering from constipation as having one of the following types: 1) imaginary constipation, 2) spastic constipation, and 3) rectal insensibility.

In the first category are those patients whose stools appear normal by ordinary standards yet who are concerned because their bowel movements do not measure up to their expectations.

In the second category are those patients who pass hard stools with an effort and who may have an abdominal aching and a sense of incomplete evacuation. They are in the spectrum of irritable bowel syndrome. It is rationalized that the sigmoid is spastic in these patients and the colonic contents are thus delayed in their passage from the colon to the rectum for evacuation. The stools are usually small and hard and may be covered with mucus. With these patients, it is important to exclude painful anal disorders as the inciting cause for the constipation.

The third category consists of patients with rectal insensibility. On examination the rectum is often found to be full of soft feces, without the patients' having any urge to defecate.

In the young person an attempt should be made at bowel training in order to minimize the patient's dependence on laxatives.[188] This is successfully accomplished by the following procedure: 1) have the patient arise early enough to allow half an hour between breakfast and starting off for the day's activities; 2) take a bulk laxative (hydrophilic colloid) with each meal; and 3) take a colonic stimulant, such as a senna capsule, at bedtime. When a normal bowel pattern is established, the laxative first and then the hydrophilic colloid should be slowly decreased in a stepwise fashion. Dietary bran has become a popular and effective means of increasing stool bulk and softness. In the older patient, the restoration of a reasonable defecation pattern is reassuring, but because the constipation is long-standing it may not be possible to maintain normal defecation without the continued use of pharmacologic aids. Some laxatives, such as oxyphenisatin, may act by decreasing nutrient and fluid absorption in the small bowel thus producing a bulk fluid load. Epsom salts and nonabsorbable materials cause an osmotic diarrhea. Others, such as senna alkaloids, have an irritative action on the colon.[150] A regular, well-rounded, nutritionally adequate diet suited to the patient's tastes is preferable to a rigid, restrictive dietary regimen.

Although chronic constipation is an extremely common complaint and patients receive considerable relief from its correction, with the exception of hypothyroidism, it is rarely a productive clue to important organic disease. A change in bowel habits, however, is frequently an important clue to serious disease, not in the colon only but elsewhere as well—for example, carcinoma of the pancreas, lead poisoning, and porphyria. Every patient who complains of the appearance of constipation or of constipation alternating with diarrhea must be evaluated by proctosigmoidoscopy, and stool examination.

CHAPTER 61
Malabsorption
THOMAS R. HENDRIX AND THEODORE M. BAYLESS

Remarkable advances have been made in the past two decades in the ability to define the cause and to provide rational, effective therapy for intestinal malabsorption. Impaired absorption, i.e., malabsorption, may involve the absorption of a single compound such as lactose in lactase deficiency or vitamin B_{12} in pernicious anemia or may involve all elements of the diet as encountered in a diffuse mucosal abnormality such as celiac disease. Malabsorption may present with voluminous, malodorous stool and weight loss, hence no diagnostic uncertainty. At the other extreme, the presentaion may be subtle and associated with no diarrhea and only nonspecific complaints of weakness, fatigue, and abdominal bloating and be erroneously attributed to psychosomatic causes.

The clinical manifestations of intestinal malabsorption include: 1) caloric deficiency resulting in weight loss; 2) specific deficiencies causing anemia, tetany, glossitis, or bleeding; and 3) intestinal dysfunction leading to diarrhea and/or steatorrhea.

To treat malabsorption effectively, the deranged step or steps in the digestive-absorptive process must first be identified. The digestive-absorptive process involves three phases: 1) intraluminal phase during which the chemical and physical states of the nutrients are altered in preparation for absorption; 2) epithelial phase concerned with surface hydrolysis at the brush border, uptake, and preparation for extrusion into the lamina propria; and 3) the transit phase during which absorbed material is removed from the lamina propria by lymph and blood flow.

PHYSIOLOGY OF DIGESTION AND ABSORPTION
An understanding of the normal physiology of digestion and absorption[3,207,209,210,217] is necessary to classify the cause of malabsorption and plan rational therapy.

The preparation of food for absorption begins in the mouth with the partial conversion of starch to dextrins and maltose by salivary amylase. In the stomach, food is homogenized and emulsified and pepsin exerts its proteolytic action by cleaving proteins to peptides.

In the duodenum, the arrival of acidified chyme from the stomach causes the release of the hormones cholecystokinin (CCK) and secretin which, in turn, stimulate the gallbladder to contract and empty bile into the duodenum and stimulate the release of digestive enzymes and bicarbonate by the pancreas. Conjugated bile salts help emulsify fats in the duodenum and facilitate the lipolysis of triglycerides into fatty acids and monoglycerides by pancreatic lipase. Conjugated bile salts form micelles which carry the products of lipolysis, cholesterol, and lipid-soluble vitamins in micellar solution to the absorbing surface of the intestine. The lipids pass into the epithelial cells while the bile salts remain in the lumen to continue to transport lipids. Finally, the bile salts are absorbed by the ileum and carried in the portal blood to the liver to be excreted again into the bile. This enterohepatic circulation of bile salts is 95 percent efficient so each day the liver has only to synthesize enough bile acid to replace the small amount lost into the colon. In the process of absorbing a meal, the bile salt pool completes two or more enterohepatic cycles.

Pancreatic amylase continues the hydrolysis of polysaccharides to disaccharides. The hydrolysis of disaccharides to monosaccharides is accomplished by enzymes (disaccharidases) on the brush border of the small-intestinal epithelium. Glucose absorption releases Gastric Inhibitory Peptide (GIP) from the intestinal mucosa which in turn stimulates insulin release and inhibits gastric secretion. The pancreatic proteolytic enzymes are secreted in an inactive form. An intestinal enzyme, enterokinase, converts trypsinogen into active trypsin which in turn converts the other proteolytic proenzymes into their active forms—chymotrypsin, elastase, carboxypeptidases, etc. The major products of intraluminal protein digestion are small polypeptides and amino acids. Brush border peptidases hydrolyze large peptides to di- and tripeptides, which are actively absorbed by a peptide transport carrier. In addition there are amino acid transport carriers.

The motor activity of the small intestine mixes and churns the chyme and the digestive enzymes and brings the products of digestion in contact with the absorbing surfaces of the intestine. The normal propulsive activity prevents stasis of the intestinal contents and consequent multiplication of bacteria that interfere with absorption in part, by deconjugating bile salts. Overgrowth of bacteria also interferes with the absorption of vitamin B_{12} because the bacteria utilize the vitamin before it reaches its site of absorption in the ileum.

The second phase of the absorptive process is the actual transfer of the products of digestion from the intestinal lumen to the blood and lymph. The absorption of nutrients occurs chiefly in the duodenum and jejunum whereas bile salts and vitamin B_{12} are absorbed in the ileum.

The epithelial cells of the villi are the functional units in intestinal absorption, with those at the tips playing the major role. Some materials such as some water-soluble vitamins, nucleic acid derivatives, and urea pass through the intestinal cells by simple diffusion. Lipids enter the cells by nonionic diffusion. The majority of foodstuffs, however, are absorbed by more efficient and often highly specialized active transport processes. For example, glucose and galactose share the same active transport mechanism whereas fructose enters through another pathway by carrier-facilitated diffusion. Although there are at least four specific amino acid transport mechanisms, most amino acids are absorbed as peptides with hydrolysis to amino acids being completed within the absorbing cell. The intestinal absorption of some materials, such as iron, copper, calcium, and magnesium involves specific and complex regulatory systems.

The portal blood is the primary route for all absorbed materials except lipids. The absorbed fatty acids and monoglycerides are reesterified within the absorbing cells. These triglycerides, along with other absorbed lipids, are packaged with a protein coat and extruded from the cell as chylomicrons which are carried from the intestine by the lymphatics.

CLASSIFICATION OF MALABSORPTION

The specific diseases are grouped according to the alterations in the normal digestive and absorptive physiology that cause malabsorption (Table 61–1).

Clinical Manifestations

The clinical manifestations of malabsorption result from the following: 1) unabsorbed food substances affecting other intestinal functions, such as fat and fatty acids producing foul, bulky diarrhea; 2) secondary deficiencies of specific nutrients that, although eaten, are not absorbed, as exemplified by tetany secondary to calcium and vitamin D malabsorption; and 3) systemic symptoms, including anorexia and weight loss.

DIARRHEA. Diarrhea is usually a major complaint of the patients with malabsorption but, at times, those with mild steatorrhea may notice no change in their stools. Since the reservoir capacity of the colon is intact and there is no rectal disease to cause urgency or tenesmus, the patient with celiac disease or pancreatic insufficiency may have only a few bowel movements per day. However, there may be exacerbations of diarrhea, with 6 to 12 movements per day, especially when there are intercurrent respiratory or intestinal infections. Patients with gastrocolic or gastroileal fistulas may have frequent diarrhea and the passage of undigested food in the stool several minutes to several hours after eating. Because bloating (caused by unabsorbed gas and liquid) and

TABLE 61-1
**Pathophysiologic Classification
of Malabsorption**

I. **Failure of Digestion (Intraluminal Phase)**

A. Decreased pancreatic enzymes
1. Pancreatic insufficiency (pancreatitis, cystic fibrosis, protein deficiency, and pancreatic cancer)
2. Inactivation of pancreatic enzymes by gastric hypersecretion (Zollinger-Ellison syndrome and ileal resection)
3. Failure to convert proenzyme to active form (enterokinase and trypsinogen deficiencies)
B. Impaired bile acid micelle formation
1. Impaired bile acid synthesis (severe hepatocellular disease)
2. Interrupted enterohepatic circulation (ileal resection, bile duct obstruction, or biliary cirrhosis)
3. Bile acid deconjugation (bacterial overgrowth)
a. stasis due to motor abnormality (scleroderma, intestinal pseudo-obstruction, diabetic visceral neuropathy)
b. stasis due to anatomic abnormalities (multiple diverticula, strictures, and blind loops including long afferent loop of a gastrojejunostomy)
c. small bowel contamination (gastrocolic and jejunocolic fistula)
C. Inadequate mixing of food, bile, and pancreatic enzymes (gastrojejunostomy)

II. **Failure of Absorption (Mucosal Phase)**

A. Inadequate absorptive surface (intestinal resection, intestinal bypass for obesity, inadvertent gastro-ileostomy)
B. Damaged absorbing surface (celiac disease, tropical sprue, hypogammaglobulinemia, giardiasis)
C. Biochemical defect without anatomic alteration
1. Disaccharide deficiency (lactase and sucrase deficiency)
2. Transport deficiency
a. carbohydrate (glucose-galactose malabsorption)
b. lipid (a-β-lipoproteinemia)
c. amino acids (cystinuria, Hartnup's disease, methionine malabsorption)
d. vitamin B_{12} malabsorption
D. Infiltration of intestinal wall (Whipple's disease, lymphoma, amyloid, Crohn's disease)

III. **Impaired Lymph and Blood Flow (Transit Phase)**

A. Developmental abnormality (intestinal lymphangiectasia, Milroy's disease)
B. Lymphatic obstruction (lymphoma, Whipple's disease, tuberculosis)
C. Mesenteric vascular insufficiency (rare if ever)

diarrhea may be accentuated by eating, some patients voluntarily decrease their food intake in order to avoid discomfort.

Unabsorbed fats and fatty acids cause the stools to be bulky and voluminous. In addition, fatty acids, particularly after bacterial hydroxylation, stimulate colonic fluid secretion, thus increasing the water content of the stools, and producing diarrhea.[146] If increased amounts of bile salts enter the colon due to ileal dysfunction or resection, fecal water is increased because bile salts also stimulate colonic fluid secretion.[216] Patients may note an oil skim in the toilet bowl or that the toilet must be reflushed. Rancid fats impart a particularly offensive odor to flatus and feces. In patients with disaccharidase deficiencies unabsorbed carbohydrates act as an osmotic load which interferes with fluid reabsorption in the ileum and colon. It is important to inspect the stool personally, since the patient's description is rarely adequate. If there ever was a situation in which one look is worth a thousand words, it is in the evaluation of abnormal stools.

WEIGHT LOSS. Weight loss and weakness are often the patient's chief complaints and occur in part because calories are lost, especially in the form of fats, but also because anorexia is an accompaniment of malabsorption. Prolonged and severe malabsorption states, such as Whipple's disease, intestinal fistulas, and celiac disease, may manifest themselves as an advanced malnutrition, often with secondary hypopituitarism and amenorrhea. These cachectic patients have been mistakenly considered to have a neoplasm.

EDEMA. Hypoalbuminemia and peripheral edema result from the prolonged malabsorption of protein and from the increased loss of serum proteins into the lumen of the intestine. This latter form of protein loss accompanies intestinal lymphangiectasia, constrictive pericarditis, portal hypertension, and a variety of diseases involving the mucosa such as Crohn's disease, Whipple's disease, and tropical sprue. Gastric neoplasms and hypertrophic gastritis may also cause excess protein loss and edema.[236]

TETANY AND BONE DEMINERALIZATION. Tetany from the prolonged malabsorption of vitamin D, calcium, and magnesium may occur but are uncommon. Trousseau's and Chovstek's signs are seen more often. In patients with extensive ileal resections magnesium depletion appears to be the major factor in the production of tetany. Serum phosphorus is low in primary malabsorptive disorders, in contrast to elevated values in hypoparathyroidism. Osteoporosis and osteomalacia with bone pain and pathologic fractures may be the presenting features of celiac disease, postgastrectomy steatorrhea, or chronic obstructive jaundice. Secondary hyperparathyroidism may complicate chronic hypocalcemia with a resultant osteitis fibrosa cystica.

BLEEDING. Patients with steatorrhea may present with a bleeding diathesis, usually manifested by ecchymoses, but occasionally by melena or hematuria. This is secondary to malabsorption of fat-soluble vitamin K and the resultant hypoprothrombinemia. In megaloblastic anemia, as seen in tropical sprue, thrombocytopenia does occur but is rarely a cause of bleeding. Retinal hemorrhages can occur with any severe anemia. The parenteral administration of vitamin K corrects a prothrombin deficiency caused by malabsorption.

ANEMIA. In the malabsorption syndrome anemia may be caused by the impaired absorption of iron, folic acid, or vitamin B_{12}, singly or in combination.

RENAL CALCULI.[200,206] Patients with malabsorption and diarrhea frequently have concentrated urine. In addition, they tend to have hyperoxaluria because they absorb a larger proportion of dietary oxalate than normal. These two findings explain the greater than expected incidence of renal calculi in patients with steatorrhea. Normally, much of the dietary oxalate is precipitated in the lumen as calcium oxalate. In the presence of steatorrhea, calcium soaps are formed leaving oxalate in solution to be absorbed.

OTHER MANIFESTATIONS. Other clinical manifestations include peripheral neuropathy, presumably secondary to vitamin deficiency; night blindness secondary to a lack of vitamin A; and nocturia caused by the delayed absorption of water. Skin pigmentation and chronic arthritis are common in Whipple's disease.

Milk (lactose) intolerance, characterized by bloating, cramps, and watery frothy diarrhea, may result from a genetically determined lactase deficiency or deficiency secondary to mucosal damage, as encountered in celiac disease and tropical sprue.

Other items in a patient's history that should alert the physician to the possibility of malabsorption include the following: chronic cholestatic liver disease; chronic alcoholism; recurrent upper or midabdominal pain; diabetes with or without peripheral neuropathy; previous surgery, especially gastrectomy, gastroenterostomy, vagotomy, or intestinal resection; severe peptic ulcer diathesis with watery diarrhea; sudden onset of diarrhea and weight loss after prolonged peptic ulcer activity; childhood history of diarrhea, anemia, potbelly or failure to thrive; previous residence or travel in a tropical area where sprue or giardiasis is endemic; and previous antibiotic therapy, especially with broad-spectrum antibiotics.

Diagnostic Procedures in Suspected Malabsorption[231]

The symptoms, appearance of the stool, evidence of secondary deficiencies, or an abnormal small bowel x-ray should lead to the suspicion that malabsorption is present, but confirmation of the diagnosis requires diagnostic tests. The investigative steps used are outlined in Figure 61-1.

ROENTGEN EXAMINATION OF THE SMALL BOWEL.[235] An abnormal small bowel pattern discovered during roentgen examination of the upper gastrointestinal tract may provide the first clue that malabsorption is the basis for the patient's symptoms. In addition a small bowel roentgen series may be useful in suggesting which category of disorders is the most likely cause of the intestinal malabsorption. Dilated small bowel loops are common in celiac disease and scleroderma. Nodular thickened folds are common in Whipple's disease, intestinal lymphoma, amyloidosis, and granulomatous diseases. In most instances the small bowel barium study only indicates the likelihood of a diagnosis but does not establish or exclude it. For example, the small bowel series is usually normal in pancreatic insufficiency but an occasional patient with pancreatic insufficiency has a clearly abnormal roentgen study.

PROVING THE PRESENCE OF STEATORRHEA. The presence of excess fecal fat, or steatorrhea, is the most commonly accepted criterion for diagnosing a disordered intestinal absorption. Microscopic examination of stools for fat is a useful screening procedure as are breath tests after ^{14}C fat ingestion.[224,228]

The determination of the blood level of fat-soluble materials, such as carotene, is also a useful screening test. Ninety percent of the patients with steatorrhea have subnormal levels. A low serum carotene does not prove malabsorption is present because it is also found when the intake of carotene-containing foods (vegetables) is decreased. Subnormal blood levels of other materials such as vitamin A, cholesterol, prothrombin, calcium, phosphorus, albumin, iron, folic acid, and vitamin B_{12} may be clues to the presence of malabsorption. In order to accurately assess fat absorption, all stools are collected for 3 days and an average daily value determined. In addition, the patient should be ingesting a normal amount of fat (70 to 120 g per day), prior to and during the collection period. Normal fecal fat with this intake is less than 6 g per day.

DISTINGUISHING MALDIGESTION FROM MALABSORPTION (D-XYLOSE TEST). The ability of the intestine to absorb specific substances can be evaluated by measuring the appearance of an orally administered test substance in the blood or in the urine. The pentose d-xylose is used most commonly to distinguish maldi-

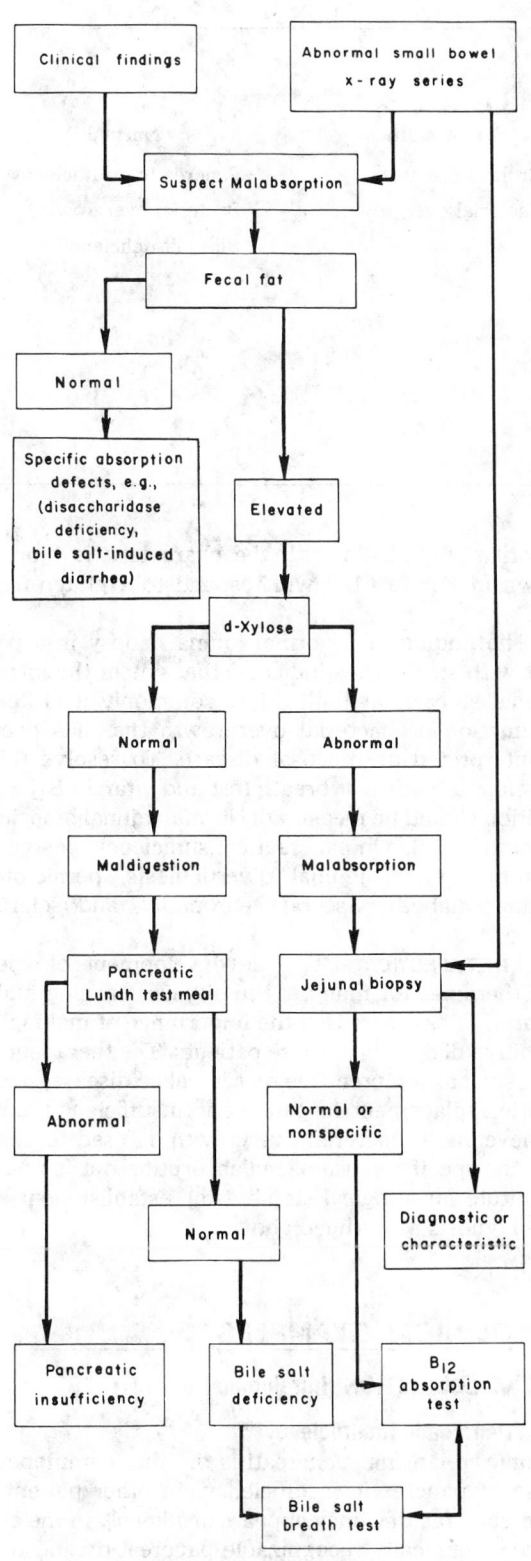

FIGURE 61-1. Evaluation of malabsorption.

gestion from malabsorption because it does not require digestion prior to absorption and a large portion of the absorbed sugar is excreted unmetabolized in the urine. If the liver and renal functions are normal and there is no delay in gastric emptying, the determination of the urinary excretion after an oral load of d-xylose is an adequate clinical measure of the absorbing capacity of the upper small intestine. The normal 5-hour urinary excretion after 25 g of d-xylose orally is greater than 4.5 g. The test is clearly abnormal in almost all symptomatic patients with malabsorption caused by diffuse mucosal disease of the duodenum and jejunum, such as in celiac disease or tropical sprue. In contrast, normal results are obtained if the defect is in intraluminal digestion, as in chronic pancreatitis with pancreatic insufficiency or bile acid deficiency.

PANCREATIC (LUNDH) TEST MEAL.[238]   The Lundh test meal is the simplest and most physiologic method to determine whether pancreatic insufficiency is the explanation of the maldigestion. In this test, after the jejunum is intubated, a 300 ml test meal containing protein, carbohydrate and fat is drunk. The jejunal contents are aspirated in 4 half-hour samples and concentration of pancreatic enzymes are measured. Failure of pancreatic enzymes to rise in response to a meal may be due to: 1) to inadequate release of hormonal stimulants (secretin and cholecystokinin) most frequently encountered in gastrojejunostomies because the meal does not come in contact with the duodenum and upper jejunum which contain the highest concentration of cells that release these hormones; 2) obstruction of the pancreatic duct by a tumor or stone; 3) pancreatic exocrine insufficiency due to pancreatitis, cystic fibrosis or pancreatic atrophy; and 4) inactivation of pancreatic enzymes by low duodenal pH, most commonly encountered in the Zollinger-Ellison syndrome but occasionally found in patients with gastric hypersecretion following ileal resection. Pancreatic function can also be measured by the secretin test in which the volume and bicarbonate content of duodenal aspirate is measured after parenteral administration of secretin.

BILE SALT BREATH TEST.[232]   The second intraluminal step in lipid assimilation is micellar solubilization. If the intestinal concentration of conjugated bile salts is below the critical micellar concentration (2 to 3 mM per liter) lipids are not solubilized and as a consequence diffusion to the absorbing surface is severely limited. Bile salt deficiency may be caused by 1) impaired hepatic synthesis and secretion of bile salts in severe chronic liver disease;[227] 2) interruption of the enterohepatic circulation of bile salts by obstruction of the common bile duct; ileal disease, most

---

TABLE 61–2
Interpretation of Jejunal Biopsies

Diagnostic	Characteristic	Nonspecific Abnormalities	Normal
Whipple's disease	Celiac disease	Crohn's disease	Pancreatic insufficiency
Giardiasis	Tropical sprue	Bacterial overgrowth	Bacterial overgrowth
Amyloidosis	Eosinophilic gastroenteritis		Bile salt deficiency
a-β-lipoproteinemia	Dermatitis herpetiformis		
Lymphoma	Dysglobulinemia		
Coccidiosis			
Mast cell disease			
Lymphangiectasia			
Macroglobulinemia			

---

often Crohn's disease or resection; or intraluminal precipitation of bile salts.[216] The latter is caused by 1) deconjugation and hydroxylation by overgrowth of bacteria in the small intestine;[214] 2) low intestinal pH due to extreme gastric hypersection;[222] or 3) binding to drugs such as neomycin and cholestyramine. The role of interruption of the enterohepatic circulation of bile salts in the pathogenesis of steatorrhea can be assessed clinically by the bile salt breath test. The test is performed by measuring $^{14}CO_2$ in the expired air after the oral administration of glycocholate with the glycine moiety labelled with ^{14}C. If the enterohepatic circulation is intact, less than 5 percent of the bile salt escapes reabsorption and enters the colon where bacteria remove the glycine and convert it to the carbon dioxide which is absorbed and excreted in the breath. If there is ileal dysfunction or overgrowth of bacteria in the small intestine, the increased deconjugation of glycocholate will be manifested by increased appearance of $^{14}CO_2$ in the breath.

PERORAL SMALL BOWEL BIOPSY.[233] The development of techniques for obtaining biopsies of the small-intestinal mucosa by the oral route was a major advance in the diagnostic approach to malabsorption. The procedures are safe and well tolerated.

The jejunal biopsy has diagnostic features in a group of disorders, most of which are rare (Table 61–2). The characteristic abnormality may be missed in some of these disorders such as intestinal lymphoma, amyloidosis, etc., because the lesion does not involve the intestine uniformly. Whipple's disease and giardiasis, the two diseases on the list for which there is the most successful therapy, can always be identified by jejunal biopsy.

The jejunal biopsy associated with celiac disease is not diagnostic, but in temperate regions the vast majority of patients with the characteristic biopsy shown in Figure 61–2 will respond to a gluten-free diet.

The finding of a normal jejunal biopsy in a patient with steatorrhea indicates that one of the intraluminal steps is at fault. Most commonly it is ileal dysfunction or bacterial overgrowth that has been misinterpreted as mucosal disease. To resolve this question, the bile salt breath test and vitamin B_{12} absorption should be measured. Normal jejunal biopsies are obtained also in pancreatic insufficiency, postgastrectomy states, jejunal diverticulosis, pernicious anemia, diabetic visceral neuropathy, and scleroderma.

THERAPEUTIC TRIAL. The development of specific therapies for many of the diseases causing malabsorption has increased the importance of making a definitive diagnosis in these patients. The therapeutic trial, such as a gluten-free diet in celiac disease, pancreatic replacement in pancreatic insufficiency, and tetracycline in bacterial overgrowth, is used to confirm the specific cause of malabsorption but is not a substitute for a logical step-by-step establishment of the diagnosis as outlined above.

CLINICAL EXAMPLES

MALDIGESTION (Intraluminal Defects)

Pancreatic Insufficiency[205]

Chronic relapsing pancreatitis is the commonest cause of pancreatic insufficiency. In other patients, pancreatic insufficiency appears insidiously in the absence of clinically recognizable pancreatitis and has been called silent pancreatitis or idiopathic pancre-

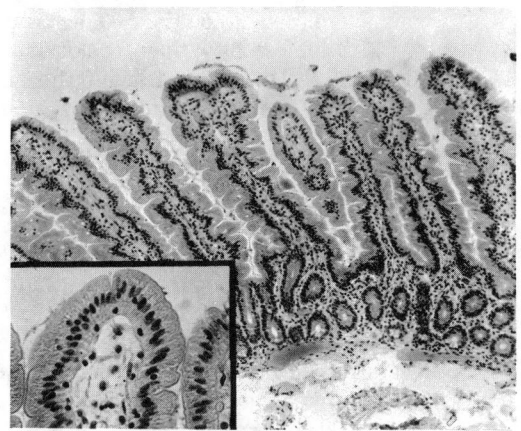

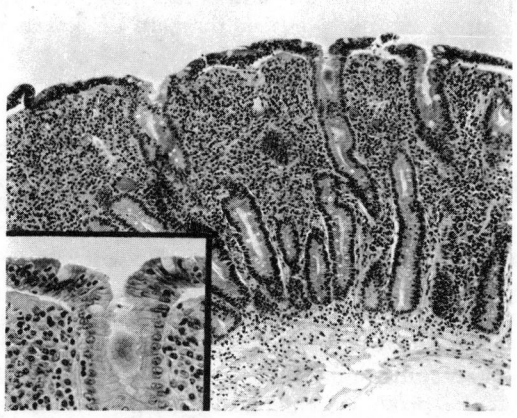

FIGURE 61-2. Jejunal biopsy. A normal jejunal biopsy is shown at top. The villi are long and slender covered by tall columnar epithelium (shown in detail in the insert). A typical biopsy from a patient with celiac disease is shown below. There are no recognizable villi and there is apparent lengthening of the crypts of Lieberkühn. The lamina propria is infiltrated with plasma cells and lymphocytes. The surface epithelium is flattened and infiltrated with lymphocytes while the crypt epithelium is normal (shown in insert).

atic atrophy. In still others, it is one of the presenting manifestations of carcinoma of the pancreas. In children, cystic fibrosis is the most frequent cause of pancreatic insufficiency. In children and young adults with pancreatic insufficiency, a sweat test should be performed to determine if cystic fibrosis is the underlying cause.

The main clinical manifestations of exocrine pancreatic insufficiency are steatorrhea, abdominal bloating, and weight loss. Steatorrhea may be massive. Some patients excrete over 80 g of fat per day, (normal less than 6 g). A helpful distinguishing feature from patients with other malabsorptive disor-

ders, such as celiac disease and Whipple's disease, is the excellent appetite and lack of cachexia that might otherwise be expected with this degree of steatorrhea.

The methods of differentiating maldigestion and malabsorption are outlined in Figure 61-1. A flat plate of the abdomen will show pancreatic calcification in 40 to 50 percent of the patients with pancreatic steatorrhea; 25 percent will be diabetic, and an additional 60 percent will have a diabetic glucose tolerance test. On upper gastrointestinal x-rays, a distortion of the pattern of the second and third portions of the duodenum may be seen with chronic pancreatitis or with a carcinoma of the head of the pancreas. Neoplasms or pseudocysts are best demonstrated by sonography or CAT scan. A therapeutic trial with pancreatic enzyme replacement is also a useful diagnostic procedure. With adequate replacement, steatorrhea will decrease but rarely disappears.

The management of pancreatic insufficiency includes the replacement of insulin and digestive enzymes.[230] There are several types of pancreatic extracts that contain varying amounts of trypsin, amylase, and lipase. The most potent are marketed as Viokase, Cotazyme and Pancrease. They are best given at least three to six times a day and probably have their optimum effect if given just before meals. For maximal effect, it is suggested that up to 12 g per day be given. The simultaneous administration of cimetedine will lessen the peptic destruction of the enzymes during their passage through the stomach. As steatorrhea decreases and nutrition improves, pancreatic function often improves and the need for pancreatic replacement may diminish.

Bile Salt Deficiency

ILEAL INSUFFICIENCY.[214,216] Extensive ileal inflammation (particularly Crohn's disease), surgical resection or bypass of the ileum interrupts the enterohepatic circulation of bile salts, and interferes with vitamin B_{12} absorption. With small resections, less than 100 cm, the liver is able to replace most of the bile acids lost, steatorrhea is mild, less than 10 g per day, and the diarrhea is primarily due to bile salts stimulating fluid secretion by the colon. Diarrhea in this circumstance can be controlled by the use of cholestyramine, a resin that binds bile salts. With larger resections, the liver is unable to synthesize sufficient bile salts to compensate for that lost into the colon. In these patients with a diminished bile salt pool, the bile salt concentration in the upper intestine exceeds the critical micellar concentration only at breakfast. Fat absorption after the other meals is greatly impaired. Increased fatty acids passing into the colon also stimulate colonic fluid secretion. Limitation of fat intake will control diarrhea but may lead to caloric deficiency and weight loss. Supplementation of the diet with medium-chain triglycerides (MCT, fatty acid chain length C8-C10) may help. These fats are water soluble hence do not require bile salts for the solubilization necessary for absorption of long chain fatty acids.[212]

Massive resection of the small bowel, usually necessitated by infarction, presents a major therapeutic challenge. Patients have survived with as little as 6 to 18 inches of jejunum beyond the ligament of Treitz especially if the ileocecal sphincter and right colon can be preserved.[237] In some patients in whom oral alimentation does not meet the caloric needs, long-term parenteral alimentation has been successful.

BACTERIAL OVERGROWTH SYNDROMES (BLIND-LOOP OR STASIS SYNDROME).[208,219] Bacterial deconjugation of bile salts in the small bowel is the second major cause of bile salt deficiency. The normal small intestine is sparsely populated with bacteria in part because the acid environment of the stomach is lethal to many bacteria, but more important is the motility of the fasting intestine that keeps it swept clean. Abnormalities of the intestine conducive to stasis of small bowel contents favor the massive proliferation of bacteria to levels in excess of 10^6 organisms per ml intestinal contents. The bacterial population is a colonic flora, including obligate anaerobes in large numbers as well as facultative anaerobes such as *E. coli* and *Streptococcus fecalis*. Situations that cause stasis include blind loops; a single, large, or multiple small intestinal diverticula; strictures; afferent loop obstruction after a gastrojejunostomy; entero-enteric anastomoses or fistula; gastrocolic fistula; radiation enteritis and generalized atony of the upper small bowel as in scleroderma or diabetic visceral neuropathy. In addition to steatorrhea from bile salt deficiency, the bacterial overgrowth syndromes are characterized by vitamin B_{12} malabsorption which is not corrected by the addition of intrinsic factor. Vitamin B_{12} is used by the bacteria before it reaches the absorptive site in the ileum.

The bile salt breath test is positive in these patients. In addition, many have a low d-xylose excretion which is the consequence of two factors: 1) metabolism of d-xylose by the abnormal intestinal flora; and 2) spotty nonspecific epithelial damage which may be found in the bacterial overgrowth syndrome.

Therapy for bacterial overgrowth includes eliminating the cause of stasis, if this is readily correctable, or, if not, antibiotic administration to decrease or change the bacterial flora. The responses to treat-

ment are variable and depend on the extent, location, and severity of the abnormality; the types of bacteria present; their sensitivity to antibiotics; and the extent of the bile salt deconjugation. Antibiotics that have been most useful are tetracycline and ampicillin. Neomycin should not be used because it precipitates bile salts.

The malabsorption that follows subtotal gastric resection and gastroenterostomy is of multiple origins. First, food may be emptied into the jejunum before the release of pancreatic enzymes and bile. Second, release of bile salt and pancreatic enzymes may be suboptimal since the duodenum and upper jejunum which contain the greatest concentration of secretin and CCK-secretory cells is bypassed. And, finally bile salts may be precipitated and pancreatic enzymes may be inactivated because the rate of gastric emptying may exceed the rate of bicarbonate production by the pancreas.

MALABSORPTION (Mucosal Defects)

Celiac Disease[229]

Celiac disease (gluten-induced enteropathy) is a chronic, probably hereditary, illness of unknown etiology occurring in both children and adults and manifested clinically by steatorrhea and deficiencies produced by intestinal malabsorption. The disordered absorption results from damage to the proximal small-intestinal mucosa by the digestion products of gluten, a protein contained in grains, especially in wheat but not in corn or rice. When food derived from these grains are avoided (gluten-free diet), a complete remission with improvement in the jejunal lesion occurs. Reintroduction of gluten causes a relapse and a worsening of the of the jejunal mucosa.

It has been postulated that the mucosa of patients with celiac disease lack one or more peptide-hydrolyzing enzymes that normally digest gluten peptides and that the unhydrolyzed peptides are injurious to the absorbing epithelial cells of the small intestine. To date no specific defect in gluten hydrolysis has been identified. A second hypothesis suggests that there is abnormal binding between a specific receptor on the absorbing columnar cell and a gluten peptide in the celiac patient results in damage to the epithelium. The mechanism of this gluten-induced damage has not been established. Possibilities include a direct toxic effect or an immunologic reaction. The likelihood that the latter plays a role is strengthened by the observation that antibodies to gluten fractions are produced locally and that prednisone will lessen the damaging effect of gluten on the surface epithelial cells.

Celiac disease has been recognized chiefly in temperate climates. Females outnumber males in most reports. Almost all of these patients are Caucasian, but we have seen two blacks with celiac disease. There is a 10 percent incidence of celiac disease in the siblings and relatives of celiacs, and a dominant inheritance with incomplete penetration has been suggested. A striking relation between celiac disease and HLA-B8 and W3 tissue antigens has been found. The highest prevalence of celiac disease is in Ireland, where the rate has been projected to be 1 in 300 live births.

Diabetes mellitus or a history of diabetes in a close relative is common in celiac disease. Patients with dermatitis herpetiformis have been found to have a high incidence of a celiac-like lesion on intestinal biopsy which is healed by removing gluten from the diet. On the other hand, these patients do not have clinical malabsorption.[204] Since patients with typical celiac disease do not have an increased incidence of dermatitis herpetiformis, it is possible that the gluten-induced lesion in dermatitis herpetiformis is caused by a defect at a different step in gluten handling than is the celiac lesion.

CLINICAL MANIFESTATIONS. The symptoms and signs of celiac disease may first appear in childhood, as early as 8 to 12 months of age.

Diarrhea, weight loss, failure to thrive, wasting of the musculature, potbelly, and anemia are the main clinical features. The disease may remit spontaneously in the middle of the first decade. Careful study shows that these children may have diarrhea occasionally, an abnormal jejunal mucosa, malabsorption and some delay in growth and body development. Most patients with celiac disease are asymptomatic in the late teens and early twenties. Some stay in apparent remission, but others have a return of symptoms in their late twenties or thirties. Other patients first develop the clinical manifestations of malabsorption between the third and sixth decades without a childhood history of celiac disease. In some adults the disease first becomes clinically apparent after gastric surgery. All these patients have the same jejunal biopsy lesion and a similar excellent response to a gluten-free diet. The main symptoms in adults include bulky, light-colored stools, abdominal bloating, weight loss, weakness, and easy fatigability. Before specific deficiencies appear, these patients are frequently considered to have a functional bowel disease. As the effects of malabsorption become more pronounced, iron deficiency or megaloblastic anemia, bleeding tendencies, peripheral edema, or tetany may occur. Milk intolerance has also been noted in some patients because lactase levels are decreased in the damaged epithelium of the jejunum. An increased incidence of adenocarcinomas and lymphomas of the small intestine has been reported in celiac disease. Intestinal ulceration and perforation have also been seen as fatal complications of celiac disease.

DIAGNOSIS. At the time of the initial diagnosis, most patients have steatorrhea, low serum carotene levels, abnormal d-xylose absorption, and an abnormal small bowel x-ray pattern. The diagnosis is verified by the finding of a flattened mucosa on jejunal biopsy and by the subsequent clinical and histologic improvement on a gluten-free diet.

TREATMENT.[203,234,239] Adults and children with celiac disease improve rapidly on a diet free of wheat, rye, oats, and barley gluten. The improvement is clinical, biochemical, and histologic. Symptoms usually decrease in the first week and most patients are in remission within two months. Weight gain is rapid, averaging over 20 pounds in the first two months. The absorption of fat and xylose returns to normal. The absorption of all food substances improves rapidly and secondary deficiencies are corrected eventually without specific replacement. If needed, calcium, potassium, vitamin K, iron, folic acid, or vitamin B_{12} can be given as emergency supportive therapy. The surface epithelium of the jejunum improves very rapidly, reaching the normal height in 7 to 10 days. Later, the villus pattern improves, and after a year or more the mucosa approaches a normal appearance if the patient continues to follow his diet. Minor dietary indiscretions may be tolerated without producing symptoms, but, if continued, mucosal damage and malabsorption reappear. Adrenal corticosteroids produce improvement of the surface epithelium despite continued gluten ingestion, but the remission obtained is usually incomplete.

Tropical Sprue[202,223]

Tropical sprue is an endemic disease of unknown etiology occurring in certain tropical areas of the world. The signs and symptoms are the result of malabsorption caused by a lesion of the small-intestinal mucosa. Although some of the clinical manifestations resemble those of celiac disease, they are two distinct diseases. Tropical sprue is common in India, the Far East, Puerto Rico, and Cuba but is not encountered in Jamaica.

Recently, patients with tropical sprue have been recognized in temperate areas, such as New York, Boston, and London. These patients were either natives or former residents in endemic tropical areas, but their illness did not appear until several months or years after leaving the tropics.[220]

An episode of viral enteritis or enterotoxic diarrhea may set the stage for the onset of tropical sprue. In addition, a role for intestinal microorganisms in the pathogenesis of this disorder is suggested by the favorable response following broad-spectrum antibiotics and the observation that enterotoxin-producing bacteria may be found in cultures of jejunal fluid.

Folic acid or vitamin B_{12} therapy leads to some improvement in intestinal absorption and the intestinal lesion. However, folic acid deficiency cannot be assigned a primary role in the pathogenesis of tropical sprue, since pure dietary deficiency of folic acid does not produce malabsorption nor a mucosal lesion like sprue. The histologic abnormalities found in intestinal biopsies from patients with tropical sprue include damage to the surface epithelium, shortening of the villi, lengthening of the crypts, and inflammation in the lamina propria.[202] In severely ill patients, the histologic changes are similar to but rarely as severe as those seen in celiac disease.

DIAGNOSIS.   The diagnosis in an endemic area is based on history, evidence of malabsorption, exclusion of giardiasis, and response to therapy. Jejunal biopsy and bone marrow abnormalities are usually present. Subclinical malabsorption and intestinal biopsy abnormalities can be found in at least one-third of the "healthy" general population of many developing countries where tropical sprue is endemic. This "tropical malabsorption" may affect the nutritional status of major population groups.

TREATMENT.[213]   Optimum therapy includes broad-spectrum antibiotics, such as tetracycline and folic acid. Vitamin B_{12} supplements are usually given in long-standing cases. Antibiotic therapy (tetracycline, 500 mg per day) for several months will correct persistent malabsorption and result in an improvement in intestinal histology. The duration of "cure" with antibiotics has not yet been established. A few patients with long-standing, severe malabsorption have relapsed soon after discontinuing treatment.

LYMPHATIC OBSTRUCTION

Whipple's Disease[215,226]

Whipple's disease has been converted from a progressive, fatal disease of unknown etiology to one that is known to be caused by a bacterium, can be readily diagnosed by jejunal biopsy and can be successfully treated by antibiotics.

CLINICAL MANIFESTATIONS.   Whipple's disease occurs predominantly in white males, and the average age at the time of diagnosis is 43 years. Migratory arthritis or arthralgia, affecting large joints and usually without deformity, occurs in 60 percent of the patients. The arthritis may be part of a generalized polyserositis, and precedes the onset of diarrhea and steatorrhea. Other manifestations in the prodromal stage may include pleuritis, low-grade fever, abdominal swelling, uveitis, ascites, and central nervous system disorders.

The effects of malabsorption often dominate the picture when the disease enters a progressive phase. Weight loss, emaciation, and asthenia may be severe. Skin pigmentation, usually sparing the buccal membranes, occurs in two-thirds of these patients. This combination of chronic ill health, weakness, hypotension, diarrhea, and skin pigmentation may result in an erroneous diagnosis of Addison's disease. Other findings include a chronic cough (30 percent) and fever (25 percent). Lymphadenopathy, either generalized or localized, is noted in 50 percent of the patients. Enlarged mesenteric and retroperitoneal nodes cause palpable abdominal masses in some patients. Uveitis, ocular palsies, dementia, and other central nervous system manifestations occasionally are the presenting symptoms or may be the major symptoms of relapse after antibiotic therapy.[221]

Laboratory tests in the period of clinical activity may show leukocytosis, normocytic or hypochromic anemia, increased erythrocyte sedimentation rate, occult blood in the stools (30 percent), steatorrhea, low serum carotene and cholesterol, hypoalbuminemia, prolonged prothrombin time, and decreased d-xylose absorption. Small bowel x-rays often show marked coarsening of the mucosal folds, especially in the jejunum, as well as the alterations associated with malabsorption caused by mucosal disease, for example, flocculation, segmentation of the barium column, and dilatation of the lumen.

Impaired lymphocyte transformation has been found in some patients in remission suggesting that an impaired host response to the infection may be a factor in the pathogenesis of the disease.

DIAGNOSIS AND TREATMENT.   Although the characteristic PAS-positive macrophages are found in many tissues, including the lymph nodes and rectal mucosa, Whipple's disease is most readily and conclusively diagnosed by intestinal biopsy. The characteristics of the intestinal biopsy are 1) infiltration of the lamina propria with the foamy PAS-positive macrophages, with the infiltrate sometimes so dense that the villi are distorted; 2) lymphatics in the villi often grossly dilated with fat; and 3) a normal intestinal epithelium. Malabsorption results, in part, from the blockage of the lamina propria and the lymphatic channels by the granule-laden macrophages.

Electronmicroscopic studies have demonstrated

bacterial structures in the intestinal mucosa and have shown that the PAS-positive granules are derived from ingested "bacillary bodies." The bacteria and the PAS-positive granules disappear after successful antibiotic treatment. Immunofluorescent studies show that the bacteria in intestinal biopsies from different patients are antigenically as well as morphologically similar so that one, as yet unidentified, organism seems to be responsible for this unusual infection.

Treatment should consist of two weeks of penicillin 1.2 million units and streptomycin 1 g IM followed by maintenance therapy with a broad-spectrum antibiotic such as tetracycline (1 g per day for 8 to 12 months). The adequacy of the therapy is best gauged by continued absence of bacteria and disappearance of the PAS macrophages from the lamina propria of the intestine.

Protein-Losing Gastroenteropathy[236]

This term is used for disorders in which there is an excessive loss of serum protein, into the stomach or intestinal tract. The albumin loss can be documented by the intravenous administration of isotopic chromium-labelled albumin followed by the measurement of the amount of radioactivity appearing in the stool. If the albumin loss exceeds the rate of synthesis by the liver, hypoalbuminemia, and edema result. This weeping of protein occurs with 1) localized inflammation, as with hypertrophic gastritis or gastric carcinoma; 2) diffuse inflammatory conditions of the bowel, including Crohn's disease, ulcerative colitis, celiac disease, and tropical sprue; 3) increased pressure in the lymphatics draining the bowel, including Whipple's disease, intestinal lymphangiectasia, congestive heart failure, constrictive pericarditis, and cirrhosis with portal hypertension.

Intestinal lymphangiectasia, a developmental abnormality of the intestinal lymphatics, is seen in adults and young children and may present with peripheral edema, at times asymmetric, serous, and chylous effusions; hypoalbuminemia; and diarrhea. Some of the patients also have mild steatorrhea. There may be a family history of Milroy's disease. On small bowel x-rays there is seen a coarsening of the folds of the jejunal mucosa and hypersecretion of fluid. Jejunal biopsies characteristically reveal dilated lymphatic channels in the mucosa with distortion of the villi. Lymphangiograms may reveal a generalized extraintestinal lymphatic involvement, and at laparotomy abnormalities of the lymphatic channels are seen.

The use of a low-fat diet or a medium-chain tri-

glyceride as the fat source has been shown to be an effective method of decreasing protein loss by decreasing intestinal lymph flow in the inadequate abnormal lymphatics.[218]

Lactase Deficiency and Milk Intolerance[201]

Some people experience gastrointestinal symptoms if they drink even moderate quantities of milk. One to four hours after consuming one or two glassfuls, they note abdominal bloating, gaseousness, and cramps although they can tolerate small amounts of milk, as in cereal or coffee. Some develop diarrhea. Most are otherwise healthy, and were able to drink milk as infants and children. Milk intolerance can increase the symptoms in patients with organic bowel disease, postgastrectomy diarrhea, or with the irritable bowel syndrome.

This milk intolerance is the result of failure of the small intestine to adequately hydrolyze and absorb the lactose in milk. The symptoms can be reproduced by several glasses of milk or by giving 50 g of lactose in a tolerance test. Inadequate digestion of lactose is documented by failure of the blood glucose to rise during the tolerance test, or by a rise in breath hydrogen which is produced when unabsorbed carbohydrate from the small intestine is metabolized by anaerobic bacteria in the colon,[225] or by demonstration of low levels of lactase activity by in vitro assay of intestinal biopsy tissue.

Intestinal lactase levels may be low if the intestinal epithelium which contains lactase and other disaccharidases is damaged, e.g., in celiac disease or tropical sprue. Congenital deficiencies of lactase are rare. The commonest cause of low lactase levels is the genetically determined decrease in lactase activity after infancy or early childhood. There are marked differences in the prevalence of this phenomenon in different ethnic groups. Lactose intolerance is found in 2 to 8 percent of adults of Scandinavian or Western European extraction, whereas the prevalence is over 60 percent in American Indians, African Bantus, Japanese, Thais, Formosans, Philippinos, American blacks, Greek Cypriots, Arabs, and Ashkenazi Jews. Although many people are potentially milk intolerant, they either drink very little or no milk or they consume it in a fermented form, such as yogurt or cheese, in which the lactose has been converted to lactic acid and hence is tolerated by a lactase-deficient person.

Milk intolerance should be suspected if symptoms appear when a patient's milk intake has been increased, as in the treatment of a peptic ulcer and in patients with unexplained abdominal distension, cramps, or diarrhea. It can be a contributing factor in the symptoms of patients with ulcerative colitis, Crohn's disease, irritable-colon syndrome and post-gastrectomy diarrhea. Treatment involves decreasing the intake of milk and ice cream to amounts that can be tolerated or using fermented dairy products.

Sucrase deficiency and sucrose intolerance have been documented in a small number of individuals and in some Eskimo tribes as a congenital inherited defect.[211] The intolerance of sucrose usually decreases with increasing age but a few adults previously thought to have an irritable-colon syndrome have been demonstrated to have their symptoms on this basis.

REFERENCES

General References

1. Davenport, H.W. Physiology of the Digestive Tract, 4th ed. Chicago, Year Book Medical Publishers, 1977.
2. Greenberger, N.J. and Winship, D.H. Gastrointestinal Disorders: A Pathophysiological Approach. Chicago, Year Book Medical Publishers, 1976.
3. Hendrix, T.R. The absorptive function of the alimentary canal; The Secretory function of the alimentary canal; The motility of the alimentary canal. In Mountcastle, V.B. (ed.), Medical Physiology, Vol. II. St. Louis, Mosby, 1974.
4. Mendeloff, A.I. and Dunn, J.P. Digestive Disease. Cambridge, Harvard University Press, 1971.
   An epidemiologic approach.

5. Morson, B.C. and Dawson, I.M.P. Gastrointestinal Pathology. Oxford, Blackwell, 1972.
6. Sleisenger, M.D. and Fordtran, J.S. Gastrointestinal Disease. Philadelphia, Saunders, 1973.
7. Spiro, H.M. Gastroenterology, 2nd ed. New York, Macmillan, 1976.
8. Truelove, S.C. and Reynell, P.C. Diseases of the Digestive System, 2nd ed. Oxford, Blackwell, 1972.
9. Yardley, J.H., Morrown, B.C., and Abell, M.R. The Gastrointestinal Tract. Baltimore, Williams & Wilkins, 1977.

Dysphagia and Heartburn

10. Adams, C.W.M., Brain, R.H.F., Ellis, F.G., Kauntze, R., and Trounce, J.R. Achalasia of the cardia. Guy's Hosp. Rep., 110:191, 1961.
11. Atkinson, M. Disorders of oesophageal motility. Clin. Gastroenterol., 5:1, 1976.
12. —— and Van Gelder, A. Esophageal intraluminal pH recording in the assessment of gastroesophageal reflux and its consequences. Am. J. Dig. Dis., 22:365, 1977.
13. Bayless, T.M. Management of Esophageal Diseases. Modern Treatment, Vol. 7. New York, Harper & Row, 1971.

14. Behar, J., Biancine, P., and Sheahan, D.C. Evaluation of esophageal tests in the diagnosis of reflux esophagitis. Gastroenterology, 71:9, 1976.
15. Bennett, J.R. and Atkinson, M. The differentiation of oesophageal and cardiac pain. Lancet, 2:1123, 1966.
16. —— and Hendrix, T.R. Diffuse esophageal spasm: a disorder with more than one cause. Gastroenterology, 59:273, 1970.
17. —— and Hendrix, T.R. Treatment of achalasia with pneumatic dilatation. Modern Treatment, 7:1217, 1970.
18. Brand, D.L., Martin, D., and Pope, C.E., II. Esophageal manometrics in patients with angina-like chest pain. Am. J. Dig. Dis., 22:300, 1977.
19. Cauthorne, R.T., Vanhoutte, J.J., Donner, M.W., and Hendrix, T.R. A study of patients with lower esophageal ring by simultaneous cineradiography and manometry. Gastroenterology, 49:632, 1965.
20. Cohen, S. and Harris, L.D. Does hiatus hernia affect competence of the gastroesophageal sphincter? N. Engl. J. Med., 284:1053, 1971.
21. —— and Hughes, W. Role of gastrin supersensitivity in the pathogenesis of lower esophageal hypertension in achalasia. J. Clin. Invest., 150:1241, 1971.
22. —— and Lipshutz, W. Lower esophageal dysfunction in achalasia. Gastroenterology, 61:814, 1971.
23. DiMarino, A.J. and Cohen, S. Characteristics of lower esophageal sphincter function in symptomatic diffuse esophageal spasm. Gastroenterology, 66:1, 1974.
24. Farrell, R.L., Roling, G.T., and Castell, D.O. Cholinergic therapy of chronic heartburn. Ann. Intern. Med., 80:573, 1974.
25. Goyal, R.K. Symposium on esophageal motility. Arch. Intern. Med., 136:511, 1976.
26. Hamilton, S. and Yardley, J.H. Regeneration of cardiac-type mucosa and acquisition of Barrett mucosa after esophago-gastrostomy. Gastroenterology, 72:669, 1977.
27. Hendrix, T.R. and Yardley, J.H. Consequences of gastro-oesophageal reflux. Clin. Gastroenterol., 5:155, 1976.
28. Hutcheon, D.F. and Hendrix, T.R. Esophageal reflux—diagnosis and treatment. Postgrad. Med. J., 61:131, 1977.
29. Kilman, W.J. and Goyal, R.K. Disorders of pharyngeal and upper esophageal sphincter motor function. Arch. Intern. Med., 136:592, 1976.
30. Kramer, P. and Ingelfinger, F.J. Esophageal sensitivity to mecholyl in cardiospasm. Gastroenterology, 19:242, 1951.
31. Lowe, W.C. Survival with carcinoma of esophagus. Ann. Intern. Med., 77:915, 1972.
32. Marchard, P. Acute caustic injuries of the esophagus. S. Afr. Med. J., 29:195, 1955.
33. Silbiger, M.L., Pikielney, R., and Donner, M.W. Neuromuscular disorders affecting the pharynx: cineradiographic analysis. Invest. Radiol., 2:442, 1967.
34. Stevens, M.B., Hookman, P., Siegel, C.I., Esterly, J.R., Shulman, L.E., and Hendrix, T.R. Aperistalsis of the esophagus in patients with connective tissue disorders and Raynaud's phenomenon. N. Engl. J. Med., 270:1218, 1964.

35. Vantrappen, G. and Hellemans, J. Diffuse muscle spasm of the oesophagus and the hypertensive lower esophageal sphincter. Clin. Gastroenterol., 5:59, 1976.

Abdominal Pain

36. Ackerman, N.B. The continuing problem of perforating appendicitis. Surg. Gynecol. Obstet., 139:29, 1974.
37. Banks, P.A. Acute pancreatitis. Gastroenterology, 61:382, 1971.
38. Becker, W.F., Powell, J.L., and Turner, R.J. A clinical study of 1,060 patients with acute cholecystitis. Surg. Gynecol. Obstet., 104:491, 1957.
39. Bricker, J., Bartholomew, L.G., Cain, J.C., and Adsow, M.A. Syndrome of intestinal arterial insufficiency (abdominal angina). Arch. Intern. Med., 117:632, 1966.
40. Burack, W.R. and Hollister, M. Tuberculous peritonitis. Am. J. Med., 28:510, 1960.
41. Cameron, J.L., Capuzzi, D.M., Zuidema, G.D., and Margolis, S. Acute pancreatitis with hyperlipidemia: the incidence of lipid abnormalities in acute pancreatitis. Ann. Surg., 177:483, 1973.
42. ———, Capuzzi, D.M., Zuidema, G.D., and Margolis, S. Acute pancreatitis with hyperlipidemia: evidence for a persistent defect in lipid metabolism. Am. J. Med., 56:483, 1974.
43. Chaudhary, N.A. and Truelove, S.C. The irritable colon syndrome. Q. J. Med., 31:307, 1962.
44. Child, C.G., III, Frey, C.F., and Fry, W.J. A reappraisal of removal of ninety-five percent of the distal portion of the pancreas. Surg. Gynecol. Obstet., 129:49, 1969.
45. Corday, E., Irving, D.W., Gold, H., Bernstein, H., and Skelton, R.B. Mesenteric vascular insufficiency. Intestinal ischemia induced by remote circulatory disturbances. Am. J. Med., 33:365, 1962.
46. Creutzfeld, W. and Schmidt, H. Aetiology and pathogenesis of pancreatitis (Current Concepts). Scand. J. Gastroenterol. (Suppl.), 6:47, 1970.
47. Davidoff, F., Tishler, S., and Rosoff, V. Marked hyperlipidemia and pancreatitis associated with oral contraceptive therapy. N. Engl. J. Med., 289:552, 1973.
48. Esler, M.D. and Goulston, K.J. Levels of anxiety in colonic disorders. N. Engl. J. Med., 288:16, 1973.
49. Fleischner, F.G. Diverticular disease of the colon. New observations and revised concepts. Gastroenterology, 60:316, 1971.
50. Glenn, F. and Thorbjarnason, B. The surgical treatment of acute cholecystitis. Surg. Gynecol. Obstet., 116:61, 1963.
51. Gross, J.B., Gambill, E.E., and Ulrich, J.A. Hereditary pancreatitis. Description of a fifth kindred and summary of clinical features. Am. J. Med., 33:358, 1962.
52. Gullick, H.D. Carcinoma of the pancreas, a review and critical analysis of 100 cases. Medicine, 38:47, 1959.
53. Gunn, A. and Kiddie, N. Some clinical observations on patients with gallstones. Lancet, 2:239, 1972.
54. Haff, R.C., Wise, L., and Ballinger, W.F. Biliary-enteric fistulas. Surg. Gynecol. Obstet., 133:84, 1971.
55. Hill, O.W. and Blendis, L. Physical and psychological evaluation of non-organic abdominal pain. Gut, 8:221, 1967.
56. Hinkell, C.L. and Moller, G.A. Correlation of symptoms, age, sex and habits with cholecystographic findings: 1000 consecutive examinations. Gastroenterology, 32:807, 1957.
57. Hofkin, G. Course of patients with perforated duodenal ulcer. Am. J. Surg., 153:911, 1961.
58. Holdstock, D.J., Misiewicz, J.J., and Waller, S. Observations on the mechanism of abdominal pain. Gut, 10:19, 1969.
59. Johnston, S.G., Ellis, C.J., and Levitt, M.D. Mechanism of increased renal clearance of amylase/creatinine in acute pancreatitis. N. Engl. J. Med., 295:1214, 1976.
60. Kappelman, N.B. and Saunders, R.C. Ultrasound in the investigation of gallbladder disease. JAMA, 239:1426, 1978.
61. Kirschner, P.A. Occlusion of the mesenteric arteries and veins with infarction of the bowel. Mt. Sinai J. Med. N.Y., 21:307, 1955.
62. Lasser, R.B., Bond, J.H., and Levitt, M.D. The role of intestinal gas in functional abdominal pain. N. Engl. J. Med., 293:524, 1975.
63. Lund, J. Surgical indications in cholelithiasis. Ann. Surg., 151:153, 1960.
64. Marston, A., Pherls, M.T., Thomas, M.L., and Morson, B.C. Ischaemic colitis. Gut, 1:1, 1966.
65. McClelland, H.A., Lewis, M.J., and Naish, J.M. Idiopathic steatorrhea with intestinal pseudo-obstruction. Gut, 3:142, 1962.
66. Mellinkoff, S.M. Systemic causes of abdominal pain. Am. J. Dig. Dis., 4:642, 1959.
67. Mittelpunkt, A. and Nora, P.F. Current features in the treatment of acute appendicitis: an analysis of 1000 consecutive cases. Surgery, 60:971, 1966.
68. Moore, H.D. Treatment of acutely perforated ulcers. Lancet, 1:163, 1955.
69. Morson, B. The muscle abnormalities in diverticular disease of the sigmoid colon. Br. J. Radiol., 36:385, 1963.
70. Nadrowski, L.F. Pathophysiology and current treatment of intestinal obstruction. Rev. Surg., 31:381, 1974.
71. Painter, N.S., Truelove, S.C., Adrian, G.M., and Tuckey, M. Segmentation and the localization of intraluminal pressures in the human colon, with special reference to the pathogenesis of colonic diverticula. Gastroenterology, 49:169, 1965.
72. Parks, T.G. Diverticular disease of the colon. Postgrad. Med. J., 44:680, 1968.
73. Ross, F.P., Boggs, J.D., and Dunphy, J.E. Studies on acute cholecystitis. The pathologic process in relation to the clinical management of the disease; the fallacy of the "critical period." Surg. Gynecol. Obstet., 91:271, 1950.
74. Salmon, P.R. Endoscopic retrograde choledochopancreatography in the diagnosis of pancreatic disease. Gut, 16:658, 1975.
75. Salt, W.B. and Shenker, S. Amylase–its clinical significance: a review of the literature. Medicine, 55:269, 1976.
76. Schuffler, D., Lowe, M.C., and Bill, A.H. Studies of idiopathic intestinal pseudo-obstruction. I. Hereditary visceral myopathy-clinical and pathological studies. Gas-

troenterology, 73:327, 1977.

77. Small, D.M. and Rapo, S. Source of abnormal bile in patients with cholesterol gallstones. N. Engl. J. Med., 283:53, 1970.

78. Stanley, R.J., Sagel, S.S., and Levitt, R.G. Computed tomographic evaluation of the pancreas. Radiology, 124:715, 1977.

78a. Steinheber, F.U. Medical conditions mimicking the acute surgical abdomen. Med. Clin. North Am., 57:1559, 1973.

79. Taylor, H. The non-surgical treatment of perforated peptic ulcer. Gastroenterology, 33:353, 1957.

80. Thistle, J.L. and Hofmann, A.F. Efficacy and specificity of chemodeoxycholic acid therapy for dissolving gallstones. N. Engl. J. Med., 289:655, 1973.

81. van der Linden, W. and Sunzel, H. Early versus delayed operation for acute cholecystitis: a controlled clinical trial. Am. J. Surg., 120:7, 1970.

82. Vlahcevic, Z.R., Bell, C.C., Jr., Buhac, I., Farrar, J.T., and Swell, L. Diminished bile acid pool size in patients with gallstones. Gastroenterology, 59:165, 1970.

83. Wenchert, A. and Robertson, B. The natural course of gallstone disease. Gastroenterology, 50:376, 1966.

84. Williams, L.F. Vascular insufficiency of the intestine. Gastroenterology, 61:757, 1971.

85. Zuidema, G.D., Reed, D., Turcotte, J.C., and Fry, W.J. Superior mesenteric artery embolectomy. Ann. Surg., 159:548, 1964.

Peptic Ulcer and Dyspepsia

86. Black, T., Hole, D., and Rhodes, J. Bile damage to gastric mucosal barrier: the influence of pH and bile concentration. Gastroenterology, 61:178, 1971.

87. Buchman, E., Kaung, D.T., Dolan, K., and Knepp, R.N. Unrestricted diet in the treatment of duodenal ulcer. Gastroenterology, 56:1016, 1969.

88. Deering, T.B. and Malagalada, J.R. Comparison of an H_2 receptor antagonist and a neutralizing antacid on postprandial acid delivery into the duodenum in patients with duodenal ulcer. Gastroenterology, 73:11, 1977.

89. Feldman, M., Richardson, C.T., and Peterson, W.L. Effect of low-dose propantheline on food-stimulated gastric acid secretion: comparison with an "optimal effective dose" and interaction with cimetidine. N. Engl. J. Med., 297:1427, 1977.

90. Finkelstein, W. and Isselbacher, K.J. Cimetidine. N. Engl. J. Med., 299:992, 1978.

91. Fordtran, J.S. Acid rebound. N. Engl. J. Med., 279:900, 1968.

92. ——— and Collyns, J.A. Antacid pharmacology in duodenal ulcer. Effects of anatacid on postcibal gastric acidity and peptic activity. N. Engl. J. Med., 274:921, 1966.

93. ——— and Grossman, M.I. (eds.). Third symposium on histamine H_2-receptor antagonists. Clinical results with cimetidine. Gastroenterology, 74:339, 1978.

94. ———, Mosawski, S.G., and Richardson, C.T. In vivo and in vitro evaluation of liquid antacid. N. Engl. J. Med., 288:923, 1973.

95. Fung, W.P., Karim, S.M., and Tye, C.Y. Effect of 15 (R) 15 methyl prostaglandin E_2 methyl ester on healing of gastric ulcers: controlled endoscopic study. Lancet, 2:10, 1974.

96. Geall, M.G., Phillips, S.F., and Summerskill, W.H.J. Profile of gastric potential difference in man. Effects of aspirin, alcohol, bile, and endogenous acid. Gastroenterology, 58.437, 1970.

97. Gilliland, I. Tri-potassium di-citrato bismuthate. Postgrad. Med. J., 51(Suppl. 5):1, 1975.

98. Goldberg, H.L. Roentgen diagnosis of ulcerative diseases. In Sleisenger, M.H. and Fordtran, J.S. (eds.), Gastrointestinal Disease. Philadelphia, Saunders, 1973.

99. Grossman, M.I. Basal and histolog-stimulated gastric secretion in control subjects and in patients with peptic ulcer or gastric cancer. Gastroenterology, 45:14, 1963.

100. Gudmand-Hoyer, E., Jensen, K.B., Krag, E., Rask-Madsen, J., Rahbek, I., Rune, S.J., and Wulff, H.R. Prophylactic effect of cimetidine in duodenal ulcer disease. Br. Med. J., 1:1095, 1978.

101. Ippoliti, A.F., Sturdevant, R.A.L., Isenberg, J.I., Binder, M., Camacho, R., Cano, R., Cooney, C., Kline, M.M., Koretz, R.L., Meyer, J.J., Samloff, M., Schwabe, A.D., Strom, E.A., Valenzuela, J.E., and Wintroub, R.H. Cimetidine versus intensive antacid therapy for duodenal ulcer. A Multicenter trial. Gastroenterology, 74:393, 1978.

102. Isenberg, J.I., Walsh, J.H., and Grossman, M.I. Zollinger-Ellison syndrome. Gastroenterology, 65:140, 1973.

103. Ivey, K.J. Anticholinergics—do they work in duodenal ulcer? Gastroenterology, 68:750, 1975.

104. Kolts, B.E., Herbst, C.A., and McGuigan, J.E. Calcium and secretin stimulated gastrin release in the Zollinger-Ellison syndrome. Ann Intern. Med., 81:758, 1974.

105. Kreel, L. and Ellis, H. Pyloric stenosis in adults: a clinical and radiological study of 100 consecutive patients. Gut, 6:253, 1965.

106. Lennard-Jones, J.E. and Bobouris, N. Effect of different foods on the acidity of the gastric contents in patients with duodenal ulcer. A comparison between two "therapeutic" diets and freely-chosen meals. Gut, 6:113, 1965.

107. LeQuesne, L.P., Hobsley, M., and Hand, B.H. The dumping syndrome. I. Factors responsible for symptoms. Br. Med. J., 1:141, 1960.

108. McCarthy, D.M. Report on the United States experience with cimetidine in Zollinger-Ellison syndrome and other hypersecretory states. Gastroenterology, 74:453, 1978.

109. McMillan, D.E. and Freeman, R.B. The milk-alkali syndrome; a study of the acute disorder with comments on the development of the chronic condition. Medicine. 44:485, 1965.

110. Mitty, W.F., Jr., Grossi, G., and Mealon, T.F., Jr. Chronic afferent loop syndrome. Ann. Surg., 172:996, 1970.

111. Morrissey, J.F. Gastrointestinal endoscopy. Gastroenterology, 68:980, 1972.

112. Myhill, J., Piper, D.W., and Fenton, B.H. Antacid therapy of peptic ulcer. Gut, 5:581, 1964.

113. Oi, M., Oshida, K., and Sugimura, S. The location of gastric ulcer. Gastroenterology, 26:45, 1959.

114. Rhodes, J. Etiology of gastric ulcer. Gastroenterology, 63:171, 1972.

115. Sheiner, H.J. Gastric emptying in man. Gut, 16:235, 1975.

116. Sircus, W. Carbenoxolone sodium. Gut, 13:816, 1972.

117. Snyder, N., Scurry, M., and Hughes, W. Hypergastrinemia in familial multiple endocrine adenomatosis. Ann. Intern. Med., 80:321, 1974.

118. Wise, L. and Ballinger, W.F. The elective surgical treatment of chronic duodenal ulcer. A critical review. Surgery, 76:811, 1975.

Gastrointestinal Bleeding

119. Anderson, D. The use of measurement of central venous pressure in the selection of patients with massive gastroduodenal haemorrhage for emergency operation. Scand. J. Gastroenterol., 5:25, 1970.

120. —— and Klebe, J.G. Measurement of central venous pressure. Its use in the transfusion treatment of patients with gastroduodenal haemorrhage. Scand. J. Gastroenterol., 3:113, 1968.

121. Athanasoulis, C.A., Baum, S., Waltman, A.C., Ring, E.J., Imbembo, A., and VanderSalm, T.J. Control of acute gastric mucosal hemorrhage. N. Engl. Med., 290:597, 1974.

122. ——, Waltman, A.C., Novelline, R.A., Krudy, A.G., and Sniderman, K.W. Angiography. Its contribution to the emergency management of gastrointestinal hemorrhage. Radiol. Clin. North Am., 14:265, 1976.

123. Balint, J.A., Sarfek, I.J., and Fried, M.B. Gastrointestinal Bleeding: Diagnosis and Management. New York, Wiley, 1977.

124. Baum, S., Athanasoulis, C.A., Waltman, A.C., Galdabini, J., Schapiro, R.H., Warshaw, A.L., Ottinger, L.W. Angiodysplasia of the right colon: a cause of gastrointestinal bleeding. Am. J. Roentg., 129:789, 1977.

125. Bean, W.B. Enteric bleeding in rare conditions with diagnostic lesions of the skin and mucous membrane. Gastroenterology, 2:807, 1958.

126. Cararella, W.J., Galloway, S.J., Taxin, R.N., Follett, D.A., Pollack, E.J., and Seaman, W.B. "Lower" gastrointestinal tract hemorrhage—new concepts based on angiography. Am. J. Roentg., 121:357, 1974.

127. Chalmers, T.C., Sebestyen, C.S., and Lee, S. Emergency surgical treatment of bleeding peptic ulcer: an analysis of the published data on 21,130 patients. Trans. Am. Clin. Climatol. Assoc., 82:188, 1970.

128. Devitt, J.E. Upper gastrointestinal bleeding with special reference to peptic ulcer. Gastroenterology, 57:89, 1969.

129. Eisenberg, D. and Sherwood, C.E. Bleeding Meckel's diverticulum diagnosed by enteroscopy and radioisotope imaging. Am. J. Dig. Dis., 20:573, 1975.

130. Fenoglio, C.M. and Lane, N. The anatomic precursor of colorectal cancer. Cancer, 34:819, 1974.

131. Greegor, D.H. Occult blood testing for detection of asymptomatic colon cancer. Cancer, 28:131, 1971.

132. Katon, R.M. and Smith, F.W. Panendoscopy in the early diagnosis of acute upper gastrointestinal bleeding. Gastroenterology, 65:728, 1973.

133. Kaufman, S.L., Harrington, D.P., Barth, K.H., Maddrey, W.C., and White, R.I., Jr. Control of variceal bleeding by superior mesenteric artery vasopressin infusion. AJR, 128:567, 1977.

134. Kemeny, N. and Yogoda, A. Chemotherapy of colorectal cancer: A critical analysis of response criteria and therapeutic efficacy. In Lipkin, M. and Good R. (eds), Gastrointestinal Tract Cancer. New York, Plenum, 1978, p. 551.

135. Luk, G.D., Bynum, T.E., and Hendrix, T.R. Gastric aspiration in localization of gastrointestinal hemorrhage. JAMA, 241:576, 1979.

136. McHardy, G., Bechtold, J.E., and McHardy, R.J. Hemorrhage from primary disease of the mesenteric small intestine: a review of the literature and analysis of 216 cases. Gastroenterology, 28:17, 1955.

137. Moertel, C., Hill, J., and Dockety, M.B. The routine proctoscopic examination: a second look. Mayo Clin. Proc., 41:368, 1966.

138. Northfield, T.C. and Smith, T. Central venous pressure in clinical management of acute gastrointestinal bleeding. Lancet, 2:584, 1970.

139. ——. Hematemesis as an index of blood loss. Lancet, 1:990, 1971.

140. Palmer, E. The vigorous approach to upper gastrointestinal tract hemorrhage (1400 cases). JAMA, 207:1477, 1969.

141. Pavlides, G.P., Milligan, F.D., Clarke, D.N., Cohen, S.B., Wennstrom, C.J., Burbige, E.J., Krush, A.J., and Murphy, E.A. Hereditary polyposis coli I: the diagnostic value of colonoscopy, barium enema, and fecal occult blood. Cancer, 40:2632, 1977.

142. Tibbs, D.J. Blood volumes in gastro-duodenal hemorrhage. Lancet, 1:266, 1956.

143. Tudhope, G.R. The loss and replacement of red cells in patients with acute gastrointestinal hemorrhage. Q. J. Med., 27:543, 1958.

144. Turnbull, R.B., Jr. Cancer of the colon: the five-and ten-year survival rates following resection utilizing the isolation technique. Ann. R. Coll. Surg. Engl., 46:243, 1970.

145. White, R.I., Jr., Strandberg, J.D., Gross, G.S., and Barth, K.H. Therapeutic embolization with long-term occluding agents and their effects on embolized tissues. Radiology, 125:677, 1977.

Diarrhea and Constipation

146. Ammon, H.V. and Phillips, S.F. Inhibition of colonic water and electrolyte absorption by fatty acids in man. Gastroenterology, 65:744, 1973.

147. Bartlett, J.G., Chang, T.W., Gurwith, M., Gorbach, S.L., and Onderdouk, A.B. Antibiotic-associated pseudomembranous colitis due to toxin-producing clostridia. N. Engl. J. Med., 298:531, 1978.

148. Bayless, T.M., Boitnott, J.K., Belitsos, N.J., and Saba, G.P. Clinical Pathologic Conference. Johns Hopkins Med. J., 141:224, 1977.

149. ——, Yardley, J.H., Huang, S.S., and Greene, C.C. Crohn's disease. South. Med. J., 71:825, 1978.

150. Binder, H.J. Pharmacology of laxatives. Annu. Rev. Pharmacol. Toxicol., 17:355, 1977.

151. Bull, D.M., Peppercorn, M.A., Glotzer, D.J., Joffe, N., Goldman, H., and Silen, W. Crohn's disease of the colon. Gastroenterology, 76:607, 1979.

152. Burbige, E.J., Huang, S.S., and Bayless, T.M. Clinical manifestations of Crohn's disease in children and adolescents. Pediatrics, 55:866, 1975.

153. ———— and Milligan, F.D. Pseudomembranous colitis associated with antibiotics and therapy with cholestyramine. JAMA, 231:1157, 1975.

154. Cummings, J.H. Progress report: dietary fibre. Gut, 14:69, 1973.

155. deDombal, F.T., Burton, I.L., Clamp, S.E., and Goligher, J.C. Short-term course and prognosis of Crohn's disease. Gut, 15:435, 1974.

156. Dissanayake, A. and Truelove, S.C. A controlled therapeutic trial of long term maintenance treatment of ulcerative colitis with sulfasalazine. Gut, 14:818, 1973.

157. Dobbins, J. and Binder, H.J. Importance of the colon in enteric hyperoxaluria. N. Engl. J. Med., 296:298, 1977.

158. Eade, M.N. Liver disease in ulcerative colitis. Ann. Intern. Med., 72:475, 1970.

159. Edwards, F.C. and Truelove, S.C. The course and prognosis in ulcerative colitis. I. Short term. II. Long term. III Complications. IV. Carcinoma of colon. Gut, 4:299, 1963; 5:1, 1964.

160. Farmer, R.G. and Brown, C.H. Ulcerative proctitis: course and prognosis. Gastroenterology, 51:219, 1966.

161. Gelernt, I.M., Bauer, J.J., and Kreel, I. The reservoir ileostomy: early experience with 54 patients. Ann. Surg., 185:179, 1977.

162. Goligher, J.C., Hoffman, D.C., and deDombal, F.T. Surgical treatment of severe attacks of ulcerative colitis with special reference to the advantages of early operation. Br. Med. J., 2:703, 1970.

163. Grahame-Smith, D.G. Natural history and diagnosis of the carcinoid syndrome. Clin. Gastroenterol., 3:575, 1974.

164. Greenstein, A., Janowitz, H., and Sachar, D. The extraintestinal complications of Crohn's disease and ulcerative colitis: a study of 100 patients. Medicine, 55:401, 1976.

165. ————, Sachar, D.V., and Pasternack, B. Reoperation and recurrence in Crohn's colitis and ileocolitis. N. Engl. J. Med., 293:685, 1975.

166. Harris, J.C., Dupont, H.L., and Hornick, R.B. Fecal leucocytes in diarrheal illness. Ann. Intern. Med., 76:697, 1972.

167. Hendrix, T.R. and Bayless, T.M. Digestion: intestinal secretion. Annu. Rev. Physiol., 32:139, 1970.

168. Hutcheon, D.F., Bayless, T.M., and Gadacz, T.R. Postcholecystectomy diarrhea. JAMA, 241:823, 1979.

169. Isaacs, P., Whittaker, S.M., and Turnberg, L.A. Diarrhea associated with medullary carcinoma of the thyroid. Gastroenterology, 67:521, 1974.

170. Kirsner, J.B. Problems in the differentiation of ulcerative colitis and Crohn's disease of the colon: the need for repeated diagnostic evaluation. Gastroenterology, 68:187, 1975.

171. Kramer, P., Kearney, M.M., and Ingelfinger, F.J. The effect of specific foods and water loading on the ileal excreta of ileostomized human subjects. Gastroenterology, 42:535, 1962.

172. Krejs, G.J., Walsh, J.H., Morawski, S.G., and Fordtran, J.S. Intestinal perfusion studies in patients with intractable diarrhea due to pancreatic cholera and serreptitious ingestion of laxatives and diuretics. Am. J. Dig. Dis., 22:280, 1970.

173. Krogstad, D.J., Spencer, H.C., Jr., Healy, G.R., Gleason, N.W., Sexton, D.J., and Herron, C.A. Amebiasis: epidemiologic studies in the United States, 1971–1979. Ann. Intern. Med., 88:89, 1978.

174. Lennard-Jones, J.E., Morson, B.C., Ritchie, J.K., Shove, D.C., and Williams, B.M. Cancer in colitis: assessment of the individual risk by clinical and histological criteria. Gastroenterology, 73:1280, 1977.

175. Luk, G.D. and Hendrix, T.R. Microscopic examination of stool as a screening test for steatorrhea. Gastroenterology, 74:1134, 1978.

176. Marston, A, Pherls, M.T., Thomas, M.L., and Morson, B.C. Ischaemic colitis. Gut, 7:1, 1966.

177. Mekhjian, H.S., Phillips, S.F., and Hofmann, A.F. Colonic secretion of water and electrolytes induced by bile acids in man. J. Clin. Invest., 50:1569, 1971.

178. Mendeloff, A.I., Monk, M., Siegel C.I., and Lilienfeld, A. Illness experience and life stresses in patients with irritable colon and with ulcerative colitis. N. Engl. J. Med., 282:14, 1970.

179. Moss, J.D. and Knauer, C.M. Tuberculous enteritis. a report of three patients. Gastroenterology, 65:959, 1973.

180. Norland, C.C. and Kirsner, J.B. Toxic dilatation of colon (toxic megacolon): etiology, treatment, and prognosis in 42 patients. Medicine, 48:229, 1969.

181. Owen, R.L. and Hill, J.L. Rectal and pharyngeal gonorrhea in homosexual men. JAMA, 220:1315, 1972.

182. Phillips, S.F. Diarrhea: a current review of the pathophysiology. Gastroenterology, 63:495, 1972.

183. Pittman, F.E., El-Hashimi, W.K., and Pittman, J.C. Studies of human amebeasis. I. Clinical and laboratory findings in eight cases of acute amebic colitis. Gastroenterology, 65:581, 1973.

184. Rambaud, J.C. and Matuchansky, C. Diarrhoea and digestive endocrine tumors. Clin. Gastroenterol., 3:657, 1974.

185. ————, Modigliani, R., Matuchansky, C., Bloom, S., Said, S., Pessayve, D., and Brenier, J.J. Studies on humoral secretions and pathophysiology of diarrhea. Gastroenterology, 69:110, 1975.

186. Sachar, D.B. and Present, D.H. Immunotherapy in inflammatory bowel disease. Med. Clin. North Am., 62:173, 1978.

187. Said, S.I. and Falcona, G.R. Elevated plasma and tissue levels of vasoactive intestinal polypeptide in the watery-diarrhea syndrome due to pancreatic, bronchogenic, and other tumors. N. Engl. J. Med., 293:155, 1975.

188. Schuster, M.M. Constipation. In Conn, H.F.(ed.), Current Therapy-1976. Philadelphia, Saunders, 1976, p. 349.

189. Singer, H.C., Anderson, J.G.D., Frischer, H., and Kirsner, J.B. Familial aspects of inflammatory bowel disease. Gastroenterology, 61:423, 1971.

190. Singleton, J.W. National Cooperative Crohn's Disease Study (NCCDS). Results of drug treatment. Gastroen-

terology, 72:1133, 1977.

191. Truelove, S.C. Medical management of ulcerative colitis. Br. Med. J., 2:539, 605, 1968.

192. Turell, R. Sigmoidoscopy. Surg. Clin. North Am., 37:261, 1957.

193. Vantrappen, G., Agg, H.O., Ponette, E., Geboes, K., and Bertrand, P. Yersinia enteritis and enterocolitis: gastroenterological aspects. Gastroenterology, 72:220, 1977.

194. Verner, J.V. and Morrison, A.B. Endocrine pancreatic islet disease with diarrhea. Report of a case due to diffuse hyperplasia of nonbeta islet tissue with a review of 54 additional cases. Arch. Intern. Med., 133:492, 1974.

195. Whalen, G.E., Soergel, K.H., and Grennen, J.E. Diabetic diarrhea. A clinical and pathophysiologic study. Gastroenterology, 56:1021, 1969.

196. Whittington, P.F., Barnes, H.V., and Bayless, T.M. Medical management of Crohn's disease in adolescence. Gastroenterology, 72:1338, 1977.

197. Yardley, J.H., Bayless, T.M., and Diamond, M.B. Cancer in ulcerative colitis. Gastroenterology, 76:221, 1979.

198. ———— and Donowitz, M. Colo-rectal biopsy in inflammatory bowel disease. In Yardley, J.H. and Morson, B.C. (eds.), The Gastrointestinal Tract. Baltimore, Williams & Wilkins, 1977, pp. 50–94.

199. Young, S.J., Alpers, D.H., Norland, C.C., and Woodruff, R.A., Jr. Psychiatric illness and the irritable bowel syndrome: practical implications for the primary physician. Gastroenterology, 70:162, 1976.

Malabsorption

200. Barilla, D.E., Notz, C., Kennedy, D., and Pak, C.Y. Renal oxalate excretion following oral oxalate loads in patients with ileal disease and with renal and absorptive hypercalcurias: effect of calcium and magnesium. Am. J. Med., 64:579, 1978.

201. Bayless, T.M., Rothfeld, B., Massa, C., Wise, L., Paige, D., and Bedine, M.S. Lactose and milk intolerance: clinical implications. N. Engl. J. Med., 292:1156, 1975.

202. ————, Wheby, M.S., and Swanson, V.L. Tropical sprue in Puerto Rico. Am. J. Clin. Nutr., 21:1030, 1968.

203. ————, Yardley, J.H., and Hendrix, T.R. Adult celiac disease: treatment with a gluten-free diet. Arch. Intern. Med., 111:83, 1963.

204. Brow, J.R., Parker, F., Weinstein, W.M., and Rubin, C.E. The small intestinal mucosa in dermatitis herpetiformis. Gastroenterology, 60:355, 1971.

205. DiMagno, E.P., Go, W.L.W., and Summerskill, W.H.J. Relation between pancreatic enzyme outputs and malabsorption in severe pancreatic insufficiency. N. Engl. J. Med., 288:813, 1973.

206. Dobbins, J.W. and Binder, H.J. Importance of the colon in enteric hyperoxaluria. N. Engl. J. Med., 296:298, 1977.

207. Gardner, J.D., Brown, M.S., and Laster, L. The columnar epithelial cell of the small intestine: digestion and transport. N. Engl. J. Med., 283:1196, 1970.

208. Gorbach, S.L. and Tabaqchali, S. Bacteria, bile and small bowel. Gut, 10:963, 1969.

209. Gray, G.M. Carbohydrate digestion and absorption. Gastroenterology, 58:96, 1970.

210. ———— and Cooper, H.L. Protein digestion and absorption. Gastroenterology, 61:535, 1971.

211. ————, Conklin, K.A., and Toconday, R.R.W. Sucrase-1 somaltase deficiency. N. Engl. J. Med., 294:750, 1976.

212. Greenberger, N.J. and Skillman, T.G. Medium chain triglycerides. Physiologic considerations and clinical implications. N. Engl. J. Med., 280:1045, 1969.

213. Guerra, R., Wheby, M.S., and Bayless, T.M. Long-term antibiotic therapy in tropical sprue. Ann. Intern. Med., 63:619, 1965.

214. Hardison, W.G.M. and Rosenberg, I.H. Bile salt deficiency in the steatorrhea following resection of the ileum and proximal colon. N. Engl. J. Med., 277:337, 1967.

215. Hendrix, T.R. and Yardley, J.H. Whipple's disease. In Card, W.I. and Creamer, B. (eds), Modern Trends in Gastroenterology, Vol. 4. London, Butterworth, 1970, p. 229.

216. Hofmann, A.F. Role of bile acid malabsorption in pathogenesis of diarrhea and steatorrhea in patients with ileal resection. I. Response to cholestyramine or replacement of dietary long chain triglyceride by medium chain triglyceride. Gastroenterology, 62:918, 1972.

217. ———— and Small, D.M. Detergent properties of bile salts: correlation with physiologic function. Ann. Rev. Med., 18:333, 1967.

218. Jefferies, G.H., Chapman, A., and Sleisenger, M.H. Low-fat diet in intestinal lymphangiectasia: its effect on albumin metabolism. N. Engl. J. Med., 270:761, 1964.

219. Kahn, I.J., Jeffries, G.H., and Sleisenger, M.H. Malabsorption in intestinal scleroderma. Correction by antibiotics. N. Engl. J. Med., 274:1339, 1966.

220. Klipstein, F.A. and Falaiye, J.M. Tropical sprue in expatriates from the tropics living in continental United States. Medicine, 48:475, 1969.

221. Knox, D.L., Bayless, T.M., and Pittman, F.E. Neurologic disease in patients with untreated Whipple's disease. Medicine, 55:467, 1976.

222. Krone, D.L., Theodor, E., Sleisenger, M.H., and Jeffries, G.H. Studies on the pathogenesis of malabsorption. Lipid hydrolysis and micelle formation in the intestinal lumen. Medicine, 47:89, 1968.

223. Lindenbaum, J. Tropical enteropathy. Gastroenterology, 64:637, 1973.

224. Luk, G.D. and Hendrix, T.R. Microscopic examination of stool as a screening test for steatorrhea. Gastroenterology, 76:1189, 1979.

225. Metz, G., Jenkins, D.J.A., Peters, T.J., Senkins, D.J.A., Newman, A., and Blendis, L.M. Breath hydrogen as a diagnostic method for hypolactasia. Lancet, 1:1155, 1975.

226. Maizel, H., Ruffin, J.M., and Dobbins, W.O., III. Whipple's disease: a review of 19 patients from one hospital and a review of the literature since 1950. Medicine, 49:175, 1970.

227. Marin, G.A., Clark, M.L., and Senior, J.R. Studies of malabsorption occurring in patients with Laennec's cirrhosis. Gastroenterology, 56:727, 1969.

228. Newcomer, A.D., Hofmann, A.F., DiMagno, E.P., Thomas, P.J., and Carlson, G.L. Triolein breath test. A

sensitive and specific test for fat malabsorption. Gastroenterology, 76:6, 1979.

229. Pena, A.S., Mann, D.L., Hague, J.A., Heck, J.A., Van Leeuwen, H.A., van Rood, J.J., and Strober, W. Genetic basis of glutensensitive enteropathy. Gastroenterology, 75:236, 1978.

230. Regan, P.T., Malagelada, J.R., DiMagno, E.P., Glanzman, S.L., and Go, V.L. Comparative effects of antacids, cimetidine, and enteric coating on the therapeutic response to oral enzymes in severe pancreatic insufficiency. N. Engl. J. Med., 297:854, 1977.

231. Russell, R.I. and Lee, F.D. Tests of small intestinal function: digestion, absorption, secretion. Clin. Gastroenterol., 7:277, 1978.

232. Sherr, H.P., Sasaki, Y., Newman, A., Banwell, J.G., Wagner, H.N., Jr., and Hendrix, T.R. Detection of bacterial deconjugation of bile salts by a convenient breath analysis technique. N. Engl. J. Med., 285:656, 1971.

233. Trier, J.S. Diagnostic value of peroral biopsy of the proximal small intestine. N. Engl. J. Med., 285:1470, 1971.

234. ———, Falchuck, Z.M., Carey, M.C., and Schreiber, D.S. Celiac sprue and refractory sprue. Gastroenterology, 75:307, 1978.

235. Tully, T.E. and Feinberg, S.B. A roentgenographic classification of diffuse diseases of the small intestine presenting with malabsorption. Am. J. Roentgen., 121:283, 1974.

236. Waldmann, T.A. Protein-losing enteropathy. Gastroenterology, 50:422, 1966.

237. Weser, E. The management of patients after small bowel resection. Gastroenterology, 71:146, 1976.

238. Wormsley, K.G. Tests of pancreatic secretion. Clin. Gastroenterol., 7:529, 1978.

239. Yardley, J.H., Bayless, T.M., Norton, J.H., and Hendrix, T.R. Celiac disease: a study of the jejunal epithelium before and after a gluten free diet. N. Engl. J. Med., 267:1173, 1962.

SECTION TEN
Diseases of the Liver
WILLIS C. MADDREY: SECTION EDITOR

INTRODUCTION

The liver is the largest organ in the body weighing some 1500 g and accounting for approximately 2 percent of normal adult body weight. Situated in the right upper quadrant of the abdomen and bordered by the diaphragm, abdominal wall, and other intra-abdominal organs, the liver is inaccessible to direct palpation except over its lower anterior surface. The many metabolic functions of the liver are facilitated by its rich blood supply, its extensive reserve capacity, and its position between the absorptive surface of the intestinal tract and the systemic circulation.

In this section, the broad range of normal and abnormal hepatic function and methods of study of liver disease will be considered (Chap. 62). The principal manifestations of liver disease—hepatic cell failure, jaundice, hepatomegaly, portal hypertension with bleeding esophageal varices, ascites, and hepatic encephalopathy—are discussed in Chapters 63 and 64. Thereafter the major categories of hepatic disease are presented: circulatory and focal liver disease (Chap. 65); acute hepatocellular disease (Chap. 66); and chronic liver disease (Chap. 67).

CHAPTER 62

Normal and Abnormal Hepatic Physiology, Liver Function Tests, and Classification of Diseases of the Liver
WILLIS C. MADDREY

NORMAL HEPATIC PHYSIOLOGY AND ITS INVESTIGATION

In normal man, the liver receives approximately 1500 ml blood per minute. This rich blood supply is consistent with the central role of the organ in metabolism. Two-thirds of the blood flow to the liver is via the portal vein and the remainder by way of the hepatic artery. The portal vein is a unique conduit linking the capillary bed of the splanchnic system to that of the hepatic sinusoids. Arterial blood flow to the splanchnic system transports the products of absorption from the gut to the liver by the portal vein. Blood in the portal vein normally has a slightly higher pressure and increased oxygen content than that found in systemic veins. Once in the hepatic sinusoids, the portal blood is mixed with hepatic arterial blood and exposed to the extensive highly permeable sinusoidal surfaces of the hepatic cells. After traversing the sinusoids, blood leaves the liver by the hepatic veins.

In addition to an abundant blood supply, each liver cell has access to an excretory system through small bile canaliculi. Bile, which is the principal hepatic secretory product, is produced at a rate of 1000 to 1500 ml per day.

Table 62–1 enumerates several of the functions of the normal liver and their derangements in disease. Carbohydrate, protein, and lipid metabolism are all intimately dependent upon proper hepatic function. The maintenance of serum glucose concentration either from breakdown of glycogen stores or gluconeogenesis is a vital hepatic anabolic function. The normal liver contains 5 to 7 percent glycogen by weight. Hypoglycemia may be seen in severe acute liver damage as a result of impaired gluconeogenesis and decreased glycogen reserves.

Both body growth and regulation of intravascular volume are dependent on hepatic synthesis of albumin. Certain proteins participating in the coagulation process (Factors II, V, VII, IX, and X) are manufactured by the liver and reduced synthesis is indicated by a prolongation of the prothrombin time and a bleeding tendency.[9] Amino acid metabolism by the liver is important in protein synthesis and in the conversion of amino acids to carbohydrates and lipids.

TABLE 62–1

Selected Normal Functions of the Liver and Clinical Manifestations in Disease

Function	Clinical Manifestations in Liver Disease
I. Metabolic	
A. Anabolic	
1. Maintenance of serum glucose	Hypoglycemia
a. Glycogenolysis	
b. Gluconeogenesis	
2. Synthesis of proteins	
a. Albumin synthesis	Hypoalbuminemia ($\downarrow$ oncotic pressure)
	Retarded body growth
b. Synthesis of coagulation proteins (II, V, VII, IX, and X)	Bleeding diathesis
c. Manufacture of haptoglobin, fibrinogen, ceruloplasmin, etc.	
3. Lipid metabolism	
a. Uptake of plasma free fatty acids and conversion to triglycerides	Fatty liver (multifactorial)
b. Lipoprotein synthesis and release	Hypercholesterolemia in obstructive jaundice
c. Cholesterol synthesis and production of lecithin cholesterol acyl transferase (LCAT)	$\downarrow$ Cholesterol esters in hepatocellular disease
d. Synthesis of bile salts	Steatorrhea—malabsorption syndrome ($\downarrow$ bile salts in gut)
	Pruritus ($\uparrow$ bile salts in serum)
B. Catabolic	
1. Conjugation, solubilization, and deamination of drugs	Acute liver injury—generally prolonged duration of drug action
	Chronic administration of certain drugs (e.g., phenobarbital) leads to induction of drug metabolizing enzymes and $\uparrow$ clearance
2. Conjugation and excretion of bilirubin	Jaundice
3. Conversion of ammonia to urea	$\uparrow$ Blood ammonia; $\downarrow$ Urea
4. Steroid metabolism	
Decreased degradation of aldosterone	Hyperaldosteronism
5. Processing of antigens (bacterial, dietary) absorbed from the gut	Hyperglobulinemia
II. Storage Activities	
A. Fat-soluble vitamins (D, A, and K)	D deficit—osteomalacia
	A deficit—night blindness
	K deficit—coagulation defect
B. Vitamin B$_{12}$	Decreased B$_{12}$ reserve
C. Metals	
1. Iron (Fe^{++})	Increased storage in hemochromatosis and hemosiderosis
2. Copper (Cu^{++})	Increased hepatic Cu^{++}—Wilson's disease; primary biliary cirrhosis
III. Reticuloendothelial Function	
Phagocytosis	Abnormal hepatic scan (^{99}Tc)
IV. Maintenance of Plasma Volume and Electrolyte Concentrations	
A. Water homeostasis	Decreased renal free water clearance
B. Sodium excretion	Increased sodium reabsorption
C. Plasma volume	Increased in chronic liver disease with portal hypertension

The conversion of ammonia to urea occurs in the liver (Krebs-Henseleit Cycle), and excess ammonia and other nitrogenous products in the blood are associated with the development of hepatic encephalopathy. Amino acid utilization is also decreased in severe liver disease and the concentrations of many amino acids are altered in both the blood and cerebrospinal fluid.

The liver contains lipids in many forms including cholesterol, free fatty acids, triglycerides, and phospholipids. It participates broadly in lipid metabolism by converting free fatty acids to triglycerides, manufacturing cholesterol and the enzyme LCAT (lecithin cholesterol acyl transferase) which esterifies cholesterol in the bloodstream, producing bile salts, and synthesizing lipoproteins. Abnormalities at any of these steps may lead to the accumulation of fat in the liver. Abnormal lipid metabolism as evidenced by fatty liver is an important manifestation of liver disease produced by ethanol, and other toxic agents.

The catabolic functions of the liver are of equal importance in hepatic metabolism. The liver is an important site for detoxification of drugs and hormones. The decreased conversion of aldosterone to its tetrahydro derivative is associated with an increased distal renal tubular reabsorption of sodium (hyperaldosteronism).

The role of the liver in the metabolism of drugs is complex and variable. The liver conjugates many water-insoluble drugs to water-soluble compounds which can then be excreted into bile or urine. Other metabolic steps include drug inactivation by oxidation, reduction, and hydroxylation. A prolongation of drug action is observed in patients with acute liver cell injury (e.g., viral hepatitis). Many drugs (e.g., phenobarbital), however, induce a proliferation of the smooth endoplasmic reticulum and its drug metabolizing enzymes and thereby increase their own rate of metabolism as well as that of other drugs.

The liver serves as a storage depot for the fat-soluble vitamins (A, D, and K), and in chronic liver diseases, especially those associated with cholestasis, deficiency syndromes of these vitamins may develop. The absorption of fat-soluble vitamins is dependent on hepatobiliary function in another way in that bile salts are necessary for their intestinal absorption. A decrease in vitamin K absorption with its concomitant bleeding tendency is the most frequent and clinically important vitamin deficiency encountered.

The reticuloendothelial cells (Kupffer cells) lining the hepatic sinusoids have an important phagocytic role. Abnormal reticuloendothelial function is detected by hepatic scintiscanning with ^{99}Tc (technetium).

Hepatic Regeneration[5]

Among the most important characteristics of liver tissue is its ability to regenerate. When liver cells are damaged by toxins, by interference with blood supply, or by obstruction to biliary flow, the remaining cells rapidly regenerate. The exact stimulus to regeneration is unknown, but several studies suggest a humoral agent is in part responsible. In the rat, surgical removal of two-thirds of the functioning liver is followed by nearly complete restoration in a matter of days. Similar regeneration occurs in humans subjected to partial hepatectomy following trauma or in an attempt to eradicate tumor. When only parenchymal cells are damaged (as in viral hepatitis), restoration of normal architecture can be obtained, but when the major blood vessels and bile duct scaffold of the liver are damaged complete restoration is not possible. In this circumstance the reticulin fibers coalesce, active fibrogenesis is promoted, and scar tissue is formed. Hypertrophy of remaining cells occurs in nonuniform fashion forming nodules of regenerating liver. The regenerative nodule obtains its blood supply from vessels that encircle its periphery much like fingers around a ball. As the nodule enlarges, pressure constriction of the blood supply develops which may limit the extent of regeneration and also result in the development of portal hypertension (see Chap. 64).

The blood flow to areas of regenerating nodules is predominantly arterial and, therefore, the regenerating nodule is more vulnerable to fluctuations in arterial pressure than is normal liver and is more likely to fail in situations associated with a decrease in the arterial blood pressure as, for example, following gastrointestinal hemorrhage.

Liver Function Tests (Table 62-2)

Numerous biochemical and radiologic tests are available to study hepatic function. These tests, properly employed, are of value in the detection of hepatic disease, in evaluating the nature and extent of dysfunction, in following the progression of disease, and in assessing the effects of therapy. The spectrum of functions performed by the liver is so broad that no one test is sufficient. The proper use of the biochemical tests of liver function requires a knowledge of the specificity and sensitivity of tests designed to evaluate several functions. Of particular importance is the recognition that impairment of function in hepatic disease may be nonuniform. For example, a reduced ability to synthesize urea is a manifestation of late and very severe dysfunction, whereas the ability to take up, conjugate, and excrete sulfobromophthalein (BSP) dye is impaired with early injury. Repeated ob-

---

TABLE 62–2

Appropriate Tests for the Study of the Hepatic Circulation, Biliary Tract, and Parenchymal Disease of the Liver

I. Hepatic circulation

A. Portal circulation	Anatomic evidence of portal vein patency	Splenoportovenogram; umbilical venogram; venous phase of superior mesenteric arteriography
	Evidence of portal to systemic collaterals	Barium esophagogram Esophagoscopy Splenoportovenogram; umbilical venogram
	Pressure measurements	Wedged hepatic venous pressure (WHVP) (indirect) Percutaneous intrasplenic pulp pressure or umbilical vein pressure (direct)
B. Hepatic venous circulation	Anatomic evidence of patency and determination of pressure	Hepatic venous catheterization with measurement of the WHVP
C. Hepatic artery	Anatomic evidence of patency and distribution	Celiac arteriography

II. Biliary Tract

A. Gallbladder function	Anatomic evidence	Oral cholecystography
B. Common bile duct patency	Anatomic evidence	Intravenous cholangiography Endoscopic retrograde cholangiography Transhepatic cholangiography
	Functional evidence	Urine urobilinogen determination Serum alkaline phosphatase and 5′ nucleotidase measurement Duodenal aspiration for bile

III. Parenchymal Disease

A. Acute liver cell disease	Anatomic evidence	Liver biopsy
	Functional evidence	
	a. Synthetic ability	Serum albumin and prothrombin
	b. Ability to conjugate and excrete	Bilirubin, BSP
B. Evidence of inflammation	Functional	Aminotransferase enzymes

---

servations over a period of time and a critical interpretation of results for technical error are important. Clinical decisions should not rest on one unconfirmed study. In the following section selected individual tests are described. Determination of serum bilirubin and its interpretation is discussed in Chapter 63.

SAFETY OF TESTS. Discussion of liver function tests must begin with a comment concerning safety to the patient. The examination of blood, stool, and urine is of no risk to the patient. The utilization of BSP or cholangiographic dye, however, has been associated with severe reactions including anaphylaxis and death. Liver biopsy and percutaneous transhepatic cholangiography are occasionally complicated by the occurrence of intraperitoneal hemorrhage, bile peritonitis, or sepsis and, in patients with cholangitis, liver abscesses. There is a risk of septicemia associated with retrograde endoscopic cannulation of the bile ducts.

SULFOBROMOPHTHALEIN (BSP) TEST. BSP is a brominated phthalein dye which, when injected intravenously, binds mainly to albumin and is transported to the liver where it is taken up by the hepatocyte, conjugated predominantly to glutathione in the cytoplasm, and subsequently excreted into bile. Conjugation of BSP to glutathione is not obligatory for biliary secretion. The clinical BSP test most often employed involves the administration of 5 mg/kg of BSP over a 5-minute period and measurement of the percentage of dye remaining in the blood at 45 minutes. Normal subjects retain less than 7 percent of the injected dose of the dye at 45 minutes. The BSP test is a sensitive indicator of hepatic dysfunction and is of particular value in detecting hepatic dysfunction when other studies of liver function are equivocal. The test is not without risk. The dye is very irritating if extravasated into tissues and reactions including anaphylaxis have been reported. The test is of no use in the presence of jaundice. Falsely high values for BSP are obtained in obese persons and in elderly normal individuals. The uptake and excretion of the dye is interfered with by the presence of certain organic anions including some gallbladder dyes. Falsely low BSP retention values may be found in patients with hypoalbuminemia because of decreased BSP binding to the protein and more rapid clearance of unbound dye.

AMINOTRANSFERASE ENZYMES. The serum oxaloacetic acid (SGOT) and glutamic pyruvate (SGPT) aminotransferases are enzymes present in high concentrations in liver cells and released into the bloodstream following cell injury. Cell death is not required for enzyme release, and elevated levels may result from altered cell permeability. Serum aminotransferase determinations are most helpful in the diagnosis of early or nonicteric hepatitis and in serially following the course of acute liver injury. A prolonged elevation of the aminotransferases may be the first indication of nonresolving or chronic hepatitis. A precipitous drop in the level of aminotransferase enzymes in a patient who is clinically deteriorating may be indicative of such severe necrosis of liver cells that no more enzymes are available to be released. In patients with obstructive jaundice, the aminotransferase levels are rarely greater than 10 times normal. SGOT is also present in high concentration in heart and skeletal muscle, but differential diagnosis of hepatitis and myocardial disease is seldom difficult. SGPT is more specific for the liver. The gamma glutamyl transpeptidase (GGTP) is an additional highly sensitive index of hepatocellular damage. Other enzymes such as lactic dehydrogenase (LDH) and xanthine oxidase offer no advantage over the aminotransferases in diagnosis.

SERUM PROTEINS. The liver produces the majority of serum proteins including all the albumin, fibrinogen, certain coagulation factors (II, V, VII, IX, and X), and most of the alpha and beta globulins. Gamma globulins are produced by the cells of the reticuloendothelial system lining the hepatic sinusoids, in the spleen, and in the bone marrow.

SERUM ALBUMIN.[10] Albumin is quantitatively the most important liver-produced protein. The serum albumin concentration is an important regulator of body growth and intravascular volume. The normal albumin level of 3.5 to 5.0 g/dl is maintained by hepatic synthesis in the endoplasmic recticulum of approximately 120 to 200 mg/kg per day. The half-life of serum albumin is 14 to 20 days. The serum albumin is usually decreased in patients with chronic liver disease. In patients with cirrhosis and portal hypertension, at least part of the decreased serum level is explained by an expansion of the plasma volume.

SERUM GLOBULIN. The serum globulins are made in the reticuloendothelial system and are elevated in many liver diseases associated with continuing cell necrosis. In diffuse hepatocellular diseases such as cirrhosis or chronic active hepatitis, the serum albumin is depressed and the globulin elevated. Occasionally in chronic active hepatitis, levels of serum globulin over 5 g/dl such as are encountered in sarcoidosis, myeloma, and kala-azar are found. The absolute levels of albumin and globulin are of importance in following the course of hepatic diseases. The albumin/globulin ratio is of no value. Little additional specificity in diagnosis is obtained by determining the levels of alpha and beta globulins.

IMMUNOGLOBULINS. Many chronic liver disorders have associated abnormalities in serum immunoglobulins. While not often of specific use in differential diagnosis, an elevation in IgG is characteristic of chronic active hepatitis; elevated IgA of alcoholic liver disease; and elevated IgM of primary biliary cirrhosis.

SERUM PROTHROMBIN TIME. The one-stage prothrombin time is a measure of multiple clotting factors of which factors II, V, VII, IX, and X are proteins manufactured by the liver.[9] A persistently long prothrombin time after the parenteral administration of vitamin K is usually indicative of liver cell disease. Prolongation of the prothrombin time to more than twice normal is an ominous prognostic sign in severe hepatic necrosis and is correlated with a fatal outcome.

SERUM ALKALINE PHOSPHATASE.[6] The serum alkaline phosphatases (SAP) are a group of isoenzymes manufactured by bone, liver, intestine, and placenta. Forty to 75 percent of the normal SAP is derived from bone. Although isoenzyme analysis is available, it is not routinely employed in clinical practice. The SAP level is most frequently elevated in diseases associated with obstruction of the bile ducts or bone destruction and remodeling. Obstruction to bile flow causes an increased synthesis of alkaline phosphatase within the liver with subsequent regurgitation of the newly formed enzyme into the serum. The SAP is a sensitive test for determining bile duct obstruction, and normal SAP activity is unusual in obstructive biliary disease. An elevation of the SAP of hepatic origin and a normal or near normal serum bilirubin is characteristic in granulomatous diseases of the liver such as sarcoidosis or tuberculosis, and is often present in metastatic tumors, and amyloidosis.

SERUM 5′ NUCLEOTIDASE. 5′ nucleotidase is an enzyme that catalyzes the hydrolysis of nucleotides and is found predominantly in the bile canaliculi and sinusoidal membranes of the liver. The enzyme is also present in the placenta but not in bone. In liver diseases, 5' nucleotidase has a similar spectrum as does the serum alkaline phosphatase.[7] The test is most useful in determining whether an elevated SAP is of bone or liver origin.

OTHER BIOCHEMICAL TESTS. Serum iron and iron binding capacity are necessary in the diagnosis of hemochromatosis and hemosiderosis. Serum iron levels are often elevated in acute viral hepatitis. Blood ammonia levels are useful in separating hepatic encephalopathy from other causes of coma and shall be discussed in detail in Chapter 63.

RADIOLOGIC, ENDOSCOPIC, AND LAPAROSCOPIC PROCEDURES.[12] Barium studies of the upper gastrointestinal tract are useful in the demonstration of esophageal varices, and may provide the first indication of portal hypertension in a patient with chronic liver disease.

Esophagogastric endoscopy in patients with liver disease often provides the earliest evidence of the presence and extent of varices in the lower esophagus and stomach. Endoscopic procedures also allow assessment of other gastrointestinal lesions which often are found in patients with liver disease—peptic ulcer, gastritis, and Mallory-Weiss tears.

The development of the technique for endoscopic retrograde cannulation of the ampulla of Vater is useful in evaluation of the pancreatic and common bile ducts. Endoscopic cannulation has the advantage of allowing determination of bile duct patency without making surgery mandatory.[11] Direct visualization of the surface of the liver and guided biopsy of focal lesions is available with laparoscopy allowing the additional opportunity to examine the peritoneal surface for tumor implants or tuberculosis and an assessment of the other intra-abdominal organs (e.g., gallbladder).

Percutaneous transhepatic cholangiography is a worthwhile adjunct in the differential diagnosis of extra- versus intrahepatic obstructive jaundice. A long thin needle is inserted into the liver and slowly withdrawn until bile is aspirated. Cholangiographic dye is then injected outlining the biliary system. Bile ducts which have become dilated as a consequence of obstruction are easily punctured. In the presence of intrahepatic obstruction, the bile ducts are small and less easily entered. The procedure should be performed in conjunction with a surgeon and an immediate operation may be required to decompress the biliary tract.

Splenoportography with determination of the splenic pulp pressure is useful in documenting the presence of portal hypertension and in demonstrating patency of the portal vein. The procedure is of low risk when performed by trained personnel in a cooperative patient with no bleeding tendency. Umbilical vein catheterization (through the vestigial umbilical vein) also allows determination of portal pressure and patency of the portal venous system.

Oral cholecystography and cholangiography are employed in the evaluation of a patient with recurrent jaundice but seldom are successful if the serum bilirubin is greater than 2 mg/dl.

ANGIOGRAPHY. Selective angiography of the celiac, hepatic, and superior mesenteric arteries is useful in the evaluation of mass lesions within the liver; in defining vascular lesions such as hemangiomas; and in allowing direct administration of pharmacologic agents. Pitressin given intravenously or via the superior mesenteric artery is used in the management of bleeding esophageal varices. The direct administration of antitumor agents is under investigation.

RADIOISOTOPE LIVER SCANS. Several gamma emitting radioisotopes selectively taken up by the liver are available and are employed in determining hepatic size, configuration, or the presence of filling defects. Colloidal gold (^{198}Au) and ^{99}Tc are both taken up by the reticuloendothelial (Kupffer) cells. The principal role for hepatic scans is in the detection of hepatic tumors and abscesses. Hepatic scans are not accurate in determining nodules of less than 3 cm and false positive scans for filling defects are frequently found in the presence of alcoholic liver disease and cirrhosis. ^{131}I Rose Bengal is taken up by the liver cells with subsequent excretion into the bile. In patients with complete obstruction of the extrahepatic biliary system, no Rose Bengal appears in the intestine in 24 hours making the test of some diagnostic importance. ^{67}Gallium is a radionuclide which is concentrated in liver abscesses and hepatocellular carcinomas.

NEEDLE BIOPSY OF THE LIVER.[8] Needle biopsy of the liver is a safe, simple procedure of considerable importance in the diagnosis of liver disease. In addition to providing material for light microscopy, specimens for electron microscopy, tissue culture, and heavy metal analysis may be obtained. The liver biopsy is particularly useful in the differential diagnosis of hepatomegaly and jaundice, in the search for hepatic neoplasms, in the evaluation of prolonged fevers, and in evaluating the course and effect of therapy in liver disease (Table 62–3). The procedure is contraindicated in an uncooperative or stuporous patient, in the presence of a bleeding tendency, or in the absence of available blood (Table 62–4). When performed by experienced physicians, less than one biopsy in 500 should be associated with a serious complication.

―TABLE 62-3―
Clinical Usefulness of Liver Biopsy

1. Differential diagnosis
   a. Hepatomegaly
   b. Jaundice
   c. Abnormal liver function tests
2. Detection of intrahepatic neoplasm
3. Recognition of systemic inflammatory or granulomatous disorders
   a. Tuberculosis
   b. Sarcoidosis
   c. Brucellosis
   d. Evaluation of prolonged fever of unknown origin
4. Evaluation of effectiveness of therapy
   a. Removal of copper (Wilson's disease) or iron (hemochromatosis)
   b. Effect of corticosteroid or immunosuppressive therapy in management of liver disease

―TABLE 62-4―
Liver Biopsy

Contraindications

Absolute

1. Uncooperative patient
2. Bleeding tendency
   a. Prothrombin time <50 percent
   b. Bleeding time prolonged
3. Unavailability of blood transfusion support

Relative

1. Obstruction to the extrahepatic biliary system
2. Infections in right lower lobe of the lung
3. Ascites

Complications

Minor

1. Pain at site of biopsy needle entry
2. Epigastric discomfort
3. Vasovagal reaction

Serious

1. Intraperitoneal hemorrhage—usually within 24 hours—rare
2. Bile peritonitis—rare

―TABLE 62-5―
Classification of Liver Diseases

I. Disorders of Circulation
   A. Passive congestion from heart failure and cardiac cirrhosis
   B. Hepatic vein thrombosis (Budd-Chiari syndrome)
   C. Portal vein thrombosis
   D. Disorders of the hepatic artery (e.g., polyarteritis nodosa, hepatic artery aneurysms)

II. Disorders Secondary to Biliary Obstruction
   A. Extrahepatic biliary obstruction
      1. Tumors of the bile duct, gallbladder, pancreas, ampulla of Vater, duodenum
      2. Choledocholithiasis
      3. Bile duct strictures, diverticulae, etc.
      4. Sclerosing cholangitis
   B. Intrahepatic biliary obstruction
      1. Intrahepatic bile duct stone or tumor
      2. Cholangitis
      3. Intrahepatic cholestasis (e.g., drugs)
      4. Primary biliary cirrhosis

III. Parenchymal Disorders
   A. Focal liver disease
      1. Abscess (pyogenic, amebic); other suppurative processes (e.g., actinomycosis)
      2. Neoplasms (primary and secondary)
      3. Cysts (e.g., echinococcal, congenital), gummas
      4. Granulomas (sarcoidosis, tuberculosis, berylliosis, histoplasmosis, etc.)
   B. Diffuse liver disorders
      1. Inborn errors of bilirubin metabolism
         a. Gilbert syndrome
         b. Dubin-Johnson and Rotor syndromes
      2. Hepatitis
         a. Viral hepatitis (A; B; non-A, non-B)
         b. Leptospirosis
         c. Drug-induced hepatitis
         d. Chronic active hepatitis
      3. Cirrhosis
         a. Portal (Laennec's)
         b. Postnecrotic
         c. Hemochromatosis
         d. Wilson's disease
         e. Primary biliary cirrhosis
         f. Alpha$_1$-antitrypsin deficiency
      4. Infiltrative diseases
         a. Fatty liver
         b. Amyloidosis, Gaucher's disease, Neimann-Pick disease
         c. Leukemia, lymphoma

Use of Liver Function Tests

All patients with definite or suspected liver abnormalities should have the following tests performed:

1. Serum bilirubin—total and direct reacting fractions
2. Serum aminotransferase—SGOT and/or SGPT
3. Serum alkaline phosphatase
4. Total serum protein with determination of albumin and globulin
5. Prothrombin time
6. Urine for bilirubin

A BSP test is useful in nonjaundiced patients in whom equivocal results are obtained from the initial studies. In patients with an isolated elevation of alkaline phosphatase, a 5′ nucleotidase level may provide added specificity that the rise is associated with disease of the biliary tract. The urine test for urobilinogen is important in deeply jaundiced patients, with the persistent absence of urinary urobilinogen often indicative of bile duct obstruction. After the initial clinical and laboratory assessment of liver function, liver biopsy is the single most useful test for differential diagnosis. Percutaneous transhepatic cholangiography, endoscopic retrograde cholangiography, laparoscopy, and laparotomy are reserved for special instances in which the differential diagnosis of extra- versus intrahepatic biliary tract obstruction is not possible by the use of simpler and more conventional means.

CLASSIFICATION OF LIVER DISEASES (Table 62–5)

Diseases of the liver are classified most satisfactorily on the basis of etiology (often presumed) or, lacking a specific etiologic agent, on the basis of morphologic changes. Three major categories of liver disease will be considered: disorders secondary to circulatory abnormalities; disorders secondary to biliary obstruction; and disorders secondary to parenchymal liver disease.

CHAPTER 63
Principal Manifestations of Liver Disease: Jaundice and Hepatomegaly
WILLIS C. MADDREY

The more dramatic manifestations of liver disease include jaundice, ascites, bleeding from esophageal varices secondary to portal hypertension, and the mental changes of hepatic encephalopathy. Often, however, even significant liver disease may present with nonspecific constitutional symptoms such as anorexia, fatigue, weight loss, nausea or fever. In Table 63–1 several common systemic symptoms and signs are enumerated with the proposed mechanism. The general deterioration of health so often encountered in liver disease cannot usually be explained by the failure of any single hepatic cell function. Associated disease (such as carcinoma) or nutritional deficits (such as in chronic alcoholism) may be of more importance in the production of the patient's symptoms than is the liver disease itself.

JAUNDICE

Jaundice (icterus) is the clinical expression of an accumulation of bilirubin in tissues and is associated with an increase in serum bilirubin. When the serum bilirubin exceeds 2 to 4 mg/dl visible staining of tissues, especially skin, mucous membranes, and sclerae, becomes detectable. Lesser elevations of serum bilirubin are detected only by biochemical means and are designated subclinical or latent jaundice.

Bilirubin may be present in plasma and tissues in both unconjugated and conjugated forms. Unconjugated bilirubin accumulates predominantly in adipose tissue and is best seen in the subcutaneous fat of the abdomen or extremities. Conjugated bilirubin preferentially stains tissues with high elastin content such as the sclerae or mucous membranes. Jaundice is more easily detected in sunlight than in artificial light and is less apparent in edematous areas because of the low protein and bilirubin content of the edema fluid. The yellow color of jaundice must be distinguished from that due to several other chemical substances (e.g., carotene) and drugs (quinacrine, picrates) which have a similar color. Neither carotene nor quinacrine causes scleral icterus. Occasionally with prolonged jaundice particularly of the conjugated type, the patient has a greenish color reflecting the oxidation of tissue bilirubin stores to biliverdin.

METABOLISM OF BILIRUBIN[20]
Eighty to ninety percent of serum bilirubin is derived from the breakdown of aged or injured red blood cells in the reticuloendothelial system (Fig. 63–1). A small proportion (10 to 20 percent) of serum bilirubin is derived from nonerythropoietic sources such as the cy-

┌─TABLE 63-1───
Systemic Signs and Symptoms in Hepatic Disease

Manifestation	Possible Mechanisms	Differential Diagnosis
Constitutional		
Anorexia; weight loss Weakness, fatigue	Overall hepatic failure	Other systemic disease (neoplastic, cardiovascular, endocrine, etc.)
Nausea	Splanchnic congestion Ascites	
Fever	Hepatic inflammation Reduced resistance to infection	
Fetor hepaticus	Abnormal methionine metabolism	
Cardiovascular		
Hyperdynamic circulation Bounding pulses; wide pulse pressure; increased cardiac output	? Hormonal induced general vasodilatation	Beri-beri, arteriovenous fistulae, anemia, thyrotoxicosis
Increased plasma volume	Associated with portal hypertension and splanchnic congestion	
Cyanosis	Arteriovenous anastomoses (lung, liver, systemic)	Chronic obstructive pulmonary disease Chronic congestive heart failure
Clubbing	Arterial oxygen unsaturation	Chronic pulmonary or cardiac disease
Cutaneous and Endocrine		
Spider telangiectases Palmar erythema	Abnormal metabolism of estrogens and androgens	Pregnancy, rheumatoid arthritis, scleroderma
Menstrual irregularities Impotence		Chronic disease
Gynecomastia		Starvation, testicular tumors, spironolactone therapy
Hematologic		
Petechiae	Decreased platelet count often associated with leucopenia and anemia	Idiopathic thrombocytopenia, drug induced thrombocytopenia
Ecchymoses	Impaired production of coagulation proteins	

tochrome enzymes, catalases, peroxidases, or abortive preerythrocytic precursors in the bone marrow. Bilirubin is released from hemoglobin breakdown as a water insoluble unconjugated compound. Unconjugated bilirubin is rapidly and tightly bound to serum albumin to provide solubilization and transport. The unconjugated bilirubin-albumin complex is not filtered by the glomerulus. At the hepatic cell membrane, bilirubin is separated from its albumin carrier and is taken up by the cell (Fig. 63-2). The mechanisms of hepatic cell membrane dissociation of the bilirubin-albumin complex and uptake of bilirubin are poorly understood. The work of Arias and his colleagues[17] has demonstrated the presence in the

cytoplasm of the hepatic cell of two basic acceptor proteins (Y and Z) which bind and store the unconjugated bilirubin. The concentration of Y and Z in the cytoplasm may determine the rate of transfer of bilirubin and other organic anions across the hepatic cell membranes. Bilirubin is subsequently conjugated to a water-soluble diglucuronide. Bilirubin is secreted into bile predominantly as a diglucuronide. Recent studies suggest bilirubin monoglucuronide is produced in the smooth endoplasmic reticulum by the enzyme UDP-glucuronyl transferase. Bilirubin monoglucuronide is subsequently converted to diglucuronide in a subcellular fraction rich in plasma membranes. The conjugated bilirubin is then actively secreted into the bile

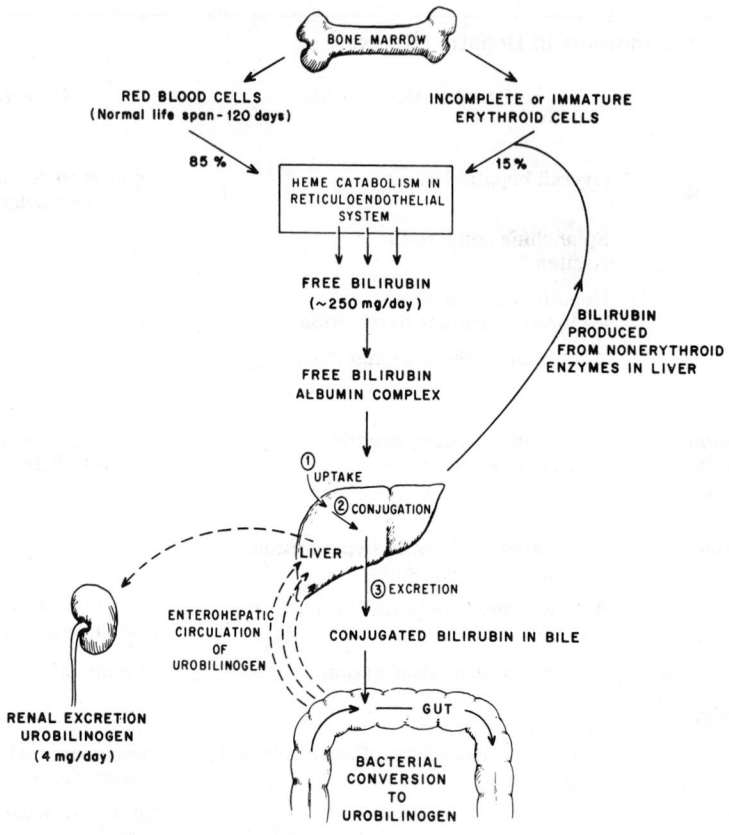

FIGURE 63–1. The metabolism of bilirubin. The breakdown of aged or injured red blood cells in the reticuloendothelial system accounts for 80 to 90 percent of bilirubin production. A small percentage of bilirubin (10 to 20 percent) is derived from immature erythroid cells in the bone marrow or from nonerythroid enzymes in the liver. Bilirubin released from hemoglobin is water insoluble (free or unconjugated bilirubin) and is transported in serum as a bilirubin-albumin complex which is not filtered at the renal glomerular membrane. At the hepatic cell membrane, the bilirubin-albumin complex is dissociated with selective uptake of the bilirubin, conjugation in the smooth endoplasmic reticulum and plasma membranes (see text) to a diglucuronide, and active secretion into bile (Fig. 63–2). Once in the intestine, the conjugated bilirubin is catabolized by bacteria to urobilinogens which are reabsorbed into an enterohepatic circulation with the majority excreted by the liver into bile. A small amount (about 4 mg per day) of urobilinogen is filtered at the glomerular membrane and excreted into the urine.

canaliculi and is transported to the duodenum. The active transport of conjugated bilirubin from the hepatic cell into the bile canaliculus is the rate-limiting step in bilirubin metabolism. If conjugated bilirubin is regurgitated into the serum, it is bound to albumin but much less tightly than is unconjugated bilirubin. Conjugated bilirubin is filtered by the glomerulus. In the gut, conjugated bilirubin is acted upon by bacteria and is catabolized first to colorless urobilinogens which are subsequently oxidized to colored urobilins. Urobilinogen is efficiently reabsorbed by an enterohepatic circulation with the majority reexcreted in the bile. Reduction of the intestinal bacteria count by an-

tibiotic treatment or ileostomy leads to excretion of conjugated bilirubin into the stool.

In normal man approximately 6.25 g of hemoglobin is released from aged red blood cells each day with the formation of some 250 mg of bilirubin. An additional 10 to 30 mg of bilirubin is produced from nonerythropoietic sources. The reserve capacity of the normal liver to handle bilirubin is considerable, and a markedly increased pigment load is required to produce hyperbilirubinemia. Approximately 50 to 250 mg urobilinogen is produced in the gut each day with some 4 mg excreted in the urine via the enterohepatic circulation.

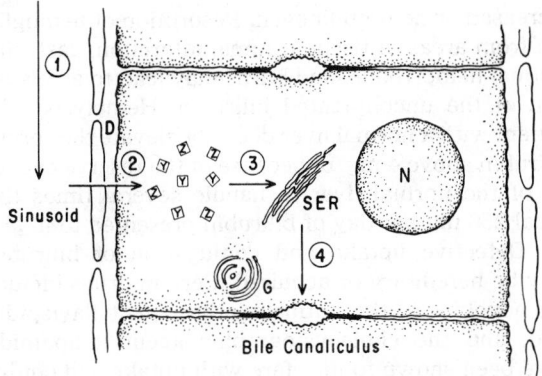

D = space of Disse ; Ⓨ Ⓩ = cytoplasmic binding proteins ;
SER = endoplasmic reticulum ; N = nucleus ; G = golgi apparatus

FIGURE 63-2. Pathway for movement of bilirubin through the liver cell. Unconjugated bilirubin tightly bound to albumin is delivered to the hepatic sinusoidal membrane where the unconjugated bilirubin is separated from the albumin and selectively taken up into the cytoplasm of the hepatic cell. Once in the cell, the free bilirubin is bound to cytoplasmic acceptor proteins (Y and Z). Subsequently the bilirubin is conjugated to a diglucuronide in the smooth endoplasmic reticulum and plasma membranes (see text). The conjugated bilirubin is then secreted by an active process into the bile canaliculus. Jaundice may occur from 1) overproduction of free bilirubin; 2) defective uptake and cell storage; 3) defective conjugation; 4) defective excretion of conjugated bilirubin. (Relate to Table 63-2.)

BLOOD, URINE, AND STOOL TESTS OF BILIRUBIN METABOLISM

Serum Bilirubin

The van den Bergh reaction is the most frequently employed test for serum bilirubin. Carotene, picrates, and quinacrine do not affect this reaction.

In the van den Bergh reaction the tetrapyrrole bilirubin molecule combines with diazotized sulfanilic acid to form chromogenic dipyrroles. The *total serum bilirubin* is determined by performing the diazo reaction in the presence of alcohol achieving reaction with both conjugated and unconjugated bilirubin compounds. Performance of the diazo reaction in an aqueous medium measures only the water soluble conjugated bilirubin and is designated the *direct reacting* fraction. The *indirect reacting* (unconjugated) bilirubin is determined by subtracting the direct reacting fraction from the total bilirubin. The separation of bilirubin into direct and indirect reacting fractions is often clinically useful but not quantitatively accurate.

Urine Bilirubin

The demonstration of bilirubinuria indicates an increase in serum conjugated bilirubin. Bilirubinuria may be easily demonstrated by vigorously shaking a tube of urine (foam test). The development and persistence of a yellow foam is a reflection of the detergent properties of bilirubin. Normal urine similarly treated forms a small white, nonpersistent foam. Bilirubinuria may also be demonstrated by use of the Ictotest or the Harrison spot test.

Urine Urobilinogen

Small amounts of urobilinogen (less than 4 mg per day) are found in the urine and may be detected by the Watson-Schwartz test. An increased urine urobilinogen is found in patients with an increased pigment load from hemolysis and in those who have had a gastrointestinal hemorrhage. The urine urobilinogen is increased in hemolytic anemias because of the increased production of bilirubin and in hepatocellular disease presumably because its normal removal from the blood by hepatic cells is impaired. The absence of urobilinogen from the urine suggests an interruption of the enterohepatic circulation of bile pigments and is found in common duct obstruction. The urine urobilinogen level may be decreased when antibiotic therapy suppresses gut flora.

Stool Pigments

Bile pigments are responsible for the normal brown color of stool. In the absence of bile, stool becomes bulky and gray both from the lack of bile pigments and the increased fat content. There is little clinical usefulness in the determination of stool urobilinogen or bilirubin.

CLASSIFICATION OF JAUNDICE

A classification of jaundice on the basis of present knowledge of bilirubin production, metabolism, and excretion is presented in Table 63-2. Investigations into bilirubin metabolism in patients with hereditary disorders which cause hyperbilirubinemia, such as the Gilbert, Crigler-Najjar, and Dubin-Johnson syndromes, with the discovery of the cytoplasmic binding proteins Y and Z, quantitation of hepatic microsomal glucuronyl transferase, and the introduction of radioactive labeling of bilirubin and its precursors have greatly expanded knowledge of the mechanisms of jaundice.

Jaundice with Predominantly Unconjugated Hyperbilirubinemia

The presence of predominantly unconjugated hyperbilirubinemia suggests either an increase in the pigment load presented to the liver (e.g., hemolysis) or a defect in the uptake and conjugation of bilirubin. Laboratory studies in such patients indicate an increased serum bilirubin with the increase in the indirect reacting fraction and no bilirubinuria. Severe

---
TABLE 63-2
Classification of Jaundice in Relation to Bilirubin Metabolism

Unconjugated Hyperbilirubinemia

I.   **Overproduction of Bilirubin**
   A. Hemolytic disorders
     1. Hereditary (e.g., sickle cell anemia; spherocytosis)
     2. Acquired (e.g., Coombs positive anemia)
     3. Liver disease (e.g., hepatitis and cirrhosis)
   B. Ineffective erythropoiesis (e.g., pernicious anemia)

II. **Defective Uptake and Storage of Bilirubin**
   A. Idiopathic unconjugated hyperbilirubinemia
     1. Hereditary—Gilbert syndrome
     2. Acquired
       a. postviral hepatitis (?)
       b. postportacaval shunt (?)
   B. Decreased availability of cytoplasmic binding proteins (Y and Z) in newborn and premature infants
   C. Drugs (e.g., flavispidic acid)

III. **Deficient Glucuronyl Transferase Activity**
   A. Deficiency
     1. Immature glucuronyl transferase system in newborn and premature infants
     2. Crigler-Najjar syndrome
     3. Gilbert syndrome
   B. Inhibition
     1. Abnormal steroids in breast milk or maternal plasma (Lucey-Driscoll type)
     2. Drugs (e.g., novobiocin)

Conjugated Hyperbilirubinemia

IV. **Defective Excretion of Conjugated Bilirubin**
   A. Hereditary
     1. Dubin-Johnson syndrome
     2. Rotor syndrome
   B. Obstructive
     1. Intrahepatic cholestasis
       a. Cirrhosis (occasionally)
       b. Hepatitis (often)
       c. Alcoholic liver disease (occasionally)
       d. Drugs (e.g., chlorpromazine and methyltestosterone)
       e. Primary biliary cirrhosis
     2. Extrahepatic obstruction of bile ducts
       a. Gallstones
       b. Carcinoma of the bile duct, pancreas, ampulla of Vater
       c. Bile duct stricture
       d. Biliary atresia
       e. Sclerosing cholangitis

---

hemolysis is of course associated with anemia but low grade compensated hemolytic anemia may only be detected by ^{51}Cr red cell life span studies. Additional evidence of hemolysis is found in an elevated reticulocyte count, decreased serum haptoglobin, and increased urine urobilinogen. Resorption of hemoglobin from areas of tissue trauma, infarction, gastrointestinal hemorrhage, and burns may lead to an elevation of the unconjugated bilirubin. Hemolysis in a patient with a normal liver does not elevate the serum bilirubin above 4 mg/dl because of the reserve capacity of the normal liver to handle several times the usual 250 mg per day of bilirubin presented to it.

Defective uptake and conjugation of bilirubin may be hereditary or acquired. Certain drugs including novobiocin, the antihelminthic agent flavispidic acid, and the cholecystographic agent iodipamide have been shown to interfere with uptake and conjugation. In the unconjugated hyperbilirubinemia characteristic of newborn and premature infants, immaturity of both the glucuronyl transferase conjugating system and the Y and Z cytoplasmic protein acceptors are of apparent importance as is the enterohepatic circulation of bilirubin deconjugated in the newborn intestinal tract by β-glucuronidase. The unconjugated hyperbilirubinemia found in infants of some nursing mothers may be related to the presence in breast milk of a factor which inhibits glucuronyl transferase activity. The factor or factors are yet to be identified but may be abnormal steroid products or fatty acids. Unconjugated hyperbilirubinemia in some neonates has been attributed to a factor in maternal serum (presumably a steroid hormone) during the last trimester of pregnancy which inhibits conjugation (Lucey-Driscoll type).

IDIOPATHIC UNCONJUGATED HYPERBILIRUBINEMIA (GILBERT SYNDROME).   An inherited, benign unconjugated hyperbilirubinemia (Gilbert syndrome) is transmitted as an autosomal dominant. An elevation in the unconjugated bilirubin was found in 16.1 percent of parents and 27.5 percent of siblings of patients with the disorder.[19] The hyperbilirubinemia (usually less than 6 mg/dl) is mild and often first noted on routine physical examination or blood tests. The jaundice is intermittent and more pronounced in young males. The bilirubin level fluctuates and may be increased by fasting or intercurrent infection. Liver biopsy and other liver function tests are normal. The pathogenesis of the hyperbilirubinemia in Gilbert syndrome is apparently a defect in the uptake and conjugation of bilirubin and reduction in the hepatic glucuronyl transferase activity.[14] The serum bilirubin can be lowered by phenobarbital therapy administration but is unaffected by corticosteroid therapy. The condition is benign and reassurance that serious liver disease is not present is most important. Gilbert syndrome must be differentiated from the asymptomatic unconjugated hyperbilirubinemia found in a variety of disorders including alcohol-induced fatty liver, cirrhosis, cardiac failure, and following apparently uncomplicated viral hepatitis and portacaval shunt operations.[18] Underlying many of the associated conditions is a mild compensated hemolytic anemia.

CRIGLER-NAJJAR SYNDROME. The Crigler-Najjar syndrome is a rare form of severe unconjugated, nonhemolytic hyperbilirubinemia found in infants and associated with an absence of glucuronyl transferase, deposition of the unconjugated bilirubin in the basal ganglia (kernicterus), and early death. Arias has examined 16 patients with chronic unconjugated hyperbilirubinemia and their families and presents evidence for two clinically similar but genetically distinct entities.[13] Group I patients had an apparent autosomal recessive pattern of inheritance with severe hyperbilirubinemia (20 to 31 mg per dl), kernicterus, and colorless bile. These patients showed no clinical response to phenobarbital therapy and are similar to those described by Crigler and Najjar. Group II patients had a lower serum bilirubin (9.1 to 17 mg/dl), did not get kernicterus, had some bile color, and apparently have an autosomal dominant pattern of inheritance. The serum bilirubin in the Group II patients does respond to the administration of phenobarbital suggesting that there is some glucuronyl transferase present which is inducible.

Jaundice Associated with Predominantly Conjugated Hyperbilirubinemia

An elevation in the serum conjugated bilirubin and bilirubinuria is characteristic of several hereditary disorders, hepatocellular disease, and biliary obstruction (Table 63-2).

The most important clinical problems in evaluating a patient with jaundice and elevated, mixed, or predominantly conjugated bilirubin are: 1) differentiation between hepatocellular and obstructive jaundice, and 2) once having decided the jaundice is due to biliary obstruction, determining whether the obstruction is intrahepatic ("medical jaundice") or extrahepatic ("surgical jaundice").

Hepatocellular disease with jaundice is more frequently associated with malaise, anorexia, fatigue, a history of hepatitis exposure, and other signs of liver disease such as evidence of ascites and portal hypertension (Table 63-1). The patient with predominantly obstructive jaundice may feel well, have an excellent appetite, and complain only of pruritus. Liver function tests other than bilirubin are useful in the differentiation of patients (Table 63-3) with elevated aminotransferases (>10 times normal) suggesting hepatocellular disease and near normal transaminases (<10 times normal), and elevated alkaline phosphatase suggesting bile duct obstruction. Urine

urobilinogen is often elevated in hepatocellular disease and is decreased or absent in patients with bile duct obstruction.

The distinction between hepatocellular disease and biliary obstruction occasionally cannot be made with certainty even after extensive clinical and laboratory examinations. This distinction is important because of the danger of precipitating acute liver failure and death by anesthesia and surgery in a patient with hepatocellular disease.

Formerly in patients in whom the clinical distinction between jaundice due to mechanical obstruction or hepatocellular disease was difficult, a period of 2 to 6 weeks of observation was recommended. With time the diagnosis often became apparent. The development of techniques for endoscopic cannulation of the bile ducts and percutaneous transhepatic cholangiography now allows earlier more accurate differentiation (see Chap. 62).

CHRONIC IDIOPATHIC JAUNDICE (DUBIN-JOHNSON SYNDROME). The Dubin-Johnson syndrome is a chronic intermittent jaundice characterized by an increase in the serum conjugated bilirubin, bilirubinuria, and the deposition of a characteristic black or yellow-brown pigment in the hepatic cells.[15] The Dubin-Johnson syndrome is apparently inherited as an autosomal recessive. The defect in the Dubin-Johnson syndrome is in the excretion of conjugated bilirubin and certain other organic anions, including BSP and cholangiographic dyes. Bile salt excretion is unimpaired and therefore pruritus is not present. There is a diagnostic abnormality in urinary coproporphyrin excretion in the Dubin-Johnson syndrome with affected patients excreting 90 percent of their urinary coproporphyrins as coproporphyrin isomer 1 whereas in normals at least 70 percent of urinary coproporphyrin is in the isomer III form.

A seemingly identical animal model of the Dubin-Johnson syndrome has been described in mutant Corriedale sheep. The hepatic pigment is grossly visible in the liver biopsy and is an accumulation of melanin.

The Dubin-Johnson syndrome is benign with no associated liver function abnormalities and may be first diagnosed in women when estrogen-containing birth control pills or the later stages of pregnancy overtax hepatic excretory reserve and produce overt jaundice. Intercurrent infections, alcohol excess, and surgery may precipitate jaundice. An aid to diagnosis is observation of serum BSP retention at 45, 90, and 135 minutes. An initial fall to normal or near normal is found with a subsequent rise in serum BSP level so that later determinations are higher than those observed early. These observations are compatible with normal conjugation of BSP but an inability to excrete

TABLE 63–3

Laboratory Studies in Adult Patients with Jaundice

Disorder Causing Jaundice	Hematology		Urine		Stool		Liver Function Studies				
	Hct	Wbc	Bilirubin	Urobilinogen	Color	Blood	TB	DRB	SAP	SGOT	Chol
I. Overproduction (e.g., hemolytic anemia)	N or ↓	N	0	↑	N	0	↑	N	N	N	N
II. Defective uptake and storage (e.g., Gilbert syndrome)	N	N	0	N or ↓	N	0	↑	N	N	N	N
III. Hepatocellular disease, viral hepatitis (usual)	N	↓	↑	↑	N or ↓	0	↑	↑	N or ↑	↑↑	N
IV. Defective excretion of bilirubin											
A. Intrahepatic cholestasis (e.g., chlorpromazine reaction)	N	N	N or ↑	↓	N or ↓	0	↑	↑	↑	N	N or ↑
B. Extrahepatic biliary obstruction	N	N or ↑	↑	↓	↓	+/−	↑	↑	↑↑	N or ↑	↑
C. Hereditary (e.g., Dubin-Johnson syndrome)	N	N	↑	N	N	0	↑	↑	N	N	N

N = normal
↑ = increased
↑↑ = markedly elevated
↓ = decreased
Hct = hematocrit
Wbc = white blood cell count
TB = total bilirubin
DRB = direct reacting bilirubin
SAP = serum alkaline phosphatase
SGOT = serum glutamic oxaloacetic transaminase
Chol = cholesterol

the conjugated dye into the bile. In most patients, neither oral nor intravenous cholangiography visualizes the gallbladder. The Rotor syndrome is a similar disorder to the Dubin-Johnson syndrome, the major difference being absence of hepatic pigment in the Rotor syndrome. No treatment is necessary in either condition.

EXTRAHEPATIC BILIARY OBSTRUCTION. Gallstones, bile duct strictures, and tumors are the most frequent causes of extrahepatic bile duct obstruction. Rarer causes include choledochal cysts, sclerosing cholangitis, and enlarged nodes in the porta hepatis.

The characteristic clinical findings in extrahepatic (mechanical) obstruction of the bile ducts are hepatomegaly, right upper quadrant pain, presumably from stretching of the hepatic capsule, and occasionally a palpable gallbladder. Fever and chills may indicate a suppurative cholangitis. Liver biopsy is not adequate for distinguishing intra- and extrahepatic bile duct obstruction and may reveal dilated bile ducts ("bile lakes"), bile duct proliferation, and periportal cellular degeneration in either. Long-standing bile duct obstruction leads to periportal fibrosis and subsequent biliary cirrhosis. The liver biopsy is particularly useful in excluding hepatitis. The antimitochondrial antibody test is negative in extrahepatic bile duct obstruction as compared to its >90 percent positivity in primary biliary cirrhosis (Chap. 67).[68] Exploratory laparotomy may occasionally be required for diagnosis, but in most instances should be preceded by a transhepatic cholangiogram or endoscopic retrograde cannulation of the ampulla of Vater.

Once extrahepatic obstruction is surgically relieved, the liver size, serum bilirubin, and alkaline phosphatase return to normal over a period of days to weeks.

Jaundice Associated with Hepatitis and Cirrhosis

Multiple mechanisms may be responsible for jaundice in hepatitis and cirrhosis. A shortened erythrocyte survival time is present in most hepatocellular diseases. Although difficult to quantitate, both impaired uptake and conjugation of bilirubin secondary to hepatocellular disease are important. The rate-limiting step of biliary excretion is most affected by liver injury and contributes to an increase in serum conjugated bilirubin. In acute viral hepatitis both decreased uptake and excretion of BSP have been demonstrated with a more rapid return of the ability to take up and store dye than the ability to excrete.

Biliary Obstruction and Cholestasis

The obstruction to bile excretion (cholestasis) may lie: 1) in the energy-requiring processes by which conjugated bilirubin is excreted across the biliary ductular epithelium into the bile canaliculus; 2) in the small canalicular bile ducts themselves; or 3) in the major bile ducts. Clinical symptoms of cholestasis are similar regardless of the level of obstruction to flow. The results of failure of bile flow include: 1) an accumulation of conjugated bilirubin in the blood; 2) bilirubinuria; 3) an enlarged liver which is often tender; 4) elevated serum lipids with the late development of xanthomas; 5) an increase in stool bulk and fat content (steatorrhea) and a decrease in stool pigments; 6) deficiency in absorption of fat soluble vitamins leading to night blindness (vitamin A), osteomalacia (vitamin D), and prolonged prothrombin time with a bleeding tendency (vitamin K). Pruritus apparently results in part from retention of bile salts.

Anatomic changes in the hepatic cells in cholestasis are related to the duration of obstruction to bile flow. The earliest changes are degeneration of cells in the centrilobular regions with bile plugging. Electron microscopic studies reveal vacuolization of the Golgi apparatus, flattening and disappearance of biliary epithelial microvilli, and an increase in lysozomes and pericanalicular vesicles. If obstruction goes on for several weeks, necrotic cells in the periportal region are replaced by fibrous bands which may slowly progress to first a biliary and later a macronodular cirrhosis. Relief of the cholestasis within a month or six weeks is usually associated with a gradual and often complete return to normal.

Complete obstruction to bile flow leads to a gradual accumulation of bilirubin in the serum for a period of two to three weeks after which time the bilirubin level stabilizes usually between 15 and 30 mg/dl.[21] At this level urinary excretion of bilirubin and alternate pathways of bilirubin excretion (mainly renal) effect a constant level. Drugs such as chloramphenicol which are predominantly excreted in the bile may accumulate in the serum and must be used with caution.

Intrahepatic Cholestasis

Intrahepatic cholestasis occurs in certain instances of viral, alcoholic, drug-induced, and chronic liver disease. The distinction between intrahepatic cholestasis and extrahepatic obstruction is often difficult (Table 63–4). Viral hepatitis is suggested by the history of a prodromal illness with malaise, fatigue, elevated aminotransferase activity, or history of exposure to needles or to jaundiced patients. Occasionally viral hepatitis presents as a predominantly cholestatic illness. Patients with alcoholic hepatitis and cholestasis usually have other evidence of chronic alcoholism and liver disease. Drug-induced cholestasis (such as is caused by methyltestosterone or chlorpromazine) may be overlooked unless a meticulous history of drug ingestion is taken (Chap. 66). Cholestatic jaundice in the postoperative period is a problem of mixed etiology with hypotension, shock, use of vasopressors, infection, and blood transfusions all important contributors.[16]

Cholestatic jaundice may be the principal manifestation of chronic active hepatitis and postnecrotic cirrhosis. The occurrence of persistent cholestatic jaundice in a middle-aged female is often the initial presentation of primary biliary cirrhosis. Intrahepatic cholestasis occasionally occurs during pregnancy especially for susceptible females during the third trimester and apparently results from increased sensitivity to estrogenic compounds. The cholestatic jaundice of pregnancy is often reproduced by the administration of birth control pills, and a careful history of complications of pregnancy should be taken in any female developing jaundice while on oral contraceptives. The family history coupled with liver biopsy demonstration of the characteristic black pigment allows the diagnosis of Dubin-Johnson syndrome to be established.

———TABLE 63–4———
Differentiation of Intrahepatic and Extrahepatic Bile Duct Obstruction

	Intra-hepatic Cholestasis	Extra-hepatic Bile Duct Obstruction
Clinical		
1. Jaundice as an early manifestation	+	+ +
2. Fever, sweats, chills	+	+ +
3. Right upper quadrant pain	0 to +	+ +
4. Hepatomegaly	+	+ +
5. Palpable gallbladder	0	+
6. History of exposure to jaundiced patients, raw shellfish, drugs	+	0 to +
Laboratory		
1. Alkaline phosphatase		
a. Normal		
b. Elevated	0 to +	0
	+	+ +
2. SGOT		
a. <300 MIU	+	+ +
b. >300 MIU	0 to +	0 to +
3. Elevated amylase	0	+
4. Blood in stool	0	+
5. Leukocytosis	0 to +	+
Course		
Acholic stools with absent urine urobilinogen	0 to +	+

0 = unusual
+ = occasional
+ + = frequent

HEPATOMEGALY

Although the most frequent explanation for a mass in the right upper quadrant is an enlarged liver, the physician must be aware of alternative causes of masses in this region. Tumors of stomach, colon, and kidney may simulate hepatomegaly as may enlargement of the gallbladder or a pancreatic pseudocyst. The normal liver may be palpable 1 to 2 cm below the costal margin in thin persons or displaced downward in patients with chronic lung disease and a depressed diaphragm. The normal upper edge of hepatic dullness determined by percussion is at the level of the fifth rib or intercostal space. A liver scan is occasionally required to determine both the size and position of the liver.

The consistency and configuration of the en-larged liver are useful in differential diagnosis. The firm, irregular edge of cirrhosis and the gross nodularity of the liver filled with metastatic tumors are diagnostically useful. The liver in congestive heart failure often presents an ill defined and often tender edge. Hepatic tenderness may also be present in hepatic abscess or metastatic disease. A rub is occasionally heard over the liver harboring tumor nodules or an abscess, and a bruit may be encountered over a tumor or in a patient with alcoholic hepatitis.

The causes of hepatomegaly are outlined in Table 63–5. A systematic consideration of whether the organ is enlarged from congestion, infiltration, infec-

———TABLE 63–5———
Causes of Hepatomegaly

I. **Venous Congestion of the Liver**
   A. Congestive heart failure
   B. Constrictive pericarditis
   C. Tricuspid insufficiency
   D. Obstruction of the hepatic veins (Budd-Chiari syndrome) with or without obstruction of the inferior vena cava

II. **Diffuse Hepatomegaly Without Infection**
   A. Cirrhosis
   B. Hepatitis secondary to drugs or toxins
   C. Infiltrative processes
      1. Fatty liver
      2. Amyloidosis
      3. Hemochromatosis
      4. Sarcoidosis (occasionally)
      5. Metabolic defects (glycogen storage diseases)
   D. Primary biliary cirrhosis

III. **Hepatomegaly Associated with Infection**
   A. Abscess (may be localized enlargement)
      1. Amebic
      2. Pyogenic
   B. Viral hepatitis (A; B; non-A, non-B)
   C. Leptospirosis
   D. Other infections (syphilis, tuberculosis, brucellosis, actinomycosis, echinococcosis, schistosomiasis)

IV. **Obstruction to Bile Ducts**
   A. Gallstones
   B. Common bile duct stricture
   C. Tumors (pancreas, ampulla of Vater, bile ducts)
   D. External pressure (enlarged lymph nodes, pancreatitis)
   E. Sclerosing cholangitis

V. **Neoplasms**
   A. Lymphomas and leukemia
   B. Metastatic tumors
   C. Primary tumors (hepatocellular carcinomas, cholangiocarcinomas)

tion, or obstruction to the flow of bile is useful. Massive hepatomegaly (greater than 10 cm below the right costal margin) suggests: tumor (primary or secondary), fatty infiltration, congestive heart failure, or amyloidosis. Cirrhosis is an occasional cause of massive enlargement but, in the later stages of known cirrhosis, rapid enlargement of the liver suggests a complication such as hepatocellular carcinoma or hepatic vein thrombosis. Liver biopsy is particularly useful in the differential diagnosis of hepatomegaly.

CHAPTER 64

Principal Manifestations of Liver Disease: Ascites, Hepatorenal Syndrome, Portal Hypertension, and Hepatic Encephalopathy

WILLIS C. MADDREY

ASCITES

Accumulation of fluid in the peritoneal cavity (ascites) may present as an isolated clinical finding or in a setting of generalized fluid retention with edema. The most common disorders associated with ascites are chronic liver disease (especially cirrhosis), tumors, nephrosis, and congestive heart failure (Table 64–1). Tuberculous peritonitis and pancreatitis are less frequent causes. Small amounts of ascites (less than 1000 ml) often go undetected. Both a high index of suspicion and careful physical examination are necessary for diagnosis. Bulging of the flanks and shifting dullness of the abdomen when the patient turns to one side are important physical signs. Ultrasonography of the abdomen is helpful in determining the presence of ascites and determining the best site for paracentesis.

Examination of the ascitic fluid by a diagnostic paracentesis (50 ml) should be performed when ascites is initially detected. Complete fluid analysis includes determination of the specific gravity, protein content, cell count, bacteriology, cytology, and fluid amylase. On the basis of the protein concentration, ascitic fluids may be separated into two broad categories: *transudates* in which the protein content is less than 2.0 g/dl and *exudates* in which the protein concentration is greater than 2.0 g/dl. Disorders associated with inflammatory reactions such as tuberculosis, tumors, and peritonitis are most frequently exudative in nature. Liver disease as well as nephrosis are common causes of transudates. The profile of fluid analysis in commonly encountered conditions is outlined in Table 64–2.

In patients with liver disease, especially portal cirrhosis, ascites is common and represents an intraperitoneal expansion of the extracellular fluid compartment.[23] The two factors of most importance in the pathogenesis of the ascites are an elevation in the portal venous pressure and a decrease in the serum colloid osmotic pressure as evidenced by a decreased serum albumin.[22] The low serum albumin reflects both impaired protein synthesis by the liver and the dilutional effect of a marked expansion of the plasma volume. The combination of portal hypertension and low serum albumin serves to drive fluid out of the splanchnic bed into the peritoneal cavity (Starling's Law).[30] Rarely is the elevation of portal pressure alone sufficient to cause ascites. In extrahepatic obstruction of the portal vein, a disorder characterized by portal hypertension and a normal serum albumin, ascites is unusual.

Hepatic lymph production is increased in patients with chronic liver disease and may contribute to the formation of ascites. The thoracic duct is often dilated to 5 to 10 times normal size with a corresponding elevation of lymph flow.[27] Chylous ascites may result from rupture of lymphatic channels in the splanchnic bed.

Additional factors contributing to ascites in chronic liver disease include abnormalities of salt and water metabolism characterized by increased sodium reabsorption in the proximal renal tubule, decreased free water clearance, and hyperaldosteronism. Patients with liver disease and ascites usually have increased reabsorption of sodium in the proximal tubules. The factor or factors responsible for enhanced proximal sodium reabsorption has not been identified but a humoral agent is suspected. Free water clearance is markedly reduced and inappropriate release or decreased degradation of antidiuretic hormone has been suggested. Hyperaldosteronism with an increased distal reabsorption of sodium is a near constant factor in patients with chronic liver disease and ascites. An impaired metabolism of aldosterone with decreased rate of degradation is present. As a result of these complex derangements in portal pressure, plasma colloid osmotic pressure, hepatic lymph production, and abnormalities in salt and water balance,

---TABLE 64–1---
Causes of Ascites

I. **Exudative Ascites**
   A. Inflammatory diseases of the peritoneum—peritonitis
      1. Ruptured viscus with or without intra-abdominal abscess: peptic ulcer, diverticulitis, appendicitis, cholecystitis, intestinal infarction, etc.
      2. Tuberculous peritonitis
      3. "Spontaneous" bacterial peritonitis
      4. Pancreatitis
      5. Bile peritonitis (secondary to ruptured gallbladder, needle penetration of dilated bile duct, etc.)
   B. Tumors
      1. Metastatic to the liver and/or peritoneal lining
      2. Leukemia, lymphoma, myeloid metaplasia
      3. Primary hepatocellular carcinoma, and cholangiocarcinoma

II. **Lymphatic Obstruction with Chylous Ascites**
   A. Trauma to the thoracic duct in the chest
   B. Mediastinal tumors
   C. Filariasis
   D. Tuberculosis (occasionally)
   E. Cirrhosis (occasionally)

III. **Transudative Ascites**
   A. As part of generalized fluid retention with hypoalbuminemia
      1. Nephrotic syndrome
      2. Protein-losing gastroenteropathy
   B. Failure of return of blood to the right side of the heart
      1. Congestive heart failure (some)
      2. Tricuspid insufficiency (occasionally other valvular lesions)
      3. Constrictive pericarditis
   C. Blockage of the hepatic veins and/or vena cava
      1. Budd-Chiari syndrome, tumor, webs, etc.*
      2. Veno-occlusive disease
   D. Diffuse hepatic disease with portal hypertension
      1. Cirrhosis—all forms (Table 67–1)
   E. Infiltrative processes of the liver
      1. Tumors, lymphomas, myeloid metaplasia, etc.*
      2. Granulomatous diseases (occasionally sarcoidosis, schistosomiasis)
   F. Portal vein obstruction (rare)

IV. **Conditions That May Mimic Ascites**
   A. Pregnancy
   B. Ovarian cyst
   C. Pancreatic cyst
   D. Mesenteric cyst

*Ascites may have characteristics of an exudate.

---TABLE 64–2---
Laboratory Analysis of Ascitic Fluid

Examination	Result	Suggested Diagnosis
Character	Clear, straw-colored	Cirrhosis
	Thick, odoriferous, cloudy	Infection or ruptured viscus
	Milky	Ruptured lymphatics
	Fibrin clots	Inflammation
	Bloody	Tumor, tuberculosis
Total protein	<2g/dl (transudate)	Cirrhosis, nephrosis
	>2 g/dl (exudate)	Tumor, tuberculosis, and other infections
Microscopic	Up to 300 WBC/mm³ (usually <100 WBC/mm³)	Noninflammatory transudate—cirrhosis, congestive failure
	>1000 WBC/mm³	Inflammatory
	RBC (>100/mm³)	Tumor, tuberculosis (or traumatic paracentesis)
Amylase		Pancreatic ascites
Cytology	Bizarre cells, large nuclei	May be reactive mesothelial cells in chronic ascites
	Malignant cells	Tumors
Bacteriology	Bacteria including tuberculosis	Ruptured viscus, peritonitis, tuberculosis

the total extracellular volume is increased, the plasma volume is expanded, and ascites develops.

Edema commonly accompanies ascites in patients with liver disease particularly in the presence of severe hypoalbuminemia. The ascites usually precedes the appearance of edema. Pleural effusion occurs in some 5 percent of patients with ascites. The pleural effusion is usually right sided and occurs in part from the direct escape of ascites from the peritoneal cavity into the chest via anatomic defects in the diaphragm.

The appearance or worsening of ascites in a patient with known cirrhosis does not necessarily signify a deterioration in the status of the underlying liver disease. The complications of cirrhosis that in themselves may cause ascites include: 1) hepatocellular carcinoma, 2) tuberculous peritonitis, and 3) spontaneous bacterial peritonitis. Abdominal pain and increased ascites may be the initial evidence of hepatocellular carcinoma. Fever with ascites may result from the underlying liver disease but should alert the clinician to the development of tuberculous or bacterial peritonitis.[23] Diagnostic paracenteses of the ascites are useful in following such patients.

Spontaneous Bacterial Peritonitis[26]

Spontaneous bacterial peritonitis is a well-recognized often fatal complication of chronic liver disease with ascites. While bacterial infection of ascites may occur from many causes including empyema of the gallbladder, rupture of a colonic diverticulum, or perforation of a peptic ulcer, the entity most often encountered is designated as "spontaneous" in that no entry site from the gut to the peritoneal cavity is found. The bacteria causing spontaneous bacterial peritonitis are predominantly of enteric origin and may be aerobic or anaerobic. Spontaneous bacterial peritonitis may result from septicemia with gut bacteria entering the portal vein and bypassing the liver or from direct movement of gut bacteria across the edematous gut wall into the ascites. Although spontaneous bacterial peritonitis is often characterized by rapidly accumulating ascites, fever, and abdominal pain, it is important to recognize that the disorder may appear with little or no fever and none of the usual signs of peritoneal inflammation.[26] The ascitic fluid is characteristically cloudy with an increased white blood cell count ($>300/mm^3$) with predominantly polymorphonuclear cells.

Management of Ascites and the Complications of Diuretic Therapy

The recognition that ascites is a result of deranged hepatic function and portal hypertension and not a disease entity itself is prerequisite to effective management. There is little to be gained but trouble if an effort is made to clear the ascites at a time when there has been no improvement in the underlying liver disease. The initial steps in management of these patients are careful assessment of the status of the liver, bedrest, and restriction of dietary sodium (Table 64-3). Hospitalization is recommended for beginning therapy in most patients. A careful search must be made for precipitating causes of the ascites with particular reference to occult gastrointestinal hemorrhage, increased dietary sodium intake, and excess

alcohol. The aid of a professional dietitian is helpful in explaining the new and quite restrictive diet to the patient.

A diagnostic paracentesis (50 ml) is recommended to document the composition of the ascites and to exclude complicating hepatocellular carcinoma, bacterial peritonitis, or tuberculous peritonitis. Unless there are compelling reasons for removing the ascites, such as respiratory embarrassment or danger of umbilical rupture, paracenteses of larger volumes should not be performed. Hypovolemia and shock may follow large (usually >1000 ml) paracenteses. Repeated paracenteses serve to further deplete total body albumin.

Many patients with ascites respond to bed rest and salt restriction with an adequate diuresis ($\frac{1}{2}$ to $1\frac{1}{2}$ pounds per day). It has been observed that determination of the urinary sodium is an accurate predictor of these early responders with >10 mEq Na^+ per liter of urine a good prognostic sign. The studies of Shear and his associates indicate that the maximum amount of ascites that can be mobilized in 24 hours is limited to only 700 to 900 ml.[37] Edema can be mobilized faster, and a greater weight loss can be safely maintained in patients with both ascites and edema.

If after two days of observation, bed rest, and dietary sodium restriction, an adequate diuresis has not been initiated, diuretic therapy should be instituted. Table 64-3 outlines an approach to the management of ascites in which several diuretic regimens are suggested. The "mildest" regimen commensurate with a $\frac{1}{2}$ to $1\frac{1}{2}$ pounds per day weight loss should be employed. It is important throughout the course of management to reassess the dietary intake of sodium frequently. Restriction of total fluid intake to 1000 ml or less is often required especially in patients with hyponatremia. Investigation of an inadequate weight loss or even weight gain during treatment often yields evidence of surreptitious salt and water ingestion.

Complications from diuretic therapy are frequent and are commensurate with the potency of the diuretic used (see Chap. 18).[38] Combinations of large doses of diuretics (furosemide and spironolactone) must be employed with extreme care. Management of the principal complications of diuretic therapy is outlined in Table 64-3. With the advent of more powerful diuretics, the former problems of "resistant" ascites have to a large degree been replaced by problems of diuretic complications.

Infrequently employed regimens for the treatment of ascites include the use of intravenous albumin infusions to initiate a diuresis but this has the danger of precipitating bleeding from esophageal varices by overexpansion of the intravascular volume.

┌───┐
TABLE 64-3

Management of Ascites in Patients with Liver Disease

I. **Determine That the Ascites Is Secondary to the Liver Disease** (rule out tuberculosis, bacterial peritonitis, neoplasm, etc.)

II. **Direct Management To Improve the Underlying Liver Disease**

III. **General Management**
   A. Bed rest
   B. Restrict sodium content of the diet
      1. Severe ascites 400 mg Na^+/day, in hospital (1 g NaCl)
      2. Moderate ascites: 400–1000 mg Na^+/day, (1–3 g NaCl) (hospital or outpatient)
   C. Appraise improvement by daily weights
      1. Loss of ½–1½ lb./day satisfactory
      2. If no weight loss in 2 days
         a. Reassess diet closely
         b. Proceed to diuretic therapy

IV. **Diuretic Therapy (Assess Progress as in III-C-2)**
   A. Initial management
      1. Spironolactone (50 mg). If no effect in 48 hours increase dose to 100 mg
      2. Spironolactone doses may be gradually increased 50 mg every 2 days to 200 mg (or more)/day
   B. If these measures fail, reassess sodium intake again and cautiously add *one* of the following regimens:
      1. Restrict total fluid intake to 1000 ml/day or less
      2. Furosemide 40–200 mg/day
      3. Intravenous albumin (25–50 g/day)
      4. Alternative diuretics include chlorothiazide 500–1000 mg or ethacrynic acid 50–200 mg
   C. If combinations of spironolactone and furosemide do not initiate a satisfactory diuresis, one of the following may be considered:
      1. Intravenous reinfusion of ascites
      2. Peritoneojugular shunt (LeVeen Shunt)
      3. Triamterene 100–300 mg/day

V. **Complications of Diuretic Therapy**
   A. Hyponatremia
      1. Nearly always from overretention of water (total body sodium normal or increased)
         a. Record intake–output and avoid overhydration intravenously or orally
         b. Restrict fluids to 500 ml/day or less
         c. Mannitol (IV) may promote water loss (beware making hyponatremia worse if not excreted)
      2. If prolonged diarrhea, losses from fistulas or overvigorous diuresis may indicate total body sodium depletion and need for salt
   B. Hypokalemia—total body K^+ usually decreased in liver disease
      1. Spironolactone minimizes losses
      2. Supplementation of 60–150 mEq/day K^+ often required
└───┘

┌───┐
TABLE 64-3 (cont.)

   C. Hypochloremic alkalosis
      Replace with chloride in form of KCl or lysine monochloride
   D. Progressive rise of serum urea nitrogen and oliguria ("hepatorenal syndrome")
      1. Stop all diuretics
      2. Use intravenous mannitol and albumin to keep urine output >500 ml/day
      3. Monitor venous pressure, prevent overexpansion
   E. Miscellaneous complications of diuretics
      1. Drug rash
      2. Agranulocytosis
      3. Pancreatitis—rarely with thiazides
      4. Gynecomastia—from spironolactones
      5. Deafness—from ethacrynic acid or furosemide
└───┘

Reinfusion of ascitic fluid intravenously is associated with many side effects especially febrile reactions and has a limited role at best. The peritoneojugular shunt (LeVeen Shunt) is a surgical approach to the management of chronic ascites with good early results.[29] In this procedure, ascites is siphoned from the peritoneal cavity through a long silastic subcutaneous tube to the jugular vein. The device is equipped with a one-way pressure operated valve and when the intra-abdominal pressure from ascites is greater than 3 cm over the venous pressure, the valve opens and ascites flows from the peritoneal cavity to the jugular vein. The effects of the peritoneojugular shunt may be dramatic in reducing ascites. Complications of the procedure include clotting of the silastic tube with blood or debris, infection, and hypervolemia with congestive failure or bleeding from esophageal varices if the reinfusion of ascites exceeds the ability of the kidney to excrete the excess fluid. Side-to-side portacaval shunts are used occasionally for resistant ascites and may be quite effective but are followed by a high incidence of hepatic encephalopathy.

PROGRESSIVE RENAL FAILURE IN LIVER DISEASE (Hepatorenal Syndrome)[32]

Progressive renal failure with azotemia and oliguria usually associated with hyponatremia and hypotension is a frequent terminal event in patients with decompensated hepatic disease. The renal failure may follow a gastrointestinal hemorrhage, an overvigorous diuresis or paracentesis, an intercurrent infection, or may occur without an obvious precipitating cause. The pathogenesis of the renal failure is unknown. The kidneys are histologically normal and have been used successfully as donor organs in human renal transplantation. Abnormalities in the volume and distribution of the renal blood flow have been demonstrated with a marked decrease in renal cortical perfusion suggesting active intrarenal vasoconstriction. The treatment of the hepatorenal syndrome is most unsatisfactory. Plasma expansion with dextran and albumin, whole blood infusions, and vasoactive drugs have all generally failed to reverse the disorder. Treatment must be directed to underlying abnormalities, maintenance of salt and water balance, and attempts early in the course to initiate a diuresis with plasma expansion. A few patients have survived following construction of a portal-systemic shunt or insertion of the LeVeen peritoneojugular shunt.

PORTAL HYPERTENSION (Table 64-4)

The portal vein is formed by the joining of the superior mesenteric vein which drains the intestinal capillaries and the splenic vein. Portal hypertension results from anatomic or functional obstruction to blood flow in the portal venous system at any point from its origin in the splanchnic bed to its exit into the systemic circulation via the inferior vena cava. Blood in the portal vein is normally at a slightly higher pressure (5 to 10 mm Hg) and higher oxygen content than that of systemic veins. Portal hypertension is considered present when the portal pressure exceeds 15 mm Hg. Once the portal vein reaches the liver it divides into many small branches which deliver the blood to the large sinusoidal system. The hepatic artery usually arises from the celiac axis and enters the liver adjacent to the portal vein. The arterial blood supply also perfuses the hepatic sinusoids. After percolating through the sinusoids, the blood is recollected by the hepatic veins and discharged into the inferior vena cava by the hepatic veins.

Obstruction to flow may be from compression or thrombosis of the extrahepatic portal vein, inflammatory obliteration of intrahepatic, portal and hepatic vein radicles, or distortion of intrahepatic architecture by collapse, infiltrations, and regenerating nodules. Rarely the major hepatic veins are occluded (Budd-Chiari syndrome) often in conjunction with obstruction to the inferior vena cava.

An increased blood flow rate in the portal system may be of importance in producing portal hypertension in patients with ma...

TABLE 64-4
Classification of Portal Hypertension

I. Portal Hypertension Secondary to Increased Resistance to Blood Flow

　A. Prehepatic (presinusoidal)
　　1. Portal venous thrombosis
　　　a. Idiopathic
　　　b. Neonatal sepsis
　　　c. Tumor compression
　　　d. Blood dyscrasias (e.g., polycythemia vera)

　B. Hepatic
　　1. Presinusoidal
　　　a. Congenital hepatic fibrosis
　　　b. Schistosomiasis
　　　c. Sarcoidosis (rare)
　　　d. Myeloproliferative disorders (rare)
　　2. Sinusoidal and postsinusoidal*
　　　a. Cirrhosis
　　　　1) alcoholic
　　　　2) postnecrotic
　　　　3) hemochromatosis
　　　　4) biliary
　　　b. Hepatitis
　　　c. Veno-occlusive disease (VOD)

　C. Posthepatic (postsinusoidal)
　　1. Hepatic vein obstruction (Budd-Chiari syndrome)
　　2. Constrictive pericarditis
　　3. Congestive heart failure

II. Portal Hypertension Secondary to Increased Flow in the Portal Vein

　A. Arteriovenous anastomoses
　B. Increased flow: massive splenomegaly

* In patients with cytotonic liver and postsinusoidal hepatitis or cirrhosis of both ...onal patients with portal hypertension m...ent ... cirrhosis develop a port...

...d patients with other and arteriove... ...patic cirrhosis and chronic liver... ...is c... ...ently divided into hepatic sa... on the ba... of whether the obcurs before ...f ...(sinusoidal) or in Portoidal and posts... ...soidal) the hetwo ...ble 64-4). To deter...ne the classifividual patient both th... portal venous sty) and the wedged hepatic venous presmeasured. The portal pressure must be measured by: 1) direct needle puncture of the ...sly in the spleen; 2) placing a needle percu... at laparotomy; and 3) catheterization of the ...ical vein allowing pressure measurement in the ...branch of the portal vein. The WHVP is deterned by wedging an endhole catheter, usually introduced percutaneously via a femoral vein into a peripheral hepatic venule. The catheter in the wedged position presumably creates stasis in the hepatic vasculature which extends to the point of anastomotic collateral run-off at the level of the hepatic sinusoids. An elevation in WHVP suggests increased resistance to collateral flow in the hepatic sinusoid.[34]

Presinusoidal portal hypertension is characterized by an elevated portal venous pressure and a normal WHVP. Portal vein thrombosis, ... and arteriovenous fistulae in the sp... are examples of presinusoidal portal ... The contribution of increased blood flow ... venous system to presinusoidal hyp... may be considerable, especially in pati... massive splenomegaly.

An elevated portal pressure and WHVP are characteristic of sinusoidal or ... sinusoidal obstruction to portal flow and ... commonly encountered in cirrhosis. St... has demonstrated a close correlation between WH... the portal pressure measured directly with both alcoholic liver disease and ... cirrhosis. A classification of the causes ... tension based on the site of obstruction ... in Table 64-4.

The physiologic con... portal hypertension are in many instances ... decrease in the blood supply to the liver ... vein and to the shunting of products ... gin around the liver into ... systemic ... The decrease in the portal component of ... blood flow is associated with a compensa... ease in the hepatic artery component at or near normal ... to maintain total flow ... cells thereby become relatively more de... arterial blood flow for their nutrition.

The most im... ... ension are the sequences of portal hypertension in an attempt ... of a collateral circulation in ... venous systems ... portal and systemic products of int... ... the shunting of ... velopment of s... ood ves... liver, the development ... Collateral commonly ... mation of ascites. ... Systemic vein ... the portal ... portal and coronary vein of the ... val system in ... the left veins of the ... and upper ... azygos lower esophagus (esophagogastric ... the walled vessels ... by the underlying ... supported ... are a frequent site of major hemo... in... with portal hypertension. Bleeding ... gastric varices accounts for death in ... one-third of patients with cirrhosis of ... gastroesophageal varices most often re...

elevation in the portal pressure, an occasional patient may have varices from superior vena cava or azygos vein obstruction.

The diagnosis of esophagogastric varices, an important consideration in all patients with chronic liver disease, becomes of utmost importance in the management of patients with liver disease and upper gastrointestinal bleeding (Table 64-5). The clinical evidence of chronic liver disease such as spider angiomas, palmar erythema, and a history of alcoholism or hepatitis may be minimal or absent. Barium swallow examination is an easily and safely performed procedure for demonstrating esophagogastric varices but is often associated with false negative results and suffers from being an indirect examination. Esophagogastroscopy is a more accurate determinant of the presence of esophagogastric varices and may be diagnostic in identifying varices as the cause of upper gastrointestinal bleeding. Observer variation (and experience) is an important limitation of the procedure. A combined assessment of the clinical setting, barium swallow, and esophagoscopy is recommended in a search for esophagogastric varices. Splenoportovenography, umbilical portography, and the venous phase of superior mesenteric arteriography are occasionally useful in the demonstration of esophagogastric varices. Other collateral channels between the portal and systemic circulations are found in the submucosa of the rectum (internal hemorrhoids), in the anterior and posterior abdominal walls, and occasionally in such unusual sites as the vagina and in ileostomies. Bleeding of clinical importance is rare from these sites.

Abdominal collateral vessels are prominent in some patients with portal hypertension and are arranged radially from the umbilicus like the spokes of a wheel (caput medusae). Occasionally these collaterals are large and are associated with a vascular bruit (Cruveilhier-Baumgartner syndrome). Dilated abdominal vessels may also appear secondary to obstruction of either the superior or inferior vena cava, and observation of the direction of blood flow in the collaterals is of particular importance in accurate diagnosis. In superior vena cava obstruction, the flow in the collaterals is downward from the chest toward the lower half of the body with the converse true for inferior vena cava obstruction. In abdominal collaterals associated with portal hypertension, the blood flow is away from the umbilicus.

Splenomegaly is common in patients with an elevated portal venous pressure, but the size of the spleen often does not correlate with the degree of the ... hypertension. In massive splenomegaly an ... ed blood flow from the spleen has been dem-

---

TABLE 64-5

Diagnosis of Esophagogastric Varices and Variceal Bleeding in Patients with Hematemesis

Question	Evidence	Comment
Are esophagogastric varices present?	Clinical	Presumptive—none need be present to have esophagogastric varices
	Evidence of chronic liver disease (history of alcoholism, hepatitis, previous upper gastrointestinal hemorrhage) in patient with splenomegaly, ascites without edema, abdominal collateral blood vessels	
	Radiographic demonstration	
	Barium swallow	Indirect—many false negatives, better for large varices
	Splenoportography	Filling of the coronary veins from the portal or splenic vein: definite evidence; added advantage of often demonstrating entire portal system; occasionally false negative
	Umbilical portography	
	Venous phase of superior mesenteric arteriography	
	Operative portography	
	Esophagogastroscopy	Direct evidence—observer variation important
		Better for small varices than radiographic techniques
	Confirmation of portal hypertension	
	Intrasplenic pressure	
	Umbilical catheter pressure	
Are varices responsible for hematemesis in a patient with hematemesis?	Esophagoscopic visualization of bleeding	Definitive information
Varices known to be present (see above)	Cessation of bleeding following vasopressin	Of limited diagnostic value
	Cessation of bleeding following Blakemore-Sengstaken tube	Presumptive
Varices not known to be present	Known diagnosis of cirrhosis	In many patients, the bleeding is from another site (gastritis, Mallory-Weiss syndrome, peptic ulcer); alternate sites particularly prevalent in patients with alcoholic liver disease

onstrated. Thrombocytopenia and leukopenia are common accompaniments of splenomegaly (hypersplenism), but do not correlate well with the size of the spleen.

MANAGEMENT OF BLEEDING ESOPHAGOGASTRIC VARICES

Upper gastrointestinal hemorrhage in a patient with liver disease is a true medical emergency. The cirrhotic liver with its regenerating nodules is more dependent on arterial flow than is normal liver and,

therefore, more liable to undergo extensive necrosis as a result of any fall in blood pressure. Secondary effects of hemorrhage include a reduction in plasma proteins at a time when the liver is unable to adequately manufacture new protein. The resulting hypoproteinemia favors the formation of ascites. The presence of blood in the gut and the absorption of nitrogenous products promotes hepatic encephalopathy.

Once the diagnosis of bleeding from esophagogastric varices is established, a vigorous program of support and therapy must be immediately instituted[24] (Table 64–6). Ice water lavage (and the passage of time) may be sufficient to stop the bleeding. Occasionally in patients with tense ascites, therapeutic paracentesis is associated with a cessation of the bleeding presumably through a decrease in intra-abdominal and portal pressures. If ice water lavage is unsuccessful, vasopressin may be administered. There are three approaches to the use of vasopressin in the management of bleeding esophagogastric varices. A large bolus of 20 units of vasopressin may be given intravenously in 100 ml of 5 percent dextrose in water over a 5- to 10-minute period. This rapid infusion may lessen or stop the hemorrhage but has several side effects including intestinal cramps and blanching of the skin. Of more importance is constriction of the coronary arteries; both angina pectoris and myocardial infarction have been observed. Lower doses of vasopressin (0.1 to 0.4 units/minute) may be infused either intravenously or directly into a superior mesenteric artery catheter. While the latter route has the appealing advantage of directly constricting the splanchnic circulation, its superiority over the intravenous route is not established.

TABLE 64–6
Management of Bleeding Esophageal Varices

A. Establish diagnosis

B. Supportive measures
1. Blood transfusion—preferably fresh blood
2. Replace vitamin deficiencies—especially vitamin K
3. Prevent hepatic coma
    a.   Clean gastrointestinal tract with magnesium citrate
    b.   Neomycin 4–6 g/day or lactulose
4. Correct electrolyte deficiencies—especially hypokalemia
5. Antacids for esophagitis

C. Measures to stop bleeding
1. Gastric ice water lavage
2. Paracentesis if tense ascites present
3. Then if bleeding persists, vasopressin 20 units in 100 ml and 5 percent dextrose in water intravenously over 20–30 minutes *or* vasopressin may be infused directly into the superior mesenteric artery or peripheral vein (0.1–0.4 units/minute).
4. Then Blakemore-Sengstaken tube-endotracheal intubation may be required
    a.   Inflate gastric balloon alone first
    b.   Inflate esophageal balloon
5. If bleeding recurs after 24 hours of tamponade, reinflate balloons for 24 hours more
6. If bleeding persists, surgery indicated:
    a.   Transthoracic ligation of varices *or*
    b.   Emergency portacaval shunt (generally preferable)

If the bleeding persists after the use of vasopressin, the Blakemore-Sengstaken tube is inserted. This double-ballooned tube is effective in stopping hemorrhage from varices in most patients by direct tamponade of the bleeding sites. Endotracheal intubation or tracheostomy prior to the positioning of the tube is often important in preventing the frequent and serious complications of aspiration and/or airway obstruction. Once the tube is in place, the position of the gastric balloon should be verified radiographically following instillation of 10 ml of a soluble radiopaque contrast media. The gastric balloon is then inflated with approximately 200 ml of air or saline and pulled snugly against the gastroesophageal junction. The tube is held in place by 1 to 2 pounds of traction applied via a pulley system or by taping the tube to rubber bands attached to the abdomen. If bleeding persists after the gastric balloon has been inflated, the esophageal balloon is inflated in a stepwise fashion starting at 25 mm Hg until control of bleeding is obtained (up to 40 mm Hg may be required). After 24 hours of tamponade, both the esophageal and gastric balloons should be deflated and the tube left in place for an additional 24 hours before removal. Complications of the Blakemore-Sengstaken tube are to a large extent related to the length of time the balloons are inflated and include lower esophageal rupture or erosion, asphyxiation from the gastric balloon sliding up into the esophagus and pharynx compressing the airway, and the ever present dangers of aspiration.

Once hemorrhage from esophagogastric varices is stopped by ice water lavage, vasopressin, or the Blakemore-Sengstaken tube, careful attention to preventive measures is necessary to guard against rebleeding in the initial posthemorrhage period. The patient must not be overtransfused lest the expansion of intravascular volume lead to renewed bleeding from the varices. Because of the possible contribution of peptic erosion to the initiation of bleeding, antacids should be used regularly and the patient should have the head of the bed elevated on blocks. Tense ascites should be tapped. Careful attention to clotting parameters are important and vitamin K should be administered. If further transfusion is required, every effort should be made to provide freshly collected blood containing platelets and clotting factors. Diuretic therapy to decrease the plasma volume, while admirable in intent, is quite dangerous and should be used with caution. Prophylactic measures to prevent the development of hepatic encephalopathy include cleansing of the gut with cathartics and enemas and the administration of either lactulose or neomycin.

Should all these more conservative measures of stopping bleeding from esophagogastric varices fail, then emergency surgical therapy is indicated.

SURGICAL MANAGEMENT OF PORTAL HYPERTENSION[31]

There are basically two surgical approaches to the management of portal hypertension and bleeding esophagogastric varices. The first is a direct attack on the varices with transthoracic or transabdominal interruption by ligation. Although temporarily effective in the majority of patients, ligation procedures have the disadvantage of generally requiring more definitive surgery later. A more satisfactory approach to surgical management is the creation of an anatomic shunt between the hypertensive portal system and the low pressure systemic venous system. As a result of the shunt, the splanchnic bed is decongested and the portal pressure drops. Hepatic blood flow is often further diminished following portacaval shunts, and the liver becomes even more dependent on its arterial blood supply. Esophagogastric varices and abdominal collaterals gradually disappear over a period of months, the spleen shrinks, and hypersplenism may lessen. The end-to-side portacaval shunt, introduced into clinical medicine by Blakemore and Whipple in 1945, is the most widely employed shunt. In this operation, the portal vein is severed and its distal end anastomosed to the side of the inferior vena cava. Alternative construction of portacaval shunts include side-to-side, splenorenal, and mesocaval. A recently developed procedure is the distal splenorenal shunt (Warren Shunt). In this operation, the coronary vein, which connects the portal vein to the esophagogastric varices, is ligated. Blood flows from the varices via the short gastric veins to the spleen and from the spleen to the renal vein and ultimately the vena cava through a surgically created splenorenal anastomosis. This procedure may be associated with a lesser incidence of subsequent hepatic encephalopathy than other decompressive operations.

The clinical usefulness of portacaval shunts remains controversial despite extensive experience.[25,31,35] It is established that technically satisfactory shunts decrease portal pressure and prevent the recurrence of bleeding from esophageal varices. These operations find their greatest application in patients with a history of severe or repeated variceal hemorrhage.

The role of the emergency portacaval shunt in the management of acutely bleeding patients remains an area of controversy. Prophylactic shunts in patients with demonstrated cirrhosis and esophageal varices who have not had a variceal hemorrhage have not been demonstrated to prolong life.[25] The decrease in mortality from the prevention of variceal hemorrhage in the shunted group was offset by an increase in the number of deaths from hepatocellular failure in the operated patients. Patient selection and prediction of

outcome for any but emergency shunt operations is related to liver function and general physical condition. Ideally, the serum bilirubin should be less than 2.0 mg/dl; the serum albumin greater than 3.0 g/dl; and there should be an absence of any history of hepatic encephalopathy. Often, of course, bleeding occurs in patients with advanced active liver disease and mortality related to the blood and the surgery may exceed 50 percent. In general the portasystemic shunt operations should not be performed in patients over the age of 50 years. Necrosis and inflammation on liver biopsy are bad prognostic signs.

The complications of portacaval shunts are formidable (Table 64–7). Thrombosis of the shunt itself may occur and is more likely in children and in operations utilizing small vessels (e.g., splenorenal anastomoses). Approximately one-fourth of all shunted patients develop significant hepatic encephalopathy. The incidence is higher in older patients. The inci-

---

TABLE 64–7
Consequences of Portacaval Shunt Procedures

Desirable	Undesirable
Early Effects	

1. Decreased portal pressure
2. Decongest splanchnic bed
	1. Operative mortality
	   Elective operation—5 percent
	   Emergency operation—>50 percent
	2. Thrombosis of shunt with rebleeding (5 percent with end-to-side shunt)
	3. Impaired hepatocellular function—transient in all
	4. Decreased hepatic blood flow (majority)
	5. Transient encephalopathy (frequent)

Late Effects	

1. Decrease in:
  a. esophagogastric varices (gradual)
  b. abdominal collaterals
  c. size of spleen
  d. hypersplenism (some)
2. Relief of ascites (best accomplished with side-to-side shunt)
	1. Recurrent or permanent encephalopathy (15–25 percent)
	2. Progressive hepatocellular failure (10 percent)
	3. Possible undesirable effects: Increased iron absorption and hepatic deposition

dence of encephalopathy is less in patients who have had splenorenal shunts or in those with near normal liver function (congenital hepatic fibrosis or extrahepatic obstruction of the portal vein). Peptic ulcers are frequent in patients who have had portacaval shunts but no controlled study has demonstrated an increase in ulcer over a similar group of cirrhotic patients who have not been shunted. Increased iron absorption and deposition in the liver is occasionally found.

HEPATIC ENCEPHALOPATHY

Hepatic encephalopathy is a complex neuropsychiatric disorder occurring in patients with acute and chronic liver disease and characterized by disturbances in consciousness, personality, behavior, and neuromuscular function.[33,36] The individual components of the syndrome are nonspecific. Early manifestations ("precoma") include reversal of sleep patterns, hypersomnia, irritability, neglect of personal appearance, and forgetfulness. In later or more fulminant phases, delirium and deep irreversible coma may both occur and lead to death. Neurologic signs include hyperreflexia, generalized rigidity, and a nonrhythmic flapping tremor of the wrist and metacarpalphalangeal joints called *asterixis* which is best demonstrated with the arms outstretched and the hands dorsiflexed. Asterixis is not specific for hepatic encephalopathy and may be found in uremia, chronic respiratory disease, and chronic cardiac disease. There are no specific liver function test abnormalities in hepatic encephalopathy, and the cerebrospinal fluid is usually normal. Abnormalities in plasma amino acid concentrations are frequent with elevations in methionine and phenylalanine and decreased concentrations of the branched chain amino acids valine, leucine, and isoleucine. Pathologic changes in the brain are likewise nondescript with only a generalized increase in protoplasmic astrocytes observed. The electroencephalogram is of value in diagnosis with a characteristic slow wave activity (delta waves less than 4 cps) found predominantly over the frontal regions.

Factors of importance in the pathogenesis of hepatic encephalopathy are the shunting of blood around the liver cells and the presence of hepatocellular dysfunction.[36] In most patients, both factors are present. The shunting of portal blood around the liver cells may be through extrahepatic or intrahepatic shunts. It is assumed that the neurologic syndrome is produced by presentation to the systemic circulation of one or more toxic products of intestinal origin normally metabolized by the liver.

Abnormalities of ammonia metabolism are most frequently incriminated in the pathogenesis of hepatic encephalopathy.[28] Ammonia is produced in the gut by bacterial ureolysis and is transported via the portal vein to the liver. Evidence in favor of ammonia as the toxin in most instances of hepatic encephalopathy includes 1) an elevated arterial or cerebrospinal fluid ammonia in approximately 90 percent of patients with this disorder; 2) induction of hepatic encephalopathy in susceptible patients by giving ammonium salts (e.g., ammonium chloride as a diuretic or by the infusion of intravenous ammonia); 3) relief of the syndrome following therapy directed toward reduction of blood ammonia (dietary protein restriction, catharsis, antibiotics to decrease gut bacteria).

Evidence marshalled against ammonia as the toxin includes the absence of a close correlation between blood ammonia levels and the clinical degree of encephalopathy and the occurrence of the disorder in some patients in whom blood ammonia is not elevated. Other compounds implicated as possible toxins in producing hepatic encephalopathy include short-chain fatty acids, mercaptans derived from methionine metabolism, and accumulation of false neurochemical transmitters (e.g., octopamine) in the brain. Most likely there are several toxins acting alone or in combination which cause hepatic encephalopathy.

Hepatic encephalopathy may arise spontaneously in the course of acute or chronic hepatic disease or may have a clearly identifiable precipitating factor. Exogenous factors of importance include an increased protein in the diet, the administration of certain drugs (morphine and barbiturates in particular), overzealous use of diuretics leading to hypovolemia and hypokalemia, vigorous paracentesis, azotemia, and gastrointestinal hemorrhage. Blood in the gut is a rich source of ammonia and gastrointestinal hemorrhage is a most important precipitating cause of hepatic encephalopathy. The particular susceptibility of patients with hypokalemia and alkalosis to hepatic encephalopathy may be a reflection of the enhanced transfer of ammonia from blood into the cells in alkalotic patients. Ammonia moves across membranes in its nonionic form (NH_3). With its pK at 9.1 only a small percentage of ammonia in the blood is in the nonionic form. When the patient becomes alkalotic more ammonia is present in the NH_3 form and therefore available for translocation into cells. Endogenous factors are less well understood, but it is clear that the patient with liver disease is more susceptible to drugs and metabolic alterations that tend by themselves to depress consciousness. Hypoxia, electrolyte abnormalities, and intercurrent infections have all been implicated in precipitating full blown coma. The increased response of the brain to drugs may be demonstrated by giving many susceptible patients a small dose of parenteral morphine. A rapid and marked disorganization of the EEG occurs with slow wave activity over the frontal areas. These EEG abnormalities may precede the onset of any clinical symptoms or signs and are useful in the differential diagnosis of other causes of altered consciousness in the patient with liver disease (e.g., subdural hematoma).

MANAGEMENT OF HEPATIC ENCEPHALOPATHY

The objective of management in hepatic encephalopathy is lowering of blood ammonia and levels of other toxic substances by the reduction or exclusion of protein from the diet, by cleansing of nitrogenous materials from the gut, and by reduction of the colonic bacterial population with nonabsorbable antibiotics[36] (Table 64–8). Meticulous general support of the confused and often comatose patient combined with aggressive efforts to detect factors such as gastrointestinal hemorrhage, dietary indiscretion, and drugs which may have precipitated or worsened the syndrome is required. Alternative explanations for coma and depressed mentation in patients with liver disease which should be considered include subdural hematoma, hypoglycemia, and misuse of sedatives or tranquilizers.

Cleansing of the gut with enemas may dramatically improve the patient. All protein should be excluded from the diet until control of the encephalopathy has been obtained. Constipation should be avoided by use of laxatives and stool softeners. The most frequently employed nonabsorbable antibiotic is neomycin in doses of 4 to 6 g per day. The dangers of long-term administration of neomycin are well documented and include ototoxicity, malabsorption, and renal tubular toxicity. The potential hazard of all drugs in patients with liver disease must be recognized with morphine, short-acting barbiturates, and tranquilizers especially dangerous. Hypokalemia if found should be rapidly corrected. A plan of management based on these principles and effective in most patients is outlined in Table 64–8.

The use of lactulose, a synthetic disaccharide that is degraded by intestinal bacteria to produce acidification of the lower gut along with an osmotic, fermentative diarrhea has been a major advance in the management of hepatic encephalopathy. Lactulose regularly reduces blood ammonia levels and is associated with a reduction in the frequency of episodes of encephalopathy in patients with chronic disease. An advantage of lactulose therapy is avoidance of the renal, auditory, and intestinal side effects of neomycin.

Other therapeutic approaches in the management of hepatic encephalopathy include attempts to increase the low levels of branched-chain amino acids by administration of those compounds either as the amino acid or as its keto-analogues. Levodopa therapy has been used to arouse deeply comatose patients but the clinical usefulness of this approach is not established.

In patients with prolonged, resistant encephalopathy, total colectomy to remove the major site of

---

TABLE 64–8

Management of Hepatic Encephalopathy

I. Careful Search for Precipitating Factors
  A. Excess nitrogen load
    1. Gastrointestinal hemorrhage
    2. Excess protein in diet
    3. Increased enterohepatic circulation of urea in azotemia
  B. Electrolyte abnormalities
    1. Hypokalemia (especially hypokalemic alkalosis induced by diuretics)
    2. Hypovolemia (gastrointestinal hemorrhage, paracentesis, diuresis)
  C. Drugs
    1. Narcotics and sedatives (morphine particularly dangerous)
    2. Diuretics
      a. Via hypovolemia and hypokalemia
      b. Increased renal production of ammonia
  D. Infection
  E. Surgical procedures

II. Management
  A. For minimal encephalopathy
    1. Reduce dietary protein to 20–40 g/day
    2. Neomycin 1.0 g orally every 6 hours or lactulose 30 ml every 4–6 hours (to promote two soft bowel movements per day)
    3. Additional use of stool softeners or other laxatives and enemas if neomycin used
    4. Follow patient with:
      a. Handwriting chart
      b. Mental status examination
      c. Repeated search for precipitating factors in I
  B. For moderate to marked encephalopathy
    1. Stop all dietary protein
    2. Vigorous catharsis—enemas and oral magnesium citrate
    3. Provide calories—1000–1500/day as carbohydrate (orally or intravenously)
    4. Neomycin 1–2 g orally or per rectum every 6 hours or lactulose 30 ml every 4–6 hours as in II–A–2
    5. Follow patient as in II–A–4 with additional observation of deep tendon reflexes
  C. Once improvement occurs
    1. Reinstitute dietary protein in 10 g increments every 3–5 days
    2. Continue neomycin or lactulose until patient can tolerate a 40–50 g protein diet

toxin production has been employed with variable success. The operation is rarely used because of the excessive operative mortality in already very ill patients.

In patients with encephalopathy developing as part of an acute fulminant hepatic failure, the approach outlined in Table 64–8 is generally employed but with less success. The other manifestations of fulminant hepatic failure (hypoglycemia, brain swelling, and secondary infection) are of more importance. Exchange transfusions are not of proven benefit in these patients.

CHAPTER 65
Circulatory and Focal Diseases of the Liver
WILLIS C. MADDREY

CIRCULATORY DISORDERS

Obstruction to the outflow of hepatic blood in congestive heart failure is the most frequent circulatory abnormality affecting the liver. The major hepatic veins enter the inferior vena cava just below the diaphragm and any elevation in right atrial pressure is associated with an increase in hepatic venous pressure. Constrictive pericarditis is an infrequent but important cause of congestive liver disease because of its potential reversibility. Obstructive lesions in the inferior vena cava and hepatic veins (Budd-Chiari syndrome) and in the small hepatic veins (veno-occlusive disease) are even less frequent causes of hepatic congestion.

As a result of a decreased outflow of blood from any cause, the liver enlarges and dilatation of both the central veins and centrilobular sinusoids occurs. Anoxia associated with decreased hepatic perfusion contributes to cell damage in the vulnerable centrilobular region. Long-standing or severe recurrent congestion with episodes of ischemia leads to fibrosis and in some instances a nonportal cirrhosis ("cardiac cirrhosis").

The clinical manifestations of congestive liver disease include hepatomegaly which is often tender and right upper quadrant abdominal pain.[41] In tricuspid insufficiency, the enlarged liver may pulsate. Ascites occurs frequently and may be an exudate with high protein content. Liver function abnormalities include mild (< 5 mg/dl) hyperbilirubinemia and an increase in the BSP retention. A moderate elevation of the serum aminotransferases (100 to 300 MIU) is common in acute congestion. Moderate elevation in alkaline phosphatase is usual. A low serum albumin may reflect a decrease in hepatic cellular synthesis or be the result of a protein-losing gastroenteropathy.

Hepatic Vein Thrombosis (Budd-Chiari Syndrome)

Thrombosis of the major hepatic veins thereby blocking outflow of blood from the liver (Budd-Chiari syndrome) is a rare disorder which may occur alone or in association with inferior vena cava thrombosis. In most patients no etiology for the thrombosis is found but associations with polycythemia vera, use of oral contraceptives, ulcerative colitis, renal cell carcinoma, and hepatocellular carcinoma are all established.[40] Membranous webs in the inferior vena cava obstructing the ostia to the hepatic veins which may be surgically removed have been a reported cause of hepatic vein obstruction in Japan. Hepatic vein thrombosis may present acutely with a rapidly enlarging liver, ascites, abdominal pain, and often watery diarrhea rapidly followed by hepatocellular failure and coma. The chronic form usually presents with progressive prominent ascites which often has the characteristics of an exudate and may be bloody. Portal hypertension with hematemesis from bleeding esophageal varices may occur. Liver biopsy reveals intense central congestion with atrophy of pericentral hepatocytes and large hemorrhagic areas. Technetium (^{99}Tc) liver scans may reveal no uptake in those areas behind the blocked veins. Inferior vena cava and hepatic venography establish the diagnosis.[40] Anticoagulants have been employed in acutely developing cases but with little success and most patients die with hepatocellular failure and hepatic coma. Side-to-side portacaval or mesocaval shunt operations may be helpful in allowing the portal vein to become an outflow vessel relieving part of the intrahepatic congestion.

Veno-Occlusive Disease

In Jamaica, an acute obstruction of the small hepatic veins in the hepatic lobule (veno-occlusive disease) has been found in both man and animals exposed to native medicinal teas containing pyrrolozidine alkaloids derived from *Senecio* or *Crotalia* species.[39] The disorder is found predominantly in children and the clinical illnesses encountered are quite similar to those found in the Budd-Chiari syndrome. Both an acute form with hepatomegaly, ascites, and early death, and a chronic nonportal cirrhosis with portal hypertension and bleeding esophagogastric varices have been observed. Liver biopsy reveals intense centrilobular congestion with thickened obstructed small hepatic veins. In contrast to the Budd-Chiari syndrome, the large hepatic veins are unaffected. No treatment is available. Repeated paracenteses may be required to relieve discomfort. Many patients make a prompt clinical recovery whereas others develop cirrhosis, portal hypertension, and continued ascites.

PORTAL VEIN THROMBOSIS

Extrahepatic obstruction of the portal venous system is often a disease of children and young adults and is usually of uncertain etiology.[45] Neonatal umbilical sepsis, pylephlebitis, abdominal trauma, pancreatitis, hepatocellular carcinoma, and cirrhosis have all been recognized in association with portal venous obstruction. The usual presentation for such patients is with a sudden, unheralded massive hematemesis. Recurrence of such bleeding over a long period of time is the general pattern. Splenomegaly is a constant feature. Liver function is usually normal, and in general these patients do not develop significant ascites or hepatic encephalopathy after a hemorrhage. When portal vein thrombosis occurs as a complication of cirrhosis, ascites may occur. The end-to-side portacaval shunt procedure is precluded by the obstructed portal vein and alternative operations including mesocaval shunts are employed.

OTHER CIRCULATORY DISORDERS

Sinusoidal packing with abnormal red blood cells leads to focal intrahepatic thromboses in patients with sickle cell anemia.[46] Diseases of the hepatic arteries are rare and include occasional instances of polyarteritis nodosa, aneurysms of the hepatic artery, embolism from subacute infective endocarditis, or inadvertent ligation of the artery at surgery.

FOCAL LIVER DISORDERS

Focal inflammation of the liver is common in many systemic disorders and often is discovered only incidentally during the investigation of a patient with fever, weight loss, or malaise. Slight hepatomegaly and moderately deranged liver function tests are found in the course of many systemic viral and bacterial infections. The pathogenesis of the liver abnormalities is often obscure and may result from transient invasion of the liver by the organisms or occur in response to the production of toxic products by the agents. Suppurative processes may involve the liver singly or in the context of multiple disseminated systemic infections. It is remarkable that the liver with its rich blood supply is not the site of more such processes. The more important of the hepatic suppurative disorders and their proposed pathogenesis are presented in Table 65-1.

Pyogenic Liver Abscess

Many liver abscesses occur in a setting of biliary tract obstruction with cholangitis secondary to either gallstones, tumors, or bile duct stricture.[44,47] Because of the age association of biliary tract disease, the majority of these patients are elderly. These abscesses are frequently multiple. In the preantibiotic era, the majority of liver abscesses occurred in young patients as a result of portal septicemia (pylephlebitis) from appendicitis and other intra-abdominal septic conditions. Other less common causes of liver abscesses include septicemia such as in subacute infective endocarditis (SIE) and liver trauma. Both blunt and penetrating injuries may be associated with hepatic

---

TABLE 65-1
Suppurative Infections of the Liver

Suppurative Process	Pathogenesis or Etiology
Bacterial abscesses	Obstructed biliary tract with cholangitis
	Portal septicemia (pylephlebitis) 1. appendicitis 2. diverticulitis
	Systemic septicemia (e.g., subacute infective endocarditis)
	Trauma (penetrating and blunt)
Amebiasis	Portal invasion secondary to intestinal amebiasis
Tuberculosis	Bloodborne granulomas frequent in miliary tuberculosis
	Tuberculous cholangitis and pylephlebitis (rare)
Actinomycosis	Portal vein spread from involved intestinal tract
	Direct extension from contiguous viscera

abscess formation. In approximately one-half of patients with liver abscesses no definite etiology for the abscess is discovered, but transient septicemia or biliary tract obstruction is usually suspect. The resistance of the normal liver to infection suggests that local interference with blood supply, impaired biliary drainage, or decreased systemic resistance to infection are important in pathogenesis. The bacteriology of liver abscesses is complex with many containing a mixed flora of *E. coli, A. aerogenes,* proteus species, and anaerobic streptococci. Improved culture techniques have led to an increased recognition of anaerobes in the pathogenesis of liver abscess.

The clinical manifestations of hepatic abscesses encompass a broad spectrum ranging from a nondescript general feeling of malaise, nonlocalized vague abdominal discomfort, low grade fever, weight loss, and anemia to an acutely or chronically recurrent septic state with spiking fevers, chills, and prostration. The liver is usually enlarged and tender. Percussion over the lower rib cage often elicits pain. A friction rub may be present over the liver. Jaundice is often present but is usually mild. Ascites is rare. Leukocytosis, moderate elevation of the serum alkaline phosphatase, and minimal elevations of the SGOT are frequent.

The diagnosis of an hepatic abscess is occasionally quite difficult. Even large abscesses may present little local evidence of their presence. The diagnosis should be considered in any patient with a wasting febrile illness, especially if associated with abdominal pain and liver function abnormalities. Recurrent chills, fever, and jaundice may be the initial manifestations of cholangitis. A plain abdominal x-ray on occasion reveals a gas-filled cavity when infection with *E. coli, Clostridia,* or other gas-forming organisms are present. The advent of both hepatic scintiscan and ultrasonography have been an important adjunct to diagnosis and serve as an aid in initial evaluation and follow-up of therapy. When the abscess is high in the liver abutting on the diaphragm, chest fluoroscopy may reveal an immobile diaphragm with atelectasis in the lung.

The management of liver abscess consists of recognition and treatment of predisposing conditions such as obstructed biliary tract disease, SIE, or other intra-abdominal abscess. The mortality from multiple liver abscesses remains high. Surgical drainage is recommended for large solitary abscesses. Broad antibiotic coverage often for a prolonged time may be required, but is seldom effective unless drainage is performed. Selection of antibiotics should include consideration of anaerobes as causative agents. Liver abscesses often heal with scarring and in an occasional patient portal hypertension may result.

Amebic Abscess

Entameba histolytica is an important worldwide cause of both dysentery and liver abscess.[44] Although improved sanitation practices have decreased the incidence of the disease in North America, a significant number of persons harbor the protozoa in their colons and are liable to develop hepatic involvement. The pathogenesis of liver abscess in amebic infections is transport of the infective vegetative forms from the gut to the small portal radicles in the liver. Upon reaching the portal areas, the amebae release proteolytic enzymes that cause local tissue destruction. Multiple abscesses may occur, but amebiasis is not a cause of hepatitis. The clinical onset of hepatic amebiasis is usually insidious with low grade fever and occasionally right upper quadrant pain. It is impossible clinically to definitely distinguish amebic from pyogenic abscesses, and patients with amebic abscesses may have bacterial superinfection. Liver function tests are often normal. The white blood cell count is usually only moderately elevated in contrast to the frequently high counts in pyogenic abscess. Indirect hemagglutination tests using purified antigen are positive in almost all patients with amebic abscess of the liver. Amebic dysentery is infrequent at the time of diagnosis of liver abscess, although some 25 percent of patients will give a history of previous dysentery. For unknown reasons, most patients with amebic abscess of the liver are male. Most of the abscesses are in the posterosuperior aspect of the liver and occasionally point tenderness over the lower right posterior ribs is present. The abscess may attain a large size and rupture into the pleura, pericardium, or peritoneum. Aspiration of the cavity reveals an "anchovy paste" material consisting of hepatic cell debris, red blood cells, and white blood cells. Amebic abscesses of the liver generally respond well to therapy with both emetine and chloroquine or metronidazole.

Secondary Tumor of the Liver

Metastatic tumors in the liver are common and occur approximately 20 times more frequently than does primary hepatocellular carcinoma.[42] From one-third to one-half of all neoplasms with the exception of tumors of the brain metastasize to the liver. Dissemination of tumor to the liver is most often by the bloodstream with contiguous or lymphatic spread less frequent. When the liver is involved with metastatic tumor, multiple lesions are the rule. The liver harboring metastatic tumor may attain gigantic size ($>$ 10,000 g).

Clinical features of secondary tumors in the liver may be overshadowed by symptoms of the primary tumor but often hepatomegaly, abdominal pain, or an abnormal liver function test is the first indication of the presence of tumor. Systemic symptoms of lassitude, weight loss, and anorexia are frequent. A dragging sensation in the right upper quadrant is common, and pain in the region of the liver occurs particularly if the metastases abut on the capsule of the liver. Portal hypertension as manifested by splenomegaly, abdominal collaterals, and esophagogastric varices may develop but are usually of no clinical importance. Bile duct obstruction or portal venous thrombosis by the tumor may occur.

Surprisingly few liver function abnormalities are encountered in even large massively replaced livers. The most constant changes are retention of BSP, elevation of serum alkaline phosphatase, and moderate increases in SGOT. Jaundice, when present, is usually mild. The diagnosis is often apparent when an enlarged, nodular liver occurs in a setting of a known tumor, but massive hepatic replacement may foreshadow any evidence of primary tumor (e.g., malignant melanoma). Hepatic scintiscanning is of value in the evaluation of the presence and extent of metastatic tumor. Liver biopsy is often a productive diagnostic procedure. The liver biopsy is positive in approximately 70 percent of patients with hepatomegaly and clinical evidence of liver disease. Even in patients with no signs or symptoms suggesting hepatic involvement, liver biopsy uncovers approximately 20 percent of metastases. A directed liver biopsy at laparoscopy may improve the diagnostic yield. Liver biopsy in the staging of tumors may save the patient an unnecessary laparotomy.

Management of these patients is largely supportive. An occasional solitary metastasis has been successfully removed by hepatic lobectomy. Results with arterial infusion of chemotherapeutic agents are unsatisfactory. Primary tumors of the liver are discussed in Chapter 67.

Granuloma of the Liver

Granulomas are found in from 3 to 10 percent of all biopsies performed in large series.[43] The differential diagnosis of these granulomas may require extensive investigation encompassing bacterial, viral, fungal, allergic, physical, and neoplastic processes. The histologic pattern of an individual granuloma is not of enough specificity to allow diagnosis. Special stains and culture of liver biopsy material for acid-fast and fungal organisms may assist in making an exact diagnosis. Table 65–2 presents several of the more common disorders associated with granulomas with an outline of principal associated features and diagnostic methods. An elevated serum alkaline phosphatase and BSP retention are frequent in granulomatous liver disease, but other liver function tests are often normal. The discovery of granulomas in liver biopsy material may be a focal point of significant value in the investigation of patients with unexplained fever, hepatomegaly, lymphadenopathy, pulmonary infiltrates, or weight loss.

TABLE 65–2
Granulomatous Liver Disease

Etiology*	Associated Features	Diagnostic Procedures
Tuberculosis	Chest infiltrates; hemoptysis; pericarditis; meningitis; etc.	Tuberculin skin tests (OT or PPD), sputum, and biopsy examination and culture for acid-fast organisms
Sarcoidosis	Bilateral hilar adenopathy; chest infiltrates; lymphadenopathy, uveitis	Diagnosis of exclusion Kveim test positive in 80% Demonstration of noncaseating granulomas in two tissues in patient with compatible history
Histoplasmosis	Residence in endemic area Chest infiltrates	Histoplasmin complement fixation test Fungal stains and culture of sputum, liver, bone marrow
Brucellosis	Occupational exposure (farmer, packing house worker, veterinarian) Acute or chronic febrile illness often with hepatosplenomegaly	Brucella skin test Complement fixation test Culture of blood, liver, bone marrow
Berylliosis	Occupational exposure	Skin patch test Urinary beryllium

* All these disorders may present with a similar clinical picture of wasting, malaise, and fever. Pulmonary involvement is frequent and often is the major manifestation of disease.

Liver biopsy is of considerable value in the diagnosis of sarcoidosis with positive specimens in approximately 75 percent of patients with the disease. The granulomatous liver disease in sarcoidosis has on occasion been associated with severe hepatocellular involvement, portal hypertension, and bleeding esophageal varices.[45] The usefulness of liver biopsy in investigating miliary tuberculosis is likewise established with virtually all these patients having granulomas on biopsy. Granulomas of the liver are common in patients with both histoplasmosis and brucellosis. A disorder characterized by hepatosplenomegaly and hepatic granulomas is found in workers exposed to beryllium compounds in the aircraft manufacturing and metallurgy industries. The diagnosis may be proved by determination of urinary beryllium.

CHAPTER 66
Acute Diffuse Hepatocellular Disease
WILLIS C. MADDREY

The most common acute hepatic diseases are viral hepatitis and drug-induced hepatitis including alcoholic liver disease. Less frequent causes of acute liver disease are leptospirosis, infectious mononucleosis, and exposure to direct hepatotoxins such as carbon tetrachloride. The mode of onset of disease, course, physical manifestations, and laboratory findings are often similar in acute liver diseases of diverse causes. Jaundice, malaise, anorexia, and weakness are frequent early symptoms of little differential diagnostic value. Evaluation of acute hepatocellular disease should include a meticulous history of possible contact with jaundiced patients, evidence of use of illicit drugs, or contact with known drug abusers, use of alcohol, exposure to therapeutic agents, place of work, recent hospitalization or dental procedures, and travel experience. The test for hepatitis B antigen (HBsAg) is mandatory.

VIRAL HEPATITIS

Viral hepatitis is an acute systemic disease caused by several viruses with predominant clinical and pathologic manifestations related to hepatic cellular necrosis. Studies of transmission of viral hepatitis have demonstrated at least three clinically similar but epidemiologically somewhat distinct types (hepatitis A, hepatitis B, and hepatitis non-A, non-B). Hepatitis A was formerly known as infectious hepatitis or short incubation hepatitis, and hepatitis B as serum hepatitis or long incubation hepatitis. Major advances in virology have identified and characterized the viruses that cause hepatitis (A and B; Table 66–1), and an agent (or agents) that causes hepatitis non-A, non-B has been successfully transmitted to primates.

HEPATITIS A
Hepatitis A virus is basically a fecal–oral transmitted disease with an incubation period of 15 to 40 days and is associated with shedding of 27nM particles (HA Ag) in the feces for one to two weeks before the appearance of elevated serum aminotransferases and symptoms. HA Ag has been demonstrated by electron microscopy of ultrafiltrates of feces mixed with the antibody containing blood from patients convalescing from hepatitis A. HA Ag particles usually disappear within several days of the onset of symptoms. HA Ag titers in the blood are generally low and transient. Antibody to hepatitis A virus (HA Ab) appears during the acute infection and reaches a peak in two to three months. HA Ab persists in the blood after infection. The prevalence of HA Ab in the population increases with age and is inversely correlated with socioeconomic status. Spread of hepatitis A is predominantly through contamination of food and water supplies with infected feces. Hepatitis A may be transmitted by raw or partially cooked clams from contaminated waters.

HEPATITIS B
Hepatitis B has a longer incubation (50 to 160 days) than hepatitis A and infection with this virus is detected by identifying the hepatitis B surface antigen (HbsAg) in serum by radioimmunoassay or hemagglutination inhibition tests. Electron microscopic studies of serum from patients with hepatitis B reveal several different particles.[62] Most abundant are the HBsAg particles which are 20 to 22nM spheres and are apparently defective viral surface coat material made by infected hepatocytes. The serum concentration of HBsAg may be enormous with levels as high as 50 mg/dl. Larger particles (Dane particles) measure 42 to 44nM and represent the complete virion

─TABLE 66-1─

Clinical, Epidemiologic, and Immunologic Features of Hepatitis A, Hepatitis B, and Hepatitis Non-A, Non-B

	Hepatitis A	Hepatitis B	Hepatitis Non-A, Non-B
Incubation period	15–40 days	50–160 days	15–180 days
Age group affected	Children and young adults predominate	All ages	All ages
Type of onset	Usually acute	Acute or insidious	Usually insidious
Seasonal variation	Peak in winter	Any season	Any season
Route of infection			
Oral	Yes	Yes	Unknown
Parenteral	Rare	Yes	Yes
Virus in blood			
Incubation	Yes	Yes	Probably Yes
Acute	Yes	Yes	Probably Yes
Convalescence	No	Occasional	Probably Yes
Carrier state	No	Yes	Probably Yes
Immunity			
Homologous	Yes	Yes	Unknown
Heterologous	No	No	Unknown

with HBsAg on the surface and a core antigen (HBcAg) in the center. Adequate tests for HBcAg are not yet widely available. Both DNA polymerase and DNA are present in the inner core but assays for these are not widely available. An additional antigen associated with hepatitis B infection is designated *e* antigen (HBeAg). The exact nature or location within the virion for HBeAg is unknown. HBeAg is only found in the serum of patients positive for HBsAg.[63]

There are several subtypes of the HB virus.[56] Hepatitis B antigen has one group specific surface determinant designated *a*. The particles generally carry two allelic subspecific determinants designated *d* or *y* and *w* or *r*. All four possible antigenic determinants— *adw, adr, ayw,* and *ayr*—have been found with considerable geographic differences in their distribution. No differences in virulence or tendency to cause chronic hepatitis have been found for any subtype. Blood containing the hepatitis B antigen has been proven to regularly transmit hepatitis to recipients. Particles morphologically identical to HBsAg have been found in feces, urine, saliva, semen, and bile of patients with hepatitis.

Hepatitis B was earlier thought to be transmitted only by parenteral routes (e.g., blood transfusions, tattoos, contaminated needle sticks), but through the widespread use of tests for HB Ag, it is now estab-

lished that many patients with hepatitis B have no history of an apparent parenteral route of infection. Such nonparenteral or inapparent parenterally transmitted cases are frequent and account for the majority of hepatitis encountered in urban adults. Oral ingestion of very small amounts of blood containing hepatitis B virus definitely can transmit hepatitis. Oral transmission of HBsAg is associated with a longer incubation period than when HBsAg is given parenterally. Hepatitis B may be transmitted by ingestion of the small amounts of blood which may come through close association with an infected person such as in kissing, sexual contact, or sharing of utensils (e.g., toothbrush). Spread of hepatitis B by arthropods, especially mosquitoes, has been suggested. Acquisition and transmission of hepatitis is a special hazard to medical personnel especially surgeons, dentists, and those working in renal dialysis.

The appearance of HBsAg in the serum is the first evidence in the serum of hepatitis B infection. HBcAg, DNA polymerase, and HBeAg often appear transiently in the serum of patients with acute hepatitis B. Antibodies to HBsAg (HBsAb) usually are detectable only after full recovery whereas HBcAb may be found during the acute illness. Once present HBsAb does persist and its presence is an indication of prior infection and immunity. HBsAg is not detected by present methods in a few patients with hepatitis B and the diagnosis must be established by determining the presence of HBsAb or HBcAb.

Persistence of hepatitis B antigen (HBsAg) occurs in patients with Down syndrome, leukemia (especially lymphocytic), lepromatous leprosy, and in patients undergoing chronic renal hemodialysis. An altered immunologic response to the virus may explain the persistence. Such patients are generally anicteric but have abnormal BSP retention, and evidence of mild hepatitis on liver biopsy. Hepatitis B antigen is more prevalent in the serum of heroin addicts most likely as a result of repeated exposure to infection. An occasional individual will be found to have persistent HBsAg on routine screening such as in blood donor programs. If HBsAg persists for more than 6 months, the individual is designated a chronic carrier. Most HBsAg chronic carriers are asymptomatic and have no history of acute hepatitis. The majority do have elevated serum aminotransferases. Liver biopsy in chronic carriers may reveal normal liver, minimal inflammation, acute hepatitis, chronic active hepatitis, or even cirrhosis. There may be considerable discrepancy between the asymptomatic clinical presentation and the liver biopsy. Chronic hepatitis B carriers must be presumed infectious to others by their blood and other body secretions. Studies have suggested that chronic HBsAg carriers who are also HBeAg positive are more likely to be infectious. If an individual has serum HBsAg for longer than 6 months, the likelihood of the antigen subsequently disappearing is low.

Although the incidence of hepatitis B antigen positive persons is extremely rare in a normal North American population (0.1 percent), population studies in the tropical countries of southeast Asia have demonstrated the antigen in a significant number (4 to 20 percent) of persons who often have no signs of liver disease.

HEPATITIS NON-A, NON-B[51]

The agent or agents causing hepatitis non-A, non-B have not yet been identified. The clinical illness of hepatitis non-A, non-B is similar to hepatitis B (Table 66–1). Hepatitis non-A, non-B became widely recognized when routine testing of all blood products before transfusion markedly reduced the incidence of posttransfusion hepatitis B but only reduced by approximately half the overall incidence of posttransfusion hepatitis. Although the viral agent causing non-A, non-B has not been identified, hepatitis has now been transmitted to a chimpanzee by the blood of an infected patient. Hepatitis non-A, non-B is occasionally associated with the development of a carrier state and the development of chronic hepatitis.

CLINICAL FEATURES OF VIRAL HEPATITIS

The typical course of hepatitis begins with a prodromal phase of 2 to 14 days' duration which is characterized by flulike symptoms of malaise, fatigue, myalgias, headache, and nausea and is followed by the development of jaundice. Anorexia, right upper quadrant abdominal pain, pruritus, loss of taste for cigarettes, and arthralgias may be prominent features. Conjunctivitis, coryza, and pharyngitis are common. Fever of 100 to 102°F is usual but shaking chills are uncommon. Physical examination early in the icteric phase reveals tender hepatomegaly in addition to jaundice. Transient enlargement of the spleen is found in 10 to 20 percent of patients and enlargement of the posterior cervical lymph nodes may be present. Occasionally transient spider angiomas appear during acute hepatitis. In many patients with hepatitis B, the prodromal and early icteric phases of hepatitis are characterized by polyarthritis, urticaria, angioneurotic edema, and a diffuse maculopapular rash. Such manifestations generally subside soon after the onset of jaundice and are most likely the result of formation and deposition of immune complexes of hepatitis B antigen and antibody.[64] This serum-sickness-like presentation is rare to nonexistent in hepatitis A or in hepatitis non-A, non-B.

The diagnosis of hepatitis is often not considered prior to the onset of dark urine and jaundice. Once jaundice appears, it increases rapidly in intensity over a week to 10 days, reaches a peak, then progressively subsides. The fever and other prodromal symptoms gradually disappear in the first week of the icteric phase and the patient may begin to feel better with an improved appetite at a time when the bilirubin is still rising.

The prognosis in acute hepatitis occurring in young, previously healthy persons is excellent. In almost all patients with hepatitis A, all clinical and biochemical evidence of disease is gone in 3 months. The case mortality rate in hepatitis A is extremely low (less than 1 per 1000 cases).

Hepatitis A does not apparently cause chronic hepatitis or cirrhosis. Approximately 10 percent of patients with hepatitis B have not completely recovered by 3 months after the onset of symptoms.[59] Both chronic persistent hepatitis and chronic active hepatitis may result from hepatitis B (Chap. 67). A prolonged cholestatic illness with persistent jaundice, light stools, and pruritus may occur in some patients with hepatitis B. The consequences of hepatitis non-A, non-B are less certain but chronic hepatitis and cirrhosis does develop in some patients.[51]

Abnormalities in liver function appear early in the prodromal phase of hepatitis and are characterized by an increase in the serum aminotransferase activity. The peak serum aminotransferase activities are found at the time jaundice appears or within a few days of this event. The serum bilirubin rarely exceeds 15 to 20 mg/dl. The serum alkaline phosphatase is usually only moderately elevated. Bilirubinuria and increased urine urobilinogen may precede the onset of jaundice by several days. The stools are often clay colored early in the icteric phase and regain their color as the jaundice subsides. The white blood cell count is normal or low during acute hepatitis and leukopenia may be observed.

Anicteric Hepatitis

In many patients with both hepatitis A, B and non-A, non-B, prodromal symptoms may be minimal or absent and may not be followed by the development of jaundice. These anicteric patients are often diagnosed only when compatible prodromal symptoms occurring during an epidemic of hepatitis lead to the detection of liver abnormalities by laboratory tests. Anicteric hepatitis is frequent in children and estimates of the ratio of anicteric to icteric cases range from 1:1 in adults to 10:1 in children. The lack of specificity of the prodromal symptoms and the frequency of anicteric hepatitis add to the difficulties in control of spread of hepatitis.

Relapsing Hepatitis

An occasional patient with acute viral hepatitis makes an apparent complete recovery and then experiences a recurrence of symptoms and signs of liver disease within 6 months of the onset of the first episode. The relapses are in general clinically milder than the initial attack and heal without the development of chronic liver disease. Relapses must be distinguished from progressive liver disease such as is found in chronic active hepatitis. Liver biopsy is often necessary in the evaluation of these patients.

Fulminant Hepatitis

Fulminant hepatic failure is a rare disorder manifested by deepening jaundice and coma appearing within a few days after the onset of hepatitis. Fulminant hepatitis may occur after viral hepatitis, exposure to hepatotoxins, and in severe idiosyncratic drug reactions. The clinical picture of rapidly deteriorating hepatic function is similar regardless of the etiology of the liver injury. The liver may rapidly decrease in size on physical examination. Liver biopsy when available reveals large areas of necrosis and collapse. There is a greater than 75 percent mortality associated with the development of such massive necrosis with death occurring in less than a week. The development of a prolonged prothrombin time ($<$ 50 per-

cent), markedly elevated bilirubin ($>$ 20 mg/dl) and leukocytosis are bad prognostic signs in patients with acute hepatocellular disease.[61] Survival from fulminant hepatitis is age-dependent with much higher survival in patients less than 20 years of age regardless of etiology or therapy. Therapy for fulminant hepatitis is directed toward support of the often comatose or combative patient. Hypoglycemia, severe generalized bleeding, cerebral edema, superimposed bacterial infections, and renal failure are frequent and require constant vigilance. There is no evidence to support the use of corticosteroids, exchange transfusions, or gamma globulin in therapy.

Posthepatitis Syndromes

Occasionally patients with viral hepatitis experience prolonged fatigue and malaise for months after apparent recovery. Reinvestigation of these patients usually reveals normal liver function and with time and reassurance the symptoms abate. Restriction of activity is not necessary.

Prolonged elevation of aminotransferases after recovery from hepatitis in an otherwise healthy patient is often associated with a minimal increase in cells in the portal triads (chronic persistent hepatitis) (Chap. 67). A number of these patients with persistently elevated aminotransferases acquired their hepatitis by intravenous use of illicit drugs. There is no evidence that chronic liver disease develops in these patients and often the aminotransferase slowly returns to normal.

Hyperbilirubinemia, often with a predominant elevation of the indirect-reacting bilirubin, may follow viral hepatitis and be unassociated with other abnormal liver function tests. Except for a history of hepatitis these patients are indistinguishable from those with Gilbert syndrome. No treatment is necessary for this benign condition.

A serious posthepatitis syndrome is the development of aplastic anemia. The aplastic anemia usually follows the viral hepatitis and may be associated with hepatitis A or B infection.

MANAGEMENT OF ACUTE HEPATITIS

No proven specific treatment is available in acute viral hepatitis. Patients with hepatitis tend to get well given time, rest, and an adequate diet. Hospitalization is often advisable to carry out diagnostic procedures, to provide the proper environment for adequate rest and nutrition, and to allow close observation of the course of the disease. There is no evidence that gamma globulin given once symptoms have begun modifies the course of the viral hepatitis regardless of the type of infection.

Rest

Bed rest is a time-honored therapy in viral hepatitis. Patients with hepatitis are often weak and both their mood and appetite are improved by rest. Controlled studies in previously healthy military personnel, however, demonstrate no deleterious effects of moderate or even forced exercise in the ultimate recovery of patients with hepatitis.[60] This study in previously healthy young patients may not apply to an older and more heterogeneous civilian population. A reasonable approach to rest therapy in the management of hepatitis is to encourage rest during the active phases of liver cell damage with gradual ambulation as the patient's symptoms subside and strength returns. Rest after meals is encouraged.

Diet

An adequate supply of calories and protein is important in the management of acute liver cell disease. In one study, patients with acute viral hepatitis who were forced to eat a 3000 calorie, 150 g protein diet were found to have a reduction in the duration of illness compared to patients on an ad lib diet.[50] Greater quantities than these of protein, calories, or amino acid supplements were not of proven benefit. To insure an adequate calorie intake for patients with hepatitis, parenteral supplementation with 10 percent glucose may be required especially when nausea and vomiting are present. Adjustment of calorie intake to provide 40 percent of the diet in the morning when nausea is often less may be useful. A mild antiemetic such as diphenhydramine is occasionally helpful in controlling nausea and thereby promoting food intake. Caloric intake takes precedence over provision of dietary protein but an intake of 1 to 1.5 g/kg of body weight of protein is desirable. Should signs of hepatic encephalopathy develop, all dietary protein must be removed.

Specific vitamin deficiencies must be corrected, but there is no need for routine vitamin supplementation in acute hepatitis. In patients with deep, prolonged jaundice, parenteral vitamin K therapy is indicated.

Adrenal Corticosteroids

The role of adrenal corticosteroid therapy in acute viral or drug induced hepatitis remains controversial. No controlled study is available demonstrating the usefulness of these agents in patients with acute viral hepatitis. In one large uncontrolled study patients *not* given corticosteroids did better than the group given the drugs.[49] Corticosteroid administration does result in a feeling of well-being, improved appetite, and more rapid resolution of the serum bilirubin and transaminase levels. There is, however, no evidence that such therapy slows the rate of liver cell necrosis or promotes regeneration of the liver in acute hepatitis. In patients with prolonged jaundice with hepatitis (cholestatic hepatitis), corticosteroids may be useful in reducing the degree of jaundice. Once introduced into the therapy of any acute liver disease, corticosteroids must be tapered slowly to avoid a recrudescence of both symptoms and liver function abnormalities.

Prevention and Prophylaxis of Viral Hepatitis

Both feces and blood from patients with hepatitis A contain virus during the prodromal and early icteric phases of the disease. Hepatitis A is spread by close personal contact and by fecally contaminated water supplies, fruits, and vegetables. General hygienic measures and stool isolation are desirable throughout the infectious phase but are of limited usefulness. The shedding of virus during the prodrome and the frequency of anicteric cases make prevention of spread difficult. Special care should be taken for adequate sewage disposal in high risk environments such as camps for children, mental institutions, and military facilities. Raw shellfish (clams and oysters) are established vectors, and control of sewage pollution in supply areas for these shellfish is necessary.

Immune serum globulin (ISG, 0.01 to 0.02 ml/kg) given to contacts of patients with hepatitis A does provide protection against development of overt hepatitis but not against subclinical infection. ISG should be given to close personal contacts of patients with hepatitis A and for travelers to tropical countries and other areas in which sanitation facilities are likely to be inadequate.

The development of tests for hepatitis B antigen allows detection of a large proportion of carriers of the hepatitis B virus and their exclusion as blood donors. The exclusion of donors particularly likely to carry hepatitis such as drug abusers has further reduced the incidence of posttransfusion hepatitis. Blood products derived from single donor sources such as whole blood and packed red cells are of less risk than blood derived from pooled plasma concentrates. Frozen blood carries a possibly decreased risk of transmitting hepatitis. Human serum albumin and gamma globulin do not transmit hepatitis. Use of disposable hypodermic and blood administration equipment and adequate cleaning of dental instruments should be required.

The role of ISG in the prophylaxis of hepatitis B is less certain with trials yielding conflicting results. It is established that in recent years the titer of HBsAb in ISG has been increasing and part of the discrepancy in results may be explained by variation in antibody titer. It is widely accepted that ISG is of little or no use in preventing posttransfusion hepatitis. Immune serum globulin with high titers of HBsAb (hyperimmune globulin; hepatitis B immune globulin; HBIG) is now available. HBIG (0.05 to 0.07 ml/kg immediately and repeated in 25 to 30 days) appears effective in reducing the incidence of hepatitis B developing after a single needlestick or mucosal exposure (as in a clinical chemistry laboratory). Furthermore, HBIG is useful in reducing the incidence of hepatitis in neonates born to mothers with acute hepatitis B in the third trimester. There is no indication HBIG is useful if the recipient already has HBsAb in the serum. The usefulness of HBIG in reducing hepatitis in household contacts of either patients with acute hepatitis B or chronic HBsAg carriers is uncertain.

The exclusion of the use of commercial blood has markedly reduced the incidence of posttransfusion hepatitis presumably through reduction in the incidence of hepatitis non-A, non-B. Whether the use of ISG or HBIG will further decrease the incidence of posttransfusion hepatitis is under study.

Goals for the future in hepatitis research include cultivation of the hepatitis viruses in tissue culture systems and development of safe effective vaccines. Preliminary trials of vaccines to inactivated HBsAg are underway and the early results are encouraging.

Infections with both hepatitis A and B appear to confer homologous but not heterologous immunity to subsequent infection.

DRUG- AND OTHER CHEMICAL-INDUCED HEPATIC INJURY

Many drugs and other chemical agents produce hepatic injury when inhaled, ingested, or administered parenterally (Table 66–2). Reactions to these agents can be divided into two broad categories: dose-dependent hepatic toxicity and idiosyncratic reactions.[53] Many therapeutic agents damaging the liver fall into the latter category. The major features of dose-dependent reactions include: 1) production of a predictable, reproducible reaction when given to man or animal; 2) a dose-related severity of reaction; 3) the appearance of clinical manifestations of reaction at a predictable interval after exposure (usually less than 48 hours); 4) laboratory features compatible with hepatocellular damage and liver biopsy findings of zonal (usually centrilobular) necrosis with little parenchymal inflammation; 5) evidence of damage to other organs (especially kidney) by the agents. Important

TABLE 66-2

Drugs and Environmental Agents Producing Hepatic Injury

Class	Specific Agents
I. Dose-Dependent Hepatotoxins	
A. Mushroom poisoning	*Amanita phalloides*
B. Industrial chemicals	Carbon tetrachloride, benzene derivatives, vinyl chloride
C. Metal intoxication	Yellow phosphorus
II. Idiosyncratic Reactions	
A. Hepatocellular reactions	
1. Anesthetic agents	Halothane, methoxyflurane
2. Antiarthritis agents	Phenylbutazone
3. Antibiotics	Rifampin, sulfonamides, isoniazid
4. Anticonvulsants	Diphenylhydantoin
B. Cholestatic reactions	
1. Oral contraceptives	All
2. Oral hypoglycemics	Chlorpropamide
3. Tranquilizers	Chlorpromazine and other phenothiazines
III. Elements of Both Dose-Dependent Hepatotoxins and Idiosyncratic Reactions	Methyltestosterone toxicity

hepatotoxins include carbon tetrachloride, benzene derivatives, and intoxication by the mushroom *Amanita phalloides.*

Idiosyncratic reactions characteristically: 1) produce hepatic injury in only a small number of persons receiving the drug; 2) do not produce injury when administered to animals; 3) demonstrate no relation between dose of the drug and extent of reaction produced; 4) have an unpredictable interval from exposure to onset of reaction; and 5) may exhibit other signs of hypersensitivity such as eosinophilia, fever, arthralgias, and rashes. The pathogenesis of idiosyncratic reactions is largely unknown. In some cases immunologic sensitization is most certainly important. In others, metabolism of the agent to a toxic product is likely. The occurence and extent of injury may be determined by individual differences in metabolism related to genetic and environmental factors.

There are two general forms of hepatic reaction to drugs: hepatocellular injury (drug hepatitis) and cholestasis. Hepatocellular reactions are usually indistinguishable from viral hepatitis on the basis of clinical, laboratory, or biopsy evidence. No specific test for drug sensitivity reactions is available. Determination of HBsAg is useful in excluding hepatitis B but in many instances the diagnosis remains presumptive. Rechallenge with suspected sensitizing drugs is the most certain approach to diagnosis but often is not justified.

Cholestatic hepatitis may be caused by drug reactions. Jaundice, pruritus, light stools, absence of urine urobilinogen, and an increase in serum alkaline phosphatase activity characterize these reactions. The predominant finding on liver biopsy is cholestasis but minor evidence of cellular damage is usually found. The phenothiazine drugs are among the most commonly encountered causes of cholestatic hepatitis. The prognosis for cholestatic drug reactions is in general excellent with the jaundice subsiding over several weeks to months.

Cholestatic reactions to methyltestosterone and other C-17 alkyl substituted steroids have characteristics of both toxic and hypersensitivity reactions. Dilatation of the bile canaliculi with flattening and loss of microvilli and a defect in the excretion of BSP and bilirubin are found in many patients given these drugs suggesting a direct toxic reaction. There is minimal parenchymal damage associated with the abnormalities in the bile canaliculi and extrahepatic manifestations of hypersensitivity are absent. The canalicular changes are usually reversible within 3 months of withdrawal of the drugs and fatalities are rare.

Carbon Tetrachloride Poisoning

Carbon tetrachloride is a cleaning solvent used in the home and industry. Poisoning may result from accidental or purposeful ingestion of the agent, inhalation in closed environments, and possibly by skin absorption. Alcoholics appear to have increased susceptibility to the poisoning. Jaundice appears 2 to 4 days after exposure and is generally associated with evidence of renal toxicity. The diagnosis should be suspected in any patient with rapidly developing azotemia and jaundice. Liver biopsy reveals centrilobular necrosis and widespread fat deposition but surprisingly little inflammation. Severe liver involvement leads to death generally within the first week after intoxication. Cirrhosis does not develop in survivors.

Vinyl Chloride-Associated Liver Disease

An increased incidence of hepatic fibrosis, portal hypertension, and angiosarcomas of the liver have been found in workers in the plastic industry, especially those exposed to vinyl chloride monomer gas during the process of polymerization.[48] The hepatic fibrosis involves the portal areas and subcapsular regions and is also found in a focal intralobular distribution. These fibrotic changes are similar to those found in patients exposed to trivalent arsenical compounds. The mechanisms by which vinyl chloride might lead to hepatic injury are unknown but may result from accumulation of reactive products during the metabolism of the compound.

Halothane-Induced Hepatic Necrosis

Idiosyncratic reactions ranging from a mild subclinical derangement of liver function tests to fulminant hepatic failure have been associated with administration of the fluorinated hydrocarbon anesthetic agent halothane. A large body of evidence has now accumulated implicating this agent in hepatic necrosis. The frequency of the reaction is low and it is apparently a hypersensitivity reaction. Although 25 percent of cases occur after the first exposure to the agent, the importance of multiple administration of halothane in the development of liver injury is established. Approximately three-fourths of patients who have developed fulminant hepatic failure following halothane anesthesia give a history of postoperative fever, often occurring from 1 to 2 weeks following an earlier exposure to the agent.[54] The adverse reactions to halothane do not appear to be related to the type of surgery. There is no greater incidence following operations on the liver or biliary tract. Liver biopsy is of particular value in separating these patients from those with postoperative jaundice from shock or sepsis. Therapy is mainly supportive. Cirrhosis may occur from repeated bouts of halothane hepatitis. The idiosyncratic nature of the reaction suggests the usefulness of corticosteroids, but the effectiveness of this therapy is unproven. Similar hepatic necrosis has been observed with the related compound methoxyflurane.

Isoniazid-Induced Hepatic Necrosis

Isoniazid (INH) has been extensively administered in both the treatment and chemoprophylaxis of tuberculosis. Approximately 10 percent of patients receiving INH alone in chemoprophylactic programs develop moderate increases in serum aminotransferases and have minimal, nonspecific inflammation on liver biopsy. A few patients (< 1 percent) develop clinically apparent hepatitis from INH.[57] The duration of therapy before the onset of symptoms may be several weeks to 6 months. Prodromal symptoms of hepatitis such as malaise, fatigue, nausea, and vomiting are usual and continuation of the drug after appearance of these symptoms may worsen the hepatitis. As in other instances of drug hepatitis, there is often a discrepancy between a relatively well-appearing patient and liver biopsy changes of bridging and multilobular necrosis. The pathogenesis of INH-induced hepatitis is uncertain and may result from production of toxic metabolic products in susceptible individuals or from a sensitization reaction. Management of INH-induced hepatitis is drug withdrawal and supportive care. Corticosteroids are not of proven benefit.

Chlorpromazine Jaundice

Clinically apparent cholestatic hepatitis occurs in some 1 to 2 percent of patients taking the phenothiazine tranquilizer chlorpromazine.[52] Serial biopsy and biochemical studies have revealed minor hepatic morphologic and functional changes in many patients receiving this agent. The syndrome of overt hepatitis characteristically appears in the second to fourth week after institution of the drug and has a prodromal phase of fever, chills, malaise, and anorexia similar to that found in viral hepatitis. Pruritus, arthralgias, and lymphadenopathy may dominate the clinical picture. Several days following the onset of constitutional symptoms, jaundice supervenes. It is unusual for liver damage to be manifest in the first week of drug administration or to appear after the patient has taken the agent for more than 5 weeks. Both liver function tests and liver biopsy reveal a cholestatic hepatitis. The course of the disorder is one of gradual resolution of liver function abnormalities over a 2- to 8-week period following withdrawal of the drug, but progression of the cholestatic reaction even to frank biliary cirrhosis has been reported. Resolution of the hepatitis while the patient continued to take the drug suggests occasional spontaneous desensitization. Instances of cross reactions to other phenothiazine derivatives have been observed.

REYE SYNDROME (Fatty Liver with Encephalopathy)

Reye syndrome is a rare acute disease in children and characterized by rapidly developing fatty infiltration of both the liver and the renal tubules.[58] The pathogenesis of the illness is unknown. The disorder often has its onset with and following an acute upper respiratory infection (occasionally after chickenpox) in an otherwise healthy child. Outstanding clinical features include stupor, headache, coma, and persistent vomiting. Hepatomegaly is usual; hypoglycemia is common, but jaundice is rare. The serum aminotransferase enzymes and blood ammonia levels are usually very high. Metabolic acidosis may occur. Many patients die in 2 to 4 days but an occasional child survives if supportive care, glucose supplements, and efforts to lower the blood ammonia level are provided.

CHAPTER 67
Chronic Diffuse Liver Disease: Cirrhosis
WILLIS C. MADDREY

Diffuse hepatic diseases characterized by: 1) evidence of present or past hepatic cell necrosis; 2) fibrosis involving all parts of the liver; and 3) the presence of regenerating nodules are grouped under the term *cirrhosis*. By definition nonuniform liver diseases such as hepatic abscesses are excluded.

Classifications of cirrhosis are based either on morphologic criteria or on the basis of presumed etiology. Neither system of classification is adequate because of the nonspecificity of the pathologic responses and the frequency with which no apparent cause for the cirrhosis can be established. The morphologic classification is of limited usefulness and divides cirrhosis into small nodular (micronodular, portal) or large nodular (macronodular, postnecrotic) varieties. Leading known causes of cirrhosis include alcohol, viral hepatitis, toxic or idiosyncratic drug reactions, biliary obstruction, long-term hepatic congestion, hepatolenticular degeneration (Wilson's disease), and hemochromatosis (Table 67–1). Many patients with cirrhosis do not have a clearly demonstrable cause for their disease. The assumption that the majority of such illnesses are caused by unrecognized viral hepatitis, while plausible, is without firm basis.

The clinical manifestations of cirrhosis are variable and may reflect the loss of hepatic cells with jaundice, wasting, hypoalbuminemia, and a bleeding tendency or may be secondary to scarring and architectural distortion of the liver resulting in portal hypertension. Occasionally cirrhosis is completely asymptomatic and discovered only at autopsy.

TABLE 67–1
Causes of Cirrhosis

I. Acquired
- A. Alcohol
- B. Hepatitis viruses (B and non-A, non-B)
- C. Hepatotoxins (e.g., vinyl chloride)
- D. Drug reactions (e.g., methyldopa)
- E. Biliary cirrhosis
    1. Primary biliary cirrhosis
    2. Secondary biliary cirrhosis
        a. Sclerosing cholangitis
        b. Bile duct stricture
        c. Bile duct tumors
- F. Cardiac cirrhosis
- G. Infiltrative diseases (sarcoidosis—rare)
- H. Infectious diseases
    1. (?) Schistosomiasis
    2. Brucellosis—rare

II. Genetically Determined
- A. Hepatolenticular degeneration (Wilson's disease)
- B. Hemochromatosis
- C. Galactosemia
- D. Cystic fibrosis
- E. Alpha$_1$-antitrypsin deficiency

The major problems facing the clinician in the management of a patient with cirrhosis are to: 1) establish an exact etiologic diagnosis and remove, insofar as possible, the inciting agent; 2) assess the nature and extent of complications; 3) estimate prognosis. The most common causes of cirrhosis and methods utilized to establish the etiology are listed in Table 67–2. In this chapter the major types of cirrhoses (alcoholic, postnecrotic, biliary, hepatolenticular degeneration [Wilson's disease] and hemochromatosis) are presented along with a discussion of chronic active hepatitis and hepatocellular carcinoma.

ALCOHOLIC LIVER DISEASE

Alcohol ingestion in man is related to the development of: 1) fatty liver; 2) alcoholic hepatitis; and 3) alcoholic (Laennec's) cirrhosis.[70] Cirrhosis related to chronic alcoholism is the most common form of chronic liver disease seen in the United States and its incidence has roughly paralleled the per capita consumption of alcohol. During the Prohibition era, deaths from cirrhosis decreased and following the repeal of the law began to rise again. The majority (80 to 90 percent) of patients with alcoholic cirrhosis give

a history of years of alcohol use and individual susceptibility to the development of cirrhosis shows considerable variability. In epidemiologic studies, only a small percentage (approximately 1 in 12) of chronic alcoholics develop cirrhosis. While the amount of alcohol ingested is established as the most important factor in the development of alcoholic cirrhosis, several observations suggest that unknown constitutional or genetic factors are also of importance.

MECHANISM OF ALCOHOL-INDUCED LIVER DISEASES

The relative contributions of alcohol as a hepatotoxin and the protein-vitamin deficient diet so characteristic of the chronic alcoholic to the development of cirrhosis are areas of continuing study. Malnutrition of proteins or vitamins per se has not been demonstrated to lead to cirrhosis in man. Cirrhosis does not develop in the most severe form of protein malnutrition, kwashiorkor. In addition, patients with alcoholic cirrhosis may improve rapidly on a very low protein diet once alcohol intake is stopped. The work of Rubin and Lieber[76] has demonstrated direct hepatotoxicity of alcohol apart from any dietary deficiencies. In their studies, short-term administration of alcohol to volunteers induced both fatty changes and ultrastructural abnormalities with electron microscopic demonstration of distorted mitochondria and vesiculated rough endoplasmic reticulum. Direct toxic effects of alcohol on liver cells are the most likely mechanisms of injury, but associated malnutrition may contribute to the liver damage. The inflammatory lesion alcoholic hepatitis and not the mere presence of fat is the precursor of alcoholic cirrhosis.

CLINICAL FEATURES

Fatty liver is the most frequent hepatic abnormality noted in alcoholics.[69] A combination of increased influx of fatty acids from adipose stores, enhanced hepatic synthesis of triglycerides from fatty acids derived from the diet, decreased fatty acid oxidation, and impaired hepatic lipoprotein synthesis are all of apparent importance in pathogenesis.

Fatty liver in the alcoholic may be clinically silent or may mimic more severe hepatic disease. Hepatomegaly often associated with hepatic tenderness is frequent. Abnormal BSP retention and an elevated serum alkaline phosphatase are common laboratory abnormalities. Jaundice is unusual, but an occasional patient may present with cholestatic jaundice and hepatic tenderness which mimic extrahepatic biliary obstruction. Liver biopsy is required to make the diagnosis of fatty liver and to assess the stage of the alcoholic liver disease. Fatty liver without concomi-

TABLE 67-2
An Approach to Establish the Etiology of Cirrhosis

Presumed Etiology	History	Histology	Additional Diagnostic Tests
Alcohol	Long-term (years) heavy ingestion of alcohol	Fatty infiltration; alcoholic hyaline; portal (usual) or postnecrotic pattern	None
Hepatitis virus(es)	Exposure to jaundiced persons or drug addicts, history of blood transfusions; intravenous drug abuse	Postnecrotic pattern with areas of collapse; often active hepatocellular necrosis	Presence of HBsAg
Hepatotoxic or drug idiosyncratic reactions	Exposure	Postnecrotic cirrhosis Biliary cirrhosis	None
Cardiac congestion	Recurrent congestive failure; tricuspid and mitral valve disease	Centrilobular congestion and fibrosis	Demonstration of elevated venous pressure
Biliary obstruction			
Primary biliary cirrhosis	Middle-aged females; pruritus	Chronic nonsuppurative destructive cholangitis	Presence of antimitochondrial antibodies ($>$ 85 percent)
Secondary	History of biliary tract surgery	Biliary cirrhosis	Visualization of the extrahepatic duct system by endoscopic retrograde bile duct cannulation, transhepatic cholangiography, or surgical exploration
Metabolic disorders			
Hepatolenticular Degeneration	+ family history; neurologic disturbances	Postnecrotic cirrhosis; increased hepatic copper	Serum ceruloplasmin; hepatic copper
Hemochromatosis	+ family history; diabetes; hyperpigmentation	Portal (usual) or postnecrotic cirrhosis; increased hepatic iron	Serum iron and iron binding capacity
Granulomatous disorders	(rare causes of cirrhosis)		
Schistosomiasis	Endemic areas	Pipestem fibrosis; granulomas	Demonstration of ova in liver or rectal biopsy
Sarcoidosis	Pulmonary disease, skin rash, lymphadenopathy	Diffuse granulomas and inflammation	Kveim test of occasional use

tant alcoholic hepatitis has an excellent prognosis with the fat resolving over a 4- to 6-week period of adequate diet and abstinence from alcohol.[69] Although both fatty liver and cirrhosis are found in the alcoholic, progression of the fatty lesion alone to cirrhosis has not been demonstrated.

Alcoholic liver disease with cell necrosis (alcoholic hepatitis) may present as an acute illness occurring during a prolonged bout of heavy alcohol intake or may be discovered when a liver biopsy is performed in an otherwise asymptomatic alcoholic with liver function test abnormalities. Abdominal pain, an enlarged tender liver, nausea, vomiting and jaundice are common presentations of alcoholic hepatitis. Fever is present with active hepatic necrosis in the ab-

sence of infection. Other manifestations of alcoholism such as pancreatitis, gastritis, peripheral neuritis, Wernicke's encephalopathy, malnutrition, or intercurrent infection often first lead the patient to seek medical attention.

Laboratory abnormalities may include hyperbilirubinemia, elevated SGOT (100 to 300 MIU), and a decrease in serum albumin. The degree of aminotransferase elevation does not reflect the extent of hepatocellular injury. SGPT is usually much lower than the SGOT in patients with alcoholic hepatitis. Leukocytosis may be pronounced. Hypokalemia is frequent in these patients and may represent gastrointestinal losses, decreased oral intake, or increased urinary excretion through acquired renal tubular acidosis. The serum IgA is often remarkably elevated. Liver biopsy reveals fatty infiltration and cell necrosis. Perinuclear eosinophilic inclusions designated alcoholic hyaline or Mallory bodies are typical. Occasionally acute alcoholic disease presents with fever, pruritus, and a predominant elevation in the serum conjugated bilirubin suggesting extrahepatic obstruction of the biliary system. Bouts of alcoholic hepatitis occurring in patients with established cirrhosis are designated florid cirrhosis or active Laennec's cirrhosis.

Alcoholic cirrhosis is most often a disease of middle-age with a history of alcohol use for 5 to 15 years. Although malnutrition and a past history of pancreatitis, gastritis, neglect, and previous bouts of acute alcoholic hepatitis are common, advanced alcoholic cirrhosis may develop in asymptomatic, well-nourished patients. In many patients cirrhosis has an insidious onset and is recognized only after the development of weight loss, ascites, confusion, or the occurrence of an upper gastrointestinal hemorrhage.

Physical examination reveals the signs of hepatocellular failure such as palmar erythema, spider angiomas, jaundice, Dupuytren's contractures, peripheral neuritis, and enlargement of the parotids and lacrimals. Clinical evidences of hypogonadism and overt feminization with gynecomastia and development of a female escutcheon and body habitus is frequently found in men with cirrhosis. The pathogenesis of these changes is complex. Male cirrhotics do have a decreased production of testosterone and a slight increase in circulating estrogen levels but these changes do not correlate well with the clinical manifestations. There is evidence to suggest a hypothalamic defect with abnormal hypothalamic-pituitary secretion of gonadotropins.[81]

The liver is generally enlarged and firm early in the course of cirrhosis but later may be of normal size or even small. Abnormalities in liver function are variable and depend on the activity of the disease. Anemia, leukopenia, and thrombocytopenia are often present. Liver biopsy is important in establishing the diagnosis and in staging the disease. The histologic pattern may be that of fatty infiltration, present or past cell necrosis, diffuse fine scarring linking portal triads and central veins, inflammatory infiltrates or any combination of these. Occasionally the liver in patients with long-standing alcoholic cirrhosis has a postnecrotic pattern with large irregular nodules. Histologically significant cirrhosis may be discovered only incidentally ("compensated cirrhosis") when abnormal liver function tests are observed and liver biopsy performed in the course of evaluating other complaints. A number of instances of alcoholic cirrhosis are discovered for the first time at autopsy.

PROGNOSIS AND SURVIVAL IN ALCOHOLIC CIRRHOSIS

The course and prognosis in alcoholic as well as other forms of cirrhosis is dependent on the ability of the liver to heal and regenerate itself. The most important determinant of healing and survival in patients with Laennec's cirrhosis is abstinence from alcohol. In a study of 278 patients with biopsy-proven Laennec's cirrhosis, Powell and Klatskin[74] observed a 63 percent overall 5-year survival in the 93 patients who stopped drinking as opposed to a 40.5 percent 5-year survival in the 185 patients who continued to drink.

The overall improved survival of patients with cirrhosis in the past 30 years may relate to emphasis on abstinence from alcohol, nutritious diet, improved understanding of the management of fluid and electrolyte disturbances, antibiotics for control of intercurrent infections, and more successful treatment of hepatic encephalopathy and bleeding esophageal varices (Chap. 64).

Abstinence from alcohol is the cornerstone of therapy for the patient with alcohol-related liver disease. Associated vitamin deficiencies are more common in these patients, and liver biopsy often reveals evidence of coexisting acute and chronic disease. Patients with jaundice and liver function abnormalities developing in a setting of acute alcoholism often benefit from evaluation in the hospital. Other complications of alcoholism such as decreased resistance to infection, electrolyte abnormalities, gastritis, and delirium tremens further complicate management. Corticosteroids have been investigated in patients with alcoholic hepatitis with varying degrees of success.

POSTNECROTIC CIRRHOSIS AND CHRONIC ACTIVE HEPATITIS

POSTNECROTIC CIRRHOSIS (PNC)

Grouped under the heading of postnecrotic cirrhosis are a number of liver diseases of both known and unknown etiology. Postnecrotic cirrhosis is the most frequent form of cirrhosis worldwide and is characterized pathologically by large areas of collapse suggesting previous significant but nonuniform liver cell damage, broad scars, and regenerating nodules of up to several centimeters in diameter. Injury to the liver by hepatitis virus as in chronic active hepatitis (see below), hepatotoxins (e.g., vinyl chloride), idiosyncratic drug reactions (e.g., methyldopa), and hepatolenticular degeneration are among the diverse processes implicated in the etiology of postnecrotic cirrhosis. In the majority of patients, no etiology can be established. The pathologic pattern of postnecrotic cirrhosis may be predominant in many patients with long-standing alcoholic liver disease.

Postnecrotic cirrhosis may be a clinically silent disorder or present with hepatocellular insufficiency and the complications of portal hypertension.[72] Patients with active cell disease are indistinguishable from the later stages of chronic active hepatitis with predominant manifestations of jaundice, ascites, and hepatic encephalopathy. In a patient with a small shrunken liver and no history or physical evidence of hepatocellular disease, the cirrhosis may first be diagnosed after an episode of hemorrhage from esophagogastric varices. These patients may also have unexplained bouts of abdominal pain or ascites. Hepatocellular carcinoma develops in 15 to 20 percent of patients with postnecrotic cirrhosis and should be considered whenever there is clinical deterioration in a previously stable patient.

CHRONIC HEPATITIS

Chronic hepatitis may be defined as an unresolving inflammatory liver disease lasting more than 3 months.[66] All ages and both sexes may be affected. Within the designation chronic hepatitis are two broad groups, *chronic persistent hepatitis* (CPH) and *chronic active hepatitis* (CAH). While the distinction between CPH and CAH can often be suggested on clinical and laboratory evaluation, liver biopsy is required to adequately define the illness.

Chronic Persistent Hepatitis

Chronic persistent hepatitis is a basically benign condition often detected when routine blood testing or follow-up after a bout of viral hepatitis reveals an elevation in serum aminotransferases. Chronic persistent hepatitis may result from hepatitis B infection often with persistence of HBsAg or be of unknown etiology. These patients are often asymptomatic. Liver function studies other than the elevated aminotransferases are generally normal. The liver biopsy reveals an intact lobular architecture and the major abnormality is predominantly a lymphocytic portal inflammation. The limiting plate around the portal triad may be eroded slightly and there may be focal inflammation throughout the hepatic parenchyma. There is little or no fibrosis. The prognosis for CPH is excellent and no treatment other than reassurance that no progressive liver disease is present is indicated.

Chronic Active Hepatitis

Chronic active hepatitis (CAH) is the designation for a group of liver diseases of various etiologies characterized by a prolonged course with continuing or episodic bouts of cell necrosis, fibrosis, and usually progression to postnecrotic cirrhosis. Knowledge of the frequency, pathogenesis, clinical manifestations, and treatment of these important disorders has rapidly expanded in the past decade.

There are several established etiologies for the syndrome of chronic active hepatitis with marked geographic variations in the incidence of the various types (Table 67–3).

The most frequently encountered group of patients with CAH have no established cause for their illness and are designated as *idiopathic*. Several clinical and laboratory features suggest that many of these idiopathic cases of chronic active hepatitis are the result of altered immune reactivity. No viral agent has been identified and the HBsAG is uniformly absent. The majority of this group (75 percent) are women with many having the onset of disease during adolescence. Gradual, often insidious appearance of jaundice and fatigue are major manifestations. Hyperglobulinemia is usually found; the L.E. cell preparation is occasionally positive (15 percent); and smooth muscle and antinuclear antibodies are frequent. Antimitochondrial antibodies occur in some patients (10 percent). Extrahepatic manifestations of disease including amenorrhea, Hashimoto's thyroiditis, pleurisy, polyarthritis, Coombs positive hemolytic anemia, Sjögren syndrome, and chronic diarrhea may dominate the presentation and further suggest a role for altered immunity. There is an apparent increased incidence of idiopathic chronic active hepatitis in patients with histocompatibility antigens HLA-A1 or HLA-A8. On physical examination these patients usually have hepatomegaly and often splenomegaly and ascites. Jaundice, acne, diffuse rashes, and a bleeding tendency with purpura may be apparent.

Idiosyncratic drug reactions involving the liver are recognized causes of a chronic active hepatitis-like illness.[55] Such reactions produce liver biopsy changes indistinguishable from CAH of other etiologies and the diagnosis can be established only by identification and withdrawal of the inciting drug. Methyldopa and isoniazid are both agents that have produced these biopsy changes. Another drug, oxyphenisatin, that was a component of several widely

---

TABLE 67–3
Etiologic Factors in Chronic Active Hepatitis

1. Idiopathic
2. Hepatitis B
3. Hepatitis non-A, non-B
4. Wilson's disease
5. Alpha$_1$-antitrypsin deficiency
6. Therapeutic drugs (e.g., methyldopa)

used laxatives has been established through rechallenge studies to produce CAH. Several of these patients in addition to the hepatitis developed L.E. cells, and smooth muscle and antinuclear antibodies. A careful search for possible inciting drugs should be part of the evaluation of every case of CAH.

Hepatitis B virus is an established cause of chronic active hepatitis accounting for 30 to 40 percent of the patients diagnosed in the United States. In these patients HBsAg tends to persist in the blood and an abnormal immune response to infection with HBsAg is suggested in the pathogenesis. The HBsAg-associated cases more often occur in men and often have an abrupt clinical onset with an acute bout of viral hepatitis which subsequently does not resolve. Chronic active hepatitis associated with HBsAg, however, may be found in asymptomatic patients discovered on routine blood testing to have the antigen and abnormal liver function tests. Extrahepatic manifestations of diseases often found with idiopathic CAH, such as thyroiditis, hemolytic anemia, and Sjögren syndrome, are unusual in CAH associated with HBsAg. Hyperglobulinemia is unusual and L.E. cells are not found. There is no evidence hepatitis A virus leads to chronic active hepatitis or cirrhosis. The agent or agents of hepatitis non-A, non-B, however, can produce CAH and result in postnecrotic cirrhosis.

Wilson's disease (p. 742) may present in an adolescent or young adult as a chronic active hepatitis with little or no evidence of neurologic damage. Furthermore, patients with hereditary deficiency of alpha$_1$ antitrypsin may have a clinical course and liver biopsy indistinguishable from CAH of other etiologies.

The pathologic features of CAH are variable. In all there is evidence of ongoing cell necrosis with portal and periportal inflammation with mononuclear and plasma cells, diffuse fibrosis, and often widespread focal hepatitis. In many patients, bridging areas of necrosis interconnecting portal and central areas of the lobule are the dominant features. Whole lobules may be collapsed (multilobular necrosis). Postnecrotic cirrhosis is already present at the time of diagnosis in many patients and develops subsequently in the majority.

The course of CAH, regardless of etiology, is variable and in untreated patients may be one of continuous deterioration with early death or intermittent bouts of acutely active hepatitis with interspersed temporary apparent remissions. Treatment with corticosteroids is clearly indicated in patients with idiopathic chronic active hepatitis.[67,79,80] Treatment with corticosteroids should be promptly instituted once the diagnosis is established and the drugs slowly ta-

pered following the clinical state of the patient, the serum aminotransferases, and the serum albumin. Repeated liver biopsies are most helpful in determining the effectiveness of therapy. Immunosuppressant drugs (e.g., azathioprine) have not been demonstrated to be as effective in therapy alone as are the corticosteroids but may be useful adjunctive agents particularly in patients who develop severe side effects from corticosteroids.[79] In patients with drug-induced disease, recognition of the inciting drug and withdrawal usually is sufficient and corticosteroid therapy not indicated. The role of corticosteroids in patients with hepatitis B virus-induced chronic active hepatitis is uncertain. In these patients a trial of corticosteroids is warranted with withdrawal of the drug if no clinical and histologic improvement is obtained.

Patients with postnecrotic cirrhosis and no evidence of ongoing necrosis often present with bleeding from esophagogastric varices, and the prognosis is dependent on the success in managing hematemesis and its sequelae. These patients often are suitable candidates for a portal systemic shunt operation.

BILIARY CIRRHOSIS

Prolonged stasis of bile is often associated with portal and periportal inflammation which over a period of months to years leads to fibrosis. Biliary cirrhosis results from linkage of these periportal areas of fibrosis. The biliary obstruction may lie in the major extrahepatic ducts (secondary biliary cirrhosis) or in the small intrahepatic biliary radicles as in primary biliary cirrhosis. The characteristic clinical features of biliary cirrhosis develop slowly and are direct consequences of the interruption of bile flow.

PRIMARY BILIARY CIRRHOSIS

This is a disease predominantly of middle-aged females (ages 30 to 55), who present with pruritus, dark urine, hepatomegaly, and evidence of steatorrhea.[78] The disorder occasionally has its onset during pregnancy. Pruritus may precede other symptoms by many months and occasionally years. Most patients feel well during the early years of the disorder complaining only of pruritus and the adverse cosmetic effects of jaundice. From its insidious beginnings, the disease slowly progresses to a characteristic picture of xanthomata, bone pain, hyperpigmentation, and cirrhosis. Most patients die in 5 to 10 years from the onset of jaundice of hepatic cellular insufficiency. Signs of hepatocellular insufficiency such as angiomas, palmar erythema, ascites, and bleeding from esophagogastric varices are late occurrences.

The etiology of primary biliary cirrhosis is not known. No virus has been isolated and an increased incidence of hepatitis B antigen has not been found. Occasionally patients have had the onset of clinically typical primary biliary cirrhosis while taking phenothiazine drugs with continuing activity of the liver disease after the drugs are stopped. An observed association with the CRST syndrome (calcinosis, Raynaud's phenomenon, sclerodactyly, and telangiectasia) and with Sjögren syndrome suggests links with other disorders of presumed disturbed immunity.[75] Certain laboratory findings strongly suggest altered immune responses in primary biliary cirrhosis. The serum immunoglobulin M (IgM) level is elevated in 80 percent and plasma cells in the portal and periportal region have been demonstrated to contain IgM. Circulating immune complexes containing cryoglobulins have also been found. Immunofluorescent studies have demonstrated a circulating antibody directed against mitochondria (antimitochondrial antibody) in greater than 85 percent of patients with primary biliary cirrhosis.[68] These antibodies are rarely positive in patients with extrahepatic obstruction of the bile ducts but are found in 10 to 15 percent of patients with chronic active hepatitis and postnecrotic cirrhosis. The interrelation of these disorders remains uncertain.

Laboratory features of primary biliary cirrhosis include hyperbilirubinemia with the serum bilirubin usually from 4 to 10 mg/dl. The alkaline phosphatase is markedly elevated and hypercholesterolemia of an extreme degree (2000 mg/dl) may be present. The serum aminotransferase enzymes are usually only slightly (100 to 200 units) increased. Liver biopsy in primary biliary cirrhosis characteristically shows portal inflammation and nonsuppurative destruction of bile ducts in the portal triads. Ductular proliferation may be a dominant feature and granulomas are often found in and around the damaged ducts. Bile stasis and periportal fibrosis may be prominent, but actual cirrhosis is a late finding.

The major complications of primary biliary cirrhosis are bone pain and fractures secondary to vitamin D deficiency and osteomalacia and occasional bleeding disorders associated with decreased absorption of vitamin K. Xanthomatous involvement of peripheral nerves may cause neuritis. The management of the disorder is supportive. Cholestyramine may be useful in controlling pruritus. Vitamin D or its derivative 25-hydroxycholecalciferol may be useful in the management of bone pain. Corticosteroid therapy is not useful in primary biliary cirrhosis and may accel-

erate osteomalacia. Preliminary trials of D-penicillamine have shown encouraging results. This agent may act by removing the excess copper characteristically found in the liver or by directly inhibiting fibrosis.

SECONDARY BILIARY CIRRHOSIS

Secondary biliary cirrhosis may result from choledocholithiasis, bile duct strictures developing after biliary tract surgery, or slow growing carcinoma of the bile ducts. It is most important to rule out a secondary, possibly correctable, cause of bile duct obstruction in any patient with biliary cirrhosis. In most instances, transduodenal cholangiography or percutaneous transhepatic cholangiography is required. The immunofluorescent tests are of considerable value in differential diagnosis of patients with a positive antimitochondrial antibody test, providing strong evidence when positive for primary biliary cirrhosis.

SCLEROSING CHOLANGITIS

Sclerosing cholangitis is a rare cause of chronic obstructive jaundice characterized pathologically by diffuse thickening and obliteration of the major bile ducts. Sclerosing cholangitis may result from recurrent cholangitis often associated with recurrent choledocholithiasis or may follow bile duct injury during surgery. Sclerosing cholangitis with no previous history of choledocholithiasis or surgery (primary sclerosing cholangitis) is a disorder of unknown etiology which may be associated with Crohn's disease, ulcerative colitis, or retroperitoneal fibrosis. The diagnosis of sclerosing cholangitis is established by demonstration of irregular diffusely narrowed bile ducts by endoscopic retrograde cholangiography or transhepatic cholangiography. It is generally difficult or impossible to distinguish sclerosing cholangitis from slow-growing carcinomas of the bile ducts. There is no satisfactory therapy for sclerosing cholangitis. Vitamins D, A, and K and cholestyramine may be useful in managing complications. Corticosteroid therapy, long-term antibiotics, and attempts at reconstructive surgery are all of doubtful value.

HEMOCHROMATOSIS

Hemochromatosis is a rare disorder of iron metabolism characterized by the gradual accumulation of excessive tissue iron stores associated with parenchymal damage and fibrosis.[71] The principal organs involved are the liver, pancreas, heart, and gonads. Total body iron stores are increased from the normal 4 g to as much as 60 g. The pathogenesis of hemochromatosis is apparently an increase in iron absorption from the gut with both genetic and environmental factors of importance. Family studies suggest that some instances of hemochromatosis are transmitted as an autosomal dominant with variable penetrance. Environmental factors associated with an increased iron uptake include ingestion of alcoholic beverages (especially wine); cooking in iron pots; and long-term administration of medicinal iron in refractory anemias.

The majority of patients with hemochromatosis are males (80 percent) and in 70 percent the disease becomes manifest between the ages of 40 and 60. The disorder is rare under the age of 20. Constitutional symptoms of lassitude and weakness are frequent. The liver is large, firm, and frequently tender. The spleen is usually enlarged. Esophagogastric varices and other signs of portal hypertension are less common than in alcoholic or postnecrotic cirrhosis. Ascites and hepatocellular failure are late manifestations. Diabetes mellitus occurs in the majority of patients and insulin therapy is required. Cardiac involvement may be manifested by congestive heart failure or by arrhythmias from involvement of both the myocardium and the cardiac conduction system (particularly the A-V node). The congestive failure in hemochromatosis may be resistant to digitalis therapy. Increased skin pigmentation is the result of melanin deposition in the basal layers of the thinned epidermis and is best seen over exposed areas, in the axillae and groin, and in scars. In some patients iron deposited in the corium adds to the pigmentation. Impotence is frequent and associated with testicular atrophy and fibrosis. Less common manifestations include arthritis from synovial deposition of iron and evidence of anterior pituitary insufficiency which may also contribute to the impotence. Chondrocalcinosis (pseudogout) is frequently found.

The goal of therapy in hemochromatosis is removal of the excess tissue iron and this is accomplished by repeated phlebotomy. Removal of 500 ml of blood rids the body of 250 mg of iron and mobilizes iron from the tissue stores. Because the amount of tissue iron may be 20 to 60 g, phlebotomy of 500 ml per week is required for up to 2 years. The effectiveness of the therapy is ascertained by determining the serum iron, iron binding capacity, and follow-up liver biopsy. For patients with hemochromatosis secondary to chronic refractory anemic states, phlebotomy is not possible and the less satisfactory therapy of

chelating agents (desferrioxamine) is instituted. Only 10 to 15 mg iron per day can be mobilized by chelation therapy. Therapy to remove iron should be instituted in asymptomatic relatives of patients with hemochromatosis when an elevation in iron stores is found.

The diagnosis of hemochromatosis is established by finding an elevation of the serum iron ($>$ 220 μg/dl), saturation of the serum iron binding capacity (greater than 90 percent), an elevated serum ferritin, and demonstration of increased tissue iron stores on liver biopsy. Liver function tests are often near normal even when considerable tissue damage is present. Diagnostic tests with iron chelating agents such as desferrioxamine are useful in demonstrating increased body stores of iron but are seldom required for diagnosis.

Hepatocellular carcinoma develops in up to 20 percent of patients with hemochromatosis.

HEPATOLENTICULAR DEGENERATION (Wilson's Disease)

Wilson's disease is a rare inherited disorder of metabolism characterized by accumulation of copper in the liver, central nervous system, cornea, kidneys and other tissues.[82] The disorder is inherited as an autosomal recessive and becomes apparent most frequently during adolescence. Liver and neurologic disease, separately or in combination, usually dominate the clinical manifestations. Wilson's disease may present with modest liver function abnormalities or as a chronic active hepatitis in an adolescent with no evidence of neurologic disease.[77] Neurologic symptoms usually present after the liver disease with the most frequent signs being those of basal ganglia damage especially rigidity, choreoathetoid movements, and ataxia. Less common presentations include hemolytic anemia or renal disease with aminoaciduria, uricosuria, and phosphaturia (acquired Fanconi syndrome). The persistent phosphaturia may cause osteomalacia. Of particular diagnostic importance is the presence of Kayser-Fleischer rings which are brownish rings of pigment at the periphery of the cornea secondary to copper deposition in Descemet's membrane, and are pathognomonic of Wilson's disease.

The pathogenesis of Wilson's disease is most likely an inability to excrete copper into the bile possibly through abnormalities in hepatic lysosome function. The major biochemical manifestations of Wilson's disease are a deficiency in ceruloplasmin, the plasma copper binding protein, an increase in hepatic copper, and an increase in urinary copper excretion. The total serum copper is generally reduced but the free (unbound) copper is markedly increased.

The diagnosis of Wilson's disease is established by the demonstration of a reduced plasma ceruloplasmin (< 20 mg/dl) and an increased hepatic copper (> 250 µg/g dry weight). These abnormalities should be sought in relatives of affected patients since excess copper stores can be reduced by the copper chelating agent D-penicillamine.

HEPATOCELLULAR CARCINOMA

Hepatic cell tumors generally arise from areas of long-standing liver injury with necrosis and repair. The majority of hepatocellular carcinomas occur in cirrhotic livers, although the number of these tumors developing in the absence of cirrhosis is apparently increasing. Marked geographic variations are found with hepatocellular carcinomas accounting for only 1 to 2 percent of all malignant tumors in North America but up to 30 percent of malignant tumors in certain parts of Africa and Asia. The demonstration that aflatoxins, food contaminants derived from *Aspergillus flavus,* are hepatic carcinogens has led to speculation that these compounds may explain in part the geographic variations.[65] An increased incidence of persistent hepatitis B viremia in patients with hepatocellular carcinomas with or without cirrhosis has been reported.

The diagnosis of hepatocellular carcinoma may be difficult to establish clinically and the tumor may be initially found at postmortem. Hepatocellular carcinoma should be considered whenever a patient with known cirrhosis has an accelerated deterioration with weight loss, rapidly enlarging liver, right upper quadrant abdominal pain, and accumulation of ascites especially when blood-tinged. Both friction rubs and hepatic bruits may be heard over the surface of the liver. Hepatocellular carcinomas may initially present with one of several paraneoplastic syndromes including erythrocytosis, porphyria cutanea tarda, virilizing syndromes, hypercalcemia, and dysproteinemias.[73] Hypoglycemia is common and most often relates to the large metabolic requirements of the tumor.

The majority of patients with hepatocellular carcinoma have increased concentrations of serum fetoglobulin and detection of this fetoprotein may confirm a suspicion of hepatocellular carcinoma. Elevated alpha-fetoprotein is rare in other tumors except in embryonal teratoblastomas and in some patients with hepatitis—conditions not likely to cause diagnostic confusion. Alpha-fetoglobulin is detected in approximately half of hepatocellular carcinomas in North America but in much higher percentages in those found in Africa. Celiac arteriography and liver scans using [67]Gallium are additional diagnostic aids.

Treatment of hepatocellular carcinoma is almost universally unsuccessful. Chemotherapy has had little success. Occasional successful partial hepatectomies have been reported especially in children with hepatoblastomas. Liver transplantation has not proven successful.

REFERENCES

General References

1. Child, C.G., III. Portal Hypertension. Philadelphia, Saunders, 1974.
2. Popper, H. and Schaffner, F. Progress in Liver Diseases. New York, Grune & Stratton, 1962, 1965, 1970, 1972, Vols. 1, 2, 3, and 4.
   Excellent series of monographs reviewing areas of liver disease under present investigation.
3. Sherlock, S. Diseases of the Liver, 5th ed. Philadelphia, F. A. Davis, 1975.
   Concise, authoritative text. Selected references.
4. Schiff, L. Diseases of the Liver, 4th ed. Philadelphia, Lippincott, 1975.

Normal and Abnormal Hepatic Physiology, Liver Function Tests, and Classification of Diseases of the Liver

5. Bucher, N.L.R. Experimental aspects of hepatic regeneration. N. Engl. J. Med., 277:686,738, 1967.
6. Kaplan, M.M. Alkaline phosphatase. N. Engl. J. Med., 286:200, 1972.
7. Kowlessar, O.D., Haeffner, L.J., Riley, E.M., and Sleisenger, M.H. Comparative study of serum leucine aminopeptidase, 5'-nucleotidase and nonspecific alkaline phosphatase in diseases affecting the pancreas, hepatobiliary tree and bone. Am. J. Med., 31:231, 1961.
8. Menghini, G. One-second biopsy of the liver—problems of its clinical application. N. Engl. J. Med., 283:582, 1970.
9. Roberts, H.R. and Cederbaum, A.I. The liver and blood coagulation: physiology and pathology. Gastroenterology, 63:297, 1972.
10. Rothschild, M.A., Oratz, M., and Schreiber, S.S. Albumin metabolism. Gastroenterology, 64:324, 1973.
11. Vennes, J.A., Jacobson, J.R., and Silvis, S.E. Endoscopic cholangiography for biliary system diagnosis. Ann. Intern. Med., 80:61, 1974.
12. Wise, R.E. and Scholz, F.J. Radiology of the liver and biliary tract. Gastroenterology, 65:967, 1973.

Principal Manifestations of Liver Disease: Jaundice and Hepatomegaly

13. Arias, I.M., Gartner, L.M., Cohen, M., Ben Ezzer, J., and Levi, A.J. Chronic nonhemolytic unconjugated hyperbilirubinemia with glucuronyl transferase deficiency. Am. J. Med., 47:395, 1969.
14. Black, M. and Billing, B.H. Hepatic bilirubin UDP-glucuronyl transferase activity in liver disease and Gilbert's syndrome. N. Engl. J. Med., 280:1266, 1969.
15. Dubin, I.N. Chronic idiopathic jaundice. A review of fifty cases. Am. J. Med., 24:268, 1958.
16. Kantrowitz, P.A., Jones, W.A., Greenberger, N.J., and Isselbacher, K.J. Severe postoperative hyperbilirubinemia simulating obstructive jaundice. N. Engl. J. Med., 276:591, 1967.
17. Levi, A.J., Gatmaitan, Z., and Arias, I.M. Two hepatic cytoplasmic protein fractions, Y and Z, and their possible role in the hepatic uptake of bilirubin, sulfobromophthalein, and other anions. J. Clin. Invest., 48:2156, 1969.
18. Levine, R.A. and Klatskin, G. Unconjugated hyperbilirubinemia in the absence of overt hemolysis. Am. J. Med., 36:541, 1964.
19. Powell, L.E., Hemingway, E., Billing, B.H., and Sherlock, S. Idiopathic unconjugated hyperbilirubinemia (Gilbert's syndrome). N. Engl. J. Med., 277:1108, 1967.
20. Schmid, R. Bilirubin metabolism in man. N. Engl. J. Med., 287:703, 1972.
21. Wollaeger, E.E. and Gross, J.B. Complete obstruction of the extra-hepatic biliary tract due to carcinoma as determined by the fecal urobilinogen test: incidence and effect on serum bilirubin concentrations. Medicine, 45:529, 1966.

Principal Manifestations of Liver Disease: Ascites, Hepatorenal Syndrome, Portal Hypertension, and Hepatic Encephalopathy

22. Atkinson, M. and Losowsky, M.S. The mechanism of ascites formation in chronic liver disease. Q. J. Med., 30:153, 1961.
23. Burack, W.R. and Hollister, R.M. Tuberculous peritonitis. Am. J. Med., 28:510, 1960.
24. Conn, H.O. The prognosis and management of bleeding esophageal varices. Ann. N.Y. Acad. Sci., 170:345, 1970.
25. ———, Lindenmuth, W.W., May, C.J., and Ramsby, G.R. Prophylactic portacaval anastomosis. Medicine, 51:27, 1972.
26. Correia, J.P. and Conn, H.O. Spontaneous bacterial peritonitis in cirrhosis: endemic or epidemic. Med. Clin. N. Am. 59:963, 1975.
27. Dumont, A.E., Witte, C.L., and Witte, M.H. Interrelationship of vascular and lymphatic changes in liver injury. Ann. N.Y. Acad. Sci., 170:127, 1970.
28. Gabuzda, G.J. Ammonium metabolism and hepatic coma. Gastroenterology, 53:806, 1967.
29. Kinney, M.J., Wapnick, S., Ahmed, N., Ip, M., Grosberg, S., and LeVeen, H.H. Cirrhosis, ascites, and impaired renal function: treatment with the LeVeen-type chronic peritoneal-venous shunt. In Epstein, M. (ed.),

The Kidney in Liver Disease. New York, Elsevier, 1978, pp. 349–364.
30. Losowsky, M.S., Jones, D.P., Lieber, C.S., and Davidson, C.S. Local factors in ascites formation during sodium retention in cirrhosis. N. Engl. J. Med., 268:651, 1963.
31. Malt, R.A. Portasystemic venous shunts. N. Engl. J. Med., 295:24, 80, 1976.
32. Papper, S. Renal failure in cirrhosis (the hepatorenal syndrome). In Epstein, M. (ed.), The Kidney in Liver Disease. New York, Elsevier, 1978, pp. 91–112.
33. Read, A.E., Sherlock, S., Laidlaw, J., and Walker, J.G. The neuropsychiatric syndromes associated with chronic liver disease and an extensive portal-systemic collateral circulation. Q. J. Med., 36:135, 1967.
34. Reynolds, T.B., Ito, S., and Iwatsuki, S. Measurement of portal pressure and its clinical application. Am. J. Med., 49–649, 1970.
35. Resnick, R.H., Chalmers, T.C., Ishihara, A.M., Garceau, A.J., Callow, A.D., Schimmel, E.M., O'Hara, E.T., and the Boston Inter-Hospital Liver Group. A controlled study of prophylactic portacaval shunt: Final report. Ann. Intern. Med., 70:675, 1969.
36. Schenker, S., Breen, K.J., and Hoyumpa, A.M., Jr. Hepatic encephalopathy: current status. Gastroenterology, 66:121, 1974.
37. Shear, L., Ching, S., and Gabuzda, G.J. Compartmentalization of ascites and edema in patients with hepatic cirrhosis. N. Engl. J. Med., 282:1391, 1970.
38. Sherlock, S., Senewirathe, B., Scott, A., and Walker, J.G. Complications of diuretic therapy in hepatic cirrhosis. Lancet, 1:1049, 1966.

Circulatory and Focal Diseases of the Liver

39. Bras, G. and Hill, K.R. Veno-occlusive disease of the liver: Essential pathology. Lancet, 2:161, 1956.
40. Clain, D., Freston, J., Kreel, L., and Sherlock, S. Clinical diagnosis of the Budd-Chiari syndrome. Am. J. Med., 43:544, 1967.
41. Dunn, G.D., Hayes, P., Brien, K.J., and Schenker, S. The liver in congestive heart failure: a review. Am. J. Med. Sci., 265:174, 1973.
42. Fenster, L.F. and Klatskin, G. Manifestations of metastatic tumor of the liver. A study of eighty-one patients subjected to needle biopsy of the liver. Am. J. Med., 31:238, 1961.
43. Guckian, J.C. and Perry, J.E. Granulomatous hepatitis. An analysis of sixty-three cases and review of the literature. Ann. Intern. Med., 65:1081, 1966.
44. Lamont, N.M. and Pooler, N.R. Hepatic amoebiasis. Q. J. Med., 27:389, 1958.
45. Maddrey, W.C., Johns, C.J., Boitnott, J.K., and Iber, F.L. Sarcoidosis and chronic hepatic disease: a clinical and pathologic study of twenty patients. Medicine, 49:375, 1970.
46. Rosenblate, H.J., Eisenstein, R., and Holmes, A.W. The liver in sickle cell anemia. Arch. Pathol. Lab. Med., 90:235, 1970.
47. Rubin, R.H., Swartz, M.N., and Malt, R. Hepatic abscess: changes in clinical, bacteriologic and therapeutic aspects. Am. J. Med., 57:601, 1974.

Acute Diffuse Hepatocellular Disease

48. Berk, P.D., Martin, J.F., Young, R.S., Creech, J., Selikoff, I., Falk, H., Watanabe, P., Popper, H., and Thomas L. Vinyl chloride-associated liver disease. Ann. Intern. Med. 84:717, 1976.

49. Blum, A.L., Stutz, R., Haemmerli, U.P., Schmid, P., and Grady, G.F. A fortuitously controlled study of steriod therapy in acute viral hepatitis I. Acute disease. Am. J. Med., 47:82, 1969.

50. Chalmers, T.C., Eckhardt, R.D., Reynolds, W.E., Cigarroa, J.H., Jr., Deane, N., Reifenstein, R.W., Smith, C.W., and Davidson, C.S. The treatment of acute infectious hepatitis. Controlled studies of the effects of diet, rest, and physical reconditioning on the acute course of the disease and on the incidence of relapses and residual abnormalities. J. Clin. Invest. 34:1163, 1955.

51. Dienstag, J.L., Purcell, R.H., Alter, H.J., Feinstone, S.M., Wong, D.C., and Holland, P.V. Non-A, non-B post-transfusion hepatitis. Lancet, 1:560, 1977.

52. Ishak, K.G. and Irey, N.S. Hepatic injury associated with the phenothiazines: Clinicopathologic and follow-up study of 36 patients. Arch. Pathol. Lab. Med., 93:283, 1972.

53. Klatskin, G. Toxic and drug-induced hepatitis. In Schiff, L. (ed.), Diseases of the Liver, 3rd ed. Philadelphia, Lippincott, 1969, pp. 498–601.

54. Klion, F.M., Schaffner, F., and Popper, H. Hepatitis after exposure to halothane. Ann. Intern. Med., 71:467, 1969.

55. Maddrey, W.C. and Boitnott, J.K. Drug-induced chronic liver disease. Gastroenterology, 72:1348, 1977.

56. Mazzur, S., Burgert, S., and Blumberg, B.S. Geographical distribution of Australia antigen determinants d, y and w. Nature, 247:38, 1974.

57. Mitchell, J.R., Zimmerman, H.J., Ishak, K.G., Thorgeirsson, U.P., Timbrell, J.A., Snodgrass, W.R., and Nelson, S.D. Isoniazid liver injury: clinical spectrum, pathology and probable pathogenesis. Ann. Intern. Med. 84:181, 1976.

58. Partin, J.C. Reye's syndrome (encephalopathy and fatty liver). Gastroenterology 69:511, 1975.

59. Redeker, A.G. Viral hepatitis: clinical aspects. Am. J. Med. Sci., 270:9, 1975.

60. Repsher, L.H. and Freebern, R.K. Effects of early and vigorous exercise on recovery from infectious hepatitis. N. Engl. J. Med., 281:1393, 1969.

61. Ritt, D.J., Whelan, G., Werner, D.J., Eigenbrodt, E.H., Schenker, S., and Combes, B. Acute hepatic necrosis with stupor or coma: an analysis of thirty-one patients. Medicine, 48:151, 1969.

62. Robinson, W.S. and Lutwick, L.I. The virus of hepatitis, type B. N. Engl. J. Med., 295:1168, 1976.

63. Trepo, C.G., Magnius, L.O., Schaefer, R.A., and Prince, A.M. Detection of a e antigen and antibody: correlations with hepatitis B surface and hepatitis B core antigens, liver disease, and outcome in hepatitis B infections. Gastroenterology 71:804, 1976.

64. Wands, J.R., Alpert, E., and Isselbacher, K.J. Arthritis associated with chronic active hepatitis: complement activation and characterization of circulating immune complexes. Gastroenterology, 69:1286, 1975.

Chronic Diffuse Liver Disease: Cirrhosis

65. Alpert, M.E. and Davidson, C.S. Mycotoxins: a possible cause of primary carcinoma of the liver. Am. J. Med., 46:325, 1969.

66. Boyer, J.L. Chronic hepatitis—a perspective on classification and determinants of prognosis. Gastroenterology, 70:1161, 1976.

67. Cook, G.C., Mulligan, R., and Sherlock, S. Controlled prospective trial of corticosteroid therapy in active chronic hepatitis. Q. J. Med., 40:159, 1971.

68. Klatskin, G. and Kantor, F.S. Mitochondrial antibody in primary biliary cirrhosis and other diseases. Ann. Intern. Med., 77:533, 1972.

69. Leevy, C.M. Fatty liver: a study of 270 patients with biopsy proven fatty liver and a review of the literature. Medicine, 41:249, 1962.

70. Lieber, C.S. Pathogenesis and early diagnosis of alcoholic liver injury. N. Engl. J. Med. 298:888, 1978.

71. MacDonald, R.A. Primary hemochromatosis: inherited or acquired? In Brown, E. B. and Moore, C. V. (eds.), Progress in Hematology, Vol. V. New York, Grune & Stratton, 1966, pp. 324–353.

72. ——— and Mallory, G.K. The natural history of postnecrotic cirrhosis. Am. J. Med., 24:334, 1958.

73. Margolis, S. and Homcy, C. Systemic manifestations of hepatoma. Medicine, 51:381, 1972.

74. Powell, W.J., Jr. and Klatskin, G. Duration of survival in patients with Laennec's cirrhosis. Am. J. Med., 44:406, 1968.

75. Reynolds, T.B., Denison, E.K., Frankl, H.D., Lieberman, F.L., and Peters, R.L. Primary biliary cirrhosis with scleroderma, Raynaud's phenomenon and telangiectasia. Am. J. Med., 50:302, 1971.

76. Rubin, E. and Lieber, C.S. Alcohol-induced hepatic injury in nonalcoholic volunteers. N. Engl. J. Med., 278:869, 1968.

77. Scott, J., Gollan, J.L., Samourian, S., and Sherlock, S. Wilson's disease, presenting as chronic active hepatitis. Gastroenterology 74:645, 1978.

78. Sherlock, S. and Scheuer, P.J. The presentation and diagnosis of 100 patients with primary biliary cirrhosis. N. Engl. J. Med. 289:674, 1973.

79. Soloway, R.D., Summerskill, W.H.J., Baggenstoss, A.H., Geall, M.G., Gitnick, G.L., Elveback, L.R., and Schoenfield, L.J. Clinical, biochemical, and histological remission of severe chronic active liver disease: a controlled study of treatments and early prognosis. Gastroenterology, 63:820, 1972.

80. Summerskill, W.H.J. Chronic active liver disease reexamined: prognosis hopeful. Gastroenterology, 66:450, 1974.

81. Van Thiel, D.H. and Lester, R. Alcoholism: its effect on hypothalamic-pituitary-gonadal function. Gastroenterology 71:318, 1976.

82. Walshe, J.N. Wilson's disease, a review. In Peisach, J. et al. (eds.), The Biochemistry of Copper. New York, Academic Press, 1966.

SECTION ELEVEN
Endocrinology
T. H. HSU AND TURNER BLEDSOE: SECTION EDITORS

CHAPTER 68
Some Endocrinologic Principles
T. H. HSU AND TURNER BLEDSOE

In man perception of and reaction to stimuli are mediated primarily through the nervous and endocrine systems. Ultimately, secretion of humoral factors is involved. Hormones (the word is from Greek, meaning "I excite") are transported in blood to specific sites for their action. Hormones do not initiate new cellular biochemical processes, but rather regulate preexisting enzymatic and chemical reactions. The cascade of events may be illustrated by the response to fear. When fear is appreciated by the nervous system, neural impulses stimulate the hypothalamus and adrenal medulla, and hypothalamic factors and catecholamines are secreted. The anterior pituitary, its target organs, and subsequently every cell in the body are activated by a chain reaction until a new homeostatic state is achieved. Since the function of the central nervous system (CNS) itself is hormone-dependent, control of human behavior requires a constantly integrated and regulated neural and humoral signal.

The principal endocrine glands include the hypothalamus, pituitary, thyroid, parathyroids, adrenals, gonads, and pancreatic islet cells. In addition, nonendocrine organs are capable of producing hormones. For example, the mucosa of the gastric antrum produces gastrin, and the kidney produces renin and erythropoietin. Endocrinology encompasses the study of the normal and disordered function of the hormone-secreting cells of these organs and their metabolic consequences. Metabolism is a discipline within endocrinology concerned with the biochemistry of intermediary metabolism of carbohydrates, proteins, lipids, and nucleic acids.

PHYSIOLOGIC PRINCIPLES

Structure and Transport of Hormones
Chemically the human hormones can be classified into 1) lipid hormones, such as steroids derived from cholesterol and prostaglandins (cyclic fatty acids) derived from arachidonic and linolenic acid; 2) amine compounds such as thyroxine and catecholamines, both derived from tyrosine; and 3) peptide and glycoprotein hormones secreted by the hypothalamus, pituitary, parathyroids, pancreas, and cells of the gastrointestinal tract.

Hormones are usually present in the circulation in concentrations of the order of 10^{-9} to 10^{-12}M. Some, in addition to affecting their specific distant target tissues, may have played important roles in the tissues of their origin. For example, testosterone concentrations in testicular plasma are 50- to 100-fold greater than that of peripheral venous blood. These high local concentrations are required for normal spermatogenesis. Similarly, high concentrations of cortisol in the adrenal medulla are critical for the normal synthesis of epinephrine.

Except in the thyroid, storage of hormones in the endocrine glands is limited. Polypeptide hormones are initially synthesized as large molecular weight prohormones. Subsequently they are enzymatically cleaved into smaller molecules prior to their release into the bloodstream. Occasionally under normal circumstances but more frequently when hormones are autonomously secreted, these prohormones may appear in the circulation. These precursors are usually relatively inert biologically but may be immunologically active. In addition some sterols, steroids, and thyroid hormones are modified by the liver, kidney, and other organs. These organs can, therefore, function not only to degrade these hormones but to regulate their activity.

Once released into circulation, steroids and thyroid hormones are bound to specific carrier proteins. Only free unbound hormone is biologically active and subject to degradation, the bound hormone remaining as a metabolically inert reservoir. While total hormone, including that bound to protein is usually measured, an assay of free hormone provides a better index of biologic activity. In contrast, peptide hormones are not bound to specific transport proteins. However, intrinisic segments of their molecules often serve to protect their biologically active cores against degradation.

Mechanism of Action[3,6]

Since hormones are widely distributed by circulation, their selective action is determined by specific receptors. Receptors for polypeptide hormones are located on the plasma membrane of target cells. In contrast, steroid and thyroid hormones penetrate the cell membrane and bind with specific intracellular receptors.

Cell membrane receptors for peptide hormones are proteins which bind the hormones rapidly and reversibly, producing acute and transient actions. The mechanism of action depends upon the activation of one or more intracellular enzyme systems which in turn generate a second messenger. In most instances the enzyme is adenyl cyclase, a component of the cell membrane, and the second messenger is cyclic 3', 5' - adenosine monophosphate (AMP). Cyclic AMP triggers appropriate cellular responses by activating protein kinase. The nature of the second messenger for some peptide hormones such as growth hormone and insulin remains uncertain. Disruption of any event in this sequence may cause disease, e.g., Graves' disease, and insulin-resistant diabetes mellitus.

There is evidence that other secondary messengers exist. In many instances, neither hormone nor cyclic AMP can initiate the cellular response without calcium. The concentrations of intracellular calcium are themselves mediated by hormones and cyclic AMP. In thyroid tissue, prostaglandin E may also play a role as a messenger.

Steroid hormones enter the cell by diffusion or facilitated transport. Intracellularly they bind to specific cytoplasmic receptors and are translocated to the nucleus as hormone-receptor complexes. Formation of these complexes is critical to the transport of steroid hormones to their sites of action in the nucleus. Within the nucleus the complex binds to "acceptor sites" in DNA and nonhistone protein. After this interaction transcription of genes takes place and synthesis of messenger RNA (mRNA) is initiated. The mRNAs are exported to cytoplasmic ribosomes where hormone-induced proteins are synthesized. In contrast to steroid hormones, intracellular thyroid hormone transport does not require formation of a hormone-receptor complex. The nuclear binding sites for thyroid hormone, particularly T_3, are localized in the chromatin. An inherited abnormality in the androgen receptor has been demonstrated in patients with the testicular feminization syndrome.[5]

Regulation of the Secretion of Hormones

Each endocrine system requires a precise and sensitive regulatory mechanism to maintain homeostasis. This is most often accomplished by a closed-loop feedback system. An example is shown in Figure 68–1. Gland A produces hormone X to regulate organ B. Organ B in turn regulates gland A by secreting a substance Y, usually a hormone, which alters the function of gland A. If constancy of Y is the aim of the system, negative feedback control is needed. In our example, hormone X stimulates B to produce more Y, and substance Y when it reaches the normal concentration inhibits further production of hormone X. However, the secretion of most hormones is regulated by more complex systems. These may include multiple interrelated feedback loops, autoregulatory processes, and variable influences (usually concentration-dependent) on the system by a given substance.

The hypothalamus-pituitary-target organ axis is an example of a complex negative feedback loop. The basic principle for this system is illustrated in Figure 68–2. Information from higher centers in the CNS is integrated in the hypothalamus and relayed to the pituitary via hypothalamic hormones. The small peptides of the hypothalamus traverse the pituitary portal system and act upon the responsive pituitary cells to regulate the synthesis and release of tropic hormones. If the hypothalamic signal is to reduce the inhibitory factor or enhance the releasing factor output, the pituitary hormone is then released into the general circulation to stimulate target gland to secrete its hormone. The latter, in turn, suppresses its regulators in the hypothalamus and pituitary. Homeostasis is thereby achieved. There is also evidence that pituitary hormones may exert short circuit feedback inhi-

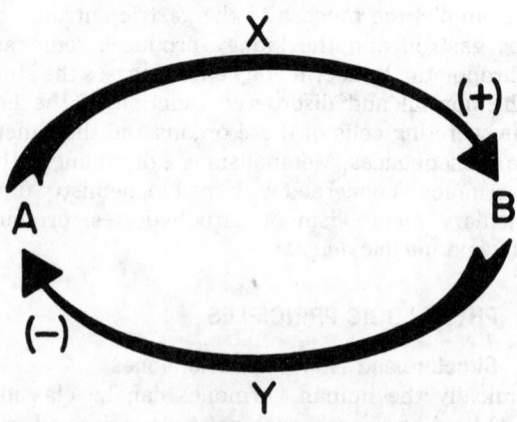

FIGURE 68–1. Closed-loop feedback system.

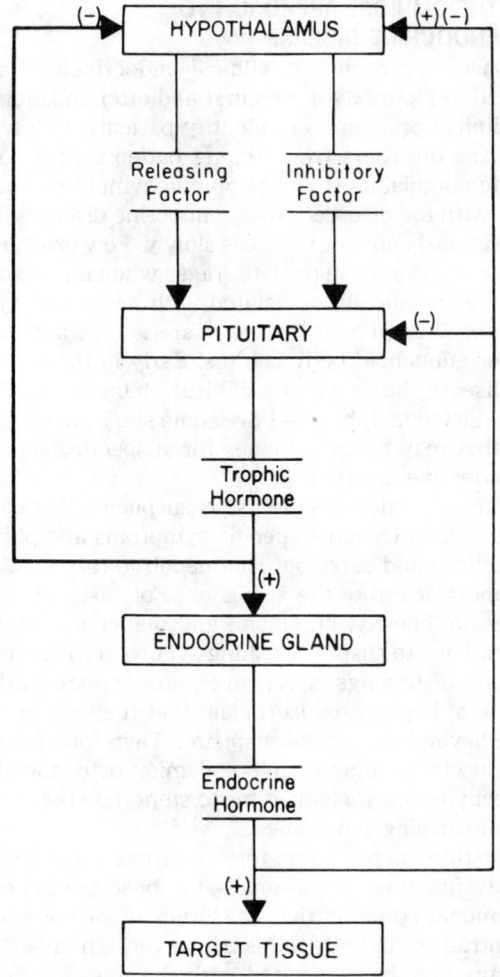

FIGURE 68-2. Schematic representation of control pathway from hypothalamic signal to release of hormone and effect on target tissue.

bition upon their own secretion or secretion of their hypothalamic releasing factors.

Extrinsic stimulation by pain, physical trauma, psychic stress, infection, fever, and hypoglycemia may produce signals to the hypothalamus to increase secretion of many of the tropic hormones until a new level of homeostasis is accomplished.

In addition to negative feedback control mechanisms and extrinsic influences, this regulatory system has an intrinsic rhythmicity. The diurnal variation in the secretion of growth hormone, ACTH, and prolactin is an example.[8] In normal man serum growth hormone rises rapidly during the first 2 hours of regular sleep. The rate of ACTH secretion, as reflected by plasma cortisol levels, is low at the time of this

growth hormone peak. Toward the end of sleep, the plasma cortisol level rises and reaches a peak between 6 and 8 A.M. (Fig. 68-3). The relationship of these two diurnal rhythms is probably not fortuitous. Since cortisol antagonizes the systemic effects of growth hormone, the combination of high growth hormone and low cortisol permits maximum growth effects. Another example is prolactin. In adults serum prolactin levels have an initial increment 1 to 2 hours after the onset of sleep; subsequently further major secretory episodes occur toward the end of sleep. The circadian rhythms in the secretion of these hormones are mediated by the hypothalamus, are dependent upon sleep–wake activity, and can be modified by altering the sleep–waking cycle.

Most pituitary and target organ hormones are elaborated episodically, and no hormone may be released between these secretory intervals. Consequently the blood levels of hormones with short half-lives fluctuate (Fig. 68-3). This has a significant effect on the interpretation of hormone measurements in blood.

The relationship between negative feedback control, intrinsic rhythmicity, and extrinsic influences is complex. These regulatory mechanisms are constantly in operation and the net effect determines the rate of hormone secretion.

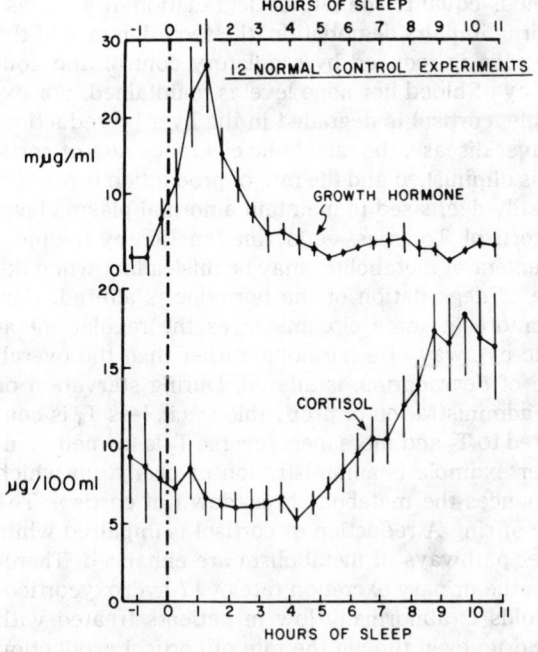

FIGURE 68-3. Diurnal variation of plasma cortisol and growth hormone (GH) in man.

Not all endocrine organs are directly under the control of the hypothalamic-pituitary axis. Activity of the parathyroid glands, pancreatic islet cells, thyroid C-cells, and zona glomerulosa of the adrenal cortex is modulated largely by nonpituitary influences.

Hormone Degradation

Degradation of hormones takes place primarily in the liver and kidney. Most degradative processes reduce the size of the hormone molecule thereby making the hormones more soluble in water and facilitating their excretion in urine. Usually hormones lose their biologic activity during degradation but in some instances biologic activity is increased or altered. Examples of the latter are the conversion of testosterone to dihydrotestosterone and estrogen, thyroxine to triiodothyronine, and cholecalciferol to 1,25 $(OH)_2$ cholecalciferol. The peripheral metabolic fate of the hormone may be the major determinant of its potency. Therefore, measurement of parent hormone levels may not suffice for evaluation of some endocrine disorders.

The rate of hormonal degradation may be variable. Starvation reduces the peripheral conversion rate of thyroxine to triiodothyronine.[2] Diseases of liver, kidney, or target tissue may also alter the rate of hormone degradation. The plasma level of a hormone is held constant when the rate of secretion of the hormone is equal to the rate of degradation. If a disease or drug impairs degradation, the secretion rate of the hormone is reduced by regulatory control and constancy of blood hormone level is maintained. For example, cortisol is degraded in the liver by reduction. In liver disease, the metabolic clearance rate of cortisol is diminished and the rate of production is proportionally decreased to maintain a normal plasma level of cortisol. To assess endocrine function by the measurement of metabolites may be misleading when the rate of degradation of the hormone is altered. Furthermore in some circumstances the regular metabolic pathway of a hormone, rather than the overall rate of degradation, is altered. During starvation or the administration of propylthiouracil, less T_4 is converted to T_3 and more inert reverse T_3 is formed.[2] Another example is administration of phenytoin which influences the metabolic breakdown of cortisol. The rate of ring A reduction of cortisol is impaired while other pathways of metabolism are enhanced. Therefore, the urinary excretion rate of 17-hydroxycorticosteroids is abnormally low in patients treated with this drug even though the rate of cortisol production is normal.[9]

THE CLINICAL APPROACH TO ENDOCRINE DISEASE

The basic approaches in clinical endocrinology are outlined in Figure 68–4. The first and often most difficult clinical problem is to identify patients with true endocrine disorders from among patients with nonspecific complaints that may mimic symptoms associated with the disorder. Many endocrine diseases begin insidiously and/or progress slowly. Few problems of recognition exist in the late stages when manifestations are specifically associated with endocrine dysfunction. Examples of the latter are goiter, amenorrhea, or eunuchoid body habitus. Early in the course of a disease, however, the clinical changes may be subtle. Listed in Table 68–1 are some signs and symptoms that may be useful clues for suspecting an occult endocrine disorder.

Once an endocrine disease is suspected, the next step is to identify more specific symptoms and physical findings and carry out routine laboratory studies to support or refute the suspicion. For instance, hypertension, obesity, hirsutism, and diabetes mellitus may lead one to suspect Cushing syndrome. This constellation of findings is, however, so common in the absence of hyperadrenocorticism that they are of little use beyond raising the suspicion. Therefore, proximal muscle weakness, hypokalemia, osteoporosis, and ecchymoses are looked for to stengthen the diagnosis of Cushing syndrome.

The third step is laboratory confirmation of endocrine dysfunction. Theoretically the best assessment of hormonal status is the measurement of hormone concentrations in body fluids. However, a number of problems may be associated with the interpretation of the values. First, for hormones with short half-lives, concentrations in the blood may fluctuate widely as a consequence of episodic secretion. Second, even in the absence of endocrine dysfunction, abnormal levels of binding proteins may influence "total" hormone concentrations (protein bound plus unbound) that are usually measured. Third, the levels of hormone in the blood do not always reflect the rate of hormone production. Therefore, multiple assessments of hormone or free hormone concentrations or determination of 24-hour urinary excretion rates are often necessary for the purpose of clinical evaluation.

Hormones are most commonly measured by radioimmunoassay. The techniques used in these assays are sensitive, specific, accurate, and relatively inexpensive. Many of the initial problems, particularly those associated with producing specific antibodies to small polypeptide and nonprotein hormones, have been resolved. Others, however, remain. Two have

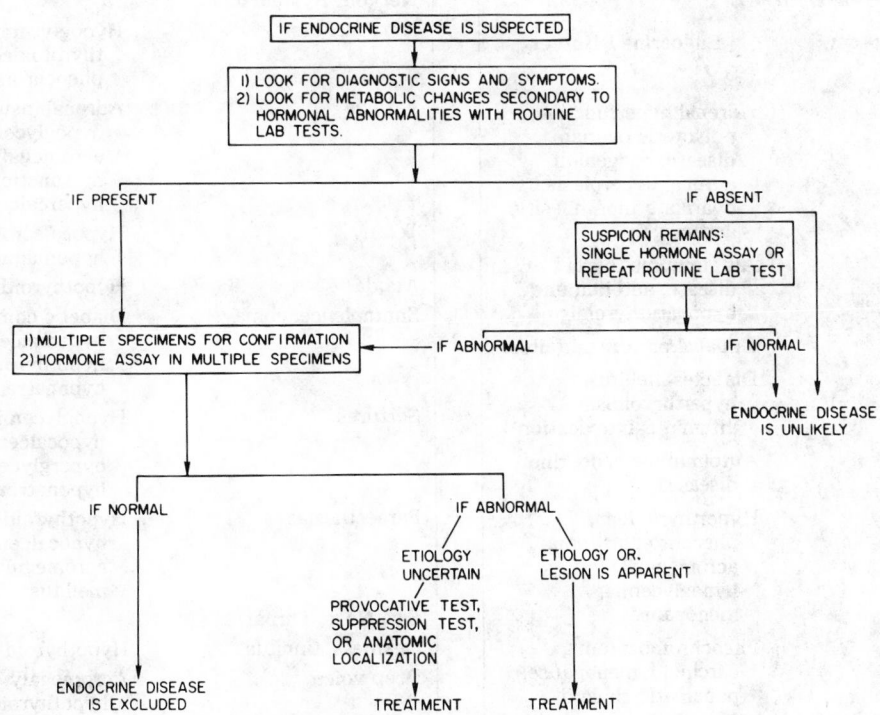

FIGURE 68-4. Basic diagnostic approaches in clinical endocrinology.

been especially troublesome: First, the immunogenic segments of the hormone molecules usually do not correspond to the biologically active segments. Consequently the result of immunoassays may measure biologically inert fragments. Furthermore the concentration of the fragments can be appreciably affected by changes in the rate of hormone degradation or the clearance rate of fragments. Second, an endocrine gland may produce an abnormal hormone which is biologically inactive but possesses immunogenic activity that is similar to the natural hormone. Discrepancies between laboratory results and clinical findings are clues to this phenomenon. Radioreceptor assays may solve these problems in the future. Unfortunately, bioassays, while specific for assessing biologic activity, are usually too insensitive to measure hormones in biologic fluids. However, modifications which permit the measurement of redox responses in cells to hormone have also been applied.[4]

An unequivocal diagnosis may be difficult to make in patients with minimal clinical manifestations and marginal abnormalities in the levels of hormone. In questionable cases pharmacologic manipulation is often useful for demonstrating alterations in physiologic control, as well as localization of the site of dys-

function. For example, the T_3-suppression test or TRH stimulation test is used to identify patients with questionable hyperthyroidism, and the dexamethasone suppression test to define the etiology of Cushing syndrome. As a rule, overactivity of a gland can be recognized by demonstrating autonomous secretion. This is done by assessing whether exogenous hormone will suppress it. Conversely hypofunction of a gland is confirmed by demonstrating that the gland cannot respond to physiologic stimulation or that its tropic hormone is elevated in the blood. Provocative tests are also useful to assess the reserve capacity of a gland since such information is not obtainable by measurement of basal plasma levels of hormone.

Whenever hormonal assay values fail to support the clinical impression, interfering drugs or laboratory error should be considered. If excessive exogenous administration of hormone is suspected, demonstration of hypofunction of the gland which normally produces the hormone is critical.

Measurements of biochemical changes secondary to hormone abnormality may also provide ancillary information. These tests are often readily available and inexpensive. They are particularly useful when direct measurement of the hormones concerned

TABLE 68-1
Useful Clues to the Presence of Endocrine Dysfunction

Sign or Symptom	Endocrine Disorder
Skin	
Hirsutism	Adrenal hyperfunction, polycystic ovarian disease, congenital adrenal hyperplasia, ovarian tumor, obesity, acromegaly
Hair loss	Autoimmune thyroid disease, autoimmune hypoparathyroidism
Sparse body hair	Gonadal or adrenal failure
Pruritis	Diabetes mellitus, hyperthryoidism, vitamin D intoxication
Vitiligo	Autoimmune endocrine diseases
Hyperhidrosis	Hyperthyroidism, pheochromocytoma, acromegaly, hypoglycemia, menopause
Flushing	Pheochromocytoma, carcinoid, menopause, pancreatic cholera
Hyperpigmentation	Addison's disease, thyrotoxicosis, ectopic ACTH syndrome
Thin, pale with fine wrinkles	Hypopituitarism
Cold skin	Hypothyroidism, pheochromocytoma
Ecchymoses	Cushing syndrome
Acanthosis nigricans	Diabetes mellitus, adrenal insufficiency, autoimmune thyroid disease, acromegaly, Cushing syndrome
Café-au-lait and other localized hyperpigmentation	Pheochromocytoma, polyostotic fibrous dysplasia
Neurofibroma, mucosal neuroma	Pheochromocytoma, medullary thyroid carcinoma
Xanthoma	Lipid disorders
Nervous System	
Headache	Pituitary tumor, hypoglycemia, pheochromocytoma, hyperaldosteronism
Psychosis	Hypoglycemia, thyrotoxicosis, hypothyroidism, Cushing syndrome, hyponatremia, hypercalcemia

TABLE 68-1 (cont.)

Sign or Symptom	Endocrine Disorder
Nervous System (cont.)	
Nervousness	Hypoglycemia, thyrotoxicosis, pheochromocytoma
Fatigue	Adrenal insufficiency, hypoglycemia, acromegaly, thyroid dysfunction, hypercalcemia
Tetany	Hypocalcemia, hypomagnesemia
Ataxia	Hypothyroidism
Somnolence, coma	Diabetic coma, hypercalcemia, hypothyroidism, hyponatremia
Seizures	Hypoglycemia, hypocalcemia, hyperglycemia, hyponatremia
Paraesthesias	Hypothyroidism, hypocalcemia, acromegaly, diabetes mellitus
Ear, Nose, Throat	
Deafness, tinnitus	Hypothyroidism
Deep voice	Acromegaly, hypothyroidism, androgen excess in female of adrenal or ovarian origin
Enlargement of salivary glands	Acromegaly, diabetes mellitus
Ocular	
Exophthalomus	Graves' disease, Hashimoto's thyroiditis, Cushing syndrome
Diplopia	Graves' disease, diabetes mellitus, pituitary tumor
Bitemporal hemianopsia	Pituitary tumors
Periorbital swelling	Hypothyroidism, Graves' disease
Cardiovascular	
Hypertension	Hyperaldosteronism, Cushing syndrome, pheochromocytoma, hypothyroidism, hypercalcemia
Orthostatic hypotension	Hyperaldosteronism, pheochromocytoma, adrenal insufficiency, diabetes mellitus
Tachycardia or tachyarrhythmia	Hyperthyroidism, pheochromocytoma
Congestive failure	Hyperthyroidism, pheochromocytoma, Cushing syndrome
Pericardial effusion	Myxedema
Bradycardia	Hypothyroidism
Premature atherosclerosis	Hyperlipidemia

TABLE 68-1 (cont.)

Sign or Symptom	Endocrine Disorder
Gastrointestinal	
Dyspepsia, anorexia	Adrenal insufficiency, hypercalcemia, hypothyroidism
Peptic ulcer	Hypercalcemia, islet cell tumor
Diarrhea	Hyperthyroidism, diabetes mellitus, carcinoid tumor, islet cell tumor, adrenal insufficiency, medullary thyroid carcinoma
Weight loss	Adrenal insufficiency, hyperthyroidism, pheochromocytoma, diabetes mellitus
Constipation	Hypothyroidism, hypercalcemia, pheochromocytoma
Ascites	Myxedema
Abdominal pain	Adrenal insufficiency, hyperlipemia, hypercalcemia, carcinoid, hyperthyroidism, diabetes mellitus
Urologic	
Polyuria, polydipsia	Hypercalcemia, hyperaldosteronism diabetes insipidus, diabetes mellitus
Kidney stones	Hyperparathyroidism, acromegaly, Cushing syndrome, hyperuricuria, hypercalciuria, cystinuria
Musculoskeletal and Extremities	
Weakness	Hyperthyroidism, Cushing syndrome, acromegaly, hypercalcemia, hyperaldosteronism, hypocalcemia
Arthralgia	Hypothyroidism, acromegaly
Bone pain	Hyperparathyroidism, osteomalacia
Fractures	Cushing syndrome, hyperparathyroidism
Edema of extremities	Cushing syndrome
Enlargement of extremities	Acromegaly, Graves' disease, hypothyroidism
Brachydactyly	Pseudohypoparathyroidism, Turner syndrome

TABLE 68-1 (cont.)

Sign or Symptom	Endocrine Disorder
Reproductive	
Menorrhagia	Hypothyroidism
Scanty menstruation	Hyperthyroidism
Loss of libido and potentia	Hypogonadism, acromegaly, hypothyroidism, diabetes mellitus, hyperprolactinemia
Amenorrhea	Hypogonadism, hyperthyroidism, Cushing syndrome, acromegaly, pituitary tumor, Sheehan syndrome, hyperprolactinemia
Gynecomastia	Hypogonadism, thyroid dysfunction, pituitary tumor, ectopic production of LH or HCG
Nonpuerperal galactorrhea	Pituitary tumor, hyperprolactinemia, hypothyroidism
Body Habitus	
Marfanoid	Type III multiple endocrine adenomatosis
Eunuchoid	Hypogonadism
Round face	Pseudohypoparathyroidism
Short stature	Turner syndrome, growth hormone deficiency, hypothyroidism, pseudohypoparathyroidism
Routine Laboratory Findings	
Hyponatremia	Adrenal insufficiency, hypopituitarism, hypothyroidism, ADH excess
Anemia	Thyroid dysfunction, hypopituitarism, adrenal insufficiency, hyperparathyroidism
Hypokalemia	Hyperaldosteronism, Cushing syndrome
Hyperkalemia	Adrenal insufficiency, hypoaldosteronism
Hypocalcemia	Hypoparathyroidism, hypomagnesemia
Hypercalcemia	Hyperparathyroidism, hyperthyroidism, adrenal insufficiency, malignancy

(Continued)

753

TABLE 68–1 (cont.)	
Sign or Symptom	**Endocrine Disorder**
Routine Laboratory Findings (cont.)	
Hypoglycemia	Islet cell tumor, early diabetes mellitus, adrenal insufficiency, growth hormone deficiency, functional hyperinsulinism
Hyperlipemia	Hypothyroidism, Cushing syndrome
EKG:	
Low voltage and heart rate	Hypothyroidism, Addison's disease
Flat T-wave and prominent U-wave	Hyperaldosteronism, Cushing syndrome
Short Q-T interval	Hypercalcemia
Prolonged Q-T interval	Hypocalcemia, Addison's disease

is not feasible. Usually, however, such tests are not sufficiently specific to confirm the diagnosis. Diabetes mellitus is an exception to this rule. Evaluation of glucose tolerance is a better index of clinically significant diabetes mellitus than measurement of plasma insulin levels.

When the diagnosis of an endocrine disorder is established, it is important to demonstrate its etiology. Autoimmune destruction of an endocrine gland may forewarn of other autoimmune disorders. The cause of glandular hyperfunction may dictate its treatment. Lastly, but importantly, many endocrine disorders have a high familial incidence; therefore it is often mandatory to obtain a detailed family history or examine other family members.

There are three main principles in the treatment of endocrine disorders. First, except in life-threatening emergencies, it is advisable to correct abnormalities slowly in order to permit organ-systems to adjust gradually to changes. Second, the patient should be treated to restore hormonal levels as closely as possible to normal. Third, the dose of hormones which normally are secreted in response to stress should be appropriately increased when the patient is under stress.

In the following sections, relatively specific signs and symptoms, laboratory tests, diagnostic maneuvers, pitfalls in the interpretation of laboratory results, and management of endocrine disorders will be discussed.

CHAPTER 69
The Hypothalamus–Pituitary Axis
T. H. HSU

The physiology and pathophysiology of the hypothalamus and the pituitary gland will be discussed together because of the intimate relationship of these two structures. The hypothalamus, together with the posterior pituitary, is a small complex organ composed of nerve cells and their axons. In contrast, the anterior pituitary consists of cells derived from the primitive foregut, although its secretory function is greatly influenced by the hypothalamus.

HYPOTHALAMIC NEUROSECRETORY UNIT
Hypothalamic endocrine neurons have both neural and secretory activities. Some hypothalamic neurons form discrete nuclei such as supraoptic and paraventricular nuclei which synthesize vasopressin and oxytocin, respectively. Hypothalamic hormones which control the function of the anterior pituitary on the other hand are produced by neurons distributed in less well-defined areas.

The secretory activities of these neurons are regulated by at least two mechanisms: 1) synaptically transmitted information from higher centers in the central nervous system; and 2) hormones that are produced by the specific endocrine target organs and whose synthesis and release is directly regulated by the secretions of the anterior pituitary.

Neurotransmitters, such as dopamine, norepinephrine, and serotonin, participate in the transmission of information from CNS centers to hypothalamic neurons. These neurotransmitter systems are of clinical importance. For example, stimulation of the dopaminergic pathways by exogenously administered L-dopa may increase growth hormone secretion but inhibit prolactin release. Serotonin antagonism induced by cyproheptadine administration will block the normal rise in growth hormone (GH) caused by hypoglycemia and also normalize excessive ACTH production in certain patients with pituitary Cushing's disease. A given neurotransmitter, for instance, serotonin, may exert a stimulatory action at the level of the limbic system and an inhibitory effect at the hypothalamic level. Because neurotransmitters have multiple actions, neuropharmacologic interventions must be made with caution.

The Hypothalamic Hormones and Their Effects

The hypothalamus–pituitary interaction is analogous to a "distant" synapse. Neuromuscular synaptic transmission activities involve the release of effector substances, norepinephrine and acetylcholine, and their activation of local receptors. In the hypothalamus–pituitary synapsis, the effectors are small peptides, and the distance between the nerve endings and their target cells of the anterior pituitary is relatively great. The problem of distance between neurosecretory nerve endings and the cells of the anterior pituitary is resolved by the hypothalamus–pituitary portal circulation. In this portal venous system, the median eminence of the hypothalamus is the final common pathway for the delivery of hypothalamic factors to pituitary cells.

Three hypothalamic hormones have been isolated and chemically characterized: thyrotropin-releasing hormone (TRH) (3 amino acids), gonadotropin-releasing hormone (GRH) (10 amino acids), and growth-hormone-releasing-inhibiting hormone (somatostatin) (14 amino acids). It was formerly believed that the secretion of each pituitary hormone was under the influence of a single specific hypothalamic releasing or inhibiting factor. It is now recognized that TRH, at a dose needed to stimulate thyroid-stimulating hormone (TSH), stimulates prolactin as well, and somatostatin in addition to inhibiting GH secretion also decreases the secretion of prolactin. The action of hypothalamic hormones appears to be mediated through cyclic AMP. In addition to their effects on the anterior pituitary, they have many extrapituitary effects. For example, somatostatin inhibits the secretion of insulin, glucagon, and gastrin.

THE ANTERIOR PITUITARY AND ITS HORMONES

During embryologic development the anterior pituitary arises from Rathke's pouch, an evagination from ectodermal tissue in the roof of the oral cavity. Cells migrate upward to the sella turcica, a cavity in the sphenoid bone. The anterior pituitary gland secretes at least six physiologically important hormones. They can be classified into three groups according to their chemical structure: 1) Growth hormone (GH) and prolactin (PRL) are polypeptides with intramolecular disulfide bonds. They and chorionic somatomammotropin (placental lactogen) have extensive similarities in amino acid structure. 2) ACTH and ACTH-related hormones are single-chain peptides.[24] ACTH consists of 39 amino acids. (Beta-melanocyte-stimulating hormone [β-MSH] is a fragment of human gamma-lipotropin (γ-LPH) that is artificially produced during extraction. Beta-lipotropin is believed to be the parent substance not only of γ-LPH and β-MSH but also of β-endorphin and the encephalins as well.[14,24,28]) 3) Pituitary hormones in the remaining group are glycoproteins. They include TSH, follicle-stimulating hormone (FSH), and luteinizing hormone (LH). The glycoprotein hormones consist of two nonidentical subunits, referred to as α and β. The α subunits are identical in each of the three hormones. However, the β subunits differ and are responsible for target organ and immunologic specificity. Chorionic gonadotropin, though not pituitary in origin, is chemically similar to these hormones.

Early light microscopic studies revealed that the anterior pituitary contains acidophil cells, which possess granules that react with acidic dyes; basophilic cells, whose granules stain with basic dyes; and chromophobe cells, which lack apparent granules. Subsequently it was shown histochemically that the basophilic cells contain predominantly glycoprotein. The secretory products of these cells have been identified by immunocytologic techniques, and electron microscopy has shown their secretory granules to differ morphologically. Furthermore, electron microscopy shows that chromophobe cells contain granules.

Somatotropic or GH-secreting cells are present in the posterolateral wings of the anterior pituitary. Lactotropic or PRL-secreting cells are similar in distribution and contain the largest granules of any pituitary cells. Thyrotropic or TSH-secreting cells are polyhedral in shape and have the smallest granules. Gonadotropin-secreting cells are distributed throughout the pituitary. Whether LH and FSH are elaborated by different cells remains uncertain. ACTH secreting cells are present in the anteromedial regions of the pituitary.

Sensitive and specific radioimmunoassays are available for measuring each pituitary hormone. However, results may not conform to biologic activity. For example, the full biologic activity of ACTH depends on the integrity of the first 20 amino acids. Since the peptide segment containing amino acids 22 to 39 is the most potent immunologic determinant, a discrepancy between radioimmunoassay and biologic activity is not unexpected.

GROWTH HORMONE, PROLACTIN, AND DISORDERS OF THE PITUITARY GLAND

Aberrations in the secretion of the growth hormone and prolactin are the most common endocrine abnormalities associated with disorders of the pituitary gland.

Growth Hormone

Growth hormone, a single chain polypeptide, is synthesized and secreted by acidophil cells of the anterior pituitary throughout life. Its production is under both stimulatory and inhibitory hypothalamic control. Hypothalamic growth-hormone-inhibiting hormone, or somatostatin, is a tetradecapeptide and is now available for clinical use. A decapeptide which stimulates GH release in rats has been isolated, but is inactive in man.

The activity of mediobasal hypothalamic neurons that secrete GH regulatory factors are mediated by at least three higher neurocenters: the ventromedial and arcuate nuclei of the hypothalamus and the limbic system of the brain. A number of important physiologic or pharmacologic agents affect GH secretion (Fig. 69-1).[33] Episodic release of GH has now been documented in man. A prominent burst of GH secretion occurs during the early part of deep sleep. Such fluctuations are more pronounced in children than in adults, and more in women than in men. These episodic secretions probably reflect intrinsic episodic changes in neurosecretory activities. In acromegalics or patients with pituitary tumors, GH secretory responses may be grossly abnormal, including paradoxic changes.

Pituitary GH reserve is evaluated by induction of hypoglycemia, administration of L-dopa or arginine, or performance of exercise.[25] In the absence of obesity, a patient who fails to demonstrate a rise in GH following provocation by two of these stimuli is considered as having GH deficiency.

Growth hormone affects skeletal growth. Before

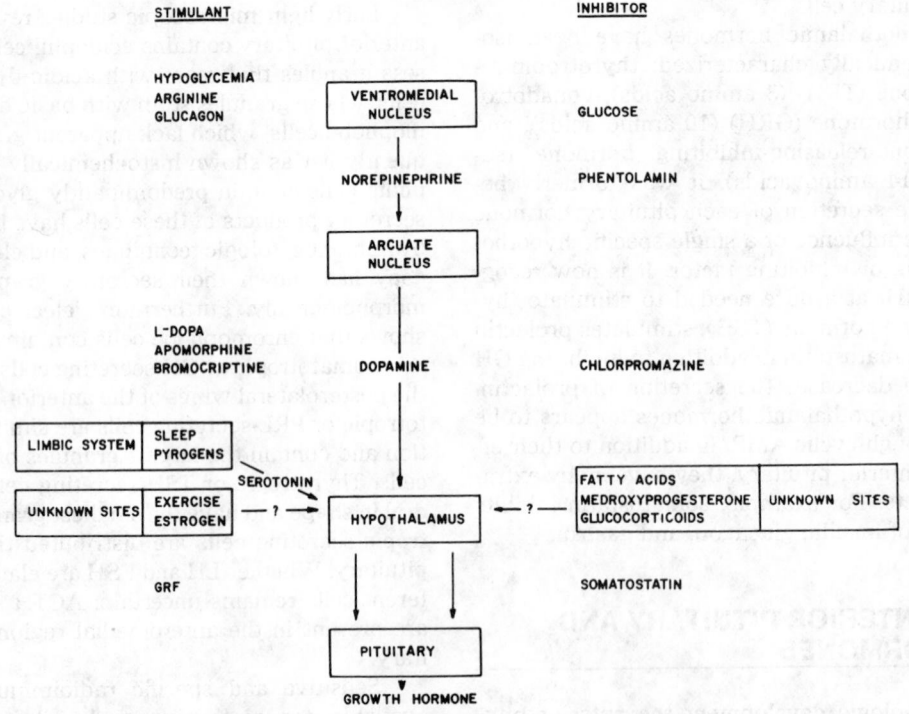

FIGURE 69-1. Major physiologic and pharmacologic factors that affect the secretion of human growth hormone and their site of action.

closure of the epiphyses, excessive production of GH produces gigantism, whereas deficiency of the hormone causes dwarfism. Although present in the human fetal pituitary around the eighth week, GH appears essential for growth only during the final stages of fetal development. Its effect on the skeleton is mediated by intermediary substances generated by liver, known as somatomedins (sulfation factor). Their activity is assayed either by measuring incorporation of radiosulfur into chondroidin sulfate of cartilage in vitro or by radioimmunoassay.

Somatomedin is present in normal man and absent in growth-hormone-deficient patients. In the latter its activity can be restored to near normal by treatment with human GH. GH acts by stimulating somatomedin production which, in turn, affects skeletal growth. Failure to form somatomedins occurs in Laron dwarfism, a clinical condition indistinguishable from that produced by GH deficiency.

Plasma somatomedin activity resides in proteins with molecular weights of 6000 to 9000 daltons. At least four chemically different peptides with somatomedin activity have been purified: somatomedins A, C, nonsuppressible insulin-like activity (NSILAS), and multiplication stimulating activity (MSA). Somatomedins A, C, and NSILAS account for most of the "sulfation" activity and they share many common properties.[43]

In addition to its growth stimulating effects, GH has an important role in the regulation of metabolism. It enhances hepatic glucose output, blocks glucose translocation into muscle and adipose tissue, enhances mobilization of free fatty acid (FFA), and stimulates uptake of FFA by skeletal muscle. Its net effect is to maintain blood glucose by mobilizing readily oxidizable fatty acids when carbohydrate deficiency is present. Growth hormone may play an important role in short-term protection against hypoglycemia. Following administration of GH, excretion of urinary peptides containing hydroxyproline is increased as a consequence of an increase in the rate of collagen synthesis and turnover. GH increases glomerular filitration rate, renal plasma flow, and tubular reabsorption of phosphate. The last is thought to be the cause of hyperphosphatemia in acromegalic subjects. Hypercalciuria is induced by GH and may contribute to renal stone formation in acromegalic patients. Finally, GH has intrinsic prolactin activity, an expected finding since these hormones have peptide sequences in common.

Basal plasma GH levels are 1 to 5 ng/ml in adults. In the newborn, they are elevated but decline to normal within 3 weeks. Levels do not rise in adolescence. The half-life of GH is 20 to 30 minutes. Such relatively rapid degradation permits levels to alter appropriately in response to acute changes in blood glucose.

Prolactin (PRL)[39]

Prolactin is a single chain polypeptide secreted by acidophilic cells. These are scattered throughout the anterior pituitary lobe. Hypertrophy typically occurs in pituitaries of neonates and lactating women.

The secretion of PRL is regulated mainly through tonic suppression by a prolactin-inhibiting factor, probably dopamine. With destruction of the hypothalamus or interruption of the hypothalamic connection by destruction of the pituitary stalk, hyperprolactinemia occurs. Agents that decrease brain dopamine concentrations or block its action increase PRL secretion. Conversely, agents that increase catecholamine concentration or mimic its effect decrease PRL secretion (Table 69–1). Cholinergic stimuli usually inhibit secretion whereas serotoninergic ones stimulate secretion of PRL. Nocturnal and nipple suckling-induced rises of PRL secretion appears to be regulated through serotoninergic fibers. Thyrotropin-releasing hormone (TRH) is also a potent pituitary stimulus for PRL secretion. However, its physiologic importance remains to be demonstrated. Estrogens increase PRL secretion by increasing the number of PRL-secreting cells and their ability to secrete PRL.

Like GH, PRL is secreted episodically and in a characteristic diurnal rhythm related to the sleep–waking cycle. Sixty to ninety minutes following the onset of sleep PRL levels rise, reaching a peak before waking, generally at 5:00 to 7:00 A.M.

TABLE 69–1

Principal Physiologic and Pharmacologic Factors or Conditions That Affect the Secretion of Prolactin in Humans

	Stimulant	Inhibitor
Physiologic factors or conditions	Sleep Stress Pregnancy Hypoglycemia Midmenstrual cycle Breast nursing	
Pharmacologic factors	Phenothiazine and other tranquilizers	L-dopa
	Morphine Estrogens TRH	Ergot derivatives

Most of the metabolic actions of PRL are permissive: PRL alone may not exert an effect, but does so indirectly by modifying the response of tissue to other hormones. The major function of PRL in man is initiation and maintenance of lactation. In addition it may 1) alter the transport of water and salt by the placenta; 2) interfere with reproductive function in both males and females;[11] and 3) enhance the production of 1,25 dihydroxycholecalciferol by the kidney thereby facilitating calcium absorption from the gut during pregnancy and lactation.[38]

INTRASELLAR AND PARASELLAR TUMORS[18,22]

Pituitary tumors come to medical attention because of neurologic symptoms, hormonal disturbances, or both. However, tumors may be asymptomatic in approximately 25 percent of cases. Since pituitary tumors often have only minor symptoms and because enlargement of the sella turcica does not always mean that a pituitary tumor is present, diagnosis of pituitary tumor requires the close collaboration of the endocrinologist, neuroradiologist, neurosurgeon, and ophthalmologist (Fig. 69–2).

The incidence of pituitary adenoma is less than 1 per 100,000 population per year. Most occur in patients over 40 but recently a significant increase in the incidence of pituitary adenoma among women of childbearing age has been observed.

Pituitary tumors may present with symptoms only after many years. Headaches and visual disturbances are the most common early manifestations. Headaches are often supraorbital and retro-orbital and can be aggravated by jarring or by physical effort, suggesting that stretched dura mater contributes to its cause.

Because of the anatomic location of the pituitary, optic nerve compression frequently occurs when the tumors enlarge. About 70 percent of patients with pituitary tumors have ocular symptoms. These symptoms include blurred vision which is difficult to correct, visual field defects, diplopia, or ptosis. Typically, but not invariably, the tumor impinges on the central portion of chiasm producing loss of vision in both upper temporal quadrants. This is followed by loss in the lower temporal quadrants. Nasal field defects rarely occur. The visual loss is often asymmetric, with loss of vision occurring primarily in one eye. Surprisingly many patients are unaware of visual impairment. Quantification and detection of early changes require perimetric studies using red objects.

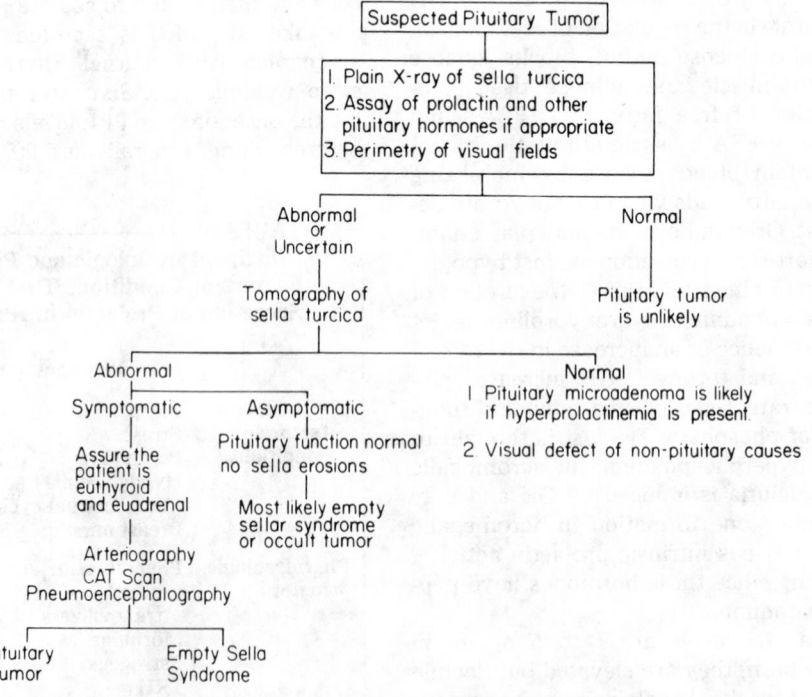

FIGURE 69–2. Evaluation of suspected pituitary tumor.

Sequential visual field evaluations at 3- to 6-month intervals provide useful information regarding the progression or regression of a pituitary tumor.

Extraocular muscle palsies, when present, commonly involve the IIIrd to the VIth cranial nerves. Usually symptoms are present only in patients with large tumors that extend laterally or into the cavernous sinus. Diplopia occurs occasionally without demonstrable palsies of cranial nerves. This is due to complete bitemporal hemianopsia; the right eye deviates to the right in an effort to see more with the retained nasal field and the left eye deviates to the left, with creation of double images. Visual symptoms can be precipitated by bleeding into the tumor, head trauma, or a physiologic enlargement of the pituitary such as occurs during pregnancy. Other symptoms that suggest the presence of extrasellar extension include the following: 1) Severe headaches, vomiting, and papilledema result from increased intracranial pressure caused by obstruction to outflow of the third ventricle. This complication is particularly common in craniopharyngioma. 2) Drowsiness, polydipsia, polyuria, hyperphagia, temporal lobe or psychomotor seizures, frontal lobe memory disturbance, and anosmia occur when the tumor extends superiorly and involves the hypothalamus.

Hormone-related symptoms may result either from deficiency or from an excess of one or more pituitary hormones. Complete destruction of the pituitary produces panhypopituitarism. Occasionally pituitary dysfunction results from tumor invading areas of the hypothalamus that regulate pituitary function. The clinical manifestations of hypopituitarism depend on the age and sex of the patient. (See section on hypopituitarism, p. 764). Growth hormone deficiency is common and occurs early. Usually it produces no symptoms in adults. Serum prolactin levels above 100 ng/ml are found in approximately 60 percent of patients with "nonfunctional" pituitary tumors, whether or not galactorrhea is present.[21] Hyperprolactinemia can be due to either prolactin-secreting adenomas or tumor invasion of the hypothalamus. It may cause galactorrhea or hypogonadism in both sexes. Hypogonadism can also result from impaired gonadotropin secretion. Overt evidence of thyroid and adrenal failure usually occurs late in the course. Elevations of pituitary hormones in CSF may indicate local extension of tumor. Serial measurements may be useful to monitor changes in the suprasellar region.[19]

"NONSECRETING" PITUITARY TUMORS

Pituitary adenomas occur most commonly during the third and fourth decades; rarely are they found before adolescence. While basophilic and acidophilic pituitary cells can give rise to adenomas, 90 percent of pituitary tumors are chromophobe adenomas. Chromophobe adenomas usually do not secrete hormones. However, because they may interfere with inhibition of prolactin secretion, prolactin levels are frequently high even when galactorrhea is not present.

Chromophobe adenomas usually grow larger than other pituitary tumors, often erode downwardly and laterally through the sella turcica, and produce local pressure effects. In at least 80 percent of patients, there are signs or symptoms of hypopituitarism, most commonly hypogonadism. As the tumor enlarges the pressure produces cell atrophy that may cause sudden or insidious panhypopituitarism.

Only about 2 percent of chromophobe tumors are actually invasive and behave as carcinomas. However, when present, they usually are massive and rapidly invasive to adjacent structures, but rarely metastasize to distant sites.

Pituitary adenomas may be associated with adenomatosis of other endocrine organs in the so-called multiple endocrine adenomatosis syndromes. Failure to treat endocrine deficiencies, particularly primary thyroid deficiency, predisposes to sellar enlargement and formation of adenomas.[45] Most likely this is due to chronic overstimulation of pituitary cells by the hypothalamic factors in the absence of regulatory suppressor.

CRANIOPHARYNGIOMA

Craniopharyngiomas develop from remnants of Rathke's pouch in the hypophysis and occur predominantly in children. Most arise in the suprasellar region but may occur in the sella as well. Characteristically they grow slowly, and are calcified in three-quarters of cases in children but infrequently in adults. The tumors are usually large by the time of presentation. Clinical symptoms include disturbances of growth and maturation, hypothalamic dysfunction, central scotomas and visual involvement when the tumor impinges on the posterior aspect of the optic chiasm, epilepsy, hemiparesis, signs of raised intracranial pressure, and mental deterioration. Complete excision of craniopharyngiomas is often difficult because of their location. As much tumor as possible should be removed and radiotherapy given.

MISCELLANEOUS TUMORS

Other space-occupying lesions that may simulate pituitary tumors include cysts of Rathke's pouch, dermoid tumors, gliomas of the optic chiasm, meningiomas of the tuberculum sellae, nasopharyngeal tumors with local invasion, and parapituitary carotid aneurysms. Metastases, particularly of breast cancer, may also affect the pituitary.

EMPTY SELLA SYNDROME

In the patient with an enlarged sella turcica but without symptoms empty sella syndrome must be considered. This entity, occurring particularly in obese women, is due to nontumorous enlargement of the sella. The pituitary is frequently pressed against the walls of the sella but its function is usually normal. It is displaced by CSF which is present due to the absence of the diaphragm above the sella permitting communication with subarachnoid space above. Definitive diagnosis requires pneumoencephalography and demonstration of air in the sella. Computerized tomographic demonstration of a large sella filled with density compatible with CSF also suggests the diagnosis. Relatively few patients have endocrine symptoms. Pituitary reserve testing may reveal minor abnormalities, however, in half of the cases. The patient with an enlarged sella turcica without symptoms, endocrine abnormalities, evidence of optic nerve compression, or bony erosion usually needs no further diagnostic studies. However, since tumors can occur also in patients with empty sella syndrome, periodic follow-up is important.

MANAGEMENT OF PITUITARY TUMOR

The first step in the management of pituitary tumor is to correct adrenal insufficiency and hypothyroidism if present. Patients undergoing stressful diagnostic procedures, such as arteriography and pneumoencephalography, or surgery for removal of the tumor should be treated with glucocorticoids (200 to 300 mg cortisol per day) even if adrenal insufficiency has yet to be confirmed.

When tumor is uncomplicated by visual impairment or extrasellar spread, transsphenoidal microsurgery is generally preferred. Major complications of this approach include cerebrospinal fluid rhinorrhea, wound infection, and diabetes insipidus. Alternatively, external irradiation with 4000 to 5000 rads to the tumor may be administered over a 5- to 6-week period. Radiotherapy is also preferred in patients with high operative risk. When treatment is initiated early, menstruation and ovulation may be restored to normal in females. Irradiation, however, can sometimes provoke edema of the tumor resulting in decrease in visual acuity. Fortunately this is usually only transitory. As a rule, radiotherapy is not the initial treatment of choice when progressive loss of vision is present. Most neurosurgeons would agree that using sophisticated surgical equipment, suprasellar extensions can be safely removed by the transsphenoidal

approach. The intracranial operative route is indicated only when the adenoma has invaded the frontal or temporal lobe. When tumors recur, surgery is usually indicated since additional irradiation may damage adjacent normal tissue.

SECRETING PITUITARY TUMORS

Functioning pituitary adenomas secrete all types of pituitary hormones. However, increased secretion of polypeptide tropic hormones is distinctly more common than that of glycoprotein hormones. It is still uncertain whether the basic functional defect is in the hypothalamus or in the pituitary. Clinically such tumors present with signs and symptoms of excessive hormone production rather than space-occupying lesions. In fact, endocrine syndromes often precede detectable sellar enlargement.

Galactorrhea with or Without Hypogonadism

Nonpuerperal galactorrhea may indicate the presence of a pituitary tumor. Galactorrhea due to pituitary tumor is almost always associated with elevations in serum prolactin[40] whereas elevations in serum prolactin are not always associated with galactorrhea. Pituitary tumors are found in nearly 30 percent of women with nonpuerperal galactorrhea accompanied by hypogonadism, menstrual abnormalities, and hyperprolactinemia. The causes of galactorrhea are outlined in Table 69–2. Serum prolactin should be measured in any patients with unexplained galactorrhea,

---

TABLE 69–2
Major Causes of Galactorrhea

I. **Drug (Including Hormone) Induced**
    A. Tranquilizers
    B. Antidepressants
    C. Antihypertensives (rauwolfia, alpha-methyldopa)
    D. Sex steroids
    E. Gonadotropins

II. **Primary Hypothalamic**
    A. Postpartum
    B. Destructive lesion of hypothalamus

III. **Pituitary Tumor and Endocrine Disorders**
    A. Prolactin-secreting pituitary tumor
    B. Other pituitary tumors (functioning or nonfunctioning)

IV. **Nonendocrine Malignancy with Ectopic Production of Prolactin**

V. **Neurogenic**
    A. Nipple stimulation
    B. Chest wall lesions

VI. **Idiopathic Variety**

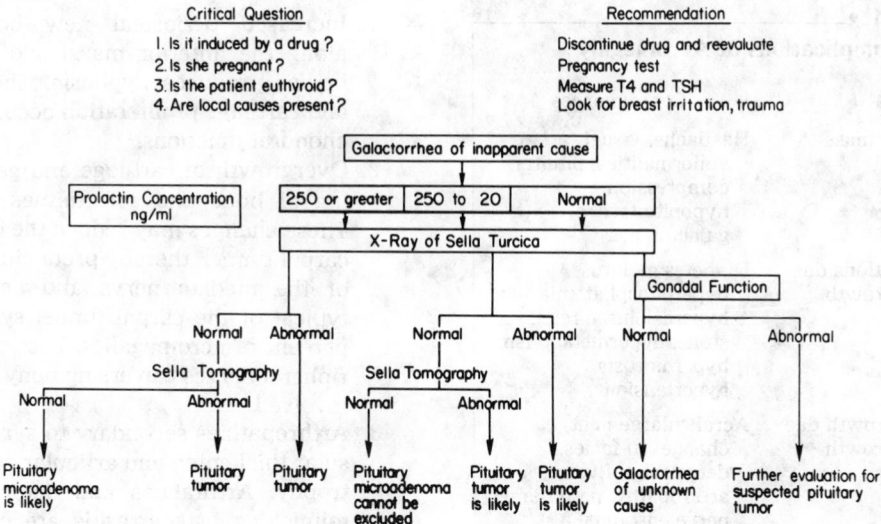

FIGURE 69-3. Evaluation of galactorrhea of unapparent cause.

amenorrhea, hypogonadism, and suspected hypotha-lamic–pituitary lesions (Fig. 69-3). Pharmacody-namic studies and stimulation and suppression tests do not help to identify the significance of prolactin elevations. The likelihood of pituitary tumor is best correlated to the magnitude of the serum prolactin concentrations.[22] Above 300 ng/ml, virtually all pa-tients harbor pituitary tumors; from 150 to 300 ng/ml, the likelihood of tumor is great; below these lev-els, there is significant overlap with other causes of hyperprolactinemia.

In many women with galactorrhea there is con-comitant amenorrhea due to suppression of the nor-mal midcycle surge of gonadotropins. Amenorrhea may occur in patients with either pituitary tumors or idiopathic galactorrhea. It is still uncertain whether prolactin interferes with reproductive functions at the level of the hypothalamus, pituitary, or gonads, and whether its effects differ in men and women. Bromo-criptine effectively suppresses prolactin in this syn-drome with restoration of normal menses and fertil-ity. Pituitary tumors, however, must be excluded since their growth may be accelerated should preg-nancy intervene.

GH-Secreting Tumors of the Pituitary: Acromegaly and Gigantism

Acidophil and some chromophobe tumors of the pitu-itary may sustain hypersecretion of GH producing ac-romegaly in adults, gigantism in children, and both disorders in teenagers. The onset is usually so insidi-ous that the condition is unrecognized until it is well advanced. The clinical features of acromegaly fall into three major groups: 1) symptoms caused by tu-mor mass, inclusive of those induced by altered se-cretion of other pituitary hormones secondary to compression of the pituitary; 2) metabolic changes produced by excessive GH secretion; and 3) symp-toms due to enlargement of skeleton, soft tissues, and visceral organs (Table 69-3).

METABOLIC CONSEQUENCES OF EXCESSIVE GH. Since GH directly inhibits peripheral glucose uptake and antagonizes the effects of insulin, increased se-cretion produces hyperglycemia. As a consequence serum insulin concentrations are elevated in most pa-tients and insulin resistance is present. Glucose intol-erance is present in 50 percent of affected patients but overt diabetes mellitus, due to exhaustion of the pancreatic islets, occurs in only 10 percent. The usual symptoms of diabetes mellitus, including polyuria, thirst, and ketoacidosis, occur, but vascular compli-cations are strikingly rare.

GH increases renal tubular reabsorption of phos-phate and mild hyperphosphatemia is common. Be-fore radioimmunoassays for GH, serum phosphate was used as a marker for GH secretion. Hypercalci-uria, which occurs in about 60 percent of acromegal-ics, is due to increased GFR and changes in renal han-dling of calcium. The increased incidence of renal stones in acromegaly may be secondary to this effect.

GH also increases basal metabolic rate, causes hypertrophy of the sweat glands, and commonly pro-duces hyperhidrosis which is often distressing. Ap-proximately 30 percent of patients with acromegaly

TABLE 69–3
Clinical Complications of Acromegaly

Causes	Consequences
Effects of tumor mass	Headache, visual abnormalities, pituitary compression, hypopituitarism, galactorrhea
Metabolic alterations due to excessive growth hormone	Diabetes mellitus, hyperphosphatemia, hypercalciuria, renal stone, hypermetabolism, hyperhidrosis, hypertension
Anatomic overgrowth due to excessive growth hormone	Acral enlargement, changes in facies, deepening of voice, arthropathy, peripheral nerve entrapment, myopathy, myocardopathy, visceromegaly

have hypertension, the pathogenesis of which remains unknown.

"OVERGROWTH SYNDROME" OF EXCESSIVE GH. Enlargement of skeleton, muscle, soft tissue, and visceral organs and thickening of the skin are the characteristic consequences of hypersomatotropism. These changes evolve so slowly that they are often unrecognized until they are rather advanced. Comparison of old pictures of the patient with his present appearance is often useful in assessing progress of the disease. There may be a history of progressive increases in shoe and glove sizes, and the patient may have noticed that rings have become increasingly tight.

The patient is large and overweight but usually not obese. Acral enlargement, increased soft tissue mass, coarse features, and prognathism are well-known features of GH excess in adults. The skin is oily, thickened, and rugose with a rubbery texture, and hypertrichosis is common. The incidence of acanthosis nigricans and fibroma molluscum is increased. When the syndrome occurs before epiphyseal fusion, the continuous growth of long bones produces gigantism.

In acromegaly, bony overgrowth of the skull is most striking. The calvaria is thickened and bony ridges are often prominent. The laryngeal cartilages are enlarged and the vocal cords thickened with deepening of the voice in 50 percent of patients. Other clinically significant osseous changes include the following:

1. Increased periosteal new bone formation along the anterior margins of the vertebral bodies produces kyphosis. The ribs thicken and cartilage proliferation occurs at the costochondral junctions.
2. Overgrowth of cartilage and general thickening of bone and soft tissues takes place.[35] These changes may reduce the capacity of the carpal tunnel, thereby producing compression of the median nerve and acroparesthesias typical of the carpal tunnel syndrome, in 30 percent of acromegalics. Less often other peripheral nerves traversing bony canals may be involved.
3. Arthropathies secondary to synovial and capsular thickening and articular cartilage hypertrophy. Arthralgias and deforming arthritis mimicking osteoarthritis are common. Joint effusions occasionally occur but stiffness is unusual.

Skeletal abnormalities of acromegaly are probably not reversible. Osteoporosis is not increased in acromegaly. Cortical bone content is normal or even increased.[35]

Hypertrophy of skeletal muscles with weakness and fatigue are common findings in acromegaly. Histologically there is hypertrophy of Type I fibers and atrophy of Type 2 fibers. Patients complain of difficulty climbing stairs and performing physical work. In about 10 percent of patients there is atrophy of large muscle groups. Quadriceps, gluteal, and deltoid wasting are often noticeable. Myopathy when present is usually a late manifestation of the disease occurring 10 to 15 years after its inception. In these patients minimal elevations of muscle enzymes in serum are not unusual.[34]

GH causes enlargement of many visceral organs including the heart, brain, lungs, salivary glands, thyroid, and kidneys. However, when hepatomegaly and splenomegaly are present a second disease must be excluded.

The heart can be disproportionately enlarged relative to other organs, with serious consequences. In fatal cases, there are hypertrophy and fragmentation of muscle fibers with diffuse fibrous hyperplasia, and moderate atherosclerosis. Cardiac decompensation is usually a late manifestation. ECG abnormalities characteristic of left ventricular hypertrophy, intraventricular conduction defects, and ventricular ectopic beats are common. Acromegalic patients tolerate hypertension and coronary insufficiency poorly, and there is an increased incidence of death due to cardiovascular and respiratory disease.

Since most acromegalic patients have sellar enlargement when first seen, symptoms produced by the expanding tumor are usually prominent. Headaches and hypopituitarism may be the presenting complaints.

DIAGNOSIS OF ACTIVE ACROMEGALY. The diagnosis of florid acromegaly in patients in whom the disease has been present for years usually is not difficult since the physical characteristics are striking and unique. However, the disease has a tendency to become quiescent, presumably due to infarction of the tumor. Therefore, measurement of serum growth hormone is essential, not only to detect occult disease but to evaluate activity in advanced cases.

Measurement of serum growth hormone by the radioimmunoassay is the most sensitive and specific method for diagnosing acromegaly, even though the GH values do not always correlate with the severity of the disease. Basal levels are always elevated and cannot be suppressed to the normal range by administration of glucose. Even when basal GH levels are only marginally higher than normal, autonomous secretion of GH can be demonstrated with glucose load. In addition, the secretion of GH from pituitary tumor responds inappropriately or paradoxically to some stimuli. Specifically, GH is promptly released following administration of TRH or GRH in acromegalic but not in the normal subjects, and L-dopa stimulates GH secretion in the normal individuals but suppresses it in acromegalics. These abnormal responses of GH may also be employed to demonstrate acidophil tumor activity. When the diagnosis of acromegaly is in doubt, it is accepted practice to follow the patient without treatment, since the disease progresses slowly.

MANAGEMENT OF ACROMEGALY. Patients with hypopituitarism and ocular symptoms due to acromegaly are treated like those with other types of sellar tumors. The principal objective is to normalize serum GH levels without affecting normal pituitary function. Unfortunately no single therapeutic modality is uniformly effective and all have inevitable and significant complications.

When tumor has extended beyond the sella, a surgical approach is recommended. Transsphenoidal microsurgery is popular because of the relatively low incidence of complications. However, selective removal of adenoma is rarely effective in lowering GH unless the tumor is small. Panhypopituitarism often occurs when complete removal of the pituitary is attempted. Cryosurgery and radiofrequency techniques are now infrequently employed.

When successful, surgery results in debulking of the tumor and rapid lowering of serum GH levels.

However, the incidence of hypopituitarism is high and success rates are largely dependent on the skill of the surgeon and selection of patients.

The pituitary gland and its tumors are relatively insensitive to irradiation. Conventional doses of 4500 rads usually give only temporary relief from headaches and paresthesias. Additional irradiation may result in damage to adjacent nerve tissues. With sophisticated equipment, narrow beams can be directed to the pituitary, significantly decreasing morbidity.

Proton beams generated from a cyclotron permit delivery of 9000 rads to the sella turcica, sparing the nearby structures.[20] Reportedly up to 90 percent of patients so treated are in satisfactory remission after 5 years.[26] Radioactive seeds of ^{90}Y or ^{198}Au can be implanted under fluoroscopic guidance directly into the pituitary to induce radionecrosis. This technique, however, has no advantage over other modes of irradiation and carries a high risk of producing cerebrospinal fluid rhinorrhea and meningitis.

The principal disadvantage of radiation therapy is that maximal benefits may not be apparent for 3 to 5 years. Proton beam treatment requires expensive equipment presently available in only two centers in the United States. To administer proton beam irradiation, precise localization of the tumor frequently requires invasive techniques. Furthermore, hypopituitarism, which occurs rarely following conventional external irradiation, occurs in about 20 percent of proton beam treated patients. Oculomotor palsies and temporal lobe damage have been occasionally observed in irradiated patients.

A number of pharmacologic agents have been used to suppress GH.[16] Unfortunately most are unsuited for prolonged use. Bromocriptine is the most promising for the long-term management of acromegaly. L-Dopa exerts a paradoxic inhibition of GH in acromegalic subjects but its effects are transitory. It may be useful, however, in controlling distressing hyperhidrosis in selected patients. Somatostatin lowers GH but is impractical since it must be given by continuous intravenous infusion and the secretion of other hormones is also inhibited. Other agents, including medroxyprogesterone, chlorpromazine, and antiserotonins, are at best variably effective. At the present time pharmacologic agents can be recommended only for use with other forms of therapy or in patients in whom surgery and radiation are inappropriate.

A substantial number of patients, mostly with far advanced disease, continue to hypersecrete GH despite all treatment. In these patients, GH-producing cells may exist outside the sella turcica or the primary defect is situated in the hypothalamus.

ACTH-Secreting and Other Functioning Pituitary Tumors. Most patients with pituitary Cushing's disease probably have radiographically undetectable microadenomas.[41] Sellar enlargement in association with Nelson syndrome (hyperpigmentation and pituitary tumor) develops in 10 percent of cases treated by bilateral adrenalectomy. Histologically most are due to chromophobe-like adenomas. Their growth can probably be retarded by irradiation to the pituitary before removal of the adrenal glands.

Clinically the patients present with ocular symptoms secondary to tumor compression or progressive Addisonian-like hyperpigmentation. Large amounts of ACTH and MSH are found in the serum.

This tumor is often locally invasive but occasionally distant metastases occur. Like other pituitary tumors, a combination of surgical hypophysectomy and irradiation is the most effective treatment.

Other Functioning Pituitary Tumors. Increased secretion of TSH by a pituitary tumor, leading to hyperthyroidism, is extremely rare. Likewise, excessive production of LH and FSH by pituitary adenomas has been documented in few cases.[12] Despite elevations of blood testosterone levels, affected patients may present with sexual hypofunction.

Pituitary Apoplexy[27]

Acute massive hemorrhage or infarction of a pituitary tumor is a rare event. Its clinical manifestations are protean and may mimic subarachnoid hemorrhage or pyogenic meningitis. Characteristically there is sudden severe headache (often retro-orbital or frontal), altered consciousness, and ocular symptoms (visual field defects, impaired vision, or ocular palsies). Sella abnormalities are usually demonstrable in plain skull x-rays. The infarction of pituitary tumor is more apt to occur in patients whose pituitaries have been previously irradiated. Precipitating causes include sudden changes of air pressure during air travel or diving. With conservative management, pituitary apoplexy may resolve without serious sequelae, and panhypopituitarism is not an inevitable complication. When it is suspected, however, the patient must be treated with glucocorticoids during the acute crisis.

HYPOPITUITARISM

Hypopituitarism may develop from destruction of the pituitary by tumors, granulomatous lesions, trauma, irradiation (including radiotherapy for head and neck tumors), surgery, and necrosis. The hypertrophied pituitary gland during pregnancy is particularly susceptible to necrosis as a consequence of postpartum hemorrhage and obstetric shock (Sheehan syndrome). It may occur antepartum in diabetics or as a complication of puerperal sepsis. Other unusual causes are autoimmune diseases and infiltrative processes which include hemochromatosis, amyloidosis, and lipidosis.

Pituitary insufficiency may also occur secondary to hypothalamic failure; any lesion that destroys the pituitary can involve the hypothalamus. In addition, psychic disturbances may produce apparent but usually reversible hypothalamic failure. A striking example is growth failure in children with the maternal deprivation syndrome. Low growth hormone levels revert to normal with change of environment. Psychogenic amenorrhea is another such disorder. Here the degree and type of gonadotropin deficiency is variable.

As a rule, pituitary failure due to the hypothalamic dysfunction is more prevalent in patients with monotropic hormone deficiency and children with hypopituitarism without readily demonstrable pituitary lesions.

Clinical Features

The clinical manifestations depend on the age of the patient when the disease first occurs (prepubertal or postpubertal), the type of hormone deficiency present, and the rapidity of the onset of the illness. Not all patients with pituitary failure develop hyposecretion of all tropic hormones. In polytropic hormone deficiency, growth hormone and prolactin are likely to be affected first. The clinical features of prepubertal hypopituitarism are often dominated by short stature, hypoglycemia, and poor sexual maturation. In adults, hypopituitarism is typically characterized by the failure of the peripheral endocrine glands which are intimately regulated by the pituitary. However, the severity of cortisol deficiency may be reduced by hypothyroidism by virtue of the decreased rate of cortisol catabolism, and aldosterone secretion is relatively undisturbed. The complete syndrome of hypopituitarism usually develops insidiously and may not be apparent for many years.

Most patients with chronic panhypopituitarism present with easy fatigability and mental asthenia. They lack appetite and sex drive and are often unable to cope with regular social duties. The skin is thin, appears pale out of proportion to anemia, and is dry and atrophic with fine wrinkling over the face and around the eyes. Hair is dry, brittle, and readily lost. The body temperature, blood pressure, and pulse rate tend to be low. Clinical evidence of hypothyroidism is usually present. There may be recurrent episodes of hypoglycemia or hyponatremia frequently associated with bizarre mental symptoms. Features of hypogonadism in females include amenorrhea, failure of lactation, scanty pubic hair, atrophic external genitalia, and involuted secondary sexual characteristics; in males, impotence, soft testes, small prostate, and slow growth of facial hair are common.

Regardless of the etiology of the pituitary failure, selective deficiencies of pituitary hormone may occur, and the clinical presentation may be dominated by hypogonadism, thyroid failure, or adrenal insufficiency. Isolated deficiency of TSH or ACTH is extremely rare. In children, isolated GH deficiency results in sexual ateliotic dwarfism. Growth is normal in utero but retarded in childhood. Puberty may be delayed but full sexual maturation is attained and patients become fertile. Body proportions are nearly normal. GH deficiency is only one of many causes of dwarfism. GH-related dwarfism can be classified into four major types: 1) GH deficiency associated with insulinopenia and insulin hypersensitivity; 2) GH deficiency associated with hyperinsulinism and normal insulin sensitivity; 3) normal or elevated immunoreactive GH levels and low somatomedin levels (Laron dwarf); and 4) normal immunoreactive GH and somatomedin levels, presumably due to peripheral unresponsiveness to GH.[30]

Hypopituitary Crisis

Hypopituitarism may present with sudden profound weakness and disturbed consciousness which varies from fainting attacks, inattention, and confusion to frank and sometimes irreversible coma. The syndrome is seen in severe panhypopituitarism and may be precipitated by stress induced by infection, surgery, trauma, emotional crisis, prolonged fasting, or exposure to cold. Other causes include the administration of CNS depressants, e.g., morphine and barbiturate, to which the hypopituitary patient is exquisitely sensitive, severe hyponatremia from excessive fluid intake, and administration of thyroid hormone to patients with limited adrenal reserve.

The principal clinical features are hypotension secondary to adrenal insufficiency, hypothermia and bradycardia, hypoglycemia, shallow and slow respirations, all of which contribute to severe metabolic derangements and cerebral anoxia. Although the foregoing abnormalities are not unique to hypopituitarism, usually other physical signs and the history of the patient lead to the recognition of the syndrome. Therapy is instituted as outlined in the treatment section as soon as the disease is suspected.

Differential Diagnosis

Overt hypopituitarism is usually not difficult to diagnose, but must be distinguished from primary failure of target glands. Rarely, its clinical presentation is dominated by psychiatric and hematologic abnormalities, which can be manifested as paranoia or manic depression, or refractory normocytic or microcytic anemias, respectively.

Anorexia Nervosa

Organic hypopituitarism must also be distinguished from the partial pituitary failure of anorexia nervosa. This condition is characterized by profound emaciation due to voluntary refusal to eat, usually in young girls with psychoneurosis and no demonstrable organic lesion.

Typically, patients fear becoming obese, have distorted concepts of body habitus, and manifest bizarre behavior and ideation about food. Some feel guilty when eating; others equate food with filth and dirt; still others pretend to eat but secretly discard food. The patient is often child-like, demanding, seclusive and has difficulty in forming adult relationships.

Despite considerable weight loss patients are strikingly unconcerned about their condition and appear cheerful and hyperactive. Vomiting, often self-induced, is characteristic and laxative abuse is common. Amenorrhea is usually present in females and males have loss of libido. In contrast to hypopituitarism, axillary and pubic hair are retained and breast tissue is surprisingly well preserved. There is no evidence of premature senility and skin atrophy but lanugo may present over the back, limbs, and face. Other common findings include hypothermia, bradycardia, hypotension, dry skin, and sometimes prolonged relaxation of deep tendon reflexes, an important sign found also in patients with hypothyroidism.

Patients with anorexia nervosa have striking metabolic and hormonal changes, some resulting from malnutrition and others from hypothalamic dysfunction.[29] Typically they are unable to maintain their body temperature when subjected to varying degrees of external temperature. Basal serum growth hormone concentrations may be normal or elevated and GH reserve tests are normal, an important distinguishing feature from hypopituitarism. Serum estrogen and gonadotropin levels are usually low. Characteristically in adult women a pubertal-type or even prepubertal-type of LH secretion release pattern during sleep with low or no spikes are found. Responses to hypothalamic releasing factors are quantitatively normal but abnormally delayed.[44] These findings suggest that the pituitary abnormalities found in anorexia nervosa are secondary to hypothalamic dysfunction.

Serum triiodothyronine concentrations are consistently low; thyroxine levels are usually in the lower range of normal while serum TSH levels are nearly always normal. These changes are characteristic of starvation in which peripheral conversion of T_4 to T_3 is decreased by increased conversion of T_4 to reverse T_3, a usual metabolite of thyroxine.

Hypothalamic dysfunction best explains the abnormalities in eating habit, sexual behavior and gonadal dysfunction, body temperature regulation, and water diuresis. However, it is uncertain whether this hypothalamic dysfunction is secondary to psychic stress or anorexia nervosa itself is a consequence of reversible idiopathic primary hypothalamic dysfunction.

This syndrome is potentially fatal. The treatment consists of refeeding, occasionally requiring tube-feeding or intravenous infusion, and intensive psychotherapy (see Chap. 73).

Diagnosis

When pituitary insufficiency is suspected laboratory investigation can proceed as outlined in Figure 69–4 and the performance of each test is noted in Table 69–4. One first identifies which target glands are hypofunctioning, then proceeds to look for evidence of compensatory elevations of pituitary tropic hormones, and finally, carries out studies to distinguish pituitary from hypothalamic failure if target organ hormone deficiency is not associated with elevated

pituitary hormones. The latter is accomplished by administration of hypothalamic-releasing hormones. Anatomic evaluation of the hypothalamic-pituitary region, if indicated, is made in collaboration with a neuroradiologist, neurosurgeon, and ophthalmologist.

The GH reserve test is the most sensitive index of hypofunctioning of the pituitary. In affected patients limited GH reserve is usually demonstrated. Less commonly prolactin deficiency is found. GH reserve is best evaluated by measuring GH response to insulin-induced hypoglycemia or to L-dopa.[25] In the presence of adrenal or thyroid failure, induction of hypoglycemia can be hazardous; therefore, L-dopa is the agent of choice in these patients. GH levels may fail to rise following stimulation in more than 50 percent of obese patients. Therefore, this test may not be helpful in overweight patients with the empty sella syndrome.

The function of thyrotropic cells is measured by administrating TRH. Normally this stimulates TSH release from the thyrotropic cells unless the latter are suppressed by exogenous thyroid hormone or by endogenous thyroid hormones produced by an autonomously functioning hyperactive thyroid. Totally or partially impaired responses occur in euthyroid patients with pituitary tumors or on high doses of glucocorticoids.

Gonadotropin reserve can be assessed by the ad-

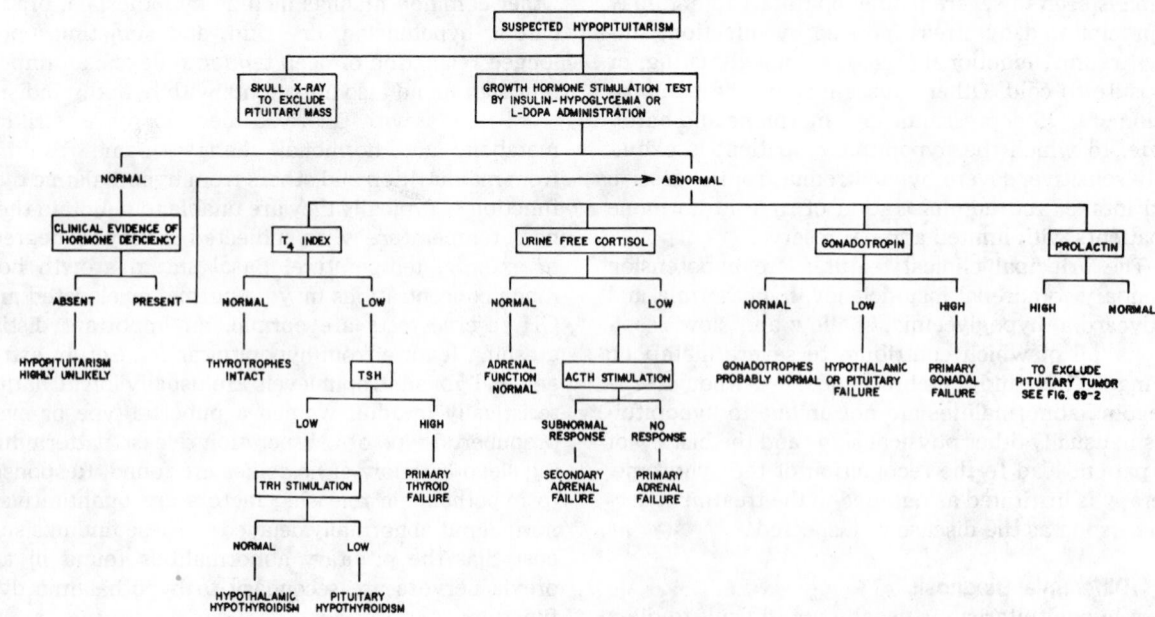

FIGURE 69–4. Evaluation of suspected hypopituitarism.

TABLE 69-4

Commonly Used Methods for Evaluation of the Function of the Anterior Pituitary

Hormone	Method of Study	Sampling Intervals	Normal Responses	Coments
GH	Hypoglycemia (CZI 0.1 to 0.15U/kg BW IV) L-dopa 0.5 g P.O.	Basal and 15 min × 4 Basal and 30 min × 4	Basal: 0–5 ng/ml Peak: >10 ng/ml	Poor response in obesity. Phenothiazine, progesterone, and high dose steroid therapy cause blunted response
TSH	TRH 500 μg IV	Baseline and 20 min × 3	Basal: 0–7 μu/ml Peak: 8 μu/ml, or 2 × basal value	Poor response in hyperthyroidism, exogenous use of thyroid hormone, autonomous thyroid, gluco-corticoid, or L-dopa therapy and renal failure
Prolactin	TRH 500 μg IV	Baseline and 10 min × 3	Basal: 0–20 ng/ml Peak: 2 × basal values	Poor response in hyperthyroidism
ACTH (reflected by cortisol changes)	Hypoglycemia	Baseline and during hypoglycemia	Basal: 8 to 16 μg/dl Peak: 20 μg/dl or 2 × basal values	Patient under stress may have high basal value and poor response to hypoglycemia
	Metyrapone 750 mg 4 hourly for 6 doses	24 hr urine the day before, the day of, and the day after metyrapone	Urine 17-OHCS 2 × basal values	
LH and FSH*	GRH 100 μg	0, 15, 30, 45, 60, and 90 min	Peak: 2 × basal values	Interpretation of GRH test may be difficult. May require a prolonged infusion of GRH

* Gonadotropin deficiency is best proven by showing low to normal immunoassayable gonadotropin in the presence of low serum testosterone and oligo- or azoospermia. GRH-stimulation test does not always differentiate hypothalamic failure from pituitary deficiency.

Other remarks: Insulin (CZI 0.1 to 0.15 U/kg body weight), 500 μg of TRH, and 100 μg of GRH may be given together, with sampling of blood at 0, 5, 15, 30, 45, 60, 90, and 120 min for assay of GH, TSH, prolactin, cortisol, FSH, and LH.

---

ministration of GRH or clomiphene. GRH stimulates secretion of both gonadotropins, with more LH than FSH being released under normal circumstances. The influence of exogenous sex steroids on the gonadotropin response to GRH is complex. For this reason, the test is best done when the patient is not on sex steroids. The GRH stimulation test cannot distinguish between hypothalamic and pituitary disease, since absent, subnormal, or normal response may be found in both conditions. Functional capacity of gonadotropic cells can be assessed by using clomiphene, an antiestrogen that blocks hypothalamic receptors for estrogen, thereby preventing normal feedback inhibition by estrogen. In normal subjects GRH levels rise

and stimulate secretion of gonadotropin. Conversely in hypothalamic or hypopituitary hypogonadism and prepubertal subjects or patients with severe anorexia nervosa, gonadotropin levels do not rise.

Evaluation of the reserve capacity of the pituitary-adrenal axis is particularly important in patients with suspected hypopituitarism. Normal basal cortisol levels do not exclude partially impaired ACTH secretion. Only when such patients are stressed may adrenal insufficiencies become evident. To evaluate the effects of stress, hypoglycemia produced by administration of insulin is used. If cortisol levels rise normally, adequate ACTH secretory reserve is presumed. ACTH reserve can also be evaluated using the metyrapone test. Metyrapone blocks the normal synthesis of cortisol by inhibiting 11-beta-hydroxylation in the adrenal cortex. As the plasma cortisol levels fall, there is in normal man increased ACTH output and consequently increased steroidogenesis to the point of blockage. Accumulation of the cortisol precursor, 11-desoxycortisol (compound S), in plasma and urine is expected. Since metabolites of compound S are measured in the urine as 17-OHCS, no rise in urine 17-OHCS after the administration of metyrapone and an increase after exogenous ACTH administration is good evidence for impaired ACTH reserve.

Treatment of Chronic Hypopituitarism

Treatment of chronic hypopituitarism consists of treating the cause of pituitary failure when appropriate and hormone replacement. The common treatable pituitary lesions are tumor and infection. Even when the underlying disorder is curable, pituitary function is rarely restored. Hormone replacement depends on the endocrine status of the patient. When the patient has panhypopituitarism, adrenal failure is treated first, then thyroid deficiency, and finally gonadal dysfunction. Cortisone acetate, 10 mg per day, is given by mouth for 3 to 5 days and then over 10 days gradually increased to the usual replacement dose, 25 to 35 mg per day. Abrupt use of full replacement doses is to be avoided since it may precipitate acute psychoses in hypopituitarism. In the event of major surgery or intercurrent severe illness, the dosage must be increased to 200 to 250 mg per day. Usual precautions for patients with adrenal insufficiency must be taken (see p. 785). Thyroxine is the preferred preparation to restore hypothyroidism to normal. Initially 0.05 mg of L-thyroxine sodium is given daily; this dosage is increased by 0.025 mg or 0.05 mg every 2 weeks until the daily dosage is 0.15 to 0.25 mg. The treatment of gonadal failure depends on the patient's needs. In males, libido and sexual function can usually be restored with injections of depot-testosterone (200 to 300 mg of testosterone enanthate) administered every 3 to 4 weeks. Smaller doses (50 mg) should be used initially to avoid priapism. Testosterone is inappropriate in the elderly patient. The restoration of fertility is more difficult. Combined therapy with human menopausal gonadotropin (100 to 200 IU) and varying amounts of human chorionic gonadotropin is only occasionally successful. In young females sexual function and secondary sex characteristics can be maintained by small doses of estrogen (either ethynyl estradiol 0.02 to 0.04 mg or stilbestrol 0.5 to 3 mg a day) given in a cyclic manner. Ovulation can be induced with gonadotropin therapy but conception must be discouraged in patients with pituitary tumors. In older women estrogen replacement is generally unnecessary. Hypopituitarism may mask the full expression of coexisting diabetes insipidus. Once deficiencies of adrenal and thyroid are corrected, symptoms of diabetes insipidus may become apparent.

Treatment of Hypopituitary Crisis

The management of hypopituitary crisis consists of intravenous administration of cortisol hemisuccinate (100 mg initially and every 4 to 6 hours) and glucose (50 to 100 ml of 50 percent solution). If the patient has hypothyroidism the dose of glucocorticoid should be reduced as soon as the patient is stable until euthyroidism is achieved. Electrolyte disturbances are usually not severe but water intoxication is a hazard in the patient with hypopituitarism. Therefore, fluids must be administered sparingly with great caution. Respiratory care and cardiac support are vital and specific treatment of the precipitating cause is mandatory. Severe hypothermia secondary to hypothyroidism is managed with slow rewarming, 0.3°C per hour, with thermal blankets and administration of 0.1 to 0.2 mg of thyroxine intravenously. Subsequent doses depend on individual circumstances.

POSTERIOR PITUITARY

The posterior lobe of the pituitary is the distal portion of a neurosecretory system that includes the supraoptic and paraventricular nuclei of the hypothalamus. The supraoptic nucleus is the main source of vasopressin whereas the paraventricular nucleus produces predominantly oxytocin. These hormones are bound to specific carrier proteins, the neurophysins. They traverse nerve fibers to their site of storage in the posterior pituitary and subsequently are selectively secreted on demand into the blood together with their respective carrier proteins.

Regulation of ADH Secretion

Arginine-vasopressin, or human antidiuretic hormone (ADH), is an octapeptide whose primary function is the regulation of water metabolism. The most important physiologic determinant of its secretion is plasma osmolality. Release is controlled by osmoregulators in the anterior hypothalamus. The normal threshold for ADH secretion is 280 mOsm/kg. An increase of only 1 percent above this in the plasma perfusing the osmoregulators is sufficient to evoke ADH release.[36] When plasma osmolality falls below the threshold, for example, after a water load, secretion is suppressed and excess water is excreted in urine. Normally, the plasma osmolality is effectively regulated by ADH within the range of 281 to 295 mOsm/kg. Nonosmotic factors such as blood volume and blood pressure may also alter ADH secretion. However, volume reduction, without a change in osmolality, must exceed 10 percent or isovolemic reduction of blood pressure be greater than 5 to 10 percent of the resting recumbent value to stimulate secretion. Therefore, under normal circumstances, volume and blood pressure are not important secretory determinants. In contrast, in pathologic states the rate of ADH release may depend upon summation of excitatory and inhibitory stimuli from receptors for plasma osmolality, volume, and blood pressure.

The hypothalamic osmoregulatory centers are intimately related to the thirst center both anatomically and functionally. Stimulation of the thirst center with hypertonic serum induces polydipsia and antidiuresis. Stimulation of the supraoptic nuclei promotes antidiuresis by increasing ADH secretion and without provoking polydipsia. Plasma osmolality (Posm) and intravascular volume (IVV) are maintained in the manner shown in Figure 69–5.

The secretion of ADH is also affected by a variety of chemical agents. Barbiturates, morphine, nicotine, histamine, acetylcholine, and other cholinergic drugs stimulate release of ADH. Emotional disturbances, pain, and vomiting also can stimulate ADH release. Alcohol and phenytoin in high doses may inhibit release of ADH. Glucocorticoids increase the stimulatory threshold for the release of ADH. Patients with adrenal insufficiency may have inappropriately high levels of ADH which impair their ability to excrete a water load.

Transport in Plasma and Degradation

The average concentration of plasma ADH in healthy adults in a normal state of hydration and supine position is 2.7 ± 1.4 pg/ml. The half-life of ADH in plasma is 10 to 20 minutes.

Metabolic Effect

ADH plays an important role in the homeostatic regulation of osmolality and body water volume. In cells of the distal renal tubules, ADH stimulates the formation of cyclic AMP which increases the permeability of tubular cells to water. In the absence of ADH, the distal convoluted tubules are almost impermeable to water whereas active reabsorption of solutes continues. Consequently fluid which enters the distal collecting duct becomes excessively hypotonic, possibly between 15 and 30 mOsm/kg. Since the collecting ducts are also relatively impermeable to water without ADH, voluminous amounts of hypotonic urine are excreted by individuals who have inadequate ADH or are refractory to the effect of the hormone. Conversely, in the presence of maximal ADH activity, active solute reabsorption by distal tubular cells is accompanied by sufficient passive reabsorption of water to make the intraluminal fluid isotonic. As this fluid passes through the collecting ducts, it can be maximally concentrated by back diffusion of water along its osmotic gradient into the hypertonic periductal tissue to concentrations as high as 1200 to 1400 mOsm/kg.

ADH is not the sole determinant of the capacity of the kidney to concentrate urine. Prolonged overhydration impairs the renal concentrating mechanism, and chronic water deprivation enhances it. These changes probably result from alterations of medullary tonicity rather than changes in the renal response to ADH. Other physiologic factors that may

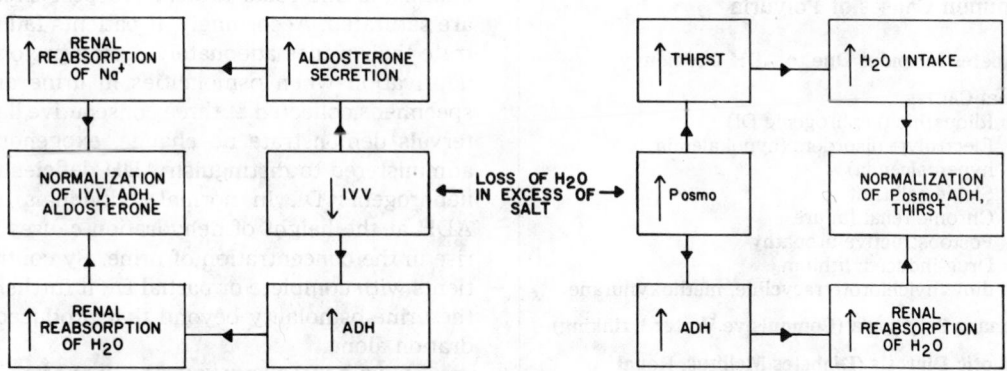

FIGURE 69–5. The role of ADH in the regulation of water homeostasis.

influence the maximal concentrating capacity of the kidney include the rate of solute excretion and intake, glomerular filtration rate, the rate of medullary blood flow, and the protein content of the diet. Glucocorticoids and thyroid hormone increase renal blood flow and glomerular filtration. Glucocorticoid deficiency also increases the permeability of the distal collecting ducts to water. Therefore, ADH deficiency may not produce large quantities of dilute urine in patients with total failure of anterior pituitary function.

DISORDERS OF THE POSTERIOR PITUITARY

Diabetes Insipidus[13]

Diabetes insipidus (DI) is a pathologic condition characterized by the excretion of large quantities of dilute urine and secondary polydipsia. The disease is usually due to inadequate synthesis or release of ADH. Occasionally, DI results from a primary defect in the renal tubular response to ADH (nephrogenic DI). The diagnosis of DI should be suspected in patients who excrete more than 3 liters per day of dilute urine with specific gravities less than 1.010 and osmolalities less than 300 mOsm/kg. Some patients with ADH deficiency, however, do not produce large volumes of dilute urine. For example, coexisting anterior pituitary deficiency may mask the full expression of DI or the degree of ADH deficiency may be too mild to be recognized.

DIFFERENTIAL DIAGNOSIS OF POLYURIA. Not all patients who excrete excessive amounts of urine lack ADH. As shown in Table 69–5, polyuria occurs in many other conditions. Iatrogenic causes should be excluded. Abnormalities in the urine and blood chemistries listed in Figure 69–6 will usually lead to the recognition of diabetes mellitus, chronic nephritis,

---

TABLE 69–5
Common Causes of Polyuria

I. **Diabetes Insipidus Due to ADH Deficiency**

II. **Renal Causes**
   A. Idiopathic (nephrogenic DI)
   B. Electrolyte disorders (hypokalemia, hypercalcemia)
   C. Sickle cell trait
   D. Chronic renal failure
   E. Postobstructive uropathy
   F. Drug-induced: lithium, dimethylchlorotetracycline, methoxyflurane

III. **Primary Polydipsia (Compulsive Water Drinking)**

IV. **Osmotic Diuresis (Diabetes Mellitus, Renal Glycosuria, Diuretic Therapy)**

---

and electrolyte derangements associated with an inability to concentrate the urine. The initial step in the evaluation of patients with polyuria requires distinguishing those with DI, nephrogenic DI, or primary polydipsia from those with polyuria due to other causes.

If another cause of polyuria can be identified, ADH deficiency is unlikely. Diabetes insipidus is virtually excluded when correction of polyuria follows control of diabetes mellitus, electrolyte abnormalities, or treatable renal disorders. A water deprivation test is carried out only when the initial evaluation fails to establish the cause of polyuria, or an etiologic factor known to cause DI is present (Table 69–6). It is almost impossible to diagnose ADH deficiency in patients with coexistent irreversible nephrogenic DI without directly measuring ADH by radioimmunoassay.

Urine specific gravity is a crude index of urine concentration. It is significantly affected by urea, protein, glucose, and radiopaque dyes which contribute little to osmolality. Urine osmolality is less than serum osmolality in most but not all patients with DI. Since glomerular filtration is decreased following severe dehydration, urinary osmolality may exceed plasma osmolality in some patients with partial DI. However, they are unable to concentrate their urine maximally without receiving exogenous ADH. This observation has been adopted as a test to determine partial ADH deficiency.[31] The principles underlying this test are as follows: In the absence of an ADH radioimmunoassay, the effect of fluid deprivation on ADH secretion can only be inferred from changes in urine production and urinary osmolality. These changes are related not only to ADH concentrations but also to the renal tubular response to ADH and the rate of solute output. During fluid deprivation in normal subjects the secretion of ADH is maximally stimulated and renal tubular receptor sites for ADH are saturated. Accordingly, if patients fail to concentrate their urines adequately during prolonged water deprivation when osmolalities in urine and plasma specimens collected at three consecutive half-hour intervals demonstrate no change, exogenous ADH is administered to distinguish ADH deficiency DI from nephrogenic DI. In normal individuals, exogenous ADH at the height of dehydration causes no further rise in the concentration of urine. By contrast, in patients with complete or partial DI, it further increases the urine osmolality beyond that produced by dehydration alone.

DI VS. PRIMARY POLYDIPSIA. It is often difficult to differentiate between DI and primary polydipsia or

Critical Question	Recommendation
1. Is it drug induced ?	Appropriate history
2. Is the patient diabetic ?	2 hr pc blood glucose, urine glucose
3. Are there renal abnormalities ?	SUN creatinine urine analysis
4. Are electrolytes derangements involved ?	Serum Ca, K
5. Is sickle cell anemia involved ?	Hemoglobin electrophoresis

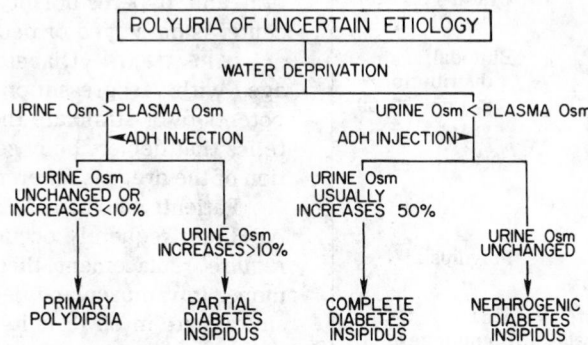

FIGURE 69-6. Differential diagnosis of polyuric syndrome.

compulsive water drinking, which can result from a central neurologic lesion, but is more commonly associated with an emotional disturbance. The difficulty is due to the fact that prolonged excessive water intake may cause a transient loss in the ability to excrete a maximally concentrated urine, probably because of decreased tonicity of the renal medullary concentrating apparatus. Clinical features are usually not helpful (Table 69-7). However, after fluid restriction, blood levels of arginine–vasopressin are normal, relative to plasma osmolality, in patients with primary polydipsia but are low in patients with true DI. Radioimmunoassay of ADH is, therefore, the best means to distinguish true diabetes insipidus from primary polydipsia. Unfortunately, the assay is not yet generally available for clinical use. The approach to establishing a diagnosis in patients with suspected DI is summarized in Figure 69-6.

THE ETIOLOGY OF ADH DEFICIENCY DI. Vasopressin deficiency DI can be primary or secondary (Table 69-6). Primary or idiopathic DI is present in nearly half of affected patients, occurs in both sexes at any age after infancy, is diagnosed only by exclusion, and is more common in males. Females often develop their symptoms during pregnancy. In some cases, there is unexplained atrophy of the supraoptic nuclei, or often of the hypothalamicohypophyseal tract, or abnormalities of secretory granules in the posterior pituitary. Daily urine output in these patients usually exceeds 5 liters and may be relatively constant, because the daily solute load to the kidney remains

fairly constant. Reducing the solute load may ameliorate the polyuria.

Diabetes insipidus may be secondary to pituitary stalk transsection or granulomatous, inflammatory, or neoplastic processes, or trauma involving the parasellar region. It may be suspected by demonstration of a space-occupying intracranial mass, abnormal function of the anterior pituitary or hypothalamus, or symptoms and signs of the underlying systemic disease. Scrutiny should be directed toward those systemic processes that may involve the neurohypophysis.

Histiocytosis X often produces diabetes insipidus secondary to lipoid deposits in the hypothalamus. Lipoid deposits also occur in the orbit producing exophthalmos, in other areas of the skull, and in long bones occasionally resulting in pathologic fractures.

TABLE 69-6
The Etiology of Diabetes Insipidus

I. Primary Diabetes Insipidus
 A. Idiopathic (most common)
 B. Familial (rare)

II. Secondary Diabetes Insipidus
 A. Therapeutic hypophysectomy
 B. Neoplasia, primary or metastatic, leukemia
 C. Head trauma
 D. Granulomata, sarcoidosis, tuberculosis, syphilis, histiocytosis X
 E. Postencephalitic complication

TABLE 69–7

Comparison of DI and Primary Polydipsia (PP)

	DI	PP
Polyuria, polydipsia	Present	Present
Mode of onset	Acute	Gradual or "stuttering"
Age of onset of illness	Any age	Bimodal distribution: 8–18 or 35–59 years
Sex	M/F = 1	80% females
Preference for ice-cold water	+ +	±
Basic disturbance	polyuria	Polydipsia
Response to ADH	Correction of polyuria, relief of thirst	Thirst continues, may develop water intoxication
Initial serum sodium and osmolality	High to high normal	Low normal to low
Psychiatric or emotional disturbance	±	+ + +
Etiologies	Organic, familial, or idiopathic	Psychogenic

A variety of skin lesions are encountered, and otitis media is common. Diabetes insipidus due to metastases is most commonly caused by carcinoma of the breast. Small and asymptomatic primary tumors may be overlooked. Sarcoid, tuberculosis, and syphilis may also produce the syndrome when the lesions are strategically located.

An increasingly important cause of either transient or permanent diabetes insipidus is damage due to trauma, surgery, or radiation of the pituitary region. Characteristically, polyuria occurs first and may last hours or days. This is followed by a normal urine output or even oliguria due to release of vasopressin from injured tissue. Within a week or so polyuria recurs and may remain permanently. The ultimate outcome is dependent upon the extent of neurohypophyseal damage. Most of the cells which elaborate ADH are located at the base of the hypothalamus or are high in the stalk. Occasionally regeneration of damaged cells may lead to amelioration of DI.

In mild DI, as long as the patient's thirst mechanism is intact, no untoward sequelae occur. The osmolality of extracellular fluid is maintained at the expense of polydipsia and a large daily fluid turnover. When volumes of 10 liters or more are imbibed and excreted daily, there is often weight loss, exhaustion, constipation, and hydronephrosis. Profound dehydration and hyperosmolality develop when the thirst center is destroyed or becomes insensitive.

TREATMENT. Diabetes insipidus can be managed with vasopressin or its derivatives, agents that potentiate or stimulate the release of ADH, and diuretics that deplete body solute. Since the mode of action of the drugs is different, their effects are additive.

Patients who have total or near total deficiency of ADH, as frequently occurs in idiopathic DI, usually require replacement therapy with exogenous hormone. Intramuscular injection of long-acting pitressin tannate in oil (5 units per ml in arachis oil) provides the most satisfactory results. Usually 5 units two to three times a week is sufficient; however, the dose must be adjusted to the individual. It is important to instruct the patient that the contents of the ampule should be warmed to body temperature and shaken thoroughly just before drawing it into a syringe; otherwise active hormone may remain adherent to the wall of the container. The effects of aqueous vasopressin are brief; therefore, this drug is impractical for long-term use in patients with chronic DI. However, it is an agent of choice when there are reasons to believe that the disease may be transient, or for unconscious patients receiving intravenous fluids. Lysine-vasopressin is available for intranasal administration. Unfortunately it frequently causes local irritation and its antidiuretic effect lasts only 4 to 6 hours. Recently a superior synthetic analogue, 1-desamino-8-D-arginine-vasopressin (DDAVP), has been introduced for the management of ADH deficiency. It is also administered nasally but in contrast to lysine-vasopressin, is effective for 10 to 24 hours and has no significant pressor side effect. Most patients respond satisfactorily to 2.5 to 15 μg twice a day.

Chlorpropamide potentiates the action of vasopressin on the renal concentrating mechanism. Use of this agent has become increasingly popular in patients with partial vasopressin deficiency. Patients with normal glucose tolerance usually tolerate up to 500 mg per day without developing symptomatic hypoglycemia. Blood glucose levels are prone to be markedly lowered in patients with concomitant deficiencies of growth hormone, glucocorticoids, or thyroid hormone. In some instances, chlorpropamide is effective in restoring derangement in the thirst mechanism to normal. Clofibrate and carbamazepine (Tegretol) have no intrinsic antidiuretic effect nor do they potentiate the peripheral action of ADH but both augment the release of ADH from the neurohypophysis. Chlorothiazide has proved useful in controlling polyuria resulting from ADH deficiency by reducing solute load.

Most patients with incomplete DI can be successfully managed with chlorpropamide alone or combined with either chlorothiazide or clofibrate 1.5 to 2.0 g per day in divided doses. Carbamazepine, because of its toxicity, is now seldom used.

Syndrome of Inappropriate Secretion of Antidiuretic Hormone (SIADH)[32]

When ADH is secreted excessively in the absence of an osmotic or other physiologic stimulus, renal excretion of water is impaired. Ingestion of water is not followed by appropriate excretion and patients develop dilutional hyponatremia secondary to expansion of body fluids. The syndrome of inappropriate secretion of ADH (SIADH) was originally reported in patients with bronchogenic carcinoma; now many other conditions associated with this syndrome have been recognized (Table 69–8). Increased fluid volume and hypotonicity increase glomerular filtration rate

---

TABLE 69–8
Causes of Syndrome of Inappropriate ADH

I. Ectopic Production of ADH
  A. Lung carcinoma, particularly oat-cell
  B. Carcinoma of GI tract
  C. Pancreatic carcinoma
  D. Thymoma
  E. Lymphoma
  F. Tuberculosis

II. Hypersecretion of ADH from Supraoptic-Hypophyseal System
  A. Trauma, especially head injury
  B. Hemorrhage
  C. Pulmonary disease: TBC, cavitation, pneumonia
  D. CNS disorders: Brain abscess, meningitis, subarachnoid hemorrhage, brain tumor, viral infection, psychosis
  E. Metabolic-endocrine disease, myxedema, Addison's disease, hypopituitarism, acute intermittent porphyria
  F. Idiopathic

III. SIADH Associated with Drug Administration
  A. Vasopressin, oxytocin, vincristine, chlorpropamide, thiazide, clofibrate, cyclophosphamide, carbamazepine

---

and decrease aldosterone secretion. Consequently, SIADH is frequently associated with increased excretion of salt. Although urinary sodium excretion in SIADH may not be excessive, the urine osmolality is almost always inappropriately high for the degree of serum hypo-osmolality. Inappropriately excessive production of ADH leads to the development of 1) hyponatremia associated with hypo-osmolality of the serum and extracellular fluid; 2) urine that is hypertonic relative to plasma; and 3) sustained urinary excretion of sodium despite hyponatremia. Similar features can occur in individuals with adrenal insufficiency or renal disease. Therefore, the following additional criteria are necessary to establish the diagnosis of SIADH: 1) normal renal and adrenal function; 2) absence of dehydration or azotemia; 3) reversal of renal sodium loss and hyponatremia by fluid deprivation.

When all the foregoing criteria are met, the diagnosis of SIADH is made easily. However, one or more criteria are often absent. Hyponatremia, the hallmark of the syndrome, is apparent only when the patient is in positive free water balance. For example, patients with terminal carcinoma are often anorectic and dehydrated. When they have excessive circulating ADH, hyponatremia develops only after parenteral hydration or forced fluids by mouth. Although urine is typically hypertonic relative to plasma in classic SIADH, under some circumstances osmolality of urine may be less than that of plasma. When the patient's solute load is extremely low, a positive free water balance is achievable with urine that is hypotonic to plasma. When the patient is on a low sodium diet, at later stages of the illness, the urine sodium may be low.

Since the hypo-osmolality of SIADH involves both the intracellular and extracellular compartments, clinical edema is usually absent. Unless there is profound hyponatremia, signs and symptoms are conspicuously absent. When hyponatremia occurs abruptly or is severe, confusion, stupor, muscle twitching, seizures, or coma may develop.

DIFFERENTIAL DIAGNOSIS OF HYPONATREMIA. Once the presence of hyponatremia is established by at least two separate sodium determinations, pseudohyponatremia due to hyperlipidemia, hyperproteinemia, or profound hyperglycemia must be excluded. True hyponatremia occurs in many situations (Table 69–9). The history and examination often provide useful clues in the differential diagnosis. The recognition of cardiac failure, cirrhosis, Addison's disease, or profound dehydration is generally not difficult. For the initial laboratory evaluation of hyponatremia, the

---TABLE 69–9---
Major Causes of Hyponatremia

True sodium depletion (deficiency of total body sodium)
    Addison's disease
    Salt-losing nephropathy
    GI loss
    Diuretic therapy
    Rigid prolonged sodium restriction

Dilutional hyponatremia (excessive body water)
    SIADH
    Psychogenic water drinker
    Inappropriate fluid therapy

Hyponatremia associated with increased total body
  sodium
    Cardiac failure
    Cirrhosis

following studies are recommended: 1) serum electrolytes (SUN, Na, K, Cl, CO_2) and glucose; 2) liver and renal function tests; 3) examination of serum for turbidity; and 4) chest and skull x-rays if indicated.

The laboratory tests and examinations are usually sufficient to establish or exclude heart failure, cirrhosis, pseudohyponatremia, or renal insufficiency. When hypothyroidism or adrenal insufficiency is suspected, additional tests are required to establish the diagnosis. To confirm SIADH, determination of urine osmolality, sodium excretion, and serum osmolality are indicated. When hyponatremia is mild and when the diagnosis is in doubt, a water loading test may be helpful (Fig. 69–7).

Normal subjects respond to a water load with a prompt diuresis of dilute urine that is more hypotonic than plasma. Because of high circulating ADH levels, patients with SIADH are unable to form free water. Consequently, despite a water load and plasma hypo-osmolality, their urine osmolalities are often higher than those of plasma. This test does not distinguish between excessive hypothalamic or ectopic ADH production. It should not be administered to patients with profound hyponatremia, since seizures may develop when hyponatremia is further aggravated by a water load. The test is performed as follows:

1. The bladder is emptied and the urine discarded.
2. Hourly urine specimens are collected for 5 hours.
3. As soon as the first urine specimen collection is completed, 1000 ml of water is given orally over a period of 20 minutes.
4. Five milliliters of plasma is obtained at the midpoint of each urine collection period for measurement of osmolality.
5. The volume and osmolality of each urine specimen as well as the osmolality of each plasma sample is recorded.

In normal subjects, at least 60 percent of the water load is excreted within 4 hours, urine osmolality is usually less than 180 mOsm/kg, and urine osmolality is less than that of plasma. Even with a water load, urine osmolality in patients with SIADH is often greater than 230 mOsm/kg, which is usually greater than plasma osmolality.[32] Defective water excretion occurs in Addison's disease, hypopituitarism, heart failure, cirrhosis, certain types of nephrosis, acute re-

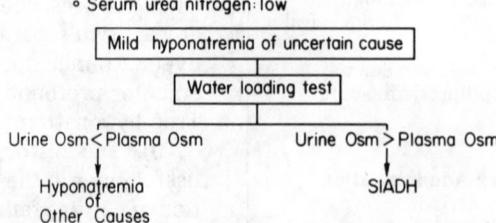

Critical Question	Recommendations
1. Is it pseudohyponatremia?	Examine serum turbidity, measure glucose, protein
2. Are liver and kidney functions normal?	SUN, creatinine, LFT
3. Is the patient euthyroid?	Measure serum T_4, TSH
4. Is adrenal function normal?	Measure plasma cortisol or ACTH stimulation test if appropriate

Usual Findings in Inappropriate ADH Syndrome

  • Urine osmology > serum osmology
  • Urine sodium excretion: high
  • Serum urea nitrogen: low

Mild hyponatremia of uncertain cause

Water loading test

Urine Osm < Plasma Osm   Urine Osm > Plasma Osm

Hyponatremia of Other Causes   SIADH

FIGURE 69–7. Evaluation of hyponatremia.

nal failure, and hypothyroidism and following shock, hemorrhage, or dehydration. If these conditions have been excluded, the diagnosis of SIADH can be made if defective water excretion is proven.

TREATMENT. Most patients can be managed by fluid restriction alone. However, if hyponatremia persists or fluid restriction is not tolerated, 600 to 1200 mg of demeclocycline per day given orally often restores serum sodium concentrations within 2 weeks. Both lithium and demeclocycline inhibit the peripheral action of ADH and produce nephrogenic diabetes insipidus. For the management of SIADH, demeclocycline appears to be superior to lithium.[14]

In life-threatening hyponatremia associated with serious mental disturbances, rapid infusion of 300 to 500 ml of hypertonic (3 to 5 percent) saline may be necessary to alleviate the symptoms; this is then followed by water restriction. Alternatively, potent diuretics such as furosemide may be administered. Fluid balance is regulated closely and losses are replaced with hypertonic saline and potassium. The syndrome of inappropriate ADH secretion is often transient; the prognosis is usually determined by the underlying disease.

POLYGLANDULAR SYNDROMES

Either because of common origin or functional interaction, cells of different endocrine tissues may simultaneously or in succession function abnormally. The changes vary from hypersecreting or inert adenomas in two or more glands to concomitant failure of multiple endocrine organs.

Multiple Endocrine Adenomatosis (MEA) Type I (Wermer Syndrome)[37]

Although this entity may occur sporadically, it is usually inherited as an autosomal dominant trait with considerable phenotypic variation. Adenomas of parathyroid glands, pancreatic islets, and pituitary occur in association. The parathyroid adenomas are usually multiple. Nearly 90 percent of patients with this syndrome have hyperparathyroidism but the consequences of hypercalcemia are usually inconspicuous. Diffuse hyperplasia of the pancreatic islets occurs and multiple adenomas may be present. They commonly secrete gastrin producing the Zollinger-Ellison syndrome. In addition, they produce insulin, glucagon, or vasoactive intestinal peptide (VIP). Zollinger-Ellison syndrome occurs in about 60 percent of patients with pancreatic adenomas, and insulinoma in 30 percent of them. The glucagonoma syndrome includes glucose intolerance, stomatitis, anemia, and characteristically necrolytic migratory erythema. Vasointestinal polypeptide-secreting tumor (VIPoma) causes the Verner-Morrison syndrome, which consists of watery diarrhea, hypokalemia, achlorhydria, acidosis, and occasionally episodic hypercalcemia. Most pituitary adenomas are nonfunctional chromophobe tumors. However, one-third of them may produce hormones which lead to acromegaly, Cushing syndrome, or hyperprolactinemia. Other lesions less commonly associated with this syndrome include carcinoid, multiple lipomas, schwannomas, thymomas, and probably thyroid tumors. Not infrequently, recognition of these uncommon tumors leads to the diagnosis of the MEA I syndrome.

The basic defect remains uncertain. One hypothesis is that this syndrome is a form of neuroectodermal dysplasia. According to this theory, neural crest cells of the APUD series, characterized by their *amine precursors uptake* and *decarboxylation* (hence the acronym) migrate to the primitive foregut derivatives that are destined to become endocrine glands. When inherited dysplasia occurs, they may secrete excessive amount of hormones. More recently the view has been advanced that these tumors manufacture a common hormone-precursor and the hormone liberated is dictated by the specific enzyme system in the well differentiated cells.[26]

Multiple Endocrine Adenomatosis Type II (MEA II or Sipple Syndrome)

The inheritance of the MEA II syndrome is also autosomal dominant. The syndrome comprises medullary carcinoma of thyroid (MCT), pheochromocytoma, and occasionally hyperparathyroidism. MCT is often asymptomatic, but may be metastatic. The tumors are rich in calcitonin secreted by the parafollicular C-cells of the thyroid and are recognized by measuring serum calcitonin levels before and after stimulation with calcium or pentagastrin. Pheochromocytomas occur bilaterally in well over 50 percent of cases, but extra-adrenal tumors are rare. Familial pheochromocytomas are likely to contain large amounts of epinephrine. Their clinical manifestations are indistinguishable from sporadically occurring tumors except that patients are more likely to be asymptomatic and normotensive. This syndrome is also thought to result from a defect of the neuroectodermal system.

Occasionally mucosal neuromas, a marfanoid habitus, intestinal ganglioneuromatosis, and thick "bumpy" lips occur in patients with this disorder. This combination probably constitutes a separate entity, MEA III.

Autoimmune Polyglandular Dysfunction[42]

Organ-specific autoimmunity of an endocrine gland usually results in failure of its function but may induce hyperfunction. Multiple endocrine glands tend to be affected. Nonendocrine organ-specific autoimmune diseases including myasthenia gravis, pernicious anemia, rheumatoid arthritis, Sjögren syndrome, and vitiligo often occur in patients with autoimmune endocrinopathies. Endocrine diseases considered to result from autoimmune processes include Hashimoto's thyroiditis, "idiopathic" Addison's disease, Graves' disease, "idiopathic" hypoparathyroidism, lymphocytic oophoritis and orchitis, diabetes mellitus, and probably hypopituitarism. The autoimmune nature of these disorders can be established by demonstrating serum antibodies specific to the involved tissue.

Autoimmune polyglandular dysfunction is often familial and is associated with an increased frequency of HLA-A1, B8 in affected persons.[42] The pathogenesis remains uncertain; however, defective immune surveillance has been incriminated. Autodestruction of tissue is normally suppressed by a subpopulation of thymic lymphocytes. Autoimmunity may occur when there is a relative deficiency of these suppressor cells.

CHAPTER 70
Disorders of the Adrenal Gland
TURNER BLEDSOE

Disorders of the adrenal glands are infrequently encountered in clinical practice. Nonetheless, each is closely mimicked by commonly occurring, less serious conditions. Because the morbidity of these adrenal disorders is significant and treatment is available, it is important that no case go unrecognized by reason of its similarity to a more benign problem.

The outermost zone of the adrenal cortex is the glomerulosa, where aldosterone, the dominant mineralocorticoid, is formed. This zone is normally under the control of the kidney via the renin–angiotensin system. Next is the middle zona fasciculata, where the glucocorticoid cortisol is formed. Various adrenal androgens also arise from the zona fasciculata as well as from the innermost zona reticularis. The zona fasciculata and zona reticularis are normally under the control of the pituitary through ACTH. Whether or not pituitary gonadotropins stimulate the zona reticularis is not certain. The differences between the steroid biosynthetic pathways of these zones are shown in Figure 70–1.

Finally, the center of the adrenal gland, the medulla, produces catecholamines rather than steroid hormones, as a part of the sympathetic nervous system. The medulla is the principal site for epinephrine production. The enzymes which convert norepinephrine to epinephrine are induced by high cortisol levels in blood. Because blood flows inwardly in the adrenal from the cortex through the medulla, the latter is uniquely situated for coordination of cortisol and epinephrine synthesis.

ABNORMALITIES OF MINERALOCORTICOID PRODUCTION

HYPERALDOSTERONISM

Under normal conditions, aldosterone participates in the daily fluctuations of sodium balance. The physiologic stimulus of standing upright leads sequentially to:

1. Pooling of blood in the venous system
2. Baroreceptor stimulation of the sympathetic nervous system
3. Stimulation of renin release by the kidney
4. Generation of angiotensins I and II
5. Stimulation of aldosterone secretion
6. Retention of sodium by the kidney
7. Expansion of effective blood volume

The plasma levels of renin, angiotensin, and aldosterone usually rise progressively over the first 4 hours of the upright position, thereafter declining as dietary sodium and water are retained. With sodium deprivation or loss of salt, this system increases its function over 3 to 5 days to greatly reduce the concentration of sodium and raise the concentration of potassium in both urine and sweat.

Secondary Hyperaldosteronism

In certain disorders the renin–angiotensin–aldosterone system becomes chronically activated. High renin levels and elevated aldosterone production may

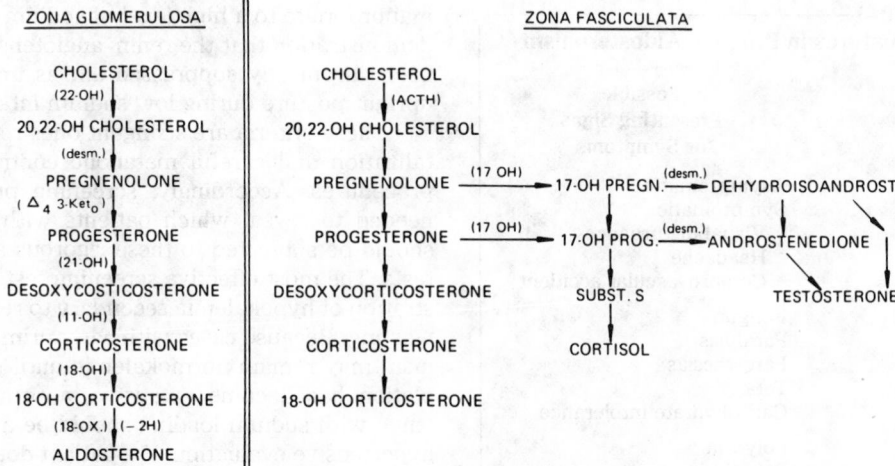

FIGURE 70-1. An outline of the synthetic pathways for glucocorticoids, mineralocorticoids, and adrenal androgens. Since pregnenolone is a common precursor for all three classes, relative or absolute blockade of one pathway results in overflow synthesis of the other adrenal steroids.

be associated with low effective blood volume such as that seen with chronic liver disease or chronic diuretic therapy. With severe renal ischemia, such as is seen in malignant hypertension, this same stimulation of renin and aldosterone commonly occurs. In all of these circumstances, potassium deficiency with hypokalemia is likely to develop. This syndrome of potassium deficiency related to high levels of renin and aldosterone is frequently referred to as "secondary hyperaldosteronism."

While the renin–angiotensin system normally dominates the control of aldosterone biosynthesis, ACTH and potassium excess also can provide this stimulus by different mechanisms. Hence one may find excessive aldosterone production associated with Cushing syndrome.

Primary Hyperaldosteronism (Conn Syndrome)[53]

Clinically, primary hyperaldosteronism is frequently indistinguishable from essential hypertension. Hypokalemia with hypertension is the typical presentation of primary aldosteronism. Moderate hypokalemia is, however, not rare with diuretic therapy for essential hypertension. For this reason it is important to measure serum electrolytes before diuretic therapy is started. If symptomatic hypokalemia develops after diuretic therapy has been instituted, repeat measurements are important after 2 to 4 weeks off these agents.

The hypertension of primary aldosteronism is usually moderate but any of the symptoms listed in

Table 70–1 may be present. Despite the role of sodium retention in the genesis of the hypertension, edema is almost invariably absent. Because the hypokalemia may become profound, the symptoms in Group II are common and may be the first clue to the presence of the disorder.

Asthenia, weakness, and fatigue may be pronounced, occasionally progressing to frank paralysis of all four limbs. Characteristically this constellation of symptoms is intermittent and may either occur spontaneously or be provoked by kaliuretic agents. The potassium ion is located principally intracellularly. When potassium deficiency becomes pronounced, sodium and hydrogen ions move into the cell to replace lost cation. There is accordingly an intracellular acidosis and an extracellular alkalosis. The alkalosis provokes symptoms ranging from mild paresthesias to frank tetany. Examination may reveal positive Trousseau and Chvostek signs. Latent tetany may be precipitated by brief hyperventilation or excitement. Deep tendon reflexes may be absent. Carbohydrate intolerance after an oral glucose meal is demonstrable in about half the patients.

The symptoms described in Group III of Table 70–1 are, at least in part, also attributable to potassium deficiency, which produces the following changes in the kidney: Morphologically, there is vacuolar degeneration of the proximal tubules; physiologically, the capacity of the kidney to concentrate urine and to excrete hydrogen ion is impaired. Urine osmolality and specific gravity approach those of a

TABLE 70-1
Clinical Features in Primary Aldosteronism

Grouped Category	Possible Presenting Signs or Symptoms

Group I Hypertension	Asymptomatic
	Symptomatic
	  Visual disturbances
	  Headache
	  Cerebrovascular accident

Group II Hypokalemia	Fatigue Paralysis Paresthesias Tetany Carbohydrate intolerance
Group III Renal	Polyuria Polydipsia Nocturia

plasma ultrafiltrate. Polyuria and polydipsia are the commonest symptoms arising from the disturbance. Patients complain of nocturia, consequent upon a reversal of the diurnal rhythm of water excretion. The potassium-depleted kidney seems prone to infection, and the manifestations of pyelonephritis may develop. The pH of the urine is usually 7.0 or higher. Urinary specific gravity is approximately 1.010, and proteinuria is present in most patients. Significant urinary potassium loss may be encountered despite hypokalemia. The ability to produce an acid urine after a standard acid load is subnormal, and there is an impairment of the urinary concentrating mechanism that can be demonstrated either by water deprivation or by vasopressin administration. A moderate reduction in the concentration of serum potassium can usually be demonstrated at some time. Although serum sodium concentration and carbon-dioxide-combining power are occasionally elevated, normal or high-normal values are usually observed.

The pathophysiologic basis of this disorder is a persistent excessive secretion of aldosterone despite the suppression of the renin–angiotensin system by the resultant blood volume expansion. In most cases this disorder is caused by a solitary benign adrenal adenoma of the zona glomerulosa. From 15 to 20 percent of cases, however, have been found to be caused by idiopathic bilateral nodular hyperplasia of the glomerulosa cells.

Diagnosis (Table 70-2)

The minimal requirements for the diagnosis of primary aldosteronism include: 1) demonstration of a supranormal aldosterone secretion or excretion rate

inappropriate to a high level of sodium intake; and 2) demonstration that the renin–angiotensin system has been chronically suppressed and is unresponsive to upright posture during low sodium intake.[54]

These criteria are stringent ones requiring hospitalization and careful metabolic control of the test procedures. Accordingly, screening procedures are needed to reveal which patients with hypertension should be subjected to these rigorous and expensive tests. The most effective screening test is the demonstration of hypokalemia secondary to renal potassium wasting. Because cases with early primary aldosteronism may remain normokalemic until potassium depletion has become extensive, a provocative challenge with sodium loading should be a part of every hypertensive evaluation. If a patient does not develop either hypokalemia or alkalosis after 4 days of added sodium chloride (2 g three times daily plus regular diet), then no further work-up for hyperaldosteronism is warranted at that time. Autonomous

TABLE 70-2
Diagnosis of Hyperaldosteronism

Critical Questions	Specific Tests	Comments
Can low serum K^+ be demonstrated?	Sodium loading (NaCl 2 g three times daily)	Reexamine every 1–2 years
Are other causes of low K^+ present?	Thiazides, licorice diarrhea, laxatives	Stop all medications for 2 weeks
Is there renal K^+ wasting?	Serum K^+ <3 mEq/L with urine K >50 mEq/day	
Is there mineralo-corticoid excess?	Spironolactone reversal of K^+ wasting	400 mg/day 4 days
Is aldosterone high?	Measure on Day 5 300 mEq Na diet	Correct hypokalemia before testing
Is renin activity suppressed?	Measure on Day 5 of 10 mEq Na diet, 4th hr. of ambulation	Or after furosemide IV
Is there bilateral hyperplasia?	Postural study of plasma aldosterone Adrenal scan	Adrenal cath. venogram or assay

hyperaldosteronism may develop in patients with essential hypertension. Therefore, this possibility should be reconsidered on an annual basis.

If hypokalemia is demonstrable before or after sodium loading, several critical questions must be answered. Can other causes of hypokalemia be excluded? The important causes of hypokalemia to be excluded are thiazide diuretics, diarrhea or chronic laxative use, chronic licorice ingestion (glycyrrhizinic acid has a mineralocorticoid action), and estrogen treatment (causes secondary hyperaldosteronism). The patient should be studied further 3 weeks after cessation of potassium-wasting drugs. If at this time hypokalemia is present one must ask, is this due to renal potassium wasting? If the patient has a serum potassium under 3 mEq/L and a simultaneous 24-hour urinary potassium excretion in excess of 50 mEq per 24 hours, then renal potassium wasting is present and further studies are mandatory. Spironolactone administration at this point (400 mg per day in divided doses for 4 days) should cause an increase in serum potassium and a fall in urinary potassium to under 20 mEq per 24 hours. This test will establish that a mineralocorticoid is responsible for the renal potassium wasting.

If renal potassium wasting is present, one must exclude Cushing syndrome, as well as Liddle syndrome[67] (exaggerated distal tubular Na^+-K^+ exchange without mineralocorticoids), and one must differentiate between primary hyperaldosteronism and hyperaldosteronism secondary to elevated plasma renin activity. Conditions associated with secondary hyperaldosteronism and hypertension include malignant or accelerated hypertension, estrogen or contraceptive pill induction of high renin substrate levels, unilateral renal ischemia, and diuretic therapy. If one of these conditions is not obvious, aldosterone measurements should be made after 5 days on a 300 mEq sodium intake and plasma renin activity should be measured on the fifth day of a 10 to 20 mEq sodium diet after 4 hours of active ambulation. If aldosterone levels are high and renin activity is low, autonomous hyperaldosteronism is established. If the spironolactone test has been positive, and renin activity and aldosterone measurements are low, hyperdesoxycorticosteronism should be suspected.[50]

Once the high aldosterone, low renin combination has been established the diagnostic work is not complete. The important surgically correctable form of hyperaldosteronism is a benign aldosterone-producing adrenal adenoma. These are unilateral and patients usually have a marked improvement in their hypertension postoperatively. A significant number of patients, however, prove to have bilateral adrenal hyperplasia which is usually nodular.[47,49] In these cases the hypertension does not respond well even to bilateral adrenalectomy. This surgery does ameliorate the hypokalemia but spironolactone administration will do this effectively as well. A rare form of aldosteronism is due to abnormal hyperresponsiveness of the aldosterone pathway to ACTH stimulation. These patients can be cured by physiologic suppression of the pituitary–adrenal axis with dexamethasone.[76]

Bilateral nodular hyperaldosteronism can be firmly established by measurement of adrenal venous aldosterone levels after bilateral catheterization studies or at surgical exploration. It is usually possible to predict this diagnosis from the following observations: First, the degree of metabolic abnormality is greater in patients with a unilateral aldosteronoma. The aldosterone production and serum bicarbonate are higher.[48,57] The serum potassium and plasma renin are lower. Second, in patients with unilateral adenoma, the plasma aldosterone measurement follows the diurnal variation of ACTH and cortisol. The patient with bilateral hyperplasia shows a postural rise in plasma aldosterone.[73] Plasma aldosterone, measured with cortisol at 7 to 8 A.M., is compared to the values obtained at 12 noon after 4 hours of ambulation. If the plasma aldosterone and cortisol fall during ambulation, unilateral adenoma is likely. If the cortisol falls and the aldosterone rises, bilateral hyperplasia is likely.

Other important features of the diagnostic workup include the observation that potassium depletion will suppress the hypersecretion of aldosterone so that correction of hypokalemia will assure the finding of high aldosterone levels.[52] If the hyperaldosteronism is due to a hypovolemic stimulus to renin synthesis, the parallel vasopressin stimulation will produce modest hyponatremia (130 to 140 mEq/L). In primary hyperaldosteronism, the volume expansion suppresses vasopressin slightly and moderate hypernatremia is common (140 to 150 mEq/L). Alternatives to the measurement of plasma renin activity include attempts to exclude secondary hyperaldosteronism by demonstrating that the high values of aldosterone will not be suppressed by administration of mineralocorticoid. Patients with secondary hyperaldosteronism given 0.4 mg of 9 α-fluorohydrocortisone (Florinef) in divided doses for 4 days, or desoxycorticosterone acetate 10 mg every 12 hours for 4 days, will show a 50 percent decrease in aldosterone excretion. Alternatives to a 5-day, low sodium diet for stimulating renin activity include measurement of plasma renin activity after intravenous administration of furosemide, ethacrynic acid, or diazoxide.[65]

A number of techniques are available for visualizing tumors of the adrenal glands. The most commonly used involves venous catheterization with selective sampling of the right and left adrenal veins. Measurement of plasma aldosterone and the performance of selective venography in skilled hands can usually clarify the type and localization of the lesion. More recently, iodocholesterol radioisotopic scanning of the adrenal glands has been introduced. Approximately 5 to 7 days of equilibration is necessary before the adrenals can be selectively visualized. Adenomas as small as 1.0 cm have been detected. Finally, equipment for body scanning with computerized axial tomography using a "rapid scan" capability has greatly improved the resolution power of this approach to adrenal visualization.

All cases in which a solitary adenoma is not apparent should have plasma aldosterone measurements after 10 days of dexamethasone suppression of the pituitary–adrenal axis to rule out the rare case of ACTH-dependent hyperaldosteronism.

Therapy

Therapy of an aldosteronoma is surgical. Biochemical abnormalities in the plasma revert to normal within the first 2 weeks. The blood pressure usually falls more slowly and may not return completely to normal. Renal abnormalities correct themselves between a fortnight and several months postoperatively, there is an increase in the titratable acidity in the urine to above 20 mEq per day, and the ability to concentrate to 1.020 and above is restored. If there has been irreversible kidney damage secondary to hypertension or pyelonephritis, the return to normal will be incomplete. A recurrence of the syndrome must make one suspect adrenal cancer.

In some cases, particularly when symptoms are not severe, moderate salt restriction and the administration of an aldosterone antagonist can produce complete amelioration of this syndrome.

Low Renin Essential Hypertension[72]

For a number of years there has been growing awareness that a considerable number of cases with essential hypertension fall into a category that involves in some way mineralocorticoid production by the adrenal. The most convincing data include 1) the finding of a suppressed renin–angiotensin system analogous to the situation found in primary hyperaldosteronism; and 2) significant amelioration of hypertension with the administration of the aldosterone antagonist spironolactone or the adrenal biosynthetic inhibitor aminoglutethimide. Absent in this syndrome, however, is significant hypokalemia and the finding of excessive amounts of a known mineralocorticoid.[59]

Implication of a number of mineralocorticoids has been suggested, including 18-hydroxy-DOC, 16-beta-hydroxy-DHEA, and aldosterone itself. None of the nonaldosterone mineralocorticoids mentioned appears to be sufficiently potent to be implicated at the levels at which they are produced. Intriguingly, however, there are occasional patients with dramatic evidence of mineralocorticoid excess but none of the known steroids can be implicated. Equally interesting is the observation in many patients with low renin hypertension that aldosterone levels, while not in excess, appear to be inappropriately normal when one takes into account the very low levels of activity of the renin–angiotensin system. These relatively excessive amounts of aldosterone may be sufficient to support the hypertensive state in susceptible individuals.

More clear-cut are those very rare cases of mineralocorticoid excess relating to excessive production of desoxycorticosterone, a mineralocorticoid with about one-half the strength of aldosterone. Usually these are related to a specific tumor of the adrenal.

HYPERCORTISOLISM: CUSHING SYNDROME

The presentation of a patient with the triad of hypertension, obesity, and diabetes mellitus often raises the suspicion of Cushing syndrome. This triad, however, appears frequently in obese patients who do not have a true excess of cortisol secretion by the adrenal. Accordingly, this rare disorder must be considered in the differential diagnosis of many patients.

Under normal circumstances, cortisol output by the adrenal is regulated through the negative feedback system involving pituitary secretion of ACTH. To interpret measurements of cortisol or ACTH, one must take into account the diurnal fluctuation of ACTH and cortisol secretion which is based largely on the individual's sleep–wake pattern of activity. Plasma cortisol is usually lowest at the midpoint of the sleep period (1:00 to 2:00 A.M.) and rises in episodic bursts to a peak in the period just after the usual hour of awakening. Less frequent bursts of secretion lead to a decline in cortisol levels over the remainder of the day. Diurnal changes in exposure to light will also influence the timing of these peak cortisol levels.

In addition to this normal diurnal fluctuation in ACTH and cortisol production, the pituitary–adrenal axis is subject to activation by stresses of many kinds. Psychic stress, such as fear or personal loss, will stimulate ACTH and cortisol output. Acute intercurrent infections, bacterial or viral, also provoke increases in this system. These stress responses take precedence over the negative feedback system. Without stress, administering a potent glucocorticoid such as dexamethasone will suppress ACTH output. With stress, however, ACTH and cortisol output will remain high even when exogenous glucocorticoid is administered to the patient.

Clinical Features[75]

The basic common denominator of all types of spontaneous Cushing syndrome is excessive cortisol production by the adrenal. The metabolic effects of cortisol are responsible for the salient clinical features outlined in Table 70-3.

The typical patient with florid Cushing syndrome presents with a round plethoric face, truncal obesity, and wasting of the extremities. The skin is thin, ecchymoses appear with subtle trauma, wide purple striae follow rapid weight gain. Hypertension is likely to be present. The patient is emotionally labile, and may complain of weakness and symptoms of overt diabetes. Amenorrhea and hirsutism are common in women.

The metabolic consequences of cortisol excess readily explain the spectrum of clinical features. Lipid mobilization leads to redistribution of adipose stores. Truncal obesity, mediastinal widening, and exophthalmos will follow. The hypercholesterolemia is ultimately life-threatening since undiagnosed Cushing syndrome leads to early atherosclerotic death. The catabolic effects of cortisol lead to protein wasting. Muscle weakness is a prominent consequence and the skin manifestations relate also to this effect. The enhanced gluconeogenesis leads to carbohydrate intolerance. Cases with ACTH excess commonly have elevations of the mineralocorticoid desoxycorticosterone and in some aldosterone is also high. This change will lead to hypertension and potassium wasting. This feature may dominate the picture in the ectopic ACTH syndrome.

The secondary endocrine effects in Cushing syndrome are varied. Cortisol antagonizes the effects of 1,25-dihydroxycholecalciferol on intestinal calcium absorption and inhibits activation of bone cells. The net result is secondary hyperparathyroidism and the development of osteopenia. Collapse of the vertebrae constitutes a most crippling complication in untreated cases. Growth hormone release and peripheral effectiveness are inhibited by cortisol excess. Growth failure in children results and the protein catabolic effects are reinforced. Alpha-MSH is usually secreted in excess with ACTH so pigmentation may develop. This is more likely to appear after adrenalectomy in pituitary Cushing syndrome or earlier in the ectopic ACTH syndrome. ACTH excess and malignant neoplasia are commonly associated with androgen excess, hence the amenorrhea and virilism in women. The effects of cortisol excess on the psyche may be very prominent. In some cases psychic stress is thought to precipitate the development of the syndrome. In most circumstances there is emotional lability, euphoria, irritability, and occasionally frank psychosis.

TABLE 70-3
Clinical-Metabolic Correlates in Cushing Syndrome

I. Metabolic Effects

  A. Fat metabolism
    Truncal obesity, widening of mediastinum
    Hypercholesterolemia, accelerated atherosclerosis

  B. Protein metabolism
    Muscle wasting with proximal myopathy
    Fragility of skin—ecchymoses, striae
    Growth hormone unresponsiveness

  C. Carbohydrate metabolism
    Latent or overt diabetes mellitus

  D. Electrolyte balance
    Aldosterone or DOC excess with hypertension,
    hypokalemic alkalosis

II. Endocrine Effects

  A. 1,25 Dihydroxycholecalciferol antagonism—
    secondary PTH excess and osteopenia

  B. Growth hormone suppression—growth failure

  C. MSH excess—hyperpigmentation

  D. Androgen excess—hirsutism, amenorrhea, and infertility

III. Neurologic

  A. Psychosis or emotional lability

Etiologic Considerations

In about 70 percent of patients, the adrenals are found to have bilateral hyperplasia, and measurements of plasma ACTH reveal values that are usually in the high normal range despite cortisol levels which would otherwise completely suppress normal pituitary secretion of ACTH. This form of Cushing syndrome is related to abnormal ACTH secretion by the pituitary. Ten percent of such cases show evidence of enlargement of the sella turcica at the time of presentation. In these cases, pituitary adenomas are readily shown to be etiologic. A significant number of patients with this form of Cushing syndrome, without sellar enlargement, can be shown to have microadenomas of the pituitary whose selective removal can completely normalize pituitary function.[74,79] An alternate etiologic theory holds that this form of the disorder may actually be caused by excessive hypothalamic corticotropin-releasing factor (CRF) which stimulates ACTH excess and leads to development of microadenomas. To support this latter theory was the finding that certain drugs, e.g., cyproheptadine, which is capable of antagonizing the serotoninergic system in the brain, may be very effective in normalizing ACTH production in about half the patients with this disorder. This agent can, however, be effective in patients with overt ACTH-secreting tumors of the pituitary.[64]

Further studies are needed to confirm the reports that pituitary–adrenal physiology returns to normal after removal of causative pituitary microadenomas.[74] If cyproheptadine is shown to be effective in a significant number of these cases with microadenomas, then a tenable etiologic hypothesis would be that these microadenomas are collections of cells that develop abnormal sensitivity to corticotropic-releasing factor or other substances in the hypothalamic–pituitary axis.

Adrenal tumors account for about one in four cases of Cushing syndrome. The tumor may be an adenoma, usually single, and surrounded by a narrow rim of atrophic cortical tissue acting as a capsule. The contralateral gland is atrophic. The cell type of the adenoma is uniform, and usually of the fasciculata variety. Or the tumor may be a carcinoma, which has a tendency to invade the adrenal vasculature, seeding out functional metastases to the liver and lung.

The remaining cases of Cushing syndrome occur in association with carcinomas of the lung, ovary, testis, thymus, exocrine and endocrine pancreas, and argentaffin and chromaffin systems. In some cases, an analysis of the tumor has yielded an ACTH-like material which is thought to stimulate adrenal-corticoid production.

Diagnosis

Whereas the diagnosis in the most glaring cases offers little challenge, the distinction between mild Cushing syndrome and simple obesity is often difficult. Not infrequently, obese subjects are hypertensive, have fine skin, develop amenorrhea, and are prone to develop psychiatric disorders. Diabetes is not unusual in such patients. Similarities between these two conditions also extend into the chemical arena in that elevated 17-hydroxycorticosteroid (17-OHCS) excretion frequently accompanies obesity. It is essential, therefore, to emphasize those clinical features which serve to differentiate the patients who will prove to have Cushing syndrome from those who merely appear to have it (Table 70–4).

The most useful clinical clues to the diagnosis of Cushing syndrome are: 1) muscle weakness; 2) ecchymoses due to thinning of the skin; 3) radiologic evidence of osteoporosis; and 4) hypokalemic alkalosis. The presence of obesity in the arms and legs is against the diagnosis. The finding of extremity obesity as evidence against the diagnosis is more helpful than the presence of truncal obesity to indicate the diagnosis of Cushing syndrome.

LABORATORY CONFIRMATION.   Once the suspicion has been raised the minimal criteria for laboratory confirmation must be met. All forms of Cushing syndrome demonstrate some degree of autonomous secretion of excessive amounts of cortisol. If the administration of slightly supraphysiologic amounts of a glucocorticoid will not suppress the pituitary–adrenal axis in an otherwise unstressed individual then the diagnosis is secure. Two methods of doing this screening procedure are equally effective.

DEXAMETHASONE SUPPRESSION.   Dexamethasone is a synthetic glucocorticoid thirtyfold as potent as cortisol and not measured by the chemical procedures which measure cortisol. If given at a dose of 0.5 mg every 6 hours for 2 days, normal adrenal function will be suppressed during the second day and urinary 17-OHCS will fall to less than 2.0 mg. It has also been shown that there is a diurnal variation in suppressibility of the pituitary ACTH output. If 1 mg of dexamethasone is administered orally between 11 P.M. and midnight, plasma cortisol at 8 A.M. the next morning will be subnormal.[69] If a 24-hour urinary steroid measurement is used with the overnight suppression test it must be collected from midnight to midnight or the dose must be repeated on two successive nights. One of these suppression tests is necessary to establish the diagnosis.

URINARY FREE CORTISOL.   Measurements of urinary 17-OHCS excretion or of cortisol secretion rates are elevated in obesity, acromegaly, and hyperthyroidism without there being true hyperadrenocorticism. In these conditions, the rise in cortisol secretion is compensatory for the increased rate of destruction of cortisol. Accordingly, plasma cortisol is normal. Measurement of urinary free cortisol is uninfluenced by compensated changes in metabolic degradation rates because it is a reflection of unbound plasma cortisol filtered by the kidney. This measurement is a more reliable index of cortisol excess under these circumstances. Because cortisol binding globulin becomes saturated at the upper limit of normal for plasma cortisol, patients with Cushing syndrome have a disproportionate increase in unbound plasma cortisol. This peculiarity is reflected in a disproportionate rise in urinary free cortisol excretion. There-

TABLE 70–4
Diagnosis of Cushing Syndrome

Critical Questions	Specific Tests	Comment
Is hypercorticism possible?	Cushingoid habitus Hypertension Diabetes mellitus	Not selective criteria
Is hypercorticism likely?	Ecchymoses Muscle weakness Hypokalemia Osteoporosis	Obesity of arms or legs is against the diagnosis
Laboratory confirmation	Abnormal low dose or overnight dexamethasone suppression tests	Suppression urinary 17-OHCS above 2 mg per 24 hours, urinary free cortisol above 20 μg per 24 hours 8 A.M. plasma corticoids above 10 mg/dl
	High urinary free corticoids	Control urinary free cortisol above 80 μg per 24 hours
	Absent diurnal variation of plasma cortisol	8 P.M. plasma cortisol more than 50% of 8 A.M. value

Etiologic Classification

	High Dose Dexamethasone Response	Metyrapone Response	ACTH Response	17-OH Excretion	17-KS Excretion	Other
Pituitary lesion	50% fall urinary 17-OH steroids	Rise	Exaggerated	High	High	? enlarged sella turcica
Benign adenoma	None	None	Variable	High	Normal	
Adrenal carcinoma	None	None	None	High	Very high (4x)	Variable baseline
Ectopic ACTH syndrome	None	Variable	Minimal	Very high (4x)	High	Variable baseline

fore, this index of adrenal function is nearly as good a discriminant as the dexamethasone suppression test in the diagnosis of Cushing syndrome. Other suggestive laboratory evidence includes demonstration that the normal diurnal variation of plasma cortisol is missing. False positives to all of these tests are observed if the patient is suffering from an intercurrent infection, psychic stress, or post-traumatic or post-surgical stress.

ETIOLOGIC DIAGNOSIS. Once the diagnosis of Cushing syndrome has been confirmed, its etiology must be established. As immunoassay of ACTH becomes available, this etiologic diagnosis will be simplified. When plasma ACTH is normal or slightly elevated the etiology is probably related to abnormal ACTH production by the pituitary. If plasma ACTH is strikingly elevated the diagnosis is most probably that of ACTH excess produced by an extrapituitary

malignancy. If ACTH is absent, the diagnosis is either a benign adrenal adenoma or an adrenal carcinoma.

If ACTH assay is not available, a reasonably secure diagnosis can be established through study of the steroid excretion pattern and the response of the pituitary-adrenal axis to physiologic manipulation.[69] The important principles used in making this analysis are outlined here and in Table 70–4.

In patients with Cushing syndrome due to oversecretion of ACTH from the pituitary gland, the negative feedback control behaves as though it is merely set at a high level of circulating cortisol. It is not usually a totally "fixed" hypersecretion. Therefore, if large doses of dexamethasone are administered, some suppression of cortisol synthesis will be seen. The standard procedure to test this hypothesis is to give 2 mg of dexamethasone every 6 hours. If urinary 17-OHCS excretion falls to 50 percent of the control value, the most likely etiology is pituitary disease. Some exceptions to this concept have been seen. If hypercorticism is severe, as much as 32 mg of dexamethasone may be needed to produce 50 percent suppression. Adrenal neoplasms and ACTH secreting carcinomas usually do not suppress with this test. A rare pituitary tumor may be more responsive to a fall in cortisol (induced by the adrenal inhibitor metyrapone) than it is to the administration of dexamethasone. In pituitary Cushing syndrome the metyrapone test will cause an exaggerated rise in urinary 17-OHCS. Adrenal neoplasms show no response to metyrapone.

A second principle in the etiologic diagnosis of Cushing syndrome relates to the pattern of steroid excretion. If the Cushing syndrome is caused by ACTH excess (pituitary or carcinoma), the steroidogenic pathway is stimulated at an early step. Accordingly, both androgens and cortisol metabolites are significantly increased. In ACTH-secreting neoplasms, the adrenals are often maximally stimulated and the excess 17-OHCS excretion is greater than fourfold. 17-ketosteroid excretion is high also but the increment is less dramatic. In pituitary Cushing syndrome modest elevations of both 17-OH steroid and 17-ketosteroid excretion are found. If the Cushing syndrome is due to a benign adrenal adenoma, ACTH is low, the androgen pathway is not stimulated, and 17-ketosteroid excretion may be normal. In adrenal carcinoma the biosynthetic sequence is more deranged than with the adenoma. In this case, exaggerated secretion of adrenal androgens is common. If the urinary 17-ketosteroids are increased fourfold with a less significant increase in 17-OH steroids, adrenal carcinoma is the likely diagnosis.

A third principle in this diagnostic search is that adrenal carcinomas are sufficiently undifferentiated that they do not respond to ACTH administration. Half of the benign adenomas respond to ACTH. Therefore, a positive response to ACTH administration (40 units over 8 hours) in the presence of "fixed" adrenal function (dexamethasone and metyrapone) suggests a benign adenoma. Absence of this response is not helpful.

The certain diagnosis of the "ectopic ACTH" syndrome caused by occult carcinomas can be difficult. Some of these tumors may retain sensitivity to pharmacologic manipulation. It is not unusual for these tumors to make more ACTH during the administration of metyrapone. Rarely, suppression of urinary 17-OH steroid excretion is seen during dexamethasone administration.[69] Accordingly, the differentiation from pituitary Cushing syndrome may be unclear. Useful clues include the observation that day to day fluctuations of urinary 17-OH steroid values are much greater in the ectopic ACTH syndrome. In more typical forms of this disorder adrenal stimulation is often maximal, 17-OH steroids are very high, hypokalemia is a prominent abnormality, and the malignant growth produces cachexia without Cushing habitus.

Treatment

Cushing syndrome is a serious disorder, with about a 50 percent mortality in 5 years when untreated.[71] The appropriate treatment depends to a certain extent on the underlying pathology. In the patient with adrenal neoplasia unilateral adrenalectomy is the treatment of choice. Since there has usually been profound suppression of the pituitary–adrenal axis these patients should be managed for many months as though they suffered from pituitary ACTH insufficiency. Steroid therapy during any surgical operation is also important.

In the cases with pituitary ACTH excess, a number of therapeutic approaches can be used.[70] These include:

1. Pharmacologic suppression of ACTH (or possibly CRF) production
2. Transsphenoidal (or transethmoidal) surgical approach to pituitary tumors or microadenomas
3. Pituitary irradiation
4. Pharmacologic suppression of adrenal steroidogenesis
5. Bilateral adrenalectomy

No one of these procedures has proved to be so universally applicable or successful as to supersede the others.

For a typical case of pituitary Cushing disease with or without sellar enlargement, the simplest first step is to initiate suppression of ACTH secretion using the antiserotoninergic agent cyproheptadine. If the patient improves significantly over the course of 1 to 4 months then the tissues in general will become stronger and ablative procedures may later be more safely pursued. Spontaneous remission is rare and most patients controlled by cyproheptadine will rebound quickly when the drug is withdrawn.

Pituitary irradiation is a relatively benign approach to pituitary ablation but runs some risk of radiation damage to overlying brain tissue with epilepsy or late development of intracranial sarcomas being among the rare delayed complications. Remission is achieved in about 25 percent of irradiated cases. Other pituitary functions usually remain normal after irradiation with 4000 to 5000 rads despite successful elimination of ACTH excess.

Neurosurgical removal of any existing pituitary tumor seems a logical approach for pituitary Cushing syndrome, particularly when tumor is evidenced by sellar enlargement. Furthermore, recent experience with transsphenoidal microsurgery in the hands of a few skilled teams of neurosurgeons, otolaryngologists, and pathologists has shown it to be possible to selectively find and remove small microadenomas from the pituitary. Normalization of pituitary function (including ACTH dynamics) has been accomplished in a significant number of cases.[74,79] However, even complete removal of the pituitary does not always guarantee a cure of the disorder. It would appear that occasionally patients may have functional pituitary tissue sequestered outside the sella turcica during embryonic development.[68]

Occasionally patients with Cushing syndrome will present with such intense hypercortisolism and such poor tissue strength that the rapid cure offered by direct intervention at the adrenal level is the most appropriate approach. In such circumstances, early bilateral adrenalectomy may be the most prudent therapy. One alternative is the use of the adrenal inhibitors o-p'DDD[77] or trilostane (WIN 24,540).[61] These drugs, while usually effective, may have unpleasant side effects and unknown long-term complications (especially o-p'DDD). At some point an ablative procedure is usually necessary.

When remission occurs, strength increases gradually, bone pain disappears, and the striae lose their purple color and atrophic appearance. Menses return in the female, and pregnancy is not unusual. Hypertension may persist if there has been irreversible renovascular damage, and in the adrenalectomized patient requirement for a subnormal mineralocorticoid replacement is occasionally found. Such patients also may require twice the replacement therapy usual for other forms of Addison's disease. This increased requirement for glucocorticoid usually resolves over the course of several months if the replacement dose is gradually tapered into the physiologic range.

ADRENAL INSUFFICIENCY (Addison's Disease)[78]

Adrenal insufficiency is another rare disorder which frequently must be considered in the differential of more common presentations. The clinical features of Addison's disease are listed in Table 70–5. In the severely ill patient a presentation with fever, hypotension, nausea, and vomiting must raise the suspicion of adrenal insufficiency. More commonly acute sepsis or

some other disorder will be found to be the cause; however, prompt recognition and treatment of adrenal crisis is crucial when it is present. In less seriously ill patients, adrenal insufficiency should be considered as the explanation of asthenia, anorexia, and weight loss. Chronic illness and depression are frequently the basis of these symptoms, but insidious development of adrenal insufficiency should be considered.

Clinical Features

Cortisol is known as the "hormone of well-being," and the syndrome of cortisol deficiency is characterized by a gradual decline in general health. Weight loss is characteristic. The patient loses his appetite or develops food idiosyncrasies. Nausea, vomiting, abdominal pain, and recurrent diarrhea are common. Acute prostration often follows a relatively minor intercurrent infection.

In Addison's disease there are deficiencies both of mineralocorticoid (aldosterone, which enhances sodium reabsorption by the kidney) and of glucocorticoid (cortisol, which plays a role in the internal support of the blood sugar). The consequences of salt deficit and of hypoglycemia may thus be prominent.

TABLE 70–5
Clinical Features in Addison's Disease

Grouped Category	Possible Presenting Signs or Symptoms
Group I. Asthenia	Decrease in strength and work capacity Irritability, drowsiness, and restlessness Paralysis (hyperkalemic)
Group II. Cardiovascular	Hypotension, small heart
Group III. Gastrointestinal disorder	Weight loss Food idiosyncrasy, poor appetite Anorexia, nausea, vomiting, diarrhea, abdominal pain
Group IV. Salt wastage	Salt craving Muscle cramps Dizziness and syncope (hypotension)
Group V. Hypoglycemia	Coma
Group VI. Pigmentation	Recent scars, buccal mucosa, knuckles, elbows, palmar creases
Group VII. Miscellaneous	Loss of sex characteristics in female Vicarious calcification

With the former the patient complains of muscle cramps and, particularly in children, there is often a history of salt craving. Dizziness and syncope occur secondary to hyponatremia and hypotension. Hypoglycemia in Addison's disease is usually seen when the patient has had a prolonged food-free interval, but it may come on several hours after a glucose meal.

The patient is underweight but not cachectic. The characteristic hyperpigmentation is caused by MSH overproduction. There may be a diffuse tan over nonexposed as well as exposed parts of the body. The skin has a dirty look, particularly over the knees, elbows, and other pressure points. Common sites of increased pigmentation are the anogenital region, the areolae, and recent scars. The hair often deepens in color. Small, black freckles appear, especially over the forehead, face, and neck. In the patient with autoimmune adrenal insufficiency there may be islands of vitiligo in the areas of greatest pigmentation. Pigment also extends over the mucous membranes, and there may be a bluish-black discoloration of the lips and gums and the buccal, rectal, and vaginal surfaces.

Axillary and pubic hair become scanty in the female, but secondary sex characteristics are not greatly affected in the male; the testes and the prostate gland are usually well preserved. The blood pressure is low (unless hypertension antedated the onset of Addison's disease), postural hypotension is demonstrable, and the heart is small. Muscle wasting is often severe. Muscle weakness is virtually always demonstrable, and with hyperkalemia there may be frank paralysis with loss of tendon jerks, a picture simulating that of Landry's ascending paralysis.

Pathophysiology

The most frequent cause of adrenal insufficiency is autoimmune destruction of the adrenal cortex through invasion by sensitized lymphocytes. Antiadrenal antibodies can be detected circulating in the blood of such individuals, if sought early in the course of the disease.[82] Occasionally such patients have a positive family history for adrenal insufficiency. These patients and their families may also develop autoimmune disorders involving thyroid and gonads as well. Diabetes mellitus, vitiligo, and rarely hypoparathyroidism with cutaneous candidiasis may complicate the disorder.

The next most frequent etiology for adrenal insufficiency is destruction of the gland by tuberculosis. Tissues with high cortisol concentrations are susceptible to invasion by the tubercle bacillus; hence destruction of the adrenal gland is common in tuberculosis. Some epinephrine reserve is usually present in autoimmune adrenal insufficiency—a point that has been used to differentiate between the two using an insulin hypoglycemic provocative test and measuring catecholamine excretion as the end point.[81] Additional destructive lesions of the adrenal include fungal diseases such as histoplasmosis, amyloidosis, hemochromatosis, or invasion by carcinomas.

Hemorrhagic destruction of the adrenal may arise iatrogenically as a complication of anticoagulant therapy, or it may occur as a consequence of severe fulminating infections such as meningococcal or staphylococcal septicemia (Waterhouse-Fredericksen syndrome). Hemorrhagic destruction of the adrenal as a complication of anticoagulant therapy may appear suddenly early after myocardial infarction. In this setting the acute onset of hypotension, nausea, and vomiting may be mistaken for an extension of the infarction.[46]

Laboratory Abnormalities

The laboratory findings provide evidence for glucocorticoid and mineralocorticoid deficiency—electrolyte disturbances, hemoconcentration, and hypoglycemia (Table 70–6). As a consequence of reduced glomerular filtration rate the patient is incapable of excreting a water load. Indeed, a large water load should be administered with caution, since symptoms of water intoxication may be provoked; cortisol corrects this defect. Often electrolyte values are within normal limits, although sodium and chloride wastage in the urine can be demonstrated, and hypercalcemia is occasionally present. The white blood count is elevated, with relative or absolute lymphocytosis and eosinophilia. Anemia and azotemia occur frequently.

Diagnosis

The final diagnosis is established by demonstrating a low secretion rate of adrenal steroids that does not respond to ACTH stimulation (Table 70–6). The simplest measurement is the 24-hour urinary excretion of 17-ketosteroids and 17-hydroxycorticosteroids. Low values suggest the diagnosis of Addison's disease, but they are not pathognomonic, being encountered in hypothyroidism, liver disease, malignancy, and other cachectic states. These low steroid excretions in the absence of adrenal disease occur because of alterations in cortisol degradation. In many diseases cortisol degradation is slowed. A normal pituitary negative feedback mechanism will then reduce cortisol synthesis so that elevated cortisol levels are avoided. When cortisol degradation is slowed cortisol synthesis is slowed and the patient remains "euadrenal." If

TABLE 70-6

An Approach to the Diagnosis of Addison's Disease

Critical Question	Primary Laboratory Evidence	Ancillary Evidence
Is output of adrenocortical steroids reduced?	Low values for Urinary 17-OHCS and, in the female, 17-KS Cortisol secretion rate Plasma 17-OHCS level	Elevated serum potassium level Reduced serum sodium and CO$_2$-combining power Low blood sugar concentration Inability to excrete a water load restored by cortisol
Is there normal response to ACTH administration? If so, are the low urinary 17-OHCS levels due to causes other than pituitary adrenal disease?	Evidence of Hypothyroidism Liver disease	Slow cortisol turnover rate Failure of degradation of 17, 21-dihydroxy, 20-keto compounds, and subsequent failure of conjugation with glucuronide
	Generalized malignancy	Caution: Malignant deposits in pituitary or adrenal
Pituitary insufficiency?	Ancillary evidence usually present of other trophic hormone deficiencies (TSH, FSH)	Evidence of a pituitary lesion Caution: Schmidt syndrome (primary thyroid and adrenal failure)
Does ACTH fail to induce an increase in adrenocortical steroid output?	This constitues evidence for adrenal insufficiency	
What is the etiology?	Tuberculosis Fungal (histoplasmosis) Hemochromatosis Amyloid Malignant deposits Autoimmune Hemorrhagic	

kidney function is normal the urinary free cortisol, which reflects the blood level of unbound cortisol (rather than cortisol secretory rate), will remain normal. In some diseases and with some drugs, a smaller proportion of cortisol is converted to urinary 17-hydroxysteroids. Hence, low urinary 17-hydroxysteroids may be found with normal cortisol secretion rates. This is particularly true of patients taking phenytoin. Urinary free cortisol, again, will remain normal.[60]

An ACTH stimulation test should be performed in all suspected cases of Addison's disease. A 1-hour ACTH stimulation test measuring plasma cortisol before and 1 hour after an intravenous dose of β1-24 synthetic ACTH (250 μg) has proved to be a convenient and reliable outpatient screening test. If plasma cortisol rises by an increment of 10 μg/dl then adrenal insufficiency is excluded. This single dose is sufficiently small and transient that it usually will not stimulate the atrophic adrenal of hypopituitarism. It is, therefore, a useful test in screening for ACTH sup-

pression or deficiency. If an unresponsive adrenal is found, a more prolonged ACTH stimulation test should be performed. Three or four days of sequential ACTH administration (ACTH gel intramuscularly, 20 units twice daily or aqueous ACTH intravenously for 8 hours) will reawaken an atrophic gland. A normal response to the prolonged ACTH stimulation is at least a twofold rise in urinary 17-hydroxysteroid excretion. Anaphylactic reactions to ACTH have been described with the use of aqueous, depot, and synthetic preparations. These reactions, however, are exceedingly rare.

In hypopituitarism, the patient is pale rather than pigmented, and signs of mineralocorticoid deficit are minimal. Occasionally dilutional hyponatremia may occur because of cortisol deficiency and water loading. Low serum urea nitrogen will differentiate this feature from the hyponatremia of aldosterone deficiency. There is usually evidence of other tropic hormone deficiencies, particularly gonadal and thyroidal. Occasionally, primary adrenocortical and thyroid deficiencies are associated (Schmidt syndrome). In these patients a goiter is usually palpable, diabetes is common, and thyroid and adrenal antibodies can be demonstrated.

Therapy

Patients with Addison's disease can be satisfactorily treated by the oral administration of cortisone, usually in a dose of 12.5 mg twice daily. A salt-retaining steroid, e.g., 9 α-fluorocortisol (0.1 mg daily), is usually added, particularly in the patient who manifests significant hypotension. It is advisable to increase salt intake by an extra 5 g of sodium chloride daily. Some prefer desoxycorticosterone acetate by daily intramuscular injection (0.5 to 1.0 mg) to 9 α-FF. Patients rapidly attain a sense of well-being after being placed on therapy. Some patients with preexisting renal disease or hypertension may require no mineralocorticoid replacement if cortisone is used. Prednisone can also be used in place of cortisone in doses of 5 to 10 mg per day. When prednisone is used, a mineralocorticoid is usually required.

In the initial stage of glucocorticoid therapy patients may exhibit hyperkinetic manifestations associated with overactivity, euphoria, and manic behavior. Usually these symptoms abate with the continued use of glucocorticoid in physiologic doses. The Addisonian patient should wear an identifying label and be instructed to increase his daily cortisone dose by 75 to 100 mg whenever he develops an infection. Some patients will require increased steroid for psychic stress as well. At home, the patient should keep injectable steroid available in the event that intercurrent illness with vomiting might prevent taking oral steroid supplement. If such a patient requires surgery, pretreatment with supraphysiologic amounts of glucocorticoid may be needed. Oral cortisone acetate (100 mg per day) or an intravenous preparation of soluble steroid (methylprednisolone, etc.) should be used. Intramuscular cortisone acetate, once a popular preparation, has been shown to produce inadequate blood levels. A useful alternative regimen is dexamethasone phosphate (4 mg intramuscularly) 30 minutes before anesthesia. Six-hourly doses of 2 mg are given for the operative day and each day the total dose is reduced by one-half until physiologic levels are achieved.

ADDISONIAN CRISIS. Patients with untreated or inadequately treated Addison's disease may present in crisis following minor infections or surgical procedures. This acute complication is characterized by fever, prostration, nausea, vomiting, circulatory collapse, cyanosis, and pulmonary edema. It may be fatal. The factors responsible for its precipitation include wastage of sodium with depletion of plasma volume, potassium intoxication, acidosis, and hypoglycemia. Addisonian crisis is a medical emergency. Methylprednisolone hemisuccinate (30 mg) and 50 g of glucose (50 percent solution) should be administered intravenously immediately. Sodium deficit may be restored by intravenous isotonic saline. If rapid restoration appears desirable this can be achieved by using 5 percent sodium chloride solution (100 to 300 ml), and 9 α-fluorohydrocortisone hemisuccinate (5 mg) should be added to the intravenous drip. A broad-spectrum parenteral antibiotic is often administered as a prophylaxis against the development or spread of an intercurrent infection. If the patient's blood pressure remains low, plasma and a pressor amine (e.g., metaraminol bitartrate, 200 mg in 500 ml of 5 percent glucose, intravenously) should be administered. Cortisol in a dosage of 300 mg within the first 24 hours may be required to reverse the crisis. As the patient improves and as dehydration and shock are corrected, oral medication can be started.

ADRENAL VIRILISM

Except in extreme forms, virilism relating to excessive adrenal androgen production is a problem that presents as excessive hirsutism in females with or without menstrual abnormalities. This is not a rare clinical problem but one which can be difficult to document and treat adequately. Part of the difficulty relates to the following features:

1. Tissue responsiveness to androgen varies widely in individual patients.
2. Many weak androgens secreted by the adrenal can be converted to more active androgens in the tissues which respond to them.
3. Temporary hypersecretion of androgens may induce irreversible changes in the hair follicle leading to permanent coarsening and darkening of the hair.
4. The implications of measurements of plasma androgens may be obscured by the level of androgen-binding proteins that are not usually measured.
5. The measurement of androgen metabolites in urine may or may not reflect secretion of active hormones.
6. The ovaries and adrenals often share in the androgen hypersecretory disorder.

Probably many patients suffering from mild virilism suffer from mild defects in the steroid biosynthetic pathways (analogous to those in the adrenogenital syndromes, see below) or from enhanced enzymatic activity in the androgen pathways.

THE ADRENOGENITAL SYNDROMES

The adrenogenital syndromes form a general category of diseases in which genital abnormalities can be traced to abnormal steroidogenesis in the adrenal gland.[51,66] The most common abnormalities are those which produce virilism in the female. Rarely feminization of the male or precocious puberty may be the mode of presentation.

The steroidogenesis of the adrenal cortex is uniquely arranged to promote androgen secretion when steroidogenesis is abnormal. The principal features of this arrangement, as shown in Figure 70–1, relate to the locus of action of ACTH. This tropic hormone has its major action at the earliest steps of steroidogenesis. ACTH stimulates the 20,22 dihydroxylation of cholesterol thus speeding the conversion of cholesterol to Δ_5-pregnenolone. Beyond this step five major branches of steroidogenesis occur.

The earliest branches are the four parallel pathways leading to androgen synthesis. Both Δ_5-pregnenolone and progesterone are good substrates for the 17-hydroxylase enzyme. In turn, both of the 17-hydroxyl derivatives of these steroids are good substrates for the desmolase enzymes which cleave the carbon 20,21 side chain to produce dehydroisoandrosterone (DHA) and Δ_4-androstenedione, respectively. Although these two steroids are only weak androgens they are readily converted by liver and other tissues into testosterone, dihydrotestosterone, and the biologically active androstenediols.

In parallel with this double pathway to androgen synthesis is the sulfate pathway within the adrenal gland. A unique feature of the sulfoconjugated steroids is their secretion by the adrenal as biologically inactive conjugates. These sulfated steroids can be hydrolyzed in peripheral organs to release active steroids. Both Δ_5-pregnenolone and 17-hydroxypregnenolone can be readily sulfated on the 3-hydroxyl position. These sulfated steroids are then protected from conversion to progesterone and 17-hydroxyprogesterone. Transformations of the carbon 20,21, however, are uninhibited by this conjugation on the other end of the molecule. Accordingly, dehydroisoandrosterone-sulfate is an "obligate" end product of the sulfate pathway. This steroid is a major contributor to the 17-ketosteroids excreted in the urine. In the pregnant state this steroid is converted to estradiol by the placenta. In nonpregnant subjects it may contribute to the active androgens by peripheral hydrolysis and metabolic transformation. The sulfokinase enzymes apparently become active progressively up to the time of normal puberty. Hence, this may explain why some forms of the adrenogenital syndrome may present during or shortly after puberty.

Because these three androgen pathways branch off in the "steroidogenic road map," any distal defects in steroidogenesis which cause a rise in ACTH are likely to exaggerate androgen production by the adrenal. A considerable variety of specific inborn errors of steroid synthesis have been identified. Each presents with unique abnormalities depending upon the site of the lesion. Many of these present with virilization in utero causing ambiguous genitalia at birth. Some of the milder defects, however, may present later in childhood with precocious puberty or pubertal virilism in the female.

The defects of steroidogenesis taken in order of their position in the steroid road map are outlined in Table 70–7.

Diagnosis of Adrenogenital Syndromes

Diagnosis of the adrenogenital syndromes involves the following critical questions: Is the steroid excretion pattern suggestive of an adrenal abnormality (elevated total plasma testosterone, dihydrotestosterone, androstenedione, and unbound 17 beta-*ol*-androgens, and elevated urinary 17-ketosteroid or 17-hydroxysteroids)?[51] Is this steroid excess under control of ACTH (tested by dexamethasone suppression)? Is there evidence of a specific enzyme defect (ambiguous external genitalia, hypertension, salt wasting, hyperpigmentation, adrenal insufficiency)? Is there any chemical evidence of steroid precursor accumulation (plasma progesterone, 17-hydroxyprogesterone, pregnenolone, 17-hydroxypregnenolone, urinary pregnanetriol, pregnanediol, tetrahydrodesoxycorticosterone)? Occasionally minor enzymatic defects can be revealed only by finding an abnormal precursor production to ACTH stimulation.

If androgen excess is not suppressed by dexamethasone, one must differentiate between adrenal tumor and gonadal androgen source. (See discussion in Chap. 77.) Rarely an adrenal tumor will cause feminization in the male, which results in gynecomastia and loss of libido. In the female this may produce precocious puberty or amenorrhea. An occasional adrenal tumor has been found to secrete unusual steroids (such as substance S) in conjunction with estrogen excess. Hence, high 17-hydroxysteroid excretion with feminization and no Cushing syndrome would suggest this diagnosis. Finding low gonadotropins and high estrogens will differentiate this condition from the more common causes of gynecomastia (see Chap. 77). Nephrotomograms during an intravenous pyelogram, adrenal arteriography or venography, comput-

TABLE 70–7
Enzyme Defects in the Adrenogenital Syndrome

Critical Defect	Accumulating Precursor	Clinical Features	Urinary Steroids		Other
			17-Keto	17-Hydroxy	
? Cholesterol desmolase	Cholesterol	Incompatible with life			
? 20, 22-hydroxylase			?	?	?
3-β-ol-dehydrogenase	Δ^5 pregnenolone, DHA	High fatality Virilism in utero	High	Low	↑ Δ_5 Pregnanetetrol
21-hydroxylase	Progesterone 17 OH-progesterone	Mild-simple virilism	High	Low	↑ Pregnanetriol
		Severe-virilism and salt wasting	High	Low	↑ Pregnanetriol Low aldosterone
11-hydroxylase	Desoxy-corticosterone Substance S	Virilism and hypertension	High	High	↑ Tetrahydro S ↑ Tetrahydro DOC
18-oxidase	Corticosterone 18-OH corti-costerone	Salt wasting	Normal	Normal	Low aldosterone ↑ 18-OH corti-costerone ↑ Corticosterone
17-hydroxylase	Corticosterone Desoxy-corticosterone	Hypertension Undervirilized Underestrogenized	Low	Low	↑ Tetrahydro-corticosterone ↑ Tetrahydro DOC

erized axial tomography, and ultrasound are in many circumstances complementary approaches in exploring the possibility of an adrenal tumor. Ovarian tumors can be identified by pelvic examination, laparoscopy, or laparotomy.

Treatment of Virilizing Adrenal Hyperplasia

In patients with an enzyme defect leading to inefficient cortisol synthesis, the androgen excess is corrected by suppression of the pituitary–adrenal axis with physiologic doses of glucocorticoid.[62] The hypertensive forms should receive treatment with synthetic steroids, these being less likely to cause sodium retention. Care must be used in the growing child to ensure growth to normal stature by avoiding glucocorticoid excess and preventing premature puberty with epiphyseal closure. Divided doses of glucocorticoid should be used to take advantage of the increased suppressibility of pituitary ACTH later in the day. In non-salt-wasting forms of virilizing adrenal hyperplasia, adding physiologic amounts of exogenous mineralocorticoid supplement appears to improve suppression of the androgen pathways. During episodes of intercurrent illness, trauma, or surgery, steroid supplement should be added as for patients with adrenal insufficiency. For patients with salt wasting lesions mineralocorticoid replacement with Florinef (0.05 to 0.1 mg per day) may be needed. In some cases high salt intake will suffice.

THE ADRENAL MEDULLA

The adrenal medulla is a specialized division of the paraganglion system, which is an extension of the sympathetic nervous system. The principal disorder of the adrenal medulla is pheochromocytoma. The medullary production of epinephrine, however, plays a critical role in protecting the individual from hypoglycemia and prepares him for the energy demands of perceived danger. Accordingly, any condition which predisposes a patient to hypoglycemic episodes will produce symptoms which may be confused with those of a pheochromocytoma.

Physiology and Metabolism of Catecholamines

Epinephrine may be released from the medulla in bursts triggered by stress or emotion acting through the sympathetic nervous system, by hypoglycemia acting directly on the gland, and probably by a fall in blood pressure such as may be induced by histamine. Epinephrine output becomes negligible under basal conditions with the patient recumbent. This is not the case with norepinephrine, which is released "tonically" from sympathetic nerve endings close to blood vessels and adipose tissue. These differences in the mode of release of the two hormones underline differences in their actions and functions in man.

Epinephrine is the hormone of "fight and flight" (Fig. 70–2). It reacts chiefly with beta-receptors, which are, in general, metabolic and inhibitory recep-

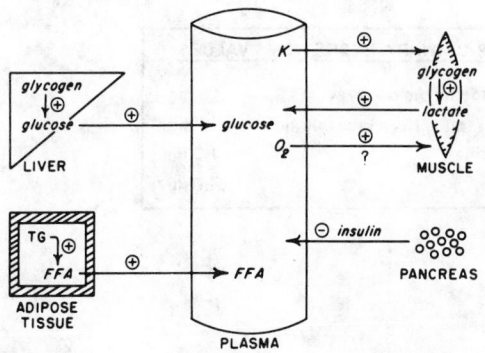

FIGURE 70-2. Schematic view of the actions of epinephrine. Epinephrine enhances (+) glucose release from the liver, FFA release from adipose tissue, and lactate output from skeletal muscle. Epinephrine inhibits (−) insulin release from the pancreas. Epinephrine induces net movement of potassium into muscle.

tors. The hemodynamic actions of epinephrine are positive chronotropic (increase in heart rate) and positive inotropic (increase in force of cardiac contraction) on the heart and productive of vasodilatation in skeletal muscle beds. Epinephrine is the hormone that makes available "instant energy": glucose for use by nervous tissue and FFA for use by skeletal muscle. It inhibits insulin release from the pancreas in response to glucose, tolbutamide, or glucagon. Epinephrine also increases lactate production by muscle. Lactate released into the circulation in part serves as a fuel for cardiac muscle, and, cycling through the liver, it is reconverted to glucose. Since the hormone is degraded rapidly in plasma, its action is not sustained after the physiologic need has passed.

Norepinephrine[80] is produced in the adrenal medulla and also at peripheral sympathetic nerve endings. It is found in at least two sites peripherally, a storage site and an effector site. Reserpine depletes storage sites of catecholamine, whereas tyramine liberates catecholamine from these sites. In pheochromocytoma there may be large peripheral stores of catecholamine, and tyramine may provoke hypertension, presumably by releasing the catecholamine, thus forming the basis of a provocative test for the presence of the tumor.

Norepinephrine acts chiefly on alpha (excitatory) receptors. Accordingly, it produces overall vasoconstriction, and its metabolic effects are weak. The following exceptions to these generalizations are important: norepinephrine produces dilatation of the coronary vascular bed and induces lipolysis of adipose-tissue triglyceride with resulting hyperlipacidemia. The role of norepinephrine in man may be to act as a local hormone, exerting a tonic effect on vas-

cular tone and on lipolysis. After adrenalectomy, urinary levels of norepinephrine do not change appreciably.

METABOLISM OF CATECHOLAMINES. The degradation of epinephrine and norepinephrine is illustrated in Figure 70-3. Of the two alternative routes, o-methylation is more important quantitatively, about 70 percent of the catecholamine being o-methylated prior to deamination. When labeled catecholamine is infused into man, about 55 percent is recovered in the urine as metanephrine, about 30 percent as vanillylmandelic acid, and less than 4 percent as the free amine. That vanillylmandelic acid forms about 75 percent of urinary catecholamine metabolites reflects the significant in situ metabolism of norepinephrine within the neuron and at the effector end plate. The great majority of the norepinephrine released from the secretory granules at the nerve ending undergoes reaccumulation at the end plate. Normal urinary values for free amine and metabolites are indicated in Figure 70-3.

PHEOCHROMOCYTOMA

The pheochromocyte can give rise to both benign and malignant tumors. About 10 percent of these tumors arise from extra-adrenal paraganglion tissue. Many of the tumors are functional, that is, they produce signs and symptoms of catecholamine overproduction. Since paraganglion tissues share a common embryologic origin with sympathetic ganglion cells, tumors arising from the latter may also produce catecholamine. The identification of the syndrome is determined by the pharmacologic effects of catecholamines in man, by whether predominantly norepinephrine or predominantly epinephrine is secreted by the tumor, and by whether the tumor shows intermittent or persistent function. Norepinephrine overproduction is more common than epinephrine excess. The latter suggests an adrenal site of origin. The former can, of course, be found with either adrenal or extra-adrenal tumors.

Small adrenal-medullary tumors have a limited storage capacity for amine. Thus they have a relatively low tissue concentration of norepinephrine and a high rate of turnover. The patient is, therefore, exposed to a high plasma concentration of norepinephrine that provokes symptoms early. These tumors usually produce only norepinephrine. An examination of the urine reveals elevated levels of free amine but usually less elevated levels of metabolites. Large tumors have a high storage capacity for amine, the turnover rate in the gland is slow, and a substantial portion of the catecholamine synthesized is degraded locally to inactive metabolites. This tumor produces both epinephrine and norepinephrine. Symptoms de-

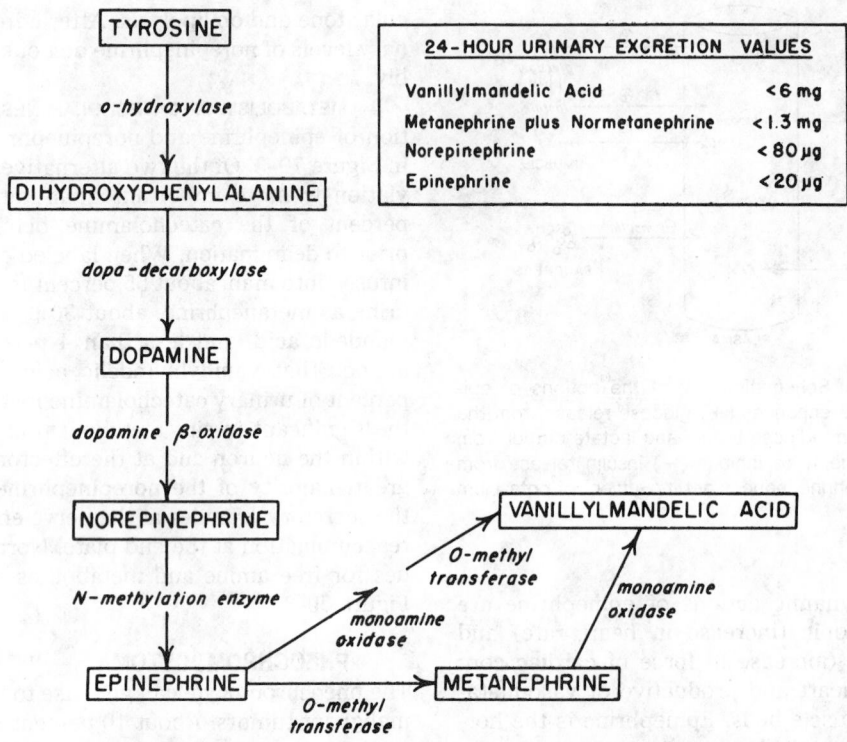

FIGURE 70-3. Synthesis and degradation of catecholamines.

velop only when the tumor is very large. Examination of the urine may show a modest elevation of free amine, but there is usually a significant increase in urinary catecholamine metabolites in most cases. There is at least a twofold increase in both free amines and their metabolites.

Clinical Features

The clinical features and differential diagnosis of pheochromocytoma are listed in Table 70–8. Patients may present with symptoms secondary to hypertension without any of the other distinguishing features found in groups II, III, and IV. Suspicion should be aroused if the hypertension is intermittent, if the blood pressure shows a paradoxical response after the administration of ganglion-blocking agents, if a precipitous elevation of the blood pressure is provoked during the induction of an anesthesia or on abdominal palpation, and if the patient shows an otherwise unexplained tendency to develop cardiac arrhythmias.

An important clinical clue that separates patients with sustained hypertension due to pheochromocytoma from other causes of hypertension is the finding of orthostatic hypotension. This is present in two-

thirds of the cases and is due to atrophy of the usual sympathetic postural reflexes. With other types of sustained hypertension, untreated, there is elevation of blood pressure on standing erect.[56]

In the rare, predominantly epinephrine-producing tumor the patient may present with hypotension. This is consequent upon peripheral vasodilation with hypovolemia and hemoconcentration. Although hematocrit values are elevated, true polycythemia is rare. Patients in this category almost invariably have, in addition, symptoms belonging to groups II and III (Table 70–8).

The most classic presentation is with intermittent "spells" or "attacks." The attack may commence with a feeling of nervousness and apprehension, often a feeling of impending doom. Headache is prominent and severe palpitations and profuse sweating are common. Nausea and vomiting are accompanied by abdominal pain, penile pain, and dysuria, symptoms probably provoked by sphincteric spasm. Angina pectoris, dyspnea, and cerebrovascular accidents are not infrequent. The patient is often very tremulous, complains of paresthesias, and may have frank tetany. The trigger for an attack can be an emotional event or a physical upset, such as a change in posture,

TABLE 70-8
Pheochromocytoma: Presenting Features and Differential Diagnosis

Presenting Features	Differential Diagnosis
Group I. Hypertension	
Episodic	Essential
Headache	hypertension
Paroxysmal	Renal hypertension
dyspnea	Other causes of
Persistent	endocrine
Cerebrovascular	hypertension
episodes	
Group II. Spells	
Excessive perspiration	Other causes of
Palpitations	catecholamine
Pain (headache, angina,	release, e.g., hypo-
abdominal pain)	glycemia
Nervousness and apprehension	5-hydroxy-tryptamine
Paresthesia	over-production
Pallor	Carcinoid
	Mastocytosis
	Menopausal
	symptoms
	Cervical spondylosis
	Horton's headaches
	Associated with use
	of monoamine
	oxidase inhibitors
Group III. Metabolic Diabetes	
Loss of weight	Diabetes mellitus
Fever	Hyperthyroidism
Group IV. Hypotension (rare)	
Hypovolemia	Other causes of
Shock	shock
Polycythemia	

count for the clinical picture, which has also been seen when methamphetamine and MAO inhibitors are taken together. Patients complain of forceful increases in the heartbeat, throbbing in the neck, choking sensations, and profuse sweating. They may be pale or flushed and are apprehensive; there is often extreme sweating, and loss of consciousness can occur. Bradycardia and various cardiac arrhythmias are seen. At some stage the patient is hypertensive, but he can become profoundly hypotensive and hyperpyrexic. The resemblance to pheochromocytoma crisis is close, and the importance of excluding any drug ingestion must be emphasized.

The spells seen in association with malignant carcinoid tumors and generalized mastocytosis bear a superficial resemblance to those seen with catecholamine release. There is usually an accompanying flush, also encountered in the female with menopausal symptoms and in the individual with Horton's cephalalgia. During a pheochromocytoma spell, pallor of the face, tachycardia, tremulousness, and cold and clammy skin occasionally accompanied by Raynaud's phenomenon may be observed.

Just as patients in group I (Table 70-8) may resemble patients with essential hypertension, so may patients in group III mimic patients with diabetes mellitus. Two important clues which suggest the diagnosis are 1) loss of weight disproportionate to the degree of glucosuria and ketonuria; and 2) symptoms of hypermetabolism, such as heat intolerance, diarrhea, and nervousness. With respect to these features, thyrotoxicosis may be suspected, and, indeed, thyroidectomy has been performed in some patients.

The physical examination may reveal only hypertension. Café-au-lait spots, neurofibromas, and retinal angiomas should be sought, since all of these have been described in association with pheochromocytoma. Inexplicable beefy red hands have also been observed in a few patients. There is an association between multiple pheochromocytomas and amyloid-producing thyroid carcinomas. This syndrome is familial—type II multiple endocrine adenomatosis.

Diagnosis and Therapy
An approach to the diagnosis of pheochromocytoma is shown in Table 70-9. It is based upon the finding of excessive catecholamines or their metabolites in the urine. Most clinical laboratories now have reliable assays for the metabolites of the catecholamines. The most discriminatory is the total metanephrine determination. The VMA in the past has been unreliable. Fluorometric methods whose upper limit of normal is above 10 mg per 24 hours should not be used. Most reliable colorimetric methods for VMA have an upper

gastric distension, a full bladder, or straining at stool.

These spells are, in the main, consequent upon the excessive secretion of catecholamine. There is, therefore, considerable resemblance between them and the symptoms provoked by hypoglycemia (Chap. 72). Similar episodes have been reported in some individuals taking the monoamine oxidase (MAO) inhibitors, tranylcypromine, and phenelzine. These attacks have often been provoked by the ingestion of cheese. Cheese contains a variable quantity of tyramine, as well as other amines. The hypertensive effect of tyramine, produced by the release of peripherally stored catecholamine, is greatly augmented in the presence of MAO inhibitors. This interplay may ac-

TABLE 70–9
Diagnosis of Pheochromocytoma

Critical Questions	Special Tests	Comments
Is the index of suspicion high?	Hypertension, headache, sweating, palpitations	R/o reactive hypoglycemia
Are reliable metabolite assays abnormal? (use two assays)	Metanephrine VMA (normal <6.8 mg/day) Free catecholamines	Values should be twice upper limit of normal
Is a provocative test needed?	Measure urine after spontaneous episode	
Provocative testing	Histamine (10 μg) Tyramine (500 μg) Glucagon (1 mg)	Dangerous in elderly Pretreatment with Dibenzyline if suspicion high; using urinary metabolite end point
Alpha blockade	Phentolamine	Improved accuracy with insulin assays during IV glucose load
Localization	Oblique x-rays of spine	
	Arteriography Surgical exploration	Keep phentolamine with patient

limit of normal less than 6.8 mg per 24 hours. If one metabolite is found elevated it should be confirmed by measurement of one of the others. Interfering drugs seldom influence more than one of these tests. Medications to be avoided include: 1) α-methyldopa (Aldomet), sympathomimetics (raise free catecholamines), 2) monoamine oxidase inhibitors (lower metanephrines, increase VMA), 3) clofibrate (Atromid S) (lowers VMA), and 4) nalidixic acid (increases VMA).

The traditional provocative tests to excite a pheochromocytoma should be reserved for unusual circumstances. Stroke and myocardial infarction are complications to be avoided. In young patients, in whom the index of suspicion is low and for whom a negative diagnosis is urgently needed, these tests may be used. It is possible to use the urinary metabolite excretion as the end point of these provocative tests. Pretreatment with phenoxybenzamine (Dibenzyline) will then prevent a hypertensive paroxysm and makes the testing procedure safer. Propranolol may be needed if unopposed β-adrenergic effects produce an arrhythmia.

Localization of the tumor preoperatively is important. Selective arteriography has the distinct advantage of revealing for the surgeon anomalies of blood supply. Since an active tumor may be stimulated during arteriography, the radiologist must be prepared to treat an intercurrent paroxysm or the patient should be pretreated with phenoxybenzamine. Computerized axial tomography and ultrasound are useful adjuncts for tumor localization. Oblique films of the sympathetic chain can be important to rule out extra-adrenal tumor.

Because of functional atrophy of neurogenic cardiovascular reflexes, all patients should undergo pharmacologic control of their symptoms for at least 1 week before surgery. Adrenergic blockade with phenoxybenzamine starting at 20 to 30 mg per day and increasing by 10 to 20 mg increments will often control the hypertension. Occasionally orthostatic hypotension or tachycardia may develop. In epinephrine-secreting tumors, combined therapy with β-adrenergic blockade will be necessary to avoid exaggerated responses to either agent. During surgery rapid injection of phentolamine intravenously (5.0 mg) is the best way to treat episodic hypertension which may occur despite adequate pretreatment.

Following successful removal of the tumor, profound shock may occur. This shock may be unresponsive to norepinephrine infusion. Prophylactic transfusion during the surgical procedure and before the tumor removal, designed to replace carefully all fluid losses during the procedure, can prevent this disaster. Overtransfusion with plasma expanders to sustain a systolic pressure of 100 mm Hg is the best treatment once it has occurred. Arrhythmias developing during the operation are treated with intravenous propranolol (1 to 3 mg).

For inoperable tumors, phenoxybenzamine has been used. More recently the competitive inhibition of tyrosine hydroxylase with α-methyl paratyrosine (2.5 mg four times daily) has proven successful.

CHAPTER 71

Diabetes Mellitus

THADDEUS E. PROUT

Diabetes mellitus[93] is a complex metabolic disease resulting from inadequate concentrations or ineffectiveness of circulating insulin. This insulin-deficient state can be caused by defects in insulin production and/or release or by resistance to insulin actions on the cell.

Insulin is produced in the endoplasmic reticulum of the beta cell as a single polypeptide chain of 86 amino acids, called proinsulin. During its storage in the beta cell, proinsulin is cleaved into an alpha chain containing 21 amino acids and a beta chain of 30 amino acids, the two being connected by two disulfide bridges. In the process of prohormone cleavage, a connecting strand (C-peptide) is removed. Insulin and the C-peptide remnant are packaged in membrane-bound granules, which migrate toward the cell membrane, and are discharged by an emiocytosis (or exocytosis) process upon demand. Since equimolar amounts of insulin and C-peptide are secreted, C-peptide levels accurately reflect insulin secretion.

Glucose is the most potent stimulus for insulin secretion, but fructose, amino acids, ketones, and hormones are also involved (Table 71-1). The response of the pancreatic beta cells to glucose is biphasic. The initial rapid secretory burst results from the release of preformed insulin from storage granules, while the basal and steady-state release is derived primarily from a newly synthesized pool. The beta cell of the pancreas detects the concentrations of these substances by a process not yet understood. A selective defect in insulin response to glucose, with preservation of the response to beta-adrenergic stimulation confirms the existence of the sensor mechanism.[147] The final common path of the release of insulin, however, involves a calcium-dependent contraction of intracellular microfilamentous structures.

To be effective at the cell membrane, insulin released by the beta cells[121] must not only survive proteolytic degradation during passage through the hepatic and renal circulation but also must overcome specific antagonists. Furthermore, insulin effect is directly related to the availability of receptor sites; for example, the altered glucose tolerance of obesity is caused by a decrease in receptors.[88] Membrane reactivity[125] depends not only on the interaction of insulin and its receptors but also on specific electrolytes.[119] If all of these mechanisms are operative, metabolites may enter through the membrane of the cell for utilization, thereby decreasing the stimulation of insulin release by a feedback mechanism.

PATHOGENESIS OF DIABETES MELLITUS

In insulin-deficient diabetes, the secretion of the hormone is either totally defective or severely impaired. The failure of the pancreatic beta cells probably involves genetic,[146] viral, and autoimmune processes, among others. If the index monozygotic twin develops diabetes before age 40, the unaffected twin has a 50 percent chance of becoming diabetic, but after 40, the chance is 90 percent. Insulin-deficient diabetes shows association with specific HLA haplotypes; the presence of BW 15, BW 3, or BW 4 gives a relative risk for diabetes of 2.4, 6.4, and 3.7, respectively, above that in the general population.[134] Viral infections are capable of damaging the pancreas, and at least eight viruses are implicated.[113] To become diabetic, an individual must not only be affected by one of these viruses but must also develop antibodies to islet cells.[87] Evidence for this thesis is provided by the presence of antibodies to islet cells in patients with diabetes following a viral illness and by the association of diabetes with other autoimmune syndromes.

Diabetes mellitus can also be caused by resistance to insulin actions on the cell. In this form of diabetes, which usually occurs in obese adults, the beta-cell defect involves only the initial rapid secretory burst. Although basal insulin level is usually normal or increased, level is below that observed in nondiabetic subjects who are obese. Furthermore, at the cellular level a reduction in insulin receptors decreases insulin binding and contributes to the insulin-deficient state. In unusual states, such as certain patients with acanthosis nigricans or lipoatrophic diabetes, extreme deficiency of insulin receptors is the dominant cause of diabetes mellitus. Thus, the insulin-deficient state is caused by lack of insulin as in juvenile diabetes, deficient or defective receptor sites as in acanthosis nigricans, or intermediate deficiencies in both as seen in obese adult diabetics.

Glucagon, a product of the alpha cell in the islets, has been implicated as a contributing factor. This hormone promotes hepatic glucose production by both gluconeogenesis and glycogenolysis. Under normal conditions, elevation of blood glucose suppresses glucagon secretion and hypoglycemia stimulates re-

TABLE 71-1
Agents Affecting Insulin Secretion[138]

	Stimulatory	Inhibitory
Metabolites	Glucose Mannose Fatty acids Ketones Arginine Leucine	Manohepulose 2-Deoxyglucose
Hormones	Secretin Gastrin Glucagon Growth hormone ACTH	Insulin Somatostatin Epinephrine Norepinephrine
Drugs	Beta-agonists Sulfonylureas	Alpha-agonists Diazoxide Catecholamines Beta-blockers (e.g., propranolol)

lease of the hormone. It is becoming increasingly apparent, however, that glucagon is inappropriately elevated in diabetics. The relative contribution of abnormal glucagon levels to the development of diabetes mellitus remains unanswered. Pathophysiologic role of somatostatin, a secretory product of the delta cell of the pancreatic islets, awaits further clarification.

FEEDING, FASTING, AND THE ROLE OF INSULIN

The normal control of glucose is best illustrated by a brief review of homeostatic mechanisms in intermediary metabolism during feeding and fasting. When normal subjects eat, the metabolites and hormones listed in Table 71-1 participate in regulation of insulin secretion. Intestinal hormones also play a role in initiating insulin secretion after food ingestion and before metabolites reach the bloodstream. Elevation in the levels of blood metabolites results in both an early and late phase of insulin secretion. The initial rapid release of insulin, presumably from granules stored near microvilli, may develop within minutes and begins to decline equally rapidly. If the level of substrate remains elevated, insulin secretion again rises, reaching a peak between 47 and 90 minutes.

In a state of high insulin secretion, the liver takes up glucose, synthesizes glycogen, shuts off gluconeogenesis and ketogenesis, and begins the process of lipogenesis. Excess calories, including those derived from carbohydrate, stimulate synthesis of fatty acids and triglycerides by the liver and subsequent storage in adipose tissue. In the muscle there is glucose uptake and probably glycogen synthesis to a modest ex-

tent. With increased availability of amino acids from the diet, the protein synthesis can begin. Similarly, in adipose tissue high levels of insulin in the fed state stimulate glucose uptake and lipid synthesis.

Following fasting in normal subjects, the levels of insulin are low and, as a result, release of free fatty acids from adipose tissue, and probably of amino acids from muscle, occurs. The continuous insulin secretion is not sufficient to retard glycogenolysis and glyconeogenesis by the liver. Thus, there is maintenance of blood sugar at levels needed by non-insulin-dependent tissues, especially the brain, and at the same time, profound lipogenesis and ketogenesis are avoided. In general, ketone production appears to parallel gluconeogenesis, but there is sufficient insulin output to prevent ketoacidosis in normal subjects, even in states of severe starvation. At the same time, glucose uptake is curtailed in muscle in order to conserve glucose for non-insulin-dependent tissues without significant proteolysis or amino acid release. Muscle glycogen may be slowly released for energy, but the principal energy store during fasting is free fatty acid. There is also an absence of glucose and triglyceride uptake in adipose tissue, and in the absence of exercise, only modest lipolysis and fatty acid release occur.

As diabetes develops and insulin deficiency progresses, normal controls gradually break down, first after feeding and eventually in periods of fasting as well. There is first a failure of translocation of glucose from serum to the intracellular compartment of insulin sensitive tissue. Fatty acids and amino acids are released from adipose tissue and muscle, respectively, leading to even more gluconeogenesis of liver. Without increase in utilization, plasma glucose rises above normal. When insulin deficiency is severe, glucose levels rise to exceed the ability of the kidney to reabsorb all glucose in the filtrate, and glycosuria develops. Loss of glucose in the urine causes loss also of water, minerals, and calories. The clinical manifestation of further deterioration in metabolism can be recognized when the diabetic begins to lose weight in spite of normal or above normal food intake. Glycosuria intensifies, and ketonuria appears as fat is mobilized. Since small amounts of insulin are needed to prevent lipolysis and ketogenesis, total decompensation of insulin effectiveness eventually leads to marked ketogenesis and to ketoacidosis. At the same time, there is an efflux of potassium from muscle, a rise in serum amino acids, and muscle wasting. Thus, the onset of carbohydrate intolerance and the further progression of diabetes are determined by the level of insulin effectiveness and, conversely, the level of glucose intolerance is used to define the presence of diabetes.

CLINICAL PRESENTATION

Two main types of diabetes are recognized on the basis of insulin need (Table 71–2). Non-insulin-dependent diabetes (NIDD) is insidious in onset and resistant to ketosis. Insulin-dependent diabetes (IDD) is usually associated with severe symptoms of recent onset, simultaneous onset of ketonemia, and, if untreated, ketoacidosis.

Non-Insulin-Dependent Diabetes

This type of diabetes is associated with obesity or a past history of obesity, in roughly 85 percent of cases. This is by far the largest group of diabetic patients whom the internist treats. The diagnosis of diabetes is frequently made while they are asymptomatic, yet evidence indicates that the disorder is longstanding. History may reveal reactive hypoglycemia at an earlier time, and in females, poor fetal survival or the birth of babies weighing more than 10 pounds. At the time of diagnosis, many patients already have complications attributed to diabetes;[157] up to 15 percent have significant retinopathy and abnormal electrocardiograms, slight decrease in renal function with or without hypertension, or clinical evidence of coronary artery disease.

Most NIDD patients have levels of circulating insulin that are above normal. They fail to translocate glucose into tissue stores because of a decrease in insulin receptors. Restriction of calories to reduce weight results in an increase in cell receptors for insulin and is thus the basic therapy for these patients. Failure to control blood glucose by dietary means may lead to the use of an oral hypoglycemic agent or insulin. Exhaustion of endogenous insulin stores in this group can lead to development of true insulin-dependent diabetes.

Although NIDD is generally associated with onset of adulthood, this form of diabetes is recognized with increasing frequency in youth. Some of these cases represent "maturity-onset diabetes of the young" (MODY),[107] which is inherited as an autosomal dominant.[115] NIDD in youth is commonly seen with long-standing juvenile obesity. Patients may develop symptoms of blurred vision, polyuria, and polydipsia without weight loss. Vaginitis in young females sometimes leads to this diagnosis. Acne is common, although diabetes is an uncommon cause for acne in the usual teen-age population. In the young patient, as in the adult with diabetes associated with obesity, loss of effectiveness of insulin results in hyperglycemia, but lipogenesis continues and ketosis is uncommon.

Insulin-Dependent Diabetes (IDD)

This type of diabetes constitutes only about 10 to 12 percent of all diabetes. It is most common in youth but may develop acutely at any age, with all of the problems of management found in the younger age group. When there is an insidious onset, the well-known symptoms and signs of polyuria and polydipsia may be attributed to a urinary tract infection, and the weight loss, lack of energy, and need for increasing rest may be ascribed to emotional problems. More frequently, however, IDD develops with alarming rapidity requiring emergency hospitalization for ketoacidosis. In no other diabetic condition can the rapid effects of insulin deficiency be seen so clearly. One often obtains a history of the progressive metabolic deterioration of the patient from normality through symptomatic hyperglycemia to inanition and a final stage of rapidly progressive ketogenesis and ketoacidosis, before the diagnosis is made.[126]

Transient Diabetes Mellitus of Infancy

This type is a unique clinical condition. It is characterized by hyperglycemia, hyperosmolality, severe dehydration, and relative resistance to ketoacidosis occurring within the first few days of life. It may es-

---

TABLE 71–2
Metabolic Presentations of Diabetes Mellitus

Class	Presentation
Non-insulin-dependent diabetes (NID-Diabetes)	Commonest form (85%) of diabetes; may be asymptomatic or present with pathologic complications. Also seen in youth (includes group designated MODY)[115]
	Symptoms of thirst and nocturia are related to amount of urine glucose, beginning at 10–20 g/24 hr
	Caloric loss may be compensated Negative balance of 50–60 g/24 hr results in weight loss of 1/2 lb./week
Insulin-dependent-diabetes (ID-Diabetes)	10–12% of all diabetes. Commonest in youth but seen at all ages
	Presents with increasing symptoms of calorie loss and dehydration. Ketonemia begins with fat mobilization, continuing to ketoacidosis as insulin falls. Viral, autoimmune etiology in susceptible HLA types postulated

cape recognition because of its rarity. Cautious administration of insulin is indicated and is effective. The diabetic state persists for only a few weeks. Such children do not go on to develop insulin-dependent diabetes.

Diabetes mellitus may be associated with many other conditions as noted in Table 71–3. These include autoimmune diseases, endocrine disorders affecting insulin secretion or its peripheral action, genetic disorders, and an enlarging list of miscellaneous conditions including those associated with impaired binding between insulin and insulin cell receptors. Characteristic skin changes, termed acanthosis nigricans (Table 71–3), are associated with deficiency in

---

TABLE 71–3
Disorders Associated with Diabetes Mellitus

Autoimmune Disorders[87]

Thyrotoxicosis
Hashimoto's disease
Primary hypothyroidism
Hypoparathyroidism
Addison's disease
Schmidt syndrome
Myasthenia gravis
Pernicious anemia
Polyendocrine disorders

Other Endocrine Disorders

Cushing syndrome
Acromegaly
Primary aldosteronism
Pheochromocytoma
Toxic nodular goiter
Somatostatinoma

Genetic Disorders[146]

Hemochromatosis
Turner syndrome
Werner syndrome
Klinefelter syndrome[280]
Optic atrophy–
    diabetes mellitus–
    diabetes insipidus syndrome
Laurence-Moon-Biedl
    syndrome
Friedreich's ataxia
Ataxia-telangiectasia
Refsum syndrome
Glycogen storage I
Myotonic dystrophy
Down syndrome

Miscellaneous

Acanthosis nigricans
Lipodystrophic syndromes
Chronic pancreatitis
Cancer of the pancreas

---

insulin receptors in virilized young females (Type A) and with antibodies to insulin receptors in older patients in association with hyperglobulinemia (Type B).[88]

DIAGNOSIS

Elevation of the blood sugar above 200 mg/dl, in either the fasting or the fed state, indicates diabetes mellitus. Furthermore, elevation of fasting blood glucose above 150 mg/dl also indicates diabetes mellitus. (Because of the widespread use of automated equipment, tests are usually performed on plasma or serum. Plasma and serum glucose levels are about 15 percent higher than those obtained from whole blood and vary only slightly with hematocrit.) If the blood sugar, especially fasting, is at the most equivocally elevated, a provocative test is indicated. The one most often used, indeed overused, is the oral glucose tolerance test (OGTT).[139,150]

A physician should perform an OGTT only if he has a clear understanding of the indications and limitations of the test. Indications for OGTT include borderline glucose values in the nonfasting state or by screening procedures, glycosuria in the absence of diagnostic hyperglycemia, a risk of glucose intolerance (obesity, family history) with or without positive screening tests, and symptoms suggesting hypoglycemia. It may also be used in patients who have unexplained neuropathy, retinopathy, peripheral vascular disease, or coronary heart disease, and in women with unexplained fetal loss, large babies, or suspected gestational diabetes.

Glucose tolerance tests are not useful in following overt diabetes or testing the efficacy of therapy. In performance of the test (Table 71–4) and interpretation of its results, dietary preparation, physical activity, and the state of the patient's health, drugs that can alter the OGTT (Table 71–5), the time of testing, and the size of the glucose load are all important considerations.[97] Standard sampling times are 0 (fasting), 1, and 2 hours.

The fasting blood glucose is relatively insensitive to age and increases an average of only 2 mg/dl per decade. The average increase for the 2-hour value is about 6 mg/dl per decade after the age of 30 in patients who have no evidence of diabetes or family history of same.[85]

The range of normality of the OGTT is difficult to establish. In addition to the normal elevation of post-challenge values with age, the rising prevalence of diabetes with age must be considered. One approach to differentiation between normality, impaired glucose tolerance, and diabetes can be based on the sum of the fasting 1- and 2-hour glucose values (Fig. 71–1).

─TABLE 71-4─
Glucose Tolerance Test

Conditions of Test

No food for 10 to 16 hours; water is permitted
Subject should be in good health, not hospitalized
Drugs known to affect glucose tolerance should be
   omitted, if not essential to health, for 2 weeks
Subject should be seated and not smoke during test

Glucose Load

The dose of glucose recommended is 75 g in 300 ml of
   flavored water, drunk in 5 minutes. In children a dose
   of 1.75 g/kg up to 40 kg with the standard dose over
   40 kg

Sample Times

Samples drawn at fasting, and 1, 2, and 3 hours after
   start of glucose load are standard.
Five-hour tests are used to document reactive
   hypoglycemia

Interpretation

See references 97, 133, 143, for discussion.
Glucose intolerance is based on fasting and 2 hr plasma
   glucose or Sum 2 hr OGTT
Reference plasma* glucose values are:
Normal: Fasting and 2 hour 140 mg/dl
Impaired Tolerance: Fasting 140 mg/dl 2 hr. 140 mg/dl
   to 170 mg/dl (at 70 years)
Diabetes mellitus: Fasting 140 mg/dl 2 hr. 200 mg/dl to
   230 (at 70 years)
Gestational diabetes: Fasting 105 mg/dl 2 hr. 165 mg/dl
   (100 g load)

* Plasma glucose 15% higher than whole blood.

─TABLE 71-5─
Classes of Drug Reported to Affect Glucose Tolerance*

Hyperglycemia

1. Diuretics (thiazides, furosemide)
2. Antihypertensives (clonidine)
3. Psychoactive drug (tricyclics, phenothiazines)
4. Beta-blockers (propranolol)
5. Miscellaneous (diphenylhydantoin, L-dopa, morphine, marihuana)

Hypoglycemia

1. Analgesics (salicylates)
2. Antiinflammatory drugs (phenylbutazone)
3. Antituberculous drugs (PAS, INH)
4. Alcohols (methyl, ethyl)
5. Miscellaneous (probenecid, thiouracil)

* The list of drugs affecting glucose tolerance is continually expanding. The categories and examples cited here are intended to illustrate some of the many drugs implicated.

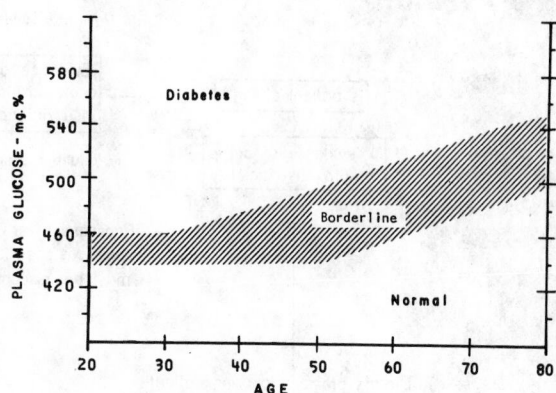

FIGURE 71-1. Diagnostic levels of SUM OGTT/2 hr (F + 1+ 2 hr) after glucose-challenge for various ages. The "SUM 2-HR OGTT" utilizes the sum of the fasting, 1- and 2-hour values of plasma glucose, and the age of the patient to determine whether the patient should be considered normal, borderline, or diabetic.

Other tests that have been utilized in the diagnosis of diabetes include the intravenous glucose tolerance test,[151] the tolbutamide tolerance test,[155] and the cortisone-glucose tolerance test.[106] These are used primarily as research tools, but may be useful in patients who have a disorder believed to be related to glucose intolerance but have a normal OGTT. The level of serum insulin following glucose challenge has also been proposed as a means for authenticating the diabetic state.[154] It has been found that only those patients who fail to have an elevation of plasma insulin above 60 μU/dl following glucose challenge are at risk for retinopathy, nephropathy, and other microvascular complications of diabetes. This observation reconfirms the fact that adult diabetic patients with obesity and elevated levels of serum insulin are not only resistant to ketosis but also relatively resistant to degenerative complications. A low or flat OGTT, defined as one in which peak serum glucose rises less than 20 mg above the fasting level, has no unique physiologic significance and is observed in 15 to 20 percent of normal adults.

TREATMENT

General (Fig. 71-2)

Once the diagnosis of diabetes has been established, the illness must be explained to the patient in a manner that will avoid misconceptions as to the effect that diabetes may have on his life. It is important that the explanation be realistic, but implications that ear-

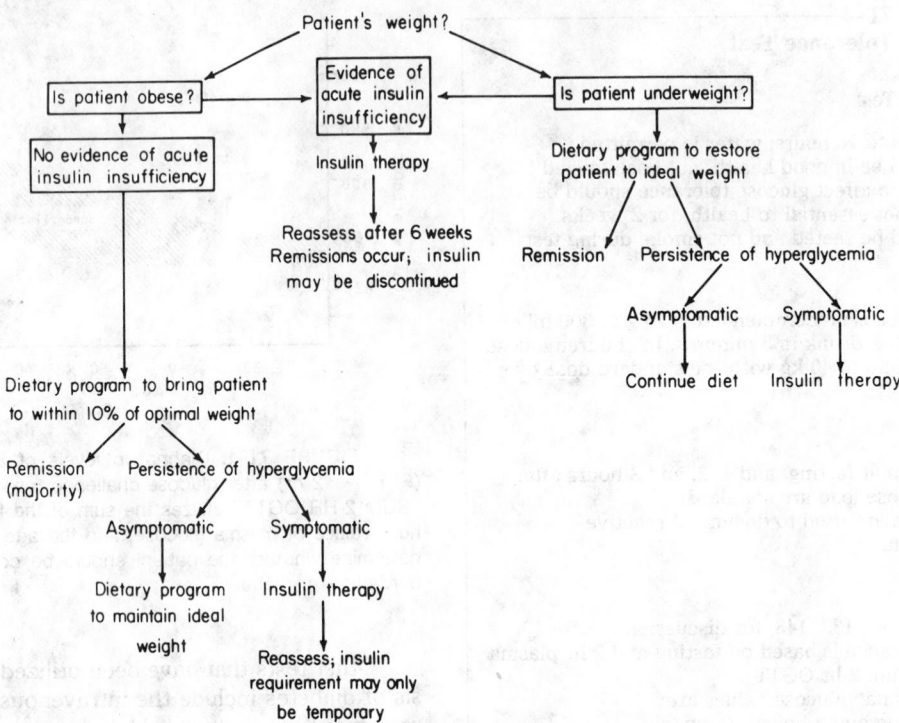

FIGURE 71-2. An approach to the selection of treatment of diabetes mellitus.

ly degenerative changes are inevitable must be avoided. No other chronic disease illustrates better the need for cooperation between patient and physician. The patient must be a coequal with the physician in the day-to-day management of his illness. The newly diagnosed diabetic frequently wishes to take a passive attitude toward his illness, leaving his care to others. On the contrary, the roles of the physician, dietitian, and nurse as counselors and of the patient as the primary manager of his condition must be firmly established from the outset.[104]

In most instances, education of the diabetic patient is best accomplished in a special clinic, so that adequate personnel, including volunteer help, is available. Teaching films covering general knowledge, insulin use, home testing, diabetic diets, and avoidance of complications are now available.[129]

About 85 percent of newly diagnosed diabetics are overweight, non-insulin-dependent, and non-ketosis-prone (Table 71-2). Weight reduction is the cornerstone of management (Table 71-6). Most are asymptomatic or only mildly symptomatic. A few are seen first because of vascular problems, and diabetes is discovered through a screening laboratory procedure. If there has been no significant recent or unexplained weight loss, it may be presumed that this pa-

tient still has sufficient effective insulin to prevent lipolysis, and the physician may proceed with dietary treatment on an ambulatory basis without concern that the patient will develop ketoacidosis, even when fasting blood glucose levels are in the range of 300 to 400 mg/dl.

Diet

This plays the key role in therapy of all diabetics. Use of either oral hypoglycemic agents or insulin without proper dietary management is improper care of a diabetic. A diet should provide adequate calories and essential nutrients for normal body weight and for the individual's level of daily activity. The diet is expected to promote weight loss in the obese patient and weight gain in the underweight patient. The American Diabetes Association recommends a diet that contains about 50 percent of its calories as carbohydrates, 20 percent as protein, and 30 percent as fat.[91] Fats may be further specified as to the percent of saturated fats and cholesterol.

The diet prescription for diabetes is given in practical terms in Table 71-7. Although this table provides a simple and easy formula which can be administered by any practitioner, every new diabetic should be seen by a dietitian for complete instructions. Dis-

TABLE 71-6

Principles of Diabetes Management:
Noninsulin Dependent Diabetes

1. Diet remains the keystone of therapy in all diabetics. It is potentially the only therapy needed in 85% of diabetes associated with obesity

2. A reduction in the caloric load in diabetics who are above ideal weight improves the levels of glucose, cholesterol, and triglycerides, even when normal body weight is not attained

3. With reduction in caloric loads, insulin receptor sites increase and insulin resistance is reduced

4. As shown by hemoglobin A1c, elevation of blood glucose causes irreversible glycosylation of body proteins which may alter protein function

5. Blood glucose levels after a glucose challenge rise increasingly with age after 50 years. For persons above the age of 50, blood glucose may normally be higher than levels considered normal for younger persons

6. Plasma glucose levels, 3 hours after eating, at or below renal threshold, or approximately 200 to 220 mg/dl, indicates adequate control in non-insulin-dependent patients with diabetes above the age of 50. Negative preprandial urine tests for glucose are a practical measure of this control

7. Hypoglycemic agents are rarely indicated up to a blood glucose level of 250 mg/dl in the postprandial period in diabetes complicated by obesity

8. Evidence that oral agents may be associated with an increased death rate due to cardiovascular disease precludes their use in patients with present or suspected coronary heart disease, without vigorous attempts at weight reduction. If lowering of blood glucose is desired, insulin is the therapy of first choice because it is more uniformly effective and perhaps safer

tribution of calories should be consistent from day to day. Mealtime should also be kept the same. Three meals are usual, but it is sometimes essential to add a midafternoon or bedtime snack.

A physiologic explanation for the importance of diet in the management of obese patients is now available.[88] The basic cause for hyperglycemia in obese diabetics is deficiency of cell receptors for insulin. Reduction in body weight not only increases the availability of insulin receptors, thereby improving insulin sensitivity, but also lowers blood sugar, cholesterol, and triglycerides. Reduction of cholesterol is important because Type IV hyperlipidemia is prevalent among diabetics. Dietary management must be coupled with regular exercise. The initial education of the obese diabetic with more than 30 percent excess

body weight should always include instructions for physical activity.

The patient in whom diabetes is associated with obesity must be given adequate time to understand and practice good dietary habits before other modes of therapy are introduced. Failure to establish the primacy of dietary management at the onset is a frequent shortcoming in the treatment of diabetes. Elevations of blood glucose in the insulin-dependent diabetic during this initial period are not life-threatening, and the use of hypoglycemic agents in the uncomplicated diabetic before good food habits are developed is to be discouraged.

The underweight diabetic is likely to have an unrecognized need for insulin. These patients often strive to avoid insulin therapy through starvation. Therapy cannot be considered successful until they have been returned to normal body weight, usually with the addition of insulin.

If the obese diabetic is unable to adhere to diet or if diet fails to control hyperglycemia, an oral hypoglycemic agent or insulin should be considered.

Oral Hypoglycemic Agents (OHA)[116]: Sulfonylureas

These agents should not be used in insulin-dependent patients, or in non-insulin-dependent patients until they have failed in dietary control. OHA are contraindicated also in patients in whom there is no significant effect on plasma glucose, either on first use ("primary failure") or after a period of presumed effectiveness ("secondary failure"). OHA should be discontinued periodically to test their effect on blood glucose.

The sulfonylureas probably have a common mode of action and differ only in relative potency and duration of action. They provoke liberation of endogenous insulin. The manner in which this is accomplished appears to differ from that of glucose. Certain pharmacologic agents (diazoxide) inhibit insulin secretion induced by glucose but have no effect on the action of sulfonylureas. In addition, these hypoglycemic agents stimulate insulin secretion only, whereas glucose enhances both synthesis and secretion of the hormone.

A long-term prospective study[158,159,160] designed to evaluate the effectiveness of hypoglycemic treatments in the prevention of vascular complication casts doubts on the usefulness of sulfonylureas in the treatment of diabetes mellitus. Consequently, the American Diabetes Association, the AMA Council on Drugs, and the Food and Drug Administration have recommended that pending further studies the use of sulfonylureas be limited to patients with symptoma-

─TABLE 71-7─
Diet Calculation for Diabetic Patients

1. Determine normal body weight (NBW), either from standard tables or by calculation using the following aids:

    Males: 115 base weight; add 5 pounds for each inch over 5 feet
    Females: 100 base weight; add 5 pounds for each inch over 5 feet
    (±10% for age, body habitus, or other individual consideration)

2. Calculate basal calories by determining NBW × 10. Add additional calories dependent upon degree of activity (0 = basal; 25% = moderate activity, 8-hour day; 50% = heavy, prolonged labor)

    To reduce obesity, subtract 500 calories from estimated caloric needs
    To gain weight, add 500 calories

3. Food allocations may be expressed in grams

    Carbohydrate: Divide total calories by 10 (50% calories)
    Protein (adult): 1/2 g protein per pound NBW (approximately 20% calories)
    Fat: Remainder of calories divided by 9 (approximately 30% calories); for low fat diet, eliminate all free fat, substitute low-fat proteins, increase CHO accordingly)

4. More conveniently, food may be expressed in servings by food class

Class	1	2	3	4	5	6
Food	Milk	Veg	Fruit	Bread	Meat*	Fat
Cal/Serving†	80	25	40	70	55	45

5. Determine number of total servings of various foods for total number of calories prescribed by chart[105] Examples are

Calories	Food Servings					
	1	2	3	4	5	6
1800	3	3	5	7	10	5
1500	2	4	6	4	8	6
1000	1	4	2	2	6	4

6. Distribute servings into exchange meal plan by tenths, utilizing spaces for 3 meals and 3 snacks. Example: 1800 calories, Distribution: 2/10-(0)-2/10-(1/10)-4/10-(1/10)

* Lean meat = 55 cal/serving. Add 1/2 fat equivalent for medium-fat and 1 fat equivalent for high fat protein. Adjust the total accordingly.
† Dietary examples are expressed in servings. See also "A Guide for Professionals: The Effective Application of 'Exchange List for Meal Planning' "[105]

─TABLE 71-7 (cont.)─

Distribution	BK 2/10	SN (0)	LU 2/10	SN (1/10)	DN 4/10	SN (1/10)	Total
Class (Cal)							
1. Milk (80)	1			1		1	3
2. Veg (25)					3		3
3. Fruit (40)	1		1		1	2	5
4. Bread (70)	1		2	1	3		7
5. Meat (55)	2		2	1	5		10
6. Fat (45)	1		1		3		5

7. Instruct patient in use of exchange lists to translate meal plans into actual meals[105]

tic maturity-onset diabetes who cannot be controlled by diet and in whom the addition of insulin is impractical and unacceptable. The recommendation and results of the study have been challenged by some diabetologists but have withstood critical impartial analysis.[96] At the very least this study should encourage the physician to apprise the patient of possible hazards of OHA (Table 71–8), to be more vigorous in promoting a proper dietary regimen, and not to reserve insulin therapy for the last possible moment.

Special mention should be made of the patient presently "controlled" on oral agents. Since experience has shown that long-term treatment with OHA may lead to so-called secondary failures or that the diabetic state may undergo amelioration after proper diet and weight adjustment, it is advisable to withdraw oral drugs from time to time to determine their actual usefulness. Such withdrawal is not expected to create metabolic catastrophe or precipitate ketoacidosis since these agents are unsuitable for therapy in patients who are insulin dependent.

Tolbutamide can be given orally or intravenously. It is rapidly absorbed from the upper gastrointestinal tract, reaches a peak concentration in the plasma in 3 to 5 hours, and has a half-life of 4 to 5 hours. It is metabolized in the liver to a carboxy derivative, which is inactive. Side effects such as leukopenia, skin reactions, and gastrointestinal complaints are occasionally seen. The usual dosage is 0.5 g three times a day, administered with meals, and no greater therapeutic effect is obtained by giving doses greater than 2 g per day.

Chlorpropamide is more potent than tolbutamide. It is rapidly absorbed from the gut, reaches a peak concentration in 2 to 4 hours, and is excreted unchanged very slowly, with a half-life in plasma of 35 to 50 hours. A single daily dose between 0.1 and

TABLE 71-8
Extrapancreatic Effects of Sulfonylureas

Organ or System	Effects
Thyroid	Hypothyroidism
Skin	Photosensitivity
Eyes	Corneal opacity
Blood	Blood dyscrasias Fibrinolytic activity
Kidney	Hyponatremia Water retention
Liver	Jaundice Enzyme inhibition
Cardiovascular	Microgranulomata Inotropic effect Increased oxygen need Elevated blood pressure
Brain	Alters the EEG in epilepsy
Stomach	Stimulates acid secretion

0.5 g is usually given in the morning. In addition to side effects similar to those reported with tolbutamide, cholestatic jaundice and purpura can develop. Side effects, especially hypoglycemia, increase when a dose of 0.5 g per day is exceeded. Chlorpropamide potentiates the action of antidiuretic hormone. A syndrome consisting of water retention, dilutional hyponatremia, and mental confusion occurs in some diabetic patients given this drug.

Acetohexamide is said to have effects intermediate between tolbutamide and chlorpropamide. The recommended dose is 0.25 to 0.5 g daily. Its degradation product, an acetylated compound, is also biologically active, and troublesome hypoglycemia can therefore result.

Tolazamide has an onset of action between 4 and 6 hours, and peak blood levels occur within 4 to 8 hours after oral administration. A single daily dose of 0.25 g is recommended. Some of the metabolic products have hypoglycemic effects but are less potent than the parent compound.

Hypoglycemia is not commonly seen in sulfonylurea-treated patients but may be a hazard in the elderly diabetic or in newborn infants of diabetic mothers ingesting these agents during the last trimester of pregnancy. Patients with restricted food intake, hepatic disease, or renal disease are also more prone to develop hypoglycemia while receiving sulfonylureas. Furthermore, the effect of these compounds may be prolonged or augmented when given simultaneously with drugs such as sulfisoxazole, bishydroxycouma-rin, phenylbutazone, alcohol, salicylate, and monoamine oxidase inhibitor.[148]

Insulin Therapy

Important characteristics of commonly used insulin preparations are given in Table 71-9. Preparations of insulin now available are 98 to 99 percent pure. "Monocomponent insulin" is even more highly purified. All patients in need of insulin for the first time should be started on the U100 preparation so that the simple decimal calibration can be used in teaching. Patients on insulins of other strength should be transferred to U100.

Patients poorly controlled on diet, or on diet and OHA, may be started on insulin without hospitalization. A small dose of insulin is used (e.g., 10 U NPH) at the start while patients are learning injection techniques and later raised to obtain control.[99] Newly discovered diabetics with rapid onset of acute symptoms, particularly those in childhood, adolescence, or early adulthood should be hospitalized for optimal care. After the patient has been treated for acute insulin deficiency and placed on a diet, steps must be taken to establish the insulin dosage appropriate for ambulatory care. Utilization of four urine collection periods over the day can provide estimates of urinary glucose loss. These estimates can be useful in calculating the amount of regular insulin to be given initially and serve as further guides to therapy (Table 71-10). As a rule of thumb, the amount of intermediate insulin to give initially is equal to three-quarters of the regular insulin used on the previous day. The intermediate insulin can be increased daily until excess glycosuria is controlled, usually by the third or fourth day of treatment. Plasma glucose values taken fasting and 3 hours after each of the regular meals are valuable to determine the need for adjustment in insulin dosage. If the total daily insulin dosage is less than 60 units, control can usually be achieved by giving two-thirds to three-quarters as intermediate insulin and the remainder as regular insulin, in a single injection. Above 60 units, twice-daily injections are recommended. Hospitalization should not be prolonged for the purpose of perfect regulation. An additional safeguard against hypoglycemia on returning home, particularly if the patient has been closely controlled while in hospital, is either to increase the diet or to decrease the insulin by 10 percent to balance the effect of increased activity.

A small group of "brittle" diabetics requiring 25 units of insulin daily or less show exquisite delicacy in their insulin requirements and swing from hypoglycemia to severe ketonemia or ketoacidosis in short periods, with trivial changes in insulin dosage or ex-

TABLE 71-9
Onset and Duration of Effects of Various Insulins

Onset	Nomenclature	Remarks
Early	Crystalline zinc insulin (CZl, regular crystalline, soluble) Maximal effect: 4–6 hours Duration: 6–8 hours	Compatible with all other insulins in mixture Used as supplement to other insulins, in acute illness, in examples of insulin resistance
	Semi-lente Maximal effect: 4–6 hours Duration: 12–16 hours	Action similar to CZl but duration is slightly longer Compatible with other members of lente family Not used intravenously
Intermediate	Neutral protamine (Isophane, NPH) Maximal effect: 8–12 hours Duration: 18–24 hours	Most commonly used insulin for daytime needs May cause hypoglycemia in late afternoon, if taken in morning
	Globin Maximal effect: 6–10 hours Duration: 12–18 hours	Duration of action may be shorter than others in this group
	Lente Mixture of 3 semi-lente and 7 ultra-lente Maximal effect: 8–12 hours Duration: 18–24 hours	Quite similar to NPH Mixes with others of lente family Produces maximum effect in late afternoon, if taken in morning
Delayed	Protamine zinc (PZl) Maximal effect: 16–18 hours Duration: 24 hours or longer	Termination of action difficult to time Action of CZl delayed when mixed with this preparation (May lead to early morning hypoglycemia)
	Ultra lente Maximal effect: 16–18 hours Duration: 30 hours or longer	Maximum action and duration of action similar to PZl

ercise. Short-acting insulin usually makes control of these patients more difficult. Careful control of diet, physical exercise, and optimal insulin therapy using several small injections of an intermediate preparation daily are often successful.

COMPLICATIONS OF INSULIN THERAPY. Hypoglycemia is more commonly a risk of insulin therapy than of OHA, but the seriousness of this problem with long-acting sulfonylureas is more likely to be misinterpreted or overlooked. Patients taking either of these medications must know not only how to recognize hypoglycemia but also how it is prevented and treated. They should be cautioned about the effects of

TABLE 71-10
Stabilization of Insulin-Requiring Diabetic Patient in Hospital

1. Start patient on an appropriate diet. Arrange for 4 daily urine collections, 6:00 A.M. to 11:00 A.M.; 11:00 A.M. to 4:00 P.M.; 4:00 P.M. to 9:00 P.M.; 9:00 P.M. to 6:00 A.M.

2. Test entire fractional specimen with Clinitest. Multiply glucose (in g/dl) by urine volume (in dl) for a semiquantitative estimate of glucose loss

3. Give regular insulin four times daily, the dose being determined by urinalysis, beginning with 3 units soluble insulin per g of glucose voided

4. If improvement is not obtained, increase insulin schedule to 4 or 5 units per g of glucose voided

5. Continue this process until moderate control is achieved, i.e., total daily glucosuria less than 5 g

6. Now change to an intermediate acting preparation. Use 75% of the previous day's total insulin dose and continue supplementation with regular insulin as before. Increase the intermediate insulin daily by ½ to ⅓ of the units of regular insulin used the day before

7. If regular insulin requirements exceed 80 units daily, divide the intermediate insulin, giving ⅔ before breakfast and ⅓ at night

8. Encourage early ambulation and activity

9. Modify insulin dosage to achieve control without hypoglycemia. After getting maximal control with intermediate insulin, it may be necessary to add short-acting insulin or long-acting insulin to cover hyperglycemia and glycosuria occurring at times of maximal effects of the respective insulin preparations

10. Final control will only be established after discharge. Do not prolong hospitalization unnecessarily for the purpose of final regulation

unusual exercise and the use of common drugs such as aspirin, phenylbutazone, or propranolol, which enhance or mask hypoglycemic symptoms.

The symptoms of hypoglycemia (Chap. 72) are likely to occur in one of two forms: 1) adrenergic symptoms with sweating, tachycardia, and a constellation of sensations including hunger, irritability, headache, apprehension, and nervousness; and 2) central nervous system symptoms including lack of concentration, progressing through unawareness of the surroundings to coma. Repeated episodes of hypoglycemia may lead to a diagnosis of "brittle diabetes," but care should be taken to recheck the fundamentals of therapy, consider abuse of insulin, and rule out some other condition that may have decreased insulin need.[131] All patients should understand that atypical symptoms should be presumed to be due to hypoglycemia and treated appropriately especially whenever failure to do so could be life-threatening (e.g., while shopping alone or driving). Ready supplies of syrup, sweetened juice, or candy should be available in office and automobile as well as at home. In some instances the physician will wish to instruct the patient on the use of glucagon and to have this available in the home for administration by another person, though not needed unless the patient will not respond to oral command and cannot take sugar. Patients who do not respond immediately to oral treatment for hypoglycemia must be treated with intravenous glucose and admitted to hospital if it is suspected that the period of hypoglycemia has been long and brain damage or vascular events may have occurred.

Many diabetic patients have brief episodes of asymptomatic hypoglycemia yet have physiologic responses to the low blood glucose. These include secretion of glucocorticoids, glucagon, catecholamines, and growth hormone. The net effect of the secretion of these hormones may be to elevate blood glucose markedly. This phenomenon of hypoglycemia-induced hyperglycemia ("Somogyi effect") should be strongly considered in the following conditions:[92]

1. Asymptomatic periods with urine free of sugar and acetone followed within a few hours by marked glycosuria and ketonuria
2. Wide swings of plasma glucose levels, unrelated to meals, over short periods
3. Significant glycosuria or hyperglycemia early in the day with morning hypothermia, nocturnal sweating, and headaches
4. Significant ketonuria without glycosuria
5. Increased insulin requirements for unexplained reasons

The unwary physician who sees the patient at the time of hyperglycemia and glycosuria may inadvisedly administer more insulin. Correct diagnosis of this syndrome often requires a diligent search for short periods of hypoglycemia, using plasma and urine glucose determinations at night and in the early morning hours. Treatment consists of reducing the daily insulin dosage until hypoglycemia no longer occurs. This may be necessary, even when hypoglycemia is suspected but not documented.

UNUSUAL DEGREES OF INSULIN RESISTANCE. Insulin resistance is not always triggered by a specific event but often develops without a known antecedent factor. Typically, such patients, admitted in ketoacidosis, are successfully treated and discharged in a few days only to be readmitted within a brief period, again in ketoacidosis without known cause. It is then evident that a much larger amount of insulin than the "maintenance dose" is needed. Insulin resistance has been arbitrarily defined as a daily insulin requirement of 200 units or more for 2 consecutive days without discernible cause; however, it is clear that insulin needs of the diabetic population form a continuous curve.

Insulin resistance can be divided into two classes according to the presence or absence of immune mechanisms. Among the nonimmune causes, one must mention technical problems of injection (especially the injection of insulin into scar tissue), cryptic endocrinopathies including excess adrenal steroids, thyroid hormone and growth hormone, and emotional stress. Absence of receptor sites is now offered as an explanation for insulin resistance in some patients. The group of patients with acanthosis nigricans, seen in young females with virilization and growth problems, is an example.[109]

The immune causes of insulin resistance include antibodies to receptors and insulin-binding antibodies. Patients with acanthosis nigricans associated with arthralgias, hypergammaglobulinemia, anti-DNA antibodies in the serum, and decreased serum complement levels have receptor antibodies. Insulin resistance due to insulin binding antibodies can develop in species injected with homologous insulins.[124] This suggests 1) that the isolation and crystallization of insulin may create or expose antigenic sites not found in endogenous insulin; and 2) that insulin antibodies will be formed in treated patients despite use of highly refined products or even human insulin. Not all cases of resistance have been satisfactorily classified into one of these major categories. The cause of insulin resistance in infection is still unknown, and although most evidence points to the loss of receptor sites as a cause for resistance in obesity, some question has been raised as to whether this is the sole explanation.[125]

In the face of insulin resistance, the goal of treatment is clearly to supply sufficient insulin to permit glucose uptake by cells. In some instances, this is difficult to accomplish and may require as much as 26 units of insulin per hour intravenously for as long as 5 days. On occasion, intramuscular injections of 50 to 100 units of regular insulin three to four times daily has provided adequate control for the patient outside the hospital. Sulfated pork insulin or soluble fish insulin also hold promise but are not yet readily available.[100] Steroid therapy has been advocated in patients known to have immunologic causes for resistance, either to decrease antibody production or to decrease the binding of insulin by antibodies.[161] This should be considered only when simple methods are not feasible, since it may create new problems and only postpone the problem of resistance to be solved when steroids are discontinued. Immunosuppressants have been advocated, but have not been shown to be practical.

Episodes of "insulin resistance" alternating with "insulin sensitivity" suggest either factitious manipulation of the insulin therapy or paradoxic hyperglycemia following insulin reaction, as described earlier. The latter invariably calls for reduction of the insulin and a new therapeutic program. If the motivation of the patient is in doubt or if malingering is suspected, psychiatric intervention should be considered.

OTHER REACTIONS TO INSULIN. Local reactions to insulin, probably related to IgE antibodies, usually disappear with continued use of insulin as a result of desensitization. Infrequently, insulin allergy may present as an urticarial reaction requiring immediate treatment with antihistamines. Anaphylactic shock has been recorded rarely, but requires very careful desensitization of the insulin-requiring patient.

Local changes in adipose tissue following use of impure insulins may be related to an allergic reaction. Lipoatrophy, the most common change, gives a hollowed-out appearance that may be misinterpreted as muscle atrophy. This occurs most frequently in children and young women, and may be almost completely reversed by injections of highly purified insulin into the atrophic site. A localized hypertrophy of adipose tissue at the site of insulin injection is commonly seen in young males. The skin overlying this "tumor" becomes relatively insensitive to pain, encouraging repeated injections into the same site. Since insulin absorption tends to be irregular from such areas, rotation to other sites for injection is recommended.

A rare and less well understood effect of insulin is "insulin edema." Classically, it occurs as hyperglycemia is brought rapidly under control; it may be characterized not only by generalized edema but also by ascites and blurred vision. It is usually corrected spontaneously by fluid restriction for a few days. Edema following the use of OHA is not well documented. Until this problem is better understood and particularly in view of the possible effects of OHA on water retention, the term "insulin edema" should be reserved for that state for which no other explanation is yet available.

DIABETIC COMA

The term "coma" is used in decompensated diabetes to describe the state of awareness often more correctly characterized as apathetic, somnolent, or perhaps stuporous. True coma with failure to respond to all stimuli is uncommon, with the possible exception of that related to hypoglycemia. Diabetic patients may, of course, present with any of the other nonmetabolic causes of coma which can be recalled by utilizing the memonics AEIOU and TIPS (Chap. 147). Only the types of coma that are diabetes related will be dealt with here. In the differential diagnosis of an altered state of consciousness specifically related to diabetes, there are four main conditions: 1) hypoglycemia, 2) diabetic ketoacidosis, 3) lactic acidosis, 4) hyperosmolality (Fig. 71–3).

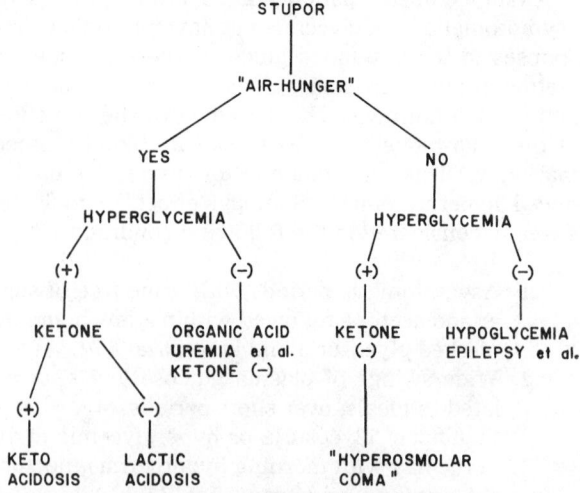

FIGURE 71–3. A schematic representation of the differential diagnostic steps in diabetic patients in "coma."

There should be no confusion between the two conditions which account for over 95 percent of metabolic coma in patients with diabetes, hypoglycemia and ketoacidosis. Patients with hypoglycemia may indeed be deeply comatose, but they exhibit none of the dehydration and neglect of patients with ketoacidosis. As noted previously, prompt response to IV glucose is expected in uncomplicated hypoglycemia. Patients who have been comatose for several hours may not respond promptly, and a complete examination should be done as soon as possible to exclude other causes of coma. Elderly patients suffering from hypoglycemia associated with oral hypoglycemic agents must be monitored for several days so that hypoglycemia does not recur.

Having disposed of the cause of coma that is easiest to diagnose and treat, one must proceed in stepwise fashion to differentiate between ketoacidosis, lactic acidosis, and hyperosmolality (Fig. 71-3). The first clinical fact of differential importance is the state of respiration. One should learn quickly to differentiate between the deep breathing associated with acidosis (Kussmaul breathing, or air hunger) and simple tachypnea. Air hunger implies uncompensated metabolic acidosis. Patients with elevated blood glucose and strong ketonemia are presumed to have ketoacidosis. Occasionally, a patient with a very low bicarbonate does not show acidotic breathing because of compensated pH.

A spot test for ketonemia utilizing nitroprusside powder or tablet should be available in every Emergency Room. In a 1:1 solution of plasma in normal saline (½ dilution), about 0.5 mM of acetoacetate is required to register a purple color on a crushed nitroprusside tablet. The positive test implies a total ketone of about 4.0 mM/L since the ratio of acetoacetate to 3-hydroxybutyrate (which does not cause a color change) is about 1:3 in uncomplicated ketoacidosis. Further serial dilutions (of 1:2, 1:4, etc.) can be used to estimate the total ketones. Since bicarbonate is displaced by ketones in equimolar amounts, this can be a rough measure of the total anion gap.

Air hunger or a large anion gap without significant ketonemia indicates the presence of other organic acids. Although lactic acidosis is likely under these circumstances, this diagnosis is made by exclusion since plasma lactate usually cannot be determined on an emergency basis. The commonest organic acids other than lactic acid to be considered include salicylates, methanol, ethylene glycol, and chloral hydrate. A small amount of organic acid associated with prerenal azotemia is common in ketoacidosis and must be differentiated from the metabolic acidosis of uremia. Patients without air hunger but with a high blood glucose and stupor most likely have hyperosmolality as the cause of their altered state of consciousness.

Diabetic Ketoacidosis (DKA)[89,108]

Ketoacidosis stems from an absolute insulin lack combined with elevated levels of growth hormone, glucagon, cortisol, and catecholamines, and comprises a series of biochemical derangements. The disturbances in normal physiology include hyperglycemia, excessive FFA release from adipose tissue, hypergluconeogenesis, and escape of amino acids and potassium from cells. The clinical picture reflects loss of water, sodium, and potassium with hydrogen-ion accumulation.

Normally, free fatty acids released from adipose tissue are degraded to acetate in the liver. In the absence of insulin, resynthesis of long-chain fatty acids is impaired, and the intermediates of fatty acids are converted to strongly acidic, four-carbon ketones, which exist as cationic salts at the physiologic pH range and displace bicarbonate on an equimolar basis.

With increasing serum concentrations of ketones, the amount filtered at the glomerulus increases. The ketone bodies, being strong acids, are excreted as sodium and potassium salts in the urine. Because of osmotic diuresis, hypovolemia and prerenal azotemia develop. The elevated plasma hydrogen-ion concentration is a potent stimulus for respiration. Hyperventilation lowers arterial P_{CO_2}, but does not decrease total body hydrogen-ion content.

The nonavailability of insulin also causes potassium loss from skeletal muscles into the blood. Before the glomerular filtration rate decreases, the kidney eliminates potassium and the sodium-potassium concentration in the plasma generally remains normal, but the patient is in negative potassium balance at the expense of muscle potassium. With dehydration and a decrease in GFR, hyperkalemia results.

CLINICAL PRESENTATION. Patients seen with ketoacidosis mainly complain of extreme thirst, weakness, fatigue, and air hunger; abdominal pain, nausea, and vomiting are also common. Examination shows signs of dehydration. The breath has a characteristic "Juicy Fruit" odor, and the patient is drowsy and inattentive or, rarely, comatose. The skin may be warm, but the body temperature is often subnormal, and an elevated temperature suggests an infection that may have precipitated decompensation. The patient has deep respirations accomplished entirely through the open mouth with marked drying of the mucous membranes. The eye globe feels soft, and opacities in the crystalline lens caused by capsular folding give an appearance of wavy lines. The pulse is rapid and weak, and arterial hypotension is present especially with upright posture. Hepatomegaly resulting from fatty infiltration may be present, particularly after long periods of poorly controlled diabetes. The liver capsule may be distended, accounting for the frequently encountered abdominal pain.

In patients with low renal blood flow, urinary findings may be misleading, but usually glycosuria, ketonuria, and a high specific gravity are present. Dehydration is further evidenced by an elevated hematocrit, SUN, and serum protein concentration, and there is a low plasma pH and bicarbonate (less than 10 mM/L). Leukocytosis up to 20,000/μl is not unusual. The serum potassium is usually normal but may be elevated despite depletion of body potassium, and the serum sodium may be normal or elevated depending upon the relative losses of sodium and water and the degree of plasma lipid increase. With an increase in plasma lipids, a sodium concentration expressed by the laboratory as 150 mEq/L may represent 170 mEq/L of plasma water. This mechanism may cause a similar error in the measurement of other plasma solutes. Plasma uric acid is frequently increased as the result of a decreased urate excretion. In severe diabetic ketoacidosis, the mean deficits of water, sodium, and potassium are 6 liters, 500 mEq, and 160 mEq, respectively.

TREATMENT. Diabetic ketoacidosis is a medical emergency. Treatment must be started promptly, as outlined in Table 71–11. The first steps are to administer insulin and to correct water and sodium deficits. As soon as the diagnosis of DKA is established, the patient should receive a bolus intravenous injection of 12 to 20 units of regular insulin followed by continuous intravenous infusion delivering about 0.1 unit of insulin per kilogram per hour. As the blood glucose returns to normal or below 250 mg/dl, 5 percent dextrose in water is begun. The insulin infusion is continued at least until the ketones are no longer detectable in serum or until the serum bicarbonate and pH are again normal. Equally good results may be obtained with intramuscular injections of 5 to 10 units of insulin at intervals of 30 to 60 minutes.[84] In using the low dose insulin regimen as outlined above, the physician in charge must make certain that an insulin effect has been seen within the first 2 to 4 hours, i.e., a fall in glucose to one-half of its admission value, or to a level below 250 mg/dl. In this way, the occasional instance of insulin resistance can be recognized.

TABLE 71–11

Management of Diabetic Ketoacidosis

1. Into a suitable vein, insert a venous catheter capable of taking a 20-gauge needle

2. Draw blood for initial plasma glucose and urea nitrogen, and for plasma bicarbonate, potassium, sodium, chloride, and protein determinations; run bedside tests for glucose and acetoacetate; measure hematocrit; record ECG

3. Commence intravenous therapy with 75 mM sodium chloride running the solution at 10–15 ml per minute. Do not delay therapy in order to prepare special solutions. Normal saline is administered if shock is present

4. Administer insulin intravenously, 10–20 U by bolus injection and 0.1 U/kg/hour by constant infusion of in normal saline thereafter

5. Keep a log of the state of consciousness, reflexes, level of hydration, fluid intake, and output. Monitor hematocrit, venous pressure, urine, plasma glucose, and ketones

6. Ensure that urine can be checked regularly. Catheterize if the patient is unable to void

7. With second liter of fluid, change to 155 mM sodium chloride. Alternate this with 75 mM sodium chloride. If the carbon-dioxide-combining power is below 8 mEq/L, add sodium bicarbonate to the intravenous therapy (1 ampule = 44.6 mEq/50 ml). Repeat if indicated

8. Maintain blood pressure; use supportive measures if necessary

9. Insert a stomach tube and aspirate contents. Occasionally acute dilatation of the stomach contributes to shock

10. Search for intercurrent infection and other causes for ketoacidosis

11. Monitor ECG regularly. Look for change from hyperkalemia to hypokalemia pattern. With evidence of hypokalemia with the third bottle of fluid, administer potassium dihydrogen phosphate at rate of 15–20 mEq/hour if urine flow is adequate. Total potassium by the intravenous route should not usually exceed 100 mEq

12. Check urine at 60-minute intervals when glucosuria drops to 1% or plasma glucose is below 250 mg/dl by Dextrostix

13. To avoid relapse, continue careful surveillance until the patient is fully conscious and ready for oral liquids

14. Proceed with hospital regulation (Table 71–10)

HYDRATION AND ELECTROLYTE REPLACEMENT.
Water losses exceed sodium losses and for this reason hypotonic saline should be employed. An intravenous solution containing 75 mEq/L of sodium chloride is satisfactory. The most severely affected patients with diabetic acidosis rarely exhibit deficits exceeding 500 mEq requiring replacement. The hematocrit and venous pressure should be repeatedly monitored. A steadily rising venous pressure dictates a reduction in the infusion rate in order to prevent pulmonary edema. If hypotension is present, normal saline should be administered intravenously, but plasma or whole blood may be required to correct shock. Occasionally shock is associated with gastric dilatation, which may be dramatically relieved by nasogastric suction. Gastric suction should be performed routinely if nausea is present to obviate the danger of gastric content aspiration.

In patients with normal renal function, therapy with sodium bicarbonate is usually not necessary for the correction of acidosis since the kidneys can retain sodium when sodium chloride is administered. In severe cases of diabetic acidosis, however, the stimulus to conserve sodium is so great that chloride is also retained, and significant hyperchloremia may be found following correction of the acidosis. For this reason the sodium can be given as a chloride-bicarbonate mixture to restore the sodium/chloride ratio in the patient's blood, but excessively vigorous treatment with intravenous sodium bicarbonate to the point of metabolic alkalosis may be deleterious to the patient.[140] The cerebrospinal pH is normal in diabetic acidosis but becomes acidotic following rapid reversal of serum pH because of translocation of CO_2 but not bicarbonate into the CSF. Confusion and disorientation on this basis have been observed with bicarbonate administration. The dangers of bicarbonate therapy should, however, not be exaggerated.[86]

The physician should appraise the clinical picture every 30 minutes. Table 71–11 provides a useful guide for intravenous therapy. After several hours of insulin therapy, the dangers of hypoglycemia and hypokalemia become prominent. Hypoglycemia can be avoided by instituting the intravenous administration of 5 percent glucose when plasma glucose drops below 250 mg/dl or when the concentration of glucose in the urine drops to 1 percent or less. Although the total body potassium deficit in diabetic acidosis may exceed several hundred mEq, early correction is not necessary unless ECG evidence of hypokalemia is present initially. At the outset of treatment, the plasma potassium concentration is usually normal (or high), and potassium administration at this stage is

hazardous. However, the diabetic in whom control has been chronically inadequate, with a low degree of acidosis present for several days or weeks, or who has some other reason for potassium loss (e.g., chronic diarrhea or diuretic use) is very likely to need potassium supplementation early in therapy. In such patients, hypokalemia may be present initially or may appear within the first hour of treatment. The ECG is a good bedside monitor for hypokalemia, and if there are ECG signs of low serum potassium the intravenous administration of potassium should be started at a rate of 15 to 20 mEq per hour. With the administration of insulin, potassium moves into cells, and hypokalemia may develop abruptly with tingling, paresthesias, decreased tendon jerks, or depression of respiratory muscles. Even in the absence of these signs, it is advisable to commence potassium repletion in the second or third hour of therapy provided urinary output is adequate. In contrast to sodium replacement, it is not necessary to attempt complete replacement of potassium parenterally. Total body phosphates are also depleted in this condition, and both hypokalemia and hypophosphatemia may be treated or prevented by potassium dihydrogen phosphate with each liter of fluid.

As soon as the patient's level of conciousness is adequate and if nausea is not a problem, oral intake of fluids may be commenced. The urinary catheter, if used at all, should be removed as soon as the patient is able to void. Patients who do not appear to be responding adequately to this regimen should be examined carefully for some complicating illness such as pneumonia, meningitis, or other infections. Urinary tract infections, upper respiratory infections, sinusitis, and otitis media are all common in diabetics and may easily be overlooked in the initial haste to begin therapy for uncontrolled diabetes.

Following recovery, a diet calculated on the basal caloric need and monitored physical activity is ordered, and instruction in personal management is started. Over the next few days while the new diabetic is learning about diabetes, urine testing, and fundamentals of diet, the dosage of insulin designed to allow mild glycosuria is worked out as previously described (Table 71–10). Patients who are well regulated on insulin before this event may be returned to their previous dosage if no obvious reasons exist to make this untenable.

The mortality from diabetic ketoacidosis is still 1 to 6 percent. In a review of severe diabetic ketoacidosis,[89] there were 32 deaths in 482 episodes. The death rate was highest in the older patients and those who had the highest serum glucose, SUN, and osmolality.

TABLE 71–12
Mortality in Diabetic Ketoacidosis

Cause	Contributing Factors
Hypovolemic shock	Inadequate fluid replacement Rapid fall in blood glucose Silent myocardial infarction
Cardiac arrhythmia	Hypokalemia—late recognition Silent myocardial infarction
Aspiration	Gastric dilatation
Cerebral edema	Aggressive bicarbonate therapy
Hypoglycemia	Delayed glucose addition
Sepsis	Underlying infection

Patients with infection and myocardial infarction in addition had an especially poor prognosis. Death in diabetic acidosis that occurs after therapy has begun calls attention to the potential iatrogenic factors in this mortality. Diabetic ketoacidosis is still accompanied by significant and often needless mortality. Table 71–12 lists the causes of fatal outcome.

Lactic Acidosis[120]

Lactic acidosis in the diabetic must be attributed to a failure to the redox system whereby excess NADH (reduced nicotinamide adenine dinucleotide) over NAD favors lactate production. This excess can be caused, for example, by ethanol ingestion. The reaction also favors the production of excess lactate when production of pyruvate is increased, as for example, with exercise, glucose administration, or excess of catecholamines.

Experimental evidence indicates that excess lactate production is not caused by uncompensated diabetes or decrease in insulin levels alone and that both resting blood lactate concentration and oral lactate tolerance tests are normal in diabetic patients. Many instances of lactic acidosis are due to shock or to some other cause of tissue anoxia. Phenformin, a biguanide no longer available for routine prescription in the United States, caused lactic acidosis, but since withdrawal of this agent, lactic acidosis is rare.[116]

The clinical presentation of lactic acidosis in the diabetic closely resembles that of severe ketoacidosis. Air hunger without ketonemia, a large anion gap, and a plasma bicarbonate below 10 mM suggest lactic acidosis. The diagnosis is confirmed by demonstration of elevated blood lactate. Blood lactate expressed in mg/dl must be divided by a factor of 9 to convert to mEq/L, to determine whether the lactate level accounts for the anion gap. Normal lactate levels of 1 to 2 mEq/L may be raised to 5 mEq/L without significant shift in the plasma bicarbonate.

Therapy of diabetic lactic acidosis has been at the best only partly successful, with a high mortality rate. The basic therapeutic aims in lactic acidosis include the following:

1. Removal of the source(s) of lactate overproduction. In the case of shock, this is accomplished by maintaining an adequate cardiac output.
2. Correction of acidosis with alkalinizing solutions. The quantity of base necessary to correct the acidosis may be roughly calculated by multiplying the bicarbonate deficit in mEq/L by a factor of 50 percent of the total body weight in kg. Usually one-half of the calculated deficit is infused during the initial 3 to 4 hours of management. Since sodium is given concomitantly, rapid bicarbonate therapy may be complicated by pulmonary edema. In patients who cannot tolerate a sodium load, administration of another alkalinizing agent, THAM (trishydroxymethyl-amino-methanol), has been advocated. The danger of hypokalemia upon correction of acidosis must be recognized.
3. Removal of excess lactate. Mechanical removal of lactate from the body by means of hemodialysis is theoretically sound, but not uniformly successful.
4. The use of intravenous glucose and insulin to increase the turnover of normal metabolic pathways has been an effective mode of therapy. This could theoretically increase lactate production, but success may be related to the fact that pyruvate generated by the glycolytic pathway begins to flow preferentially through the tricarboxylic acid cycle. (Too long for a rare state and too long for treatment that does not work anyway, witness almost 100% fatality.)

The Hyperosmolar Syndrome[110]

The fundamental difference between this syndrome and ketoacidosis is the biochemical mechanism that leads to altered consciousness. Blood glucose may rise as high as 1000 to 2000 mg/dl, to contribute 55 to 110 mOsm, without ketogenesis or shift in serum pH. The hyperosmolar syndrome usually occurs in adult-onset diabetes. This disorder again illustrates that low insulin levels in patients with NIDD are sufficient to prevent lipolysis but not adequate to allow entrance of glucose into cells. Marked hyperglycemia leads to intense glycosuria, loss of plasma volume, and further increase in serum osmolality. Typically this occurs in the elderly who do not restore their depleted fluids normally and frequently have underlying renal disease. Precipitating events are usually not identified but acute infection, pancreatitis, or cerebrovascular events may be associated. Drugs, including diuretics, phenytoins, and propranolol, may play a role. Physical findings, in addition to dehydration, relate to the precipitating cause. Hypotension and deep stupor are consistent features. Laboratory abnormalities are those of hemoconcentration, with leukocytosis, but a normal bicarbonate. Approximate serum osmolality can be calculated from the formula:

$$Posm\ (mOsm/KgH_2O) = 2 \times Na(mEq/L) + \frac{glucose\ (mg/dl)}{18}$$

The principal therapy must be restoration of fluid volume since hypovolemic shock is the immediate threat to life. Insulin administration may be given by the same method used for ketoacidosis with similar monitoring to avoid hypoglycemia and hypokalemia.[98] Plasma osmolality should be lowered slowly after reaching a level of about 320 mOsm/L, to prevent cellular overhydration and especially cerebral edema. Restoration of fluid volume must be monitored by venous pressure in view of the frequently precarious cardiovascular status of the patients.

LATE COMPLICATIONS OF DIABETES MELLITUS

The late complications of diabetes are related to both large and small vessel disease. The atherosclerosis of diabetics is qualitatively not different from that of nondiabetics. Small vessel disease is, however, nearly unique to diabetes; it is characterized by accumulation of PAS-stainable material in vessel walls, to endothelial proliferations, and to basement membrane thickening.

The renal glomerular basement membrane contains hydroxylysine-linked disaccharide units containing glucose, the synthesis of which is dependent on an enzyme, glycosyltransferase.[152] The level of this enzyme reflects the quantity of basement membrane synthesized. Diabetic animals have significant elevations of glycosyltransferase, the activity of which can be restored to normal with early insulin treatment. Studies of human glomerular basement membranes have shown increases in hydroxylysine and disaccharides.

Sorbitol, the alcohol of glucose formed by the catalytic action of aldose reductase and an immediate precursor of fructose, may play a role in the development of cataracts and the neuropathy in diabetes.[111] Once synthesized within cells, sorbitol and fructose penetrate cell membranes poorly and, thus trapped within the cell, act as an osmotic force to draw water into the cell. During incubation of the rabbit lens in a high-glucose medium, the sorbitol and water content increases linearly with time and the lens becomes leaky to sodium influx and potassium efflux. When the sodium-potassium pump can no longer compensate for the difference in tonicity between intralenticular and ambient fluids, sodium concentration increases in the lens with further swelling, lens disruption, and development of cataracts. In vitro cataract formation is prevented by incubating lenses with an inhibitor of aldose reductase. Orally administered inhibitors of aldose reductase, furthermore, delay the appearance of cataracts in rats fed high galactose diets.[112] Significantly, the sorbitol pathway becomes operative only at high plasma glucose concentrations. Observations relating sorbitol metabolism to abnormalities have been made also in peripheral nerves. Nerves of diabetic rats have increased concentrations of glucose, sorbitol, and fructose, and decreased conduction velocities, presumably due to increase in water content of nerve. These changes can be reversed by insulin treatment.[94,111]

The role of the glycosylation of proteins in the late complications of diabetes is not fully elucidated. Glycosylation of hemoglobin in hyperglycemia to form Hb A1c is a nonenzymatic process.[118] To what extent similar glycosylation occurs in other proteins, e.g., basement membrane collagen, is not clear.

Plasma viscosity is abnormal in patients with diabetes mellitus and increases with poor control.[128] High plasma viscosity may alter the pliability of red cells making them less capable of passing through capillaries. Occlusion of capillaries in the retina leads to nonperfusion of retinal tissue and sets up a stimulus for neovascularization.

Coronary Artery Disease

The prevalence of coronary artery disease in the diabetic of 10 or more years' duration is about twice that of the nondiabetic. Thus, cardiovascular disease is the commonest cause of death in the middle-aged non-insulin-dependent diabetic. The higher risk of coronary artery disease in males disappears when males and diabetic postmenopausal females are compared. Coronary artery disease causes symptoms at an earlier age and progresses more rapidly in the diabetic population. Obesity and elevated cholesterol accompanying diabetes do not emerge as additional risk factors, however.[137]

Two points concerning the clinical manifestations of coronary artery disease in the diabetic should be emphasized: 1) myocardial ischemia may be less symptomatic in diabetes; and 2) diabetic patients with myocardial infarction have a greater incidence of heart failure and higher mortality rates than do nondiabetics.[136] This increase in the frequency of coronary death may be related to endothelial proliferation in the small vessels of the myocardium in diabetics.[123]

Diabetic Cardiomyopathy

Although the basis of heart disease in diabetics has been presumed to be related to coronary artery disease, primary heart muscle abnormalities may also be present. In diabetic animals, glycoproteins are deposited with a decrease in diastolic compliance.[145] In human diabetics who develop cardiac decompensation in the absence of another specific cause, autopsy may reveal interstitial accumulation of collagen and glycoprotein similar to that observed in diabetic animals.

Peripheral Vascular Disease[161]

The most important clinical manifestations of peripheral vascular disease involve the feet and lower limbs. In the adult-onset diabetic, up to 15 percent have evidence of arterial vascular disease with calcification at the time the diagnosis of diabetes is made.[157] As in coronary artery disease, peripheral vascular disease also occurs at a younger age, but the Mönckeberg type of atherosclerosis is most common and leads eventually to medial calcification in approximately 80 to 85 percent of patients with IDD for 20 or more years. Amputation accounts for 50 percent of operations in the diabetic population. Although it has been shown that gangrene is now rarely the cause of death in diabetic patients, the presence of severe peripheral vascular disease with amputation delineates a population only 36 percent of which will be alive in 5 years.

The care of the lower limbs in patients with diabetes must include recognition of the combination of neuropathy and infection as well as vascular insufficiency.[122] Ischemia is more easily accepted than neuropathy in the pathogenesis of foot lesions, but neuropathy is equally important. In the latter, the change in weight bearing due to muscle atrophy and failure of sensation combine to increase the likelihood of painless trauma, ulceration, infection, gangrene, and ultimate amputation.

Simple but vigorous lower limb hygiene is vital for the diabetic. The feet should be inspected daily, washed in tepid water, carefully dried, and massaged with lanolin. Fungus infection will usually respond to the application of a fungicide. Proper care of the nails requires careful pedicure with sharp scissors utilizing a straight line cut for all toenails in order to avoid ingrowth. Deformities (ingrown nails, bunions) must be diligently dealt with by orthopedists, podiatrists, or general surgeons with an interest in the care of the foot in cooperation with the primary care physician. Patients are advised against going barefoot and are required to wear well-fitted stockings and shoes that are adequate for support. Most major cities have facilities for the fitting of shoes molded to the weight-bearing surface. This is especially important in patients with partial amputations of the foot or toes and in all patients with uneven distribution of weight on the foot surface.

The use of vasodilators is disappointing in the care of patients with vascular insufficiency due to either large or small vessel disease. Some studies have demonstrated that circulation may be preferentially diverted to the lesser involved of the two extremities due to the fact that there is fixed circulation in the more involved side. On the other hand, Buerger's exercises may serve to increase peripheral circulation and be a useful therapeutic and preventive measure. Sympathectomy is rarely of help in ischemic problems from large vessel disease, but bypass grafts are successful for discrete areas of arterial disease associated with a relatively open vessel below the obstruction.

Every care should be given to the preservation of the foot if at all possible including long-term supportive care without weight bearing.[122] Few, if any, patients beyond 65 years of age are capable of mastering orthopedic appliances without prolonged personal care and supervision. There can be no justification for early amputation before it is clear that attempts to save the foot for weight-bearing have been unsuccessful.

Renal Disease

The major renal complications in the diabetic are glomerulosclerosis (nodular, diffuse, and exudative), pyelonephritis (acute, chronic, and fulminant), and renal artery arteriosclerosis and arteriolosclerosis.[90]

The prevalence of diabetic glomerulosclerosis is directly related to the duration of the disease. An abnormal mucopolysaccharide is deposited that penetrates the capillary endothelial cell. A laminated nodule results that increases in size, pushing capillaries ahead of it. There is an involvement of the basement membrane and epithelial cells, and the nodule becomes totally hyalinized. The lesion is often silent clinically. Less than 10 percent of the patients with the nodular lesion develop the nephrotic syndrome. No relation appears to exist between the severity of nodular glomerulosclerosis and clinical evidence of renal disfunction.

Diffuse glomerulosclerosis is a more sinister lesion. There is a thickening of capillary walls caused by the deposition of a mucopolysaccharide complex. The capillary lumen narrows and is eventually occluded. The clinical picture is defined by the following features: proteinuria, hypertension, nephrotic syndrome, or azotemia.

With the onset of renal disease there is often an amelioration of the glucose intolerance with a fall in insulin requirements.[101] The kidney plays an important role in degrading circulating insulin. In severe renal disease, insulin degradation is retarded which has the effect of increasing the potency of the given insulin dose. Contributory factors may include loss of insulin antibodies in the urine, decrease in food intake, and decreased renal gluconeogenesis.

The diabetic patient is prone to attacks of pyelonephritis. Care must be taken not to catheterize these patients unnecessarily and to have repeated follow-up for urinary tract infection in all patients. The appearance of leukocytes in urine sediment should suggest infection even in the absence of symptoms. Urinary tract infections are often resistant to therapy until the patient becomes aglucosuric. In necrotizing renal papillitis, ischemic necrosis of the renal papillae is secondary to severe pyelonephritis. The patient is severely ill, there is hematuria, and portions of the sloughed papillae can be detected in the urine. Intravenous therapy to correct shock and treatment with antibiotics are necessary to allay the progress of this fulminant disease.

Both chronic dialysis and transplantation for the end stage diabetic kidney are life saving.[117,144] Chronic dialysis may, however, accelerate atherosclerosis with intermittent episodes of increased retinopathy, peripheral ischemia, and gangrene resulting in patients ultimately dying of myocardial infarction, congestive failure, or stroke. It is likely that histologic changes associated with diabetes will eventually develop in the transplanted kidneys.

Eye Disease

Diabetic retinopathy is the most common cause of newly developed blindness in the 40- to 60-year age group, and second only to congenital defects in the age group 20 to 40 years. This complication and its treatment[102] are discussed in Chapter 154.

Neurologic Disease

Diabetic neuropathy[95] can be categorized according to the anatomic site of involvement:

1. Nerve roots producing a segmental neuropathy
2. Single cranial or spinal nerve causing a mononeuropathy
3. Ganglia causing derangements of autonomic function
4. Motor end plates causing a loss of muscle and referred to as amyotrophy
5. Peripheral nerves usually symmetric and called simply polyneuropathy (this is the most common site)

Nerve root or segmental neuropathy is uncommon. The lesion may be found as a result of the patient's complaint of loss of sensation in a limited area. On occasions segmental pain and burning suggesting herpes zoster without eruption will be manifest. No specific therapy is known.

Mononeuropathies, especially those affecting extraocular muscles, are common. They are usually self-limited and may last only 1 to 2 weeks. During this period diplopia must be treated by placing an opaque lens or patch over one eye. Similar mononeuropathies of the laryngeal nerve, facial nerve, or, occasionally, spinal nerves including the median or peritoneal have been described. These have been attributed to microinfarcts and are also self-limited.

Disturbances of autonomic function are longstanding if not permanent, and rarely respond to metabolic control. Impotence, a common complaint in diabetic males over 40 years, may be an exception to this generalization. This form of impotence is usually not helped by testosterone. In all instances of impotence, hidden depression relating to a difficult life situation should be considered.

Other autonomic changes include gustatory sweating, failure of pupillary response, loss of peripheral sweating especially in the lower limbs, nocturnal diarrhea, and postural hypotension. Loss of sweating may be documented by placing the patient in a warm room and doing a starch-iodine test. Nocturnal diarrhea will often respond to a short course of oral antibiotics, and postural hypotension may require either the use of support stockings or salt-retaining hormones such as fluorocortisone acetate in doses of 0.1 mg per day.

Diabetic neuropathy in some form probably affects most diabetics at some time. This may be in the form of pressure-induced neuropathies, distal blunting of sensory modalities, decrease or loss of peripheral reflex arcs, or repetitive short episodes of burning discomfort in the lower limbs, frequently at night. In 10 to 15 percent of the patients, polyneuropathy will be more severe. Pain may be of a deep, boring distress coming on at night and preventing sleep. Since this discomfort responds poorly to analgesics, narcotics should be avoided. Trial of phenytoin or carbamazepine is warranted, with due care in warning the patient against overdosage and side effects. In other patients peripheral neuropathy may be insidious, with virtually complete loss of all sensory perception, leading to unrecognized fractures and Charcot joints.

Treatment of the diabetic is undertaken with the tacit assumption that return of the plasma glucose to or toward normal will lessen or prevent complications. What methods are available for monitoring control of plasma glucose? Can close control be expected to reduce or prevent late complications of diabetes?

Long-term control can be monitored by measurement of hemoglobin A1c.[118] An irreversible bond between glucose and hemoglobin is formed by a nonenzymatic process through simple exposure. One product of this process is called A1c, being a derivative of normal adult hemoglobin, Hb A1. The concentration of Hb A1c is proportional to the duration and degree of hyperglycemia. Thus, hemoglobin A1c reflects adequacy of diabetes control.

Whether close control of blood glucose levels prevents late complications is debatable.[127,132,142] A study of adult-onset diabetes[158] could demonstrate no difference in the frequency of complications between a group treated with diet alone and one treated with insulin in quantities designed to normalize blood glucose. The results may not be applicable to patients with an earlier onset (mean age at which patients entered the study was 53 years) or those who are insulin-dependent. Furthermore, studies in some special groups suggest a relationship between hyperglycemia and complications. In the Pima Indians, complications were found only in patients whose blood glucose rose above 200 mg/dl after a standard glucose challenge.[103]

PREGNANCY AND DIABETES MELLITUS (Table 71-13)[130]

Pregnancy imposes a major stress on carbohydrate metabolism and, as a result, diabetes mellitus may then be detected for the first time. The changes in

---

TABLE 71-13
Principles of Diabetes Management: Pregnancy

1. Encourage the young diabetic to begin her family early, before vascular pathology becomes evident. With good control, the outcome of the pregnancy should not differ from that of the nondiabetic patient

2. Management of a diabetic patient during pregnancy requires continuous cooperation of patient, obstetrician, and internist

3. Hyperglycemia in the mother leads to fetal islet hyperplasia and hyperinsulinemia, causing excess fetal weight

4. Efforts should be made to maintain the postprandial plasma glucose in the range that occurs in nondiabetic pregnant women, i.e., 70 to 100 mg/dl and not above 120 mg/dl

5. Management is facilitated by multiple injections of insulin, usually AM and PM only, and by monitoring the blood glucose several times weekly until the patient is stabilized at the appropriate glucose level

6. Hospitalization with careful surveillance may be needed when control cannot be achieved on an outpatient basis. Leaves of absence between hospital and home before discharge may facilitate the transition without loss of control

7. Ketonemia should be avoided even in the obese pregnant female. Weight reduction should be accomplished before pregnancy

8. Under these circumstances pregnancy may be safely carried with appropriate monitoring to 38 weeks or longer and thereby lessen the pulmonary immaturity characteristic of the premature infant

9. Insulin is delayed after delivery until there is a demonstrated need as shown by an increased plasma glucose or significant glycosuria after restoring the caloric needs of the patient

10. Insulin requirements are frequently decreased during breast feeding. Patients should be encouraged to relax their previously rigorous control and avoid hypoglycemia as a result of their erratic work–sleep schedule during the postpartum period

---

carbohydrate metabolism during pregnancy are probably the summation of effects of several gestational hormones. Elevated levels of estrogen and glucocorticoids, in addition to the presence of placental lactogen and increased insulin degradation by the placenta, account for the rise in insulin requirements seen in the pregnant diabetic.

Diabetes increases the complications of pregnancy and may be associated with considerable fetal wastage. Toxemia and hydramnios are important complications if regulation of the diabetes is not achieved. A suitable diet for the pregnant patient should provide a weight gain of 24 pounds during a pregnancy. A caloric intake of no less than 30 calories per kg, containing 200 g of carbohydrate, 100 g of protein, and 40 to 50 g of fat, is recommended. Sodium restriction to 4 g per day and the use of thiazides are indicated only if toxemic signs of hypertension and pathologic edema appear.

Insulin therapy should be adjusted so that hyperglycemia is strictly avoided (Table 71–13). Every effort should be made to maintain the postprandial plasma glucose in the range that occurs in the nondiabetic pregnant woman. Hypoglycemia is avoided if possible, but emphasis has moved from tolerance of hyperglycemia a decade ago to the opposite extreme at the present time. Insulin requirements tend to be the same or lower than usual during the first trimester but increase markedly during the latter half of pregnancy. Infection, dehydration, and acidosis are uncommon but, if present, should be corrected promptly. The timing of delivery is the most critical decision to be made by the obstetrician. Fetal deaths occurring before the 35th week of gestation are associated with poorly controlled diabetes while those occurring later are usually due to errors in obstetric judgment. In general, the patient is allowed to reach the 35th week, and if metabolic control and fetal well-being are satisfactory, the pregnancy is continued on a day-to-day basis. Some interest in taking carefully controlled pregnancies to term is now emerging, but delivery at the 38th week remains the usual practice. At this time labor is induced, and if progress is not satisfactory at 6 hours, the baby is delivered by Caesarean section.

SURGERY AND DIABETES MELLITUS

The diabetic patient may have two conditions relevant to surgery that can trap the unwary. First, abdominal discomfort and leukocytosis are commonly seen in diabetic ketoacidosis. Elevation of the serum amylase is also not uncommon in this circumstance. Fortunately, the abdomen in such patients is usually soft except for epigastric or right upper quadrant guarding, and bowel sounds are present. Nasogastric

suction is indicated in any case, and gastric atony is commonly found.

Second, in older persons with longstanding diabetes, serious intra-abdominal events may be masked by diabetic neuropathy. Peritonitis, for example, may be present without obvious signs.

Experience with intravenous and intramuscular insulin[83,84] in the treatment of diabetic coma (as described earlier) has simplified the management of the diabetic at surgery. With frequent monitoring of blood glucose and an open intravenous line, any diabetic showing hyperglycemia as the only complication can be carried through surgery without difficulty.

With minor surgery or ambulatory procedures for which a patient may ordinarily be admitted for only one day, little change in insulin therapy is needed. Some caution should be exercised about unduly anxious patients, for unless they are given reassurance and sedation before surgery, a well controlled patient facing relatively minor surgery may develop significant hyperglycemia and ketonuria on the day of operation. Procedures should be done early in the day to prevent a mismatch between the usual insulin dosage and the calories for the day. Following minor surgery, eating is allowed as soon as the procedure is completed and the patient is fully awake. An IV line is kept open to add glucose if eating is not possible.

For more complicated elective surgery, a number of regimens may be used in patients requiring insulin. Patients rarely need less insulin on the day of surgery. Thus, if one elects to give only two-thirds or three-quarters of their usual intermediate insulin, as is commonly done, one should be prepared to supplement this later in the day with soluble or crystalline insulin. When the surgical procedure requires a stomach tube, intravenous fluids with glucose are recommended, monitored by blood glucose determinations at 6-hourly intervals and intramuscular insulin as needed. The usual insulin dose is 5 to 10 units at 6-hourly intervals unless the patient is known to be insulin resistant to some degree.

Emergency surgery in the diabetic can be handled from the metabolic point of view with careful monitoring and continual adjustment of fluids, electrolytes, glucose, and intravenous insulin. Low serum pH, poor fluid balance, hyperglycemia, and cardiovascular/respiratory problems must be corrected. Greater confidence in management with newer techniques is not an excuse to begin a procedure on an inadequately prepared patient. When a seriously ill patient needs protracted surgery, a palliative procedure is preferred until the patient achieves an optimal condition.

CHAPTER 72

Hypoglycemia

SIMEON MARGOLIS

Chemical hypoglycemia, often defined arbitrarily as a plasma glucose level less than 50 mg/dl, is not uncommon, particularly in women. Less frequently, low plasma glucose triggers symptomatic hypoglycemia. Evaluation of a patient for possible hypoglycemia poses two diagnostic problems: demonstration that hypoglycemia produces the patient's symptoms and identification of the underlying cause for the abnormally low plasma glucose.

The degree of hypoglycemia required to produce symptoms varies widely, as do the clinical manifestations reported by different patients. However, a similar pattern of symptoms generally recurs in any one individual. The symptoms of hypoglycemia result from catecholamine release from the adrenal medulla and impaired function. Symptoms consequent to epinephrine excess are more common when plasma glucose falls rapidly. They include sweating, palpitations, tremor, nervousness, acral and perioral numbness, faintness, and weakness. Hypoglycemia also impairs the central nervous system, which requires an adequate supply of glucose for normal function. Central nervous system symptoms, which can mimic a wide variety of neurologic and psychiatric abnormalities, usually predominate when plasma glucose levels decline slowly. Common symptoms include headache, diplopia, confusion, inappropriate affect, motor incoordination, and with extreme hypoglycemia, seizures, coma, and ultimately death. Convulsions are particularly common in children. Signs of severe hypoglycemia include hypothermia, conjugate deviation of the eyes, extensor rigidity of the limbs, trismus, and Babinski sign. In patients with cerebral vascular disease, symptoms may occur at higher plasma glucose levels and localized neurologic findings may correlate with underperfused regions of the brain. The symptoms and signs of hypoglycemia are generally reversible, but permanent brain damage can result from prolonged, severe hypoglycemia.

Glucose values vary with the method of measurement. Although many reports are based on values obtained from whole blood, most laboratories now employ automated methods to measure *plasma glucose,* which is 10 to 15 percent higher than blood glucose values. Thus, a blood glucose of 50 mg/dl corresponds to a plasma glucose of about 57 mg/dl, and such differences are significant in the definition of chemical hypoglycemia. Only plasma glucose values will be used in this chapter.

MAINTENANCE OF GLUCOSE HOMEOSTASIS[164,167]

Hypoglycemia results when the removal of glucose from the bloodstream by peripheral tissues exceeds glucose delivery from the diet or the liver. In the normal state, a number of hormones, through their actions on both the exit and entry of glucose, maintain the level of plasma glucose within fairly constant and narrowly defined limits.

Immediately after food intake, absorbed glucose and amino acids together with hormones from the intestinal mucosa promote insulin secretion by pancreatic beta cells. Insulin stimulates glucose translocation into muscle and adipose tissue cells where glucose is utilized for energy or stored after conversion to glycogen or triglycerides. As much as 70 percent of ingested glucose is retained by the liver where insulin promotes glycogen storage and inhibits the synthesis of glucose (gluconeogenesis) from amino acids, lactate, and glycerol. As blood glucose falls, prompt cessation of insulin secretion, along with increased release of glucagon and growth hormone, normally prevents a fall in plasma glucose to hypoglycemic levels. If hypoglycemia occurs despite these hormonal changes, other hormonal responses are triggered. These include the release of glucocorticoids and catecholamines; the latter are responsible for most symptoms of postprandial hypoglycemia. Catecholamines act rapidly to stimulate glycogen breakdown and fatty acid mobilization and to inhibit insulin secretion and glucose uptake in peripheral tissues.

Early in fasting, plasma glucose levels are maintained through increased glucose production, almost exclusively by the liver. Glycogen breakdown predominates in the first 24 hours of fasting. During a more prolonged fast, peripheral glucose utilization is decreased and hepatic gluconeogenesis becomes the sole source of plasma glucose. Gluconeogenesis is regulated by hormonal control of the activity of hepatic enzymes as well as the release of substrates from muscle (amino acids) and adipose tissue (glycerol). The most significant hormonal alteration is a marked reduction in levels of circulating insulin. Insulinopenia decreases peripheral glucose utilization; allows mobilization of glycerol, fatty acids (the major energy source during fasting), and amino acids; diminishes hepatic glycogen synthesis; and permits glycogenolysis and gluconeogenesis in the liver. Secre-

TABLE 72-1
Causes of Hypoglycemia

I. **Postprandial State**
Reactive hypoglycemia
Maturity-onset diabetes mellitus
Alimentary hypoglycemia
Hormonal

II. **Fasting State**
Hepatic—reduced glucose release
Liver disease
Alcohol ingestion
Enzyme defects
Hormonal—combination of reduced glucose
release and excessive glucose
utilization
Insulin excess
Insulinoma
Insulin injection
Sulfonylurea ingestion
Growth hormone deficiency
Glucocorticoid deficiency
Extrapancreatic tumors

tion of counterregulatory hormones also helps to maintain plasma glucose levels. Thus, glucagon promotes glycogen breakdown in the liver; glucagon and cortisol stimulate hepatic gluconeogenesis; growth hormone and cortisol impede glucose entry into muscle. Glucocorticoids also increase the availability of amino acids for gluconeogenesis, and, along with growth hormone, stimulate triglyceride breakdown in adipose tissue.

Based on their relation to food intake, two major patterns of hypoglycemia can be defined: 1) hypoglycemia provoked by food ingestion; and 2) hypoglycemia during the fasting state. Although symptoms may occasionaly follow a meal in those conditions that are usually characterized by fasting hypoglycemia, patients with the postprandial forms of hypoglycemia never develop symptomatic hypoglycemia in the fasting state. The major recognized etiologies of hypoglycemia are listed in Table 72-1.

SYMPTOMATIC HYPOGLYCEMIA OCCURRING ONLY IN THE POSTPRANDIAL STATE[166,169]

Although hypoglycemia has become a popular diagnosis to explain a wide variety of often vague complaints, symptoms from postprandial hypoglycemia are uncommon. Symptoms of hypoglycemia induced by food ingestion generally occur within 1 to 5 hours after a meal. In rare hereditary abnormalities seen in children, hypoglycemia may follow the ingestion of galactose, fructose, or leucine; in adults, hypoglycemia is usually related to glucose intake. Symptoms of postprandial hypoglycemia are caused by catecholamine release. Significant CNS symptoms are uncommon in the adult; seizures and coma are rare. The symptoms usually subside within 30 minutes even if no therapy is undertaken. The diagnosis of postprandial hypoglycemia is often suggested by the repetition of a particular constellation of symptoms in a fairly constant relationship to food intake, most commonly in the late morning or afternoon.

Although a poor substitute for a regular meal, the 5-hour glucose tolerance test is the procedure of choice to provoke postprandial hypoglycemia. Blood samples are obtained at 30-minute intervals throughout the test. In addition, the patient is instructed to record the time and nature of any symptoms and to notify the technician so that an immediate blood sample can be obtained. While no single value is uniformly accepted as evidence of chemical hypoglycemia, plasma glucose levels less than 50 mg/dl, in association with appropriate symptoms, strongly suggest a diagnosis of symptomatic hypoglycemia. Values below 50 mg/dl, without symptoms, may be seen in normal individuals.

The glucose tolerance test may also help to distinguish between the types of postprandial hypoglycemia (Fig. 72-1). In most patients, the pattern of the glucose tolerance test discriminates between reactive hypoglycemia and early diabetes mellitus. However, the glucose responses in a single individual often vary considerably on serial testing. As a consequence, the pattern may change over the years from reactive hypoglycemia to that of early diabetes mellitus. Alimentary hypoglycemia usually presents with the most characteristic clinical picture and test results. In addition to these well-recognized causes of postprandial hypoglycemia, deficiencies of growth hormone, cortisol, and thyroxine may also cause postprandial symptoms.

Reactive, Functional, or Idiopathic Hypoglycemia

This syndrome is the most common of the postprandial hypoglycemias. Although abnormalities in the secretion of a number of hormones have been suggested by various investigators, the pathogenesis remains unknown. The glucose tolerance test tends to be flat with a blunted early rise in plasma glucose. Serum insulin levels are heterogeneous. In some, serum insulin responses are appropriate for the plasma glucose (Fig. 72-1). Occasionally, serum insulin levels are excessively high; most often the insulin response is delayed in onset but normal in magnitude. Symptoms, which usually appear 3 to 5 hours after a meal,

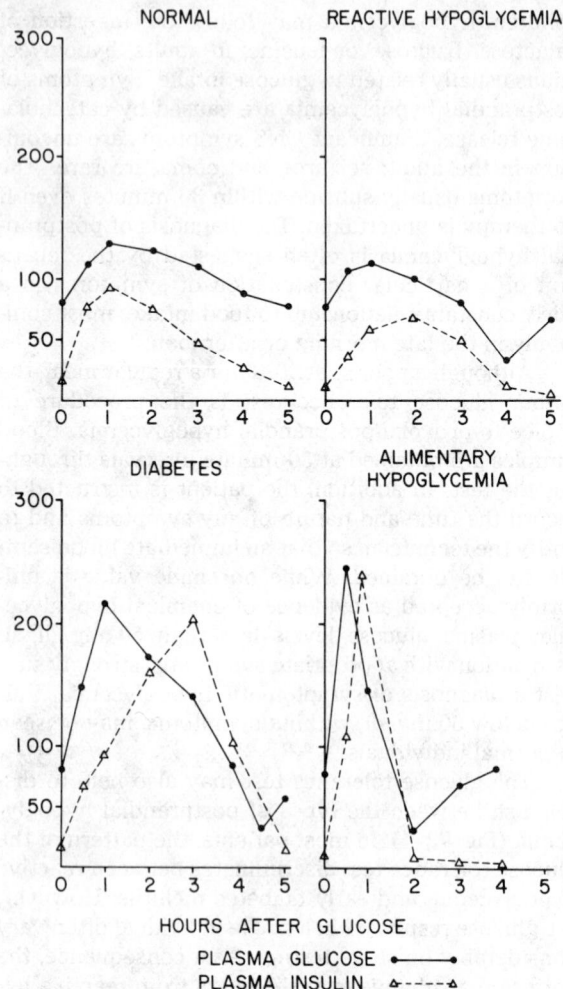

FIGURE 72–1. Comparison of glucose and insulin levels in normal subjects and individuals with various types of postprandial hypoglycemia during a 5-hour glucose tolerance test.

may be limited to mild anxiety and restlessness, but some patients describe more severe complaints associated with blatant epinephrine excess. Consequently, the diagnosis of functional hypoglycemia is often confused with psychoneurotic anxiety states. Conversely, many individuals with psychoneurotic syndromes are, incorrectly, thought to have functional hypoglycemia. It has long been stressed that individuals who develop reactive hypoglycemia tend to be asthenic, hyperkinetic, obsessive-compulsive persons who are tense and often emotionally labile. However, psychological tests showed similar personality profiles in patients with all types of symptomatic postprandial hypoglycemia.[166]

Maturity-Onset Diabetes Mellitus

In some patients with maturity-onset diabetes mellitus, a hyperglycemic response to glucose precedes symptomatic hypoglycemia by 3 to 4 hours. Such hypoglycemic episodes occur during early stages of diabetes when fasting plasma glucose is usually within the normal range. Hypoglycemia in diabetics is attributed to their delayed insulin response to a glucose load. As a consequence, excessive insulin levels at a time of falling glucose (Fig. 72–1) may produce late hypoglycemia after glucose ingestion. However, a similar pattern of abnormal insulin secretion is typically observed in adult-onset diabetics without hypoglycemic symptoms.

Alimentary Hypoglycemia

Alimentary hypoglycemia may occur in patients with thyrotoxicosis or rapid gastric emptying of unknown cause, but most often the syndrome follows gastrectomy, gastrojejunostomy, or vagotomy and pyloroplasty. As demonstrated in Figure 72–1, a precipitous rise in plasma glucose levels, resulting from rapid entry of large amounts of glucose into the small intestine, provokes dramatic secretion of insulin and subsequent hypoglycemia, which occurs earlier than in the other forms of postprandial hypoglycemia. The dumping syndrome (Chap. 58) rather than hypoglycemia may cause symptoms in many individuals following gastrointestinal surgery.

Treatment of Postprandial Hypoglycemia[169,180]

The management of patients with postprandial hypoglycemia is hampered by a lack of controlled clinical trials and objective measures to quantify therapeutic effectiveness. Therapy has included both dietary modification and drugs. Multiple small feedings may be helpful in any type of postprandial hypoglycemia. High protein, restricted carbohydrate diets were stressed in the past, but available studies suggest little benefit, and possibly increased symptoms, from a low carbohydrate intake. Instead, emphasis should be placed on the intake of complex carbohydrates (such as starches) and elimination of simple sugars. Reduction to ideal body weight is an important dietary measure in patients with hypoglycemia due to maturity-onset diabetes.

If dietary treatment is not totally satisfactory, anticholinergic drugs may help to control symptoms by slowing gastric emptying and intestinal motility as well as inhibiting vagal stimulation of insulin release. Tincture of belladonna (10 to 15 drops), atropine sulfate (0.5 to 1 mg) or Pro-Banthine (7.5 mg) 30 minutes before each meal have all proved effective in some patients. Most success has been achieved in reactive hypoglycemia, but symptoms may also respond in alimentary hypoglycemia. The sulfonylurea hypoglycemic agents, which stimulate the early secretion of insulin, may ameliorate hypoglycemic symptoms in early diabetes as well as in patients with reactive hypoglycemia. In a few patients, symptoms are relieved with phenytoin or propranolol. The latter is more effective in blocking symptoms than in preventing the hypoglycemia. Psychotherapy has long been recommended for patients with reactive hypoglycemia, and symptoms may abate in these patients with improved psychiatric status. Considering the evidence for abnormal personality profiles in patients with other types of postprandial hypoglycemia, psychiatric treatment may prove equally beneficial in them.

SYMPTOMATIC HYPOGLYCEMIA IN THE FASTING STATE[165]

The overnight fasting glucose level, rather than a glucose tolerance test, is the most useful screening test for fasting hypoglycemia. Fasting plasma glucose values must be interpreted carefully, especially in women, since prolonged fasting causes a much greater fall in plasma glucose in healthy young females than in males.[165,178] Even when fasted for 72 hours, no male had a plasma glucose concentration less then 50 mg/dl. In contrast, the mean plasma glucose in asymptomatic women fell to 40 mg/dl after a 72-hour fast; plasma glucose in the great majority was less than 50 mg/dl and fell as low as 22 mg/dl in one subject. Thus, a fasting plasma glucose level below 50 mg/dl in a male should raise strong suspicion of significant hypoglycemia. In women the lower limit of plasma glucose is not defined with certainty. Plasma glucose levels were 10 to 20 mg/dl lower in women 16 to 22 weeks pregnant than in nonpregnant women. In all individuals, concomitant symptoms are more important for the diagnosis of hypoglycemia than is the absolute level of plasma glucose.

Since the underlying disorder is more serious in the fasting than in the postprandial hypoglycemias, it is imperative to identify the abnormality. The major causes of fasting hypoglycemia are listed in Table 72-1.

HEPATIC

Liver Abnormalities

A slight lowering of fasting glucose levels and a greater than normal rise, followed by a delayed fall in plasma glucose, are often seen after glucose ingestion

by patients with significant parenchymal liver disease. However, liver disease is an infrequent cause of symptomatic hypoglycemia. Unless preventive measures are taken, severe hypoglycemia usually occurs immediately after extensive surgical resection of the liver. Hypoglycemia also follows acute, fulminant hepatic necrosis of viral or toxic origin. Transient hypoglycemia occasionally complicates congestive heart failure or pericardial disease, presumably because poor perfusion of the liver limits the supply of amino acids needed for gluconeogenesis. Recognition of hypoglycemia can be difficult in this situation where symptoms may be misinterpreted as evidence of cerebral anoxia.

Symptomatic hypoglycemia may occur in some severe cirrhotics, but the physician should be especially alert to the presence of a hepatoma when repeated hypoglycemia is noted in the course of cirrhosis. Most commonly a poorly differentiated hepatoma is associated with severe anorexia, marked weight loss, and hypoglycemia as a late complication. In a few patients with well-differentiated hepatomas, hypoglycemia begins many months before their death, whereas loss of appetite and weight develop late in their illness. The cause of the hypoglycemia in these patients is not clear. Massive replacement of normal liver may diminish hepatic glucose production, but in many cases other factors must play an important role in the hypoglycemia.[175]

Alcohol Ingestion[173]

Most commonly, ethanol causes hypoglycemia in chronically malnourished alcoholics who stop their intake of food and alcohol 10 to 20 hours earlier. However, neither liver disease nor hepatic glycogen depletion is necessary since hypoglycemia can follow a short drinking spree in healthy adults or children. Normal amounts of liver glycogen provide some protection against alcoholic hypoglycemia which results mainly from blockage of hepatic gluconeogenesis by products of ethanol metabolism. Reduced nicotinamide-adenine dinucleotide (NADH) accumulates in the liver during ethanol oxidation. The consequent increase in the ratio of NADH to NAD prevents the entry of substrates, such as alanine, lactate, and glycerol, into the gluconeogenic pathway. Obese subjects are less sensitive to the hypoglycemic effects of ethanol. Diabetic patients using insulin or sulfonylureas are especially susceptible to induction of low plasma glucose levels by ethanol.

Ethanol ingestion is probably the most frequent cause of fasting hypoglycemia, especially in urban centers, but its manifestations are often mistakenly attributed to drunkenness. To improve the recognition of alcoholic hypoglycemia, plasma glucose should be determined in all symptomatic patients with a history of significant alcohol intake. Although hypoglycemic symptoms usually respond promptly to intravenous glucose infusions, glucose administration must be continued for a number of hours to prevent recurrence of hypoglycemia.

Enzyme Defects

Hypoglycemia also occurs in several rare disorders, each resulting from deficiency of a specific hepatic enzyme required for normal carbohydrate metabolism. In these diseases, which include glycogen storage diseases, galactosemia, and hereditary fructose intolerance, hypoglycemic symptoms usually begin in infancy and are less prominent in affected adults.

HORMONAL

Insulinoma and Other Functioning Islet Cell Tumors

As shown in Table 72–2, a variety of clinical syndromes result from functioning islet cell tumors. Most commonly, the tumors secrete insulin, with resultant hypoglycemia, or gastrin, which causes the Zollinger-Ellison syndrome (Chap. 58). Diarrheal syndromes (Chap. 60) may result from tumor production of vasoactive intestinal peptide (VIP), gastrin, secretin, or prostaglandin E. ACTH secretion by islet cell tumors may cause Cushing syndrome. Some pancreatic tumors produce serotonin and consequently the carcinoid syndrome.

TABLE 72–2
Functioning Islet Cell Tumors

Product	Cell Type	Clinical Manifestations
Glucagon	α	Hyperglycemia, skin lesions, weight loss
Insulin	β	Fasting hypoglycemia
Somatostatin	D	Hyperglycemia
ACTH	?	Cushing syndrome
Gastrin	?	Gastric hypersection, peptic ulcer, diarrhea
Vasoactive intestinal peptide (VIP)	?	Watery diarrhea, hypokalemia, hyperglycemia
Secretin	?	Pancreatic hypersecretion, diarrhea
Serotonin	?	Carcinoid syndrome
Prostaglandin E	?	Diarrhea

Several types of islet cell tumors are associated with hyperglycemia. Glucagon-secreting tumors[174] have been documented in numerous instances. The most common clinical manifestations of glucagonoma include glucose intolerance, dermatitis, and weight loss without accompanying anorexia. Glossitis or stomatitis occurs in about one-third of the patients and a few have diarrhea. The tumor occurs more commonly in women and is malignant in about 80 percent of reported cases. When suspected on clinical grounds, the diagnosis is made by demonstrating high levels of circulating glucagon; the tumor may be localized by angiography. A few case reports have described hyperglycemia resulting from somatostatin secretion by D-cell tumors of the pancreas.[168] VIP-producing tumors, in addition to causing watery diarrhea, may cause hyperglycemia and hypercalcemia.

Symptoms caused by the simultaneous production of other hormones by islet cell tumors may complicate the recognition of insulinoma-induced hypoglycemia. Moreover, insulinomas may coexist with other nonpancreatic tumors as part of the syndrome of multiple endocrine adenomatosis (MEA).[162] Three major forms of MEA are now recognized. In MEA-type I (Wermer syndrome), islet cell tumors and parathyroid adenomas or hyperplasia occur in 80 to 90 percent of patients. About one-third of the pancreatic tumors secrete insulin; the remainder produce diarrhea or the Zollinger-Ellison syndrome. Pituitary tumors are identified in about two-thirds, nonfunctioning adrenal cortical adenomas in one-third, and thyroid adenomas in one-fifth of these patients. Medullary thyroid carcinoma occurs in virtually all patients with the other two forms of MEA. One-half the patients with MEA-type II (Sipple syndrome) also have pheochromocytomas and 25 percent exhibit hyperparathyroidism. MEA-type III (mucosal neuroma syndrome) is characterized by mucosal neuromas, intestinal ganglioneuromas, and medullary thyroid carcinoma. Pheochromocytomas are present in about one-half the patients; hyperparathyroidism is not a feature of this syndrome. MEA-types I and II are almost always familial (autosomal dominant) whereas type III is sporadic in about one-half the cases.

Insulinomas[172] are rare tumors that occur at all ages and with equal frequency in males and females. They are diagnosed most commonly in individuals in the fourth through seventh decades. Multiple insulinomas are present in approximately 10 percent of the cases and a similar number are malignant.

Since nonspecific complaints, such as malaise, profound fatigue, confusion, or headaches upon arising, often predominate in early stages of the disorder, symptoms have generally been present for a long time before correct diagnosis. With increasing size of the tumor, symptoms of acute hypoglycemia become more prominent. Hunger and compulsive eating occasionally lead to weight gain. In addition to autonomic alterations, the patient may develop reversible paralysis or a seizure disorder. Because the clinical picture can mimic a wide variety of neuropsychiatric disorders, patients are often admitted to neurologic or psychiatric wards. In one series, 40 percent of patients with insulinomas had neuropsychiatric deficits. After successful removal of the tumor, half of the patients had persistent, irreversible neuropsychiatric complaints which were thought to be related to the duration of symptoms before appropriate therapy.

The diagnosis of an insulinoma requires the demonstration of insulin levels that are inappropriately high for the plasma glucose concentration. During continued fasting by normal individuals, plasma glucose and insulin decline together. As a result, the ratio of immunoreactive insulin (IRI) to glucose (G) remains constant. IRI/G was less than 0.3 units/mg in all healthy nonobese men tested.[178] In the great majority of insulinomas, an abnormal ratio of insulin to glucose is apparent after 12 to 14 hours of fasting. Because tumor secretion may be episodic and insulin half-life is short, IRI/G should be measured several times. Occasionally, demonstration of fasting hypoglycemia with inappropriate insulin levels may require as long as 72 hours of fasting. If an abnormality is not established by then, subjects should be exercised for 2 hours since exercise raises low plasma glucose in normals but decreases glucose levels further in patients with an insulinoma.[178] In addition to observations during fasting, other diagnostic tests may be useful. The sensitivity of insulinomas to glucose is generally no greater than that of normal beta cells, but insulinomas may release more insulin when challenged with tolbutamide, glucagon, leucine, or calcium[171,177] (Table 72–3). An excessive insulin response to provocative tests with such agents may, therefore, prove helpful in difficult cases. Suppression tests have been used to distinguish between autonomous (nonsuppressible) insulin production and β–cells under normal physiologic control. Suppression is assessed following insulin-induced hypoglycemia. Measurements are made of serum insulin after injection of fish insulin or of serum C-peptide following administration of commercial insulins.[177,181] C-peptide levels may be particularly valuable when an insulinoma is suspected in an insulin-dependent diabetic in whom accurate plasma insulin determinations are not possible because of insulin antibodies. Proinsulin levels are often elevated in individuals with insulinomas. Serum levels of chorionic gonadotropin, or its α or β subunits, are also elevated in about two-thirds of patients

with malignant functioning insulinomas, but not in those with benign or inactive tumors.[170]

When the diagnosis of insulinoma is strongly suspected and surgery is anticipated, efforts to locate the tumor should be undertaken. Tumors larger then 2 to 3 cm can be detected by ultrasonography or computerized axial tomography, but angiography is more sensitive for small tumors. About one-half of the tumors can be identified before surgery by celiac and superior mesenteric arteriography. If the tumor cannot be located by radiography or direct palpation, progressive pancreatic resection is advised, beginning at the tail and proceeding toward the body, with frequent monitoring of blood glucose levels as well as the pathologic specimens.

If surgery fails to restore normoglycemia or a malignant tumor has spread, attempts are made to control hypoglycemic episodes with medical therapy. Management may require only frequent high-carbohydrate feedings. In cases of more profound hypoglycemia, pharmacologic agents have been used with variable success. Diazoxide, 200 mg daily in three equal doses, may help to control intractable hypoglycemia in some patients with insulinoma. The hyperglycemic effect of diazoxide is believed to result from inhibition of insulin release and enhanced secretion of catecholamines. Diazoxide may also increase hepatic glycogenolysis through direct effects on the liver. Serious side effects include sodium and fluid retention which may precipitate congestive heart failure, as well as diabetic ketoacidosis and hyperosmolar nonketotic coma. The antibiotic streptozotocin destroys beta cells of the pancreas. In one study,[163] intravenous administration of streptozotocin, 1 g/m² body surface area per week for 4 weeks, gave relief and improved survival in about one-half of those treated. Almost all patients had significant symptomatic complications, however; most serious was irreversible renal failure. Administration of zinc glucagon or glucocorticoids reduces hypoglycemic manifestations, but their action is short-lived and accompanied by undesirable side effects.

Insulin Administration

Insulin overdosage in diabetics is the most common cause of hypoglycemia. Most diabetics learn to recognize their own particular symptoms and to abort attacks by carbohydrate ingestion. Occasionally a nondiabetic may self-administer insulin and produce symptoms of recurrent hypoglycemia. Such is most commonly observed either in family members of insulin-dependent diabetics or in hospital personnel, such as nurses, who have ready access to insulin and syringes. An individual suspected of this type of malingering must be examined carefully for injection

---

TABLE 72-3

Diagnostic Approach to Hypoglycemia

Prove that hypoglycemia is responsible for symptoms:	During spontaneous or provoked attack show: 1. Typical symptoms 2. Plasma glucose less than 50 mg/dl 3. Prompt relief of fasting symptoms by glucose ingestion or infusion
a. When symptoms are related to food ingestion	Obtain 5-hour glucose tolerance test 1. Measure plasma glucose every 30 min 2. Ask patient to keep record of any symptoms 3. Obtain additional plasma glucose at time of symptoms
b. When symptoms occur during fasting	Measure plasma glucose levels after overnight fast Save aliquot of frozen plasma for insulin determination if glucose is less than 50 mg/dl
If fasting hypoglycemia is demonstrated,	
a. Eliminate causes other than insulinoma	History and physical examination Liver function tests Urinary or plasma cortisol levels Plasma growth hormone response to arginine infusion Insulin antibodies
b. Determine ratio of plasma insulin/glucose after overnight fast. If the ratio of insulin/glucose after an overnight fast is not diagnostic of insulinoma and this disorder is strongly suspected	Begin 72-hour fast with repeated determinations of plasma insulin/glucose ratio Exercise patient at the end of the fast when hypoglycemia is not documented Provocative tests: measure glucose and insulin response to tolbutamide, leucine, and/or glucagon. Administer 1 g tolbutamide in 20 ml sterile water IV or 150 mg/kg leucine p.o. in orange juice and collect aliquots at 0, 15, 30, 45, 60, 90, and 120 minutes. Give 1.0 mg glucagon IM with sampling at 0, 5, 10, 15, 30, 60, 90, and 120 minutes[14] Suppression test: administer fish or commercial insulin and measure insulin or C-peptide response
Once chemical tests establish the diagnosis of insulinoma	Selective celiac angiography

marks, and his hospital room should be searched for hidden insulin and syringes. The detection of insulin antibodies in a nondiabetic supports the suspicion of self-administration of insulin, but insulin autoantibodies occur in some individuals who have not received exogenous insulin. Another useful laboratory test is measurement of serum levels of C-peptide, which will be low relative to serum insulin in patients with factitious insulin injection.[181]

Oral Hypoglycemic Agents[182]
All of the sulfonylureas have produced hypoglycemia, but the longer acting drugs, such as chlorpropamide, are more commonly the causative agents. Nondiabe-

tics may use oral hypoglycemic agents to induce hypoglycemia. Clinical settings that favor the development of drug-induced hypoglycemia include decreased food intake or malnutrition, impaired liver or renal function that prolongs the action of sulfonylureas, decreased adrenocortical activity, and extremes of age. Concomitant use of ethanol or other drugs, especially salicylates, also augments the hypoglycemic effect of the sulfonylureas. Sulfonylurea ingestion can cause protracted and severe hypoglycemia. After an initial injection of 50 percent glucose, the patient should be hospitalized and plasma glucose levels maintained over 100 mg/dl with continous intravenous glucose. Glucose infusions are cautiously slowed and finally discontinued when the patient's plasma glucose level is stable on an oral intake of at least 300 g of carbohydrate daily.

Pituitary Disorders

Growth hormone and ACTH are the pituitary hormones that play important roles in the regulation of glucose metabolism. Growth hormone acts directly on both the liver and peripheral tissues whereas ACTH deficiency produces hypoglycemia through the resultant secondary adrenal insufficiency. Since available evidence indicates that the peripheral actions of insulin are antagonized by growth hormone, deficiency of this hormone probably produces hypoglycemia because of peripheral glucose overutilization when insulin effects are unopposed by growth hormone. Absence of both growth hormone and ACTH can lead to hypoglycemia in patients with all types of acquired pituitary insufficiency. Hypoglycemia can also occur in patients with isolated deficiencies of either growth hormone or ACTH. Thus, attacks of hypoglycemia may occur in cases of pituitary dwarfism caused by a genetic defect in the secretion of growth hormone, although many such patients have a compensatory insulinopenia. Patients with growth hormone deficiency may have hypoglycemic symptoms in either the fasting or postprandial state. With glucocorticoid replacement, episodes of symptomatic hypoglycemia are uncommon in adults but occur in about 10 percent of cases of panhypopituitarism that begin in childhood.

Glucocorticoid Deficiency

Patients with diminished glucocorticoid secretion commonly manifest low levels of plasma glucose, and symptomatic hypoglycemia may follow a period of fasting. The low plasma glucose probably results from diminished glucose output during fasting since cortisol is required for optimal hepatic gluconeogenesis. Occasionally, patients with glucocorticoid deficiency exhibit hypoglycemic symptoms late in the postprandial period. Adequate steroid replacement completely prevents attacks of hypoglycemia.

EXTRAPANCREATIC TUMORS[176]

Hypoglycemia can occur in patients with tumors of virtually any histopathologic type. Most frequently described are mesenchymal tumors, massive fibromas, or sarcomas located (in decreasing order of frequency) in the retroperitoneal, intrathoracic, and intra-abdominal spaces. Hypoglycemia may also complicate the course of other non-islet-cell tumors, including hepatoma, adrenocortical tumors, and gastrointestinal, bronchial, and exocrine pancreatic car-

cinomas. In most patients, the low plasma glucose results from a combination of decreased glucose production and inappropriately high glucose utilization. The cause of hypoglycemia is not known and probably varies from case to case. It is clear that these tumors do not synthesize or store insulin, and circulating insulin levels are found to be low during hypoglycemic episodes. Some attribute hypoglycemia to elevated levels of nonsuppressible insulin-like activity (NSILA), measured by radioimmunoassay;[179] but NSILA levels are normal in a sizable fraction of these hypoglycemic patients, while others have described elevated NSILA in cancer patients without hypoglycemia. Some tumors are thought to lower plasma glucose by converting large amounts of glucose to lactate while other investigators have suggested that the tumors secrete a substance that inhibits hepatic gluconeogenesis.

Extrapancreatic tumors are usually distinguished from an insulinoma by the presence of a large abdominal mass, radiologic evidence of a tumor, cachexia, and absence of elevated plasma insulin levels. In some cases, however, the clinical picture in patients with extrapancreatic tumors may closely resemble the hypoglycemia of islet cell tumors.

Because of their size, these tumors are generally not resectable and management has been directed toward raising blood glucose levels through frequent feedings, glucose infusions, and diazoxide therapy.

DIAGNOSTIC APPROACH TO SYMPTOMATIC HYPOGLYCEMIA

The most important step in the diagnosis of symptomatic hypoglycemia (Table 72–3) is to document that chemical hypoglycemia and typical symptoms occur at the same time during a spontaneous attack or a provocative test. Moreover, prompt relief of symptoms, especially those provoked by fasting, following glucose ingestion or infusion may provide a valuable clue.

POSTPRANDIAL HYPOGLYCEMIA

A 5-hour glucose tolerance test should be performed if symptoms occur in postprandial periods. Since the plasma glucose nadir is often quite transient, plasma glucose should be measured every 30 minutes; and an additional sample must be obtained as soon as the patient reports symptoms. Historical information and the pattern of the plasma glucose during the test usually permit distinction between reactive hypoglycemia, maturity-onset diabetes mellitus, and alimentary hypoglycemia. Measurement of growth hormone, cortisol, and thyroxine may uncover a rare patient with postprandial hypoglycemia resulting from abnormal levels of one of these hormones.

Patients and physicians alike are inclined to attribute a great variety of symptoms to hypoglycemia. Lack of energy, chronic anxiety, lethargy, mental dullness, and similar complaints rarely result from hypoglycemia. Yet a large number of patients persistently blame hypoglycemia for such symptoms which they attempt to control by a variety of dietary measures.[183] The physician performs a valuable service when he demonstrates that symptoms have been incorrectly attributed to hypoglycemia. He must recognize that plasma glucose may fall below 50 mg/dl during a glucose tolerance test in normal individuals and insist on the concurrence of chemical hypoglycemia and characteristic symptoms before making a diagnosis of symptomatic hypoglycemia.

FASTING HYPOGLYCEMIA

When suggestive symptoms occur during the fasting state, efforts should be made to document hypoglycemia by measurement of glucose and insulin levels after an overnight fast. Once fasting hypoglycemia is demonstrated, the physician must distinguish between an insulinoma, where operative intervention is necessary, and other causes of fasting hypoglycemia. When clinical evidence suggests hypoadrenalism or hypopituitarism, measurement of growth hormone and cortisol are obtained. Alcohol ingestion, the use of sulfonylureas, severe liver disease, or insulin self-administration can generally be distinguished by history, physical examination, liver function tests, and insulin antibody measurements. If the clinical findings and specific laboratory tests do not support the presence of one of these conditions, the differential diagnosis generally lies between insulinoma and extrapancreatic tumor. Severe wasting or an abdominal mass favors the diagnosis of extrapancreatic tumor. An elevated ratio of plasma insulin to glucose following an overnight fast, as well as increased concentrations of C-peptide or proinsulin, strongly suggest insulinoma.

When glucose and insulin levels fail to establish a diagnosis after a 12–hour fast, these measurements can be continued during a prolonged period of starvation (48 to 72 hours). These measures will establish the diagnosis in most patients. On occasion, recognition of an insulinoma may require measurement of plasma glucose and insulin responses to stimulation with tolbutamide, leucine, glucagon, or calcium, or suppression by insulin injection. During such tests the physician must monitor the patient closely and intervene promptly if symptomatic hypoglycemia occurs. After chemical tests have established the diagnosis, appearance of an abnormal collection of vessels or a tumor blush during selective angiography may localize the insulinoma. Despite all diagnostic efforts, laboratory tests may yield equivocal results in some patients. Under these circumstances, the physician has the option of continued observation and retesting the patient after an interval, or proceeding immediately to exploratory laparotomy. This decision must be based in part upon the intensity of the patient's symptoms.

CHAPTER 73

Eating Disorders: Obesity and Anorexia Nervosa

ARNOLD E. ANDERSEN AND SIMEON MARGOLIS

Obesity, a descriptive term for excess body fat, is the most common chonic medical problem in this country. There is considerable information on the hormonal and metabolic consequences of obesity, but little progress has been made in detecting any metabolic aberration that causes obesity. Moreover, the normal physiologic controls of body weight are incompletely understood. As a consequence, the medical management of obesity is directed largely toward promotion of weight loss, using approaches based on experience rather than rationally derived from a scientific understanding of the pathophysiology. Inadequate attention has been paid to prevention or to the underlying social, cultural, and emotional factors responsible for obesity. Overconcern about obesity leads to excessive fasting and the syndrome of anorexia nervosa in some young subjects.

OBESITY

Definition

Gross obesity is evident on inspection. Lesser degrees are generally recognized when the patient's weight exceeds the normal range in tables relating weight to height, sex, age, and body build. This procedure, in fact, defines overweight, which may result from an excessive mass of muscle, bone, or fat, whereas obesity specifically requires the presence of increased amounts of fat. The distinction between overweight and obesity is sharpened by measurement of body fat content. Most methods for quantitation of body fat are too complicated for routine clinical use. One exception is skinfold thickness measurements which are simple to perform and provide a fairly accurate estimate of total body fat. The triceps skinfold thickness, the most commonly employed measurement, is determined with a caliper at a point midway between the shoulder and elbow with the arm hanging freely. Obesity is diagnosed when the triceps skinfold thickness is greater than 20 mm in men or 30 mm in women. Other methods that provide more quantitative estimates of percent body fat, without the need for special equipment, utilize various ratios of weight to height, such as the Body Mass Index (weight/height^2).

Classification

No uniform method for classifying obesity exists, but several categorical distinctions may be useful. Obesity can be classified by age of onset, distribution of fat, severity, familial pattern, etiology, and the presence or absence of medical or psychosocial problems. Childhood obesity is generally characterized by both adipocyte hyperplasia and hypertrophy (see below) as well as both peripheral and central fat distribution. Patients with adult-onset obesity, in contrast, have predominantly adipocyte hypertrophy and central obesity. Rare patients have lipodystrophy with very unusual patterns of fat deposition. Individuals may also be classified by the severity of their weight problems, i.e., as having mild, moderate, severe, or morbid obesity where they exceed ideal body weight by 15 to 30, 30 to 50, 50 to 100, or more than 100 percent, respectively.

For physicians, obesity is most conveniently divided into primary (idiopathic) and secondary varieties. Although few patients have secondary obesity resulting from a known medical disorder, most of our understanding of the pertinent physiology of body weight and feeding is derived from study of these identified causes of obesity. Such information can then be applied to treatment of the more common primary variety. A multifactorial classification of obesity may, in the last analysis, be the most useful.

Epidemiology

Obesity correlates with many epidemiologic variables, such as socioeconomic status, age, sex, religion, national origin, and number of generations lived in the United States.

In the United States, the strongest correlation is with social class; obesity is six times more common in women of lower socioeconomic status than in women of the upper class.[189] Women who are upwardly mobile are less obese than women who are downwardly mobile. In contrast, obesity is associated with increased socioeconomic class in developing countries. The second strongest correlation is with age. Both men and women gain weight slowly but steadily with increasing age. While 25 percent of men and women between the ages of 30 and 39 are more than 20 percent overweight, this figure increases to 32 percent for men and 40 percent for women between the ages of 40 and 49. Obesity declines with increasing number of generations a family has lived in the United States. Nine percent of American women of British origin were obese, compared to 27 percent of Italian origin, a difference partly, but not completely, explained by social class. Morbid obesity may be a separate category that does not correlate with these epidemiologic variables.

Adipose Tissue in Obesity

In an average adult, adipose tissue mass ranges from 11 to 17 kg and provides the storage of 100,000 to 150,000 calories.[186] Among average-weight young adults who do not participate regularly in vigorous physical activity, adipose tissue constitutes approximately 15 percent of total body weight in males and 25 percent in females. In most adults, weight gain means an increase in adipose tissue.

Two factors finally determining total adipose tissue mass are the number and size of fat cells. Experimental work suggests that the number of fat cells is largely fixed during the early years of childhood.[192] During this period, obesity results primarily from an increased number (hyperplasia) of fat cells. Thereafter, until adolescence, the rate of hyperplasia continues to decrease. Accretion of adipose tissue mass during adult life occurs mostly by increasing the size (hypertrophy) of existing fat cells. Thus, the time of onset of obesity determines the relative contribution made by increased number *vs.* size of fat cells.

Animal studies suggest that the potential for massive obesity requires the presence of fat cell hyperplasia which results from excessive caloric intake during childhood. Morbid obesity occurs much more commonly in individuals with early onset obesity. Their obesity is relatively refractory to dietary control and is often associated with a perceptual distortion of body image. Fewer than 5 percent of extremely obese individuals with early onset will return to near ideal body weight. Adult-onset obesity is more responsive to weight reduction by dietary measures and is seldom associated with distortion of body image.

Physiologic Control of Weight, Feeding, and Satiety

Animals allowed to feed freely from a variety of nutrients will choose well-balanced diets containing adequate calories to maintain body weight at a steady level. Various concentrations of any nutrients are delivered from the stomach into the duodenum at exactly the rate of 1.2 calories per minute until the concentration of nutrients becomes very dense, at which point the control of caloric release breaks down and excess calories leave the stomach.[194] Thus, both feeding behavior and gastric emptying are very carefully controlled. The neural, gastrointestinal, and endocrine controls for feeding, satiety, and gastric responses to food are multiple, overlapping, integrated, and precise. Therefore, abnormalities of weight and eating result from either a disorder in the anatomy and physiology of the eating controls, which is rare, or from other factors, usually psychosocial, which override these controls.

Neurophysiologic experiments in several animal species have reported localizing a "feeding center" in the ventrolateral hypothalamus and a "satiety center" in the ventromedial hypothalamic nucleus. While these nuclei are important in the neural control of appetite and weight, they are actually part of a much more extensive system, involving the limbic system and cortex. It is, therefore, an unwarranted oversimplification of neurophysiology to attribute the regulation of feeding and satiety to the hypothalamus alone.

Etiology and Physiology of Obesity

Genetics, increasing age, and psychosocial factors appear to be most important in producing obesity. As with many other disorders, the greatest effect occurs when environmental factors are added to a physiologic predisposition. Further, the relative contributions of these etiologic factors may vary significantly with the type of obesity. Although rigorous evidence is lacking, age and psychosocial factors probably play the greatest role in mild to moderate obesity whereas genetic factors probably make the major contribution in severe to extreme obesity. The increased frequency of obesity in children of obese parents almost certainly results from both learning and inheritance.

Physicians occasionally have a role in producing obesity through the type of medication, diet, and activity they prescribe. The smallest contribution to obesity is probably from underlying medical diseases (see below), but it is important to recognize and treat secondary obesity with appropriate specific measures.

Etiologic studies in the past have tended toward unitary hypotheses such as the "lipostat," "glucostat," "thermostat," or "calorostat" theories. Each probably describes aspects of pathophysiologic change in some or all obese patients, but none satisfactorily offers a causal explanation for obesity.

While the possible etiologic role of hormonal or metabolic abnormalities remains unclear, obesity regularly provokes several hormonal and metabolic alterations that are generally reversible with return to normal weight.[197] These include increased glucocorticoid production, hyperinsulinism, and diminished release of growth hormone in response to stimuli. Glucagon levels are unaffected. In obesity, basal insulin levels and the insulin response to glucose or amino acid loads are markedly increased. Elevated insulin levels coupled with normal carbohydrate tolerance, as well as direct evidence, suggest that liver, muscle, and adipose tissue are at least partially resistant to the actions of insulin. The larger size of the fat cell in obesity is a contributing factor to the resistance of adipose tissue. In addition, the relative proportions of dietary fat and carbohydrate can alter insulin sensitivity.[199] Diminished cellular receptors for insulin may be partly responsible for the resistance. In patients with a genetic predisposition for diabetes mellitus, the stress of obesity is likely to unmask the defect and produce glucose intolerance. These responses no doubt account for the high association between obesity and maturity-onset diabetes, and for the improvement in carbohydrate tolerance frequently seen when the obese diabetic patient loses weight.

The Psychology and Behavior of Obese Individuals

No simple psychological explanations for obesity have proven valid. Obesity appears to result from psychological conflicts in some individuals; more commonly, obesity is the cause of much psychological suffering. In many, psychological issues are not prominent causes or consequences of obesity. Although no single pattern characterizes the psychology and behavior of all obese individuals, certain statements can be made about groups of obese individuals. Shachter[200] explored the idea that obese people are stimulated by external cues and are relatively unresponsive to internal physiologic signals for eating and satiety. He suggested that obese people act in many ways like animals with hypothalamic hyperphagia. They eat more than controls, but work less hard for food; they eat more sweetened food than controls, but are "finicky" about less palatable food. Obese individuals eat more food in general, specifically more food per meal, fewer meals, and faster meals. It is uncertain whether these behavioral characteristics are causes or effects of obesity.

No personality characteristics are unique to obese patients. Many obese people have difficulty in identifying mood states and use food when experiencing dysphoria of any kind.

Stunkard[202] described several specific behavioral syndromes of obesity. In the "night-eating syndrome" evening hyperphagia and nocturnal insomnia are followed by morning anorexia. This occurs in about 10 percent of obese patients, especially women, when experiencing continuing stress. Less than 5 percent of obese patients have the "binge eating syndrome," characterized by a subjective sense of compulsion and the eating of large amounts of food, usually in the setting of an identified stressful precipitant. Finally, eating without satiation is often associated with neurologic damage.

Weight loss after ileal bypass surgery is usually accompanied by improved psychological state, including improved mood, increased self-esteem,[201] and decreased food intake. Thus, psychological distress, such as depression and anxiety, which often occurs during weight loss from dieting, may be more related to the accompanying severe hunger than to the weight loss itself.

OBESITY SECONDARY TO MEDICAL ILLNESS

Central Nervous System Diseases

Obesity associated with central nervous system disease is generally mediated by destructive lesions in the ventromedial nucleus of the hypothalamus. Both hyperphagia and reduced activity may play a role in hypothalamic obesity. Solid tumors, particularly craniopharyngiomas, are the most common lesion. Inflammatory diseases or trauma may also produce hypothalamic obesity. While uncommon, obesity may also result from increased intraventricular pressure.

Several genetic disorders of the central nervous system are associated with obesity. The syndrome of idiopathic adiposogenital dystrophy consists of early childhood obesity and genital hypoplasia. It has been incorrectly called the Fröhlich syndrome, which originally referred to obesity, retarded growth, and genital hypoplasia associated with a hypothalamic tumor. The Prader-Willi syndrome consists of moderate to extreme obesity, beginning early in life, extreme hyperphagia, short stature, hypotonia, hypogonadism, small hands and feet, and mental retardation. The insatiable feeding behavior of these patients, as well as the medical consequences of their obesity, causes their families to bring these patients to physicians. They appear extremely sensitive to the effects of haloperidol or the phenothiazines, which are occa-

sionally used to control their behavior, and they may develop a delirious state even when given small doses.

Endocrine Disorders

Although many patients ask physicians if their obesity is due to an endocrine problem, relatively few people develop obesity on this basis. In hypothyroidism, added adipose tissue and myxedema fluid may contribute to weight gain, but few hypothyroid patients are truly obese. Obesity occurs commonly in Cushing syndrome, but the central distribution of fat in these patients is a distinguishing feature. Significant obesity results only occasionally from the hyperphagia caused by high insulin levels in patients with an insulinoma. A similar mechanism may contribute to the maintenance of obesity in adult-onset diabetics treated with insulin. Although eunuchoid males, and women with the Stein-Leventhal syndrome, tend to be obese, gonadal deficiency is not a common cause of obesity.

Iatrogenic Obesity

Obesity may result from prescribed medical treatments. Neuroleptic agents, such as phenothiazines and butyrophenones (haloperidol), used to treat schizophrenia and other disorders, are often associated with weight gain.[198] Tricyclic antidepressants not only improve the anorexia often accompanying the depressed phase of manic-depressive illness, but may in addition promote excessive weight gain. Corticosteroids, in high doses, may produce Cushing syndrome with severe obesity. Women using birth control pills may gain weight for a variety of reasons, including increased appetite and fluid retention. Cyproheptadine, a serotonin and histamine antagonist, promotes weight gain, but to a lesser degree than the steroids or neuroleptics.

Prescribed diets may lead to obesity when the total calories exceed the patient's nutritional requirements. Some physicians still prescribe frequent small feedings of bland foods, especially dairy products, for peptic ulcer disease, and obesity may result. Frequent small meals are often recommended for gastroesophageal reflux, especially for hiatal hernia, and also for reactive hypoglycemia, often diagnosed for nonspecific symptoms in young women.

Other Medical Disorders Associated with Obesity

Adiposis dolorosa (Dercum's disease) is a disorder of painful irregular masses of subcutaneous fat, peripheral neuropathy, endocrine adenomas, and sometimes generalized obesity. In addition, several lipodystrophies are characterized by regional lipid deposits, for example in the legs, with deficiency of fat of the trunk, arms, and cheeks.

MEDICAL CONSEQUENCES OF OBESITY

Although serious limitations are recognized in the data, life insurance statistics show an association between obesity and early mortality, especially when obesity is marked. As indicated in Table 73–1, a number of diseases occur with increased frequency in obese subjects. Moreover, the presence of obesity complicates the management and diminishes the likelihood of recovery from many other illnesses. On the average, the frequency and severity of medical complications are proportional to the degree of obesity.

Extreme adiposity in the thoracic and abdominal regions can interfere with the mechanics of ventilation to the extent that cardiorespiratory failure occurs. This is referred to as Pickwickian syndrome characterized by alveolar hypoventilation with extreme obesity. The clinical features of this syndrome are obesity, somnolence, periodic breathing, cyanosis, secondary polycythemia, right ventricular hypertrophy, and cor pulmonale. Prompt recognition of this syndrome is imperative since sudden respiratory arrest commonly occurs in the presence of an apparently stable clinical condition. In addition to weight reduction and therapy for cardiac failure, other measures should be taken especially if CO_2 narcosis is present. The patient must be closely observed and vigorous attempts made to keep the patient awake and breathing. Controlled oxygen administration is frequently necessary; if severe hypoxemia persists, artificial respiration should be employed. A greater willingness to employ artificial respiratory therapy in recent years has reduced the mortality of this syndrome.[193] The usefulness of respiratory stimulants such as aminophylline is uncertain. Prophylactic anticoagulant therapy is recommended.

EVALUATION OF THE PATIENT WITH OBESITY

The physician should carry out a complete medical and psychological history, physical examination, and appropriate laboratory studies. Table 73–2 presents a suggested evaluation which integrates medical, psychological, and behavioral factors. The following areas should receive special attention.

Medical

The weight history of the patient allows delineation of the pattern of weight gain and differentiation between early- and late-onset obesity. Though seldom present, medical diseases which cause obesity should be carefully excluded. Identification of medical complications of obesity helps to document expected changes with treatment and may motivate the patient to follow a plan of therapy.

Psychological

An understanding of the psychological history of patients is essential to the treatment of their obesity. Important considerations include their strengths and vulnerabilities, psychiatric symptoms, psychotropic medications, use of food to alleviate dysphoric need states or as a reward, and appreciation of the daily life situation, including marriage, family, occupation, and financial status. After their motivation and insight are assessed, the benefits and hazards of weight reduction should be frankly discussed.

General Considerations

Upon completion of the history and examination, and before the initiation of treatment, conclusions should be reached regarding the following:

1. Obesity vs. simple overweight
2. Type of obesity
3. The patient's rationale for losing weight
4. Presence or absence of severe medical or psychological symptoms secondary to excess weight
5. Degree of medical concern for weight loss, i.e., medically urgent (severe congestive heart failure, respiratory failure), medically beneficial (adult-onset diabetes mellitus), or psychologically beneficial (demoralization, social stigmatization, job disability)

TABLE 73–1
Complications of Obesity*

Pulmonary	Pickwickian syndrome
	Respiratory tract infections
Cardiovascular	Hypertension
	Coronary artery disease
	Congestive heart failure
	Varicose veins
Endocrine and metabolic	Diabetes mellitus
	Amenorrhea
	Hirsutism
	Fatty liver
	Hypertriglyceridemia
Gastrointestinal	Cholecystitis and cholelithiasis
Psychiatric and social problems	Dyspepsia
Miscellaneous	Skin infections
	Osteoarthritis
	Toxema of pregnancy

* More than 20 percent overweight.

TABLE 73-2
Suggested Work-Up of Obesity*

	Medical	Psychological	Behavioral
Weight and food	Weight at birth, 1 year, 1st grade, puberty, high school graduation, and each decade thereafter	Chart age of significant events (marriage, pregnancy, etc.)	History of eating patterns, especially in response to stress and depression
	Note age of onset of obesity and chart serial weights	Significant current stresses (job, family, children, finances)	Note if specific behavioral syndromes of eating are present
	Results of previous attempts at dieting		
Etiologic factors	Weight of parents at age 25 and currently	Use of food as a reward or as treatment of dysphoric states	Activity level
	History of diabetes mellitus		Family and cultural patterns of eating
	Use of weight-producing medications, alcohol intake		
Examinations	Weight, height, skin fold thickness	Assessment of patient's personality	Examine records of patient's food intake, time of day, location, mood state, ongoing events
	Medical causes of obesity	Presence of depression, anxiety	If possible, observe patient eating a meal
	Medical consequences of obesity (congestive heart failure, hypertension, osteoarthritis, etc.)	Estimation of insight, motivation for weight loss	
Laboratory	Appropriate endocrine tests	General Health Questionnaire, SCL–90, or other assessment of psychological symptoms	

* The suggested work-up should be used in addition to a thorough medical and psychiatric history, physical examination, and laboratory studies.

6. The patient's psychological preparedness for weight reduction
7. Choice of the optimal method of treatment, considering the urgency of weight loss, severity of obesity, and physical and psychological state of the patient

If simple dietary limitation with exercise, behavioral relearning, and an ethical weight reduction organization have not been successful, consideration should be given to pharmacologic, surgical, or behavioral methods to produce weight loss.

TREATMENT OF SECONDARY OBESITY

The treatment of secondary obesity focuses on management of the underlying medical disorder rather than on treatment of the obesity itself. Some nonremediable disorders, such as the Prader-Willi syndrome, may respond to a limitation of food intake and the prescription of fenfluramine.[185] The physician should also be alert to the weight-producing tendencies of prescribed medications or dietary regimens.

TREATMENT OF MILD-TO-MODERATE OBESITY

Mild-to-moderate obesity may require no treatment unless accompanied by a medical disorder worsened by the presence of obesity or associated with persisting demoralization related to the weight. Even if treatment is desirable, there is little evidence that medical doctors produce better results than ethical lay organizations, such as Weight Watchers or TOPS (Take Off Pounds Sensibly). Nonetheless, physicians are often called on to treat this class of obese patients.

The goals in the treatment of mild-to-moderate obesity are listed in Table 73–3. All too often attention is focused on the weight loss itself rather than on long-term maintenance of weight loss. In fact, temporary weight decrease can be accomplished by a wide variety of means, but maintained by very few. Table

┌───┐
TABLE 73–3

Goals in the Treatment of Mild-to-Moderate Obesity

I. Medical and Behavioral
A. Weight loss to within 15 percent of Ideal Body Weight
B. Loss of adipose tissue rather than muscle mass
C. Long-term maintenance of weight loss
D. Improved nutritional understanding
E. Increased physical activity
F. More healthy patterns of eating behavior

II. Psychological
A. Avoid psychological distress of unphysiologic diet methods
B. Acceptance of a different body image and changes in social functioning resulting from weight loss
C. Eliminate the use of food as a type of medication for psychological distress
└───┘

73–3 emphasizes goals related to maintenance of weight loss.

The essential feature of ordinary programs for weight loss is reduction in calories below the amount required for energy expenditure. To maintain weight with only basal activity, an average adult needs 1500 to 1800 calories per day. Ordinary physical activity or a cold environment increases this need to approximately 2500 calories per day. Therefore, mild or moderate food restriction, to 1200 to 1500 or 900 to 1200 calories, respectively, with ordinary physical activity will promote gradual weight loss. It is seldom effective to provide a patient with general advice to ingest a certain number of calories. Instead specific instructions are needed, such as:

1. Printed or preferably personal instruction from a dietitian about the major food groups required for adequate nutrition
2. A diary of food eaten, time of day, location, and emotional state, in order to increase accountability and obtain a pattern of eating behavior
3. A printed sample menu with a week of meals

An approximate, but useful, rule of thumb is that about 15 calories per pound are necessary to maintain weight. Therefore, one method of calculating a diet is to multiply the desired weight by 15 and begin that number of calories. For example, a woman who begins an 1800-calorie diet at any weight above 120 will asymptotically approach 120 pounds.

Foods with lower density and increased nonabsorbable residue, such as whole grains, vegetables, and fruits result in a more rapid transit time through the intestinal tract. This principle reflects the previously mentioned finding that gastric control of caloric metering breaks down with very concentrated fats or sugars.

Moderate exercise (for example, a half-hour brisk walk a day) plus encouragement of a generally less sedentary life-style is a valuable adjunct to calorie control. The insulin resistance of obese individuals diminishes with exercise even before weight falls. Exercise helps to prevent the undesirable loss of muscle mass during weight loss. Finally, a moderate increase in physical activity, if calories are not increased proportionately, will help maintain weight loss over a long period of time.

Some patients pursue weight reduction through strenuous exercise. Young women, often joggers, who decrease their percentage of body fat significantly, even without a change in weight, may develop amenorrhea. Body weight in general, and percentage of lipid tissue in particular, must exceed specific limits for menses to occur.[188]

A few principles of behavioral relearning can be accomplished without specialized consultation with behavioral therapists. These general principles include: 1) eating more slowly, noting the taste of each bite of food; and 2) eating in a specified place with a full place setting and no distracting activities. Obese people eat less when they can see themselves during a meal.

Patients may be discouraged when the loss of several pounds, largely water, in the first week is followed by a significantly slower rate of weight loss. They should be informed about this sequence so that they will expect modest continued weight loss. Likewise, when patients discontinue a diet, they may initially experience a sudden gain of several pounds from water retention. If they are aware of these facts, and especially if they begin a maintenance diet a few pounds below their weight goal, they will be less surprised and discouraged.

TREATMENT OF SEVERE TO EXTREME OBESITY

Dietary

Prolonged complete fasting effectively lowers weight in the morbidly obese, but a year later 80 percent of patients have regained their former weight or more. In addition to its ineffectiveness, prolonged fasting may cause multiple medical complications, including ketosis, weakness, renolithiasis, vitamin deficiencies, and negative nitrogen balance. Small quantities of high-quality dietary protein will spare tissue protein dissolution during fasting, but the process still is accompanied by an apparent increase in cardiomyopathy and sudden death. Moreover, fasting provides no long-term learning of improved patterns of nutrition and eating behavior. Nonetheless, fasting may have a role in cases of obesity associated with severe medical complications when accomplished as part of a supervised inpatient program, with adequate hydration, electrolyte replacement, and vitamins. Liquid protein diets are especially hazardous.

Diets that stress a single item, i.e., protein, fat, or specific foods such as brown rice or grapefruit are medically dangerous, only temporarily effective, and usually unpalatable, and they produce no long-term learning of improved nutritional patterns.

Pharmacologic

Several anorexic pharmacologic agents produce weight loss, but none, except possibly fenfluramine and its congeners, have a safe and proven role in the treatment of obesity.[203] If fenfluramine is used, blood levels should be obtained regularly to insure correct dosage. The amphetamines cause anorexia, but rebound hyperphagia after cessation may negate their effects. Psychiatric sequelae of chronic amphetamines include dependence, depression, hallucinations, and delusions. Methylphenidate is similarly contraindicated.

Various ineffective, over-the-counter preparations employ the mild anorexic side effects of caffeine and sympathomimetic agents.

Thyroid medication reduces weight by accelerating metabolism and causing the loss of a high percentage of muscle mass as weight falls. Diuretics produce spurious weight loss by removing fluids, at the cost of electrolyte abnormalities, without changing adipose tissue mass.

Surgical Procedures

Several surgical procedures have been attempted for the treatment of obesity. The most common indications are chronic morbid obesity, intractable to several years of dietary management, the presence of significant medical symptoms that will not improve without weight loss, and continuing demoralization due to excess weight.

The most widely used procedure, intestinal bypass, is an end-to-side jejunoileal anastomosis which connects 14 inches of jejunum to 4 inches of ileum. The procedure has produced loss of more than half of the original weight in 15 percent of patients, and a third of body weight in a larger percentage. Weight reduction results from both the expected malabsorp-

tion and from diminished food ingestion without an apparent change in appetite. Decreased hypertension, improved glucose tolerance, and profound falls in serum lipids have resulted. Unfortunately, in one series, 58 percent of patients experienced either a life-threatening complication or required surgical revision.[191] The most serious complication is liver dysfunction from progressive fatty metamorphosis and fibrosis, leading to hepatic encephalopathy and/or ascites, peripheral edema, and hypoprothrombinemia. Other common complications are cholelithiasis, nephrolithiasis, arthralgias, nausea and vomiting, diarrhea, electrolyte disturbances, general weakness, and neuromyopathy. The mortality in several series is around 5 percent.

A more promising procedure is the gastric bypass where the upper 10 percent of the stomach is connected to the small intestine through a 1.5 cm channel.[196] The incidence of stomal ulcers is only about 2 percent, and almost no diarrhea results. Liver function improves rather than worsens. Median weight loss is 36 percent. The operating time is considerably longer than for the ileal bypass, and mortality (19 percent) is high for patients over 50 years of age. A longer follow-up is needed to evaluate the true results of this operation, but it should be considered for patients with morbid obesity.

A variety of this gastric operation is the gastroplasty, in which the stomach is narrowed into a small channel with sutures in the middle. Operating time is less than with the gastric bypass, but results are more variable because the channel may either be too wide to be effective or so narrow that obstruction results.

PREVENTION OF OBESITY

Wherever possible, good medical practice stresses prevention rather than treatment. The nutrition of infants is a balance between avoidance of adipocyte hyperplasia and the dangers of overly restrictive diets. Thirty-six percent of infants in the 90th percentile of weight or greater become overweight adults. In contrast, only 14 percent of those who are average or below average in weight as infants become obese adults.

In most cases, treatment of overweight infants is best postponed until after 1 year of age. Although the use of skim milk appears to be a healthy dietary habit, it should be avoided too early in life because of its low fat content, unphysiologically high concentration of protein, and excessive solute load. Beginning at about 1 year of age, however, a gradual transition may be started to dairy products with reduced fat content. Especially to be encouraged is the use of social praise for good nutritional habits, the avoidance of concentrated sweets and fats, and the use of food for nutritional purposes only, rather than as a reward for good conduct or a substitute for affection.

During childhood, realistic teaching of "survival skills" in fast food chains is helpful. Adolescents have special needs because of the social pressures to conform to idiosyncratic patterns of eating. The fact that 80 percent of obese adolescents become obese adults emphasizes the need for attention to weight problems of adolescence.

ANOREXIA NERVOSA

The syndrome of anorexia nervosa is most common in adolescent women whose profound weight loss is associated with fear of fatness and amenorrhea. The disorder was clearly defined in 19th-century societies which did not value slimness. Thus, the current emphasis on slimness may have increased the incidence of anorexia nervosa, but its fundamental basis is more than a cultural fad.

Anorexia nervosa is a serious disorder. The mortality is 5 to 15 percent, and considerable morbidity results from both emaciation and the abnormal behavior of these patients. The urgency to make a correct diagnosis is highlighted not only by the serious consequences of the disorder but also by its potentially treatable nature. Patients with anorexia nervosa usually present to internists and family doctors, rather than to psychiatrists, with medical symptoms. The multiple guises of the disorder lead to referrals to various specialists. Gynecologists are often consulted for secondary amenorrhea. Physically active, thin, intense young women may present to endocrinologists with hyperthyroidism as a presumed explanation of their weight loss. Gastroenterologists consider malabsorption and often carry out a full radiologic evaluation of the gastrointestinal tract. Neurologists are consulted for symptoms that suggest a hypothalamic tumor.

Diagnosis

The diagnosis of anorexia nervosa (Table 73–4) should be based on the clinical presentation and direct examination of the patient's mental state. Medical illness must be excluded, but failure to recognize the characteristic features of anorexia nervosa often leads to unnecessary tests and considerable delay in diagnosis. Early diagnosis and treatment improves the outcome by decreasing the time during which symptoms become firmly and chronically fixed. The three essential diagnostic criteria are:

1. Significant weight loss that is self-induced and unexplained by medical illness or other psychiatric disorders, usually in a woman 10 to 30 years of age, but occasionally in older individuals, and in males in about 10 percent of cases[184]
2. Fear of losing control of eating and becoming fat
3. Amenorrhea. Diagnostic criteria are presented in more detail in Table 73–4.

When these diagnostic criteria are used, a medical disorder is rarely if ever found to explain weight loss.

Clinical Presentation

The typical adolescent patient with anorexia nervosa starts to diet when 5 to 10 kg overweight. As the diet proceeds, the patient seeks ever lower weights and becomes increasingly fearful of losing control and becoming overweight. Many, but not all, patients have

---

TABLE 73–4
Criteria for Diagnosis of Anorexia Nervosa

A. Onset between the age of 10 and 30

B. Weight loss of at least 20% of original body weight

C. A distorted attitude toward eating, food, or weight, for example:
1. Fear of fatness, especially associated with fear of loss of control of eating
2. Desire to produce lower and lower body weight, especially associated with change in body image manifested by thin or cachectic patients considering themselves normal or overweight
3. Denial of illness and nutritional needs
4. Preoccupation with thoughts of food, and increased food-related activities
5. Unusual behavior related to food: secretive disposal, hoarding, food fads, starvation, extreme limitation of calories, or self-induced vomiting

D. Amenorrhea

E. At least one of the following:
1. Excessive physical activity
2. Food binges
3. Use of diuretics or laxatives to lower weight
4. Bradycardia
5. Lanugo hair

F. No known prior medical illness associated with significant weight loss

G. No known prior psychiatric illness of which serious weight loss is a regular symptom, especially:
1. Primary depressive illness
2. Obsessive-compulsive disorders
3. Schizophrenia with delusions related to eating

the perceptual distortion that they are normal or overweight even when emaciated. Weight loss is induced by a variety of techniques. More than half of patients simply decrease their caloric intake. They first eliminate foods with a high sugar or fat content, then decrease all foods, and finally reach weights as low as 25 kg. They often assist the weight loss by strenuous exercise; as a consequence, they appear more energetic than patients who attain low weights through medical illness. Diuretic or laxative abuse in some patients may produce severe hypokalemic alkalosis. Serum potassium levels below 2 mEq/L may occasionally lead to cardiac arrest. Some eat normal, or even greatly excessive amounts of food, but induce vomiting which may add severe metabolic abnormalities to their weight loss. Anorexia-producing drugs are rarely employed.

The end results of starvation, bingeing, vomiting, exercising, and abuse of medications produce a variety of confusing manifestations which are a blend from four different origins. The direct effects of starvation may produce hypotension, inanition, hypothermia, anemia, weakness, difficulty in intellectual concentration, and constipation. The particular means of inducing weight loss confer other symptoms, for example, the hypokalemia of diuretic abuse or vomiting. The reduced weight of patients with anorexia nervosa makes them more vulnerable to certain medical disorders. They often respond poorly to mycotic or bacterial infections, but are surprisingly resistant to viral infections. Lastly, and speculatively, certain symptoms may be unique to anorexia nervosa. This possibility is suggested by the fact that about one-third of women with anorexia nervosa lose their menses before their weight falls. Extensive endocrinologic investigations by Vigersky[204] suggest that the dysfunction in temperature control and the partial diabetes insipidus of these patients may be unique. Bradycardia, found in most patients, appears to result from a combination of factors: the decreased activity of the sympathetic nervous system common in starvation, extreme exercise, and perhaps a factor specific for anorexia nervosa since the bradycardia is especially prominent in these patients. Other studies, however, conclude that all symptoms are due to starvation.

Etiology

The cause of anorexia nervosa is unknown, but it is probably multifactorial in origin. Most adolescent women patients have a perfectionistic and sensitive temperament before illness, but they are not introspective. They are often model students and children as evidenced by high grades, obedience, and compli-

ance toward parents. The highest incidence of anorexia nervosa occurs in families of upper-middle socioeconomic status. Only a few cases have been reported among non-Caucasians. Some experts believe that the family is the primary cause of anorexia nervosa, but this hypothesis has not been borne out empirically. However, the families are often stressed by internal or external conflicts, such as divorce, separation, or a change of location. Compared to controls, the families of these patients have a greater frequency of weight disorders.[190] In the absence of convincing etiologic data, it is presently best to view the disorder as occurring when weight loss from dieting (occasionally from a medical illness or romantic disappointment) occurs in a person with vulnerable temperament, stressed family, and perhaps preexisting dysfunction of biologic regulation. Although clear evidence for a hypothalamic origin has not been found, hypothalamic and pituitary consequences of anorexia nervosa are well documented (see Chap. 69).

Treatment

All treatment programs seem to work better when patients are younger, less severely ill, acutely rather than chronically ill, motivated to improve, and have a relatively normal temperament and family structure before the onset of illness. The prognosis is less favorable in those with atypical features, such as maleness, older age of onset, and the presence of more severe and enduring features of illness. In addition to weight gain, goals for treatment include achieving a relative absence of preoccupation with food and weight, normal menstrual function, return to school or work, and good working relationships with parents or other family members.

A variety of treatment approaches has been tried, but none has been uniformly successful. Strict psychoanalytic psychotherapy, independent of weight gain, has been classically used without demonstrable improvement in weight or psychological function. Strict behavior modification, based on rewarding weight gain in a systematic way, produces short-term weight gain, but long-term benefits are unknown. The phenothiazines, tricyclic antidepressants, and to some extent cyproheptadine encourage weight gain, but stimulation of appetite without alleviating the fear of fatness may produce only increased distress in patients with anorexia nervosa where there is no true loss of appetite. Nonetheless, these medications may be helpful in selected patients. Family therapy is currently employed by those who believe that the etiology is familial, but it is not clear that results are superior with this method.

Perhaps the most effective management employs an empirical team approach to this multifactorial disorder of unknown origin. Four stages are involved, beginning with nutritional rehabilitation which employs 24-hour nursing care but no nasogastric tubes or intravenous alimentation. On rare occasions, such treatment may be necessary in patients with life-threatening inanition. Psychological treatment is not effective in the very starved person; concentration is poor and symptoms result from a mixture of starvation and pertinent psychological issues. During this period, exercise is limited and the patient's nutritional needs are prescribed like medication. After nutritional status has improved, individualized psychotherapy is begun. The issues discussed in individual, group, and family therapy arise from the individual's personality, life situation, and experiences rather than from a theoretical construct. The next stage of therapy attempts to return the control for food, weight, and exercise to the patient's own choice. This period provides a chance for the patient to practice, under supervision and with encouragement, the information learned and explored in the second stage of treatment. Finally, the patient is followed after leaving the hospital. Reintroduction of the patient to the environment that spawned the initial symptoms results in predictable stresses and, occasionally, a return to the previous symptoms. Close follow-up and attention to structured programs of everyday activities and eating schedules increase the probability of maintained improvement.

Prognosis

Although mortality and morbidity are decreased when the disorder is recognized quickly and treated appropriately, few patients recover completely.[195] Most are substantially improved by treatment but are left with some continuing preoccupation with issues of food and weight, especially at times of stress. Menses may not return until the patient's weight exceeds by several kg her weight at the menarche; sometimes amenorrhea persists for months after the attainment of normal weight. Between 25 and 35 percent of patients remain chronically ill, with lowered weight and severe psychological distress.

CHAPTER 74

Hyperlipidemia
SIMEON MARGOLIS

The primary clinical manifestation of hyperlipidemia, defined as an elevation of serum cholesterol and/or triglycerides, is premature atherosclerotic vascular disease. In addition, severe hypertriglyceridemia may cause recurrent attacks of acute pancreatitis. Xanthelasma and cutaneous and tendinous xanthomas, the only nonlaboratory clues to the presence of hyperlipidemia, may pose cosmetic problems.

The major serum lipids, cholesterol, cholesterol esters, triglycerides, and phospholipids, are all transported in combination with proteins to form the serum lipoproteins. Hyperlipidemia is always associated with an increased concentration of one or more of these lipoproteins (hyperlipoproteinemia). As a guide to therapy, it is useful to identify the type of hyperlipoproteinemia by determining which lipoproteins are present in excess.

LIPOPROTEIN NOMENCLATURE AND COMPOSITION (Table 74-1)[215,217]

The serum lipoproteins are named from their density properties during ultracentrifugation or from their mobility on electrophoresis. Lipoproteins with the most lipids have the lowest density; as the percentage of lipid decreases and protein increases, the lipoproteins become more dense. Based on these principles, four classes of lipoproteins have been separated by ultracentrifugation (Table 74-1). Largest and least dense are the chylomicrons; progressively smaller in size and greater in density are the very low density (VLDL), low density (LDL), and high density (HDL) lipoproteins. The common clinical use of lipoprotein electrophoresis has led to a second nomenclature for the lipoproteins based on their electrophoretic mobility. VLDL is identical with pre-β, LDL with β, and HDL with α lipoproteins.

Each lipoprotein has a characteristic composition (Table 74-1). Triglycerides are the major component of chylomicrons (85 to 90 percent) and VLDL (55 to 65 percent). Cholesterol, about two-thirds as esters, comprises about half of LDL. Except for chylomicrons, each lipoprotein contains about 20 percent phospholipids. The protein content varies from about 2 percent in chylomicrons to 50 percent in HDL. Recently, investigators have purified and sequenced most of the protein components, or apoproteins, each

―TABLE 74-1―
Lipoprotein Classes[214,215]

Density Classification	Electrophoretic Mobility	Components (%)	Apolipoproteins (%)	Important Features
Chylomicrons	Remain at origin	Triglycerides 85–95, derived from dietary fat	Apo A—12 Apo B—22 Apo C—66	Float if refrigerated overnight
		Cholesterol 2–7		Synthesized in intestinal mucosal cells to transport dietary fat
		Phospholipid 3–6 Protein 1–2		Not present after overnight fast in normal individuals
Very low density lipoprotein (VLDL)	Pre-beta	Triglycerides 55–65, derived from endogenous synthesis Cholesterol 10–15 Phospholipids 15–20 Proteins 5–10	Apo A—5 Apo B—35 Apo C—50 Apo-glu Apo-ser Apo-ala	Synthesized mainly in the liver, to transport triglycerides formed from fatty acids and carbohydrates, but also in the intestine Apo-glu is activator of the enzyme lipoprotein lipase
			Apo E(arginine-rich)—10	
Low density lipoprotein (LDL)	Beta	Triglycerides 15 Cholesterol 45 Phospholipids 20 Protein 20	Apo B	Mainly arises from breakdown of VLDL in the circulation
High density lipoproteins (HDL)	Alpha	Triglycerides 5 Cholesterol 15 Phospholipids 30 Proteins 50	Apo A 95 Apo-Gln-I—75 Apo-Gln-II—25 Apo C-s	Apo-Gln-I is activator of LCAT enzyme May transport cholesterol from peripheral tissues to liver

named by its C-terminal amino acid. The apoprotein content differs in each lipoprotein class. HDL contains the two Apo A peptides, Apo-Gln-I and Apo-Gln-II. The peptide of LDL is termed Apo B. VLDL has the most complex composition. The small Apo C peptides comprise about half its protein mass, while Apo B, Apo A, and Apo E comprise 35, 5, and 10 percent of VLDL protein, respectively. Apo A and Apo C peptides exchange readily between HDL, VLDL, and chylomicrons.

Chylomicrons are synthesized exclusively in the intestine. Although the liver is the main site for VLDL and HDL production, both of these lipoproteins are also formed in the intestine. LDL arises primarily through the catabolism of VLDL.

PHYSIOLOGY OF LIPID TRANSPORT
(Figs. 74-1, 74-2)[207,208]

Almost all cells can synthesize cholesterol, but its major sites of synthesis are the liver and intestinal mucosa. Between 300 and 500 mg of cholesterol per day are absorbed from the usual American diet. He-

patic cholesterol synthesis is reduced by dietary cholesterol and stimulated by interruption of the enterohepatic recirculation of bile acids, such as by T-tube drainage of bile or cholestyramine treatment. Cholesterol is eliminated from the body only by the liver. Excretion is achieved by direct secretion into the bile and by hepatic conversion of cholesterol to bile acids, which is stimulated by thyroid hormone. Cholesterol is an important component of cell membranes, the precursor of steroid hormones, and an essential structural component of the circulating lipoproteins.

Triglyceride transport is the major recognized function of the serum lipoproteins; chylomicrons carry triglycerides from the intestine and VLDL transports triglycerides from the liver. The major digestion products of dietary triglycerides, fatty acids and monoglycerides, are resynthesized to triglycerides within mucosal cells of the small intestine. These triglycerides are combined with small amounts of other lipids and proteins to form chylomicrons. Endogenous triglycerides are synthesized mainly in the liver

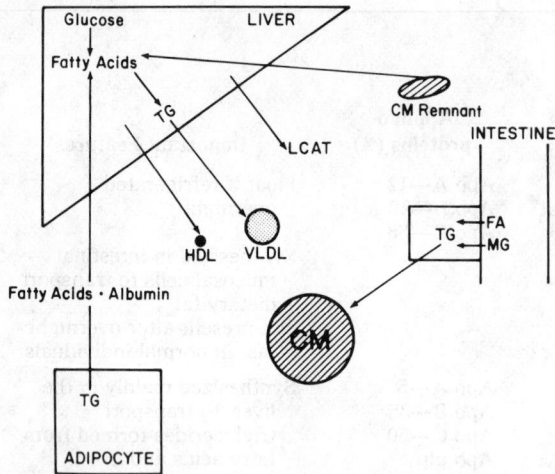

FIGURE 74-1. Overall scheme for lipoprotein formation. Ingested fats are broken down in the intestinal lumen to form fatty acids (FA) and monoglycerides (MG) which are absorbed into the mucosal cell. Triglycerides (TG) are resynthesized and released into the lymphatics on chylomicrons (CM) which enter the general circulation. Removal of TG in peripheral tissues (see Fig. 74-2) converts CM to CM remnants which are removed by the liver. Following a meal, hepatic FA, derived from CM remnants and synthesized from glucose, are used to form TG. During fasting periods, FA released from adipose tissue are the source of hepatic TG. TG are released from the liver on VLDL. The intestine also synthesizes VLDL and HDL, though both lipoproteins are primarily formed in the liver, which also secretes LCAT.

Lipoprotein lipase requires Apo-Glu for activation. After triglyceride removal, VLDL and chylomicrons contain redundant cholesterol and phospholipids on their surface. Working together, HDL and the enzyme lecithin:cholesterol acyltransferase (LCAT), released into the blood from the liver, form cholesterol esters and lysolecithin from the excess cholesterol and lecithin, which are thus removed from the surface of chylomicrons and VLDL. The action of LCAT promotes a structural rearrangement of the lipoprotein, which allows further triglyceride removal by lipoprotein lipase. The concerted action of these two enzymes produces chylomicron "remnants" which are rapidly removed from the circulation by the liver. These enzymatic reactions, accompanied by the loss of the Apo A and Apo C peptides, also convert VLDL to LDL (Fig. 74-2). Thus, LDL mostly arises as a product of VLDL catabolism; it is not known whether LDL is secreted as such by the liver. LDL functions to control the rate of cholesterol synthesis and esterification in some tissues.

Recent evidence suggests that HDL is secreted from both liver and intestine as a "nascent" lipoprotein that is disc-shaped and has a high ratio of phospholipids to cholesterol.[213] The newly formed HDL picks up cholesterol from peripheral tissues and transports it to the liver for excretion. Apo-Gln I of HDL also activates LCAT. The combination of added

from fatty acid sources that vary with the dietary state of the individual. Postprandially, fatty acids are derived mainly from de novo hepatic synthesis from carbohydrates as well as from chylomicron triglycerides. Hepatic fatty acid synthesis is enhanced by dietary carbohydrates, alcohol intake, and elevated insulin levels. During fasting, unesterified fatty acids, bound to serum albumin after release from the adipose stores, are the major energy source for most tissues except the brain. When their mobilization greatly exceeds energy demands, much of the fatty acids are esterified to form triglycerides in the liver. Triglycerides are exported from the liver bound to VLDL (see Fig. 74-1). Failure of lipoprotein synthesis or excessive movement of fatty acids to the liver may produce fatty liver.

Circulating triglycerides may be stored in adipose tissue or utilized directly as an energy source by peripheral tissues, such as muscle. The enzyme lipoprotein lipase, located in the capillary endothelium of adipose tissue and muscle, splits circulating triglycerides into their constituent fatty acids and thus removes triglycerides from chylomicrons and VLDL.

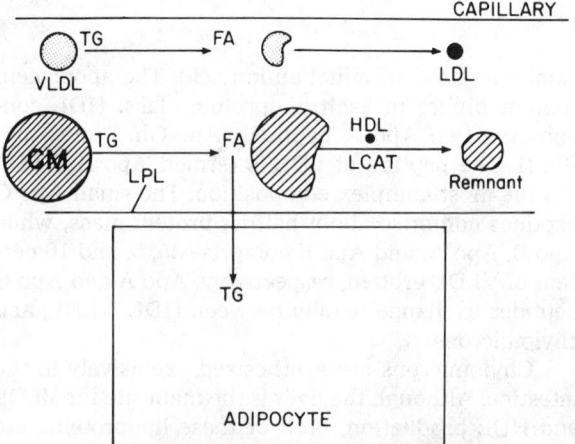

FIGURE 74-2. Chylomicron (CM) and VLDL metabolism in peripheral tissues. As CM and VLDL traverse adipose tissue (or muscle), lipoprotein lipase (LPL) bound to the capillaries splits their triglycerides (TG) to form glycerol and fatty acids (FA). FA enter the adipocyte where TG are resynthesized. LCAT and HDL together remove excess cholesterol and phospholipids from the surface of the lipoprotein. In concert, LPL and LCAT convert CM to CM remnants and VLDL to LDL.

cholesterol and LCAT action converts discoidal HDL to a larger spherical particle. HDL may exert its protective effects against atherosclerosis by partially blocking the uptake of LDL cholesterol by endothelial or smooth muscle cells of large arteries. Large amounts of dietary cholesterol produce HDL_c, an abnormal HDL which contains apo E and excessive cholesterol.[218]

The regulation of serum lipoprotein levels is complex. Synthesis may be altered by factors which influence availability or production of lipids, formation of the peptide portion of the lipoprotein, coupling of lipid to peptide, or secretion of the completed lipoprotein. The removal of lipoproteins from the serum involves metabolism of both the lipid and protein portions of the molecule. Although the precise pathogenesis is unknown for many forms of hyperlipidemia, as indicated later, considerable progress has been made in Type I hyperlipoproteinemia and in familial hypercholesterolemia. In general, hyperlipidemia must result from either increased synthesis or diminished removal of serum lipoproteins and their constituent lipids. The complex nature of lipoprotein metabolism and the hormonal regulation exerted at several steps may account for the frequency of secondary hyperlipoproteinemia as a complication of other diseases.

CLASSIFICATION OF HYPERLIPIDEMIA (Table 74-2)[208]

One popular classification proposed by Fredrickson and co-workers,[208] has used the electrophoretic separation of lipoproteins to delineate five general types of hyperlipoproteinemia. Each results from increased serum concentrations of chylomicrons, VLDL or LDL, either alone or in combination. The structure and composition of the lipoproteins are normal in each of the hyperlipoproteinemias except Type III ("broad beta disease") in which patients accumulate an abnormal lipoprotein, probably an intermediate in the conversion of VLDL to LDL. Elevated HDL levels have not been reported as a cause of hyperlipidemia.

An isolated elevation of chylomicrons is designated Type I. Type II, characterized by increased concentrations of LDL, is divided into two distinct subtypes. In Type IIA, only cholesterol and LDL levels are increased. Type IIB patients, in addition, have hypertriglyceridemia due to an elevated concentration of VLDL. Hypertriglyceridemia results from increased levels of VLDL alone in Type IV and both VLDL and chylomicrons in Type V. The salient features of each type of hyperlipoproteinemia are outlined in Table 74-2.

Although assignment of the correct type for each involved subject is an aid to appropriate prognosis and management, each type may be caused by any one of several different genetic defects or represent a secondary manifestation of various disease states. Classification is further complicated by changes in the lipoprotein pattern as a consequence of treatment with diet or hypolipidemic agent, administration of certain drugs, and several endocrine abnormalities. In addition, some genetic disorders may produce different patterns in members of the same family. Thus, a Type IIA parent with familial hypercholesterolemia may have affected children with either Type IIA or IIB patterns. Combined hyperlipidemia, in which affected family members may have either Type IIA, IIB, IV, or V patterns, may be the most common form of familial hyperlipidemia.[212] Familial Types II and IV are also fairly common in the United States, occurring with an estimated frequency of 0.1 to 0.2 and 0.2 percent, respectively.

The clinical clues that lead to a suspicion of hyperlipidemia include the presence of xanthomas, premature coronary or peripheral vascular disease, recurrent pancreatitis, and a family history of hyperlipidemia. Xanthelasmas are the most common indicators of Type II, but about 60 percent of patients with xanthelasma have normal serum lipids. Patients with Type II may also have premature arcus senilis and tendinous xanthomas, which are almost always indicative of familial hypercholesterolemia. Type III is characterized by planar xanthomas in the palmar creases. Tuberous xanthomas can occur in Types II, III, and IV. When serum triglycerides reach especially high levels and chylomicronemia is present, patients may develop hepatosplenomegaly, eruptive xanthomas, and severe abdominal pain, often due to pancreatitis. Types II, III, and possibly IV are associated with a high risk of premature coronary heart disease. Peripheral vascular disease is especially common in Type III. Hyperuricemia occurs in more than half the patients with hypertriglyceridemia.

APPROACH TO DIAGNOSIS (Table 74-3)

Because of the serious consequences of coronary heart disease and the availability of effective therapy for most hyperlipidemic patients, a strong argument can be made for screening serum lipid values in all patients. At the very least, serum cholesterol and triglycerides should be measured in those with xanthomas, a family history of hyperlipidemia, evidence of atherosclerotic vascular disease, or other "risk factors" for coronary heart disease. Since prevention of atherosclerosis is the goal, testing of serum lipids is especially urgent in young subjects.

TABLE 74-2
Classification of Hyperlipidemia[208]

Type	Prevalence	Appearance of Plasma on Overnight Refrigeration	Major Fraction Elevated		Clinical Manifestations		Other Features
			Lipid	Lipoprotein	Signs and Symptoms	CHD Risk	
I	Rare	Creamy layer over clear infranatant	TG	CM	Bouts of abdominal pain, hepatosplenomegaly, eruptive xanthomas, and recurrent pancreatitis	Low	Sensitive to dietary fat Deficient lipoprotein lipase activity causes inability to utilize dietary fat Symptoms begin in infancy or childhood
IIA	Common	Clear	CH	LDL	Tendinous and tuberous xanthomas; xanthelasma; corneal arcus	Very high	One genetic form, familial hypercholesterolemia, is inherited as an autosomal dominant trait and can be diagnosed at time of birth
IIB	Common	Clear or cloudy	CH and TG	LDL and VLDL			
III	Uncommon	Clear or cloudy	CH and TG	Abnormal "broad beta" lipoprotein	Palmar xanthomas Risk of peripheral-vascular disease is high	Very high	Abnormal glucose tolerance common Abnormal conversion of VLDL to LDL
IV	Common	Clear or grossly cloudy	TG	VLDL	Tuberous xanthomas	Probably high	Abnormal glucose tolerance common Usually not manifest until early adulthood
V	Uncommon	Creamy layer over cloudy infranatant	TG	VLDL and CM	Bouts of abdominal pain, hepatosplenomegaly, eruptive xanthomas, and recurrent pancreatitis	Probably low	Sensitive to dietary fat Abnormal glucose tolerance common Symptoms begin in adult life

Serum lipid analysis should be done during a period when the patient maintains a stable weight and continues his usual diet and intake of alcohol. After the patient has fasted overnight, blood is obtained for determination of both cholesterol and triglycerides.

About 2 ml of serum from the same blood sample is refrigerated, examined the next morning for turbidity, and saved for further tests that may be needed when triglycerides are elevated. Because serum cholesterol and triglyceride levels tend to increase with

TABLE 74-3
Approach to the Diagnosis of Hyperlipidemia

Question	Comments
I. Is hyperlipidemia present?	Unless xanthomas are present diagnosis usually not suspected on clinical grounds Turbid fasting serum is always abnormal and diagnostic of elevated triglycerides Serum may be clear despite severe hypercholesterolemia
A. Who should be tested?	Patients with xanthomas, hypertension, obesity, diabetes, premature coronary or peripheral vascular disease, family history of hyperlipidemia, or premature atherosclerotic vascular disease
B. What tests should be done?	Fasting serum triglycerides and cholesterol Examine serum after overnight refrigeration Serum lipoprotein electrophoresis if triglycerides are elevated
C. When are tests abnormal?	Since lipid values rise with age in the United States, patient's values must be compared with normal range in subjects of the same age (see Table 74-4)
II. What is the type of hyperlipidemia?	Depends upon delineation of lipoprotein present in excessive concentration (see Table 74-2)
III. Is hyperlipidemia primary or secondary?	See text for causes of secondary hyperlipidemia
IV. Are other family members affected?	Since hyperlipidemia is often genetically determined, other family members are likely to be affected Familial hypercholesterolemia can usually be detected at birth or shortly thereafter Familial hypertriglyceridemia (Type IV) is usually not manifest until late teens or early twenties

age in the American population, the results are considered abnormal when they exceed the 95th percentile for individuals of the same age and sex. From a recent survey of almost 50,000 white subjects, the values indicated in Table 74-4 were calculated as the upper limits of normal for serum cholesterol and triglycerides.[206] The triglyceride values, particularly in men, are much higher than those cited in earlier studies. Ideally, at least three lipid determinations, obtained at weekly intervals, are needed to confirm the diagnosis and to establish a pretreatment baseline.

When serum cholesterol is distinctly high and triglycerides are normal, a diagnosis of Type IIA can be made without further tests. In patients with borderline values of serum cholesterol, direct measurement of LDL cholesterol levels is helpful, but this test requires ultracentrifugation and is available in only a few laboratories. The pathogenesis of familial hypercholesterolemia, one form of Type II hyperlipoproteinemia, has been clarified.[211] Familial hypercholesterolemia is inherited as an autosomal dominant trait. Marked elevations of serum cholesterol (300 to 500 mg/dl in heterozygotes), tendinous xanthomas, and premature coronary heart disease characterize this disorder, which has a frequency of about 1 in 500 in the United States. Studies of fibroblasts from patients with familial hypercholesterolemia have demonstrated defects in membrane interactions with LDL. Normal fibroblasts specifically bind and internalize LDL. Within fibroblast lysosomes, LDL protein and cholesterol esters are hydrolyzed. The rise in intracellular free cholesterol stimulates cholesterol esterification and slows cholesterol synthesis by inhibiting hy-

TABLE 74-4
"Upper Limits of Normal" (95th percentile) for Fasting Plasma Cholesterol and Triglycerides in White Subjects[206]

Cholesterol (mg/dl)			Triglycerides (mg/dl)		
Age (yrs)	Men	Women*	Age (yrs)	Men	Women*
0–19	200	200	0–9	100	108
20–24	218	216	10–19	136	128
25–29	244	222	20–24	201	131
30–34	254	230	25–29	249	144
35–44	269	247	30–34	266	150
45–49	276	265	35–44	320	184
50–54	277	285	45–54	323	224
55–69	275	300	55–69	286	262

* Values are for women not taking sex hormones. Plasma cholesterol values are somewhat higher before the age of 50 and lower after the age of 50 in women taking sex hormones. Plasma triglyceride values are higher in women less than 50 years of age taking sex hormones.

droxymethyl glutaryl coenzyme A reductase, the rate-limiting step in cholesterol formation. In fibroblasts from patients with familial hypercholesterolemia, cell membrane receptors for LDL are absent or defective (Chap. 41). Resultant failure of specific LDL binding, or rarely an internalization defect, interferes with LDL degradation in peripheral tissues and results in uncontrolled overproduction of cholesterol. Studies of fibroblasts from suspected patients will allow diagnosis of familial hypercholesterolemia by a specific test that is independent of serum cholesterol. The receptor assay is not widely available as a diagnostic tool. When both parents have familial hypercholesterolemia, the offspring may be homozygous, a condition with a frequency of about one per million persons. The disorder is much more severe in homozygotes; serum cholesterol often exceeds 800 mg/dl and death from coronary artery disease usually results before age 20.

The presence of hypertriglyceridemia dictates further studies to determine the type of abnormality. Examination of overnight refrigerated serum will often delineate the type of hypertriglyceridemia. A floating creamy layer demonstrates the presence of chylomicrons, which indicate either that the patient was not fasting at the time blood was drawn or has Type I or V hyperlipoproteinemia. Chylomicrons float on top of otherwise clear serum in Type I and above a turbid infranatant in Type V. When patients with Types IIB, III, or IV have significant hypertriglyceridemia, the serum shows diffuse turbidity without a chylomicron layer. Lipoprotein electrophoresis may also help to distinguish between the types of hypertriglyceridemia. Type I hyperlipoproteinemia may be suspected by a failure to demonstrate increased lipoprotein mobility on electrophoresis of serum obtained ten minutes after an injection of heparin. Special tests are required to make a certain diagnosis of Type I or III. Although measurement of postheparin lipolytic activity (PHLA) was used to identify deficient lipoprotein lipase (LPL) activity in Type I, PHLA is not an accurate measure of LPL because heparin also releases a triglyceride lipase from the liver. A more accurate measure of LPL activity in postheparin plasma is provided by physical separation of the two lipases, addition of inhibitors of LPL, or the use of specific antisera to LPL. Alternatively, LPL activity can be measured in a needle biopsy of adipose tissue. Type III is strongly suspected when VLDL, isolated by ultracentrifugation, exhibits the electrophoretic mobility of LDL or has a cholesterol-to-triglyceride ratio greater than 0.3.[209] Deficiency of E-III, one of the subfractions of Apo E, may be the specific biochemical abnormality in most patients with Type III.[221]

In addition to its occurrence as a primary inherited disorder, hyperlipidemia may present as a complication of the following conditions: diabetes, pancreatitis, nephrotic syndrome, chronic renal failure, hypothyroidism, excessive alcohol intake, pregnancy, use of oral contraceptives or glucocorticoids, glycogen storage disease, acute intermittent porphyria, and dysproteinemias (multiple myeloma, macroglobulinemia, systemic lupus erythematosus).[217] Secondary hyperlipidemia may present as any of the five types, but Type IV is most common. An abnormal, cholesterol-rich lipoprotein ("lipoprotein X") may be present in patients with hypercholesterolemia resulting from obstructive liver disease. Chylomicron levels may be increased due to a deficiency in the activity of tissue lipoprotein lipase in hypothyroidism, severe insulin deficiency, or chronic glucocorticoid administration. Since treatment of the underlying disorder in patients with secondary hyperlipidemia may return serum lipid values to normal, appropriate studies should be carried out to eliminate these conditions as a possible cause of the hyperlipidemia.

Although severe degrees of hyperlipidemia are invariably the result of a metabolic abnormality or are secondary to some demonstrable disease, modest elevations of serum lipids may occur in subjects who ingest large amounts of calories or animal fat. Such diet-induced hyperlipidemia is more frequent in countries with a high standard of living. In general, the hyperlipidemia in such subjects responds well to dietary measures.

Finally, since all types of hyperlipidemia may be genetically determined, family members, especially children, should be screened for elevated serum lipid levels so that treatment can be initiated before irreversible vascular changes occur. Familial hypercholesterolemia can be detected in affected children at the time of birth. In contrast, Type IV hyperlipoproteinemia is often not manifest until the late teens or early twenties.

MANAGEMENT (Table 74-5)

Rationale for Treatment

The major goal in the treatment of hyperlipidemia is the prevention of premature vascular disease. Prospective epidemiologic studies have shown that hypercholesterolemia is a major risk factor for coronary heart disease.[216] In fact, complications of coronary heart disease parallel cholesterol levels even within the "normal range" of serum cholesterol. Although studies have not yet proved that reduction of serum cholesterol slows development of atherosclerosis or increases longevity, the strong correlation between

TABLE 74-5

Treatment of Hyperlipidemia

Type of Hyperlipidemia	Dietary Treatment				Drugs
	Total Calories	**Fat Intake**	**Restriction of Specific Fats**	**Alcohol**	
I	Not restricted	25–30 g	None	Not recommended	
IIA	Not restricted	30% of calories	Replace saturated with polyunsaturated fats Cholesterol < 300 mg	Not restricted	Cholestyramine or colestipol 4 g, 4–5 × daily D-thyroxine 4 to 8 mg daily
IIB	Reduce to and maintain ideal body weight	30–35% of calories	Replace saturated with polyunsaturated fats Cholesterol < 300 mg	Not recommended	Cholestyramine or colestipol 4 g, 4–5 × daily (if cholesterol especially high) Clofibrate 1 g, 2 × daily (if triglycerides especially high)
III	Reduce to and maintain ideal body weight	30% of calories	Replace saturated with polyun-saturated fats	Limited	Clofibrate 1 g, 2 × daily
IV	Reduce to and maintain ideal body weight	30–35% of calories	Replace saturated with polyun-saturated fats	Limited	Clofibrate 1 g, 2 × daily Nicotinic acid initial dose 100 mg, 3 × daily; maintenance dose 1–2 g, 3 × daily
V	Reduce to and maintain ideal body weight	25–30% of calories	None	Not recommended	Clofibrate 1 g, 2 × daily Nicotinic acid final dose 1–2 g, 3 × daily Norethindrone acetate 5–10 mg daily (in women) Oxandrolone 2.5 mg, 3 × daily (in men)

cholesterol levels and coronary heart disease suggests that we should initiate efforts to lower serum cholesterol while we await final proof of beneficial effects. Completed studies have not shown that triglycerides are an independent risk factor for premature coronary artery disease. However, the potential risk of hypertriglyceridemia has not been fully addressed.

The epidemiologic evidence cited above demonstrates that LDL is, and VLDL probably is, atherogen-

ic. In contrast, HDL protects against coronary heart disease.[219] Therefore, our efforts should be directed toward measures that reduce serum LDL and VLDL or increase levels of HDL. Intensive exercise and modest alcohol intake raise HDL levels, whereas obesity and cigarette smoking lower HDL.

A decision on whether to lower serum lipid levels in individual patients depends on their age and enthusiasm for preventive measures and the philosophy of the physician. When cholesterol levels exceed the

95th percentile for the individual's age and sex, or serum triglycerides are greater than 300 mg/dl, therapy is clearly indicated. It is desirable to reduce serum cholesterol in individuals positive for other major risk factors, such as hypertension, cigarette smoking, or diabetes mellitus, even when their serum cholesterol is in the "normal range." The strictness of these efforts to prevent premature vascular disease should be inversely proportional to the patient's age. Lipid lowering measures are usually limited to patients less than 60 years of age.

A second reason for treating hyperlipidemia is prevention of acute pancreatitis.[205] Severe hypertriglyceridemia, usually associated with the chylomicronemia of Type I or V, can provoke attacks of acute pancreatitis; reduction of serum triglyceride levels may completely prevent further attacks in these patients.

General Measures

Dietary management, the keystone of therapy for all hyperlipidemic patients, is more likely to succeed when a trained nutritionist explains the diet. Drugs are employed, usually in combination with dietary measures, only when the diet is ineffective or cannot be followed by the patient. Since a 6- to 8-week period is generally sufficient to determine the effectiveness of a dietary or drug regimen, a drug may be started if dietary measures fail over such a time period. If serum lipids do not fall adequately in the next 6 to 8 weeks, the initial drug is discontinued and another is tried in a similar manner. A combination of lipid-lowering agents may be required in some hyperlipidemic patients. Because patients should not be maintained for long periods on an ineffective drug or combination of drugs, there is a clear need for adequate baseline lipid values before institution of therapy.

Reduction of Serum Cholesterol Levels

The most effective dietary approach to lower serum cholesterol levels involves reduced intake of saturated fat, achieved by restriction of total fats to about 30 percent of calories and partial replacement of saturated fats with polyunsaturated ones. These measures will also reduce cholesterol intake, but it is difficult to lower serum cholesterol by further restriction of dietary cholesterol. If dietary cholesterol is lowered from the amounts present in the average American diet (500 to 800 mg/day) to levels often recommended (300 mg/day), the reduction in serum cholesterol is small. However, restriction of dietary cholesterol to about 100 mg/day does significantly decrease serum cholesterol. Reduction to ideal body weight also produces a modest fall in serum cholesterol. These die-

tary measures usually reduce serum cholesterol by 10 to 20 percent. Drugs should be added when levels remain in the hypercholesterolemic range.

Cholestyramine and colestipol, resins which reduce cholesterol levels by 20 to 30 percent, are drugs of choice. Although these agents are inconvenient to take and often produce minor gastrointestinal side effects, major adverse reactions are rare. D-Thyroxine lowers cholesterol levels by 15 to 25 percent, but serious cardiovascular side effects limit its use to subjects with no evidence of coronary artery disease. Beta-sitosterol is safe but only lowers serum cholesterol by about 10 percent. Probucol decreases cholesterol levels by 10 to 15 percent. Although nicotinic acid lowers serum cholesterol by 15 to 25 percent, its efficacy is counterbalanced by a high frequency of troublesome side effects, such as flushing. In contrast, clofibrate is well tolerated and lowers serum cholesterol by about 10 percent; recently recognized chronic side effects dictate limiting the use of this drug for reduction of serum cholesterol to those patients who fail to respond to or are unable to tolerate other medications.

Partial ileal bypass should be considered in severely hypercholesterolemic patients who fail to respond to the measures outlined above. By interfering with the reabsorption of bile acids, ileal exclusion lowers serum cholesterol by 25 to 35 percent in most patients. Some are troubled by persistent diarrhea, usually controlled with cholestyramine. Hypercholesterolemia is not relieved in homozygotes for familial hypercholesterolemia. Serum cholesterol levels may also be lowered by repeated plasmapheresis. Portocaval shunt surgery lowers serum cholesterol but must be considered experimental.

Treatment of Hypertriglyceridemia

The goal in the treatment of Types IIB, III, and IV is the prevention of premature vascular disease. In Types I and V efforts are made to reduce serum triglycerides sufficiently to prevent episodes of acute pancreatitis. Weight reduction and maintenance of ideal body weight are the most important dietary measures for the treatment of all forms of hypertriglyceridemia except Type I. Drugs should be started only after maximal efforts to control triglyceride levels by dietary measures.

Diabetes is often associated with Types III, IV, or V. In these subjects insulin treatment may help control hypertriglyceridemia. When insulin deficiency is profound, often during periods of prolonged treatment with oral hypoglycemic agents, some diabetics may accumulate excessive chylomicrons and convert from a Type IV to a Type V pattern. Insulin treatment will rapidly clear the chylomicronemia in such patients. Many diabetics also have inherited a predisposition to primary hypertriglyceridemia which requires additional specific therapy. Because of their high risk of coronary and peripheral vascular disease, reduced intake of saturated fat is recommended in all diabetics.

Oral contraceptives should not be prescribed for women with Type IV or V. Depression of lipoprotein lipase activity by estrogen causes chylomicronemia and appearance of a Type V pattern in patients with Type IV, and accentuates the hypertriglyceridemia in those with Type V. Attacks of acute pancreatitis may complicate the severe hypertriglyceridemia resulting from poorly controlled diabetes or oral contraceptive use.

TYPE I. This disorder is treated by restricting fat intake to about 30 g daily. The diet can be made more palatable by adding 30 to 40 g of commercially prepared medium chain triglycerides which are absorbed directly into the portal blood rather than as chylomicron triglycerides. These patients should avoid alcohol. Drugs are unnecessary.

TYPES IIB AND III. As indicated in Table 74–5, the main elements in dietary management of both Types IIB and III are maintenance of ideal body weight, restricted intake of saturated fat, along with a relative increase in polyunsaturated fats in the diet, and limited alcohol use. When combined with dietary measures, clofibrate is highly effective in lowering serum lipid levels in patients with Type III. Drug treatment in patients with Type IIB depends on the relative levels of serum cholesterol and triglycerides. When serum cholesterol is particularly high and triglycerides are only modestly elevated, cholestyramine or colestipol is the drug of choice, as in Type IIA patients. Clofibrate may be tried in those with markedly increased triglycerides and only slightly raised cholesterol. Nicotinic acid is often effective in patients with Type IIB. Some experts advise the combination of a resin with clofibrate.

TYPE IV. Dietary management is identical with that of Types IIB and III. Alcohol must be severely limited since it may increase VLDL levels drastically in some patients with Type IV. Weight loss lowers triglyceride levels in almost all obese patients with Type IV, but drugs may be indicated if substantial hypertriglyceridemia persists. Clofibrate is the most effective drug, but serum triglycerides respond less in Type IV than in Type III. Nicotinic acid usually decreases triglycerides in Type IV patients.

TYPE V. Dietary measures include maintenance of ideal weight, restriction of fat intake to 25 to 30 percent of calories, and avoidance of alcohol. Fat intake can be supplemented with 30 to 40 g of medium chain triglycerides. Although clofibrate or nicotinic acid reduces serum triglyceride levels only modestly, attacks of pancreatitis are usually prevented when one of these agents is added to the appropriate diet. When these drugs are ineffective or poorly tolerated, triglyceride levels can often be controlled with progestational agents in women and anabolic steroids in men.

Lipid-Lowering Drugs[222]

Cholestyramine and colestipol are ion exchange resins which bind bile acids and remove them in the stools, thus increasing the conversion of cholesterol to bile acids. Although cholesterol synthesis is also enhanced, the net effect is a reduction in serum cholesterol levels. Constipation, a troublesome side effect in about 20 percent of patients, is often ameliorated by a stool softener. Epigastric discomfort and bloating usually disappear after a few days on the drug. The usual dose for both resins is 16 to 20 g per day. Malabsorption of fat and fat-soluble vitamins occurs only if a daily dosage greater than 28 g is required. Since resins may impair the absorption of other drugs, such as coumadin, digoxin, thyroxine, and antibiotics, other medications should be taken at least one hour before cholestyramine or colestipol. Resins may also reduce folate absorption.

D-Thyroxine lowers cholesterol levels by enhancing the conversion of cholesterol to bile acids. Treatment is started with 2 mg daily and slowly raised to 4 to 8 mg a day. Serious side effects limit its utility. These include occasional symptoms of thyrotoxicosis, aggravation of diabetes, and precipitation of arrhythmias or angina in patients with coronary heart disease. The drug is contraindicated in these patients and in those with congestive failure, arrhythmias, significant hypertension, and advanced renal or liver disease. The use of this agent is largely limited to young patients. Since D-thyroxine potentiates their action, the dose of warfarin anticoagulants should be reduced by 30 percent.

Clofibrate, 2 g daily, is the drug of choice for most patients with hypertriglyceridemia. Since chronic clofibrate administration causes long-term side effects, including increased gallstone formation, this drug should be used only when a significant degree of hypertriglyceridemia persists after optimal dietary management.[220] The most important action of clofibrate may be to reduce the synthesis or release of VLDL by the liver. Weight gain, mild nausea, diarrhea, or a skin rash may occur in a few patients. Rarely, a reversible myositis may require discontinuation of the drug. Since clofibrate potentiates warfarin anticoagulants, the dosage of these drugs should be halved when clofibrate is started and prothrombin time must initially be monitored closely.

Nicotinic acid usually lowers both cholesterol and triglyceride levels. The dosage is increased slowly over a two-week period from 300 mg daily to a full therapeutic dose of 1 to 2 g three times daily. Flushing occurs within two hours of taking the drug, but this side effect usually disappears by the time the patient is on a full dose of the drug. Other common problems include gastrointestinal symptoms, abnormal liver function tests, glucose intolerance, and hyperuricemia. Nicotinic acid augments the hypotensive effects of ganglionic blocking agents.

Sitosterols are plant sterols which probably lower serum cholesterol by interfering with its absorption from the intestine. The usual dosage is 3 to 6 g before each meal. Diarrhea is the major side effect.

Probucol is a new agent for reduction of serum cholesterol. About 10 percent of patients have diarrhea at the recommended dose of 500 mg twice daily. Flatulence, abdominal pain, nausea, and vomiting are less common and transient side effects.

Progestational agents, such as norethindrone acetate or medroxyprogesterone acetate, probably lower serum triglycerides by activating the enzyme lipoprotein lipase. These drugs are only recommended in adult women. The usual dose is 5 to 10 mg daily. Fluid retention is common; unusual side effects are cholestatic jaundice, nausea, anorexia, and tenderness and enlargement of the breasts.

Oxandrolone is an anabolic steroid which probably increases the activity of lipoprotein lipase. Use of the drug is limited to adult men because it may cause virilism in women. At a dose of 2.5 mg three times daily, the drug is usually well tolerated; side effects include leukopenia, retention of sodium and water, and disturbances of liver function. The drug should not be given to patients with prostatic carcinoma. Oxandrolone may be effective in Type IV as well as Type V hyperlipoproteinemia.

UNUSUAL FORMS OF DYSLIPIDEMIA

Deficiency of a serum lipoprotein or one of the lipid-removing enzymes is recognized as the cause of four rare conditions. Tangier disease (HDL deficiency) and a betalipoproteinemia have characteristic clinical pictures. Type I hyperlipoproteinemia results from lipoprotein lipase deficiency (discussed earlier). An absence of LCAT has also been identified in several families.

Tangier disease,[214] analphalipoproteinemia, results from an excessive rate of catabolism of the Apo-Gln-I component of HDL. The normal ratio of Apo-Gln-I to Apo-Gln-II in HDL is 3:1; in Tangier disease the ratio is 1:12. Transmitted as an autosomal recessive trait, the disease is recognized by very low levels of HDL and cholesterol, along with slightly increased serum triglycerides.

Deposition of cholesterol esters in reticuloendothelial tissues may produce hepatosplenomegaly and lymphadenopathy, but the most dramatic clinical finding is grossly enlarged, orange-colored tonsils. Lipid deposits are also found in skin, cornea, and blood vessels. Systemic manifestations are generally minor although some families have neurologic symptoms and premature coronary heart disease may occur.

In a betalipoproteinemia,[214] both cholesterol and triglyceride levels are quite low and chylomicrons are not formed in response to a fatty meal. Since the basic defect is an inability to synthesize the Apo B peptide of LDL and VLDL, the disease is diagnosed by the complete absence of these two lipoproteins. The clinical manifestations include fat malabsorption with steatorrhea and triglyceride deposition in cells of the intestinal mucosa, fatty liver, growth retardation, severe neurologic deficits, acanthocytosis, and pigmentary retinal degeneration.

In patients with *familial LCAT deficiency* (Norum's disease),[210] abnormal particles, rich in unesterified cholesterol and lecithin, are present in the circulation. These particles are thought to arise from incomplete degradation of chylomicrons and VLDL. Hemolytic anemia is associated with an increased content of cholesterol in red blood cells. Lipids are deposited in the cornea and glomeruli. Proteinuria is an early finding and patients ultimately develop renal failure. The disorder has been found mainly in Norway.

CHAPTER 75

Disorders of Calcium and Metabolic Bone Diseases

T. H. HSU AND GIRAUD V. FOSTER

INTRODUCTION

Comprising 2 percent of the human body weight, calcium is the most abundant cation. Almost all of it is present in the skeleton (99 percent) where much of it is in dynamic equilibrium with the remaining 1 percent in soft tissue and blood. The equilibrium is such that plasma levels are normally maintained within the range of 9 to 10.5 mg/dl. This precise control of blood levels may be necessary to provide the proper environment for many important physiologic functions. These include maintenance of cell permeability, blood coagulation, cardiac rhythmicity, nervous excitability, muscle contraction, and regulation of cell division. The calcium blood level is regulated within narrow limits to facilitate these functions despite wide variations in dietary intake, the demands of the skeleton during growth, and loss during pregnancy and lactation. Control is maintained largely by the actions of parathyroid hormone (PTH), calcitonin, and vitamin D.

CALCIUM HOMEOSTASIS[228,230,237]

Calcium is absorbed by the small bowel by a combination of active transport and facilitated diffusion (Fig. 75-1). The average daily intake is between 600 and 1200 mg but this may vary day to day between far greater extremes. To accommodate the needs of the organism and prevent wide oscillations in plasma calcium, a greater proportion of calcium is absorbed when the diet is deficient and a lesser proportion when intake is high. This control is largely mediated by a specific calcium binding protein in the intestine whose production is regulated by 1,25-dihydroxy-vitamin D (1,25(OH)$_2$D).

Of the calcium absorbed, approximately 100 mg is excreted into the intestinal tract in saliva and biliary secretions. At present it is not known whether hormones play a role in this process. It is known, however, that a number of nonhormonal factors affect net absorption. Absorption of calcium is increased by acid conditions which permit greater solubility of calcium salts, excessive lactose which forms soluble complexes with calcium, and high protein

diet. Conversely, absorption is impaired by a high intake of fats, oxalates, and alkali (all of which promote the formation of insoluble compounds) and of ions, including strontium, magnesium, and phosphate, which may affect vitamin D metabolism.

Calcium is lost from the body primarily in the feces as a result of both nonabsorption and active secretion. This loss constitutes approximately 70 to 90 percent of the dietary intake when the body is in normal calcium balance. The remaining 10 to 20 percent is excreted in the urine. Urinary loss, however, is critical and is under exacting control. Of the approximately 10 g of calcium handled by the renal tubules a day, 97 to 99 percent is reabsorbed.

When plasma values fall below 8 mg/dl, little is excreted; and when plasma levels are excessive, losses may be high. These changes are largely mediated by parathyroid hormone. The equilibrium between calcium in the skeleton and in the body fluids is likewise hormonally regulated (Fig. 75-1). Of the 900 mg of calcium in the extracellular fluid, about 250 mg is in the plasma where the concentration of calcium is approximately 40 percent greater. The increased concentration can be explained on the basis of binding to plasma proteins. Only 65 percent of the plasma calcium is freely diffusible; 52 percent is ionic calcium and 13 percent is calcium complexed with citrated, carbonate, phosphate, and possibly sugars and some amino acids. Of the remaining 35 percent, approximately 7 percent is bound to globulins and 27 percent to albumin. Aberrations in serum proteins, especially albumin, readily cause changes in the total calcium value in plasma, while not affecting the concentration of ionic calcium.

The exchangeable calcium in bone and the calcium in the extracellular fluid are in continual interchange. The kinetics of this flux are mediated by all three of the calcium regulating hormones, PTH, calcitonin, and vitamin D. Not only are these humoral factors responsible for homeostasis of ionic calcium, but ionic calcium, in turn, regulates their rates of production.

Finally, any discussion of ionic calcium must take into consideration the three common calcium complexing ions, HPO$_4^-$, citrate and HCO$_3^-$. Changes in concentration of these can affect the concentration of calcium. Bone contains approximately 70 percent of all citrate in the body and 90 percent of all HPO$_4^-$.

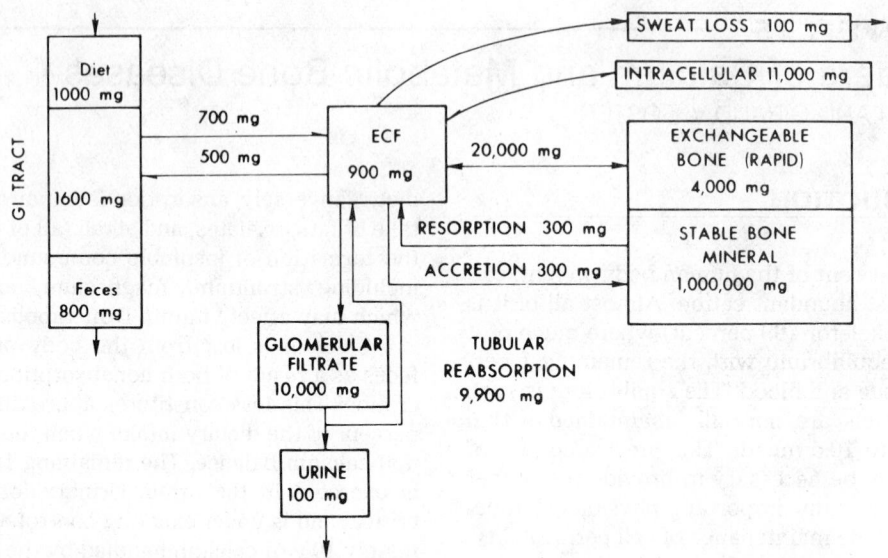

FIGURE 75–1. Shown above are the various functional pools of calcium distribution (ECF = extracellular fluid). The size of the pools and the magnitude of flux between them are as indicated.

Factors that affect calcium movement in bone produce similar changes in these ions as well.

BONE METABOLISM[225]

Chemically bone consists of approximately 65 to 70 percent crystalline hydroxyapatite. The remaining 30 to 35 percent is organic matrix composed of 95 percent collagen and 5 percent proteins and carbohydrates and polymers of these with hexosamines and glucuronic acid. Studies of the ultrastructure have shown collagen to be a rigid rod-shaped molecule approximately 2800A° long and 14A° wide. Collagen I ("collagen vulgaris" of bone, tendon, and skin) is composed of three polypeptide chains. One of these differs from the other two. Characteristically, collagen contains a constant 33 ±5 percent glycine and approximately 25 percent of the amino acids, proline and hydroxyproline. The presence of large numbers of γ-glutamyl peptide linkages may be an important determinant of the secondary and tertiary structure. The three polypeptide chains are left-handed helices oriented to one another in a right-handed superhelix.

Bone collagen is capable of initiating nucleation of crystals of hydroxyapatite. These crystals are small hexagonal rods, distributed over the surface of the collagen. Total bone crystal surface in man has been estimated to be as great as 100 acres. All this surface, however, is not in equilibrium with the surrounding fluid. As crystals of hydroxyapatite form on collagen, they displace the water molecules which make up the sphere of hydration surrounding individual collagen fibrils. As the crystal population increases and the sphere of hydration decreases, the facility with which ions can enter is impaired and crystal formation stops. The structural characteristics of the relationship of hydroxyapatite crystals to collagen account for why less than 1 percent of bone mineral is freely exchangeable. Presumably only those collagen fibrils which do not have their full complement of crystals are capable of presenting surfaces upon which exchange can readily take place. Conditions which interfere with either collagen synthesis, the (Ca^{++}) (HPO_4^-) solubility coefficient, or mucopolysaccharide formation will likewise affect hydroxyapatite deposition and the ability of mineral ions to participate in exchange reactions.

The collagen molecules are longitudinally oriented within the basic microscopic unit of bone, the osteon or Haversian system. The osteon is an irregular cylindrical structure about 150 μ in external diameter. Within its center is a narrow lumen, the Haversian canal, which has its own nutrient artery. Branching from the Haversian canal are multiple interconnecting canalicules. These serve as conduits for the microcirculatory system connecting the central Haversian canal with the lucunae, or concentrically located housing units for the bone cells.

The bone cells are of three types: osteoblasts, osteocytes, and osteoclasts. The osteoblasts derive from mesenchymal precursor cells during early development of the skeleton. They synthesize the collagen and glycoproteins of bone matrix. With growth, the osteoblasts become surrounded by uncalcified matrix, called osteoid, and develop into osteocytes. The osteocytes continue to lay down matrix which eventually becomes mineralized. The osteocytes remain connected with the osteoblasts covering the external surface of bone by cytoplasmic processes which extend radially from each cell in the canalicules. The osteocytes are arranged concentrically within the Haversian systems and maintain already formed bone by local resorption, accretion and transport of nutrients and waste products. Additional bone resorption is carried out by multinucleated osteoclasts which promote local bone dissolution by the elaboration of lytic enzymes and organic acids. Osteoclasts probably develop from osteoblasts, macrophages, or more primitive progenitor cells. They line the surface of the marrow cavity. By their action, the medullary cavity is enlarged during growth at a rate appropriate to the external apposition of new bone. The activity and possibly the differentiation of all three types of bone cells—osteoblasts, osteocytes and osteoclasts—is, at least in part, hormone dependent.

Physiologic factors which alter bone resorption and accretion include:

1. Hormones: In addition to those with specific effects on calcium metabolism, those with generalized anabolic or catabolic activity affect bone cells and therefore influence bone growth.

2. Changes in blood vessels: Alterations in blood supply, produced by anatomic, nervous, or biochemical processes, will alter the nutrition of the osteons.

3. Nutrients in the blood: Since bone matrix is composed of collagen and mucopolysaccharides, protein deficiencies may have adverse effects on bone formation.

4. Ions: Increases in plasma phosphate promote deposition of calcium in bone and inhibit bone resorption. As a consequence, plasma calcium and phosphate are inversely related. Other ions may affect crystalization of hydroxyapatite. Of particular note is fluoride which may affect both crystal size and solubility leading to friable bones.

5. Pyrophosphate: Naturally occurring pyrophosphate plays a role as an inhibitor of both bone accretion and resorption. It acts by replacing phosphate in the crystal surface thereby altering exchange properties. Its physiologic importance is poorly understood due to its rapid intracellar degradation.

6. Mechanical stress: Weight bearing and the functional activity of muscles as they relate to the forces they exert on bone at their insertions generate local differences in piezoelectric fields in bone. These play a causative role in the distribution of osteoclasts and osteoblasts in bone thereby altering the effects of hormones on bone determining morphology and the rate of bone remodeling.

In general bone is of two types: cortical bone which is highly calcified, but relatively inactive metabolically, and spongiosa, which is more metabolically active, and composed of trabeculae. Both are surrounded by an endosteal membrane consisting of osteoblasts and their precursors which act as calcium pumps in controlling the local concentration of calcium in the fluid surrounding bone and, therefore, the concentration of calcium in plasma as well.

From the preceding considerations the following clinically relevant conclusions concerning the actions of hormones on bone can be drawn:

1. Hormonally induced changes in the rate of bone resorption can be quantified by measuring changes in the rate of urinary excretion of hydroxyproline and changes in the rate of bone accretion by measuring changes in serum alkaline phosphatase.

2. Because bone is composed of collagen and mucopolysaccharides, hormones which affect protein and carbohydrate metabolism may also affect the skeleton.

3. Since the extent to which bone is mineralized, and therefore the degree to which calcium ions can readily exchange, is age dependent, hormones are more likely to produce effects in young than old bone. For similar reasons, hormones will affect metaphyseal bone more readily than diaphyseal bone.

4. Hormones and hormone-like substances, such as histamine and prostaglandins, may affect bone metabolism by altering the circulation to the skeleton, an increase favoring resorption and a decrease hindering resorption.

5. As a consequence of the inverse relationship between calcium and phosphate in plasma, changes in phosphate, by producing reciprocal changes in calcium, can alter the secretion of calcium-regulating hormones whose rates of secretion are dependent upon the ionic calcium concentration.

6. Hormones which have an effect either on the activity of bone cells or upon their number affect calcium metabolism.

7. Since osteoblasts or osteoblast-like cells forming limiting membranes for bone act as calcium pumps, hormones that affect these cells may acutely alter the bone-plasma calcium equilibrium.

CALCIUM-REGULATING HORMONES

Of the three principal hormones that affect calcium metabolism, the earliest to evolve were calcitonin and vitamin D. Their initial function may have been to conserve phosphate. With the development of terrestrial forms of life, they were probably adapted to regulate calcium homeostasis. To facilitate more efficient remodeling of the skeleton, parathyroid hormone evolved later as an adjunctive control.

Parathyroid Hormone (PTH)

PTH is synthesized in the parathyroid glands as a pre-prohormone, converted to a prohormone by intracellular enzymes, and released principally as a single chain 84 amino acid peptide at a rate inversely proportional to the ambient serum ionic calcium concentration. Evidence indicates that changes in calcium as little as 1 percent acutely affect secretion. Since the parathyroid glands contain relatively little stored PTH, changes in the rate of secretion reflect changes in synthesis.

Magnesium, $1,25(OH)_2D$, glucocorticoids, vitamin D, and epinephrine may also modulate elaboration of PTH. While less effective than calcium, high concentrations of magnesium inhibit secretion. However, in magnesium deficiency, hypocalcemia paradoxically develops due to impaired synthesis and possibly altered end-organ response. Glucocorticoids transiently augment PTH secretion, indirectly by lowering plasma calcium as a consequence of inhibiting bone resorption and decreasing calcium absorption from the gut as well as directly by stimulating the parathyroid glands. Like glucocorticoids, vitamin D also may have a direct and indirect effect. Indirectly they inhibit secretion by inducing hypercalcemia consequent to increasing bone resorption and calcium absorption. Current evidence suggests a direct inhibitory effect. Finally, epinephrine stimulates PTH secretion. While this may not be of physiologic significance it could explain the association between pheochromocytoma and hypercalcemia.

In the peripheral circulation, PTH is rapidly degraded by the liver and kidney. Liver degradation may play a role in the production of active fragments. Biologic activity resides in the first 27 amino acids in the N-terminal portion of the molecule. High and low calcium concentrations, respectively, inhibit and stimulate generation of fragments containing this active moiety. As a consequence of both secretion and degradation, marked heterogeneity of PTH is present in blood; characteristically, however, biologically active fragments containing the N-terminal portion of the molecule, when present, are found in only low concentrations. The predominant form is a biologically inert carboxy-terminal fragment with a molecular weight of 7000 daltons. It is against this carboxy-terminal portion of the molecule that most antisera used in currently available radioimmunoassays are directed. As a consequence, such assays while having the capacity to measure intact hormone, prohormone, and preprohormone, in fact measure predominantly biologically inactive fragments, when applied to blood.

PTH acts on bone, kidney, and gut. Separately and together these actions raise serum calcium levels.

The effects of the hormone on bone are twofold. PTH directly affects the activity of osteoclasts by increasing their ruffled borders. This is associated with an increase in citric acid, through a decrease in its degradation, and an increase in synthesis of many lytic enzymes. Both citrate and enzymes presumably play a role in bone resorption. In addition, PTH regulates the size and number of osteoclasts. It has not yet been resolved whether this action is brought about by retarding the transformation of osteoclasts into osteoblasts, or stimulating de novo proliferation of osteoclasts from progenitor cells. Indirectly, PTH promotes bone accretion by augmenting production of $1,25(OH)_2D$ which, in turn, promotes intestinal absorption of phosphate. However, the rate of accretion is usually less than the rate of absorption so that net bone loss results. The increase in both functions leads to an increase in the rate of bone turnover and this accounts for the PTH-induced increases in urinary hydroxyproline excretion and plasma alkaline phosphatase activity.

PTH has three effects on the kidney. It enhances renal tubular reabsorption of calcium; increases urinary excretion of phosphorus, bicarbonate, potassium, sodium, and amino acids; and enhances conversion of $25(OH)D$ to the more active $1,25(OH)_2D$. The hormone appears to have different actions in different parts of the renal tubule, the predominant effect on phosphate being mediated by changes in the proximal tubule whereas the main effects on calcium are mediated through changes in the distal tubule.

PTH promotes the absorption of calcium indirectly on the gut through its action on the metabolism of vitamin D.

The mode of action of PTH on all three major organ systems presumably is the same. The hormone binds to a specific cell receptor thereby activating adenylate cyclase, and increasing the entry of calcium into the cells. Increases in intracellular calcium augment the production of appropriate kinases that bring about specific enzymatic reactions that characterize the cell type affected.

Vitamin D

This sterol increases bone resorption and absorption of both calcium and phosphate from the intestine. These actions are mediated by its most polar metabolite, 1,25-dihydroxycholecalciferol $(1,25(OH)_2D)$, the production of which is exquisitely controlled in order to effect regulation of serum calcium, facilitate growth, and maintain the normal skeleton. The production of $1,25(OH)_2D$ is dependent upon the availability of precursors and the subsequential hydroxylation of these, first in the liver and then in the kidney.

The daily requirement for vitamin D is about 400 IU In the United States, this is obtained principally in the diet as ergocalciferol (vitamin D_2) in fortified milk, breads, and cereals, and cholecalciferol (vitamin D_3) in animal products, notably butter, eggs, and fish oils. Absorption of these from the intestinal lumen requires micelle formation. If bile production is impaired, vitamin D deficiency may result. Once internalized, vitamin D is incorporated into chylomicra and transported via the lymphatics to the liver. Solubilization of the lipophylic sterol is facilitated in the circulation by a specific binding protein, transcalciferol, an alpha$_2$ globulin also known as Gc (for "group-specific component") protein. In countries where food products are not fortified with vitamin D, the precursor requirements are met primarily by conversion of 7-dehydroxycholesterol in the skin under the influence of ultraviolet light, the amount of sunlight being a critical determinant of the availability of cholecalciferol.

In the liver, vitamin D is hydroxylated to 25-hydroxycholecalciferol (25(OH)D) by a microsomal enzyme. This conversion is precursor dependent and unaffected by serum calcium, phosphorus or PTH. 25(OH)D is the major circulating metabolite of vitamine D. Some, conjugated in the liver and excreted in bile, is reabsorbed from the gut. However, larger amounts can be lost in malabsorption states. The principal known role of 25(OH)D is that of substrate for conversion to $1,25(OH)_2D$. Since only a small fraction of 25(OH)D is converted to $1,25(OH)_2D$, extensive liver damage must be present before impaired production becomes apparent.

In the renal cortex, 25(OH)D is further hydroxylated by two mitochondrial enzymes, 25(OH)-1-hydroxylase and 25(OH)-24-hydroxylase. The reaction mediated by 25(OH)-1-hydroxylase is stringently regulated such that output of $1,25(OH)_2D$ is commensurate with the needs of the organism. Its activity is enhanced by 1) hypophosphatemia directly; and 2) hypocalcemia mediated by PTH, and inhibited by $1,25(OH)_2D$ itself by feedback regulation. Each of these initiates appropriate correction of plasma calcium, phosphate, and $1,25(OH)_2D$ levels toward normal. The effect of this metabolite on intestinal calcium reabsorption is at lest fivefold greater than either vitamin D_3 or 25(OH)D and 100-fold greater on bone absorption.

The second renal cortical enzyme (which is also present in the gut) converts 25(OH)D to 24,25-dihydroxy cholecalciferol ($24,25(OH)_2D$), a biologically inactive metabolite. The production of $1,25(OH)_2D$ and $24,25(OH)_2D$ are conjointly regulated by the ambient calcium and phosphate levels such that when either is low, $1,25(OH)_2D$ is elaborated and, conversely, when either is high, $24,25(OH)_2D$ is produced. In this way, the appropriate product is secreted to maintain normal serum calcium and phosphate levels. Under normal conditions, approximately 100 times more $24,25(OH)_2D$ is present in the circulation than $1,25(OH)_2D$.

Vitamin D and its biologically active metabolites, 25(OH)D and $1,25(OH)_2D$, act on bone and intestine. Whether or not they alter renal tubular transport of calcium or phosphate is not known. Calcium is absorbed by the gut primarily in the distal portion of the small bowel by passive diffusion. However, a significant amount is actively absorbed in the duodenum. This process requires energy and is mediated by a specific calcium-binding protein whose synthesis is directly regulated by $1,25(OH)_2D$.

The active metabolites of vitamin D directly increase the rate of bone resorption. This effect, while not requiring the presence of PTH, is less marked in its absence. In vitro, $1,25(OH)_2D$ has no effect on the rate of bone formation, unlike in vivo where an increase in bone resorption is followed by an increase in the rate of mineral accretion.

Calcitonin

Calcitonin is secreted in man by the parafollicular or "C" cells of the thyroid. In lower species, the hormone is elaborated by cells of the ultimobranchial bodies. Secreting cells originate from the neural crest and migrate during early development to the last pharyngeal pouch which subsequently participates in the formation of the thyroid gland. Structurally the hormone is a 32 amino acid single-chain polypeptide containing a 1-7 disulfide bond and a C-terminal proline amide.

In contradistinction to PTH, calcitonin is secreted in response to elevations in plasma calcium, its rate of secretion being directly proportional to the concentration of this cation. It acts to inhibit bone resorption. Since calcium ions in blood and bone are in constant interchange, by preventing the egress of calcium from bone while allowing calcium from blood to enter bone, hypocalcemia is induced. Secretion of calcitonin may, in part, be mediated by gastrin under physiologic conditions. In experimental animals, gastrin is secreted in response to a calcium meal. Since the gastrin is a calcitonin secretagogue, the secretion of calcitonin is stimulated before a rise in plasma calcium due to calcium absorption thereby protecting against postprandial hypercalcemia. Other secretagogues for calcitonin include secretin, glucagon, strontium, and magnesium. However, the physiologic significance of these in man remains in doubt.

In bone, calcitonin has a direct and immediate effect on osteoclasts. Within minutes after its administration the ruffled border of these cells retracts from the surface of adjacent bone undergoing resorption. Subsequent effects of hormone include a reduction in the rate of production of osteoclast progenitor cells and an increase in the modulation of osteoclasts to osteoblasts. For this reason, calcitonin is a useful therapeutic agent in reducing increased osteolysis in such conditions as Paget's disease of bone.

Calcitonin in pharmacologic doses promotes the renal excretion of phosphate, sodium, and potassium. However, to date no evidence suggests a direct physiologic effect on the handling of calcium by either the kidney or gut. The mechanism of action of calcitonin remains unknown. Following administration of the hormone, a transient elevation in plasma calcium is observed. This may reflect release of calcium from bone cells. This intracellular depletion of calcium may inhibit the release of citric acid and osteolytic enzymes from the osteoclasts and osteocytes.

In animals, calcitonin subserves three functions. First, it protects against postprandial hypercalcemia. This protection is indirectly mediated by calcium-induced release of gastrin. Second, it protects the skeleton against demineralization during times of excessive demands for calcium. Presumptive evidence exists that calcitonin secretion in animals is augmented during pregnancy and lactation. Third, by counterbalancing the effects of vitamin D and parathyroid hormone, calcitonin modulates plasma calcium homeostasis and bone remodeling. This activity may be particularly important during growth by permitting the calcium conserving activity of vitamin D and PTH on gut and kidney, respectively, while preventing excessive bone resorption. Finally, calcitonin may have physiologic functions still unrecognized. The recent observation that the hormone is present in the brain suggests that it may participate in neuroregulatory activity.

In contrast to animals, a physiologic role of calcitonin in man remains to be demonstrated. Two observations suggest that the hormone is not of importance in calcium homeostasis. First, in patients with medullary carcinoma of the thyroid in whom high concentrations of plasma calcitonin are present, little or no aberrations in plasma calcium levels are seen. Second, following thyroidectomy without obvious impairment of PTH secretion, deficiency of calcitonin does not lead to overt impairment of handling of calcium loads. These findings, however, do not constitute definitive proof that calcitonin is inactive in man since it can be argued that in medullary carcinoma the effects of excessive amounts of the hormone are prevented by concomitant increases in PTH secretion. In patients who are thyroidectomized, the fall in plasma calcium following a calcium infusion may be delayed and this delay may result in excessive renal loss of the ion leading ultimately to a deficiency of calcium. The present view is that if calcitonin is physiologically active in calcium regulation in man, it plays a lesser role than either PTH or vitamin D.

Other Factors Which May Affect Mineral Metabolism

In addition to PTH, vitamin D, and calcitonin, other hormones and metabolically active substances alter calcium and phosphate metabolism. These include somatomedins, glucocorticoids, insulin, estrogens, androgens, thyroid hormone, osteoclast-activating factor, and prostaglandins.

The growth-promoting effects of growth hormone on the skeleton are indirectly mediated through the production of somatomedins. These substances are peptides produced primarily in the liver, which stimulate DNA and RNA synthesis in osteoblasts and promote the uptake of amino acids and sulfate required by these cells for the production of collagen. When in excess they may induce gigantism or acromegaly; conversely, deficiencies of these substances or end organ failure in children may result in short stature.

Glucocorticoids are essential for normal skeletal growth. When in high concentration, however, they promote loss of bone mass. Multiple factors may be involved including impaired generation of somatomedins, interference with vitamin D metabolism, and inhibition of intestinal calcium transport independent of vitamin D.

Insulin likewise is required for normal development of the skeleton. It promotes the rate of collagen synthesis. The osteoporosis in patients with diabetes mellitus has been attributed, in part, to insulin deficiency. While glucagon in animal experiments inhibits bone resorption directly and indirectly by stimulating calcitonin secretion, in man its physiologic role in the regulation of calcium metabolism remains uncertain.

Estrogens and androgens affect epiphyseal closure at puberty and inhibit bone resorption. High plasma levels prior to puberty prevent attainment of full growth potential and low levels in postmenopausal women may contribute to the development of osteoporosis by leaving the effects of PTH on the skeleton unopposed.

Thyroid hormones increase the rates of both bone accretion and bone resorption thereby augmenting bone turnover. Deficiencies in these hormones in early childhood may result in dwarfism.

Prostaglandins, principally PGE_2, stimulate bone resorption. They may play a significant role in the genesis of hypercalcemia associated with some malignant tumors.

Osteoclast-activating factor likewise is a potent stimulator of bone resorption. It is present in leukocytes and may induce hypercalcemia in lymphoproliferative disorders, especially multiple myeloma.

DISORDERED CALCIUM HOMEOSTASIS

HYPERCALCEMIA

The signs and symptoms of hypercalcemia are nonspecific. Three major organ systems, neuromuscular, gastrointestinal, and genitourinary, are affected by chronic elevation of serum calcium. In addition, most patients have symptoms directly related to the disease underlying the hypercalcemia.

Neurologic symptoms include somnolence, memory deficits, personality disturbances, irritability, and other nonspecific complaints often indistinguishable from psychoneurosis. Occasionally a patient may present in stupor or even coma following an acute rise in plasma calcium. Muscle weakness, specifically proximal muscle weakness, related to the effects of hypercalcemia on neuromuscular transmission is often prominent. Hypokalemia induced by hypercalcemia may contribute. The principal gastrointestinal complaints are anorexia, nausea, vomiting, constipation, and occasionally abdominal pain.

The incidence of peptic ulcer is increased, seemingly as a consequence of calcium-induced hypergastrinemia which stimulates secretion of gastric acid. Hypercalcemia usually leads to hypercalciuria, which may contribute to nephrolithiasis. Hyposthenuria and polyuria may occur secondary to osmotic diuresis, calcium nephropathy, reduction in the medullary osmolarity gradient, and inhibition of antidiuretic hormone-dependent cyclic AMP formation in the renal medulla by calcium itself. Physical examination is rarely helpful in recognizing hypercalcemia except when band keratopathy is observed.

Reproducibly elevated serum total calcium concentrations in excess of 12.5 mg/dl presents little or no challenge to the diagnosis of true hypercalcemia.

However, when serum calcium values are only slightly or intermittently elevated, their interpretation in the absence of symptoms may be difficult. Several artifacts may spuriously affect the measurement of serum calcium. Hemoconcentration secondary to prolonged application of a venipuncture tourniquet, profound dehydration and prolonged fasting can result in high serum calcium estimation but usually no greater than 0.5 mg/dl above true values. Conversely, prolonged contact of serum with red cells can produce low values. Since serum calcium is largely bound to serum proteins, mainly albumin, changes in the concentration of albumin can also produce changes in serum calcium. Adjusted approximation can be made since an elevation of the albumin of 1 g/dl will increase total serum calcium by 0.8 mg/dl. However, direct measurement of ionized calcium is preferred when serum protein abnormalities are present. When the serum calcium is only marginally elevated multiple samples should be obtained. Once true hypercalcemia is established, its cause (Table 75-1) should be determined.

Since excessive parathyroid hormone, in addition to raising serum calcium, produces a number of chemical abnormalities in the blood and urine, useful information can be obtained by relatively simple initial screening tests (Table 75-2). Later steps in the

---

TABLE 75-1
Causes of Hypercalcemia

I. **Excessive Production of Humoral Substances**
  A. PTH
    Primary hyperparathyroidism
    Hyperparathyroidism of renal failure
    Ectopic production of PTH by nonparathyroid tumor
  B. Prostaglandins
    Excessive production by nonparathyroid tumor
  C. "PTH" like bone resorbing factor
    Osteoclast-stimulator produced by tumors

II. **Excessive Vitamin D or Vitamin D Hypersensitivity**
  A. Vitamin D intoxication
  B. Sarcoidosis
  C. Certain hypercalcemia of childhood

III. **Drug-Induced (Vitamin A, Estrogen, Thiazide, Magnesium, etc.)**

IV. **Miscellaneous Causes—May Also Be Associated with PTH Excessiveness**
  A. Hyperthyroidism
  B. Immobilization
  C. Adrenal insufficiency
  D. Milk-alkali syndrome
  E. Pheochromocytoma

TABLE 75–2
Diagnostic Screening Tests of Hypercalcemia

Serum Tests
1. Fasting calcium and phosphate × 3
2. SUN and creatinine
3. Na, K, Cl, CO_2
4. Total protein with albumin/globulin
5. Alkaline phosphatase
6. Magnesium

Urine Tests
1. 24-hour urinary calcium

Radiographic Evaluations
1. Chest x-ray
2. Intravenous pyelogram
3. Bone x-ray when serum alkaline phosphatase is elevated

---

differential diagnosis are more complex and are dictated by the initial results (Fig. 75–2).

Primary Hyperparathyroidism

Primary hyperparathyroidism is due to excessive secretion of parathyroid hormone. It is a common disease, occurring in 1 in 1000 persons. Signs and symptoms, when present, are secondary to hypercalcemia and include two specific complications of excessive secretion of parathyroid hormone, kidney stones and bone disorders. Its etiology is most commonly a solitary adenoma of one of the parathyroid glands (90 percent). Multiple adenomas are found in about 4 percent of patients. Chief cell or clear cell hyperplasia of the parathyroid glands constitute 5 percent of cases and may occur as a familial disorder. Carcinoma of the parathyroid is rare. Parathyroid adenomas may be located outside of the cervical region, often in the mediastinum, and usually occur in patients with more than four glands. Secretion of parathyroid hormone by adenomas is not totally autonomous, since it is commonly suppressible by calcium infusion. Many patients with mild hypercalcemia are asymptomatic and are discovered only as a result of routine multichannel automated testing.

Renal calculi may occur in any patient with hypercalcemia and hypercalciuria but it is commonest in those with primary hyperparathyroidism. In one review of 57 cases, 30 percent presented initially with renal colic, and 23 percent were discovered fortuitously.[234] Kidney stones and their symptoms continue to be the best clinical clue to the recognition of patients with primary hyperparathyroidism.

Parathyroid-hormone-induced osteomalacia, or osteitis fibrosa cystica, may be accompanied by nonspecific bone pain, arthralgia, or myalgia. Neuromus-

cular, gastrointestinal tract, and genitourinary complaints have been mentioned. Other symptoms and complications include pruritis, paresthesias, headache, loose teeth, gout, pathologic fractures, and pancreatitis. In addition, parathyroid adenomas may occur with other endocrinopathies, especially with multiple endocrine adenomatosis.

Objective physical findings are few and nonspecific. Hypertension is common (40 percent). Neuromuscular findings are not rare. In order of frequency, proximal muscle weakness, cranial nerve abnormalities (especially fasciculations of the tongue), and reduced acral vibratory appreciation are found. Progressive kyphoscoliosis is seen only in far advanced disease. Band keratopathy is a result of chronic hypercalcemia. Radiologic evaluation of the skeletal system is useful, particularly when serum alkaline phosphatase levels are elevated. The most specific bone change is subperiosteal resorption found in the phalanges, lateral ends of clavicles, long bones, and pelvis. Bone cysts are less frequent and not specific.

The diagnosis of hyperparathyroidism is best supported by serum PTH values that are elevated relative to the concentration of ionized calcium. However, the fact that PTH exists in heterogeneous forms in the peripheral circulation has created uncertainties. The biologically active "N-terminus" fragment of the hormone has a short half-life and is rapidly cleared from plasma. Therefore, peripheral venous blood contains predominantly carboxy-terminal fragments which possess no biologic activity. Therefore, measurement of PTH using antisera directed to the carboxy-terminus only indirectly reflects secretory rate. In most circumstances, abnormally elevated levels suggest hyperparathyroidism. Values of PTH measured by antisera directed primarily at the amino-terminus are difficult to interpret because they are low in the peripheral circulation due to rapid degradation of the N-terminal fragments. However, the assay of N-terminal fragment is the method of choice for selective venous catheterization to localize adenomas since relatively high concentrations of N-terminal fragments may be found in the venous effluent from tumors.

The most difficult problem in the diagnosis of primary hyperparathyroidism is the exclusion of ectopic production of PTH by an occult malignancy. Furthermore, in rare instances, patients with malignancies may also have concomitant primary hyperparathyroidism. In such patients, PTH assay of multiple samples obtained during selective venous catheterization of the major cervical veins and the veins draining the thyroid may be useful for identifying the site of abnormal PTH production.

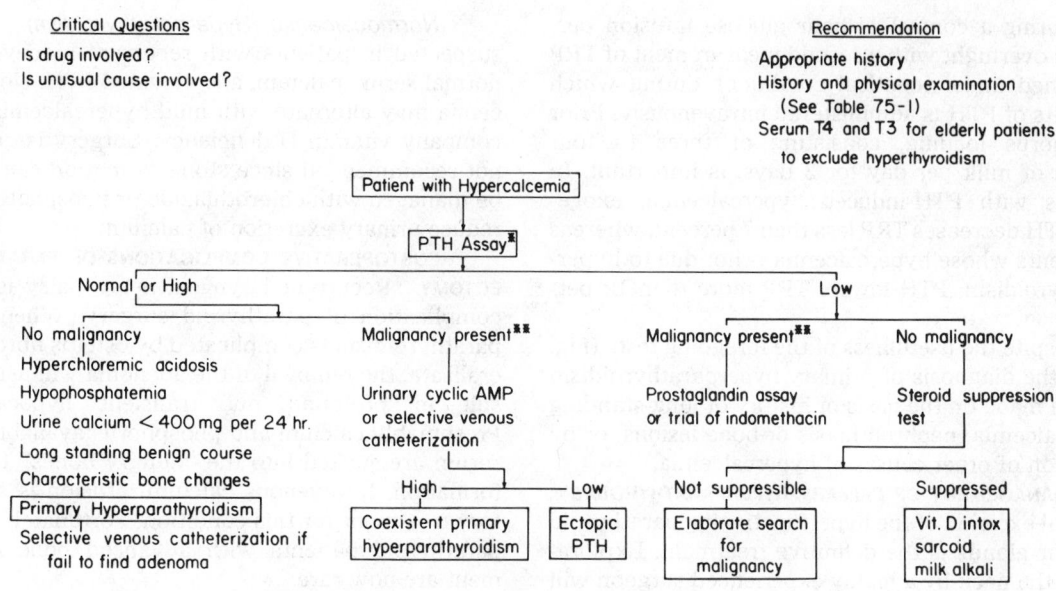

FIGURE 75-2. An approach to differential diagnosis of hypercalcemia.

Measurement of nephrogenic cyclic AMP, though not widely available, is also a helpful adjunct in the diagnosis of hyperparathyroidism. Patients with paraneoplastic hypercalcemia with increased nephrogenic cyclic AMP in the urine are likely to have primary hyperparathyroidism.[229] The prevalence of primary hyperparathyroidism among these patients whose hypercalcemia is labelled as paraneoplastic is probably higher than generally appreciated.

Since total reliance upon immunoassay of PTH is unwise, it is often necessary to diagnose primary hyperparathyroidism on the basis of biochemical changes and clinical presentation and by exclusion of other causes of hypercalcemia.

In uncomplicated primary hyperparathyroidism, biochemical abnormalities include:

1. Hypercalcemia which may be intermittent
2. Hypophosphatemia (50 percent of patients)
3. Bicarbonate less than 24 mEq/L (24 percent)
4. Serum chloride greater than 107 mEq/L (39 percent)
5. Uric acid greater than 6.8 mg/dl (62 percent)

These abnormalities are consequences of the enhanced urinary excretion of phosphate and bicarbonate produced by PTH. In the ectopic PTH syndrome,

hyperchloremic acidosis may not be apparent but hypokalemia is common.

In the absence of renal failure, urinary calcium excretion is increased. However, since PTH enhances calcium reabsorption by the renal tubules, excretion of calcium is less in hyperparathyroidism than in hypercalcemia due to other causes.

The corticosteroid suppression test may be useful in distinguishing patients with sarcoid, vitamin D intoxication, and milk-alkali syndrome, whose hypercalcemia is in part secondary to increased absorption of calcium from the gastrointestinal tract. The levels of serum calcium in these patients may decrease substantially in 7 to 10 days with administration of 100 to 120 mg of cortisone acetate or its equivalent. Rarely a case of primary hyperparathyroidism or malignancy-associated hypercalcemia will show a similar response. These exceptions are usually patients with severe osteitis fibrosa.

In addition to raising serum calcium, PTH promotes urinary excretion of phosphate. Assessment of the phosphaturic effects of exogenously administered hormone by measuring tubular reabsorption of phosphate (TRP) or renal clearance of phosphate is often employed to assess whether the receptor sites in the renal tubules have already been saturated by excessive endogenous hormone. The test compares the

TRP during a control 11-hour glucose infusion performed overnight with a second measurement of TRP performed under identical conditions during which 200 units of PTH is administered intravenously. Prior phosphorus loading, consisting of three to four glasses of milk per day for 3 days, is important. In patients with PTH-induced hypercalcemia, exogenous PTH decreases TRP less than 7 percent, whereas in patients whose hypercalcemia is not due to hyperparathyroidism, PTH lowers TRP more than 12 percent.

Despite the usefulness of the foregoing tests (Fig. 75-2), the diagnosis of primary hyperparathyroidism is often made on the basis of history of long-standing hypercalcemia, nephrolithiasis or bone lesions, or by exclusion of other causes of hypercalcemia.

MANAGEMENT OF PRIMARY HYPERPARATHYROIDISM. Surgical excision of the hyperfunctioning parathyroid gland or glands is the definitive treatment. Exploration of the neck by a highly experienced surgeon will locate the tumor in 90 to 95 percent of patients. If the initial operation is unsuccessful, venous catheterization studies and selective arteriography should be carried out.

If surgery is contraindicated and hypercalcemia is significant, the patient can be managed with oral neutral phosphorus (1 to 1.25 g of phosphorus per day as Neutra-Phos). This treatment if maintained will usually prevent renal calculi and lower serum calcium. Careful follow-up of renal function is, however, essential since progressive renal failure is the principal complication of this therapy.

SPECIAL PROBLEMS ASSOCIATED WITH THE MANAGEMENT OF PRIMARY HYPERPARATHYROIDISM. *Hypercalcemic Crisis.* Occasionally patients with hyperparathyroidism may present with serum calcium in excess of 15 mg/dl. When it is accompanied by mental deterioration, it should be vigorously treated medically to reduce the serum calcium before surgery.

Asymptomatic Mild Hypercalcemic Hyperparathyroidism. When the serum calcium is less than 10 percent above the upper limit of normal and the patient is asymptomatic, management should be individualized. As a rule, surgery is recommended in patients less than 60 years of age. Older patients can usually be followed untreated, even for an extended period of time, since the disease rarely progresses rapidly.

Chlorothiazide-associated Hypercalcemia. The mechanism is unknown. Sustained and significant hypercalcemia is unusual. The drug should be discontinued and an alternative diuretic used. If hypercalcemia persists, other causes of hypercalcemia should be sought.

Normocalcemic Hyperparathyroidism. This is suspected in patients with recurrent kidney stones, normal serum calcium, and elevated PTH. Normocalcemia may alternate with mild hypercalcemia or accompany vitamin D deficiency. Surgery is generally not recommended since stone formation can usually be managed with chlorothiazide or phosphate, which reduce urinary excretion of calcium.

POSTOPERATIVE COMPLICATIONS OF PARATHYROIDECTOMY. Recurrent laryngeal nerve palsy is a rare complication of parathyroid surgery. When hyperparathyroidism is complicated by osteitis fibrosa generalisata, the removal of the adenoma will usually result in profound but transient hypocalcemia. Presumably calcium and phosphorus available in the serum are sucked into the "hungry bones" for bone formation. Intravenous calcium infusion is satisfactory treatment for this condition. Fortunately, hyperparathyroid patients with advanced bone involvement are now rare.

Transient mild hypocalcemia is common, is usually well tolerated, and seldom requires treatment. Permanent hypoparathyroidism occurs in less than 20 percent of cases. Persistent hypophosphatemia and profound hypophosphaturia are excellent indices of successful surgery, but phosphatemia in excess of 5.8 mg/dl developing within 14 days postoperatively is highly suggestive of permanent hypoparathyroidism. Its management is outlined in the section on hypoparathyroidism. Severe hyperchloremic metabolic acidosis may develop postoperatively, usually within the first 24 hours. Bicarbonate may be administered judiciously if careful control of serum calcium is also maintained. Predisposing factors in the development of this complication are impaired renal function and significant bone involvement. Other postoperative complications may include hypomagnesemia, hypoparathyroidism secondary to hypomagnesemia, pancreatitis, and gout.

Secondary Hyperparathyroidism

The pathogenesis of secondary hyperparathyroidism is a low serum calcium or more precisely, a low serum ionized calcium, in individuals with initially normally functioning parathyroid glands. Precipitating conditions include insufficient vitamin D intake or production, calcium malabsorption, 1,25-dihydroxycholecalciferol-deficiency secondary to renal disease, vitamin D malabsorption from the gut, and inborn errors of vitamin D metabolism. Prolonged stimulation of the parathyroids by persistent hypocalcemia may result in hypertrophy of all the glands.

The pathogenesis of hyperparathyroidism secondary to renal failure is complex. With progressive loss of nephrons, there is retention of phosphate. Hyperphosphatemia causes hypocalcemia both by reciprocal reduction in serum calcium by physiochemical mechanisms and by inhibition of the synthesis of $1,25(OH)_2D$, which is already decreased because of loss of functioning renal tissue. Prolonged hypocalcemia leads to hypersecretion of PTH and hypertrophy of the glands. Treatment consists of oral aluminum hydroxide or aluminum carbonate to bind phosphate in the gut and hence lower serum phosphate, restriction of dietary phosphate intake, administration of $1,25(OH)_2D_3$, dialysis if necessary, and management of the underlying renal disease. In a few patients, sustained hypercalcemia develops after the renal failure is corrected, especially following renal transplantation. In these instances, involution of the secondary hyperparathyroidism may be incomplete and autonomous parathyroid adenoma may develop (tertiary hyperparathyroidism). Parathyroidectomy may be necessary but only in less than 10 percent of patients.

Hypercalcemia Associated with Malignant Disease

Hypercalcemia is a common complication of malignant disease. In a survey of 438 patients admitted for radiotherapy of cancer, 9.1 percent had hypercalcemia.[243] The elevated calcium may be due to

1. Production of PTH or a PTH-like substance (ectopic hyperparathyroidism)
2. Secretion of prostaglandins, osteoclast-activating factor, or a vitamin D-like sterol by the tumor
3. Osteolytic metastases
4. Coexistent primary hyperparathyroidism

In most instances, the hypercalcemia appears abruptly and late in the course of the disease when the diagnosis is already obvious. In some patients, however, tumor may be occult, and a careful search for the neoplasm is necessary. Malignancies that cause hypercalcemia include squamous carcinoma of lung, hypernephroma, lymphoma, breast cancer, multiple myeloma, cancer of gastrointestinal tract, and nasopharyngeal cancer. Osteoclast-activating factor is often produced by myeloma cells. The patient with prostaglandin-associated hypercalcemia has low serum PTH and is characteristically responsive to usual therapeutic doses of indomethacin (25 mg four times daily) or salicylates.[239] To distinguish ectopic PTH syndrome from hyperfunction of the parathyroids is difficult. Increased urinary excretion of cyclic AMP favors the diagnosis of primary hyperparathyroidism. Screening studies should include x-ray of the lung and IVP and, if indicated, x-rays of the gastrointestinal tract, bone marrow studies, protein electrophoresis, and analysis for Bence Jones protein in the urine.

Vitamin D Intoxication

This disorder is now rare. If daily doses of vitamin D in excess of 50,000 IU per day are given to normal individuals, vitamin D poisoning may occur. The sequence of events may be as follows: 1) increased calcium absorption; 2) increased serum calcium; 3) suppression of PTH; 4) decreased urinary phosphorus excretion and, when renal function deteriorates; 5) hyperphosphatemia; and 6) ectopic calcification in soft tissue and visceral organs. The clinical picture is usually one typical of hypercalcemia. Nausea, vomiting, and dehydration may be prominent, and pruritis is common. Rarely, except in severe cases, will hypercalcemia persist as long as 1 year after vitamin D has been stopped. Response to glucocorticoids is usually prompt.

Milk-Alkali Syndrome

An unusual complication of peptic ulcer therapy is hypercalcemia consequent to excessive intake of milk (1.5 quarts or greater a day) and absorbable alkali, usually as calcium carbonate. In advanced cases significant renal failure, phosphate retention, and ectopic calcification may be present. The renal damage is usually reversible following exclusion of milk and alkali. When hypercalcemia is severe enough to cause alteration of consciousness, glucocorticoids may be required in addition to hydration.

Both the milk-alkali syndrome and vitamin D intoxication are diagnosed by taking a careful history of dietary habits and medications. Medicines obtainable without prescriptions, such as Tums, Rolaids, and vitamin preparations, are often not regarded as "medicine" by patients. When possible, family members should be questioned since hypercalcemia can affect the patient's memory and state of consciousness.

Sarcoidosis

Hypercalcemia and hypercalciuria may be associated with sarcoidosis. The mechanism remains obscure, although evidence suggests hypersensitivity to normal amounts of vitamin D. Patients behave as though they had hypervitaminosis D: calcium absorption from the gut is enhanced and urinary calcium excretion exaggerated. It is unusual to find sarcoidosis in the process of evaluating a patient with cryptic hypercalcemia. More often, the patient has typical lesions of the skin and lungs, mediastinal adenopathy, or cystic changes in bones, characteristically in the hands. Suspicion of the disorder is raised by finding hyperglobulinemia and hypercalciuria. The diagnosis is confirmed with Kveim test and biopsy of the involved organ. Glucocorticoid therapy is effective.

Hyperthyroidism

Rarely, hypercalcemia is associated with hyperthyroidism as a result of accelerated turnover of bone. When present it is often accompanied by hypercalciuria, phosphaturia, and elevation of the serum alkaline phosphatase. Calcium homeostasis is restored when thyrotoxicosis is controlled, and coexistent hyperparathyroidism need be considered only if hypercalcemia persists after euthyroidism is achieved.

Acute Adrenal Insufficiency

Acute adrenal insufficiency may be accompanied by hypercalcemia and hypophosphatemia. The clinical picture is dominated by that of adrenal crisis. The cause of the hypercalcemia is not known but profound dehydration is one of the contributing factors. Hypercalcemia may also appear with acute withdrawal of exogenous corticoids. It usually resolves with steroid treatment.

Hypercalcemia of Immobilization

Hypercalcemia and hypercalciuria may occur when patients with active turnover of bone are immobilized. This can be observed in young people and patients with thyrotoxicosis, Paget's disease, or hyperparathyroidism, occasionally unmasking previously unsuspected disease. Surprisingly, serum parathyroid hormone levels are usually elevated and return to normal with mobilization.[233] If bed confinement is unavoidable, calcium restriction, hydration and oral phosphorus supplementation should be instituted.

Other Conditions Associated with Hypercalcemia

The coexistence of pheochromocytoma and primary hyperparathyroidism is well known (Type 2 multiple endocrine adenomatosis). Some patients with pheochromocytoma, especially those with the familial type, have mild hypercalcemia that is readily corrected by removal of the tumor.[241] Mild elevations of serum calcium also have been observed in patients with the watery diarrhea (pancreatic cholera) syndrome. The cause is unexplained but resection of tumor results in the reestablishment of normocalcemia.

Treatment of Acute Hypercalcemic Crisis

Since hypercalcemia can be life-threatening, management constitutes a medical emergency. The most important therapeutic measure, irrespective of the cause, is hydration. Rapid rehydration with normal saline (usual recommendation, 3 liters over 9 hours) is important. Sodium enhances calciuria by competitively inhibiting tubular reabsorption of calcium. Calcium excretion can be further enhanced by furosemide infusion (60 to 80 mg per hour) after loading with 1 to 2 liters of saline and with continued fluid and electrolyte replacement.

If cardiac and renal functions are poor, hydration alone is ineffective and may be hazardous. Mithramycin, a cytotoxic antibiotic, has been used with increasing frequency in the management of severe hypercalcemia. The usual dose is 15 to 25 μg/kg body weight given intravenously as a single bolus injection. It strikingly inhibits bone resorption, producing within 48 hours its hypocalcemic effect which may persist for several days. If necessary, repeated doses can be given but toxic effects on bone marrow, liver, and kidney are more likely to develop.

High doses of glucocorticoids (200 mg cortisone or greater per day) are most effective in treating the hypercalcemia of vitamin D intoxication, sarcoidosis, milk-alkali syndrome, lymphoma, breast cancer, multiple myeloma, and certainly adrenal insufficiency. Generally the onset of action of the steroid is slow. Calcitonin is another hypocalcemic agent which has some use in the management of hypercalcemia. It exerts its hypocalcemic effect by inhibiting bone resorption. The usual dose is 50 to 100 units given subcutaneously at 12-hour intervals. Its effect is short-lived and often not marked unless the rate of bone turnover is unusually high. When hypercalcemia is associated with hyperphosphatemia, it may be the agent of choice since it also promotes urinary phosphate excretion.

Intravenous infusion of phosphate (1500 mg phosphorus given over 6 to 8 hours) can effectively and reliably reduce serum calcium, primarily by precipitating calcium into bone. However, undesirable ectopic deposits of calcium salts can also occur. Since fatal arrhythmias and irreversible renal damage have been reported as complications of this treatment, it should be used only as a last resort.

EDTA administered intravenously effectively lowers ionized calcium by chelation. It too may cause severe renal toxicity. Since therapeutic alternatives are available, its use is no longer warranted. Indomethacin and salicylates in usual therapeutic doses are effective in controlling malignancy-induced hypercalcemia due to prostaglandin production.

The major agents which lower plasma calcium are listed in Table 75–3. In general, a combination of hydration with one of these agents is recommended to manage hypercalcemic crisis.

Patients with far-advanced, well-documented, incurable neoplasms may present with life-threatening hypercalcemia. In such patients, the somnolence induced by hypercalcemia may be a welcome develop-

TABLE 75-3

Commonly Used Agents for the Management of Hypercalcemia

	Onset of Action	Dosage	Comments
Saline hydration and furosemide	Rapid	3 liter/9 hr 60 to 80 mg/hr	Reduce serum calcium 2 to 3 mg/dl but rarely normalize serum calcium, may precipitate CHF
Mithramycin	Rapid	25 µg/kg/body weight, IV push	Effective in all types of hypercalcemia associated with increased bone resorption; toxic to bone, liver, and kidney
Calcitonin	Rapid but not sustained	50–100 MRC U, subcutaneously; aqueous form can be given IV	Ideal for hypercalcemia associated with hyperphosphatemia
Phosphate	Rapid	1500 mg phosphorus given IV 6–8 hrs (In-Phos or Hyper-Phos-K)	Effective but may cause soft tissue calcification
Glucocorticoid	Slow	200 to 300 mg cortisone acetate	Most useful for vitamin D intoxication, milk alkali, myeloma lymphoma, breast cancer, leukemia
Indomethacin	Slow	100 to 150 mg/day	Effective for prostaglandin-associated hypercalcemia

ment. Therefore, the decision to treat should depend upon the relative advantages and disadvantages of alternative palliatives and the patient's immediate prognosis. Mild hypercalcemia of malignancy may be left untreated since it may serve as a marker to assess the effects of chemotherapy.

HYPOCALCEMIA[238]

Hypocalcemia develops when either PTH or vitamin D is deficient or defective, or their end organs fail to respond. Proof of sustained hypocalcemia requires multiple serum calcium determinations. Since serum albumin levels and serum pH can influence the values of serum calcium, they should be measured concomitantly for meaningful interpretations. If serum albumin is normal, symptoms of hypocalcemia may not be apparent until serum calcium falls below 7.5 mg/dl. The cardinal clinical manifestation is tetany. Characteristically an attack of tetany is heralded by perioral or acral paresthesias. This may be followed by a feeling of stiffness in the limbs that will be involved. Muscle cramps and carpopedal spasm next develop. The hands assume a characteristic form with the thumbs forced into adduction while the fingers are firmly pressed together with the metacarpophalangeal joints flexed (obstetrician's hand). Rarely laryngeal stridor and seizures may occur. Psychoneurotic manifestations associated with hypocalcemia include emotional lability, anxiety, delirium, and a variety of frank psychoses. Symptoms of extrapyramidal or cerebellar lesions, tremor, athetosis, and ataxia have been reported. Papilledema with or without increased CSF pressure may occur. Long-term complications of untreated hypocalcemia include changes in the texture of the skin (dry and scaly), monilia infection, alopecia, cutaneous moniliasis, cataracts, growth and mental retardation, osteosclerosis, and metastatic calcification. With mild hypocalcemia, spontaneous tetany is usually absent; however, carpopedal spasm may be elicited in the arm by a sphygmomanometer by compression of nerves inflated above the systolic pressure for at least 3 minutes (Trousseau's sign). Increased neuromuscular irritability can also be demonstrated by eliciting twitching of facial muscles by tapping the facial nerve (Chvostek's sign). Latent tetany may also be precipitated by menstruation, pregnancy, lactation, and exercise. It is important to appreciate that Chvostek's sign is present in 10 percent of the normal population. Therefore, serial examinations, including preoperative evaluations of hyperparathyroid patients, are often helpful.

Symptoms of overt or latent tetany are dependent on altered muscle membrane stability which may be mimicked by systemic alkalosis. Accordingly,

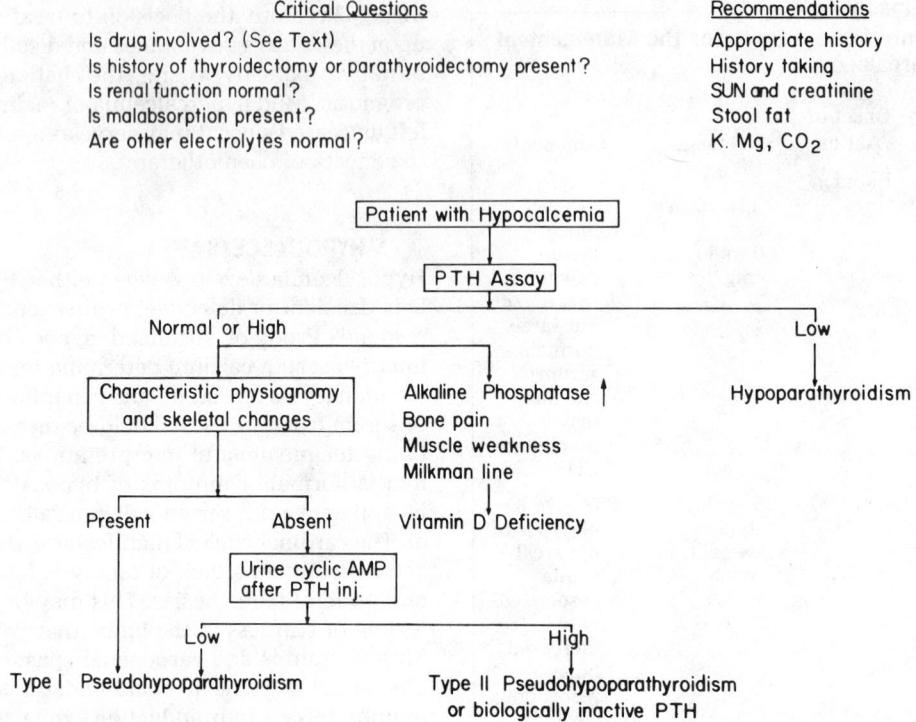

Critical Questions

Is drug involved? (See Text)
Is history of thyroidectomy or parathyroidectomy present?
Is renal function normal?
Is malabsorption present?
Are other electrolytes normal?

Recommendations

Appropriate history
History taking
SUN and creatinine
Stool fat
K, Mg, CO_2

FIGURE 75–3. Differential diagnosis of hypocalcemia. Extensive study is usually not necessary in patient with surgical hypoparathyroidism.

tetany may also occur with hyperventilation syndrome, alkali ingestion, hypokalemia, and magnesium deficiency. Serum electrolytes and a careful history usually suffice to differentiate the causes (Fig. 75–3).

Causes of Hypocalcemia

Hypocalcemia secondary to low serum albumin does not present a clinical problem since ionized calcium levels are usually normal. Simultaneous measurement of serum proteins should always be obtained to exclude such pseudohypocalcemia. A normal ionized serum calcium excludes true hypocalcemia. Hypocalcemic agents, such as mithramycin, calcitonin, phosphate, EDTA can cause hypocalcemia when used inappropriately. Acute pancreatitis, by depositing calcium ion in the alkaline pancreatic tissue and by causing relative PTH deficiency, can cause hypocalcemia.[227] Low serum calcium levels occur in a significant number of patients with advanced carcinoma of the breast. In other malignancies, resistance to vitamin D may develop. The precise mechanisms for hypocalcemia in these disorders remains unclear.

HYPOPARATHYROIDISM. Primary hypoparathyroidism occurs most commonly following surgery

and in patients who develop idiopathic disease. Transient hypocalcemia is frequent after parathyroidectomy and thyroidectomy, especially in patients with markedly hyperfunctioning parathyroid glands. Spontaneous recovery is the rule but hypocalcemia may recur and become permanent many months or years later. The incidence of surgical hypoparathyroidism is decreasing and in experienced hands is probably less than 2 percent. Idiopathic hypoparathyroidism may be an autoimmune phenomenon analogous to autoimmune thyroiditis and adrenal failure, since antibodies to parathyroid tissue have been demonstrated. This entity is usually detected in childhood. It has been reported in sibs and may be associated with moniliasis, diabetes mellitus, hypothyroidism, Addison's disease, pernicious anemia, and hypogonadism. In some families, this syndrome is associated with the HLA-A1, B8 haplotype. Congenital absence of the parathyroids and thymus, due to maldevelopment of the third and fourth branchial arches, occurs in the DiGeorge syndrome. Rarely the parathyroid glands are affected by infiltrative processes, metastatic disease, or hemochromatosis.

In the absence of PTH, serum phosphorus rises and both factors contribute to impaired 1-hydroxylation of 25-hydroxycholecalciferol. In these circumstances, calcium absorption from the gut is low, the rate of bone resorption is decreased, and calcium fails to be normally resorbed by the renal tubules. As a consequence hypocalcemia results.

HYPOPARATHYROIDISM DUE TO DEFECTIVE PTH. This disorder apparently results from production of an immunogically active but biologically inactive form of PTH. Clinically it is indistinguishable from hypoparathyroidism except that PTH is detected by radioimmunoassay. This condition is not associated with autoimmune endocrinopathies.[235]

SECONDARY HYPOPARATHYROIDISM. Hypomagnesemia reversibly inhibits PTH secretion.[223] When profound it produces typical hypocalcemia with hyperphosphatemia and tetany may result. An element of peripheral resistance to PTH and vitamin D may also be present in some patients. Measurement of serum magnesium is, therefore, essential in the evaluation of all hypocalcemic patients.

PSEUDOHYPOPARATHYROIDISM. This disease is mendelian and probably transmitted as an X-linked dominant. It is found occasionally in association with hypothyroidism (often due to isolated TSH deficiency), impaired prolactin secretion, and diabetes mellitus. Impaired taste and olfaction have been reported in this disorder.

In contrast to hypoparathyroidism, immunoassayable parathyroid hormone concentrations are high but biochemical abnormalities associated with the absence of a physiologic effect of PTH, namely hypocalcemia and hyperphosphatemia, are present. Furthermore, the patients usually have a peculiar somatotype characterized by round face, short stature, strabismus, brachydactyly of the fourth and fifth metacarpal and metatarsal bones, early closures of epiphyses, soft tissue and CNS calcifications (especially of the basal ganglia), and mental retardation. In rare instances the metabolic abnormalities are present without the skeletal changes.

The basic pathophysiologic defect in pseudohypoparathyroidism is failure of bone and kidney to respond to PTH. However, the degree of PTH unresponsiveness may vary and the lesions in the two organs and the subcellular levels may be different. Consequently there are variants of this disorder.

The commonest and best understood variant is one in which renal cells are unable to synthesize cyclic AMP in response to PTH. Normal phosphate excretory mechanisms are impaired and hyperphosphatemia ensues. This is referred to as Type I pseudohypoparathyroidism. The hallmark of this disorder is 1) inability of exogenous PTH to increase cyclic AMP and phosphate excretion; and 2) elevated

blood PTH concentrations. There is failure of 1-hydroxylation of 25(OH)D in this disease.[240] As a result, absorption of calcium is decreased and osteomalacia may develop. The impaired formation of 1,25(OH)$_2$D from 25(OH)D suggests that the suppressive effects of hyperphosphatemia can override the stimulatory effects of PTH on the 1-hydroxylation or the tissue responsiveness to PTH which includes a refractoriness of the renal 1-hydroxylase activity. The fact that osteomalacia, osteitis fibrosa, or subperiosteal resorption may develop in a small number of patients indicates that bone cells are not always totally refractory to PTH. This conclusion is supported by the observation that administration of 1,25(OH)$_2$D$_3$ to patients with pseudohypoparathyroidism restores the normal skeletal response to PTH.

A second variant is one in which patients respond to PTH by a brisk increase in urinary cyclic AMP but fail to increase their excretion of phosphate. These patients are probably refractory to cyclic AMP. This disorder is called Type II pseudohypoparathyroidism. Patients have neither the skeletal stigmata nor the pattern of inheritance of Type I.

Pseudo-pseudohypoparathyroidism is a condition in which the skeletal abnormalities of pseudohypoparathyroidism are present but serum calcium, phosphorus and PTH levels are normal.

Vitamin D and Hypocalcemia

Vitamin D deficiency, due to diet or impaired conversion of vitamin D to 1,25(OH)$_2$D, can result in failure of bone to mineralize normally. Profound hypocalcemia is unusual in vitamin D deficient disorders since compensatory hyperparathyroidism occurs. Severe forms may present with diffuse bone pain and muscle weakness. Suggestive laboratory findings include hypophosphatemia, hyperphosphatasia, and low to low-normal serum and urinary calcium. Radiologically, osteopenia or biconcave-shaped vertebrae may be evident but the most characteristic finding is the presence of Looser zones, also known as pseudofractures or Milkman lines. The major conditions related to vitamin D deficiency are listed in Table 75–4. In the United States, dietary vitamin D deficiency is not a major cause of osteomalacia. However, it is a well recognized complication of intestinal malabsorption, gastric surgery, chronic laxative abuse, hepatic disease, renal failure, and long-term treatment with either phenytoin or barbiturates.

TREATMENT OF HYPOCALCEMIA. Acute severe hypocalcemia associated with tetany or seizures requires intravenous administration of calcium. In the adult, symptoms are usually relieved by a single bolus of 10 to 20 ml of 10 percent calcium gluconate

TABLE 75-4
Causes of Osteomalacia Syndromes

I. **Disorders of Vitamin D**
  A. Inadequate vitamin D supply
    1. Dietary deficiency
    2. Malabsorption syndrome (gastric surgery, laxative abuse, pancreatic insufficiency, cholestyramine)
  B. Impaired metabolism of vitamin D
    1. 25-hydroxylation defect
      a. Phenytoin, barbiturate administration
      b. Cholestatic liver disease
    2. 1-hydroxylation defect
      a. Hypoparathyroidism and pseudohypoparathyroidism
      b. Renal failure
      c. Hereditary vitamin D-dependent rickets
      d. Oncogenic osteomalacic syndrome
  C. Target organ resistant to 1,25 (OH)$_2$ D
    1. Uremia
    2. Phenytoin and barbiturate administration
    3. Primary resistant to 1,25 (OH)$_2$ D

II. **Phosphate Deficiency**
  A. Familial hypophosphatemic rickets
  B. Acquired hypophosphatemic rickets

III. **Hypophosphatasia**

IV. **Defects in Formation of Bone Matrix**

V. **Drug Induced**
  A. Fluorides
  B. Diphosphonate

injected slowly intravenously. Thereafter 15 mg calcium/kg body weight may be infused over 4 to 6 hours with serum calcium closely monitored.

Chronic hypoparathyroidism is treated with a combination of oral calcium and vitamin D. Elemental calcium, 1.5 to 2.0 g per day, is given as lactate, gluconate, or chloride salts. To provide 1 g of elemental calcium, 8 g of calcium lactate, 11 g of calcium gluconate, or 5.5 g of calcium chloride must be administered. In the absence of PTH and in the presence of hyperphosphatemia, pharmacologic doses of vitamin D in the order of 50,000 IU (1.25 mg)/day (but this may vary from 25,000 to 200,000 IU/day) are required to control hypocalcemia. The daily therapeutic dosage of 1,25(OH)$_2$D$_3$ is much lower: 0.5 to 1 μg. The dose of vitamin D may have to be reduced if the patient is concomitantly receiving thiazide diuretics or if hyperthyroidism or adrenal insufficiency is present. Higher doses may be necessary when the patient is on a diet rich in phosphate, or is taking tranquilizers or estrogen preparations.[224]

The therapeutic goal is to maintain serum calcium in the low normal range (8.5 to 9.5 mg/dl). In the absence of PTH, tubular reabsorption of calcium

is diminished and nephrocalcinosis and deterioration of renal function subsequent to massive hypercalciuria may occur if the treatment is too vigorous. To maintain eucalcemia without inducing hypercalciuria, 50 mg a day of chlorthalidone orally plus a low salt diet (50 mEq per day) appears to be an effective alternative to vitamin D in some patients with hypoparathyroidism.[236]

Acute hypomagnesemia can be managed by the intravenous administration of 1 to 2 g of magnesium (usually in the form of magnesium sulfate) as a 10 percent solution. Oral magnesium is best given in the form of magnesium oxide, 35 to 70 mEq per day. Dietary vitamin D deficiency can be treated with as little as 100 IU of vitamin D per day. Osteomalacia in epileptics taking anticonvulsants is best managed with at least 2 μg of 1,25(OH)$_2$D$_3$, daily.

METABOLIC BONE DISEASE

Bone is an active metabolic organ. It is constantly being remodeled, a process whereby old bone is resorbed and replaced with new bone. This requires continous production of new cells whose function and differentiation are closely regulated.

Disorders which alter this remodeling process lead to abnormal bone structure. Therefore, metabolic bone disease can be produced by abnormalities of any of the following: 1) 1,25 dihydroxycholecalciferol; 2) parathyroid hormone; 3) phosphorus metabolism; 4) calcium metabolism; 5) collagen synthesis; 6) osteoprogenitor cell activity; 7) osteocyte activity; and, probably, 8) calcitonin.

In most instances there is a single principal cause of a metabolic disorder. The interrelationships between factors controlling bone and mineral metabolism, however, may obscure this cause when homeostatic mechanisms come into play that produce their own biochemical abnormalities.

CLASSIFICATION

Metabolic bone disease includes any disorder in which the process of bone remodeling is altered to the extent that abnormal bone structure results. Radiographically it may present as porous or dense bone. Osteopenia is a generic term for radiologically porous bone. The commonest osteopenic conditions include osteoporosis (loss of bone mass), osteomalacia (failure of calcification of osteoid), and osteitis fibrosa cystica. The latter is a condition characterized by excessive bone resorption, cyst formation, and secondary fibrosis. It is most frequently associated with long-standing hyperparathyroidism. Radiographically, dense bone is observed in osteopetrosis, osteosclerosis, and Paget's disease.

Since the radioimmunoassays of PTH and vitamin D metabolites are still in a state of rapid changes, an attempt to classify metabolic bone disease according to humoral changes is premature.

Polyostotic fibrous dysplasia is a disease of unknown etiology. Radiologic examination of bone characteristically shows patchy cyst-like lesions in the cortex or ground-glass appearance in the expanded cortex.

LABORATORY EVALUATION[225]
Metabolic bone disease can be evaluated:

1. Radiographically to demonstrate gross alterations in bone
2. Histologically if a bone biopsy is available
3. Biochemically by measuring serum and urine calcium, phosphorus, and magnesium
4. By measuring serum levels of osseous alkaline phosphatase (index of the pyrophosphatase activity of the osteocyte) to assess bone formation, and urinary hydroxyproline excretion rate to evaluate bone resorption
5. By measuring humoral factors that regulate bone remodeling such as vitamin D and its metabolites, PTH, calcitonin, and prostaglandins

The serum alkaline phosphatases are enzymes which originate in liver, bone, kidney, gut, and placenta. Elevated alkaline phosphatase activity is found in normal growing children and in pregnancy but when due to disease, it is most commonly from liver or bone. The most satisfactory way to distinguish hepatic from osseous alkaline phosphatase is the measurement of 5′nucleotidase. The hepatic alkaline phosphatase cross-reacts in the routine assay for 5′nucleotidase activity. Accordingly, an increased serum alkaline phosphatase and a normal 5′nucleotidase indicate that the alkaline phosphatase activity originates from bone.

Hydroxyproline is released and excreted in the urine as a consequence of collagen breakdown. As the skeleton contains 55 to 60 percent of total body collagen, increased bone resorption is invariably associated with an increase in the rate of urinary hydroxyproline excretion. Care in the interpretation of values is essential. Excretion normally varies with age, being greatest in the first year and at puberty and lowest in adulthood (15 to 50 mg/24 hours). It may be raised when dietary intake of gelatin or collagen is high or with increased extraskeletal collagen

turnover secondary to burns, Cushing syndrome, or psoriasis.

OSTEOMALACIA AND RICKETS[231]
In the adults, failure to mineralize bone is known as osteomalacia. An increase in noncalcified bone matrix results in soft and pliable bones. In children, this condition is called rickets and frequently results in clinically recognizable bony deformities. Since bone growth has ceased in the adult, gross skeletal abnormalities are rare. The clinical manifestations of osteomalacia are subtle and often difficult to recognize. Moderate to severe forms may present with diffuse muscle weakness and bone pain. In the elderly, it may occur concomitantly with senile osteoporosis. Since uncomplicated osteoporosis is usually painless, the presence of pain in a patient with radiographic evidence of osteoporosis is suggestive that osteomalacia may also be present. Laboratory findings are usually normal but in some patients with severe active disease, serum calcium and phosphate may be low and alkaline phosphatase and PTH elevated, while urinary calcium excretion is low but urinary hydroxyproline excretion is high. Radiographically, generalized porosity of bone and biconcave-shaped vertebral bodies may be present; however, Looser zones are almost pathognomonic of osteomalacia. Looser zones are linear decalcification along the course of large blood vessels frequently found symmetrically distributed in the scapulae, pelvis, and proximal long bones. When hypocalcemia persists, bone changes such as subperiosteal erosions, cysts, and osteitis fibrosa cystica due to secondary hyperparathyroidism may occur. In children, there is widening and irregularity of the epiphysis. Cupping of the metaphysis, fractures, and bowing of bones may develop. Definitive diagnosis of osteomalacia is made by bone biopsy and the demonstration of an excess of osteoid.

The radioimmunoassays for vitamin D and its active polar metabolites have greatly contributed to our understanding of the pathogenesis of osteomalacia. The defect in mineralization that occurs in osteomalacia may arise from lack of $1,25(OH)_2D$ or its effects, deficiency of phosphate, or a defect in production of alkaline phosphatase and bone matrix (Table 75-4).

Nutritional Osteomalacia
The daily requirement of dietary vitamin D is approximately 400 IU. In the United States, nutritional deprivation of this vitamin has not been regarded as an important cause of osteomalacia. However, in elderly persons who have eaten sparingly and have little or no exposure to sunlight, it may be more common than generally appreciated. Clearly, vitamin D deficiency occurs in patients with intestinal mal-

absorption, gastrectomy, pancreatic insufficiency, chronic obstructive jaundice, laxative abuse, and long-term administration of cholestyramine. Interruption of enterohepatic circulation of 25(OH)D may be an important mechanism of vitamin D deficiency associated with gastrointestinal and hepatobiliary disease.

Disorders of Vitamin D Metabolism

Abnormalities that impair the availability or effectiveness of $1,25(OH)_2D$, the active metabolite of vitamin D, can arise in three organs:

1. The liver, where 25-hydroxylation of cholecalciferol occurs
2. The kidney, where 1-hydroxylation of 25(OH)D takes place
3. In the intestine, where $1,25(OH)_2D$ stimulates calcium absorption.

Defects of 25-Hydroxylation of Vitamin D

The serum concentration of 25(OH)D is dependent primarily on diet and exposure to sunlight. Severe hepatic disease can diminish the production of 25(OH)D in one of two ways: by disrupting its enterohepatic circulation or by destruction of tissue that normally produces 25-hydroxylase. Osteomalacia is an infrequent complication of liver disease but serum 25(OH)D concentrations are low in some patients with parenchymal and cholestatic disease. Although the diseased liver is usually able to convert administered vitamin D to its 25-hydroxylated metabolite, complete healing of undermineralized osteoid may require oral administration 25(OH)D.

Patients on long-term anticonvulsant treatment with phenytoin and phenobarbital may develop osteomalacia. In many, circulating levels of serum 25(OH)D are decreased, presumably because of accelerated metabolic destruction of both cholecalciferol and 25(OH)D. However, serum levels of $1,25(OH)_2D$ are usually normal. Therefore, osteomalacia is most likely secondary to either a direct suppressive effect of anticonvulsants on the action of $1,25(OH)_2D$ on gut absorption of calcium or a deficiency of 25(OH)D which may be required to promote normal mineralization of bone.

Defects of 1-Hydroxylation of 25(OH)D

Renal 1-hydroxylase activity is regulated by PTH, serum phosphate, and probably the $1,25(OH)_2D$ itself. Of these, the principal direct stimulus is low serum phosphate.

Renal Osteodystrophy

Metabolic bone disease is inevitable in patients with chronic renal failure. In approximately 50 to 80 percent of patients, the bones show pathologic changes that are a complex mixture of varying degrees of osteomalacia, osteitis fibrosa generalisata and osteosclerosis. The pathogenesis of renal osteodystrophy remains unclear but unquestionably impaired metabolism of vitamin D and secondary hyperparathyroidism play a role.

Plasma levels of 25(OH)D are normal in most patients with renal failure, but the concentrations of $1,25(OH)_2D$ are usually low. Chronic hyperphosphatemia inhibits 1-hydroxylation of 25(OH)D. Furthermore, the severely damaged kidney synthesizes insufficient amounts of $1,25(OH)_2D$. As a result, intestinal calcium absorption is decreased, hypocalcemia develops, and PTH secretion is stimulated. While this cascade of events accounts for the presence of osteomalacia and osteitis fibrosa in renal osteodystrophy, it does not explain why osteomalacia is inconsistently observed. That a defect in 1-hydroxylation of 25(OH)D persists is consistent with the dramatic improvement in uremic man following administration of $1,25(OH)_2D_3$. Near physiologic doses of $1,25(OH)_2D_3$ (about 1 μg per day) will correct calcium malabsorption and return serum calcium and PTH to normal; however, osteomalacia only partially improves. In some patients with sufficient functioning renal tissue, vigorous control of hyperphosphatemia may result in return of $1,25(OH)_2D$ levels to normal.

As uremia progresses, muscle weakness, bone pain, and arthralgias may become prominent, parathyroid hyperplasia develops, and serum calcium may become inappropriately elevated relative to phosphate levels. As a consequence, there is a predisposition for metastatic calcification to occur in subcutaneous tissues and conjunctivae. Calcium phosphate crystals in the conjunctivae are responsible for the "red eyes" observed in patients with far advanced uremia. Successful renal transplantation results in a return of $1,25(OH)_2D$ levels to normal, but parathyroid hyperplasia may persist and cause posttransplantation hypercalcemia. Whether pretreatment with $1,25(OH)_2D_3$ to restore calcium homeostasis to normal can prevent the occurrence of hypercalcemia after transplantation remains to be seen.

Hypoparathyroidism and Pseudohypoparathyroidism

Osteomalacia is not usually produced by PTH deficiency. Low levels of PTH reduces the 1-hydroxylation of 25(OH)D and concomitant hyperphosphatemia suppresses the production of $1,25(OH)_2D$.

Decreased blood levels of $1,25(OH)_2D$ measured by radioimmunoassay have been reported in both hypo- and pseudohypoparathyroidism. These aberrations in vitamin D metabolism probably account for the fact that patients with these conditions are relatively resistant to vitamin D and require pharmacologic doses to prevent hypocalcemia. Despite the fact that $1,25(OH)_2D$ production is low, osteomalacia is rare in this disorder. Conceivably full expression of the bone lesion requires the presence of PTH.

Vitamin D-Dependent Rickets

This disorder is clinically indistinguishable from dietary vitamin D deficient rickets except for its autosomal recessive inheritance and the massive doses of exogenous vitamin D or 25(OH)D needed for its treatment. Minute amounts of $1,25(OH)_2D_3$ (1 μg), however, are sufficient to restore the metabolic abnormalities. These findings together with the observation that blood levels of $1,25(OH)_2D$ are low in these patients, suggest that the basic defect in this disorder is the failure of 1-hydroxylation of 25(OH)D.

Tumor Osteomalacia

A number of neoplasms, including giant cell, mesenchymal, angiomatous, and granulomatous tumors, produce hypophosphatemic rickets and osteomalacia clinically indistinguishable from hereditary hypophosphatemic rickets. Usually the tumors are benign. The metabolic bone lesions heal upon their removal, but also regress with administration of high doses of vitamin D. Characteristically, blood levels of 25(OH)D are normal but $1,25(OH)_2D$ values are low. These tumors of connective-tissue origin may produce a substance that inhibits 1-hydroxylation of 25(OH)D.

Target Tissue Resistant to $1,25(OH)_2D$

Osteomalacia may result from target tissue (intestine, bone, and kidney) unresponsiveness to $1,25(OH)_2D$. In uremic patients, in addition to deficient production of $1,25(OH)_2D$, intestinal response to $1,25(OH)_2D$ is diminished. Another example of end-organ unresponsiveness to vitamin D is in patients treated with phenobarbital and phenytoin. Both drugs, in addition to altering the metabolism of vitamin D, inhibit bone resorption that is normally stimulated by PTH and $1,25(OH)_2D$. Finally, rickets with normal serum 25(OH)D levels and markedly elevated $1,25(OH)_2D$ levels has been reported. This disorder may result from primary end-organ hyporesponse to $1,25-(OH)_2D_3$.[226]

Therapeutic Implications of Metabolic Disorders of Vitamin D Metabolism

Administration of $1,25(OH)_2D_3$ has thus far been found clinically effective in most vitamin D-resistant conditions. This compound has the following advantages:

1. Its onset of action is rapid (normocalcemia may be restored in 3 to 7 days in contrast to 4 to 8 weeks for vitamin D).
2. Its toxic effects subside faster than other vitamin D preparations (3 to 5 days in contrast to 6 to 18 weeks for vitamin D and 4 to 12 weeks for 25(OH)D.
3. It bypasses vitamin D hydroxylation abnormalities that may exist in the liver or kidney.

Only in patients with end-organ resistance and in some patients with renal osteodystrophy are suboptimal responses observed.

The recommended daily dose of $1,25(OH)_2D_3$ is 0.25 μg. This, however, may be increased to 1 to 2 μg a day depending on the clinical indications.

Another useful agent is synthetic dihydrotachysterol (DHT or AT 10). This substance is a sterol which has a 3-hydroxyl group that is sterically positioned in such a way that it mimics the position of the 1-hydroxyl of 1(OH)D and 1, $25(OH)_2D$. It has proved to be a useful substitute for the active derivatives of cholecalciferol. A daily dose of 1 mg of DHT is usually sufficient.

Osteomalacia of Phosphorus Deficiency

Chronic hypophosphatemia may lead to florid rickets or osteomalacia. Pure hypophosphatemia is often a result of X-linked renal tubular disorder. Serum concentrations of both 25(OH)D and $1,25(OH)_2D$ are normal. However, the levels of $1,25(OH)_2D$ might be expected to be elevated in the presence of hypophosphatemia. Therefore, the possibility of a partial defect in intermediary metabolism of vitamin D cannot be totally excluded. X-linked hypophosphatemia usually presents in childhood with growth failure and rickets. Nonfamilial adulthood hypophosphatemic osteomalacia is rare. In contrast to X-linked hypophosphatemia, myopathy is often present. Presenting symptoms include muscle weakness, bone pain, and frequent fractures of long bones. Since slow-growing tumors such as angiomas, sarcomas, and hemangiomas can produce a similar condition, even when small, a search should be carried out to exclude them. The treatment is phosphorus supplement and vitamin D to correct phosphate-induced hypocalcemia.

Phosphatase Deficiency

This genetic disorder is inherited as an autosomal recessive trait. Radiographically and histologically it resembles rickets; it differs from rickets in that there is premature synostoses of the skull, dental abnormalities, and excretion of abnormal quantities of phosphoethanolamine and inorganic pyrophosphate in the urine. The alkaline phosphatase is low in bone, plasma, and leukocytes but normal in other nonskeletal tissues. Hypophosphatasia should be suspected prenatally when ultrasonography fails to visualize a fetal head by the 16th week of gestation. This is due to deficient mineralization of the fetal head.

Calcium-Wasting Osteomalacia

Intestinal malabsorptive states commonly are complicated by insufficient absorption of both calcium and vitamin D. Occasionally hypomagnesemia is also present and magnesium replacement may be required to facilitate restitution of calcium homeostasis.

Osteomalacia occurs in patients with hypercalciuria, Fanconi syndrome, and renal tubular acidosis. Multiple factors may be involved in its cause. Loss of calcium is one. The hallmark of Fanconi syndrome and renal tubular acidosis is the renal phosphate loss which may also contribute to failure of calcification of osteoid. Systemic acidosis augments the rate of bone resorption producing hypercalciuria and hyperparathyroidism as a consequence. Experimental evidence suggests that renal 1-hydroxylase activity is decreased in Fanconi syndrome. This may explain why large doses of vitamin D may be required to maintain normal calcium levels. In patients with these disorders, phosphate therapy is indicated not only to inhibit renal stone formation but to enhance bone accretion as well.

The pathogenesis of so-called "idiopathic" hypercalciuria has been partially resolved.[232] It is now thought that excessive excretion of calcium can have two causes. In one form, the primary defect is inability of the kidney to conserve calcium. With loss of calcium, secondary hyperparathyroidism develops. Excess PTH, in turn, promotes phosphaturia and enhances 1-hydroxylation of 25(OH)D and hence intestinal calcium absorption. The cause of calcium wasting by the kidney is unknown. Patients with this disorder usually present with renal stones and are found to have normal serum calcium, low phosphorus, increased intestinal absorption of calcium, hypercalciuria, increased urinary cyclic AMP, and reduced tubular reabsorption of phosphorus. Radiologic evidence of osteopenia is rare. Their stone-forming tendency can be managed with chlorothiazide and neutral phosphate.

The second cause of idiopathic hypercalciuria is increased intestinal absorption of calcium that is unrelated to secondary hyperparathyroidism. Two subpopulations of patients have been identified: one with normal levels of 1,25(OH)$_2$D and the other with high levels. Those with normal levels probably have a primary intestinal defect which is responsible for hyperabsorption of calcium. Those with high levels of 1,25(OH)$_2$D invariably have hypophosphatemia secondary to unexplained renal phosphate-wasting. The hypophosphatemia stimulates formation of 1,25(OH)$_2$D which enhances the intestinal absorption of calcium. Low serum PTH concentration reduces tubular reabsorption of calcium thereby further promoting hypercalciuria and renal stone formation. In those patients with hypophosphatemia, oral phosphate is effective therapy since it reduces circulating 1,25(OH)$_2$D and therefore urinary calcium excretion. Osteomalacia is not a feature of this disorder, since presumably osteoid is mineralized in the presence of excess 1,25(OH)$_2$D.

Involutional Osteoporosis

Osteoporosis is defined as loss of bone mass and is the commonest osteopenic disorder. Almost every organ loses some of its functional capacity with age, and the human skeletal system is no exception. With time, bone mass is lost and osteoporosis develops. After maturity in women, the rate of bone loss is about 8 percent per decade, in men 3 percent. Unlike osteomalacia, the ratio of mineral to organic matrix in osteoporosis does not change; rather both are decreased in the same proportion.

It is the commonest bone disease affecting the elderly, occurring in 15 to 50 percent of persons over age 65. Up to 80, women are affected four times more often than men. The sex incidence is the same after age 80. Caucasians and Northern Europeans are particularly susceptible.

Osteoporosis is clinically significant only when bone mass is reduced to the extent that the skeleton is insufficient to perform its normal function. It is usually painless. The coexistence of osteomalacia or other underlying disease should be considered in patients with pain and radiographic evidence of "osteoporosis" without apparent fractures. Common complications of osteoporosis include compression fractures of vertebral bodies with the development of kyphosis and back pain. Fractures of the proximal femur, wrist, and lower thoracic and first lumbar vertebrae are frequent occurrences.

Serum calcium, phosphorus, alkaline phosphatase, and PTH are nearly always normal. Mild hypercalciuria may be found in some patients but usually the rates of excretion of urinary calcium and hydroxyproline are normal. Histologically, the number of bone cells involved in the remodeling process are decreased. Bone trabeculae are reduced in number and more widely separated. The osteoclasts have fewer nuclei and bone turnover is decreased. In concert with this decreased remodeling, the rate of development of bone cells appears to be retarded. The result is a relative increase in the area of bone undergoing resorption as the existing osteoclasts delay their maturation into osteoblasts.

The pathogenesis of involutional osteoporosis remains unclear. It has been suggested that age-related bone loss is a universal phenomenon. Subjects most likely to develop osteoporosis are those who reach skeletal maturation with less than normal amount of bone. Consistent with this view is the observation that males and blacks, who normally have a greater bone mass than Caucasian women, are less susceptible to osteoporosis. This bone disorder can be secondary to a number of systemic diseases (Table 75–5).

Recognition of osteoporosis is based on roentgenologic evidence of bone rarefaction. Typically, changes involve all bones but are often most prominent in the axial skeleton. Roentgenologic estimation of bone quantity is rather insensitive, since as much as 30 percent of bone tissue may have to be lost before density changes are apparent. The mineral content of bone can be more accurately measured using low-energy photons emitted from a radioactive source. Such photon absorptiometry has proven quite reproducible and can provide an accurate means of following response to therapy. It is not useful in distinguishing osteoporosis from osteomalacia.

Management of Osteoporosis

Successful measures to prevent or to treat involutional osteoporosis remain elusive. Patients who suffer from fractures and are in acute pain usually require hospitalization. Here collaboration between internist, orthopedist, and physical therapist is essential. Programmed exercise to increase muscle tone and tailor-made braces to correct postural abnormalities are useful. When obesity is present, weight control is always recommended. It must be kept in mind that not every pain in the area where osteoporosis is present, necessarily arises from this condition.

Calcium supplements, vitamin D, estrogen, calcitonin, and fluoride have been used to treat osteoporosis, with variable results. Estrogen and calcitonin, while inhibiting osteoclastic activity, retard the maturation of osteoprogenitor cells. Therefore, temporary improvement in negative skeletal balance is achieved, but long-term restoration of bone mass is difficult. Fluoride stimulates new bone formation but also prevents normal calcification. Fluoride treated bone is dense but fragile. If fluoride is used the doses should not exceed 20 to 25 mg/day.

A regimen which appears to hold greater promise includes physical activity, vitamin D (50,000 IU every other day), and inorganic phosphorus (1 to 1.5 g per day). Phosphate diminishes bone resorption and enhances formation. Vitamin D is added to prevent the development of secondary hyperparathyroidism from chronic use of phosphate and to treat possible coexistent osteomalacia. Physical exercise increases circulation to the skeleton and prevents loss of bone mineral associated with inactivity.

Glucocorticoid-Associated Osteoporosis

Glucocorticoid therapy and adrenal hypercorticism commonly produce osteoporosis. Radiographic evidence of skeletal loss is found in about 50 percent of patients with obvious Cushing syndrome. Postmenopausal women, immobilized subjects, adolescents, and patients with emphysema appear more susceptible to the adverse skeletal effects of glucocorticoids. Glucocorticoid excess accelerates catabolism of $1,25(OH)_2D$, decreases calcium absorption from gut, and prolongs the time necessary for completion of each bone modeling unit. Catabolic effects of glucocorticoid lead to inadequate formation of bone matrix and delay in healing of bone fractures.

TABLE 75–5
Conditions Associated with Osteoporosis

Primary
Involutional
Osteoporosis of juveniles

Secondary
Cushing syndrome
Hyperthyroidism
Hypogonadism
Diabetes mellitus
Hyperparathyroidism
Malnutrition
Chronic liver disease
Immobilization
Heparin therapy
Alcoholism
Myeloma, lymphoma
Calcium deficiency
Scurvy
Chronic obstructive pulmonary disease

Heritable disorders
Homocystinuria
Osteogenesis imperfecta

Management of glucocorticoid-associated osteoporosis should be directed to correction of the endogenous cause or reduction of the dose of steroid. Since it is not always possible to reduce the dose of glucocorticoid because of the underlying illness, 50,000 IU of vitamin D per day and programmed exercise should be given to those patients requiring long-term treatment. The use of $1,25(OH)_2D_3$ may prove to be more effective.

Other Hormone-Related Osteoporosis

The rate of bone turnover is increased in thyrotoxic patients. Hypercalciuria is common. Serum alkaline phosphatase and urinary hydroxyproline excretion are increased. Marked bone resorption can occur in some patients producing mild hypercalcemia. Clinically significant bone loss may occur in patients with long-standing unrecognized hyperthyroidism.

Osteoporosis is associated with the Klinefelter and Turner syndromes. Sex steroids replacement may be effective in decreasing the rates of bone loss in patients with these conditions. The incidence of osteoporosis is also increased in patients with diabetes mellitus. When insulin secretion is deficient, collagen synthesis is impaired.

Disuse Osteoporosis

Mechanical stress plays an important role in the maintenance of normal bone mass. Immobilization leads to rapid mobilization of bone mineral which produces hypercalciuria, an increase in urinary excretion of hydroxyproline, and occasionally elevations of serum PTH and hypercalcemia. Loss of skeletal mass results from a decrease in osteoblastic bone formation and an increase in osteoclastic resorption. When a limb is immobilized by a cast, local osteoporosis may develop.

Patients must be mobilized as soon as conditions permit. Hydration is essential since hypercalciuria is common. Oral phosphate may be used when hypercalcemia needs treatment.

Osteoporosis of Deficient Collagen Synthesis

In severe malnutrition, scurvy and chronic illnesses complicated by protein wasting, osteoporosis may develop. In these conditions newly formed bone may be defective.

A number of heritable disorders of connective tissue may be associated with osteoporosis. In osteogenesis imperfecta deficient bone mass may be severe. In this disorder, of which several forms are recognized, the synthesis and organization of collagen in bone and skin are abnormal. The bones may be severely deformed and fragile. The numbers of osteoblasts and osteoclasts are normal but turnover of bone is high with the balance favoring resorption.

Osteoporosis is also a common finding in patients with homocystinuria. The diagnosis is established by determining homocystine in urine. Homocystine or its metabolites interfere with the formation of intermolecular cross-links that are necessary to stabilize collagen.

Idiopathic Osteoporosis

This disorder is seen primarily in males under 40 years of age. It differs from involutional osteoporosis in several respects: hypercalciuria is common, urinary hydroxyproline may be elevated, and histologically there appears to be increased activity of bone cells. The etiology of this disorder is unknown.

INCREASED DENSITY OF BONE

Osteopetrosis

Increased density of bone is observed in only a few diseases. The term "osteopetrosis" is usually reserved for Albers-Schönberg disease (marble bone disease), an inherited disorder characterized by generalized and marked increase in bone density. In its most severe form, there may be obliteration of the bone marrow cavity, severe deformities of the skull and compression of the cranial nerves. Death occurs in childhood from severe anemia, bleeding disorders, extramedullary hematopoiesis, and increased intracranial pressure. In mild cases that survive, there is short stature, a propensity to develop fractures, and increased density of bone radiographically. Patients are prone to develop osteomyelitis, particularly in the mandible. Histologically, there is evidence of reduced bone resorption and osteoclasts are absent. Serum calcium, phosphate and alkaline phosphatase are normal but acid phosphatase activity is often elevated. The basic defect is unknown. In mice with a disorder apparently homologous to the severe autosomal recessive form of osteopetrosis, there is evidence that a stem-cell defect results in deficiency of osteoclasts. Bone marrow transplantation is an experimental method for restoring osteoclasts in cases of this "malignant" form of osteopetrosis. The differential diagnosis of osteopetrosis includes vitamin A intoxication, fluorosis, and myelosclerosis.

Osteosclerosis is occasionally observed in patients with renal osteodystrophy. This condition is characterized by increased bone density which is particularly prominent in the metaphyseal regions of the vertebrae. Its etiology remains unknown, although some evidence suggests that PTH or elevated serum phosphate may be causative factors. More commonly, aberrations in phosphate, PTH, and vitamin D lead to the development of osteomalacia and osteitis fibrosa cystica which may be present concomitantly with osteosclerosis.

Paget's Disease of Bone (Osteitis Deformans)

Paget's disease is a disorder of locally increased bone remodeling. The clinical manifestations depend upon the extent and location of the lesions as well as the presence of associated complications. Many patients are asymptomatic, and their lesions are usually detected during radiographic evaluation of unrelated illness. Local pain and joint stiffness, often described as rheumatic, gouty, or neuralgia, are common complaints. As the spine, pelvis, skull, and femur are the usual sites of involvement, hip pain, low back pain, headaches, and tinnitus are frequent symptoms. Pathologic fractures may be the initial presentation. Basilar skull invagination in advanced cases may lead to progressive ataxia and tetraplegia, as a result of compression of the cerebellar tonsils. Paraplegia is probably due to concentric narrowing of the spinal canal. The most common neurologic complication is hearing loss secondary to eighth nerve compression by involved temporal bone. A marked increase in bone blood flow is well recognized. Cardiac output may be markedly increased when involvement of the skeleton is extensive. Hyperkinetic circulation may aggravate preexisting cardiac dysfunction and hasten the development of congestive heart failure in the elderly.

Physical findings when present, include an enlarged skull with prominent superficial veins, hearing impairment, progressive kyphosis with shortening of stature, and deformity of long bones. The skin temperature overlying a lesion may be elevated, and flow murmurs are sometimes audible. Angioid streaks of the retina have been observed in some patients.

Paget's disease is more common in the elderly than generally appreciated. The true incidence is difficult to estimate. European autopsy and radiographic studies suggest that about 3 percent of adult population are affected by this disease. By the ninth decade, the incidence may be as high as 5 to 11 percent. The basic pathologic process is an accelerated resorption of bone due to excessive osteoclastic activity, followed by osteoblastic regeneration, and formation of new bone. The newly formed bone under these circumstances, however, is defective and often deformed. Sarcomatous degeneration of the bone lesions occurs but fortunately affects no more than 1 percent of the patients. The etiology of this disorder remains obscure. Attention has been drawn to the occasional hereditary nature of the disease. Recently,

linkage of Paget's disease with HLA haplotypes has been demonstrated in the familial form.

Serum calcium and phosphorus are normal but hypercalciuria is common. During immobilization for severe pain or fractures, excessive bone resorption continues, whereas the rate of new bone formation is diminished. Such a distortion of the balance between bone resorption and formation occasionally leads to hypercalcemia.

The laboratory approach to the diagnosis of Paget's disease can be divided into two major categories: 1) anatomic delineation of the lesion, and 2) assessment of the activity of the disease. In the absence of bone histology, the anatomic evaluation can be made by conventional radiography and radioisotopic scanning. The bone changes noted on x-rays need not reflect active disease. The majority (85 percent) of bone lesions are detectable by both radiography and scan; 10 percent are visualized by radiograph alone; and the remaining by the scan alone. Pagetic lesions detected by bone scan are usually symptomatic lesions.

Measurements of serum alkaline phosphatase activity and total urinary hydroxyproline are both sensitive indices of the activity of Paget's disease of bone. They are also useful "markers" to assess treatment. Elevation of serum acid phosphatase activity also occurs in severe Paget's disease.

TREATMENT OF PAGET'S DISEASE.   Paget's disease is usually amenable to treatment with pharmacologic doses (50 to 100 MRC units per day) of calcitonin given subcutaneously. Salmon calcitonin, by virtue of its long half-life in man, has proved to be more effective than the porcine hormone. In some instances in which remission has not been sustained, development of neutralizing antibodies to calcitonin or an escape of the bone cells from the effects of the hormone have been incriminated. Calcitonin restores normal bone remodeling, is safe for long-term use and has only trivial side effects. Its principal disadvantage is that it can be given only by injection.

Sodium editronate is also available for the management of this disease. This compound binds strongly to crystals of hydroxyapatite to slow bone turnover rate. The usual dose is 5 mg/kg/day given orally. The effectiveness of this agent is similar to that obtained by calcitonin injection. The duration of treatment generally should not exceed 6 months since significant impairment of mineralization of both normal and diseased bone occurs thereafter. Other agents that have been used include mithramycin, actinomycin D, and glucagon.

Mild Paget's disease may be managed with salicylate or indomethacin. The indications for more specific treatment include significant bone pain, prevention of further deformity, operative preparation for joint replacement, hearing loss, and high output congestive heart failure.

Polyostotic Fibrous Dysplasia (Albright Syndrome)[242]

This is a disease of unknown etiology. The classic triad of this syndrome consists of skin pigmentation, bone lesions, and precocious sexual development. The brownish skin pigmentation tends to be unilateral, flat, and multiple with irregularly indented margins. The bone lesions are results of fibrous dyplasia.

Radiologically, they appear as cystic lesions in the cortex or ground-glass change in an expanded cortex. Like the skin lesions, these bone involvements are usually unilateral, often on the same side as the skin pigmentation. Precocious puberty is the best known endocrine disorder associated with this syndrome, but other reported conditions include goiter, hyperthyroidism, acromegaly, Cushing syndrome, gynecomastia, and parathyroid enlargement. It has been postulated that a congenital abnormality of the hypothalamus causes excessive production of hypothalamic-releasing hormones in this syndrome.

CHAPTER 76
The Thyroid Gland
ROBERT I. GREGERMAN

Disturbances of thyroid growth and function are among the disorders most commonly encountered in practice.[248,268] Excessive production of the thyroid hormones, thyroxine (T4) and triiodothyronine (T3) (Fig. 76–1), results in the syndrome of hyperthyroidism, or thyrotoxicosis; decreased function is responsible for hypothyroidism. Generalized enlargement of the thyroid, regardless of cause, is termed goiter. Focal enlargement of the thyroid is usually benign. Either goiter or focal enlargement may be associated with abnormal thyroid function. Goiter can produce anatomic changes ranging from the simply cosmetic to disturbance in the structure and function of contiguous structures such as the trachea and esophagus.

ANATOMY AND PHYSIOLOGY[269]

EMBRYOLOGY AND ANATOMY

Embryologically, the thyroid develops from the entodermal cells of the pharyngeal floor. During early gestation these cells migrate caudad from an area at the base of the tongue to the level of the thyroid cartilage, forming the two lateral lobes and the connecting midline isthmus anterior to the trachea. The small cephalad extension of the isthmus is known as the pyramidal lobe, a structure not usually discernible unless the gland is pathologically enlarged. Abnormalities in migration occasionally result in malpositioning of the gland, usually sublingually or in the nasopharyngeal area. Such ectopic glandular tissue is rarely sufficient in function to meet hormonal demands. The migra-

tory tract normally involutes during gestation, though on occasion its remnants give rise to midline cyst(s) that can present clinically at any time during life.

Histologically, the thyroid is made up primarily of follicles or acini lined with cuboidal epithelium and filled with colloid which contains thyroglobulin. This protein, unique to the thyroid, contains T4 and T3, as well as their iodinated amino acid precursors, mono-iodo- and diiodotyrosine (MIT and DIT). Between the follicles is a highly vascular stroma containing the parafollicular or "C" cells. These secretory cells, of neural crest origin, produce thyrocalcitonin (Chap. 75).

THYROID REGULATORY MECHANISMS

The principal regulatory mechanisms of the thyroid are 1) the hypothalamic–pituitary–thyroid negative feedback control system; and 2) an intrathyroidal autoregulatory system.

The hypothalamus secretes thyrotropin-releasing hormone (TRH), which travels via the hypophyseal portal system to the pituitary, where it stimulates release of thyroid-stimulating hormone (TSH). The latter is a glycoprotein composed of two subunits; the α subunit being common to the other glycoprotein hormones, while the β subunit is unique to TSH. Acting at least in part via activation of thyroidal adenylate cyclase and production of the "second messenger," cyclic AMP, TSH stimulates many aspects of thyroid activity: hormone synthesis, synthesis of nucleic acids and proteins, release of thyroid hormones, and growth of follicles. Secretion of TSH by the pituitary

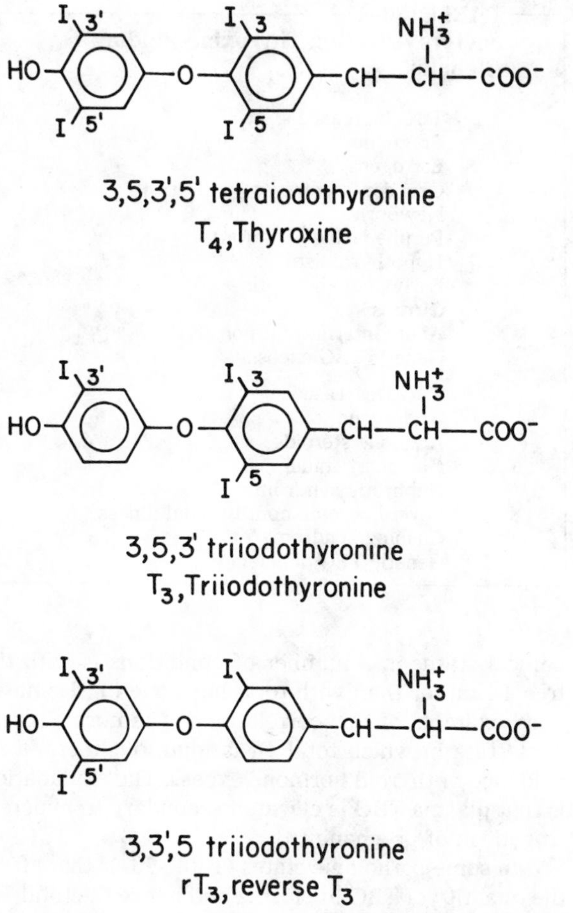

FIGURE 76-1. Chemical structures of major thyroid hormones.

is inhibited by the thyroid hormones, thus the term "negative feedback loop."

Autoregulation of thyroid activity is not well understood, but in some manner intrathyroidal iodine serves to control iodine accumulation and other aspects of the metabolic activity within the thyroid. These influences are independent of TSH.

Thyroid Hormonogenesis and Secretion[263]
Iodide from plasma is concentrated by an active process (iodide "pump") which can maintain a thyroid/plasma iodide ratio as high as 500 to 1. Iodide is thereafter converted through the action of a peroxidase to another form, the nature of which is still unknown, followed by iodination of tyrosine to form monoiodo- and diiodotyrosines. The coupling of these iodoamino acids results in the formation of T3 and T4 bound within the thyroglobulin sequence. The release of these hormones occurs by pinocytosis of follicular colloid at the apical margin of the cells, producing droplets which fuse with lysosomes in which hydrolysis of thyroglobulin by proteases occurs. T4 and T3 are then secreted into the circulation, but MIT and DIT are, in the main, deiodinated intrathyroidally and their iodide reutilized. Normally, only a small proportion of this iodide excess enters the circulation (iodide leak), but under some pathologic circumstances, the loss may be large.

The iodide pump actively transports a number of anions other than iodide, e.g., thiocyanate and perchlorate, a phenomenon which has been exploited diagnostically and therapeutically. For example, perchlorate was once used as an antithyroid drug to interfere with thyroid hormone synthesis. The pertechnetate anion, as the radioactive isotope ^{99m}Tc, is widely used for thyroid imaging.

Iodide Metabolism
The normal thyroid contains 5000 to 8000 μg of iodine, almost all of it organically bound. The minimum daily requirement of iodide is only about 100 to 200 μg, an amount which is determined by obligatory loss through the kidney and to a lesser extent through the gastrointestinal tract. The minimal daily requirement is enormously exceeded by dietary intake; for example iodinated salt provides about 1,000 μg in a normal 10 g daily intake. Thus, iodide deficiency, once common in the United States and elsewhere, is essentially unknown except in remote areas of the underdeveloped world.

Any chemical substance that interferes with thyroid hormone formation or release to lower blood hormone concentration induces compensatory hypertrophy of the gland (goiter) via stimulation of TSH secretion. Certain substances are known to prevent iodide accumulation by impairment of the iodide trapping mechanism ("pump"). Other substances interfere with hormone synthesis or inhibit hormone release. Clinically useful agents which have been employed for therapeutic effects in states of excess hormone production (hyperthyroidism) are known to act at one or another of these points. Perchlorate, no longer commonly used therapeutically, inhibits the iodide pump. The thiocarbamide drugs interfere with hormone synthesis by blockade of incorporation of iodide into the tyrosines ("organification") and the coupling reactions in iodothyronine formation, but have more effect on coupling than on organification. Lithium ion interferes with thyroglobulin proteolysis and hormone release. Iodide itself in pharmacologic amounts interferes with hormone formation and release; the effect on hormone synthesis is usually of short duration.

METABOLIC EFFECTS OF THYROID HORMONE

The thyroid hormones exert their actions through a variety of mechanisms.[261,267] A classic thyroid hormone effect is on basal metabolic rate (BMR), the basis for the first laboratory method for clinical assessment of thyroid status. The numerous known actions of thyroid hormone range from specific stimulation of mitochondrial oxidative metabolism to the nuclear regulation of protein synthesis. Thyroid hormones also exert specific regulatory effects on membrane physiology, e.g., potentiation of catecholamine induced lipolysis in fat cells. The molecular mechanism of some of these effects is through control of the number of plasma membrane beta-adrenergic receptors or modulation of the linkage between the catecholamine receptors and adenylate cyclase.[244] Elucidation of this latter action of thyroid hormones provides an understanding of the exaggerated sympathetic activity in hyperthyroidism and its therapy by beta-adrenergic blockade.

Thyroid hormone effects are age-dependent. The normal development of the brain of the fetus and infant is dependent on the presence of adequate quantities of thyroid hormones. Thyroid hormone deficiency at this stage can result in irreversible mental retardation. During childhood, retardation of somatic growth is the major effect. At the other end of the normal life span, the myocardium of the elderly person is especially susceptible to the deleterious effect of thyroid hormone excess. Elderly persons with hyperthyroidism are prone to develop tachyarrhythmias and heart failure.

Hormone Transport

The thyroid hormones in the blood are T4 and a much smaller quantity of T3. They are tightly but reversibly bound to several plasma proteins, mainly thyroid hormone binding globulin (TBG). In the normal person 65 to 70 percent of the thyroid hormones are bound to TBG, about 15 percent to the secondary carriers, thyroxine-binding prealbumin (TBPA), and about 15 percent to albumin. Variations of TBG are common and account for most of the changes in T4 concentration in plasma that occur in clinical states other than hypo- and hyperthyroidism. The small quantities of T4 (0.03%) and T3 (0.3%) that are not protein-bound (unbound or "free") are in rapid equilibrium with the protein-bound fraction. Total T4 in plasma is 50 times that of T3, but because T3 is less tightly bound than T4, the relative concentrations of the unbound hormones are about 5:1.

The concentrations of unbound ("free") T4 and T3 in plasma are thought to reflect the amount of hormone exerting an effect upon tissues. Correlation of

---

TABLE 76–1
Factors Affecting Thyroxine-Binding Globulin

TBG Increased
Pregnancy
Estrogens
Oral contraceptives
Newborn
Perphenazine (Trilafon)
Hypothyroidism
Early acute hepatitis
Cirrhosis
Acute intermittent porphyria
Genetic TBG excess

TBG Decreased
Androgens
Anabolic steroids
Glucocorticoids
Nephrotic syndrome
Severe chronic nonthyroidal illness
Cushing syndrome
Genetic TBG deficiency

---

clinical status in a number of conditions is with the free T4 rather than with total hormone in plasma. A good example of this correlation is the normal pregnant state in which total T4 is high, but there is no evidence of thyroid hormone excess. The explanation is that plasma TBG is elevated secondary to hyperestrogenism of pregnancy.

In some pathologic states (Table 76–1) that affect the quantity of TBG in plasma and hence the total T4, the absolute concentration of free T4 may not adjust to a normal value. During illness, factors other than the concentration of TBG and TBPA appear to determine the free hormone concentration, presumably by affecting the affinity of the TBG-T4 interaction.[251]

Metabolism and Interconversion of the Thyroid Hormones

Practically all tissues metabolize and degrade the thyroid hormones, but the liver is quantitatively most important and a site at which regulation of hormone degradation occurs. T4 metabolism is the major source (80 percent) of circulating T3 in the normal individual.[248] The normal thyroid secretes mainly T4 and only a small amount of T3. Only in hyperthyroidism, iodine deficiency, and certain other pathologic circumstances is T3 sometimes the predominantly secreted hormone (Fig. 76–2).

Most of the T4 secreted (about 85 percent) is ultimately deiodinated and further degraded. The physiologically most important pathway involves conversion of about 35 percent of the T4 to metabolically active T3, which is itself further deiodinated. About

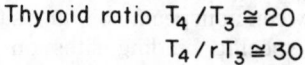

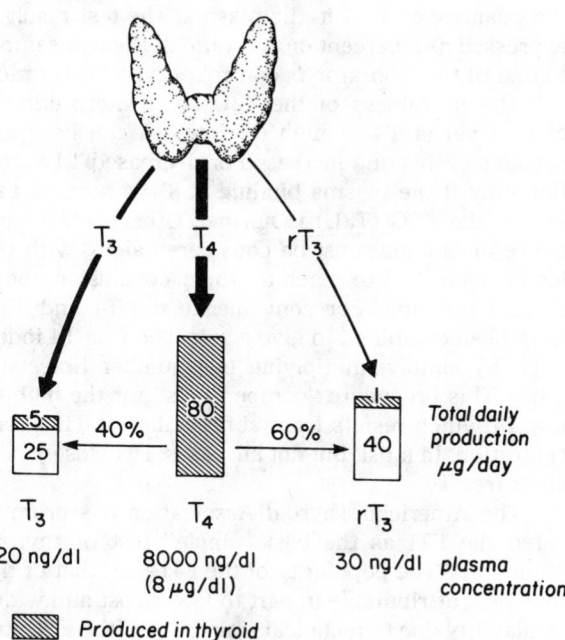

FIGURE 76-2. Production rates and sources of thyroid hormones.

an equal amount of T4 is converted to reverse T3 (rT3) (Fig. 76–1). Although not active in calorigenesis, rT3 does antagonize a number of the effects of T3 and may thus have some physiologic importance. In a variety of pathologic states the formation of T3 is inhibited whereas that of rT3 is reciprocally enhanced. The

deiodination of T4 is accomplished, in part, by the enzymes of the hepatic smooth endoplasmic reticulum. Drugs, such as phenobarbital, which enhance activity of these enzymes, accelerate the metabolic disposal of T4. About 10 to 15 percent of secreted T4 is not deiodinated but is excreted in the stool in the form of conjugates, while small quantities undergo oxidative deamination to the acetic acid analogs, tetra-, and triiodoacetic acids.

LABORATORY TESTS OF THYROID FUNCTION AND OF THYROID DISEASE

Most thyroid "function" tests assess gland secretory activity only indirectly. Measurements of blood hormone concentrations, the most commonly used tests, cannot be equated directly with hormone production rate although they *reflect* that rate when plasma binding of hormones is normal. However, a variety of illnesses, drugs, and alterations of physiologic state affect plasma binding. Accordingly, proper interpretation of plasma hormone concentrations demands concomitant assessment of plasma binding. Thyroid gland function can be assessed somewhat more directly by measurements of thyroidal iodide accumulation ("uptake"; RaIU) using isotopes of iodide (^{131}I, ^{123}I). These tests also must be properly interpreted, since uptake of tracer is only an approximation of the accumulation of stable iodide and of hormone synthesis.

Other laboratory tests are useful in the assessment of thyroid status and the diagnosis of thyroid disease but are not, strictly speaking, tests of thyroid function. Such tests include measurements of the integrity of the physiologic feedback control system, thyroid autoantibodies, and the immunoglobulins related to Graves' disease.

TABLE 76-2
Thyroid Function Tests

	Plasma T4 (μg/dl)	Plasma T3 (ng/dl)	Plasma rT3 (ng/dl)	T3U* (%)	T3UR*	TSH (mU/ml)	FT4* (ng/dl)	FTI*
Normal mean	8	120	30	30	1	—	1.5	2.4
Normal range	5–12	80–160	25–35	25–35	0.85–1.15	0–6	1.0–2.0	1.5–3.6
Confidence limits	±1	±20	±8	±2	±0.05	±2	±0.3	—

Abbreviations: T3U, T3 resin uptake; T3UR, T3 resin uptake ratio; FT4, free thyroxine; FTI, free thyroxine index. See text for limitations of interpretation of normal ranges. Confidence limits (95 percent) of a single value are approximate and depend on both the laboratory and the level within the range.

Measurements of Plasma Hormones: Plasma T4, T3, and rT3

The commonly used and important tests are T4 and T3 determined by radioimmunoassay or other specific methods. Unlike older techniques, no interference is produced by drugs or iodine containing substances. rT3 is also used in differential diagnosis. Normal values of the common tests are given in Table 76–2.

THE "FREE T4": MEASUREMENT OF NON-PROTEIN-BOUND THYROID HORMONE IN PLASMA. The "free T4" of plasma is estimated by separate measurements of the non-protein-bound T4 (equilibrium dialysis) and the total T4; their arithmetic product equals the free T4. The dialyzable (non-protein-bound) T4 normally approximates only 0.03 percent of the total.

The free T4 hypothesis has been helpful as a physiologic concept. Determination of the free T4 for clinical purposes is often useful, but the measurement has serious limitations. In some states, such as pregnancy or during estrogen therapy, both T4 and TBG are elevated and thyroid status is accurately reflected by the free T4. The dialyzable fraction is decreased, but since the T4 is elevated the free T4 is normal. In hyperthyroidism, free T4 reflects thyroid status better than total T4, since the altered metabolic state itself lowers TBG; in some cases a normal or borderline elevation of T4 is associated with an elevated free T4. In hypothyroidism, TBG is often elevated and the free T4 decreased more than is the total T4.

Problems of interpretation of the free T4 arise in many seriously ill patients. A variety of nonthyroidal diseases ranging from acute infections to liver disease can result in elevation of the free T4. In these situations, the patient is usually euthyroid with a normal T4; the free T4 is elevated only because the dialyzable fraction is increased. An explanation for this phenomenon is not readily available. Altered concentrations of neither TBG or TBPA account for the increased free T4. The appearance of a factor in plasma which interferes with protein binding of T4 has been postulated. Thus, an elevated free T4 is *not* a specific finding related solely to thyroid status.

ESTIMATES OF TBG: T3 RESIN UPTAKE AND THE "FREE T4 INDEX" (FTI). The T3 uptake test (T3U) is not to be confused with the concentration of T3 in plasma. The T3U is not a thyroid function test but merely provides an indirect estimate of the concentration of plasma TBG. To some extent, T3U is also influenced by the quantity of T4 in plasma, i.e., by the degree of saturation of the T4- (and T3) binding sites on TBG. The T3U may be replaced by direct quantitation of TBG. Technically the T3U is measured by adding a tracer quantity of T3 and a nonspecific T3 binding absorbent resin to the sample of plasma to be tested. The tracer distributes itself between nonspecific binding sites on the absorbent and specific binding sites on TBG. Resin-bound tracer is therefore reciprocally related to the quantity of TBG in the plasma. The test result is expressed as a percent or as a ratio of the test sample to that of the laboratory's control plasma (T3U ratio).

The usefulness of the T3U is in interpreting a given level of T4. A high (or low) T4 can be interpreted as reflecting increased or decreased T4 secretion only if the plasma binding of T4 is normal, i.e., only if the TBG (T3U) is normal. Otherwise, disturbance of binding must be considered along with the high (or low) T4 to reach a proper conclusion about thyroid function. For convenience the T4 and T3U have been combined to give a so-called free T4 index (FTI) by simply multiplying one number times the other. This procedure "compensates" for the high or low T4 which results from abnormality of TBG concentration. In most, but not all, cases, FTI closely parallels free T4.

The American Thyroid Association has promulgated the FTI as the best "single" test of thyroid "function." The popularity of the FTI over that of the free T4 is attributable in part to lower cost and wider availability due to technical simplicity of the FTI. Another advantage of the FTI is its freedom from spurious elevation in nonthyroidal illness. However, both the FTI and free T4 tests must still be interpreted with caution in the patient with severe nonthyroidal illness.

Tests of the Negative Feedback System

THYROID STIMULATING HORMONE (TSH). Plasma TSH is invariably elevated in primary hypothyroidism because of reduced feedback inhibition by the decreased concentrations of the thyroid hormones. The measurement of plasma TSH is important both in the diagnosis of primary hypothyroidism and in monitoring the adequacy of thyroid hormone replacement therapy. Elevation of plasma TSH is the most sensitive indicator of hypothyroid status. Elevations of TSH are reliably measured by radioimmunoassay techniques currently available. However, by most assay methods plasma TSH of normal subjects is below the sensitivity of the method; many of the values reported to be within the normal range may be nonspecific, and in fact abnormally low. A diagnosis of secondary hypothyroidism (pituitary TSH deficiency) should not be discarded because of a "normal" TSH.

SUPPRESSION TESTS USING T4 AND T3. In several thyroid diseases gland function becomes independent of TSH, i.e., nonsuppressible by amounts of exogenous thyroid hormone that inhibit normal pituitary secretion of TSH. Nonsuppressibility is seen in hyperthyroidism due to any cause, in cases of hyperfunctioning adenoma ("hot nodule") with or without hyperthyroidism, and in some cases of nontoxic nodular goiter. About one-half of patients with Graves' ophthalmopathy without hyperthyroidism also have nonsuppressible thyroid function. Return of suppressibility in the course of Graves' disease indicates clinical remission, and the test is therefore a useful guide to therapy as well as diagnosis. Testing for suppressibility is done with T3 or T4 using a 50 percent decrease of RaIU as the endpoint. T4 is given as a single 3 mg dose or 25 μg of T3 is given every 8 hours. RaIU is measured during the eighth day.

THE TRH TEST. Parenterally administered TRH produces release of TSH from the pituitary. Response to TRH is abnormal in several clinical circumstances and is of diagnostic use. In theory the test should distinguish hypothalamic ("tertiary") from pituitary ("secondary") hypothyroidism, but the test is unreliable for this purpose. Confirmation of a diagnosis of primary hypothyroidism is possible when the plasma TSH elevation is borderline, since an exaggerated plasma TSH response will be seen. The most common use is as an alternative to the T3 suppression test in the diagnosis of hyperthyroidism. Hypersecretion of thyroid hormones producing even minimal elevation of blood hormone levels blunts or abolishes the normal response to TRH. The TRH test is also useful in the differential diagnosis of severely ill patients with low plasma T4 (see p. 885). The TRH test is of limited use in the elderly in whom lack of TRH response is normal.

THYROIDAL RADIOIODIDE UPTAKE (RAIU) TESTS. The rate of tracer iodide accumulation (^{131}I, ^{123}I) in the thyroid can be measured using times ranging from a few minutes to the plateau of accumulation (24 hours). These procedures, although still in wide use, have been rendered almost obsolete by the simpler and less expensive measurements of hormone concentrations in plasma. The diagnostic usefulness of the RaIU is also seriously limited by the "saturation" of western diets with iodide. This has resulted in RaIU values that are now too low to discriminate normal function from hypofunction. Results are also "normal" in up to 50 percent of cases of hyperthyroidism. The RaIU is also subject to interference by chemical agents and clinical circumstances that produce both false positive and false negative results. The RaIU should no longer be used for the *routine* evaluation of thyroid function.

Immunologic Tests
Assay of antibodies to thyroidal antigens (thyroglobulin, microsomes), so-called thyroid autoantibodies, are useful in determining the presence of au-

toimmune thyroiditis (Hashimoto's disease). Measurement of thyroid-stimulating immunoglobulins (TSI) (see Graves' disease) may be useful in the pregnant patient. High levels in pregnant women are associated with increased likelihood of neonatal hyperthyroidism.

Other Tests Related to Thyroid Diseases
A variety of scintiscan or imaging techniques are available to delineate the anatomy of the thyroid and to distinguish functional from nonfunctional tissue, a consideration in the differential diagnosis of thyroid neoplasms. Currently, ^{99m}Tc pertechnetate (TcO$_4^-$) is most widely used, but ^{123}I is the imaging agent of choice. In some thyroid diseases the organification process is impaired while the pump mechanism remains intact. Perchlorate anion (ClO$_4^-$) competes with iodide and can be used diagnostically to discharge nonorganified iodide. Ultrasound imaging (sonography) is a useful procedure which clearly distinguishes cystic from solid enlargements. Needle biopsy and needle aspiration have also assumed the status of routine procedures in some centers.

Thyroid Function and Thyroid Hormone Economy in Nonthyroidal Illness
The preceding discussion alludes to some of the clinical states other than thyroid disease *per se* in which thyroid "function" tests may be altered. A brief summary is given here of the numerous clinical circumstances in which alterations of thyroid function tests can be encountered; a more detailed discussion can be found elsewhere.[268]

GONADAL AND ADRENAL HORMONES. Estrogens (pregnancy, contraceptives) raise and androgens lower T4 by altering plasma TBG. Glucocorticoids inhibit thyroid activity acutely by interfering with TSH secretion and affect the pituitary's responsiveness to TRH. The plasma T4 is lowered during chronic glucocorticoid therapy, due mainly to a decrease of TBG. When dexamethasone is given acutely, the plasma T4 decreases slightly, T3 falls sharply, and rT3 rises as the pathways of T4 metabolism are shifted.

LIVER DISEASES. A variety of alterations of thyroid function tests are produced by liver diseases. Early in infectious hepatitis, the T4 is elevated secondary to an increase of TBG. Chronic liver disease produces many abnormalities in an unpredictable fashion. T4 may be increased or decreased in parallel with TBG and the T3U. Free T4 is often elevated with no obvious relationship to the TBG. T3 is usually low and rT3 is increased. A frequent and unexplained abnormality is elevation of TSH, although the response to TRH is not exaggerated as in hypothyroidism. RaIU is often elevated in acute alcoholic hepatitis with or without cirrhosis and in some cases of cholangitis. These changes have been attributed both to iodide depletion and to acceleration of T4 metabolism.

RENAL DISEASES.   The nephrotic syndrome is often associated with depressed T4, but the decrease is not always explained by lowered TBG. In chronic renal disease, the *means* of T4, TBG, and the FTI are not significantly different from normal, but the range is greater and values may exceed the usual normal limits. Some patients with severe chronic renal failure receiving long-term dialysis show a progressive decrease of T4. These patients and those with the nephrotic syndrome may represent examples of the recently recognized "euthyroid sick syndrome" (see p. 885). As one would expect in any chronic illness, the plasma T3 is depressed.[252]

INFECTIONS, MALNUTRITION, AND DRUGS.   The T4 may drop early in the course of acute infection and free T4 rises. Neither change is accounted for by an alteration of TBG. During starvation, plasma T3 falls and rT3 increases. Free T4 is often increased without relation to the TBG. Plasma T3 is often decreased in the elderly, a change which has to be attributed to aging but is in fact due to diminished food intake and nonspecific illness.[260] Closely correlated alterations of T3U and plasma TBG have been reported in protein–calorie malnutrition. Some pharmacologic agents affect the thyroid hormones of plasma. Phenytoin (Dilantin) lowers the T4 and free T4, often into the hypothyroid range. Although plasma TSH may be somewhat elevated, clinical hypothyroidism is not seen. Heparin acutely elevates the free T4. The mechanisms of these changes are not known. Propranolol decreases plasma T3 by inhibition of the normal T4 deiodination route; rT3 is increased. A similar effect is produced by some radiopaque contrast media used for visualization of the gallbladder.

Statistical Considerations in the Interpretation of Thyroid Function Tests

No single numerical value divides normal from abnormal in any thyroid function test. The upper and lower limits of normal for plasma T4, free T4 index, and T3 are set at ±2 standard deviations from the mean. By definition, therefore, 2.5 percent of normal persons will have abnormal values at each end of the distribution. To complicate the issue, a small number of hyperthyroid or hypothyroid persons have values that fall within the normal range. In addition to the statistical overlap, one must recall that both biologic day-to-day variation and unavoidable analytic error further obscures the dividing line between normal and abnormal. For example, 95 percent confidence limits of a single T4 measurement are ±1 μg/dl at the

upper and lower limits of the normal range. For all of these reasons, and because of the occasional instance of laboratory or reporting error, a single determination can neither establish nor exclude a diagnosis with anything more than reasonable statistical certainty.

HYPERTHYROIDISM (Thyrotoxicosis)

Hyperthyroidism, the clinical state resulting from an excess of thyroid hormone, is the commonest functional disorder of the thyroid. Although essentially the same clinical picture results from any of several distinct pathologic processes (Table 76–3), selection of proper therapy demands that the correct diagnosis be established. The most common variety of hyperthyroidism is Graves' disease, an autoimmune process also known as diffuse toxic goiter. Somewhat less commonly, hyperthyroidism is due to a hyperfunctioning nodular goiter (toxic nodular goiter). Occasionally hyperthyroidism is due to a solitary hyperfunctioning adenoma. Rarely, hyperthyroidism is seen as a transient phenomenon in the evolution of thyroiditis; as a manifestation of metastatic thyroid carcinoma; or as a complication of trophoblastic tumors such as malignant hydatidiform mole or choriocarcinoma of the testis. Occasional cases of factitious hyperthyroidism are sometimes seen, usually due to surreptitious consumption of thyroid hormone or inappropriate administration. A few cases of hyperthyroidism due to excess TSH secretion have been de-

---

TABLE 76–3
Causes of Hyperthyroidism*

1. Graves' disease
2. Toxic nodular goiter (TNG)
    Multinodular
    Uninodular
3. Hyperthyroidism in association with thyroiditis
    Chronic lymphocytic thyroiditis
    Acute nonsuppurative thyroiditis
4. Hyperthyroidism induced by exogenous iodide
5. Thyrotoxicosis due to TSH or TSH-like stimulator
    Pituitary tumor or TSH excess
    Choriocarcinoma or hydatidiform mole
    Embryonal cell carcinoma of testis
6. Toxic thyroid carcinoma
7. Hyperthyroidism due to exogenous thyroid hormone
    Factitia
    Medicamentosa
8. Toxic struma ovarii

* Listed in approximate order of frequency.

---

scribed, some due to pituitary tumors and others to hypersecretion of TSH in the absence of demonstrable tumor.[254]

GRAVES' DISEASE

Graves' disease is a complex disorder comprising toxic goiter, ophthalmopathy, and occasionally dermopathy. At any given time during the course of the disease, one of these manifestations may be an isolated finding. Graves' ophthalmopathy and Graves' dermopathy can occur independently of thyroid hormone excess[265,269] and are almost certainly the pathologic effects of certain immunoglobulins present in this disease.

Excessive TSH is not the basis of Graves' disease. Evidence for its autoimmune or immunoglobulin basis is now substantial. A variety of abnormal immunoglobulins are found in the plasma of patients with Graves' disease. Some of these immunoglobulins have TSH-like activity, and are currently designated thyroid-stimulating immunoglobulins (TSI). The first such immunoglobulin recognized was termed long-acting thyroid stimulator (LATS), since in the bioassay in which it was quantitated, its action was of longer duration than that of TSH. TSI/LATS are antibodies to the normal receptor sites for TSH. TSI not only bind to thyroid membranes but, like TSH, activate adenylate cyclase, increase thyroidal iodide accumulation and induce thyroid hyperplasia.[258] A reasonable hypothesis for at least part of the Graves' disease syndrome can now be formulated.[265] For unknown reasons, one or more thyroidal constituents become antigenic. Production ensues of a variety of immunoglobulins, some of which have stimulator properties similar to that of TSH. Thyroid overactivity may then occur, depending on the bioactivity and quantity of TSI present.

The plasma of patients with Graves' ophthalmopathy contains a factor (exophthalmos-producing substance (EPS)), which produces exophthalmos and other abnormalities of orbital tissues in suitable test animals. This material resembles in its action a naturally occurring glycoprotein present in the normal pituitary gland. This protein, of unknown function but biochemically similar to TSH, produces both deposition of mucopolysaccharides in orbital fibro-fatty tissues and exophthalmos in test animals. The stimulus for the production of the EPS of Graves' disease is unknown, but the material itself may be an immunoglobulin with a relationship to the normal pituitary material analogous to that of TSI to TSH. On the other hand, thyroglobulin or its breakdown products have been immunologically identified as deposits in the orbital tissues of patients with Graves' ophthal-

mopathy. Thus, the orbital pathology may be a tissue hypersensitivity reaction to deposited thyroglobulin.

Dermopathy, a unique, albeit unusual, finding of Graves' disease, consists of more or less circumscribed areas of mucopolysaccharide deposition, typically on the shins, hence the term "pretibial myxedema." This unfortunate designation unjustifiably suggests a relationship between the process of generalized mucopolysaccharide disposition in hypothyroidism and the localized deposition in Graves' disease.

Pathology

In classic Graves' disease, the thyroid is diffusely enlarged and highly vascular. Both hyperplasia and hypertrophy of the follicles are seen. The follicular walls are infolded, colloid is depleted, and there is cytologic evidence of overactivity. Frequently, there is also cellular infiltration by lymphocytes. In some cases, this infiltration is so extensive as to suggest Hashimoto's thyroiditis. When Graves' disease is present over many years the gland may become nodular.

In Graves' ophthalmopathy, the extraocular muscles show interstitial edema, increased connective tissue, fatty infiltration, and infiltration with lymphocytes. Eventually, gross degenerative changes such as fibrosis may occur. Generalized lymph node enlargement and splenomegaly, occasionally seen in Graves' disease, may be a reflection of the autoimmune nature of the disease process.

The pathology of Graves' disease includes, in addition to the effects of the immunoglobulins, the consequences of long-standing thyroid hormone excess. The heart may show generalized enlargement. Fatty infiltration of the liver and generalized loss of skeletal muscle mass and adipose tissue are common. Skeletal demineralization is also noted at times.

Clinical Presentation

The presentation of the patient with Graves' disease is highly variable (Table 76–4). The severity of the thyrotoxic aspect is determined not only by the degree of hormone excess but also by its rapidity of onset, its duration, and the age of the patient. The thyroid is palpably enlarged in 95 percent of cases. Asymmetric enlargement is frequent. Extreme vascularity of the gland may result in palpable or audible blood flow, a bruit, usually heard over the enlarged lobes but occasionally best heard over the superior thyroidal arteries. Finding a bruit is diagnostic of hyperthyroidism, except when the gland is hypervascular because of iodide deficiency or goitrogen ingestion.

TABLE 76-4

Signs and Symptoms of Hyperthyroidism

Groups	Signs and Symptoms
Adrenergic manifestations	Excess sweating, heat intolerance palpitations, tachycardia, tremor, nervousness, and excitability
Hypermetabolism and catabolism	Increased appetite, weight loss
One system predominance	
Eyes	Stare, periorbital edema exophthalmos, chemosis, ophthalmoplegia, papilledema
Cardiac	Arrhythmia, congestive heart failure
Muscle	Fatigue and weakness, muscle wasting, proximal myopathy, periodic paralysis
Gastrointestinal	Increased frequency of bowel movements, pernicious vomiting
Bone	Acropachy, osteoporosis, hypercalcemia
Reproductive	Infertility, abortion, scanty menses, testicular atrophy, gynecomastia
Mental	Anxiety, irritability, apathy, psychosis, insomnia
Skin	Onycholysis, myxedema, circumscripta, hyperpigmentation

As the disease progresses in severity, skeletal muscle wasting may occur, which tends to involve especially the limb girdle musculature producing a proximal myopathy. Even young patients with relatively mild disease may develop severe myopathy with inability to climb stairs or to arise from a squatting position without using their arms. Exertional dyspnea, without evidence of cardiac failure, is common.

The cardiovascular findings include sinus tachycardia, atrial fibrillation, systolic flow murmurs, and wide pulse pressure. The apex impulse is often prominent and forceful. A to-and-fro, rough sound in the pulmonic area may mimic a pericardial friction rub. Cardiac failure may develop in severe cases of long duration, especially in elderly persons.

Diagnosis

Recognition of Graves' disease in a typical case is not difficult, but, because of its frequently insidious onset, diagnosis may be long delayed. Especially with no eye findings and minimal thyroid enlargement, the diagnosis may not be readily apparent.

The usual thyroid function tests will substantiate the diagnosis in most cases. In doubtful cases the laboratory results should be repeated and confirmed before therapy is undertaken. If the results of the usual thyroid function tests (T4; free T4 index) are borderline or normal, the plasma T3 should be measured. Hyperthyroidism due to elevation of T3 alone, T3-toxicosis, occurs in less than 5 percent of cases. Elevation of T3 alone is more common early in the evolution of Graves' disease.

Occasionally, all the tests of thyroid hormone levels are borderline. If the clinical suspicion of thyrotoxicosis is strong, every effort should still be made to obtain laboratory confirmation by measurement of RaIU, the T3 suppression test or the TRH test.

Differential Diagnosis

The usual patient with disease of mild to moderate severity presents with the following symptoms or signs: "nervousness" (irritability or, less commonly, emotional lability), weight loss, excessive sweating, and heat intolerance. Palpitations occur intermittently or the patient develops a persistently rapid pulse. A fine tremor of the outstretched hands is common. Appetite is usually increased. The combination of normal or increased appetite with weight loss should certainly alert the physician to the likelihood of hyperthyroidism. A few patients develop anorexia early in the disease; if anorexia develops late, the patient's clinical state is likely to be precarious. Overt muscle weakness is a late sign, although many patients complain of easy fatiguability. Increased frequency of defecation up to several times daily is common, but diarrhea is not ordinarily seen. In women, prolonged intermenstrual intervals or even amenorrhea may be noted.

Physical examination may show a variety of subtle changes. Hair loss is common, usually appearing as diffuse thinning of scalp hair. The silky hair of thyrotoxicosis is infrequent. Occasionally hyperpigmentation occurs which may be diffuse but is usually most marked over the extensor surfaces of elbows or knees and the small joints of the hands. The face may be diffusely pigmented and a pregnancy-like chloasma may be evident. The skin may show excessive sweating and typically the hands are warm. Clubbing of the fingers and toes is rare (thyroid acropachy) and distinguishable radiographically from that seen in pulmonary disease. A common sign is separation of the distal portion of one or more fingernails from its nailbed (onycholysis). The dermopathy of Graves' disease occurs most commonly on the legs ("pretibial myxedema"), but also can be seen on the dorsum of the foot, the back, the hands, or even the face. The plaque usually has a sharp, raised margin and may have an orange-peel-like appearance. The affected areas are often intensely pruritic.

The eye findings can be separated into those that occur as a result of thyroid hormone excess and those that are part of the ophthalmopathy of Graves' disease. Excessive thyroid hormone enhances sympathetic tone. The innervation of the eyelids is partially under such control. Lid retraction with increased scleral visibility above and below the iris along with infrequent blinking leads to the "stare" so commonly seen. Failure of the lid to follow promptly movements of the globe ("lid lag") is another manifestation of the same process. When Graves' ophthalmopathy is present, there is forward protrusion of the globe. This process may be unilateral at first and is often asymmetrical. Such protrusion represents true proptosis and contributes an additional component to the stare produced by increased sympathetic tone. Extraocular muscle weakness results in limitation of ability to converge and to perform extreme movements of gaze. Strabismus and diplopia are more severe manifestations. The most serious complications of Graves' ophthalmopathy are infiltrative and will be discussed later.

In some patients, particularly elderly ones,[246] the clinical picture may not suggest hyperthyroidism and only an astute clinician will promptly consider the correct diagnosis. Such patients may present with only unexplained weight loss or weakness. Occult neoplasm may first be suspected and the diagnosis of hyperthyroidism missed entirely or considered only after extensive evaluation fails to yield a diagnosis.

Congestive heart failure or atrial fibrillation may be the presenting manifestation. So-called thyrocardiac patients have been incorrectly thought to be resistant to ordinary doses of digitalis. This is occasionally true, but a normal response to conventional therapy for cardiac failure or an arrythmia should not be considered incompatible with the diagnosis of hyperthyroidism.

Some patients with anxiety may present with tachycardia, tremor, irritability, and weakness simulating hyperthyroidism. The "anxiety" of thyrotoxicosis is more likely to appear as irritability and hyperkinesis than as an expressed feeling of anxiety. The typical anxiety state often exhibits features of depression which are usually absent in hyperthyroidism. In depression, weight loss is invariably accompanied by anorexia. Anorexia sometimes occurs in hyperthyroidism, especially in elderly patients. Pheochromocytoma is a rare disease, but patients with that disorder may be mistakenly thought to have hyperthyroidism.

The characteristic ophthalmopathy of Graves' disease may offer the first clue to the diagnosis. However, ophthalmopathy may not be accompanied by hyperthyroidism and may be unilateral. The T3 suppression test or TRH test will substantiate the diagnosis in most but not all cases of euthyroid Graves' ophthalmopathy.[265] Without evidence of either thyroid hyperfunction, disturbance of the negative feedback system, or dermopathy, the diagnosis of Graves' ophthalmopathy cannot be made with absolute assurance. Indeed, other diseases of the orbit or retro-orbital space must be considered. Computerized axial tomography of the skull and the orbital contents and high resolution sonography have been useful diagnostic tools. These procedures can visualize the enlarged extraocular muscles of Graves' ophthalmopathy, although such enlargement is also seen in pseudotumor. In many cases of Graves' ophthalmopathy, other aspects of the Graves syndrome eventually become apparent.

When hyperthyroidism is found in a patient without goiter or exophthalmos, suspicions of factitious hyperthyroidism may be warranted. An RaIU test and scan will establish whether the thyroid is functional and sometimes will give evidence for enlargement that is not palpable. A very low uptake suggests that thyroid hormone is being ingested or being ectopically produced, e.g., by an ovarian struma. Hyperthyroidism due to ingestion of levothyroxine or desiccated thyroid will be accompanied by an elevated T4 index. If triiodothyronine is being taken, the plasma T3 will be elevated briefly, since its half-life is about 24 hours. Hyperthyroidism with low radioiodide uptake in the thyroid occurs also in functioning metastic thyroid carcinoma. Usually, however, the metastatic disease is obvious, or the patient gives a history of thyroid surgery for carcinoma.

Tumors of trophoblastic origin (malignant hydatidiform mole or choriocarcinoma of the uterus or testis) sometimes produce hyperthyroidism. Such tumors produce huge quantities of chorionic gonadotropin (HCG) which has intrinsic thyroid stimulating (TSH-like) activity.

Therapy

Hyperthyroidism due to Graves' disease is sometimes a self-limited process that terminates within a year or two in about one-half of cases. This natural history of Graves' disease strongly influences selection of therapy. Other therapeutic considerations relate to the age of the patient and the presence or absence of complications.

Since we presently have no means of controlling the underlying cause of the disease, presumably TSI production, therapy is designed to interfere with thyroid hormone synthesis by drugs or by ablation of thyroid tissue by radioiodide or surgery. Opinions differ on approaches, but the views expressed here probably closely approximate a consensus of conservative medical opinion. Each form of therapy has advantages and disadvantages; none provides a simple, definitive solution and none is truly curative. The objective of therapy is to assure minimal morbidity from both the therapy and the disease.

THERAPY WITH THIOCARBAMIDE ANTITHYROID DRUGS. These agents will predictably control excessive production of thyroid hormones in essentially all cases. Restoration of the clinically euthyroid state requires at least 4 to 8 weeks, although clinical improvement is usually seen much sooner. Antithyroid drugs are the preferred *initial* treatment for children, adults below age 40 without complications or other medical problems, and the pregnant patient. The antithyroid drugs are also routinely used as preliminary therapy in patients who are to be treated by surgery. The objective in these cases is to insure euthyroid status at the time of operation. Patients who are to be treated with radioiodide are also sometimes treated with an antithyroid drug pre- and/or postablation. Radioiodide is slow in producing its effect and may have to be given in multiple doses. Use of an antithyroid drug prior to or following such therapy is a temporary but useful adjunct.

In the United States, only two such drugs are available, propylthiouracil and methimazole (Tapazole). Propylthiouracil may have an advantage when speed in restoration of euthyroid status is an urgent consideration. Propylthiouracil, unlike methimazole, in addition to its effects in inhibiting thyroid hormone synthesis, also inhibits conversion of T4 to T3 in peripheral tissues. Methimazole is longer acting than propylthiouracil and may be given on a less frequent dosage schedule. In most adults with hyperthyroidism, 100 to 150 mg of propylthiouracil every 8 hours or 20 to 30 mg of methimazole every 12 hours will usually suffice as initial therapy, whereas maintenance is often possible with 50 to 100 mg of propylthiouracil twice daily or 5 to 10 mg of methimazole once or twice daily. Some physicians prefer to continue the initial dosage and to add thyroxine when the patient's plasma T4 falls into the hypothyroid range. This approach is simple and avoids the need for titrating the dosage of antithyroid drug, a tedious and frequently unsuccessful procedure.

SPECIAL CONSIDERATIONS IN THE USE OF ANTITHYROID DRUGS. Although the recommended doses will control the disease in the vast majority of cases, some individuals clearly need higher doses. If the patient is severely ill, larger doses should be given from the beginning. The risk of an adverse drug effect may be increased, but this is not established and should not be a consideration under such circumstances. In order to achieve total blockade of hormone synthesis, as much as 200 mg of propylthiouracil every 4 hours may be necessary. Methimazole has a longer duration of action, and need not be given so often, but 30 to 40 mg three times daily may be needed in some cases.

Occasionally an individual has a good response to an ordinary dose of either drug and continues for many months with a stable clinical response. Unpredictably, the disease then appears to exacerbate and an increase of dose is required. Sometimes lack of patient compliance is responsible. Compliance is frequently professed when, in fact, exacerbation is due to discontinuation or erratic use of the drug.

A once-a-day drug schedule is probably satisfactory for many patients with mild disease, but its routine use will result in needless morbidity for some patients unless larger than customary doses are used. For example, single doses of methimazole may have to be as large as 80 to 120 mg. The use of a twice daily schedule with conventional doses of drug will almost invariably control the disease and usually wins excellent patient compliance.

Conventional and time-honored treatment schedules suggest that a period of 12 to 18 months of therapy be used before consideration is given to discontinuation of the drug. When considering discontinuation, a few indicators are helpful in predicting success or failure of the outcome. Patients who have continued to require large doses of drug are almost certain not to have achieved remission. On the other hand, reduction in thyroid mass during therapy is often predictive of lasting clinical remission. A test for restoration of the normal negative feedback system (thyroid suppressibility) is sometimes helpful. To perform this test, the antithyroid drug is discontinued. The patient is given 75 μg of T3 daily or a single 3 mg dose of T4; RaIU is then determined after 1 week. Low postsuppression 24 hour uptake (<10%) predicts reasonably accurately that the patient will remain in remission. An uptake above the normal range almost invariably indicates continuation of active disease. Intermediate values are not useful. If continued disease activity seems to be present, discontinuation of therapy is inadvisable and will almost certainly result in clinical relapse and needless morbidity.

If a suppression test or other signs suggest that remission has been reached, antithyroid drug therapy is terminated and the patient observed. If the status is indeterminate, antithyroid drug may be reduced to one-half the maintenance level for 3 to 4 months in the expectation that recurrence, if it occurs, will be blunted. Prophylactic use of propranolol during withdrawal of antithyroid drug therapy is a useful maneuver that prevents emergence of symptoms of overt hyperthyroidism should relapse occur. Routine determination of plasma T4 or T3 every 3 to 4 weeks allows recognition of return of thyroid overactivity.

If the hyperthyroid state recurs, treatment with antithyroid drug may be reinitiated for another course or alternative therapy undertaken (^{131}I or surgery). A second course of antithyroid drug has a significant chance of inducing remission. In selected patients, prolonged or even indefinite drug therapy is reasonable, but with most patients such an approach is not desirable.

Minor side effects of drug therapy occur in about 10 percent of patients. Skin rashes, the most common, are usually seen in the first months of therapy, and often disappear even if therapy is continued. Antihistamine drugs are useful in controlling urticaria and pruritus. Leukopenia is not uncommon but is usually not severe and is dose related. If the absolute number of polymorphonuclear leukocytes falls below 2000, the dose should be reduced or the drug discontinued. If the side effects are not tolerated, a switch to another agent will allow continuation of therapy in about half the cases. For the rare case in which neither of the thiocarbamides is satisfactory, perchlorate can be used. Major complications of drug therapy occur in less than 0.1 percent of cases. Agranulocytosis is the most dreaded complication. Unlike leukopenia, agranulocytosis from thiocarbamides is not dose related and is of such sudden onset that routine blood counts are of no help in prevention. The patient should, however, be instructed to contact the physician promptly if severe sore mouth or throat and fever occur. Fortunately, most cases recover, albeit after a stormy course. Other toxic reactions include drug fever and arthralgias, both of which appear to be dose related. Elevations of alkaline phosphatase are commonly seen in patients receiving propylthiouracil. If other liver enzymes are normal, the drug may be continued, but persistent laboratory evidence of hepatocellular damage is an indication for discontinuation of therapy. White blood count should be monitored after several weeks of therapy and following increases of drug dose. Liver enzymes should be measured every 3 to 6 months.

ADJUNCTIVE DRUG THERAPY. *Iodide.* Iodide in the treatment of hyperthyroidism should be reserved for cases with specific indications. Occasionally, iodide therapy produces severe dermatitis. Use of iodide will also predictably preclude for many weeks the use of radioactive iodide, the thyroid uptake of which will be greatly diminished.

Iodide, the best agent available for inhibiting hormone release, is useful in patients who need rapid correction of the hyperthyroid state. Iodide should, however, not be administered until several hours after initiation of therapy with an antithyroid drug sufficient to block hormone synthesis. Otherwise the iodide may act to increase thyroid hormone synthesis, exacerbate the hyperthyroidism and delay restoration of the euthyroid state. Iodide also has a time-honored place in preoperative preparation for thyroidectomy to reduce vascularity of the gland. When given following radioiodide therapy, iodide seems especially effective in accelerating restoration of euthyroid status.

The dose of iodide is one drop of a saturated solution (50 mg) of potassium iodide two times a day; larger doses are often given but are unnecessary. Lugol solution is a pharmacologic concoction containing iodine and iodide which has no virtue over iodide alone.

Adrenergic Antagonists. The symptoms and signs of thyrotoxicosis that are related to sensitization of the sympathetic nervous system are in large measure abolished by β-adrenergic blocking drugs. The current agent of choice is propranolol. The indications for its use are severe tachycardia, tremor, sweating, and agitation. Propranolol is effective for relief of these manifestations of hyperthyroidism, but does not appreciably affect excessive metabolic rate or reverse the catabolic state of severe cases. Propranolol does lower plasma T3 (and increase rT3). This effect may contribute to its therapeutic benefit, especially in mild cases. Propranolol has occasional undesirable side effects and is relatively contraindicated in some individuals (e.g., those with asthma). Concern is often expressed that patients with heart disease may be thrown into congestive heart failure or that heart failure if present may worsen. On the other hand, some patients with congestive heart failure may respond well to the drug when excessive heart rate is a major contributing factor. Guanethedine and practolol have been used successfully in hyperthyroidism with refractory congestive heart failure and may be the preferred agents in this situation.[249] Postural hypotension, a troublesome side effect of guanethedine in the euthyroid patient, is hardly ever seen in the hyperthyroid individual. Propranolol has been used as the sole agent to prepare patients with mild hyperthyroidism for surgery, including thyroidectomy, although ideally the patient should be euthyroid at the time of thyroid surgery. Other uses for propranolol are in the prevention of symptoms during trial withdrawal of an antithyroid drug and while awaiting the effects of ^{131}I therapy. Most patients require propranolol in doses of at least 160 mg daily, but doses up to 720 mg may be necessary. The drug should be discontinued as soon as the patient is rendered euthyroid by other therapy.

Radioactive Iodide. Radioactive iodide (^{131}I) is uniformly effective therapy, simple to administer, and inexpensive. The single disadvantage of radioactive iodide is that hypothyroidism is a frequent consequence. For many years, concern was expressed over the possibility of producing carcinoma of the thyroid, leukemia, or genetic damage in the future offspring of women in their childbearing years. All of these concerns have been shown to be groundless. Although *low* doses of external radiation do produce carcinoma of the thyroid, the doses used for treatment of hyperthyroidism do not. Long-term follow-up of treated patients over the past 30 years has failed to substantiate any such risk or any increased risk of leukemia. The amount of radiation to the ovaries from therapeutic doses of radioiodide used for therapy of hyperthyroidism are lower than those delivered by diagnostic x-ray procedures and can be expected to produce no genetic effects. Thus, radioiodide therapy for hyperthyroidism can be considered for any adult patient.

Hypothyroidism follows radioiodide therapy in the immediate few months post-therapy in a more or less dose-related fashion. Large doses predictably eliminate hyperthyroidism with certainty but totally ablate the thyroid with great regularity. Small, single doses render the patient euthyroid with 50 to 70 percent likelihood but unavoidably still produce hypothyroidism within a year in about 10 percent of cases. Furthermore, of the cases rendered euthyroid, 3 to 4 percent *per year* develop hypothyroidism over the ensuing 20 years.

One may question whether the high frequency of post-treatment hypothyroidism constitutes a significant disadvantage of radioiodide therapy. The answer is that for the majority of those who become hypothyroid, replacement therapy with thyroxine is a trivial inconvenience. For these patients, the advantages of radioiodide therapy far outweigh the one disadvantage. Unfortunately, a few patients, despite warnings to the contrary, discontinue their required life-long replacement therapy, become lost to follow-up, and suffer all the consequences of long-standing hypothyroidism and myxedema.

Some physicians advocate the use of deliberately ablative doses of ^{131}I. This approach to therapy certainly greatly simplifies patient management and is reasonable in view of the high probability of post-therapy hypothyroidism regardless of dose. Nonetheless, most physicians do not advocate deliberate ablation unless the patient has experienced a major complication of hyperthyroidism (e.g., severe heart disease) or has complicating medical problems that demand prompt control. In young patients who are tolerating their disease reasonably well, most physi-

cians prefer to use small doses of ^{131}I, repeated if necessary, until the patient is euthyroid. Such an approach does not, of course, guarantee that hypothyroidism will be avoided.

In the past, elaborate schemes have been used to estimate the required dose of ^{131}I. Unfortunately, none of these has proven helpful, since the biologic sensitivity to radiation effect, the most important variable, is not measurable. Currently, in a typical "low dose" treatment scheme patients with small glands are given 2 to 3 mC, while those with moderately enlarged to large glands are given 5 to 10 mC. Ablative doses approximate 15 mC. Because of the unpredictable response with nonablative doses, antithyroid drugs are often used initially to render the patient euthyroid. Antithyroid drug therapy is then interrupted for 48 hours before the ^{131}I is given and reinstituted 24 hours afterward. A similar approach combining antithyroid drug and ^{131}I is almost routinely used in patients with severe or complicated hyperthyroidism, e.g., thyrocardiac disease.

The undocumented notion has long persisted that radiation thyroiditis may produce excessive release of thyroid hormone 7 to 14 days after therapy with the possibility of consequent worsening of the clinical state. This complication, if it occurs at all, must be rare. Nonetheless, prudence dictates a conservative approach in precarious patients, e.g., those in congestive heart failure, who are best brought to euthyroid status or are at least significantly improved by antithyroid drug therapy before ablation with ^{131}I. At 3 months following ^{131}I, when the short-term radiation effect reaches maximal, the antithyroid drug can be discontinued or tapered.

SURGICAL THERAPY. For many years surgical ablation of the thyroid, e.g., subtotal thyroidectomy was a main therapy for hyperthyroidism. This procedure still has its advocates, especially for young adults and for children who cannot be successfully treated with antithyroid drugs. In the hands of experienced surgeons, subtotal thyroidectomy is certainly effective therapy attended by minimal morbidity. However, complications include the small but real risk of anesthesia/operative mortality, recurrent laryngeal nerve damage with vocal cord paralysis, permanent hypoparathyroidism, and, most commonly, hypothyroidism. The latter two complications are, to a certain extent, unavoidable and are not merely the consequence of poor surgical technique. In addition to about a 10 percent occurrence of immediate postsurgical hypothyroidism, 2 to 3 percent of patients become hypothyroid each year following surgery, a figure only slightly lower than that following therapy with ^{131}I. A higher complication rate must be expected when the operation is performed by surgeons with limited experience in thyroid surgery. Surgery also is followed by a significant (5 percent) rate of recurrent hyperthyroidism, sometimes occurring many years later. In this case, even the most enthusiastic supporters of surgical treatment agree that recurrent hyperthyroidism should not be treated by a second operation, since the frequency of major complications rises to an unacceptable level. Radioiodide is the clear choice in cases of hyperthyroidism recurrent after surgery.

When subtotal thyroidectomy is used as therapy, standard practice employs an antithyroid drug to bring the patient to euthyroid status before surgery, iodide therapy for 10 to 14 days preoperatively to reduce gland vascularity, and propranolol as adjunctive therapy.

TREATMENT OF HYPERTHYROIDISM DURING PREGNANCY. Hyperthyroidism during pregnancy, almost invariably due to Graves' disease, should be treated with an antithyroid drug. Surgery has been used successfully during pregnancy, but has no advantage and may be associated with increased fetal losses. Radioactive iodide is contraindicated. Therapy with antithyroid drug during pregnancy is guided by two considerations. First, the antithyroid drugs freely cross the placenta and can, in large doses, produce goiter and hypothyroidism in the infant. Second, thyroid hormones do not cross the placenta from mother to fetus. The dose of antithyroid drugs should be the minimal amount adequate to control the hyperthyroidism. A dose of drug which totally blocks hormone synthesis along with a replacement amount of thyroxine is not appropriate during pregnancy. When ordinary doses of antithyroid drug are used, the fetus is usually born without goiter, but as a precaution the dose is often reduced, if possible, during the last month of pregnancy. Iodide should not be used during pregnancy, since the fetal thyroid is especially susceptible to the goitrogenic effect of iodide. Monitoring the plasma hormone level requires determination of free T4 or the free T4 index, since T4 is normally elevated during pregnancy in association with the increased TBG.

TSI of Graves' disease cross the placenta and enter the fetal circulation. Occasionally, the newborn infant is hyperthyroid as a result of this passive transfer. Neonatal hyperthyroidism subsides in a few weeks, but the disease may be severe and even fatal. Therapy is with antithyroid drugs and propranolol.

OPHTHALMOPATHY

The exact frequency of opthalmopathy in Graves' disease is not known, but most cases have either no obvious eye involvement or show only minimal to moderate proptosis. Severe exophthalmos occurs in no more than a few percent of cases. Proptosis becomes more than a cosmetic concern when the eyelids fail to close, setting the stage for corneal ulceration. Paresis of the extraocular muscles producing diplopia can also be troublesome and may require use of an eyepatch or corrective surgery. The most disturbing and rarest eye involvement is chemosis or marked inflammation and edema of the conjunctivae and periorbital soft tissues. Ophthalmopathy of this severity is termed malignant or infiltrative exophthalmos. Rarely optic neuritis leading to blindness occurs.

A variety of therapeutic maneuvers are helpful. Elevation of the head of the bed during sleep may reduce soft tissue swelling, including that which leads to proptosis. Protective eyeglasses may be useful. Methylcellulose solution helps prevent drying of the exposed cornea, but in some cases plastic shields or taping of the eyelids at night may be necessary. When chemosis is marked, high-dose glucocorticoid therapy may be necessary and is usually effective, at least in controlling the gross inflammatory process. Surgical approaches are reserved for the most severe cases. Tarsorrhaphy is useful both cosmetically and for relief of corneal exposure. Orbital decompression may be necessary when proptosis is severe or sight is threatened by optic neuritis. Strictly cosmetic surgery should be reserved for a stage when the ophthalmopathy is stable. In most cases, the infiltrative aspect of even severe ophthalmopathy subsides eventually, but some degree of residual proptosis almost always remains.

Graves' ophthalmopathy follows a temporal course which may be totally dissociated from the hyperthyroidism, the treatment of which should be independent of and uninfluenced by the eye disease. Despite claims to the contrary, no form of treatment of hyperthyroidism has any advantage for control of the ophthalmopathy. All manner of combinations, including total thyroid ablation by surgery and radioiodide, have been used without any convincing evidence of improvement in the course of the ophthalmopathy. The notion persists that induction of hypothyroidism may aggravate exophthalmos. Development of clinical hypothyroidism should be avoided especially when exophthalmos is present.

HYPERTHYROIDISM ASSOCIATED WITH NODULAR GOITER (Toxic Nodular Goiter)

Toxic nodular goiter is usually seen in adults in midlife or in the elderly. While the typical patient with Graves' disease usually relates symptoms extending over a few months to a year, the history in toxic nodular goiter is often much longer. Many years may pass before diagnosis. Because of the patient's age and the duration of illness, severe cardiac or musculoskeletal involvement is common.

Toxic nodular goiter appears to arise in the pathologic evolution of some cases of nodular goiter. Most nodular goiters are initially TSH dependent, i.e., suppressible with exogenous thyroid hormone. Eventually, some of these goiters develop autonomous areas with other regions of relatively decreased activity. Nodular goiters at this stage of evolution do not secrete enough hormone to produce clinical hyperthyroidism but show nonsuppressible function. A few of these autonomously functioning goiters evolve to a stage where excessive production of hormone and clinical hyperthyroidism ensue. Pathologically, one cannot distinguish the nontoxic from the toxic nodular goiter. The scintiscan also fails to provide distinguishing features; the usual case merely shows irregular iodide uptake. In those cases of multinodular goiter in which most of the uptake is confined to a single area and the remainder of the gland appears hypofunctional, one presumes that a discrete adenomatous area has become autonomous. True solitary adenomas may also be autonomous and hyperactive, but in these cases the remainder of the thyroid is not involved in the goitrous process.

If the usual laboratory tests (T4, free T4 index) are borderline, special tests such as measurement of the T3, suppression with thyroid hormone, or TRH stimulation should be considered. The suppression test can be undertaken cautiously in the elderly patient without overt heart disease, but should not be used if heart disease is obvious. The test is more helpful in excluding the diagnosis than in establishing a state of hormone excess, since a significant number of cases of nontoxic nodular goiter are also not suppressible. The TRH test is of limited value in the elderly.

Therapy of toxic nodular goiter is best accomplished with [131]I. Rather large doses, in the range of 10 to 30 mC, are usually necessary. Hypothyroidism occurs much less frequently following ^{131}I therapy for nodular goiter than for Graves' disease. If the clinical situation demands prompt relief of the hyperthyroidism, an antithyroid drug can be used following the therapeutic dose of ^{131}I, since the response to radioiodide is often slow and multiple doses may be needed. Otherwise ^{131}I given alone is simple therapy, without side effects, and easily monitored by measurements of plasma T4. Other therapeutic considerations including the use of adjunctive therapy follow those outlined for the therapy of Graves' disease with one exception. In hyperthyroidism due to toxic nodular goiter, antithyroid drugs alone cannot be expected to produce a lasting remission.

HYPERTHYROIDISM DUE TO EXCESSIVE SECRETION OF T3; "T3 TOXICOSIS"

In most cases of hyperthyroidism, the thyroid secretes excessive quantities of both T4 and T3. However, in perhaps 5 percent of cases, T3 is the predominant hormone secreted. The patient who appears clinically hyperthyroid but whose T4 is normal should have plasma T3 measured. T3 toxicosis sometimes occurs early in the course of hyperthyroidism due to Graves' disease and can be seen during therapy with an antithyroid drug.

THYROID STORM (Thyrotoxic Crisis)

This dreaded complication of hyperthyroidism is now only rarely encountered. When thyroid storm does occur, it is usually in the setting of a severe medical or surgical stress imposed on a patient with uncontrolled or unrecognized hyperthyroidism. In the era before the antithyroid drugs were used to prepare the patient for surgery, thyroid storm was frequently seen as a postoperative complication of thyroidectomy. Clinical features of full-blown thyroid storm include fever, sometimes to the level of extreme hyperpyrexia, marked tachycardia, great irritability, diarrhea, and hypotension. Thyroid storm often progresses rapidly to delirium and coma. Occasionally, fever may be minimal and the patient sinks into coma with little other change to suggest the diagnosis. Vascular collapse may ensue. Obviously, the clinical picture is nonspecific. When a patient with known hyperthyroidism develops a postoperative complication or superimposed illness producing fever and gastrointestinal symptoms, the differential diagnosis may be difficult or impossible. In this situation, the patient should be treated as having thyrotoxic crisis, since the mortality of storm is high.

Treatment of thyroid storm includes control of extreme hyperpyrexia with a cooling blanket. Hypotension is treated by correction of volume deficit and with vasopressor agents, if absolutely necessary. Glucocorticoids are always used. The original basis for the use of glucocorticoids was the concept of relative or absolute adrenal insufficiency in hyperthyroidism. Although no good evidence exists to support this notion, high doses of dexamethasone (8 to 16 mg/day) inhibit the conversion of T4 to T3 and acutely lower both T4 and T3 in plasma. High doses of antithyroid drug are also used, e.g., 200 mg propylthiouracil every 4 hours; since no parenteral preparation is available, a nasogastric tube may have to be used. Propylthiouracil has a theoretical advantage over methimazole since it inhibits the peripheral conversion of T4 to T3. A few hours after starting a fully blocking dose of antithyroid drug, 500 mg of iodide should be given orally or intravenously. Propranolol is useful and can be given intravenously or orally. Digitalis preparations should be used in conventional doses. Attempts to control heart rate or heart failure with larger than normal doses of digitalis may lead to toxicity. A number of days may be needed before visible improvement occurs. During this time, attention should be given to maintenance of adequate nutrition including calories, amino acids, and vitamins. Fever, hypermetabolism, and diarrhea contribute to greatly increased requirements for fluids and electrolytes, as well as to caloric requirements. Parenteral hyperalimentation should be considered. In patients who may already be severely depleted, these supportive measures together with optimal nursing care may be of critical importance and as important as specific therapy.

HYPOTHYROIDISM

Hypothyroidism, the metabolic state resulting from deficient thyroid hormones, is relatively common. Most cases can be diagnosed even when symptoms and signs are minimal, provided that the physician considers the diagnosis and seeks appropriate laboratory confirmation. The manifestations of hypothyroidism are varied and to a large measure age-dependent. Myxedema is a severe form of hypothyroidism which results in deposition of mucopolysaccharides in the skin and other tissues producing a characteristic appearance and a constellation of physical findings. The term *myxedema* is commonly but incorrectly used interchangeably with hypothyroidism. *Primary hypothyroidism* is the term used to indicate that the hormone deficiency results from a disease or other process within the thyroid gland. Secondary hypothyroidism, much less common, results from lack of thyrotropin (TSH) secretion, a result of pituitary or, rarely, hypothalamic disease. Hypothyroidism due to hypothalamic disease is now recognized, at least in theory, through use of the TRH test and has been termed "tertiary" hypothyroidism.

ETIOLOGY

Currently, the commonest cause of hypothyroidism is iatrogenic, i.e., the result of therapy of hyperthyroidism with radioiodide or by surgery. Spontaneous cases occur as an idiopathic process of thyroid atrophy or in association with Hashimoto's thyroiditis. Hypothyroidism from other causes is uncommon. A clinical classification is given in Table 76-5.

Idiopathic hypothyroidism may in most cases be the result of long-standing Hashimoto's thyroiditis. This conclusion is based mainly on the frequent oc-

---

TABLE 76–5
Clinical Classification of Hypothyroidism*

I. **Hypothyroidism Without Goiter (Decrease of Thyroid Tissue Mass)**
   a. Postablative for hyperthyroidism (radioiodide therapy or surgery)
   b. Idiopathic atrophy
   c. Developmental defect (congenital)

II. **Hypothyroidism with Goiter**
   a. Chronic thyroiditis (Hashimoto's disease, etc.)
   b. Drug induced (antithyroid drugs, iodide, lithium, etc.)
   c. Iodide deficiency (remote geographic areas)
   d. Genetic biosynthetic defects

* Hypothyroidism in the United States is now most commonly the consequence of therapy for hyperthyroidism. Hypothyroidism due to idiopathic atrophy of the thyroid is second in frequency. Developmental defects (e.g., lingual thyroid) are rare. Hypothyroidism with goiter is nearly always due to Hashimoto's thyroiditis, rarely to a drug. Genetic biosynthetic defects are rare and usually become manifest in childhood.

---

currence of high titers of autoantibodies to thyroid antigens in both circumstances. In addition, both occur frequently in association with other autoimmune diseases such as pernicious anemia. As a clinically encountered thyroid abnormality, Hashimoto's thyroiditis is second in frequency only to nontoxic nodular goiter and is by far the commonest cause of goitrous hypothyroidism. Impairment of hormone synthesis is easily demonstrated. The iodide trap often remains intact, as can be shown by the perchlorate discharge test, but organification is impaired and abnormal iodoproteins are secreted.

DRUG-INDUCED HYPOTHYROIDISM

A variety of drugs can produce hypothyroidism that is invariably associated with goiter formation. Overtreatment of hyperthyroidism with an antithyroid drug will, of course, produce hypothyroidism. Iodide in pharmacologic amounts is an antithyroid drug and will also occasionally produce goiter and hypothyroidism as in patients given long-term iodide therapy for asthma or other chronic lung disease. However, most adults who are susceptible to the antithyroid action of iodide have an underlying thyroid abnormality, such as Hashimoto's thyroiditis or radioiodide-treated Graves' disease. In contrast, the thyroid of the normal fetus is very sensitive to the antithyroid effects of iodide excess. Therefore, the use of iodide during pregnancy, even as adjunct therapy of hyperthyroidism, should be avoided. A number of drugs no longer commonly used in clinical medicine have weak antithyroid action and have occasionally produced hypothyroidism, e.g., p-aminosalicylic acid, cobalt salts, and sulfonylureas. Lithium, currently in wide use for the treatment of manic-depressive illness, occasionally produces hypothyroidism.

When hypothyroidism results from a defect of the pituitary or hypothalamus, decreased TSH secretion is the immediate cause. The thyroid is usually smaller than normal and not palpable. Almost invariably the hypothyroidism is part of a generalized decrease in pituitary function that has resulted from postpartum necrosis, pituitary tumor, pituitary apoplexy, or, rarely, granulomatous disease or other causes.

CLINICAL FEATURES

The manifestations of hypothyroidism are dependent not only on the degree of thyroid hormone deficiency but also on age of onset. When the thyroid hormone deficiency is present in utero, cretinism may be apparent at birth but more often becomes evident in the first few months. Prompt recognition and institution of replacement therapy at the earliest possible time is essential if mental retardation is to be avoided or minimized. Introduction of mass screening programs for detection of hypothyroidism in the newborn reflects this concern. Such programs, using measurements of plasma T4 or TSH, are detecting one case in about 4000 newborns. When hypothyroidism becomes manifest after the first few years, mental retardation does not occur and the disease is less obvious. Usually growth retardation or, rarely, delayed onset of puberty calls attention to the diagnosis. Characteristically bone age is retarded relative to chronologic age.

Hypothyroidism in the adult is highly variable in its presentation. Usually, onset is insidious, often occurring over many years, with the result that the symptoms go unappreciated by patient and physician alike. The nonspecificity of the symptoms also contributes to the delayed diagnosis. No predictable progression of symptoms is apparent, but easy fatiguability, lethargy, increased sleep requirement, cold intolerance, muscle aching, and stiffness are perhaps the commonest early symptoms. The skin is dry and scaling. Hair loss is frequent. The eyebrows become sparse, and the face "puffy," i.e., full, with edema of the periorbital areas. The voice often becomes low pitched and rough. Constipation is common and may be severe enough to produce megacolon; sometimes the diagnosis is suggested by the radiologist from the results of a barium enema. Diminished hearing, especially in old persons, is easily overlooked or attributed to "aging." Ordinarily, the affected individual becomes abnormally placid, but agitation and frank psychosis occur rarely. Paresthesias of the hands due to carpal tunnel syndrome are common. Diminished sexual function is the rule. Women often experience menorrhagia. Rarely, galactorrhea may be seen in women of childbearing age. Fertility is diminished, but pregnancy may occur and normal delivery is possible. The newborn is euthyroid, unless the mother's hypothyroidism is drug-related or the hypothyroidism is of the rare familial athyreotic variety.

Severe Hypothyroidism with Myxedema

In spontaneous cases of hypothyroidism, only with severe, long-standing disease does extensive deposition of mucopolysaccharide occur, producing the clinical state of myxedema. Rarely, myxedema may develop rapidly after radioiodine or surgical ablation of the thyroid for hyperthyroidism.

In myxedema, a variety of manifestations can be appreciated on physical examination and, of course, vary with the severity and duration of the disease. The skin, in addition to being dry and scaling, is typically cool. The scaling may be extensive so that large flakes are shed over the elbows and knees. The subcutaneous tissues may be infiltrated by mucopolysaccharides so that the skin appears to be "thickened" or "doughy." In the elderly, atrophy of the epidermis may occur simultaneously producing a stiff, translucent, parchment-like appearance. Yellow-orange discoloration of the skin may be evident, especially in the palms. The presence of edema is not obvious, since pitting is not noted except in extreme cases complicated by hypoproteinemia. An exception is the collection around the eyes of "bags of water." This finding is not, however, specific for hypothyroidism. The tongue is sometimes enlarged. The heart rate is usually slow (sinus bradycardia). The heart may appear enlarged, due either to dilatation of the myocardium or pericardial effusion. Pleural effusions and ascites may also be present, sometimes even in cases that are otherwise not clinically severe. Dilutional hyponatremia, clinically indistinguishable from the syndrome of inappropriate antidiuretic hormone excess, may be present. Altered renal hemodynamics has been thought to be the basis for the impairment of water handling in these patients, but an abnormality in secretion of antidiuretic hormone is demonstrable.[264] The deep tendon reflexes characteristically show a delay in their relaxation phase, the so-called "hung-up reflex." This is a highly suggestive finding but may be seen occasionally in other diseases. Mental functioning is slowed, as reflected in the characteristically slow speech. The reading speed may be greatly reduced. Hearing loss may be severe or of a degree apparent only on audiometric testing. Cerebellar dysfunction, if present, is usually evident only on extensive neurologic testing but in rare cases is grossly apparent as ataxia.

Myxedema Coma

This severe, often fatal event is an infrequent complication of long-standing disease and is typically seen in the elderly patient. Myxedema coma is often associated with or precipitated by pneumonia, peritonitis, or some other serious infection. The patient is frequently hypothermic, but fever should not mislead the physician into neglecting the possibility of coma being related to hypothyroidism. Severe respiratory failure is a major feature and can be due to a variety of factors ranging from upper airway obstruction to impaired chest wall mechanics.[245]

Since elderly patients often become hypothermic on exposure to cold or during sepsis, the diagnosis of myxedema coma is more frequently raised than actually encountered. However, if the diagnosis is seriously entertained, therapy should be promptly instituted, even before laboratory confirmation is at hand, since delay may ensure a fatal outcome.

LABORATORY FINDINGS

In primary hypothyroidism, the combination of low plasma T4, free T4 index (or free T4), and high TSH is diagnostic. Diagnostic difficulties are encountered only in occasional cases. The plasma T3 is usually low in hypothyroidism, but T3 is not a useful diagnostic test because of its decrease in a variety of nonthyroidal illnesses ranging from malnutrition to liver disease. Furthermore, it is normal in many cases of mild hypothyroidism. In hypothyroidism due to pituitary or hypothalamic disease the TSH is low or "normal." The TRH test is ordinarily not necessary.

In addition to the definitive diagnostic tests, a variety of other laboratory abnormalities are encountered, although they serve no useful diagnostic purpose. Urinary cortisol metabolite excretion is low (17-keto and 17-hydroxysteroids) but only as a result of slowed metabolism of cortisol; plasma levels of cortisol are normal. Plasma prolactin is increased. Plasma cholesterol and triglycerides are commonly elevated. Elevation of plasma carotene in hypothyroidism contributes to the yellow-orange color of the skin. The mechanism of this phenomenon is inadequate conversion of ingested carotene to vitamin A during absorption through the gut mucosa; the activity of carotene cleaving enzyme is regulated by thyroid hormone.

A common laboratory finding is elevation of plasma enzymes which originate in skeletal muscle: creatine phosphokinase (CPK), glutamic oxaloacetic transaminase (SGOT), glutamic pyruvic transaminase (SGPT), and lactic dehydrogenase (LDH). Frac-tionation studies show that these enzymes when elevated in hypothyroidism do not have their origin in cardiac muscle. Other abnormalities include electrocardiographic changes (such as flattened or inverted T waves, minor ST segment depressions, and low amplitude QRS complexes) and abnormalities of blood gas measurements due to hypoventilation.

DIFFERENTIAL DIAGNOSIS

The most difficult problem in diagnosis is the simple clinical appreciation of the possibility that the patient may be hypothyroid. Once that process occurs, the subsequent history, physical examination, and laboratory findings will easily establish the diagnosis in all but a few cases. However, some special problems may be encountered. Any elderly patient who is sick, pale, and puffy-faced becomes a suspect for the diagnosis, especially if an adequate history cannot be obtained. The patient with atypical chest pain, nonspecific electrocardiographic abnormalities, and elevated CPK or SGOT is not infrequently labeled as having ischemic heart disease and myocardial infarction; the proper diagnosis may be hypothyroidism. The patient with the nephrotic syndrome might be mistaken for one having hypothyroidism. However, although the plasma T4 may be low (TBG is low in some nephrotic patients), the free T4 index (or free T4) is normal. More important, the patient with the nephrotic syndrome will have features characteristic of that disorder, e.g., massive proteinuria, hypoalbuminemia.

The "Euthyroid Sick Syndrome" Versus Hypothyroidism

The diagnosis of hypothyroidism in severely ill patients presents special problems.[252,253,266] Patients with the simulating "euthyroid sick syndrome" are usually elderly and often have sepsis. The possibility of hypothyroidism is usually raised by the patient's appearance, a finding such as hypothermia, or a nonspecific laboratory finding. When confirmation of the diagnosis is sought by measurement of T4 and T4 index, the result may be low, well into the hypothyroid range. However, a diagnosis of hypothyroidism cannot be made on the basis of these results alone. Further studies in such cases often show the free T4 to be normal or elevated; if low, the value may be disproportionately high for the level of T4. In all such cases the TSH is normal, a finding that rules out primary hypothyroidism but does not exclude the rare possibility of secondary hypothyroidism. The TRH test is normal in these cases, a finding that excludes pituitary hypothyroidism. One other useful differential finding is elevation of serum reverse T3 (rT3) in some but not all cases. Increase of rT3 and decrease of T3 is due to alteration of the degradative pathways of thyroxine metabolism during acute and chronic illness.

Since TSH or rT3 results may not be immediately available, clinical circumstances may make it necessary to treat the patient for severe hypothyroidism, i.e., for myxedema coma. If clinical recovery ensues, the exception rather than the rule in such cases, the T4 returns to normal. To date this syndrome has been recognized only in very severely ill patients, but may occur in less seriously ill persons. Unfortunately, the clinical determinants of this syndrome have not yet been defined, nor has the possible role of replacement therapy.

TREATMENT

The best preparation for ordinary use is T4 (levothyroxine; sodium L-thyroxine). T3 (liothyronine, Cytomel) is also effective and sometime preferable for treatment of goiter, but has no special advantage for routine therapy of hypothyroidism and has the distinct disadvantage that one cannot monitor the plasma T4 to determine adequacy of replacement. Combinations of T4 and T3 offer nothing but increased cost. Although desiccated thyroid is still available, and some preparations are reliably standardized, this relic of therapeutics should no longer be used.

Traditionally, initiation of thyroid hormone replacement therapy has been cautious and conservative and has utilized dosage schedules that ensure slow restoration of a normal metabolic state. While the principle is rational, the practice is often faulty. Therapy should be adjusted to the individual case, with several points in mind. If the patient is not elderly and has never had overt cardiac disease, overcautious initiation of therapy will result only in needless prolongation of the hypothyroid state with its attendant morbidity. Serious suspicion of hypothyroidism with coma demands emergency therapy, without waiting for laboratory confirmation. If the patient has evidence of preexisting cardiac disease, therapy should be started slowly, but unnecessary delay should be avoided. Only rarely will serious heart disease, such as angina pectoris, prevent at least partial therapy sufficient to eliminate myxedema, if not full correction of hypothyroidism.

The ordinary case of hypothyroidism without complicating medical problems may be started on full daily replacement dosage. Even with this therapeutic schedule, the clinical response will be very slow. One can expect several months to pass before restoration of the normal metabolic state. If a conservative approach is elected, i.e., if the patient is elderly or has known cardiovascular disease, a daily dose of 0.025 to 0.05 mg of T4 can be started with 0.05 mg increases at 2 weekly intervals.

The objective of therapy is to regain the euthyroid state. Enough thyroxine is given daily (0.1 to 0.2 mg) to maintain the plasma T4 at the upper range of normal, or, ideally, to the point where the TSH is restored to normal. Most persons need about 0.15 mg per day; only rarely is as much as 0.3 mg necessary. Determination of plasma T3 during therapy with T4 is unnecessary; the value will parallel that of T4.

Treatment of myxedema coma is an emergency that requires intravenous therapy with 200 to 400 μg of thyroxine as a single dose followed by 100 μg (0.1 mg) every day or every other day. In the United States, the only thyroid hormone currently available for intravenous use is T4 (levothyroxine). Some prefer T3 (liothyronine) because of its more rapid onset of action, but it is not clear that this offers any advantage.

Hypothyroid patients who require surgery are poor risks until their thyroid status is corrected, a process that requires 3 to 4 weeks with ordinary oral therapy. Elective surgery is best delayed in such patients. In an urgent situation, an intravenous dose of T4 is probably warranted to prepare for surgery in a few days. The increased susceptibility of hypothyroid persons to respiratory depression by conventional doses of many CNS active drugs should be borne in mind. This increased drug sensitivity has been responsible for precipitation of myxedema coma.

GOITER

A goiter is an enlarged, although usually benign, thyroid gland. The term implies nothing about the functional state of the gland. Goiter is the commonest thyroid abnormality. *Diffuse goiter*, also called simple goiter, is a gland that is uniformly and symmetrically enlarged without apparent irregularities. (Some use the term *simple goiter* to denote any nontoxic or nonhyperfunctioning gland, regardless of its anatomy.) In some areas of the world thyroid enlargement is so common as to be termed *endemic goiter*. Before the widespread introduction of iodized salt these areas were common, but this is no longer the case. Endemic goiter, for practical purposes synonymous with iodine deficiency goiter, is now found only in selected geographically isolated areas, e.g., certain parts of central Africa and the highlands of New Guinea. The term *sporadic goiter* refers to thyroid enlargement as now encountered in the United States and other developed areas. Sporadic goiter is seen in a few percent of the population and increases in frequency with age.

CAUSES

Any process that prevents the synthesis of normal quantities of thyroid hormones will produce goiter. If impairment of hormone synthesis is severe enough, goiter formation is associated with reduction of blood hormone levels, eventually to be followed by clinical hypothyroidism. The mechanism of the thyroid enlargement in this situation is increased pituitary TSH secretion via activation of the feedback system. The resulting increased thyroid mass is a compensatory mechanism which may allow sufficient hormone synthesis to occur so that the patient remains euthyroid.

In the past, widespread iodide deficiency was the commonest cause of goiter (endemic goiter). Iodide deficiency results in decreased hormone synthesis, and promotes a shift in the synthetic mechanism away from T4 and toward T3. Thus, endemic goiter may be seen with normal or even elevated levels of plasma T3 and low plasma T4. Clinical hypothyroidism sometimes is associated with such a hormone pattern. This observation argues strongly that T4 is not merely a prohormone but also has a major role of its own in maintaining the euthyroid state.

Interference with hormone synthesis can, of course, also be produced by a variety of chemical agents. Only one well-defined, naturally occurring compound is known, L-5-vinyl-2-thio-oxazolidone. This substance, with a mechanism of action much like that of the thiocarbamides, occurs in cabbage, turnips, soybeans, and several other vegetables. Other goiter-producing substances have been detected in the food and water supplies of some areas. However, no environmental factor has been incriminated as a cause of sporadic goiter, the etiology of which remains obscure.

As mentioned earlier, drugs that interfere with thyroid hormone synthesis include the thiocarbamides, sulfonylureas, lithium, and iodides. These can lead to goiter. Withdrawal of a goitrogenic drug results in regression of the goiter, as will administration of enough T4 or T3 to suppress endogenous TSH secretion. Goiter is almost invariably seen in hyperthyroidism due to Graves' disease. Here the gland enlargement is not due to excessive TSH but to the presence of TSH-like thyroid stimulating immunoglobulins (TSI).

PATHOLOGY

The following considerations apply to both endemic and sporadic goiter. The duration of thyroid gland hypertrophy appears to determine the gross and microscopic pathologic anatomy. The normal thyroid gland consists of collections of 20 to 40 follicles surrounded by scanty connective tissue forming lobules. During goiter formation there is initially uniform hypertrophy and hyperplasia of follicles and increased vascularity. As time passes, the normal architecture becomes distorted, micronodules form and eventually coalesce forming macronodules. Involution occurs in small or large areas coincident with hypertrophy elsewhere. Cellular infiltration, cysts, focal hemorrhage, and calcification develop.

RECOGNITION

A mass in the base of the neck recognized by the patient or physician is the usual mode of presentation of goiter. Occasionally a scintiscan shows enlargement that cannot be readily appreciated on physical examination. Rarely, an enlarged thyroid is neither visible nor readily palpable but is incidentally found by x-ray of the chest or esophagus when either a retrosternal mass is noted or the trachea or esophagus is found to be deviated. Except in subacute thyroiditis, pain is not a usual symptom but can develop during cyst formation or hemorrhage, a fairly frequent event in multinodular goiter.

Obstruction of the trachea or esophagus can be produced, but dysphagia should not be readily attributed to minor degrees of thyroid enlargement. Hoarseness may occur due to involvement of the recurrent laryngeal nerve, but this is rare in benign enlargement, and its occurrence suggests thyroid neoplasm.

DIFFERENTIAL DIAGNOSIS

Clinical and laboratory assessment of thyroid function should be made in all cases of goiter. The clinician must recognize that the functional state may change with time, sometimes rather rapidly, and hence the precise diagnosis may not be possible on a single examination. Goiter in association with hyperthyroidism suggests Graves' disease, toxic nodular goiter, or a hyperfunctioning ("hot") nodule. Hypofunction in association with goiter is likely to represent Hashimoto's thyroiditis, but other possibilities may have to be excluded. These range from drug ingestion to such rarities as an infiltrative process (amyloid disease, metastatic neoplasm) and the inherited defects of hormone synthesis (organification or coupling defects).

If the clinical and laboratory assessments suggest normal thyroid function, the diagnosis of euthyroid goiter is made. Multinodular enlargement almost always indicates a process of many years standing. Differentiation of diffuse enlargement from nodular enlargement may require scintiscanning, since small nodules may be missed on physical examination. When only small, nonpalpable nodules are present, an optimally performed scan may show irregular ("patchy") uptake of tracer. Thyroid autoantibodies are diagnostically elevated in most goiters due to Hashimoto's thyroiditis. A proper history will point to possible drug-related goiter. Rapidity of enlargement may help differentiate benign from malignant lesions, while the presence or absence of pain will help in identifying inflammatory thyroiditis.

TREATMENT

Although thyroid enlargement is idiopathic in sporadic goiter, the process is nevertheless dependent on the presence of TSH. Administration of a physiologic quantity of thyroid hormone results in suppression of TSH release. When TSH secretion is chronically suppressed, the enlarged thyroid eventually regresses or at least ceases to enlarge. This suppression therapy may be accomplished with thyroxine (T4; sodium-L-thyroxine; levothyroxin) or triiodothyronine (T3; liothyronine; Cytomel). The dose should not be excessive. T4 at a dose of 0.15 mg $\pm$ 0.05 mg daily is ample. T3 is given at a dose of 50 to 75 μg daily. Some evidence suggests that T3 may be effective in a greater proportion of cases.

Suppression therapy must be monitored. One must be certain that the gland is suppressible, since perhaps as many as 20 percent of nontoxic nodular goiters are autonomous. Other goiters may represent inapparent euthyroid Graves' disease. These patients may, if not monitored, develop iatrogenic hyperthyroidism due to the exogenous thyroid hormone. Monitoring therapy also assures that an adequate amount of hormone is being given. Regression of goiter is, of course, evidence of adequacy of therapy, but one wishes to be certain that the dose is adequate in those cases that do not show obvious regression. Theoretically, plasma TSH should be a useful index but limitation of sensitivity of the current assays in the "normal" range do not permit such an approach. Suppression of RaIU was once the standard method of assessing adequacy of dose and suppressibility, but is less useful now because of the low RaIU so often seen in normal persons.

Suppression therapy with T3 has the advantage that the plasma T4 falls to a level below normal if suppression is adequate, thus obviating the need for RaIU testing. When T4 is used for suppression therapy, a plasma T4 which is not in excess of normal provides assurance that the dose is not excessive.

If the treated gland is diffusely enlarged, obvious regression by 6 months is to be expected. Nodular glands are less likely to respond and any response that occurs is slower. Several years may be necessary to discern regression of a long-standing multinodular goiter, and during that time one or more nodules may become more easily palpable as the relatively normal portions of the gland regress. Some confusion may occur if the physician interprets this as progression of the disease or as the appearance of a malignant area.

Suppression therapy is often performed for cosmetic reasons. Even if complete regression is not accomplished, prevention of further gland enlargement can be expected. Suppression therapy is clearly indicated for individuals with many years of life expectancy during which mechanical problems may develop. However, little is to be gained by treatment of patients whose glands are known not to have changed in size over many years and who are, therefore, unlikely to develop such difficulties. A clear and unequivocal indication is found in the patient who has already had surgery for goiter. Recurrence of goiter is frequent in such persons but can predictably be prevented with suppression therapy.

Once started, suppression therapy is usually continued indefinitely but can be terminated or withdrawn if regression occurs. Some cases do not recur; in those that do, therapy can be reinstituted. Suppression therapy does not lead to permanent loss of TSH secretion, even after decades of thyroid hormone administration, although rare individuals may manifest a brief period of hypothyroidism when prolonged therapy is withdrawn.

Goiter so large as to produce significant tracheal compression (not merely deviation) and interfere with swallowing is now a rarity. In these cases, surgery, although attended by significant morbidity, should be considered, since suppression therapy is unlikely to be effective in significantly reducing the size of such large goiters. Radioiodide therapy can be considered in these cases, especially in the elderly or individuals with other serious medical problems. Multiple doses are usually required. While the response is slow, useful reduction in the size of the goiter may be achieved.

The frequency of carcinoma in multinodular goiter has been debated for years. Unwarranted concern has resulted in countless unnecessary operations.

THYROID NEOPLASMS

One of the commonest abnormalities of the thyroid is a localized area of enlargement commonly known as a nodule. In evaluating the thyroid nodule, the possibility of malignancy is the main concern. About 90 percent are benign adenomas or cysts; the remaining ones are lesions of varying degrees of malignancy.

BENIGN THYROID NEOPLASMS: THE SOLITARY NODULE

Many solitary nodules are true adenomas and are encapsulated. Histologically, three main types are seen, follicular, papillary, or Hürthle cell. Follicular adenomas, the most common, are subdivided into three subgroups: colloid (macrofollicular), fetal (microfollicular), and embryonal. While most benign adenomas are relatively hypofunctioning, follicular adenomas may exhibit normal or greater than normal function, i.e., they take up iodine and elaborate thyroid hormone. The growth of most benign adenomas, hypofunctional though they may be, is dependent on endogenous TSH. Adenomas whose function is independent of TSH, are termed *autonomous*.

Benign thyroid nodules are present in at least 5 percent of the population, but clinically aggressive thyroid carcinoma is rare. In a group of over 200 patients with thyroid nodules identified in the Framingham Study (4 percent of 5000 patients examined, ages 30 to 60) and followed for 15 years, none developed clinically evident malignancy. In that population, new thyroid nodules continued to appear at a rate of about 1 per 1000 persons per year, about twice as frequently in women as in men.

CLINICAL APPROACH TO THE PATIENT WITH A SOLITARY NODULE

The first point to be established is whether the patient really has only a single nodule. Palpation by an *experienced* examiner is essential. Frequently, the "solitary" nodule turns out to be one of several nodules in a nontoxic nodular goiter. A single nodule in a clearly enlarged thyroid has a similar connotation, since the enlarged gland is likely to be harboring many small, nondiscrete nodules. Although most patients with a nodule are euthyroid at presentation, T4 index should be determined for confirmation. If any question about the clinical status exists, plasma T3 should also be measured.

The next essential question is that of the functional state of the nodule relative to the remaining thyroid tissue, since the hyperfunctioning nodule is almost invariably benign. When scintiscanning with pertechnetate or preferably ^{123}I, is performed, accumulation of isotope in the nodule can approximate that of the surrounding gland tissue ("warm" nodule), be greater ("hot" nodule), or be less ("cold" nodule). A "hot" nodule can be considered benign (98 percent likelihood with pertechnetate; 99.8 percent with ^{123}I). "Warm" nodules are far more likely to be benign than not, but the statistics are not so unequivocal as for the hot nodule.

The "Hot" Nodule

Management of the hot nodule depends on whether an excessive amount of thyroid hormone is being produced. The autonomous hot nodule, if it produces an amount of hormone equal to or greater than that of normal gland output, suppresses TSH; the remaining normal tissue then becomes relatively inactive and may not be visible, or is only poorly visible, by scintiscan. In cases in which the nodule is hyperactive but has not clearly suppressed the remaining thyroid tissue, demonstration of autonomous function may depend on a suppression test with administered thyroid hormone.

If the amount of hormone produced by the adenoma considerably exceeds normal, thyrotoxicosis should be clinically apparent. Usually T4 and T3 are produced in excess. However, hyperthyroidism due to T3 alone (T3 toxicosis) is fairly frequent with such hyperactive nodules.

The natural history of the hot nodule is variable. Over a 10-year interval about one-third will show little change, one-third will become frankly hyperactive, and the remainder will become "cold," sometimes with obvious hemorrhagic infarction and cystic degeneration. Treatment of the hot nodule that is producing hyperthyroidism can be satisfactorily accomplished with radioactive iodine or surgery. Prophylactic ablative therapy is not indicated for hot nodules. Suppression therapy with thyroid hormone is, of course, not effective and will lead to iatrogenic hyperthyroidism.

The "Cold" Nodule

In the evaluation of the cold nodule, one should bear in mind that 90 percent of such lesions are benign; only 10 percent are malignant and almost all of these are very slow growing and of low grade malignancy.

Two additional procedures, now widely available, can provide a diagnosis and avoid unnecessary surgery. They should be performed sequentially, if possible. 1) Ultrasound (sonography) examination accurately identifies about 10 percent of all "cold" nodules as cystic. Almost all (98 percent) predominantly cystic lesions represent benign adenomas; mixed cystic-solid lesions are less certainly benign. A large proportion of "cold" nodules can be spared surgery by this simple, noninvasive technique. 2) Several needle biopsy techniques have gained wide favor in recent years, as has fine needle aspiration with cytologic examination.[259]

Thyroid Hormone Suppression Therapy for Nodules

A conservative approach to the cold nodule, involving a trial of suppression therapy with thyroxine, is recommended. Lesions less than 2.5 cm diameter can be handled in this way with great safety. Regression of the nodule over a 6-month period indicates benign disease; such patients can be followed indefinitely with continued suppression therapy. Some physicians are satisfied when a nodule at least does not grow larger during suppression therapy. Considering the probability that 90 percent of cases treated in this way represent benign disease in the first place and the low grade malignancy of almost all of the remaining cases, this approach is reasonable. However, close follow-up is necessary to insure that appropriate therapy is instituted should the lesion enlarge further during suppression therapy or lymph nodes become palpable.

THYROID CARCINOMAS

General Considerations

About 95 percent of thyroid carcinomas are of the papillary or follicular variety; of these 80 to 90 percent are papillary carcinomas. Anaplastic and medullary carcinomas probably account for no more than 5 percent of the total. The relative frequency of the various types of thyroid carcinomas is markedly age-dependent.

At autopsy, occult thyroid carcinoma (defined as lesions with the histologic appearance of carcinoma, but less than 1.5 cm in diameter) is found in 5 to 10 percent of U.S. and European populations and 30 percent for Japanese samples. Clearly, occult carcinoma behaves as a benign disease and does not warrant aggressive management.

In the United States, about 10,000 new cases of thyroid carcinoma are seen each year, but only about 1000 persons die of thyroid carcinoma. Most of these deaths result from the aggressive forms of the disease, i.e., anaplastic lesions, the unusually aggressive follicular carcinomas, and a few from the very uncommon aggressive papillary lesions.[250] Only rare deaths are attributable to medullary carcinoma.

Therapeutic Considerations in Thyroid Carcinoma

PAPILLARY CARCINOMA. Enough information[256] is now available to provide support for a middle-of-the-road approach, one which falls between that which advocated thyroid hormone suppression therapy without surgery and that which has employed radical surgery alone. Long observations have now also reasonably defined the role of radioiodide ablation therapy[255,257].

Surgery for Papillary Carcinoma. Follow-up at 10 years[256] indicates a recurrence rate of about 20 percent for subtotal resection versus 10 percent for total removal of the gland. Deaths due to carcinoma are 1.5 and 0.5 percent, respectively. The differences are statistically significant. However, the complication rate for total thyroidectomy (hypoparathyroidism, vocal cord paralysis) remains high. As a result, many surgeons have now adopted a modified or "near total" thyroidectomy. In this procedure the affected side is completely removed; most of the contralateral lobe is also removed but the posterior capsule is left together with the tip of the upper pole. Visibly involved lymph nodes are always removed, but radical neck dissection is not justified even in the presence of obviously involved nodes.

The presence of cervical node metastases at operation or the type of lymphadenectomy does *not* seem to influence recurrence rate or death rate. The death rate in lesions under 2.5 cm without local invasion and without evident distant metastases at the time of surgery is less than 1 percent in 10 years and 4 to 8 percent in the less favorable categories.[256]

Postoperative Therapy: TSH Suppression and Ablation with Radioiodine. Postoperative therapy with full replacement doses of thyroxine will suppress endogenous TSH and reduce recurrence of papillary carcinoma. In addition, postsurgical ablative therapy with radioactive iodide has a role, although not all cases of localized disease need such therapy.[256] The patient with a minimal papillary lesion needs no additional therapy but the patient with a large, locally invasive lesion should receive ablative therapy. In cases with an intermediate-sized lesion, without invasion of the thyroid capsule and without lymph node metastases, the recurrence rate is greatly reduced by treatment with radioiodine, and deaths from recurrent disease may be completely abolished.[255] The hesitation to use radioiodine routinely stems from fear of radiation-induced leukemia. Doses of ^{131}I smaller than those customarily recommended may be equally effective.[257] In contrast to the constraints on radioiodide therapy of localized disease, known metastatic disease should always be treated vigorously.

FOLLICULAR CARCINOMA. This tumor is often more aggressive than papillary carcinoma, tends to be angioinvasive, and to metastasize to bones and lungs. In contrast, the tumor seldom spreads to regional lymph nodes, a marked difference from papillary disease. The most important prognostic feature is invasion, either through the tumor capsule or into blood vessels. Unlike papillary carcinoma, primary tumor size at presentation does not appear to influence prognosis.[256]

The clinical presentation may be very different from papillary disease; the patient may present with metastatic disease involving lungs, bone, brain, or spinal cord. In these cases the primary may be small and initially overlooked. Only rarely do the metastases produce sufficient thyroid hormones to cause thyrotoxicosis.

The surgical approach to follicular carcinoma should be that taken for papillary carcinoma. Suppression therapy with thyroid hormone replacement is routine. Vigorous postoperative ablative therapy with radioiodine appears warranted, especially for those patients with invasive disease. However, the removal of a histologically benign, noninvasive follicular lesion allows a less aggressive approach to ^{131}I iodine ablation therapy.

ANAPLASTIC CARCINOMA. This carcinoma is relatively uncommon; its frequency depends on the age structure of the population. Anaplastic carcinoma is very rare in children and in adults under the age of about 35. By age 50, as many as 10 percent of cases of thyroid carcinoma are due to anaplastic disease and by age 80 nearly half of the cases are of this variety.[256] The disease is locally invasive in a highly aggressive fashion and quickly produces pain, dysphagia, hemoptysis, and hoarseness. Death usually occurs within 6 to 12 months. Surgically resectable disease without evidence of metastases, even if it has extended outside the thyroid capsule, can be associated with a long-term survival (20 to 30 percent). It is important to distinguish the small cell type from lymphoma of the thyroid. This rare disease, unlike anaplastic carcinoma, is radiosensitive and amenable to chemotherapy.

MEDULLARY CARCINOMA. Medullary carcinoma accounts for only 1 to 2 percent of all thyroid cancers. The tumors arise from the parafollicular or C-cells and produce thyrocalcitonin. Both sporadic and familial varieties are known. The sporadic case typically presents as a solitary nodule, while the familial variety is often multifocal and part of a multiple endocrine adenomatosis syndrome. Diarrhea occurs in some patients. Thyrocalcitonin in plasma is elevated in the basal state or after stimulation with calcium or pentagastrin infusion. When surgical excision is performed before regional nodes have become involved, 90 percent of patients survive to 10 years. Once the nodes are involved, only 40 percent survival can be expected. Medullary carcinoma does not appear to respond to suppression therapy with thyroid hormone.

The Question of Carcinoma in the Multinodular Thyroid

While the approach to the single nodule is reasonably straightforward, opinion regarding the risk of carcinoma in a nontoxic nodular goiter is divided. Occult carcinoma will be found in a significant proportion of such cases. However, the approach to such occult lesions is no different from that to occult carcinoma in the non-nodular gland. Demonstration of multinodularity by palpation or its suggestion by scan leads some physicians to a firm recommendation against surgical intervention. Suppression therapy is recommended, but only for prevention of further gland enlargement and not out of concern for malignancy. Others feel that large nonfunctioning nodules within multinodular goiters should be treated with suppression therapy for a period of 6 months. Failure to regress is considered an indication for surgical excision. Most large nodules in multinodular goiters do not regress within such a period of time, while a significant number may actually become more prominent as less abnormal tissue regresses. Serial sonographic estimates of nodule size may prove useful in such cases.

Radiation-Associated Thyroid Carcinoma

Low-dose irradiation of the thyroid is a stimulus to thyroid carcinogenesis, with a latency period of one to several decades.[247]

Thyroid carcinomas have been noted in greatly increased incidence in patients who received radiation therapy some years earlier for enlarged tonsils, adenoids, or thymus; acne; cervical lymphadenopathy, etc. A distinction must be made between treatment with penetrating external radiation and local irradiation with point sources (radium rod or plaque treatment). Thyroid carcinoma has not been related to such limited exposures.

As many as one-third of irradiated individuals may develop thyroid carcinoma. Papillary and follicular carcinomas are seen in about the same proportion as in nonirradiated cases, but a relationship to medullary carcinoma and anaplastic carcinoma has not been established. The carcinomas are multifocal in about half the cases. The biologic behavior of radiation-induced carcinomas is similar to those that appear spontaneously.

The approach to the patient with a history of irradiation to the head and neck is not presently standardized. If no thyroid abnormality is palpable, re-examination of the patient at intervals of one to two years should suffice. The place of routine scanning procedures for patients with nonpalpable lesions is controversial, but experience suggests that many nonpalpable lesions (0.5 to 1.0 cm) can be detected by optimal use of methods now available. Also the frequency of carcinomas in irradiated patients with abnormalities on scan alone is probably similar to that with palpable disease. The issue at stake here is the natural history of such small lesions. Lesions too small to be palpable are clinically, if not pathologically, benign, and should be managed conservatively. Prophylactic suppression therapy with thyroxine for patients known to have been irradiated is not defined, but has a sound experimental basis. Parathyroid adenomas also may occur with increased frequency in irradiated persons.[262]

THYROIDITIS

Pyogenic or suppurative thyroiditis, also known as acute thyroiditis, is very rare. The thyroid infection usually follows bacteremia, but can occur as an isolated, primary event. The organism is often diplococcus or staphylococcus. Pain and swelling are the hallmarks and eventual suppuration may occur. Treatment is with antibiotics and, if necessary, surgical drainage.

Riedel's thyroiditis is another rare but indolent form of thyroiditis. The process is one of chronic fibrosis which often involves not only the thyroid but also contiguous structures. The intense induration makes the clinical differentiation from infiltrating neoplasm difficult. Hashimoto's thyroiditis is common.

Subacute thyroiditis, also known as granulomatous or de Quervain's thyroiditis, is common. Many mild cases are probably never diagnosed. The term subacute is often deceiving and sometimes inappropriate. Although the onset may be insidious, it is perhaps just as often acute over several days. Many cases give a history of recent antecedent upper respiratory tract infection.

The earliest symptom may be referred pain, usually to the ear, but pain can appear to originate in the jaw or occiput. This phase may last a few hours or days before tenderness and discomfort in the thyroid area becomes apparent. Rarely, the patient is concerned only with the referred pain and unaware of thyroidal tenderness until examination makes it apparent. When the onset is acute the symptoms and signs are more likely to be severe. Initially, pain and swelling of the thyroid are often unilateral, but the process usually does not remain localized for more than a few days. Systemic symptoms include fever, especially in acute cases, and a sensation of intense fatigue and malaise. The course may be protracted with symptoms persisting for months, although usually symptoms subside within a week or two. Erythrocyte sedimentation rate may be elevated. Early in the disease, the thyroidal radioiodide uptake is depressed, while plasma T4 is elevated. More striking is elevation of the plasma protein-bound iodine (PBI), a consequence of the release from the thyroid of iodinated proteins. This event results in a larger than normal gap between the T4 and PBI. Although these tests are likely to show the described abnormalities in typical cases, they are not recommended as routine diagnostic aides. Typical cases can be diagnosed clinically, while mild cases have only borderline abnormalities of the tests. Significant titers of thyroid autoantibodies are not usually seen.

Clinical hyperthyroidism is occasionally seen with this syndrome. Rarely hypothyroidism occurs and lasts for several months. Permanent hypothyroidism is unusual.

Therapy is directed toward relief of local and systemic symptoms. In mild cases, aspirin in doses sufficient to maintain therapeutic blood levels may be effective, but glucocorticoid therapy (30 to 60 mg prednisone or equivalent) may be necessary. Therapy can usually be gradually withdrawn after several weeks, although relapse is frequent.

CHAPTER 77

The Gonads
PATRICK C. WALSH, JOHN E. A. TYSON, AND T. H. HSU

Disorders of the reproductive system present a wide clinical spectrum. They can usually be related to abnormalities occurring at various milestones in sexual maturation. Abnormalities in utero present with abnormal sexual differentiation. Abnormalities occurring between infancy and puberty may present as precocious maturation with appropriate or inappropriate secondary sexual characteristics. At the time of puberty, the commonest presentations are related to delay of puberty or abnormalities in the maturation process (gynecomastia in men, asymmetry of breast development, or virilization in women). Postpubertal gonadal disorders include menstrual abnormalities, infertility, inappropriate virilization or feminization, and premature gonadal failure.

The great variety and complexity of gonadal disorders stem from the fact that the male and female reproductive organs develop from the same fetal anlage, respond to the same pituitary tropic hormones, and synthesize their steroidal hormones in similar fashion. Understanding these disorders is facilitated if each is approached with a proper background in the known effects of sex hormones, the complex reciprocal pituitary-gonadal relationships, and the normal sequence of reproductive development.

SEXUAL DIFFERENTIATION[281]

The undifferentiated fetal gonad, which is formed between 3 and 5 weeks of gestation, is bipotential in sexual differentiation. Early in the gestation both wolffian and müllerian ducts are present. Further male sexual development requires the presence of testes whereas femaleness represents the innate tendency of the fetal sex organ and does not require ovarian influence.

Normal sexual differentiation is the result of a series of individual steps that occur in an orderly fashion. During embryogenesis, any disturbances of the various steps may be reflected clinically as a disorder of intersexuality. Consequently, a complete understanding of the progression of these normal sexual differentiations is essential for evaluation and management of sexual disorders.

Development of Male Sex Organs[279]

Once an indifferent gonad is formed, chromosomal determinants direct the subsequent differentiation into either an ovary or a testis.[285] Then the fetal testis, acting via humoral factors, is responsible for differentiation of the internal ducts and external genitalia.

For the formation of a testis, factors on the Y chromosome, X chromosome, and possibly an autosomal chromosome are necessary.[277,286,309] The testis-determining gene on the Y chromosome is presumably located on the short arm near the centromere. A locus for a histocompatibility antigen (H-Y antigen) is linked so closely with the testis-determining gene to suggest that it may represent the testis determining factor.[306,309]

Beginning at six weeks of gestation, the primordial germ cells in the male fetus are incorporated into testicular cords, and by 9 weeks Leydig cells are formed.

The fetal testes secrete two factors, müllerian-inhibiting factor and testosterone, which act ipsilaterally to direct the development of internal ductal system to maleness. Müllerian-inhibiting substance, which is produced by the fetal Sertoli cells,[273] causes regression of the müllerian ducts,[271] and testosterone promotes differentiation of the wolffian duct structures.[305] The proximal wolffian duct becomes elongated and convoluted to form the epididymis, and the remainder of the duct gives rise to the vas deferens and the seminal vesicle. In the absence of a normal fetal testis, as in the normal female, müllerian ducts persist and differentiate into the fallopian tubes, the uterus, and the upper vagina. Without the influence of testosterone, wolffian ducts regress spontaneously.

The fetal external genitalia, consisting of the urogenital sinus, genital tubercle, genital folds, and genital swellings, are also sexually bipotential. In the male, between 10 and 15 weeks of gestation under the influence of androgen, the urogenital sinus, gives rise to the prostate, the genital tubercle forms the glans penis, and the genital swellings merge and migrate inferiorly to form the scrotum. For testosterone to exert this effect, it must be converted to dihydrotestosterone by the 5α-reductase enzymes located in the urogenital sinus and external genitalia.[305] In the absence of androgen, they differentiate into female external genitalia.

Development of Female Sex Organs

For the formation of normal ovaries, the 46 XX chromosomal makeup is necessary. Ovarian development does not begin however, until the 13th week of gestation, when the first mitotic activity begins in the germinal cells. Follicles appear near the center of the ovary at about the 16th week.

In the absence of testes, whether the ovaries are present or not, the wolffian ducts regress spontaneously and the müllerian ducts differentiate to form the fallopian tubes, uterus, and upper portion of the vagina during the third month of fetal life. The fetal testicular factors responsible for differentiation of wolffian ducts act locally. Therefore, when a female fetus is exposed to androgens from other sources, e.g., congenital adrenal hyperplasia or maternal medication, male internal ducts do not develop even though the external genitalia may be markedly virilized.

In the absence of androgen, the urogenital sinus forms the lower vagina, the genital tubercle becomes the clitoris, the genital folds develop into the labia minora, and the genital swellings form the labia majora. When the female fetus is exposed to excessive androgens, various degrees of ambiguity of external genitalia occur.

ABNORMAL SEXUAL DIFFERENTIATION

During embryogenesis, any disturbance of the various steps in normal sexual differentiation may be reflected clinically as a disorder of intersexuality. However, the three most common classes of disorders are: 1) sex chromosomal anomalies, 2) defective androgen production or action in the male, producing feminization of the genitalia (male pseudohermaphroditism; Table 77–1), and 3) excessive androgen production in the female producing virilization of the external genitalia (female pseudohermaphroditism).

Disorders of Male Sexual Differentiation

CHROMOSOME ABNORMALITIES (See also Chap. 40). The Klinefelter syndrome (47, XXY) is the most common disorder of gonadal differentiation in men affecting 0.2 percent of males.

In its classic form, defective spermatogenesis, azoospermia, small firm testes, and gynecomastia are present. Plasma LH and FSH levels are high, and plasma testosterone levels are only 50 percent of normal. In addition to the classic form, about 30 other karyotypic varieties have been described, including XXYY, XXXY, XXXXY, and a variety of mosaics, such as XY/XXY. In the classic form, a diagnosis can be made from the buccal smear which shows a nuclear chromatin clump (Barr body) inappropriate for the male cell, while the mosaic forms require chromosomal analysis to confirm the diagnosis.

The presence of both ovarian and testicular tissue is a condition known as true hermaphroditism.[279,312] Although differentiation of the external genitalia is variable, 75 percent of patients have been reared as males because of the size of the phallus. Eighty percent of the patients are chromatin-positive and the most common karyotype is 46, XX; however, since these patients are H-Y antigen positive, Y-chromosomal material was presumably translocated to another chromosome.[309] Patients with mixed gonadal dysgenesis have a streak gonad on one side and a testis on the other.[279] All patients have a uterus and at least one fallopian tube, with wide variability in the appearance of the external genitalia. However, most patients are poorly virilized, and consequently more than 50 percent have been reared as females. The most common karyotype is 45,XO/46,XY. In adulthood, the seminiferous tubules lack all germinal elements and more than 25 percent of the patients develop testicular tumors, typically gonadoblastomas.

MALE PSEUDOHERMAPHRODITISM.   In this disorder genetic males (46,XY) with bilateral testes differentiate partially or completely as phenotypic females.[308,312] This disorder can result from defects in androgen synthesis, defects in androgen action, or defective müllerian regression. Five enzymatic steps are necessary for the conversion of cholesterol to testosterone. A defect in any one of these enzymes may give rise to inadequate testosterone synthesis in utero resulting in incomplete virilization with ambiguous genitalia in male infants. The diagnosis is based on the demonstration of inadequate testosterone synthesis, elevated gonadotropin secretion after puberty, and the presence of elevated steroids that accumulate proximal to the particular metabolic block.

Four distinct familial forms of defective androgen action can be identified (Table 77–1).

1. Patients with the testicular feminization syndrome are phenotypic females with absent pubic and axillary hair but with normally developed breasts and a shallow blind-ending vagina. This disorder, which is inherited as an X-linked recessive trait, represents the most complete form of androgen resistance. Although testosterone synthesis is normal, the primary defect in this disorder is an inherited abnormality in the amount or function of the androgen receptor.

2. The term familial incomplete male pseudohermaphroditism type 1 has been applied to a group of disorders in which the usual presentation is that of a

---

TABLE 77-1
Classification of Intersexuality

Disorder	Gonads	Internal Ducts	External Genitalia	Sex Chromatin	Karyotype
Disorders of Gonadal Differentiation					
Klinefelter syndrome	Bilateral testes	Wolffian	Male	Positive	47,XXY
Turner syndrome	Bilateral streaks	Müllerian	Female	50% Negative	45,XO
True hermaphroditism	Testis + ovary	Mixed	Variable	80% Positive	46,XX; 46,XY; mosaics
Mixed gonadal dysgenesis	Testis + streak	Mixed	Variable	Negative	45,XO/46,XY; 46,XY; other mosaics
Female Pseudohermaphroditism					
Congenital adrenal hyperplasia	Bilateral ovaries	Müllerian	Variable virilization	Positive	46,XX
Prenatal virilization from drugs					
Virilizing disorder of mother					
Idiopathic					
Male Pseudohermaphroditism					
Defective androgen production	Bilateral testes	Wolffian	Variable virilization	Negative	46,XY
3β-hydroxysteroid dehydrogenase deficiency					
17-hydroxylase deficiency					
17-ketosteroid reductase deficiency					
20,21-desmolase deficiency					
17,20-desmolase deficiency					
Defective androgen action					
Testicular feminization	Bilateral testes	Absent	Female	Negative	46,XY
Incomplete testicular feminization	Bilateral testes	Wolffian	Variable virilization	Negative	46,XY
Incomplete male pseudohermaphroditism type I					
Lubs syndrome	Bilateral testes	Partial wolffian	Variable virilization	Negative	46,XY
Gilbert-Dreyfus syndrome	Bilateral testes	Partial wolffian	Variable virilization	Negative	46,XY
Reifenstein syndrome	Bilateral testes	Wolffian	Variable virilization	Negative	46,XY
Rosewater syndrome	Bilateral testes	Wolffian	Male	Negative	46,XY
Incomplete male pseudohermaphroditism type II	Bilateral testes	Wolffian	Variable virilization	Negative	46,XY
Defective Müllerian Regression					
Persistent müllerian duct syndrome	Bilateral testes	Müllerian and wolffian	Male	Negative	46,XY

male with hypospadias, azoospermia, incomplete virilization at the time of puberty, gynecomastia, and a family history consistent with X-linked inheritance (Reifenstein syndrome). In this disorder the level of the cytoplasmic receptor protein for androgen is low.

3. Incomplete male pseudohermaphroditism type 2 (pseudovaginal perineoscrotal hypospadias) is a disorder in which phenotypic females present with normal wolffian duct structures, severe perineal hypospadias, masculinization to a variable extent at puberty, and a family history consistent with autosomal recessive inheritance. A defect in dihydrotestosterone formation because of deficiency of 5α-reductase is the fundamental defect in this disorder.

4. Persistent müllerian duct syndrome (hernia uteri inguinale) is a condition in which phenotypic males with cryptorchism are found to have a rudimentary uterus, bilateral fallopian tubes, and variable development of the vasa deferentia. The exact defect in this disorder is uncertain, but there are three possible explanations: 1) failure of the fetal testis to produce müllerian-inhibiting substance, 2) poor timing of the release of müllerian-inhibiting substance, or 3) failure of the tissues to respond to this hormone.

Disorders of Female Sexual Differentiation

CHROMOSOME ABNORMALITIES (See also Chap. 40). In the female, the most common disorder of gonadal differentiation is the Turner syndrome (gonadal dysgenesis) in which the most common karyotype is 45,XO.[279] Classically, these patients have nonfunctional streak gonads and usually one or more associated somatic abnormalities such as short stature, wide (shield) chest, brachydactyly, cubitus valgus, web neck, low hairline, lymphedema, coarctation of the aorta, or intestinal telangiectasia. In addition, some other X chromosome abnormalities are associated with gonadal dysgenesis; about 40 percent are mosaics, of which XX/XO is the most common.

In the classic form, the external genitalia are unambiguously female but remain immature even in adulthood unless the patient is treated with estrogen. The internal genitalia consist of bilateral fallopian tubes, a small but normally formed uterus, and bilateral streak gonads. Diagnosis of the classic syndrome can be made on buccal smear, from the absence of Barr bodies. Diagnosis of mosaic Turner syndrome requires a chromosomal analysis, since the buccal smear may be normal. Pure gonadal dysgenesis is a closely related disorder. These patients are phenotypic females of normal stature who have bilateral streak ovaries but no other stigmata of the Turner syndrome. It occurs in familial 46,XX and 46,XY forms.

FEMALE PSEUDOHERMAPHRODITISM.[279] Patients with this disorder are genetic females (46,XX) with bilateral ovaries who have virilization of the external genitalia produced by intrauterine exposure to excessive androgen. However, because they have normally developed ovaries and müllerian derivatives, they are all potentially fertile. Depending on the stage of differentiation at the time of exposure to androgen, the degree of masculinization varies from clitoral hypertrophy to true phallic-urethral formation with labioscrotal fusion. The most common cause is congenital adrenal hyperplasia in which cortisol synthesis is impaired (Chap. 70). In attempting to compensate for lowered cortisol levels, ACTH stimulates the adrenal to secrete excess androgen. The two most common

enzyme defects that give rise to congenital adrenal hyperplasia are the 21-hydroxylase disorder, which in the complete form is associated with severe salt loss, and the 11-hydroxylase deficiency, which is associated with the accumulation of the potent salt retaining hormone desoxycorticosterone, resulting in hypertension. The other causes of female pseudohermaphroditism include prenatal virilization from drugs, maternal virilizing tumors, and an idiopathic form.

GONADAL PHYSIOLOGY

Testis

The adult testis normally measures 4.6 cm in longest diameter (range 3.6 to 5.5 cm) and 2.6 cm in width (range 2.1 to 3.2 cm) and weighs about 21 g. The arterial supply to the testis arises from three sources (the internal spermatic artery, the deferential artery, and the cremasteric artery) and the venous collaterals from the testis and epididymis join to drain into the internal spermatic vein which empties into the inferior vena cava on the right and the renal vein on the left. The intimate relationship of the arteries and veins in the spermatic cord provides a mechanism for precooling arterial blood before it reaches the testis. This factor, coupled with the anatomic location of the testis within the scrotum, provides a cooler environment for the seminiferous tubules; in man, the abdominoscrotal temperature difference averages 2.2°C.

Beneath the white outer capsule of the testis, the seminiferous tubules are separated by fibrous septa into 250 pyramidal lobules each containing several coiled, U-shaped tubules. The seminiferous tubules have a central lumen, stratified epithelium four to eight cells in thickness composed of Sertoli cells and spermatogenic cells, and an outer thin basement membrane. Because the seminiferous tubules occupy over 75 percent of the total mass of the testis, when isolated damage to the tubules occurs, the testes become small and soft.

The Leydig cells, which are found in the loose connective tissue stroma between the tubules, constitute about 12 percent of the testicular volume and are the principal source of testosterone, secreting about 7 mg per day. Once formed, testosterone traverses the myoid cell layer to enter the seminiferous tubules or leaves by the capillary venous or lymphatic route to enter the systemic circulation. In plasma, testosterone is transported bound to protein, largely to albumin and to a specific steroid hormone transport protein, testosterone–estradiol-binding globulin. Less than 1 percent of testosterone circulates in the free form.

The testes are regulated by two pituitary gonadotropins: luteinizing hormone (LH) and follicle-stimulating hormone (FSH). These hormones are synthesized and stored in the anterior pituitary and their release is regulated by the hypothalamic decapeptide, gonadotropin-releasing hormone (GRH).[274] LH and FSH are secreted from the pituitary into the general circulation in an episodic fashion. This results in rhythmic elevations in serum LH levels that occur at 60- to 100-minute intervals and vary from 20 to 400 percent.[298] The slower metabolic clearance rate of FSH is reflected by more constant serum levels of this hormone. LH acts on the Leydig cell to stimulate the secretion of testosterone. FSH binds to the Sertoli cell and by some mechanism facilitates the maturation of mature spermatids to spermatozoa.[270] In addition, FSH may augment testosterone secretion, possibly by regulating the number of LH receptors on the Leydig cell.

The hypothalamus–pituitary gonadal system consists of a closed-loop feedback control mechanism directed at maintaining normal reproductive functions. In this manner, hormones produced by the testes have inhibitory effects on the secretion of LH and FSH. Testosterone is the primary regulator of gonadotropin secretion in men. Although castration results in an elevation of both LH and FSH, selective germ cell damage produces an elevation of serum FSH but not LH.[291] Consequently, it has been assumed that the testes produce a second hormone, which is a product of spermatogenic tissue. This substance, termed inhibin, appears to be a nonsteroidal, polypeptide hormone.

Ovary

The mature ovary measures about $3.5 \times 2 \times 1.5$ cm, although there is considerable variation. Its principal components are surface epithelium, follicles in different stages of maturation, stroma, and vascular structures. The main functions of the ovary are the production of ova and the secretion of estrogen and progesterone. The ovarian follicle is the principal functional unit of the adult ovary.

During each menstrual cycle of a sexually mature woman, groups of immature follicles are stimulated to grow under the influence of FSH. While numerous follicles develop simultaneously, only one or two achieve maturity, expand and rupture, and extrude a mature ovum into the abdominal cavity to be soon enveloped by the fallopian tube and transported toward the uterus. As follicular maturation progresses, estrogens, predominantly estradiol, are secreted by the theca cells. Following ovum maturation and ovulation, the follicle is transformed into a corpus luteum. The luteinized granulosa cells secrete predominantly progesterone.[276] The functional life of the corpus luteum is about two weeks unless stimulated anew by HCG from an embedded trophoblast. The cause of its regression is unknown. Presence of both granulosa and theca cells in the ovary enhances production of both estrogen and progesterone beyond the synthetic capabilities of either cell alone. In vitro incubation of preovulatory granulosa cells leads to progesterone production, implying indirectly the presence of a luteinization inhibitor in the ovary. In addition to ovarian granulosa and theca cells, stroma cells under the stimulation of LH produce significant amounts of dehydroepiandrosterone and androstenedione.

The physiologic functions of the sex steroids are many and varied. They are responsible for the phenotypic expression of female sex, and have particular effects on the female genitalia, endometrium, the cervical mucus, vaginal mucosa, and breasts. Estrogens, in particular, function in the feedback control of the secretion of gonadotropin. However, the regulation of gonadotropin secretion by nonsteroidal ovarian substances has been suggested. Such a substance, called inhibin, has been isolated from bovine and porcine follicles and inhibits further growth of other follicles.[276]

THE MENSTRUAL CYCLE.[294] Normally 28.2 days in length on the average, the menstrual cycle is marked by a dynamic balance between stimulation of pituitary gonadotropin secretion by GRH and the subsequent stimulation of ovarian steroidogenesis with negative feedback. Plasma FSH rises at the end of the luteal phase of the previous cycle to initiate the maturation of a group (usually 6 to 12) of primary follicles. These developing follicles begin to produce increasing amounts of estradiol, which reach a peak 12 to 24 hours before the LH ovulatory surge. The progressively rising blood estrogen initially exerts a negative feedback effect on FSH secretion. Thus, there is a reciprocal decline of FSH levels throughout the follicular phase until the ovulatory LH-FSH surge occurs. The abrupt increase of estrogen serves as an ovarian signal to trigger the gonadotropin surge via a positive feedback mechanism by acting at a hypothalamic cyclic center (Fig. 77–1).

The process of ovulation then occurs in an orderly manner. Following ovulation, serum levels of FSH, LH, and estradiol fall rapidly, but as the follicle is transformed into the corpus luteum, estradiol production again increases concomitantly with the pro-

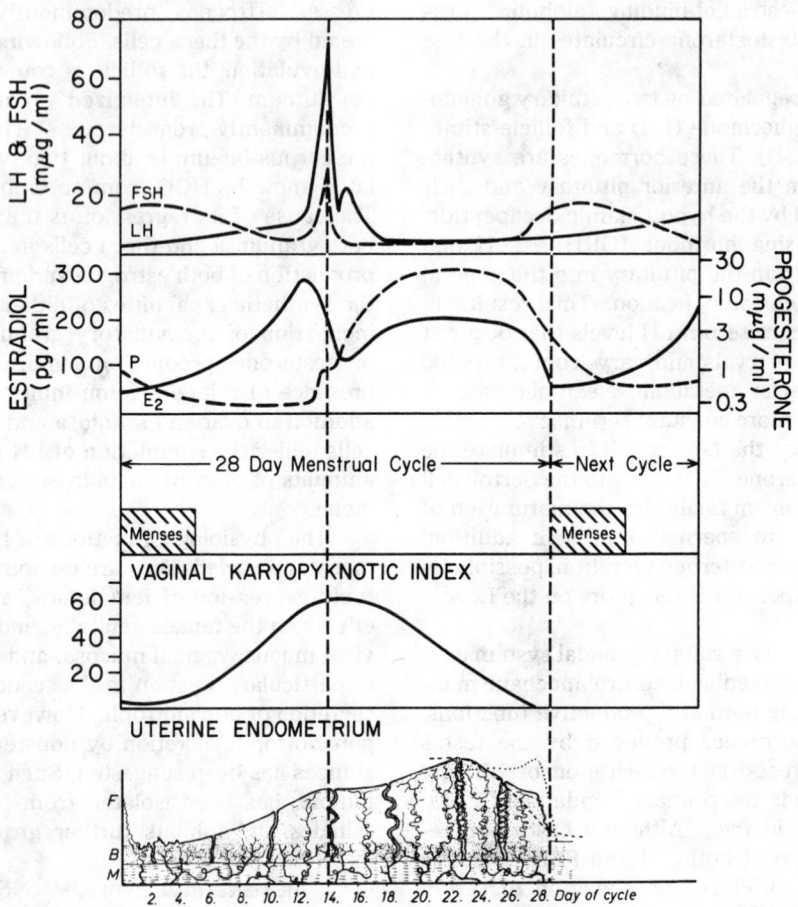

FIGURE 77-1. Changes in blood LH, FSH, progesterone (P), and estradiol (E₂) throughout a normal menstrual cycle. Changes in Vaginal Karyopyknotic Index and in uterine endometrium are also shown schematically. Reproduced from W. D. Odell.[294]

duction of luteal progesterone. These rise to a peak at midluteal phase and then steadily fall at the end of the phase. This fall in both blood estradiol and progesterone is the immediate cause of "withdrawal" bleeding from the endometrium—menstruation. Should conception occur, human chorionic gonadotropin production may be detectable in 8 to 10 days. The rapidly rising concentration of HCG prolongs the life of the corpus luteum and stimulates its steroid production.

Other hormonal factors, such as ovarian androgens, intrafollicular estrogen concentrations, and small amounts of progesterone from the developing follicle, may also participate in regulation of the menstrual cycle. A reciprocal relationship probably exists between the levels of serum prolactin and follicular progesterone. When PRL rises, ovarian progesterone production decreases.[293] Appropriate amounts of PRL may be necessary for normal ovarian function. Hyperprolactinemia, on the other hand, interferes with a normal secretion of gonadotropin and prolongs the follicular phase of the menstrual cycle.

PUBERTY AND ITS DISORDERS[272,298]

Puberty is a complex process of attainment of reproductive capacity accompanied by maturation of gonads, acceleration of somatic growth, and hormonal and psychological changes (see Chap. 152). The factors which control the initiation of puberty are uncertain. In prepubertal children, levels of gonadotropin and sex hormones are low. Toward the beginning of puberty, an increased secretion of LH and FSH occurs during sleep.[274] This event augments the secretion of testosterone in boys and estrogen in girls to promote pubertal changes. The onset of puberty is both genetically predetermined and environmentally influenced. The age of onset and rate of progression vary widely. The "average" pattern of sexual maturation is listed in Table 77–2.[308] Adolescent spurt occurs some 2 years earlier in girls than in boys. About 95 percent of girls experience their menarche between their 11th and 13th birthday. Boys usually reach full development between the 13th and 18th birthday.

Isosexual Precocious Puberty

The attainment of sexual maturity before the sixth birthday in girls and the eighth birthday in boys is abnormal. Sexual prematurity associated with a mature hypothalamic-pituitary-gonadal axis is defined as complete sexual precocity. A patient with this condition, if untreated, will reach complete sexual maturity except for their psychosexuality. Pathologically accelerated puberty where the reproductive system is only partially mature is defined as incomplete sexual precocity.

COMPLETE SEXUAL PRECOCITY.   In this condition, sexual development follows the usual pattern of normal puberty. In the majority of patients, the cause is unknown. Of identified causes, cerebral lesions (hamartoma of the hypothalamus, hydrocephalus of the third ventricle, pineal tumors) are most common. Damage in the posterior parts of the diencephalon by tumor compression probably abolishes sexual-inhibiting impulses and results in prematurity of the reproductive system. Other causes include polyostotic fibrous dysplasia (Albright syndrome) and untreated juvenile hypothyroidism.

Biochemically their serum and urine concentrations of FSH, LH, sex steroids, and 17-ketosteroids are consistent with their stage of maturity but exceed those for chronologic age. Approaches to differential diagnosis of precocious puberty are shown in Tables 77–3 (male) and 77–4 (female). The treatment of complete precocious puberty depends upon the cause. Removal of CNS tumors may be curative but they are usually located in areas such that they are not easily excisable. Prognosis is, therefore, usually poor. Drug therapy of "idiopathic" complete precocious puberty consists of the administration of a progestational agent to suppress gonadotropin secretion. Depo-medroxyprogesterone acetate, 100 to 300 mg, injected twice a month is effective.

ISOSEXUAL INCOMPLETE PRECOCIOUS PUBERTY.   In this condition sexual maturity is not accompanied by a mature hypothalamic-pituitary-gonadal axis. It is usually caused by humoral factors that are secreted without the regulation of the pituitary-gonadal system or extrinsic to this axis. In females, excess androgens from the adrenogenital syndrome cause heterosexual precocity but in males premature masculinization occurs. Despite advanced sexual maturation, testes are characteristically infantile unless hyperplastic aberrant adrenocortical tissue is located in the testes. Assay of urinary steroids makes the distinction of this condition possible.

TABLE 77–2
Stages of Adolescent Sexual Development

Stage	Mean Age +2 SD	Male	Mean Age +2 SD	Female
I		Preadolescent		Preadolescent
II	11.5 ±2	Growth of testes and scrotum; areolae darken; scanty pubic hair	11.5 ±2	Breast bud formation; areolar size increases; hips widen; scanty labial hair
III	13.5 ±2	Testes enlarge further; penis enlarges; pubic hair increases; facial hair appears and voice begins to deepen	12.5 ±2.2	Breast 2–11 cm, pubic hair increase, estrogenic vaginal mucosa
IV	14.5 ±2.2	Axillary hair appears; penis enlarges in circumference; first ejaculate often occurs in this stage	13 ±2	Menarche occurs; axillary hair appears
V	15.5 ±2	Maturation reaches adult stage	15 ±2.5	Maturation reaches adult stage

TABLE 77–3
Sexual Precocity in Males

	Testicular Size for Stage	Urine 17-KS for Stage	Serum Gonadotropin for Stage
Constitutional	N	N	N
Hypothalamic	N	N	N
Adrenal hyperplasia*	Small	H	L
Adrenal tumor†	Small	H	L
Testicular tumor†	Asymmetric	N or H	L
HCG-producing tumor	Enlarged	H	H
Exogenous androgen	Small	L or N	L

N = normal; H = high; L = low.

* Urine pregnanetriol is often elevated.
† Dehydroisoandrosterone is usually elevated.

TABLE 77–4
Sexual Precocity in Females

	Ovarian Size	Urine 17-KS for Stage	Estrogen Excretion for Stage	FSH and LH for Stage
Constitutional	Adolescent	N	N	N
Hypothalamic*	Adolescent	N	N	N
Adrenal tumor	Infantile	H	H	L
Ovarian tumor	Asymmetric	H	H	L
Ovarian cyst	Asymmetric	N	H	L
Albright syndrome†	Adolescent	N	N	N
Exogenous estrogen	Infantile	N	H	L

N = normal; H = high; L = low.

* CNS symptoms often present.
† See Chapter 75 for characteristic features.

Other causes of incomplete sexual precocity include hepatoblastoma, producing a LH-like substance, Leydig cell and other functioning testicular tumors producing testosterone in boys, and trophoblastic tumor producing HCG in boys and girls. Ovarian tumors, especially the granulosa-theca-cell tumors, produce excessive estrogen and may result in early sexual maturation in girls. Therapeutic use of gonadotropin and sex hormones may also accelerate sexual maturation.

Delayed Puberty
Puberty is medically considered delayed in boys when the first enlargement of the testes does not occur by 13.9 years, pubic hair is absent by 15.2 years, penile enlargement is lacking by 15.5 years, or peak height growth velocity is not reached by 15.2 years. The corresponding values for girls are first budding of breast by 13.4 years, appearance of pubic hair by 12.7 years, menarche by 15.6 years, and peak height growth velocity by 14.4 years. Wide normal variations must be considered in defining delayed puberty.

Causes of slow onset of puberty are many, but none of them occurs commonly. Disturbances of the hypothalamic-pituitary-gonadal axis, insufficiencies of gonads or thyroid, and diabetes mellitus are major endocrine causes. Others include chronic systemic disease, particularly malabsorption, chronic asthma, psychic deprivation and the like. By far the commonest cause is constitutional delay of puberty. Its diagnosis can be reasonably established from 1) showing lack of evidence for systemic illness; 2) a normal physical examination (except the presenting problem), including a normal upper-lower body segment ratio, arm span, and euosmia; 3) a normal nutritional status; 4) a normal radiograph of the sella turcica; 5) linear growth rate of at least 3.75 cm per year; 6) a reasonably normal psychic background; and 7) a family history of delayed puberty. Their bone age is usually delayed 1.5 to 4.0 years behind chronologic age.

Treatment beyond reassurance is rarely needed in any patients in whom the diagnosis of constitutional delayed puberty is certain. However, if the patient's anxieties and psychosocial factors are pressing, short-term testosterone or human chorionic gonadotropin may be given to boys. The preferred regimen is 100 mg depo-testosterone IM initially and then 200 mg in monthly intervals for 4 to 6 months, or 2000 units of HCG IM twice a week for 3 to 4 months. In girls, the hormonal therapy is highly conjectural. Low dose (0.02 mg) oral ethinylestradiol given daily for few months may initiate breast growth and menses in some patients.

GONADAL DISORDERS IN MEN

General Considerations

Men with gonadal dysfunction may present with a variety of primary complaints: infertility, impotence, symptoms of hypogonadism, e.g., lack of beard, gynecomastia, undescended testes, hypospadias, or scrotal masses. In taking a history detailed questions should be asked about subjective as well as objective changes. Specifically, information should be obtained on the following: congenital anomalies (hypospadias, undescended testes), age at onset of puberty, adequacy of the four elements of male sexual function (libido, erection, ejaculation, orgasm), exposure to physical agents that may alter testicular function (radiation, alkylating agents, high temperatures), ingestion of drugs (alcohol, estrogen, spironolactone, antihypertensive drugs), and fertility. In addition, a search should be made for endocrine diseases such as hypothyroidism or hypopituitarism, other organic derangement such as uremia, and significant psychic disturbances.

In the examination, the extent of virilism must be judged, the presence or absence of subclinical gynecomastia should be evaluated, and the size, consistency, and normality of the phallus, testes, and prostate should be documented. The sense of smell should be tested (see Table 77–6, Kallmann syndrome). If pituitary disease is suspected, careful attention must be given to the ocular examination to exclude papilledema, optic atrophy, and visual field defects.

If hypogonadism is under consideration, measurement of serum levels of LH, FSH, and testosterone can be helpful (Table 77–5). Episodic fluctuations of serum LH and testosterone levels cause the range of normal values to be broad. In patients with symptoms and signs of androgen deficiency who have low plasma testosterone levels, the measurement of serum LH and FSH can differentiate hypogonadotropic hypogonadism from primary testicular disease. If plasma gonadotropin levels are elevated, the patient has primary testicular disease. If plasma gonadotropin levels are low or borderline normal, a diagnosis of hypogonadotropic hypogonadism can be made. Occasionally if the results are equivocal, the clomiphene stimulation test may be useful. Clomiphene, which is a nonsteroidal compound with antiestrogenic activity, interferes with the negative feedback of testicular steroids on the pituitary and hypothalamus. Consequently in normal patients serum LH and FSH levels increase. Following the administration of 50 mg of clomiphene twice a day for seven days, the minimal normal response should be an increase over control levels of 30 percent for LH and 22 percent for FSH.[296] To determine whether the cause of hypogonadotropism is a defect in the hypothalamus or pituitary, treatment with GRH (100 μg intravenously) has been advised. Unfortunately, this test does not reliably distinguish between these two disorders, because in patients with hypothalamic deficiency, the pituitary must be exposed to GRH for prolonged periods of time before a normal adult response occurs.

Hypospadias and Cryptorchidism

Hypospadias occurs in 0.2 percent of newborn males. The disorder is classified according to the location of the urethral meatus: coronal, penile, penoscrotal, or perineal. Most cases are sporadic and are not associated with genetic or endocrine abnormalities. However, if both hypospadias and cryptorchidism are present, 25 to 50 percent of these patients will have a disorder of sexual differentiation.[299]

Cryptorchidism is the most common disorder of male sexual differentiation, occurring in 0.8 percent of men.[301] A careful examination is necessary to differentiate true cryptorchidism from the more common condition of retractile testes, which exist in approximately 6 percent of boys age 5 to 9 years. Although retractile testes have no long-term serious sequelae, patients with cryptorchidism have an increased incidence of infertility and malignant testicular tumors. Consequently, to assure the greatest potential for future fertility and to place the testis in a site where it is assessable for routine examination, placement of the testis into the scrotum is desirable at an early age (before 5 years). Unless the testis is ectopically placed in the subcutaneous pouch, a trial of therapy with chorionic gonadotropin is wise before orchiopexy.

TABLE 77–5
Serum Gonadotropin and Testosterone Levels in Male Hypogonadism*

	LH	FSH	Testosterone
Primary testicular failure	H	H	N or L
Gonadotropin deficiency	N or L	N or H	L
Isolated seminiferous tubular failure	N	H	N

* N = normal; H = high; L = low.

Hypogonadism

Hypogonadism in the male may present as delayed puberty, incomplete virilization at puberty, postpubertal gonadal failure, or merely infertility. Because androgens have a major influence on sexual desire in men, the presenting complaint may be loss of libido. A decrease in libido may indicate androgen deficiency arising from either hypogonadotropism or faulty testosterone secretion by the testes. This possibility can be tested easily by plasma testosterone and gonadotropin measurements. However, because the testosterone required to maintain libido is often less than the amount necessary for full stimulation of the prostate and seminal vesicles, if the loss of libido is on an endocrine basis, the patient should also complain of decreased semen volume. Conversely, if patients have normal libido and normal semen volume, it is highly unlikely that endocrine factors are responsible for the sexual dysfunction.

On physical examination, hypogonadism is suggested by feminine habitus (narrow shoulders, wide hips, fat chest), absence of beard and poor secondary sex hair growth, arm span greatly exceeding height (this is a normal racial characteristic of blacks), small phallus, atrophic testes (< 4 cm), small prostate, and gynecomastia. The broadest classification of hypogonadism is based on the absence or presence of pituitary gonadotropin (Table 77–6).[296] Evaluation of patients includes measurement of serum gonadotropins and testosterone (Table 77–5), karyotype analysis, and sperm count. In patients with gonadotropin deficiency, virilization and fertility may be induced by treatment with GRH or gonadotropins.

Infertility

About 15 percent of marriages in the United States are barren and, another 10 percent have fewer children than desired.[270] In these marriages, the husband is the significant factor in 30 percent of the cases and in another 20 percent he plays a contributing role. When a history is obtained from the male partner in a barren marriage, information should be obtained about the duration of infertility, fertility in other marriages of either the husband or wife, acquired or congenital disease that may lead to infertility (Table 77–7), technique and frequency of intercourse, and family history of infertility. The examination should evaluate the distribution of body hair, the presence of gynecomastia, the development of the scrotum and penis, the location of the urethral meatus, and the presence of normal vasa deferentia and epididymides. The size of each testis should be estimated with care. Because the seminiferous tubules account for more than 75 percent of the testicular mass, a reduction in

TABLE 77–6
Male Hypogonadism

Abnormalities in Hypothalamus-Pituitary Function

Kallmann syndrome	Anosmia or hyposmia, familial GRH deficiency
Fertile eunuch	Forme fruste of Kallmann syndrome
Panhypopituitarism	
Prader-Willi syndrome	Obesity, mental retardation, diabetes mellitus, neonatal muscle hypotonia
Laurence-Moon-Biedl syndrome	Retinitis pigmentosa, obesity, mental deficiency, polydactyly
Cerebellar ataxia (one form)	Nerve deafness, cerebellar ataxia
Hyperprolactinemia	Impotence, pituitary tumor

Abnormalities in Testicular Function

Klinefelter syndrome	XXY and mosaics
Sertoli-cell-only syndrome	Azoospermia, ↑ FSH
Congenital anorchia	Delayed puberty, phenotypic male, absent testes
Male Turner syndrome (Noonan syndrome)	46,XY Somatic stigmata of Turner syndrome
Postorchitis testicular failure	Bacterial or viral (mumps)
Myotonia dystrophica	Frontal baldness, cataracts
Idiopathic oligospermia	

testicular size (< 4 cm in length) indicates a severe deficiency in the spermatogenic function of the testis. Finally, with the patient standing in the upright position, the Valsalva maneuver should be used to test for varicocele.

The next step in the evaluation of the male partner is the semen analysis. This provides a semiquantitative estimation of the severity of the dysfunction. The findings are usually considered normal if the semen coagulates and then liquefies, the volume is 2 to 5 ml, the count is > 20 million/ml, more than 60 percent of the sperm are actively motile, and more than 60 percent have normal morphology. If no sperm are present, the term azoospermia is used; if sperm are present, but the count is < 20 million/ml, the patient is considered to have oligospermia. In the azoospermic male, the differential diagnosis includes hyalin-

┌───┐
TABLE 77–7
Causes of Male Infertility

Gonadotropin deficiency, e.g., Kallmann syndrome
Chromosomal disorders
   Klinefelter syndrome
Drugs
Physical agents
   Heat (cryptorchidism)
   Radiation
Sertoli-cell-only syndrome
Varicocele
Renal failure
Idiopathic oligospermia
└───┘

ization of the seminiferous tubules, the Sertoli-cell-only syndrome, gonadotropin deficiency, ductal obstruction, or maturation arrest. Plasma testosterone and serum LH and FSH measurements are helpful in separating these conditons. In patients with hyalinization of the seminiferous tubules, LH and FSH are elevated and plasma testosterone is low or borderline normal. Patients with the Sertoli-cell-only syndrome usually have normal LH and testosterone levels, but characteristically FSH levels are elevated. In gonadotropin deficiency, LH, FSH, and testosterone are low. In ductal obstruction or maturation arrest, all studies are normal. To differentiate between the last two disorders, a testicular biopsy is necessary. In oligospermic patients, if the history and examination are normal, further laboratory investigations are not likely to be useful in defining the etiology. These patients are usually classified in the large group termed idiopathic oligospermia.

Gynecomastia

The normal male breast contains scattered ducts with strands of collagenous tissue supporting them. Gynecomastia, or enlargement of the male breast, is associated histologically with either 1) an increase in ductal elements accompanied by lobule formation, or 2) proliferation of the stroma, often associated with ductal hyperplasia. When lobular formation is present, a source for excess estrogen or androgen is usually found, while stromal proliferation is generally present in conditions where serum testosterone and estrogen are normal. The enlargement may be unilateral (more frequently on the left than the right) or bilateral. It is usually asymptomatic, but sometimes the breasts are tender. The hormonal milieu that produces adolescent gynecomastia may be rapid changes in hormone levels and/or an inappropriate androgen-estrogen ratio. The breast is a target organ for both androgens

and estrogens. Normally, in men, androgen secretion exceeds estrogen production, and consequently the breast fails to enlarge. In conditions where there is a decrease in androgen production or an increase in estrogen secretion, however, gynecomastia occurs. In men with gynecomastia, the only common hormonal denominator that can be identified is a decreased ratio of androgen to estrogen.[304]

The diagnosis of gynecomastia is based on the palpation of subareolar glandular tissue while in the pseudogynecomastia of obesity there is no palpable subareolar glandular tissue so that pressing down on the nipple gives an impression of placing the finger into a hole. Pseudogynecomastia is far more common than gynecomastia.

Transient gynecomastia occurs in about 50 percent of normal males at puberty. This is also a time at which gynecomastia may occur in various disorders of gonadal function such as true hermaphroditism, the Klinefelter and Reifenstein syndromes, and primary hypogonadism. If the patient at puberty has a normal phallus and testes and is otherwise virilizing properly, no further evaluation is necessary. Gonadotropin and sex steroid levels are normal for the development stage in benign adolescent gynecomastia. These and other causes of gynecomastia are shown in Table 77–8.

Scrotal Masses

Based on the findings of a careful physical examination, the examiner should be able to classify a scrotal mass into one of four major categories: 1) mass in the spermatic cord; 2) fluid within the tunica vaginalis (hydrocele); 3) mass in the epididymis; 4) mass in the testis. Hydroceles are the most common cause of scrotal swelling. The mass usually obscures all normal anatomic landmarks within the scrotum and transillumination is usually necessary to confirm the diagnosis. The most common abnormality in the spermatic cord is a variocele. Retrograde filling of the internal spermatic vein and pampiniform plexus produces a "worm-like" mass in the scrotum that is present in the upright position and disappears in the recumbent position. Ninety percent of varicoceles are on the left side. The sudden development of a varicocele in an adult male should suggest inferior vena caval obstruction. Frequently, this is secondary to invasion of the renal vein by renal cell carcinoma.

As a rule, a mass in the epididymis is benign, whereas a mass in the testis is malignant until proven otherwise. The most common epididymal abnormalities include epididymal cyst, spermatocele, epididymitis (bacterial or tuberculosis), and rare benign tumors. The malignant germinal tumors of the testis, in

┌─────────────────────────────────────┐
TABLE 77-8
Gynecomastia

Adolescent Gynecomastia

Gynecomastia in Association with Gonadal Disorders
Klinefelter syndrome
Reifenstein syndrome
True hermaphrodite

Gynecomastia in Association with Systemic Disease
Cirrhosis of the liver
Ulcerative colitis
High spinal cord lesions
Hodgkin's disease
Bronchogenic carcinoma
Testicular tumors: Choriocarcinoma, mixed cell,
   interstitial cell adenomas
Adrenal tumors: Feminizing adrenal carcinoma
Refeeding following malnutrition
   tuberculosis, diabetes mellitus, cirrhosis
Thyroid dysfunction, hyperthyroidism, and
   hypothyroidism

Isolated Gynecomastia
Familial
Drug induced: Estrogens, testosterone, phenothiazine,
   meprobamate, reserpine, spironolactone, digitalis,
   marihuana
Mammary carcinoma
Renal failure on chronic hemodialysis
Idiopathic
Pseudogynecomastia of obesity
└─────────────────────────────────────┘

order of decreasing prognosis, are seminoma, teratocarcinoma, embryonal carcinoma, and choriocarcinoma. Although sonography may provide some help in evaluating testicular masses, most patients require surgical exploration. The prognosis of testicular tumors has improved with the development of new diagnostic and therapeutic techniques:[278] tumor markers (β-chain HCG and α-fetoprotein), accurate staging techniques (chest tomography, lymphangiography, CAT scanning), improved surgical procedures for lymphadenectomy, new chemotherapeutic agents, e.g., cis-platinum.

Treatment of Androgen Deficiency

In the treatment of hypogonadal patients with primary testicular failure, the intramuscular administration of the long-acting esters of testosterone (cypionate or enanthate) appears to be the most effective means for both induction of sexual maturation and maintenance of virilization. Unfortunately, testosterone, because of its rapid metabolism by the liver, is not very effective when taken orally. To reduce the rapid metabolic clearance of orally administered tes-

testosterone, a variety of 17α substitutions have been utilized, for example, 17α-methyltestosterone. However, the serum half-life of 17α-methyltestosterone is only 2.7 hours, and when administered in doses of 75 to 100 mg per day this agent is associated with cholestatic jaundice. In addition, peliosis hepatis or hepatic carcinoma may develop in patients receiving 17α-substituted androgens. Consequently, the injectable forms of testosterone appear to be the safest effective agents for the induction and maintenance of virilization. An obvious disadvantage of this form of therapy is the necessity for intramuscular administration. However, when testosterone enanthate is administered intramuscularly in a dose of 200 mg, blood levels of testosterone are maintained for 2 to 4 weeks. Treatment is usually initiated with bimonthly injections of 200 mg until the desired result is achieved. At this time, the interval between doses can often be left to the discretion of the patient, since these patients are sensitive to the subtle alterations in libido and aggressive behavior as the blood level of testosterone falls. Based on these subjective feelings, they can usually titrate themselves appropriately.

GONADAL DISORDERS OF THE FEMALE

THE AMENORRHEAS[271]

Absence of menstrual flow in females of childbearing age is amenorrhea. It is the most common symptom of female gonadal disorders. Since regular menstruation requires a normal hypothalamic-pituitary-ovarian axis, endometrium, and outflow tract, disruption at any level of this complex system may lead to abnormality of menstruation. Amenorrhea in a patient who has never menstruated after age 18 is defined as primary. In contrast, cessation of menstruation that occurs after the onset of spontaneous postpubertal menstruation is classified as secondary amenorrhea. Many conditions that usually cause primary amenorrhea may occasionally produce secondary amenorrhea.

Primary Amenorrhea

WITH POOR SECONDARY SEXUAL CHARACTERISTICS.
Patients with primary amenorrhea caused by ovarian failure have deficiency of sex hormone, and, therefore, show underdeveloped secondary sexual characteristics. Ovarian abnormalities are commonly caused by failure of the gonad to differentiate or to function normally. The Turner syndrome (Chap. 40) is the most common cause, accounting for 10 to 25 per-

cent of cases. The recognition of a typical patient—short stature, webbed neck, shield chest, cubitus valgus, and genital infantilism—is not difficult. Other gonadal abnormalities that cause primary amenorrhea include true hermaphroditism (Chap. 40), congenital absence of ovaries, hypoplastic, or polycystic ovaries. The treatment of these conditions is limited to the administration of estrogens beginning at the time of puberty to promote the development of secondary sexual characteristics.

Hypogonadotropic amenorrhea may occur with or without evidence of other tropic hormone deficiencies. Measurement of gonadotropin at puberty distinguishes this condition from primary ovarian failure. Craniopharyngioma, pituitary tumors, and chronic systemic illness inclusive of malnutrition, renal, cardiovascular, or hepatic disease and unusually delayed puberty must be considered in the patient with hypogonadotropic amenorrhea.

The clinical consequences of the congenital adrenogenital syndrome (Chap. 70) depends on the age of onset and the degree of exposure to androgens. Severe cases present as ambiguous genitalia in infants or early childhood. Mild cases are often not detected until puberty. They constitute 5 to 10 percent of all patients with primary amenorrhea. Because premature closure of epiphyses resulted from excessive androgens, patients are short, muscular, and masculine. Their hypothalamic-pituitary-ovarian axes are immature from chronic suppression by androgens. There are no clinical signs of cyclic function of the ovaries and the female sexual characteristics are poorly developed. Androgen-producing ovarian or adrenal tumors can produce features similar to that of the adrenogenital syndrome but they are extremely rare in puberty.

WITH NORMAL SECONDARY SEXUAL CHARACTERISTICS. Abnormality of outflow tract or endometrium, or dysgenesis of the müllerian ducts must be considered in girls with primary amenorrhea associated with normal secondary sexual characteristics. Gynecologic examination and laparoscopy are essential to diagnose such disorders including vaginal agenesis, imperforate hyman, uterine agnesis, or müllerian dysgenesis.

The testicular feminization syndrome is not a disorder of the female gonad, but the affected patients often present for the evaluation of primary amenorrhea. The diagnosis of this syndrome must be considered in a phenotypic female with proper secondary sexual development except for absent or scanty pubic axillary hair and a shallow blind-ending vagina, often with palpable inguinal masses (testes). A diagnostic approach to a patient with primary amenorrhea is listed in Table 77–9.

TABLE 77-9
Evaluation of Primary Amenorrhea*

Critical Questions	Special Tests	Comment
Are genital and pelvic organs normal?	Gynecologic evaluation	Ambiguous genitalia, imperforated hymen, agenesis of uterus or vagina can be excluded
Are features of Turner syndrome present?	Buccal smear, karyotype	
Are secondary sexual characteristics normal?	Use Table 77–1	If sexual development is poor, primary or secondary ovarian failure or adrenal hyperplasia is likely
Are pubic and axillary hair unusually scanty or absent?	Look for "inguinal mass," shallow-ending vagina; serum testosterone determination	Testicular feminization syndrome must be excluded
Is a pituitary tumor present?	Skull x-ray, visual field, assay of prolactin	See Figure 69–2
Is the patient hirsute or virilized?	Serum testosterone, androstenedione; urine 17-KS	To exclude adrenogenital syndrome, polycystic ovary, ovarian or adrenal tumor
Are CNS symptoms present?	Evaluation of hypothalamic region	
Is drug involved?		Tranquilizers, MAO inhibitor, drug addiction may cause amenorrhea
Is the patient under stress?		Stress-related amenorrhea is common in young girls

* If there is no apparent cause of amenorrhea, progesterone withdrawing test is carried out as outlined in Figure 77–2.

Secondary Amenorrhea[283] (Table 77–10)

Two important rules for the evaluation of secondary amenorrhea are 1) in women of childbearing age, the commonest cause of secondary amenorrhea is pregnancy; and 2) when conception is not responsible for amenorrhea, extensive evaluation is not indicated until the patient has had amenorrhea for at least 8 to 10 months. Exclusion or establishment of early pregnancy can be accomplished by the measurement of urinary chorionic gonadotropin. Typically, it reaches a level detectable by immunoassay 35 to 40 days after the last menstrual period.

HYPOTHALAMUS-PITUITARY DYSFUNCTION. Pituitary tumor, regardless of its functional capacity, may cause amenorrhea (Chap. 70). Galactorrhea is frequently seen in these patients. In fact amenorrhea, galactorrhea, and hyperprolactinemia may proceed detectable parapituitary lesions. Hyperprolactinemia leads to menstrual abnormalities by interfering with both hypothalamic and ovarian function, including that of the corpus luteum. As many as 30 percent of women complaining of amenorrhea and galactorrhea have pituitary tumor.

TABLE 77–10
Causes of Secondary Amenorrhea

I. **Physiologic**
   Pregnancy
   Breast feeding
   Spontaneous menopause

II. **Pathologic**
   A. Hypothalamic-pituitary dysfunction
      1. Tumors
      2. Congenital absence of gonadotropins
      3. Functional aberration:
         Acute and chronic systemic illness
         Nutritional (starvation, anorexia nervosa)
         Nongonadal endocrinopathies
         Psychogenic stress
         Pharmacologic causes (antifertility agents)
         Hyperprolactinemia of any causes
         Continuous estrus (polycystic ovary syndrome)
   B. Primary ovarian disorders
      1. Congenital dysgenesis
      2. Acquired:
         Autoimmune destruction
         Surgical oophorectomy
         Radiation
         Infection
      3. Functioning ovarian tumors (feminizing or masculinizing)
   C. Uterine disorder
      1. Hysterectomy
      2. Asherman syndrome
      3. Endometrial destruction (tuberculosis, radiation)

Acute and chronic systemic illness, notably tuberculosis, renal failure, and liver disease often cause amenorrhea by interfering with function of CNS-pituitary-ovarian axis. Malnutrition from starvation or anorexia nervosa causes profound weight loss. There is a critical body weight below which menstruation does not occur.

Amenorrhea is known to occur in nongonadal endocrinopathies. About 50 percent of patients with juvenile diabetes mellitus have menstrual abnormalities. Dysfunction of thyroid or adrenal is also often associated with amenorrhea. Usually menstruations are restored by controlling the underlying disease. Amenorrhea may occur in stressed young women who have no demonstrable organic lesions. It probably arises from functional disturbances in the hypothalamus, and usually is transient. Certain tranquilizers, such as phenothiazines and reserpine, may inhibit menses and ovulation.

About one percent of women lose their menstrual function after discontinuation of oral contraceptives. Amenorrhea may persist for extended period, but a quarter of them recover spontaneously without intervention. Others need pharmacologic induction, most commonly with clomiphene.

Polycystic ovarian disease is characterized by hirsutism, polycystic ovaries, amenorrhea, and obesity. The basic derangement seems to be an abnormal hypothalamic-pituitary-ovarian axis exhibited by high levels of serum LH and sex steroids, but low or normal FSH.

PRIMARY OVARIAN DISORDERS. Amenorrhea caused by primary ovarian failure is characterized by evidence of hypoestrogenism (atrophy of the breasts and vaginal epithelium and presence of noncornified vaginal epithelium) accompanied by high levels of serum gonadotropins. Normally, the ovaries cease to function at about age 45 to 50. Causes of premature ovarian failure include autoimmune destruction, surgical removal, irradiation, antimetabolite chemotherapy, and rarely infection. The management of ovarian failure is limited to relief of symptoms by administration of estrogen.

Functioning ovarian tumors produce excess sex steroid to suppress gonadotropin and produce amenorrhea. Granulosa-theca-cell tumors tend to produce estrogen, whereas arrhenoblastomas, gonadoblastomas, and adrenal rest tumors cause virilization and amenorrhea by producing excess androgen. These tumors are rare, but are often amenable to surgical resection.

UTERINE DISORDER. With the increasing use of suction curettage for the termination of unwanted pregnancies, intrauterine fibrosis or synechiae (Asherman syndrome) has become common. Vigorous curettage results in total loss of functioning endometrial glands and fibrous tissue obliterates the uterine cavity. In spite of normal ovarian function, no menstruation occurs. The endometrial cavity of women suffering from the Asherman syndrome has a characteristic hysterogram. Treatment consists of repeated dilation and curettage to lyse adhesions, administration of steroids (5 mg Premarin daily for 21 days, followed by 10 mg medroxyprogesterone for 5 days for three cycles) to stimulate the endometrium, and insertion of an intrauterine device to keep the uterine walls separated. Finally, endometrium may be destroyed by tuberculous infection or radiation.

DIAGNOSIS. Pregnancy must be excluded by measurement of chorionic gonadotropin in urine. Assay of serum prolactin is useful when galactorrhea is present. Further evaluation of secondary amenorrhea of inapparent cause may be carried out according to Figure 77–2. The occurrence of uterine bleeding following the oral administration of 10 mg medroxyprogesterone daily for 5 days or 100 mg of progesterone in oil indicates that 1) the outflow tract is normal, 2) the endometrium is normal and has been adequately stimulated by endogenous estrogen, and 3) estrogen production is normal, which indirectly implies a normal hypothalamic-pituitary-ovarian axis. The conclusion is that lack of progesterone most likely resulted from anovulation.

Failure to bleed in the progesterone withdrawal test indicates inadequate estrogen production, impaired pituitary-ovarian axis, an endometrial defect, or obstruction of the outflow tract.

Further challenge with initial administration of estrogen to induce endometrial proliferation followed by a progesterone withdrawal bleeding test is useful to distinguish an endometrial defect from one of the hypothalamic-pituitary-ovarian axis. If no bleeding occurs, the cause of amenorrhea is endometrial failure. When bleeding occurs, the implication is that hormonal deficiency resulted from a defect along the hypothalamic-pituitary-ovarian axis. Information on serum levels of gonadotropin is obtained to identify the defective site. To differentiate hypothalamic failure from pituitary deficiency is difficult, however.

TREATMENT. Correct diagnosis of the cause for secondary amenorrhea is the key to the appropriate treatment. The purpose of treatment and the patient's wishes should also be considered in selecting the mode of therapy. If the amenorrhea has no apparent

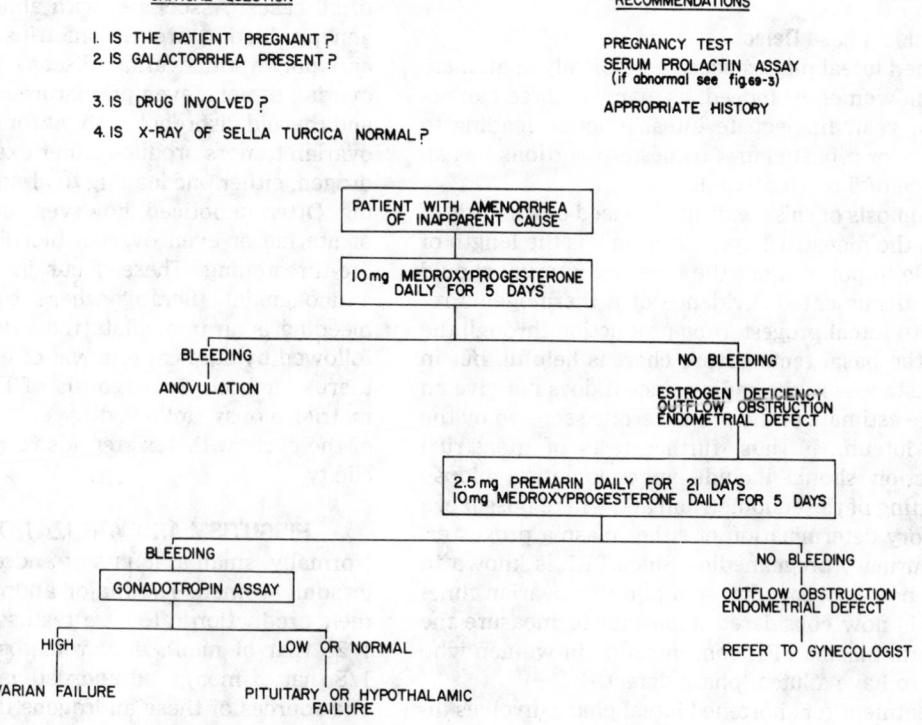

CRITICAL QUESTION

1. IS THE PATIENT PREGNANT?
2. IS GALACTORRHEA PRESENT?

3. IS DRUG INVOLVED?
4. IS X-RAY OF SELLA TURCICA NORMAL?

RECOMMENDATIONS

PREGNANCY TEST
SERUM PROLACTIN ASSAY
(if abnormal see fig.69-3)
APPROPRIATE HISTORY

PATIENT WITH AMENORRHEA
OF INAPPARENT CAUSE

10 mg MEDROXYPROGESTERONE
DAILY FOR 5 DAYS

BLEEDING — ANOVULATION

NO BLEEDING
ESTROGEN DEFICIENCY
OUTFLOW OBSTRUCTION
ENDOMETRIAL DEFECT

2.5 mg PREMARIN DAILY FOR 21 DAYS
10mg MEDROXYPROGESTERONE DAILY FOR 5 DAYS

BLEEDING

GONADOTROPIN ASSAY

NO BLEEDING
OUTFLOW OBSTRUCTION
ENDOMETRIAL DEFECT
REFER TO GYNECOLOGIST

HIGH — OVARIAN FAILURE

LOW OR NORMAL — PITUITARY OR HYPOTHALAMIC FAILURE

FIGURE 77–2. Evaluation of secondary amenorrhea.

cause, reassurance and follow-up are all that is needed. The management of amenorrhea secondary to pituitary tumor is described in Chapter 69. Amenorrhea in a patient with hyperprolactinemia can be treated with a dopamine agonist, bromocriptine. The usual dosage is 2.5 mg 3 or 4 times a day administered orally. It is, however, not easy to exclude the existence of microadenoma of the pituitary in a patient with elevation of prolactin. Restoration of fertility and subsequent pregnancy may stimulate growth of tumor. Patients should be warned of this possibility and mechanical contraception is advised in cases with particularly high prolactin levels. When restoration of fertility is the aim of the treatment in patients with hypogonadotropic amenorrhea, ovulation can be induced by gonadotropins, provided that a pituitary tumor is excluded.

When the patient is producing sufficient estrogen but is anovulatory, spontaneous menstruation and ovulation may be restored by giving 10 mg medroxyprogesterone orally for 5 days every 6 weeks.

In young patients with premature ovarian failure or menopausal women with symptoms of estrogen deficiency, 0.6 to 1.2 mg of conjugated estrogen (Premarin) is administered daily. To give a fully physiologic replacement with menstrual bleeding, 10 mg medroxyprogesterone is added daily on days 20 to 24 of monthly period.

Luteal Phase Defect

Shortened luteal phases occur periodically in all menstruating women.[307] Indeed, as many as three can occur in a year. Inadequate luteal function leading to infertility or repeated first trimester abortions has an incidence of 5 to 10 percent.

Diagnosis of this condition is based on analysis of data on the menstrual cycle. Not only is the length of the cycle important, but the bleeding interval should also be documented. Evidence of a thermogenic response to luteal progesterone production through the use of the basal temperature chart is helpful, but in some instances is misleading since it does not give an accurate estimate of the progesterone secreted by the corpus luteum.[284] Thus, further tests of menstrual dysfunction should include an endometrial biopsy with dating of the endometrium and where possible, a laboratory determination of either plasma progesterone or urinary pregnanediol. Since PRL is known to modify not only gonadotropin but also ovarian function, it is now considered important to measure the peripheral plasma PRL concentration in women who appear to have a luteal phase defect.[303]

Treatment for shortened luteal phase involves increasing luteal progesterone production by either lowering plasma PRL or by stimulating a more appropriate follicular maturation through the use of minute amounts of estrogen during the first 14 days of the follicular phase of the menstrual cycle. The application of topical progesterone via vaginal suppositories is successful in the treatment of this condition.[284]

A rare, yet easily recognized abnormality of ovarian function, which is the exact opposite of luteal phase defect, is that of the persistent corpus luteum. Ovarian progesterone production persists more than 16 days and menstruation fails to occur, yet endometrial biopsy indicates the patient has adequate amounts of progesterone. Clinicians should exclude pregnancy but also biopsy the endometrium.

Dysfunctional Uterine Bleeding (DUB)

While amenorrhea accounts for 50 percent of all infertility investigations, dysfunctional uterine bleeding (DUB) is also a frequent disorder related to endocrine abnormality. In most cases, DUB must be diagnosed by endometrial curettage, especially in women in the perimenopausal age group, to rule out abnormal endometrial proliferation which is related to the subsequent development of endometrial carcinoma. Pituitary-ovarian dysfunction can also lead to excessive estrogen production and breakthrough bleeding of the endometrium will occur. This is most common in women who fail to ovulate, and represents 70 percent of all cases. Associated with abnormally high estrogen production are endometriosis, uterine fibroids, and polycystic ovarian disease (PCO), functioning ovarian tumors, even premature menopause. Adrenal and thyroid disorders account for others. Functioning ovarian tumors produce either excess estrogen or androgen, either one leading to abnormal uterine bleeding. Often unnoticed, however, are iatrogenic causes of uterine or even ovarian bleeding which could be life-threatening. These occur in women on chronic anticoagulant therapy where the management of bleeding is an immediate reduction in anticoagulant followed by surgical removal of either the ovary, the uterus, or both.[302] Diagnosis of DUB includes endometrial biopsy, followed by endocrine manipulation of the cycle with sex steroids to restore pituitary cyclicity.

HIRSUTISM AND VIRILIZATION

Normally, small amounts of androgens are produced in adult women. The major androgenic steroids and their production rates are testosterone (300 μg/day; 1/25 that of men), dihydrotestosterone (60 μg/day; 1/8 that of men), and androstenediol (2000 μg/day). The sources of these androgens in women are three: 25 percent each directly from ovary and adrenal gland and the remaining 50 percent from the peripheral conversion of prehormones Δ^4-androstenedione, dihydroepiandrosterone (DHEA) and Δ^5-androstenediol, products of both adrenals and ovaries.[287]

When androgen is excessive in women, defeminization (hirsutism, amenorrhea, decreased breast size, and loss of female body contour) first occurs followed by virilization (clitoral hypertrophy, deepening of the voice, and temporal balding). The triad of obesity, mild hirsutism, and menstrual abnormalities is commonly encountered in practice, but endocrinopathy is rarely found in them. Virilization, however, always reflects a serious underlying disease, usually tumor of adrenal or ovary.

Major causes of hirsutism and virilization are listed in Table 77–11. Hirsutism caused by the disorders of the hypothalamus or pituitary are usually mild. Clinical manifestations are predominantly those of the underlying disorders. Excessive hair growth may occur in long-standing hyperprolactinemic amenorrhea. Prolactin appears to stimulate the adrenal to produce dehydroepiandrosterone sulfate

---

TABLE 77–11
Etiology of Hirsutism and Virilization

I. **Central**
  A. Hypothalamic
    1. Postencephalitis
    2. Hyperostosis frontalis interna
    3. Polycystic ovarian disease
    4. Obesity-stress syndrome
  B. Pituitary
    1. Prolactin secreting adenoma
    2. Acromegaly
    3. Achard-Thiers syndrome ("hairy diabetic")
    4. Basophil adenoma (Cushing syndrome)

II. **Adrenal Disease**
  A. Adrenogenital syndrome
  B. Cushing syndrome

III. **Ovarian Disease**
  A. Ovarian tumor
    1. Hilar cell adenoma
    2. Luteoma
    3. Arrhenoblastoma
    4. Adrenal rest tumor
  B. Polycystic ovarian disease

IV. **Iatrogenic**
    1. Phenytoin
    2. Progestins, androgens
    3. Vitamin-hormonal compounds (anabolic steroids)

V. **Constitutional Factors**
  A. Familial
  B. Menopausal
  C. Idiopathic

(DHEAS), a weak androgen. DHEAS in sufficiently high concentrations will stimulate hair growth.[275,300]

Adrenal Androgen Excess

Adult onset adrenal virilism may result from a mild 21-or 11-β hydroxylase deficiency (Chap. 70) which becomes evident after puberty. Although these conditions are rare, they must be considered since they are amenable to glucocorticoid therapy. Cushing syndrome also causes hirsutism (Chap. 70). Characteristically hyperandrogenemia of adrenal origin is associated with marked elevation in urinary 17-ketosteroid that is usually suppressible with exogenous glucocorticoid except when it is caused by functioning adrenal tumor.

Ovarian Androgen Excess

Androgen-secreting ovarian tumors are rare. They usually secrete large amounts of testosterone and cause not only hirsutism but virilization. The commonest types are arrhenoblastoma and hilus cell tumor. Despite markedly elevated serum testosterone, urinary 17-ketosteroid excretion is typically normal or only moderately elevated. Localization of tumor is usually accomplished by ultrasonography, laparoscopy, or ovarian vein catheterization.

Polycystic ovarian disease (PCO) is a common disorder that causes hirsutism and in some instances virilization. A disorder of young women, PCO is characterized clinically by hirsutism, infertility, amenorrhea, obesity, and often palpably enlarged polycystic ovaries. It is uncertain whether the basic defect is primarily in ovarian steroidogenesis or whether the hypothalamus initiates abnormal gonadotropin release which in turn leads to cystic changes in the ovary and abnormal steroidogenesis. In most patients, serum LH levels are inappropriately elevated, but FSH is low or normal.[300] In response to this change, ovarian androgen and estrogen production is usually increased.

Laparoscopy permits early diagnosis of PCO. The ovaries are usually enlarged, multilobular, and sclerocystic with a pearl-grey avascular surface. Biopsy demonstrates numerous primordial follicles in various stages of arrested maturation. PCO women over the age of 35 years should have endometrial biopsies to insure that abnormal changes in the endometrium have not occurred as a result of unopposed estrogen stimulation to their uterus. Treatment of polycystic ovarian disease varies. Wedge resection of the ovary was thought to be effective therapy by lowering production of sex steroids and leading to decreased plasma testosterone. Thus treatment is often associated with infertility, related to postoperative surgical adhesions to the operative site, especially to the fallopian tubes. Moreover, restoration of normal ovarian function in PCO has been achieved merely by laparotomy. For these reasons, wedge resection of the ovary for PCO has been largely abandoned.[310] PCO can be treated effectively with clomiphene citrate, a nonsteroidal compound generically related to diethylstilbestrol (DES). It acts by binding to the estrogen receptor in hypothalamic sites, and brings about augmented secretion of GRH.[314] When clomiphene citrate is administered in PCO, plasma FSH and LH gradually rise. As clomiphene citrate is removed from the system, circulating estrogen replaces it, stimulating a gonadotropic surge which induces ovulation in 70 percent of cases.[289]

Mixed Adrenal and Ovarian Androgen Excess

In nearly 30 percent of hirsute women, data suggest that both the adrenal and ovary are responsible for excessive androgen production.[288] The same defect may exist in both organs, or a primary defect in one may affect the function of the other.

Diagnosis

Diagnostic approaches for hirsute women include tests 1) to establish that excess androgen is present, 2) to identify the origin of excess androgens by hormonal studies and pharmacologic manipulations, and 3) anatomic localization of the lesion.

Excessive production of androgens can be inferred by showing an elevated plasma level of testosterone and/or androstenedione. In some instances, elevation of these androgens is obscured by a low level of androgen-binding proteins, a consequence of excessive androgens. Free (unbound) testosterone, although difficult to measure, is a superior index. If the levels of plasma androgens are normal, hirsutism may be caused by increased sensitivity of hair follicles to androgens.

Once it is established that hirsutism is associated with abnormally high androgens, further studies include measurements of urinary free cortisol excretion to exclude Cushing syndrome, and assays of urinary 17-ketosteroids and pregnanetriol. Markedly elevated urinary 17-KS usually suggests that the excessive androgens come from the adrenals. In contrast, it is often normal in androgen-producing ovarian tumors. Congenital adrenal hyperplasia is likely when pregnanetriol is increased in the urine.

The low dose dexamethasone suppression test also provides some information regarding the origin of excess androgens. In the absence of Cushing syndrome, resistance of urine 17-KS and plasma testosterone to dexamethasone suppression makes the ovary the likely site of abnormal androgen production. Suppression of these substances does not necessarily indicate the adrenal is at fault, since similar changes occur in some patients with PCO syndrome. Finally, ovarian and adrenal vein catheterization studies have been employed to identify the lesion but it is not uniformly useful.[288,311]

Anatomic localization of the lesion can be accomplished by ultrasonography, computerized tomography, venography, or laparoscopy.

Treatment

Tumors of adrenal or ovary are usually resectable. Cushing syndrome is managed as outlined in Chapter 70. Congenital adrenal hyperplasia is responsive to glucocorticoids.

The management of hirsutism in the remaining group (which includes most patients) is difficult. From the beginning, the patient should be informed of the limitations of treatment, so she can accept a realistic goal. Since most patients have excessive androgen production from both ovary and adrenal, concomitant use of glucocorticoids (usually 5 mg of prednisone) and estrogens (0.6 to 1.2 mg of Premarin) is recommended. In most cases, however, hormonal therapy does not produce appreciable changes in the excessive hair growth. Local cosmetic removal by electrolysis is usually needed in severe cases. The value of vigorous weight reduction for obese patients should be stressed. In patients with PCO syndrome, administration of 50 mg clomiphene citrate daily for 5 days in cyclic manner often restores menstruation, ovulation, and some reduction of androgen production.

Cyproterone, an antiandrogenic, competes with biologically active androgens for receptor proteins to block their effects.[282] This drug is, however, not yet available for routine use in the treatment of hirsutism.

REFERENCES

General References

1. Bondy, P.K. and Rosenberg, L.E., Duncan's Disease of Metabolism-Endocrinology, 7th ed. Philadelphia, Saunders, Co. 1974.
2. Cavalieri, R.R. and Rapoport, B. Impaired peripheral conversion of thyroxine to triiodothyronine. Annu. Rev. Med., 28:57, 1977.
3. Chan, L. and O'Malley, B.W., Steriod hormone action: recent advances. Ann. Intern. Med., 89:694, 1978.

4. Chayen, J. General introduction to cytochemical hormone bioassay. Clin. Endocrinol., 3:303, 1974.

5. Jacobs, S. and Cuatrecasas, P. Current concepts: cell receptors in disease. N. Engl. J. Med., 297:1383, 1977.

6. Kahn, C.R., Megyesi, K., Bar, R.S., et al. Receptors for peptide hormones. Ann. Intern. Med., 86:205, 1977.

7. Stanbury, J.B. Wyngaarden, J.B., and Frederickson, D. S. (eds.). The Metabolic Basis of Inherited Disease, 4th ed. New York, McGraw-Hill, 1978.

8. Weitzman, E.D. Circadian rhythms and episodic hormone secretion in man. Annu. Rev. Med., 27:225, 1976.

9. Werk, E.E., Jr., MacGee, J., and Sholiton, L.J., Effects of diphenylhydantoin on cortisol metabolism in man. J. Clin. Invest., 43:1824, 1964.

10. William, R.H. (ed.). Textbook of Endocrinology, 5th ed., Philadelphia, Saunders, 1974.

The Hypothalamus–Pituitary Axis

11. Carter, J.N., Tyson, J.E., Tolis, G., et al. Prolactin-secreting tumors and hypogonadism in 22 men. N. Engl. J. Med., 299:847, 1978.

12. Demura, R., Kubo, O., Demura, H., et al. FSH and LH secreting pituitary adenoma. J. Clin. Endocrinol. Metab., 45:653, 1977.

13. Edwards, C.R.W. Vasopressin and oxytocin in health and disease. Clin. Endocrinol. Metab., 6:223, 1977.

14. Edwards, C.R.W. and Besser, G.M. Disease of the hypothalamus and pituitary gland. Clin. Endocrinol. Metab., 3:495, 1974.

15. Forrest, J.N., Jr., Cox, M., Hong, C., et al. Demeclocycline versus lithium for inappropriate secretion of antidiuretic hormone. N. Engl. J. Med., 298:173, 1978.

16. Goldfine, I.D. Medical treatment of acromegaly. Annu. Rev. Med., 29:407, 1978.

17. Gomez-Pan, A. and Hall, R. Somatostatin. Clin. Endocrinol. Metab., 6:181, 1977.

18. Hankinson, J. Pituitary and Parapituitary Tumors. Philadelphia, Saunders, 1976.

19. Jordan, R.M., Kendall, J.W., Seaich, J.L., et al. Cerebral fluid hormone concentration in the evaluation of pituitary tumors. Ann. Intern. Med., 85:49, 1976.

20. Kjellberg, R.N. and Kliman, B. Bragg-peak proton treatment for pituitary related conditions. Proc. R. Soc. Med., 67:32, 1974.

21. Kleinberg, D.L., Noel, G.L., and Frantz, A.G. Galactorrhea: a study of 235 cases, including 48 with pituitary tumor. N. Engl. J. Med., 296:589, 1977.

22. Kohler, P.O. and Ross, G.T. (eds.). Diagnosis and Treatment of Pituitary Tumors. New York, Elsevier, 1973.

23. Krieger, D.T., Amorosa, L., and Linick, F. Cyproheptadine-induced remission of Cushing's disease. N. Engl. J. Med., 293:893, 1975.

24. Krieger, D.T. and Ganong, W.F. (eds.). ACTH and related peptides: structure, regulation, and actions. Ann. N.Y. Acad. Sci., 297:1, 1977.

25. Lin, T. and Tucci, J.R. Provocative tests of growth hormone release. Ann. Intern. Med., 80:464, 1974.

26. Lips, C.J.M. and Van der Sluys, J. Common precursor molecules as origin for the ectopic-hormone-producing-tumor syndrome. Lancet, 1:16, 1978.

27. Lloyd, M.H. and Belchetz, P.E. Clinical features and management of pituitary apoplexy. Postgrad. Med. J., 53:82, 1977.

28. Mains, R., Eipper, B., and Ling, N. Common precursor to corticotropins and endorphins. Proc. Natl. Acad. Sci. USA, 74:3014, 1977.

29. Mecklenburg, R.S., Loriaux, D.L., Thompson, R.H., et al. Hypothalamic dysfunction in patients with anorexia nervosa. Medicine, 53:147, 1974.

30. Merimee, T.J. Isolated growth hormone deficiency and related disorders. Annu. Rev. Med., 25:137, 1974.

31. Miller, M., Dalakos, T., Moses, A.M., et al. Recognition of partial defects in antidiuretic hormone secretion. Ann. Intern. Med., 73:721, 1970.

32. Moses, A.M., Miller, M., and Streeten, D.H.P. Pathophysiology and pharmacologic alterations in the release and action of ADH. Metabolism, 25:697, 1976.

33. Muller, E.E. Nervous control of growth hormone secretion. Neuroendocrinology, 11:338, 1973.

34. Pickett, J.E.B., III, Layzer, R.B., Levine, S.B. et al. Neuromuscular complications of acromegaly. Neurology, 25:638, 1975.

35. Riggs, R.L., Randall, R.V., Wahner, H.W., et al. The nature of the metabolic bone disorders in acromegaly. J. Clin. Endocrinol. Metab., 34:911, 1972.

36. Robertson, G.L. Vasopressin in osmotic regulation in man. Annu. Rev. Med., 25:315, 1974.

37. Schimke, N. Multiple endocrine adenomatosis syndromes. Adv. Intern. Med., 21:249, 1976.

38. Spanos, E., Colston, K.W., Evans, I.M.S., et al. Effect of prolactin on Vitamin D metabolism. Mol. Cell. Endocrinol., 5:163, 1976.

39. Thorner, M.O. Prolactin. Clin. Endocrinol. Metab., 6:201, 1977.

40. Carter, J.N., Tyson, J.E., Tolis, G., et al. Prolactin-secreting tumors and hypogonadism in 22 men. N. Engl. J. Med. 299:847, 1978.

41. Tyrrell, J.B. Brooks, R.M., Fitzgerald, P.A., et al. Cushing's disease: selective transsphenoidal resection of pituitary microadenomas. N. Engl. J. Med., 298:753, 1978.

42. Valper, R. The role of autoimmunity in hypoendocrine and hyperendocrine function. Ann. Intern. Med., 87:86, 1977.

43. Van Wyk, J.J. and Underwood, L.E. Relation between growth hormone and somatomedin. Annu. Rev. Med., 26:427, 1975.

44. Vigersky, R.A., Loriaux, D.L., Anderson, A.E., et al. Delayed pituitary hormone response to LH releasing factor (LRF) and TSH releasing factor (TRF) in patients with anorexia nervosa and with secondary amenorrhea associated with simple weight loss. J. Clin. Endocrinol. Metab., 43:893, 1976.

45. Yamada, T., Tsukui, T., Ikeziri, K., et al. Volume of sella turcica in normal subjects and in patients with primary hypothyroidism and hyperthyroidism. J. Clin. Endocrinol. Metab., 42:817, 1976.

Disorders of The Adrenal Glands

46. Amador, E. Adrenal hemorrhage during anticoagulant therapy. Ann. Intern. Med., 63:559, 1965.

47. Baer, L., Sommers, S.C., Lawrence R.K., Newton, M.A., and Laragh, J.H. Pseudoprimary aldosteronism.

An entity distinct from true primary aldosteronism. Circ. Res., 26–27:1, 1970.

48. Biglieri, E.G., Schambelan, M., Brust, N., Chang, B., and Hogan, M. Plasma aldosterone concentration: further characterization of aldosterone producing adenomas. Circ. Res., 34, (Suppl). (1), 23:175, 1974.

49. ———, Schambelan, M., Slaton, P.E., and Stockigt, J.R. The intercurrent hypertension of primary aldosteronism. Circ. Res. 26–27:I, 1970.

50. ———, Slaton, P.E., Schambelan M., and Kronfield, S.J. Hypermineralocorticoidism. Am. J. Med., 45:170, 1968.

51. Bongiovanni, A.M. and Root, A.W. The adrenogenital syndrome. N. Engl. J. Med., 268:1283, 1963.

52. Cannon, P.J., Ames, R.P., and Laragh, J.H. Relation between potassium balance and aldosterone secretion in normal subjects and in patients with hypertensive or renal tubular disease. J. Clin. Invest., 45:865, 1966.

53. Conn, J.W., Knopf, R.F., and Nesbitt, R.M. Clinical characteristics of primary aldosteronism from an analysis of 145 cases. Am. J. Surg., 107:159, 1974.

54. ———, Rovner, D.R., Cohen, E.L., Bookstein, J., Cerny, J., and Lucas, C.P. Preoperative diagnosis of primary aldosteronism. Arch. Int. Med., 123:113, 1969.

55. Cooke, C.R., Brown, T.C., Zacherle, B.J., and Walker, W.G. The effect of altered sodium concentration in the distal nephron segments on renin release. J. Clin. Invest., 49:1630, 1970.

56. Engelman, K. Pheochromocytoma. In Landsberg, L. (ed.), Clinics in Endocrinology and Metabolism-Catecholamines, Vol. 6. Philadelphia, Saunders, 1977, p. 767.

57. Ferriss, J.B., Brown, J.J., Fraser, R., Kay, A.W., Neville, A.M., O'Muircheataigh, I.G., Robertson, J.I.S., Symington, T., and Lever, A.F. Hypertension with aldosterone excess and low plasma renin preoperative distinction between patients with and without adrenocortical tumor. Lancet, 2:995, 1970.

58. Gifford, R.W., Kvale, W.F., Maher, F.T., Roth, G.M., and Priestley, J.T. Clinical features, diagnosis and treatment of pheochromocytoma. A review of 76 cases. Mayo Clin. Proc., 39:281, 1964.

59. Guthrie, G.P. Jr., Genest, J., Nowaczynski, W., Boucher, R., and Kuchel, O. Dissociation of plasma renin activity and aldosterone in essential hypertension. J. Clin. Endocrinol. Metab., 43:446, 1976.

60. Hsu, T.H. and Bledsoe, T. Measurement of urinary free corticoids by competitive protein binding radioassay in hypoadrenal states. J. Clin. Endocrinol. Metab., 30:443, 1970.

61. Komanicky, R., Spark, R.F., and Melby, J.C. Treatment of Cushing's syndrome with Trilostane (WIN 24,540), and inhibitor of adrenal steroid biosynthesis. J. Clin. Endocrinol. Metab., 47:1042, 1978.

62. Korth-Schutz, S., Virois, R., Soenger, P., Chow, D.M., Levine, L.S., and New, M.I. Serum androgens as a continuing index of adequacy of treatment of congenital adrenal hyperplasia. J. Clin. Endocrinol. Metab., 46:452, 1978.

63. Krieger, D.T., Amorosa, L., and Linick, F. Cyproheptadine-induced remission of Cushing's disease. N. Engl. J. Med., 293:893, 1975.

64. Krieger, D.T. and Condon, E.M. Cyproheptadine treat-ment of Nelson's syndrome: restoration of plasma ACTH circadian periodicity and reversal of response to TRF. J. Clin. Endocrinol. Metab., 46:349, 1978.

65. Kuchel, O., Fishman, L.M., Liddle, G.W., and Mishelakis, A. Effect of diazoxide on plasma renin activity in hypertensive patients. Ann. Intern. Med., 67:791, 1967.

66. Lee, P.A., Plotnick, L.P., Kowarski, A.A., and Migeon, C.J. (eds.). Congenital Adrenal Hyperplasia. Baltimore, University Park Press, 1977.

67. Liddle, G.W., Bledsoe, T., and Coppage, W.S. Jr., A familial renal disorder simulating primary aldosteronism but with negligible aldosterone secretion. Trans. Assoc. Am. Physicians, 76:199, 1963.

68. Lindholm, J., Korsgrand, O., Rassmussen, P. Ectopic pituitary function. Acta Med. Scand., 198:299, 1975.

69. Nichols, T., Nugent, C.A., and Tyler, F.H. Steroid laboratory tests in the diagnosis of Cushing's syndrome. Am. J. Med. 116:172, 1965.

70. Orth, D.N. and Liddle, G.W. Results of treating Cushing's syndrome. N. Engl. J. Med., 285:243, 1971.

71. Plotz, C.M., Knowlton, A.I., and Regan, C. The natural history of Cushing's syndrome. Am. J. Med., 13:597, 1952.

72. Re, R.N., Sancho, J., Kliman, B., and Haber, E. The characterization of low renin hypertension by plasma renin activity and plasma aldosterone concentration. J. Clin. Endocrinol. Metab., 46:189, 1978.

73. Schambelan, M., Brust, N.L., Chang, B.C.F., Slaton, P.E., and Biglieri, E.G. Circadian rhythm and effect of posture on plasma aldosterone concentration in primary aldosteronism. J. Clin. Endocrinol. Metab., 43:115, 1976.

74. Schnall, A.M., Brodkey, J.S., Kaufman, B., Pearson, O.H. Pituitary function after removal of pituitary microadenomas in Cushing's disease. J. Clin. Endocrinol. Metab., 47:410, 1978.

75. Soffer, L.J., Iannaccone, A., and Gabrilove, J.L. Cushing's syndrome: a study of 50 patients. Am. J. Med., 30:129, 1961.

76. Sutherland, D.J.A., Ruse, J.L., and Laidlaw, J.C. Hypertension increased aldosterone secretion and low plasma renin activity relieved by dexamethasone. Can. Med. Assoc. J., 95:1109, 1966.

77. Temple, T.E., Jr., Jones, D.J., Jr., Liddle, G.W., and Dexter, R. Cushing's disease: correction of hypercortisolism by o,p'DDD. N. Engl. J. Med., 281:801, 1969.

78. Thorn, G.W. The Diagnosis and Treatment of Adrenal Insufficiency. Oxford, Blackwell, 1949.

79. Tyrrell, J.B., Brooks, R.M., Fitzgerald, P.A., Cofoid, P.B., Forsham, P.H., and Wilson, C.B. Cushing's disease: selective trans-sphenoidal resection of pituitary microadenomas. N. Engl. J. Med., 298:753, 1978.

80. von Euler, U.S. Noradrenaline: Chemistry, Physiology, Pharmacology and Clinical Aspects. Springfield, Ill., Charles C Thomas, 1956.

81. Wegienka, L.C., Grasso, S.G., and Forsham, P.J. Estimation of adrenomedullary reserve by infusion of 2-desoxy-d-glucose. J. Clin. Endocrinol. Metab., 26:37, 1966.

82. Wuepper, K.D., Wegienka, L.C., and Fudenberg, H.H. Immunologic aspects of adrenocortical insufficiency. Am. J. Med., 46:206, 1969.

Diabetes Mellitus

83. Alberti, K.G.M.M., Hockaday, T.D.R., and Turner, R.C. Small doses of insulin in treatment of diabetic "coma." Lancet, 1:951, 1973.

84. ———, Hockaday, T.D.R., and Turner, R.C. Small doses of intramuscular insulin in the treatment of diabetic "coma." Lancet, 2:515, 1973.

85. Andres, R. Aging and diabetes. Med. Clin. North Am., 55:835, 1971.

86. Assal, J.P., Aoki, T.T., Manzano, F.M., and Kozak, G.P. Metabolic effects of sodium bicarbonate in management of diabetic ketoacidosis. Diabetes, 23:405, 1974.

87. Autoimmune diabetes mellitus. Lancet, 2:1549, 1974.

88. Bar, R.S. and Roth, J. Insulin receptor status in disease states in man. Arch. Intern. Med., 137:474, 1977.

89. Beigelman, P.M. Severe diabetic ketoacidosis (diabetic "coma"): 482 episodes in 257 patients; experience of three years. Diabetes, 20:490, 1971.

90. Bell, E.T. A postmortem study of vascular disease in diabetics. Arch. Pathol. Lab. Med., 53:444, 1952.

91. Bierman, E.L., Albrink, M.J., Arby, R.A., Connor, W.E., Dayton, S., Spritz, N., and Steinberg, D. Principles of nutrition and dietary recommendations for patients with diabetes mellitus. Diabetes, 20:633, 1971.

92. Bloom, M.E., Mintz, D.H., and Field, J.B. Insulin induced post-hypoglycemic hyperglycemia as a cause of "brittle" diabetes. Am. J. Med., 47:891, 1969.

93. Cahill, G.F., Jr. Diabetes mellitus: a brief overview. Johns Hopkins Med. J., 143:155-159, 1978.

94. Clements, R.S., Jr. and Rynertson, R. Myoinositol metabolism in diabetes mellitus: effect of insulin treatment. Diabetes, 26:215, 1977.

95. Colby, A.G. Neurologic disorders of diabetes mellitus I, II. Diabetes, 14:424, 516, 1965.

96. Committee for the Assessment of the Biometric Aspects of Controlled Trials of Hypoglycemic Agents. Report. JAMA, 231:583, 1975.

97. Committee on Statistics, American Diabetic Association Standardization of the glucose tolerance test. Diabetes, 18:299, 1969.

98. Dandona, P., Healey, F., Foster, M., Greenbury, E., and Beckett, A.G. Low-dose insulin infusions in diabetic patients with high insulin requirements. Lancet, 2:283, 1978.

99. Danowski, T.S. and Sunder, J.H. Jet injection of insulin during self-monitoring of blood glucose. Diabetes Care, 1:27, 1978.

100. Davidson, J.K. and Debra, D.W. Immunologic insulin resistance. Diabetes 27:307, 1978.

101. DeFronzo, R.A., Andres, R., Edgar, P., and Walker, W.G. Carbohydrate metabolism in uremia: a review. Medicine, 52:469, 1973.

102. Diabetic Retinopathy Study Research Group. Preliminary report on effects of photocoagulation therapy. Am. J. Ophthalmol., 81:383, 1976.

103. Dorf, A., Ballantine, E.J., Bennett, P.H., and Miller, M. Retinopathy in Pima indians. Diabetes, 25:554, 1976.

104. Etzwiler, D.D. Who's teaching the diabetic? Diabetes, 16:111, 1967.

105. Exchange list for meal planning. New York, American Diabetes Association, 1976.

106. Fajans, S.S., Cloutier, M.C., and Crowther, R.L. Clinical and etiologic heterogeneity of idiopathic diabetes mellitus. Diabetes, 27:1112, 1978.

107. Fajans, S.S. The diagnosis and natural history of diabetes in 20th postgraduate course syllabus, San Francisco. New York, American Diabetes Association, 1973, p. 38.

108. Felts, P.W. Diabetic ketoacidosis. In Sussman, K.E. and Metz, R.J.S. (eds.), Diabetes Mellitus, 4th ed. New York, American Diabetes Association, 1975, p. 161.

109. Flier, J.S., Kahn, C.R., and Roth, J. Receptors, antireceptor antibodies and mechanisms of insulin resistance. N. Engl. J. Med., 300:413, 1979.

110. Foster, D.W. Insulin deficiency and hyperosmolar coma. Adv. Intern. Med., 19:159, 1974.

111. Gabbay, K.H. The sorbitol pathway and the complications of diabetes. N. Engl. J. Med., 288:831, 1973.

112. Gabbay, K.H. and Kinoshita, J.H. Mechanism of development and possible prevention of sugar cataracts. Isr. J. Med. Sci., 8:1557, 1972.

113. Ganda, O.P. and Soeldner, J.S., Genetic, acquired and related factors in the etiology of diabetes mellitus. JAMA, 137:461, 1977.

114. Grodsky, G.M. A threshold distribution hypothesis for packet storage of insulin and its mathematical modeling. J. Clin. Invest., 51:2047, 1972.

115. Johansen, K. and Gregersen, G. A family with dominantly inherited mild juvenile diabetes. Acta Med. Scand., 201:567, 1977.

116. Karam, J.H. Oral hypoglycemic drugs. In Sussman, K.E. and Metz, R.L.S. (eds.), Diabetes Mellitus, 4th ed. New York, American Diabetes Association, 1975, pp. 93–101.

117. Kjellstrand, C.M., Shideman, J.R., Simmons, R.L., Buselmeier, T.J., von Hartitzch, B., Goetz, F.C., and Najarian, J.S. Renal transplantation in insulin-dependent diabetic patients. Kidney Int., 6:515, 1974.

118. Koenig, R.J., Peterson, C.M., Jones, R.L., Saudels, C., Lehrman, M., and Cerami, A. Correlation of glucose regulation and hemoglobin A1c in diabetes mellitus. N. Engl. J. Med., 295:417, 1976.

119. Krahl, M.E. Insulin action at the molecular level fact and speculations. Diabetes, (Supp 2) 21:695, 1972.

120. Lactic acidosis. Lancet, 2:27, 1973.

121. Lacy, PE. Beta cell secretion from the standpoint of a pathologist. Diabetes, 19:895, 1970.

122. Levin, M.E. and O'Neal, L.W. The Diabetic Foot. St. Louis, Mosby, 1973.

123. Liebow, I.M. and Badger, G.F. Myocardial infarction in the practice of a group of private physicians. A comparison of patients with and without diabetes. J. Chronic Dis., 16:1013, 1963.

124. Lockwood, D.H. and Prout, T.E. Antigenicity of heterologous and homologous insulin. Metabolism, 14:530, 1965.

125. ———, East, L.E., Kane, M., and Livingston, J.N. Effects of fasting on insulin binding and glucose transport by fat cells. Diabetes, 25 (Suppl 1):321, 1976.

126. Ludvigsson, J., Hedding, L.G., Larsson, Y., and Leander, A. C-peptide in juvenile diabetes beyond the post-initial remission period. Acta Paediatr. Scan., 66:177, 1977.

127. McMillan, D.E. Deterioration of the microcirculation in diabetes. Diabetes, 24:944, 1975.

128. ———. Plasma protein changes, blood viscosity and diabetic microangiopathy. Diabetes, 25 (Suppl 2):858, 1976.

129. Milner-Fenwick, Inc. Diabetes Teaching Films. 2125 Greenspring Drive, Timonium, Md., 21093.

130. Mintz, D.H., Skyler, J.S., and Chez, R.A. Diabetes and pregnancy: a clinical review. Diabetes Care, 1:49, 1978.

131. Molnar, G.D. Clinical evaluation of metabolic control. Diabetes 27 (Suppl):216, 1978.

132. Najarian, J.C. Islet cell transplantation in treatment of diabetes. Hosp. Prac. 12:63, 1977.

133. National Committee for Diabetes. Report of the work group on the definition and diagnosis of diabetes mellitus. 3:45, 1977.

134. Neel, J.U. The genetics of juvenile-onset type diabetes mellitus. N. Engl. J. Med., 297:1062, 1977.

135. O'Sullivan, J.B. and Mahan, C.M. Criteria for the oral glucose tolerance test in pregnancy. Diabetes, 13:278, 1964.

136. Partamian, J.O. and Bradley, R.F. Acute myocardial infarction in 258 cases of diabetes: immediate mortality and five-year survival. N. Engl. J. Med., 273:455, 1965.

137. Pell, S. and D'Alonzo, C.A. Factors associated with long-term survival of diabetics. JAMA, 214:1833, 1970.

138. Petrides, P., Weiss, L., Löffler, G., and Wieland, O.H. Diabetes Mellitus, Theory and Management. (Trans. Williamson, D.H.) Baltimore, Urban and Schwarzenberg, 1978.

139. Pickens, J.M., Burkeholder, N.J. Womach, W.N. Oral glucose tolerance test in normal children. Diabetes, 16:11, 1967.

140. Posner, J.B. and Plum, F. Protection of CSF pH and brain function during severe metabolic acidosis. Trans. Am. Neurol. Assoc., 91:38, 1966.

141. Prout, T.E. Heart disease and diabetes: contributions of clinical trials. In Scott, R.C., (ed.), Diabetes and the Heart. Futura, Mt. Kisco, N.Y., 1979.

142. ———. The role of diabetic control in diabetic retinopathy. Int. Ophthalmol. Clin. 18:73, 1978.

143. ———. The use of screening and diagnostic procedures: The oral glucose tolerance test. In Sussman, K.E. and Metz, R.S.S. (eds.), Diabetes Mellitus, 4th ed. New York, American Diabetes Association, 1975, pp. 57–66.

144. Recker, L., Haymond, M., Goetz, F.C., and Willmert, J. Rehabilitation status: 175 diabetic kidney transplant recipients. Diabetes, 26 (Suppl):371, 1977.

145. Regan, T.J., Ettinger, P.O., Khan, M.I., Jesrani, M.Y., Lyons, M.M., Oldewurtel, H.A., and Weber, M. Altered myocardial function and metabolism in chronic diabetes mellitus without ischemia in dogs. Circ. Res., 35:222, 1974.

146. Rimoin, D.L. The genetics of diabetes mellitus. In Ellenberg, M. and Rifkin, H. (eds.), Diabetes Mellitus: Theory and Practice. New York, McGraw-Hill, 1970.

147. Robertson, R.P. and Port, D., Jr. The glucose receptor: a defective mechanism in diabetes mellitus distinct from the β-adrenergic receptor. J. Clin. Invest., 52:870, 1973.

148. Seltzer, H.S. Drug induced hypoglycemia. A review based on 473 cases. Diabetes, 21:955, 1972.

149. Shipp, J.C., Cunningham, R.W., Russell, R.O., and Marble, A. Insulin resistance: clinical features, natural course and effects of adrenal steroid treatment. Medicine 44:165, 1965.

150. Siperstein, M.D. The glucose tolerance test. In Stollerman, G.H. (ed.), Advances in Internal Medicine, Chicago, Year Book Medical Publishers, 1975, p. 297.

151. Soeldner, J.S. The intravenous glucose tolerance test. In Fajans, S.S. and Sussman, K.E. (eds.), Diabetes Mellitus, Diagnosis and Treatment. Vol. III. New York, American Diabetes Association, 1971, pp.107–113.

152. Spiro, R.G. Biochemistry of the renal glomerular basement membrane and its alterations in diabetes mellitus. N. Engl. J. Med., 288:1337, 1973.

153. Tattersall, R.B. and Pyke, D.A. Diabetes in identical twins. Lancet, 2:1120, 1972.

154. Turkington, R.W. and Weindling, H.K. Insulin secretion in the diagnosis of adult-onset diabetes mellitus. JAMA, 240:833, 1978.

155. Unger, R.H. and Madison, L.L. Comparison of response to intravenously administered sodium tolbutamide in mild diabetic and non-diabetic subjects. J. Clin. Invest., 37:627, 1958.

156. US Public Health Service Cooperative Study: long-term therapy for chronic bacturia in men. Ann. Intern. Med., 83:133, 1975.

157. University Group Diabetes Program. Effects of hypoglycemic agents on vascular complications in patients with adult onset diabetes. I. Design, methods and baseline results; II. Mortality results. Diabetes, 19 (Suppl 2):747, 1970.

158. University Group Diabetes Program. Effects of hypoglycemic agents of vascular complications in patients with adult onset diabetes. VII. Report on insulin treatment. Mortality and selected non-fatal events. JAMA, 240:37, 1978.

159. University Group Diabetes Program. Effects of hypoglycemic agents on vascular complications in patients with adult onset diabetes. V. Evaluation of Phenformin therapy. Diabetes 24 (Suppl. 1):65, 1975.

160. The UGDP Controversy: Clinical trials vs. clinical impressions. Diabetes 21:1035, 1972.

161. West, K.M. Special types of diabetes. In Epidemiology of Diabetes and its Vascular Lesions. New York, Elsevier, 1978, pp. 289–338.

Hypoglycemia

162. Baylin, S.B. The multiple endocrine neoplasia syndromes: implications for the study of inherited tumors. Semin. Oncol., 5: 35, 1978.

163. Broder, L.E. and Carter, S.K. Pancreatic islet cell carcinoma II. Results of therapy with streptozotocin in 52 patients. Ann. Intern. Med., 79:108, 1973.

164. Exton, J.H. Gluconeogenesis. Metabolism, 21:945, 1972.

165. Fajans, S.S. and Floyd, J.C., Jr. Fasting hypoglycemia in adults. N. Engl. J. Med., 294:766, 1976.

166. Ford, C.V., Bray, G.A., and Swerdloff, R.S. Psychiatric

study of patients referred with a diagnosis of hypoglycemia. Am. J. Psych., 133:290, 1976.

167. Freinkel, N. and Metzger, B.E. Oral glucose tolerance curve and hypoglycemias in the fed state. N. Engl. J. Med., 280:820, 1969.

168. Ganda, O.P., Weir, G.C., Soeldner, J.S., Legg, M.A., Chick, W.L., Patel, Y.C., Ebeid, A.M., Gabbay, K.H., and Reichlin, S. "Somatostatinoma": a somatostatin-containing tumor of the endocrine pancreas. N. Engl. J. Med., 296:963, 1977.

169. Hofeldt, F.D. Reactive hypoglycemia. Metabolism, 24: 1193, 1975.

170. Kahn, C.R., Rosen, S.W., Weintraub, B.D., Fajans, S.S., and Gorden, P. Ectopic production of chorionic gonadotropin and its subunits by islet-cell tumors: a specific marker for malignancy. N. Engl. J. Med., 297:565, 1977.

171. Kaplan, E.L. and Rubenstein, A. Calcium infusion—a provocative test for insulinomas. Endocrine Society, 59th Annual Meeting. 105, 1977.

172. Laurent, J., Debry, G., and Floquet, J. Hypoglycemic Tumors. Amsterdam, Exerpta Medica Foundation, 1971.

173. Madison, L.L. Ethanol-induced hypoglycemia. Adv. Metab. Disord., 3:85, 1968.

174. Mallinson, C.N., Bloom, S.R., Warin, A.P., Salmon, P.R., and Cox, B. A glucagonoma syndrome. Lancet, 2: 1, 1974.

175. Margolis, S. and Homcy, C. Systemic manifestations of hepatoma. Medicine, 51:381, 1972.

176. Marks, V. Hypoglycemia. 2. Other causes. Clin. Endocrinol. Metab., 5: 769, 1976.

177. Marks, V. and Alberti, K.G. Selected tests of carbohydrate metabolism. Clin. Endocrinol. Metab., 5:805, 1976.

178. Merimee, T.J. and Tyson, J.E. Stabilization of plasma glucose during fasting: normal variations in two separate studies. N. Engl. J. Med., 291:1275, 1974.

179. Megyesi, K., Kahn, C.R., Roth, J., and Gorden, P. Hypoglycemia in association with extrapancreatic tumors: demonstration of elevated plasma NSILA-S by a new radioreceptor assay. J. Clin. Endocrinol. Metab., 38: 931, 1974.

180. Permutt, M.A. Postprandial hypoglycemia. Diabetes, 25:719, 1976.

181. Rubenstein, A.H., Kuzuya, H., and Horwitz, D.L. Clinical significance of circulating C-peptide in diabetes mellitus and hypoglycemic disorders. Arch. Intern. Med., 137:625, 1977.

182. Seltzer, H.S. Drug-induced hypoglycemia. Review based on 473 cases. Diabetes, 21:955, 1972.

183. Yager, J. and Young, R.T. Non-hypoglycemia is an epidemic condition. N. Engl. J. Med., 291:907, 1974.

Eating Disorders: Obesity and Anorexia Nervosa

184. Andersen, A.E. Atypical anorexia nervosa. In Vigersky, R.A. (ed.), Anorexia Nervosa. New York, Raven Press, 1977, pp.11–19.

185. Bistrian, B.R., Blackburn, G.L., and Stanbury, J.B. Metabolic aspects of a protein-sparing modified fast in the dietary management of Prader-Willi obesity. N. Engl. J. Med., 296:774, 1977.

186. Cahill, G.F., Jr. Starvation in man. In Albrink, M.J. (ed.), Clinics in Endocrinology and Metabolism. London, Saunders, 1976, pp. 397–415.

187. Charney, E., Goodwin, H.C., McBride, M., Lyon, B., and Pratt, R. Childhood antecedents of adult obesity. N. Engl. J. Med., 295:6, 1976.

188. Frisch, R.E. and McAuthur, J.W. Menstrual cycles: fatness as a determinant of minimum weight for height necessary for their maintenance or onset. Science, 185: 949, 1974.

189. Goldblatt, P.B., Moore, M.E., and Stunkard, A.J. Social factors in obesity. JAMA, 192:1039, 1965.

190. Halmi, K.A., Struss, A.L., and Goldberg, S. An investigation of weights in the parents of anorexia nervosa patients. J. Nerv. Ment. Dis., 166:358, 1978.

191. Halverson, J.D., Wise, L., and Ballinger, W.F. Jejuno-ileal bypass for morbid obesity. Am. J. Med., 64:461, 1978.

192. Hirsch, J. and Batchelor, B. Adipose tissue cellularity in human obesity. In Albrink, M.J. (ed.), Clinics in Endocrinology and Metabolism. London, Saunders, 1976, pp. 299–311.

193. MacGregor, M.A., Block, A.J., and Ball, W.C., Jr. Serious complications and sudden death in the Pickwickian syndrome. Johns Hopkins Med. J., 126:279, 1970.

194. McHugh, P.R., Moran, T.H., and Barton, G.N. Satiety: a graded behavioral phenomenon regulating caloric intake. Science, 190:167, 1975.

195. Morgan, H.G. and Russell, G.F.M. Value of family background and clinical features as predictors of long-term outcome in anorexia nervosa: a four-year follow-up study of 41 patients. Psychol. Med., 5:355, 1975.

196. Printen, K.J. and Mason, E.E. Gastric surgery for relief of morbid obesity. Arch. Surg., 106:428, 1973.

197. Rabinowitz, D. Some endocrine and metabolic aspects of obesity. Annu. Rev. Med., 21:241, 1970.

198. Robinson, R.G., McHugh, P.R., and Bloom, F.E. Chlorpromazine induced hyperphagia in the rat. Psychopharmacol. Commun. 1:37, 1975.

199. Salans, L.B., Bray, G.A., Suchman, S.W., Danforth, E., Jr., Glennon, J.A., Horton, E.A., and Sims, E.A.H. Glucose metabolism and the response to insulin by human adipose tissue in spontaneous and experimental obesity. Effects of dietary composition and adipose cell size. J. Clin. Invest., 53:848, 1974.

200. Schachter, S. Some extraordinary facts about obese humans and rats. Am. Psychol., 26:129, 1971.

201. Solow, C., Silberfarb, P.M., and Swift, K. Psychosocial effects of intestinal bypass surgery for severe obesity. N. Engl. J. Med., 290:300, 1974.

202. Stunkard, A.J. Obesity. In Freedman, A.M., Kaplan, H.I., and Sabock, B.J. (eds.), Modern Synopsis of Comprehensive Textbook of Psychiatry/II (2nd ed.). Baltimore, Williams & Wilkins, 1976, pp. 805–810.

203. Stunkard, A., Rickets, K., and Hesbacher, P. Fenfluramine in the treatment of obesity. Lancet, 1:503, 1973.

204. Vigersky, R.A., Loriaux, D.L., Andersen, A.E., and Lipsett, M.B. Anorexia nervosa: behavioural and hypothalamic aspects. Clin. Endocrinol. Metab., 5:517, 1976.

Hyperlipidemia

205. Cameron, J.L., Capuzzi, D.M., Zuidema, G.D., and Margolis, S. Acute pancreatitis with hyperlipidemia. The incidence of lipid abnormalities in acute pancreatitis. Ann. Surg., 177:483–489, 1973.

206. Epidemiology Committee. The Lipid Research Clinics Program. Plasma lipid distributions in selected North American populations: The Lipid Research Clinics Program Prevalence Study. Circulation, 60:427, 1979.

207. Eisenberg, S. and Levy, R.I. Lipoprotein metabolism. Adv. Lipid Res., 13:1, 1975.

208. Fredrickson, D.S., Goldstein, J.L., and Brown, J.S. The familial hyperlipoproteinemias. In Stanbury, J.B., Wyngaarden, J.B., and Fredrickson, D.S. (eds.), The Metabolic Basis of Inherited Disease. New York, McGraw-Hill, 1978, pp. 604–655.

209. Fredrickson, D.S., Morganrath, J., and Levy, R.I. Type III Hyperlipoproteinemia: an analysis of two contemporary definitions. Ann. Intern. Med., 82:150, 1975.

210. Gjone, E., Norum, K.R., and Glomset, J.A. Familial lecithin: cholesterol acyltransferase deficiency. In Stanbury, J.B., Wyngaarden, J.B., and Fredrickson, D.S. (eds.), The Metabolic Basis of Inherited Disease. New York, McGraw-Hill, 1978, pp. 589–603.

211. Goldstein, J.L. and Brown, M.S. Atherosclerosis: the low-density lipoprotein receptor hypothesis. Metabolism, 26:1257, 1977.

212. Goldstein, J.L., Schrott, H.G., Hazzard, W.R., Bierman, E.L., and Motulsky, A.G. Hyperlipidemia in coronary heart disease. II. Genetic analysis of lipid levels in 176 families and delineation of a new inherited disorder, combined hyperlipidemia. J. Clin. Invest., 52:1544, 1973.

213. Hamilton, R.L., Williams, M.C., Fielding, C.J., and Havel, R.J. Discoidal bilayer structure of nascent high density lipoproteins from perfused rat liver. J. Clin. Invest., 58:667, 1976.

214. Herbert, P.N., Gotto, A.M., and Fredrickson, D.S. Familial lipoprotein deficiency (abetalipoproteinemia, hypobetalipoproteinemia, and Tangier disease). In Stanbury, J.B., Wyngaarden, J.B. and Fredrickson, D.S. (eds.), The Metabolic Basis of Inherited Disease. New York, McGraw-Hill, 1978, pp. 544–588.

215. Jackson, R.L., Morrisett, J.D., and Gotto, A.M., Jr. Lipoprotein structure and metabolism. Physiol. Rev., 56:259, 1976.

216. Kannel, W.B., Castelli, W.P., Gordon, T., and McNamara, P. Serum cholesterol, lipoproteins and the risk of coronary heart disease: the Framingham Study. Ann. Intern. Med., 74:1, 1971.

217. Lewis, B. The Hyperlipidaemias: Clinical and Laboratory Practice. Oxford, Blackwell, 1976, pp. 292–340.

218. Mahley, R.W., Bersot, T.P., Innerarity, T.L., Lipson, A., and Margolis, S. Alterations of human high-density lipoproteins, with or without increased plasma-cholesterol, induced by diets high in cholesterol. Lancet, 2:807, 1978.

219. Miller, G.J. and Miller, N.E. Plasma high density lipoprotein concentration and development of ischemic heart disease. Lancet, 1:16, 1975.

220. Oliver, M.F., Heady, J.A., Morris, J.N., and Cooper, J. A co-operative trial in the primary prevention of ischaemic heart disease using clofibrate. Br. Heart J., 40:1069, 1978.

221. Utermann, G., Jaeschke, M., and Menzel, J. Familial hyperlipoproteinemia Type III: deficiency of a specific apolipoprotein (apo E-III) in very low density lipoproteins. FEBS Lett., 56:352, 1975.

222. Yeshurun, D. and Gotto, A.M., Jr. Drug treatment of hyperlipidemia. Am. J. Med., 60:379, 1976.

Disorders of Calcium and Metabolic Bone Diseases

223. Anast, C.S., Winnacker, J.L., Forte, L.R., et al. Impaired release of parathyroid hormone in magnesium deficiency. J. Clin. Endocrinol. Metab., 42:707, 1976.

224. Avioli, L.V. The therapeutic approach to hypoparathyroidism. Am. J. Med., 57:34, 1974.

225. Avioli, L.V. and Krane, S.M. (eds.). Metabolic Bone Disease. Vol. 1. New York, Academic Press, 1977.

226. Brooks, M.H., Bell, N.H., Love, L., et al. Vitamin-D-dependent rickets type II: resistance of target organ to 1, 25-dihydroxy-vitamin D. N. Engl. J. Med., 298:996, 1978.

227. Condon, J.R., Ives, D., Knight, M.J., et al. Etiology of hypocalcemia in acute pancreatitis, Br. J. Surg., 62:115, 1975.

228. Deftos, L.J. Calcitonin in clinical medicine. In Stollerman, G.H. (ed.), Advances in Internal Medicine. Vol. 23. Chicago, Year Book Medical Publishers, 1978.

229. Drezner, M.K. and Lebovitz, H.E. Primary hyperparathyroidism in paraneoplastic hypercalcemia. Lancet, 1:1004, 1978.

230. Favus, M.J. Vitamin D physiology and some clinical aspects of the vitamin D endocrine system. Med. Clin. North Am., 62:1291, 1978.

231. Habener, J.F. and Mahaffey, J.E. Osteomalacia and disorders of vitamin D metabolism. Annu. Rev. Med., 29:327, 1978.

232. Haussler, M. R. and McCain, T.A. Basic and clinical concepts related to vitamin D metabolism and action. N. Engl. J. Med., 297:974, 1977.

233. Lerman, S., Canterbury, J.M., and Reiss, E. Parathyroid hormone and the hypercalcemia of immobilization. J. Clin. Endocrinol. Metab., 45:425, 1977.

234. Mallette, L.E., Bilezikian, J.P., Heath, D.A., and Aurbach, G.D., Primary hyperparathyroidism: clinical and biochemical features. Medicine, 53:127, 1974.

235. Nusynowitz, M.L. and Klein, M.H. Pseudoidiopathic hypoparathyroidism and ineffective parathyroid hormone. Am. J. Med., 56:667, 1973.

236. Porter, R.H., Cox, B.G., Heaney, D., et al. Treatment of hypoparathyroid patients with chlorthalidone. N. Engl. J. Med., 298:577–581, 1978.

237. Raisz, L.G., Mundy, G.R., Dietrich, J.W., and Canalis, E.M. Hormone regulation of mineral metabolism. In McCann, S.M. (ed.), International Review of Physiology, Endocrine Physiology II. Vol. 16. Baltimore, University Park Press, 1977.

238. Schneider, A.B. and Sherwood, L.M. Pathogenesis and management of hypoparathyroidism and other hypocalcemic disorders. Metabolism, 24:871, 1975.

239. Seyberth, H.W., Segre, G.V., Morgan, J.L., et. al. Pros-

taglandins as mediators of hypercalcemia associated with certain types of cancer. N. Engl. J. Med., 293: 1278, 1975.

240. Sinha, T.K., DeLuca, H.F., and Bell, N.H. Evidence for a defect in the formation of 1, 25-dihydroxyvitamin D in pseudoparathyroidism. Metabolism, 26:731, 1977.

241. Swinton, N.W., Jr., Clerkin, E.P., and Flint, L.D. Hypercalcemia and familial pheochromocytoma: correction after adrenalectomy. Ann. Intern. Med., 76:455, 1972.

242. Warrick, C.K. Some aspects of polyostotic fibrous dysplasia: possible hypothesis to account for associated endocrinologic changes. Clin. Radiol., 24:125, 1973.

243. Warwick, O.H., Yendt, E.R., and Olin, J.S. The clinical features of hypercalcemia associated with malignant disease. Can. Med. Assoc. J., 85:719, 1961.

The Thyroid Gland

244. Bilezekian, J.P., Loeb, J.N., and Gammon, D.E. The influence of hyperthyroidism and hypothyroidism on the adrenergic responsiveness of the turkey erythrocyte. J. Clin. Invest., 63:184, 1979.

245. Blum, M. Myxedema coma. Am. J. Med. Sci., 264:432, 1972.

246. Davis, P.J. and Davis, F.B. Hyperthyroidism in patients over the age of 60 years. Medicine, 53:161, 1974.

247. DeGroot, L.J., Frohman, L.A., Kaplan, E.L., and Refetoff, S. (eds.). Radiation Associated Thyroid Carcinoma. New York, Grune & Straton, 1977.

248. DeGroot, L.J. and Stanbury, J.B. The Thyroid and Its Diseases, 4th ed. New York, Wiley, 1975.

249. Epstein, S. and Pimstone, B. Practolol in hyperthyroid cardiac failure. S. Afr. Med. J., 45:812, 1971.

250. Franssila, K.O. Prognosis in thyroid carcinoma. Cancer 36:1138, 1975.

251. Gregerman, R.I. and Davis, P.J. In Werner, S.C. and Ingbar, S.H. (eds.), The Thryoid, 4th ed. New York, Harper & Row, 1978, pp. 223–246.

252. Kaptein, E.M., Kamiel, M.B., Spencer, C.A., Hall, T.D., and Nicoloff, J.T. Suppression of thyroid function with severe illness. Program 60th Annual Meeting of the Endocrine Society, 1978, Abstract No. 74, p. 111.

253. Kaptein, E.M., Wheeler, W.S., Hall, T.D., and Nicoloff, J.T. Thyroid hormone economy in severe illness. Clin. Res., 27:21A, 1979.

254. Kourides, I.A., Ridgway, E.C., Weintraub, B.D., Bigos, S.T., Gershengorn, M.C., and Maloff, F. Thyrotropin-induced hyperthyroidism: use of alpha and beta subunit levels to identify patients with pituitary tumors. J. Clin. Endocrinol. Metab., 45:534, 1977.

255. Krishnamurthy, G.T. and Blahd, W.H. Radioiodine I-131 therapy in the management of thyroid cancer. A prospective study. Cancer 40:195, 1977.

256. Mazzaferri, E.L., Young, R.L., Oertel, J.E., Kemmerer, W.T., and Page, C.P. Papillary thyroid carcinoma: the impact of therapy in 576 patients. Medicine, 56:171, 1977.

257. McCowen, K.D., Adler, R.A., Ghaed, N., Verdon, T., and Hofeldt, F.D. Low dose radioiodide thyroid ablation in postsurgical patients with thyroid cancer. Am. J. Med., 61:52, 1976.

258. Mehdi, S.Q. and Kriss, J.P. Preparation of radiolabeled thyroid-stimulating immunoglobulins (TSI) by recombining TSI heavy chains with ^{125}I-labeled light chains: direct evidence that the product binds to the membrane thyrotropic receptor and stimulates adenylate cyclase. Endocrinology 103:296, 1978.

259. Miller, J.M., Hamburger, J.I., and Kini, S. Diagnosis of thyroid nodules. Use of fine needle aspiration and needle biopsy. JAMA, 241:481, 1979.

260. Olsen, T., Laurberg, P., and Weeke, J. Low serum triiodothyronine and high serum reverse triiodothyronine in old age: an effect of disease not age. J. Clin. Endocrinol. Metab., 47:1111, 1978.

261. Oppenheimer, J.H. Thyroid hormone action at the cellular level. Science, 203:971, 1979.

262. Roudebush, C.P., Asteris, G.T., and DeGroot, L.J. Natural history of radiation associated thyroid cancer. Arch. Intern. Med., 138:1631, 1978.

263. Schimmel, M. and Utiger, R.D. Thyroidal and peripheral production of thyroid hormones. Review of recent findings and their clinical implications. Ann. Intern. Med., 87:760, 1977.

264. Skowsky, W.R. and Kikuchi, T.A. The role of vasopressin in the impaired water excretion of myxedema. Am. J. Med., 64:613, 1978.

265. Solomon, D.H., Chopra, I.J., Chopra, U., and Smith, F.J. Identification of subgroups of euthyroid Graves' ophthalmopathy. N. Engl. J. Med., 296:181, 186, 1977.

266. Spector, D.A., Davis, P.J., Helderman, J.H., Bell, B., and Utiger, R.D. Thyroid function and metabolic state in chronic renal failure. Ann. Intern. Med., 85:724, 1976.

267. Sterling, K. Thyroid hormone action at the cell level. N. Engl. J. Med., 300:117, 173, 1979.

268. Werner, S.C. and Ingbar, S.H. (eds.). The Thyroid, 4th ed. New York, Harper & Row, 1978.

269. Williams, R.H. (ed.) Textbook of Endocrinology, 5th ed. Philadelphia, Saunders, 1974.

The Gonads

270. Amelar, R.D., Dubin, L., and Walsh, P.C. Male Infertility. Philadelphia, Saunders, 1977.

271. Bettendorf, G. and Leidenberger, S. Amenorrhea and dysfunctional uterine bleeding in puberty. Clin. Endocrinol. Metab., 4:89, 1975.

272. Bierich, J.R. Sexual precocity. Clin. Endocrinol. Metab., 4:107, 1975.

273. Blanchard, M.D. and Josso, N. Source of the anti-müllerian hormone synthesized by the fetal-testis: müllerian inhibiting activity of fetal bovine Sertoli cells in tissue culture. Pediatr. Res., 8:968, 1974.

274. Boyar, R.M. Control of the onset of puberty. Annu. Rev. Med., 29:509, 1978.

275. Carter, J.N., Tyson, J.E., Warne, G.L., McNeilly, A.S., Faiman, C., and Friesen, H.G. Adrenocortical function in hyperprolactinemic women. J. Clin. Endocrinol. Metab. 45:973, 1977.

276. Channing, C.P., Anderson, L.D., Batta, S.K. Follicular growth and development. Clin. Obstet. Gynecol., 5:375, 1978.

277. Espiner, E.A., Veale, A.M.D., Sands, V.E., and Fitzgerald, P.H. Familial syndrome of streak gonads and nor-

mal karyotype in five phenotypic females. N. Engl. J. Med., 283:6, 1970.

278. Fraley, E.E. (ed). Testicular tumors. Urol. Clin. North Am., 4:343, 1977.

279. Grumbach, M.M. and Van Wyk, J.J. Disorders of sex differentiation. In Williams, R.H. (ed.), Textbook of Endocrinology. Philadelphia, Saunders, 1974, pp. 423–501.

280. Hsueh, W.A., Hsu, T.H., and Federman, D.D. Endocrine features of Klinefelter's syndrome. Medicine, 57:447, 1978.

281. Imperato-McGinley, J. and Peterson R. Male pseudohermaphroditism: the complexities of male phenotypic development. Am. J. Med., 61:251, 1976.

282. Ismail, A.A.A., Davidson, D.W., Souka, A.R., et al. The evaluation of the role of androgens in hirsutism and the use of new anti-androgen "cyproterone acetate" for therapy. J. Clin. Endocrinol. Metab., 39:81, 1974.

283. Jewelewicz, R. The diagnosis and treatment of amenorrheas. Fertil. Steril., 27, 1347, 1976.

284. Jones, G.S., Aksel, S., and Wentz, A.C. Serum progesterone levels in luteal phase defects. Obstet. Gynecol., 44:26, 1974.

285. Jost, A., Vigier, B., Prepin, J., and Perchellet, J.P. Studies on sex differentiation in mammals. Recent Prog. Horm. Res., 29:1, 1973.

286. Kasdan, R., Nankin, H.R., Troen, P., Wald, N., Pan, S., and Yanaihara, T. Paternal transmission of maleness in XX human. N. Engl. J. Med., 288:539, 1972.

287. Kirschner, M.A. and Bardin, C.W. Androgen production and metabolism in normal and virilized women. Metabolism, 21:667, 1972.

288. Kirschner, M.A. and Jacobs, J.B. Combined ovarian and adrenal vein catheterization to determine the site(s) of androgen overproduction in hirsute women. J. Clin. Endocrinol. Metab., 33:199, 1971.

289. Kistner, R.W. Sequential use of clomiphene citrate and human menopausal gonadotropin in ovulation induction. Fertil. Steril., 27:72, 1976.

290. Kleinberg, D.L., Gordon, L.N., and Frantz, A.G. Galactorrhea: A study of 235 cases including 48 with pituitary tumors. N. Engl. J. Med., 296:589, 1977.

291. McCann, S.M. A hypothalamic luteinizing hormone-releasing factor. Am. J. Physiol., 202:395, 1962.

292. McNatty, K.P., Hunter, W.M., McNeilly, A.S., and Sawers, R.S. Changes in the concentration of pituitary and steroid hormone in the follicular fluid of human graafian follicles throughout the menstrual cycle. J. Endocrinol., 64:555, 1975.

293. McNatty, K.P., Sawers, R.S., McNeilly, A.S. A possible role for prolactin in control of steroid secretion by the human graafian follicle. Nature, 250:653, 1974.

294. Odell, W.D. Physiology of the reproductive system in women. In DeGroot, L.S. (ed.), Textbook of Endocrine Physiology. New York, Grune & Stratton, 1978.

295. Odell, W.D. and Swerdloff, R.S., Male hypogonadism. West. J. Med. 124:446, 1976.

296. Paulsen, C.A. The testes. In Williams, R.H. (ed.), Textbook of Endocrinology, 5th ed. Philadelphia, Saunders, 1974, pp. 323–367.

297. Penny, R., Guyda, H.J., Baghdassarian, A., et al. Correlation of serum follicle stimulating hormone (FSH) and luteinizing hormone (LH) as measured by radioimmunoassay in disorders of sexual development. J. Clin. Invest., 49:1847, 1970.

298. Prader, A. Delayed adolescence. Clin. Endocrinol. Metabol., 4:143, 1975.

299. Rajfer, J. and Walsh, P.C. The incidence of intersexuality in patients with hypospadias and cryptorchidism. J. Urol., 116:769, 1976.

300. Rebar, R., Judd, H.L., Yen, S.S.C., et al. Characterization of the inappropriate gonadotropin secretion in polycystic ovary syndrome. J. Clin. Invest., 57:1320, 1976.

301. Scorer, C.G. and Farrington, G.H. Congenital Deformities of the Testis and Epididymis. New York, Appleton, 1971.

302. Semchyshyn, S. and Zuspan, F.P. Ovarian hemorrhage due to anticoagulants. Am. J. Obstet. Gynecol., 131:837, 1978.

303. Seppala, M., Hirvonen, E., and Ranta, T. Hyperprolactinaemia and luteal insufficiency. Lancet, 1:229, 1976.

304. Siiteri, P.K. and MacDonald, P.C. Role of extraglandular estrogen in human endocrinology. In Geiger, S.R., Astwood, E.B., and Greep, R.O. (eds.), Handbook of Physiology, Section 7, Endocrinology. Washington, D.C., American Physiology Society, 1973, pp. 615–629.

305. Siiteri, P.K. and Wilson, J.D. Testosterone formation and metabolism during male sexual differentiation in the human embryo. J. Clin. Endocrinol. Metab., 38:113, 1974.

306. Silvers, W.K. and Wachtel, S.S. H-Y antigen: behavior and function. Science, 195:956, 1977.

307. Strott, C.A., Cargille, C.M., Ross, G.T., and Lipsett, M.G. The short luteal phase. J. Clin. Endocrinol. Metab., 30:246, 1970.

308. Tanner, J.M. Growth at adolescence, 2nd ed. Oxford, Blackwell, 1962.

309. Wachtel, S.S., Koo, G.C., Breg, W.R., et al. Serologic detection of a Y-linked gene in XX males and XX true hermaphrodites. N. Engl. J. Med., 295:750, 1976.

310. Weinstein, D. and Polishuk, W.Z. The role of wedge resection of the ovary as a cause for mechanical sterilization. Surg. Gynecol. Obstet. 141:417, 1975.

311. Wentz, A.C., White, R.I., Hsu, T.H, et al. Differential ovarian and adrenal vein catheterization. Am. J. Obstet. Gynecol., 125:1000, 1976.

312. Wilson, J.D. and MacDonald, P.C. Male pseudohermaphroditism due to androgen resistance: testicular feminization and related syndromes. In Stanbury, J.B., Wyngaarden, J., and Fredericksen, D.S. (eds.), Metabolic Basis of Inherited Disease. New York, McGraw-Hill, 1978.

313. Wilson, J.D. and Walsh, P.D. Disorders of sexual differentiation. In Harrison, J.H., Gittes, R.F., Perlmutter, A.D., Stamey, T.A., and Walsh, P.C. (eds.), Campbell's Urology, 4th ed. Philadelphia, Saunders, 1974, pp. 1484–1532.

314. Wyss, R.H., Karsznia, R., Heinrichs, W.L., and Herrmann, W.L. Inhibition of uterine receptor binding of estradiol by antiestrogens (clomiphene and CL-868). J. Clin. Endocrinol. Metab., 28:1824, 1968.

SECTION TWELVE
Infectious Diseases
ALBERT H. OWENS, Jr.: SECTION EDITOR

CHAPTER 78
Infectious Diseases: General Considerations
PATRICK A. MURPHY

The Normal Flora

All of us become colonized with bacteria shortly after birth, and we carry large populations of organisms with us throughout life. Different regions of the body have highly characteristic floras, and there is comparatively little variation from one person to another. Certain species of bacteria are invariably cultured from a particular region. All humans always carry alpha hemolytic streptococci in the throat, diphtheroids on the skin, and *Bacteroides fragilis* in the bowel. These constant organisms are collectively known as the autochthonous flora. Other bacteria are not constant but are commonly found on body surfaces in the absence of disease. These organisms are included along with autochthonous organisms in the term "normal flora."

It was once possible to draw a distinction between the normal flora and the pathogens that cause disease. The normal flora was regarded as harmless in itself, and useful because it protected the host from colonization and disease caused by pathogenic species. It is now clear that the normal flora is far from harmless. Dental caries and periodontal disease are universal; they appear to be entirely caused by the bacteria that normally live on and around teeth. Healthy people may develop infections with their normal flora. Most are minor, such as boils and urinary tract infections, but lethal infection may follow a ruptured appendix. Lastly, modern medicine has created great numbers of people with impaired host defenses. Such people are very susceptible to infection, and the infections are characteristically caused by organisms from the normal flora or from the environment that seldom or never produces disease in the normal population.

Essentially, any organism can be pathogenic if it enters the tissues in large numbers. Organisms gathered in one site cause the formation of a local abscess; organisms disseminated in the bloodstream cause septicemia, shock, and death. The pathogens which cause disease in healthy people are those bacteria that can multiply from a small inoculum. By and large, these infections kill or are cured; the pathogen does not persist in the body for a long time. Thus, immunosuppressed people usually become infected with staphylococci and gram-negative rods because these organisms are always available to initiate infection, whereas the pneumococcus or *Haemophilus influenzae* are transient visitors.

The nonpathogenicity of the normal bacteria is, thus, strictly relative. They seldom cause disease in healthy people, but this is only because of the continuous operation of host defenses. However, the normal flora does exert significant protective effects; examples have been found in all sites investigated. Some of the bacteria that normally live in the throat make bacteriocines which kill the β-hemolytic streptococcus. In an epidemic situation, children carrying these bacteria were shown to be protected from streptococcal pharyngitis.[3] Similarly, *Bacteroides fragilis* produces acetate, proprionate, and butyrate as fermentation products, and these inhibit shigellae and salmonellae. Staphylococci and diphteroids on skin break down the triglycerides of sebum to free fatty acids, which are bactericidal for streptococci and gram-negative rods which happen to alight there.

It is clear that the normal flora is not essential for life; mice can be maintained in the germ-free state, and humans with Swiss-type agammaglobulinemia have been raised to adolescence in plastic enclosures. Patients with acute leukemia can be rendered free of virtually all organisms with intensive regimens of local and systemic antibiotics, provided that exposure to new organisms is prevented by putting the patient into a laminar flow room or plastic enclosure.

Effects of Antibiotic Therapy

The equilibrium between man and his microbes is most frequently disturbed by antibiotic therapy. In ordinary clinical practice, it is rare to prescribe antibiotic regimes that are sufficiently broad in spectrum and intensive in application to inhibit all the organisms of the normal flora. And almost never is the patient so efficiently isolated that organisms from the environment cannot contaminate him. Because of this, when antibiotics are prescribed, there is always a risk that the patient will develop an overgrowth of antibiotic resistant organisms, either survivors from his normal flora or invaders from outside. Most of the time, such changes in flora are symptomless and resolve spontaneously when the antibiotic is stopped. This outcome is likely when the spectrum of the antibiotic is narrow, the dose is low, the duration of therapy is short, and the patient is basically healthy. However, even in healthy people, syndromes such as diarrhea and vaginal candidiasis are common after antibiotic therapy. Sick old people may develop serious or lethal superinfections such as gram-negative rod pneumonias.

Colonization with Pathogenic Bacteria

It is not possible to draw a precise distinction between infection and colonization with bacteria. Infection implies that the presence of the organisms is abnormal, that they have caused disease or are likely to, and that one ought to do something about it. Colonization implies that the organisms are to be expected in that situation, that they are unlikely to cause trouble in their host or to spread to other people, and that treatment will do more harm than good. Thus, a symptomless girl with gonococci in her cervical secretions should be regarded as infected because she might develop disseminated infection and because she is a danger to her male friends. On the other hand, staphylococci in the nose or the axilla would usually be regarded as normal flora because the risk of boils and other staphylococcal infections is very low. However, if the host was a nurse in the pediatric intensive care unit and the infants were being infected with her staphylococci, one would take a different view. Sometimes the decision that the presence of an organism is merely colonization reflects an inability to do anything useful about the situation. An elderly man with chronic bronchitis may have pneumococci or *Haemophilus influenzae* in the tracheobronchial tree. This is clearly abnormal, and he may develop pneumonia due to either organism. But if he is treated with antibiotics, something more unpleasant, such as pseudomonas or Klebsiella, may move into the vacuum.

MECHANISMS OF MICROBIAL DISEASES

A thorough knowledge of how microorganisms cause disease is essential to good medical practice. In individual patients, the clinical features may be suggestive of infection with a particular organism. This information is the basis for selecting the right initial treatment. A well-taken history may uncover items such as a tick bite or the fact that the patient works in a slaughterhouse. The diagnoses of Rocky Mountain spotted fever and brucellosis then become easy, and early treatment may be life saving. In many cases, the organism responsible for an infection is never isolated and serologic investigations are negative or confusing. Under these circumstances, the correct interpretation of the clinical features of the illness becomes the only diagnostic resource.

EPIDEMIOLOGIC CONSIDERATIONS

Any organism can cause disease or death under special circumstances. However, when one considers the behavior of infectious diseases in populations, it is useful to maintain the old distinction between pathogens and opportunistic pathogens.

Pathogenic Organisms

Pathogenic organisms are capable of causing disease in a substantial proportion of the normal population. For these persons, the main determinant of disease is the establishment of conditions under which many people become infected. In general, they are found only in man but can survive for only a limited time in any one person and are dependent upon a succession of new hosts for their long-term survival. Diseases such as pneumococcal pneumonia, dysentery, measles, and smallpox fit this pattern. A second type of pathogen is not at all dependent on man for survival but is adapted to some other vertebrates and is transmitted by biting insects. Arbovirus infections, most rickettsioses, and plague are examples.

Opportunistic Pathogens

Opportunistic pathogens are either part of the normal flora of all individuals or are widely disseminated in the environment. Colonization by these organisms is universal, and disease is mostly determined by some special circumstance causing a general or specific impairment of host defenses. At one end of the spectrum is *Staphylococcus aureus*, which causes minor disease in everyone from time to time and, on occasion, causes severe disease in people who are ostensibly normal and have no obvious defect in their defenses. In the middle is *Bacteroides fragilis,* which can cause severe disease, but only when some obvious circumstance, such as a ruptured appendix or an infected placental site, has allowed the organism entry to the tissues. And at the other end is *Pneumocystis carinii,* which causes pneumonia in premature babies, children with various congenital immune deficiency syndromes, and grossly immunosuppressed adults. Also at this end of the spectrum is *Aspergillus fumigatus,* which cannot even maintain itself in the flora of normal individuals but is so widely disseminated in nature as a free-living organism that it is always available to infect those members of the population who are immunosuppressed. A special case arises when huge numbers of organisms are introduced directly into the tissues by intravenous infusions, bladder irrigations, and the like. Under these circumstances, organisms such as *Pseudomonas cepacia* and *Serratia marcescens,* which have virtually no pathogenic potential by themselves, may cause severe disease.

MODES OF TRANSMISSION

The major routes by which infection passes from one person to another are detailed in Table 78-1. It should be noted that while organisms generally spread by one route, they will grow wherever they have the opportunity, and many variations are possible. Thus, syphilis is normally a venereal infection, but it can be acquired transplacentally or by blood transfusion.

Inhalation

Organisms that cause infection by inhalation can be classified into two main types. Streptococci and meningococci are unable to initiate an infection once they have been dried. They are, therefore, spread only by fairly close contact which permits the exchange of moist respiratory droplets. They are typically diseases of the winter months, when people huddle together indoors, or of close, crowded populations such as those in military training camps. Organisms which can survive in dust are not so dependent and cause diseases throughout the year whenever a susceptible host inhales a sufficient dose of organisms. Epidemics of these diseases arise when many people are exposed simultaneously, for example, when a battalion of troops acquires Q fever from being quartered in a barn where the hay contains *Coxiella burneti.*

Ingestion

Organisms causing infection by ingestion also fall into two main groups. One group, exemplified by typhoid and cholera, is usually water-borne but some-

---

TABLE 78–1
Modes of Transmission of Infection

I. **Direct Contact**
  A. Venereal infections—syphilis, gonorrhea
  B. Inoculation of wounds—tetanus, rabies, sporotrichosis
  C. Penetration of intact skin—schistosomiasis, hookworm
  D. Skin-to-skin contact—staphylococcal infections, ectoparasites

II. **Contamination of Food and Water**
  A. Fecal-oral spread from other humans—poliomyelitis, dysentery, amoebiasis, ascariasis
  B. Naturally occurring contamination of food by parasites which can infect man—salmonellosis, trichinosis, tapeworms
  C. Milk-borne diseases—brucellosis, tuberculosis

III. **Respiratory Spread**
  A. By droplet infection only—streptococci, pneumococci, influenza
  B. By inhalation of dried material containing spores or resistant forms—tuberculosis, pulmonary mycoses, anthrax

IV. **Arthropod Vectors**
  A. From man to man—yellow fever, relapsing fever, malaria, filariasis
  B. From animal to man—plague, most rickettsioses

V. **Transmission by Medical Procedures**
  A. Blood transfusion—viral hepatitis
  B. Wound infections—staphylococci, klebsiella, etc.
  C. Associated with urologic instrumentation—various gram-negative rods
  D. Associated with respirators and ancillary equipment—various gram-negative rods
  E. Associated with intravenous therapy
    1. Infected catheters—candida, klebsiella
    2. Infected fluids—various organisms

VI. **Congenital Infections**
  A. Transplacental—syphilis, rubella, toxoplasmosis
  B. From the birth canal—*Herpes simplex,* group B streptococci

---

times may also spread by gross contamination of food. The second group, typified by amebic and bacillary dysentery, are spread by people's hands and are classic infections of mental institutions or military camps where soap and toilet paper are in short supply. Here, the difference may lie in the number of organisms required to establish an infection. Typhoid and cholera need upwards of 10^6 organisms and are best transmitted by some dietary component, such as water, which is consumed in large quantity. Shigellosis can be initiated by as few as 200 organisms, and there is a report that only 10 virulent *Shigella dysenteriae* may suffice.

Arthropod Vectors

Diseases spread by arthropod vectors are greatly influenced by geography and climate because these determine the prevalence of the vectors and intermediate hosts. The epidemic of encephalitis in Venezuela in 1962 probably occurred because heavy rain and flooding both increased the mosquito population and crowded rodents together. Drought may sometimes promote encephalitis if a normally dominant mosquito is eliminated and a more effective vector takes over. Epidemics are also greatly influenced by man's activities. Nomadic peoples, or populations forced to move by war or famine may take their arboviruses or malarial parasites with them into new communities where the local mosquito populations promptly transmit the disease. Alternatively, the new arrivals may be decimated by infections to which the resident population is immune. The crowding of people in shanty towns is associated with pools of water in storage jars, old tires, cans, and wheel ruts in which *Aedes aegypti* can breed. Epidemics of yellow fever, chikungunya, and dengue follow. *Culex fatigans* flourishes in sewage and has led to a dramatic increase in bancroftian filariasis in many Indian cities. In rural areas, irrigation projects often lead to huge increases in mosquito populations and their associated diseases, exemplified by recent outbreaks of Western equine and St. Louis encephalitis in southern California.

VARIATIONS IN THE ORGANISM

Communicability

Any organism which is to cause epidemics must clearly be virulent, but this alone is not sufficient. The organism must also be able to pass easily from one person to another. Evidence of unusual communicability of human pathogens is hard to come by, but the notorious 80/81 strain of *Staphylococcus aureus* could displace other strains from the nose, multiplied there to higher titers, persisted longer in the nose, and survived longer in air and floor dust than less successful strains. *Vibrio cholerae* has recently sustained a mutation which enables the carrier state to persist longer than formerly. The cholera in those afflicted with the disease is apparently of average severity, but the increased efficiency of transmission is responsible for the spread of these strains into parts of Africa and Europe which had been cholera-free for 50 to 100 years.

Virulence

Animal data show clearly that different strains of the same organism may vary strikingly in their ability to cause disease on parenteral challenge, and it is, thus, reasonable to believe that some epidemics in humans arise because the organism responsible has changed into a form which can initiate disease from a smaller inoculum. This is known to be the cause of pandemics of Influenza A, which occur when the virus acquires a hemagglutinin which most of the population has not encountered previously. In bacteria, phenotypic changes which enhance virulence occur when the organisms are passed rapidly from one person to another. The evidence that "epidemic strains" of capsulated organisms do exist is clearest with β-hemolytic streptococcal infections.[14] When a soldier is experimentally infected with material from a sick comrade's throat, he develops a sore throat associated with the presence of large numbers of heavily capsulated streptococci. In the absence of treatment, the streptococci may persist for many weeks, but their infectivity declines steadily and this is associated with a phenotypic change whereby most of the organisms secrete little or no M protein and are nontypable. There is solid experimental evidence that M protein is the major virulence factor for the streptococcus. In naturally acquired streptococcal infections, the severity of disease and the incidence of complications are very variable. In army camps where there is a constant supply of susceptible new recruits, there is intense transmission of streptococci. Disease is common and severe, and rheumatic fever follows about 3 percent of the infections. The streptococci are heavily capsulated and almost all are typable with anti-M sera. In civilian practice, disease is milder, rheumatic fever infrequent, and fully half of the streptococci are nontypable. Analogous but more fragmentary observations exist for pneumococcal, meningococcal, and *H. influenzae* infections.

Evidence of genotypic changes in bacteria which enhance virulence for humans is lacking. There certainly are major differences in virulence between different strains of staphylococci. In a surgical ward which was carefully observed for a year, one strain succeeded in colonizing 80 patients, but did not cause a single case of wound infection. Another strain infected only 12 patients but caused 3 wound infections and 1 case of septicemia. The nature and number of the genes which control these differences are unknown. However, it is clearly possible that hypervirulent strains could arise either by mutation or by any of the methods by which bacteria exchange genes. Plasmid gain or loss would be a particularly attractive explanation of sudden changes in virulence.

VARIATIONS IN THE HOST

Crowding

The commonest and simplest type of epidemic occurs when large numbers of susceptible hosts are crowded together. As discussed above, there is sometimes evidence of increased virulence of the organism. However, epidemics of mycoplasmal and adenovirus pneumonia are also characteristic of military camps, and there is no evidence that these organisms are more virulent than average. During World War I, Glover was able to halt epidemics of meningitis by the simple expedient of spacing the soldiers' beds 6 feet apart instead of the 9 inches which had been customary.[7]

Genetic Differences

When an organism is being transmitted widely in a population, there are often measurable differences between those who fall ill and those who do not. A good example is the tendency of tuberculosis to be extremely severe when it is introduced into a population and to ameliorate within a couple of generations as the genetically susceptible members are killed off.[13] Webster was able to produce two strains of mice, one almost totally resistant to *Salmonella typhimurium* and one almost totally susceptible, by selective breeding from an original population of intermediate sensitivity. If a cage full of equal numbers of sensitive and resistant mice was infected by introducing a new mouse excreting *S. typhimurium,* the resulting epidemic would pick out only the sensitive mice, leaving the resistant ones unharmed. The virulence of the organism, as measured in a third strain of mice, was unaltered.[20]

In general, we do not know how genetic factors make one person susceptible to a particular infection whereas another is not. Most familial infections in humans are to be explained by common exposure to infection, but there are examples of families where several members from two or three generations have died at different times from meningococcal meningitis. Other members of the same families have developed disseminated gonococcemia, and a few persons have developed both types of infection at different times. This specific inability to handle Neisseria is due to deficiency of one of the late acting complement components; familial deficiency of C6, C7, or C8 can cause this syndrome.

Phenotypic Differences

Any phenotypic change which suppresses the inflammatory response or the immune system will render an individual susceptible to infectious conditions which happen to be prevalent at the time. The change may be a general one, such as corticosteroid treatment predisposing to all infections, or a local one, exemplified by the prevalence of all forms of pneumonia in those with chronic lung disease. The most important phenotypic determinant of infectious disease on a world-wide scale is malnutrition. Malnutrition predisposes to infectious disease, and infectious disease compounds the malnutrition. The resulting vicious cycle is responsible for the enormous childhood mortalities in developing countries, and in adult populations the well-fed members generally escape with much lower mortality than those less fortunate.

Acquired Immunity

Assuming that an organism is being widely transmitted in a population, another major determinant of individual susceptibility is acquired immunity. In almost all diseases, a substantial amount of immunity develops during childhood as a consequence of prior experience with small doses of the same organisms or with cross-reacting antigens of other organisms. The efficiency of the protection provided to the individual varies with the organism concerned. Opsonizing antibody against the common gram-negative rods develops within a few weeks of birth, and fairly solid protection ensues. Similarly, many pneumococci cross-react with throat streptococci of the normal flora, and a substantial degree of immunity is obtained. Substantial levels of resistance to *Mycobacterium tuberculosis* can be produced by prior exposure to atypical mycobacteria, which themselves are of low virulence. On the other hand, organisms that have very great strain differences are little affected by previous experience of the population with anything other than the epidemic strain. It should be noted that minor degrees of immunity may be useful in populations where exposure to infection is random and inocula are often low. In fact, "herd immunity" may be substantial when formal challenge of individuals shows no measurable protection.

An important public health question is whether immunizing one part of a population protects the other, unimmunized part. The answer seems to vary from one disease to another. In diphtheria, the bacillus is unable to maintain itself adequately in the throats of immunized persons; so that when more than 75 percent of the population is immunized, carrier rates decline and the organism may disappear from a community. Since the nonimmunized people are not exposed to the organism, they are also protected. However, if the vaccine does not reduce transmission of the agent, but merely prevents the disease, nonimmunized individuals are not at all protected.

There has been a recent epidemic of 108 cases of poliomyelitis in the Netherlands in a religious group that eschews vaccination.[2] This occurred despite the fact that more than 95 percent of the general population had been immunized with killed polio vaccine. Immunity of the general public was proved because not a single case was seen in a vaccinated person. In the United States, only about 65 percent of the population has been immunized against polio, but the live vaccine is used. This has two effects; it blocks the enteric transmission of wild type polioviruses, and because the vaccine is alive, it may spread to members of the population who have not been formally immunized. At any rate, the present incidence of polio in the United States, is less than 10 cases per year.

CONTROL OF INFECTIOUS DISEASES

Control of infectious diseases in populations may be approached in three general ways: to interfere with the mode of transmission of the organism, to rely on case-finding and isolation procedures, and to artificially induce immunity. The first is the most certain: typhoid and cholera have disappeared because we have been reasonably successful in separating drinking water from sewage; most people do not carry body lice, so we do not see typhus or relapsing fevers; pasteurization of milk has reduced brucellosis to a slaughter house problem. The second is only rarely of value because in most diseases the ratio of asymptomatic carriers to obvious cases is high, and even in an infection such as measles, where almost everyone gets the disease, the most infectious period occurs before the rash comes out. Smallpox has been totally eradicated because its only host is man, serious infectivity does not precede the rash, there are no asymptomatic or chronic carriers, and the spread of disease can be checked by isolation of cases and the vaccination of contacts. The efficacy of immunization varies from one disease to another. Diphtheria and tetanus toxins are single, well-characterized proteins which are good immunogens. These diseases have, therefore, been essentially eliminated in developed countries. Antibacterial immunity is usually much less effective; typhoid vaccine is only marginally useful. However, as mentioned above, less than perfect immunity may still be very useful on a population scale; BCG is only 80 percent effective in preventing tuberculosis, but if tuberculosis is responsible for 10 percent of all deaths, a large reduction in mortality and morbidity can be obtained by the use of BCG.

Diseases where the mode of transmission is secure, the number of asymptomatic carriers is high, and no effective immunity can be developed are not controllable by present methods. Good examples are gonorrhea and most upper respiratory tract infections.

THE MECHANISMS OF MICROBIAL DAMAGE

Bacteria

Occasionally, bottles of intravenous fluids become contaminated by bacteria. Most of these organisms are of low pathogenicity; they have been selected by the ability to grow at 4°C, to survive boiling, to grow in the water in which autoclaved bottled are cooled, and similarly irrelevant criteria. Some of them cannot even be identified by conventional means. And yet the introduction of these nonpathogens into the bloodstream causes high fever and shock, and if the infusion is not terminated rapidly, death may ensue. Gram-negative organisms are much more likely to cause death than are gram-positive ones. The deaths almost all occur within a few hours of the contaminated transfusion and are not influenced by antimicrobic therapy. There is no evidence that the organisms have multiplied after introduction into the bloodstream. Indeed, the patients' blood and internal organs are usually sterile.

Similar observations have been made by injecting dead bacteria into the skin of man; the number of gram-negative organisms required to cause an abscess is the same whether or not the organisms are pathogenic. Dead gram-positive organisms must be injected in much larger doses to produce the same effect, and again, nonpathogens are just as effective as pathogens.[8]

Thus, the introduction of large numbers of bacterial bodies into the bloodstream of man causes shock and death; injection into skin causes abscesses. In the skin experiments, bacterial multiplication and exotoxin production were excluded as washed dead bacteria were used. In blood transfusion accidents, multiplication and exotoxin production are improbable explanations. In both cases, "nonpathogenic" organisms are just as damaging as are "pathogens." Therefore, there must be properties common to all bacterial bodies which cause disease.

In the case of gram-negative organisms, the principal inflammatory component is the endotoxin. Injection of large doses of endotoxin produces fever, hypotension progressing to shock, hypercoagulability of the blood, and death. The portion of the endotoxin molecule which is responsible for these effects is lipid A; there are only minor structural variations in this substance between one gram-negative organism and another, and all endotoxins are roughly equal in toxicity on a weight basis. The weight of endotoxin per bacterial cell does vary somewhat, but not by more than one log. Thus, any gram-negative organism will cause disease if a large enough population is achieved.

In the case of gram-positive bacteria, the toxic structural component common to all organisms is the peptidoglycan. This produces many of the effects of endotoxin, but the dose required is between 1 and 4 logs higher. Teichoic acids also contribute to the inflammatory effect. Gram-positive cell walls are particularly effective at causing local abscesses; many peptidoglycans cannot be digested efficiently by phagocytes, so that the inflammatory stimulus is long lasting.

With all bacteria, many of the features of disease occur because of overstimulated host responses. Fever, elevated sedimentation rate, and other acute phase reactions are known to be caused by proteins liberated from neutrophils and macrophages in inflammatory sites. These proteins reach the circulation through the lymph and alter the function of organs, such as the hypothalamus and the liver, in a quasi-hormonal way.[4] Abscesses are largely caused by digestion of host tissue by proteases liberated from phagocytic cells, primarily neutrophils. These enzymes are released by the cells to some extent during phagocytosis, and the total content is released if the cell dies. Inhibitors of proteolytic enzymes are present in normal serum, so that release of small amounts of proteases do no damage. However, large numbers of bacteria attract large numbers of phagocytes. The local protease concentration rises to levels which overwhelm the serum inhibitors, and suppuration follows.

Immunologic reactions may also contribute to tissue damage. One organism weighs about 1 picogram, far below the weight threshold for any immunologic reaction, so that large populations of bacteria are required to cause damage. All organisms fix complement by the alternate pathway; this may cause activation of the Hageman factor and promote blood clotting. Thromboplastic substances liberated from neutrophils and platelets are thought to contribute, and the process may go on to disseminated intravascular coagulation. Antigen–antibody complexes are responsible for some unusual features of disease such as erythema nodosum, glomerulonephritis, and the arthritis of meningococcemia.

Involvement of other mechanisms is speculative. Anaphylaxis is probably not important in most infections, although there is a suggestion that it causes the spreading edema of pneumococcal pneumonia. It is possible that cells which have adsorbed bacterial antigens might be subject to cytotoxic attack by macrophages and lymphocytes. Lastly, cell-mediated immunity may be involved. The internal antigens of bacteria do not vary greatly, and delayed skin reactions to them can be elicited in the majority of the normal population. Furthermore, intense cell-mediated immune reactions lead to tissue destruction, as in tuberculosis. One can only guess how far cell-mediated immunity accounts for damage in ordinary infections, but intravenous injection of antigens to which CMI is established is one of the few immunologic reactions which can cause rapid death.

The features discussed so far apply to all bacteria; they explain why any bacterium is pathogenic under special circumstances. However, some organisms have special features which enable them to cause death or tissue damage at less than the usual concentrations. The most important of these is exotoxin production. In some cases, infection may not be necessary; the toxin is produced in food and remains toxic even if the bacteria are subsequently killed. Staphylococcal and other bacterial food poisonings are produced in this way. In other cases, such as diphtheria and tetanus, infection is necessary, but a local lesion suffices as a depot in which a lethal dose of exotoxin can be made. Some bacteria which do cause septicemia may kill because of exotoxin production; anthrax and *Pseudomonas aeruginosa* are examples.

Many pathogenic bacteria produce extracellular enzymes and short-range toxins which enhance local tissue destruction. Leukocidins cause damage indirectly by killing phagocytes with subsequent release of lysosomal enzymes into the tissue. Bacterial proteases and other destructive enzymes cause damage directly; one particularly clear example is the digestion of the cornea by the elastase of *Pseudomonas aeruginosa*.

Viruses

The most obvious way in which viruses cause disease is by multiplying inside cells and killing them. In the case of infection of neurons by poliomyelitis or of respiratory epithelium by influenza, this may be the whole explanation of the disease state. However, immunologic reactions to viral antigens are important in many diseases. Complexes of hepatitis B surface antigen and immunoglobulin M have been found in the arterial walls of some patients with polyarteritis nodosa. It is strongly suspected that viral antigen–antibody complexes may cause some cases of glomerulonephritis and may partially explain the pathology of systemic lupus erythematosus. Cells infected by enveloped viruses may display viral antigens on their membranes. They are then subject to cytolytic attack, either by macrophages and K cells which need antibody to identify the infected cell as a target, or by cytotoxic T cells which recognize viral antigens directly. Cytotoxicity mediated by T cells is known to underlie the fatal outcome of lymphocytic choriomeningitis in mice, and some workers think that the overt phase of viral hepatitis represents destruction of infected hepatocytes by T cells.

Fungi and Parasites

The mechanisms by which these organisms cause disease are the same as those discussed above—various combinations of direct damage and overstimulated immune reactions. Further details should be sought in textbooks of mycology and parasitology.[6,15]

DEFENSES AGAINST INFECTION

When an infectious agent reaches a new host, the outcome is determined by events occurring at a series of defense lines starting at epithelial surfaces and ending with the bloodstream. Mechanisms at individual epithelial surfaces are all different because of the very different chemical and physical circumstances which obtain there and because of great local variations in the established bacterial and protozoal floras. Once the tissues have been breached, responses are more stereotyped; there is little histologic difference between a dental abscess and an appendix abscess. Because bacterial infections are still the most common cause of severe or lethal disease, much of the discussion will center on them, but many of the principles apply also to viral, protozoal, and helminthic diseases, and digressions will be made where it seems appropriate.

MECHANICAL FACTORS

The most important host defenses are the chemical and biologic factors which prevent colonization of epithelial surfaces by pathogenic bacteria, the integrity of the skin and mucous membranes, and the mechanical arrangements by which normally sterile areas of the body are protected from the huge bacterial populations in the upper airway and in the gastrointestinal tract. These mechanisms function by keeping the inoculum size of invading microorganisms at levels which other body defenses can cope with. In experimental animals, there are very few organisms which can establish a lethal infection when a single

bacterium breaches the defenses. Conversely, almost any organism can establish a lethal infection if introduced intravenously, intraperitoneally, or subcutaneously in adequate numbers. Similarly, experimental pyelonephritis or pneumonia can easily be produced by injecting organisms into the kidney or down the trachea. Clinical analogues of these experiments can be seen on any hospital ward.

Skin

Normal skin is dry and has a pH of about 5. Very few organisms grow well under these conditions, and usually the skin flora is restricted to a few corynebacteria, propionibacteria, and *Staphylococcus albus*. These organisms make life even more difficult for competitors by splitting the triglycerides of sebum into unsaturated fatty acids (chiefly oleic), which are bactericidal. Hemolytic streptococci and *Escherichia coli* die on skin within 20 minutes. The vital importance of normal skin is underlined by the effects of destroying it. Extensive burns are often lethal because many organisms can multiply in the wet, dead tissue and from this base can cause cellulitis and septicemia. Before antibiotics were available, death was usually due to infection with staphylococci and streptococci; nowadays, it tends to follow infection with pseudomonas or Candida species. Other diseases leading to extensive skin loss, such as exfoliative dermatitis, pemphigus, and mycosis fungoides, are also eventually lethal because of uncontrollable infection. Minor impairment in the skin defenses is commonly seen in housewives who constantly have their hands in water and, in addition, remove their skin lipids with detergent. Dermatitis and paronychia due to Candida species commonly result. More seriously, overuse of detergents has been implicated in outbreaks of pyoderma in newborn nurseries.

Wound Infections

Wound infections do not normally follow a simple incision which is rapidly repaired, even though contamination of the deeper tissues undoubtedly occurs. Some other factor which enables the initial inoculum to multiply is required, and the commonest are accumulations of blood or serum or the presence of dead tissue or a foreign body in the wound. These facts underly the established surgical management of wounds—adequate debridement, removal of foreign material, complete hemostasis, and the use of nonirritant sutures. *Why* foreign bodies promote infection has never been made clear; *that* they do is solidly proved experimentally[5] and exemplified clinically by abscesses around splinters and sutures, infection of metal screws and plates in orthopedic practice, and infections in deeper tissues containing foreign materials such as prosthetic valves and dacron vascular grafts.

Mucous Membranes

The bowel contains staggering numbers of potential pathogens. Under normal circumstances the mucosa is an extremely efficient barrier, but it seems probable that it is not quite as complete as is the skin. Small numbers of bacteria have been cultivated from the portal blood of normal people, and in cirrhotics, systemic bacteremia is not unusual;[18] presumably shunts take portal blood around the liver, and bacteria are not filtered out by Kupffer cells. In mice, even nonpathogens like *Bacillus cereus* can be recovered from the liver after oral challenge, and in man, various anerobes have been found circulating after sigmoidoscopy. Other mucous surfaces are likewise not entirely impermeable to bacteria—mouth streptococci may be found circulating after dental procedures or vigorous chewing, organisms in the urinary tract may cause bacteremia after instrumentation or spontaneously, pneumococci and meningococci can apparently cross the nasal mucous membrane in small numbers, and so on. This all underlines the point made earlier that small inocula of almost any organism can be coped with and may, in fact, give rise to useful degrees of immunity. Many people have antibody to the Type I pneumococcus without ever having had pneumonia. A second point is that these small leaks may lead to significant disease in an otherwise normal person if there is a site suitable for colonization such as a stenotic mitral valve. In persons whose defenses are defective, generalized sepsis may result.

Peritonitis

Normal people develop serious infections with their own flora when some kind of breach occurs in an epithelial surface and massive and continuing contamination of the tissues occurs. In the abdomen, perforated peptic ulcer, appendicitis, and postoperative anastomotic leaks are common examples of through and through communications that allow gut flora to directly infect the peritoneal cavity. The inocula are huge, and even though the organisms are not particularly virulent, large and continuing leaks lead inevitably to fatal general peritonitis. Small leaks lead to localized abscesses at the site of perforation or perhaps to transperitoneal spread to the subphrenic spaces or the pouch of Douglas. The normal peritoneum can destroy very large numbers of bacteria if these are injected all at once and in pure culture. 10^8 *Escherichia coli* or *Streptococcus fecalis* disappear without trace when injected into the peritoneal cavity of a normal

dog. Experimental peritonitis with one organism can only be established if some kind of particulate matter is also injected or if blood is present in the peritoneal cavity. A different mechanism for establishing experimental peritonitis is to use mixtures of organisms. In the dog, 10^6 *Escherichia coli* plus 10^6 *Streptococcus fecalis* causes lethal peritonitis.

The clinical correlates of this are clear: by far the most important therapeutic maneuver is to close the leak, and if that cannot be accomplished, cure is improbable. The best that can be hoped for is that by draining the site to the outside, a fistula will form which will prevent local abscess formation and which later may close spontaneously. The peritoneum should be cleansed of food particles, feces, and blood, and a drain should be inserted to prevent local accumulations of blood or serum which subsequently might become infected. If antibiotics are to be given, it is not necessary to treat every organism found in the peritoneal cavity because many of the infections are synergic. Altemeier[1] has pointed out that the mortality of general peritonitis secondary to a ruptured appendix dropped sharply when penicillin became available and has not subsequently changed very much. It is hardly necessary to say that most of the bowel flora is not susceptible to penicillin.

Mouth

In the mouth, there are also large populations of organisms, and local sepsis related to dental caries and periodontal disease is common. Again, the susceptibility to infection should not be exaggerated; it is in fact surprising that people with the poorest oral hygiene may go for years without problems. Similarly, although osteitis of bone adjoining the nasal sinuses or the middle ear cavity is common and important, it is uncommon when compared to the total incidence of acute otitis media and sinusitis.

Respiratory Tract

The respiratory tract below the level of the larynx is usually sterile. Aspiration of small quantities of material from the upper airway is probably a normal occurrence during sleep, but the organisms are mopped up by alveolar macrophages or physically removed by the ciliary blanket, and no harm results. Aspiration of larger quantities of material is exceedingly frequent during unconscious states such as strokes or drug overdoses. Any neurologic disease causing bulbar palsy, such as motor neuron disease or poliomyelitis, may lead to aspiration when the patient is fully conscious. Achalasia and other causes of esophageal obstruction are classically associated with bilateral basal pneumonitis. Aspiration during anesthesia is commonplace even when the anesthetist has noticed nothing amiss and an endotracheal tube has been in place.

Aspiration pneumonia may occur in people with a normal swallowing mechanism in any situation where cough is ineffective, when the ciliary movement is inhibited by irritant gases such as tobacco smoke or nitrogen dioxide, or when there are localized areas of inefficient drainage due to bronchial obstruction or bronchiectasis. It may also occur when there is some defect of the patients' immune system as a whole, as in myeloma or granulocytopenic states. Most aspiration pneumonias and lung abscesses are due to mixtures of anaerobic organisms.

Secretory Glands

All the glands of external secretion open onto heavily infected surfaces but are themselves sterile. Most secretions contain various bacteriostatic and bactericidal substances, such as lysozyme and lactoperoxidase, but a major defense mechanism is the constant flow of secretion. Obstruction of any gland duct by a calculus or stricture is sooner or later followed by infection behind the block. In addition to the stagnant pool of nutrient material provided to the organism, leucocytes have difficulty emigrating into the area because of the increased pressure, which in the case of the salivary glands may exceed the arterial pressure. Ascending cholangitis is a good example of this type of infection and may be impossible to eradicate without removing the stone.

The Urinary Tract

The urinary tract is a special case because of its anatomic complexity. In the male, the urethra is long and the ingress of bacteria is further prevented by potent bactericidal substances in prostatic fluid. Contamination of the bladder by microbes is, therefore, common, and even in the presence of prostatic obstruction or a urethral stricture with considerable residual urine, infection is uncommon unless the patient has been catheterized. By contrast, in females the urethra is short, and the external opening is deeply buried in the introitus. Bowel flora often flourish in the moist skin folds, and may easily ascend to the bladder. "Spontaneous" infections are common, and if there is residual urine because of uterine prolapse or some other disorder, the frequency of infection becomes very high. In both sexes, obstruction of the upper urinary tract by stone or idiopathic hydronephrosis is rarely complicated by infection if the patient has not been instrumented. Once the urinary tract is infected, the infection will persist despite therapy unless the obstruction is corrected and may persist even then because of the ability of organisms to survive in protected enclaves such as the renal medulla.

HOSPITAL ORGANISMS

The last few paragraphs have dealt with circumstances which allow the normal flora to establish infections. In general, such infections are relatively easily managed because the organisms are susceptible to antibiotics. But persons in hospitals may be colonized in various sites with "hospital organisms" which are at once unusually communicable, unusually capable of displacing the normal flora, and may be more virulent than average. This type of colonization is potentiated by antibiotic therapy, and the larger the dose, the broader the spectrum, and the more drugs used, the more likely is colonization by a resistant organism. However, this is not the only factor. Sanford has clearly shown that normal, healthy hospital employees do not colonize their upper airway with Klebsiella species, nor do physically healthy patients on the psychiatry service. But sick patients develop spontaneous colonization within a few days of admission, and the "sicker" they are (as measured by hypotension, fever, etc.), the more probable this is. Patients so colonized frequently go on to develop frank infections with the same organism.[10]

ANTIMICROBICS

Antimicrobics may also encourage the growth of members of the normal flora which are usually present in numbers too small to cause disease. Thrush and staphylococcal enteritis are good examples of the diseases which may ensue. The pathogenesis cannot be simple, however, because only a minority of patients given broad-spectrum oral antimicrobics develop these complications, and both are seen occasionally in the absence of antibiotic therapy.

DEFENSES OF MUCOUS MEMBRANES

The Bowel

Enteric pathogens must succeed in establishing residence on the intestinal mucosa and often must multiply there to provide a population with which a successful tissue invasion can be mounted. We know almost nothing of the factors involved here, but they must be one important determinant of whether or not disease develops following colonization. At least in some cases, protection appears to be predictable statistically but not individually, which suggests the operation of many random variables. Hornick showed that some men can develop shigellosis following challenge with only 200 organisms, whereas others remained well after 10^5 organisms. If he now took these "resistant" men and rechallenged them with an intermediate dose causing illness in about 50 percent of an unselected group, about 50 percent of them would develop infection.

One important defense against enteric pathogens is gastric acid. Gastric juice is very damaging to both *Salmonella typhi* and *Vibrio cholerae,* and both tend to infect members of the population who are taking antacids, have had gastrectomies, or are for other reasons achlorhydric. The established normal flora of the bowel is a powerful defense against both shigella and salmonella infections because acetic, propionic, and butyric acids produced by bacteroides species are lethal to the pathogens. Experimentally, in man, broad-spectrum antibiotics increase susceptibility to *Salmonella typhi* many-fold. Clinically, antimicrobic therapy for nontyphoidal salmonelloses leads an increased incidence and duration of the carrier state. Lastly, the normal motility of the bowel may also be an important defense; there is at least one clinical trial in which patients with shigellosis who were given diphenoxylate developed a much more severe infection than those left untreated.

The Respiratory Tract

Respiratory pathogens must also establish residence in an upper airway thickly populated with well-adapted organisms of the normal flora. However, one rarely sees antibiotic therapy predisposing to streptococcal or meningococcal infections because these organisms are themselves susceptible to most of the common antibiotics.

Secretory Antibody

Acquired immunity is presumably responsible for the termination of carrier states, although again we know almost nothing of the mechanisms involved. One factor is probably secretory antibody because protection against reinfection is type specific or strain specific. Attachment to receptors on epithelial cells is a necessary preliminary for organisms which must penetrate into cells to establish infection. Secretory antibody is known to block attachment of salmonella and shigellae. Mycoplasmal and chlamydial infections are also prevented by secretory antibody, but here the mechanism seems to be destruction of the organisms once they get inside epithelial cells.

TISSUE DEFENSES

Nonspecific Mechanisms

Once organisms enter the tissues, many factors determine whether or not they will be able to grow there. A few are unable to grow at an elevated temperature,

and this confines them to cooler regions of the body. Rhinoviruses and certain mycobacteria infecting the skin are examples. Others are unable to grow at the oxidation-reduction potential of normal tissues. Neither *Clostridium tetani* nor *Clostridium perfringens* cause disease when injected intramuscularly into animals, but each causes lethal infection 1) if other organisms in the injection, themselves nonpathogenic, scavenge the local oxygen; 2) if the infection contains an agent promoting local death of muscle; or 3) if the local blood supply is temporarily shut off by including epinephrine in the injection. The clinical parallels are obvious. It seems likely that many other anaerobic infections get their start in these ways. Some organisms are unable to find an essential nutrient in normal tissue, and it must be supplied by another organism growing synergically. The mouth flora found in lung abscesses are good examples: *Treponema microdentium* needs at least three growth factors which are supplied by other components of the mix, and doubtless reciprocal benefits obtain.

Although most organisms grow well on various soups and digests of animal tissue; the nutrients they need may not be available to them in the living host with undenatured proteins. Iron is bound so tightly by the transferrin in normal serum that the free concentration is estimated at 10^{-18} M. In animals, the most diverse infections can be potentiated by many orders of magnitude by saturating transferrin with intravenous iron. In kwashiorkor, most deaths are due to infection, and there is some suggestion that those children with reduced serum transferrin are the most likely to die and that rapid intravenous repletion of iron stores may actually be detrimental.

Phagocytosis

Pathogenic organisms are not susceptible to the nonspecific defense mechanisms discussed above and can be destroyed only by phagocytic cells. They can be divided into two classes: the vast majority are incapable of surviving phagocytosis and are dealt with by polymorphonuclear neutrophil leukocytes which are mobilized by the acute inflammatory response. Local macrophage populations and monocytes mobilized from the blood assist in this process. This type of infection is a race between the proliferating organism and the phagocytic defenses. If the host does not die of septicemia, the organism loses the race as soon as anticapsular antibody has been synthesized. The only way it can survive for an extended period is by establishing some protected enclave, such as an abscess, osteomyelitis, or endocarditis, where the host defenses are ineffective. Infections with the pyogenic cocci and aerobic and anaerobic gram-negative rods are of this type. A smaller group is little affected by polymorphs and is initially capable of surviving also in monocytes and macrophages. However, during the course of infection, macrophages acquire new capacities that enable them to kill organisms which were at first capable of growing in their cytoplasm. This process takes time and is not always effective, so that infections of this type tend to chronicity and are characterized by granulomatous inflammation. Examples are tuberculosis and most systemic fungal infections.

The immune system is involved in defense to both types of organism; antibodies (secreted by B cells) with or without assistance from complement opsonize extracellular parasites and allow neutrophils to ingest and destroy them; for the second group, sensitized T lymphoid cells convert normal macrophages to activated "killer" macrophages which can destroy their contained parasites ("cell-mediated immunity"). Both the nature of the process by which T cells instruct macrophages and the mechanism by which the macrophages kill the organisms, are currently obscure.

Some bacteria appear to be intermediate in their properties. Thus, *Staphylococcus aureus* can survive intracellularly in small numbers. Salmonellae and brucellae are intracellular parasites, but it is easy to show experimentally that antibody does add a certain degree of protection.

Abscesses

Although the evidence is hard to obtain, it seems likely that the overwhelming majority of infections are disposed of without ever causing enough local inflammation to arouse symptoms. Only some combination of unfortunate circumstances allows an extracellular parasite to achieve a substantial local bacterial population. If it does, however, the resulting abscess provides conditions under which it is much easier for the organisms to survive. Many organisms produce toxins which are specifically able to kill phagocytic cells. Streptolysins O and S and the Panton-Valentine leukocidin of staphylococci are examples. The amount of these toxins produced by a single organism is inconsequential, but the concentrations may become very significant in abscess cavities; certainly it can be seen histologically that phagocytes which attempt to invade the area die before they reach it. Abscesses also contain large amounts of enzymes which are derived from the granules of dead polymorphs; these break down and liquify the tissue to produce a menstruum in which phagocytosis would be very inefficient even if phagocytes could survive. Chemotaxis cannot occur in a liquid medium, and proteolytic enzymes would destroy anti-

body and complement opsonins. As will be mentioned again later, many organisms cannot be killed in the absence of oxygen even if they could be phagocytosed: because of the very high bacterial population, growth is slow or nonexistent. Antibiotics which inhibit cell wall synthesis and rely on continued growth to burst the organism are therefore ineffective, and antibiotics which inhibit growth are also useless. The upshot of all this is that abscesses cannot be expected to heal spontaneously, nor can they be treated effectively with antibiotics. If spontaneous or surgical drainage does not occur, the best that can be hoped for is encapsulation and eventual walling off by fibrous tissue.

Spread of Infection

Meantime, the abscess provides a base from which further invasions can occur. Because of the extensive breakdown of macromolecules, the osmotic pressure is high and the pus is under tension. Abscesses, therefore, tend to enlarge and to dissect along or between fascial planes. This accounts for many classical syndromes such as the groin abscess secondary to vertebral caries or the tendency of infections of the little finger to involve all the tendon sheaths anterior to the wrist joint.

Not all organisms excite such a pronounced inflammatory response that they become localized at the site of entry. Pneumococci, streptococci, and clostridia excite a more exudative reaction, and organisms can travel far as the infected edema fluid dissects tissue planes. This is the type of infection seen in lobar pneumonia, cellulitis, and gas gangrene. If the infected tissue dies, as in necrotizing fasciitis or gas gangrene, the inflammatory response becomes completely ineffective, and very extensive surgery may be required.

Organisms not immediately localized tend to spread through lymphatics to the local nodes. As a rule, the lymphatics themselves are not inflamed, but lymphangitis is classical in streptococcal infections. Lymph nodes contain large numbers of macrophages with their processes strung across the sinusoids and are very efficient filters. This efficiency is soon greatly increased by the arrival of polymorphonuclear cells from the blood. Swelling and tenderness of lymph nodes draining infected areas are common, but abscesses are quite unusual. A fully inflamed lymph node may remove and destroy all but 0.001 percent of the organisms presented to it.

Bacteremia

There are two main types of bacteremia. The first occurs when the last lymph node in a chain allows organisms access to the thoracic or right lymphatic ducts.

This type of bacteremia is usually intermittent. It is not uncommon in pneumonias of all types, presumably because the lymph node chains are short, but is uncommon with localized infections of the extremities or abdomen. The second type of bacteremia occurs as a consequence of the penchant of some organisms such as bacteroides or pseudomonas to invade blood vessels and set up a septic thrombophlebitis. Infected emboli break off and establish a hematogenous pneumonia or pylephlebitis, and from these organs further spread may occur by a similar mechanism. Bacteremia also occurs occasionally by displacement of organisms into the circulation from small or trivial abscesses with no evidence of lymphatic spread or venous thrombosis. Sometimes recognizable factors can be elicited from the history, as in the case of the man who had high fever and shaking chills every time he had a bowel movement and proved to have a paracolic abscess.

Bacteremia is usually associated with spectacular symptoms; fever, shaking chills, prostration, and shock. Very large numbers of organisms can be cleared from the bloodstream by the liver and spleen macrophages, and even capsulated pneumococci cannot maintain themselves in the circulating blood. Continuous bacteremia can only occur when organisms are continually fed into the circulation, typically when there is an intravascular focus such as endocarditis or septic thrombophlebitis. This is the idea behind the clinical rule that continued bacteremia with *Staphylococcus aureus* is probably due to endocarditis and should be treated as such.[19]

Metastatic Infections

Occasionally, organisms localize in the meninges, joints, bones, or other sites during bacteremia and set up metastatic infections. We have no clear idea of how the penetration is effected, but presumably similar mechanisms during subclinical bacteremia account for the otherwise inexplicable osteomyelitis or brain abscess occurring in a setting of perfect health or when the local lesion seems trivial.

DEFECTS IN THE INFLAMMATORY RESPONSE

Because inflammation is such a complex process, many different types of defect may cause it to be inefficient and predispose to infection. Here, a series of circumscribed defects will be described, each of which increase susceptibility to infection in single, understandable ways. They are mostly rare, but useful as illustrations. The common clinical conditions predisposing to infection, such as diabetes, starvation, and malignancy, act at more than one point and will be discussed in Chapter 91.

Blood Supply

Inflammation cannot occur in the absence of a blood supply, as exemplified by the tendency to gangrene in an ischemic foot. Similarly, pneumonia and osteomyelitis in sickle-cell disease appear to be attributable to blockage of small vessels with masses of sickled cells.

Neutropenia

Any condition in which there is a deficiency of circulating neutrophils predisposes to infection. The susceptibility to infection becomes measurable when the neutrophil count falls below $1000/\mu l$ and becomes very severe as the count drops toward zero. If a pneumonia or septicemia occurs in a patient with <100 neutrophils$/\mu l$, recovery is improbable unless the count rises spontaneously or the patient is given granulocyte transfusions.[9] Only mature neutrophils are efficient phagocytes; leukemic cells are not mobilized into inflammatory sites. Most neutropenias are due to bone marrow depression, which also affects the rate at which monocytes can be delivered to the tissues; if the monocyte count is >500, as in some congenital neutropenias, susceptibility to infection may not be marked.

Chemotactic Defects

Once in the tissues, neutrophils must seek out the organisms. Most bacteria produce directly acting chemotactic factors, but other factors are derived from C3 and C5. Congenital deficiency of either of these proteins is known to predispose to infection, but it is improbable that the lowered levels of C3 in nephritis, liver disease, or systemic lupus erythematosus are low enough to be significant. Some congenital defects in which leukocytes do not respond to chemotactic factors have been described ("lazy leukocyte syndrome"), and the patients have had recurrent gingivitis and otitis media. Serum inhibitors of chemotaxis have been described in cirrhosis of the liver and as a congenital abnormality. Lastly, abnormalities of overall neutrophil motility have been described and attributed to a defective actin molecule.

Phagocytic Defects

Once the organisms come within range, they must be phagocytosed. Most nonpathogens can be phagocytosed in liquid media containing no serum; mere contact between cell and organism is enough. Pathogens usually have capsules and other surface structures that make phagocytosis difficult, but they can be taken up by being trapped against tissue surfaces. Any cause of pulmonary edema predisposes to pneumonia, and interference with surface phagocytosis is thought to be the mechanism. Almost all bacteria can fix complement through the alternate, or properdin pathway, and the C3 fixed on the bacterial surface is a useful opsonin. Two men with different defects of this pathway have been described; both had many episodes of sepsis with pneumococci, staphylococci, meningococci, and *Haemophilus influenzae*. Since there is no corresponding increase in susceptibility to infection in people with congenital defects of C2 or C4, it seems at present that complement fixation by the early components of the classical pathway is less vital to antibacterial defense.

The most efficient opsonin is specific antibody, especially IgM antibody. This is because a single molecule of IgM on a bacterial surface will fix many hundred molecules of C3b, but many IgG molecules must bind before two of them happen to take up the right alignment. "Natural antibody" to all common pathogens is present in normal serum and much of it is of the IgM class. It arises from prior experience with the organism or with cross-reacting antigens, and its importance is likely to be very great. Any condition in which immunoglobulin synthesis is impaired is associated with an increased frequency and severity of infection with extracellular parasites.

Defective Killing of Phagocytosed Bacteria

Once neutrophils have phagocytosed organisms, degranulation normally occurs and lysosomal enzymes are delivered onto the surface of the organism, which is subsequently killed. The neutrophil contains at least two types of granules, one of which contains myeloperoxidase. In the presence of oxygen, normal cells generate hydrogen peroxide, and peroxidase uses this to kill the organisms by mechanisms which are still uncertain. Children with chronic granulomatous disease are unable to make hydrogen peroxide, and they commonly fall prey to staphylococcal infections at an early age. Other, less crippling defects of this system have been described, and acquired varieties may cause increased susceptibility to infection in adult life. The neutrophil does have a second set of granular enzymes which do not require oxygen for their action; however, a few organisms are not susceptible to them. When these organisms (staphylococci, candida, and some gram-negative rods) are phagocytosed under anaerobic conditions, they are not killed.

None of these defects in chemotaxis, opsonins, phagocytosis, or intracellular bacterial killing is as devastating as total absence of neutrophils. Even an untreated child with chronic granulomatous disease survives for a year or two, whereas a person with complete agranulocytosis rarely lasts a week. The reason probably is that so many of these mechanisms

are multiple, and while absence of a given factor may make infection more probable, it does not make it either inevitable or uncontrollable.

DEFECTS IN CELL-MEDIATED IMMUNITY

Congenital defects of cell-mediated immunity may or may not be associated with immunoglobulin deficiency and may be of several grades of severity. The simplest is perhaps chronic mucocutaneous candidiasis, in which there seems to be a more or less pure inability to establish delayed hypersensitivity to *Candida albicans*. More severe disorders, such as the DiGeorge syndrome, are associated with intractable infections with mycobacteria, various fungi, many viruses, especially *Herpes simplex* and *Pneumocystis carinii*. Severe combined immunodeficiency ("Swiss agammaglobulinemia") is almost inevitably fatal because when neither B or T cell systems are working, the patient is susceptible to all kinds of infectious agents. The only children with this defect who have survived have been treated by being raised in the germ-free state or by bone marrow transplantation.

In adults, deficiency of the T cell system occurs naturally in old age, although usually the anergy is partial rather than total. Various lymphomas and nonneoplastic diseases of lymphoid tissue, such as sarcoidosis and leprosy, may produce it. It is also a common complication of radiation, corticosteroid, and cytotoxic therapy for leukemia and other neoplasms. The infections which commonly result are those listed above.

STATISTICAL CONSIDERATIONS

Finally, it should be admitted that any account of the pathogenesis of bacterial infections can only be statistical. At several points in this chapter it has been noted that a particular predisposing factor cannot be of primary importance because not all people possessing it become infected. One could go on further, and state positively that so many factors are involved in the genesis of any infection that the statistical laws governing random behavior are applicable. We saw that this was true in men challenged with *Shigella flexneri*, and in mice there is quite solid evidence that salmonella infections follow statistical laws. The consequences of this line of thought are interesting; one is that if it were possible to replay the scenario, the result would not necessarily be the same. Another is that each individual organism has a small but finite chance by itself of establishing a lethal infection. None of the body defenses is absolute; there is room for error at many points, and while lethal infection is very improbable, it is not impossible. Therefore, it must occasionally happen, and this is a useful explanation of otherwise inexplicable overwhelming infections in people who are ostensibly normal.[12]

DETERMINANTS OF VIRAL INFECTIONS

Variations in the Organism

Most virus species have many strains, each with an immunologically unique outer layer. As in bacteria, infection by one strain confers protection only against the homologous strain, so that multiple attacks of infection are possible. Viruses with stable outer layers, such as measles and smallpox, characteristically cause a single attack of disease, which is followed by permanent immunity. The influenza virus is unusual in that its outer layers continually change by mutation, so that the new variants can reinfect people who had influenza only a year or two before. A few viruses can cause chronic disease. The majority of people infected with hepatitis B virus develop antibodies to the surface antigen; when this happens the virus is permanently cleared from the blood. Some people do not form antibodies to the surface antigen (although they may form antibodies to the core or other components), and in them viremia may continue indefinitely. Slow virus infections of the nervous system are sometimes caused by conventional viruses and sometimes by uncharacterized agents such as that which causes scrapie in sheep. The mechanisms by which these organisms can persist in humans are poorly understood.

Avirulent mutants of most viruses are prepared easily in the laboratory and are useful as vaccines. Mutants of unusual virulence probably evolve under natural conditions and account for unusually severe epidemics.

Host Factors

As far as the host is concerned, the susceptibility to a particular virus of the cells of different tissues may vary markedly and accounts for characteristic clinical syndromes such as jaundice in yellow fever and parotitis in mumps. Even the cells of a particular tissue may show striking changes of susceptibility with age; usually cells from newborn animals are much more susceptible than those of adults. Herpes simplex type 2 is a trivial disease (leaving out the possibility of carcinogenesis) except in newborn infants, who often develop progressive generalized infection, which is usually fatal. Similarly, intrauterine infection with rubella or cytomegalovirus may lead to fetal death or severe congenital anomalies. For most viruses, these differences in cellular sensitivity correspond with the presence or absence of receptors to which the virus can bind, but some differences appear to arise be-

cause of changes in the rate of interferon production, or in the rate of viral replication.

Antibody is the most important single factor in preventing viral infections; for those infections where viremia is part of the pathogenesis, serum antibody is protective. Respiratory and presumably enteric infections are prevented by secretory IgA antibody. Many successful virus vaccines have been shown to work by inducing antibody synthesis, and the degree of protection induced is proportional to the antibody titer. Viral infections with long incubation periods, such as infectious hepatitis, may be attenuated by the use of gamma globulin, and in rabies even immunization of the patient is often effective.

However, it is less clear that antibody plays a part in the recovery from most viral infections. There is usually little relationship between antibody titers and the progress of the infection, and there are many examples of progressive infection despite high antibody titers, e.g., *Herpes zoster* or *Vaccinia gangrenosa.*

Cell-mediated immunity is very clearly responsible for the control of many viral infections. Children with thymic defects who were accidentally vaccinated developed progressive gangrene of the local site with secondary infections of minor skin breaks elsewhere and a rapidly fatal course. Adults with defective cell-mediated immunity may develop reactivation of herpes viruses which they have carried without incident for upwards of 50 years. *Herpes zoster, Herpes simplex,* and cytomegalic inclusion disease are all common and serious problems. When cell-mediated immunity is depressed deliberately in patients with renal transplants or systemic lupus erythematosus, these infections may become life threatening, and discontinuing the immunosuppression may be the only possible course, even if the kidney rejects or the disease exacerbates.

DETERMINANTS OF PARASITIC INFESTATIONS

Parasitic infestations can be roughly divided into those due to protozoa and those due to worms. In general, protozoa multiply in the human host, and disease may follow trivial exposure—a single mosquito bite may induce malignant tertian malaria. However, most worms do not multiply in humans, and so usually, the intensity of infection is a very important variable. One tapeworm constitutes the disease, but this is exceptional; a single hookworm, schistosome, or filarioid worm would hardly be noticed.

The immunology of parasitic infestations is still in its infancy, but since parasites are large it is hard for them to hide, and any which live in host tissues must strike an accommodation with the immune system. Malaria parasites appear to exist in a very large, but finite number of strains, and parasitemia is maintained over periods of years by successive reinfections. Trypanosomes, on the other hand, appear to mutate successively during the infection. Schistosomes probably make themselves invisible by adsorption of host antigens. In those infections where larval stages must migrate through the tissues for a prolonged period before maturing into the adult worm, such as ascariasis and schistosomiasis, substantial immunity against the larvae may develop and may prevent any further addition to the parasite burden. Many of these diseases appear to be actually caused by immunologic reactions to the worms or their eggs, e.g., filariasis, schistosomiasis. It is not yet possible to integrate all these threads into a coherent whole, far less to explain precisely how a few unfortunates out of an exposed population develop clinical disease while the rest continue in fair health.

DETERMINANTS OF FUNGAL INFECTIONS

The fungi causing systemic mycoses are free living organisms that infect man only accidentally. Most of the population in endemic areas acquire the infection, but clinical disease is exceptional, and the main control mechanism appears to be cell-mediated immunity. The organisms persist in old scars and may reactivate if the patient becomes immunosuppressed for any reason.

Opportunistic fungi are special problems in hospitals for a number of reasons. They may be present in the environment in large numbers (aspergilli in air conditioners) and may even be introduced directly into the tissues (*Torulopsis glabrata* in intravenous fluids). Antimicrobic treatment may suppress the normal flora and allow the fungi to grow to much higher titers than normal (candida in the throat and bowel). Corticosteroid treatment, radiation, and cytotoxic drugs may be used in the treatment of diseases which already produce some suppression of cell-mediated immunity. General diseases, such as diabetes, may predispose to infection (phycomycosis), and local abnormalities may provide a site where defenses are ineffective (aspergilli in damaged lungs with old cavities). These diseases do not respond to blind antibacterial chemotherapy and may be hard to diagnose unless they are sought after aggressively.

THE RECOGNITION OF INFECTIOUS DISEASES

Clinical Features

Most infectious diseases are initially suspected because of the symptoms and signs that they cause. In general, these occur at the portal of entry; there is a sore throat, a pneumonia, diarrhea, evidence of cystitis, and so on. The diagnosis of infection is particularly likely if the onset is acute or if there is an acute change in the patient's chronic symptoms. Serious infections are also associated with general symptoms such as fever, rigors, and shock. Occasionally, the initial complaints are caused by a metastatic infection such as meningitis or osteomyelitis.

However, suggestive symptoms and signs can be produced by many noninfectious processes, and the only way of proving that an illness is due to infection is to demonstrate the responsible organism. Ordinarily, this is done by culture, sometimes by direct demonstration of the organism in the lesions. These methods are definitive but have a number of problems. Often, one does not have access to the specimen one would like to culture or examine. Thus, in pneumonia the lung is inaccessible, so one cultures blood and sputum. Blood cultures are helpful if positive, but most are sterile. Sputum cultures may be overgrown with mouth flora, and even if positive, they require careful interpretation. Many pathogenic bacteria are difficult to grow on ordinary media, and cultures will be sterile or confusing unless the correct diagnosis has been suspected initially and the right cultural conditions employed. Some viruses and a few bacteria cannot be cultured at all. A proportion of cultures become contaminated with irrelevant organisms from the patient's skin or from the personnel in the clinical microbiology laboratory. Many patients have been treated with antibiotics before a microbiologic diagnosis is attempted, and cultures from them are, therefore, sterile. Lastly, even under the best conditions, positive cultures cannot be expected in less than 24 hours, and for some organisms the processing time will be days or weeks.

For all these reasons, attempts have been made to find alternative means of diagnosing infectious diseases. Three principles have been involved: infected people show characteristic responses, organisms produce characteristic metabolic products, and organisms are foreign to the body and act as antigens. In the last case, one may either use the organism or its antigens to search for antibody formation in the patient, or one can use preformed antibody from some suitable animal to search for antigens in the patient's body fluids.

Host Responses to Infection

Infected persons show a collection of rather stereotyped responses which are generally all found together and in proportion to one another. In fact, there is some evidence that all these responses are caused by a single protein secreted by neutrophils which was originally found to cause fever and was therefore called endogenous pyrogen.[11] They are fever, elevated ESR, raised levels of serum fibrinogen, haptoglobins, ceruloplasmin, and C-reactive protein, depression of the serum iron and zinc, and mobilization of neutrophils from the bone marrow reserve. The elevated ESR is simply a manifestation of the increased serum fibrinogen. The mobilization of neutrophils is initially expressed by a raised WBC with a high percentage of neutrophils and a left shift. In severe infections, toxic granules, Dohle bodies, and vacuoles may be seen in blood smears; vacuoles are particularly suggestive of bacteremia.[21] In very severe infections, the consumption of neutrophils in infected areas outruns the bone marrow reserves; the WBC drops to normal or even to leukopenic levels, but the shift to the left is retained. Most of the proteins which show an elevated concentration are α_2 globulins; serum electrophoresis therefore shows increased protein in this region. The low serum iron reflects a diversion of iron from the bone marrow to the reticuloendothelial system, and if the infection has been of some duration, the normocytic, normochromic "anemia of infection" develops.

None of these responses is specific, all may be seen in noninfectious conditions such as rheumatoid arthritis or myocardial infarction. Nonetheless, in a patient whose clinical condition suggests the presence of infection, they offer useful confirmatory evidence. In clinical practice one would take the appropriate samples for culture and Gram staining and initiate antibiotic therapy.

A more sophisticated test of the neutrophils in infection is the NBT test. During phagocytosis, neutrophils reduce the blue dye to blue-black deposits, which can be seen in their cytoplasm. Blood neutrophils from normal people develop very few (about 3 percent) of these deposits when incubated with NBT. Neutrophils from infected people show a much higher percentage (15 to > 50 percent). Unless the test is meticulously performed, artifactual positive tests develop, and several workers have reported that the test is useless. However, it clearly can work in some laboratories, and has, for example, been found useful in the differentiation of pneumonia and pulmonary embolism.[16]

Metabolites of Bacteria

Although the above tests may suggest the presence of infection, they give no hint of what the organism may be. Most bacteria ferment glucose and other substrates to products which are not formed by mammalian cells. The pattern of metabolites is often characteristic of particular species, and very small amounts can be detected in serum or CSF by gas–liquid chromatography (GLC). However, great skill and experience are necessary to detect tiny quantities of metabolites with GLC equipment, and the method has not been made suitable for general use.

Metabolite patterns are routinely used to speciate anaerobic and other bacteria. In this case, GLC is performed directly on a culture filtrate, and plenty of material is available. Bacterial metabolism has also been used to diagnose positive cultures before growth becomes obvious macroscopically. The simplest such system measures the evolution of $^{14}CO_2$ from ^{14}carbon-labeled glucose, and may be clearly positive within 2 hours of inoculating the tubes. If some tubes contain antibiotics, failure to evolve $^{14}CO_2$ in those tubes is evidence of sensitivity to the antibiotics.

Serologic Diagnosis

The serologic diagnosis of infectious illnesses is extremely reliable for some organisms and much less so for others. If the organism is not found in normal people, the presence of antibody in any titer is evidence of present or previous infection with the organism. For some unculturable agents, such as *Treponema pallidum* or the virus of hepatitis B, serum antibody may be the only way to establish the diagnosis. For other organisms, such as rickettsiae, chlamydiae, most viruses, *Francisella tularensis,* and other organisms which are difficult and/or dangerous to culture, serology is also the best way to confirm the diagnosis. Unfortunately, when the patient is acutely ill, antibody titers are often low or negative. If a second serum sample taken 2 to 3 weeks after the first shows a four-fold or greater rise in titer, that is presumptive evidence of recent infection with the organism concerned. This information is rarely useful clinically because of the delay, and it is subject to confusion because antibody titers to several different organisms may all rise to some degree. This "anamnestic response" to infection used to be mysterious but has become less so with the discovery that several organisms make polyclonal B cell mitogens such as endotoxin. Because of the possibility that a four-fold or greater serologic response is merely anamnestic, it is usual to require that the convalescent serum attains some minimal titer, which varies with the organism concerned, and that one of the responses is much larger than the others.

Some organisms are found in all normal people, and others are frequent causes of infection in normal people. Some level of antibody is universal. Systemic infection with these organisms is associated with greatly increased antibody titers. Arbitrary antibody levels have been set which have been claimed to be diagnostic of various diseases such as rheumatic fever, staphylococcal endocarditis, or disseminated candidiasis. Unfortunately, no one level of any antibody absolutely distinguishes between normal and infected people. Furthermore, many infections with normal flora occur in people who for one reason or another are unable to mount antibody responses, and antibody levels are consequently of no diagnostic value. For these reasons, high antibody levels are merely suggestive of infection rather than diagnostic, and low antibody levels do not always exclude infection.

The Significance of Antibody Class

In some illnesses, the initial serum presents an elevated antibody titer, which does not subsequently increase. If it can be shown that most of the initial antibody is of the IgM class, that is strong support for the diagnosis of recent infection. This is particularly useful in brucellosis. In the diagnosis of transplacental congenital infections, the presence of antibody in cord blood is not helpful because it could be maternal. However, if some antibody is of the IgM class, that could only have been made by the fetus, and transplacental infection is, therefore, proved.

Antigen Detection

The detection of foreign antigens in body fluids has the great advantage of providing certainty of diagnosis. No normal person has cryptococcal polysaccharide in the cerebrospinal fluid (CSF) or pneumococcal capsular antigens in the blood or urine. These antigens can be detected by any appropriate immunologic technique, but because of its rapidity, the most commonly used is counterimmunoelectrophoresis (CIE). Most experience has been obtained with CSF, and here the technique appears to be highly reliable, with very few cross-reactions and essentially no false positives. It is not as sensitive as culture, which in theory can detect one organism, but it remains positive even in patients who have been treated with antibiotics before admission to hospital. Tests for antigens in serum have, in general, been positive only in bacteremic infections, and in a minority of them.[17]

One bacterial antigen which can be detected by nonimmunologic means is endotoxin. The amebocytes of the horseshoe crab contain a protein which can be coagulated by minute amounts of endotoxin. The limulus lysate test has been used with success in the early diagnosis of gram-negative meningitides; it is somewhat more sensitive than CIE and also remains positive after antibiotic treatment. However, the sensitivity of the test and the ubiquity of gram-negative organisms produce many false positive responses. Furthermore, the basis of the test is not understood, and some workers think that it is not specific for endotoxin. Whatever the reason, the test has

not given consistent results in serum in most peoples' hands.

Both CIE and the limulus test have one other advantage over culture. They cannot only show that organisms are present, but give a rough estimate of how many there are. In all bacterial infections, increased levels of antigen in body fluids correlate well with increases in the clinical severity of the illness, mortality, and long-term sequelae. Antibiotics do not influence this poor prognosis because they cannot prevent tissue damage due to bacterial products synthesized before treatment begins.

Direct Demonstration of Organisms

Protozoal and helminthic parasites are sufficiently differentiated to allow them to be characterized on morphologic grounds alone. Furthermore, in most cases of clinical illness due to parasites, enough organisms are present to make recognition of them or their eggs a relatively easy matter. Morphology is also the traditional mode of diagnosis in early syphilis, where culture is not available and serology may be negative. In this case, the dark field microscope must be used because the organisms are too thin to see with the light microscope. *Treponema pallidum* has a characteristic length, thickness, tightness of coil, and motility which make it easily recognizable by experts.

In ordinary bacterial infections, the Gram stain is a traditional source of immediate information. If the tissue or fluid is normally sterile, identification of organisms by Gram stain is proof positive of disease. Unfortunately, artifacts are common unless the personnel doing the test are very experienced. It is particularly unwise to attempt to diagnose the species of bacteria on the basis of Gram stain appearances. For example, to assume that the cause of a meningitis is the meningococcus because gram-negative cocci have been seen in a Gram stain may lead to tragedy if only penicillin is given as initial treatment and the organism turns out to be *Haemophilus influenzae*.

Pus taken from abscesses at the time of opening usually gives Gram stain appearances which are reliable. However, a lesion which has been draining for some time may have become colonized by all kinds of secondary invaders which are of no pathologic significance. Similarly, Gram stains of material from areas with large resident bacterial populations, such as the mouth, the bowel, or the vagina, are usually valueless.

Some organisms have very unusual properties which enable a microscopic diagnosis to be made with assurance. The tubercle bacillus, its close relatives, and nocardia are the only common causes of pulmonary infection which are acid-fast. Similarly, *Yersinia pestis* is the only common cause of acute lymphadenitis which appears as small gram-negative rods with bipolar staining.

Because Gram stain appearances may be misleading, there have been recurrent attempts to increase the precision of diagnosis by the use of organism-specific fluorescent antisera. In principle, any organism could be demonstrated in this way, and in practice, the method has been shown to work for gonococci, streptococci, influenza A, adenoviruses, and many other organisms. Artifacts can develop with fluoroscopic microscopes, and positive and negative controls must be included with every batch of specimens. The method is very attractive because it provides quick diagnosis of viral diseases and because it can detect bacterial antigens when the bacteria themselves will not grow.

In summary, the mainstays of infectious disease diagnosis are still Gram stain appearances, cultures, and serologic tests. A great many tests based on newer technology offer greater speed and specificity in diagnosis. However, all require considerable expertise on the part of the operator, and many require expensive equipment. It is not clear whether the benefits to be obtained by implementing this technology on a large scale will outweigh the cost.

CHAPTER 79
Infections in Patients with Impaired Defenses
PATRICK A. MURPHY

Most of the common clinical conditions which predispose to infection such as old age, malnutrition, diabetes mellitus, and neoplastic diseases, can be shown to affect several of the defense mechanisms discussed in Chapter 78. Because no one defect is predominant, the infections are variable with respect to their site, the causative organisms, and the outcome. Furthermore, a given patient may suffer from several conditions simultaneously; a man may be an old diabetic convalescing from a resection for carcinoma of the stomach. Since our methods of measuring defects in host defenses are crude, it becomes difficult to describe the situation in anything other than general terms.

OLD AGE
The commonest single disorder predisposing to infection in this country is old age. Old people have usually accumulated various structural defects ranging from emphysematous lungs and prostatic enlargement to ischemia of the feet. Neurologic disorders may produce inanition leading to aspiration pneumonia and bedsores. Because of the prevalence of noninfectious, chronic medical illness, old people are commonly admitted to the hospital, where they are exposed to large numbers of hospital-adapted pathogens, are subjected to all kinds of invasive procedures, and may have their normal flora ablated by ill-considered "prophylactic" antibiotic therapy. Most surgical procedures are performed in old people, and many of them are extensive. All these things provide portals of entry for microorganisms.

Old people usually have neutrophil counts and gammaglobulin levels in the normal range. However, there is clear evidence that old animals have many fewer hemopoietic stem cells than young ones and that the ability to mobilize granulocytes in response to an infection is defective. Not many old people produce leukocytosis in the 30 to 40,000 range as young people do. Similarly, the antibody response to a new antigen is defective in old animals, even though secondary responses may be intact. In man, there is fairly definite evidence that cell-mediated immunity wanes with age. Young healthy people show delayed hypersensitivity reactions when tested intradermally with antigens of organisms most people have met such as mumps, candida, and trichophyton. Old people may fail to react to one or more of these and may also lose reactivity to tuberculin, histoplasmin, etc. when these tests were previously known to be positive. Reactivation of quiescent tuberculosis in old people is now much the commonest form of the disease, and *Herpes zoster* is another example of a disease due to revival of a long-dormant organism which is repressed by cell-mediated immunity.[37]

There is no specific infection associated with old age; rather, the incidence and severity of all types is increased. Surgical anastomoses leak and cause peritonitis; klebsiella bacteremia develops from a simple urinary tract infection; staphylococcal pneumonia follows an attack of influenza. The inflammatory response is often defective, pus is thin, and infections are not well localized but tend to spread progressively. Healing of wounds and ulcers is noticeably slow. Patients tend to remain prostrated much longer than younger people would, and commonly a new infection supervenes before the first has resolved. The mortality of all infections steadily increases with age beyond 70; when the cause of death is examined, no constant pattern is seen. People die of congestive heart failure, pulmonary emboli, hepatic and renal failure, stroke, and various other noninfectious conditions as well as undiagnosed or uncontrollable infections. Old age is the example par excellence of a condition where nothing works very well.

MALNUTRITION

Malnutrition and infectious disease compound one another. On a population scale, chronically ill people have little interest in work or physical stamina when they do work, so agricultural productivity is low and a vicious circle is closed. Social customs, such as prolonged breast feeding, or even worse, weaning onto starchy food providing calories but little protein, produce particularly severe nutritional defects in young children. Heavy loads of intestinal parasites contribute to protein deficiency; especially important is the steady blood loss due to hookworm. On an individual level, infection causes fever, which wastes calories, and a strongly negative nitrogen balance, which wastes irreplaceable protein. Lack of appetite promotes a low food intake, and diarrhea produces malabsorption of what food is eaten. Frank kwashiorkor and various vitamin deficiencies, such as beri-beri and scurvy, are commonly precipitated by the increased metabolic demands of an intercurrent infection.

On the other side of the coin, there is reasonably good evidence in animals that protein and vitamin deficiencies decrease the resistance to all bacterial infections, especially tuberculosis, and to most viral infections. In humans, there is not a single report of a nutritional deficiency state which leads to an increased resistance to any infection.

Many host defense mechanisms are impaired by malnutrition and especially by protein deficiency. Specifically, it has been shown 1) that serum transferrin is grossly reduced; 2) that neutrophil reserves and tissue mobilization are <10 percent of normal; 3) that phagocytosis per neutrophil is reduced; 4) that bacteria taken into neutrophils are killed less efficiently; 5) that antibody response is reduced, especially to new antigens; and 6) that there is a serious defect in cell-mediated immunity. These may all be understood as

the consequence of the inability to synthesize new protein; cell proliferation cannot take place as normally, and what cells are made contain low amounts of granules and other proteins needed for normal function. Field studies in malnourished populations in Guatemala and the Punjab have shown that supplementing the diet is more useful than medical care.[34] It was shown in a recent study that American patients who were malnourished as a consequence of various diseases of the gut had gross defects of both B and T cell systems. These were greatly improved by intravenous feeding, while the defects in a control group were unaffected.[27] Malnutrition is not simply a condition that one sees in Bangladesh.

Naturally, one would not expect a uniform pattern of infections in malnourished patients. Nonetheless, if one had to pick one of the defects as most "important," it would have to be the defect in cell-mediated immunity. Children with kwashiorkor have low counts of circulating small lymphocytes, are commonly anergic when tested intradermally with the usual antigens, and at autopsy show gross atrophy of the thymus and the paracortical areas of lymph nodes. Measles, *Herpes simplex*, gram-negative rod infections, and tuberculosis are all of unusual severity. Measles changes its behavior in a very revealing way. The rash in normal children is thought to be the result of cell-mediated immunity eliminating virus and virus-infected cells in the skin. In malnourished children, the rash is often not prominent, but involvement of the lungs with giant cell pneumonia is frequent.

DIABETES MELLITUS

Diabetes mellitus probably affects 4 percent of the population, and the incidence rises with age. A number of mechanisms predisposing to infection have been demonstrated. Neutrophil mobilization in skin windows is less than normal, especially in the presence of ketosis; phagocytosis is impaired by raised serum osmolarity; bacterial killing is defective in ketotic serum and can be returned to normal by putting the cells in normal serum. The immune and complement systems appear to be normal.[35]

Infection of the feet is common and may show different behavior from that in other sclerotic patients, in that spreading cellulitis and wet gangrene occurs in a foot where the arterial pulses are normal, and antibiotic therapy results in healing. Because prevention is much easier than cure, all patients should be carefully instructed in how to care for their feet. Other spreading skin infections are common in diabetics; staphyloccal boils rapidly progress to carbuncles, and minor varicose eczema gives way to cellulitis of the leg. Urinary tract infections are frequent, may be of unusual severity, and may lead to renal papillary necrosis.

There are several specific infections which are seen more commonly or even exclusively in the diabetic. The most frequent is candidiasis of the vulva and vagina, usually attributed to glycosuria. Others include malignant otitis externa (due to *Pseudomonas aeruginosa*) and phycomycosis, an aggressive sinusitis due to several species of normally saprophytic fungi.

ALCOHOLISM

Alcoholics frequently suffer from infections, and the commonest is pneumonia. One obvious reason is the liability to aspiration while intoxicated. A factor of probably equal importance is that alcohol in intoxicating doses blocks the emigration of neutrophils from the blood, and it also blocks the ability of alveolar macrophages to phagocytose and destroy microorganisms. Alcoholics are often malnourished, suffering from protein deficiency and/or specific deficiency states such as beri-beri. Folate deficiency is thought to be the cause of the leukopenia and inadequate granulocyte reserves commonly seen in alcoholics, but there may also be a specific toxic effect of alcohol on the bone marrow.[29] Most pneumonias are pneumococcal, but occasionally one sees klebsiella pneumonia, which usually affects an upper lobe, produces a state of severe prostration, and tends to chronicity and abscess formation. Tuberculosis is also relatively frequent.

CIRRHOSIS

Hepatic cirrhosis is most common in alcoholics, but may occur independently. There is probably a general susceptibility to all infections, which has been tentatively related to a failure to mobilize neutrophils in inflammatory sites or to an alleged defect of cell-mediated immunity. Two infections are referable to the local abnormalities. Gram-negative bacteremia is fairly frequent, as already discussed, and occasionally gram-negative infection of the ascitic fluid occurs.[23,30]

ADRENOCORTICOSTEROIDS

Adrenocorticosteroids are now used for the treatment of many illnesses, and there is no doubt that high doses increase the liability to infection.[26] Susceptibility to infection is also seen in Cushing's disease. Corticosteroids impair the emigration of neutrophils from the blood; this is shown both by high counts and low turnover times in the peripheral blood and by grossly inadequate mobilization at Rebuck skin window sites. There are other effects on neutrophils, but this seems to be the main one. There is a variable suppression of cell-mediated immunity, probably due to lysis of T lymphocytes. Antibody synthesis is usually normal.

Some patients can be treated satisfactorily by giving corticosteroids on alternate days. When this is done, the abnormalities of neutrophil mobilization are less marked on the second day. It has not yet been shown that patients so treated actually do have lower infection rates than those given corticosteroids every day.

The infections seen are a "mixed bag," as would be expected. Especially common is staphylococcal skin infection. More sinister are tuberculosis and various systemic mycoses, which may be far advanced before they are diagnosed. Diagnosis of any infection in a corticosteroid-treated patient is difficult; fever may be suppressed, the patient may not look or feel very ill, the usual inflammatory symptoms at the local site may not be prominent, and leucocytosis is "normal" for the patient. In addition, there may be confusing local or systemic manifestations of the disease for which steroids were prescribed. It is necessary to be unusually meticulous about doing blood cultures whenever one even thinks they might be indicated and to take seriously any pulmonary symptoms.

SPLENECTOMY

Patients without spleens have a tendency to develop sudden overwhelming septicemias, most commonly with the pneumococcus.[22,23] Two mechanisms appear to operate; the spleen is a major site for clearance of circulating particles, and it is also the major site for synthesis of antibody against antigens presented by the intravenous route. The risk appears to be greatest for about 2 years following splenectomy, and then declines. It is also greatly influenced by the reason for which the splenectomy was done; overwhelming septicemia is seen only occasionally after removal of the spleen because of trauma, but is quite common (up to 10 percent of cases) after removal of the spleen for Cooley's anemia and various disorders of lipid storage. In the traumatic cases, it is known that accessory spleens may regenerate from cells spilled into the peritoneum at the time of splenic rupture. In the latter cases, there is usually no source from which splenic regeneration could occur, and it is thought that the liver macrophages are too busy dealing with erythrocytes and lipids, respectively, to function as effective phagocytes. Cases of septicemia have occurred in patients splenectomized to stage their lymphomas. At present, it is not clear whether the extra information gained is worth the risk. Since pneumococci cause about 90 percent of overwhelming septicemias, it would seem reasonable to attempt to protect all splenectomized patients with the pneumococcal vaccine.

NEOPLASTIC DISEASES

Infection is probably the commonest immediate cause of death in patients with malignant neoplasms, and intercurrent, nonfatal infections contribute greatly to morbidity. However, it is misleading to say that malignancy per se predisposes to infection. There are many different types of neoplasm and each predisposes to infection in its own particular way. In addition, the methods used for treating neoplastic conditions are various, and each type of treatment carries its own risk. Finally, neoplasms may lead to malnutrition or to failure of specific organs, and either may increase the liability to infection still further.

The Type of Neoplasm

Most carcinomas arise in the gastrointestinal tract, and the infections which they cause are related to ulceration or perforation of the primary tumor with invasion by the intestinal flora. Similarly, portals of entry are provided by carcinomas of the breast and the female genital tract. Another mechanism is obstruction of a drainage pathway, as when pneumonia develops behind a carcinoma of the lung. Carcinoma of the kidney, which is not directly exposed to infection, may reach a huge size without any infectious complication, as may bone and soft tissue sarcomas. However, leukemias and lymphomas do specifically predispose to infection. In acute leukemia, the number of functional neutrophils is greatly reduced, and a spectrum of infections similar to those in agranulocytosis is seen. In chronic myeloid leukemia, there are usually plenty of mature neutrophils, and infection is not a problem until acute blastic transformation occurs. Chronic lymphatic leukemia is not associated with any defect until late in its course, but then there may be a failure to synthesize antibodies, especially against new antigens, and infections with pneumococci and other extracellular parasites occur. Myeloma is characteristically associated from an early stage with infections caused by extracellular parasites, and for the same reason. Hodgkin's disease was classically associated with tuberculosis, and for years an argument raged over whether the defective cell-mediated immunity which was demonstrable was due to the disease or to its treatment. It has now been clearly shown that cutaneous anergy and inability to develop contact dermatitis on challenge with DNCB

are present in some untreated patients.[28] The degree of anergy is seldom absolute, and it is most marked in patients with advanced disease. Patients with untreated Hodgkin's disease may present with other infections normally repressed by cell-mediated immunity such as *Herpes zoster* and salmonellosis. As Hodgkin's disease progresses, hypogammaglobulinemia may become apparent; often IgM is more depressed than IgG. Hypogammaglobulinemia may also be seen in other lymphomas. Depressed globulin levels are presumably one factor contributing to infections with conventional bacteria like pneumococci, staphylococci, and gram-negative rods.

The Treatment of Neoplasm

Most cancer operations are extensive, and since the patient is in the hospital, he is exposed to many sources of infection while in his weakened state. They include anastomotic leaks, wound infections, pneumonia, exposure to hospital organisms, broad spectrum antibiotic therapy, and invasive procedures. Radiation therapy may create portals of entry through dermatitis or damage to an internal viscus; and extensive radiation produces bone marrow failure and atrophy of lymphoid tissues. Neutrophils, antibody formation, and cell-mediated immunity may all be defective to some extent. The effect of chemotherapy varies from one drug to another. Many regimens include high doses of prednisone, and the bad effects of this have already been discussed (Chap. 54). In acute leukemias, a deliberate attempt is made to render the bone marrow aplastic with cytotoxic drugs, and this is often an unwanted side effect of the chemotherapy of solid tumors. Neutrophil counts and reserves are thus reduced to levels which make infection very probable. The endothelium of the gastrointestinal tract may be severely damaged by cytotoxic drugs, and widespread ulcers in small or large bowel may allow bacteria to enter and cause septicemia. Cytotoxic drugs have no effect on antibody levels already in the serum, but since they poison dividing cells, they reduce or abolish the response to new antigens. Furthermore, since plasma cells have a life span of a week or less, and since the half-life of gammaglobulin is only a few weeks, levels of preexisting antibody will decline if chemotherapy is long continued. Cell-mediated immunity is also dependent on the ability of lymphocytes to multiply; it is known that the populations of lymphocytes which mediate it are short lived, and that in the absence of continuous stimulation by products of lymphocytes, activated macrophages lose their ability to kill intracellular parasites. Patients with cancer sometimes have demonstrable defects of cell-mediated immunity before any treatment is given, but it is clear that gross anergy is much more common in patients who have received chemotherapy.

Malnutrition

Patients become malnourished for many reasons. The primary tumor is often in the gastrointestinal tract and leads to anorexia, vomiting, or diarrhea. Chronic bleeding and purulent drainage cause small but steady protein losses and major amounts of protein can be removed in pleural fluid or ascites. Any surgical operation produces a catabolic state whose intensity is proportional to the extent of the surgery, and recovery may be impeded because major sections of the gut have been removed. The increased metabolic demands of intercurrent infections contribute. Radiation therapy causes a catabolic state, and both radiation and cancer chemotherapy commonly cause nausea and vomiting. Steroids cause breakdown of protein in muscle and bone, with a strongly negative nitrogen balance. All these things lead to wasting and protein deficiency, which predispose to infection.[24]

CLINICAL FEATURES OF INFECTIONS IN NEUTROPENIC PATIENTS

Infections in neutropenic patients become noticeably more frequent when the peripheral neutrophil count drops below 1000/µl.[32] Infection appears to be a random process; there is no one count which guarantees protection from infection, and infection is not inevitable even when there are no circulating neutrophils. However, reasonably accurate statistical predictions can be made about groups of patients; when the peripheral neutrophil count is between 100 and 500, patients have clinically obvious infections about 30 percent of the time.

The vast majority of the infections are bacterial, and most are caused by gram-negative rods. *Staphylococcus aureus* is the commonest gram-positive pathogen. In the case of the gram-negative rods, colonization ususally precedes infection, and survey cultures done when the patient is well may give useful preliminary information when they become ill. The commonest infections are septicemia without an obvious source and pneumonia. However, all manner of local infections of the skin or mucous membranes may occur, especially at sites of intravenous catheters, in intertriginous areas, and in the perirectal region. All these infections share common characteristics. There may be few or no local symptoms, apparently because the heat, redness, swelling, and pain of bacterial infections in normal people are due

to the host response to infection rather than to the bacteria themselves. For similar reasons, there is little or no pus formation. In pneumonia, the chest x-ray may be normal and may remain so until the death of the patient. There is small tendency for the infection to localize; trivial initial lesions progress steadily to spreading cellulitis and wet gangrene, and postive blood cultures may progress to frank septicemia. Curiously, when sepsis does supervene, the patient almost always responds with fever, and this may be the only abnormality early on.

Bacteria not only account for at least 90 percent of diagnosed infections in neutropenic patients, but of all the possible pathogens they pose the most immediate threat to life. Both sepsis and pneumonia progress with appalling speed in these people; death in 24 hours is not unusual. Since about half of all febrile (T >101°F) episodes in neutropenic patients are due to infection, each episode must be treated as a medical emergency. The patient should be rapidly examined for sources of sepsis, such as intravenous catheter sites, the urine, and the lungs. Cultures should be made of blood, urine, sputum, and any other material likely to provide useful information. Within an hour, antibacterial therapy should be started. Various regimens have been tried, and no one of them is clearly superior to the others. Indeed, one would expect that the best combination will vary from one place to another and in the same place from time to time because of fluctuations in species and antibiotic susceptibility of the local gram-negative rods. It is, therefore, important to know what has been working locally recently. Most regimens are combinations of a cell-wall acting antibiotic such as carbenicillin or cephalothin with an aminoglycoside such as gentamicin or amikacin. It is best to tailor the regimen so that both halves of the combination are likely to be effective against the dominant local gram-negative rod. *Staphylococcus aureus* is an important pathogen in these people, but it seems that theoretically unsuitable regimens, such as carbenicillin and gentamicin, will in practice hold it in check until cultural information is available. Other bacterial pathogens, such as pneumococci and streptococci, are distinctly rare in this setting and are so susceptible to antibiotics that almost any regimen will be adequate. Attempts have been made to broaden coverage so that every conceivable pathogen is covered by a first choice antibiotic. Combinations of three, four, and even five antibiotics have been subjected to controlled clinical trial. The survival rates have not been obviously better than with two drug regimens, and renal and other toxicity has been a major problem.

In addition to antibiotics, the patient may need intravenous fluids, colloids or red cells, vasopressors, and attention to the airway and to oxygenation. If he survives for 48 hours, the situation should be reassessed. By this time, blood cultures are usually positive if they are ever going to be positive, and the fever either has or has not responded to therapy. If cultures are positive, the antibiotics are appropriate and the patient is better; it is merely necessary to continue therapy for about 7 days. If the antibiotics are appropriate but the patient has not responded, a reason should be sought. The commonest are that the dosage of antibiotic is inadequate, or that there is some continuing source of sepsis, such as an infected intravenous line, or septic thrombophlebitis in a vein previously cannulated. Pneumonia or an extensive cellulitis may respond very slowly to adequate treatment, and persistence of fever at 48 hours does not necessarily demand a change of regimen. If blood cultures are negative but the patient clearly responded to therapy, antibiotics should also be continued for about 7 days.

Difficulties arise when the patient remains febrile and cultures are negative. The first step should be to completely reexamine the patient, looking for evidence of local sepsis which might have been missed the first time. Examination should be thorough, including areas such as the ears, nasal sinuses, mouth, throat, vagina, and rectum. The fundi should be examined for the white spots diagnostic of disseminated candidiasis, and the urine should be examined for small numbers of yeasts and hyphae which may have the same significance. New blood cultures and a new chest x-ray should be made. If no other source of fever can be identified, it is well to change and culture all intravenous lines.

Assuming that all the above leads to no immediately useful information, what should be done depends on the appearance of the patient. If he is clinically deteriorating or frankly septic, a new antibacterial regimen should be tried, including a new aminoglycoside such as amikacin. If there is no response and no evidence of bacterial infection after a further 48 hours, amphotericin B should be started empirically. Patients who have disseminated candidiasis usually have positive candida cultures at many peripheral sites, such as the throat, sputum, stool, or vagina, but they may not have positive blood cultures until late in the disease.

Patients who are febrile but not particularly ill are commonly found to have a nonbacterial cause of fever such as tumor, a drug reaction, or localized fungal infection. Therapy must be individualized, but it is not good practice to maintain antibacterial antibiotics indefinitely in a patient who is persistently culture-negative. Most such patients do not have bacterial infections, and the danger of superinfection with resistant bacteria or with fungi mounts steadily as antibiotics are continued.

The incidence of infections in neutropenic patients can be reduced in several ways, and each oncology center has its own practices. Reverse isolation will protect the patient from external contamination; the most efficient systems are the laminar-flow room and the plastic life island, but simple glove, mask, and gown techniques work if conscientiously used. Infection by the patient's own organisms can be reduced by nonabsorbable antibacterial antibiotics such as vancomycin and neomycin. It is usual to add Nystatin to prevent candida overgrowth. Some centers have used prophylactic antibiotic regimens, with which patients are treated for as long as the neutrophil count is below $1000/\mu l$. The antibiotics are changed regularly to minimize the emergence of resistant forms. The transfusion of histocompatible granulocytes is known to be effective as therapy for infections in neutropenic patients; studies to test its efficiency as prophylaxis are in progress. All these measures involve a great deal of time, effort, and money, and it remains to be seen whether what is theoretically the best management will be economically feasible.

Pneumonia in neutropenic patients is usually due to bacteria, and in the absence of therapy progresses rapidly to the death of the patient.[36] The physical signs of pneumonia may be limited to a few areas of harsh breath sounds and an occasional moist sound. The chest x-ray may be normal or nearly so. However, in most cases there is obvious consolidation on examination and an infiltrate on the x-ray. In either case, progressive dyspnea and cyanosis give the diagnosis away and can be confirmed by deteriorating blood gases. Cultures of blood and sputum should be done immediately. If the sputum Gram stain suggests that the specimen is not satisfactory (epithelial cells or mixed flora), then a transtracheal aspirate should probably be done unless the patient is thrombocytopenic. Therapy should be started immediately with antibiotics covering staphylococci and gram-negative rods. It can be refined later when cultures are available.

Sometimes, the onset of pneumonia is subacute or even chronic; pulmonary infiltrates develop slowly while the patient becomes steadily more anoxic and febrile. The pneumonia may be caused by viruses, such as CMV, by common bacteria such as gram-negative rods, by specialized bacteria such as *M. tu-*

berculosis or nocardia, by fungi such as aspergillus or cryptococcus, or by the protozoan *Pneumocystis carinii.* It may also reflect invasion by tumor or a reaction to a drug such as busulfan or bleomycin.

There is no therapy which could cover all of the above possibilities. Furthermore, unless the correct therapy is chosen, the patient will probably die. Therefore, correct diagnosis is vital and should be urgently pursued before the patient's condition becomes critical. If routine measures, such as examination of sputum, are unhelpful, one should proceed to transtracheal aspiration, fiberoptic bronchoscopy with brushings and biopsy and finally, open lung biopsy.[25] Needle biopsy of the lung has largely been abandoned because the specimens were commonly inadequate and because pneumothorax and hemothorax were so common. However, some centers have had good luck with needle aspiration of the lung, especially for *P. carinii* infections. The presence of thrombocytopenia may influence the choice of diagnostic procedure—transtracheal aspiration is distinctly more hazardous in this situation even if platelet transfusions are given. However, the important thing is to obtain a firm diagnosis, and open lung biopsy has proved to give excellent diagnostic specimens with surprisingly little morbidity even in the presence of thrombocytopenia, provided compatible platelets are available. Once the diagnosis is established, therapy becomes automatic, but one should not forget that these patients commonly are infected by more than one pathogen.

INFECTION IN RECIPIENTS OF TRANSPLANTED ORGANS

Kidney transplantation is now commonplace, and unless the donor and the recipient are identical twins, immunosuppression will be required more or less permanently to prevent graft rejection. The infections of transplant recipients can be conveniently divided into those which occur shortly after the operation and those which occur later.[31]

Early infections include all those which commonly plague surgical patients such as infections of intravenous lines, wound infections, and pneumonia. In addition, the transplant itself is at special risk. Sometimes the patient's old kidneys are left in, although they are known to be pyelonephritic. Infection of the transplant with the same organism usually follows. Occasionally, wound infection is deep, involving mainly the transplant bed with very little superficial involvement. Sonography is particularly useful for showing such infected fluid collections. If the patient is catheterized, infection of the urine may be introduced from outside and may be perpetuated if there is some obstructive lesion, such as a stenosis, at the ureterovesical junction.

As a general rule, transplant patients do not develop the severe degrees of neutropenia seen in patients undergoing chemotherapy for malignant disease. If neutropenia is induced, witholding azathioprine for a day or two will ordinarily return the count to the safe range. Overwhelming bacteremia or pneumonia do occur in this population, but are on the whole uncommon. Unexplained fever in a recent transplant recipient should be vigorously investigated as described for leukemics, and blind antibacterial coverage is probably indicated until the situation resolves. However, if there is no clinical or laboratory evidence of bacterial infection after a reasonable time, antibiotics should be discontinued and another explanation sought. A common alternative explanation is transplant rejection, but this usually is made obvious by a fall in urine volume and increased serum creatinine. Antirejection treatment with methylprednisolone and/or local irradiation often leads to defervescence.

Fungal infections in recent transplant recipients are mainly due to Candida species. The source is usually the patient, in which case throat and stool cultures are likely to be positive and there may be clinically obvious thrush or esophagitis. Another common source is an infected intravenous line. Aspergillus infections are also relatively common; they usually arise from inhalation and cause fungal pneumonia. Sometimes, sources of aspergillus spores are found in the environment; contaminated air conditioners and asbestos fire-proofing have been implicated.

As time passes after transplantation, acute bacterial infections become less common, and a series of infections of insidious onset begin to appear. Generalized fungal infections with candida, aspergillus, or cryptococci may be seen. There may also be localized fungal infections such as aspergillus pneumonitis, cryptococcal meningitis, or mucormycosis of the nasal sinuses. Bacterial infections tend to involve unusual organisms such as listeria or nocardia. Herpes virus infections may cause hepatitis or pneumonitis which last for months and may end fatally. The syndrome of progressive and unexplained pulmonary infiltrate is also relatively common.

These infections are to be expected in a population given large doses of corticosteroids and whose cell-mediated immune responses are deliberately suppressed. They are especially common when antilymphocyte globulin is used, and some centers have discontinued its use for this reason. Little can be done to prevent them because, in general, the agents are ubiquitous. It is usual to recommend that transplant recipients with a positive tuberculin test should be given a year's treatment with isoniazid. Immunosup-

pression should be reduced to the lowest level compatible with survival of the graft, and neutropenia should be avoided if possible. Otherwise, one can only wait for infection to occur, diagnose it early, and treat it aggressively.

CHAPTER 80
Management of Infectious Diseases
PAUL S. LIETMAN

The rational treatment of bacterial and fungal diseases involves a mixture of science and empiricism. Perhaps in no other area of therapeutics is the biochemical mechanism of drug action so precisely known and yet the clinical use of the same drug so often based on far less firm scientific evidence.[38] Perhaps in no other area of therapeutics are drugs so effective and yet so misused. The goal of antimicrobial chemotherapy is the eradication of the infection, and this can be accomplished most efficaciously if a knowledge of the principles of chemotherapy is combined with a familiarity for the drugs used. Some of the major principles of chemotherapy will be reviewed and a synopsis of the chemotherapeutic agents in current use will be provided (Table 80–1). Several excellent recent references are available dealing with the rational use of antimicrobial agents.[39-43]

In approaching the patient with an infectious disease, the precision with which the diagnosis is made is of utmost importance in the design of an effective therapeutic regimen. In an optimal situation one would know all of the following facts prior to the initiation of therapy:

1. The adequacy of the host defense mechanisms
2. The site of infection
3. The offending organism
4. The antibiotic sensitivities of the organism
5. The usual resistance pattern exhibited by the organism in the context of conditions existent in the host
6. The severity of infection
7. The natural history of the infection if untreated
8. The pharmacokinetics of the drug
9. The toxicity of the drug

Seldom is all of this information available at the time therapy is initiated. Nevertheless, it is a useful exercise to review this list and to bring as much infor-

mation as possible to bear on the construction of a therapeutic regimen.

GENERAL SYMPTOMATIC AND SUPPORTIVE CARE

The therapeutic approach to the patient with an infectious disease must include an overall concern for the relief of the patient's suffering, an effort to correct the pathophysiologic consequences of the infection, and a specific attack on the offending microorganism. The proper balance between these three facets of management often demands considerable clinical judgment. The exercise of such judgment should include attention to the principles considered in this section.

Fever

The presence of fever should not evoke a reflex prescription for an antipyretic. Some thought should be given to both the disadvantages and the advantages of fever. The disadvantages include the detrimental effects of hyperpyrexia (over 105.8°F) per se and the augmentation of metabolic demands that accompany temperatures of even less than 104°F. These increases in metabolic demands may be hazardous to a patient with coronary insufficiency or congestive heart failure. In most patients, however, temperatures of 104°F or less produce no harm and, in fact, may be beneficial. Not only may fever serve as a valuable clinical sign that permits evaluation of a patient's response to antimicrobial therapy, but fever may also be useful as a part of the host's defense mechanism. An elevated body temperature has been shown to enhance phagocytosis, to cure a few bacterial infections in animals and in man, to inhibit the replication of some viruses in cell culture, and to prevent the pathogenesis of some viral infections in animals. While the evidence in behalf of fever as a de-

TABLE 80-1
Antimicrobial Agents in Current Clinical Use

	Mechanism of Action	Mechanism of Resistance	Serious Toxicity	Usual Daily Dose Range	Usual Dosage Interval (hours)
Penicillins	Inhibition of bacterial cell wall synthesis by inhibiting the cross-linking reaction (transpeptidation)	Beta-lactamases of staphylococci and gram-negative organisms	Anaphylactic shock		
Penicillin G			Allergic reactions	1.2–24 million units	4–6
Procaine penicillin G			Seizures	1–2 million units	12
Benzathine penicillin				1.2 million units	Monthly
Penicillin V				1–2 g	6
Ampicillin				1–12 g (R)	6
Carbenicillin			Bleeding diathesis Sodium overload	4–40 g (R)	4–6
Ticarcillin				2–20 g (R)	4–6
Methicillin		Inherent undefined resistance	Interstitial nephritis	6–12 g (R)	4–6
Dicloxacillin		Inherent undefined resistance		2–4 g (R)	6
Cephalosporins	Same as penicillins	Beta-lactamases of gram-negative organisms	Anaphylactic shock		
Cephalothin			Allergic reactions	2–12 g	4–6
Cephalexin			Thrombophlebitis	1–4 g (R)	6
Cephazolin			Renal damage	1–4 g (R)	6
Erythromycin	Inhibition of bacterial protein synthesis at step of translocation	Decreased ribosomal binding	Rare	1–4 g (H,R)	6
Clindamycin	Inhibition of bacterial protein synthesis at step of peptide bond formation	Decreased ribosomal binding Impermeability	Colitis	600–1200 mg (H)	6
Chloramphenicol	Same as clindamycin	Decreased ribosomal binding. R factor acetylation	Aplastic anemia Transient bone marrow suppression	2–4 g (H)	6
Tetracyclines	Inhibition of bacterial protein synthesis at attachment of new amino acids to ribosomes via tRNA	Impermeability	Superinfection		
Tetracycline			Hepatic damage	1–2 g (H,R)	6
Doxycycline				100–200 mg (Loading dose = 200 mg)	12–24
Aminoglycosides	Inhibition of bacterial protein synthesis at initiation		Renal damage Neuromuscular paralysis		
Kanamycin		R factor adenylylation, phosphorylation, acetylation	Ototoxicity (primarily auditory)	1–1.5 g	6–8

(R)—Dosage adjustment needed in renal disease.
(H)—Dosage adjustment needed in hepatic disease.

(Continued)

─────TABLE 80–1 (cont.)─────

	Mechanism of Action	Mechanism of Resistance	Serious Toxicity	Usual Daily Dose Range	Usual Dosage Interval (hours)
Aminoglycosides (cont.)					
Gentamicin and Tobramycin		R factor adenylylation, acetylation	Ototoxicity (primarily vestibular)	80–360 mg	6–8
Amikacin		R factor acetylation	Ototoxicity (primarily auditory)	0.3–1.5 g	6–8
Streptomycin		R Factor adenylylation phosphorylation	Ototoxicity (primarily vestibular)	0.5–2 g	12–24
Polymyxins	Damage to bacterial cell membranes		Renal damage		
Polymyxin B			Neurotoxicity	150–200 mg	8
Colistin				300–360 mg	8
Rifampicin	Inhibition of bacterial RNA synthesis	Altered RNA polymerase	Hepatotoxicity Thrombocytopenia	450–900 mg	8–12
Vancomycin	Inhibition of bacterial cell wall synthesis		Ototoxicity (primarily deafness). Renal damage. Allergic reactions	2–4 g	6–12
Sulfonamides	Inhibition of bacterial folic acid synthesis at step of PABA insertion		Drug fever		
Sulfisoxazole			Allergic reactions	2–8 g	6–8
Cotrimoxazole			Transient bone marrow suppression		
Trimethoprim	Inhibition of bacterial dihydrofolate reductase			160–480 mg	6–12
Sulfamethoxazole	Same as other sulfonamides		Same as sulfonamides	800–2400 mg	6–12
Nitrofurantoin	Unknown	Unknown	Peripheral neuritis Pulmonary reactions	200–400 mg	6

fense mechanism is not yet compelling, it is sufficient to justify careful thought prior to the use of antipyretics or other temperature reducing maneuvers.

If the decision is made to lower the temperature, several antipyretics are available, of which acetaminophen is the drug of choice. Acetylsalicylic acid (aspirin) has an anti-inflammatory action as well as an antipyretic and analgesic action, while acetaminophen has only antipyretic and analgesic action. However, there are few situations in the management of infectious diseases in which the anti-inflammatory action of aspirin is an advantage. Acetaminophen causes less toxicity except in massive overdoses. Thus, gastrointestinal and other bleeding is far less frequent following the use of acetaminophen, as is gastrointestinal irritation. The relief of pain and malaise may also be accomplished with the antipyretics.

Pain and Malaise

Both codeine and propoxyphene in adequate doses are effective in relieving pain without having any effect on body temperature. If more potent analgesia is needed, narcotics may be used since addiction is seldom a problem with short-term use of these agents. Adequate dosage is essential if one is to achieve effective relief of pain.

Shock

The presence of shock as a consequence of septicemia or endotoxemia demands immediate and effective therapy. The principles of managing this type of shock are discussed in Chapter 145. The current approach to shock accompanying an infectious disease combines the general approach to tissue hypoperfusion with the specific attack on the underlying infection as described below.

Surgical Intervention

Localized infections usually require surgical debridement or drainage in addition to adequate antimicrobial therapy. Not only does the walled-off abscess present a barrier for penetration of the antibacterial agent, but the cell debris encountered in the interior of the abscess can bind or inactivate some antibiotics, notably the aminoglycosides. Furthermore, the acidic environment of the abscess cavity can destroy some antibiotics and diminish the activity of others that require a neutral or basic milieu. Necrotic tissue, even in the absence of abscess formation, provides an excellent medium for the growth of anaerobes with the danger of gas gangrene or tetanus.

AN APPROACH TO CHEMOTHERAPY

Several steps are required in the therapeutic approach to an infectious disease. After the initial decision as to the necessity of treatment is made, an antimicrobial agent is selected, a therapeutic regimen is designed, and a plan for monitoring its effectiveness is formulated.

THE DECISION TO TREAT OR NOT TO TREAT

While this decision is easy in the presence of a severe or life-threatening illness, it becomes more difficult with less severe or trivial infections and still more so when the therapy is aimed at preventing rather than curing an infectious disease.

Since infections by organisms, such as the pneumococcus, which are highly sensitive to antimicrobial agents, may proceed rapidly toward an irreversible state, one must begin treatment as early as possible in the course of infection that could be life threatening. The manifest seriousness of some infections demands the immediate initiation of specific antimicrobial therapy without waiting for cultural proof of the specific organism involved and without knowing the sensitivities of that organism. Here the choice of an appropriate antimicrobial regimen depends on a sophisticated clinical estimate of the etiologic agent most likely to be involved, as a base for the selection of the most logical antimicrobial agent or agents. This type of decision is essential in most patients with a local infection judged to be proceeding towards septicemia, septicemia itself, most cases of meningitis, and many cases of pneumonitis.

More difficulty is encountered with less immediately serious infections. Here one is often justified in withholding treatment while collecting as much information as possible on which to base a rational decision. An example is the patient with a urinary tract infection who has an indwelling catheter in place or has a structural abnormality. In this situation one may first identify the organism and determine its sensitivities before initiating therapy. This is a situation in which any regimen selected is unlikely to successfully eradicate the organism. Faced with this knowledge, it may be best to refrain from subjecting the patient to the potential toxicity of the drug.

Perhaps the greatest misuse of antibiotics is in the treatment of viral or presumed viral illnesses. It has been stated that greater than 50 percent of common colds that are brought to the attention of a physician are treated with antibiotics. While the argument is sometimes made that the antibiotic may prevent the occasional bacterial superinfection, this concept lacks documentation. Clearly, this is a situation where even a remote chance of serious toxicity from the drug is unacceptable.

The use of antimicrobial agents to prevent infections is of proven value in only a few situations. These include the prevention of streptococcal infections in patients with rheumatic heart disease or past rheumatic fever (penicillin, a sulfonamide, or erythromycin), the prevention of meningococcal infection in close contacts of infected patients in epidemic situations (a sulfonamide if the meningococcus is sensitive, or minocycline or rifampicin if not), the prevention of exacerbations in a setting of chronic bronchitis (ampicillin or a tetracycline), the prevention of postoperative infections after vaginal hysterectomy (a cephalosporin), the prevention of postoperative infections after major bowel surgery (oral neomycin and a tetracycline), the prevention of tuberculous disease in tuberculin-positive patients receiving steroids (isoniazid), the prevention of influenza A (amantidine), and the prevention of smallpox (methisazone). Although of unproven value, the use of penicillin and an aminoglycoside is recommended by the American Heart Association for the prevention of infective endocarditis in patients with rheumatic or congenital heart disease who undergo dental manipulations or oral surgery. Similarly unproven is the widely advocated use of antibiotics in the presence of penetrating wounds, skull fractures, and other compound fractures.

THE CHOICE OF AN ANTIMICROBIAL AGENT

Without specific knowledge of the antimicrobial sensitivities of the organism involved in a particular infection, one must proceed on the basis of the usual sensitivities of similar organisms. With the emergence of resistance due to plasmid transfer between organisms of different species, one must be aware of the ecology of resistance in the particular population of patients being treated. Even within a single institution there may be wide divergences in the sensitivities of a group of organisms. A tabulation of drugs of choice and alternative drugs is presented in Table 80–2. One must emphasize, however, that the "drug of choice" may be determined on grounds other than clinical effectiveness. If several drugs are equally effective, selection of the "drug of choice" may be on the basis of less toxicity, less cost, convenience of administration, or some combination of these factors. Individual consideration, including those presented below, may therefore alter one's "drug of choice" in a particular situation.

Bacterial Sensitivities

Sensitivity and resistance are relative terms based on the ability of a selected concentration of drug to inhibit bacterial growth (minimum inhibitory concentration or MIC) or to kill bacterial cells (minimum bactericidal concentration or MBC). The selected level separating sensitivity from resistance is somewhat arbitrarily chosen based on some relationship with the attainability of an effective level, usually in plasma. Several features of bacterial sensitivity testing should be kept in mind when evaluating the laboratory results and planning therapy. An organism may be "resistant" as defined by a lack of growth inhibition at concentrations achievable in plasma and yet be quite "susceptible" to the higher concentrations of antibiotic achieved in urine. Conversely, an organism may be "sensitive" to the selected plasma level but "resistant" because the infection is in the

meninges, where the concentration of the drug in question is less. It should also be noted that the MIC or MBC chosen is based on having that level of antibiotic constantly in contact with the bacterial cell over a 24- to 48-hour period. Consequently, one must consider the MIC or MBC as a minimal antibiotic concentration to be exceeded all of or at least a great proportion of each dosing interval.

The rate of killing of bacteria probably increases in some relation to the concentration of drug in the bacterium's environment. This is true for penicillin up to some plateau level, beyond which no further increase in killing rate occurs. For other antibiotics the plateau phenomenon does not appear to exist, and an increased rate of killing is associated with increasing concentrations of the antibiotic. Thus, for most antibiotics the dosage used for a serious infection is limited only by its toxicity. One must always weigh the toxicity of the antibiotic against the severity of the illness. It may be reasonable to risk some vestibular dysfunction or even hearing deficit as a result of gentamicin's ototoxicity in order to prevent death from a pseudomonas septicemia.

Finally, it should be recognized that the conditions under which the sensitivity is determined in vitro differ considerably from those existing at the site of infection. For example, protein binding is usually not considered in the determination of an MIC or MBC.

As a result of these considerations, the MIC or MBC should be viewed only as a rough guide to the likelihood of success or failure of treatment with the antibiotic tested against that particular organism. It is, however, unlikely that a systemic infection due to an organism shown to be resistant to a given agent in vitro will be effectively treated by that agent.

Resistance Patterns

The ability of microorganisms to develop resistance to antibiotics and chemotherapeutic agents is truly remarkable, and the construction of a rational therapeutic regimen is greatly influenced by this phenomenon. For example, the mechanism of resistance that develops to erythromycin (an "induced resistance" in which low erythromycin levels encourage an increased resistance to the erythromycin) extends as well to clindamycin. Consequently, in treating an erythromycin-resistant organism one should not use clindamycin. Conversely, erythromycin would be poorly advised in an infection due to a clindamycin-resistant organism.

Resistance to the tetracyclines is usually on the basis of reduced permeability of an organism to the antibiotic. This resistance is shared by all of the

TABLE 80-2
Antimicrobial Selection Based on Organisms

	Drug of Choice	Alternative Drugs
Gram-Positive Cocci		
Staphylococcus aureus		
Non-penicillinase producing	Penicillin G	A cephalosporin Erythromycin Clindamycin Vancomycin
Penicillinase producing	Methicillin Dicloxacillin (p.o.)	A cephalosporin Erythromycin Clindamycin Vancomycin
Streptococcus pyogenes (Groups A,B,C, and G)	Penicillin G	Erythromycin Clindamycin A cephalosporin
Streptococcus viridans	Penicillin G plus an aminoglycoside	A cephalosporin Erythromycin Vancomycin
Streptococcus, anaerobic	Penicillin G	Erythromycin A tetracycline Clindamycin
Enterococcus	Penicillin G plus an aminoglycoside	Vancomycin
Pneumococcus	Penicillin G	Erythromycin Clindamycin Chloramphenicol (in meningitis)
Gram-Negative Cocci		
Neisseria meningitidis	Penicillin G	Chloramphenicol A tetracycline
Neisseria gonorrhoeae	Penicillin G	Spectinomycin (local infections only) A tetracycline
Gram-Positive Bacilli		
Bacillus anthracis	Penicillin G	Erythromycin Chloramphenicol A tetracycline
Listeria monocytogenes	Penicillin G	Erythromycin A tetracycline
Clostridium welchii and *tetani*	Penicillin G	Erythromycin A tetracycline
Corynebacterium diphtheriae	Penicillin G	Erythromycin A tetracycline
Gram-Negative Bacilli		

*Escherichia coli**	Gentamicin
	  or Tobramycin
		Kanamycin
		Amikacin
		Ampicillin
		Chloramphenicol
		Trimethoprim-
		  Sulfomethoxozole

*Klebsiella pneumoniae**	Gentamicin or Tobramycin	Chloramphenicol Amikacin Kanamycin A cephalosporin Polymyxin
Enterobacter*	Gentamicin or Tobramycin	Kanamycin Amikacin Chloramphenicol Polymyxin Carbenicillin

* Resistance to antimicrobics is often determined by genetic information coded by plasmids and will be variable. Patterns must be determined for each treatment setting.

(Continued)

TABLE 80-2 (cont.)

	Drug of Choice	Alternative Drugs
Gram-Positive Bacilli (cont.)		
Serratia*	Gentamicin or Tobramycin	Kanamycin Amikacin Chloramphenicol Co-trimoxazole Carbenicillin
Proteus mirabilis*	Ampicillin	Gentamicin Kanamycin Amikacin A cephalosporin
Proteus, others*	Gentamicin or Tobramycin	Kanamycin Amikacin Chloramphenicol Carbenicillin A cephalosporin
Pseudomonas aeruginosa*	Carbenicillin and/or either Gentamicin or Tobramycin	Polymyxin Amikacin
Bacteroides, respiratory	Penicillin G	Chloramphenicol A tetracycline Clindamycin
Bacteroides, gastrointestinal	Clindamycin	Chloramphenicol
Salmonella	Chloramphenicol	Ampicillin Co-trimoxazole
Shigella	Ampicillin	A tetracycline Chloramphenicol Co-trimoxazole
Haemophilus influenzae	Chloramphenicol	Ampicillin A tetracycline Co-trimoxazole
Haemophilus ducreyi	A tetracycline	Ampicillin
Bordetella pertussis	Erythromycin	Ampicillin A tetracycline
Pseudomonas pseudomallei	A tetracycline	Chloramphenicol
Brucella	A tetracycline	Chloramphenicol Streptomycin
Actinobacillus malei	A tetracycline plus streptomycin	Chloramphenicol plus Streptomycin
Francisella tularensis	Streptomycin	A tetracycline
Yersinia pestis	Streptomycin	A tetracycline
Vibrio cholerae	A tetracycline	Furazolidone Chloramphenicol
Fusobacterium fusiforme	Penicillin G	A tetracycline Erythromycin
Calymmatobacterium granulomatis	A tetracycline	Ampicillin Streptomycin
Spirochetes		
Treponema pallidum	Penicillin G	A tetracycline Erythromycin
Treponema pertenue	Penicillin G	A tetracycline Erythromycin
Leptospira	Penicillin G	A tetracycline
Spirillum minor	Penicillin G	Erythromycin Streptomycin
Borrelia recurrentis	A tetracycline	Penicillin G

* Resistance to antimicrobics is often determined by genetic information coded by plasmids and will be variable. Patterns must be determined for each treatment setting.

TABLE 80-2 (cont.)

	Drug of Choice	Alternative Drugs
Acid-Fast Bacilli		
Mycobacterium tuberculosis	Isoniazide plus Ethambutol	Rifampin PAS Streptomycin Pyrazinamide Cycloserine
Atypical mycobacterium	Isoniazid, Ethambutol, and Streptomycin	Rifampin PAS Pyrazinamide Cycloserine
Mycobacterium balnei	Cycloserine	Isoniazid Rifampin
Myobacterium leprae	A sulfone	Amithiozone
Actinomycetes		
Actinomyces israelii	Penicillin G	A tetracycline Erythromycin
Actinomyces muris ratti	Ampicillin	Erythromycin Streptomycin
Nocardia	A sulfonamide plus streptomycin	A tetracycline plus cycloserine; A sulfonamide plus ampicillin; Co-trimoxazole
Fungi		
Histoplasma capsulatum	Amphotericin B	
Candida albicans	Amphotericin B	Flucytosine
Aspergillus	Amphotericin B	Flucytosine
Cryptococcus neoformans	Amphotericin B	Flucytosine
Mucor	Amphotericin B	
Coccidioides immitis	Amphotericin B	
Blastomyces dermatitidis	Amphotericin B	Hydroxystilbamidine
Blastomyces brasiliensis	Amphotericin B	A sulfonamide
Sporotrichum schenckii	An iodide	Amphotericin B Griseofulvin
Fonsecaea	Amphotericin B	
Dermatophytes	Griseofulvin	
Viruses		
Variola	Methisazone (prophylactic)	
Herpes simplex	Idoxuridine (topical) Adenosine arabinaside	
Influenza A	Amantadine (prophylactic)	
Inclusion conjunctivitis	A tetracycline Chloramphenicol	
Filterable Agents and Chlamydiae		
Mycoplasma pneumoniae	Erythromycin	Tetracycline Chloramphenicol
Psittacosis	A tetracycline	Chloramphenicol
Lymphogranuloma venereum	A tetracycline	Chloramphenicol
Chlamydia trachomatis	A tetracycline	Erythromycin Chloramphenicol A sulfonamide
Other		
Legionella pneumophila	Erythromycin	Rifampin

numerous tetracycline derivatives and, consequently, one should change categories of antibiotics if resistance to a tetracycline is seen.

Resistance to chloramphenicol is often mediated by an R factor and simultaneously acquired resistance to multiple antibacterial agents is commonly seen. This acquired resistance to multiple drugs is due to the ability of the R factor DNA to carry into the bacterium information coding for several gene products capable of modifying several antibiotics. Thus, in addition to promoting the acetylation of chloramphenicol, the sulfonamides may be acetylated, kanamycin may be phosphorylated, gentamicin may be adenylylated, and the tetracyclines may be poorly transported into the bacterium. All of these resistances may be simultaneously conferred upon a cell by the same R factor. As noted above, R factors may be transferred between bacterial species.

Resistance to the aminoglycosides (streptomycin, kanamycin, gentamicin, tobramycin, and amikacin) is usually via an R factor-mediated modification of the antibiotic. This modification may be by phosphorylation, adenylylation, or acetylation. The specificity of the R factor-mediated enzymes catalyzing these three modifications allows the modification of one of the aminoglycosides without necessarily conferring resistance simultaneously on the others. Thus, resistance to one aminoglycoside does not necessarily mean that resistance will be seen to the others. Individual sensitivities must be performed to each clinically useful aminoglycoside (currently gentamicin, kanamycin, tobramycin, and amikacin).

The β-lactamases inactivate penicillins and cephalosporins by catalyzing hydrolysis of the β-lactam ring contained within these two antibiotic structures. A variety of β-lactamases differing in substrate specificity exist in both gram-positive and gram-negative organisms. In general, the staphylococcal β-lactamases are usually meant when the term penicillinase is used. These β-lactamases inactivate penicillin G, penicillin V, ampicillin, amoxycillin, carbenicillin, and ticarcillin but fail to inactivate methicillin, nafcillin, oxacillin, cloxacillin, dicloxacillin, and the cephalosporins. Among the gram-negative organisms, the β-lactamase of the pseudomonas is capable of hydrolyzing penicillin, ampicillin, amoxycillin, and the current cephalosporins but not carbenicillin or ticarcillin. The resistance of carbenicillin and ticarcillin to the pseudomonas β-lactamase accounts in part for their usefulness in treating pseudomonas infections.

The sulfonamides are inactivated by acetylation and this activity is often conferred by an R factor-mediated mechanism.

Resistance to trimethoprim is usually due to a mutation in the dihydrofolate reductase of the bacterium so that trimethoprim no longer binds to nor does it inhibit the mutant enzyme of the resistant species.

The Site and Extent of Infection

Occasionally, the selection of a specific antimicrobial agent is based primarily on this criterion and often the selection is influenced by it.

Urinary tract infections clearly can be eradicated by many chemotherapeutic agents that achieve adequate urinary levels but fail to achieve adequate plasma or tissue levels. From such observations one relates the effectiveness of therapy in urinary tract infections to the urinary levels of drugs and not to plasma or tissue levels. With some chemotherapeutic agents the urinary levels are adequate in spite of plasma and tissue levels that are never effective (such as nitrofurantoin, nalidixic acid, oxolinic acid and mandelamine). This approach also is useful in considering the appropriate dosage regimens of other drugs, such as penicillin, ampicillin, and carbenicillin, where even "resistant" organisms may succumb to the enormous levels achieved in the urine. The concentration of penicillins in the urine allows for the administration of much smaller doses than are required for systemic infections.

A second site of infection that often modifies the selection of an antibiotic is the cerebrospinal fluid (CSF) or meninges. Here the entry of the drug into the CSF becomes of critical importance and several chemotherapeutic agents that are effective elsewhere are impotent in treating meningitis. Examples include cephalothin (and presumably other cephalosporins), clindamycin, erythromycin, and probably the highly protein-bound, semi-synthetic, penicillinase-resistant penicillins such as nafcillin, oxacillin, cloxacillin, and dicloxacillin. Chloramphenicol assumes an increased importance in the treatment of meningitis since its cerebrospinal fluid (CSF) levels are one-third to one-half those in simultaneously measured plasma. Both trimethoprim and sulfamethoxazole also enter the CSF well.

The localization of bacteria within fibrin often requires the use of high doses of antibiotics in order to achieve penetration to the microorganism. This situation is seen with infective endocarditis.

An intracellular localization of organisms may require the drug to enter the cell. Chloramphenicol, rifampicin, and trimethoprim are effectively distributed into cells while most of the others are not. In rare cases, such as in patients with chronic granulomatous disease where the cells own bacteriocidal activity is impaired, the use of one of these drugs may be indicated in preference to a drug with greater in vitro sensitivity.

The Adequacy of Host Defense Mechanisms

The selection of an antimicrobial agent is often influenced by the adequacy or inadequacy of the host defense mechanisms. Although this seems to be of documented value in relatively few situations, it is wise to consider host defense factors in choosing an appropriate drug.

In general, it is believed that "bactericidal" drugs should be used in preference to "bacteristatic" drugs in patients with compromised host defense mechanisms including immune deficiencies, granulocytopenia, chronic granulomatous disease, patients after splenectomy, and in patients who are immunosuppressed. Such "bactericidal" drugs include the penicillins, cephalosporins, and aminoglycosides while erythromycin, the tetracyclines, chloramphenicol, and the sulfonamides are usually considered bacteristatic. It should be recognized, however, that the terms "bactericidal" and "bacteristatic" are not entirely clear in their meanings. Often, a drug is considered "bacteristatic" at low concentrations and "bactericidal" at high concentrations, as claimed for clindamycin, chloramphenicol, and erythromycin. The bactericidal action of a drug is usually not a property of the drug itself but of the interaction between the drug, the microbe, and the environment. Penicillin, for example, is "bactericidal" if the microbe is in a hypotonic environment but not so if in a hypertonic milieu or in an abscess cavity. Trimethoprim is bacteristatic if the organism is grown in a minimal medium but bactericidal if an exogenous supply of amino acids and purines is present. Chloramphenicol is bacteristatic for *E. coli,* but bactericidal for *S. pneumonide, N. meningitidis,* and *H. influenzae.* Thus, the usefulness of these terms in clinical practice must not be overemphasized.

As cited above, the penetration of a chemotherapeutic agent into host cells may be far more important than the categorization of the drug as "cidal" or "static."

The Pharmacokinetics of the Drug

Occasionally, the selection of an antimicrobial agent is based on the pharmacokinetics of the drug. For example, in patients with impaired renal function, most of the tetracyclines are retained with an enhanced risk of drug toxicity. Doxycycline, however, is excreted into the gut and its kinetics do not change appreciably in the presence of diminished or changing renal function.

The individual kinetics of sulfamethoxazole and trimethoprim differ considerably in patients with severely compromised renal function and, the rational use of this fixed-dose combination then becomes difficult.

In the presence of liver dysfunction, chloramphenicol cannot be efficiently detoxified by glucuronidation, and dose-related toxicity is seen more frequently unless the plasma levels are followed to ensure a subtoxic concentration. Similarly, the plasma levels of gentamicin, kanamycin, and tobramycin should be followed in the patient with marked renal dysfunction in order to attain adequate levels with a minimum of toxicity.

The Benefit-to-Risk Ratio of the Drug

Both an estimation of benefit and an estimation of risk should be considered in the selection of any appropriate antimicrobial agent.

In general, greater risks are acceptable in the treatment of more severe infections and no serious risks are acceptable in the treatment of minor infections. However, this axiom is violated frequently. For example, there is often concern about ototoxicity associated with the use of high doses of gentamicin even in the presence of a life-threatening pseudomonas septicemia. Clearly, it is the proper choice to preserve life even at the expense of complete loss of vestibular function. Conversely, it has been estimated that about 50 percent of the use of clindamycin in a recent year was for self-limited upper respiratory infections. Yet clindamycin is occasionally associated with a pseudomembranous colitis and at least two dozen deaths have been attributed to the colitis. Surely no mortality as a result of drug therapy is acceptable in the treatment of a trivial viral illness.

The proper estimation of a benefit-to-risk ratio requires accurate information quantifying the benefits attributable to the drug and accurate incidence figures with respect to the adverse reactions associated with it. Usually, neither of these is available in as firm a form as we would like. Consider, for example, the choice between ampicillin and chloramphenicol for the treatment of a serious *Haemophilus influenzae* infection. Usually, one would consider the two to provide about equal effectiveness and consequently, the choice usually rests on the relative risks associated with the two drugs. Invariably, ampicillin has been chosen on grounds of lesser toxicity. But the available estimates of the incidence of fatal anaphylaxis associated with penicillin (1:10,000 to 1:100,000) and by inference also with ampicillin are in about the same range as the estimates of fatal aplastic anemia associated with chloramphenicol (1:15,000 to 1:60,000). Furthermore, the incidence of fatal thromboembolic phenomena associated with oral contraceptives is in the same range. Yet we find it acceptable to give oral contraceptives to normal women and we fear the administration of chloramphenicol even to the seriously ill.

Combinations of Antimicrobial Agents

Often two or more antimicrobial agents are used simultaneously. Such combination chemotherapy is advantageous in several common clinical situations. The initial treatment of a serious infection in the absence of an identified bacteriologic agent constitutes the usual justification for the simultaneous use of two drugs. In this situation, one wishes to maximize one's chances of success by covering the most likely possibilities. In general, one assumes that the risk involved in the use of a second (or even third) drug is less than the risk associated with failure to appropriately attack the offending organism. One usually further assumes that the use of two or three "specific" antibiotics is preferable to the use of a single broad spectrum antibiotic. Evidence for such an assumption is meagre indeed. Nevertheless, this indication is reasonable on logical grounds and clinically acceptable.

A second indication for combination chemotherapy takes advantage of the synergistic effect of some combinations on some bacteria or fungi. Although the situations with proven synergism are rare, they are of sufficient clinical importance to be considered. Perhaps the most commonly encountered example of synergism is in the combination of trimethoprim with sulfamethoxazole. In vitro synergism has been clearly demonstrated with this combination against a number of bacterial species. This synergism is based on the inhibition of two sequential steps in tetrahydrofolic acid biosynthesis by the two components. The combination of sulfamethoxazole with trimethoprim is also likely to be advantageous because of the rapid emergence of resistance that might be seen with trimethoprim alone and the diminution of this development with the simultaneous administration of a sulfonamide. Carbenicillin and gentamicin are synergistic against many strains (perhaps 30 percent of all strains) of *Pseudomonas aeruginosa.* About the same percentage of strains of *E. coli* are susceptible to a synergism between ampicillin and gentamicin. *Streptococcus viridans,* even though sensitive to penicillin, often shows synergism between penicillin and an aminoglycoside. Some fungi are inhibited in a synergistic fashion by amphotericin B and flucytosine given concurrently.

A third rationale for the use of combinations of chemotherapeutic agents involves the simultaneous treatment of infections caused by multiple organisms. This may be thought of as particularly relevant in the treatment of contaminated gastrointestinal surgery after trauma or the rupture of a viscus. In this situation, there is experimental evidence for the effectiveness of clindamycin combined with an aminoglycoside to aim at both anaerobes and aerobic gram-negative bacilli.

A fourth indication for combination chemotherapy is in an attempt to forestall the emergence of resistance to a single drug. This indication has been cited above with respect to the combination of trimethoprim with sulfamethoxazole. It is also frequently invoked in antituberculous chemotherapy in an effort to delay the emergence of resistance to isoniazid.

Although some significant advantages may accrue with the use of combinations of chemotherapeutic agents, some disadvantages are also apparent. The cost of therapy usually increases, the incidence of adverse reactions is compounded, a sense of security may be falsely engendered, and there may occasionally be antagonism between the components of the combination. Antagonism, although commonly considered, is rarely encountered at a clinical level. Two examples have been well documented. The combination of chlortetracycline with penicillin in the management of pneumococcal meningitis was associated with an increased mortality over that seen with the use of penicillin alone. No refutation of the conclusions of this study exists. However, the conclusions should not be extrapolated to other clinical infections since no antagonism was seen with the simultaneous use of these two agents in the treatment of pneumococcal pneumonia.

The second situation of proven antagonism involves the inactivation of gentamicin by high concentrations of carbenicillin. This inactivation has been clearly demonstrated in vitro, and the two drugs should not be added to the same intravenous bottle. The inactivation does not appear to occur in vivo in the usual case but in the patient with markedly impaired renal function this inactivation may be realized.

Drug Interactions

The selection of a chemotherapeutic agent is at times influenced by drug interactions. These interactions may be at many different levels ranging from direct chemical interactions, as noted above for the inactivation of gentamicin by carbenicillin, through interactions affecting absorption, distribution, metabolism, and excretion. The absorption of the tetracyclines is impaired in the presence of iron salts, and the absorption of rifampicin is significantly diminished if PAS is concurrently administered. Both of these interactions are of clinical significance. Many chemotherapeutic agents are tightly bound to plasma proteins and the potential certainly exists for displacing these drugs by simultaneously administering other bound drugs. Conversely, the bound chemotherapeutic agent may displace other drugs leading to elevated levels of the free drug. The metabolism of many drugs by way of microsomal, drug-metabolizing enzymes is inhibited by chloramphenicol and the metabolism of diphenylhydantoin is inhibited by isoniazid. The metabolism of theophyllin is inhibited by erythromycin. Conversely, the metabolism of many drugs is enhanced by inducers of microsomal enzymes, and rifampicin has been shown capable of such induction. This latter interaction has been shown to be clinically significant with respect to oral anticoagulants and to oral contraceptives as well. This type of interaction should be considered when selecting any chemotherapeutic agent that is significantly metabolized by the hepatic microsomal system. Drug interactions affecting excretion include the well-known effect of probenecid on the renal secretion of penicillins and the influence of amphotericin-induced renal damage on the elimination of 5-fluorocytosine and the aminoglycosides.

THE RATIONAL ADMINISTRATION OF THE CHOSEN AGENT

Once the chemotherapeutic agent is chosen, the physician's next obligation is to provide the drug by way of an optimal regimen. Many of the considerations here are similar to those utilized in the selection of the drug. Several additional considerations are also important.

THE ROUTE OF ADMINISTRATION. Usually, if alternative routes of administration are available, the choice lies between oral, intramuscular, intravenous, and, occasionally, intrathecal routes.

Clearly, the oral route has many advantages and should be selected when possible for relatively minor infections. However, several disadvantages are also inherent in the oral administration of a drug. On an ambulatory basis this is usually the only feasible route, but one should recognize that compliance is a major problem with any orally administered drug. Careful attention to compliance is in order in every patient since it is notoriously difficult to predict compliance or noncompliance. A second disadvantage is the unpredictability of absorption of many orally given drugs. While this problem may be overemphasized, it seems reasonable to use parenteral routes preferentially in the treatment of serious infections whenever feasible.

The intramuscular route obviates the need for a continuous intravenous line with its own propensity to serve as a nidus for infections. Furthermore, it is considerably less expensive considering the added cost of intravenous fluids. However, the seriously ill patient will usually have an intravenous line installed for other reasons and its use for antimicrobial administration saves the patient from repeated intramuscular injections.

The intravenous route is frequently the route chosen in the seriously ill patient. In addition to the hygiene associated with an indwelling intravenous line, one has the additional problems of drug incompatabilities and drug stabilities. The list of incompatabilities is extensive and, as a generalization, one should attempt to deliver each drug singly and at its own time via the intravenous line. The delivery of drugs in an intermittent fashion allows this single drug administration and in addition attends to the problem of drug instability. The latter is particularly important with ampicillin and methicillin administration.

The intrathecal route is seldom used but is occasionally indicated in the treatment of difficult cases of meningitis. The problem arises here because of the severity of gram-negative meningitis and because of the inability of the aminoglycosides (usually the drugs of choice in such serious gram-negative infections) to enter the CSF. Although the usual method of delivery involves the administration following a lumbar puncture, the flow of CSF prevents the antibiotic from entering the ventricles and the intraventricular administration of the drug via a surgically placed reservoir has recently been advocated. Although this constitutes a major decision, the continuing high mortality associated with gram-negative meningitis demands that we continue our search for better treatment regimens.

The Relationship Between in-Vivo Antimicrobial Levels and in-Vitro Minimal Inhibitory Concentration (MIC)

The MIC has been described above as it pertains to our selection of a therapeutic agent. Now we consider it again with regard to the relationship that should exist between the concentration of antimicrobial agent at the site of infection and the MIC of the organism. Since the MIC is performed by exposing the microbe to the drug continuously for the period of assay (usually 24 and sometimes 48 hours), a logical conclusion would be that this level of antimicrobial agent should be exceeded continuously. Exceptions can be immediately cited. For example, penicillin can be quite effective even though the concentration falls to suboptimal levels for a part of each dosing interval. The same is certainly true of isoniazid. These exceptions may suggest that the above generalization applies less stringently to situations in which an irreversible interaction occurs between the drug and the organism. Nevertheless, even in these situations, it is advantageous to exceed the MIC for at least a large part of each dosing interval. The next decision is by how much to exceed the MIC. This question has been addressed in a formal manner for penicillin G but far less information exists with other drugs. With increasing concentrations of penicillin G above the MIC the bacteria are killed more rapidly and more effectively up to a point. Beyond this point the continued increase in concentration adds no more effectiveness to the system. Thus, a plateau is reached beyond which more drug is of no advantage. This plateau is usually seen at a multiple of about 10 times the MIC of an organism. Other antimicrobials do not show this same plateau phenomenon, however, and increasing concentrations lead to increasing rates of bacterial killing. From this information one can tentatively suggest that the rate of bacterial growth inhibition or bacterial killing increases with increasing concentrations of an antimicrobial agent with the exception of the penicillins. In most cases, then, there should be no "optimal" multiple of the MIC that should be achieved. Instead, one should give as much of an antimicrobial agent as possible, at least in the seriously ill patient, without producing unacceptable toxicity.

Drug Distribution

The goal of chemotherapy is the eradication of the infection. To achieve that goal one must provide an adequate concentration of drug in the immediate environment of the organisms to be eradicated. It is difficult to assess the level of drug at the site of infection since access to compartments other than blood, urine, or CSF is difficult. One can utilize the available information on the penetration of drugs into urine, CSF, and models of interstitial fluid.

Most chemotherapeutic agents are eliminated in large part by the kidneys, and even with those drugs that are highly metabolized, a generous percentage of the administered dose is eliminated into the urine as the unmetabolized drug. Thus, urinary concentrations are often high and if the drug is secreted into the urine (as are the penicillins and cephalosporins) may be enormous. Even a drug such as doxycycline, however, that may be eliminated largely by an extrarenal mechanism provides adequate urinary concentrations for the treatment of many urinary tract infections. Thus, the provision of adequate drug to the urine is rarely difficult.

Much more difficult is the provision of drug to the CSF. Although our understanding of antimicrobial penetration into the CSF is rudimentary, some information is available. Few antimicrobials enter the CSF with facility. Therefore, one is usually faced with a choice between giving high levels of the drug intravenously in hopes of driving enough into the CSF or giving the drug directly into the CSF via the lumbar route or the ventricular route. Direct instillation has received considerable recent support in the treatment

of gram-negative meningitis with gentamicin. For most other drugs the alternative choice is usually made.

The distribution of antimicrobial agent into extravascular extracellular spaces has received renewed interest recently, but the guidelines remain scanty. In general, there is probably a reasonable correlation between plasma levels and interstitial fluid levels of most chemotherapeutic agents, although the kinetics of each compartment may vary. For this reason and because of the inability to directly measure the interstitial concentrations of an antimicrobial agent, one should strive for adequate plasma drug levels as an approximation of extracellular tissue levels. A unique site of drug distribution is prostatic fluid. Two chemotherapeutic agents (erythromycin and trimethoprim) are concentrated in this fluid.

Intermittent *Versus* Continuous Administration

While this issue has been debated for many years, no clear evidence in favor of one or the other has emerged. For practical reasons, as cited above, an intermittent infusion is usually chosen. Care must be taken in using an intermittent regimen that the dosage interval is sufficiently short relative to the growth rate of the microorganism so that the microbes do not have a chance of recovering between doses. Perhaps one extreme example of this point is seen in the biweekly isoniazid regimens used in the treatment of tuberculosis. This is predicated upon the slow growth rate of the tubercle bacillus combined with the nearly irreversible interaction between isoniazid and the bacterium. A similar argument, although contracted in time, can be generated to explain the efficacy of penicillin given by intermittent dosing.

Toxicologic Restrictions

If the effectiveness of an antimicrobial agent increases with increasing concentration of the drug at the site of infection (as suggested above), then adverse drug reactions that are dose related become important as restrictions on the amount of drug to be given. Examples of such dose-related toxicities include the neurotoxicity of penicillins, the nephrotoxicity of cephalosporins, aminoglycosides, polymyxin and amphotericin B, the ototoxicity of the aminoglycosides, the gray baby syndrome and possibly a similar adult syndrome with chloramphenicol, a transient bone marrow suppression with chloramphenicol, hepatotoxicity with the tetracyclines, sodium overload and bleeding with carbenicillin, and diarrhea with most of the orally administered chemotherapeutic agents. As emphasized above, however, in each individual situation one must carefully weigh the disadvantages of toxicity with the advantages anticipated from increased dosages.

Modifications of Therapeutic Regimens

Modification of an otherwise optimal therapeutic regimen should be considered in the presence of renal or hepatic dysfunction.

Since most antimicrobial agents are ultimately eliminated by the kidneys, any significant reduction of renal function should lead to a reappraisal of one's therapeutic regimen. Although an isolated impairment of tubular secretory capacity could theoretically lead to a change in the kinetics of elimination of the penicillins and cephalosporins, it is usually an impaired glomerular filtration that leads to a clinically important prolongation of the drug's residence in the host. Consequently, the dosage adjustments that are necessary usually correlate closely with the creatinine clearance or more roughly with the serum creatinine. In principle, a dosage adjustment should probably be made for nearly every chemotherapeutic agent in the face of moderate or marked glomerular dysfunction. However, such adjustments are essential with a few drugs where dose related toxicity occurs at drug levels near to those necessary for clinical effectiveness. The most common example is seen in the use of the aminoglycosides for major systemic infections. Since the margin of safety with these antibiotics is rather narrow, one is often bordering on the toxic level in order to achieve maximal effectiveness. A moderate change in glomerular filtration can then initiate a viscious cycle with accumulation of the aminoglycoside, nephrotoxicity from the higher levels of drug, and greater accumulation of the aminoglycoside in a spiralling fashion. Nomograms and simple rules-of-thumb have been formulated in order to guide therapy in this situation, but the individual variation seen with each of the proposed guidelines makes a strong case for the monitoring of plasma aminoglycoside levels as a guide to dosage. Similar care should be taken with cephaloridine and other cephalosporins, polymyxin, the tetracyclines (excepting doxycycline whose kinetics change little even with severe renal dysfunction), and 5-fluorocytosine.

Rational modification of antimicrobial dosage is much more difficult in the presence of hepatic dysfunction, for here the mechanisms of drug metabolism are variable and there is no commonality similar to the glomerular filtration of the kidney. Thus, chloramphenicol is glucuronidated, clindamycin is demethylated and conjugated with sulfoxide, cephalothin is deacetylated, and the sulfonamides are acetylated. There is no commonly used "liver function test" that correlates well with any of these biochemical modifications. The best safeguard in the presence of liver dysfunction is to follow plasma levels if dose-related toxicity is a potential problem.

THERAPEUTIC MONITORING

In order to ensure a steady progression toward the eradication of an infection, it is essential that therapy be continually monitored after its initiation. This monitoring can be at a clinical, radiologic, microbiologic, or pharmacologic level and usually consists of some combination of these. Since the others will receive consideration in the succeeding chapters on individual infectious diseases, only the pharmacologic level of monitoring will be discussed here.

Two basically dissimilar approaches are available for antimicrobial monitoring. One can either measure the activity of a body fluid against a microorganism (and usually against the patient's own organism) or one can measure the concentration of the drug in an accessible fluid. Proponents of the former method (serum "cidal" levels) argue that the results are more indicative of the actual antimicrobial effectiveness since the determination measures the activity of the drug. Although the logic of this argument seems persuasive, there is little evidence in support of this view. Equally unimpressive is the evidence that allows a measured "cidal" level to be considered inadequate, adequate, or optimal. Usually the level is considered adequate if the serum, plasma, or fluid can be diluted eight-fold or more and still exhibit the inhibitory activity. It is also unclear when, in relation to a dose, one should seek such levels. Furthermore, it is apparent that once the serum, plasma or other biologic fluid is diluted with a buffered salt solution, it no longer resembles the original fluid and with increasing dilution the resemblence becomes even less. One of the consequences of the dilution of the fluid is the weakening of the plasma protein binding of some antibiotics. Thus, highly bound antibiotics may appear increasingly active with dilution, due to the availability of a greater percentage of the drug in the free or active state. Finally, the "cidal" level offers a composite answer in the presence of multiple antibiotics. While this may be the desired measurement, it does not aid in the manipulation of each antimicrobial agent on an individual basis.

The alternative assay that is useful for antimicrobial monitoring is the measurement of absolute drug levels in the biologic fluid. Several new approaches including enzymologic and radioimmunologic assays have added to the ease with which a few chemotherapeutic agents can be quantified and the more classical bioassay has been improved so as to provide greater rapidity and sensitivity. Although such antibiotic levels can be measured with ease, they provide only partial information and must be considered along with the tissue level of an antibiotic. The direct measurement of the concentration of the drug offers the additional advantages of providing individualized information about each drug and of allowing an assessment of the potential for dose-related toxicity.

It should be emphasized that the use of pharmacologic monitoring is of value primarily in the seriously ill patient or in the patient who has an underlying propensity to drug toxicity. Most infectious diseases can be adequately monitored at a clinical level and an additional number with the addition of radiologic and bacteriologic assistance.

Duration of Therapy

The decision to stop antimicrobial chemotherapy is usually based on a combination of empiricism, logic, and some scientific evidence.

Rarely is a regimen so standardized as to be nearly routine, but such is the case in the treatment of streptococcal pharyngitis where a 10-day course of therapy is accepted by nearly all. Other rather standard durations of therapy include 4 weeks for infective endocarditis due to *Streptococcus viridans* and 6 weeks for other endocarditides. Other clinical situations are less well defined and based, to a great extent, on the course during therapeutic monitoring as noted above. It is usually suggested that therapy continue for a few days after most evidence of infection has cleared. *Salmonella typhosa* infections should be treated longer after the patient is afebrile; perhaps for an additional 14 days and shigella infections for an additional 7 days. The duration of therapy in uncomplicated urinary tract infections is the subject of much debate.

CHAPTER 81

Infections Without Localizing Manifestations (Fever of Obscure Origin)

JOHN J. MANN

Patients are frequently encountered who do not have localizing signs or symptoms and in whom fever is the dominant feature of their illness. The cause of fever may remain obscure despite appropriate microbiologic, radiologic, and serologic studies for the detection of specific infections. The problem is often confused by the premature use of therapeutic agents that alter the course of the illness, either by producing temporary defervescence or by inducing a febrile sensitivity reaction. The problem of the patient with unexplained fever will serve to illustrate the principles outlined in the systematic approach to diagnosis (Chap. 4) and the necessity of constructing a careful plan for the management of a patient's illness (Chap. 4). The differential diagnosis in a patient with obscure fever deserves special consideration as a common and often vexing challenge to the physician.

Definition

A patient is considered to have fever of obscure origin when the cause of the temperature elevation is not clear after the initial examinations usually performed in persons presenting with fever have been completed.[51] Many common causes of fever are excluded by this definition, either because they can be readily diagnosed or because they are self-limited.

The history, physical examination, blood counts, chest x-ray, and urinalysis and initial microbiologic evaluation are sufficient to establish a presumptive diagnosis in the majority of patients.

The causes of fever of undetermined origin are so varied and numerous that it is difficult to devise any fully practical classification of them. A simple and workable classification is presented in Table 81-1. Fever may also be noted in many other conditions not listed such as heat stroke and congenital absence of the sweat glands. In these situations the cause of fever is usually obvious and the abnormal temperature is not the important feature that calls for diagnostic study.

Fever

It is important to recall that a low-grade fever does not always signify the presence of illness. The body temperature may rise above normal during exercise or excitement, particularly in a warm environment. A few individuals who are otherwise in perfect health persistently have a temperature of a degree or so above normal, a condition known as habitual hyperthermia.[4]

The normal body temperature, as measured rectally, undergoes a diurnal variation from as low as

┌─────────────────────────────────────┐
TABLE 81-1
Causes of Fever of Unknown Origin

I. **Infections**

    A. Endovascular (streptococci, enterococci, staphylococci, and many others)

    B. Extravascular focus

        1. Respiratory (lung abscess, empyema, bronchiectasis, pneumonia)

        2. Abdominal (appendiceal abscess, hepatic abscess, subdiaphragmatic abscess, psoas abscess, cholangitis)

        3. Genitourinary (renal carbuncle, perinephric abscess, kidney infection, prostatitis, pelvic abscess)

        4. Neurologic (brain abscess, epidural abscess, meningitis)

        5. Musculoskeletal (osteomyelitis, pyogenic arthritis, pyomyositis)

    C. Specific infections

        1. Salmonellosis (typhoid, paratyphoid, other)

        2. Plague

        3. Parasitic infections (malaria, filariasis)

        4. Rickettsial infections

        5. Spirochetal infections (syphilis, leptospirosis)

        6. Listeriosis

        7. Viral infections

        8. Brucellosis

        9. Tularemia

    D. Mycobacterial infections (tuberculosis, leprosy)

    E. Fungal infections

II. **Tumors (Malignant or Benign)**

    A. Hypernephroma

    B. Carcinoma of gastrointestinal tract

    C. Hepatic carcinoma (primary or metastatic)

    D. Carcinoma of lung and pleura

    E. Myxoma, simulating subacute bacterial endocarditis

III. **Diseases of the Blood-Forming Organs**

    A. Leukemia

    B. Hemolytic disorders

    C. Pernicious anemia

    D. Hodgkin's disease and other lymphomas

IV. **Liver Diseases**

    A. Hepatitis

    B. Cirrhosis

V. **Disorders Due to Toxins and Allergens**

    A. Allergenic drugs (sulfonamides, penicillin, iodides)

    B. Foreign proteins (horse serum)

    C. Products of tissue injury

        1. Myocardial infarction (including postmyocardial infarction syndrome)

        2. Pulmonary infarction

        3. Gangrene of extremities
└─────────────────────────────────────┘

┌─────────────────────────────────────┐
TABLE 81-1 (cont.)

V. **Disorders Due to Toxins and Allergens (cont.)**

        4. Tissue necrosis with remote sterile inflammation

        5. Accumulation of blood in body cavities or intestinal tract

VI. **Connective Tissue Disease**

    A. Rheumatic fever

    B. Rheumatoid arthritis

    C. Systemic lupus erythematosus

    D. Polyarteritis nodosa

    E. Polymyositis

    F. Giant-cell arteritis

VII. **Miscellaneous**

    A. Sarcoidosis

    B. Inflammatory bowel disease

        1. Regional enteritis

        2. Ulcerative colitis

        3. Whipple's disease

    C. Metabolic

        1. Porphyria

        2. Gout

        3. Hyperthyroidism

VIII. **Factitious Fever**
└─────────────────────────────────────┘

97.5°F during the early morning hours to as high as 100.2°F in the late afternoon or early evening. In most patients with fever, the temperature curve tends to follow the same pattern with higher levels occurring in the evening. The spikes of a widely swinging or hectic fever also usually occur in the evening. Rectal temperatures are about a degree higher than oral readings, and axillary temperatures are about a degree lower than oral temperatures. Rectal temperatures are preferred in patients who cannot cooperate sufficiently to obtain accurate oral readings.

PATTERN AND DEGREE OF FEVER. The heat-regulating mechanisms operating through the peripheral circulation and sweat glands usually prevent life-threatening elevations of body temperature, so that rectal temperatures exceeding 106°F are unusual. Marked hyperthermia may be observed in patients with heat stroke or central nervous system lesions (meningitis, cerebrovascular accident, encephalitis, tumor of the hypothalamus, brain surgery, and trauma to the cervical cord). Other conditions sometimes causing elevations above 106°F are lymphomas, acute yellow atrophy of the liver, thyroid crisis, fulminant pancreatitis, and drug reactions. Infections often associated with fevers above 105°F are those of the urinary tract caused by gram-negative bacilli, meningococcemia, typhoid fever, brucellosis, tularemia, tuberculosis, malaria, relapsing fever, and leptospirosis. In contrast, some infections are characterized by low-grade or even no fever. Thus, not infrequently, disseminated fungal infections are associated with only mild elevation of temperature. Apart from these generalities, the height of the fever is not usually helpful in diagnosis. Thus, sensitivity to phenobarbital may produce as much fever as pneumococcal bacteremia.[46]

Occasionally, patients present with recurrent febrile episodes over prolonged periods of time but enjoy relatively good health during the intervals. This is typical of Pel-Ebstein fever which occurs in a small percentage of patients with Hodgkin's disease. A number of other entities can be associated with this pattern including malaria, relapsing fever, rat-bite fever, some forms of granulomatous pleuritis and pericarditis, drug reactions, inflammatory bowel disease, and familial Mediterranean fever. However, the search for less esoteric entities is often rewarding. Commonly, localized pyogenic infections of the biliary, genitourinary, gastrointestinal, or respiratory tracts are responsible for obscure intermittent febrile illnesses. Intermittent biliary obstruction (Charcot's intermittent biliary fever), prostatitis, diverticulosis, or bronchiectasis are often overlooked, yet readily treatable causes.

Chills

Although shaking chills occur most frequently in bacterial infections, especially when associated with bacteremia, they may also occur with drug reactions, neoplasms, collagen disorders, viral infections, and antipyretic treatment. Chills are, therefore, of limited help in distinguishing the cause of a febrile illness.

CAUSES OF FEVER OF UNKNOWN ORIGIN

Causes of fever of unknown origin (FUO) are categorized in Table 81–1. Differential diagnosis may be exceedingly difficult, since many diseases presenting an undiagnosed fever may have similar clinical manifestations. Thus, such frequent causes of FUO as chronic infections, neoplasms, collagen-vascular disorders, drug hypersensitivity states, and granulomatous diseases may all be associated with similar physical findings, including weight loss, chills, sweats, skin eruptions, arthritis, myositis, neuritis, and enlargement of the spleen, liver, and lymph nodes. These disorders may also present with only such nonspecific symptoms as irritability, malaise, easy fatigability, headache, and anorexia.

Commonly encountered causes of FUO will now be considered, with emphasis on the clues which may lead to the proper diagnosis.[47,49,52]

INFECTIONS

Bacteremia

Multiple blood cultures should be obtained in all cases of unexplained fever. Both aerobic and anaerobic techniques should be used, and the cultures should be held for more than 2 weeks to permit recognition of slow-growing organisms such as bacteroides. In addition to obtaining blood cultures an hour before the daily temperature is expected, additional cultures spaced over the 24-hour period should be carried out since bacteremia may be intermittent. At least three cultures should be taken on the same day as well as on several subsequent days if there is a strong clinical suspicion of bacteremia.

Very often, septicemia begins without any apparent locus of origin. An insignificant skin puncture may be the starting point. It is always well to question a patient with septicemia about minor injuries, squeezing pimples, pulling hair, and so on. In the female, the pelvic organs should always be a suspected source and examined carefully.

Two particularly elusive agents which are responsible for bacteremia are bacteroides and meningococci. Infections caused by bacteroides occur more often than is appreciated and are often overlooked, particularly if cultures are discarded too soon, because the organisms usually grow slowly. One must think of bacteroides when the setting of an illness strongly suggests infection but no organism can be isolated. A wide variety of focal infections may be produced by this organism, including peritonsillitis, pylephlebitis, endocarditis, pneumonitis, osteomyelitis, empyema, and intra-abdominal abscesses.

Meningococcal infections may take a number of clinical forms, with or without meningitis. In the absence of meningitis the presentation may be disarming. Chronic meningococcemia frequently masquerades as a collagen disease because of the recurrent fever, arthritis, arthralgia, and peculiar skin lesions characteristic of the disease. In chronic meningococcemia, petechial and purpuric lesions are no more common than lesions resembling hives or mosquito bites occurring in crops. Purpura and petechiae are more characteristic of acute meningococcemia.

Antibiotic administration should be withheld until after the blood cultures have been obtained. Otherwise the correct diagnosis may never be made, and the successful management of the illness will be rendered more difficult, especially if improvement does not occur. Once the cultures have been taken, appropriate antibiotics may be indicated if the patient is seriously ill. The initial treatment regimen can be appropriately altered when the causative organism is isolated and its antibiotic sensitivity determined.

Localized Infections with or Without Abscess Formation

The observer should review systematically the possibility of there being a localized infection in the brain, meninges, pharynx, mediastinum, pericardium, endocardium, or thoracic cavity, below the diaphragm, in the liver or spleen, or in or about the kidneys, abdominal cavity, pelvis, perirectal area, prostate, bones and joints, or soft tissues. If such a systematic approach is not followed and each possible locus considered in an orderly fashion, the cause of the patient's fever may well be overlooked. Certain localized infections deserve special mention here, although they are discussed more fully in other chapters.

LIVER ABSCESS. Liver abscess often remains obscure clinically. Frequently, there is no obvious antecedent infection from which it could have originated such as colitis, ruptured appendix, and the like. The only manifestations may be fever, chills, anorexia, and malaise. The white blood cell count may be normal. The liver may be only slightly enlarged and not at all tender. The diaphragm may be high and fixed. A friction rub over the surface of the liver is only infrequently heard. Exploratory laparotomy may be the only means of discovering a liver abscess. Needle aspiration is helpful if it is positive but it carries the danger of hemorrhage or irreversible shock if the contents of an abscess is spilled into the peritoneum and does not exclude abscess when negative. Radioisotopic scanning of the liver may reveal filing defects, but small abscesses (less than 2 cm) will be missed.[48,50]

SUBDIAPHRAGMATIC ABSCESS. The subdiaphragmatic abscess can be as elusive as a liver abscess. The classical features of fixation and elevation of the diaphragm with secondary pleural reaction and ipsilateral tenderness in the shoulder muscles are not uniformly present. A subdiaphragmatic abscess may be found in patients whose histories reveal no obvious underlying cause. For example, several weeks after a seemingly uncomplicated operation, a patient developed a spiking fever, sweats, and malaise. Ultimately,

a subdiaphragmatic abscess was found, and it was realized that the operation had been complicated by an infection, which had been masked by the postoperative administration of antibiotics.[44]

CHOLANGITIS. Charcot's fever produced by intermittent blockage of the biliary ducts is a common cause of periodic fever. Success in diagnosis depends on the detection of transient elevations of the serum bilirubin or alkaline phosphatase. For this reason these determinations should be made at the onset and the peaks of febrile episodes.

APPENDICITIS AND DIVERTICULITIS. In elderly persons or in those receiving adrenal steroids, acute appendicitis or diverticulitis may be overlooked or misjudged mainly because the usual manifestations of an acute inflammatory process may not be present. A ruptured viscus with abscess formation, sometimes associated with pylephlebitis, is not rare in these settings.

PERIRECTAL ABSCESS. Perirectal abscess is a common cause of obscure fever in patients with diabetes or leukemia. It is readily diagnosed if a rectal examination is performed. Unfortunately, this is not always done. No febrile patient is too sick to have a rectal examination. Such abscesses may also complicate the course of regional enteritis, ulcerative colitis, diverticulitis, and granulomatous lesions involving the gut.

PERINEPHRIC ABSCESS. This infection is commonly mistaken for pyelonephritis or sepsis. Suggestive features are unilateral flank pain, dysuria, flank or abdominal mass, and lack of renal mobility on intravenous pyelogram. Organisms are usually aerobic, enteric, gram-negative bacilli although gram-positive cocci can be responsible.

PROSTATITIS. The prostate can contain a reservoir of pathogenic bacteria and can be the focus for repeated febrile episodes. The history of febrile episodes occurring after long periods of riding or sitting should make one suspect the diagnosis.

Specific Infections

When the characteristic manifestations of a specific infection, such as typhoid fever, have reached their full development, the diagnosis is usually evident. It is in the early stages of the illness, when the only manifestations present are common to many infections, that problems of identification arise.

SALMONELLOSIS. Salmonella infections are common and may follow typhoidal courses, with continual fever and chills for several weeks. Metastatic abscesses may be formed. There is an increased incidence of salmonella infections in thalassemia, sickle-cell disease, leukemia, cirrhosis of the liver, neoplastic disease, and postsplenectomy. The organism can localize in neoplasms, hematomas, or in ulcerated plaques in the major arteries.

MALARIA. Hundreds of millions of people live in areas where malaria still exacts a heavy toll. Physicians throughout the United States must consider malaria in the differential diagnosis of any febrile illness in patients who have travelled in endemic areas, particularly Southeast Asia. Even in patients who have never travelled to endemic areas, one should still consider the possibility of malaria acquired through artificial means such as blood transfusion or the sharing of common syringes; the latter possibility should particularly be considered in narcotic addicts.

RICKETTSIAL INFECTIONS. A careful epidemiologic history, physical examination, and appropriate serologic studies usually serve to rapidly identify the rickettsial infections and remove them from the category of fevers of obscure origin.

SPIROCHETAL INFECTIONS. Syphilis because of its protean manifestations must always be considered as a possible cause of fever (Chap. 85). Other spirochetes including leptospira can cause prolonged febrile illnesses.

VIRAL INFECTIONS. Viral infections are not usually associated with fever of unknown origin. Most common viral illnesses are of short duration. Infectious mononucleosis, however, is a viral infection that is often overlooked. About 20 percent of patients present with only fever, malaise, a refractory sore throat, and vague musculoskeletal complaints. The classical features of this illness may not be present. Although the febrile period usually lasts only 7 to 14 days, it may be prolonged for several weeks. The characteristic blood and serologic alterations may not make their appearance until late in the course, so that initially the correct diagnosis can be obscure.

In addition, an infectious mononucleosis-like illness has been described with cytomegalic inclusion disease virus particularly after open-heart surgery and the use of the extracorporeal pump system. The heterophile antibody test is negative, but diagnosis can be made by a rise in specific antibody in the serum and isolation of the organism from blood or urine. In patients with defective host defense mechanisms the cytomegalic inclusion disease virus can cause disseminated disease, with fever, hepatitis, lymphadenopathy, renal impairment, and/or pneumonia.

Prolonged fever with few localizing signs also may characterize hepatitis. Although alterations in liver functions usually lead toward the diagnosis, the occurrence of rashes and arthropathy may confuse the issue.

GRANULOMATOUS INFECTIONS. Not infrequently in the search for a diagnosis in a case of FUO, granulomas will be found in liver, lymph nodes, bone marrow, or other tissues. Although helpful, the presence of granulomas does not establish a diagnosis. Since the differential diagnosis includes many treatable conditions, it behooves the physician to make all efforts to establish a specific etiologic diagnosis. The following diseases have been associated with formation of granulomas in tissue: sarcoidosis, tuberculosis, fungal infections, brucellosis, tularemia, syphilis, leprosy, Hodgkin's disease, drug reactions, and vasculitis. Recently, attention has been called to a group of patients with prolonged hectic fevers, marked constitutional symptoms, and usually only modest signs of disease. Biopsy of the liver shows multiple hepatic granulomas and there is a good response to corticosteroid therapy. Whether this entity of "granulomatous hepatitis" represents a separate disease is not yet clear. Tuberculosis and to a lesser extent disseminated fungal infections commonly present as fever of unknown origin and will be discussed in more detail.

TUBERCULOSIS. Of all the chronic infections, tuberculosis is the one that most commonly presents as a fever of unexplained origin and is the one that is most commonly overlooked. This is a medical tragedy because it is so readily treated. Stead and others have contributed greatly to our understanding of the natural history of this complex disease.[55]

Primary Tuberculosis. Although the incidence of tuberculosis in the U.S. has decreased in the past 60 years, it is still a significant problem.[56] Early in this century, 80 percent of the population under age 20 had a positive tuberculin skin test. At present, less than 5 percent of young adults have a positive tuberculin skin test. However, in some urban centers half of the population over age 50 reacts to tuberculin.

Primary tuberculosis can be defined as the invasion of a nonimmune host by the tubercle bacillus. Most such individuals do not develop disease but show only a positive tuberculin skin test. The detection of these converters is extremely important since, if untreated, approximately 5 to 10 percent will develop significant clinical tuberculosis within 5 years and an additional 2 to 5 percent will show recrudescence of their disease at a later time. When primary tuberculosis results in significant host injury primary pulmonary tuberculosis results. Early in the disease the patient may be asymptomatic. With progression of the disease, weight loss, anorexia, fever, and mild respiratory symptoms appear. The chest x-ray shows patches of pneumonia almost always in the lower two-thirds of the lung fields. Progression of the initial lesion may lead to pleurisy, pleural effusion, and cavitation with or without hemoptysis. Occasionally, the onset of primary pulmonary tuberculosis is more dramatic with high fever, chills, marked respiratory symptoms, and leukocytosis, and may masquerade as acute bacterial pneumonia.

Prior to the development of specific immunity, it is not unusual for the tubercle bacillus to disseminate widely throughout the body. Almost always this dissemination is silent and lesions heal spontaneously with the development of immunity. Lesions tend to localize in areas characterized by high tissue oxygen tension (e.g., apex of the lung, kidney, brain, spine, long bones, etc.). Uncommonly, disease will progress in these sites shortly after the initial infection. The result will be miliary tuberculosis or tuberculosis of extrapulmonary sites (e.g., meningitis, osteomyelitis) (Table 81-2). The prognosis then is ominous and prompt, and adequate treatment is necessary to prevent a fatal outcome.

Postprimary Tuberculosis. Postprimary tuberculosis can be defined as reappearance of active tuberculosis in a previously sensitized individual. In the past, this development was thought to be due to reinfection. At the present time, the evidence strongly indicates that postprimary tuberculosis develops not because of reinfection, but because of reactivation of dormant infection. This reactivation of the disease can occur a few months or many decades after the initial infection. It is more likely to occur when the host defense mechanisms are impaired by such things as steroid treatment, diabetes, cirrhosis, pneumoconiosis, neoplasms, and blood dyscrasias.

Postprimary Pulmonary Tuberculosis. As opposed to primary pulmonary tuberculosis, spontaneous healing in postprimary pulmonary tuberculosis is unusual and tendencies to chronicity, liquefaction necrosis, and development of fibrosis are characteristic. Here again, the onset is usually insidious, and extensive lung damage has usually occurred by the time the classical symptoms of fever, night sweats, weight loss, cough, and hemoptysis are noted. On chest film, lesions are usually located in the apices of the lungs and consist of fibronodular infiltrates, cavities, and fibrosis. Pneumothorax, pleurisy, and pleural effusions develop from extension of active tuberculous lesions to the pleura.

Postprimary Extrapulmonary Tuberculosis. As mentioned previously, seeding of tubercle bacilli throughout the body can occur during the primary phase of the disease.[53] Table 81-2 lists the organs commonly involved in the recrudescence of active disease. Usually, symptoms will point to the specific organ involved. However, tuberculous peritonitis and tuberculosis of the genital tract often present with fe-

ver and nonspecific symptoms for prolonged periods of time. Diagnosis usually requires laparotomy.

Disseminated Tuberculosis. It may be particularly difficult to recognize tuberculosis in its disseminated form when there are no localized phenomena pointing to the diagnosis. Some patients can continue their work for a year or longer with active disseminated tuberculosis. The very mildness of the course may disarm the physician and delude him into excluding this possibility because the patient does not appear sick enough. In addition, disseminated tuberculosis in the adult tends to be superimposed on a variety of illnesses which impair host defense mechanisms. In such cases the tuberculous infection may be completely overshadowed by the underlying disease.

Disseminated tuberculosis can occur with the primary or with the postprimary phase. It can be an acute illness with high fever, chills, malaise, headache, and prostration. The fever is usually intermittent and well tolerated by the patient who often is unaware of its presence despite peaks to 103° or 105°F. Reversal of the normal diurnal variation or double quotidian fever patterns are sometimes seen. Pulmonary findings are usually unimpressive and sputum cultures are usually negative unless active pulmonary disease preceded the hematogenous spread. The chest film may show a miliary pattern which represents conglomeration of innumerable small miliary lesions. Hepatosplenomegaly, lymphadenopathy, and involvement of meninges, pericardium, pleura, peritoneum, eyes, and other organs may also develop. During acute miliary dissemination, polymorphonuclear leukocytosis is frequent and a leukemoid reaction with white blood counts as high as $100,000/\mu l$ may occur.

More commonly in the adult disseminated tuberculosis will take the form of a chronic illness with low-grade fever and few or no pulmonary signs or symptoms. Other symptoms are nonspecific and the physical alterations are common to a variety of disorders. Among the changes seen are hepatosplenomegaly, lymphadenopathy, muscle wasting, arthritis, chorioretinitis, hypergammaglobulinemia, hemolytic anemia or refractory anemia, leukopenia or leukocytosis, thrombopenia, or thrombocytosis. The tuberculin skin test may be negative. It is easy to understand why in these cases the diagnosis may be exceedingly difficult to establish. The most valuable diagnostic procedure is biopsy of the liver which is indicated even in the absence of clinical liver involvement. Biopsy and culture of lymph nodes and bone marrow may yield similar information. The demonstration of acid-fast bacilli on stain or culture is diagnostic. As previously mentioned, the finding of granuloma with-

---TABLE 81-2---
Extrapulmonary Tuberculosis

Site	Manifestation
I. Direct Extension from Pulmonary Tuberculosis	
Pleura	Dry pleurisy (fibrinous); pleuritic chest pain
	Wet pleurisy; effusion (often serosanguinous) with or without pulmonary involvement
	Empyema; complication of bronchopleural fistula
Larynx	Hoarseness, dysphagia
	Severe inflammation may endanger airway
	Formerly resulted in fibrosis and aphonia (now rare)
Bronchi and trachea	Cough, wheezing; bronchial obstruction (from granulation and ulceration) may lead to abscess formation or bronchiectasis
	Usually secondary to active pulmonary disease; occasionally results from rupture of caseous node into bronchus
	Responds well to chemotherapy; steroids may be dramatically beneficial
Alimentary tract	
Buccal cavity, and tongue	Painful ulcerations
	Usually late complication of chronic cavitary pulmonary disease
	Biopsy may aggravate
Tonsil	Acquired from drinking infected milk (now virtually absent in U.S.)
Esophagus and stomach	Rare; by extension from contiguous lymph nodes
Intestine	Vague abdominal pain; constipation or diarrhea
	Usually secondary to swallowing heavily infected sputum in active pulmonary disease (contaminated milk is a source outside the U.S.A.)
	Ileocecal involvement commonest form
	May be confused with regional enteritis (Crohn's disease)
	Fistula-in-ano and ischiorectal abscess formerly common with active pulmonary disease
II. Hematogenous and/or Lymphogenous Spread (or Direct Extension from Nonpulmonary Lesion)	
Disseminated hematogenous (miliary)	
Acute	In childhood, follows soon after primary infection; in adults, may occur at any time in chronic active disease

---TABLE 81-2 (cont.)---

Site	Manifestation
II. Hematogenous and/or Lymphogenous Spread (or Direct Extension from Nonpulmonary Lesion) (cont.)	
	Abrupt onset of fever, chills, headache, malaise, prostration
	Leukocytosis up to 20,000 or leukemoid reaction
	Localization may involve one or more sites; lungs (dyspnea, sometimes scattered rales); miliary (millet seed) pulmonary x-ray lesions may be visible on chest film before acute symptoms, they proceed to conglomeration and cavitation
	Pleura (pleuritic pain, effusion)
	Meninges (meningitis develops in up to two-thirds of untreated childhood cases)
	Eye (choroidal tubercles may be detected)
	Spleen (enlargement)
	Liver (hepatomegaly—increased alkaline phosphatase, bilirubin usually only minimally elevated; liver biopsy often positive for tubercles)
	Lymph nodes (enlargement)
	Peritoneum (with or without signs of peritonitis)
	Pericardium (pain, rub, tamponade)
Chronic	Dissemination occurs insidiously or in indolent intermittent episodes
	Signs and symptoms depend on organ sites predominantly involved
Nervous system Meningitis	May not be acute in onset; irritability and listlessness in children
	Headache, and bizarre behavior in older children and adults
	Change of mental state, disorientation, and finally coma
	Stiff neck, cranial nerve signs
	Spinal fluid shows predominantly mononuclear pleocytosis (up to several hundred cells per mm^3), elevated protein, and low sugar
	Organism difficult to stain, though more often culturable
	Treatment must not await results of culture
	Untreated cases almost invariably fatal
	Without early treatment, permanent sequelae may include blindness, deafness, or mental deficiency

┌─────────────────────────────────────┐
─TABLE 81-2 (cont.)─────────────

Site	Manifestation
II. Hematogenous and/or Lymphogenous Spread (or Direct Extension from Nonpulmonary Lesion) (cont.)	
Nervous system Meningitis **(cont.)**	Possible role of head trauma in localization of infection
	In addition to INH and ethambutol, corticosteroids appear to ameliorate severe acute manifestations, relieve coma
	(Prevention of late sequelae is undocumented)
Tuberculoma	Signs and symptoms of expanding intracranial mass
	Cannot easily be distinguished from neoplasm without surgical exploration
Lymph nodes	Pulmonary hilar involvement prominent in primary tuberculosis
	Mediastinal, tracheobronchial nodes may be source of spread to bronchi, pericardium, or elsewhere
	May cause cough and wheezing by pressure on bronchi
	Cervical lymphadenitis (scrofula)
	Painless swellings in the neck (single or multiple), nontender
	Tend to become matted
	May form cold abscess and chronic cutaneous sinus tracts
	Most often associated with pulmonary tuberculosis
	Some cases now caused by atypical mycobacteria
	Abdominal (mesenteric)
	May cause pain and fever or palpable abdominal masses
	Diagnosis usually requires laparotomy
Pericardium	Precordial pain, symptoms of cardiac tamponade, friction rub
	Ewart's sign (posterior dullness and bronchial breath sounds due to lung compression by massive pericardial effusion)
	Usually arises by erosion of adjacent mediastinal node into pericardium
	Effusion may be predominantly a hypersensitivity reaction to tuberculoprotein
	Mycobacterium often not detectable by smear or culture
	Pericardiocentesis may aid diagnosis and treatment
	Late complication: constrictive pericarditis

─TABLE 81-2 (cont.)─────────────

Site	Manifestation
II. Hematogenous and/or Lymphogenous Spread (or Direct Extension from Nonpulmonary Lesion) (cont.)	
Peritoneum	Acute onset with moderate abdominal pain, fever, distension from rapid accumulation of fluid
	Local abscess, adhesions, and loculations may produce doughy consistency
	Paracentesis may perforate bowel when significant adhesions present
	May be insidious in onset
	Most often secondary to old abdominal focus
	Limited laparotomy for diagnosis and evacuation of fluid often indicated
	Response to chemotherapy is good
Kidney	Hematuria (microscopic or gross)
	Secondary bladder involvement may produce symptoms of cystitis; frequency, dysuria, pyuria
	Pyuria without bacteriuria on routine smear and culture always raises suspicion of renal tuberculosis
	Nephrectomy now rarely necessary because of good response to chemotherapy
Genital Female	Salpingitis
	May be asymptomatic cause of sterility
	Menstrual irregularities may be present
	Pelvic peritonitis may be associated
	Adnexal mass usually detectable on pelvic examination
	Extension to ovaries and/or uterine endometrium may occur
	Endometrial currettage, leukorrheal discharge or menstruum may yield organism
	Surgical resection may be indicated after control of local peritonitis with chemotherapy
Male	Epididymitis most frequently seen, though prostate and seminal vesicles often involved asymptomatically
	Acute swelling and tenderness or insidious appearance of slightly tender nodule
	Excision may be indicated to establish diagnosis

(Continued)

---TABLE 81-2 (cont.)---

Site	Manifestation
II. Hematogenous and/or Lymphogenous Spread (or Direct Extension from Nonpulmonary Lesion)(cont.)	
Musculoskeletal	Spine (tuberculous spondylitis or Pott's disease)
	Starts as osteomyelitis of vertebral body
	Destruction with vertebral collapse followed by healing and ankylosis produces kyphosis (gibbus)
	Associated paravertebral cold abscess
	Treatment with decompression, currettage, and immobilization (external fusion of lateral spinous processes) plus chemotherapy
	Joints (large, weight-bearing joints; hip and knee, most common) pain, swelling
	Initial involvement usually in epiphysis of long bone or synovium
	Cartilage involvement is secondary; after destruction, anklylosis and immobilization may lead to healing
	Arthrodesis of large joints may not be required if early intensive chemotherapy is given

out positive stains on culture is not diagnostic of active tuberculosis.

FUNGUS INFECTIONS. Fungal infections can present as febrile illnesses either during the acute primary pulmonary phase or more commonly when the disease has disseminated. Some of the features of the more common systemic mycotic infections are shown in Table 81-3.

Histoplasma capsulatum is a dimorphic fungus occurring both in yeast and mycelial forms. During infection of man only the yeast form is produced. The vast majority of cases of histoplasmosis are asymptomatic. Skin test studies indicate rapid conversion to positivity during childhood in endemic areas. In some areas as many as 80 percent of children have a positive histoplasmin skin test by age 5. A certain number of asymptomatic infections result in pulmonary calcifications in the periphery of the lung parenchyma and in calcification of hilar nodes and spleen. This benign process represents over 99 percent of human infections.[54]

Acute Pulmonary Histoplasmosis. This benign and self-limited syndrome often occurs in small epidemics following exposure to contaminated chicken coops, caves, or freshly disturbed, shaded soil. The incubation period is 5 to 20 days and the illness is characterized by fever, night sweats, chills, cough, chest pain, and less frequently, shortness of breath and hemoptysis. The severity of the symptoms varies from mild respiratory symptoms to severe prostration with high fever and cyanosis. The chest film usually shows bilateral disease with discrete or diffuse nodular pneumonic infiltrates with hilar adenopathy. *Histoplasma capsulatum* may be cultured from sputum or gastric aspirates. Sometimes, even in these benign cases, the fungus can also be cultured from bone marrow or lymph node indicating that the illness is not confined to the lungs. Usually the illness lasts from 2 weeks to 3 months with spontaneous resolution. The prognosis is excellent and treatment with amphotericin B is not required. The histoplasmin skin test is almost always positive as is the serology.

Chronic Pulmonary Histoplasmosis. This illness which occurs predominantly in adults is entirely similar to chronic pulmonary tuberculosis. The symptoms are those of chronic pulmonary disease: cough, weight loss, dyspnea, recurrent fevers, hemoptysis, and chest pain.

The skin test is positive in 80 percent of cases and the serology is positive in 90 percent of cases. Treatment with Amphotericin B is effective.

Disseminated Histoplasmosis. Disseminated histoplasmosis has been observed at all ages but more commonly occurs at the extremes of life.[54] Symptoms and signs of pulmonary disease are absent in half of the patients. Ulcerative granulomatous lesions of the mouth, tongue, nose, pharynx, and larynx are suggestive of the diagnosis. Biopsy of these lesions will reveal the characteristic small intracellular yeast. The most commonly involved organs are the lungs, adrenal glands, liver, spleen, and lymph nodes. Clinically, hepatosplenomegaly is common and in almost 20 percent of cases adrenal insufficiency will develop. Hematologic and liver function test abnormalities are common but nonspecific. The most helpful tool in diagnosis is culture of bone marrow. Positive results will be obtained in 75 percent of cases. The diagnosis cannot be ruled out by skin test (which is negative in 50 percent) or by serology (which is negative in 40 percent). The mortality of the untreated disease is well over 80 percent. Treatment with intravenous amphotericin B has reduced the mortality to 25 percent.

TABLE 81–3

Common Systemic Mycotic Infections

Disease	Source of Infection	Distinguishing Features

Histoplasmosis	Soil contaminated with bird droppings
	Worldwide, Mississippi Valley, Eastern and
	  Central U.S.
	Airborne
		High incidence of subclinical infections
		Acute, subacute, or chronic pulmonary
		  infection
		Disseminated disease with
		  hepatosplenomegaly, fever, anemia, skin
		  and mucous membrane lesions
		Organism can be cultured from sputum,
		  tissue, or bone marrow
		Reliable skin tests and serology except in
		  disseminated disease (50 percent
		  negative)

Cryptococcosis	Soil contaminated with pigeon droppings
	Worldwide
	Airborne
		Primary lesion, apparent or inapparent
		  pulmonary lesion, coin lesion or
		  pneumonia
		Very high predilection for CNS infection
		  mostly in patients with lymphoma,
		  leukemia or on steroids
		Organisms frequently seen in CSF by India
		  ink examination
		Can also involve bone, skin, mucous
		  membranes, and kidneys
		Skin test not reliable
		Serology extremely useful: presence of
		  cryptococcus polysaccharide antigen is
		  diagnostic of active infection

Coccidioidomycosis	Dry desert soil, Limited geographic
	  distribution (Southwestern U.S.)
	Airborne
		High incidence of subclinical infections
		Acute, subacute, or chronic pulmonary
		  infection
		Dissemination disease with involvement of
		  skin, bones, viscera, and CNS
		Blacks and Filipinos particularly prone to
		  disseminated disease
		Meningitis extremely chronic and prone to
		  relapses
		Reliable skin test for primary disease
		Serology extremely useful: Serum or CSF
		  antibody C.F. titer of 1:16 indicates
		  serious illness

North American
  Blastomycosis
	Soil probably
	North American continent, Southwestern
	  U.S.
	Airborne
		Primary pulmonary infection usually
		  inapparent
		Disseminated disease with involvement of
		  skin, lungs, bones, and urogenital tract
		Characteristic verrucous or ulcerative skin
		  lesions with central healing
		Skin test and serology not helpful

Sporotrichosis	Worldwide
	Often follows puncture wounds by rose or
	  barberry thorns, splinters, or metal
	  particles
		Ulcerative skin lesion, usually on exposed
		  surface, such as forearm, followed by
		  lymphadenitis and lymphangitis with
		  nodular ulcerations along lymphatics
		May disseminate and produce widespread
		  skin and mucosal lesions and less
		  frequently bone, joint, and lung
		  involvement
		Visceral lesions observed rarely
		Iodide therapy effective for skin
		  involvement only
		Skin test and serology unreliable

(Continued)

—— TABLE 81-3 (cont.) ——

Disease	Source of Infection	Distinguishing Features
Candidiasis	Normal inhabitant of man Worldwide	Disseminated disease associated with debilitating illness, antibiotic and/or immunosuppressive treatment, indwelling intravenous or bladder catheters, gastrointestinal lesions, and diabetes mellitus Onset characterized by fever, chills, hypotension Organs involved are kidney, heart, lung, gastrointestinal tract, spleen, liver, skin, and mucous membranes Can present as endocarditis, meningitis, or endophthalmitis Skin test and serology unreliable
Phycomycosis (mucormycosis)	Worldwide Common in animal feces and in decaying vegetable matter Possible airborne	Orbital cellulitis and necrosis in persons with acidosis (diabetic or renal) Can also present a pulmonary or disseminated infection
Aspergillosis	Common saprophytes on decaying vegetable matter Possibly airborne	Can present picture of asthma, allergic bronchopulmonary aspergillosis, fungus ball, necrotizing pneumonia, or disseminated aspergillosis The latter is characterized by tissue and vascular invasion with thrombosis and infarction in patients with lymphoreticular or hematopoietic malignancies

NEOPLASMS AND HEMATOLOGIC DISORDERS

Tumors are among the common causes of prolonged fever.[51] Although lymphomas and tumors of the kidney and liver are most likely to present with fever any malignant tumor has the capacity to induce fever. Fever may be produced by tissue necrosis, involvement of the temperature regulating center, hemorrhage, secondary infection, or obstruction of the bronchus, ureter, or bile ducts.

The temperature may be high and swinging, may be associated with chills, and may mimic the pattern followed in an infectious process.

Tumor as a cause of obscure fever may be overlooked for a variety of reasons. The frequency with which neoplasms present with fever may not be appreciated. There may be no historical or physical data pointing to the presence of a neoplasm, and laboratory changes are usually nonspecific. The tumor is often not detectable as a mass lesion even with the aid of special radiologic techniques. Its presence may be heralded by peripheral manifestations suggesting a different type of disease. Thus, bronchogenic tumor may present initially with severe joint pains (osteoarthropathy), which can be mistaken for those of rheumatoid arthritis. A lymphoma may be associated with a variety of skin eruptions, pancreatic carcinoma with polyphlebitis, carcinoma of the breast with peculiar neurologic alterations, and gastric cancer with a polymyositis. One must be familiar with these general disturbances produced by new growths (Chap. 53).

The fever associated with neoplasms of all sorts, including the leukemias, is often due not to the new growth itself but to some accompanying infection. Patients with neoplasms may have impaired immune responses which predispose them to infection, and, once acquired, such infections may run rampant. For this reason the finding of a new growth in a patient with fever does not necessarily mean that the true cause of the fever has been located.

Benign tumors may also be the cause of fever. Patients with atrial myxoma may have a pattern of illness with fever and embolic manifestations simulating infective endocarditis.

LIVER DISEASE

Cirrhosis of the liver and hepatitis due to various agents may be associated with fever.[57] The laboratory findings associated with these disorders are often nonspecific. Even the presence of hepatitis viremia may not be related to illness (Chap. 66). Liver biopsy may be needed to distinguish granulomatous liver disease from neoplastic disorders or cirrhosis. Liver scans usually detect abscesses or tumor deposits.

DRUG FEVER

Drug reactions are an increasingly important cause of prolonged fever. The possibility of a drug reaction should always be an early consideration in dealing with puzzling fever.[46]

Although certain drugs are more likely to cause fever than others are, it must be realized that any drug has the capacity to produce fever if it is given to a person who is hypersensitive to it.

A detailed drug history for each patient is essential. It should be explained to the patient that literally any drug or toxic agent is potentially capable of producing fever and that a detailed account of every medicine ingested and of all contact with toxic materials is desired. Patients (and some physicians) fail to appreciate that a drug well tolerated for many years may abruptly induce a reaction, including fever.

In the hospital it is a good practice to examine carefully the order sheets and nursing notes for the patient with unexplained fever. Drug hypersensitivity may produce clinical changes common to the collagen disorders, neoplasms, blood dyscrasias, and granulomatous infections and can be confused with such processes. Often the problem can be clarified only by withdrawing all medications or by substituting drugs that the patient has never taken before.

CONNECTIVE TISSUE DISEASE

It is well known that the patient with systemic lupus erythematosus may not present with classical features of the disease in a readily recognizable pattern. The initial manifestations may be persistent fever which lasts for weeks before other significant abnormalities appear. Polyarteritis has also become increasingly familiar as a cause of obscure fever accompanied by weight loss and mild leukocytosis. Complicating infections and drug reactions are known to occur in this group of diseases, and it is important to rule out carefully such treatable illnesses as tuberculosis and other infections before accepting the diagnosis of a collagen disease when the classical manifestations of such a disease are not present.

MISCELLANEOUS

Among the causes of fever of obscure origin, sarcoidosis is important. This disorder may be characterized by little or no constitutional reaction or can be associated with marked wasting and a prolonged hectic fever. The distinction of this illness from tuberculosis or disseminated fungal infection is most difficult and is generally made by exclusion after special stains of biopsy specimens and cultures fail to yield an etiologic agent.

Occult inflammatory diseases of the small and large bowel may be one of the most difficult and obscure causes of fever. Frequently symptoms referable to the gastrointestinal tract are minimal and nonspecific. Contrast studies may be entirely negative and only laparotomy will finally establish a diagnosis of Whipple's disease or regional enteritis.

Occasionally, certain disorders of metabolism may present primarily with a fever, although more often than not they will declare themselves in a more familiar way. Hyperthyroidism, porphyria, and gout would be the main considerations should this possibility arise.

Familial Mediterranean fever is a disease of unknown etiology which should be recognized on the basis of history. Characteristics of this disease are as follows: frequent positive family history, marked predilection for patients of Sephardic Jewish, Armenian, or Arab ancestry, predictable cycles of fever of abrupt onset and short duration associated with severe abdominal pain, polyserositis, and less commonly, skin rash and arthritis.

FACTITIOUS FEVER

Fever is readily accepted as incontrovertible evidence of organic disease. However, factitious fever may be encountered when least expected. It is wise to give this possibility early consideration when dealing with puzzling fever.[52] It may be difficult, and at times almost impossible, to detect the manner in which the patient produced factitious fever. Such factitious fevers are most commonly seen in medical and paramedical personnel and members of their families. There are several points that may call attention to the possibility of factitious fever: failure of the temperature curve to follow the normal diurnal pattern, failure of the pulse to accelerate with sudden spikes of fever, rapid defervescence without sweating, and disparity between body and urine temperatures.

APPROACH TO THE PATIENT WITH FEVER OF UNKNOWN ORIGIN

The mainstay of the clinical approach to the patient with fever of unknown origin (FUO) remains an analysis of the data derived from an accurate, complete history and physical examination. In the history, particular attention should be paid to potential exposures, to the history of drug intake, to the details of the onset of the illness, and to the past history for clues to multisystem disease. Daily physical examination of the patient is important since changes in physical findings may give the clue to diagnosis. The following aspects of the physical examination are often neglected and yet many times prove to be rewarding: eye grounds, oral cavity, skin including palms and soles, diaphragmatic mobility, sternal tenderness, rectum, prostate, testes, pelvic organs in the female, navel, auscultation of the liver, abdomen, and painful areas, and careful palpation for nodes, nodules, and areas of tenderness.

The laboratory should be used in a logical manner as dictated by the clinical setting. When obtaining specimens for culture, all potential pathogens should be kept in mind and special cultures should be requested as indicated. Since abscesses and tumors are common causes of FUO, liver scanning, gallium scanning, computed tomography, and ultrasonography should be performed early in the evaluation. These procedures are expensive but not usually dangerous. They have a relatively high rate of success particularly when done in conjunction with each other.[48,50] To a large extent they have helped the clinician in better evaluating the need for exploratory surgery.

EXPLORATORY SURGERY

Not infrequently, in managing a patient with obscure fever, there comes a time when, despite one's best diagnostic effort, the cause of the patient's fever remains hidden. Then the difficult question has to be faced—should an exploratory laparotomy be performed? The answer to this question is extremely complex. Several guidelines have been offered and should be reviewed carefully in all cases.[44,45] In general, an exploratory laparotomy is likely to be rewarding if there are symptoms or signs clearly pointing to some type of intra-abdominal disease. Many disorders, although originating outside the abdominal cavity may be accompanied by disturbances of bowel function, nausea, abdominal distension or pain, and mild derangement of liver function tests. On the other hand, exploratory laparotomy may be successful even in the absence of any suggestive symptoms or signs. In instances in which there is no clinical evidence whatever of intra-abdominal disease, one should prolong the period of observation first and search the abdomen only if there is progressive deterioration of the patient's condition.

THERAPEUTIC TRIALS

As already stated, it is frequently difficult and sometimes impossible to detect on clinical grounds the specific cause of an illness presenting with fever, and the question of the wisdom and usefulness of a therapeutic trial often arises in such circumstances.

There are pros and cons to the use of a therapeutic trial in FUO. A therapeutic trial is no substitute for a thorough investigation of the patient's situation. Effective management of the patient's illness usually requires specific therapy, and suspicions or hunches are not sound bases for definitive therapy.

The trial usually entails the use of antibiotics, various steroids, or antitumor agents, including radiation. All have potentially deleterious side effects that may complicate an already confused problem through the production of more fever, eruptions, jaundice, alterations in the blood, and so on. Not only may the patient's course be confused by the harmful side effects of such therapy, but any nonspecific beneficial effects which these agents produce may also mislead one into a false sense of achievement. Thus, a patient with a liver abscess may be symptomatically improved by being given corticosteroids, and hence valuable time is lost in bringing definitive therapy to bear.

A therapeutic trial may have a negative psychological effect on the patient and his family. Transient improvement may induce false hopes and dampen their willingness to embark upon some more difficult course, such as a longer period of observation or an exploratory operation, which may actually be the only avenue to recovery.

A therapeutic trial can become an undesirable delaying action when pushing ahead to definitive information by biopsy or exploratory laparotomy holds the single hope of recovery.

If clinical judgment indicates that none of the organ systems (heart, kidneys, etc.) is being seriously impaired by the underlying process, there is no reason for haste in beginning a therapeutic trial. Fever alone is no cause for hurry. Too often it becomes an alarm that results in actions which would never be employed on calm second thought. As a general rule, therefore, therapeutic trials in FUO are to be avoided except in very well-delineated circumstances.

On the other hand, rapidly advancing, life-threatening disease clearly demands the use of a therapeutic trial, but even in this circumstance there is always time to secure material for important studies such as blood cultures.

In addition to life-threatening disease, there is one circumstance that may call for a therapeutic trial. This is exemplified by an elderly patient with severe cardiopulmonary disease who is believed on the basis of careful study to have either disseminated tuberculosis or metastatic carcinoma. Exploratory laparotomy is considered too risky, and liver biopsy, exfoliative cytology, and cultures have not been helpful. Giving antituberculosis therapy would seem a reasonable course of action at this juncture. Thus, it is good practice to treat the treatable possibilities when careful study is unrevealing, the patient has continuing illness, and definitive diagnosis is not feasible.

If the decision is reached to attempt a therapeutic trial, several important considerations enter into the selection of an agent. First, it should be one to which the patient is least likely to have an adverse reaction. Second, to give the therapeutic trial differential diagnostic significance, the agent should be one of limited and, if possible, specific therapeutic effectiveness. Clearly, if an agent having a broad therapeutic potential is used, the patient's response to it will be of little diagnostic value. An obvious exception to this dictum is the critically ill patient, for whom adequacy of treatment must be assured from its very inception. In such instances, the desire to establish the specific diagnosis has to yield to the need to rescue the patient from his critical state. Therefore, a broad therapeutic regimen must be devised, so that no treatable possibilities are overlooked. There may not be time for second attempts.

In addition to the most appropriate agent for the particular problem at hand being selected, it should be given in a dosage that will be effective and hence give a clear-cut, definite end point. Thus, if a patient is suspected of having systemic lupus erythematosus, it is an error to start a therapeutic trial with prednisone at a dosage level of only 20 mg, since this dosage is often inadequate. Enough of the drug must be given for the physician to be certain of its efficacy or lack of it. Clearly, it is also essential to continue the drug for a sufficient period of time.

Furthermore, it is requisite that the observer fully understand the various ways in which the therapeutic trial may affect the course of the suspected disease. Thus, a patient with tuberculosis may have a sustained temperature course converted into a swinging, septic type shortly after isoniazid is begun. This is followed by gradual defervescence. Unless one is aware of this possible effect, it might be suspected that the patient is becoming more ill or has another disease.

CHAPTER 82
Bacterial Infections of Skin, Muscle, and Bone
NATHANIEL F. PIERCE

These infections vary greatly in severity and in mechanisms of pathogenesis. They may be superficial, localized, and benign or may spread rapidly and be associated with tissue destruction, systemic "toxicity" or sepsis, and an appreciable risk of death. They are considered here according to the tissue involved and the type of clinical syndrome produced, e.g., erysipelas, cellulitis, gangrene, toxigenic infections, osteomyelitis. Particular emphasis is placed on early diagnosis and prompt treatment of infections that are surgical emergencies or pose a serious risk of systemic dissemination. Viral infections are not included because they are usually manifestations of systemic infection, e.g., the viral exanthems, although cutaneous viral infections do occur, e.g., *Herpes simplex*, warts. Fungal infections and the genital manifestations of venereal infections are considered elsewhere (Chapters 81 and 88).

SUPERFICIAL INFECTIONS OF SKIN

Pyoderma
The most common causes of superficial pyogenic infections are *Streptoccus pyogenes* and *Staphylococcus aureus* (Table 82–1). The streptococcal infections include impetigo, ecthyma, and erysipelas. They characteristically follow minor or unnoticed injuries, such as scratches, insect bites, or minor abrasions. Impetigo may occur without trauma and is restricted to the epidermis, often of the face. Vesicles form early but break and weep seropurulent fluid leading to the development of typical crusted lesions. *Staphylococcus aureus* frequently contaminates these infections but is probably not causative; it does, however, cause a bullous form of impetigo which may occur in epidemics among newborns. Ecthyma is a deeper infection which erodes the dermis to form a crusted ulcer. This occurs most commonly on the legs at the sites of minor trauma.[63]

Treatment by thorough cleansing and application of warm soaks is usually sufficient for impetigo and ecthyma. When impetigo is severe or occurs in newborns, antibiotics are indicated.

Erysipelas
Erysipelas involves progressive spread of infection through the skin and lymphatics. This may occur after a minor wound in normal skin, but is more likely when prior injury has impaired the lymphatic or venous drainage of the skin or left extensive scarring.

TABLE 82-1
Superficial Skin Infections—Pyoderma and Erysipelas

Disorder	Organism(s)	Clinical Features	Treatment
Impetigo	*Str. pyogenes; Staph. aureus* in newborn	Vesicles with erythema, then weeping and crusting; epidemics in newborns	Careful cleansing; heat and soaks; penicillin (erythromycin*); dicloxacillin for *Staph. aureus*
Ecthyma	*Str. pyogenes*	Crusted ulcer, usually on legs	As for impetigo
Erysipelas	*Str. pyogenes; Staph. aureus* in a few	Local: spreading erythema, warmth and pain, lymphangitic streaks; systemic: fever, chills, toxicity	Penicillin (erythromycin), add dicloxacillin or methicillin if severe
Folliculitis	*Staph. aureus*	Superficial pustule at hair follicle	Warm soaks, careful cleansing
Furunculosis	*Staph. aureua*	Deep pustule at hair follicle	Warm soaks, careful cleansing
Carbuncle	*Staph. aureus*	Multiple adjacent deep infected follicles with draining pus; fever sometimes	Surgical drainage, dicloxacillin or methicillin (erythromycin)

* Second choice antibiotic in parentheses.

The infection causes an enlarging superficial cellulitis with warmth, local pain, discrete erythema, and moderate swelling but lacking fluctuance or dermal necrosis. There may be purulent drainage or pustule formation at the inoculation site. Erythema may extend along superficial draining lymphatics; regional lymph nodes are often enlarged and tender. Systemic "toxicity," chills, and fever are common. If untreated, metastatic infection may occur and there is appreciable mortality. Facial infections are especially dangerous because of possible intracranial spread via draining lymphatics or veins. Ninety percent of episodes are due to *Streptococcus pyogenes* but a small portion are due to *Staphylococcus aureus* and these cannot be distinguished clinically. A small percentage of patients with streptococcal infection develop glomerulonephritis during convalescence.[63] Infections resembling erysipelas may also be caused by *Pasteurella multocida* or *Erisipelothrix rhusiopathiae* (Table 82-2). The specific cause may be suggested by Gram stain of purulent drainage and confirmed by culture of this material or by culturing sterile saline injected and withdrawn at the margin of the erythematous lesion. Blood cultures are occasionally positive. Antibiotics should be started without delay. Minor episodes may be treated with oral penicillin, dicloxacillin, or erythromycin. Extensive lesions and those of the face are best treated with parenteral antibiotics until the causative agent is known or the infection is controlled; antibiotics effective against both streptococci and staphylococci should be used (Table 82-1). Warm soaks are also beneficial. Erythema and warmth usually diminish after 1 or 2 days of therapy but treatment should continue for at least 7 days.

Furuncle

Folliculitis, furuncles, and carbuncles are increasingly severe infections of hair follicles, usually caused by *Staphylococcus aureus*. Folliculitis involves minor inflammation, often with superficial pustule formation. Deeper follicular infection causes pustular furuncles which occur commonly on hairy areas exposed to friction and maceration, e.g., buttocks, neck, face, and axillae. Carbuncles are a coalescent mass of deeply infected follicles with multiple openings for purulent drainage; the dorsum of the neck is a common location; they occur with increased frequency in diabetics. Folliculitis and furuncles may be treated with careful cleansing and warm soaks and prevented by careful skin hygiene using antibacterial soaps (e.g., those containing hexachlorophene). Carbuncles require wide surgical drainage, warm soaks, and therapy with an antistaphylococcal antibiotic (Table 82-1).

WOUND INFECTIONS

Intact dry skin is a formidable barrier to infection. Most bacteria are infective only when this barrier is breached. This occurs with obvious trauma, such as lacerations, burns, and abrasions, and also with mi-

┌───┐
TABLE 82-2
Surgical Management of Infections of Skin, Muscle, and Bone

Finding	Possible Cause(s)	Surgical Procedure*
Fluctuance, or pus aspirated from deep swelling	Abscess; multiple organisms, including: *Staph. aureus*, enteric bacilli, anaerobes	Drainage
Diminished arterial pulse; cool, mottled, or pale extremity	Streptococcal fasciitis; clostridial or mixed anaerobic gangrene	*Urgent* debridement, decompression, drainage
Gas in soft tissues	*E. coli* cellulitis, clostridial cellulitis, or gangrene, occasionally other organisms	Drainage and/or debridement, depending on findings
Closed space infection of hand	*Staph. aureus* most common	Prompt drainage
Probable acute osteomyelitis	Multiple; *Staph. aureus* common	Exploration to confirm diagnosis; aspirate subperiosteal pus for culture, Gram stain

* Pus or necrotic material should *always* be examined by Gram stain and cultured under aerobic and anaerobic conditions.
└───┘

nor defects such as scratches and insect bites. The features of the ensuing infection depend upon the nature of the wound, the infecting organism(s), and the defensive responses of the infected person. The management of wound infections should focus on:

1. Early bacteriologic diagnosis by examining gram-stained smears of pus or necrotic tissue
2. Prompt surgical intervention in necrotizing, gangrenous, or abscess-forming infections (Table 82–2)
3. Early antibiotic therapy when there is apparent spread of infection in soft tissue or by the bloodstream

Abscess

The most frequent form of cutaneous or subcutaneous wound infection is abscess formation. It occurs when infected cellular debris from a localized infection cannot drain to the outside. *Staphylococcus aureus* is the most common organism in abscesses of infected accidental wounds and "clean" surgical wounds. Its presence is suggested by thick yellow pus-containing clusters of large gram-positive cocci. Gram-negative enteric bacilli may also be seen; these, along with intestinal anaerobes, are especially common in infected wounds following intestinal or pelvic surgery. Successful treatment requires drainage. Small, superficial abscesses may drain spontaneously after application of warm soaks; otherwise, surgical drainage is needed. Infected surgical wounds must often be opened and left to heal by secondary intention. Infections of the closed fascial spaces of the hand require urgent surgical drainage to prevent irreparable

damage. Antibiotics are important adjuncts in treating abscesses if there is appreciable soft tissue inflammation or uncertainty as to the adequacy of drainage (Table 82–3). Prophylactic antibiotics, especially those effective against intestinal anaerobes, are effective in preventing wound infections during intestinal or pelvic surgery.[61]

Cellulitis

Cellulitis results from the spread of infection through soft tissues adjacent to the wound. This produces local warmth, pain, significant swelling, and induration. Necrosis of skin may occur at the wound site, and there may also be destruction of subcutaneous tissue with pus formation, especially in mixed infections. Fever and systemic toxicity are common; bacteremia may occur and cause serious metastatic infection. Animal and human bites are important causes of cellulitis; anaerobic bacteria are especially important in human bites. Exposure to animal products or sea water also suggests specific infecting agents. Enteric gram-negative bacilli, often combined with intestinal anaerobes, are an important cause of cellulitis in diabetics, in persons with leukemia (causing perirectal phlegmons), and in patients with decubitus ulcers (Table 82–3).

Successful treatment of cellulitis requires appropriate antibiotic therapy. If necrotic tissue, pus or gas are present and prompt surgical debridement is also essential. Initial antibiotic selection should be based upon organisms seen in gram-stained pus or debris. If this is unavailable, the selection should cover likely aerobic and anerobic organisms until the causative agent(s) are identified by culture of purulent drain-

TABLE 82–3
Wound Infections

Disorder	Organism(s)	Wound/Exposure	Manifestations Local	Manifestations Systemic	Treatment*
Cutaneous abscess	Mostly *Staph. aureus*	Minor injury, especially to hands and feet	Erythema and pus, paronychia or felon on fingers, abscesses elsewhere	Usually none, rarely bacteremia	Surgical drainage, warm soaks; methicillin or dicloxacillin (erythromycin) for cellulitis
Surgical wound infection	Many causes: *Staph. aureus*, gram-negative enteric rods, and intestinal anaerobes are most common. Specific organisms determined by source of contamination, prior antibiotic therapy	Contaminated surgical wound	Erythema, pus, abscess formation, poor healing	Fever in some	Warm soaks if mild; open, drain, and cleanse deep or severe infections. Antibiotics for cellulitis based on Gram stain of pus and in vitro sensitivity
Infected cutaneous ulcers	Many, including *Staph. aureus*, gram-negative enteric rods, intestinal anaerobes	Chronic vascular, neurologic, or pressure ulcer with secondary infection	Purulent drainage, superficial necrosis, surrounding cellulitis	Usually none	Debridement, warm soaks, antibiotics for cellulitis based on Gram stain and culture
Cellulitis	Enteric gram-negative bacilli, especially *E. coli*	Contaminated wound, decubitus ulcer, perirectal infection	Erythema, pain, swelling, and heat. Gas with some *E. coli*	Fever, toxicity	Antibiotic appropriate to isolated agent; surgical drainage for pus or gas
	Anaerobic cellulitis (mixed anaerobes and enteric aerobes)	Contaminated wound or human bite	Spreading subcutaneous infection, may have gas	Fever, variable toxicity	Surgical drainage, gentamicin plus chloramphenicol or clindamycin
	Bacillus anthracis	Minor wound contaminated with animal products	Painless papule, then ulcer and eschar	Fever, toxicity if sepsis occurs	Penicillin (erythromycin)*
	Pasteurella multocida	Dog or cat scratch or bite	Nonnecrotizing cellulitis; may resemble erysipelas	Fever; occasional bacteremia and metastatis infection	Penicillin (tetracycline)
	Erysipelothrix rhusiopathiae	Minor wound contaminated with animal products	Nonnecrotizing cellulitis; may resemble erysipelas	Rarely endocarditis	Penicillin (erythromycin)
	Marine vibrios (several species)	Minor wound exposed to seawater	Necrotizing cellulitis, may develop gangrene	Fever, toxicity, bacteremia	Debridement; antibiotics determined by in vitro sensitivity

* Second choice antibiotic in parentheses.

TABLE 82–3 (cont.)

| Disorder | Organism(s) | Wound/Exposure | Manifestations | | Treatment* |
			Local	Systemic	
Fasciitis	*Str. pyogenes* and/or *Staph. aureus*	Infected surgical or accidental wound	Marked firm soft tissue swelling, obliteration of arterial pulses, pale ischemia	Fever, toxicity	*Prompt* wide surgical incision for drainage and relief of swelling; penicillin
Gangrene	*Cl. perfringens, Cl. septicum, Cl. novyi*	Contaminated wound with necrotic tissue	Swelling, ischemia, serous discharge, gas, hemorrhagic bullae	Toxicity, hemolysis	Prompt extensive debridement, penicillin (chloramphenicol), hyperbaric oxygen
	Anaerobic streptococci and *Staph. aureus* or gram-negative bacilli (Meleny's gangrene)	Infected injury or surgical wound, especially in diabetics	Progressive gangrene of muscle or skin	Toxicity	*Prompt* debridement, penicillin (erythromycin)
	Anaerobic streptococci (streptococcal myonecrosis)	Infected wound, especially in diabetics	Progressive muscular destruction by spreading infection	Fever, toxicity	*Prompt* debridement, penicillin (chloramphenicol)
Burns	Many including: *Str. pyogenes, Staph. aureus*; gram-negative enteric bacilli, especially *Pseudomonas aeruginosa*	Infected burn	Purulent drainage, may be no signs of infection	Fever, bacteremia, toxicity	Antibiotic choice based on burn wound culture and/or blood culture
Wound infections which initiate systemic infection	*Pseudomonas mallei* (Glanders)	Minor wound with animal exposure (in Asia, Africa, South America)	Suppurative nodule with lymphangitis	Fever, malaise, may become bacteremic	Sulfadiazine
	Pseudomonas pseudomallei (Meliodosis)	Soil contamination of wound (in South Asia)	Suppurative nodule with lymphangitis, multiple necrotic skin lesions	Bacteremia, metastatic abscesses	Based on in vitro sensitivity tests
	Pasteurella tularensis (Tularemia)	Wound exposed to infected animal, e.g., rabbit	Nodule which ulcerates, local lymphadenopathy	Fever, prostration	Streptomycin
	Streptobacillus moniliformis	Bite of infected rat	Ulceration at bite, local adenopathy	Fever, macular rash, arthritis, endocarditis	Penicillin (erythromycin)
	Spirillum minus	Bite of infected rat	Ulceration at bite, local adenopathy	Relapsing fever, macular rash	Penicillin (tetracycline)

* Second choice antibiotic in parentheses.

age, necrotic material, or blood. Suitable antibiotic combinations in this instance are clindamycin and gentamicin or penicillin and chloramphenicol. Attention should be given to possible bacteremia and metastatic infection, including endocarditis.

Fasciitis and Gangrene

Fasciitis and gangrene are deep soft tissue infections which are usually surgical emergencies. Acute fasciitis is due to spread of infection along subcutaneous and intermuscular fascial planes. This occurs more frequently in diabetics and may complicate a variety of wounds including acute trauma, cutaneous ulcers or decubiti, and surgical wounds. Infection may be caused by *Streptococcus pyogenes* or a combination of enteric gram-negative aerobic bacilli and enteric anaerobes, principally streptococci and bacteroides. Fasciitis caused by *Streptococcus pyogenes* is especially severe, causing marked soft tissue swelling, arterial obstruction, and ischemia with progressive spread of infection and a high mortality rate.[59] Dark or purple discoloration of skin associated with a diminished or absent arterial pulse should suggest this diagnosis. Surgical intervention should be immediate with extensive fasciotomy to relieve arterial obstruction and prevent tissue death. High-dose penicillin is required but is ineffective without surgical decompression and drainage. Fascial plane infections with mixed enteric aerobic and anaerobic flora may show slower progression, pus formation, and, occasionally, gas. Fasciotomy, drainage, and appropriate antibiotics are also required for this condition.

Infected gangrene develops in tissue made anoxic by extensive trauma or vascular obstruction; anaerobic bacteria play an important causative role. This process can be largely prevented by careful wound management, including prompt removal of dead tissue and foreign bodies and careful cleansing; closure should be delayed if the wound cannot be thoroughly cleaned. Gas gangrene is due to toxin-producing clostridia but other aerobes and anaerobes are usually present.[64] Infection spreads rapidly from the wound site, usually in the lower extremity, destroying muscle and other soft tissue as it progresses. The limb becomes cold, swollen, and pulseless, and obvious gangrene ensues. Gas in soft tissues may be detected early by x-ray but is not usually palpable until the process is advanced. Patients are typically prostrate, severely toxic, and apprehensive, with a tachycardia and low-grade fever. Hemolysis may occur. Treatment requires immediate surgical debridement of devitalized tissue and nonclosure of wounds. Amputation of the affected extremity is often necessary. Hyperbaric oxygen, if available, is thought to give ad-

ditional benefit but is not a substitute for debridement or antibiotic therapy. Penicillin is the antibiotic of choice; it should be used in high dosage. Polyvalent gas gangrene antitoxin has no proven value. Gangrene may also be caused by anaerobic streptococci (anaerobic streptococcal myonecrosis) or a mixed infection with *Staphylococcus aureus* and anaerobic streptococci (Meleny's synergistic gangrene). These may complicate surgical or accidental wounds and occur with greatly increased frequency in diabetics. Prompt debridement and antibiotic therapy are required (Table 82–3).

Systemic Infections Following Wound Infection

Wound infections may also be the initial event in serious systemic infections (Table 82–3). Burns routinely become infected, the usual organisms being gram-positive cocci and gram-negative enteric bacilli. The routine use of local and systemic chemoprophylaxis allows resistant gram-negative infections to emerge, especially those due to *Pseudomonas aeruginosa*. Organisms multiply to high counts in the burn eschar and then disseminate to cause bacteremia. Symptoms may include those of bacteremic shock. Treatment of bacteremia is discussed in Chapter 85.

Specific systemic infections may also follow rat bites or wound infection with contaminated animal products or soil. These infections include rat bite fever, tularemia, glanders, and meliodosis (Table 82–3). Symptoms of systemic infection usually predominate; the cutaneous manifestation is often limited to a nodule or ulcer at the inoculation site, local lymphangitis, and regional lymphadenopathy. A history of appropriate exposure should suggest the diagnosis. Confirmation is by cultural or serologic techniques appropriate for the specific infection.

TOXIGENIC INFECTIONS

Two organisms, *Clostridium tetani* and *Corynebacterium diphtheriae,* may infect wounds and cause little or no local damage but produce serious distant sequellae by the elaboration of potent exotoxins. Highly effective toxoid vaccines are available for protection against each toxin.

Tetanus

The tetanus bacillus is noninvasive and grows only in an anaerobic environment. Infection usually occurs in contaminated superficial or deep wounds containing necrotic tissue, but may also occur in areas of chronic suppuration. After infection, a potent neurotoxin is released, enters the circulation and acts on the central nervous system to induce exaggerated motor activity with muscular rigidity and episodic severe muscular spasms. The onset is 3 to 14 days after infection, spasticity beginning in muscles of the head and neck. The first complaint is usually a painless inability to open the jaw; examination also reveals hyperactive deep tendon reflexes and rigidity of the abdominal muscles. Spasticity then spreads to the trunk and extremities. In severe cases this spread is complete in a few hours, but in milder cases it may take 6 days. Intense, painful spasms occur; these are characterized by a facial grimace with a closed jaw (risus sardonicus), opisthotonus, and rigid extension of the extremities. Laryngeal spasm, apnea, and death may occur during these spasms. The diagnosis of tetanus is based on this clinical picture. Tetanus must be distinguished from meningitis, hypocalcemic tetany, and disease of the temporomandibular joint.

Management of tetanus is outlined in Table 82–4. Initial treatment aims to prevent further fixation of toxin to nervous tissue, to remove necrotic tissue harboring the organism, and to destroy any remaining tetanus bacilli. Supportive management includes control of muscular rigidity and spasms, maintenance of adequate ventilation, and careful nursing care. Antispasmodic therapy may be required for several weeks. Combination therapy is often required but it is best to begin with a single drug and use it in full dosage before another is added. By using a muscle relaxant first, followed by chlorpromazine, then phenobarbital, it is possible to minimize respiratory depression. Most patients require a tracheostomy, which should be performed early. Assisted ventilation may be needed when sedative therapy depresses respiration. In experienced centers, paralysis with succinylcholine combined with careful ventilatory support has been used successfully in treating tetanus. Overall, mortality from tetanus is about 30 per-

cent. Prognosis is poorer in newborns, narcotic addicts, the aged, persons with severe soft tissue wounds or infections, and when the incubation period is brief (less than 3 days) or the period from first symptoms to onset of convulsive spasms is less than 24 hours.

Tetanus is completely prevented by active immunization. All persons, including patients recovered from tetanus, should be immunized. Tetanus prophylaxis in wound management is summarized in Table 82–5.[58]

TABLE 82–5
Tetanus Prophylaxis in Wound Management[1]

Previous Tetanus Toxoid Doses	Clean, Minor Wounds		All Other Wounds	
	Td*	TIG†	Td	TIG
Uncertain	Yes	No	Yes	Yes
0–1	Yes	No	Yes	Yes
2	Yes	No	Yes	No‡
3 or more	No§	No	No‖	No

* Td = Tetanus toxoid.
† TIG = Tetanus immune globulin (human) 250–500 units IM at site separate from Td.
‡ = Unless wound is more than 24 hours old.
§ = Unless more than 10 years since last dose.
‖ = Unless more than 5 years since last dose.

TABLE 82–4
Management of Tetanus

Initial Treatment
Human antitoxin (50 U/kg IM)
Penicillin (1.2 million U/day) or tetracycline (1 g/day)
Cleanse and debride wound

Supportive Measures
Control rigidity and spasms
    Muscle relaxants—diazepam (300–400 mg IM q 4 hr),
    meprobamate (0.5–1.0 mg/kg IM q 4 hr),
    chlorpromazine (25–75 mg IM q 4 hr)
    Barbiturates—phenobarbital (50–100 mg IM q 4 hr),
    amobarbital (25–30 mg IV for severe spasms)
Tracheostomy
Mechanical ventilation

Cutaneous Diphtheria

Diphtheria of the skin results from wound infection with *Corynebacteria diphtheriae* (diphtheria is discussed at greater length in Chapter 83). Cutaneous diphtheria occurs in tropical climates as a chronic cutaneous ulcer but is also found occasionally among "skid row" and other underprivileged groups in temperate zones. Typically, the chronic skin infection becomes covered with a "dirty grey" membrane; Gram stain of this lesion reveal gram-positive club-shaped bacilli; culture on Loeffler's medium yields *C. diphtheriae*. About 20 percent of persons with cutaneous diphtheria harbor the same organism in their pharynx. Toxigenic strains may cause cutaneous anesthesia in the area of the wound, but neuritis or myocarditis occur in only 3 to 5 percent of cases, possibly because of poor absorption of the toxin. Treatment involves administration of equine antitoxin, cleansing and debridement of the wound, and treatment with erythromycin or penicillin.

BLOODBORNE INFECTIONS OF SKIN

A wide variety of infectious agents produce skin lesions when bacteremia occurs (Table 82–6). In most instances, skin involvement is not the major focus of disease but it often produces typical lesions which facilitate diagnosis. These lesions may also serve as a source of infected material for culture, or in some instances for spread of infection to others. Treatment is that required for control of the systemic infection.

INFECTIONS OF BONE AND DEEP SOFT TISSUE

Osteomyelitis

A majority of cases of acute osteomyelitis are caused by *Staphylococcus aureus* and occur before 12 years of age; the disease may, however, be caused by almost any organism and occur at any age. Successful management requires early diagnosis and prompt, appropriate therapy. Delayed or inadequate therapy frequently leads to chronic osteomyelitis which may be incurable.[60,62]

TABLE 82–6
Bacteremic Infections of Skin

Str. viridans, Staphylococcus aureus, and many others which cause acute or subacute infective endocarditis	Petechiae, subungual "splinter" hemorrhages, Janeway lesions, Osler's nodes
Neisseria meningitidis	Petechiae, ecchymoses, cutaneous infarction
Neisseria gonorrheae	Hemorrhagic pustules, usually few
Pseudomonas aeruginosa	Ecthyma gangrenosum
Haemophilus influenzae	Purplish cellulitis in child, often on face
Salmonella typhosa	Rose spots in typhoid fever
Pasteurella pestis	Bubos, which may drain; petechiae and ecchymoses; occasional subcutaneous abscesses or cutaneous ulcers
Treponema pallidum	Widespread macular, papulular, or pustular syphilides, including palms, soles, face, and scalp (secondary syphilis)
Mycobacterium leprae	Hypo- or hyperpigmented macules, anesthetic patches; nodules and papules on face, ears, and pressure points; erythema nodosum leprosum

---

Osteomyelitis is usually a blood-borne infection. Possible origins include the skin (*Staphylococcus aureus*) and infection or manipulation of the genitourinary tract (gram-negative enteric rods), the lungs (*M. tuberculosis*), or enteric infection (salmonellae). Hematogenous infection is frequently preceded by blunt trauma to the affected bone. Osteomyelitis due to salmonella species occurs with increased frequency in persons with sickle cell disease. Osteomyelitis also occurs after direct inoculation of bone with infective material. *Staphylococcus aureus* is a common contaminant during "clean" bone surgery; *Pseudomonas aeruginosa* causes osteomyelitis in bones of the foot infected by puncture wounds; a variety of gram-positive and gram-negative organisms infect bone after compound fracture or by adjacent soft tissue infection; anaerobes may cause osteomyelitis, especially in the mandible or maxilla.

Clinical features of acute osteomyelitis differ in children and adults. In children, hematogenous infection usually becomes established in the metaphyseal regions of long bones. The onset of symptoms is abrupt, with chills, fever, and systemic toxicity; the affected limb rapidly becomes swollen, erythematous, and vary painful. Weight-bearing on an involved leg is difficult or impossible. A marked leukocytosis is common, and blood cultures are positive in half of cases. In contrast, hematogenous osteomyelitis in adults mostly involves bones of the spine. The onset is often insidious with pain in the neck or back being the major complaint; local bony tenderness is common and fever may occur. Blood cultures are usually negative. Osteomyelitis which follows direct infections of bone usually has a subacute course with local pain, warmth, and swelling; fever may occur and purulent drainage from the infected wound is usual.

The initial result of infection is abscess formation in the involved bone. Typically, this extends through the cortex to elevate the periosteum and eventually rupture into the adjacent soft tissue. When the spine is involved, infection may occur in the neural arch or the vertebral body. Infection tends to spread to the adjacent vertebra, resulting in vertebral fusion. Extension of the abscess into the subdural space may cause serious spinal cord compression or meningitis. Paravertebral abscess (Pott's disease) suggests tuberculous infection but also occurs with pyogenic bacteria. Destruction of bone by infection leads to formation of a devitalized sequestrum. Subsequent new bone formation is termed the involucrum.

Early diagnosis of osteomyelitis is based upon the clinical features described above. In children, the syndrome of acute fever, limb pain, leukocytosis, preceding trauma or cutaneous infection, local tenderness, and staphylococcal bacteremia is diagnostic. When bacteremia is lacking, the syndrome may resemble acute rheumatic fever. The diagnosis in adults may be more difficult but should be suggested by the combination of back pain, local tenderness, and fever, although fever and local warmth are usually absent in tuberculous osteomyelitis. Periosteal elevation in long bones may be visible on x-rays after 10 to 14 days. Rarefaction of bone and narrowing of the intervertebral disc space occur after several weeks. New bone formation is vigorous with pyogenic infections but poor with tuberculous infection. Bone scans with ^{85}Sr may become positive somewhat earlier than changes seen on x-rays. Confusing abnormalities on bone scan may be produced by other processes including metastatic carcinoma. Determination of specific etiology is of great importance and, in the absence of positive blood cultures, is done best by culture and examination of the involved tissue. This can be by careful needle aspiration through the periosteum and, if possible, into underlying softened bone (Table 82–2). Surgical exploration is appropriate when necrotic bone is seen on x-ray or when differentiation between osteomyelitis and deep soft tissue abscess (pyomyositis) is difficult. Pus or necrotic tissue should be cultured for aerobes, anaerobes, fungi and mycobacteria, and examined by Gram stain and acid-fast stain techniques.

Treatment of acute osteomyelitis includes antibiotic therapy directed at the isolated organism, drainage of pus, and debridement of necrotic bone. Prompt, appropriate therapy yields cure rates of 95 to 100 percent. Antibiotics should not be given "blindly" until thorough efforts to isolate the causative organism have been made; these include blood cultures, needle aspiration of involved bone, and surgical exploration if necrotic bone is present. Antibiotics should be given parenterally in high dosage for at least 4 weeks. A penicillinase-resistant penicillin should be used to treat staphylococcal infection and infections of undetermined etiology; clindamycin is used in persons allergic to penicillin. Other infections are treated according to the in vitro sensitivity of the infecting agent. Defervescence and gradual decline of the erythrocyte sedimentation rate to normal indicate a good therapeutic response.

Therapy of chronic osteomyelitis is much less satisfactory. Recurrence is the rule, often after years of quiescence.[60] Prolonged antistaphylococcal therapy for 6 to 12 months has yielded apparent cures in some cases.

Pyomyositis

Tropical pyomyositis is a deep staphylococcal infection of muscle, usually of the lower extremity. Infection is apparently blood-borne. The result is deep inflammation and abscess formation which may give symptoms similar to acute osteomyelitis. Needle aspiration or surgical exploration yielding thick pus containing *Staphylococcus aureus* is diagnostic. Treatment includes surgical drainage and antistaphylococcal antibiotic therapy. A similar condition caused by enteric gram-negative bacilli and anerobic bacteria may occur in diabetics.

CHAPTER 83
Upper Respiratory Infections
PATRICK A. MURPHY

Patients with upper respiratory infections often present vexing problems. Most of these infections are benign and self-limited, and many are caused by viruses for which we have no effective treatment. However, some of them are complicated by bacterial infection of the nasal sinuses or middle ear cavity, and if this is not recognized and treated, serious or lethal results, such as meningitis and septic thrombophlebitis, may follow. Some sore throats are caused by pathogens, such as *Corynebacterium diphtheriae*, which may cause serious systemic complications, and others are secondary to illnesses such as agranulocytosis or acute leukemia. Diagnostic facilities may be limited, since these patients are usually seen at home or in offices instead of in hospitals. The physician must, therefore, rely heavily on clinical features in reaching a diagnosis. Unfortunately, it is not possible to distinguish bacterial from viral infections on clinical grounds alone, since the manifestations may be the same. The physician must, therefore, have a rational plan of managing those patients whose diagnosis is uncertain.

This chapter deals with the management of the patient who presents with a cold, a sore throat, or tracheobronchitis. The common local complications, such as sinusitis, and otitis media, will be discussed and the major bacterial infections of the pharynx, streptococcal, and diphtheritic pharyngitis will be considered in more detail.

MANAGEMENT OF THE PATIENT WITH A COLD

When the major complaints are a runny nose, sneezing, and a dry cough with or without mild sore throat, viral infection can be diagnosed with reasonable confidence. A large number of viruses may cause this syndrome, and as a rule their identification by culture or serologic tests is of no great importance. The only bacterial diseases causing primarily nasal symptoms are nasal diphtheria, which is rare, and infection by *Haemophilus influenzae* or meningococci. In these cases, the discharge is purulent from the outset. Viral infections are often associated with systemic symptoms such as headache, myalgias, and mild to moderate fever. The nasal discharge is clear mucus, and while tenderness over the sinuses is common, this is not severe, and spontaneous sinus pain is unusual. The eardrums are commonly retracted because of temporary Eustachian tube blockage but are not inflamed. The cough, if present, is nonproductive, and the chest is clear to physical examination. Such a patient should be treated symptomatically.

In most colds, after a few days the nasal discharge becomes mucopurulent, signaling that secondary bacterial infections has occurred. This in itself is not a cause for alarm and usually resolves spontaneously. However, bacteria may invade either the nasal sinuses or the middle ear, especially if mucosal swelling is severe enough to lead to obstruction of the sinus ostium or Eustachian tube. Most cases of otitis media and purulent sinusitis will improve spontaneously, but this fact must not lull one into a false sense of security.

Acute Sinusitis

The symptoms of acute sinusitis are sinus pain and tenderness, nasal blockage, and frankly purulent nasal discharge, with mild to moderate fever. Sometimes the inflammation is severe enough to cause nasal bleeding. The pain is usually moderate and due to absorption of air behind a blocked ostium; less often it is severe and due to the accumulation of pus under pressure (sinus empyema). Examination of the nose shows an inflamed, swollen mucosa and purulent discharge; if the nose is cleared by blowing it may be possible to see reaccumulation of pus in a particular

area, although commonly all the sinuses are involved to a greater or lesser degree.

The main principles of treatment are to establish drainage of the sinuses and to combat the infection with antibiotics. The inhalation of steam, whether medicated or not, is effective for temporarily clearing the nasal passages and promoting drainage. Oral "cold tablets" containing antihistamines and sympathomimetic drugs are entirely useless. It is possible to achieve useful shrinkage of the nasal mucosa by nasal drops such as 0.5% ephedrine in saline provided fairly large volumes (5 to 10 ml) are used and the head is carefully positioned to ensure that the medication actually reaches the ostium of the sinus mainly affected. However, nasal sprays and drops as customarily used are without value. The bacterial flora in acute sinusitis is very varied and may include any of the organisms commonly found in the upper airway such as pneumococci, streptococci, and *Haemophilus influenzae*. In addition, sinusitis may be caused by staphylococci, gram-negative rods, and anaerobic bacteria. The antibiotics commonly used for the treatment of acute sinusitis are penicillin, erythromycin, and tetracycline, and in general they are effective. However, since drainage procedures are inadequate and since no antibiotic can cover all the possible organisms, treatment failure and the development of major complications are to be expected occasionally. Because of this it is vital that patients are warned that treatment may not be effective and that they should report back at once if deterioration or new symptoms occur and also if the symptoms continue unabated for a week. If antibiotics are clearly failing to control sinusitis, one should not hesitate to arrange for the most severely affected sinuses to be drained surgically.[67]

The major complications of sinusitis are due to erosion of bone and spread of the infection to adjacent structures. Obviously, the pathology will vary with the sinus affected, but the possibilities include orbital cellulitis, cavernous sinus thrombosis, meningitis, and brain abscess, usually in the frontal lobe. Severe local pain, headache, vomiting high fever, shaking chills, and obvious systemic illness all suggest the onset of one of these complications. They demand urgent admission to hospital, accurate diagnosis, parenteral antibiotics in high dose, and surgical consultation.

Some patients have bacterial sinusitis with every cold, and in them it is well to search for local abnormalities such as deviation of the nasal septum or nasal polyps. Surgical correction of these defects between acute attacks may lead to great improvement.

Acute Otitis Media

Infection of the middle ear cavity is easier to manage than acute sinusitis because one can see what is going on rather than infer it. The three cardinal symptoms are earache, discharge, and conductive deafness. Initially, pain may be due to lowered air pressure in the middle ear cleft, and the tympanic membrane is gray and retracted. In an established bacterial infection, the pain is due to accumulation of pus under pressure, and the drum becomes red, loses its landmarks, and bulges. If it has perforated, pus can be induced to leak from the site of perforation by lowering the air pressure in the external auditory meatus.[69]

The onset of discharge is often associated with a lessening of the pain, for obvious reasons. Deafness is not usually severe, and if it is severe it denotes an extensive infection. Abnormal bone conduction means that the infection has spread to the inner ear. Mild infections of the middle ear cavity may cause little pain and only moderate deafness, and examination shows only a few dilated vessels on the tympanic membrane and perhaps an accumulation of mucoid exudate behind the drum, with a fluid level.

The treatment of acute otitis media is antibiotics, sometimes with myringotomy in those cases where there is severe pain and the drum is as yet intact. The responsible bacteria are usually pneumococci, streptococci, or *Haemophilus influenzae,* although almost any bacterium may be responsible on occasion,[69] and in at least one-third of cases, only viruses can be grown from middle ear fluid.[66] If the drum has perforated, or if a myringotomy is done, then material for culture may be obtained which will guide antibiotic therapy; but often one must treat blindly. Because of the *Haemophilus influenzae,* it is usual to recommend the use of ampicillin for otitis media in children below the age of 8. In adults, penicillin is adequate. The important thing is to recognize that any antibiotic regime is likely to fail on occasion. Vasconstrictor nasal drops and any sort of ear drops are of very dubious value.

As in sinusitis, the chief dangers are that some narrow drainage pathway will be obstructed and pus will accumulate under pressure and lead to necrosis of the mucoendosteum, osteomyelitis, and spread of the infection to surrounding structures. Infection of the middle ear cavity alone rarely leads to intracranial extension, probably because of spontaneous drainage through the eardrum. However, infection of the mastoid antrum with occlusion of the aditus by swollen mucosa is a classic source of septic thrombosis of the sigmoid sinus, extradural abscess, pyogenic meningitis, and brain abscess in either the temporal lobe or the cerebellum. Because most patients are treated with antibiotics, it is not usual nowadays for these complications to develop directly out of the acute otitis. Rather, the patient improves substantially, but persistent low fever, pain in the mastoid area, and continuing deafness signal that all is not well, and if these warnings are neglected, disaster may ensue. If the patient is not returned completely to normal by a week of antibiotic treatment, an otologist should be consulted.

The actual onset of a major complication is marked by the symptoms discussed above; headache, vomiting, fever, shaking chills, and systemic illness. Shaking chills are particularly suggestive of septic thrombophlebitis. In addition, vertigo and nerve deafness may occur secondary to invasion of the inner ear, and there may be evidence of local abscess formation in the mastoid area. Rarely, one sees paralysis of the Vth or VIth cranial nerve due to osteitis of the petrous temporal bone. Again, urgent hospital admission, parenteral antibiotics, and surgical advice are appropriate.

Note that while intracranial complications of both sinusitis and otitis media may arise during the course of an acute respiratory infection in a person whose upper airway is basically normal, brain abscess, meningitis, and the like are actually more common as complications of chronic sinusitis or otitis media.[71]

MANAGEMENT OF THE PATIENT WITH SORE THROAT

When the major complaint is sore throat, the cause may be either bacterial or viral, and the bacterial infections often demand specific treatment. Diagnosis from clinical features alone is possible in classical cases (Table 83–1), especially when it is known that an epidemic of sore throat due to a particular organism is in progress. However, most sore throats are mild and present no distinguishing features on examination. One approach maintains that because of the danger of nephritis and rheumatic fever following streptococcal sore throat, all sore throats without exception must be cultured and any with positive streptococcal cultures should be treated. Recent evidence suggests that this approach may involve an unreasonable investment of time, money, and penicillin allergy except under special circumstances.

TABLE 83-1
Distinguishing Features of Infections Causing Pharyngitis, Tonsillitis, and Sore Throat

Etiology	Clinical Manifestations			Laboratory Findings		
	Symptoms	Local Appearance	Other Findings	Leukocyte Count	Culture	Other Findings
Group A Beta-hemolytic Streptococcus (strepto-coccal tonsillitis and pharyngitis)	Sudden onset, chills, headache, myalgia, vomiting Painful swallow-ing	Fiery red edematous pharynx, tonsillar swelling; thin whitish yellow exudate restricted to tonsils Cobblestone lymphoid hyperplasia of posterior pharynx	Fever to 103 to 105°F Patient looks ill Tender cervical adenitis Rash of scarlet fever (occasional)	10 to 15,000	Beta-hemolytic streptococci on blood agar plates	Rising titer of anti-streptolysin-0, anti-deoxyribo-nuclease B, and related antibodies
Coryne-bacterium diphtheriae (faucial diphtheria)	Gradual onset of chilliness, general malaise, mild sore throat Swallowing is relatively painless Laryngitis and airway obstruc-tion may be present	Dull red injection, yellow-white adherent spots on tonsils Dirty white or grayish yellow pseudo-membrane; when stripped away a raw bleeding surface is exposed Evidence of naso-pharyngeal or laryngeal involvement may be noted	Moderate fever (101-103°F) May be few systemic manifesta-tions until complica-tions develop	Moderate leukocytosis, up to 15,000	Throat swab onto Loeffler's, Tellurite, and blood agar	Identification of typical organisms on stained smears of the lesion is occasionally helpful
Vincent's angina (fusospirochetal pharyngitis)	Minimal save for local pain Salivation	Superficial ulceration covered with a grayish white membrane that is easily removed Foul odor	Minimal fever (up to 102°F) Submaxillary node enlargement	May have slight leukocytosis	Not useful	Typical fusiform bacilli and spirochetes rapidly motile in wet preparations, spirochetes stain poorly in fixed smears of exudate or necrotic tissue

982

Organism	Symptoms	Throat findings	Other findings	Blood count	Culture	Special tests
Candida (thrush)	Dysphagia, sore mouth and throat	Diffuse erythema, whitish mucoid exudate	May be none, but usually patient is already sick with some other disease and has been given antibiotics	No characteristic changes	Candida species	Stained smears of exudate show myriads of organisms in yeast form
Infectious mononucleosis	Gradual onset of malaise, headache, anorexia, sore throat	Edema, mild erythema Tonsillar swelling and exudate Pearly white membrane occurs which can be confused with diphtheria May have coexistent streptococcal infection	Enlargement of nodes, especially posterior cervical, low-grade fever, splenomegaly, rashes, evidence of hepatitis Illness may be prolonged	Leukopenia is common early, mild leukocytosis in second and third week Lymphocytosis, especially with atypical cells	Negative for bacterial pathogens unless streptococcal infection coexists	Heterophile agglutinins Stained smears of tonsillar exudate reveal myriads of atypical lymphocytes E-B virus antibody titer
Viruses Rhinoviruses (common cold) Adenoviruses (febrile pharyngitis) Coxsackie A viruses (herpangina) Influenza, parainfluenza	Malaise, headache, myalgia; common cold syndrome Hoarseness, cough, mild sore throat	Pharyngeal edema and injection, lymphoid hyperplasia No exudate usually, but is seen with certain uncommon viruses	Low-grade fever, rhinitis, conjunctivitis Fever to 104°F in some cases Slight regional adenopathy	Usually normal, but mild leukopenia or moderate leukocytosis is seen	Negative for bacterial pathogens	Serologic tests may be useful for epidemiologic purposes

STREPTOCOCCAL PHARYNGITIS

Streptococcal pharyngitis is seen in its most classical form during epidemics in communities where people live in close physical proximity. Examples are schools, camps, and military training centers. Under these conditions, the introduction of a new streptococcal type may lead to rapid person-to-person transmission throughout the susceptible population. The organisms are well covered with protective M protein, inocula are large, clinical disease is severe, and the incidence of sequelae is high. In the general population, many of the streptococcal carriers have established immunity to their own organism, which responds by losing much of its M protein and incidentally becoming less virulent. Disease due to these streptococci is milder, and the incidence of sequelae is much less. Under normal circumstances, about 5 percent of the asymptomatic general population and at least 10 percent of children carry Group A, β-hemolytic streptococci in the pharynx. In the winter, when families huddle together indoors, transmission occurs more frequently, organisms become more virulent, and both the carrier rate and the disease incidence are increased. It has been show conclusively that infection is transmitted by respiratory droplets; dried streptococci in bed clothes, floor dust, etc. are incapable of causing disease.

Clinical Presentation

The classic symptoms are sore throat, dysphagia which may be so severe that only liquids can be swallowed, fever, and systemic upset. Cough, laryngitis, or coryza are rare and their presence suggests some other diagnosis. On examination, the throat is intensely red and edematous, and if the tonsils are present there may be yellow flecks of exudate in the crypts which can easily be wiped away. Sometimes the exudate is confluent, but it remains yellow and easy to remove. The faucial pillars, the soft palate, and the uvula are swollen, and hypertrophy of lymphoid tissue under the posterior pharyngeal wall may produce a cobblestone appearance. The tonsillar lymph nodes are enlarged and tender, the temperature may range up to 104°F or higher, and there is a neutrophil leukocytosis. Unfortunately, many proven streptococcal infections cause only mild symptoms, and a few are entirely asymptomatic.

The clinical diagnosis may be confirmed by a number of laboratory tests. The most important is culture of the throat, which in a typical case will demonstrate large numbers of mucoid colonies of β-hemolytic streptococci. Such streptococcal colonies are not necessarily Group A, and this should be con-firmed either by capillary precipitin or fluorescent antibody, which are specific tests; or by bacitracin sensitivity which is easy and useful but has an error of about 5 percent in both directions. It is worth knowing that streptococci are delicate organisms which may easily die on cotton swabs if for any reason these cannot be plated immediately. A number of good transport media are available, and the organisms do survive well when dried on filter paper. The significance of small numbers of streptococci in the throat is less certain: many such cases are merely carriers of the organism and the sore throat is due to concomitant viral infection.

Evidence of actual tissue invasion is provided by demonstrating significant (fourfold) rises in the serum levels of antibody to various streptococcal products. Antistreptolysin O is the classic antibody studied, and in throat infections significant rises are demonstrated in over 85 percent of cases. Other antigens, such as DNAse B and NADase, may be useful as confirmatory tests in doubtful situations, although their main value is in the confirmation of streptococcal skin infections. Because streptococcal infections are universal, all normal human sera contain antibodies to streptococcal products; the mere presence of an antibody, no matter what the titer, does not prove that a current illness is due to streptococci. Serologic information is, therefore, only useful in retrospect.

The blood usually shows a neutrophil leukocytosis with white counts ranging up to about 20,000/μl in a severe infection. Higher values and gross shifts to the left would suggest some suppurative complication. Leukopenia is rare and would suggest either viral infection or perhaps that the patient has some underlying condition which has lowered the blood neutrophil count and led to increased susceptibility to disease.

Therapy

Streptococcal pharyngitis is probably best treated by a single injection of 1.2 million units of benzathine penicillin G. This ensures that streptococci will be eradicated from the throat and that rheumatic fever will be prevented. Oral regimens must be continued for 10 days to achieve the same result; probably the best currently available is phenoxymethyl penicillin 250 mg q.i.d. Patients who are genuinely allergic to penicillin should be treated with erythromycin 250 mg q.i.d. for 10 days. Culture of all family members makes little sense since streptococci cannot be demonstrated in the throats of experimentally infected individuals until about 4 hours before symptoms of sore throat begin. Eradicative therapy for family members is indicated only when the strain of streptococcus is known to be nephritogenic, and if this is the case, therapy should be given regardless of culture results because by the time symptoms and positive cultures develop it may be too late to prevent nephritis.

Complications

The complications of streptococcal pharyngitis are spread of the infection in readily understandable ways: scarlet fever (which is a systemic toxemia) and glomerulonephritis, rheumatic fever, and other less common conditions whose pathogenesis is not understood. Direct local spread of infection may produce peritonsillar abscess (quinsy), and abscesses may also develop in cervical lymph nodes or in lymphoid tissue of the posterior pharyngeal wall (retropharyngeal abscess). Acute streptococcal otitis media or sinusitis may occur, and rarely, downward spread to the lungs produces streptococcal pneumonia. Generalized streptococcal sepsis with bacteremia and metastatic infections is very uncommon except in debilitated people.

SCARLET FEVER. Scarlet fever occurs when the streptococcus in the throat is lysogenized by a bacteriophage that codes for the production of the erythrogenic toxin. It is not agreed whether the toxin produces the rash directly or whether a state of hypersensitivity is responsible. The skin shows multiple, tiny erythematous papules which produce a generalized pink or red appearance from a distance. Circumoral pallor is classical. Later the rash becomes brownish, and extensive desquamation occurs. The tongue initially shows epithelial hypertrophy leading to a thick gray coat, and subsequent desquamation leaves a red tongue with prominent fungiform papillae (the "strawberry tongue"). It is usually said that the presence or absence of scarlet fever does not affect the severity of either the supprative or the nonsuppurative complications. This may be true now that antibiotic therapy is available, but was not always so, and the fact that small doses of purified toxin can kill rabbits and monkeys would suggest that its action extends beyond vasodilatation in the skin.

A third group of complications appears not to require the presence of the organism in the lesions, and includes rheumatic fever, acute glomerulonephritis, Sydenham's chorea, and erythema nodosum. The clinical features of these illnesses are discussed elsewhere, and only their relationship to streptococcal sore throat will be discussed here.

RHEUMATIC FEVER. During epidemics of streptococcal infection, the peak incidence of rheumatic fever occurs about 3 weeks after the peak of pharyngitis, and this incubation period has been confirmed in military recruits and schoolchildren where the onset of infection could be timed precisely.[73] It does not shorten in second or subsequent attacks, even when these follow closely on a previous infection, and this long incubation period provides an opportunity for effective preventive therapy. Treatment with penicillin within 5 days of the onset of sore throat will completely prevent the subsequent onset of rheumatic fever, and treatment as late as 10 days after onset is of measureable value. Rheumatic fever may follow infection with many different streptococcal types, and no one type is especially prone to cause the disease. During epidemics, rheumatic fever was found by Rammelkamp to follow 3 percent of proved cases of streptococcal pharyngitis. However, as mentioned above, the organisms are unusually virulent in these circumstances, and in the general population the figure is 0.3 percent and sometimes lower. There is a very different situation in those who have declared themselves to be rheumatic by having had a documented attack of rheumatic fever. If a second streptococcal pharyngitis confirmed by culture and antibody rise is acquired within 6 months of an attack of rheumatic fever, the likelihood of recurrence is 50 percent. Over a 5-year period, the risk of recurrence following proved streptococcal pharyngitis slowly drops to about 10 percent and then appears to continue at that level indefinitely. The indefinite persistence of susceptibility to rheumatic fever is underlined by the fact that in Baltimore, 18 percent of all cases of rheumatic fever diagnosed between 1960 and 1964 occurred in adults and that the annual incidence in adults aged 20 to 39 was 3.1 per 100,000, or about 20 percent of the rate in children.

Although rheumatic fever follows streptococcal infection, the exact pathogenesis is unknown, and from the data above, the occurrence of proved streptococcal infection with rises in serum antibody is not by itself enough even to guarantee a recurrence in subjects with known rheumatic tendencies. Clearly, there are associated factors, and what they may be is totally obscure. Genetic differences between rheumatic subjects and the general public have been suspected from family studies but the evidence is not conclusive. Racial and socioeconomic differences are not demonstrable if the rates are corrected for the degree of crowding. There is no evidence that rheumatic patients differ in their susceptibility to streptococcal infection: indeed, a comparative study between 164 families with at least one rheumatic member and 179 normal families showed that the streptococcal isolation rates were identical for both adults and children.[74] Epidemiologic analysis suggests, in fact, that the only important determinant of the incidence of streptococcal infections is population crowding and that the rheumatic fever incidence is a simple function of the streptococcal attack rate.

There is abundant evidence that the antibody response to streptococcal infection is unusually intense in rheumatic subjects. This is a statistical phenomenon, there being extensive overlap with the normal at all ages; no level of antibody response to any antigen leads to a clear separation. There is evidence that streptococcal infections lead to the development of antibodies directed against cardiac muscle, and gammaglobulin has been demonstrated fixed to cardiac muscle in rheumatic subjects. However, similar antibodies occur also in normal people and after cardiac operations and myocardial infarctions. Furthermore, antibodies directed against vascular smooth muscle and skeletal muscle are also formed during streptococcal infections, but these tissues are not involved in rheumatic fever. In fairness, one must also add that antibodies directed against a glycoprotein in heart valves and against protoplasmic astrocytes have also been discovered and are obviously of possible pathogenetic significance. Finally, lymphocytes sensitized against streptococcal antigens can kill beating heart muscle cultures, and it has been shown that patients with rheumatic fever have many more such lymphocytes than do normal subjects infected with streptococci. However, no one has yet integrated these immunologic observations into a coherent theory of pathogenesis.

How should we go about preventing rheumatic fever and rheumatic heart disease? There are two distinct questions here; the prevention of recurrent attacks of rheumatic fever in those who have already had one attack ("secondary prevention"), and the complete eradication of rheumatic fever ("primary prevention"). About secondary prevention there is no argument; it is known that the risk of recurrence is high and that continuous treatment with small doses of penicillin will reduce the risk to very low levels. What can be achieved was shown in a 10-year study in which patients were treated with 1.2 megaunits of benzathine penicillin G once monthly. No patient without cardiac damage at the outset developed it subsequently, and 70 percent of patients with established mitral incompetence at the outset lost their murmur.[80] Daily oral penicillin is less effective than monthly injections, as patients cannot be relied on to take it. No clinically important resistance of Group A streptococci to penicillin G has occurred, and the incidence of allergic reactions seems to be low. Some

cases of endocarditis due to *Streptococcus viridans* strains moderately resistant to penicillin have been reported, but the incidence is low, and anyone who has had a clearly documented attack of rheumatic fever should be treated with intramuscular penicillin, probably for life. If the patient is allergic to penicillin, erythromycin is an acceptable substitute.

Primary prevention is a more thorny problem. Only about one-third of cases of rheumatic fever occur after a sore throat for which the patient sought medical attention. In one-third, the symptoms are mild, and in one-third there are no symptoms at all. Considering the one-third where prevention is possible, it is usually recommended that all patients complaining of sore throat should have a throat culture, and that if the culture is positive, they should be treated with penicillin. This general approach has been taken to its logical conclusion in Casper, Wyoming, where all children have monthly throat swabs and any found to be harboring streptococci are treated. Another example of total prevention is in military camps, where epidemics are halted by treating the entire population of incoming recruits with prophylactic antibiotics.

An alternative viewpoint is gaining strength in Europe.[68] Death from a first attack of acute rheumatic fever is exceedingly uncommon, and chronic cardiac damage rarely results from a single attack. Sore throat is common; about 50 percent of the population has at least one sore throat per year. Only 20 percent of sore throats harbor streptococci and only 3 percent are associated with a rise in ASO titer. Most people with positive streptococcal cultures do not have symptoms. Even if only patients with both a sore throat and a positive culture were treated, 20 percent of the entire population would receive a 10 day course of penicillin each year, and 20,000 cases of sore throat would have to be diagnosed and treated to prevent one case of rheumatic fever. The mortality of penicillin treatment is uncertain but is thought to be of the order of 1 in 100,000 patients treated.[70] The conclusion is to reserve primary prevention for well-defined epidemic situations where streptococci are known to be prevalent and virulent, where most sore throats are streptococcal, and the risk of rheumatic fever is presumably about 3 percent. Sore throats found under nonepidemic conditions in the general population should be managed symptomatically and the time, effort, and money put into ensuring that those who have already had one attack of rheumatic fever do not get a second.[77]

GLOMERULONEPHRITIS. Acute glomerulonephritis follows infection with only a few streptococcal types, and in the throat, this is usually Type 12. The incidence of nephritis per proved Type 12 streptococcal infection depends upon how hard one looks. Obvious nephritis with edema, oliguria, and hematuria occurs in about 10 percent of cases, and if abnormal urine is accepted as the criterion, the incidence is above 20 percent. By renal biopsy, nephritis can be demonstrated in up to 50 percent of cases.

Acute poststreptococcal glomerulonephritis may occur at any age and is usually severe in adults. Why nephritis is so common after infection with particular streptococcal strains is unknown: electron micrographs show lumps of material underneath the glomerular epithelium which look like antigen–antibody complexes, but the nature of the antigen is unknown.

It is not at all certain that nephritis can be prevented by penicillin treatment of an established sore throat; in the only controlled trial of this question, no effect was demonstrable.[81] If there is protection, it is only partially effective. The patient should be treated mainly to prevent spread of the nephritogenic organisms to others, and there is a strong case for prophylactic treatment of close contacts, especially if they are adult. Once a patient has recovered from nephritis second attacks are uncommon, probably because of the persistence of type-specific protective antibody. Long-term penicillin therapy is, therefore, unnecessary.

OTHER NONSUPPURATIVE COMPLICATIONS. Chorea usually occurs along with other manifestations of acute rheumatic fever, and long-term penicillin prophylaxis is indicated. What should be done in those cases where chorea is apparently an isolated manifestation is not altogether clear, because the etiology of such cases is obscure and they may not all be poststreptococcal. However, if there is serologic evidence of recent streptococcal infection, penicillin therapy would seem to be reasonable.

Erythema nodosum is sometimes due to streptococcal infection and treatment with penicillin is then indicated. Long-term therapy is not required.

DIPHTHERIA AND ITS DELAYED SEQUELAE

Dipththeria is a localized infection of the upper respiratory tract which may be associated with delayed systemic manifestations, chiefly myocarditis and peripheral neuropathy. The systemic manifestations are due to a toxin whose primary action is to block protein synthesis. Since the use of immunization on a large scale, diphtheria has become rare, but there was an epidemic in San Antonio in 1973 in a population where immunization was not practiced. The penalty for missing the diagnosis for 24 hours may easily be the patient's life, so the disease must be recognized.[79]

Clinical Presentation

The patient has commonly been ill for a day or two with headache and malaise before developing a mild sore throat without much dysphagia and slight fever. He looks ill, with a gray pallor and a pulse rate raised out of proportion to the temperature. The tonsils are enlarged and the pharynx red and edematous. The membrane is dirty white in color and spreads not only over the tonsils but over the adjacent pillars of the fauces, the soft palate, and the uvula. This extratonsillar spread is pathognomonic. The membrane may spread downward to involve the larynx, and a common termination of untreated cases used to be death from laryngeal obstruction. The symptoms of laryngeal obstruction are hoarseness, stridor, and rib retraction on inspiration. Occasionally, no membrane is visible in the throat, and only the nasopharynx is involved. In this case the patient is usually less ill, but has a blood-stained, purulent nasal discharge, which may be unilateral. This membrane is composed of necrotic epithelium, fibrin, and inflammatory cells, with the organism visible in the interstices. Because the epithelium is part of the membrane, it may be difficult to remove, and when it is removed, a raw bleeding surface is left.

The cervical lymph nodes enlarge early and this combined with extensive edema of the tissues of the neck may produce the classic "bull neck" appearance. In neglected cases, paralysis of the soft palate may lead to a nasal voice and the regurgitation of fluid through the nose. Usually, by this time the membrane has partially sloughed and hangs in shreds from the pharyngeal wall.

Laboratory studies must not only demonstrate the organism but also that it is toxigenic. Smears of material from the edge of the membrane usually show gram-positive bacilli, but confirmation by culture is required because nonpathogenic corynebacteria may have similar morphology. Corynebacteria have simple growth requirements and will grow on most media, but because they may be overgrown by pneumococci and streptococci, it is best to plate swabs on blood or chocolate agar containing potassium tellurite. In the past, the colony morphology was thought to indicate whether or not the strain was toxigenic, but the correlations are only statistical and not useful in a particular case. Toxin formation is best demonstrated either by animal inoculation or by the Elek plate immunodiffusion procedure.

Systemic Complications

These are due to infection by a strain lysogenized with B prophage, and it can be shown that the phage actually carries the structural gene for the toxin. The mode of action of the toxin explains some of the clinical features and determines the approach to therapy. The toxin is a protein which is inactive until split into two chains by proteolytic enzymes at cell surfaces. One chain is required for the attachment to cell surfaces, the other is toxic if it can gain access to cell cytoplasm. The toxic action involves the enzymatic conversion of the translocation factor EF2 into an inactive form. Inactivation of all the EF2 molecules in a cell can be produced by only one molecule of toxin, but it is a process which requires many hours for completion. Once completed, protein synthesis is brought to a standstill. Functional damage will not be evident until the preformed supply of some critical protein has been exhausted.

The most susceptible tissue is the heart, and some degree of myocarditis probably occurs in all cases. Clinical cardiac involvement occurs in about 10 percent of cases, especially when the throat disease is extensive. It is most commonly seen in the second week of illness, but may be earlier or later. Physical signs include sinus tachycardia, first degree heart block, distant heart sounds, myocardial dilatation, and low blood pressure. Severe myocarditis is indicated by congestive cardiac failure, second or third degree heart block, and ventricular tachycardias. Such patients have a bad prognosis and may die either from progressive congestive failure or suddenly from ventricular fibrillation or asystole. Treatment of the cardiac involvement with the usual regimens for congestive heart failure probably has little influence on the outcome. Pathologically, there is focal myocardial necrosis with edema, hyaline degeneration, and, sometimes, fatty change. The inflammatory response is usually minor; if recovery occurs, it is generally complete.

Peripheral neuropathy is of two distinct types. Palatal paralysis is apparently caused by direct access of the toxin to the nerves, and a similar paralysis confined to the affected segment may be seen in wound diphtheria. As would be expected, it is usually the earliest neurologic symptom, appearing the second or third week of illness. Other palsies are due to blood spread of the toxin, and paralysis of accommodation is common in the third or fourth week. Subsequently, generalized polyneuritis may develop between the fifth and seventh week. It may produce death either by pharyngeal and laryngeal palsy, with aspiration pneumonia, or by paralysis of the diaphragm and intercostal muscles with respiratory failure. Treatment, thus, should include close observation of the patient's airway and of his vital capacity, with recourse to nursing in the prone position, endotracheal tubes, tracheostomy, and artificial ventilation as they seem indicated. The lower limbs are generally more severely affected than the upper, and there may be extensive sensory involvement. The sphincters are almost always intact. If the patient survives, recovery may take many months but is usually complete.

Therapy

The most important part of the therapy of diphtheria is to give a large dose of antitoxin at the earliest possible moment. The aim is to give enough to neutralize all the circulating toxin, to neutralize any toxin that may be formed subsequently, and, hopefully, to neutralize toxin already bound to cells but not yet interiorized. The quantity given is 30 to 40,000 units in a moderately severe case, half being given intravenously and the rest intramuscularly. More is given if there is extensive involvement of the throat. The serum is raised in horses, so the possibility of anaphylaxis should be borne in mind. Toxin already within cells is not accessible to antibody, and fatal myocarditis or severe neuropathy may still develop despite serum therapy. Cases treated on Day 1 of the illness have a negligible mortality, cases treated >4 days after the onset have the same mortality as controls.[79] Hence, the need for haste; serum should be given as soon as there is reasonable suspicion of the diagnosis without waiting for bacteriologic confirmation. If an adequate dose of antitoxin has been given at the outset, there is little point in giving more when paralysis or myocarditis later develops.

Antibiotics should also be given to eradicate the organism from the throat—both for the patient's sake and because convalescent carriers are a danger to others. It is usual to use penicillin, although there are indications that erythromycin might be even better.

Because of the dangers of laryngeal obstruction, myocarditis, and neurologic involvement, the patient should always be admitted to hospital and nursed in a unit capable of dealing with cardiac and respiratory crises if they should occur.

VINCENT'S ANGINA

This is synergic infection of the pharynx by two organisms, a spirochete and a fusiform gram-negative rod, which are normal inhabitants of the gingival crevices. Other bacteria, such as anaerobic streptococci and bacteroides species, may also be present in the lesions. The infection is usually found in persons with poor oral hygiene and is associated with more or less obvious gingivitis. It is especially common in malnourished, crowded populations and in patients with agranulocytosis or acute leukemia.

The major symptom is severe pain in the throat and gums, with dysphagia, dysarthria, and trismus. The breath is foul smelling, and the throat shows a gray-brown membrane which is easily wiped off. Fever is usually modest and there is not much systemic disturbance unless the patient has an underlying condition. Motile spirochetes can be seen in wet preparations from the membrane, and several sorts of bacteria are usually demonstrable by culture under anaerobic conditions. The disease should be treated with 3 percent hydrogen peroxide mouthwashes and with systemic penicillin therapy. If a patient develops this infection despite previous good health and reasonable oral hygiene, a blood dyscrasia should be sought.

HAEMOPHILUS PHARYNGITIS

Until recently, *Haemophilus influenzae* infection was a rarity in adults because almost everyone had type-specific antibody in their serum as a result of infection in childhood. However, now a substantial number of adults do not carry protective antibody,[75] whether because of the widespread use of antibiotics in children or because of better living conditions leading to a lower incidence of infection.

The dominant clinical symptom is sore throat whose severity is out of all proportion to the visible change, coupled with dysphagia and hoarseness. The infection is commonly bacteremic, with high fever, neutrophilic leucocytosis, and positive blood cultures. Very soon, a dry, irritative cough and stridor are added, and the clinical condition deteriorates dramatically within a few hours. The patient becomes prostrated, with gross laryngeal obstruction and cyanosis and may die within 24 hours of the onset.

The throat is red and swollen, but there are no ulcers or membranes and nodes are not particularly prominent. A laryngeal mirror will show gross edema and redness of the epiglottis and aryepiglottic folds. All such patients should be admitted to hospital, and if there is any evidence of respiratory obstruction, one should proceed to tracheostomy. The best antibiotics are ampicillin or chloramphenicol in doses of 0.5 g q.i.d.

THRUSH

Candida albicans is part of the normal mouth flora and rarely causes trouble in well people. However, if the normal flora is altered by antibiotic therapy, Candida may flourish and give rise to a very characteristic syndrome. It is especially common when lozenges containing antibiotics have been prescribed but can also complicate systemic antibiotic therapy. In addition, it may be seen in sick people who have not been given antibiotics, particularly in those with leukemias or lymphomas.

The throat is sore, but often the patient does not complain about it spontaneously. On examination there are pathognomonic patches of dead white exudate on an erythematous background. Unlike food particles, they cannot easily be wiped away, and potassium hydroxide preparations show masses of yeasts and pseudohyphae. Thrush is usually merely a nuisance and responds well to mouthwashes with Nystatin or to the old-fashioned painting with gentian violet. Occasionally, however, it spreads down the esophagus and causes monilial esophagitis, which is characterized by severe pain on swallowing. It may be lethal if untreated and requires systemic antifungal chemotherapy.

SYPHILIS AND GONORRHEA

Lastly, pharyngitis may occur in both syphilis and gonorrhea. Secondary syphilis is usually accompanied by a galaxy of physical signs—papular rash involving palms and soles, lymphadenopathy involving epitrochlear nodes, splenomegaly, arthritis, alopecia, conjunctivitis, condylomata, and so on. The pharyngitis is of gradual onset and is accompanied by mild to moderate fever. Inspection may show the classic snail track ulcers, and the lesions teem with spirochetes which can be seen on darkfield examination. Serologic tests for syphilis are strongly positive. Gonococcal pharyngitis usually presents no distinguishing features on examination, and the cultural result is a surprise. Further details are contained in Chapter 88.

VIRAL PHARYNGITIS

In most viral upper respiratory infections, there is coryza or tracheobronchitis as well as sore throat. Also there may be conjunctivitis, viral pneumonia, or gastrointestinal symptoms. Some groups of symptoms can be assigned with reasonable confidence to particular viruses. Thus, "acute respiratory disease" in military recruits is characterized by high fever, headache, sore throat, and nonproductive cough. The throat is merely red, without exudate, and the causative agent is usually adenovirus type 4 or 7. "Pharyngoconjunctival fever" is the same infection with more conjunctivitis and less bronchitis. Herpangina is characterized by fever, sore throat, and a pathognomic vesicular eruption on the anterior pillars of the fauces. It is generally caused by Coxsackie Group A viruses. Primary herpetic gingivostomatitis usually occurs in children below the age of 5. However, it is occasionally seen in adults, and most such infections turn out to be due to *Herpes simplex* Type I rather than Type II. The vesicles on the throat look like herpangina, but the gingivitis is diagnostic. Upper respiratory illness associated with nausea, vomiting, and diarrhea may be caused by ECHO viruses. When sore throat is the principal complaint, adenovirus infection is most likely followed by picornavirus infections.

INFECTIOUS MONONUCLEOSIS

Infectious mononucleosis is a systemic illness, but sore throat may be the most prominent clinical feature. Usually the patient has been ill for a few days with fever and headache before the sore throat develops. The throat may be very sore, indeed, and examination then shows deep cut ulcers of the tonsils with a yellow slough at the base. Similar ulceration of the adenoids may cause a purulent postnasal discharge. In milder cases, the throat shows no specific features. Petechial hemorrhages at the posterior end of the hard palate may be seen but are not diagnostic.

Evidence of systemic illness may be provided by enlargement of cervical nodes other than the tonsillar group, generalized lymphadenopathy, splenomegaly, or hepatitis (Chap. 51). The blood shows atypical lymphocytes, and these may also be found in smears from tonsils. The Paul–Bunnel test becomes positive, as does antibody to the Ebstein-Barr virus.

MYCOPLASMA INFECTIONS

Mycoplasma pneumoniae is the exception to the general rule that multiple involvement suggests viral infection which should be managed symptomatically. Most patients have upper respiratory symptoms, including sore throat, and only a minority actually develop pneumonia. One feature which occurs in only a small proportion of cases, but is pathognomonic when it does, is hemorrhagic bullae on the tympanic membrane. The disease responds fairly well to tetracycline or erythromycin therapy.

PRACTICAL PATIENT MANAGEMENT

It is obvious that the initial management of all acute upper respiratory illnesses that include sore throat as one component should be symptomatic. As the disease progresses one should remember the possibility of secondary bacterial sinus or ear infections and the less likely possibility that the whole illness is due to *Mycoplasma pneumoniae*. Whether or not to culture the throat for β-hemolytic streptococci is a question which each person must resolve for himself. It may be inevitable under present medico-legal conditions in this country, but it is by no means clear that it is totally rational.

When sore throat is the major complaint and especially when the patient is febrile and sick rather than merely inconvenienced, the probability of bacterial infection is higher. It is most important to exclude the rare but potentially lethal *Corynebacterium diphtheriae* and *Haemophilus influenzae* infections, which are not hard to diagnose provided one thinks of them. In the presence of exudative tonsillitis of the classic streptococcal type, one can take a culture and give therapy immediately, preferably 1.2 million units of benzathine penicillin. Penicillin therapy does not measureably affect the duration of clinical symptoms, but suppurative complications do occur and therapy is indicated when high fever and leukocytosis are present. When the sore throat shows no characteristic features and does not demand instant therapy, one can take a culture and institute penicillin therapy later if it is positive for streptococci. If a nephritogenic streptococcus is known to be about, therapy should be given immediately. If the culture shows only a few streptococci, it is likely that they are not the cause of the illness, and the need for therapy is moot. Many of these organisms are not Group A, and those that are may be untypable because they have lost all or most of their M protein.

Whether antibiotics are given or not, the fever and general upset can be satisfactorily treated with aspirin, and various anesthetic lozenges may provide local analgesia. If the patient does not respond to treatment within a few days, infectious mononucleosis and blood dyscrasias should be considered.

MANAGEMENT OF THE PATIENT WITH TRACHEOBRONCHITIS

Most tracheobronchitis is caused by viruses, and recovery is rapid and spontaneous. Bacterial superinfection may occur, especially in patients with chronic obstructive pulmonary disease, asthma, bronchiectasis, and certain rare conditions such as cystic fibrosis. This may progress to severe and sometimes fatal bronchopneumonia, or may precipitate heart failure in a person with chronic cardiac disease. In addition, the viruses themselves may cause pneumonia, although this is ordinarily not severe and may only be diagnosed radiographically.

In adults, the commonest cause of tracheobronchitis without much coryza or sore throat is the influenza virus. Parainfluenza viruses, rhinoviruses, and the respiratory syncytial virus cause much less bronchitis in adults than they do in children. Exceptionally, Coxsackie and ECHO viruses may cause acute bronchitis in adults, and an occasional, but treatable, cause is *Mycoplasma pneumoniae* infection.

The symptoms usually begin with headache, myalgia, and fever, with or without coryza or sore throat. The cough is commonly spasmodic and nonproductive or there may be a small amount of whitish sputum. Dyspnea is not a feature if the lungs were previously normal, and the only pain is substernal soreness. There may be concomitant laryngitis with partial or total loss of voice. Stridor is almost unheard of in viral infections of adults and would suggest hemophilus infection or perhaps diphtheria.

Examination shows nothing very specific. The patient has mild to moderate fever but is not usually very sick, and in particular, is neither dyspneic nor cyanosed. The chest may show a few wheezes on auscultation, but there is no evidence of pulmonary consolidation.

In normal people, an annual bout of bronchitis is to be expected, and everyone has his own method of treating it. The doctor's duty is limited to excluding pneumonia and signing whatever forms the patient may need to excuse him from work. Patients with chronic pulmonary disease deserve more attention, and there is solid evidence that they should be treated with antibiotics as soon as an attack of bronchitis develops. These patients carry pneumococci, streptococci, and *H. influenzae* in the tracheobronchial tree, and a viral infection which leads to lysis of ciliated epithelial cells may start a severe bronchopneumonia. Suitable drug regimens are tetracycline or ampicillin 500 mg q.i.d. Antibiotics may also be given if a basically healthy person with acute bronchitis begins to cough up large quantities of purulent sputum. Bronchodilators may be required if there is much wheezing, especially in chronic bronchitis or asthmatics. Cough suppressants should be used judiciously, recognizing that cough is the best way of getting pus out of the airways and that respiratory depressants may precipitate respiratory failure in those with carbon dioxide retention. If the patient will listen, he should stop smoking until he is recovered. These simple measures suffice for the vast majority of cases. Laryngitis, if present, improves spontaneously along with the bronchitis.

In aged patients, patients already ill with some other disease, pregnant women, and postoperative patients, the bronchitis may progress to bronchopneumonia. Fever and general malaise become more pronounced, the cough becomes productive with large amounts of purulent sputum, and dyspnea, tachypnea, and cyanosis appear. The chest now shows generalized coarse and medium crepitations, and there may be patches of dullness to percussion and bronchial breathing. Old people may become delirious. Such patients should be admitted to hospital and treated with oxygen, pulmonary toilet, and assisted ventilation as necessary, combined with parenteral antibiotics. This is discussed more fully later. Bacterial infection of the sinuses or middle ear may also occur and is managed as discussed above.

INFLUENZA

The influenza viruses are the most important agents causing acute respiratory disease because although there is a relatively low case-fatality rate, enormous numbers of individuals are affected. During the influenza epidemic in the winter of 1962–1963, there were an estimated 80 million cases in the United States, and deaths from influenza and pneumonia increased by about 70,000. Because it is a well-studied epidemic viral disease, because of its prevalence and importance, and because it is a representative localized viral respiratory infection with prominent systemic manifestations, influenza is used here to illustrate certain general epidemiologic, clinical, and immunologic features of viral disease.[65,72]

Epidemiology

Pandemics (worldwide epidemics) of influenza have been recorded at the rate of about four per century since 1610; the most severe pandemic occurred in 1917 to 1918, when an estimated 10 million persons died. In 1933, Smith, Laidlaw, and Andrewes first isolated the virus, and serologic tests useful in diagnosis and in epidemiologic studies followed rapidly. By 1936 a practical method for the manufacture of a vaccine protective for animals had been found, and it was soon demonstrated that the vaccine offered some protection for man. However, in 1947 there was an epidemic caused by the A-1 strain, and it became apparent that a new strain of the virus against which the available vaccines offered little protection had appeared. In 1957 and in 1968, pandemics were caused by the Asian (A-2) and Hong Kong (A-3) strains.

The only important source of influenza virus is infected persons. The virus is readily found in respiratory secretions during the first few days of the illness, but is rarely detectable for longer than the first week. Persistent carriers have not been demonstrated. However, there is evidence that inapparent or mild infections are more common than clinical disease;

thus, the viruses may persist in a population by causing sporadic mild illnesses resembling the common cold.

During nonepidemic periods, the viral antigens change slowly, and peptide mapping shows that successive single-base mutations leading to single amino acid substitutions are responsible for the changes ("antigenic drift"). The outbreak of a new pandemic is associated with a major change in the viral hemagglutinin to a completely new type ("antigenic shift"). The neuraminidase may or may not shift also. The mechanism for the shift(s) is probably that the virus has a segmented genome consisting of at least eight separate pieces of RNA. If two strains of influenza virus replicate in the same cell, then major recombination is possible. Perhaps the recombination occurs in an animal, rather than a man. At any rate, a virus with a totally new hemagglutinin finds most of the world's population defenseless, with no preformed neutralizing antibody. A new neuraminidase is less dangerous because antibodies against this antigen have less influence on the outcome of infection.

The Asian strain of influenza virus was detected in China early in 1957 and possessed both a new hemagglutinin and a new neuraminidase. It was widely seeded throughout the United States by midsummer, but outbreaks of clinical disease occurred at that time only in camps, institutions, and communities in which schools were open. A substantial increase in cases occurred throughout the United States in September when schools reopened, but it was not until the onset of cold weather that the infection appeared in truly epidemic proportions. Thus, widespread seeding of influenza virus may occur without epidemics being noted until other conditions are appropriate.[65] This often leads to the simultaneous appearance of explosive outbreaks in widely distant areas. Wet weather, crowding, cold, stress, air pollution, and travel in closed vehicles are among the factors that have been proposed to explain this.

Major influenza epidemics are caused only by type A strains. No part of the world escapes for long, widespread influenza recurring every 2 to 4 years. Nearly all epidemics reach their peak in the winter, with January and February the peak months in the Northern Hemisphere. Type B usually causes less severe epidemics, often localized to schools, military camps, and other closed populations, and occurring in 4- to 6-year cycles. Type C rarely causes epidemic disease.

Epidemics in any one locality tend to last only from 6 to 8 weeks. The short incubation period (2 to 3 days), the ease of transmission, the widespread seeding of the virus prior to the outbreak, and the high attack rates (50 to 75 percent when subclinical infections are included) may account for the short, explosive nature of the epidemics.

Clinical Features

The clinical manifestations of influenza vary from those of a mild upper respiratory illness to a severe pneumonia with involvement of many organs. There is little to distinguish the illness of isolated cases from that of disease caused by other common upper-respiratory-tract pathogens (Table 83–2), but a characteristic pattern is readily discernible when groups of patients are encountered, and the knowledge that influenza infection is prevalent is a most important clue to the diagnosis.

The incubation period is usually about 2 days. The patient characteristically presents with the sudden onset of prostration, myalgia, headache, retro-orbital pain, and marked toxicity. Fever of 103° to 104°F may ensue within a few hours. Bradycardia is common, but tachycardia is usually seen in the most severely ill. A flushed face and hot, dry skin are typical. Heliotrope cyanosis (reddish purple) suggests the diagnosis of influenzal pneumonia.

Systemic symptoms predominate during the first 24 to 48 hours of illness; as they subside, respiratory symptoms become prominent. Pharyngitis alone is distinctly unusual, but combinations with coryza, conjunctivitis, nasopharyngitis, tracheobronchitis, and bronchiolitis are common. Mucosal hyperemia is always present, and this may occasionally progress to hemorrhagic necrosis of the tracheobronchial mucosa. Scattered rhonchi or moist rales in the lungs are found in as much as a third of uncomplicated cases. Radiologic evidence of pulmonary involvement is also frequent. A dry, hacking cough and retrosternal burning pain are often most distressing parts of the illness. Secondary bacterial pulmonary infections are most frequent during the late stages of the illness and are heralded by the sudden return of high fever and prostration or by the appearance of dyspnea and cyanosis. Gastrointestinal manifestations are rare in influenza. Neurologic involvement, including meningoencephalitis, is not unusual in outbreaks. Myocarditis and pericarditis have also been reported; arrhythmias, hypotension, and cardiac failure are the usual manifestations.

Secondary bacterial infections of the ears, sinuses, bronchi, and lungs are frequent and important complications, and bacterial pneumonia is responsible for many of the fatalities. Bacterial infections occurring on the third to fifth day of influenza and influenzal pneumonia are particularly troublesome in patients with rheumatic heart disease, congestive

TABLE 83-2
Common Respiratory Infection Syndromes

Infectious Agent	Rhinitis Coryza		Pharyngitis		Laryngitis		Tracheo-Bronchitis		Pneumonia		Other Features
	Child	Adult	Child	Adult	Child	Adult	Child	Adult	Child	Adult	
Influenza virus	+	+	+	+	+	+	+	+	+	+	Severe myalgia, malaise, orbital headache
Adenoviruses	+	+	+	+	−	−	+	−	+	+	Keratoconjunctivitis Pleurodynia, orchitis, aseptic meningitis in recruits
Parainfluenza viruses	+	+	+	+	+	−	+	−	+	−	Croup
Coxsackie	+	+	+	+	−	−	−	−	−	−	Pleurodynia, orchitis, aseptic meningitis, pericarditis, herpangina
Respiratory synctial virus	+	+	+	+	+		+	−	+	−	Little or no fever
Rhinoviruses	+	+	+	+	−		+	−	+	−	Little or no fever
Mycoplasma pneumoniae	+	+	+	+	+	+	+	+	+	+	Complement-fixation test positive Tetracyclines useful

heart failure, or chronic pulmonary disease and in pregnant women. Even in the absence of complications, the disease tends to be more severe in such patients. Influenzal pneumonia, which is usually diffuse and hemorrhagic, can sometimes be distinguished from secondary bacterial pneumonia in patients with influenza (Table 83–3).[72]

In most patients, recovery takes place in a few days or, at most, a week, but delayed convalescence manifested by easy fatigability, persistent cough, recurrent myalgia, malaise, and depression may follow influenza. Subjective manifestations persisting beyond 3 weeks can be frequently related to a depressive propensity of the patient.

Laboratory Findings
Leukopenia and lymphopenia are often seen early in influenza but mild leukocytosis is more common. Brisk leukocytosis (more than 15,000 cells/μl) sug-

gests a secondary bacterial infection. Virus isolation in tissue culture or embryonated eggs is most readily accomplished with throat washings obtained before the sixth day of the illness. Hemagglutination-inhibition or complement-fixation tests are useful if both acute and convalescent sera are available. Virus isolation attempts are successful in only about 50 percent of the patients who develop serologic evidence of the illness.

Management
Only supportive therapy is indicated in uncomplicated influenza. Codeine is particularly efficacious in alleviating myalgia, cough, and headache. Aspirin is useful, but may make the patient more uncomfortable because of sweating and chilliness if it is given intermittently. Antibiotics are useful when secondary bacterial complications develop, but do not influence the course of the viral illness and do not prevent bac-

---

TABLE 83-3

Comparison of Influenza Viral and Secondary Bacterial Pneumonia

	Influenzal Pneumonia	Influenza with Bacterial Pneumonia
Onset	Seen early in illness, rapidly progressive	Several days after onset of influenza
Physical findings and chest x-ray	Diffuse infiltrates	Focal infiltrates Early pleural fluid (streptococci) Multiple cavities (staphylococci)
Sputum	Bloody, sparse bacteria and leukocytes	Purulent, many bacteria and leukocytes
White blood cell count	Often normal	Usually greater than 15,000 Polymorphonuclear leukocytosis
Erythrocyte sedimentation rate	Often normal	Usually increased
Prognosis	Mortality rate high, especially in patients with underlying disease (heart disease, chronic lung disease, pregnancy)	Responds to antibiotic therapy Greatest risk in patients with underlying cardiac or pulmonary disease

---

terial complications. Sinusitis, otitis media, and purulent bronchitis are managed as discussed earlier. However, the onset of bronchopneumonia should be treated with a penicillinase-resistant semisynthetic penicillin, such as nafcillin, because many such cases are due to secondary staphylococcal infection. Cultures of the sputum and of the blood should be done at the outset to determine the responsible organism, and therapy should be modified as appropriate. Such patients will of course need to be managed in the hospital, and until it is known that they are not coughing up *Staphylococcus aureus,* they should be isolated. In addition to antibiotics, they will often require treatment for respiratory failure. Simple treatment is 24 or 28 percent oxygen by mask, humidification of the inspired air, nasotracheal suction, and postural drainage. Major crises may require tracheostomy and artificial ventilation.

Vaccination and Other Preventive Measures

It is easy to protect human volunteers against experimental challenge with influenza. Either formalinized whole virus vaccines or purified hemagglutinin ("split virus") vaccines produce useful, but not solid immunity.[78] Split virus vaccines produce fewer side effects, especially in children, but are somewhat less effective stimuli of antibody production. Antibody responses are also influenced by previous experience with influenza infection; adults and older children usually require only one injection of vaccine, children under 6 years usually need two. Provided that the vaccine virus is closely related to the epidemic strains, these vaccines also convey short-lived but useful immunity to wild-type influenza in the general population.

It is not practical to persuade the entire population every year to take a vaccine against an infection which is trivial in most people. Furthermore, in years in which the virus has a major antigenic shift, it probably would be impossible to make, test, distribute, and administer enough vaccine in time to abort the epidemic. Finally, the epidemic of Guillain-Barre syndrome following the swine flu immunization campaign of 1976 reminds us that no vaccine is free from side effects. For all these reasons, the current strategy is to vaccinate annually only that segment of the population which is likely to die of influenza. This includes all persons over the age of 65 and people of any age who have chronic disease of the heart or lungs. Some physicians vaccinate all patients with any other chronic illness, but the evidence that this is useful is meager.

An adjunct in the control of influenza epidemics is the use of amantadine. There is clear evidence that this substance protects people against most influenza A strains if it is given before infection.[76] It can be given in a dose of 200 mg daily for 3 weeks after vaccination to provide protection while the antibody response is developing. Under epidemic circumstances, this can be very useful. There are two drawbacks: amantadine is not very effective once the patient is clinically ill with influenza, and most of the clinical trials have been done in college students. Old people treated with amantadine have a fairly high incidence of (reversible) neurologic side effects.

Since the virus is widespread in a community during an epidemic, measures of isolation and quarantine are of little value. Crowding should be avoided, but measures which interfere with the normal activities of a community are not practical. Isolated populations may be protected during an epidemic by exclusion of visitors. During an epidemic, health authorities should give primary attention to minimizing complications in those who develop the disease.

CHAPTER 84

Pneumonia
PATRICK A. MURPHY

Pneumonia poses some of the most fascinating diagnostic and therapeutic challenges in medicine. Acute inflammation in pulmonary tissue is usually caused by bacteria, and more than half of such cases are due to the pneumococcus. However, even in patients presenting with pneumonia as the primary complaint, about half the cases are due to other organisms. Staphylococcal and gram-negative rod pneumonias carry a much worse prognosis than pneumococcal pneumonia and require very different treatment. Furthermore, almost any bacterium can cause pneumonia on occasion; the list of exotic bacterial causes ranges from *Bacillus cereus* to *Pasteurella multocida*.

Pneumonia may also be caused by specialized bacteria, such as rickettsia and mycoplasmas, and in some circumstances by slow-growing organisms such as tubercle bacilli or nocardia. Pneumonia due to viral infection is very common; it seems likely that most cases are undiagnosed. Most pulmonary fungal infections are chronic, but there are exceptions. Even protozoa, such as *Pneumocytis carinii,* or helminths, such as *Ascaris lumbricoides,* may cause relatively acute pulmonary symptoms.

Finally, the clinical syndrome of fever and pulmonary infiltrate can also be due to a wide variety of noninfectious causes. Pulmonary embolism, allergic reactions to drugs or inhaled substances, aspiration pneumonia, and metastatic tumor are some of the possibilities.

Almost always, the available information is insufficient to make a precise diagnosis when the patient is first seen. However, different organisms do tend to cause distinctive clinical syndromes, and a provisional diagnosis should be made on the basis of the clinical findings and rapidly obtainable laboratory results (Tables 84-1 and 84-2). Time must not be frittered away in endless diagnostic maneuvers; unless bacterial pneumonia is thought to be improbable, the patient should be on antibiotics within an hour and a half of presenting. This chapter first deals with the various clinical patterns which may be seen in pneumonia and how to make an educated guess at the etiology. Second, it deals with the various techniques which can be used to firm up or alter the provisional diagnosis and how the common pneumonias should be managed.

MODES OF PRESENTATION

Classical Lobar Pneumonia
Lobar pneumonia is a localized disease; one lobe of one lung is consolidated, the remaining lobes are normal. It is true that sometimes more than one lobe is affected ("double" or "triple" pneumonia), but almost always there are one or more normal lobes. Most such cases are caused by the pneumococcus. The earliest manifestation is usually the abrupt onset of fever, with a shaking chill. Soon cough, purulent or rusty sputum, dyspnea, and pain in the side of the chest on inspiration or coughing supervene. Sometimes diaphragmatic pleurisy produces pain in the shoulder or the upper abdomen.

On physical examination the patient appears acutely ill, febrile, often cyanotic, and has the characteristic physical signs of lobar consolidation. These include inspiratory lag and decreased respiratory excursions (splinting) of the involved hemithorax, with moderate percussion dullness, increased tactile fremitus, bronchial breath sounds, whispering pectoriloquy, and coarse inspiratory rales over the involved lobe. A pleural friction rub may also be heard over the area. Sometimes a sterile effusion develops along with the pneumonia; this will cause stony dullness to percussion and reduced to absent breath sounds. Frank empyema is unusual until the pneumonia has been established for a few days.

TABLE 84-1

Clinical Clues to Etiologic Diagnosis in Acute Pneumonia

Etiologic Agent	Fever	Chills	Cough	Sputum	Other Features
Bacterial					
Pneumococcus (*Streptococcus pneumoniae*)	102–106°F, usually sustained	Often single shaking chill at onset	Productive in 75% Pleuritic chest pain	Rusty, blood-streaked, mucopurulent	Preceding URI in many Herpes labialis frequent Lobar consolidation frequent
Staphylococcus aureus	Intermittent, hectic, or sustained, 102–105°F	Multiple	Pleuritic pain Often nonproductive when hematogenous in origin	Purulent, blood-streaked, occasionally gross hemoptysis	In infants, debilitated persons, or following influenza Lung abscess or pneumatocele
Group A Beta-hemolytic streptococcus	Hectic, 104°F or higher	Multiple	Productive Often with pleuritic pain	Purulent and bloody	Early pleural effusion and empyema common Often follows influenza or measles
Klebsiella pneumoniae (Friedländer's bacillus)	Often remittent, 102–105°F	Multiple	Productive Severe pleuritic pain	Thick, bloody, mucopurulent Gram stain very useful	Upper lobes; abscess Bulging fissure especially common in alcoholics, diabetics
Haemophilus influenzae	Variable	Usually absent	Productive Wheezing common in children	Purulent Gram stain useful	Most common in alcoholics or patients with chronic lung disease Lobar consolidation may occur
Bacteroides	101–104°F	Multiple	Often not prominent	Gram-negative bacilli may be present on smear, fail to grow on aerobic media	1. Hematogenous pneumonia secondary to pelvic thrombo-phlebitis and bacteremia in young women Empyema not prominent 2. Aspiration pneumonia in older people Empyema often massive
Escherichia coli	100–103°F	Multiple	Prominent	Thick, purulent, with gram-negative bacilli readily seen on smear	Usually associated with preexisting chronic debilitating illness Lower lobes almost always involved
Proteus	101–104°F	Multiple	Prominent	Thick, purulent, with small gram-negative bacilli on smear	Usually superimposed on chronic lung disease Dense lobar consolidation, with multiple abscess formation

TABLE 84–1 (cont.)

Etiologic Agent	Fever	Chills	Cough	Sputum	Other Features
Bacterial (cont.)					
Pseudomonas	Reversal of diurnal temperature curve	Multiple	Prominent	Copious yellow or green sputum with gram-negative bacilli on smear	Usually diffuse broncho-pneumonia in patients with underlying pulmonary or cardiac disease
Francisella tularensis	102–105°F, sustained	Variable	Often not prominent	Generally scanty Gram stain of little value	Previous exposure to rabbits, rodents, insect vectors Sometimes cutaneous ulcer Often severe toxicity
Mycoplasma					
Mycoplasma pneumoniae (Eaton's agent)	101–104°F	In less than 25%	Persistent, hacking nonproductive Pleurisy rare	Scant, mucoid	Physical findings often unimpressive Insidious onset Complement fixation test positive Tetracyclines and erythromycin effective
Viral					
Influenza	Up to 105°F	Suggestive of 2	1. Dry cough 2. Productive cough	1. Scant or bloody 2. Purulent or bloody	1. True influenzal pneumonia, heliotrope cyanosis, marked dyspnea 2. Secondary bacterial pneumonia, shaking chills, prostration
Varicella	Up to 105°F	Rare	Usually harsh, dry cough, cyanosis	Scant (bloody)	Pulmonary involvement in 10% of adults with chickenpox Lesions may be miliary
Measles	Up to 105°F	Rare	1. Dry 2. Productive	1. Scant 2. Copious, purulent	1. True measles giant cell pneumonia in persons with defective cell mediated immunity 2. Secondary bacterial infection
Respiratory syncytial virus	Often mild	Rare	Dry	Scant	Children primarily, obstructive bronchiolitis
Adenovirus	Often mild	Rare	Variable	Scant	Most frequent in military recruits, often pharyngitis also

(Continued)

TABLE 84–1 (cont.)

Etiologic Agent	Fever	Chills	Cough	Sputum	Other Features
Chlamydiae					
C. psittaci	Variable, 101–105°F	Shaking chills in one-third	Dry, hacking, pleurisy rare	Small amount blood-streaked sputum	Acquired from birds Tetracyclines effective C. F. test positive
Rickettsiae					
Coxiella burneti (Q fever)	Up to 105°F	Common	Cough and pleurisy late manifestations	Scant	Primarily a systemic illness Headache, myalgia C. F. test positive
Mycobacterial					
Mycobacterium tuberculosis	Usually under 102°F, remittent or intermittent	May occur	Variable	Varies with stage of disease	History of exposure or previous tuberculous infection
Fungal					
Histoplasma capsulatum	Variable	Rare	Usually nonproductive	Scant	Contact with bird droppings Culture and serologic evidence Self-limiting course
Coccidioides immitis	Variable	Common	Nonproductive, poorly localized chest pain	Scant	Often asympto-matic or flu-like Usually self-limited A wide range of pulmonary syndromes occur Erythema nodosum Southwestern U.S.
Cryptococcus neoformans	Usually low-grade	Rare	Often prominent	Scant	Pulmonary disease often silent, chronic, and not detected until meningitis appears Contact with pigeons
Aspergillus fumigatus	Up to 105°	Rare	Cough and pleurisy late manifestations	Scant, but smear shows diagnostic branching hyphae	Usually occurs in patients on steroid or immuno-suppressive therapy (e.g., postrenal transplant)

Atypical Presentations of Pneumococcal Pneumonia

Pneumococcal pneumonia is not always as easy to diagnose. Symptoms of fever, dyspnea, and pleuritic pain may precede physical or radiologic signs of pneumonia by as much as 24 hours. The earliest physical signs are fever and bronchial breathing; these suffice as the basis for a tentative diagnosis of pneumonia. In the elderly, pneumonia may cause little or no fever and, especially in the presence of advanced emphysema, abnormal physical signs may be difficult to detect. Often the most striking changes are delirium, stupor, congestive heart failure, or unexplained prostration. Unless pneumonia is actively sought in such patients, the diagnosis will be missed. Alcoholic patients may also present with fever and prostration out of proportion to the physical signs, or with delirium tremens. One should remember that *Klebsiella pneumoniae* is not infrequently the cause of lobar pneumonia in alcoholics.

Recurrent Pneumococcal Pneumonia

Recurrent pneumonias are often indicative of underlying diseases, either local or systemic. Repeated bouts of pneumonia in the same area and slow resolution of pneumonia suggest bronchostenosis or bronchiectasis. In this circumstance, bronchoscopy should be done first, followed by a bronchogram if necessary. If bronchostenosis is found, determination of the etiology (by sputum cytology, culture for tubercule bacilli, bronchoscopic biopsy) is of greatest importance because the condition may be an early manifestation of a curable but potentially lethal disease (e.g., bronchogenic carcinoma, tuberculosis). Bronchiectasis should usually be managed by regular postural drainage with antibiotics as needed for exacerbations. Occasionally, segmental resection may be desirable.

Recurrent bouts of pneumonia in different sites should suggest systemic disease, such as systemic lupus erythematosus (SLE), or impaired immunologic defense mechanisms, as seen in patients with multiple myeloma. Early etiologic diagnosis and therapy are especially urgent when pneumonia occurs in association with such systemic disease. Whenever there is a question whether acute disease is due to acute bacterial infection or to underlying illness (e.g., SLE, polyarteritis), it is reasonable to manage the patient as though acute bacterial pneumonia was present.

LOBAR PNEUMONIA DUE TO OTHER ORGANISMS

Occasionally, true lobar consolidation is due to bacteria other than the pneumococcus. Group A streptococci, *Haemophilus influenzae, Klebsiella pneumoniae,* Proteus species, and Herellea (Acinetobacter) do so with some frequency. Even *Staphylococcus aureus* has been associated with lobar consolidation on occasion, although it typically causes bronchopneumonia. Viruses and mycoplasmas usually cause segmental consolidation, and the patients are less ill, but some cases cannot be distinguished from bacterial pneumonias. These possibilities should be remembered if a patient does not respond to low-dose penicillin G.

Bronchopneumonia

In bronchopneumonia, organisms spread down the trachea into both lungs and cause bilateral signs. Usually the bases are more severely affected than the apices, but often there is no normal lung anywhere. Bronchopneumonia usually occurs in patients who have some other acute or chronic disease. It very commonly follows influenza, usually in old people, but sometimes in the young and healthy. Other patients susceptible to bronchopneumonia include those with neoplasms of the hemopoietic or lymphatic systems, postoperative patients, those treated with immunosuppressive drugs, and those with chronic bronchitis or emphysema. Bronchopneumonia may also supervene when normal people inhale particularly virulent pathogens, such as plague bacilli. It is rarely caused by viruses alone, although fatal bronchopneumonia due only to influenza virus does occur.

The onset of bronchopneumonia is usually gradual, but deterioration is progressive, and by the time patients present they are usually gravely ill, with some cyanosis and dyspnea. Delirium and cardiac failure may be precipitated by anoxia and acidosis. Cough, sputum, and pleurisy may be minimal because the patient is too weak to breathe effectively, and fever may be only modest.

Staphylococcal Pneumonia

Staphylococcal pneumonia is responsible for about one-quarter of severe postinfluenzal pneumonia and occurs sporadically in individuals with impaired resistance to infection.[85] Multiple chills and hectic fever are common, and the sputum is often bloody. Because the infection is necrotizing, abscesses occur early. In children, these abscesses may rupture into the pleura, producing the classic pyopneumothorax. Staphylococcal pneumonia may be hematogenous; the infiltrates being infected pulmonary emboli. The physical signs are then less prominent than the x-ray findings, and there is usually an infected skin site which was the portal of entry.

Group A Streptococcal Pneumonia

This was a common complication of influenza in the 1918 epidemic.[83] It also occurs in a minute proportion of cases of streptococcal sore throat. There is early involvement of the lymphatics, which become blocked by masses of organisms and inflammatory cells and are visible as streaks in the x-ray and as white cords at the autopsy table. Thin, bilateral pleural effusions accumulate very rapidly and usually contain streptococci. High fever, multiple chills, and severe bilateral pleural pain are characteristic.

Klebsiella Pneumonia

Klebsiella (Friedländer's) pneumonia is classically a severe necrotizing upper lobar pneumonia seen most commonly in alcoholics.[87] It may also affect diabetics and persons in left heart failure, and often there is a great deal of bronchopneumonic involvement as well as lobar. The onset is usually fulminant with very viscid sputum, often grossly bloody. Sometimes there is a subacute course of days or weeks, and the illness may be mistaken for tuberculosis. The classic x-ray signs are bulging of the fissure and central cavitation, but they are not diagnostic. Healing is slow and scarring severe.

Haemophilus Influenzae Pneumonia

This organism is the commonest bacterium associated with acute respiratory failure in chronic bronchitics.[84] Many of the strains from these patients are noncapsulated, and it is uncertain that the bacteria in the sputum really cause the acute deterioration. However, there is no doubt that *Haemophilus influenzae* causes lobar or bronchopneumonia on occasion, because it has been isolated from blood and/or empyemas in such patients. There are no distinguishing clinical features of this pneumonia.

Pneumonia Due to Other Gram-Negative Bacilli

Enterobacteria such as *Escherichia coli* or *Serratia marcescens* have caused an increasing proportion of nosocomial pneumonias in the last two decades.[91] Most patients have had major operations or suffered from grave medical illnesses. Many were being artificially ventilated or had been given antibiotics. Similar cases may be caused by other gram-negative rods such as *Pseudomonas aeruginosa* or Acinetobacter species. These organisms are endemic in hospitals, are spread from one patient to another by the staff, are commonly resistant to antibiotics, and may be introduced directly down the trachea by ventilatory equipment. Cases of primary pneumonia due to these organisms also may occur in patients with chronic lung disease or in diabetics and alcoholics. In the nosocomial cases, colonization of the throat and/or sputum by gram-negative rods usually precedes pneumonia by several days. The identity and antibiotic susceptibility pattern of the most probable organisms are, therefore, often available from the chart. Previous colonization may also occur in chronic bronchitics or those with cystic fibrosis. In primary cases, the sputum is loaded with gram-negative rods, but neither the appearance of the smear nor the x-ray changes give a reliable indication of which species of gram-negative rod is responsible for the pneumonia.

Tularemic Pneumonia

In this illness, there is usually a history of shooting and skinning rabbits. The disease is bacteremic, with high fever and severe systemic toxicity, and the pneumonia may be more evident on the x-ray than in the patient. Bilateral hilar adenopathy is very suggestive.[89]

Interstitial Pneumonia

This syndrome results from infection of the alveolar walls and the spaces between them. It usually affects segments of the lung, but can affect a whole lobe and may be generalized. Often, consolidation occurs in one segment, clears there, and then affects another segment. Because the infiltrate is interstitial, there may be little or nothing abnormal on auscultation. The most common infectious causes are viruses, especially influenza and adenoviruses. However, *Mycoplasma pneumoniae*, Q fever, and the bacillus of Legionnaires disease are all treatable causes of the syndrome.[90] In immunosuppressed patients, "interstitial pneumonia" is very suggestive of *Pneumocystis carinii* infection. The commonest x-ray finding here is "ground glass" infiltrates spreading from both hila.[96]

Most patients with interstitial pneumonia due to infection give an acute history. Fever and cough either develop abruptly or are preceded by a few days of upper respiratory symptoms. Dyspnea and cyanosis are not usually marked, and pleural pain and effusion are uncommon, although not unknown. Typically, there is a distressing, hacking cough but little or no sputum. As a group, the patients are less ill than those with bacterial pneumonias.

Under epidemic circumstances, the cause of the prevalent pneumonia may be known. Patients may give significant historical items, such as exposure to birds (*Chlamydia psittaci*) or cattle (*Coxiella burneti*). Gram stains of the sputum show few or no leukocytes and no dominant bacteria. This is useful negative information, but a positive diagnosis can only be made by isolating the organism or by serologic means. Neither is immediately helpful, and the patient must be managed by clinical judgment.

Tuberculous Pneumonia

A tuberculous focus in a node or in the lung may erode into a bronchus and result in widespread or lobar contamination with tuberculous pus. A rapid consolidation occurs, which is accompanied by high fever. However, most of the changes are due to allergy to tuberculin and other bacterial products. Acid-fast bacilli may be scarce in the sputum, and substantial or complete resolution is common even in the absence of therapy ("epituberculosis"). A more ominous illness is true tuberculous bronchopneumonia. Here the course is relentlessly downhill, and the patient dies in a matter of weeks without therapy ("galloping consumption"). The sputum is strongly positive for tubercle bacilli. Lastly, pulmonary tuberculosis of the ordinary type may be complicated with a pneumococcal or other pneumonia. Sputum from cases of pneumonia should always be stained for acid-fast bacilli.

Fungal Pneumonia

The commonest fungal pneumonia is acute primary infection with *Histoplasma capsulatum* or *Coccidioides immitis*. Other fungi, e.g., *Blastomyces dermatitidis,* may produce a similar picture. There may be a history of exposure, such as a visit to the San Joaquin Valley, or cleaning out a chicken coop. In this case, several friends or family members are often affected also.

The dominant clinical feature is a spectacularly abnormal chest x-ray with generalized nodular and linear infiltrates and unilateral or bilateral hilar adenopathy. There may be the fungal equivalent of a Ghon complex. The patient is not usually particularly ill, although fever may be high. Cough is not prominent; there is little or no sputum and dyspnea, cyanosis, and chest pain are uncommon. Many such patients never see a doctor and are diagnosed retrospectively by the presence of calcified nodules on the chest x-ray. In those with severe acute symptoms, the sputum often does not show fungi and the diagnosis must be established serologically or by culture.

Chronic fungal infections following the pattern of tuberculosis may be seen and may be complicated by bacterial pneumonias in the same way. The sputum smear usually does show fungi, spherules in coccidioidomycosis, and small intracellular yeasts in histo-

plasmosis. In immunosuppressed people, many saprophytic or commensal fungi may cause pneumonia. As a rule, the sputum is unhelpful, and diagnosis requires the examination of lung tissue.

Aspiration Pneumonia

In a sense, the vast majority of pneumonias are due to aspiration, since the pathogens are inhaled. However, the term is confined to the diseases resulting from aspiration of macroscopic quantities of material from the upper airway or of gastric contents.[82] Two distinct syndromes occur. Gastric juice causes a chemical burn of the bronchial mucosa which leads to leaky pulmonary capillaries and the loss of albuminous fluid from the plasma into the alveoli. Also, pulmonary surfactant is destroyed and there is a progressive atelectasis. These processes are noninfective and are, therefore, unaffected by antibiotics. Aspiration of gastric juice carries a high mortality, but there is experimental evidence that this can be reduced by early treatment with large doses of corticosteroids and the intravenous infusion of concentrated albumin.

The second syndrome is due to infection; it may follow the first process if the patient survives or may occur independently. The upper airway normally contains large numbers of anaerobic bacteria that are of low pathogenicity. However, if grossly infected material is inhaled, these bacteria can cause a synergic necrotizing infection. The area of the lung affected is determined by the patient's position at the time the aspiration occurs. In the supine position, the most dependent areas are the posterior basal segments of the upper lobes, and these are the areas most commonly affected. Right-sided involvement is more common than left, allegedly because the right main bronchus is more or less a direct continuation of the trachea.

Aspiration pneumonia is uncommon in normal people except following anesthesia. Alcoholics and epileptics are classic victims, as are those with neurologic diseases which impair swallowing and those with achalasia or other causes of esophageal obstruction. Patients without these predisposing features generally have grossly neglected teeth with extensive periodontal disease.

The aspiration may or may not be witnessed or remembered. The symptoms include fever, cough, sputum, dyspnea, and pleuritic pain. The course is subacute or even chronic, and the patient wastes rapidly. The sputum and breath have a characteristically foul smell. The chest shows evidence of segmental consolidation. It should be noted that an identical syndrome can follow bronchial obstruction from foreign body or tumor.

Pneumonia in Persons with Chronic Lung Disease

Persons with chronic bronchitis, bronchiectasis, cystic fibrosis, and certain other chronic lung diseases start out with grossly impaired pulmonary function. They normally have productive cough and dyspnea, abnormal physical signs in the chest, and abnormal chest x-rays. Furthermore, relatively mild infections may throw these patients into acute respiratory failure and because they have often been treated with antibiotics, they may be infected with resistant pathogens such as staphylococci or gram-negative rods. The most helpful symptoms and signs are fever, malaise, and new infiltrates on the chest x-ray.

Pneumonia in Immunocompromised Hosts

Persons with impaired host defense mechanisms include renal transplant recipients on corticosteroids and azathioprine and those with neoplastic diseases on various cytotoxic drugs, and often steroids as well. Such patients are prone to infection, and pulmonary infections form about one-quarter of the total. However, pneumonia in these patients shows many differences from pneumonia in normal people, and the management is totally different.[96]

The organisms usually responsible for pneumonia are gram-negative rods and staphylococci. Why the pneumococcus is uncommon in these people is not clear. A sizable proportion of cases is due to viruses, but many are due to herpes viruses rather than influenza and adenoviruses. A numerically minor but very important group of cases is caused by *Pneumocystis carinii*. Fungal pneumonia is much more likely to be due to Aspergilli or Candida species than to the fungi pathogenic for normal people. These patients may also have pulmonary infiltrates secondary to infarction, tumor, or sensitivity to drugs.

The symptoms and signs of pneumonia are muted. Fever is almost constant, but cough, sputum, and dyspnea are often absent. However, dyspnea, tachypnea, and cyanosis are usually present. There may be little or no dullness to percussion, and on auscultation there may be only harsh breath sounds or minor degrees of bronchial breathing. Even the x-ray may be clear and may remain so. The reason for the dearth of symptoms and signs is probably that the patients have few or no inflammatory cells and cannot mount a local response.

Lastly, bacterial pneumonia in these people progresses with appalling speed. The mortality in most large series treated in good hospitals is around 40 percent. Fungal and pneumocystis pneumonia are a little slower but are inevitably fatal without treatment. The logic of management is, therefore,

1. To culture blood, sputum, and pleural fluid if available
2. To put the patient on large doses of antibiotics covering both staphylococci and gram-negative rods
3. Unless there is clinical improvement within 48 hours, to add amphotericin B to the antibiotics and to pursue a tissue diagnosis of the infecting organism by whatever means is necessary.

It is usual to escalate from transtracheal aspiration to endobronchial brushings and biopsy to open lung biopsy. Needle biopsy of the lung has largely been abandoned because of problems with inadequate samples, bleeding, and pneumothorax. However, there are a number of centers that have obtained satisfactory results with transthoracic needle aspiration.

LABORATORY STUDIES BEFORE TREATMENT

Before treatment, all patients with pneumonia should have a Gram stain of the sputum, cultures of blood and sputum for bacteria, a white blood cell count and differential, and a chest x-ray. If the patient does well, some of these will prove superfluous but they may be invaluable if the initial diagnosis was wrong. If the patient is desperately ill, specimens can be taken immediately and examined after treatment has been started.

Sputum Smear

The specimen must be sputum; the physician should personally watch the patient cough and select a purulent sample for examination. Heat fixation of the slide is not usually necessary, and it impairs the assessment of cellular morphology. Several smears should be made and some unstained ones kept for later examination if necessary. The best indication that a specimen is sputum is the presence of alveolar macrophages; reasonable evidence is that it contains polymorphonuclear cells and a fairly uniform bacterial population. Mixed bacterial populations in genuine sputum suggest aspiration. The presence of epithelial cells and mixed bacteria means that the specimen is saliva.

In bacterial pneumonia, sheets of the responsible pathogen are usually seen. The smear is least useful for the diagnosis of pneumococcal pneumonia; this is because morphologically similar bacteria are common in the upper airway and because pneumococci disappear quickly from the sputum with antibiotic therapy. If sheets of extracellular diplococci are seen, pneumococcal pneumonia is probable, but their absence is uninterpretable. However, if polyvalent anticapsular pneumococcal antiserum is available ("Omniserum"), the diagnosis can be ruled in or out with better than 90 percent accuracy by doing a Quellung reaction on the sputum.

The real importance of doing a Gram stain of the sputum is to look for staphylococci and gram-negative rods. Staphylococci are characteristically round, occur in clumps, and are often seen inside the cytoplasm of leukocytes. Gram-negative rods are extracellular; short, fat rods suggest klebsiella; long thin ones suggest pseudomonas and cocco-bacilli suggest *Haemophilus influenzae*. However, it is unwise to rely on morphology to make a bacteriologic diagnosis; the patient should be covered for all the possibilities until cultures are available.

In pneumonia due to viruses and specialized bacteria such as mycoplasmas, the sputum shows few or no leukocytes and bacteria. As a rule, cells containing inclusion bodies or other obvious evidence of viral infection are also absent. However, such cells may be demonstrable by the use of specific fluorescent antisera.

If sputum is not available, one must use clinical judgment as to how far to pursue it. It would be absurd to do a transtracheal aspiration because a healthy young man with influenza has a segmental infiltrate. However, in an obtunded patient with bacterial pneumonia, it may be essential.

Sputum Culture

Sputum culture is usually positive in the more common bacterial pneumonias if proper cultural techniques are employed (Table 84-2). However, it must be realized that sputum is collected through the mouth and is invariably contaminated with mouth flora, which may include many of the common causes of pneumonia. In addition, many chronic bronchitics carry a resident population of bacteria in the tracheobronchial tree even when they are well. The mere presence of an organism in sputum cultures, even if the numbers are large, is not evidence of pneumonia caused by that organism.

In pneumococcal pneumonia, the sputum culture is not uncommonly negative. The pneumococcus is a relatively fragile microorganism and may die if the specimen is allowed to sit for several hours before being streaked; it may also be overgrown by other organisms if the plate is not examined within 24 hours. It disappears irretrievably if even one dose of an antibiotic has been given before the specimen was collected. Staphylococci and most gram-negative rods are less fastidious, and sputum cultures are usually positive. Special cultural techniques are required for *Francisella tularensis*, so the laboratory should be alerted if this organism is suspected. Cultures of mycoplasma and of viral respiratory pathogens rarely yield positive results in time to be of therapeutic value. Likewise, fungus cultures seldom yield useful diagnostic information in less than 4 or 5 days and are of little help in the early differential diagnosis of the pneumonia patient (Table 84-2).

Blood Cultures

The advantage of blood culture is that if an organism grows from the blood (or from pleural fluid), there is no doubt about its pathogenicity. Up to 50 percent of pneumococcal pneumonias are bacteremic; in other bacterial pneumonias the figure is 20 percent or less. Blood culture is of no value in viral or rickettsial pneumonias.

Leukocyte Count

Bacterial pneumonia is almost always accompanied by a brisk neutrophilic leukocytosis with a left shift. Low leukocyte counts occur in two circumstances: The patient may have none because of a disease or its treatment, or he may have such an overwhelming infection that the marrow reserve of granulocytes has been exhausted. In the first case, the neutrophil count is simply low; in the second, the total count of neutrophils is low, but the proportion of immature forms is very high and the left shift very marked. The combination of low total count and gross left shift is particularly likely to occur in alcoholics, old people, and others whose bone marrow reserves of neutrophils are lower than normal. It used to denote a bad prognosis, but this is less true with antibiotic therapy.

Viral, rickettsial, and fungal pneumonias are usually associated with normal or low neutrophil counts, and there is no left shift. However, exceptions occur, and neutrophil counts in excess of 20,000 with left shift have been seen in cases of pure influenzal bronchopneumonia. Traditionally, tuberculosis is associated with a normal neutrophil count, an elevated lymphocyte count if the prognosis is good, and an elevated monocyte count if the prognosis is bad.

The Chest X-Ray

In a recent study, 6 radiologists reviewed blindly the x-rays of 31 cases of pneumonia for which the diagnosis was definitely established. Sixteen pneumonias were bacterial, 9 were viral, and 6 were mycoplasmal. All 6 radiologists made the correct diagnosis in only 9 cases out of 31, and in 5 cases all 6 radiologists were agreed on an incorrect diagnosis. Overall, two-thirds of diagnoses of bacterial and viral pneumonia were correct, and only 20 percent of diagnoses of mycoplasmal pneumonia.[94]

TABLE 84-2

Laboratory Studies Performed Prior to Treatment

Etiologic Agent	Sputum Smear	Sputum Culture	Blood Culture	WBC	Chest X-Ray
Pneumococcus (*Streptococcus pneumoniae*)	Many gram-positive, lancet-shaped diplococci, often in sheets	Usually positive if sputum immediately plated on blood agar	Positive in over 20% of patients	Usually elevated (10–30,000) but leukopenia may be present (alcoholics, overwhelming infections)	May be negative in early stages despite clear-cut clinical signs and symptoms of pneumonia. Infiltrates apt to be broncho-pneumonic rather than lobar in unusually susceptible individuals
Staphylococcus aureus	Clusters of gram-positive cocci, often intracellular, usually present. May be absent if pneumonia is hematogenous	Usually positive	Frequently positive	Usually elevated (10–30,000) but leukopenia may be present in overwhelming infections	Broncho-pneumonic pattern with multiple infiltrates and early abscess formation. Pneumatoceles and pyopneumo-thorax common in children
Group A Beta-hemolytic streptococcus	Of little value, since streptococci are abundantly present in normal flora	Usually positive	Often positive	Generally very high (20–30,000)	Extensive pleural effusions often present early. Frequent confluent involvement of two lobes
Klebsiella pneumoniae (Friedländer's bacillus)	Gram stain of major value, showing gram-negative rods, often in pairs	Almost always positive	Positive in less than 20% of patients	Generally very high (20–40,000) but leukopenia may be present in overwhelming infections	Usually upper or right middle lobe involvement. Early abscess formation common
Haemophilus influenzae	Gram stain useful in showing small gram-negative coccobacilli, often in clumps, associated with gram-negative threadlike forms	Frequently positive if immediately plated on chocolate agar and incubated in CO_2 jar	Rarely positive in adults	Generally high (15–30,000)	Frequently broncho-pneumonic infiltrates, but may show lobar pattern

TABLE 84–2 (cont.)

Etiologic Agent	Sputum Smear	Sputum Culture	Blood Culture	WBC	Chest X-Ray
Bacteroides	Small, gram-negative bacilli usually seen	Negative unless anaerobic cultures carefully performed	Generally negative, except when pneumonia is associated with pelvic disease	Generally moderately elevated (15–20,000)	In older people or alcoholics, pleural effusions early, often massive, generally obscure underlying broncho-pneumonia
Escherichia coli	Gram stain of major value, consistently showing gram-negative bacilli	Almost always positive	Often positive	Generally high, with shift to left	Lower lobe broncho-pneumonic infiltrates almost always present
Proteus	Predominance of small gram-negative bacilli	Almost always positive, persisting for days after appropriate antimicrobial therapy	Rarely positive	Generally high (15–30,000)	Dense pneumonic infiltrates, generally with multiple abscesses
Pseudomonas	Gram-negative bacilli prominent	Uniformly positive, with organisms persisting during antimicrobial therapy	Initially negative May be positive later in course of illness	Often normal early in illness, with later rise to 15–20,000 range	Diffuse broncho-pneumonia with nodular infiltrates, frequently with multiple small abscesses
Francisella (Pasteurella) tularensis	Generally not helpful	Positive if plated on cysteine-blood agar Cultural material hazardous to laboratory personnel	Almost always negative	Usually within normal limits, but marked leukocytosis (>20,000) may occur	Perihilar infiltrate character-istic, often with enlarged hilar nodes
Mycoplasma pneumoniae	Not helpful	Positive in over 50% of cases if immediately plated on appropriate diphasic media, but not helpful in time to be of clinical value	Negative	Usually below 10,000, but up to 20,000 in 10% of clinical cases	Infiltrates may be perihilar or lobar Two or more lobes involved in one-third of cases
Influenza	Not helpful	Not helpful in time to be of clinical value	Negative	Moderate leukocytosis (10–20,000) may occur	Interstitial infiltrates, often in fine, widespread pattern *(Continued)*

TABLE 84–2 (cont.)

Etiologic Agent	Sputum Smear	Sputum Culture	Blood Culture	WBC	Chest X-Ray
Varicella	Not helpful	Not helpful	Negative	Usually within normal limits	Same as influenza
Rubeola	Not helpful	Not helpful	Negative	Usually within normal limits	Same as influenza
Respiratory syncytial virus	Not helpful	Not helpful	Negative	Usually within normal limits	Same as influenza
Adenovirus	Not helpful	Not helpful	Negative	Usually within normal limits	Same as influenza
Chlamydia psittaci Psittacosis Ornithosis	Not helpful	Not helpful	Negative	Usually within normal limits	Perihilar infiltrates most common
Mycobacterium tuberculosis	Acid-fast stain positive with cavitary disease, but often negative with early pneumonia	Positive, but only after 4–6 weeks incubation	Negative	Often normal with acute pneumonia or with cavitary disease	Cavitary disease: upper lobe involvement may be confused with klebsiella pneumonia
Coxiella burnetii (Q fever)	Negative	Not helpful	Not helpful	Variable	Patchy infiltrates, generally perihilar in distribution
Histoplasma capsulatum	Intracellular organisms seen on PAS stain Also seen, less clearly, on Gram stain	Positive, often 4–8 days, on Sabouraud's agar	Rarely positive	Variable, but generally within normal limits	Nonspecific, but often multiple, diffuse pulmonary infiltrates
Coccidioides immitis	Characteristic spheres with endospores after treatment with 20% potassium hydroxide	Positive on Sabouraud's agar but only after 5–10 days	Not helpful	Variable, but generally within normal limits	Multiple infiltrates and prominent hilar lymphadenopathy common Pleural effusions frequent
Cryptococcus neoformans	Often positive, with characteristic spherical yeast-forms (5–15μ) seen on India ink preparation	Positive on Sabouraud's agar but only after 5–10 days	Often positive	Variable, but generally within normal limits	Nonspecific Usually dense, localized infiltration of basilar segments

TABLE 84-2 (cont.)

Etiologic Agent	Sputum Smear	Sputum Culture	Blood Culture	WBC	Chest X-Ray
Blastomyces dermatitidis	Often positive, with characteristic, thick-walled, single budding yeast cells of variable size (4–24μ)	Positive on blood or Sabouraud's agar, but only after 5–10 days	Negative	Variable, but generally within normal limits	Nonspecific Infiltration may be fine and diffuse, or well-localized and dense Thin-walled cavities may be present
Aspergillus fumigatus	Very helpful, showing segmented mycelia bearing small round spores	Positive on Sabouraud's agar, but of diagnostic value only if obtained directly from infected segment	Negative	Generally within normal limits except with overwhelming disease	Initially multiple infiltrates, with later cavitation

The lesson from all this is that the chest x-ray can suggest or confirm an etiologic diagnosis, but by itself it is insufficient to be more than suggestive. The features which were associated with bacterial pneumonia in the study quoted were, in descending order of reliability: cavitation, pleural effusion, lobar consolidation, bulging of the fissure, multiple small abscesses, segmental consolidation, and bilateral involvement. For viral pneumonia, the features were nodular infiltrates, diffuse involvement, reticular infiltrates, prominent bronchovascular structures, perihilar pneumonia, involvement of new areas, and hilar adenopathy.

Despite the overall variability in appearances, some bacteria do produce classical x-ray changes most of the time. Pneumococcal pneumonia usually shows a homogeneous lobar or segmented consolidation. Staphylococcal pneumonia is usually bilateral, basal, and abscesses usually form sooner or later. Streptococcal pneumonia is the only pneumonia in which early massive pleural effusions are common. Klebsiella pneumonia usually occurs in the upper lobes or the right middle lobe and is particularly likely to be associated with cavitation and the bulging fissure sign.

In viral, rickettsial, and mycoplasmal pneumonias, the appearances are generally similar, as described above. Two features most unsuggestive of a viral etiology are lobar consolidation and abscess formation. However, lobar consolidation is not uncommon in mycoplasmal pneumonia.

Apical cavitation is typical of chronic tuberculous and fungal infection.

CONDITIONS WHICH MAY BE MISTAKEN FOR PNEUMONIA

A list of these conditions is given in Table 84–3, and a few are discussed below.

Pulmonary Infarction

Pulmonary infarction is very common and causes symptoms and signs which may be identical to those of bacterial pneumonia—fever, cough, bloody sputum, dyspnea, pleuritic pain, and basal consolidation. If the patient has recently had an operation or a baby or has a leg in a cast, the diagnosis may be easy. However, pulmonary infarctions may occur in young women in perfect health, especially if they use oral contraceptives.[92]

The sputum may contain leukocytes but shows few or no bacteria. Cultures of blood and sputum are negative, although this is not immediately useful. There is usually no leukocytosis in pulmonary infarction, but this cannot be relied on. The chest x-ray may show basal segmental infiltrates with pleural effusions, but commonly the appearances cannot be distinguished from pneumonia.

TABLE 84-3

Causes of Pulmonary Infiltrates Resembling Pneumonia Caused by Microorganisms

Condition	Distinguishing Features	
	Radiologic	**Other**
Pulmonary infarct	Wedge-shaped infiltrates, especially lower lobes Avascular areas	Sudden onset, sometimes hemoptysis, occasionally right heart strain
Atelectasis	Displacement of interlobar fissures, elevation of diaphragm, shift of mediastinum	Abdominal surgery, pleuritic pain, or other predisposing factor
Carcinoma, primary, or metastatic	Variable	Weight loss, signs of chronic illness Evidence of neoplasm elsewhere Cytology of sputum
Lymphoma	Variable Hilar and mediastinal adenopathy	Anemia, splenomegaly, lymphadenopathy
Chemical or lipoid pneumonia	Variable, not characteristic	History of ingestion or aspiration of oil, gasoline, kerosene
Irradiation pneumonitis	Variable	History of irradiation
Loeffler's pneumonia	Migratory, patchy infiltrates, often multiple	Eosinophilia History of drug ingestion, helminthiasis
Pulmonary edema	Butterfly pattern of diffuse perihilar infiltrates, but localized infiltrates are not unusual	Cardiac disease, inhalation of noxious gases
Pulmonary alveolar proteinosis	Bilateral infiltrates radiating from hilum in butterfly fashion, especially lower lobes	Biopsy PAS-positive alveolar material
Idiopathic pulmonary hemosiderosis	Usually miliary mottling, with evanescent patchy infiltrates	Glomerulonephritis (Goodpasture syndrome), iron-deficiency anemia
Sarcoidosis	Hilar adenopathy, fine reticular parenchymal pattern	Other signs of sarcoidosis
Collagen-vascular diseases	Variable	Other evidence of the conditions
Uremic pneumonitis	Often butterfly pattern of diffuse perihilar infiltrates	Severe azotemia
Drug lung	Variable	History of drug ingestion

The most useful investigations for differentiating pneumonia from infarction are the blood gases, the test for fibrin degradation products in the blood, and the pulmonary scan. Most patients with infarction have a low Po_2, often <60 mm Hg and enough hyperventilation to produce a low Pco_2 also. The plasma almost always contains fibrin degradation products. Segmental basal defects on the scan are associated with a high probability of pulmonary embolism. The definitive test is pulmonary angiography, but newer scans may make it of historical interest only. There are reports that [67]gallium citrate scans are positive in pneumonia and negative in infarction. An even newer and more exciting scan uses [11]carbon monoxide. This combines with hemoglobin and is normally rapidly removed from the lungs. In pulmonary infarction, the stagnant column of blood beyond the arterial block remains as a "hot spot."

If there is real doubt as to the diagnosis, it may be safest to treat the patient for both conditions until the diagnosis is clear.

Fractured Ribs

This condition causes severe pain on inspiration but few or none of the other symptoms of pneumonia. Fractures may occur secondary to coughing or to metastases and may happen spontaneously in old people. They are easily detected by local tenderness and by exacerbation of the pain when one presses on the sternum. However, they may be very difficult to see on x-ray.

Pulmonary Vasculitis

The list of conditions causing pulmonary vasculitis is very long, but only a few are likely to present with acute symptoms.[88] They include SLE and the variants of polyarteritis. It is usually wise to treat for pneumonia initially if the diagnosis is in doubt.

Sickle Cell Disease

Patients with Hgb SS disease often have attacks of fever, chest pain, and pulmonary infiltrate. Most of these episodes are probably noninfective, but again, antibiotics are a wise precaution.

Drug Lung

Most pulmonary reactions to drugs are chronic, but a few present acutely.[93] Nitrofurantoin commonly does so. Drug-induced SLE is also worth remembering; the patients have antinuclear factor and may have any of the clinical features of spontaneous SLE. Hydralazine is a common cause. Some patients with pulmonary infiltrates have eosinophilia and would come under the general category of Loeffler syndrome.

MANAGEMENT

The most important part of managing a patient with pneumonia is the selection of an appropriate antibiotic(s). One must also consider the patient's oxygenation and requirements for fluids and nutrition. Sometimes bacteria spread from the lung to other tissues; this must be recognized and treated. Later in the illness, it may become clear that the condition is not responding to treatment or that an initial improvement has been followed by deterioration.

Antibiotic Treatment

Antibiotic therapy has revolutionized the prognosis of pneumonia, but the disease remains a serious one. Pneumococcal pneumonia severe enough to require hospital admission still carries a mortality of 10 to 15 percent in most large series. Staphylococcal pneumonia mortality rates are of the order of 40 to 50 percent, and gram-negative rod pneumonias have mortalities in excess of 50 percent. Many factors are involved in these deaths, the most important being the type of patient who presents for treatment in university hospitals. They are often indigent, malnourished, or alcoholic, and frequently have other serious diseases, such as chronic lung disease or congestive heart failure. In addition, they may present for treatment at an advanced stage. In all bacteremias, there

is a "point of no return" after which antibiotic therapy does not influence the outcome—this is seen particularly clearly in pneumococcal pneumonia, where most of the deaths occur in the first 24 hours. The second type of irretrievable situation that may be produced by delay is when the lung has become honeycombed with abscesses, when local spread has produced empyema or pericarditis, or when metastatic infections, such as endocarditis, meningitis, or liver abscesses, have been established. Even if these are not immediately fatal, the patient is in for a long, drawn out illness, during which he will be liable to the illnesses of the bedridden—bedsores, pulmonary embolism, and bronchopneumonia.

In view of all this, it is important that delay is not compounded when the patient does reach the hospital. An abbreviated history covering the present illness, previous therapy, and other relevant information, such as drug allergies, can be completed in 15 minutes, and a physical examination is not much more. Chest x-ray, blood count, and blood and sputum cultures can be completed in another half hour, and treatment started. There is no excuse for the 5- or 6-hour delays which are common in most hospitals.

If the presumptive diagnosis is pneumococcal pneumonia, procaine penicillin is the drug of choice in a dose of 600,000 units twice daily intramuscularly. It is wise to give any sick patient a loading dose of 1 million units of crystalline penicillin intravenously because procaine penicillin may not produce adequate blood levels for 2 or 3 hours. Pneumococci are invariably sensitive to these doses of penicillin, and the use of larger doses merely promotes colonization by staphylococci and gram-negative organisms, which may cause secondary pneumonia. In patients allergic to penicillin, erythromycin (2 g per day) is probably the best alternative. Therapy should be continued for a week. As a rule, clinical improvement is noted within 24 hours, although sometimes the temperature may be elevated for 3 to 5 days. A patient who remains febrile after a week of treatment probably has undrained pus somewhere other than in the lung, as discussed below. However, the chest x-ray may remain abnormal for up to 3 months, and it is not necessary to continue therapy until the x-ray is normal. Resolution is normally complete.

If clinical and laboratory features (Tables 84–1 and 84–2) lead to the presumptive diagnosis of staphylococcal pneumonia, the best initial treatment is probably nafcillin in a daily dose of 6 to 9 g parenterally. If the staphylococcus turns out to be sensitive to penicillin G, this drug can be substituted in a dose of 4 to 6 million units daily. In patients said to be allergic to penicillin, skin testing should be done to confirm that anaphylactic sensitization exists. If the skin test is negative, there is no danger of death from anaphylaxis, although nafcillin therapy may later cause drug fever. If it does, cephalothin is usually tolerated. If the skin test is positive, neither penicillins nor cephalosporins should be used, and the best alternative is vancomycin 2 g daily parenterally. Whatever antibiotic is selected should be continued for at least 3 weeks. The best treatment for β-hemolytic streptococcal pneumonia is penicillin G in a dose of 2 to 4 million units daily, parenterally.

In gram-negative rod pneumonias, local knowledge is more useful than general recommendations. It may be known, for example, that the klebsiellas in a particular hospital are resistant to gentamicin or that *Serratia marcescens* is prevalent in the urology ward. It may also be known that a particular patient on a respirator was colonized 3 days ago with an *Escherichia coli* resistant to all common antibiotics except amikacin. If no information is available, the drugs suggested in Table 84–4 should be used in the first instance but must be changed in the light of the clinical progress of the patient and the results of in vitro sensitivity tests. Therapy in gram-negative rod pneumonias should be prolonged, especially for klebsiella and pseudomonas pneumonias. Tularemia is best treated with streptomycin, and the response to treatment is usually dramatic.

It is usually impossible to distinguish pneumonia due to mycoplasmas and rickettsiae from that due to viruses until serologic results become available. The treatable causes of the primary atypical pneumonia syndrome are *Mycoplasma pneumoniae*, *Coxiella burneti*, *Chlamydia psittaci*, and the bacillus of Legionnaires disease. Mycoplasmal pneumonia and Legionnaires disease respond best to erythromycin, 2 g per day. Mycoplasmal pneumonia is very common (about 5 percent of all cases), and Legionnaires disease is dangerous, so it is recommended that all cases of atypical pneumonia be treated with erythromycin in the first instance. However, tetracycline is a much

better drug for Q fever, which is fairly common, and for psittacosis, which is dangerous. If the patient fails to improve, therefore, and if there is no evidence of infection with ordinary bacteria, a switch to tetracycline may be indicated.

Blind Treatment

Often, the laboratory data gathered on the patient's admission to the hospital provide no clue to etiologic diagnosis. In this setting, initial choice of antibiotics is influenced by the patient's clinical status. If the patient is young, previously healthy, and presents with fever, tachypnea, leukocytosis, and x-ray evidence of an infiltrate in one of the lower lobes, the presumptive diagnosis of pneumococcal pneumonia can be made and the patient treated with penicillin until the specific etiologic diagnosis is established. If, on the other hand, the patient presents with hypotension, cyanosis, confusion, and predominantly upper-lobe or multilobar involvement, initial therapy should include drugs effective against staphylococcus and klebsiella as well as the pneumococcus. Appropriate therapy in such a case might be Cephalothin 8 to 12 g/day and gentamicin 5 mg/kg/day (if renal function is normal). The optimum antibiotic therapy would be determined by subsequent cultures and antibiotic sensitivity studies.

General Measures

CLOSE OBSERVATION. Ideally, patients with pneumonia should be admitted to hospital for at least 48 hours, until it is clear that they are responding to treatment. However, this is not always possible, and it is clear that many cases of pneumococcal pneumonia do perfectly well at home. A good person for outpatient management is one who is young, reasonably intelligent, has someone who cares about him, and is not very sick. He should be made to understand that response to intramuscular penicillin is not guaranteed and that he should return to the hospital promptly if he fails to improve. Patients who are old, unreliable, anoxic, or suffer from other chronic diseases should always be admitted.

REST AND HYDRATION. In general, the patient should be allowed to undertake whatever activities he wishes, but it is wise to make sure that he is accompanied to the bathroom or elsewhere until clinical improvement occurs. Sick patients usually cannot drink enough to replace the several liters per day that they lose in sweating and through the respiratory tract. If dehydration is allowed to occur, bronchial secretions may become inspissated and may lead to atelectasis. It is therefore wise to use intravenous fluids for the first day or two.

TABLE 84–4
Antibiotics Generally Effective in Gram-Negative Rod Pneumonias

Organism	Antibiotic(s)
E. coli	Gentamicin
Klebsiella	Cephalothin and gentamicin
Proteus	Carbenicillin
H. influenza	Ampicillin
Pseudomonas	Carbenicillin and tobramycin
Serratia	Gentamicin

PLEURITIC PAIN. If the pain is too severe to be managed with aspirin, it is probably better to induce local anesthesia by intercostal nerve block than to use codeine or stronger narcotics. This is because narcotics suppress the cough reflex. An agent like mepivicaine may provide anesthesia for 48 hours with only one injection, and a second may not be necessary.

COUGH. Paroxysms of coughing may be very exhausting, especially to patients with heart disease. They may also seriously interfere with oxygenation. Moderate doses of codeine (32 mg) may suppress paroxysms, but it is unwise to use large doses because the cough reflex may be totally suppressed.

Important Concurrent Problems

CYANOSIS. There are three major mechanisms by which cyanosis may develop in pneumonia. In pneumococcal pneumonia, there may be extensive blood flow through an airless consolidated lobe or lobes, so that a large fraction of the cardiac output is not oxygenated. Obviously, neither oxygen nor tracheobronchial suction is very effective for this condition, but it responds spontaneously in a day or two as the pneumonia improves. In bronchopneumonia, there are consolidated areas, but in addition, many airways are blocked by purulent secretions which add a component of ventilatory failure. Here, postural drainage, assisted coughing, and tracheobronchial suction can produce considerable improvement. Especially in exacerbations of chronic bronchitis, alveolar hypoventilation may rapidly become extreme, and severe carbon dioxide retention and hypoxemia develop. Such patients need antibiotics, bronchodilators, efficient physical therapy, tracheobronchial suction, and cautious 24 or 28 percent oxygen therapy. If these measures fail, tracheostomy and artificial ventilation may be necessary. Lastly, in extensive viral (influenzal) pneumonia there may be interstitial pulmonary edema leading to a "diffusion block" type of respiratory failure with hypoxemia and hypocapnia. This state usually responds to oxygen therapy with positive end-expiratory pressure, although high concentrations may be required. If not, there is some evidence that forced dehydration with fluid restriction and large doses of diuretics may be helpful.

SHOCK. When hypotension results from severe hypoxia, therapy is directed as discussed in the section on cyanosis above. Gastric dilatation and paralytic ileus are fairly common complications of pneumonia, especially with lower-lobe involvement. They are readily detectable on physical examination and corrected by nasogastric intubation. When neither significant hypoxia nor gastric dilatation is present, the hypotension may be the result of bacteremia, and treatment for bacteremic shock should be initiated.

ATELECTASIS. Atelectasis of all or part of a lobe may occur at any stage of acute pneumonia and usually results in increasing tachypnea and, if an entire lobe is involved, in severe dyspnea. Often the atelectatic area will clear with coughing, deep breathing, or forced expiration. If clearing is not observed in 2 to 3 hours after these respiratory maneuvers, bronchoscopic aspiration should be carried out because the affected area may become fibrotic and functionless if the atelectasis persist.

DELIRIUM. Delirium is a common complication of pneumonia, and since meningitis is a fairly common complication of bacteremia, lumbar puncture should always be done. If pyogenic meningitis is not adequately treated, all the signs of meningitis may be suppressed by the low doses of penicillin prescribed for the pneumonia, only to recur in fulminant form several days after cessation of treatment. Hypoxia is a frequent cause of delirium in the older pneumonia patient. Delirium tremens is commonly observed when alcoholics develop bacterial pneumonia. When it occurs (and meningitis and hypoxia have been excluded), it is treated with hydration and mild sedation.

COMPLICATIONS

Serious metastatic infections often occur in the pneumonia patient despite appropriate antibiotic therapy. They include empyema, lung abscess, pericarditis, brain abscess, meningitis, pyarthrosis, and endocarditis.

Pleural Effusion

Despite penicillin therapy, pleural effusion occurs in about 5 percent of patients with pneumococcal pneumonia. It is seen in a much higher proportion of patients with streptococcal pneumonia and it is almost invariably present in individuals with bacteroides infections of the lung. When significant pleural effusion is present, fluid should always be removed by thoracentesis and examined for pyogenic and acid-fast organisms. If the effusion is thick and purulent, it is best to drain it by means of intercostal tube at the outset because multiple thoracenteses usually fail eventually, and by that time more extensive surgery may be necessary. Even when the fluid is thin, it is probably wise to install a tube if it reaccumulates after one thoracentesis.

Lung Abscess

Abscess formation, always uncommon in pneumococcal pneumonia but relatively common in staphylococcal, klebsiella, bacteroides, proteus, and pseudomonas pneumonias, is common in pneumonia secondary to aspiration of gastric contents. Abscesses are treated by encouraging drainage by physical therapy and sometimes by endoscopic aspiration. Most of the pneumonias in which abscesses occur are already being treated with maximal doses of antibiotics, and there is no indication for a change in therapy unless it is shown that the organism is resistant to the drugs being used. A slow response to treatment of a necrotizing pneumonia is expected, and antibiotic therapy should be continued longer than with a simple pneumonia. Lung abscess secondary to aspiration pneumonia responds well to fairly low doses of penicillin G, 2 to 4 million units per day. Unless the abscess ruptures into the pleural cavity, surgical drainage is almost never necessary.

Pericarditis

Pericarditis usually causes precordial pain and a friction rub but may occur without either. It is especially common with empyema and should be considered in any patient who remains febrile and sick after his empyema has been drained. The chest x-ray may or may not be helpful, but echocardiography will demonstrate even small effusions. As with any other abscess, drainage is required. Needle aspiration is commonly done, but serious complications or death may result, and in a large institution it is probably best to drain the pericardium surgically.

Brain Abscess and Meningitis

Brain abscess is typically a complication of aspiration pneumonia, and the usual flora are bacteroides and anaerobic streptococci. The condition may follow an obvious lung abscess or may occur after an episode of aspiration which was clinically minor. Brain abscess also occurs occasionally following staphylococcal pneumonia. Headache, vomiting, and unusual behavior are the most common symptoms; fever is slight and may be absent. The best diagnostic test for brain abscess is computerized axial tomography; if this is not available, brain scan is almost always positive. Lumbar puncture should not be done because of the danger of coning.

Meningitis is most common with pneumococcal pneumonia and requires therapy with large doses of penicillin. If it complicates gram-negative pneumonia, intrathecal therapy with amnioglycosides will be required.

Pyarthrosis

The symptoms of a septic joint are severe local pain and inability to move the limb. On examination, the joint is hot, red, very tender to touch, and contains a purulent effusion. Usually, the organism is visible on Gram stains of the joint fluid. Antibiotics penetrate well into joints and modification of dose is not usually required. Drainage is required, however, and if the fluid accumulates despite repeated taps, the joint should be opened surgically.

PERSISTENT BACTEREMIA. When blood cultures remain positive 24 hours after therapy has started, infective endocarditis is a probable explanation. The patient may also have undrained pus in the pleural space or one of the other sites discussed above. If there is no evidence of a septic focus elsewhere, the patient should be assumed to have endocarditis whether or not there is a murmur. Antibiotic treatment should be escalated until the serum bactericidal level is satisfactory (1:8 or better), and therapy should be continued for 3 to 6 weeks, depending on the organism.

SUPERINFECTION. Superinfection with organisms resistant to penicillin is unusual in pneumococcal pneumonia if the recommended dosage is employed.[95] However, it is seen regularly with high doses or when antibiotics with an unnecessarily broad spectrum are employed, and the secondary pneumonias are more lethal than the primary. Superinfection is common in klebsiella pneumonia because of the combinations of broad spectrum antibiotics which are usually used. If respiratory signs and symptoms fail to improve after 5 to 6 days of treatment, the sputum must be cultured again. If a new organism resistant to the antibiotics employed is found and no other complications of pneumonia are detected, the antibiotic regimen should be altered as indicated by sensitivity studies.

UNFAVORABLE COURSE AND ITS MANAGEMENT

Patients with unfavorable courses fall into two main groups. In the first, the pneumonia does not respond to treatment either clinically or radiologically. In the second group, the pneumonia resolves satisfactorily, but the patient remains febrile or becomes febrile again after the initial improvement.

FAILURE OF THE PNEUMONIA TO RESOLVE. If the patient is clinically well, afebrile, eating, and walking about without discomfort, the persistence of x-ray changes is no cause for alarm. It is not necessary to increase the dose of antibiotics, change the treatment, or continue for a longer time than usual. Even pneumococcal pneumonia may take weeks to clear on the x-ray.[86] Most other bacterial pneumonias are slower to resolve and may leave permanent scarring.

If the infiltrate persists and the patient remains sick, he should be completely reassessed, starting with a new physical examination. The first consideration is to rule out infection anywhere other than in the lung. It is essential to make sure that no part of the infiltrate represents infected pleural fluid, perhaps trapped in one of the fissures. The next most likely possibility is that the bacterial diagnosis is wrong and that the antimicrobial agent used is inappropriate or being used in too small a dose. If bacteria were isolated only from the sputum, they may be irrelevant to the illness. New cultures should be obtained and the treatment altered if necessary. If the evidence for bacterial etiology is good and the antibiotics are adequate as assessed in vitro, persistence or worsening of the infiltrate suggests inadequate drainage of pus. Staphylococcal and gram-negative rod pneumonias are characteristically necrotizing, causing multiple abscesses. A common explanation is bronchial obstruction, usually due to a tumor. Failure to resolve may also be a consequence of underlying tuberculous or fungal infection.

If the infiltrate persists but there is no unequivocal evidence of bacterial infection, other possibilities should be considered. The most important in normal people are the treatable causes of the primary atypical pneumonia syndrome. In immunosuppressed people, one should be most concerned about infection with saprophytic fungi and pneumocystis. Lastly, the whole illness may be noninfectious, and the patient should be assessed for the diseases listed in Table 84-3. Since these are many and various, one should only order tests when the diagnosis under consideration is clinically plausible.

PERSISTENT FEVER. Streptococcal, staphylococcal, and gram-negative rod pneumonias are charac-teristically slow to respond, and fever may persist up to 2 weeks in uncomplicated cases. If the patient is febrile but the chest symptoms and signs are improving and the x-ray is starting to clear, then it is probable that the drugs used were appropriate and the doses adequate. The likeliest explanation for persistent fever is an undrained focus of infection, either in the chest or elsewhere, and a thorough search for empyema, pericarditis, and the other entities discussed above should be made. Sometimes, metastatic abscesses turn up in very unusual places, such as the vertebral column or the spleen, and in case of difficulty it is wise to investigate any area where the patient has even mild complaints.

RETURN OF FEVER. When fever returns after an initial improvement, the likeliest explanation is superinfection in the lung or some other site. Superinfection in the lung produces a return of respiratory symptoms and a deterioration in respiratory function. If these are not present, the commonest sources of fever are the urine and intravenous catheter sites. Recurrent fever may also be due to a metastatic infection with the original organism. Drug allergy usually develops after 7 to 10 days of treatment, but it may be earlier in sensitized patients. It is often accompanied by eosinophilia, pruritus, and skin rashes. However, the neutrophil count is commonly normal. When the drug is withdrawn, the temperature usually falls to normal within 48 hours. Very occasionally, the original organism develops resistance to the antibiotics employed and causes a relapse.

CHAPTER 85
Infective Endocarditis
JOHN J. MANN

Infective endocarditis is caused by the implantation of microorganisms on the endocardium followed by tissue damage. Infective arteritis refers to the same process in extracardiac arterial structures. This localized infection is associated with prominent systemic manifestations and sometimes dramatic structural alterations. The systemic symptoms are often manifestations of bacteremia, emboli, metastatic abscesses, or immune phenomena. Structural alterations include destruction of valves and/or other cardiac structures with the frequent development of congestive heart failure. The aim of therapy must include not only the eradication of the infection but also the repair of the structural damage. Major recent changes in the treatment of endocarditis relate to the increasingly important role of surgery in the acute phase of the illness.[115]

PATHOGENESIS
Bacterial endocarditis occurs either in patients with preexisting endocardial damage or in patients with normal heart valves in whom the bloodstream has been invaded by virulent microorganisms (e.g., staphylococci, enterococci). Transient and asymptomatic bacteremia is the usual event inciting the endocardial infection. A careful historical review for conditions predisposing to bacteremia may furnish clues to the nature of the organism. The mouth is the usual portal of entry for alpha streptococci. Dental proce-

dures, poor dental hygiene, gingivitis, tonsillectomy, and viral upper-respiratory infections have been implicated, since transient bacteremia has been demonstrated in association with these conditions. Enterococci are normal fecal inhabitants, and gastrointestinal and genitourinary factors, such as prostatitis, catheterization, urologic surgery and instrumentation, parturition, and septic abortion, frequently are responsible for transient enterococcal bacteremia. Cutaneous furuncles, cardiac surgery, infected wounds, and (occasionally) osteomyelitis are the usual sources of staphylococci. Addicts using narcotics intravenously are especially likely to develop staphylococcal endocarditis of the tricuspid valve, but may also develop α-streptococcal, enterococcal, or candida infection of the left heart valves.[112] Candidal endocarditis should be suspected in patients with embolic complications involving larger vessels. Patients with pneumococcal pneumonia, bacteremia, and meningitis occasionally develop pneumococcal endocarditis of the aortic valve. In the preantibiotic era endocarditis afflicted mostly young adults with rheumatic heart disease. Currently, the disease is most common in elderly patients with degenerative forms of cardiovascular disease or with no clinically obvious heart disease. Endocarditis has occurred on atheromatous deposits, calcifications of the mitral annulus or aortic valve, thrombi overlying areas of myocardial infarction, and surgically altered endocardium. Children who develop the disease usually have congenital heart disease. Interventricular septal defects, patent ductus arteriosus, coarctation of the aorta, bicuspid aortic valves, and the tetralogy of Fallot are the most important predisposing congenital lesions. Rheumatic, degenerative, and congenital heart diseases act similarly by producing an opportunity for deposition of platelets and fibrin on a heart valve. This results in the formation of a nonbacterial thrombotic endocarditis. Bacteremia by any of the mechanisms described above may transform this into bacterial endocarditis. Several investigations have demonstrated the repetitive production of bacterial endocarditis by intravenous injections of even nonvirulent bacteria in animals with catheter-induced nonbacterial thrombotic endocarditis.[103] In contrast, animals with normal heart valves do not develop bacterial endocarditis.

MICROBIOLOGY

Almost any microorganism may cause endocarditis; most bacteria and fungi, some viruses, and rickettsia have been implicated. Over the past 75 years there has been a decrease in the incidence of *S. viridans, N.*

gonorrhoeae, and *S. pneumoniae* and an increase in the incidence of staphylococci, enterococci, fungi, and unusual organisms. Despite the striking increase in bacteremias caused by gram-negative enteric bacilli, these organisms still account for only 1 to 3 percent of cases of endocarditis. Currently, gram-positive cocci (streptococci and staphylococci) account for 55 percent of cases.[113] In 15 to 20 percent of cases cultures are sterile. Certain clinical settings tend to be associated with specific microorganisms. Subacute endocarditis in a young person with rheumatic mitral disease is usually associated with *S. viridans.* Staphylococci cause 50 percent of cases of acute endocarditis. Endocarditis which follows genitourinary manipulation is usually due to enterococci. Prosthetic valve infections are usually due to staphylococci, less commonly to streptococci, gram-negative bacteria, and fungi. Drug addicts are particularly prone to develop either right or left-sided endocarditis secondary to staphylococci or pseudomonas. Severely compromised patients treated with intensive courses of antibiotics often develop fungal endocarditis, most commonly due to candida, less commonly due to aspergillus, histoplasma, and others.

CLINICAL FEATURES

It has been traditional to label cases of endocarditis as subacute or acute. Subacute endocarditis occurs in younger patients usually with rheumatic heart disease. The illness has been of long duration, slow progression with sterile emboli, and little change in cardiac status. The organism usually is *S. viridans.* Acute endocarditis often occurs without previous heart disease, with abrupt onset and prominent constitutional symptoms, early appearance of new murmurs, suppurative emboli, early anemia, and often marked leukocytosis. Congestive heart failure is commonly present. Obviously, the timing and choice of therapy will be influenced by the type of endocarditis.

Presentation of Endocarditis

FEVER AND HEART MURMUR. Fever is the cardinal manifestation of infective endocarditis and is the sign most frequently present. There is little that is characteristic about the fever. Generally, it is intermittent, irregular, mild, and not associated with shaking chills, but with more virulent organisms the course may be septic. Afebrile periods occur but are rarely prolonged, and fever is in all series the most frequent and reliable sign of endocarditis. Fever may be absent in cases complicated by severe congestive heart failure and/or uremia and during the administration of antimicrobial drugs.

The presence of cardiac murmur is a common but not required feature. A murmur is absent initially in up to 50 percent of patients with right-sided endocarditis.[98] Murmurs are commonly absent during the early stage of acute endocarditis. Changing murmurs are present in the minority of cases. Even when present, murmurs may be unimpressive, particularly apical systolic murmurs. If needless deaths are to be prevented, infective endocarditis should be suspected in every patient with *fever and cardiac murmur* or *fever and anemia,* especially if the fever lasts more than a week. Familiarity with all the varied manifestations of the disease and a high index of suspicion make it even more likely that an early diagnosis will be made.

The unfortunately common practice of using antimicrobial drugs in treating undiagnosed febrile disease complicates the recognition of infective endocarditis. A patient with endocarditis given a short course of antibiotics may improve and become afebrile, even when the antibiotic was merely bacteriostatic. However, when antibiotics are discontinued, the illness will recur. Recurrent febrile disease because of inappropriate diagnosis and treatment is unfortunately often seen in patients with endocarditis. Attempts to establish the diagnosis by blood culture may be unsuccessful while the antibiotics are continued. For these reasons, recurrent febrile illness with short remission induced by antibiotic treatment and associated with negative blood cultures must be suspected of being infective endocarditis, particularly in the patient with valvular or congenital cardiac disease.

The onset of endocarditis is often vague and insidious, marked by anorexia, easy fatigability, weight loss, low-grade fever, malaise, myalgia, and arthralgia. Often, it is only after treatment has been effective that the patient becomes aware that he has not felt well for several months. Such presentations are characteristic of subacute infective endocarditis, in which *Streptococcus viridans* or Group D streptococci are most frequently incriminated. Abundant serum antibodies to these relatively avirulent organisms are usually present at the time of clinical onset. Adverse effects of the interaction of antibody with bacterial antigens may account for some of the clinical manifestations. Purpura, clubbing, arthralgias, nephritis, decreased serum complements, elevated gammaglobulins, positive rheumatoid factor, and positive antinuclear antibody test are immunologic features of endocarditis that can lead to confusion in diagnosis.

EMBOLI AND VASCULAR ACCIDENTS. The manifestations of infective endocarditis are protean, since practically any organ can become involved. The most common localized manifestations of the disease are

TABLE 85-1 Manifestations of Infective Endocarditis	
General	Anorexia, weakness, malaise, fever, weight loss
Central nervous system	Emboli, mycotic aneurysms, brain abscess, meningitis, cerebrovascular accidents, paresis, diffuse encephalitis, coma, subarachnoid hemorrhage
Ocular	Roth's spots
Cardiopulmonary	Progressive valvular damage, rupture of chordae tendinae, markedly changing murmurs Pulmonary emboli and infarction, hemoptysis Congestive heart failure Coronary embolism, myocarditis, myocardial valve ring abscess
Gastrointestinal	Splenomegaly, abdominal pain Splenic infarcts, mesenteric vascular occlusion Abnormal liver function tests
Genitourinary	Albuminuria, hematuria, embolic glomerulonephritis Flank pain, renal infarction Diffuse glomerulonephritis, uremia
Dermatologic	Petechiae, splinter hemorrhages, Osler's nodes, Janeway's lesions, pallor, icterus Pustular skin rashes
Extremities	Myalgia, arthralgia, arthritis, clubbing, osteomyelitis
Hematologic	Leukocytosis, anemia, elevated sedimentation, reduced serum complement, hyperglobulinemia, antigammaglobulin factor with positive Rose or latex fixation tests, positive antinuclear antibody test

outlined in Table 85–1. Mycotic aneurysms, infarction, bleeding, and septic emboli account for most of the regional manifestations. Since friable, easily dislodged, valvular vegetations are almost invariably present in infective endocarditis, it is not surprising that embolic phenomena are seen so frequently. They may be the initial manifestation of the disease and are often fatal. Emboli can involve any organ but are most frequent in spleen, kidney, heart, brain, and, with right-sided endocarditis, lung. Suppurative pulmonary emboli are particularly common in narcotic addicts with staphylococcal infections of the tricuspid valve. It is particularly important to consider endocarditis in elderly patients with strokes. When the infective agent is the alpha streptococcus, it is rare for the embolic lesions to suppurate.

SPLENOMEGALY. Whereas splenomegaly is seen in nearly half of patients with subacute infective endocarditis, clinically apparent splenomegaly occurs in less than a quarter of individuals with acute infective endocarditis.[107] The sudden appearance of splenomegaly with left upper quadrant pain and a friction rub in the region of the spleen is suggestive of splenic infarction. The spleen is the most frequent site of recognized infarction, but renal infarcts are almost as common.

NEPHRITIS AND UREMIA. Focal embolic glomerulitis with flea-bitten kidneys is frequent in endocarditis, and repeated search for hematuria and intermittent albuminuria is important in establishing the diagnosis. A diffuse proliferative glomerulonephritis, probably caused by circulating antigen–antibody complexes and occasionally producing uremia, is sometimes the outstanding feature of the illness, especially with staphylococcal or culture negative endocarditis.[105] In this setting the illness can easily be mistaken for systemic lupus erythematosus.

NEUROLOGIC MANIFESTATIONS. Neurologic complications occur in 40 percent of patients. Cerebral embolism, mycotic aneurysm, brain abscess, purulent meningitis, and aseptic meningitis are the most common manifestations.[111]

CUTANEOUS MANIFESTATIONS. Since clubbing of the fingers and anemia are relatively late signs, they are not helpful in making an early diagnosis. Petechiae, especially those in the retina and with white centers (Roth's spots), are strongly suggestive of the diagnosis. Petechiae are most frequently seen in the oral mucosa, especially on the palate, in the retina and conjunctiva, over the upper anterior chest, and on the distal extremities. Nontender splinter hemorrhages are seen in the nail beds but are nonspecific. Erythematous macules and papules (Janeway's lesions) occur on the palms and soles and may be especially prominent and early manifestations of acute infective endocarditis. Tender, raised, erythematous lesions encountered in the pads of fingers and toes (Osler's nodes) are of great diagnostic importance but occur in less than 25 percent of cases with subacute endocarditis and are very rarely seen in acute infective endocarditis.[107] Petechiae, splinter hemorrhages, Osler's nodes, and emboli may continue to appear for several weeks during effective antibiotic therapy.

Heart Failure and Aortic Insufficiency

In the preantibiotic era, patients with endocarditis died usually from the bacterial infection. At present, congestive heart failure is the most common cause of death. The development of heart failure is associated with acute endocarditis, virulent microorganisms, and aortic insufficiency.[109] Severe valvular damage with or without rapidly changing murmurs may occur in a few days, leading to the sudden onset of heart failure in a previously healthy person. The severity of aortic insufficiency may be difficult to assess clinically because of its rapid development. The classical signs of aortic insufficiency depend on the presence of a large pulse pressure. When aortic insufficiency develops rapidly, the left ventricular end diastolic pressure rises steeply thus preventing a fall in diastolic pressure. In this setting wide-open aortic insufficiency can be present without the usual clinical findings.

Prosthetic Endocarditis

Advances in cardiac surgery have been accompanied by the creation of a new type of endocarditis, prosthetic endocarditis, with its own clinical presentation and microbiology. Cases of prosthetic endocarditis can be divided into an "early" and "late" group. In the "early" group infections develop usually within 4 weeks of surgery and are due to staphylococci, diphtheroids, fungi, and gram-negative organisms. Sources of infections are either operating room contaminations or postoperative wound, pulmonary, or genitourinary infections. The course is usually acute with changing murmurs, heart failure, valve dehiscence, high fever, and associated mediastinitis, pneumonia, or urinary tract infection. Prognosis is poor with a mortality of around 80 percent.

In the "late" group infections develop as a result of transient bacteremias and are similar to cases of classical endocarditis. The clinical picture depends on the organism involved. Staphylococci produce usually an acute infection which often requires replacement of the prosthetic valve. With *S. viridans* the infection is typical of subacute infective endocarditis. In either case the prognosis is better, 50 to 55 percent survival higher than in the early group.[103]

Physical Examination

The classical signs of endocarditis are fever, heart murmur, pallor, splenomegaly, wasting, weight loss, clubbing, splinter hemorrhages, Osler's nodes, Janeway's spots, ocular hemorrhages, Roth's spots, and petechiae. Current experience indicates that the cutaneous manifestations of subacute infective endocarditis generally occur late in the course of the disease and are present in less than half the patients at the time the diagnosis is established. Rapidly changing murmurs are common only in acute infective endocarditis, where they suggest perforation or tear of the cusp or rupture of chordae tendinae. Signs of peripheral vascular complications and congestive heart failure are frequent.

LABORATORY DIAGNOSIS

Normocytic normochromic anemia is usually present. The rapid development of anemia indicates acute infection. The sedimentation rate is almost always elevated. These two parameters are useful in judging results of therapy.

Only slight leukocytosis is expected in subacute infective endocarditis, and even this is absent in about 50 percent of patients with subacute disease. Usually increased numbers of immature granulocytes are found in the blood. Leukocytosis greater than 15,000 is common with acute infective endocarditis. When, however, leukocytosis of this degree occurs in the course of subacute infective endocarditis, it suggests a complication such as an infarct. Demonstration of immature granulocytes may be helpful in patients suspected of having endocarditis despite sterile blood cultures.

Hyperglobulinemia and significant titers of rheumatoid factor are seen in about 50 percent of patients with subacute infective endocarditis. Microscopic hematuria is common; a few patients develop the full picture of glomerulonephritis with red blood cell casts, proteinuria, and low serum complement.[105]

With proper techniques, positive venous blood cultures can be obtained in almost all patients with infective endocarditis.[99,107] The frequency of positive cultures is equally great when the focus of infection is in the right heart.[98] In most reported series, however, the blood has been sterile in about 15 percent of the cases. The bacteremia is characteristically continuous, and the usual pathogens can be readily isolated if both aerobic and anaerobic media are used and incubated for 3 weeks. Gram stains of all cultures should be made before they are discarded as negative. In many laboratories, cultures are discarded if they are negative after only 1 week's incubation. One pair of blood cultures should be incubated at room temperature. Prior antibiotic therapy may delay growth of the organism but does not necessarily preclude growth if the infection is still active. Four to six blood cultures should be obtained over the course of 12 to 72 hours. The time of day at which they are taken is of little importance. Arterial blood cultures are of no special

value, but bone-marrow cultures may be useful if unusual pathogens are suspected or when venous cultures remain sterile. If six cultures are negative, it is unlikely that additional blood cultures will be helpful. About 1 ml of blood should be used for each 10 ml of culture media, and penicillinase should be added if the patient has recently received penicillin or one of its analogues. Careful in vitro sensitivity testing of recovered organisms is crucial. Tube dilution sensitivity studies should include determinations of minimum inhibitory concentration and minimum bactericidal concentration. After the antibiotic regimen has been started, the ability of the patient's serum to inhibit or kill the infecting organism should also be determined. A serum MBC activity of 1:8 or greater is thought to be necessary for cure of infection.

MANAGEMENT OF ENDOCARDITIS

Medical Management

Synergism between cell wall active antibiotics, such as penicillin, and aminoglycoside antibiotics, such as streptomycin or gentamicin, has been well documented by in vitro experiments[106] and by studies on experimental endocarditis in animals.[102] This synergism is essential for the complete killing of even sensitive organisms such as *S. viridans*. It has also been demonstrated experimentally for more resistant streptococci and even staphylococci. Recommendations in Table 85–2 are based on this principle. Clinical support for this point of view is also becoming available.[110] A bactericidal regimen is essential if cure rather than mere suppression of infective endocarditis is to be achieved. Combinations of bactericidal and bacteriostatic drugs should be avoided in this disease, since the net effect may be bacteriostatic. The temptation to begin therapy prior to obtaining adequate blood cultures should be resisted unless the diagnosis is obvious or the patient is very ill. Once adequately spaced blood cultures have been obtained therapy may begin, directed toward the organism or organisms which appear, on clinical grounds, to be the most likely offenders. Standard regimens are indicated in Table 85–2. The recommendations are based on the concept that endocarditis is always fatal when untreated and extremely dangerous when undertreated. Modifications are made on the basis of the clinical response or on the basis of laboratory information such as final culture reports, sensitivity tests, and determination of serum activity. It is important to realize that clinical response is always the best indicator and should take precedence over the information received from the laboratory. However, it is clear

TABLE 85-2
Standard Regimens for Bacterial Endocarditis

Organism	Antibiotic	Dose/Day	Route	Duration
Penicillin-sensitive S. viridans	Penicillin + streptomycin	2.4–5.0 million units 1 g	IM-IV* IM	4 weeks 2 weeks
Penicillin-less sensitive S. viridans	Penicillin + streptomycin	10–20 million units 1–2 g	IV IM	4 weeks 2 weeks
Enterococcus, Group D streptococcus	Penicillin† + streptomycin‡	20–60 million units 1–2 g	IV IM	4–6 weeks 4 weeks
Penicillin-sensitive staphylococcus§	Penicillin + gentamicin	10–40 million units 3–5 mg/kg	IV IM-IV	6 weeks 1–2 weeks
Penicillin-resistant staphylococcus	Methicillin or nafcillin + Gentamicin	8–16 g 4–8 g 3–5 mg/kg	IV IM-IV	6 weeks 1–2 weeks

* Oral penicillin can be used but is thought less reliable.
† In some cases Ampicillin 8–12 g may be substituted.
‡ In some cases Gentamicin may be substituted.
§All staphylococci should be considered penicillin resistant until proven otherwise.

that a regimen which does not provide satisfactory in vitro levels will almost always fail. The converse is not true. A regimen may provide excellent in vitro levels but the patient may fail to improve. Penicillin combined with streptomycin or gentamicin is the regimen of choice for streptococci and staphylococci. Treatment of gram-negative organisms depends on precise sensitivity tests. Combinations of penicillin or carbenicillin and kanamycin or gentamicin are most useful. Sterilization of the blood in pseudomonas endocarditis requires this combination. Since prognosis is poor with any regimen, maximally tolerated doses should be used. Surgical removal of the infected valve is often required. This is also true in fungal endocarditis where amphotericin B alone rarely sterilizes the infection. The combination of amphotericin B and 5-fluorocytosine may be helpful in candida endocarditis.

Patients with a history of a penicillin reaction present a difficult problem. Penicillin skin testing with major and minor determinants is very useful. Patients with negative skin tests will usually not manifest serious immediate reactions and should be treated with penicillin. Delayed reactions can be controlled with antihistamines or adrenal corticosteroids. Patients with positive skin tests should either undergo desensitization or receive an alternate drug based on sensitivity testing. Erythromycin or cephalothin can be used for penicillin sensitive organisms, although cephalothin is dangerous in patients with positive penicillin skin tests. Cephalothin or vanco-

mycin combined with an aminoglycoside have been used in enterococcal endocarditis, and vancomycin has shown some success in staphylococcal endocarditis.

Surgical Management

As previously indicated, eradication of the infection is only the first step in management. Often the structural damage must be repaired surgically. Recently it has become clear that early surgery is important in the management of heart failure developing in the course of endocarditis.[109] This is particularly true when aortic insufficiency is present. Sudden death is common in this setting. When heart failure is absent medical therapy alone is effective. When heart failure is severe, i.e., requiring more than digitalis, early surgery to correct the valvular incompetence is mandatory. When heart failure is mild the decision is often difficult and must be based on an assessment of both the severity and progression of the valvular damage. This may require cardiac catheterization since clinical signs may be misleading.[115]

In addition, echocardiography can provide a rapid, noninvasive diagnosis of bacterial vegetation in some patients. It may also identify patients with more severe diseases which are likely to require surgery.[113]

Other indications for surgery include the following: failure to sterilize the bloodstream infection; recurrent significant emboli, particularly cerebral and coronary emboli; prosthetic valve infection; cardiovascular accidents such as ruptured cusps, chordae, septum; mycotic aneurysms; and possibly progressive renal failure. Recent experience has indicated that surgery can be performed in the first few days of antibiotic treatment without significant increase in subsequent infection of the prosthetic valve.[104]

Common Management Problems

NEGATIVE BLOOD CULTURES IN SUSPECTED SUB-ACUTE INFECTIVE ENDOCARDITIS. The incidence of sterile blood cultures in published series averages 10 to 20 percent. In most cases, sterile blood cultures result from prior antibiotic therapy, failure to obtain sufficient cultures, use of improper media, failure to observe the cultures for at least 3 weeks, or incorrect diagnosis. The so-called sterile phase of the disease is a distinctly unlikely explanation, especially early in the illness. Active rheumatic fever, drug fever, sterile embolization in association with congestive heart failure, rheumatic pneumonitis, the postcommissurotomy syndrome, and connective-tissue disorders are the most common conditions masquerading as endocarditis. Atrial fibrillation and congestive failure suggest sterile emboli and weigh against the diagnosis of endocarditis in such patients; anemia favors it. Atrial myxoma, tuberculosis, lymphoma, and occult neoplasm or abscess should also be considered.

It is common practice to begin therapy for infective endocarditis in such patients after six blood cultures have been obtained. Some recommend that therapy be directed against viridans streptococci; others believe the possibility of enterococci should be the determinant of therapy. Some recommend 2 weeks of therapy; others recommend 6 weeks. There is no simple answer. Since the prognosis is less favorable in patients with sterile blood cultures, vigorous therapy appears to be indicated, with 20 million units of penicillin and 1 g of streptomycin per day for 6 weeks. If therapeutic response is observed, a full course of antibiotics is indicated. Defervescence, a rising hematocrit and reticulocytosis, the return of the appetite and the leukocyte count to normal, and the appearance of sense of well-being in the patient are helpful signs. If there is no response in 2 weeks, therapy should be discontinued and the patient reevaluated. Treatment of infective endocarditis is expensive, inconvenient, and potentially dangerous and should not be undertaken lightly. Whenever possible, a therapeutic trial should be avoided, since it is rarely helpful and is often confusing.

RECURRENCE OF FEVER DURING TREATMENT OF PROVED ENDOCARDITIS. When fever recurs in patients being treated for endocarditis, inadequate antibiotic therapy is usually suspected, but it is rarely the cause when appropriate, standard, bactericidal regimens are used (Table 85–2). This is not surprising when one realizes that many forms of antibiotic therapy that are incapable of curing endocarditis are capable of suppressing most of the manifestations of the infection. It is rare for the organisms to become resistant during therapy. Drug fever, intercurrent infections, sterile abscesses at injection sites, embolization, thrombophlebitis at the site of intravenous therapy, superinfection of the valve with a resistant strain, metastatic abscesses, bleeding mycotic aneurysms, and coexisting disease should be suspected. Ancillary evidence supporting these possibilities should be sought (eosinophilia, rash, new physical findings, and so on). Nonessential drugs that may cause fever, such as sedatives, should be discontinued. More blood cultures should be obtained, and penicillinase (8000 units per ml blood) should be added to the cultures if any of the penicillin analogues are being used in treatment. Determination of the bactericidal activity of serum from the patient against the offending organism may be helpful. Some enterococcus strains may require 50 million to 100 million units of penicillin daily. If serum diluted 1:8 in broth is bactericidal, therapy is probably adequate, and there is little reason to increase the dose of antibiotics.

If drug fever is suspected and an alternative bactericidal regimen is available, it may be wise to discontinue the suspected antibiotics. If no other antibiotic regimen is suitable, the presumed allergic reaction may be treated with antihistamines, aspirin, ephedrine, epinephrine, or adrenal corticosteroids as needed.

FEVER AFTER CARDIAC SURGERY. When patients undergoing cardiac surgery develop fever in the postoperative period, a stitch abscess of the myocardium of the great vessels or at the site of a prosthesis is an all too frequent cause.[108] Blood cultures are almost always positive with this complication but may be sterile until antibiotics are discontinued. Other causes of fever should be considered; among them are drug fever, viral hepatitis, wound abscess not involving the heart, pneumonia, atelectasis, empyema, osteomyelitis, endarteritis at the site of femoral cannulation, urinary-tract infection, postcardiotomy syndrome, and cytomegalovirus infection. Intracardiac infections are more frequent in poor-risk patients undergoing long and technically difficult operations and in patients in whom it was difficult to achieve hemostasis.

If an intracardiac infection seems likely, an intensive and prolonged course of antibiotic therapy should be given. This is very hazardous unless the microbial etiology has been established. Control of the infection prepares the patient for reoperation, which is usually necessary. It is practically impossible to cure the infection unless the prosthesis or infected suture is removed, but a few patients have been cured when infection caused by very sensitive organisms was treated intensively for prolonged periods with bactericidal therapy.

PROPHYLACTIC ANTIBIOTICS. Prophylactic antimicrobial drugs should be given to patients with congenital or acquired valvular heart disease at the time of diagnostic or therapeutic manipulations involving the teeth and the upper respiratory or urinary tracts.

The experimental endocarditis model suggests that oral penicillin, erythromycin, tetracycline, ampicillin, cephalothin and many other single agents are not effective—Vancomycin or the combination of penicillin with an aminoglycoside is effective.[101] Recently, the American Heart Association has published new recommendations which are significantly different from previous regimens.[97]

CHAPTER 86
Infections of the Gastrointestinal Tract
NATHANIEL F. PIERCE

Infections of the intestinal tract are second in frequency only to those of the upper respiratory tract. They affect all ages but are most frequent among children. Cases may be sporadic, but epidemic spread is common. In developing countries, acute infectious diarrhea is a major cause of morbidity and mortality, especially among small children. Causative agents include viruses, bacteria, and protozoans. The most frequent symptoms of gastrointestinal infection are vomiting and diarrhea. Evidence of mucosal damage, including bleeding, exudate formation, and perforation, is also common.

INTESTINAL FLORA AND MUCOSAL IMMUNITY
Establishment of the complex intestinal microflora begins at birth and becomes stabilized in the early years of life. The greatest numbers of bacteria are in the distal ileum and colon where intestinal contents move slowly. Normal adult stool reflects colonic flora and contains about 10^{11} bacteria per gram; more than 99 percent are anaerobes (bacteroides, lactobacilli, and clostridia), the rest being aerobes or facultative anaerobes (coli-aerogenes, proteus, pseudomonas, and enterococci). These large and relatively stable populations reflect a balanced environment created by the various bacterial species themselves and the host immune response at the mucosal surface. The upper small intestine has far fewer bacteria, about 10^3/ml of fluid. Its colonization is probably minimized by locally produced secretory antibody and mucus which diminish bacterial adherence to the mucosa and by the continuous downstream propulsion of intestinal contents.

The normal flora may be altered by a variety of events including: damage to the mucosa (irradiation or cytotoxic drug therapy), changes in intestinal motility (diarrhea, intestinal stasis, or the presence of "blind loops" of gut), interference with bacterial growth (antibiotic therapy), or the introduction of a new viral, bacterial, or protozoan agent. Colonization with new microbial agents is usually brief, ending in a few days or weeks as the host develops a specific mucosal immune response. Most episodes of transient colonization are asymptomatic. However, when the colonizing agent is a pathogen, symptoms frequently develop. These symptoms depend upon the portion of the bowel involved and the virulence mechanisms of the pathogen.

PATHOGENESIS OF INTESTINAL INFECTIONS

Bacterial Infections
Most enteric pathogens cause disease by one of two mechanisms, 1) the production of enterotoxins, or 2) invasion and damage of the mucosa (Tables 86–1 and 86–2). With some, these mechanisms may be combined.[119] Toxigenic bacteria which colonize but do not invade the mucosa include *V. cholerae*, some *E. coli*, and possibly others. Colonization occurs in the small bowel, and the enterotoxins act directly on small bowel mucosa to cause secretion of an isotonic electrolyte solution which causes watery diarrhea. The major effect upon the host is the loss of water and electrolytes, which may cause death. *V. cholerae* and *E. coli* produce antigenically related protein enterotoxins which cause electrolyte secretion by

---

TABLE 86-1
Bacterial Infections of the Intestine

	Mechanism	Major Symptoms	Fecal Leukocytes	Common Causative Organisms
1.	Enterotoxin released in small bowel	Watery diarrhea, vomiting	No	Toxigenic *E. coli, V. cholerae V. parahaemolyticus*
2.	Preformed enterotoxin in food	Vomiting, diarrhea	No	*Staphylococcus aureus, Clostridium perfringens, Bacillus cereus*
3.	Cytotoxicity, possibly by bacterial toxin	Diarrhea with blood and/or mucus, "pseudomembranous colitis"	Yes	*Staphylococcus aureus, Cl. dificile*
4.	Mucosal invasion causing inflammation	Dysentery, blood and/or mucus in stool, fever, tenesmus, "toxicity," may have watery diarrhea at onset	Yes	Shigella, invasive *E. coli,* some salmonella, *V. parahaemolyticus*
5.	Mucosal invasion leading to bacteremia	"Enteric fever," some have watery diarrhea at onset	Yes	Salmonella, including *S. typhi*

---

stimulating adenyl cyclase activity and raising the level of cAMP in mucosal epithelium.[123,126] Some *E. coli* produce an unrelated heat-stable enterotoxin which induces secretion by increasing levels of cyclic GMP in mucosal cells.[125] Enterotoxin production in *V. cholerae* is controlled by bacterial genes, whereas in *E. coli* this genetic material is in transferable plasmids. Enterotoxin production may also be important in diarrhea caused by some strains of shigella, salmonella, aeromonas, *V. parahaemolyticus*, and noncholera vibrios. Additionally, some bacteria produce enterotoxins in contaminated food; ingestion of these preformed enterotoxins causes vomiting and diarrhea without bacterial colonization of the intestine. These bacteria, which include toxigenic strains of *Staphylococcus aureus*, *Clostridium perfringens*, and *Bacillus cereus*, are the major causes of food poisoning. Finally, colonic overgrowth of staphylococci or certain strains of clostridia may complicate antibiotic therapy, chronic illness, or surgery; the result is colitis with mucosal damage and diarrhea possibly mediated by cytotoxins of the offending organisms.

Invasive organisms include shigella, salmonella, and some nontoxigenic strains of *E. coli*. Invasion occurs in the distal ileum and colon. Shigella and invasive *E. coli* cause disruption of the mucosa and induce a vigorous inflammatory response with signs of colonic irritation (tenesmus, abdominal pain) and the appearance of blood, mucus, and pus in the stool. Bacteremia with these organisms is unusual even though systemic "toxicity" is common. In contrast, mucosal invasion by salmonellae may be the first step leading to bacteremia and the syndrome of enteric fever. Diarrhea may also occur and is possibly mediated by an enterotoxin.

Viral Infections

Acute gastroenteritis, with vomiting, diarrhea, and fever, may be caused by a variety of viral agents (Table 86–2).[117,118] The best studied is the human rotavirus, which is the major cause of acute gastroenteritis in infants. Other viruses resembling parvoviruses or coronaviruses also cause diarrhea in humans and animals. Viruses replicate in duodenal and jejunal mucosa inducing mild inflammatory changes and transient flattening of the villi. Secretion of water and electrolytes occurs during mucosal repair and may be related to the transient predominance of immature mucosal cells. Malabsorption of dietary ingredients, especially lactose, also contributes to the diarrhea.

Other viral infections of the gut produce no enteric symptoms but may lead to systemic spread with serious consequences, as occurs with poliomyelitis, other enterovirus infections, and infectious hepatitis.

Protozoan Infections

Two protozoans, *Giardia lamblia* and *Entamoeba histolytica*, are important causes of intestinal infection (Table 86–2). Each are acquired by ingestion of cysts. *Giardia lamblia* adheres to the mucosa of the

TABLE 86-2
Causes of Acute Infectious Diarrhea

	Agent	Disease Form(s)	Comments
I. Viruses	Rotavirus	Infantile diarrhea	Most common cause of infantile diarrhea in winter
	Coronaviruses, parvoviruses	Winter vomiting disease, "intestinal flu"	Epidemics, affect all ages
II. Bacteria	Toxigenic *E. coli*	Watery diarrhea	Two types of toxin, important cause of travelers' diarrhea
	Invasive *E. coli*	Dysentery	Resembles shigellosis clinically
	"Enteropathogenic" *E. coli*	Watery diarrhea	Specific serotypes which may cause infantile diarrhea by unknown mechanism
	Bacillus cereus	Food poisoning	Probable enterotoxin
	Clostridium perfringens	Food poisoning	Preformed enterotoxin in food, onset 8–14 hours
	Staphylococcus aureus	Food poisoning	Preformed enterotoxin in food, onset 1–7 hours
		Pseudomembranous enterocolitis	In chronically ill patients, especially after antibiotics or surgery
	Clostridium dificile	Enterocolitis	May complicate clindamycin therapy
	Salmonella species	Enteric fever Watery diarrhea Dysentery Focal extraintestinal infections	Organisms (except *S. typhi*) in many processed foods. Febrile enteritis is common form. Gallbladder carriers for *S. typhi*
	Shigella species	Watery diarrhea and/or dysentery Systemic complications with *S. dysenteriae*	Person to person spread. Effective inoculum may be very low
	Vibrio cholerae	Watery diarrhea	Now present in South Asia, the Mideast, and Africa
	Vibrio parahaemolyticus	Watery diarrhea or dysentery	Poorly cooked shellfish are common source. May cause sepsis
	Yersinia enterocolitica	Dysentery	Diarrhea is secondary feature; sepsis, arthritis common
III. Protozoa	*Giardia lamblia*	Watery diarrhea Chronic diarrhea with malabsorption	Spread in water supply
	Entamoeba histolytica	Dysentery and/or hepatic abscess	Often asymptomatic

upper small intestine and causes flattening of jejunal villi. Flatulence, abdominal pain, malabsorption, and watery diarrhea are common symptoms, but the mechanism by which these are produced is uncertain. Persons with immunoglobulin deficiencies have an increased risk of developing giardiasis. *Entamoeba histolytica* usually reside in the lumen of the colon but occasionally penetrate colonic or terminal ileal mucosa producing characteristic ulcerative lesions and an inflammatory exudative response, frequently with bleeding. In some instances *E. histolytica* migrate by the portal circulation to lodge in the liver or elsewhere and produce necrosis with abscess formation.

EPIDEMIOLOGY AND SUSCEPTIBILITY TO INFECTION

Most gastrointestinal infections follow ingestion of contaminated water or food. Thus they are most common in conditions of poor sanitation, especially when host susceptibility is high. The combination of poor sanitation and high host susceptibility permits epidemic spread, which can occur with almost any enteric pathogen. The mode of spread is determined largely by the inoculum required to produce disease. Agents infective in low inoculum (e.g., shigella) are readily spread by contaminated food or hands while those requiring high inocula (e.g., *V. cholerae*) are more readily spread by water.

Host susceptibility is determined primarily by prior infection, which often provides some degree of immunity. Additional determinants include malnutrition, which may impair mucosal immune mechanisms, and impaired gastric acid production, which increases susceptibility to acid-sensitive bacterial pathogens such as *V. cholerae*. Because they lack acquired immunity, children are the most frequent victims of enteric infection. This is especially true for agents that induce appreciable immunity, such as enteroviruses or the human rotavirus, but is also true for some bacterial pathogens. Adults who escape childhood exposure remain susceptible and are at high risk of infection when exposed, as may occur when traveling from areas of high to low sanitation. This explains the high incidence of travelers' diarrhea, often due to toxigenic *E. coli*, among persons traveling from developed to underdeveloped countries.[121]

Some enteric infections, especially viral ones, exhibit a seasonal pattern which is unexplained. Thus, enteroviruses cause disease primarily in the late summer and fall, while human rotavirus infections occur mostly in winter months.

CLINICAL CONSEQUENCES OF INTESTINAL INFECTION

Many episodes of intestinal infection are entirely asymptomatic. Such persons are important and unknowing sources for spread of the pathogen to others. Infection is usually terminated by immune mechanisms with resultant increased immunity for the host.

Water and Electrolyte Loss

The clinical consequences of watery diarrhea are due entirely to the loss of water and electrolytes, i.e., sodium, potassium, chloride, and bicarbonate. Watery diarrhea originates as small bowel secretion with concentrations of sodium, potassium, chloride, and bicarbonate which resemble plasma. Liquid stool is isosmotic with plasma, but its electrolyte composition is determined by the speed of passage through the gut and the presence of osmotically active derivatives of food. Electrolyte concentrations are highest when stool loss is rapid and there is no dietary intake (Table 86-3). When stool losses are combined with losses in urine, and by evaporation and vomiting, the usual net deficit is isotonic with plasma, i.e., isotonic dehydration. Water may be lost in excess of sodium, giving hypertonic dehydration; this occurs when feeding of cow's milk is sustained and water intake is inadequate.

Most important is the loss of isotonic saline. This causes extracellular volume depletion which leads progressively to hypotension, shock, and death. When this loss equals 10 percent of the body weight, death is near and the signs are obvious; poor skin turgor, cold extremities, thready or absent radial pulse, stupor, oliguria, and flat neck veins. On the other hand, loss of only half this amount, 5 percent of body weight, may appear deceptively benign, the only signs being thirst, a "washed out" feeling, and possibly accentuated postural changes in pulse. It is obviously important that patients be recognized and treated at this point since symptoms and the risk of serious morbidity and mortality increase rapidly with further unreplaced fluid losses.

Bicarbonate loss causes metabolic acidosis which may be severe; Kussmaul respirations develop as a compensatory mechanism. There is also a shift of blood volume into the pulmonary circulation. Thus, correction of hypovolemia with normal saline without correction of the acidosis risks pulmonary edema.

Acute diarrhea causes potassium depletion, but hypokalemia may not develop until the acidosis is corrected. Symptomatic hypokalemia is uncommon

---

TABLE 86-3

Electrolyte Content of Plasma and Stool During Watery Diarrhea (mEq or mM/L)

	Plasma, Normal	Watery Stool*	Plasma Severe Diarrhea†
Sodium	140	30–140	130–144
Potassium	4	10–30	3.5–5
Bicarbonate	25	10–50	7–15
Chloride	100	40–105	105–120

* Sodium and chloride content increase and potassium decreases with increasing rate of loss of stool. Bicarbonate declines with uncorrected acidosis or organic acids in stool, as occurs with lactase deficiency and continued milk intake.
† Typical values for isotonic dehydration.

in adults unless there was preexisting potassium depletion due to diuretics or other causes. Hypokalemic symptoms, including arrhythmias and paralytic ileus, are more common in children.

Intestinal Damage and Malabsorption

The most common manifestation of intestinal damage by enteritis is lactose intolerance due to loss of the brush border enzyme lactase. This enzyme splits lactose into absorbable glucose and galactose. When lactose hydrolysis fails, intestinal bacteria ferment it, producing acid, gas, and osmotically active fragments which draw more water into the intestine. Lactose intolerance occurs with all forms of infectious enteritis which involve the small intestine and may last for weeks or even months.

Other sugars, fats, and vitamins are also malabsorbed during or shortly after diarrhea. This, combined with the common practice of withholding food during episodes of diarrhea, contributes to a cycle of diarrhea–malabsorption–malnutrition which occurs among the underprivileged in all countries.

Enteric Blood and Protein Loss

Anemia and hypoproteinemia, due to intestinal loss of blood and serum proteins, may be serious consequences of any of the invasive diarrheas, especially in patients already malnourished. Both acute, fulminating, and chronic, relapsing enterocolitis may be responsible.

Fever, Toxicity, and Sepsis

Patients with diarrhea caused by invasive bacteria often have fever, headache, myalgia, abdominal pain, malaise, tenesmus, and prostration. Children with shigellosis may also develop grand mal seizures, while a syndrome including hemolytic anemia and a leukemoid reaction has been seen in children and young adults infected with *Shigella dysenteriae*. Bacteremia, however, is rare with shigella infections, but more common in salmonella infections. Salmonella may cause localized infection (osteomyelitis, aortitis, abscesses) in compromised patients such as those with sickle cell disease, immune deficiencies, or neoplastic disease. Typhoid fever is a special case of severe septicemic infection due to *Salmonella typhi* in which diarrhea is a minor feature.

DIAGNOSIS

Determining the cause of an episode of diarrhea or dysentery is important for two reasons:

1. To guide the use of specific antimicrobial therapy
2. To assist epidemiologic studies and control efforts by public health workers

Unfortunately, the etiologic agent is frequently unidentified despite thorough diagnostic efforts. It should also be emphasized that etiologic diagnosis is of secondary importance in patients with dehydrating watery diarrhea; their greatest need is prompt replacement of water and electrolyte losses.

Historical information may be of considerable value, particularly information on recent travel, similar symptoms among friends or contacts, antibiotic therapy, or gastric surgery or achlorhydria. Diagnostic studies aimed at determining the etiologic agent are summarized in Table 86–4. Direct examinations of fresh stool are of special value since they may provide rapid identification of invasive bacterial diarrhea by the presence of fecal leukocytes (Table 86–1).[120] Amebiasis, giardiasis, or staphylococcal enterocolitis may also be rapidly diagnosed. Proof of specific bacterial or viral etiology requires isolation of the agent or serologic evidence of infection, which may take several days or weeks. Moreover, some diagnostic studies are available only in reference laboratories. Isolation of shigella from stool or of salmonella from blood or urine are the most common cultural results which influence specific antimicrobial therapy. Among patients with bloody, mucoid stool, sigmoidoscopy may assist in obtaining optimal samples for detection of amebae and in differentiating amebiasis from ulcerative colitis or regional enteritis.

TREATMENT

The major objectives of treatment are: 1) replacement of water and electrolyte losses; and 2) termination of infection. Additionally, nutritional maintenance is important for malnourished patients.

Water and Electrolyte Replacement

The first step in treating patients with diarrhea is estimation of the fluid deficit. A rule-of-thumb for estimating isotonic fluid deficit is that a 5 percent loss of body weight produces minimal signs (thirst, slight tachycardia, slightly diminished skin turgor), whereas 10 percent deficit is nearly lethal (causing severe thirst, anuria, markedly decreased skin turgor, thready or absent radial pulse, hypotension, and stupor). Both situations require water and electrolyte replacement; in the latter the need is urgent.

The goals are correction of existing water and electrolyte deficits and replacement of ongoing stool losses until diarrhea stops. This can be done by two methods:

1. Intravenous infusion of electrolyte solutions with appropriate concentrations of the lost electrolytes
2. Oral replacement using a glucose or sucrose-electrolyte solution

TABLE 86-4
Tests for the Etiology of Intestinal Infection

Procedure	Comment
I. Stool Examination	
Appearance	Watery stool suggests enterotoxin or viral diarrhea; mucoid, bloody stool suggests invasive agent
Methylene blue stain for leukocytes	PMNs suggest mucosal invasion and damage. Mononuclears suggest *S. typhosa* (Table 86–1)
Fresh, 37°C wet preparation for amebae	Identification of pathogenic trophozoites requires experienced observer
Stool concentrate	For cysts of *E. histolytica, Giardia lamblia*; needs experienced observer
Gram stain	Staphylococci predominate in pseudomembranous staphylococcal enterocolitis
II. Culture	
Stool	Helpful for salmonella, shigella, vibrios, staphylococci, and yersinia. Enteropathogenic *E. coli* are of uncertain importance. Testing of *E. coli* for enterotoxin or invasiveness requires a reference laboratory
Blood, urine	Frequently positive in enteric fever due to *S. typhi* or other salmonellae; rarely positive for shigellae
III. Serology	
Typhoid fever	Rise in antibody to O antigen (Widal test); not entirely specific
Cholera, toxigenic *E. coli*	Frequent rise in antibody to cholera toxin or heat-labile *E. coli* toxin; rise in bactericidal antibody to *V. cholerae*; require reference laboratory
Viral diarrhea	Rise in antibody to specific virus; requires reference laboratory
Amebiasis	Elevated latex agglutination titer suggests extraintestinal disease

Intravenous therapy is acceptable in modern hospitals and is essential to correct hypovolemia with shock. Oral rehydration is convenient for patients who can drink and are not seriously hypovolemic; it is the most practical therapy when treatment facilities are limited as occurs during epidemics in underdeveloped countries.

For rapid intravenous rehydration, a large, secure intravenous route must be quickly established. With severe volume depletion, peripheral veins are often collapsed; initial infusion through the external jugular vein or femoral vein may be necessary. The replacement fluid should have an electrolyte content nearly isotonic with plasma and include appropriate electrolytes to correct serious existing deficits, including correction of metabolic acidosis and potassium depletion. Ringer's lactate is the best commercially available solution but requires potassium supplementation to a total of 15 mEq/L. Normal saline is the poorest electrolyte solution but is much improved if supplemented with bicarbonate (30 mEq/L) and potassium (15 mEq/L).

At least one-half the estimated fluid deficit should be infused in the first hour, the rest being given over 2 to 4 hours. Rapid replacement is most important in patients with severe hypovolemia. Ongoing losses should be replaced as they occur. When possible, stool should be measured and replaced volume-for-volume with the same intravenous fluid. Stool may be collected in a bedside commode, bedpan, or plastic-backed diapers which are frequently changed and weighed. Adequate "free" water, given by mouth or as dextrose–water infusion, is needed to replace evaporative and urinary losses. Adequate volume replacement is indicated by full peripheral pulses, adequate urine output, good skin turgor, and a stable posthydration body weight. Frequent bedside evaluation of the state of hydration and general well-being is the best method of confirming adequate water and electrolyte replacement. Persistent hypotension after adequate volume replacement may occur with some invasive enteropathogens (e.g., salmonellae or shigella). Treatment is as described for other septic hypotensive conditions (Chap. 145).

Oral therapy with a glucose or sucrose-electrolyte solution (Table 86-5) is effective for dehydrating diarrhea of bacterial or viral etiology in patients of all

TABLE 86-5
Composition of Oral Glucose or Sucrose–Electrolyte Solution

	Grams/L		Millimoles/L
NaCl	3.5	Na⁺	90
NaHCO₃	2.5	K⁺	20
KCl	1.5	Cl⁻	80
Glucose or	20	HCO₃⁻	30
Sucrose	40	Glucose or sucrose	110

ages.[122,124] The glucose or sucrose is required to facilitate sodium and water absorption. A single solution can be used safely for all patients; it can be prepared as needed using table salt, baking soda, and potassium chloride and glucose or sucrose. The solution should not be heated and need not be sterile. The advantages of oral therapy are: low cost, easily available ingredients, simple administration, and reduced need for intravenous fluids. Patients with severe dehydration, inability to drink, or paralytic ileus require initial intravenous rehydration (50 to 100 ml/kg) after which the oral solution can usually be started. Further intravenous fluids are not usually needed. Those with less serious dehydration can generally be treated with the oral solution alone from the outset. Most patients will take, ad libitum, sufficient amounts to maintain fluid and electrolyte balance. Patients with rapid continuing diarrhea may need encouragement to drink the needed amounts. To allow patients to rest, oral solutions can also be given by a thin nasogastric tube.

Vomiting usually stops after initial intravenous rehydration of severely hypovolemic patients and seldom interferes seriously with oral therapy. When vomiting occurs, the amounts are small in relation to the volumes of stool and oral solution and can be replaced by additional oral solution. Vomiting is less common when the oral solution is given by nasogastric tube. If vomiting is severe and there are signs of increasing dehydration, intravenous replacement must be used.

Antimicrobial Therapy

Antibiotics are useful in specific enteric infections (Table 86-6) but are never a substitute for adequate rehydration. Oral tetracycline benefits cholera by reducing the volume of stool, the duration of diarrhea, and the duration of excretion of the pathogen. The same is true with shigellosis. However, antibiotic sensitivity of the organism is unpredicable and must be determined to assure proper antibiotic selection. In contrast, antibiotic treatment of salmonella gastroenteritis prolongs the convalescent carrier state and is contraindicated in mild disease. Systemic salmonella infections, however, require specific therapy, e.g., typhoid fever, enteric fever, focal infections; chloramphenicol or ampicillin are usually effective but the sensitivity of the organism should be confirmed. Oral vancomycin is effective for staphylococcal enterocolitis and possibly for clindamycin enterocolitis due to *Clostridium dificile*. Antibiotics have no proven value in acute "nonspecific" diarrhea.

Other Medications

Opiates and derivatives (deodorized tincture of opium, Lomotil) relieve peristaltic cramping and stool frequency by increasing bowel tone and decreasing forward propulsion. They are useless in serious watery diarrhea and are contraindicated in invasive diarrhea because symptoms worsen and the disease is prolonged. Absorbants such as kaolin, pectin, bismuth, and charcoal are of little value and can interfere with absorption of antibiotics.

TABLE 86-6
Antimicrobial Therapy of Acute Intestinal Infections

Organism	Antimicrobial Therapy	Comment
Shigella	Ampicillin or tetracycline (Trimethoprim-sulfamethoxazole)*	Confirm sensitivity in laboratory; avoid tetracycline under 6 years of age
Salmonella	Chloramphenicol or Ampicillin (Trimethoprim-sulfamethoxazole)	Confirm sensitivity in laboratory; no antibiotics for uncomplicated enteritis
V. cholerae	Tetracycline (Nitrofurantoin)	
Staphylococcal enteritis	Vancomycin	
Clindamycin colitis	Vancomycin	Early reports suggest efficacy
Giardia lamblia	Metronidazole	
Entamoeba histolytica	Metronidazole (dihydroemetine plus chloroquine)	For dysentery and liver abscess
	Diiodohydroxyquinoline	To eliminate intestinal cysts

* Second choice therapy is shown in parentheses.

Diet

In uncomplicated cases, food intake should be determined by the patient's appetite. Foods containing lactose or a high concentration of other sugars should be resumed slowly. Boullion, chicken soup, cereals, toast, and bananas are well tolerated. Special efforts should be made to maintain nutrient intake in malnourished patients.

PREVENTION

Safe water supply, effective sewage processing, and careful food preparation have diminished enteric infections in developed nations. Enteric viral infections remain frequent, however, and salmonella species are widespread in processed foods. Lack of environmental sanitation in most developing nations makes control of enteric infections almost impossible.

Immunization

Poliovaccine is the outstanding example of effective immunoprophylaxis of an enteric infection. The oral live vaccine has the apparent advantage of inducing mucosal immunity and thus preventing asymptomatic intestinal infection. Typhoid vaccine is partially effective, but this protection is overcome by large inocula of bacteria. Cholera vaccine is ineffective in preventing intestinal colonization with *V. cholerae*

and only modestly protective against clinical cholera. Prospects are excellent for the development of effective vaccines against the newly described diarrheagenic viruses, e.g., rotavirus, and increasing knowledge of the mechanisms of intestinal immunity suggests that oral immunization against enteric bacterial infections may also be possible.

Antibiotic Prophylaxis

Recent studies in Africa and Mexico show that travelers' diarrhea is caused largely by tetracycline-sensitive strains of toxigenic *E. coli*.[121] Daily prophylaxis with doxycycline (200 mg) has proved highly effective in preventing this disease. Oral tetracycline is also effective in preventing secondary cases of cholera among persons exposed to a proven case. There are no other examples of effective antibiotic prophylaxis of intestinal infection.

Avoiding Antibiotic Abuse

Staphylococcal enterocolitis is frequently preceded by prolonged therapy with multiple antibiotics. Similarly, clindamycin colitis results from sustained therapy with this antibiotic. Reducing the incidence of these diseases and other complications of antibiotic therapy requires judicious use of antibiotics and careful observation of patients during treatment.

CHAPTER 87
Infections of the Urinary Tract
R. BRADLEY SACK

Urinary tract infections are among the most commonly recognized and defined infectious diseases in the United States, probably second in frequency only to viral upper respiratory tract infections. Furthermore, the population most susceptible to these infections has also been well defined, including females, pregnant women, individuals with structural abnormalities of the urinary tract, older people, and those with metabolic diseases such as diabetes. In spite of increasing understanding of the pathogenesis of urinary tract infections, their true potential for damage is still poorly understood. The notion that repeated urinary tract infections necessarily lead to the development of chronic pyelonephritis must still be questioned. It is well known that many acute urinary tract infections will heal without specific therapy and that autopsy studies do not show a marked increase in

chronic pyelonephritis in that segment of the population who experience most of the symptomatic acute infections. Chronic pyelonephritis is, however, most clearly associated with recurrent infections in persons with obstructive lesions in the genitourinary tract.

Urinary tract infections are the most common source of bacteremia due to gram-negative bacilli, and are, therefore, particularly important sources of generalized sepsis in hospitalized patients.

PATHOGENESIS

The bacteria responsible for urinary tract infections almost always come from the normal facultative fecal flora of the patient. Although infection may spread to the kidneys via the bloodstream, such as in staphylococcal sepsis, or by way of lymphatics, by far the most common route is the retrograde one from the urethra to the bladder and then through the ureter to the kidney.

The distal urethra normally has a commensal flora consisting of alpha streptococci, diptheroids, and *Staphylococcus epidermidis*, which rarely cause urinary tract infections. In the female particularly, however, the perineal area is also frequently colonized with facultative gram-negative bacilli similar to those found in the patient's feces. It has been well documented in females both clinically ("honeymoon cystitis") and experimentally by urethral massage that trauma to the short urethra may allow these fecal organisms access to the bladder.[128] This is even more directly evident following a single urethral catheterization in either sex which regularly leads to a small percentage (1 to 2 percent) of recognized infections.

The urethra and bladder have well-recognized but poorly defined antibacterial defense mechanisms which prevent most introduced bacteria from colonizing this area. Probably the regular, complete emptying of the bladder is one of the most important host defense mechanisms, since any interference with this process regularly leads to an increased incidence of infection.

In the male, the prostate is an anatomic area vulnerable to infection and one which may serve as a source of continuing and relapsing infection.[137]

Although it has been thought that ureteral-vesical reflux was an important predisposing factor to infection, it now seems clear that this is a frequent physiologic event and one that is certainly not a prerequisite of bacteria ascending the urinary tract.

Bacteria may remain localized to the bladder or may ascend to one or both kidneys. Unfortunately, the clinical symptomology accompanying this progression of infection is not pathognomonic, and it is perhaps wiser to think of the urinary tract as one functioning unit, vulnerable to infection in its entirety, rather than a compartmentalized one, unless specific tests have been done to localize the site of infection.

The renal medulla is particularly susceptible to infection by small inocula or bacteria; this is in marked contrast to the renal cortex which is relatively resistant. Much of the increased susceptibility of the medulla may be related to

1. A direct effect of hypertonicity, resulting in a decreased effectiveness of polymorphonuclear phagocytes and a more favorable media for persistance of cell wall defective bacterial forms
2. Inactivation of the fourth component of complement[139]

CLINICAL MANIFESTATIONS

As previously indicated, the symptoms of urinary tract infection may be relatively nonspecific and occasionally may be absent. Conversely, symptoms identical to those of urinary tract infection may be seen without bacterial infection; this situation has been called the "urethral syndrome." The sudden onset of shaking chills, fever, flank pain, and costovertebral angle tenderness classically describes acute pyelonephritis, whereas low-grade fever, dysuria, urgency, frequency, lower abdominal discomfort, and gross hematuria are more suggestive of acute cystitis. The anatomic localization of infection, however, is frequently not this clear, and, therefore, one should use the term "acute urinary tract infection" to describe this symptom complex.

The clinical patterns of urinary tract infection are varied and frequently confusing. A simplified scheme developed by Turck and Petersdorf which is useful in defining these patterns clinically, bacteriologically, and therapeutically is given in Table 87-1 in modified form.[139]

Acute Uncomplicated Urinary Tract Infections

These occur almost exclusively in women, for the reasons previously given. They occur in the absence of any predisposing anatomic or metabolic factors. The fecal organisms responsible are usually an antibiotic-sensitive strain of *E. coli*. These infections respond readily to therapy and if treated properly are probably benign.

Acute Complicated Urinary Tract Infections

These are defined as those occurring in persons with structural abnormalities of the urinary tract. These are seen frequently in young males who have congenital abnormalities of the urinary tract, elderly males with prostatic enlargement, or females who have multiple infections which accompany a structural abnormality of the urinary tract. The bacteriology and therapeutic outcome are less predictable in this group but are determined to a large extent upon early correction of the underlying obstructive lesion.

Asymptomatic Bacteriuria

Asymptomatic bacteriuria is usually discovered during an investigation of other unrelated complaints in women. There may be no definite history of urinary tract symptoms in these patients. The evaluation of these patients for structural abnormalities and the vigor of treatment should be tempered somewhat by the age of the patient and the clinical course following diagnosis. Frequently, renal function is normal in these patients. Some patients, including pregnant

TABLE 87-1
Classification of Urinary Tract Infections*

Category	History	Symptoms	Usual Pathogen	Usual Therapy
Uncomplicated, acute	Negative for previous urinary tract infections	Classic cystitis or pyelonephritis (women only)	E. coli	Sulfanamides Ampicillin Tetracycline
Complicated, acute	May be negative for previous urinary tract infections	Classic cystitis or pyelonephritis (both sexes)	Predominantly E. coli	As above, plus antibiotic sensitivity tests Relief of obstruction
Asymptomatic bacteriuria	Usually negative	None (often pregnant women, middle-aged women, and older men)	E. coli, Klebsiella-enterobacter, proteus	Based on antibiotic sensitivity testing only
Chronic bacteriuria	Repeated symptomatic episodes	Classic cystitis or pyelonephritis	E. coli (resistant), Klebsiella-enterobacter, Proteus, Pseudomonas	Gentamicin, modified according to antibiotic sensitivity tests Surgical repair when possible Suppressive therapy may be necessary
Urethral syndrome	Usually negative	Classic cystitis (primarily women)	None identified	Symptomatic

* Adapted from Wallace, J. F., and Petersdorf, R. G. Urinary tract infections. Postgrad. Med., 50:132, 1971.

women, will subsequently develop symptomatic infections at a later time and should be followed carefully.

Chronic Bacteriuria

Chronic bacteriuria describes patients who have alternating periods of symptomatic and asymptomatic bacteriuria. Many of these patients are elderly and many are male; some have underlying obstructive uropathy and others do not. The therapy in these patients is determined by the bacteriology of the repeat infections, which indicates whether relapses (infection with the same organism) or reinfection (infection with a new organism) is occurring.

Urethral Syndrome

The urethral syndrome, usually seen in females, may account for 30 to 40 percent of episodes of dysuria.[130] Symptoms may be identical to those of a bacterial infection, but urine cultures are sterile. No specific etiologic agent has been associated with the syndrome, which seems to be benign.

Chronic Pyelonephritis

The term *chronic pyelonephritis* describes a pathologic entity which leads to progressive, severe structural and functional impairment of both kidneys. Al-

though this condition seems to be initiated by infection, the role of continuing infection in the progression of the disease is not clear. These patients may have no history of acute urinary tract infections and, indeed, may have no bacteriuria. The symptoms that lead to this diagnosis are those associated with chronic renal failure.

LABORATORY DIAGNOSIS

The presence of significant bacteria and the accompanying inflammatory cells in the urine establish the diagnosis of urinary tract infection.

Examination of freshly voided, uncentrifuged, midstream urine for the presence of pus cells and bacteria is the simplest way of making a presumptive diagnosis. Because of the resolution of this method, the presence of bacteria (in stained or unstained preparation) indicates a bacterial count of 10^5 or greater per milliliter. Similarly, the presence of polymorphonuclear leukocytes in such a preparation is indicative of significant inflammatory reaction, secondary to infection.[129]

Examination of centrifuged urine is useful for detecting pyuria (greater than 10 white cells per high-power field), hematuria (which occurs most frequently with cystitis), and granular and white cell casts which indicate intrarenal inflammation. A Gram stain of centrifuged urine is less helpful because of the urethral organisms and contaminants which one can almost always find. The Gram-stain reaction may be useful if one has identified a significant number of organisms in the uncentrifuged specimen.

The confirmatory tests to establish etiology of urinary tract infections are the bacteriologic colony counts, identification of the organism, and antibiotic sensitivity testing. Normally bladder urine is sterile, and the normal urethral bacteria shed into the urine during voiding give colony counts less than 10^4 organisms/ml. During urinary tract infections, however, colony counts are usually 10^5/ml or greater. A single clean-catch midstream urine has about an 80 percent probability level of indicating infection; two samples increase this probability to 90 to 95 percent.[133] Therefore, urethral catheterization can usually be avoided in obtaining urine for culture. Suprapubic aspiration of urine completely avoids the problem of urethral contaminants and is a safe procedure. This should be the method of choice when voided urine results are inconclusive.

The use of colony counts in clean voided specimens is subject to the problems of obtaining adequate specimens and delivering them promptly to the laboratory for culturing. Falsely low counts may result from contamination of the urine with disinfectant; falsely high counts are usually the results of inadequate preparatory cleansing prior to voiding or delay in culturing, resulting in room temperature incubation. If the specimen cannot be processed promptly, it should be stored at refrigerator temperature, and this can be done for up to 24 hours without significantly altering the counts. Colony counts between 10^4 and 10^5/ml should be repeated, with these special precautions taken.

Bacteriology

The bacteria most frequently the cause of urinary tract infections are the facultative gram-negative organisms of fecal origin which may also colonize the periurethral areas in females. *Escherichia coli* is by far the most common invading organism (Table 87-2). Any *E. coli* may be pathogenic in this location but there is recent evidence to suggest that certain *E. coli* serotypes and/or strains that possess adherence factors for epithelial cells have increased virulence for the urinary tract.[134,136] Other organisms, such as enterobacter, klebsiella, proteus, and pseudomonas, are more commonly associated with repeated infections. Likewise, multiple antibiotic resistance is more commonly seen in these complicated infections.

TABLE 87-2

Frequency of Isolation of Different Bacterial Species from 360 Patients with Acute Pyelonephritis*

	Percent
E. coli	90
Klebsiella—Enterobacter species	5
Proteus	4
Enterococci	1

* Adapted from Hoeprich, P. D. (ed.). Infectious Diseases. New York, Harper & Row, 1972.

Enterococci, also a fecal inhabitant, are the most common gram-positive organisms to cause urinary tract infections. *Staphylococcus aureus* probably most often invades the urinary tract via the blood, whereas *S. epidermitis*, a rare cause of infections, probably invades by the usual retrograde route.

Curiously anaerobic organisms are almost never associated with urinary tract infections. Likewise, viruses have not been implicated as specific urinary tract pathogens. Fungi, such as candida, may be a cause of pyelonephritis, particularly in compromised hosts.

Renal Function

Acute urinary tract infections affect renal function only minimally, as can be evidenced by water loading tests. Nitrogen retention is seen only in chronic renal disease.

Radiologic Examination

Radiologic evaluation of the urinary tract is an important means of detecting potentially correctable abnormalities which may predispose to or perpetuate infection.

All male patients with newly discovered urinary tract infections, female patients with repeated or persistent infections, and any patient with unexplained impairment of renal function should have a careful evaluation of the urinary tract which includes excretory pyelography and voiding cystourethrogram. The early detection of obstructing or deforming lesions of the urinary tract is extremely important because surgical correction can be expected to alleviate this cause of recurrent infections. Moreover, the long-term prognosis in recurrent infections is excellent in the presence of a normal radiologic examination.

Differentiation of Upper and Lower Urinary Tract Infection

The differentiation of upper and lower urinary tract infections can be made by differential bladder washout techniques, and/or urethral catheterization, although this is rarely necessary. Recent studies suggest that detection of antibody on the bacterial cells in the urine may be a reliable indicator of pyelonephritis.[131] The absence of antibody coating indicates that the infection is limited to the bladder. Being able to make this differentiation may greatly facilitate antibiotic therapy, as indicated below. About half of all recognized urinary tract infections involve only the bladder.[136] Renal biopsy is of no value in assessing patient with acute urinary tract infection.

APPROACH TO MANAGEMENT OF PATIENTS WITH URINARY TRACT INFECTIONS

The therapy of acute urinary tract infection in general is twofold; antibacterial agents, of which there are many effective ones available, and relief of any obstruction present. Antibiotics can be given parenterally or orally depending upon the seriousness of the infection. Although certain antibiotics are more effective at different pH levels in the urine, it is rarely necessary to adjust urine pH, except when using mandelamine, which requires acidification in order to be effective. Likewise, water intake is not critical and should neither be restricted or unnecessarily encouraged, the only exception being its encouragement when using sulfonamides that may precipitate in the renal tubules if urine flow is markedly reduced. Whether antibiotic levels of serum or urine are the more critical for effective treatment is still debated. Clinically, however, antibiotics which achieve high urinary concentrations (in spite of low serum levels) are effective in successfully treating infections.

The historical information from the patients plus the urine culture results will usually allow the physician to categorize patients into one of the five clinical categories previously mentioned. Appropriate therapy and need for urologic evaluation will be discussed separately according to these designations.

Acute Uncomplicated Infections

Since the organisms responsible are usually always sensitive to many antimicrobial agents, the therapy is fairly simple. Sulfonamides (2 to 4 g of sulfisoxazole), ampicillin (1 to 2 g daily), or tetracycline (1 to 2 g daily) are equally effective in eradicating the organisms. A 10- to 14-day course of therapy is adequate. Alternative drugs include furadantin and the cephalo-

sporins. If one is able to localize the infection to the bladder, single dose therapy is equally effective.[131,135]

Acute Complicated Infections

The therapy is similar to that described above, except that the obstructive lesion must be adequately treated as well. It is almost impossible to terminate infection in a patient with a persistent unrelieved obstruction.

Asymptomatic Bacteriuria

This is probably the most difficult and frustrating of all the infections to treat. In some patients, a 10- to 14-day course of appropriate antibiotic may eliminate the infection. In many, however, this is almost impossible to accomplish, and one may be using multiple repeated doses of different antibiotics only to accomplish a change in the organism responsible for the bacteriuria. In the absence of any structural abnormality, it would seem reasonable to give only a single course of antibiotics. Repeat periodic urine cultures may be helpful in the treatment of a subsequent symptomatic infection.

Chronic Bacteriuria

Treatment should be based on whether the repeated episodes are due to reinfection or relapse. This differentiation can only be made bacteriologically. A bacterial isolate which is different from that which caused the previous infection establishes the diagnosis of reinfection, and a short course of antibiotics is indicated. If, on the other hand, the same species is isolated, a recurrence is likely, indicating the high probability of a focus of infection in the kidney. In this instance, a 6-week course of antibiotics might be effective in eradicating the organism.

In some patients in the latter category, in whom an indwelling catheter is mandatory or in whom corrective surgery cannot be done, there is value in giving chronic suppressive therapy with either mandelamine (associated with acidification of the urine) or nitrofurantoin. These agents prevent repeated episodes of symptomatic urinary tract infection, although bacteriuria persists.

Urethral Syndrome

No specific antimicrobial therapy is indicated.

In *severely* ill patients, therapy must be instituted before in vitro sensitivites are available. In such instances, antibiotics should be given parenterally and selected to cover the most likely pathogenic agent. For most gram-negative organisms, gentamicin (3 to

5 mg/kg per day) is adequate and for possible staphylococci, methicillin (12 g per day), or nafcillin (8 g per day) are the drugs of choice. These drugs can then be changed according to antibiotic sensitivity tests that become available later. In the presence of impaired renal function, the doses of many of the potentially toxic antibiotics must be reduced.[140]

Follow-Up Evaluation

It is necessary to ensure eradication of bacteria from all patients being treated with urinary tract infections whenever possible. This is best done with follow-up cultures done a week or so after the antibiotic has been stopped. Inability to eradicate the infection should indicate to the physician the possibility of complicating obstructive problems or possibly of the use of an inappropriate antibiotic.

SPECIAL PROBLEMS OF URINARY TRACT INFECTIONS

The Urinary Catheter

Catheterization of the urethra carries with it an infectious complication rate of 1 to 2 percent. A catheter left in place, however, for 4 to 5 days has an associated infection rate of 90 to 100 percent. This marked risk of developing infection can be minimized in several ways. Urethral catheterization should be avoided whenever possible and carried out with the utmost aseptic care when performed. For indwelling catheters, a system of closed drainage should be used to minimize organisms being introduced into the drainage system. An antibiotic solution containing polymyxin and neomycin has been shown to reduce infections when dripped continuously into a three-way closed catheter system.

Infection in Pregnancy

The increased incidence of infection begins early in pregnancy before the uterus is of sufficient size to obstruct urine flow, and may reflect hormonal influences on ureteral smooth muscle tone. The incidence of urinary tract infections in pregnant women has been determined to be approximately 10 percent. There is evidence to suggest that untreated urinary tract infections may lead to an increase of low birth weight in term infants.

Other Systemic Illness

Diabetics have an increased incidence of urinary tract infection for reasons which are not clear but probably relate to loss of normal antibacterial clearance mechanisms in the urinary tract. Acute papillary necrosis is most commonly seen in diabetics and may lead to ureteral obstruction by the necrotic papillary tissue.

Patients with hypertension also have an increased incidence of urinary tract infection, although the mechanisms responsible are not known.

Prevention of Infection

In some women, repeated urinary tract infections (several per year) seem to regularly occur for reasons previously discussed. Such infections can be significantly prevented by the regular (usually nightly) administration of an antibacterial drug such as furadantin, ampicillin, or more recently, trimethoprim-sulfamethoxazole.[127,132] This treatment should be in addition to advice about emptying the bladder after intercourse and the encouragement of sanitary precautions to minimize fecal contamination of the perineal area.

—CHAPTER 88—
Sexually Transmitted Diseases
PETER E. DANS

The new name of this group of infections and infestations, once called the venereal diseases (VD) after Venus, the goddess of love, reflects the pragmatism of our age. Love is not necessary for transmission; intimate contact is. Group membership has been expanded beyond the classic venereal diseases (see Table 88–1). Despite the commonly held myth, sexually transmitted diseases (STD) have never been limited to the socially deprived but have always traveled in the "best circles" among artists, composers, and kings.[166,175] They occur among those who are unable or unwilling to maintain a stable monogamous sexual relationship and their unwitting partners.

Since the common denominator is sexual transmission, an understanding of sexual behavior is essential.[146,174] Heterosexual sexual intercourse is practiced by some preteens and reaches a peak prevalence and frequency in the 18 to 25 age group.

┌───┐
TABLE 88-1
Sexually Transmitted Diseases

  I. **Classic Reportable Venereal Diseases**
      Gonorrhea
      Syphilis
      Chancroid
      Granuloma inguinale
      Lymphogranuloma venereum

 II. **Others Commonly Transmitted Sexually**
      Nongonococcal urethritis
      Genital herpes
      Trichomoniasis
      Nonspecific vaginitis
      Phthirus pubis ("crabs")
      Scabies
      Condyloma acuminatium
      Molluscum contagiosum

III. **Others Occasionally Transmitted Sexually**
      Cytomegalovirus
      Candidiasis
      Enteric diseases
         Amebiasis
         Giardiasis
         Shigellosis
         Typhoid fever
      Hepatitis—especially B
      Infectious mononucleosis
      Group B hemolytic streptococci
      Postcoital urinary tract infections
└───┘

Although the frequency declines thereafter, it remains the dominant sexual behavior when compared to masturbation or homosexuality. The latter increases in prevalence after adolescence, especially in higher socioeconomic groups.

There are important racial differences in sexual behavior. In a study reported in 1969, 24 percent of white women, 63 percent of black women, 40 percent of white men, and 85 percent of black men admitted to coitus before the age of 20.[146] Consistent with these findings, reported rates of STD are disproportionately greater in blacks, but the rates of STD in whites have increased as their sexual behavior has changed. The percentage of white coeds reporting premarital sex, stable at about 20 percent in studies from 1953 to 1967, has doubled in recent years, coincident with widespread availability of oral contraceptives. In fact, in this new era of sexual freedom, increasing pressure to perform sex with casual partners may have replaced pressure for sexual prohibition on college campuses, creating a new set of problems. In addition, there has been a change in sexual practices with more partners practicing fellatio, cunnilingus, anilingus, and penorectal intromission. This has influenced both the type of infections and the manner in which they present.

In managing these diseases, physicians often act simultaneously at three levels to help

1. Those directly affected, by preventing serious complications
2. Those affected secondarily, such as children or partners, by preventive or abortive therapy
3. The general public, by interrupting transmission

The purpose of this chapter is to provide a sound data base for such appropriate managment by describing the major conditions and then discussing the approach to the diagnosis of common clinical problems.

GONORRHEA

The number of reported cases of gonorrhea in the United States rose dramatically in the decade beginning in 1965, to over 1 million in 1978. Reasons usually given for this include

1. Demographic changes with an increasing number of sexually active persons at risk, i.e., more young persons, divorced, or separated, etc.
2. Change in sexual attitudes and behavior with an increase in activity with multiple partners, especially in the form of casual sexual encounters
3. The short incubation period of the infection, which averages 3 to 5 days, coupled with the increased mobility of the population, making interruption of spread difficult
4. Increased resistance of the organism to antibiotics, such as penicillin, requiring much larger doses for cure
5. The abandonment of the condom or barrier contraceptives, which may have decreased transmission
6. Better reporting of cases as more people seek help for STD in public clinics, rather than from private physicians

Except in the neonate, and some young children, gonorrhea is virtually always transmitted sexually. In prepubertal patients, older than 1 year, with gonorrhea, one must strongly consider sexual molestation.[150,152,159,160,174]

Uncomplicated Gonorrhea

The most common forms of uncomplicated gonorrhea are urethritis, cervicitis, anorectal infection, and pharyngitis. The efficiency of a single genital-to-genital transmission has been estimated to be 80 to 90 percent from infected male to exposed female, and about 20 to 50 percent from infected female to exposed male.

Urethritis, the most common manifestation of gonorrhea in males, is asymptomatic in 5 percent of newly infected patients; in the remainder, the discharge varies from slightly mucoid to very purulent. As symptomatic patients are treated, the percent of asymptomatic carriers of gonorrhea among those infected increases. Approximately 40 percent of male contacts of women with pelvic inflammatory disease (PID) have asymptomatic infection.[149]

The major site of primary infection in prepubertal girls is the vagina, and in postpubertal women, the cervix. In one study, about 80 percent of women had symptoms soon after infection, including a purulent or increased vaginal discharge, dysuria, abnormal menstrual bleeding in the first cycle after infection, lower abdominal pain, and anorectal symptoms.

Anorectal involvement occurs in approximately 40 percent of women and 50 percent of homosexual males, especially those males who play a receptor role in penorectal intercourse. Anorectal symptoms are present in up to 10 percent of infected patients. The most frequent complaints are anal itching and irritation, painful defecation, sensation of rectal fullness, and constipation. Signs include erythema and edema of the anal crypts, an anal discharge, and rarely, rectal bleeding or frank ulcerative proctitis.[157]

Gonococcal pharyngeal infection occurs principally from fellatio and rarely from cunnilingus. Up to 10 percent of women and 25 percent of homosexual men with gonorrhea have pharyngeal involvement. Although 20 to 30 percent of patients with pharyngeal infection have signs or symptoms, it is difficult in the individual case to ascribe these to gonococcal infection because sore throat is a more frequent complaint among patients who practice fellatio than those who do not and because of the possibility of other intercurrent infections.

Complicated Gonorrhea

PID occurs in 10 to 20 percent of infected women. It appears to result from direct spread of organisms from the endocervix through the uterine cavity to the fallopian tubes often during the first menstrual period after acquisition. The risk of PID is three- to ninefold greater in women with intrauterine devices, especially in the first month after insertion.

PID is generally divided into acute, chronic, and recurrent forms. Gonococcal PID should be differentiated from the nongonococcal form.[173] In one study, 89 percent of patients with no previous history of salpin-

gitis were infected with gonococci.[165] Recurrences in the first month often are due to gonococcal infection from asymptomatically infected male partners; later recurrences are more often associated with other organisms, such as anaerobic peptostreptococci, *Bacteroides fragilis*, and Chlamydia. Fewer than half the patients with a history of three or more episodes of PID have gonococcal infections.

Acute signs and symptoms include fever, chills, malaise, anorexia, nausea, and vomiting. Lower abdomial pain may vary from being a very mild discomfort (so-called "VD clinic PID"), to being very severe with peritoneal signs. There may be a yellow endocervical discharge and exquisite pain on movement of the cervix. Polymorphonuclear leukocytosis may be absent in 50 percent, and the erythrocyte sedimentation rate normal in 25 percent, again depending upon severity.

Hospitalization is usually preferable where

1. The diagnosis is uncertain and surgical emergencies such as appendicitis and ectopic pregnancy must be excluded.
2. The diagnosis is certain, but the patient is severely ill, pregnant, or unable to follow or tolerate an outpatient regimen.
3. Pelvic abscess is suspected.
4. The patient fails to respond to outpatient therapy.

Definitive diagnosis of PID may require laparoscopy. In one study of 800 patient who underwent laparoscopy, only 65 percent of the cases had the diagnosis of PID confirmed. Other disorders were detected in 12 percent, and 23 percent were visually normal. The most common conditions confused with acute salpingitis were acute appendicitis, endometriosis, ovarian cyst, and tubal pregnancy.[155]

About 15 percent of women develop unilateral obstruction of the fallopian tubes after a single episode of PID. This may lead to tubo-ovarian abscess. These patients have a greater risk of ectopic pregnancy. Lastly, perihepatitis or the Fitzhugh-Curtis syndrome is an uncommon complication occurring in women, probably from contiguous spread.

Dissemination of the gonococcus is often associated with asymptomatic carriage in all sites including the pharynx.[174] Recent studies have suggested that dissemination is more likely to occur in patients with abnormalities in complement activity. The organisms that disseminate have more fastidious nutrient requirements and are more susceptible to antibiotics. The most common form of systemic disease is the arthritis-dermatitis syndrome. Less common forms are endocarditis and meningitis. Conjunctivitis, another form of gonococcal infection, is usually due to direct inoculation.

Patients with arthritis-dermatitis syndrome often present with polyarthralgias, fever, and a tenosynovitis involving tendons around the wrist or the ankle. The arthritis develops in the wrist, ankles, and knees. Skin lesions usually begin as small papules on an erythematous base and develop a central targeting. Organisms may be seen in Gram stain of material from the lesions, and sometimes can be cultured. Fever and bacteremia occur early in the course of the disease. After the development of frank arthritis, joint effusions are usually culture-positive.

Diagnosis and Treatment

Gram stain, when performed on an adequate specimen of exudate, will show *Neisseria gonorrhoeae*, a gram-negative intracellular diplococcus, in more than 90 percent of symptomatic males with gonococcal urethritis, but only two-thirds of women with cervicitis and 30 percent of patients with rectal involvement. Gram stains of pharyngeal exudate are not useful because of confusion with neisseria in normal respiratory flora. Like other techniques, the usefulness of a Gram stain is directly proportional to the skill of the observer. Except in the case of the urethral exudate, Gram stains should not be relied upon for the diagnosis of gonorrhea.

The sensitivity (true positive rate) of a single culture swab is 90 to 98 percent in a *symptomatic* male with urethritis and 80 to 93 percent in a female with cervicitis. Rectal and pharyngeal cultures are slightly less reliable. Delay in plating or improper handling (failure to use selective media, or to incubate plates under higher CO_2 tension) may result in missing 20 percent or more of isolates.

Treatment regimens are outlined in Table 88–2.[148] None is completely effective. Despite this, most recurrent infections after appropriate treatment are due to reinfection. However, since infection by penicillinase (beta-lactamase) producing *Neisseria gonorrhoea* can occur, post-treatment isolates should be tested for penicillinase production. Spectinomycin is the drug of choice in treating anyone suspected of being a treatment failure.

Repeat culture of the infected site should be taken about 1 week after completion of therapy for test of cure. All women treated for gonorrhea should have anal canal cultures obtained routinely. In order to increase the certainty of the culture results, two separate swabs inoculated on a biplate are recommended for pharyngeal and rectal infections. In high

risk patients, e.g., recidivists, a second reculture is recommended at 4 weeks after therapy. Other important parts of the diagnostic and treatment plan include consideration of other STD, follow-up and immediate treatment of all sexual contacts, and patient education.

SYPHILIS

Syphilis illustrates how we must adapt our approach to a disease as its natural history changes. In the Middle Ages, it was called "Great Pox" because it produced larger lesions and was generally more severe than small pox.[166] Its variety of presentations led Osler to call it the "great imitator" and to state that "he who knows syphilis, knows medicine." With widespread use of penicillin and effective contact tracing, there has been a dramatic decrease in the prevalence of late untreated disease. There has also been a recent change in its epidemiology; infectious syphilis now is more common among male homosexuals or bisexuals who are more apt to have multiple anonymous and transient liaisons. They also may represent a relatively underserved population and when they do seek care, their sexual preference is more likely to remain unidentified by the health care provider.[143,150,152,160,171]

Paralleling the decline in prevalence has been a decreased ability of physicians to recognize the disease and of laboratory personnel to perform such techniques as darkfield microscopy. Of necessity, newer strategies have evolved for the use of serologic testing. Fortunately, the organism is still sensitive to penicillin, and, unlike gonorrhea, there has been no need to alter therapy. Such changes in natural history and prevalence of disease, which are not unique to syphilis, force us to adapt our knowledge and behavior accordingly.

Acquired Syphilis

Syphilis is a chronic infection with the spirochete, *Treponema pallidum*. The organism is rapidly killed on exposure to oxygen, drying, or soap and water. Transmitted by intimate sexual contact, the organism penetrates mucous membranes and apparently unbroken skin through minute abrasions. The disease is divided into different stages (Table 88–3).

PRIMARY STAGE. The chancre, characteristic of primary syphilis, is usually found in the genital area, mouth, or rectum, but may occur anywhere. Beginning as a single painless papule, it evolves into a 2- to 20-mm diameter ulcer with a clean base and heaped-up indurated edges. The thin serum overlying the ulcer contains many spirochetes. Men with genital le-

---

TABLE 88-2
Treatment of Gonorrhea*

Part A: Comparison of Treatment Schedules for Uncomplicated Gonococcal Infection†

	Aqueous Procaine Penicillin G (4 800 000 U) plus Probenecid (1 g)	Tetracycline (0.5 g Four Times Daily)	Ampicillin (3.5 g) or Amoxicillin (3 g) plus Probenecid (1 g)	Spectinomycin (2 g)‡
Route of administration	Intramuscular plus oral	Oral	Oral	Intramuscular
Duration of treatment	Single dose	5 days	Single dose	Single dose
Efficacy in gonococcal infection				
Genital	Good	Good	Good	Good
Pharyngeal	Good	Good	Poor	Uncertain
Anorectal (men)§	Good	Poor	Poor	Good
Anorectal (women)§	Good	Good	Good	Good
Aborts incubating (seronegative) syphilis	Yes	Probably	Probably	No
Effective against *Chlamydia trachomatis*	No	Yes	No	No
Prevents postgonococcal urethritis	No	Yes	No	No
Safe for use in pregnancy	Yes	No	Yes	Probably

Part B: Treatment Schedules for Complicated or Disseminated Gonorrhea

I.   Treatment of Acute Salpingitis (PID)
   A. Outpatient‖
      1. Tetracycline 0.5 g orally 4 times a day for 10 days, or
      2. Standard APPG, ampicillin, or amoxicillin regimen (above), followed by ampicillin or amoxicillin 0.5 g orally 4 times a day for 10 days
   B. Hospitalized patient
      1. Aqueous crystalline penicillin G, 20 million units IV daily until improvement, then 0.5 g ampicillin orally 4 times a day to complete 10 days, or
      2. Alternative tetracycline regimen in penicillin-allergic patients who are not pregnant, with normal renal function: 0.25 g IV 4 times a day until improvement, followed by 0.5 g orally 4 times a day to complete 10 days

II. Treatment of Arthritis-Dermatitis Syndrome
   A. In patients without known allergy to penicillin or probenecid
      1. Aqueous crystalline penicillin G, 10 million units intravenously per day for 3 days or until there is significant clinical improvement. This may be followed with ampicillin, 0.5 g 4 times a day orally to complete 7 days of antibiotic treatment, or
      2. Ampicillin, 3.5 g orally, plus probenecid 1 g, followed by ampicillin, 0.5 g 4 times a day orally for at least 7 days
   B. In patients allergic to penicillin and/or probenecid
      1. Tetracycline 0.5 g 4 times a day orally for at least 7 days. Tetracycline should not be used for complicated gonococcal infection in pregnant women because of potential toxic effects for mother and fetus, or
      2. Erythromycin 0.5 g orally 4 times a day for 7 days, or
      3. Spectinomycin 2.0 g IM twice a day for 3 days

---

* The reader must be alert to changes in recommended therapy as new drugs are discovered and tested, or micro-organisms adapt to medications in current use. See Cefoxitin treatment of Penicillinase-producing *Neisseria gonorrhoeae*. N. Engl. J. Med., 301:509–511, 1979. (This article was published after the table was prepared.)
† Part A reprinted with permission from Ann. Intern. Med. 90:845, 1979.
‡ Regimen for infection with penicillinase-producing gonococci and treatment failures.
§ Zaidi, A. A., personal communication.
‖ Same regimen for gonococcal epididymitis in the male.

TABLE 88-3
Outline of Clinical Stages of Syphilis*

Stage	Characteristic Findings	Usual Onset after Exposure	Persistence in Untreated Patients	Presence of Treponemes	Serologic Results % Reactive	
					VDRL	FTA-ABS
Primary	Chancre—may be absent or not visible (e.g., in vagina, mouth)	10–90 days (21-average)	2–6 weeks	+	78	85
Secondary	Rash—Condyloma latum	6 weeks–6 months	2–6 weeks recurrences in 25% over 2 year period	+ (Especially moist lesions)	97	99
Acute syphilitic meningitis	Headache, cranial nerve lesions, papilledema, seizures, CSF lymphocytosis, and increase protein	6 weeks–2 years	Not applicable	+ CSF	97	99
Latent Early‡ Late‡	None† Late (tertiary)	After or between above stages if they develop	May be life long— only ⅓ of untreated patients develop tertiary syphilis	–	74	95
Late (3‡) Benign	Gumma—skin, bone, cartilage, liver	2–10 years	Indolent	–	77	95
Cardiovascular	Aortic aneurysm Aortic insufficiency	10–30 years 2–3 times more common in men than in women	Progressive, may be fatal	Aorta may be +	77	95
Neurosyphilis Asymptomatic— None Meningovascular— signs of infection depending on area involved; Paresis—may be mild to severe psychosis; Tabes dorsalis— signs of posterior column degeneration; Combinations or modifications of above	CSF cell count and protein are increased in proportion to the activity of the process	5–35 years	Progressive, may be fatal	CSF or brain may be +	77	95

* Modified and reprinted with permission from Ill. Med. J. 152:499, 1977.
† For definitive diagnosis, i.e., to exclude asymptomatic neurosyphilis, a lumbar puncture may be performed (see text).
‡ Variously defined—usual division at 4 years; for epidemiologic purposes (contact tracing) 1 year is more practical.

(Continued)

┌─ **TABLE 88–3(cont.)** ──────────────────────────────

Stage	Characteristic Findings	Usual Onset after Exposure	Persistence in Untreated Patients	Presence of Treponemes	Serologic Results % Reactive	
					VDRL	FTA-ABS
Congenital Early	Rash, mucous patches, rhinitis	Up to 2 years	Neonatal onset usually severe and often fatal	+	Almost invariably positive in early stage but in neonates, passive placental transfer must be differentiated from active infection. In later stages, results are similar to those in acquired syphilis (above)	
Late	Interstitial keratitis, Hutchinson's teeth, VIIIth nerve deafness Periostitis of nose ("saddle nose") and of shin (saber shin) May be same as adults, i.e., latent or late syphilis	After 2 years	Lifetime	Usually –		

sions usually have bilateral inguinal lymphadenopathy; and women, pelvic lymphadenopathy.

SECONDARY STAGE.   The primary stage may be entirely absent. It also may overlap in 25 percent of cases with the secondary stage, which develops approximately 6 weeks to 6 months after exposure. The latter is characterized by skin lesions that are principally macular and papular, but not vesicular or bullous. Secondary syphilis can involve all areas, but lesions on the palms and soles are highly suggestive. Scalp and eyelash alopecia has been reported. A flat, wart-like lesion, condyloma latum, may develop and should be distinguished from the more common condyloma acuminatum, a pointy, fleshy wart (described later). Although all lesions are infectious, those involving the mucous membrane of the mouth or vagina (mucous patches) or moist areas of the skin, such as condyloma latum, are particularly so.

There may be associated fever, headache, rhinitis, conjunctivitis, sore throat, and arthralgia. Generalized, nontender lymphadenopathy characteristically involves the inguinal, epitrochlear, and axillary nodes. Occasionally, hepatitis, immune-complex nephropathy, deafness, or iritis may occur. Although 15 percent or more of patients with secondary syphilis may have an abnormal spinal fluid, very few develop clinical signs of meningitis. In the absence of meningeal signs or symptoms, lumbar puncture is not indicated. Virtually all patients have positive serologic tests.

The major differential consideration is pityriasis rosea, a seasonal disease thought to be caused by a virus. It is characterized by a single, large initial lesion called the herald patch. This is followed by erythematous, maculopapular lesions along the lines of skin cleavage on the trunk. In most cases, these do not appear on the soles and palms. A major distinguishing feature is intense pruritus with pityriasis rosea. Darkfield examination in this condition is negative. Other considerations in the differential diagnosis are psoriasis, lichen planus, tinea versicolor, drug eruption, condyloma acuminatum, and infectious mononucleosis.

LATENT STAGE.   In untreated patients, secondary eruptions clear within 4 to 12 weeks, but may recur over a 4-year period. Patients then enter the latent stage, i.e., true positive serology without clinical evidence of syphilis. For epidemiologic purposes, latent syphilis is divided at 1 year into early and late because retrieving contacts of patients with syphilis of greater than 1-year duration is unlikely to turn up any new infections.

TERTIARY STAGE.   In the preantibiotic era, approximately 30 percent of untreated patients went on to develop late syphilis (Table 88–3); however, tertiary syphilis is uncommon today. The three principal forms are late benign, cardiovascular, and neurosyphilis. Late benign syphilis is so called because the lesions are seldom incapacitating except when they involve the brain. The usual lesion, the gumma, does not contain organisms and appears to be a hypersensitivity reaction.

Cardiovascular syphilis is two to three times more common in untreated men than women. The basic lesion involves destruction of the elastic tissue of the media of the aorta and an endarteritis of the vasa vasorum. Clinical sequelae include aneurysmal dilatation of the aorta, usually of the ascending portion or the arch. This may be associated with calcification of the ascending aorta from superimposed atherosclerosis, which is almost pathognomonic of syphilis. Progressive dilatation of the aortic ring results in increasingly severe aortic insufficiency and heart failure. Atrial fibrillation is rarely associated with syphilitic aortic incompetence, in contrast to its frequency in rheumatic aortic regurgitation. Coronary ostial obstruction may coexist with aortic incompetence and result in angina pectoris and myocardial infarction. Treatment may arrest the disease but does not reverse it.

Neurosyphilis occurs in a variety of forms:

Asymptomatic Neurosyphilis. By definition, this applies to otherwise well patients with a reactive blood serology and an abnormal spinal fluid.

Meningovascular Syphilis. Headache, irritability, delirium, convulsions, change in personality, amnesia, or neck stiffness may be among the initial symptoms. Cranial nerve involvement, including optic neuritis, as well as papilledema are frequent. Hemiparesis may result from endarteritis and acute vascular occlusion.

Tabes Dorsalis. This is characterized by signs of posterior column degeneration with ataxia, areflexia, paresthesias, bladder disturbance, impotence, lightning pains in the extremities and severe gastric disturbance ("gastric crisis"). These patients may develop trophic joint changes (Charcot's joints). A typical finding is the Argyll Robertson pupil, i.e., one which is small, irregular, and can accommodate but fails to react to light.

General Paresis. This is characterized by the insidious onset of changes in personality, with irritability, insomnia, poor judgment, forgetfulness, and decreasing intellectual capacity. In the early stage of paresis, neurologic signs are uncommon. Progressive dementia occurs with periods of euphoria and delusions of grandeur; increasing paranoia eventually leads to incapacitation requiring institutionalization.

As the condition progresses, slurring of speech, tremors of the hands and tongue, and hyperactivity of the biceps, triceps, knee, and ankle reflexes may be noted.

Diagnosis

The diagnosis of neurosyphilis can be very difficult. Kofman has called attention to the fact that classic neurosyphilis patterns are being replaced by atypical forms.[158] Spinal fluid protein and mononuclear cells are usually increased, but the sugar is normal except in rare cases of acute syphilitic meningitis. The colloidal gold (mastic) curve is no longer used to differentiate forms of neurosyphilis. A positive cerebrospinal fluid (CSF) serology, although not invariable, clinches the diagnosis.

Syphilis In Pregnancy

Pregnancy during untreated syphilis in the first year of illness carries a risk of 80 to 90 percent chance of transmission to the fetus. Twenty-five percent of untreated fetuses infected in utero die before birth. Another 20 to 30 percent die shortly after birth if they remain untreated. Of the infected untreated children who survive infancy, 40 percent develop symptomatic syphilis. Adequate treatment before the 16th week of gestation will prevent the disease in the infant; treatment thereafter can arrest progression. The severity of persistent stigmata is proportional to the duration of uterine infection.

Congenital syphilis principally refers to infection of the fetus in utero (prenatal) but a child can be infected during the passage through the birth canal (neonatal). (Table 88–3) This condition is reviewed elsewhere.[171]

Syphilis Serology

The easiest and often the only method for syphilis diagnosis is serologic.[156] The most widely used variations of the original Wassermann test are the Venereal Disease Research Laboratory (VDRL) and the Rapid Plasma Reagin (RPR) test. These are called nontreponemal tests because they detect antibody to a nonspecific lipoprotein antigen, resulting from the combination of the organism and host tissues. They have different sensitivities (percentage of true positives detected) at different stages of the disease (see Table 88–3) and are useful as screening tests because of their simplicity, reproducibility, and low cost. Both tests are expressed in the highest dilution at which the test is fully reactive. RPR titers are generally higher than VDRL titers, so they cannot be used interchangeably when comparing test results.

Fluorescent treponemal antibody absorption test

(FTA-ABS) and the microhemagglutination test for *Treponema pallidum* (MHA-TP) tests are called treponemal tests because they detect antibody specifically directed at *Treponema pallidum*. The FTA-ABS is now the confirmatory test of choice in patients suspected of having syphilis because of its greater sensitivity and specificity under ideal conditions. Because it is more complex than the VDRL, it is more vulnerable to error, especially at low levels of reactivity.[142] The FTA-ABS test should be used only to confirm a positive VDRL, or in the case of a negative VDRL when tertiary syphilis is suspected. Patients with a previously positive FTA-ABS should not be retested since reversion to negative is uncommon except in very early treatment of primary syphilis.[169]

Treatment

The drug of choice is penicillin. Based on in vitro studies, serum concentration of 0.03 units of penicillin/ml gives several times the tissue levels needed to kill *Treponema pallidum*. This level should be maintained for at least 7 to 10 days in early syphilis. Benzathine penicillin (Bicillin LA) satisfies these criteria. *Treponema pallidum* disappears from lesions of primary syphilis in 6 to 24 hours after treatment with penicillin. In penicillin allergic patients, tetracycline and erythromycin are preferred alternatives (Table 88–4). Because of the inability to achieve adequate levels of penicillin in the CSF after treatment with benzathine penicillin, it is recommended that in active neurosyphilis, 12 to 24 million units of intravenous aqueous crystalline penicillin G be given daily for 10 days.[153]

Complications of therapy include allergic reactions and the Jarisch-Herxheimer (JH) reaction. Anaphylaxis from parenteral penicillin is the most feared reaction. Although its incidence is extremely low, one must be prepared by having an emergency cart available and cautioning the patient to remain in the waiting room for at least 30 minutes after receiving intramuscular penicillin. The JH reaction occurs in active disease and is believed to be caused by microbial lysis and the release of endotoxin. Reactions consist of fever and development of more prominent signs, such as deepening of a rash. They are transient and occur only with the first dose. Severe reactions have been rarely reported in patients with neurosyphilis or aortic disease.

Follow-Up

Follow-up is essential since 2 to 10 percent of patients with early syphilis will not respond to appropriate treatment. The indices for successful treatment are few. Clinical signs in early syphilis will disappear even without treatment. Aortic aneurysms persist and, in fact, may progress with continued stress upon the weakened wall. The effect of treatment upon the signs and symptoms of neurosyphilis is directly related to the degree of active inflammation as indicated by pretreatment CSF.

The titer of nontreponemal tests remains the most useful index of effective treatment, especially in early syphilis or where the titers tend to be higher. In patients who have sero-negative darkfield positive primary syphilis, treatment may abort the development of positive serology. After adequate treatment of sero-positive patients in primary, secondary, or early latent stage of less than a year, nontreponemal tests will usually revert to negative or show a fourfold or greater drop, i.e., 1:32 to 1:8 or lower in 9 to 12 months. In the absence of such change, retreatment is indicated. Titers are usually so low in late latent or late syphilis that a fourfold drop cannot be noted. Consequently, one must follow the patient for a

---

TABLE 88–4
Recommended Treatment Schedules for Syphilis

Syphilis Stage	Benzathine Penicillin G (Bicillin LA) Intramuscular	Major Alternatives to Penicillin—Oral Tetracycline or Erythromycin*
Primary and Secondary		
Latent† and contacts to infectious syphilis	2.4 million units single session	30 g (2 q.d. × 15)
Latent‡ and late syphilis	7.2 million units (2.4 million units weekly × 3)	60 g (2 g q.d. × 30)

* Erythromycin is preferable in penicillin-allergic pregnant patients.
† Of less than 1 year's duration.
‡ Of greater than 1 year's duration.

longer period and check for development of clinical signs or a rise in titer as an evidence of inadequate therapy.

There is no natural immunity to syphilis. Over 90 percent of reported reinfections have occurred in patients who were treated in the first 6 months of their disease. Patients treated years after acquisition of the disease have also been shown to be more resistant to experimental reinfection.

CHANCROID

Although common in tropical areas, only 455 cases of chancroid were reported in the United States in 1978.[150,160] Herpes and syphilis are sometimes misdiagnosed as chancroid. Caused by *Haemophilus ducreyi*, it characteristically starts as an inflammatory macule which progresses to a nonindurated shallow ulceration with an erythematous margin. The ulcer is ragged, undermined, and has a base covered with yellow or gray exudate. Typically, lesions are multiple and painful. Unilateral inguinal adenopathy occurs in one-half of patients after about 2 weeks.

Definitive diagnosis is extremely difficult. Gram stain reveals short gram-negative rods often in chains ("school of fish"). Culture requires special techniques and is unreliable except in expert hands. Treatment involves local hygiene and the administration of sulfathiazole or tetracycline.

GRANULOMA INGUINALE

Caused by *Calymmatobacterium granulomatis*, the disease is found in tropical or subtropical areas and is rare in the United States.[150,160] The number of cases reported in the United States in 1978 was 75. Incubation period is approximately 2 to 12 weeks. Genital lesions may progress to elevated masses of beefy granulation tissue or ulcers. Confirmation requires demonstration of intracytoplasmic gram-negative rods with polar-staining in large mononuclear cells (Donovan bodies). Recommended therapy is with tetracycline for 2 to 4 weeks.

LYMPHOGRANULOMA VENEREUM (LGV)

The number of reported cases of LGV in the United States in 1978 was 348.[150,160] Caused by serotypes of *Chlamydia trachomatis*, it has an incubation period of 1 to 12 weeks (usually 7 to 12 days). It begins as a small erosion or painless vesicle which is usually not seen when the patient presents with lymphatic enlargement. Inguinal adenopathy occurs when the clitoris, vulva, or male genitals are involved. Iliac and anorectal nodes enlarge when the rectum or vagina are involved.

The diagnosis is made by noting a fourfold rise in

Psittacosis-LGV complement fixation test and the presence of clinical signs of LGV. A single titer of 1:64 or greater is suspicious but not diagnostic. The Frei test is neither specific nor sensitive and is no longer available. Antimicrobial therapy with tetracycline or sulfathiazole is recommended.

NONGONOCOCCAL URETHRITIS

The various names of this condition are instructive: "nonspecific urethritis" (NSU), "nongonococcal urethritis" (NGU), and "postgonococcal urethritis" (PGU). The name "NSU" resulted from its once having been a disease in search of an etiology. However, it is now believed that about 50 percent of cases are caused by *Chlamydia trachomatis*, up to 30 percent by *Ureaplasma urealyticum* (T strain mycoplasma), and 1 to 2 percent by *Trichomonas hominis*, candida, and *Herpes simplex* virus. The cause of the remaining 15 to 20 percent is unknown. The name NGU reflects, however, that this is still a disease of exclusion, i.e., ruling out gonorrhea rules in NGU. PGU is so called because about 25 percent of males with gonococcal urethritis may be simultaneously infected with one of the agents causing NGU. In such cases, shortly after adequate treatment with penicillin or ampicillin (which do not affect NGU), the patient exhibits signs of NGU.[150-152,154]

NGU accounts for 30 to 90 percent of acute urethritis in males, depending upon race, socioeconomic status, type of sexual activity, and age. The percentage of patients with urethritis in whom gonococci have been isolated has varied from 8 percent in college students to 32 percent in whites attending a public clinic, to 60 percent in blacks attending a public clinic. NGU is a less common cause of urethritis than gonorrhea in men who are exclusively homosexual.

The incubation period varies from about 1 to 3 weeks. The most common presenting complaint is the appearance of a bead of pus at the urethral meatus on arising, hence the name "morning drop." The urethra is usually washed clean with urination and when the patient is seen later in the day, no discharge may be visible. On milking the urethra, about 80 percent of patients will have a discharge, which is usually scant and mucoid. Other complaints include tingling or burning with urination and meatal pruritus.

Diagnosis is principally by Gram stain of the discharge demonstrating polymorphonuclear or mononuclear leukocytes, but no gonococci. Facilities to isolate Chlamydia and T stain mycoplasma isolation are not yet routinely available.

Therapy consists of tetracycline in a dosage of 0.5 g four times a day for 1 week. This allows for coverage of the occasional patient with gonorrhea in whom the Gram stain is negative. Chlamydia infection of the cervix occurs in up to 70 percent of sexual contacts of infected men. Similarly, contacts of nonchlamydial NGU have a high yield of *Ureaplasma urealyticum*. This explains the high rate of relapse of NGU; half the patients relapse in the year following infection. Consequently, if there is a steady relationship, it is advisable to treat the partner with 250 mg of tetracycline four times a day for 7 days.

In refractory cases, the patient and his partner should be examined for Trichomonas infection. If no other etiologic agents are found, tetracycline therapy should be reinstituted for 3 weeks. About half of cases of "so-called" idiopathic epididymitis may be caused by Chlamydia. Urethral strictures are uncommon complications of nongonococcal urethritis. Since serotypes of *Chlamydia trachomatis* produce trachoma, conjunctivitis and other genital infections, these conditions are occasionally associated. One should be alert to the growing evidence that Chlamydia plays a role in nongonococcal PID.[173]

GENITAL HERPES

The most common cause of a genital sore, this condition is principally caused by herpes virus hominis serotype 2.[152,160,162,164] From 200,000–500,000 patients annually seek care for genital herpes in the United States. After an incubation period of 3 to 6 days, multiple painful vesicles appear at the site of infection with little satellite crops appearing over the next few days. The vesicles usually break, leaving a 2- to 5-mm shallow ulcer with nonindurated edges. Fever, headache, malaise, and myalgia occur in about 30 percent of patients with symptomatic primary infection. Complications include secondary infection of the lesion, dysuria with urinary retention, painful defecation and fecal retention, sacral radiculopathy, and aseptic meningitis. Because of the risk of transmission to infants during vaginal delivery, Caesarean section should be performed before rupture of membranes in women with active lesions who are about to deliver.

Examination of a Giemsa stain of fluid from an intact vesicle for multinucleated giant cells and intracellular inclusions is highly sensitive. Unruptured vesicles on the skin yield herpes virus in tissue culture more often than those from vaginal and cervical sites. Acute and convalescent herpes complement fixation antibody titers are useful for confirmation.

Primary herpes lasts 2 or 3 weeks unless there is secondary infection. About two-thirds of patients develop recurrences, which diminish in frequency and severity with time. Pain and virus shedding last about 4 days, and lesions disappear in about 11 days.

In controlled trials, there is no evidence that such therapies as idoxuridine or phototherapy shorten the course of the infection. Consequently, therapy is entirely supportive, using anesthetic ointments, Sitz baths, or betadine gel for relief of pain. The lesions should be kept dry and patients should wear cotton underwear, avoiding nylon underwear or pantyhose which facilitate spread by trapping moisture and preventing air circulation. Patients should refrain from intercourse until the lesions are completely healed. Previously infected males should be advised to use condoms in the year following infection, especially when they have prodromal symptoms, because viral shedding can precede the development of lesions. Infected women should obtain Pap smears annually because of accumulating evidence of an association between herpes virus 2 infection and carcinoma of the cervix.

GENITAL WARTS (Condyloma Acuminatum)

More than 200,000 patients in the United States are annually infected by the papovavirus responsible for genital warts.[160,174] Lesions occur on the genitalia perianal region, or urethra, 3 months after exposure to an infected patient in two-thirds of sex contacts. Growth is enhanced by vaginal discharge, heavy perspiration or poor personal hygiene. The warts sometimes enlarge during pregnancy and then regress after delivery. An uncommon form seen more in whites is the giant benign wart (Buschke-Lowenstein tumor). The development of laryngeal polyps in the first 6 months after birth and has been noted in newborns of mothers with genital warts.

Therapy consists of applying 10 to 25 percent podophyllin as a tincture or in benzoin. The skin around the base of the lesion should be protected with petrolatum jelly. Patients should wash the treated sites about 4 hours after application, to prevent the possibility of severe irritation. Podophyllin should not be used in pregnant women or on large or abraded areas due to its potential for toxicity. Lesions on moist surfaces respond best; refractory lesions often respond to therapy with liquid nitrogen, electrodesiccation, or surgical excision.

MOLLUSCUM CONTAGIOSUM

This condition is not always sexually transmitted. It is caused by a pox virus and has an incubation period of 1 to 6 weeks.[160,174] The characteristic presentation is a perigenital distribution of flesh-colored umbilicated papules, 2 to 10 mm in diameter. The clinical diagnosis can be confirmed by a potassium hydroxide (KOH) preparation of the specimen crushed between a slide and coverslip to reveal intracytoplasmic inclusions. Therapy consists of removing the central nodule by curettage, electrodesiccation, or silver nitrate treatment.[160,174]

PHTHIRUS PUBIS (Crabs)

This disease is caused by crab louse infestation of the pubic hair around the anus, abdomen, and thigh, and rarely, the axilla and eyelashes. The most pronounced symptom is itching. Diagnosis is made by locating the eggs (nits) or adult lice on the hair shaft. Therapy is with Kwell (1 percent gamma benzene hexachloride shampoo) massaged into the infected sites and applied to the hair from umbilicus to knees and left on for 10 to 15 minutes. Adherent nits should be removed with a fine tooth comb. Treatment may be repeated in 24 to 48 hours. Clothing and bedding should be washed or dry cleaned, even though the louse dies within 24 hours after separation from the host.[160,174]

SCABIES

This is caused by transfer of the itch mite *Sarcoptes scabiei* by close personal contact. The disease is usually asymptomatic for several weeks after infestation. Sensitization results in irritation and itching, especially at night. This leads to scratching and to secondary infection. The original lesions can be erythematous patches or follicular papules, vesicles, pustules, hives, or nodules. They can involve the nipples, palms, finger webs, flexor aspects of the wrist, extensor surfaces of the forearms, anterior axillary folds, the belt line, buttocks, genitalia, or borders of the feet. Definitive diagnosis is made by discovering the burrow and scraping the lesion, revealing a parasite under the microscope. The recommended therapy is the application of Kwell lotion to the affected areas and thorough rinsing after no more than 4 hours because of the potential toxicity.[160,163,174]

APPROACH TO COMMON CLINICAL PRESENTATIONS

Sexually transmitted diseases represent a special area of knowledge in general medicine. Management requires a nonjudgmental attitude on the part of the professional, an understanding of people and their behavior, and an ability to look beyond the presenting complaint. Human sexuality and problems in the genital area are among the most sensitive areas both physically and psychologically that a patient will discuss with a practitioner. Embarrassment may lead patients to be vague or to concoct a fictitious chief complaint in response to questioning by a clerk or

nurse in a public waiting room. They may be upset about a recent sexual encounter, laden with guilt or suspicion, and may express the wish for "a checkup." This is especially the case when someone has had a casual sexual encounter, outside of a steady relationship; return to the partner raises concerns about transmitting a disease.

Practitioners must overcome any embarrassment they may have and put the patient at ease. An approach that is both understanding and straightforward works best. Patients must be assured that frank questions will be asked to help ascertain their problem and that the answers will be kept strictly confidential. They should be urged to vent concerns they have about their illness before history taking. A standardized data base should then be collected in all patients.[144]

A careful history should include information about sexual preference, frequency and type of sexual practice, and number and nature of sexual partners. If the patient gives a history of STD contact, one should ascertain signs or symptoms the partners may have had and what they know about the etiology of the STD (culture results, epidemiologic referral, etc.). Sometimes "definite contacts" turn out to be those ones the patient is worried about, and the worry may have magnified into a certainty with the passage of time since the liaison.

After a careful examination with appropriate routine diagnostic procedures, such as culture for gonorrhea, wet preparation, and the like, one should explain the incubation period of the conditions with which the patients are concerned (usually gonorrhea and syphilis), discuss the likelihood of their acquisition, the signs and symptoms they should look for, and advise them concerning the use of barrier preventive measures when they do resume sexual activity with their partner. One should try to help the patient work through any difficult situation without resorting to lies, since such subterfuges undermine a relationship. Although honesty is the best policy, patients do not always wish to be straightforward, especially in the case of extramarital liaisons, because their relationship may be a tenuous one. The patient's wishes must be respected. At such times, one must resort to subterfuges such as "the need for a routine examination" to retrieve contacts. The current openness and honesty among youth about sex has made follow-up easier and more complete. Common presenting complaints are a urethral discharge, genital sore or rash, an abnormal serology, and a vaginal discharge. The purpose of this section is to discuss the approach to the definition and management of these problems.

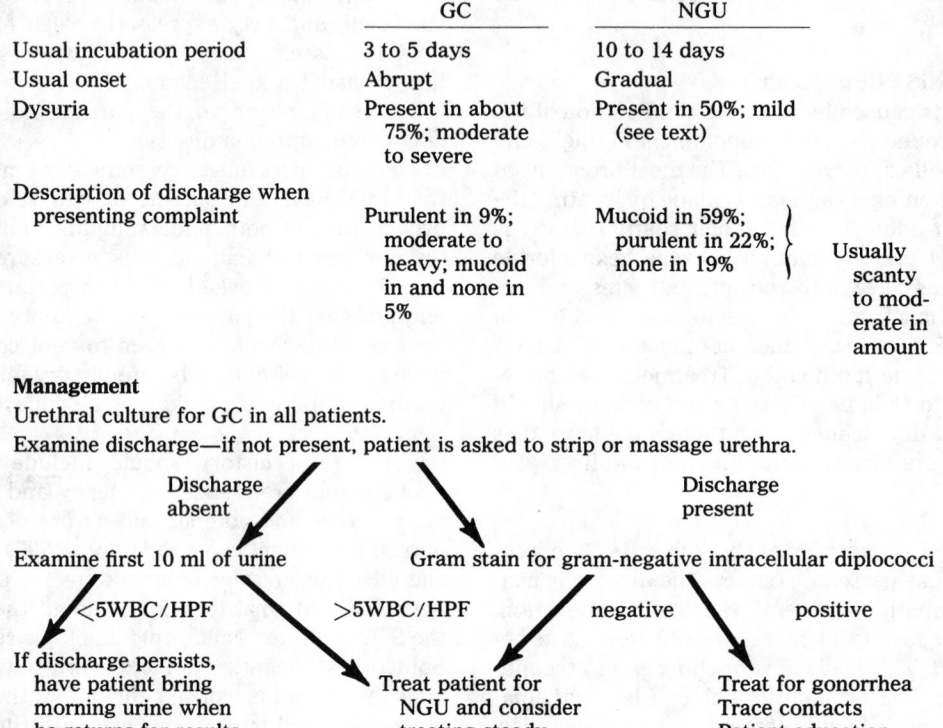

FIGURE 88-1. Approach to the diagnosis of urethritis.

URETHRAL DISCHARGE

Patients with nongonoccal urethritis (NGU) are more likely to be white, heterosexual, of higher socioeconomic status, and to have had first sexual activity at an older age, fewer sex partners, and NGU in the past. This only defines an average profile; an individual patient may not conform to this. Similarly, despite the usual features of gonorrhea or NGU outlined in Part A of Figure 88–1, patients may present with a picture varying from no symptoms to a florid urethritis.[154] Section B of Figure 88–1 outlines a management plan.

GENITAL SORE OR RASH

Sometimes the "sore" is a normal part of the person's anatomy, noticed in connection with a suspicious encounter. While it is important to always think of syphilis, the condition we cannot afford to miss, remember that other causes, such as genital herpes, are more common. Listed in Table 88–5 are the usual diagnostic considerations.

Approach to the diagnosis should include:

1. Determination of onset and likelihood that a contact within the incubation period had infectious syphilis or other condition. Availability of contacts, if limited in number, can help define the etiology in selected cases
2. Careful evaluation of the evolution and present state of the lesion. Often experienced clinicians can make a diagnosis on clinical grounds alone.
3. Use of diagnostic techniques as noted in the Table 88–5

Darkfield microscopy should be performed on all lesions where primary syphilis is suspected, e.g., indurated ulcers. Darkfield examination not only gives an immediate diagnosis, but in one-fifth of the cases may be the only positive test. Darkfield microscopy is performed in the following manner: The examiner, wearing gloves, takes a specimen by abrading the le-

―TABLE 88-5―
Approach to the Diagnosis of a Genital Sore*

	Incubation Period	Description	Number	Diagnosis
Primary syphilis (chancre)	10–90 days (usual 21 days)	Papule → painless indurated ulcer; nonvesicular; painless adenopathy	Single in at least 75%	Darkfield microscopy serology (see Table 88-3)
Genital herpes	3–6 days	Vesicular → 2–5 mm nonindurated painful ulcer; painful adenopathy	Multiple	Virus isolation, Wright's stain of vesicle fluids (see text)
Trauma	Immediate	Abrasion, tear, bite; painful initially	Single	History, presentation
Genital warts	? 3 months	Papillary flesh-colored painless wart, 10–15 mm	Multiple	Clinical
Molluscum contagiosum	? 1–6 weeks	2–10 mm umbilicated painless papules	Multiple crops	KOH preparation, (see text) clinical
Crabs	? 1–3 weeks	Excoriations, louse visible, itching	Multiple	Obtaining parasite microscopic confirmation
Scabies	3–6 weeks	Variable (see text); parasite invisible itching, excoriations	Multiple	Microscopic confirmation of organism from burrow
Chancroid	1–5 days	Soft superficial erosions, shallow ragged painful ulcers	Multiple	Very difficult (see text)
Granuloma inguinale	2–12 weeks	Masses of beefy granulation tissue usually in the inguinal area	Multiple	Gram stain for Donovan bodies
Lymphogranuloma venereum	1–12 weeks (usual, 7–12 days)	Not usually seen; transient painless erosion or vesicle	Single	Psittacosis LGV complement fixation test on paired sera

* Other considerations include candida infection, folliculitis, sebaceous cysts, seborrheic keratoses, benign papillomata, lichen planus, psoriasis, eczema, contact dermatitis, fixed drug eruption especially to phenolphthalein, and pearly penile papules.

sion in question to provoke exudate. The lesion is squeezed to allow more serum to accumulate on a slide or in a microhematocrit tube. The advantage of the latter is that the organism will remain motile in the tube until microscopic examination can be performed. Darkfield microscopy is not reliable on mouth lesions because most observers cannot differentiate *T. microdentium*, a normal inhabitant of the mouth, from *T. pallidum*. In suspect cases, the darkfield examination should be performed two or three times before findings are definitely considered nega-

tive. If the patient has used any salve, especially if it contains an antibiotic, this may be sufficient to give a false negative result. A serologic test for syphilis should be done routinely in patients suspected of having STD. An RPR can be very useful in the immediate determination of patients suspected of having primary syphilus.

A POSITIVE SEROLOGY
One of the commonest and often perplexing problems in practice is determining the significance of an ab-

normal serology. As noted in Figure 88–2, the patient's age, previous serologic results, the serologic titer, and the clinical context are the key points to focus on. When the clinical situation does not fit with the abnormal result, one should repeat the nontreponemal test because mix-up of patients' sera or laboratory error, though an infrequent event, can occur. The VDRL or RPR are highly reproducible. The next thing to focus on is the previous serologic results. If all previous serologies have been negative, one must do an FTA-ABS to differentiate a true positive from a false positive, the various resulting combinations are shown in Figure 88–2.[142,156,167]

In general, titers lower than 1 to 8 in any nontreponemal test can be seen in primary, latent, late or adequately treated serofast syphilis, and also as a false positive reaction. Titers greater than 1 to 8 are usually seen in early syphilis (primary, secondary, or early latent) and are infrequently false positive reactions. Depending upon the population sampled, as many as one-third of positive serologies may be false positive reactions. Acute false positive tests (less than 6 month's duration) are caused by recent vacci-

nations, infectious hepatitis, infectious mononucleosis, pneumonia, malaria, chicken pox, measles, leprosy, and intravenous drug abuse. Chronic false positive (greater than 6 months) occur in diseases of disordered immunity, especially systemic lupus erythematosus, rheumatoid arthritis (in some aged patients because of alteration of their immunoglobulin), in patients with long-term intravenous drug abuse, and on a hereditary basis.

About 5 in 1000 positive FTA-ABS tests will be false positive (a specificity of 99.5%). Since this test is complex, the average laboratory may have a lower specificity (i.e., a higher false positive rate) due to laboratory error. Biologic false positivity has been documented in systemic lupus erythematosus, rheumatoid arthritis, and thyroiditis. Borderline FTA-ABS tests are not considered to be positive tests; they are nondiagnostic and on repeat testing are usually negative. The approach to evaluating a positive serology is illustrated in Figure 88–2.

A common clinical situation is that of an older patient admitted to a hospital for other problems where the nontreponemal test comes back with a

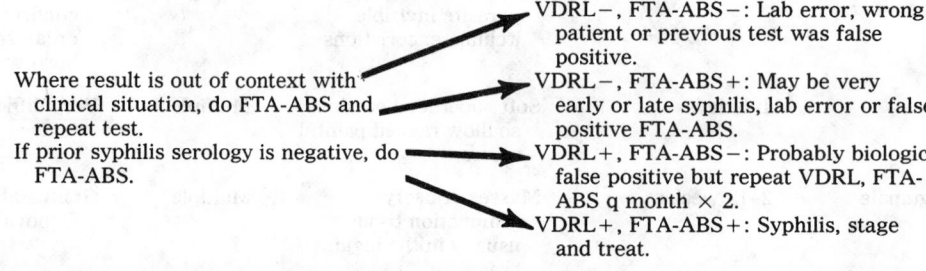

Where result is out of context with clinical situation, do FTA-ABS and repeat test.

If prior syphilis serology is negative, do FTA-ABS.

VDRL–, FTA-ABS–: Lab error, wrong patient or previous test was false positive.

VDRL–, FTA-ABS+: May be very early or late syphilis, lab error or false positive FTA-ABS.

VDRL+, FTA-ABS–: Probably biologic false positive but repeat VDRL, FTA-ABS q month × 2.

VDRL+, FTA-ABS+: Syphilis, stage and treat.

1. Note titer of VDRL; greater than 1:8 early syphilis likely.

2. Obtain results and date of previous serologic tests. In patients with prior syphilis, VDRL or RPR titer should fall at least fourfold in response to Rx. Stable or fourfold ↑ in titer indicates Rx failure or reinfection.

3. Obtain contact history (stage of contact if available); if contact to infectious syphilis within incubation period, check for primary syphilis. If negative, treat epidemiologically as "incubating syphilis."

4. Type of sexual activity and area of contact—to locate possible lesion.

5. History of sore, rash or conditions leading to false positive.

6. Physical exam: especially note sore, rash (Darkfield if present); Darkfield positive = clinical confirmation of primary or secondary syphilis stage, treat and trace contacts.

7. Latent syphilis diagnosed in absence of: a) history of recent contact to infectious case; b) prior history of adequate treatment; or c) signs of syphilis. If serology nonreactive in past year: a) classify as early latent; b) trace contacts. If serology was reactive for more than a year, and there are no neurologic signs or symptoms, CSF exam need not be performed to differentiate latent syphilis from asymptomatic neurosyphilis. In such cases, treat patient as asymptomatic neurosyphilis (3 weekly doses of 2.4 million units of Bicillin[R] LA). In penicillin-allergic patients or those whose titers of 1:4 or more remain stable after Rx, examine CSF.

FIGURE 88–2. Work-up of a positive nontreponemal test.

positive VDRL of low titer, e.g., 1 to 1 and a positive FTA-ABS. Often such patients have had previously positive titers. If syphilis has been diagnosed in the past and appropriate therapy administered, no further testing should be done. In the absence of any such history or of any signs or symptoms of syphilis, treatment for late latent syphilis should be administered. Lumbar puncture is unnecessary unless neurologic or psychiatric signs are present; but therapy should cover the possibility of asymptomatic neurosyphilis. (Table 88–4.)

A particularly knotty problem is the evaluation of serologic results in children born to syphilitic mothers. Since IgG is passively transferred across the placenta, positive VDRL and FTA-ABS tests result. Unless a child has a titer at least four times higher than that of his mother, the VDRL test is not diagnostic for active congenital syphilis. If the mother has been adequately treated, it is suggested that children with a

positive titer equal to or lower than that of the mother should be followed for 3 months, because maternal IgG will have disappeared by that time and the serology will revert to negative. This may, however, be impractical, and retreatment of the child is usually preferred because it is easy, safe and one would rather err on the side of overtreatment.

VAGINAL DISCHARGE

In defining the cause of vaginitis, one should determine the onset of discharge (relation to menses), characteristics of the discharge (color, amount, odor), and associated symptoms (itching, dysuria, labial swelling) (Table 88–6). The definitive diagnosis depends upon the pelvic examination. A speculum, which is warmed in tepid water, should be inserted into the vagina without lubrication to prevent interference with cultures and other diagnostic tests. Confirmatory diagnostic examinations include the wet

---

TABLE 88-6

Approach to the Diagnosis of a Vaginal Discharge

Cause of Vaginitis	Pruritus	Odor	Color of Discharge	Consistency of Discharge	Swelling and Erythema of Labia	Diagnostic Technique
Physiologic	No	No	Colorless	Thin	No	Clinical, but wet prep and Gram stain
Allergic	Yes	No	Colorless	Thin	Yes	shows few leukocytes and
Atrophic	No; if present, mild	No	Colorless to white	Thin	Minimal	normal flora
Foreign body (e.g., tampon)	No	Foul smelling	Watery sero-sarguinous	Thin	Minimal	(lactobacilli)
Candida	Yes (intense) often only presenting complaint—premenstrual	None to mild	White	Thick curd-like or watery sheen adherent to vaginal wall, often scanty	Yes (intense)	Organism on wet prep or Gram stain
Trichomonas	Up to 75% complain of discharge and itching during or after menses.	Foul smelling	Greenish-grey or yellow	Frothy, often profuse	Yes	Organism on wet prep
"Nonspecific"	No, but may be minimal in 30%	Foul smelling	Gray-white, sometimes yellow	Thin, adherent to vaginal wall	No	Clue cells (see text) Normal flora, and polys absent; KOH → "fishy" odor

preparation, i.e., mixing a drop of normal saline with a small amount of vaginal discharge on a slide. One can also obtain a swab of the vaginal secretion from the posterior vaginal fornix and place it in a tube holding a small amount of saline for examination after the pelvic examination is completed. A slide of the vaginal discharge for later Gram staining is also very helpful in defining some of the conditions as noted.[152,160,164,174]

Physiologic vaginal discharges may be caused by estrogen or progesterone levels at ovulation, before menses, in pregnancy, and with the use of oral contraceptives. Discharge may also result from allergic reactions to douches or feminine hygiene products. Atrophic vaginitis is seen in postmenopausal women. This is a drying and irritation of the vagina due to a lack of lubrication leading to increased friability with intercourse. A common cause of a malodorous vaginal discharge is the "forgotten tampon." This acts as a foreign body allowing overgrowth of anaerobic bacteria. The vaginitis usually clears on removing the tampon.

Candida Vaginitis

Candida is part of the normal flora of about 50 percent of women and, it is difficult to differentiate colonization from true infection. Vaginitis associated with candida is not usually sexually transmitted; however, 10 to 15 percent of regular male sex partners of women with definite candida vulvo-vaginitis can present with balanitis or discrete penile lesions secondary to candida. Pruritus or dyspareunia may occur especially during the premenstrual period. Predisposing factors include therapy with oral contraceptives, broad spectrum antibiotics or steroids, pregnancy, and hypoparathyroidism.

The combination of symptoms and signs with a large number of yeast with budding or pseudohyphae on Gram stain suggests true infection rather than simple colonization (Table 88–6). The sensitivity of a wet preparation or Gram stain varies anywhere from 30 percent to 90 percent depending upon the skill of the observer. Culture is only useful in selected cases.[167]

Therapy in symptomatic women consists of Miconazole Nitrate vaginal cream (Monistat) or Clotrimazole suppositories nightly for 7 days or Mycostatin vaginal cream or suppositories twice a day for 10 days. Patients should be asked to avoid constricting or insulating undergarments such as pantyhose.

Trichomonas Vaginitis

The most common sexually transmitted cause of vaginitis is trichomoniasis, with an estimated case rate in the United States of 2.5 to 3 million per year. Colonization is directly related to sexual activity; half of those colonized have no symptoms. Symptoms often occur after the menses. Dyspareunia has been reported in 20 percent of cases.

In skilled hands, a wet preparation can have a sensitivity of about 75 percent. The etiologic organism is a motile, pear-shaped flagellated organism about twice the size of a red cell. Culture is not generally available.

Recommended therapy is Metronidazole (Flagyl) in a single 2-g dose. Steady partners may be colonized in up to 75 percent of cases and must be treated simultaneously. Patients should be counseled to avoid alcohol for 24 hours after therapy because of the antabuse-like effect of the drug. Candida overgrowth may result from alteration in vaginal flora. Other side effects are a metallic taste in the mouth and minor gastrointestinal complaints. The cure rate is about 95 percent if both partners are treated and there is no reexposure.

Nonspecific Vaginitis

Nonspecific vaginitis is characterized by a mild to moderate vaginal discharge unrelated to menses. The condition is thought to be caused by an organism variously called *Corynebacterium vaginale* or *Haemophilus vaginalis*. Up to one-third of women in a venereal disease clinic population are colonized. The diagnosis is best made by Gram stain or wet preparation showing so-called "clue" cells (vaginal epithelial cells covered by myriads of small gram-negative rods). Conspicuously absent are polymorphonuclear leukocytes and normal flora. Gram stain can have a sensitivity and specificity as high as 95 and 90 percent, respectively, depending upon the skill of the observer. Another diagnostic technique involves mixing 10 percent KOH with the discharge, liberating a "fishy" or amine-like odor.[164]

Recent studies suggest that the drug of choice is metronidazole in doses of 500 mg b.i.d. for 7 days; however, ampicillin in doses of 500 mg, four times a day for 7 days has been efficacious in other studies. Despite recent questions about efficacy, most patients are still treated with locally applied sulfa creams. Since about 80 percent of steady male partners have urethral colonization, therapy of partners may be advisable, especially in refractory cases.[164]

MISCELLANY

The changing nature of sexually transmitted diseases is illustrated by the disparate infections listed in Group III of Table 88–1. A number of studies have demonstrated an increased prevalence of hepatitis B infection (up to 50 percent) in male homosexuals.[172] Subsequent studies have also documented an increase in other enteric disease (shigellosis, amebiasis, and giardiasis) in male homosexuals, probably as a result of anilingus (fecal ingestion during oral–anal contact).[161]

Cytomegalovirus (CMV) has occasionally been shown to be transmitted sexually. Although usually asymptomatic, it can produce an infectious mononucleosis or hepatitis-like syndrome in adults. Of greater public health importance is the transmission of CMV to the fetus during delivery, because the infant may develop a severe infection (the so-called Torch syndrome).

Lastly, new evidence is appearing about urinary tract infections in susceptible women after intercourse.[141] Studies have shown that colonization of the introitus and the urethra by bowel flora precedes infections. Trauma to the urethra during intercourse appears to allow organisms to migrate into the blad-

der. Women with recurrent infections are advised to void as soon as practicable after intercourse and to wipe front to back with toilet tissue after defecation. If refractory cases, antimicrobial prophylaxis in temporal relation to intercourse is advised.

EPIDEMIOLOGY AND PREVENTION

As previously noted, the approach to patients with STD must be nonjudgmental and free of moralizing. Otherwise, patients may not return or may refuse to report their contacts. Another important element is the maintenance of confidentiality. Many states have enacted minor consent laws to ensure confidentiality for treatment and contact tracing. Assurance of confidentiality should not be equated with failure to report. Gonorrhea and syphilis are among the reportable diseases for monitoring and epidemiologic purposes. Failure to report could have devastating ef-

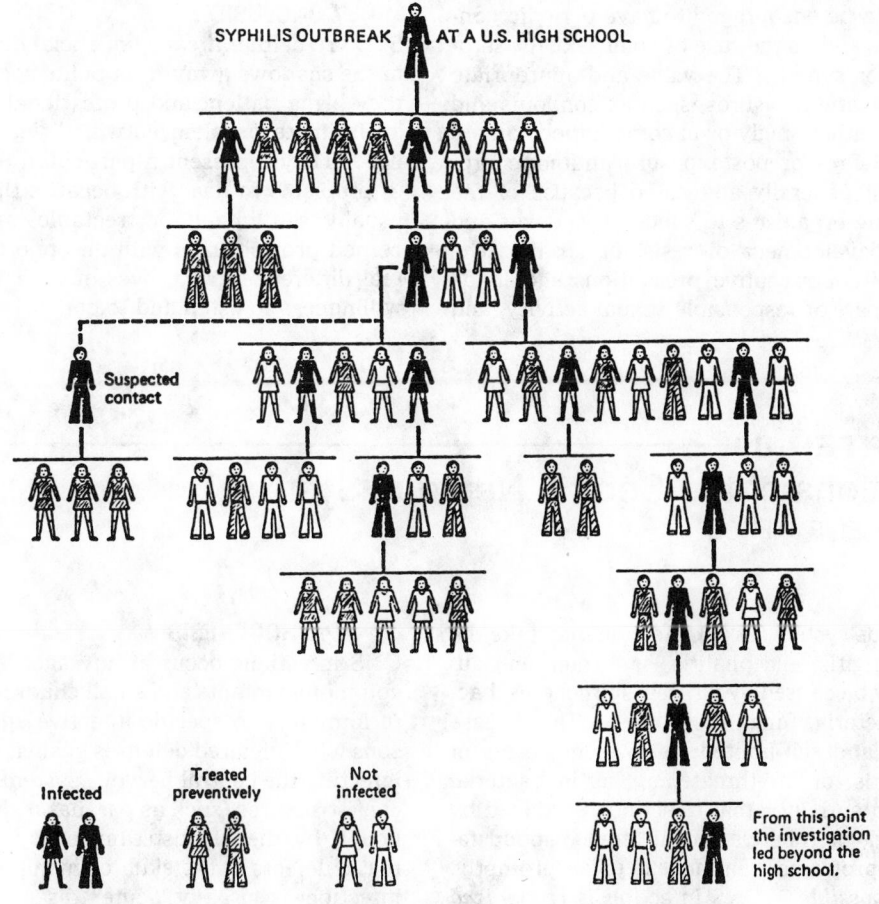

FIGURE 88–3. Epidemiology and prevention of syphilis. Syphilis outbreak at a U.S. high school. (From Medcom, Inc. World Leader in Multimedia Medical Education, 1633 Broadway, N.Y., N.Y. 10019, from *Venereal Disease: A Medcom Review for the 70s.* Produced under an education grant from Pfizer Laboratories, 1972.)

fects on unwitting or unsuspecting people if transmission chains, such as the one outlined in Figure 88–3, are not interrupted.

The examination of sexual contacts, even if they are asymptomatic, is an essential part of the treatment plan. Contacts to gonorrhea or infectious syphilis should undergo diagnostic tests and treatment where appropriate. If they have documented infection, their contacts must also be traced. Contact tracing requires diplomacy and tact. Each state has carefully trained investigators skilled at tracing contacts without revealing their sources.

Patient education should be an integral part of the treatment plan because many patients are quite ignorant, not only of STD, but of human sexuality in general. This should include a brief instruction about the diseases themselves, and a discussion of the importance of steady relationships or limitation in number and selectivity in choice of partners for decreasing risk. Patients engaging in sex with multiple partners should be encouraged to have periodic gonorrhea cultures and, in the case of homosexuals, serologic testing for syphilis. The value and appropriate use of prophylactic measures, such as condoms and vaginal foams either singly or in combination, should be stressed.[147] Pre- or postexposure antibiotic prophylaxis is not generally advocated because of the risk of exposing organisms to subcurative doses and encouraging development of resistant strains. The importance of contraceptive precautions should be stressed as a part of responsible sexual activity, and

help given to any patients with inadequate knowledge or inadequate contraceptive techniques.

When treating one infection, one should be alert to detecting other STD. Screening or case detection programs should be aimed at high-risk groups, such as contacts of women with PID, homosexuals or recidivists. Gonorrhea and syphilis screening is recommended at the first prenatal visit of all pregnant women and at 36 weeks in high-risk women, such as those with a prior history of STD, or at delivery if third trimester results are missing.

The group at highest risk, adolescents and young adults, do not seek care regularly because they are generally well. Consequently, it is useful to be alert to other problems prevalent in these age groups (Chap. 152). These include psychological maladjustment and even frank psychiatric and sociopathic problems, such as drug abuse, as well as potentially remediable medical problems such as hypertension.[145]

CONCLUSION

STD are neither arcane nor social diseases to be kept in the shadows away from polite society. Far from it; they bring patient and professional together around an intimate problem entwined with a basic human need. They represent a particularly satisfying group of problems to deal with because they are common, usually self-limited or treatable, and provide concerned professionals with an opportunity to make a real difference in the lives of their patients by their willingness to listen and to counsel.

CHAPTER 89
Infections of the Central Nervous System
NATHANIEL F. PIERCE

Central nervous system (CNS) infection may take the form of meningitis, encephalitis, or intracranial abscess and may be caused by viruses, spirochetes, bacteria, mycobacteria, fungi, or protozoa. The disease may be mild and self-limited, as in some forms of viral meningitis, or life-threatening, as in bacterial meningitis. Potentially lethal infections produced by bacteria, fungi, or tubercle bacilli often respond favorably to appropriate treatment if given promptly. *This is only possible if CNS infection is recognized early and the probable infective agent determined rapidly.* Delayed diagnosis is a major cause of increased morbidity and mortality.[180]

PATHOGENESIS

CNS infections occur at any age, but are especially common in infants and small children because of lack of immunity to specific infective agents, and in persons with impaired defenses against infection. Agents infecting the central nervous system enter from adjacent structures (such as paranasal sinuses or mastoid bone), by the bloodstream, or by surgical or traumatic defects in the skull or meninges. The resulting infection is usually acute, disease becoming full-blown in a few hours or days. Focal infections, such as abscesses, may develop somewhat more slowly over several days or weeks. The same is true for tuberculous or fungal infections. Some agents seed the CNS and become latent, causing active infection years later when host defenses decline, e.g., tubercle bacilli.

The type of CNS infection is determined partly by the nature of the infecting agent. Aerobic bacteria,

fungi, and tubercle bacilli usually produce meningitis. Viruses produce either meningitis or encephalitis. Anaerobic bacteria are common causes of intracranial abscess, although aerobes and fungi may also be responsible.

CNS infection initiates three processes which

TABLE 89-1

Spinal Fluid Findings in Central Nervous System Infections

	Cell Count (µl)	Cell Type	Glucose (mg/dl)	Protein (mg/dl)	Microscopic Examination	Culture
Normal	0–5	Lympho-cytes	40–80 or more than ½ of serum level	10–40	Negative	Negative
Meningitis						
Untreated bacterial	10–100,000	Predomi-nantly PMN's	Low	Normal to 600, usually increased	90 percent positive	90 percent positive
Partially treated bacterial	10–10,000	Predomi-nantly PMN's	Low or normal	Usually increased	Positive or negative, bacteria may stain poorly	Frequently negative
Viral	10–2,000	Early; mostly PMN's Late; mostly lymphs	Normal	Normal to 100	Negative	Negative
Tuberculous	10–1,000	30–100 percent lymphs	Low, may be normal early	Elevated, 100 to 500	Rarely positive	Usually positive
Fungal	10–1,000	Predomi-nantly lymphs	Low, occa-sionally normal	Elevated, up to 500	India ink positive for crypto-cocci	Usually positive
Encephalitis	10–2,000	Early; mostly PMN's Late; mostly lymphs	Normal	Normal to 120	Negative	Negative
Brain abscess	10–500	Early; mostly PMN's Late; mostly lymphs	Normal	Early; increased up to 500 Late; frequently normal	Negative	Negative

cause all of its manifestations: inflammation, increased intracranial pressure, and tissue necrosis. Inflammation of the meninges and cerebral cortex cause nuchal rigidity and encephalitic symptoms (e.g., headache, seizures), respectively. Increased pressure from brain abscess, subdural empyema, or diffuse brain swelling cause altered consciousness and focal neurologic deficits. Tissue necrosis results from vascular thromboses on the surface of the brain, as occurs in bacterial meningitis, and contributes to serious brain swelling and dysfunction.

CNS inflammation usually produces changes in the spinal fluid (CSF). These may include a cellular pleocytosis, increased protein content, and decreased glucose content (Table 89–1). Lymphocytes usually predominate in viral, fungal, or tuberculous infections, whereas a predominance of polymorphonuclear leukocytes is the hallmark of bacterial infections. Uncentrifuged CSF with one polymorphonuclear leukocyte or more than five lymphocytes is abnormal. In very early bacterial meningitis, bacteria may be present in CSF in the absence of a pleocytosis. The protein content of CSF increases with most infections. The increase is minimal with most viral infections but is greater with bacterial, fungal, or tuberculous infection. An increase in protein may be the only abnormality in brain abscess. CSF glucose is usually less than 40 mg/dl (or less than one-half of a simultaneous blood glucose) in untreated bacterial meningitis and frequently so in fungal and tuberculous meningitis. CSF glucose may also be depressed, however, in mumps meningitis, sarcoid or tumor of the CNS, and subarachnoid hemorrhage. Lowered CSF glucose is probably due to altered glucose transport between blood and CSF.

CLINICAL MANIFESTATIONS

Combinations of fever, nuchal rigidity, severe headache, and altered CNS function should immediately suggest a diagnosis of CNS infection.[180] However, any one of these findings in isolation also requires that CNS infection be seriously considered. Important alterations in CNS function include acute changes in personality or behavior, alterations in consciousness, cranial nerve palsies, or focal or generalized seizures. A careful examination to detect even minimal nuchal rigidity should be performed on persons with fever, an unusually severe or persistant headache, or altered CNS function.

The evidences of CNS infection may be attributed to or masked by other disease processes. Fever may be attributed to recognized infection elsewhere such as bacterial pneumonia, endocarditis, otitis, or sinusitis. Similarly, altered CNS function may be blamed on alcoholism, head trauma, stroke, brain tumor, subarachnoid hemorrhage, or senility. Treatable CNS infection, particularly bacterial meningitis, must be ruled out in such patients. This is usually done by lumbar puncture and careful CSF examination.

Physical findings will often suggest the specific cause of CNS infection. Cutaneous petechiae and purpuric lesions strongly suggest meningococcal infection. However, viral agents, such as ECHO 9, can also cause a confusing petechial rash. Meningitis in a patient with middle ear or sinus infection, CSF rhinorrhea, or pneumonia suggests a pneumococcal etiology; while varicella-zoster virus would be the likely cause of encephalitis in a child with resolving chicken pox.

There may be great overlap in the symptomatology of CNS infections. Meningitis is frequently accompanied by encephalitic manifestations, such as seizures or altered consciousness, and encephalitis may be associated with moderate nuchal rigidity. Similarly, encephalitis, brain abscess, and subdural empyema can each cause focal neurologic deficits and signs of an intracranial mass.

SPECIFIC TYPES OF CNS INFECTION

Bacterial Meningitis

The immediate differentiation of bacterial meningitis from other varieties of CNS infection depends upon spinal fluid examination (Table 89–1) and physical findings.[180] Bacterial meningitis is strongly suggested by the finding of a predominantly polymorphonuclear spinal fluid pleocytosis with the total cell count ranging from 100 to many thousand/μl and a coexistent spinal fluid glucose value of less than 40 mg/dl or less than half of the simultaneously obtained blood glucose. The demonstration of bacteria on Gram stain of centrifuged spinal fluid confirms the diagnosis and permits tentative identification of the infective agent by morphology and staining characteristics. Specific bacterial etiology is confirmed by isolation from culture of CSF.

Differentiation of bacterial meningitis from other forms of CNS infection becomes more difficult after antibiotics have been administered for several hours or days. If the antibiotic is at least partially effective, it may be impossible to visualize the organism on a stained smear of CSF or to grow it in culture. Although the CSF will be abnormal, the glucose content may be normal (Table 89–1). Such patients must be treated as having bacterial meningitis of undetermined etiology while attempting to determine the specific etiology.

Physical findings also help differentiate bacterial

meningitis from other CNS infections. While fever and nuchal rigidity suggest bacterial meningitis, persistent cranial nerve palsies or papilledema are uncommon and should suggest encephalitis or intracranial abscess.

Bacterial meningitis may be caused by almost any pathogenic bacteria. However, about 80 percent of cases are caused by either *H. influenzae* type B, *Str. pneumoniae,* or *N. meningitidis. H. influenzae* type B infections occur largely in children under 5 years of age and meningococcal infections are seen predominantly in children and young adults. Each produces acute disease in apparently normal persons. Pneumococcal infections occur at all ages, but most frequently in infants, in the elderly, and in association with alcoholism, multiple myeloma, pneumococcal pneumonia or endocarditis, CSF rhinorrhea, and infection of the middle ear, sinuses, or mastoids. Staphylococci and the gram-negative enteric rods may produce meningitis in association with systemic infection, especially in persons with altered host defense mechanisms. Staphylococci are also an important cause of meningitis associated with cranial trauma or neurosurgery. Physical examination should include a careful search for distant foci of infection which may be associated with or give rise to bacterial meningitis.

Tuberculous Meningitis

Tuberculous meningitis occurs by hematogenous spread of miliary disease, especially in children, or by rupture into the CSF of a previously latent CNS tubercle.[176] The disease is not indolent but progresses with steadily increasing symptoms over a period of several days to several weeks. The predominant clinical manifestations include nuchal rigidity, headache, lethargy, and progressive deterioration of mental function. Ocular palsies, when present, help to distinguish tuberculous meningitis from viral or bacterial meningitis. Many patients with tuberculous meningitis give a history of exposure to tuberculosis and may have demonstrable tuberculosis involving other organs. The purified protein derivative (PPD) skin test may be negative in children but is positive in more than 90 percent of adults.

Spinal fluid findings in tuberculous meningitis are shown in Table 89–1. When examined early in the course of disease, CSF glucose may be normal and other findings may be similar to those in viral meningitis or encephalitis. If so, repeat lumbar punctures to detect changes in spinal fluid glucose concentration are usually preferable to early initiation of antituberculous therapy. If spinal fluid glucose concentration falls below normal, antituberculous therapy should be initiated. If it remains normal for 7 to 10 days or if the patient improves without antituberculous therapy, the tubercle bacillus is ruled out as the cause of infection. When treatment is required, it must usually be started without having seen the organism, since they are rarely found in directly examined CSF.

Viral Meningitis

The causes of viral meningitis are varied (Table 89–2). Enteroviruses, including poliomyelitis, predominate in summer months, and mumps in winter and spring. Viral meningitis is largely a disease of children and young adults.[179]

TABLE 89–2
Clinical Features of CNS Infections

Type	Site of Primary Infection	Special Clinical Features	Treatment	Comment
MENINGITIS				
1. Gram-Positive Bacteria				
Pneumococcus*	Lung, ear, sinuses	Antecedent infection common pneumonia, endocarditis, sinusitis; previous head trauma	Penicillin G, chloramphenicol is second choice	Search for focal infection (sinuses, ears) Most frequent in infants, the elderly, alcoholics, myeloma
Staphylococcus	Endocarditis, skin, sinuses; often no primary apparent	Usually associated with septicemia, brain abscess, epidural abscess, thrombosis of venous sinuses	Penicillin G and methicillin	Abscess formation common

* Indicates most frequent etiologic agents.

(Continued)

─────── TABLE 89–2 (cont.) ───────

Type	Site of Primary Infection	Special Clinical Features	Treatment	Comment
MENINGITIS (cont.)				
1. Gram-Positive Bacteria (cont.)				
Streptococcus	Skin, sinus, wound, septicemia	Usually associated with parameningeal focus	Penicillin G, add gentamicin for Group D streptococci	Group B infections common in newborn
Listeria	Unknown ? GI tract	Common in infants, alcoholics, and debilitated states	Ampicillin, tetracycline is second choice	May be confused with dipththeroids in culture
II. Gram-Negative Bacteria				
Meningococcus*	Nasopharynx	Petechial or purpuric skin rash, arthritis, shock, disseminated intravascular coagulation	Penicillin G, chloramphenicol is second choice	May occur in epidemics, fulminant disease common
Haemophilus *influenzae*	Nasopharynx, respiratory tract	Croup, epiglottitis, subdural effusions common in infants	Chloramphenicol; ampicillin only if isolate is sensitive	Uncommon after the age of 5 years. Resistance to ampicillin is increasing
Salmonellae	GI tract, gallbladder	Associated with septicemia	Ampicillin or chloramphenicol	Rare in uncomplicated enteritis
E. coli Klebsiella Proteus Pseudomonas }	Wound, GI tract, urinary tract, bacteremia	Common in newborn. May follow neurosurgery or trauma. Also occurs in elderly and immunocompromised hosts.	Gentamicin and ampicillin. Add carbenicillin 400–500 mg/kg/day for pseudomonas. Adjust therapy for sensitivity of organism. Use chloramphenicol in adults if organism is sensitive	Aminoglycosides enter CNS poorly, may require intraventricular administration
III. Viral				
Mumps*	Salivary glands	Clinical mumps or orchitis may not occur	Supportive	Very common, CSF glucose may be low
Enteroviruses* ECHO Coxsackie Poliomyelitis	GI tract	Rashes common Pleuritis, pericarditis, paralysis (polio)	Supportive	Prevention by immunization (poliomyelitis)
IV. Mycobacteria				
*M. tuberculosis**	Lung, latent CNS tubercle	Focal neurologic signs common. Obvious pulmonary or disseminated TB often not present	INH, ethambutol, and streptomycin. Rifampin if resistance likely. Steroids if CSF pressure increased	Meningeal signs may be minimal, neurologic signs prominent

* Indicates most frequent etiologic agents.

─── **TABLE 89-2 (cont.)** ───────

Type	Site of Primary Infection	Special Clinical Features	Treatment	Comment
V. Fungi				
Cryptococcus * *neoformans*	Lung	Insidious onset suggests brain tumor; headache prominent	Amphotericin B (May need to be given intraventricularly)	Contact with birds. Underlying Hodgkins-lymphoma common
Coccidioides immitis	Lung	Disseminated disease often present	Amphotericin B	History of previous primary fungal illness. Travel in San Joaquin Valley (Coccidiodomycosis)
Histoplasma capsulatum	Lung	Complement fixing antibody increased		
Blastomyces dermatidis	Skin			
VI. Spirochetal				
Syphilis	Genital	Wide spectrum of CNS changes	Procaine penicillin G 600,000 units/day for 2 weeks or penicillin G 12–24 10^6 units IV for 10 days	Follows inadequate treatment of primary disease
Leptospirosis	?Lung or GI tract	Hepatitis, conjunctivitis, extreme muscle tenderness	Penicillin G	Exposure to urine of rodents, dogs, swine
ENCEPHALITIS				
Arboviruses* St. Louis Western equine Eastern equine Japanese B	Mosquito bite	Focal signs common Variable severity	Supportive	Animal reservoir
Herpes simplex *	Latent infection	Signs of temporal lobe tumor or other brain mass	Adenine arabinoside	Brain biopsy for diagnosis, may also cause mild meningitis
Varicella-Zoster	Skin	Cerebellar signs common	Supportive	Unusual complication of chicken pox, may occur as skin lesions clear
Rabies	Animal bite Inhaled bat excreta (caves)	Invariably fatal	Supportive	Immunization after bite; study animal's brain for Negri bodies
LOCALIZED INTRACRANIAL INFECTION				
Anaerobes* Bacteroides	Lung or pelvic abcess, or	Common in brain abscess,	Drainage, chloramphenicol	Examine smears for mixed flora;
Streptococci	no focus found	subdural empyema		anaerobic culture
Staphylococcus*	Parameningeal focus, endocarditis, neurosurgery	Common in subdural empyema, septic thrombophlebitis	Penicillin and methicillin, drainage of empyema or abscess	Search for primary site
Streptococci Pneumococcis	Sinusitis or otitis, bacteremia	Occur in subdural empyema, epidural abscess	Penicillin; drainage if possible	Drain primary site in ear or sinuses
Enteric bacteria	After surgery, trauma, or antibiotics	Occur in brain abscess, subdural empyema, epidural abscess	Chloramphenicol if sensitive, otherwise determined by sensitivity pattern; drainage of pus	Aminoglycosides enter CNS poorly, may require intraventricular administration
Nocardia, actinomycetes	Parameningeal or lung	Occasional cause of brain abscess or subdural infection	Drainage; tetracycline or sulfonamide	Anaerobes also frequently present

Spinal fluid findings are shown in Table 89–1. Cell counts are usually between 100 and 500/μl. In the first day of illness, polymorphonuclears may predominate. Thereafter, the response is largely lymphocytic. Specific etiology is determined by isolation of the virus from spinal fluid or demonstration of a significant rise in specific serum antibodies. Isolation of virus from the pharynx, stool, or rectal swab suggests but does not prove that the agent caused the episode of meningitis.

The disease is usually brief and requires no specific therapy. Headache and stiff neck are common complaints, but altered conscious is not and should suggest another diagnosis. Patients are usually much improved in 1 to 3 days. Except with poliomyelitis which is primarily a neuronitis, long-lasting significant muscular paresis is unusual.

Viral meningitis is largely a diagnosis of exclusion. CNS infections which require specific therapy and have a poor prognosis if untreated must be seriously considered and ruled out before making this diagnosis. Repeat CSF examinations may be necessary to make this differentiation.

Fungal Meningitis

The clinical picture of fungal meningitis varies widely and depends in part upon the infecting agent (Table 89–2). Fungal meningitis, especially when caused by *Cryptococcus neoformans,* candida, aspergillus, and mucor, tends to occur in chronically ill persons, especially those with diabetes or lymphoid or hematopoietic malignancies or persons receiving immunosuppressive drugs, including corticosteroids.[176]

Specific fungal agents produce differing patterns of disease. Cryptococcal meningitis, the most common form of fungal meningitis, is usually associated with fever, headache, mental aberrations, and weight loss. Physical findings commonly include altered consciousness, stiff neck, abnormal reflexes, cranial nerve palsies (especially the VIth), and papilledema. The clinical picture can easily be confused with a brain tumor or other space-occupying lesion. In contrast, meningitis caused by *Histoplasma capsulatum* may be associated only with hepatosplenomegaly, fever, lymphadenopathy, and weight loss. Neurologic findings and nuchal rigidity may be absent.

CSF findings in fungal meningitis are similar to those in tuberculous meningitis (Table 89–1). Direct examination of centrifuged spinal fluid with India ink is important for the recognition of cryptococci which may appear as mononuclear leukocytes in CSF. The use of India ink permits demonstration of their large, clear capsule and budding morphology. Multiple examinations of CSF with India ink and by culture may

be necessary to demonstrate cryptococci. Cryptococcal capsular antigen can be detected rapidly in CSF by counterimmunoelectrophoresis. This test is available in some centers and is more sensitive than the India ink method. Spinal fluid culture is usually positive in infection due to *Cryptococcus neoformans* or Candida. In other fungal infections, the organism is more likely to be recovered from or seen in bone marrow or liver biopsy (e.g., histoplasmosis) or in nasal secretions (e.g., mucormycosis). In still other infections, a rising serum titer of complement-fixing antibody (e.g., coccidioidomycosis) provides the basis for diagnosis.

Other Types of Meningitis and Meningeal Syndromes

Meningitis also occurs in two spirochetal diseases. Meningovascular syphilis is a late complication of untreated syphilis. Prominent complaints include headache, intellectual impairment, and focal neurologic deficits involving cranial nerves or sometimes producing hemiparesis. Pupillary light reflex is impaired and papilledema and nuchal rigidity may be present. CSF shows a lymphocytic pleocytosis with elevated protein and normal sugar. Serologic tests for syphilis are positive in spinal fluid and blood.

Meningitis is also a common manifestation of leptospirosis. Patients may have a variety of abnormalities including headache, fever, conjunctival infection, impairment of renal function, jaundice, and cough. The disease follows contact with infected urine of dogs, rodents, swine, cattle, or certain wild animals. In may be mild and self-limited or rapidly fatal with hepatic and renal failure. Spinal fluid findings are similar to those in viral meningitis. The diagnosis is usually made by demonstrating a rise in titer of specific complement-fixing antibody.

Free-living amebas normally found in soil may cause a severe form of meningoencephalitis in fresh water swimmers. The most prominent complaint is severe headache. Spinal fluid findings are similar to those of bacterial meningitis except that motile amebas may be identified and bacteria are absent. The disease progresses rapidly ending fatally in several days unless recognized and treated. Amphotericin B appears to be effective if started promptly.

Nuchal rigidity and spinal fluid pleocytosis may also be produced by a variety of processes which are not CNS infections such as neoplasia demyelinating diseases, and autoimmune disease. These are commonly associated with CSF cell counts of less than 200/μl which are predominantly lymphocytes, little if any rise in protein concentration, and normal glucose concentration. An important cause is a parameningeal focus of infection such as sinusitis, mastoiditis, or vertebral osteomyelitis. Other causes include hypersensitivity meningitis (i.e., secondary to sulfonamide drugs), chemical meningitis following intrathecal injection of radiopaque contrast media, air, or anesthetic agents, and neoplastic meningitis. In the latter, tumor cells may be seen in spinal fluid and CSF glucose content may be decreased.

VIRAL ENCEPHALITIS

The clinical picture of viral encephalitis varies from mild unrecognized infection to rapidly lethal disease. Severity of disease is related to specific etiology (Table 89-2), mild disease being more common with mumps, lymphocytic choriomeningitis, enterovirus, Western Equine, and St. Louis varieties of encephalitis while severe disease is common with Herpes simplex, Eastern Equine, Japanese B, and rabies infections.[179]

The clinical picture provides little help in determining etiology. Onset is typically abrupt with severe headache and fever as high as 106°F. Nuchal rigidity may be present. Mental symptoms range from confusion and apathy to delirium, hyperexcitability, tremor, ataxia, convulsions, and coma. Cranial nerve palsies are common in severe cases. *Herpes simplex* encephalitis may present clinical and radiographic evidence of a temporal or frontal lobe mass due to focal necrosis. Examination of spinal fluid gives findings identical to those in viral meningitis.

Specific diagnosis is by isolation of the etiologic agent from spinal fluid or involved tissue, or by rising titers of specific antibody in serum or CSF. Rapid diagnosis is especially important for infections which are treatable with antiviral agents. Initial reports already suggest that adenine arabinoside is effective in treating *Herpes simplex* encephalitis. Early diagnosis of this disease is possible only by culture of brain taken from the infected site. With this exception, no specific therapy is presently available and management is symptomatic. In mild disease, recovery may be complete but with severe disease surviving patients may suffer severe permanent neurologic impairment.

LOCALIZED INTRACRANIAL INFECTION

This category includes brain abscess, subdural empyema, epidural abscess, and septic thrombophlebitis of the major venous sinuses.[177,178] These bacterial infections usually develop rapidly, although brain abscess may develop over several weeks. Severe headache is often the earliest symptom with evidence of increased intracranial pressure, focal neurologic deficits, and altered consciousness being late features.

Epidural abscesses are often small and produce fewer serious neurologic signs. Specific neurologic deficits reflect the location of the process. Proptosis and ophthalmoplegia are features of cavernous sinus thrombosis. Hemiparesis and focal seizures suggest subdural empyema, while the signs of brain abscess vary with the portion of the brain involved. Most localized infections are caused by suppuration in adjacent cranial structures. This includes chronic ear or mastoid infections, purulent sinusitis, facial cellulitis, cranial osteomyelitis, or infection introduced by trauma or neurosurgery. Blood-borne infection from distant sites, such as lung abscess, pleural empyema, or pelvic abscess, is also an important cause of brain abscess. The bacteria involved reflect the flora of the infected focus of origin. In abscesses, more than one bacterial strain may be present with anaerobes (bacteroides, streptococci) being very common. Aerobic streptococci, enterobacteria, and staphylococci are also frequently present. Staphylococci are important causes of septic thrombophlebitis and neurosurgical infections.

Important diagnostic techniques to detect and differentiate these processes include careful neurologic examination, scanning by computerized axial tomography (for brain abscesses and subdural empyema), radioisotope brain scan (for brain abscess), and arteriography for subdural empyema. Lumbar puncture is of limited value and may be dangerous. CSF pressure is often elevated and may contain increased protein or cells (Table 89-1), but these findings are not diagnostic. Bacteria are not present unless the infection has extended to produce meningitis.

IMMEDIATE DIAGNOSTIC PROCEDURES

The initial goal is *rapid* determination of the type of CNS infection and, if possible, its etiology. Delayed diagnosis leads to delayed treatment, often with disastrous results.

INITIAL EXAMINATION. This should include evaluation for cranial trauma, level of consciousness, cranial nerve palsies, nuchal rigidity, and increased intracranial pressure. If papilledema is present a lumbar puncture may be contraindicated (see below). A search should be made for other foci of infection (e.g., ears, sinuses, and lungs) and for physical signs suggesting a specific microbial etiology (e.g., hemorrhagic skin rash).

LUMBAR PUNCTURE. A lumbar puncture should be done promptly in all cases of suspected CNS infection except those with signs primarily suggesting an intracranial mass with increased intracranial pressure, e.g., cranial nerve palsies and papilledema. Such patients should have intracerebral or subdural masses ruled out first to minimize the risk of herniation of the brain after lumbar puncture. Emergency computerized axial tomography is the procedure of choice, but a technetium brain scan is also suitable for intracerebral masses while arteriography is satisfactory for subdural collections.

Lumbar puncture should always be done carefully using a small bore needle and taking only the amount of fluid needed for smears, culture, and biochemical tests. If the fluid is bloody or xanthochromic, the possibility of intracranial bleeding must be investigated. Since CSF examination is of critical importance it should always be done by experienced observers.

CULTURES. Blood cultures should be obtained. CSF cultures should be placed immediately on warmed chocolate agar plates, blood agar plates, and other standard media. Cultures for fungi and mycobacteria should be done unless a bacterial agent is seen on Gram stain. Pus obtained from intracranial abscesses should be cultured carefully for strict anaerobes as well as aerobes. Material obtained from other septic foci (e.g., draining ear, sputum) should also be cultured.

CELL COUNT. The total cell count is done on uncentrifuged fluid in a counting chamber. If numerous red blood cells are present, a count should be performed before and after their lysis with dilute HCl. The ratio of white blood cell count to red blood cell count can then be compared to that in venous blood to determine if the spinal fluid contains an increased number of white blood cells. For differential cell count, a drop of fluid should be allowed to dry on a clean slide and stained with Wright's stain.

GRAM STAIN. The Gram stain of centrifuged cerebrospinal fluid should be examined before searching for acid-fast bacilli, fungi, or protozoa. Bacterial morphology and staining characteristics provide important evidence of specific etiology and may be the basis for selection of initial therapy. The most common causes of bacterial meningitis, *Haemophilus influenzae*, *Streptococcus pneumoniae*, and *Neisseria meningitidis*, can be readily distinguished from one another by examination of the Gram stain.

FURTHER TESTS ON SPINAL FLUID. If the Gram stain is negative, an India ink preparation and acid-fast smears should be done and, if indicated, a wet preparation observed for amebae. Blood glucose should be measured for comparison with the CSF glucose. The protein content, titers of specific antibodies, and assays for fungal antigens can be done on the remaining fluid. Fluid may also be sent for cytologic examination for tumor cells.

TREATMENT OF CNS INFECTIONS

Bacterial Infections

Antibiotic treatment of bacterial infections (meningitis and intracranial infections) should begin as soon as possible. Dosages of frequently used antibiotics are in Table 89–3. In *bacterial meningitis,* this should be after initial examination of the patient, examination of CSF, and obtaining necessary cultures, a process which should not require more than 30 minutes. At this point, a bacterial etiology is usually apparent. If not, it may be wise to repeat the lumbar puncture in 8 to 12 hours, at which time the CSF findings may be more diagnostic, or to consider a diagnosis other than bacterial meningitis. In an acutely ill patient, it is often necessary to treat for the most likely bacterial pathogens even if evidence of a specific etiology is lacking.

Antibiotic treatment for specific causes of bacterial meningitis is summarized in Table 89–2.[180] For *H. influenzae* meningitis, chloramphenicol is replacing ampicillin because of the appearance of ampicillin-resistant strains. Some experts recommend use of both agents until the sensitivity of the organism is known. Chloramphenicol is also the drug of choice to treat pneumococcal and meningococcal infections in

---

TABLE 89–3
Antibiotics for Bacterial Infections of the CNS

Antibiotic	Age	Dosage (IV)
Penicillin G	Adult	20–24×10^6 units/day
	Child	250,000 units/kg/day
	Neonate	100,000 units/kg/day
Ampicillin	Adult	12 g/day
	Child	300–400 mg/kg/day
	Neonate	100–200 mg/kg/day
Methicillin*	Adult	12–18 g/day
	Child	100–200 mg/kg/day
	Neonate	100–200 mg/kg/day
Chloramphenicol	Adult	3–4 g/day
	Child	75 mg/kg/day
	Neonate	25–50 mg/kg/day
Gentamicin†	Adult	5 mg/kg/day
	Child	7.5 mg/kg/day
	Neonate	7.5 mg/kg/day

* Naficillin may also be used. Dosage is two-thirds of that for methicillin in adults and the same as methicillin in children and neonates.
† Intravenous dosage is lower if renal function is impaired. Intraventricular or intrathecal gentamicin (1 mg/d in infants, 5 mg/d in adults) may be required in addition to intravenous dosage because of poor penetration of the drug to the CNS.

patients allergic to penicillin. *If the bacterial etiology is unknown,* children should receive chloramphenicol alone or in combination with ampicillin. In newborns and prematures, gentamicin is given with ampicillin because of the high incidence of meningitis due to gram-negative enteric rods. If pseudomonas is suspected carbenicillin should be added. Adults should be given penicillin or chloramphenicol. If staphylococcal infection is suspected, initial therapy should include both penicillin G and methicillin until it is known if the organism produces penicillinase. Infection caused by enteric rods in adults is treated initially with gentamicin (5 mg/kg intravenously and 5 mg intrathecally per day); subsequent therapy is guided by the sensitivity of the isolated organism and the response of the patient. Intravenous chloramphenicol is chosen if the organism is sensitive. If gentamicin therapy is sustained, it may be more effective given intravenously *and* intraventricularly.

Therapy should be continued for 10 days with meningococcal infection and at least 14 days with other agents. Longer courses may be required for staphylococcal or enteric rod infections. The patient should be afebrile at least 3 days before discontinuing treatment, and a repeat lumbar puncture should have less than 30 leukocytes/μl, none of which are polymorphonuclears. The spinal fluid glucose should be normal and the protein content only minimally elevated. Values exceeding these require search for a loculated infection or a sterile subdural fluid collection. The latter is rare in patients over the age of 2 years. Continued antibiotic therapy may be necessary.

The prognosis in bacterial meningitis is determined by the causative organism and the condition of the patient when treatment is started. Factors contributing to a poor prognosis include meningitis caused by pneumococcus, staphylococcus or enteric rods, severe neurologic deficit or coma at onset of treatment, concomitant lobar pneumonia, alcoholism, diabetes, and impaired host immunologic or phagocytic defense mechanisms. Mortality in pneumococcal meningitis is about 50 percent, while in meningococcal or *H. influenzae* meningitis it is about 5 percent.

Tuberculous Infection

Treatment of *tuberculous meningitis* involves use of three antituberculous drugs: INH 400 mg daily, ethambutol (15 mg/kg per day), and streptomycin (1 g per day).[176] Pyridoxine, 50 mg per day, should also be given. Rifampin can also be used in place of one of the above drugs. Treatment should continue for at least 18 months. Short-term use of high dosage adrenal corticosteroids may diminish cerebral edema and decrease the risk of cerebellar herniation in persons with markedly elevated intracranial pressure, but improved survival has not been proven. Response to treatment is slow and may continue for weeks or months. Most patients become afebrile in 1 to 4 weeks. Spinal fluid leukocyte count and glucose and protein content may not become normal for several months. Tuberculous meningitis has the poorest prognosis in patients less than 2 years of age and in those with severely altered central nervous system function at the onset of treatment. Even with recovery from infection, permanent neurologic sequelae are common.

Fungal Infections

Amphotericin B is the drug of choice for the most common forms of fungal CNS infections and infections due to amebae.[176] It is fungistatic and produces untoward side effects including fever, headache, nausea and vomiting, phlebitis, anemia, hypokalemia, and impairment of renal function. It is usually given intravenously, but in severe or unresponsive CNS infection it may also be given intrathecally or directly into the cerebral ventricular system. Dosage is chosen to achieve control of the infection while minimizing side effects. Maximal dosage should usually not exceed 40 mg per day, although double dosage may be given every other day with equally good results. Usually several months of therapy, with a total dose of 1 to 2 g will be necessary to achieve cure. The appearance of serious renal impairment requires reduction of dosage or, occasionally, discontinuation of amphotericin B. An oral antifungal drug, 5-flurocytosine, (100 to 200 mg/kg per day) has been useful in treating both cryptococcal and candidal infections of the CNS; it is most useful when combined with amphotericin B. Following cessation of therapy, patients require careful follow-up with examination of spinal fluid several times yearly for 2 to 4 years to permit early detection and treatment of recurrences.

Treatment of localized CNS infections depends upon the type of infection and the causative organisms.[177,178] Intracranial abscesses should be treated initially with parenteral penicillin G, methicillin, and chloramphenicol. Treatment should begin as soon as the diagnosis is considered. Early surgical drainage is crucial in treatment of subdural empyema, and early drainage by aspiration is increasingly common for brain abscess. Antibiotic therapy may be revised based upon culture of abscess fluid but should be continued for at least 3 weeks after drainage. If the origin of this infection, e.g., ear or sinus, yields other organisms on culture, the antibiotic therapy should be revised appropriately. Surgical drainage may not be necessary for small epidural abscesses. Septic thrombophlebitis is treated by antibiotics alone; many episodes are due to staphylococci and should be treated with a combination of penicillin G and methicillin in high dosage parenterally.

PREVENTION

Vaccines are available against certain viral CNS infections, including poliomyelitis and rabies and against Group A and C meningococcal infections. The latter are used to prevent disease in closed popula-

tions (such as the military) or in epidemics but are not recommended for general use. A polyvalent pneumococcal vaccine has also been released for use in persons with increased risk of pneumococcal infection. It is presumed that it will give protection against pneumococcal meningitis.

Prevention of secondary cases of meningococcal disease is also possible by antibiotic prophylaxis of close contacts. Rifampin, 600 mg a day for 4 days, is the drug of choice. Minocycline, 100 mg every 12 hours for 5 days, is also effective but may cause disturbing vestibular symptoms.

——CHAPTER 90——
Geographic Medicine
R. BRADLEY SACK AND THOMAS W. SIMPSON

Natural barriers that once served efficiently to limit diseases to certain geographic areas are gradually being eliminated in the process of world development. Time, mountains, and oceans are being surmounted by rapid and frequent movement of persons throughout the world. Meanwhile, disease patterns too are changing, often for unknown reasons and, therefore, some of the older "classical" literature in tropical and geographic medicine is now chiefly of historical interest. For these reasons it is quite probable that physicians in the United States will increasingly be coming in contact with diseases that are largely unfamiliar to them.[187]

These "obscure" diseases are, however, of major importance to the health of most of the world's population, and they provide fundamental insights into basic host–parasite relationships and microbial mechanisms of pathogenesis. As these diseases are now being studied more intensively with modern scientific methodologies, new methods of diagnosis and treatment are being developed; unfortunately, much of this information is outside the scope of knowledge of most United States-trained physicians and, therefore, is unavailable to the United States population that might benefit from it.[181]

This chapter is written primarily for physicians in the United States who will, on occasion, need to diagnose and treat these geographically determined illnesses. Some of the changing aspects of global infectious diseases will be discussed, as well as possible means to their diagnosis and treatment. Since specific details of each illness can be found from other sources, the primary aim here will be to heighten the physician's awareness for these diseases.

CHANGING PATTERNS OF GEOGRAPHIC ILLNESSES

Patterns of disease spread may be readily observed, although the causative factors may not be understood. Epidemics of shigella dysentery and typhoid fever caused by strains of bacteria carrying plasmids that confer multiple-drug resistance (R factors) have appeared and disappeared over a several-year period in Central America and Southeast Asia. Diseases usually controlled through the provision of safe water and sewerage disposal can suddenly appear when these become inadequate. The recent occurrence of cholera in the United States exemplifies this. Malaria resistant to chloroquine is spreading geographically and is of importance to physicians first encountering patients with this disease. Drug-resistant tuberculosis, now highly prevalent in certain areas of Southeast Asia, may be encountered in persons arriving from these areas. Probably the major change in worldwide disease patterns has been the elimination of smallpox through intensive circumscribed vaccination efforts.

As new bacteria and viruses are discovered to be etiologic agents of infectious diseases, our understanding of their geographic niche gradually becomes clear. Lassa fever, first thought to be a rare highly lethal disease, is now known to be a common, mild febrile illness in most persons who are infected. Rotavirus-mediated diarrheal disease, first discovered as a major cause of infantile diarrhea in temperate climates, is now known to have a worldwide distribution, including the tropics.

Geographic foci of "unusual" diseases also exist in the United States, such as those for plague (south-west), coccidioidomycosis (San Joaquin Valley in California), Rocky Mountain spotted fever (the southeastern seaboard), and even echinococcocus (Alaska).

CHANGES IN THERAPY FOR GEOGRAPHIC ILLNESSES

Improvements in therapy for some of these diseases are also of importance. Effective means for treating cholera which were developed in cholera endemic areas were not practiced during some of the recent outbreaks of cholera in Europe, resulting in an unacceptably high mortality rate. Many of the drugs now known to be effective for some of these geographically determined diseases are not available in the United States (Table 90–1); a drug presently recommended as prophylaxis against chloroquine-resistant malaria cannot be purchased in this country.[186]

DIAGNOSIS AND TREATMENT OF GEOGRAPHIC ILLNESSES

How then does the physician develop an enlightened awareness for these diseases? Probably the first, most important consideration is the recognition of a history of travel by the patient: to be aware that modern transportation which can virtually place someone in almost any geographic area within hours may 1) lead to unusual exposures; and 2) bring the person to the United States well within the incubation period of most infectious diseases. For United States physicians then, it is most important to recognize disease in travelers returning to the United States or in persons immigrating either temporarily (as students) or permanently to this country.[184,187]

Once a possible history of exposure through travel can be established, it is important to inquire specifically about exposures: animals, rural areas, insects (if known), and presumed sanitation of consumed food and water.

Then, of course, it is necessary to know which diseases are endemic to the area and their seasons of transmission. Since this information is constantly changing, standard texts may be inadequate for this purpose. This up-to-date information is most readily available through two sources: the Center for Disease Control Morbidity and Mortality weekly reports and the Weekly Epidemiologic Record of the World Health Organization. Obviously, disease patterns do

---

TABLE 90–1

Acceptable Treatment Regimens for Selected Parasitic Infections*

Disease	Pathogen	Drug of Choice	Alternatives
I. Blood and Tissue Protozoa			
Uncomplicated malaria	*Plasmodium falciparum, P. vivax, P. malariae, P. ovale*	Chloroquine phosphate (P.O.) 1 g stat, 0.5 g in 6 hours, then 0.5 g daily × 2 days (total 2500 mg)	Amodioquine dihydrochloride
Complicated, severe malaria	*P. falciparum*	Chloroquine hydrochloride (IM) 250 mg every 6 hr. until oral therapy as above can be instituted, up to same total dose	Quinine dihydrochloride (IV)
Chloroquine-resistant falciparum malaria	*P. falciparum*	Quinine sulfate (P.O.), 650 mg tid × 14 days, plus pyrimethamine (P.O.) 25 mg bid × 3 days, plus sulfadiazine (P.O) 500 mg qid × 5 days	Quinine dihydrochloride
Early stages of African trypanosomiasis	*Trypanosoma gambiense, T. rhodesiense*	Suramin† (IV)	Pentamidine
Late CNS stages of African trypanosomiasis	*T. gambiense, T. rhodesiense*	Melarsoprol† (IM)	Tryparsamide plus suramin
American trypanosomiasis	*T. cruzi*	Bayer (Nifurtimox) 2502† (IV)	None
Amebic meningoencephalitis	Naegleria sp., Acanthameba sp.	Amphotericin B (IV)	None

* Abstracted from Medical Letter 20, 17–24, 1978.
† Available from Center for Disease Control, Atlanta, Georgia.

(Continued)

┌─ **TABLE 90-1 (cont.)** ─────────────────────────────────────

Disease	Pathogen	Drug of Choice	Alternatives
II. Blood and Tissue Helminths			
Visceral larva migrans	*Toxocara canis*	(for severe symptoms only) thiabendazole plus prednisone	Diethylcarbamazine
Trichiniasis	*Trichinella spiralis*	(for severe symptoms only) thiabendazole plus prednisone	None
Filariasis	*Wuchereria bancrofti, Brugia malayi, Loa loa, Dipetalonema sp.*	Diethylcarbamazine	None
Onchocerciasis	*Onchocerca volvulus*	Diethylcarbamazine	None
Schistosomiasis	*S. mansoni*	Antimony sodium dimercaptosuccinate† or niridazole†	Stibophen
	S. hematobium	Niridazole†	Antimony sodium dimercaptosuccinate or stibophen
	S. japonicum	Antimony potassium tartrate	Antimony sodium dimercaptosuccinate
Echinococciasis	*Echinococcus granulosus* and other species	None except surgical excision	None
III. Intestinal Protozoa			
Amebiasis asymptomatic	*Entamoeba histolytica*	Diiodohydroxyquin (650 mg tid × 20 days)	Metranidazole or diloxanide furoate
mild to moderate intestinal disease		Paromomycin (25–30 mg/kg/d in 3 doses × 5–10 days) plus diiodohydroxyquin	Metranidazole plus diiodohydroxyquin
severe intestinal disease		Metranidazole (750 mg tid × 5–10 days) plus diiodohydroxyquin or paramomycin plus diiodohydroxyquin	Dehydroemetine plus paromomycin followed by diiodohydroxyquin
hepatic abscess		Metronidazole (750 mg tid × 5–10 days)	Dehydroemetine plus chloroquine phosphate
Giardiasis	*Giardia lamblia*	Quinacrine hydrochloride (100 mg tid × 5 days)	Metronidazole
IV. Intestinal Helminths			
Ascariasis	*Ascaris lumbricoides*	Pyrantel pamoate (single dose of 11 mg/kg—max 1 g), or mebendazole (100 mg bid × 3 days)	Piperazine citrate
Trichuriasis	*Trichuris trichiura*	Mebendazole (100 mg bid × 3 days)	None
Hookworm	*Necator americanus, Ancylostoma duodenale*	Mebendazole or pyrantel pamoate (same doses as above)	Thiabendazole
Strongyloidiasis	*Strongyloides stercoralis*	Thiabendazole (25 mg/kg bid × 2 days)	Pyrvinium pamoate
Tapeworm infections	*Taenia saginata, T. solium, Hymenolepis nana, H. diminuta*	Niclosamide† (single dose, 2 g)	Paromomycin

not conform to political units, the basis on which these reports are prepared, and it is necessary to realize the importance of broad ecologic regions, common because of their general aspects of geography and climate.[184] A summary of some of these diseases is given in Table 90–2. Fortunately, most diseases of travelers, because they are caused by viruses or enteric pathogens, are self-limited and may require no specific therapy.

Specific diagnosis of these diseases, once suspected through a history of travel and/or exposure, and a physical examination which may be helpful (and can be diagnostic in some situations) can be

made through 1) isolation and/or identification of the pathogen from body fluids or tissues; and 2) specific immunologic responses to the pathogen. In some cases, it is necessary to treat on the suspicion of a specific diagnosis, since laboratory confirmation may not be available for many days. Such is the case with diphtheria or rickettsial diseases such as Rocky Mountain spotted fever or suspected drug-resistant malaria.

Laboratory tests are constantly being improved, and current literature must be consulted for the most recent ones. Appropriate types of laboratory examinations for diagnosis are also listed in Table 90–2.

TABLE 90–2

Infections That May Pose a Serious Health Hazard to Travelers or Persons Living in Selected Geographic Regions or Subject to Exposure in Certain Environmental Situations

Disease	Pathogen	Usual Mode of Transmission	Incubation Period (days)	Laboratory Diagnosis	Primary Geographic Location
I. Viral, Chlamydial, and Rickettsial					
Smallpox	Variola virus	Contact, airborne	9–15	Lesion examination (antigen detection, EM), viral isolation	Eradicated (last in Africa)
Lassa fever	Lassa fever virus	Not known	Approx. 14	Viral isolation, Ab titers	Africa
Yellow fever	Yellow fever virus	Vectors (mosquitoes)	3–6	Liver biopsy, viral isolation	Central Africa, South America
Hemorrhagic fever	Tickborne arboviruses, dengue virus, arenaviruses, Marburg agent, etc.	Vectors (ticks, mosquitoes), contact	Variable	Viral isolation, Ab titer, EM for Marburg agent	Worldwide; individual species often localized to select geographic areas
Viral encephalitis	Many arboviruses, herpesvirus, myxoviruses, enteroviruses, etc.	Vectors (mosquitoes), airborne, fecal-oral	3–10 or longer	Viral isolation, Ab titer	Worldwide; individual species often localized to select geographic areas
Rabies	Rabies virus	Contact (animal bites)	10 to much longer (months)	Viral isolation, Ab titer, brain biopsy	Worldwide
Hepatitis A	Hepatitis A virus	Contact (blood), fecal-oral	15–45	Liver biopsy, enzymes, Ab titer	Worldwide
Hepatitis B	Hepatitis B virus	Contact (blood)	45–180	Liver biopsy, antigen and Ab detection, enzymes	Worldwide

(Continued)

TABLE 90–2 (cont.)

Disease	Pathogen	Usual Mode of Transmission	Incubation Period (days)	Laboratory Diagnosis	Primary Geographic Location
I. Viral, Chlamydial, and Rickettsial (cont.)					
Typhus	*Rickettsia prowazeki*	Vectors (lice, fleas)	7–15	Ab titer (incl. Weil-Felix)	Worldwide
Spotted fever	*R. rickettsi*, etc.	Vectors (ticks)	3–12	Ab titer (incl. Weil-Felix)	Eastern U.S.
Scrub typhus	*Rickettsia tsutsugamushi*	Vectors (mites)	6–12	Ab titer (incl. Weil-Felix)	Southeast Asia
II. Bacterial and Fungal					
Epidemic meningitis	*Neisseria meningitidis*	Airborne	Variable	CSF examination, culture	Africa, South America
Diphtheria	*Corynebacterium diphtheriae*	Airborne	1–7	Culture	Worldwide
Anthrax	*Bacillus anthracis*	Contact (animals, soil), airborne	1–7	Exudate examination, culture	Worldwide
Plague	*Yersinia pestis*	Vectors (fleas), airborne	1–12	Exudate examination, culture	Worldwide, Southwestern U.S., Southeast Asia
Cholera	*Vibrio cholerae*	Waterborne, foodborne	1–2	Culture, stool examination	Asia, Africa
Typhoid and paratyphoid	Salmonella sp.	Fecal-oral, waterborne	3–15 or longer	Culture, Ab titer	Worldwide, developing countries
Bacillary dysentery	Shigella sp.	Fecal-oral, waterborne	1–2	Culture	Worldwide, developing countries
Enterotoxic diarrhea	*Escherichia coli*, enterotoxigenic	Fecal-oral, foodborne	1–2	Culture	Worldwide, developing countries
Melioidosis	*Pseudomonas pseudomallei*	Contact (soil), airborne	2 or longer	Culture	Southeast Asia
Bartonellosis	*Bartonella bacilliformis*	Vectors (sandflies)	7–14	Culture, blood examination	Andes Mountains
Leptospirosis	Leptospira sp.	Waterborne, contact (animal urine)	2–20	Culture, Ab titer	Worldwide
Relapsing fever	Borrelia sp.	Vectors (lice, ticks)	4–18	Blood examination (Giemsa)	Africa, worldwide
Leprosy	*Mycobacterium leprae*	Contact (personal, soil?)	Variable but long (months)	Skin snip or blood examination	Worldwide
Tuberculosis	*M. tuberculosis*	Airborne, food (dairy products)	Variable	Sputum or exudate examination culture, biopsy	Worldwide
Coccidiodo-mycosis	*Coccidioides immitis*	Airborne (soil)	Variable	Sputum examination (KOH), culture	Southwestern U.S.

— **TABLE 90-2 (cont.)** —

Disease	Pathogen	Usual Mode of Transmission	Incubation Period (days)	Laboratory Diagnosis	Primary Geographic Location
III. Protozoan					
Falciparum malaria	*Plasmodium falciparum*	Vectors (anopheline mosquitoes)	10–14	Blood examination (Giemsa)	Tropics
Vivax malaria	*P. vivax*	Vectors (anopheline mosquitoes)	10–14	Blood examination (Giemsa)	Tropics
Quartan malaria	*P. malariae*	Vectors (anopheline mosquitoes)	18–42	Blood examination (Giemsa)	Tropics
Kala azar	*Leishmania donovani*	Vectors (sandflies)	60 to much longer (months)	Bone marrow and blood	Tropics
African sleeping sickness	*Trypanosoma brucei*	Vectors (tsetse flies)	14 or longer	Blood, LN, and CSF examination (Giemsa)	Tropical Africa
Chagas' disease	*Trypanosoma cruzi*	Vectors (reduviid bugs)	Variable	Blood and marrow examinations (Giemsa) biopsy	South America
Amebiasis	*Entamoeba histolytica*	Waterborne, fecal-oral	Variable	Stool, exudate, or tissue examination	Worldwide
Giardiasis	*Giardia lamblia*	Waterborne, fecal-oral	Variable	Stool or duodenal aspirate examination	Worldwide
IV. Helminthic					
Strongyloidiasis	*Strongyloides stercoralis*	Contact (soil)	Variable	Stool or duodenal aspirate examination	Worldwide
Eosinophilic meningitis	*Angiostrongylus cantonensis*, etc.	Food (snails, shrimp)	Variable	CSF examination	South Pacific
Filariasis	*Wuchereria bancrofti, Brugia malayi, Onchocerca volvulus, Dipetalonema* sp.	Vectors (mosquitoes, black-flies, etc.)	Variable but long (months)	Blood, urine, effusion, LN or skin snip examination	Tropics
Schistosomiasis	*Schistosoma mansoni, S. haematobium S. japonicum*	Contact (water containing cercariae from snail host)	30–60	Stool or urine examination, rectal biopsy, Ab titer	Tropics
Paragonimiasis	*Paragonimus westermani*	Food (crabs, etc.)	Variable (months)	Sputum and stool examination biopsy	Far East
Echinococciasis	Echinococcus sp.	Fecal-oral (dog feces)	Variable (months)	Ab titer, fluid examination (surgically resected cyst, non aspirate)	Worldwide

CULTURES AND MICROSCOPIC EXAMINATIONS

Cultures for bacteria and fungi and cell count and description from body fluids can often be diagnostic.[181,182] In addition, special examinations for larger parasitologic forms may be indicated. Sources of these diagnostic materials include:

Blood. Thick blood films, hemolyzed and stained by Giemsa or Fields methods, facilitate detection of malaria parasites, hemoflagellates, and microfilariae; identification can then be made in corresponding well-stained thin films.

Urine and Pleural, Ascitic Fluids. Search of centrifuged sediment from body fluids may sometimes reveal filarial worms or their microfilariae.

Cerebrospinal Fluid. Certain amebae that are usually free living (members of the genera *Naegleria* or *Acanthamoeba*) may be isolated from the cerebrospinal fluid of patients with primary amebic meningoencephalitis. Trypanosomes are present in the CSF during the later stages of African sleeping sickness. Subadult rat lungworms, *Angiostrongylus cantonensis,* may occasionally be aspirated from the subarachnoid space of human patients with eosinophilic meningitis caused by this parasite.

Tissue Aspirates and Biopsy Material. Skin snips or needle aspirates from the advancing margin of skin lesions as in the diagnosis of leprosy may be useful also in demonstrating the etiologic agents of cutaneous leishmaniasis, onchocerciasis, streptocerciasis, creeping eruption (due to canine hookworm larvae), scabies, and other cutaneous parasitic infections. Lymph node aspirates or biopsy may reveal trypanosomes or *Toxoplasma gondii;* adult filarial worms may be found on dissection or sectioning of lymph nodes from patients with bancroftian or Malayan filariasis. When searching for protozoal parasites in fresh biopsy material (lymph nodes, liver, bone marrow, lung, or other), stained tissue impressions greatly facilitate the examination and should be made in addition to the usual fixed tissue sections. Helminths are difficult to identify in tissue sections. Although an experienced parasitologist may easily recognize the higher taxonomic category to which the parasite belongs, the species may be impossible to determine. It is wise to preserve a portion of fresh tissue for crush preparations between glass slides or for tearing apart under a dissecting microscope in an effort to recover whole worms or identifiable large fragments. Biopsy of a rectal valve margin may be a useful maneuver in diagnosing schistosomal infections, especially *Schistosoma mansoni.*

Feces. Routine bacteriologic examination for shigella and salmonella may be rewarding, but the most common cause of travelers' diarrhea, enterotoxigenic *E. coli,* cannot be identified except by special techniques not now routinely available. Other specific pathogens, such as *Vibrio parahaemolyticus,* require special media for their isolation.[185]

Intestinal protozoa and helminths are usually detected by the presence of diagnostic stages in the stools. These include the motile trophozoites or thin-walled cysts of protozoa and the eggs, larvae, or adult stages of helminths, the latter either entire or as detached segments (tapeworm proglottids). Because of the enormous disparity in size of these objects, varying from several meters for the larger tapeworms and about 30 cm for a mature ascarid worm to protozoa smaller than an erythrocyte, stool examination must be conducted at several levels of magnification. After careful gross inspection, fecal suspensions in saline are scanned methodically under low-power light microscopy and critical identification then made under higher power (including the 100 × oil immersion lens for stained protozoa).

Loose, watery specimens that may contain actively motile amebic trophozoites containing ingested red blood cells should be examined promptly; specimens kept at room temperature longer than half an hour or so will usually show only inactive, rounded-up precystic stages which are quite nondiagnostic. Fresh diarrheal specimens that cannot be examined immediately should be preserved in polyvinyl alcohol solution in vials and on slides prepared for permanent staining.

All specimens should be examined in warm saline coverslip preparations, supplemented by iodine or merthiolate-iodine stained suspensions for identification of protozoal cysts.

Formed stool specimens, kept under refrigeration (not frozen) if examination is delayed more than a few hours, should also be examined by using one of the techniques for concentration of protozoal cysts and helminth eggs.

Even when concentration techniques are used to full advantage, detection of intestinal parasites is enhanced by examining a series of specimens (usually three or more) collected on different days from each individual patient. Examination of sigmoidoscopic curettings from suspected amebic ulcers aids in finding trophozoites of *Entamoeba histolytica;* material from the wall of abscesses in liver or other tissue, from the margin of abdominal or perineal skin ulcers, or from sputum may provide evidence of extraintestinal amebiasis. (Cultures of *E. histolytica* are feasible in commercially available media but cannot supplant meticulous microscopic examination.) Duodenal fluid may sometimes contain motile trophozoites of *Giardia lamblia* or rhabditiform larvae of *Strongyloides stercoralis* when examination of the feces has failed to reveal the infection.

Immunologic Tests

Serology may provide the only diagnostic evidence of infection due to viruses and rickettsia. In most bacterial and parasitic diseases, identification of the organisms rather than serology will be of most importance. However, through the development of highly specific, refined antigens and reliably sensitive techniques (especially fluorescent-antibody staining and gel-diffusion methods), serodiagnosis has become useful and practical in the recognition of several important parasitic infections. Although of greater value in surveys of disease prevalence than in individual case diagnosis, immunologic tests are currently available for diagnosis of malaria, amebiasis, American trypanosomiasis (Chagas' disease), trichiniasis, cysticercosis, and echinococcosis. The results of all serologic tests should be interpreted critically and used with discrimination in the individual patient whose "positive" test may reflect prior exposure rather than active disease. Titers of acute and convalescent sera must always be determined to identify recent exposure to the etiologic agent.

Biohazards

Attending physicians, nurses, and laboratory personnel may be at considerable risk in handling fresh specimens and living cultures taken from patients with undiagnosed disease contracted in other parts of the world. The well-documented experiences with smallpox and with the virus of Lassa fever and other related arenaviruses afforded telling examples of the hazard even to highly trained persons. Hepatitis, rabies, most arboviral and rickettsial diseases, psittacosis, anthrax, coccidioidomycosis (infectious arthrospores), plague, and tularemia may be dangerous to the unwary. Attempts to isolate the causative organism should be made only by experienced workers with special high-containment laboratory facilities.

TREATMENT OF GEOGRAPHIC ILLNESSES

The treatment of bacterial, mycobacterial, fungal, and viral illnesses has been discussed elsewhere in the text. Treatment of common parasitic infections, for example pinworm and ascarid infections in children, may be relatively safe and straight-forward. Therapy of the less familiar parasitic diseases, however, may require medications that are seldom used and may be toxic. The initial decision of whether to treat or not must be weighed carefully. Attention must be given to age, body size, nutritional status, and intercurrent disease when deciding the therapeutic regimen. Consultation should be sought if experience is lacking.[183,185]

Current therapeutic recommendations for the most important protozoal and helminthic infections are given in Table 90–1, with dosages appropriate for adults in otherwise good health. Dosages for children and debilitated adults should be determined with due care. Some immunobiologic and chemotherapeutic agents are currently available only through the Center for Disease Control, and this agency should be consulted regarding the use of these drugs.[186]

PREVENTION OF GEOGRAPHIC ILLNESSES

In addition to being able to recognize disease in persons traveling from areas where these diseases may be acquired, the U.S. physician should also be able to give advice about prevention of some of these illnesses to persons traveling abroad, particularly to developing countries.[184] Advice to travelers for prophylaxis should include

1. Avoidance of fresh fruits and vegetables (unless they can be peeled) in all areas where sanitation is in question
2. Care in drinking only water that can be ascertained as being potable
3. Immunizations appropriate to the geographic areas. These include smallpox (which may soon be unnecessary), yellow fever, and cholera. (The latter is required by certain countries even though the vaccine is probably of no value to either the traveler or the country.) Other effective vaccines may be given including those for typhoid fever and diphtheria. It is expected that most travelers will have been immunized against tetanus and poliomyelitis. Rabies immunization may be given to persons going to developing areas where exposure to animals, particularly dogs, will be great
4. Passive protection against hepatitis A which can be given with gammaglobulin injections immediately prior to travel. This should be considered for all travelers to the developing world.
5. Malaria prophylaxis for persons traveling to areas known to have malaria. Chloroquine or *Fansidar* (pyrimethamine plus sulfadoxine) prophylaxis should be given according to the known pattern of drug resistance. *Fansidar* must be obtained outside the United States.
6. Diarrhea prophylaxis for short-term travelers to developing areas of a month or less. Doxycycline can be given to prevent most cases of travelers' diarrhea, which are most commonly

caused by antibiotic sensitive strains of enterotoxigenic *E. coli*. (A specific exception to this finding is in the Far East where these strains are often resistant to antibiotics.) Advice can also be given regarding oral fluid and electrolyte replacement for those who may contract severe diarrheal disease.

REFERENCES

General References

1. Altemeier, W.A., Culbertson, W.R., and Fullen, W.D. Intra-abdominal sepsis. Adv. Surg., 5:281, 1971.
2. Bijkerk, H. Follow-up on poliomyelitis in the Netherlands. Morbidity and Mortality Weekly Report, 27:381, 1978.
3. Crowe, C.C., Sanders, W.E., and Longley, S. Role of the normal throat flora in prevention of colonization by Group A streptococcus. J. Infect. Dis., 128:527, 1973.
4. Dinarello, C.A. and Wolff, S.M. Pathogenesis of fever in man. N. Engl. J. Med., 298:607, 1978.
5. Elek, S.D. and Conen, P.E. The virulence of Staphylococcus Pyogenes (Aureus) for man. Br. J. Exp. Pathol., 38:573, 1957.
6. Faust, E.C. and Russel, P.F. Clinical Parasitology, 7th ed. Philadelphia, Lea & Febiger, 1964.
7. Glover, J.A. Observations of the Meningococcus carrier rate, and their application to the prevention of cerebrospinal fever. Medical Research Council: Special Report Series (London), 50:133, 1920.
8. Griesman, S.E. and Hornick, R.B. Cellular inflammatory responses of man to bacterial endotoxin. A comparison with PPD and other bacterial antigens. J. Immunol., 109:1210, 1974.
9. Herzig, R.H., Herzig, G.P., Graw, R.G., et al. Successful granulocyte transfusion therapy for Gram-negative septicemia. A prospective randomized controlled study. N. Engl. J. Med., 296:701, 1977.
10. Johanson, W.G., Pierce, A.K., Sanford, J.P., and Thomas, G.D. Nosocomial respiratory infections with gram-negative bacilli. Ann. Intern. Med., 77:701, 1972.
11. Merriman, C.R., Pulliam, L.A., and Kampschmidt, R.F. Comparison of leukocytic pyrogen and leukocyte endogenous mediator. Proc. Soc. Exp. Biol. Med., 154:224, 1977.
12. Moxon, E.R. and Murphy, P.A. Haemophilus Influenzae bacteremia and meningitis resulting from survival of a single organism. Proc. Natl. Acad. Sci. USA, 75:1534, 1978.
13. Pagel, W., Simmonds, F.A.H., Macdonald, N., and Nassau, E. Pulmonary Tuberculosis. London, Oxford University Press, 1964, pp. 445–462.
14. Rammelkamp, C.H. Epidemiology of Streptococcal infections. Harvey Lect., 51:113, 1956.
15. Rippon, J.W. Medical Mycology. Philadelphia, Saunders, 1974.
16. Rowan, R.M., Gordon, A.M., Chauduri, A.K.R., et al. A further application of the Nitroblue Tetrazolium Test. Br. Med. J., 3:317, 1974.
17. Rytel, M.W. Rapid diagnostic methods in infectious diseases. Adv. Intern. Med., 20:37, 1974.
18. Tisdale, W.A. Spontaneous colon bacillus bacteremia in Laennec's cirrhosis. Gastroenterology, 40:141, 1961.
19. Watanakunakorn, C., Tan, J.S., and Phair, J.P. Some salient features of Staphylococcus Aureus Endocarditis. Am. J. Med., 54:473, 1973.
20. Webster, L.T. Experimental epidemiology. Medicine, 25:77, 1946 (especially pp. 102–108).
21. Zieve, P.D., Haghshanass, M., and Krevans, J.R. Vacuolization of the neutrophil. Arch. Intern. Med., 118:356, 1966.

Infections in Patients with Impaired Defenses

22. Chilcote, R.R., Baehner, R.L., Hammond, D., et al. Septicemia and meningitis in children splenectomized for Hodgkin's disease. N. Engl. J. Med., 295:798, 1976.
23. Conn, H.O. and Fessel, J.M. Spontaneous bacterial peritonitis in cirrhosis. Medicine, 50:161, 1971.
24. Costa, G. Cachexia, the metabolic component of neoplastic diseases. Cancer Res., 37:2327, 1977.
25. Cunningham, J.H., Zavala, D.C., Corry, R.S., et al. Trephine air drill, bronchial brush and fiberoptic transbronchial lung biopsies in immunosuppressed patients. Am. Rev. Respir. Dis., 115:213, 1977.
26. Fauve, R.M. and Pierce-Chese, C.H. Comparative effects of corticosteroids on host resistance to infection in relation to chemical structure. J. Exp. Med., 125:807, 1967.
27. Law, D.K., Dudrick, S.S., and Abdou, N.I. Immunocompetence of patients with protein-calorie malnutrition. Ann. Intern. Med., 79:545, 1973.
28. Levy, R. and Kaplan, H.S. Impaired lymphocyte function in untreated Hodgkin's disease. N. Engl. J. Med., 290:181, 1974.
29. Liu, Y.K. Leukopenia in alcoholics. Am. J. Med., 54:605, 1973.
30. Martin, W.J., Spittal, J.A., Morlock, J.A., and Baggenstoss, A.H. Severe liver disease complicated by bacteremia due to gram-negative bacilli. Arch. Intern. Med., 98:8, 1956.
31. Myerowitz, R.L., Medeiros, A.A., and O'Brien, T.F. Bacterial infection in renal homotransplant recipients. Am. J. Med., 53:308, 1972.
32. Pennington, J.E. Fever, neutropenia and malignancy, a clinical syndrome in evolution. Cancer, 39:1345, 1977.
33. Singer, D.B. Postsplenectomy sepsis. Perspect. Pediatr. Pathol., 1:285, 1973.
34. Taylor, C.E. and DeSweener, C. Nutrition and Infection. World Rev. Nutr. Diet., 16:203, 1973.
35. Thornton, G.F. Infections and diabetes. Med. Clin. North Am., 55:931, 1971.
36. Valdivieso, M., Gil-Extremera, B., Zornoza, J., et al. Gram-negative bacillary pneumonia in the compromised host. Medicine, 56:241, 1977.
37. Yunis, E.J. and Greenberg, L.J. Symposium: immunopathology of aging. Fed. Proc., 33:2017, 1974.

Management of Infectious Diseases

38. Gale, E.F., Cundliffe, E., Reynolds, P.E., Richmond, M.H., and Waring, M.J. The Molecular Basis of Antibiotic Action. New York, Wiley, 1972.
39. Garrod, L.P. and O'Grady, F. Antibiotic and Chemotherapy. London, Churchill Livingstone, 1972.
40. Goodman, L.S. and Gilman, A. The Pharmacological Basis of Therapeutics, 5th ed. New York, Macmillan, 1975.
41. Kucers, A. The Use of Antibiotics. Philadelphia, Lippincott, 1975.
42. The Medical Letter on Drugs and Therapeutics. Handbook of Antimicrobial Therapy. Revised Edition, 1974. New Rochelle, N.Y., Medical Letter, 1974.
43. Weinstein, L. and Dalton, A.C. Host determinants of response to antimicrobial agents. N. Engl. J. Med., 279:467, 1968.

Infections Without Localizing Manifestations

44. Altemeier, W.A., Culbertson, W.R., Fullen, W.D., et al. Intra-abdominal abscesses. Am. J. Surg., 125:70, 1973.
45. Baker, R.R., Tumulty, P.A., and Shelley, W.M. The value of exploratory laparotomy in fever of undetermined etiology. Johns Hopkins Med. J., 125:159, 1969.
46. Cluff, L.E. and Johnson, J.E. Drug fever. Prog. Allergy, 8:149, 1964.
47. Deller, J.J., Jr. and Russell, P.K. An analysis of fevers of unknown origin in American soldiers in Vietnam. Ann. Intern. Med., 66:1129, 1967.
48. Grossman, Z.D., Wistow, B.W., Bryan, P.J., Dinn, W.M., McAfee, J.G., and Kiefer, S.A. Radionuclide imaging, computer tomography, and gray-scale ultrasonography of the liver: a comparative study. J. Nucl. Med. Allied Sci., 18:327, 1977.
49. Jacoby, G. and Swarz, M.N. Fever of undetermined origin. N. Engl. J. Med., 289:1407, 1974.
50. Kumar, B., Alderson, P.O., and Geisse, G. The role of Ga-67 citrate imaging and diagnostic ultrasound in patients with suspected abdominal abscesses. J. Nucl. Med. Allied Sci., 18:534, 1977.
51. Petersdorf, R.G. and Beeson, P.B. Fever of unexplained origin: report of 100 cases. Medicine, 40:1, 1961.
52. ——— and Bennett, I.L., Jr. Factitious fever. Ann. Intern. Med., 46:1039, 1957.
53. Rich, A.R. The Pathogenesis of Tuberculosis, 2nd ed. Springfield, Ill., Thomas, 1951.
54. Rubin, H., Furcolow, M.L., Yates, J.L., and Brusher, C.A. Seminar on mycotic infections: the course and prognosis of histoplasmosis. Am. J. Med., 27:278, 1959.
55. Stead, W.W. The pathogenesis of pulmonary tuberculosis among older persons. Am. Rev. Respir. Dis., 91:811, 1965.
56. ———, Kerby, G.R., Schlueter, D.P., and Jordahl, C.W. The clinical spectrum of primary tuberculosis in adults. Ann. Intern. Med., 68:731, 1968.
57. Tisdale, W.A. and Klatskin, G. The fever of Laennec's cirrhosis. Yale J. Biol. Med., 33:94, 1960.

Bacterial Infections of Skin, Muscle, and Bone

58. Center for Disease Control. Morbidity and Mortality Weekly Report, 26:407, 1977.

59. Collins, R.H. and Nadel, M.S. Gangrene due to the hemolytic streptococcus: a rare but treatable disease. N. Engl. J. Med., 272:578, 1965.
60. Falkner, F. Chronic osteomyelitis. Lancet, 1:415, 1976.
61. Antimicrobial prophylaxis: prevention of wound infection and sepsis after surgery. Medical Letter, 19:37, 1977.
62. Waldvogel, F.A., Medoff, G., and Swartz, M.N. Osteomyelitis: a review of clinical features, therapeutic considerations and unusual aspects. N. Engl. J. Med., 282:198, 260, 316, 1970.
63. Wannamaker, L.W. Difference between streptococcal infections of the throat and the skin. N. Engl. J. Med., 282:23, 78, 1970.
64. Weinstein, L. and Barza, M.A. Gas gangrene. N. Engl. J. Med., 289:1129, 1973.

Upper Respiratory Infections

65. Asian variant influenza. Public Health Rep., 73:99, 1958.
66. Bergland, G., Salmivalli, A., and Towanen, P. Isolation of respiratory syncytial virus from middle ear exudates of infants. Acta Otolaryngol., 61:475, 1966.
67. Evans, F.O., Jr., Syndor, J.B., Moore, W.E.C., et al. Sinusitis of the maxillary antrum. N. Engl. J. Med., 293:735, 1975.
68. Haverkorn, M.J., Valkenburg, H.A., and Goslings, W.R.O. Streptococcal pharyngitis in the general population I. A controlled study of streptococcal pharyngitis and its complications in the Netherlands. II. The attack rate of rheumatic fever and acute glomerulonephritis in patients not treated with penicillin. J. Infect. Dis., 124:339, 348, 1971.
69. Howie, V.M., Ploussard, J.H., and Luster, R.L. Otitis media: a clinical and bacteriological correlation. Pediatrics, 45:29, 1975.
70. Idsoe, O., Guthe, T., Willcox, R.R., et al. Nature and extent of penicillin side-reactions with particular reference to fatalities from anaphylactic shock. Bull. WHO, 38:159, 1968.
71. Juselius, H. and Kaltiokallio, K. Complications of acute and chronic otitis media in the antibiotic era. Acta Otolaryngol., 74:445, 1972.
72. Louria, D.B., Blumenfeld, H.L., Ellis, J.T., Kilbourne, E.D., and Rogers, D.E. Studies on influenza in the pandemic of 1958–59. II. Pulmonary complications of influenza. J. Clin. Invest., 38:321, 1959.
73. Markowitz, M. and Gordis, L. Rheumatic Fever, 2nd ed. Philadelphia, Saunders, 1972.
74. Matanoski, G.M., Price, W.H., and Ferencz, C. Epidemiology of streptococcal infections in rheumatic and non-rheumatic families. Am. J. Epidemiol., 87:179, 1968.
75. Norden, C.W., Callerance, M.L., and Baum, J. Hemophilus influenzae meningitis in an adult: a study of bactericidal antibodies. N. Engl. J. Med., 282:190, 1970.
76. O'Donoghue, J.M., Ray, C.G., Terry, D.W., Jr., et al. Prevention of nosocomial influenza infection with amantidine. Am. J. Epidemiol., 97:276, 1973.
77. Pantell, R.H. Cost-effectiveness of pharyngitis management and prevention of rheumatic fever. Ann. Intern. Med., 86:497, 1977.

78. Public Health Service Advisory Committee on Immunization Practices. Influenza vaccine. Morbidity and Mortality Weekly Reports, 26:24, 1977.

79. Russel, W.T. The epidemiology of diphtheria during the last 40 years. Medical Research Council: Special Report Series (London), 247:9, 1943.

80. Tompkins, D.G., Boxerbau, B., and Liebman, J. Long-term prognosis of rheumatic fever patients receiving regular intramuscular benzathine penicillin. Circulation, 45:543, 1972.

81. Weinstein, L. and Lefrock, J. Does antimicrobial therapy of streptococcal pharyngitis or pyoderma alter the risk of glomerulonephritis? J. Infect. Dis., 124:229, 1971.

Pneumonia

82. Bartlett, J.G., Gorbach, S.L., and Finegold, S.M. The bacteriology of aspiration pneumonia. Am. J. Med., 56:202, 1974.

83. Basiliere, J.C., Bistrong, H.W., and Spence, W.F. Streptococcal pneumonia: recent outbreaks in military recruit populations. Am. J. Med., 44:580, 1968.

84. Everett, E.D., Rahm, A.E., Adaniya, R., et al. Haemophilus influenzae pneumonia in adults. JAMA, 238:319, 1977.

85. Fisher, A.M., Trever, R., Cutron, J.A., et al. Staphylococcal pneumonia: a review of 21 cases in adults. N. Engl. J. Med., 258:919, 1958.

86. Jay, S.J., Johansen, W.G., and Pierce, A.K. The radiographic resolution of Streptococcus Pneumoniae pneumonia. N. Engl. J. Med., 293:798, 1975.

87. Lampe, W.T. Klebsiella pneumonia: a review of forty-five cases and reevaluation of the incidence and antibiotic sensitivities. Dis. Chest, 46:599, 1964.

88. Lie, J.T. Nosology of pulmonary vasculitides. Mayo Clin. Proc., 52:520, 1977.

89. Morgan, H.J. Pleuropulmonary tularemia. Ann. Intern. Med., 27:519, 1947.

90. Mufson, M.A., Manko, M.A., Kingston, J.R., et al. Eaton agent pneumonia—clinical features. JAMA, 178:369, 1961.

91. Pearce, A.K. and Sanford, J.P. Aerobic gram-negative bacillary pneumonias. Am. Rev. Respir. Dis., 110:647, 1974.

92. Poulose, K.P., Reba, R.C., Gilday, D.L., et al. Diagnosis of pulmonary embolism: a correlative study of the clinical, scan and angiographic findings. Br. Med. J., 3:67, 1970.

93. Rosenow, E.C. The spectrum of drug-induced pulmonary disease. Ann. Intern. Med., 77:977, 1972.

94. Tew, J., Calenoff, L., and Berlin, B.S. Bacterial or nonbacterial pneumonia: accuracy of radiological diagnosis. Radiology, 124:607, 1977.

95. Tillotson, J.R. and Finland, M. Bacterial colonization and clinical superinfection of the respiratory tract complicating antibiotic treatment of pneumonia. J. Infect. Dis., 119:597, 1969.

96. Williams, D.M., Krick, J.A., and Remington, J.S. Pulmonary infection in the compromised host. Am. Rev. Respir. Dis., 114:359, 1976.

Infective Endocarditis

97. AHA Committee Report—Prevention of bacterial endocarditis. Circulation, 56:139A, 1977.

98. Bain, R.C., Edwards, J.E., Scheiffey, C.H., and Geraci, J.E. Right-sided bacterial endocarditis and endarteritis: clinical and pathologic study. Am. J. Med., 24:98, 1958.

99. Bennett, I.L., Jr. and Beeson, P.B. Bacteremia: a consideration of some experimental and clinical aspects. Yale J. Biol. Med., 26:241, 1954.

100. Durack, D.T. and Beeson, P.B. Experimental bacterial endocarditis. I. Colonization of a sterile vegetation. Br. J. Exp. Pathol., 53:44, 1972.

101. ——— and Petersdorf, R.G. Chemotherapy of experimental streptococcal endocarditis. I. Comparison of commonly recommended prophylactic regimes. J. Clin. Invest., 52:592, 1973.

102. ———, Pelleher, L., and Petersdorf, R.B. Chemotherapy of experimental streptococcal endocarditis. II. Synergism between penicillin and streptomycin against penicillin-sensitive streptococci. J. Clin. Invest., 53:829, 1974.

103. Garvey, G.J. and New, H.C. Infective endocarditis—an involving disease. A review of endocarditis at the Columbia Presbyterian Medical Center 1968–1973. Medicine, 57:125, 1978.

104. Griffin, F.M., Jr., Jones, G., and Gobbs, C.G. Aortic insufficiency in bacterial endocarditis. Ann. Intern. Med., 76:23, 1972.

105. Gutman, R.A., Striker, G.E., Gilliland, B.C., and Cutler, R.E. The immune complex glomerulonephritis of bacterial endocarditis. Medicine, 51:1, 1972.

106. Hunter, T.H. The treatment of some bacterial infections of the heart and pericardium. Bull. NY Acad. Med., 28:213, 1952.

107. Lerner, P.I. and Weinstein, L. Infective endocarditis in the antibiotic era. N. Engl. J. Med., 274:199, 259, 323, 288, 1966.

108. Lord, J.W., Imparato, A.M., Hackel, A., and Doyle, E.F. Endocarditis complicating open-heart surgery. Circulation, 23:608, 1970.

109. Mills, J., Utley, J., and Abbott, J. Heart failure in infective endocarditis: predisposing factors, course and treatment. Chest, 66:151, 1974.

110. Murray, H.W., Wigley, F.M., Mann, J.J., and Arthur, R.R. Combination antibiotic therapy in Staphylococcal endocarditis. Arch. Intern. Med., 136:480, 1976.

111. Pruitt, A.A., Rubin, R.H., Karchmer, A.W., and Duncan, G.W. Neurologic complications of bacterial endocarditis. Medicine, 57:329, 1978.

112. Ramsey, R.G., Gunnar, R.M., and Tobin, J.R. Endocarditis in the drug addict. Am. J. Cardiol., 25:608, 1970.

113. Wann, L.S., Dillon, J.C., Weyman, A.E., and Fiegenbaum, H. Echocardiography in bacterial endocarditis. N. Engl. J. Med., 295:135, 1976.

114. Weinstein, L. and Rubin, R.H. Infective endocarditis. Prog. Cardiovasc. Dis., 16:239, 1973.

115. Wise, J.R., Jr., Cleland, W.P., Hallidie-Smith, K.A., Benrall, H.H., Goodwin, J.F., and Oakley, C.M. Urgent aortic valve replacement for acute aortic regurgitation due to infective endocarditis. Lancet, 2:115, 1971.

116. Wolfe, J.C. and Johnson, W.D., Jr. Penicillin-sensitive streptococcal endocarditis. Ann. Intern. Med., 81:178, 1974.

Infections of the Gastrointestinal Tract

117. Dolin, R., Levy, A.G., Wyatt, R.G., Thornhill, T.S., and Gardner, J.D. Viral gastroenteritis induced by the Hawaii agent. Jejunal histopathology and serologic response. Am. J. Med., 59:761, 1975.

118. DuPont, H.L., Portnoy, B.L., and Conklin, R.H. Viral agents and diarrheal illness. Annu. Rev. Med., 28:167, 1977.

119. Grady, G.F. and Keusch, G.T. Pathogenesis of bacterial diarrheas. N. Engl. J. Med., 285:831, 1971.

120. Harris, J.C., Dupont, H.L., and Hornick, R.B. Fecal leukocytes in diarrheal illness. Ann. Intern. Med., 76:697, 1972.

121. Merson, M.H., Morris, G.K., Sack, D.A., Wells, J.G., Feeley, J.C., Sack, R.B., Creech, W.B., Kapikian, A.Z., and Gangarosa, E.J. Travelers' diarrhea in Mexico. A prospective study of physicians and family members attending a conference. N. Engl. J. Med., 294:1299, 1976.

122. Palmer, D.L., Koster, F.T., Rafiqul Islam, A.F.M., Mizanaur Rahman, A.F.M., and Sack, R.B. Comparison of sucrose and glucose in the oral electrolyte therapy of cholera and other severe diarrheas. N. Engl. J. Med., 297:1107, 1977.

123. Pierce, N.F., Greenough, W.B., and Carpenter, C.C.J. *Vibrio cholerae* enterotoxin, and its mode of action. Bacteriol. Rev., 35:1, 1971.

124. Pierce, N.F. and Hirschhorn, N. Oral fluid—A simple weapon against dehydration in diarrhea. WHO Chron., 3:87, 1977.

125. Sack, D.A., Merson, M.H., Wells, J.G., Sack, R.B., and Morris, G.K. Diarrhea associated with heat-stable enterotoxin-producing strains of *Escherichia coli*. Lancet, 2:239, 1975.

126. Sack, R.B. Human diarrheal disease caused by enterotoxigenic *Escherichia coli*. Annu. Rev. Microbiol., 29:333, 1975.

Infections of the Urinary Tract

127. Bailey, R.R., Roberts, A.P., Gower, P.E., and deWardener, H.E. Prevention of urinary-tract infection with low-dose nitrofurantoin. Lancet, 2:1112, 1971.

128. Bran, J.L., Levison, M.E., and Kaye, D. Entrance of bacteria into the female urinary bladder. N. Engl. J. Med., 286:626, 1972.

129. Bulger, R.J. and Kirby, W.M. Simple tests for significant bacteriuria. Arch. Intern. Med., 112:742, 1963.

130. Dans, P.E. and Klaus, B. Dysuria in women. Johns Hopkins Med. J., 138:13, 1976.

131. Fang, L.S.T., Tolkoff-Rubin, N.E., and Rubin, R.H. Efficacy of single-dose and conventional amoxicillin therapy in urinary-tract infection localized by the antibody-coated bacteria technic. N. Engl. J. Med., 298:413, 1978.

132. Harding, G.K.M. and Ronald, A.R. A controlled study of antimicrobial prophylaxis of recurrent urinary infections in women. N. Engl. J. Med., 291:597, 1974.

133. Kass, E.H. Bacteriuria and diagnosis of infections of the urinary tract. Arch. Intern. Med., 100:709, 1957.

134. Mabeck, C.E., Ørskov, F., and Ørskov, I. *Escherichia coli* serotypes and renal involvement in urinary-tract infection. Lancet, 1:1312, 1971.

135. Ronald, A.R., Boutros, P., and Mourtada, H. Bacteriuria localization and response to single-dose therapy in women. JAMA, 235:1854, 1976.

136. Sanford, J.P. Urinary tract symptoms and infections. Annu. Rev. Med., 26:485, 1975.

137. Stamey, T.A. and Pfau, A. Urinary infections: a selective review and some observations. Calif. Med., 113:16, 1970.

138. Thomas, V., Shelokov, A., and Forland, M. Antibody-coated bacteria in the urine and the site of urinary-tract infection. N. Engl. J. Med., 290:588, 1974.

139. Turck, M., Anderson, K., and Petersdorf, R.G. Relapse and reinfection in chronic bacteriuria. N. Engl. J. Med., 275:70, 1966.

140. Whelton, A. Antibacterial chemotherapy in renal insufficiency. Antibiot. Chemother., 18:1, 1974.

Sexually Transmitted Infections

141. Buckley, R.M., McGuckin, M., and MacGregor, R.R. Urine bacterial counts after sexual intercourse. N. Engl. J. Med., 298:321, 1978.

142. Dans, P.E. FTA-ABS test, a diagnostic help or hindrance? South. Med. J., 70:312, 1977.

143. ———. Treatment of gonorrhea and syphilis, Parts I and II. South. Med. J., 68:1287, 1295, 1975.

144. ———. Organization and operation of a facility for sexually transmitted dieseases. Bull. NY Acad. Med., 52:955, 1976.

145. ———, Klaus, B., and Owen, M. A problem oriented approach to the venereal disease clinic patient. J. Am. Vener. Dis. Assoc., 1:158, 1975.

146. Darrow, W.W. Social and behavioral aspects of the sexually transmitted diseases In Gordon, S. and Libby, R.W. (eds.), Sexuality Today and Tomorrow. North Scituate, Mass., Duxbury Press, 1976.

147. Darrow, W.W., Wiesner, P.J. Personal prophylaxis for venereal disease. JAMA, 233:444, 1975.

148. Gonorrhea CDC Recommended Treatment Schedules. 1979. Mortality and Morbidity Weekly Report, January 19, 1979.

149. Handsfield, H.H., Lipman, T.O., Harnisch, J.P., Tronca, E., and Holmes, K.K. Asymptomatic gonorrhea in men—diagnosis, natural course, prevalence and significance. N. Engl. J. Med., 290:117, 1974.

150. Hoeprich, P.D. (ed.). Infectious Diseases, 2nd ed. Hagerstown, Md., Harper & Row, 1977.

151. Holmes, K.K., Handsfield, H.H., Wang, S.P., Wentworth, B.B., Turck, M., Anderson, J.B., and Alexander, E.R. Etiology of nongonococcal urethritis. N. Engl. J. Med., 292:1199, 1975.

152. ——— and Martin, B. Sexually transmitted diseases. Postgrad. Med., 64:121, 1978.

153. Hooshmand, H., Escobar, M.R., and Kopf, S.W. Neurosyphilis, a study of 241 patients. JAMA, 219:726, 1972.

154. Jacobs, N.F., Kraus, S.J. Gonococcal and non-gonococcal urethritis in men. Ann. Intern. Med., 82:7, 1975.

155. Jacobson, L. and Westrom, L. Objectivized diagnosis of acute pelvic inflammatory disease. Am. J. Obstet. Gynecol., 105:1088, 1969.

156. Jaffe, H.W. The laboratory diagnosis of syphilis. Ann. Intern. Med., 83:846, 1975.

157. Klein, E.J., Fisher, L.S., Chow, A.W., and Guze, L.B. Anorectal gonococcal infection. Ann. Intern. Med., 86:340, 1977.

158. Kofman, O. The changing pattern of neurosyphilis. Can. Med. Assoc. J., 74:807, 1956.

159. Litt, I.F., Edberg, S.C., and Finberg, L. Gonorrhea in children and adolescents: a current review. J. Pediatr., 85:595, 1974.

160. Mandell, G.L., Douglas, R.G., and Bennett, J.E. (eds.). Principles and Practice of Infectious Disease. New York, Wiley, 1979.

161. Mildvan, D., Gelb, A.M., and William, D. Venereal transmission of enteric pathogens in male homosexuals. JAMA, 228:1387, 1977.

162. Nahmias, A.J. and Roizman, B. Infection with herpes simplex viruses 1 and 2 (in 3 parts). N. Engl. J. Med., 289:667, 719, 781, 1973.

163. Orkin, M., Epstein, I., and Maibach, H.I. Treatment of today's scabies and pediculosis. JAMA, 236:1136, 1976.

164. Pheifer, T.A., Forsyth, P.S., Durfee, M.A., Pollock, H.M., and Holmes, K.K. Nonspecific vaginitis. N. Engl. J. Med., 298:1429, 1978.

165. Rendtorff, R.C., Curran, J.W., and Chandler, R.W. Economic consequences of gonorrhea in women: experience from an urban hospital. J. Am. Vener. Dis. Assoc., 1:40, 1974.

166. Rosebury, T. Microbes and Morals. New York, Viking, 1971.

167. Rothenberg, R.B., Simon, R., Chipperfield, E., and Catterall, R.D. Efficacy of selected diagnostic tests for sexually transmitted diseases. JAMA, 235:49, 1976.

168. Schachter, J. Chlamydial Infections (in 3 parts). N. Engl. J. Med., 298:428, 490, 540, 1978.

169. Schroeter, A.L., Lucas, J.B., Price, E.V., and Falcone, V.H. Treatment for early syphilis and reactivity of serologic tests. JAMA, 221:471, 1972.

170. Scott, W.C. Pelvic abscess in association with intrauterine contraceptive device. Am. J. Obstet. Gynecol., 131:149, 1978.

171. Syphilis—A Synopsis. Public Health Service Publication No. 1660, Washington, D.C., U.S. Government Printing Office, January, 1968.

172. Szmuness, W., Much, M.I., Prince, H.M., Hoofnagle, J.H., Cherubin, C.E., Harley, E.I., and Block, G.H. On the role of sexual behavior in the spread of hepatitis B infection. Ann. Intern. Med., 83:489, 1975.

173. Thompson, S.E. and Hager, W.D. Acute pelvic inflammatory disease. Sex. Trans. Dis., 4:105, 1977.

174. Wiesner, P.J. and Tyler, C.W., Jr. (eds.). Clin. Obstet. Gynecol., 18:1, March 1975.

175. Wright, A.D. Venereal disease and the great. Br. J. Vener. Dis., 47:295, 1971.

Infections of the Central Nervous System

176. Ellner, J.J. and Bennett, J.E. Chronic meningitis. Medicine, 55:341, 1976.

177. Heineman, H.S. and Braude, A.I. Anaerobic infection of the brain: observations on eighteen cases of brain abscess. Am. J. Med., 35:682, 1963.

178. Kaufman, D.A., Miller, M.H., and Stiegbigel, N.H. Subdural empyema: analysis of 17 recent cases and review of the literature. Medicine, 54:485, 1975.

179. Lepow, M.L., Coyne, N., Thompson, L.B., Carver, D.H., and Robbins, F.C. A clinical, epidemiologic and laboratory investigation of aseptic meningitis during the four-year period, 1955–1958. N. Engl. J. Med., 266:1188, 1962.

180. Swartz, M.N. and Dodge, P.R. Bacterial meningitis—a review of related aspects. N. Engl. J. Med., 272:725, 779, 842, 898, 954, 1003, 1965.

Geographic Medicine

181. Berman, S.J., Irving, G.S., Kunden, W.D., et al. Epidemiology of the acute fever of unknown origin in South Vietnam: effect of laboratory support upon clinical diagnosis. Am. J. Trop. Med. Hyg., 22:769, 1973.

182. Burrows, R.B. Microscopic Diagnosis of the Parasites of Man. New Haven, Yale, 1965.

183. Drugs for Parasitic Infections. The Medical Letter on Drugs and Therapeutics, 20:17, 1978.

184. Health Information for International Travel, 1977, (Supplement to 1315A Morbidity and Mortality Weekly Report, Vol. 26, Aug. 1977). U.S. Dept. of Health, Education, and Welfare. No. CDC77-8280. Center for Disease Control, Atlanta, Georgia.

185. Hunter, G.W., Swartzwelder, J.C., and Clyde, D.F. A Manual of Tropical Medicine, 5th ed. Philadelphia, Saunders, 1975.

186. Johnson, R.H. and Ellis, R.J. Immunobiologic agents and drugs available from the Center for Disease Control. Ann. Intern. Med., 81:61, 1974.

187. Warren, K.S. and Mahmound, A.A.F. Geographic Medicine for the Practitioner. Chicago, University of Chicago, 1978.

SECTION THIRTEEN
Diseases with Abnormalities of Immunity
PHILIP S. NORMAN AND LAWRENCE M. LICHTENSTEIN: SECTION EDITORS

Several clinical disorders have been grouped together in this section because they display a representative variety of commonly encountered abnormalities of immune responses. A necessarily brief and simplified consideration of the immune responses in man is also included to provide a framework on which the student may develop his

further understanding of the pathophysiologic basis for the many clinical manifestations of disordered immunity and a logical basis for their treatment. Consideration of additional diseases with abnormal immune responses may be found in various chapters in Sections Five, Seven, Eight, Nine, and Eleven.

CHAPTER 91
Immune Responses in Man
PHILIP S. NORMAN AND LAWRENCE M. LICHTENSTEIN

The immune responses observed in man are a primary function of lymphoreticular cells and constitute a portion of the phenomena collectively termed "host resistance." Immune responses are important in protecting the body from infections by various microorganisms and from the effects of toxins. The immune system also probably serves a useful internal role in the removal of abnormal neoplastic cells. However, its powerful effects may become misdirected and cause disease.[7]

ANTIGENIC STIMULI
Substances of the chemical and physical constitution capable of inducing specific immunologic responses when introduced into the body are called antigens. Exogenous antigens are encountered by man in the form of airborne particles, skin contactants, food, invasive microorganisms, drugs, and other therapeutic materials. Naturally occurring antigens are macromolecules ($>$5000 daltons) and are usually proteins, although complex large polysaccharides, e.g., pneumococcal polysaccharides, are also immunogens. In order to be immunologically potent, an antigen should be as dissimilar as possible in structure to host proteins, be large and complex, be somewhat resistant to the host's degradation enzymes, have a rigid three dimensional structure, and have a high proportion of aromatic amino acids.

Antigens may be considered to be an array of determinants bound to "carrier" substance. Small molecules (haptens), such as penicillin (penicilloyls) and

sulfadiazine, are antigenic only when combined with proteins. The hapten together with the amino acids adjacent to the coupled hapten constitute the immunologic determinant that binds to antibody, and the rest of the protein acts as a carrier. Such "synthetic antigens" are a model for naturally occurring antigens in which certain parts of the molecule (immunodominant determinants) appear to be particularly important stimulators of immune responses. A group of such determinants lies within immunodominant regions situated on the outer surface of the molecule when dissolved in an aqueous solvent.[2,3]

LYMPHOCYTES
The immune response has a humoral (antibody) arm and a cell-mediated arm. Both functions are carried out by lymphocytes with genetically determined surface receptors capable of interacting with specific antigenic determinants. Lymphocytes are either thymus derived (T cells) or differentiate under bone marrow control (B cells). Both have characteristic surface antigens and receptors. Antibody binding determinants or haptens bind to surface immunoglobulin on B cells whereas larger "carrier" determinants react with T-cell receptors, as yet incompletely characterized. B cells are the precursors of antibody forming cells, whereas T cells are the effectors of cell-mediated immunity, which includes graft injection. The immune response is initiated when the antigen interacts with those particular B and T cells which bear complementary receptor-units which "recognize" the antigen.

The result is twofold: cell proliferation enlarging that cell population (clone) which can bind the antigen, and cell differentiation, producing T- and B-effector cells.

Antigen-driven lymphocyte differentiation of both T and B cells changes the display of surface macromolecules. Some are deleted, other new ones are expressed; both types are called differentiation antigens. One set of these antigens, the Ly antigens of T cells, are expressed on different functional subpopulations and on their precursors, providing evidence that the many immunologic functions of T cells are not carried out by one cell line at different stages of its life cycle, but rather that distinctive subsets of cells have specific functions. On B cells, the class of surface immunoglobulin has been observed to change during differentiation from IgM and IgD to IgG or in some cases IgA. Antibodies are synthesized and secreted primarily by the progeny of B lymphocytes, large RNA-rich plasma cells which take 4 to 7 days to develop.[2,4]

IMMUNOGLOBULINS

Antibodies are a heterogeneous group of immunoglobulins of similar basic structure but with variations which confer different functional and antigen-combining specificities. All immunoglobulins are composed of two polypeptide chains of different size, the light and heavy chains, and a single immunoglobulin unit comprises two heavy and two light chains symmetrically arranged in a Y shape (Chap. 92). The arms of the Y are comprised of the light chains and the aminoterminal halves of the heavy chains while the carboxy-terminal halves of the heavy chains comprise the stem. The arms and stem are linked by a flexible segment of the heavy chains called the hinge region. The antigen combining sites are located at the ends of the arms, while the sites determining biologic function are on the stem.

The amino acid sequence of the amino-terminal ends of both the heavy and light chains are highly variable and together determine the specificity of the molecule toward antigen. Within each of these variable regions there are hypervariable sequences, which in some cases have been identified as containing the amino acids which contact antigen.

The amino acid sequence of the remainder of the heavy and light chains is far more constant especially within an Ig class. Depending on the structure of the constant region of the heavy chain, immunoglobulins are divided into five classes: IgG, IgA, IgM, IgD, and IgE. The biologic functions governed by the Fc (stem) end include activation of the complement system and combination with cell surface receptors on basophils,

lymphocytes, and macrophages. IgE, for instance, attaches to receptors on mast cells, whereas IgM and certain subclasses of IgG can activate complement.[1,2]

Antibody synthesis probably begins within hours, usually with IgM as the first Ig produced. With most antigens there is a subsequent shift to IgG or IgA; however, with some antigens, such as those on the surface of cells and bacteria, the antibody remains predominantly IgM. In general, most synthesizing cells seem to contain only one molecular species of antibody. Antigenic substances may also gain access to the body through mucous membranes, respiratory tract, or gastrointestinal tract and stimulate antibody responses in the lymphoid tissues associated with these organs. In this case, the response may be in the form of IgA and IgE antibodies as well as IgG. IgA antibodies are secreted actively into the lumen of these organs and play an important role in local resistance to infections, particularly with viruses. IgE antibodies mediate immediate allergic reactions but may also play a useful role in resistance to parasitic worms.[3,6]

The magnitude of the antibody response may be increased by several nonspecific factors that are unrelated to the antigen in question. Thus, antibody response may be enhanced by the nearly simultaneous administration of bacterial endotoxin or pertussis vaccine. It may also be increased by mixing the antigen with mineral oil, detergents, or other substances termed adjuvants. Many of these nonspecific factors seem to stimulate the proliferation of lymphoreticular cells.

T-Cell Functions

The end cells of T-lymphocyte clonal expansion are effector T cells which have four primary functions: 1) to kill target cells, 2) to produce lymphokines, 3) to "help" antibody production, and 4) to suppress antibody production (immunoregulation). Cytotoxic or "killer" cells, produced primarily in response to cell associated antigens or viruses, are thought to be a major mechanism for rejection of transplanted foreign tissue and may also be important in the control of neoplastic growth. When the cytotoxic T cell with receptor(s) for antigen interacts with an antigen-bearing cell, the T cell is "triggered" to cause target cell lysis. The cytotoxic ability of the cell is unaltered after the killing process and it can kill repeatedly. The action is specific: cells bearing antigen on the surface are lysed, cells lacking antigen are not. In viral systems there is further specificity in that virus bearing cells must share major surface histocompatibility antigens with the effector cell in order to be recognized for lysis. Such cells are to be distinguished from nonspecific "K" lymphocytes which effect killing with the help of antibody and complement and still other lymphocytes which can kill nonspecifically without antibody.[4]

Effector T cells also make lymphokines, soluble mediators with a variety of biologic activities, not all of which may reside in separate molecular entities. Lymphokines may be chemotactic, cytotoxic (not the major pathway to cytolysis), or inhibitory to cell movement. Migration inhibitory factors may be selective as to cell type, the best known acting on macrophages (macrophage migration inhibitory factor, MIF). Others act primarily on lymphoid cells. Lymphokine synthesis is triggered by specific antigen–receptor interaction, but the mediators themselves do not show immunologic specificity. Although there is little doubt that lymphokines collectively play an important role in host defenses, precise roles are difficult to specify. B cells may also synthesize lymphokines, and among T cells, lymphokine synthesis is not subclass restricted. T lymphocytes also mediate a delayed cutaneous hypersensitivity (tuberculin) reaction characterized by the development of erythema and induration (inflammation) at the site of application of the specific antigen after 24 to 72 hours. Delayed reactivity cannot be transferred from sensitive to normal individuals by means of serum, but it can be accomplished by intact lymphocytes, or in man, by a subcellular fraction of low molecular weight (transfer factor).

In addition to these effector functions, T cells strongly influence antibody synthesis by the progeny of B cells. Although very large molecules with repeating antigenic determinants are often capable of activating B cells in the absence of T cells, the antibody formed in most of these cases is limited to the IgM class. Most antigens require both T cells and macrophages before B cells differentiate into antibody-forming cells. It appears necessary that antigens bind to the surface of macrophages which then present antigen to T cells. The resulting activation of "helper" T cells results in the synthesis and secretion of soluble mediators which aid, in an as yet unspecified way, in B-cell differentiation.[2,4]

When there has been prior exposure to antigen, a new exposure results in more rapid development of both cellular immunity and serum antibody, thus providing evidence for immunologic "memory." Current evidence suggests that memory can reside in both T- and B-cell compartments.

Despite the variety of immunologic capabilities, an individual does not ordinarily make a detectable immune response to the constituents of his own body. The reason is usually a state of specific immunologic tolerance which requires interaction between antigen and lymphocytes bearing specific receptors for that antigen. Why some antigen–lymphocyte interactions lead to cell activation and an immune response while other apparently similar interactions lead to inactivation is not completely understood. Conditions such as a large dose of antigen and immaturity of the animal favor tolerance induction. In a mouse model, T cells require a lower antigen dose than B cells and T-cell tolerance lasts much longer than B-cell tolerance.[4]

T-cell tolerance can be partially explained by the induction of antigen-specific suppressor T cells. Regulation of antibody responses by suppressor T cells can occur for antibodies of all immunoglobulin classes. Furthermore, there may be nonantigen-specific suppressor activity for many or most antibodies in a class. IgE antibody responses provide examples of both kinds of suppression and are highly T-cell dependent, being particularly sensitive to both helper and suppressor T cells. In animals, repeated injections of antigen depress ongoing IgE antibody formation through activation of suppressor T cells specific for IgE responses to the particular antigen. Similar mechanisms may operate when desensitization for an allergic condition is attempted.

THE "AMPLIFYING" SYSTEMS

In addition to the specific elements of the immune system, immunoglobulins and lymphocytes, inflammatory processes bring into play one or more of four groups of protein effector systems in the blood plasma, i.e., the complement, coagulation, fibrinolytic, and kinin-forming systems. These effector systems circulate as precursors or zymogens which are changed by appropriate stimuli, sometimes immunologic, sometimes not, to active proteins which catalyze limited proteolysis of specific substrates, which are then capable of protein–protein interactions leading to multimolecular complexes with new activity. Controls of these systems include both feedback enhancement by products formed and control steps with dampening activity. Because of their recursive and apparent downhill nature, protein effector systems have been likened to waterfalls or cascades.

Complement

Antigen–antibody combination on cell surfaces or as free floating complexes can activate complement, an effector system of some 20 proteins which interact sequentially, producing products which can lyse erythrocytes, bacteria, platelets, viruses with a lipoprotein envelope, or lymphocytes, attract leukocytes, release histamine from mast cells, and activate kinins. Hereditary deficiency of one of the complement proteins may lead to chronic renal disease, systemic lupus erythematosus, recurrent infections, or episodes of angioedema, depending on the functions of the deficient protein, thus illustrating the importance of the system to the maintenance of normal health.

Hageman Factor Systems

A second system starting with Hageman factor can bring into play still other systems: bradykinin, clotting, or fibrinolysis. Biologic activities generated by one or another of the factors in these complexes include increased vascular permeability, chemotaxis of leukocytes, smooth muscle contraction, pain, coagulation, or hypotension. A critical role in disease processes, however, has yet to be determined.

IMMUNOGENETICS

Immune responses are under complex genetic control.[1] The major histocompatibility complex (MHC) is a multigenic system on chromosome 6 in man that determines the structure and expression of a variety of cell-surface glycoproteins known collectively as HLA (human leukocyte antigens). Originally recognized on lymphocytes by sera from normal, multiparous, multiply transfused, and specifically immunized individuals, these antigens are pertinent to the clinical results of renal homografting (Chap. 11), bone marrow transplantation, and platelet transfusion (Chap. 52) and are present on all cell membranes.

In mice, antigens (H-2) of the MHC are linked to antigen-specific immune response (Ir) genes which control the role of T cells in immune responses. Ir genes associated with HLA have yet to be identified in man, but associations between specific HLA antigens and several diseases with immune disorders have been identified. The strongest association is in ankylosing spondylitis where 90 percent of patients have HLA-B27. An increased incidence of certain HLA antigens has been noted in gluten-sensitive enteropathy, Hodgkin's disease, and leukemia. Relationships are being explored in many more conditions, particularly in respiratory allergy.[5,6]

HOMOGRAFT REACTION

Much of our knowledge of the homograft reaction is based on studies of skin grafts. When skin is transplanted from one individual to an unrelated individual, it is rejected, generally in 8 to 11 days. If after 2 to 4 weeks a second graft is exchanged between the same donor and recipient, it is rejected more rapidly, surviving 4 to 5 days. Cellular isoantigens of MHC are also responsible for similar phenomena following homografting of other tissue.

T lymphocytes are the major effectors of the homograft reaction. Humoral antibodies that react with donor cells also appear in the recipient's serum during homograft rejection. Although such antibodies are capable in the presence of complement of initiating damage to lymphoid tissue or bone marrow suspensions, they generally have little effect on other cell types. Thus, at present it is difficult to assign to serum antibody an important role in the rejection of nonhematopoietic grafts.[2,6]

IMMUNOLOGIC SURVEILLANCE

Effective immunologic self-screening mechanisms appear to serve a protective function in eliminating neoplastic cells. There is a high incidence of tumors in heritable and acquired immunodeficiencies and in patients treated with immunosuppressive agents. Careful histologic examination of organs such as adrenal, thyroid, or prostate has suggested that many normal individuals have suppressed or eliminated potential malignancies.

Macrophages, cytotoxic antibodies with complement, and T lymphocytes can accomplish the killing of aberrant cells. On the other hand, the immune system may at times elaborate "blocking" antibodies which coat tumor cells, prevent cytotoxic reactions, and thus thwart the immune surveillance system.

ADVERSE IMMUNOLOGIC RESPONSES

The immunologic reactions that have been proved responsible for the pathogenesis of clinical disorders are qualitatively similar to "normal responses" and involve either the humoral or cellular arms of the immune system.[5,7]

Disorders dependent on humoral factors may be categorized into: 1) those in which circulating cells or circulating cells combined with haptens (e.g., red cells or platelets combined with quinidine) are damaged by reaction with antibody; 2) those such as serum sickness in which the presence of circulating antigen–antibody complexes may be correlated with the evolution of tissue lesions; and 3) those such as the atopic disorders in which antibody capable of binding to mediator-containing cells is of pathogenetic importance.

Immune Complexes and Disease

Complexes of antigen and antibody may form when a critical molecular balance exists between intravascular antigen and antibody. When the ratio is around Ag_3Ab_2 or higher, soluble complexes may develop which fix complement and may localize on filtering membranes, attracting neutrophils which during phagocytosis release lysosomal enzymes which disrupt the local architecture. Filtering membranes, such as kidney and choroid plexus, are most frequently involved but blood vessel walls, skin, and synovial membranes may also be affected. Serum sickness due to horse serum is the classic example (Chap. 94), but many examples involving exogenous antigens, such as drugs or infectious agents, and endogenous (self or altered self) antigens, such as DNA or thyroglobulin, have been identified. Table 91-1 lists

TABLE 91-1
Antigens Associated with Immune Complex Disease

Exogenous	Examples	Disease
Nonreplicating		
Drugs	Quinine, quinidine, Stibophen	Drug-induced hemolytic anemia or thrombocytopenia
Hormones	Insulin, ACTH	Serum sickness syndrome
Serum proteins	Horse serum antitoxins	Serum sickness
Vaccines	Rabies, tetanus, diphtheria	Local Arthus reaction
Replicating		
Protozoa	Malaria	
Bacteria	Staphylococcus Streptococcus *Myobacterium leprae*	Glomerulonephritis
Actinomycetes		
Viruses	Hepatitis B., dengue, rubella Epstein-Barr	

Endogenous (Self and Altered Self)

Tumor associated	Carcinoembryonic	Tumor associated glomerulonephritis and polyarteritis
Specific	Renal cell	
Nuclear	Native and denatured DNA	Lupus erythematosus
Immunoglobulins	Altered IgG (rheumatoid factor)	Rheumatoid arthritis
Tissue	Renal tubular epithelium	Glomerulonephritis
	Thyroglobulin	Autoimmune thyroiditis (Hashimoto's disease)

classes of antigens with specific examples and the resulting diseases.

Mediator Release and Allergic Disease

Cytotropic antibodies fix to mediator-containing cells (mast cells and basophils), sensitizing those cells for rapid secretion or synthesis of potent mediators of physiologic responses and inflammation when subsequently exposed to antigen. Any list of mediators is necessarily incomplete because of the rapid rate of discovery of new factors but must include histamine, slow-reacting substance, bradykinin-generating enzyme(s), and eosinophil chemotactic factor. In man, the only class of antibodies recognized as cytotropic are of the IgE class, although examples from other species suggest that other classes may also occasionally be cytotropic. When the antigen is introduced rapidly by injection (drugs, diagnostic materials, insect stings) or ingestion (drugs, foods), the reaction may be rapid, generalized, and life threatening (anaphylaxis, Chap. 94). When the antigen is introduced by inhalation, the reaction may be local and involve the nose if the particle is large (hay fever, Chap. 95) or the lung if the particle is small (asthma, Chap. 35). Such reactions are characterized by smooth muscle contraction, itching, vasodilation, leakage of fluid from small blood vessels, edema, and infiltration with eosinophils. Usually the substance is otherwise innocuous and incites such reactions in a small proportion of individuals. The tendency to have immediate allergies has a familial element partially explained by a recessive gene which confers elevated IgE levels in homozygotes, acting in conjunction with other as yet undetermined but probably genetic factors.

Lymphocyte-Mediated Disease

As the cell-mediated arm of the immune system has been defined more recently, its role in disease is less well delineated. As lymphocytes elaborate antibodies both before and after differentiation, both arms are probably brought into play in the conditions discussed below.

CONTACT (ALLERGIC) DERMATITIS. Contact (allergic) dermatitis may follow exposure to a variety of chemical substances which can act as haptens by combining with skin proteins. An acute reaction is manifested by cutaneous erythema, edema, and papule and vesicle formation, whereas the chronic phase is characterized by lichenification and scaling. The response is T-cell mediated and involves recruitment of basophils to the site where they slowly release mediators.

HYPERSENSITIVITY AND INFECTIOUS DISEASES. Infection by pathogenic microorganisms will provoke a variety of immune responses, including antibody synthesis and cellular immunity. At times, after the resolution of the infection, an illness will appear with features suggestive of an immunologic disorder. As examples, one may cite acute glomerulonephritis, acute rheumatic fever, and erythema nodosum, all of which occur after streptococcal infections. In these instances, it has been postulated that tissue damage might follow: 1) the reaction of antibody with tissue-bound streptococcal antigen, 2) the circulation of antigen–antibody complexes, 3) cross reactions between streptococcal antigens and normal tissue components, or 4) tissue damage leading to autosensitization during infection.

The development of cell-mediated immunity is common in such diseases as tuberculosis, brucellosis, and those caused by various fungi. The tissue damage that may result at the site of contact between the microorganisms and sensitized lymphocytes and that may occur at distant sites in the absence of organisms is responsible for many of the manifestations of these diseases. In addition, the same mechanisms contribute to some of the systemic symptoms.

Autoimmune Disorders

Several disorders of unknown etiology with prominent immunologic manifestations have been termed "autoimmune" because of the existence of apparent autosensitivity.[7] For example, individuals with systemic lupus erythematosus (SLE) may show serum factors capable of reacting with various autologous tissue components. These include the LE-cell factor, the Wasserman antibody, and antibodies to various nuclear and cytoplasmic components. DNA is found in the glomerular lesions of lupus complexed with specific antibody and complement. At times, antibodies against red cells or blood clotting factors are responsible for other significant clinical abnormalities. Experimentally, the autoimmune process may be initiated in several ways. Viral infection and malignant transformation may result in the induction of new antigens. Cellular injury or infection can alter existing antigens to expose previously hidden antigenic sites. Small haptens, drugs for instance, may become attached to normal tissue proteins and an immune response is developed to both hapten and carrier. Finally, immunoregulatory processes that suppress immune reactions to self-proteins may fail. Induction of SLE by hydralazine in man and a virus in NZB mice along with clinical responses from both immunosuppressor and immunopotentiator drugs suggest

that SLE may be brought about by more than one mechanism and at times by several acting in concert.

Some self-antigens may exist in "privileged" sites, insulated from contact with the immune system. A process causing cell injury may release the antigen provoking an immune response which then breaches the privileged site. Thyroglobulin and lens protein are two examples of such antigens and autoimmune thyroiditis (Hashimoto's disease) and phacogenic uveitis involve immune responses to these proteins.

THERAPEUTIC CONSIDERATIONS

A simplified scheme of cellular events associated with the development of specific antibody production and delayed hypersensitivity is indicated in Table 91–2. Therapeutic considerations currently pertinent to the management of clinical immunologic disorders are noted at the level of their major loci of action.[5,7]

Since the early stages of immune responses involve cell division and protein synthesis, agents which interfere with cellular proliferation might be expected to be immunosuppressive. Indeed, under varying conditions, whole body x-ray, alkylating agents, antimetabolites, and so on have been shown to block immune responses (Chap. 54). Adrenal corticosteroids affect stimulated lumphocytes directly and lessen tissue inflammation. These drugs have been used to inhibit renal homograft rejection and in the treatment of autoimmune hemolytic anemia, rheumatoid arthritis, and similar disorders. They are highly effective in allergic disorders despite their inability to alter mediator secretion. In general, the nature of their toxicity and their narrow therapeutic margin limit the clinical utility of these agents.

The physician is most helpful in those situations where he can prevent an adverse immune response (e.g., by prompt treatment of streptococcal infections), identify an avoidable environmental allergen (e.g., a skin contactant), or sustain an individual during an unexpected anaphylactic episode. Further, the physician must remain fully aware of the possible immunologic sequelae of his diagnostic and therapeutic prescriptions and act accordingly.

Once established, immune responses are difficult to reverse. However, many are self-limited. In those situations in which histamine, serotonin, and other active agents are released (e.g., in anaphylaxis, hay fever, and asthma), a degree of symptomatic relief can be achieved through the use of drugs which suppress mediator release, such as chromolyn, or drugs which blockade mediators by interfering with inter-

Table 91-2
Therapeutic Considerations in Immunologic Disorders

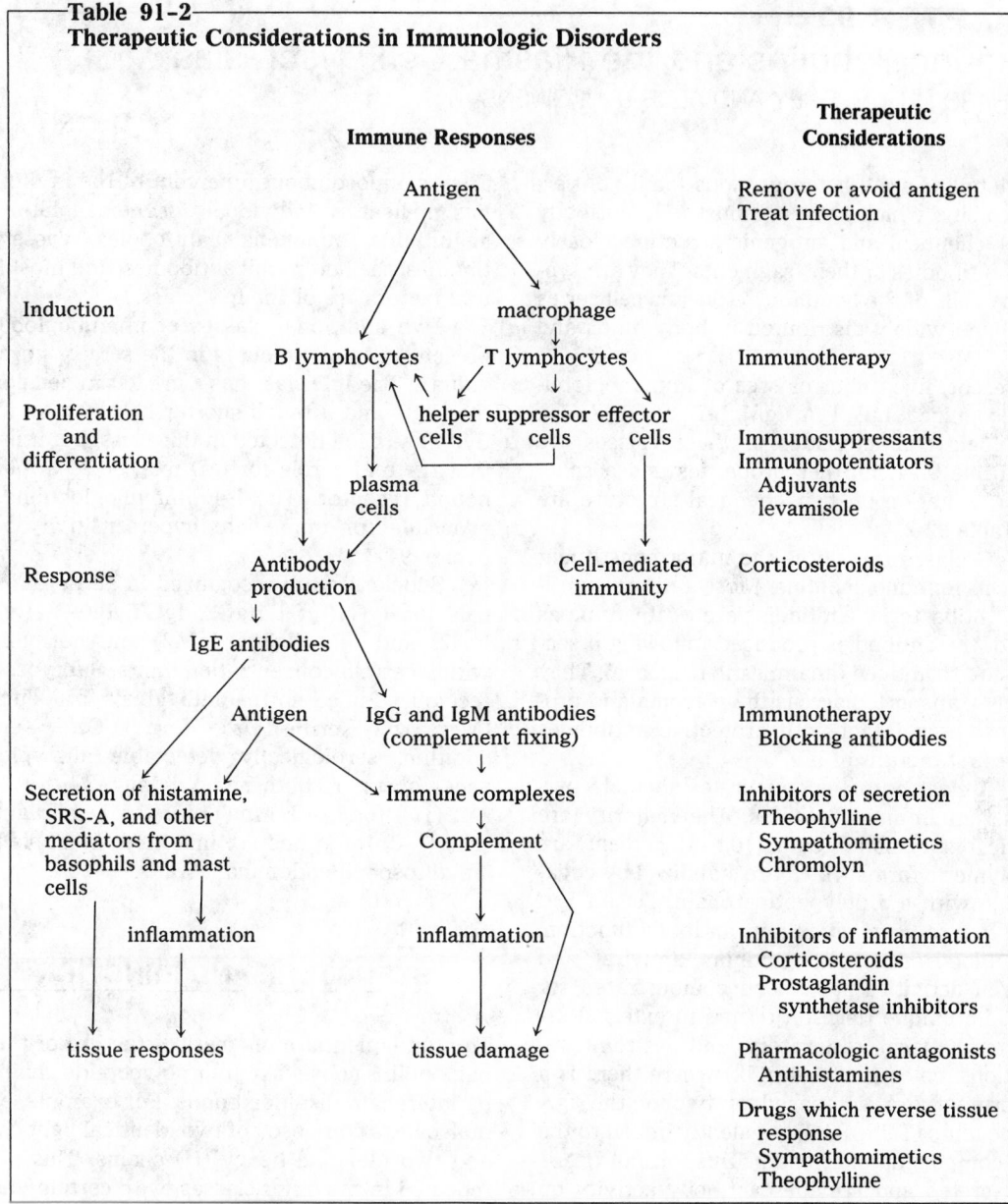

Immune Responses	Therapeutic Considerations

Antigen → Remove or avoid antigen / Treat infection

Induction

macrophage

B lymphocytes   T lymphocytes → Immunotherapy

Proliferation and differentiation

helper suppressor effector cells   cells   cells → Immunosuppressants / Immunopotentiators / Adjuvants / levamisole

plasma cells

Response

Antibody production   Cell-mediated immunity → Corticosteroids

IgE antibodies

Antigen   IgG and IgM antibodies (complement fixing) → Immunotherapy / Blocking antibodies

Secretion of histamine, SRS-A, and other mediators from basophils and mast cells   Immune complexes → Inhibitors of secretion / Theophylline / Sympathomimetics / Chromolyn

Complement

inflammation   inflammation → Inhibitors of inflammation / Corticosteroids / Prostaglandin synthetase inhibitors

tissue responses   tissue damage → Pharmacologic antagonists / Antihistamines

Drugs which reverse tissue response / Sympathomimetics / Theophylline

action with receptors such as antihistamines. Drugs which raise intracellular cyclic AMP, such as sympathomimetics or theophylline, have a dual action, both preventing mediator release and counteracting some mediator effects. The adrenal corticosteroids are widely employed to minimize the effects of all types of established immunologic responses and probably achieve this primarily because of their anti-inflammatory action.

It should be remembered that Table 91-2 presents only a simplified overview relating the stages of the immune response to available therapy. The physician must familiarize himself with the important factors in each therapeutic situation.

CHAPTER 92
Immunoglobulins and the Plasma Cell Dyscrasias
RICHARD L. HUMPHREY AND ALBERT H. OWENS, Jr.

Immunoglobulins are a heterogeneous family of vertebrate proteins which have demonstrable antibody activity or chemical and antigenic structure closely related to antibodies or their fragments. They are synthesized by cells of the lymphocyte-plasma cell series and are found widely distributed in body fluids and secretions.[7,19,22,25]

At present, five major classes of immunoglobulins are recognized: IgG, IgA, IgM, IgD, and IgE. The major biologic characteristics of these classes are given in Table 92-1. Further properties and a schematic representation of their chemical structure are given in Table 92-2.

The IgG class normally is the major constituent of the serum immunoglobulins. Most antitoxic, antiviral, and antibacterial antibodies are of this type as are most of the antibodies produced following a second exposure to antigen (anamnestic response). They are actively transported across the placenta and provide the newborn infant with protective antibodies during the first months of life.

The IgA class normally constitutes about 18 percent of serum immunoglobulins. The majority are monomeric, but a small fraction (10 to 15 percent) are larger, polymeric forms which are stabilized by covalent linkage with a J polypeptide chain. Serum IgA does not seem to have any unique antibody function. However, blood group isoagglutinins, antiviral, and antibacterial activities have been demonstrated for this class. Its unique function occurs in external secretions (tears, nasal, respiratory, and gastrointestinal secretions; colostrum and milk) where there is a special form of IgA composed of two of the IgA monomeric units (Table 92-2) covalently linked to the secretory component and J chain. This form of IgA is actively secreted and provides antibody activity on mucous membrane surfaces that is relatively resistant to proteolytic digestion.

The IgM class of immunoglobulins has a molecular weight of approximately 900,000 and because of this size, these molecules have been called macroglobulins. As a polymer (pentamer) of the basic structure (2H + 2L) they are stabilized by linkage to a J chain. They do not cross the placenta and because of their size they are contained primarily within the intravascular space. Their relative agglutinating and hemolytic efficiency is high. They are usually the first antibodies detected after primary antigenic stimulus.

They compose about 5 percent of the immunoglobulins in healthy individuals. Isohemagglutinins, cold agglutinins, salmonella O antibodies, Wasserman antibodies, the heterophil antibodies, and most rheumatoid factors are of the IgM class.

Two additional classes of immunoglobulins are present in trace amounts in the sera of normal individuals. The IgD class has a greater molecular weight than IgG and a much shorter half-life. Antibody activity has been detected in this class, but it is thought that the major role for IgD may be as a membrane-bound receptor. The IgE immunoglobulins are responsible for immediate hypersensitivity reactions (Chap. 94).

Subclasses are recognized in all normal individuals for IgG (IgG1, IgG2, IgG3, IgG4), IgA (IgA1, IgA2) and IgM (IgM1, IgM2) and normally occur within certain concentration limits. Subtypes are also recognized in all normal individuals for λ light chains (Mcg, Oz + Kern −, Oz − Kern +, Oz − Kern −). In addition, serologically detectable allotypic differences occur on both heavy [Gm(1–27) for IgG1,2,3; Am (1,2) for IgA2; Mm(1) for IgM] and light chains [Km (1–3) for κ] and are inherited as simple mendelian autosomal codominant traits.[43]

STRUCTURE AND FUNCTION

The fundamental monomeric structure of the immunoglobulins consists of four polypeptide chains linked by interchain disulfide bonds. For example, each IgG molecule is composed of two identical light (L) chains and two identical heavy (H) chains. This pattern is repeated in the other classes, with certain variations. Class specificity is determined by the nature of the H chain, which in turn determines most of the metabolic and biologic properties of the molecule (Tables 92-1 and 92-2). The L chains (κ and λ) are shared by all heavy chains, and in most cases, cooperation between an H and an L chain is necessary to create the appropriate spatial configuration for binding antigen.[44]

A vertebrate animal can make specific antibodies against an almost unlimited number of different antigenic determinants. This is explained on a molecular level by the presence of certain regions (amino termi-

TABLE 92-1
Properties of the Human Immunoglobulin Classes

Class	IgG	IgA	IgM	IgD	IgE
Metabolic Properties					
Mean adult serum concentration (mg/dl)	1200.0	280.0	80.0	3.0	0.3
% Intravascular	45.0	42.0	76.0	75.0	51.0
Half-life (days)	23.0	5.8	5.1	2.8	2.3
Antibody Function					
Placental transfer	Yes	No	No	No	No
Predominance in external secretions	No	Yes, as secretory form	No	No	Yes, saliva and nasal secretions
Skin fixation	Yes	No	No	No	Yes
Complement fixation	Yes	No	Yes	No	No
Relative hemolytic efficiency	1	0	5–10	—	0
Relative agglutinating efficiency	1	2–100	10–1000	—	0
Viral inhibition	Yes	Yes	Yes	—	—
Antibacterial activity	Yes	Yes	Yes	—	—

nal half of L and amino terminal quarter of H) in which the amino acid sequence is different between antibodies of different specificities (V or variable region). The remainder of the molecule is constant in amino acid sequence for any given class or subclass of immunoglobulin except for genetic (allotypic) variations (C or constant region). The genetic control of antibody diversity is complex and in some ways unique.

Although all antibody producing cells presumably possess the genetic potential to make any given antibody, at any one time a single cell will make only one H and one L chain. This is a dramatic example of specific gene activation and its converse, specific gene repression. This specific gene repression extends to the point that one or the other parental allele (in a heterozygote) at that locus in a given cell will be inactive (allelic or allotypic exclusion).

These mechanisms insure the functional symmetry of the immunoglobulin. Thus, an antipneumococcal antibody will have a pneumococcal antigen binding site at each end of the molecule, and "nonsense antibodies" are avoided.

However, specific allelic exclusion appears to be a random phenomenon among differentiating B cells. Consequently, each individual's serum contains immunoglobulin molecules representing his full genetic endowment. In the serum therefore, the Gm, Am, Mm, and Km factors behave as autosomal codominant alleles operating at a complex partially linked series of loci. These factors can be used like any other genetic marker to follow transplanted bone marrow cells, to study populations, and to help solve paternity or other medicolegal problems.

During early development, cells of the B-cell series are produced that carry immunoglobulin receptors on their surface capable of reacting in the aggregate with all of the antigens to which the individual can respond; but on a single cell level they respond to only a very restricted range of antigenic determinants. When antigen is introduced, it is processed and brought into contact with this pool of potentially reactive cells, stimulating only those with complementary surface receptors. These cells then undergo "blast transformation" and several cell divisions, and eventually differentiate into immunoglobulin producing cells (plasma cells), each cell line or clone making a biochemically unique (idiotypic) antibody. Since there are many cells, each committed to making a slightly different kind of antibody directed at a given antigenic determinant, the usual response to an antigen is quite heterogeneous.

Studies with antigen-free animals indicate that antigenic stimulation is essential for immunoglobulin

---

TABLE 92-2

Properties of the Human Immunoglobulin Classes

Class	IgG	IgA	IgM	IgD	IgE
Schematic polypeptide chain structure (——) of human immunoglobulins showing interchain disulfide bonds (··), secretory component (SC =▼) and J chain (J).		(a) 7S IgA1 (b) 7S IgA2 (c) 9S IgA (dimer) J (e) SECRETORY IgA secretory component (SC) J	(d) 11S IgA (trimer) J		
General molecular formula is $(H_2L_2)_n$, where H = heavy chain ($\gamma, \alpha, \mu, \delta$, or ε) and L = light chain (κ or λ). n = 1 for IgG, IgA (a and b), IgD and IgE. n = 2 to 5 for polymeric IgA (c, d,e,etc.). n = 5 for IgM.					
Heavy (H) chain terminology (confers class specificity)	(gamma) γ	(alpha) α	(mu) μ	(delta) δ	(epsilon) ε
Molecular formula (after union of H chain with kappa (κ) or lambda (λ) light chains)	$\gamma_2\kappa_2$ or $\gamma_2\lambda_2$	$(\alpha_2\kappa_2)_n$ (a,b) + J (c,d) + SC J (e) or $(\alpha_2\lambda_2)_n$ (a,b) + J (c,d) + SC J (e)	$(\mu_2\kappa_2)_5 J$ or $(\mu_2\lambda_2)_5 J$	$\delta_2\kappa_2$ or $\delta_2\lambda_2$	$\varepsilon_2\kappa_2$ or $\varepsilon_2\lambda_2$
Molecular weight	150,000	(a,b) 160,000 (c)320,000 (d)480,000 (e)380,000	900,000	180,000	200,000
Carbohydrate (%)	2–5	5–15	5–15	12	10
Number of antigen binding sites	2	2	5–10	2	2
Number of subclasses	4	2	2	—	—
Allotypic variants[38] (H chain related)	Gm (1–27)	Am (1,2)	Mm(1)	—	—
(κ chain related) Km (1–3)	+	+	+	+	+

production, and it is postulated that all immunoglobulin represents antibody, although for the most part directed at antigenic determinants that have not been identified. Gut flora, food, inhalants, contactants, and infections are the most likely sources of these antigens. Under normal circumstances, the antigenic experiences and immunoglobulin production are balanced in such a way that the many chains, classes, subclasses, etc., are kept within a fairly constant concentration range (Table 92-1).

HYPERGAMMAGLOBULINEMIA

Increased concentrations of serum immunoglobulins are seen in a variety of clinical disorders. In acute and chronic infections, sarcoid, many liver diseases, and connective tissue disorders, this increased concentration is due to increases in all or most of the immunoglobulin classes (polyclonal). This is an exaggeration of the normal situation in which antigen exposure is the driving force of the B-cell transformation to plasma cells and the resultant immunoglobulin production. However, in certain disorders, such as the plasma cell dyscrasias, there is a selective increase of a single molecular species of immunoglobulin. Not only is the immunoglobulin found to be of one class, subclass, genetic allotype, and so forth, but also, all the molecules within this population are identical. Although present in high concentration, these immunoglobulins do not differ from those present in normal sera with respect to their physical, chemical, structural, and antigenic characteristics. A few have been shown to have antibodylike activity. These homogeneous immunoglobulins are called monoclonal immunoglobulins or "M components" (M = myeloma, macroglobulinemia, or monoclonal), and the associated disorders are often called "monoclonal gammopathies."[52]

In general the monoclonal immunoglobulins are composed of intact molecules, but occasionally only a part of the immunoglobulin structure is present. When excess light chain is synthesized it is readily filtered by the glomerulus and if it exceeds the catabolic capacity of the renal tubular epithelium it will appear as a homogeneous protein in the urine. About half of these molecules display a peculiar thermal insolubility property (under acid conditions, precipitating at 40° to 60°C and redissolving at 95° to 100°C with repeat precipitation on cooling) and can properly be called Bence Jones protein. By extension, all free light chains (serum or urine) often are referred to as Bence Jones proteins whether they have this heat solubility property or not.

There are a number of different clinical syndromes in which a protein is found related to the heavy polypeptide chain of either IgG, IgA, or IgM (γ, α, μ). Collectively, these have been called the "heavy chain diseases."

The clinical circumstances in which such monoclonal immunoglobulins may be seen are diverse (Table 92–3). The diseases most commonly associated with their presence, the plasma cell dyscrasias, are multiple myeloma and its variants and Waldenström's macroglobulinemia. Various lymphoreticular neoplasms (e.g., leukemias and lymphomas),[8] malignant tumors of epithelial structures (e.g., those of the lungs, gastrointestinal, and genitourinary tracts), and other diseases (e.g., polycythemia vera, renal tubular acidosis) may also be associated with a monoclonal immunoglobulin. Occasionally, the serum of an apparently normal individual will contain such a protein, particularly among the elderly. Whether such individuals will develop other evidence of a progressive disorder or remain stable for years cannot be reliably predicted.[35]

TABLE 92–3
Monoclonal Hypergammaglobulinemias

I. Plasma Cell Dyscrasias

A. Multiple myeloma   (IgG, IgA, IgD, or IgE, ± free L chain; free L chain alone, rarely ($<$1%) no detectable immunoglobulin abnormality; very rarely bi- or oligoclonal)

B. Macroglobulinemia   (IgM ± free L chain)

C. Heavy chain diseases   (γ, α, or μ chain or fragment)

D. Primary amyloidosis   (IgG, IgA, IgM, or IgD, ± free L chain; free L chain alone, occasionally no detectable immunoglobulin abnormality)

II. Lymphoreticular Neoplasms[8]

Lymphoma, chronic lymphatic leukemia (often hypogammaglobulinemia; M component when present often IgM, occasionally IgG)

III. Nonlymphoreticular Neoplasms

Cancer of colon, prostate, breast, stomach and other sites (no consistent pattern of M components)

IV. Diseases with Autoimmune Features

A. Mixed cryoglobulinemia (homogeneous IgM acting as anti-IgG)

B. Hypergammaglobulinemic purpura (homogeneous IgG acting as anti-IgG)

C. Cold agglutinin disease   (IgM; κ predominantly)

D. Sjögren's disease   (IgM)

V. Disorders of Varying and Unknown Etiology

Chronic infections, parasitic diseases, cirrhosis of the liver, sarcoid, polycythemia vera, renal tubular acidosis (no consistent pattern of M components); Gaucher's disease (IgG), pyoderma gangrenosum (IgA), lichen myxedematosus (IgG, λ predominantly)

VI. No Associated Disease

Benign monoclonal gammopathy[35] (no consistent pattern of M components)

MONOCLONAL IMMUNOGLOBULIN IDENTIFICATION

The laboratory report of a reversed albumin/globulin ratio with hypergammaglobulinemia may be the first indication of a plasma cell dyscrasia. The first step in the evaluation of hypergammaglobulinemia is to differentiate between a monoclonal or polyclonal hypergammaglobulinemia. Zonal electrophoresis on a supporting membrane (such as agarose or cellulose acetate) will be of great value in this differentiation if it reveals the very tall, symmetrical spike of an M component, but on occasion, this distinction may be difficult. M components can be simulated on electrophoresis by an extremely high concentration of polyclonal IgG, an increased α_2 macroglobulin (chronic disease or the nephrotic syndrome), hemoglobin (hemolyzed sera), fibrinogen (plasma), increased lipoproteins, and a precipitate at the point of application of the serum to the strip. In addition, there are instances in which a monoclonal protein is electrophoretically heterogeneous (e.g., polymer formation or variable sialic acid content).

In the presence of an M component, immunoglobulin quantitation usually reveals a single class to be elevated with a reduction in concentration in one or both of the other main classes. Immunoelectrophoresis (precipitin lines are developed by specific antisera after electrophoresis of the serum in agar) often reveals the symmetrical, bowed arc of the M component, interposed in the immunoelectrophoretic arc of its "normal" counterpart.

Demonstration of a single light chain type (either all κ or all λ) is usually taken as proof of the monoclonal nature of the protein. Occasionally, though, light chain typing may not be possible and other methods may be required. Determination of molecular size (analytical ultracentrifugation or molecular exclusion gel chromatography) offers additional evidence for the presence of an IgM, although it must be remembered that monomeric IgM has been observed. Other techniques, such as determination of carbohydrate content, light chain typing after reductive cleavage of the molecule, etc., may prove helpful in selected instances in establishing the molecular homogeneity of the immunoglobulin.

CLINICAL SIGNIFICANCE

The presence of a monoclonal immunoglobulin in high concentration in the serum has two major clinical implications. The first relates to its diagnostic significance (Table 92–3), with the final diagnosis depending on careful correlation of the laboratory tests with the clinical findings. The second concerns the physiologic abnormalities that the protein itself may cause. Such abnormalities occasionally result from high concentration of IgG or IgA immunoglobulins. However, about 70 percent of patients with a monoclonal IgM increase will have symptoms attributable to the protein itself (e.g., hyperviscosity syndrome).[30,36]

Occasionally, the monoclonal IgM (most frequently) or the IgG or IgA M component will have the property of gelling or precipitating at a temperature lower than body temperature (cryoglobulinemia).[15] Patients so affected may present with purpura, Raynaud's phenomenon, or even frank vascular obstruction with gangrene. Waldenström has described a dis-

tinctive type of hypergammaglobulinemic purpura (not to be confused with his macroglobulinemia), primarily affecting young females. Their latex fixation test is positive due to the presence of small amounts of monoclonal IgG acting as an anti-IgG antibody. IgG–anti-IgG complexes are intermediate in size between the IgG and the IgM and can be resolved from the normal serum proteins by analytical ultracentrifugation. The complexes can also be detected by their reaction with the C1q component of complement, although serum complement levels are generally normal. The disease is usually benign and often spontaneous remission occurs. Therapy with corticosteroids is usually without demonstrable benefit[16] (Table 92–3, IV B).

Meltzer et al[40] have described another purpuric syndrome associated with a monoclonal IgM which acts as an antibody against IgG. This disorder also primarily affects females, although it occurs at a somewhat older age. Occasionally, immune complexes are deposited on the glomerular membranes resulting in progressive, fatal glomerulonephritis. Rarely, the amount of the monoclonal IgM may be so large as to cause hyperviscosity and require plasmapheresis. Treatment with alkylating agents, or other chemotherapeutic drugs, sulfhydryl reducing agents, splenectomy, or corticosteroids has been helpful in controlling symptoms and prolonging useful life in some instances (Table 92–3, IV A).

Another serious problem seen in patients with a monoclonal immunoglobulin relates to their severely disordered humoral immunity. Patients with multiple myeloma, malignant lymphoma, and chronic lymphatic leukemia frequently develop an increased susceptibility to infections, particularly bacterial infections.[41] This acquired immunodeficiency results from an impaired ability to synthesize specific antibody in response to antigenic challenge. This has been shown to result from the activation of phagocytic suppressor cells in the case of multiple myeloma and from suppressor T cells in chronic lymphatic leukemia.[14] Replacement therapy with gammaglobulin preparations has not proven useful nor has the prophylactic use of antibiotics. It is usually wise to treat febrile patients promptly with broad-spectrum antibiotics while awaiting specific identification of the causal organism and antibiotic sensitivity studies.

Amyloidosis of the kidneys, liver, heart, and gastrointestinal tract is also seen in association with plasma cell dyscrasias. Some forms of amyloid have been shown to be the variable end of light chains and consequently represent another way in which abnormalities of the metabolism of the immunoglobulins can result in disease.[24]

THE PLASMA CELL DYSCRASIAS

The major diseases included in the category of the plasma cell dyscrasias are multiple myeloma and its variants, Waldenström's macroglobulinemia, the heavy (H) chain diseases, and primary amyloidosis. Two major features are shared by these diseases that lead to their being considered together. The first is an uncontrolled proliferation of cells of the plasma cell or lymphocyte series, and the second is the production by these cells of an excessive amount of homogeneous immunoglobulin (or its subunits or fragments). The nature of the protein produced serves as a convenient way to classify these diseases (e.g., IgG, IgA, IgD, or IgE myeloma, and so on), but it should be emphasized that these diseases overlap to some extent, both biochemically and clinically, and an occasional patient will display clinical features that are inconsistent with the disease process as defined by the M component (e.g., IgM and skeletal lesions, IgG and hyperviscosity, etc.).

The homogeneity of the protein produced by any one patient, and yet its uniquely individual characteristics when compared with that from another patient, has led to the concept of a neoplastic transformation occurring within a single cell leading to the proliferation of a clone of cells that ultimately may destroy the patient. Hence, the differentiation between a polyclonal and a monoclonal immunoglobulinopathy is of considerable importance.

The monoclonal nature of the disease process suggests that the neoplastic transformational event operates upon a single cell. If many cells are simultaneously transformed, one cell line may have a survival advantage so that when the disease becomes clinically evident only one cell line is apparent. The infrequently observed biclonal or oligoclonal disease states therefore might reflect the rare simultaneous transformation of more than one cell with equal proliferative capacity. Alternatively, in some rare instances the rule of "one cell–one antibody" seems to have broken down and each cell is making two or more immunoglobulins.

MULTIPLE MYELOMA

Multiple myeloma,[32,51,53] a plasma cell neoplasm with an incidence of approximately 3 per 100,000, is seen with increasing frequency in individuals over the age of 40. Its occurrence in men approximates that in women, but there is evidence that blacks are more susceptible and have an earlier age of onset. Although similarities exist between multiple myeloma and syndromes experimentally produced in laboratory animals (e.g., BALB/c mice), the pathogenesis of this disorder in man largely remains unknown. However, epidemiologic studies have revealed that low-dose radiation exposure causes an increased incidence of myeloma.[38] No clear-cut role for chronic antigenic exposure has been demonstrated, although gallstones and liver disease are found with increased incidence in myeloma patients.[28]

Clinical Presentation

The onset and early course of multiple myeloma are usually insidious. Common complaints include weakness, anorexia, and weight loss and suggest a chronic progressive systemic illness. In more advanced cases, symptoms caused by bone involvement, anemia, renal insufficiency, neurologic deficits, and repeated bacterial infections may become increasingly prominent.

Skeletal Lesions

Bone pain of varying intensity is among the most frequent complaints of these patients. It is usually related to osteolytic lesions produced by focal accumulations of plasma cells. Although the lesions of myeloma are generally multiple, solitary skeletal defects are noted initially in 2 to 10 percent of cases. Their margins are sharply demarcated on radiologic examination, hence the common descriptive terms "punched out" and "soap bubble." They may be located in any part of the skeletal system but are identified most often in the red marrow bearing areas of the skeleton such as the skull, spine, ribs, and pelvis. Soft-tissue plasma cell tumors occur but are uncommon.

Diffuse demineralization of the bones is present in 60 percent or more of cases. Although it is most often associated with osteolytic defects, it may occur in their absence. The skeletal destruction has been related to the release of an osteoclast activating factor (OAF) by the malignant plasma cells.[42] Hypercalcemia can be a very severe and life-threatening problem and requires prompt treatment with saline hydration, diuresis, and mithramycin.

Pathologic fractures and the collapse of demineralized vertebral bodies are frequent occurrences, producing nerve root or spinal cord compression. Hypercalcemia is frequently encountered in this setting but is rarely associated with tissue calcification or nephrolithiasis. About 15 to 20 percent of patients will have no demonstrable skeletal lesions at the time of their initial presentation. Failure to appreciate this fact at times obscures the diagnosis of multiple myeloma.

Nephropathy

Over 50 percent of patients with multiple myeloma have free light chain (Bence Jones protein) demonstrable in their urine at the time of their diagnosis, and 80 to 90 percent of patients develop some form of proteinuria during the course of their illness. The Bence Jones protein has the unique property of becoming insoluble at acid pH between 40° and 60°C and redissolving at 95°C. On occasion, the finding of proteinuria with this characteristic on routine urinalysis leads to the diagnosis of myeloma. It should be emphasized, however, that all of the routine tests for detecting Bence Jones protein (heat solubility, salting out, para-toluene sulfonic acid precipitation, and so on) have a high failure rate with both false positive and false negative reactions. The only certain way to discriminate the true nature of the proteinuria is to perform zonal electrophoresis (e.g., cellulose acetate) followed by immunoelectrophoresis with appropriate specific antisera. Many times, the amount of protein will be insufficient for electrophoresis and concentrated samples (100 to 200×) will be required.

Light chain proteinuria will often be missed if reliance is placed upon the screening tests using a dye-impregnated strip. The isoelectric point of the light chains is such that they often fail to induce a strong color reaction. A better screening test for the presence of proteinuria is the sulfosalicylic acid (SSA) precipitation test or the heat and acetic acid test, but these also may be negative if only small amounts of light chain are present. A positive SSA reaction in the presence of a negative dip stick test is presumptive evidence of Bence Jones proteinuria.

Impairment of renal function can be either acute or chronic. The acute form[18] is almost always seen in patients with Bence Jones proteinuria whose illness is complicated by hypercalcemia and/or dehydration. These patients are candidates for aggressive support including peritoneal or hemodialysis because in many instances this acute renal failure is reversible. Acute renal failure has also been reported following intravenous pyelography, and this procedure should be avoided if possible in these patients or only performed after careful hydration.

Progressive renal insufficiency[17] is a common occurrence and has been related to the presence of light chain proteinuria. Large numbers of eosinophilic lamellated casts are frequently present in the renal tubules, and the tubular cells themselves are markedly atrophic, often containing hyaline droplets and occasionally crystalline material. Glomeruli are usually normal for the age of the patient, but the loss of tubules is prominent, sometimes accompanied by interstitial fibrosis and a nonspecific cellular infiltration.

In the past, chronic impairment of renal function was attributed to renal tubular obstruction by these proteinaceous casts. It is now known that the kidney is the principal site for catabolism of free light chains and that toxic damage may be done to the renal tubular epithelium by the absorption and attempted catabolism of some of these Bence Jones proteins. Why some are nephrotoxic and others are not is currently unknown. Additional factors contributing to renal insufficiency are amyloid deposits (seen in the blood vessels or glomeruli of 5 to 15 percent of cases), hypercalcemia (occasionally with nephrocalcinosis), and pyelonephritis.

A Fanconi-type renal tubular defect occurs infrequently in patients with multiple myeloma and results in glycosuria, aminoaciduria, renal tubular acidosis, hypokalemia, and hypophosphatemia.[23] Occasionally, this syndrome is incomplete consisting only of the renal tubular acidosis.

The relative importance of these factors varies from case to case and must be considered together with the vascular lesions and possible prostatic obstructive uropathy common in this age group. Although discrete plasmacytomas or diffuse plasma cell infiltrates are occasionally encountered in the kidneys, they are rarely responsible for functional impairment.

Neuropathy[47]

Neurologic signs and symptoms occur in about one-third of patients with myeloma. Among the several factors responsible for the development of these often distressing abnormalities are nerve root or spinal cord compression because of skeletal fractures, vertebral collapse, or compression by a localized plasma cell mass. Amyloid can infiltrate peripheral nerves and various poorly understood demyelinating syndromes can occur. This latter syndrome is often seen in conjunction with osteosclerotic skeletal change and is almost always seen with λ as the light chain type. These different factors can result in various combinations of pain, palsies, and paresthesias according to the extent and location of the lesions in the nervous system.

Bacterial Infections

At times, patients with myeloma come to medical attention because of the repeated occurrence of pneumonia, meningitis, or urinary tract infections.[41] Their peculiar susceptibility to bacterial infections, especially pneumococcal, is related to their decreased ability to synthesize normal amounts of specific antibody following antigenic exposure. They should be thought of as functionally hypo- or agammaglobulinemic even though they may be chemically hypergammaglobulinemic since the M component does not provide normal antibody protection. With antitumor chemotherapy further reducing host resistance (chiefly by inducing leukopenia), gram-negative sepis (especially pseudomonas) becomes a very serious problem.

Hematologic Abnormalities

A normochromic anemia is an almost invariable accompaniment of multiple myeloma, and complaints related to anemia often bring patients to the physician. Rouleaux formation of the red cells complicates their proper enumeration, the preparation of blood smears, and blood typing and cross-matching procedures and results in a rapid erythrocyte sedimentation rate. Rouleaux formation may provide an early clue to the diagnosis of myeloma.

In addition to severe anemia, progressive plasma cell proliferation in the marrow may result in leukopenia and thrombocytopenia. Anemia may also result from hemolysis caused by warm or cold antibodies. Furthermore, renal insufficiency and blood loss may contribute to the anemia.

Occasional plasma cells are found in the peripheral blood of about 50 percent of cases, especially if buffy coat preparations are examined. In 1 to 2 percent of individuals, plasma cells are sufficiently numerous (e.g., greater than 500 per mm^3 to suggest the term "plasma cell leukemia."[27] Plasma cell leukemia may be the way in which the disorder presents or it may be a late manifestation of an otherwise typical course for multiple myeloma. In either case, it seems to be extraordinarily resistant to chemotherapy and associated with a very short survival (median about 5 months).

Serum Protein Abnormalities

Hyperglobulinemia is observed in the vast majority of cases, and plasma cell dyscrasias are among the most common causes of serum globulin concentrations in excess of 5.0 g/dl. Excessive amounts of protein, homogeneous by electrophoretic and immunochemical techniques, are found in the serum or urine of nearly all patients (M components). IgG or IgA M components and/or free light chains are encountered most often. In a few instances the identification of a serum or urinary protein abnormality of the myeloma type has preceded the appearance of other features of the plasma cell neoplasm by months or years. In general, the nature of the M component does not predict for survival or for response to therapy but its physicochemical nature can lead to specific complications and symptoms.[45]

Infrequently the IgG or IgA M components polymerize or physically associate in vivo and result in serum hyperviscosity. Since only about 40 percent of the IgG or IgA globulin is intravascular and since the relationship between IgG or IgA concentration and viscosity is usually linear, plasmapheresis for the control of hyperviscosity in patients with multiple myeloma is much less effective than in Waldenström's macroglobulinemia.

In other infrequent cases, cryoprecipitable globulins may result in Raynaud's phenomenon or other vaso-occlusive disturbances. Proteins that precipitate at 56°C (pyroglobulins) have also been described but are of uncertain clinical significance. Certain myeloma proteins have also been observed to interact with various clotting factors, thus behaving as circulating anticoagulants and inducing a bleeding diathesis.[33]

Diagnostic Considerations

The common clinical manifestations of the plasma cell dyscrasias are compared and summarized in Table 92–4. The clinical diagnosis of multiple myeloma rests chiefly on the concurrent demonstration of compatible bone disease, characteristic monoclonal immunoglobulin in serum and/or urine, and typical plasma cell infiltration of the bone marrow or other tissue. However, care must be taken to exclude other causes of plasmacytosis such as hypersensitivity states, connective tissue disorders, cirrhosis of the liver, chronic infections, and other neoplasms. Malignant plasma cells cannot be reliably distinguished from reactive ones on their light microscopic morphology, although electron microscopic features (nuclear-cytoplasmic asynchrony) have been described.

Course and Prognosis

Untreated, median survival expectancy is approximately 12 months. Patients with several "risk factors," such as anemia (Hct < 30 ml/dl), renal insufficiency (BUN > 30 mg/dl), hypercalcemia (Ca^{++} > 12 mg/dl), or who are bedridden (poor performance status) have a median survival of only 6 to 8 months.

Other risk factors have been identified that also predict for shortened survival. These include hypoalbuminemia (< 3 g/dl), thrombocytopenia (<20,000/μl), leukopenia (< 1,000/μl), the presence of amyloidosis, the presence of plasma cell leukemia (>500 plasma cells/μl), and failure to respond to treatment or relapse after an initial response. On the other hand, patients without these risk factors can have median survival expectancy of about 2 years.

TABLE 92–4

Clinical Manifestations of the Plasma Cell Dyscrasias

Manifestation	Myeloma	Macroglobulinemia	Heavy Chain Diseases
Fever	Rare without infection	Frequent (unrelated to infection)	Common
Bacterial infection	> 50% of cases	30% of cases	Common
Amyloidosis	5–15% of cases	Infrequent (5%)	10% of cases
Lymphoreticular adenopathy and/or hepatosplenomegaly	Infrequent in absence of amyloidosis	Modest enlargement frequent (35–55%)	Tender enlargement common, waxing and waning; with edema of uvula and palate
Renal			
Proteinuria	Bence Jones > 50% of cases	Bence Jones 10% of cases	γ, α, or μ chain
Azotemia	Common	Infrequent	Infrequent
Skeletal osteolytic lesions	Solitary, 2–10% of cases Multiple circumscribed lesions common	Uncommon (8%)[30]	Rare
Osteoporosis	Common (60%) Without lytic lesions, 10% of cases	Frequent	Common
Neurologic	Root pain, cord compression Rare peripheral polyneuropathy	Bizarre encephalopathy, myelitis, neuropathy frequent	Not reported
Hematologic			
Bleeding diathesis	30% of cases	50% of cases	Not noted
Blood and marrow	Marrow and sometimes blood and tissues infiltrated with plasma cells	Lymphocytoid–plasma cell infiltration of marrow, blood, nodes, and tissues	Variable—may show lymphocytoid–plasma cell infiltration of marrow, blood, nodes, and tissues or may be normal
Monoclonal protein	IgG (~55%), IgA (~20%) Light chain alone (~25%) No serum or urine protein abnormality in < 1%	IgM > 15% total serum protein and/or > 1000 mg/dl	γ, α, or μ chain
Serum hyperviscosity	Rare	Common (75%) (50% symptomatic)	Not reported

Another important determinant of survival is the tempo or pace of the disease. This is difficult to assess by the features of the disease at the time of presentation and often will be apparent only as the patient is followed. Although multiple myeloma advances with varying degrees of rapidity in different patients and may seem to remain static for prolonged periods, complete spontaneous remissions virtually never occur and progressive disease is always an indication for treatment. Response to treatment will significantly prolong survival and improve the quality of life.

VARIANTS OF MULTIPLE MYELOMA

Light Chain Disease (Bence Jones Proteinemia)[49]

In about 50 percent of the patients with IgG and IgA myeloma, the synthesis of the H and L chains appears to be well balanced and the serum immunoglobulin abnormality consists of an increased concentration of the monoclonal immunoglobulin and a reduction in the normal classes. In approximately 30 percent of the IgG and IgA myeloma cases, however, the immunoglobulin synthesis is more deranged and an excess of L chain is produced which fails to couple with H chain, escapes from the cell, and can be found in the serum by using sensitive techniques. Because of its small molecular weight (23,000 for the monomer), it is rapidly cleared from the serum through the glomerular membrane and is found in the urine. In about 25 percent of all of the patients with myeloma, normal cellular function is even more deranged and L chain alone is synthesized. In these cases the serum abnormality is that of hypogammaglobulinemia. Overlooking this fact and not thinking of myeloma as a cause of hypogammaglobulinemia is a very common diagnostic error. An important clue, of course, is the presence of the Bence Jones protein in the urine.

With progressive renal deterioration and a failure to clear them from the serum, L chains will accumulate and may even reach a sufficiently high concentration to be visualized as a monoclonal band on electrophoresis. These cases (5 to 10 percent of all cases of multiple myeloma) have been designated as Bence Jones proteinemia. In some series, the patients synthesizing only L chains seem to have a somewhat more fulminant course with widespread bony disease, hypercalcemia, and relentless renal deterioration. This seems to be particularly true of those patients synthesizing the λ type of L chains.

IgD Myeloma[29]
Clinically, patients with IgD myeloma (about 1.5 percent of myeloma cases) are similar to those with IgG or IgA myeloma, but they seem to have a somewhat earlier age of onset and a more aggressive form of the disease. Most of the patients are male (two-thirds to three-fourths). It is of interest that some 93 percent of the reported cases have high concentrations of L chain in urine (versus 30 percent for IgG and IgA myeloma), with some 80 to 90 percent being of the λ type (in contrast to about one-third λ in the other cases of myeloma). Serum concentrations of the IgD are often low, perhaps reflecting the short half-life of this molecule, and they may not appear as monoclonal spikes and hence be missed in routine zonal electrophoresis.

IgE Myeloma[46]
Several cases of IgE myeloma have been recognized. Most of these patients had many circulating plasma cells (i.e., plasma cell leukemia) and did not have bony lesions and almost all have had λ light chains in their urine. Some of these patients have responded to melphalan or cyclophosphamide despite the poorer prognosis usually associated with plasma cell leukemia.

Nonsecretory Myeloma[37]
Rarely (<1 percent), a plasma cell neoplasm will be observed that is not accompanied by an M component in either serum or urine. Some of these cases are marked by the cells' inability to secrete the M component after synthesis in the cytoplasm. Other cases seem to represent a total loss of the ability to synthesize an immunoglobulin molecule or fragment.

Extramedullary and Solitary Plasmacytomas[55]
Patients with solitary plasmacytomas, especially if adequately treated (surgery, radiotherapy), may survive for many years. This is particularly true for those patients who have a soft-tissue plasmacytoma, many of whom are cured. It is usually observed that a solitary plasmacytoma in bone will eventually disseminate but may take years to do so.

Amyloidosis
Extracellular proteinaceous infiltrates can be found in a variety of organs in 5 to 15 percent of individuals with multiple myeloma, particularly those producing L chains, especially of the λ variety. These amyloid deposits are responsible for a variety of clinical findings depending on their extent and locations; for example, macroglossia, the carpal tunnel syndrome, congestive heart failure, the nephrotic syndrome, postural hypotension, gastrointestinal bleeding, and various neuropathies.

Management[10,12]
The major therapeutic problems in the management of patients with myeloma are bone pain and structural defects of the skeleton, hypercalcemia, bone marrow failure with refractory anemia, leukopenia and thrombocytopenia, progressive renal insufficiency, and recurrent bacterial infections. Logical supportive treatment of these abnormalities is basic to optimal patient care. The maintenance of ambulation will help forestall bone demineralization and the development of hypercalcemia. In the management of renal insufficiency, the benefits of adequate hydration cannot be overstated. Depending on the status of the underlying disease, peritoneal or hemodialysis can be justified, and some patients have even been completely rehabilitated with cadaveric renal transplants.[26]

In general, myelomatous tumors are moderately radiosensitive. Local radiation therapy used in conjunction with the appropriate orthopedic procedures, including internal fixation, often provides the best available palliation of local bone pain and permits rapid reambulation. Callus formation is commonly observed at the site of pathologic fractures, and recalcification may occur in osteolytic bone lesions following irradiation.

The alkylating agents melphalan and cyclophosphamide have been reported to induce partial remissions in about 50 percent of individuals treated over a 3- to 4-month period, with doses sufficient to produce mild leukopenia. Such responses commonly are characterized by relief of symptoms, reduction in bone marrow plasmacytosis, decrease in L chain proteinuria, decrease in the serum M component, and improvement in hematocrit, white blood cell count, and platelets. Recovery of normal immunoglobulins and recalcification of bony lesions occur but are rare. Corticosteroids (e.g., prednisone) have been commonly used in combination with alkylating agents and are clearly helpful in some patients, but their chronic use in patients with marked osteoporosis, renal insufficiency, and recurrent bacterial infections must be carefully considered because of their adverse effects on these conditions. There seems to be no relationship between the nature of the protein abnormality and the patient's response to systemic chemotherapy. Chemotherapeutic agents given at higher doses (e.g., cyclophosphamide) or in various combinations and on varying schedules are being investigated in the hope of improving their therapeutic ratio, particularly in patients with multiple risk factors and poor survival expectancy. To date, combination chemotherapy has not provided any significant improvement over the results seen with the intermittent pulsing with melphalan and prednisone. Preliminary results in small numbers of patients using interferon therapy are encouraging.[39] Patients who achieve objective responses by any of these means have extended median survival expectancy, in some studies in the range of 4 or more years.

WALDENSTRÖM'S MACROGLOBULINEMIA

Macroglobulinemia[30] is a relatively rare disorder characterized by an uncontrolled proliferation of a single clone of lymphocytes, plasma cells, or cells intermediate in morphology (lymphocytoid–plasma cells) that synthesize a homogeneous IgM. It is usually observed in individuals over the age of 50, with an incidence peaking in the sixth and seventh decades and of approximately equal frequency in men and women.

Clinical Presentation

Macroglobulinemia may be a coincidental laboratory discovery before the onset of symptoms. The common complaints of weakness, lassitude, headache, weight loss, and mild exertional dyspnea are not distinctive and may be quite insidious in onset. As the disorder progresses, prominent features develop that mimic primary abnormalities of the cardiovascular, nervous, reticuloendothelial, or hematopoietic systems (Table 92–4). Many of the distinctive clinical features are related to serum hyperviscosity.

Cardiovascular System

Mild cardiac insufficiency accompanied by peripheral edema and pulmonary congestion is often encountered. Its severity is frequently related to the existing degree of serum hyperviscosity and the associated increase in plasma volume.[36] Occasionally, low environmental temperature precipitates pain in the extremities, as in Raynaud syndrome, because of the cryoprecipitable properties of some of the Waldenström macroglobulins.[15] Rarely, purpura, ulceration, and gangrene result from the occlusion of small blood vessels.

Nervous System

Neurologic symptoms and signs occur in about one-quarter of the patients and comprise a variety of often bizarre patterns. Focal and diffuse encephalopathy, intracranial hemorrhage, myelitis, radiculitis, and peripheral neuropathy have been seen. Visual disturbances, often related to retinal hemorrhages, are common. Marked venous engorgement and segmentation of blood within the retinal vessels may be present (sausage veins).

Reticuloendothelial and Hematopoietic Systems

Generalized lymphadenopathy is frequently observed but rarely is a prominent clinical feature. The liver and spleen are often slightly enlarged. An absolute lymphocytosis is seen infrequently in the peripheral blood, but more often leukopenia is encountered with a relative lymphocytosis. Abnormal circulating cells are often intermediate between lymphocytes and plasma cells in their morphology (lymphocytoid–plasma cells). Protein synthetic and immunofluorescent studies have demonstrated that these circulating cells synthesize the homogeneous IgM.

A normochromic anemia commonly accompanies macroglobulinemia. Hemolysis is demonstrated rarely, but when present may be accompanied by cold agglutinins. Many patients complain of a bleeding tendency, especially epistaxis and gingival oozing, and they may note cutaneous purpura. At times life-threatening gastrointestinal or intracranial hemorrhage occurs. The platelet count is often normal in these cases with the coagulation abnormality related to the macroglobulin.[33]

Other Systemic Effects

Bacterial infections are seen in about a third of the patients and account for many of the febrile episodes. However, fever attributed to the disease itself is also seen, in contrast to myeloma where this phenomenon is rare. Also in contrast to patients with myeloma, patients with Waldenström's macroglobulinemia usually do not have bone lesions or skeletal pain although osteoporosis is common.[34] Hypercalcemia and renal insufficiency are also infrequent, although Bence Jones proteinuria has been reported in about 10 percent of cases.

Diagnostic Considerations[30]

The diagnosis of Waldenström's macroglobulinemia is based primarily on the coexistence of high serum concentrations of monoclonal IgM (greater than 15 percent of the total serum protein and/or greater than 1000 mg/dl, i.e., greater than tenfold increase over normal levels) and abnormal accumulations of lymphocytoid cells in the bone marrow and other tissues. The predominant cells present may appear as typical plasma cells, cells intermediate between the lymphocyte and the plasma cell (most often), or nearly normal lymphocytes. Often, there is an associated increase in marrow basophils (tissue mast cells). Similar histopathologic findings may be noted in the lymph nodes, spleen, or in soft-tissue tumors. In some instances the biopsy may resemble lymphocytic lymphoma, histiocytic lymphoma, or, when scarring is prominent, Hodgkin's disease. The liver (especially the portal areas) and the kidney may be infiltrated by these cells. PAS positive staining, if present, is helpful but it is often not prominent. Amyloidosis has been associated with macroglobulinemia but is uncommon (about 5 percent of cases).

Hyperviscosity Syndrome[36]

The IgM molecule is large and asymmetrical, having an axial ratio of about 10:1. As a consequence, it has a high intrinsic viscosity and significantly increases the viscosity of blood when it is present in high concentrations. Levels of relative viscosity 10 to 15 times that of normal sera may result. Concomitant interaction with red cells, intravascular rouleaux formation (red cell clumping) may result in hypersequestration and shortened survival of circulating red cells, in addition to aggravating the blood viscosity. Coating of platelets interferes with their function in hemostasis. Blood flow in capillaries is compromised and there may be anoxic damage and tissue hemorrhage. The work load on the heart is significantly increased.

The set of clinical features resulting from high serum viscosity has been termed the "hyperviscosity syndrome." This consists of a bleeding diathesis manifested as spontaneous bleeding from the mucous membranes into various tissues or at the sites of trauma. Visual disturbances result from intraocular hemorrhage and capillary stasis. A wide variety of neurologic symptoms, such as focal and diffuse brain syndromes, encephalopathy, and peripheral neuropathies, may also result from hemorrhage or capillary stasis. When severe, the hyperviscosity syndrome is life-threatening, leading to coma, convulsions, and fatal cerebrovascular accidents.

As a rule, hyperviscosity symptoms are not seen below a value of 3.0 (normal relative serum viscosity is 1.4 to 1.8). However, the level of serum viscosity at which symptoms of the hyperviscosity syndrome arise varies from individual to individual. The reasons for such variations are not fully understood, but the hematocrit level, the interaction of the IgM with red cells (rouleaux), and the presence of cardiovascular disease may make an individual less able to compensate for the circulatory derangements of increased blood viscosity and plasma volume. Whatever the factors are which cause this individual variation, the level of viscosity that will cause symptoms in a given individual is reasonably reproducible. This has been termed the "symptomatic threshold," and therapeutic measures (plasmapheresis or drug therapy) which maintain viscosity below this level will prevent the development of clinical symptoms.

This unique situation, in which the presence of the Waldenström's macroglobulin itself may account for significant symptomatology, has important therapeutic implications. Dramatic relief from neurologic symptoms, ocular disturbances, overt bleeding diathesis, and congestive heart failure may result from lowering serum viscosity. Since most (about 80 percent) of the IgM is retained within the vascular space and since viscosity increases exponentially with increasing concentrations of IgM, plasmapheresis is an effective way of controlling this symptomatology. Because of this nonlinear relationship between viscosity and IgM concentration, modest reduction of IgM concentration will result in a clinically important reduction in blood viscosity.

Course and Prognosis

Waldenström's macroglobulinemia may follow a relatively benign course for several years. Once major abnormalities develop, the usual prognosis for life is similar to that of patients with multiple myeloma. As the disorder progresses, its cellular proliferative aspects may become more prominent. An occasional patient may show a good response to therapy and be well controlled for several years only to succumb to a disseminated proliferative phase indistinguishable from lymphocytic or histiocytic lymphoma. This can happen without an associated change in the concentration of the IgM as though a new clone has arisen that does not synthesize an immunoglobulin. In the usual situation, however, death is related to uncontrolled serum hyperviscosity, hemorrhage, or bacterial infection.

Management

The supportive care of individuals with macroglobulinemia is similar to that employed in multiple myeloma. In addition, plasmapheresis should be used to reduce serum viscosity promptly and to correct the clotting defects caused by high serum concentrations of macroglobulin. Some patients can be managed for prolonged periods by plasmapheresis alone.

Alkylating agents, such as chlorambucil, cyclophosphamide, and melphalan, have been helpful in the more protracted treatment of Waldenström's macroglobulinemia. Clinically useful responses may be expected in about 40 percent of patients who have been treated over a 3- to 4-month period with doses sufficient to produce mild leukopenia. These responses include a decrease in neoplastic tissue masses, a reduction of organomegaly, a lowering of serum macroglobulin concentration, reduced plasmapheresis requirement, an improvement in anemia, and a related improvement in the patient's symptoms. Responders have significantly longer average survival (49 months) than nonresponders (24 months).[30] An occasional response has been produced by prednisone used alone but usually this is given in combination with an alkylating agent.

THE HEAVY CHAIN DISEASES

The heavy chain diseases[20] are characterized by the presence of an increased concentration in the serum and urine of immunoglobulin fragments related to the heavy polypeptide chains. To date it has been reported to involve the H chains of the three major immunoglobulin classes (γ, α, μ). Their clinical features overlap to some extent with other lymphoid neoplasms, but their unique biochemical features justify separate classification and a brief description.

Gamma (γ) Heavy Chain Disease[13,20]

This syndrome has been recognized in 35 cases or more. It was thought earlier to be predominantly a disease of males, but with more experience women have also been recognized to have the disease. Current ratio stands at about 1.7 males to 1 female. The average age at diagnosis is 57 years, which is lower than the other plasma cell dyscrasias. The mode of onset is usually insidious, but may be rapid. Patients survive for variable periods after diagnosis (months to years), usually succumbing to infection.

Clinically, the syndrome is characterized by fever, recurrent infections (particularly pneumonia), a peculiar (often transient) edema and erythema of the palate and uvula (attributed to lymphoid enlargement of Waldeyers' ring), waxing and waning, generalized lymphadenopathy which is sometimes painful, and hepatosplenomegaly. (One patient has been described who had a clinical picture like α heavy chain disease, but with γ chain protein.)

Laboratory findings include a normocytic, normochromic anemia (present in all cases), as well as frequent leukopenia, thrombocytopenia, and an eosinophilia (sometimes marked). Many cases have had atypical lymphocytes or plasma cells in their blood; two cases were diagnosed as plasma cell leukemia. Bone marrow plasmacytosis is common as is hyperuricemia. Skeletal lesions have been noted in only two cases.

Histologic examination of the bone marrow or lymph nodes often reveals a pleomorphic infiltration by plasma cells, reticulum cells, atypical lymphoid forms, and eosinophils. This tissue morphology has suggested the diagnosis of reactive hyperplasia, chronic inflammation, or Hodgkin's disease, and sometimes repeated biopsies or autopsy is necessary to define the process as malignant lymphoma.

By definition, the feature common to all of these cases is the presence in serum and urine of a protein having the chemical and antigenic features of free γ chains with no evidence of attachment to light chains. In only one of the cases to date has there been free L chains in either serum or urine, and this occurred in a patient with concomitant Bence Jones proteinuria and macroglobulinemia. The proteinuria is usually of marked degree and does not display the characteristic heat solubility associated with Bence Jones protein. The concentration of the normal immunoglobulins is usually reduced. On simultaneous urine and serum electrophoresis an identically migrating (γ or β region) monoclonal band is seen in both. Immunoelectrophoresis with appropriate antisera is essential to the diagnosis. Molecular weight determinations or other more specialized studies may be helpful. With more cases, the previous preponderance of γ3 subclass has changed to more nearly parallel the normal serum concentration of the subclasses.

The basic molecular defect seems to be an extensive deletion (about 200 amino acids) in the variable (V) region of the structural gene so that a major portion of the amino terminal half of the heavy chain cannot be made. How this genetic molecular lesion is related to the cellular behavior and disease manifestations remains to be clarified.

Survival in the cases thus far reported has ranged from just a few weeks to more than 5 years after the onset of symptoms. As the disease advances, recurrent bacterial infections and the progressive neoplastic growth present the main therapeutic problems. These patients require general supportive care similar to that for other lymphomas. Mechlorethamine, vincristine, procarbazine, and prednisone have been used with encouraging results. In several instances, splenic and nodal irradiation induced a partial regression in spleen size and temporary relief of systemic manifestations. Treatment of these patients with an alkylating agent (e.g., cyclophosphamide) alone has been disappointing.

Alpha (α) Heavy Chain Disease[20,48]

To date approximately 60 cases of this disorder have been recognized, predominantly in young Arabs and non-Ashkenasi Jews residing in the Middle East. It is characterized by abdominal pain and severe malabsorption due to a malignant lymphoma ("Mediterranean lymphoma") involving the whole length of the small intestine and the mesenteric lymph nodes. The bowel wall and the lymph nodes are infiltrated by lymphocytes, reticulum cells, and numerous plasma cells. Bone marrow or other organ involvement does not usually occur. Two children have been described with this protein abnormality in association with a pulmonary form of lymphoma.

On serum electrophoresis, some cases have had an abnormal band in the β region. In all cases, characteristic abnormal α1 chains have been identified on immunoelectrophoresis with no associated L chains. Diagnosis is complicated, however, by their low concentration, broad mobility, and a common tendency for IgA to fail to react with anti-L chain antisera. It is not yet known whether this represents the whole α heavy chain or only a portion. Many of these proteins have had a high carbohydrate content and a strong tendency to polymerize. The abnormal protein has been found in the urine in only about one-half of the cases, and usually in low amounts. Free L chain or Bence Jones protein has not been found in these cases. The abnormal α1 protein has not been found in the parotid saliva but is present in jejunal fluid associated with a secretory component.

Treatment has been with chemotherapy, chiefly alkylating agents or radiotherapy. About 10 percent of the patients have experienced remissions with chemotherapy, but this has also occurred with antimicrobial therapy alone.

MU (μ) Heavy Chain Disease[20,21]

Seven cases of long-standing chronic lymphatic leukemia (CLL) have been described in which an increased serum concentration of μ heavy chain has been demonstrated. Clinically, these patients are somewhat unique in that they had retroperitoneal adenopathy and hepatosplenomegaly, but peripheral adenopathy was minimal. In addition, the lymphocytoid–plasma cells were characterized by vacuolated cytoplasm. One patient was recently described with the clinical picture of lymphoma (splenic involvement and subcutaneous mass) who in addition to the μ heavy chain had a monoclonal IgA.

Serum protein electrophoresis reveals hypogammaglobulinemia with no spike, and immunoelectrophoresis is required to detect the abnormality. Five of these patients also had large amounts of free kappa chains (something not yet seen with α heavy chain disease, and rare in γ heavy chain disease). In addition, bony lesions were seen (not present in α chain disease, and rare in γ heavy chain disease), as was amyloidosis (seen in only two cases of γ chain disease). The μ chain was not found in the urine because it tended to polymerize and was, therefore, too large to pass through the glomeruli. Fluorescent staining with specific antisera revealed that most of the cells made both the μ and κ chains. Their failure to be properly assembled into the whole molecule may be related to a deletion in the μ chain but this remains to be clarified.

AMYLOIDOSIS

Amyloidosis[24,31] is a rare disorder encountered in fewer than one percent of autopsies at large general hospitals. It is characterized by the variable accumulation of an intercellular proteinaceous substance that may be found in nearly all tissues of the body. Amyloid is not starch, as the name implies, but rather a complex protein mixture dominated by a fibrillar component that can be visualized by electron microscopy.

Diagnosis

The diagnosis is made histologically, although there may be certain clinical and laboratory features that strongly suggest the disorder. There are three ways to identify amyloid specifically. By light microscopy, using hematoxylin and eosin staining, there will be an amorphous, acellular, eosinophilic material infiltrating tissues and organs. More specific is the characteristic metachromatic reaction with stains such as crystal violet and fluorescence with stains like thioflavin-S. However, the amyloid material is identified most specifically by its pink staining reaction with alkaline Congo red which undergoes a brilliant yellow–orange to apple-green birefringence when examined with polarized light. This suggests an underlying ordered structure. Indeed, when examined by the electron microscope (the second method of identification), the amorphous material appears as a mat or web of fibrils of about 80 Å diameter and unknown lengths (estimated in the thousands of Å). The third method, low angle x-ray diffraction, reveals yet another level of organization in the amyloid fibril, i.e., the polypeptide chains are largely arranged in an antiparallel β–pleated sheet. All of these methods give reactions which are largely without a counterpart in the normal individual and when taken together are highly specific for amyloid.

Classification

There have been many different attempts to subclassify this disorder based upon patterns of organ involvement, presence of associated disease or a positive family history, microscopic localization in tissue, ultrastructure of amyloid fibril, etc. The problem with each of these has been the wide overlap of features exhibited by individual patients. Currently, the most widely accepted classification is the one originally proposed by Reimann[31] based largely on clinical features:

1. Primary amyloidosis—no underlying or associated disease (about 50 to 60 percent of cases)
2. Myeloma associated—seen in about 5 to 15 percent of patients with myeloma (accounting for about 20 to 30 percent of amyloidosis cases)
3. Secondary amyloidosis—preexistent or coexisting chronic disease (e.g., rheumatoid arthritis, pulmonary tuberculosis, etc.—about 10 percent of amyloidosis cases)
4. Familial or hereditary forms (e.g., familial Mediterranean fever, hereditary neuropathic amyloidosis, etc.—percent dependent on nature of patient population being investigated)
5. Localized masses (e.g., isolated pulmonary nodule—about 5 percent or less of cases)

Amino acid sequence studies of the fibrillar component of amyloid from different patients have identified two major distinct biochemical forms.[24] In the primary and myeloma-associated forms of amyloid, the fibrillar component was found to be the variable end of light chain or intact light chain. Hence, these forms of the disease are truly forms of a plasma cell dyscrasia. In contrast, in the secondary and some of the hereditary forms (e.g., familial Mediterranean fever), the amyloid fibril is the same from patient to patient but differs from any other protein that has previously been sequenced (hence "amyloid of unknown origin" or AUO). The AUO form is clearly not homologous with any known immunoglobulin fragment, J chain, or secretory component, and so these forms of amyloidosis are not a disorder of plasma cells.

In most of the cases studied by these techniques, there has been no overlap between these two biochemical forms; however, in a few instances there is some evidence for the presence of both types of fibril or a discrepancy between the clinical and biochemical assignment. For the most part, however, the clinical and laboratory features fall into distinctive patterns. More recent information suggests that prohormones and perhaps other proteins as well may assemble in this particular form and may be responsible for rare forms of this disease.[54]

Primary Amyloidosis

Since the demonstration of the immunoglobulin nature of the amyloid fibril, it is easier to understand why the symptoms and laboratory features of patients with primary amyloidosis resemble so closely those of patients with multiple myeloma associated amyloidosis. In some cases, it is very hard to distinguish between these two possibilities, and often the major criterion for the diagnosis of myeloma is the existence of skeletal destruction. Since the amyloid protein will differ from one patient to the next (variable end of L chain), there is some latitude for variation in the clinical expression of the disease (i.e., the organ predominantly involved, presence of serum or urinary M components, etc.). These variations are attributed to the physicochemical nature of that individual amyloid fibril, i.e., its tissue/organ affinity, solubility, susceptibility to catabolism, etc. Making allowances for these individual variations, a pattern emerges that is fairly characteristic.

The disease is rare before the age of 40. Peak incidence is in the middle 60s, with males outnumbering females. Symptoms are often nonspecific and insidious in onset, but prominent is fatigue, weight loss, and paresthesias. Depending upon the organ involvement, cardiac or renal insufficiency may dominate the clinical picture. Postural hypotension can occur and sometimes is very severe and difficult to manage. Carpal tunnel syndrome, nephrotic syndrome, and a sprue-like syndrome have also been noted. Physical findings include hepatomegaly, but splenomegaly and adenopathy are less common. Macroglossia with indentations on the tongue margins due to pressure of adjacent teeth is almost pathognomonic. Purpura is sometimes prominent, especially in areas subjected to trauma or increased hydrostatic pressure. Periorbital ecchymosis from coughing, vomiting, or being placed in the inverted position (sigmoidoscopy) may be dramatic. The skin may be so fragile as to mimic epidermolysis bullosa or actually be infiltrated with nodules or plaques resembling xanthelasma. Laboratory findings may include proteinuria, sometimes in massive amounts, Bence Jones protein, serum M components, anemia, bone marrow plasmacytosis, and evidence of renal failure.

Albumin may be low and alkaline phosphatase elevated, but liver function, even with massive infiltration, usually is well preserved. In comparison with myeloma patients where kappa light chain predominates ($2/1$:κ/λ), this ratio is reversed in amyloidosis. Hence, lambda seems to be more "amyloidogenic."

The diagnosis is established by histologic examination. Biopsy material is obtained more conveniently from the rectum (mucosa and submucosa), gingiva, tongue, or a clinically involved area of skin. Crosby-capsule biopsy of the bowel and needle biopsy of the bone marrow, kidney, or liver may reveal the amyloid deposits. In centers where it is available, myocardial (endocardial) biopsy via catheter has been of growing importance in establishing amyloid as the etiology in patients who present with otherwise unexplained cardiac failure. Bleeding can be a problem, and choice of biopsy site should partly be governed by the ease with which the complication of bleeding can be recognized and controlled.

Cardiac and renal failure are prominent causes of death and median survival has been found to be about 15 months. Treatment to date has largely been supportive, but there are scattered reports of remissions induced with alkylating agents such as melphalan. Steroids given alone do not seem to have contributed to the management of these patients. Chronic hemodialysis and peritoneal dialysis have been of help in selected patients and a few patients have benefited from renal transplantation.

Myeloma Associated Amyloidosis

Most of what was said above in relation to primary amyloidosis applies here. However, these patients display skeletal destruction, more extensive bone marrow plasma cell infiltration, and greater incidence and amounts of Bence Jones proteinuria, serum M components, and more anemia, hypercalcemia, etc. In short, they seem to suffer not only the relentless damage due to the amyloid deposition, but in addition, are subject to all the difficulties of the progressive proliferation of the plasma cells themselves. Sur-

vival is accordingly less favorable than with either myeloma alone or primary amyloidosis, and median survival expectancy has been found to be about 5 months. Treatment should be pursued aggressively. The general principles of management are the same as for multiple myeloma.

Secondary Amyloidosis

This form of amyloidosis is seen in patients with coexistent chronic disease. In patients with long-standing suppurative disorders (osteomyelitis, bronchiectasis, pyelonephritis), lepromatous leprosy, paraplegia, tuberculosis, rheumatoid arthritis, or various malignancies, amyloid deposition was classically described as occurring predominantly in the liver, spleen, and lymph nodes (tissues rich in reticuloendothelial cells), as well as the kidneys and adrenal glands.

With the elucidation of the biochemical nature of the fibrillar component, it is clear that the vast majority of patients who have developed amyloidosis in this clinical setting are depositing a unique homogeneous protein (amyloid of unknown origin—AUO), which is the same from patient to patient.[50] The cell of origin of this protein is unknown as is its normal counterpart and function, but since the protein bears no relation to immunoglobulin, the plasma cell is not at fault. In large series of cases of amyloidosis, the secondary form accounts for 8 to 16 percent of the cases. In former years, tuberculosis led the list of associated diseases, but as this has come under control with effective antibiotic therapy, rheumatoid arthritis has become the most common cause with osteomyelitis second. The incidence among patients with rheumatoid arthritis ranges from 5 to 26 percent. It should be suspected if unexplained proteinuria develops in such a patient. The clinical patterns seen in patients with secondary amyloidosis include the nephrotic syndrome, malabsorption, and neuropathy.

Management consists of adequate treatment and resolution of the underlying disease process. If this can be accomplished, there are a number of documented instances (as well as animal models) in which the amyloidosis resolves.

Familial or Hereditary Amyloidosis[11]

There are perhaps eight or more distinct varieties of hereditary generalized amyloidosis, and it is thought that this probably does not exhaust the heterogeneity of these disorders.

Only with familial Mediterranean fever (FMF) is there biochemical information which reveals the amyloid in this situation to be the amyloid of unknown origin (AUO) involving primarily the kidneys, liver, spleen, and adrenals. In this setting, proteinuria is often observed to progress to the nephrotic syndrome and eventually to increasing uremia, which results in death.

Recent studies have established the utility of colchicine therapy in reducing the frequency and severity of the febrile/peritoneal attacks of FMF, but what the effects on the development of amyloidosis will be is unknown.

CHAPTER 93
The Immunodeficiency Diseases
RICHARD L. HUMPHREY

Deficiencies of immunity are being recognized with increasing frequency in a wide variety of clinical circumstances. Most commonly, impairments of cellular or humoral immunity are associated with acquired diseases of the lymphoreticular tissues (for example, myeloma, lymphoma) or with the long continued use of cytotoxic and immunosuppressive drugs. Rarely, immunodeficiencies are due to heritable disorders.[58,59,62,65,67]

Repeated infections often lead to the detection of an underlying immunodeficiency disorder. At times, these infections may be difficult to diagnose because the classic tissue responses to invading microorganisms are lacking. However, it is important to identify the invading microorganism and the patient's immunologic deficit as soon as possible so that appropriate specific antibiotic and supportive care can be provided (Chap. 80).[56]

Although the primary immunodeficiency states are rare and are recognized most commonly in childhood, they are of considerable importance for medicine in general because of the insight they give into the interrelationships and mechanisms of the normal immune response. Figure 93–1 provides a schematic representation of the development and organization of the immune system. In the yolk sac, during embryonic development, hematopoietic and lymphoid precursor cells emerge which migrate to the liver and later to primitive bone marrow. These lymphoid precursor cells come under the influence of two different organizing principles, the developing epithelial thymus and the avian bursa analogue.[67]

The thymus, derived from epithelial outpouchings in the third and fourth pharyngeal pouches, induces differentiation of the thymus-dependent lymphocytes (T cells) which circulate to peripheral lymphoid tissue and mediate cellular immune reactions. These cellular immune reactions include delayed hypersensitivity skin reactions, homograft re-

jection, and graft versus host reactivity (Chap. 92).

In birds, the bursa of Fabricius (the bursa analogue in mammals is unknown; perhaps it is the bone marrow) induces differentiation of the bursa-dependent lymphocytes (B cells) which mediate humoral immunity. B cells on encounter with antigen (in some instances macrophage processing seems required) differentiate into plasma cells which secrete specific immunoglobulin (Chap. 92). These two major divisions dominate the immune system: T-cell mediated cellular immunity and B-cell mediated humoral immunity. However, an additional set of complexities is introduced by the recognition of interactions between these systems as is illustrated by Figure 93–1: "helper T cells" and "suppressor T cells" in addition to the regulatory role of macrophages. Nevertheless, an appreciation of the fundamental organization of the immune system permits a useful framework for the classification of this very complex group of disorders and will permit a description of the clinical features useful in the preliminary screening and evaluation of patients.

CLASSIFICATION

Based upon the considerations above, the primary immunodeficiency states can be grouped broadly into four major groups: 1) humoral immunodeficiency, 2) cell-mediated immunodeficiency, 3) combined immunodeficiency, and 4) partial immunodeficiencies. The secondary immunodeficiency states would share features with these four broad categories but would be related to some underlying process such as a lymphoreticular neoplasm, immunosuppressive therapy, severe protein loss such as with intestinal lymphangiectasia, the nephrotic syndrome, severe burns, or extensive skin disease.[65]

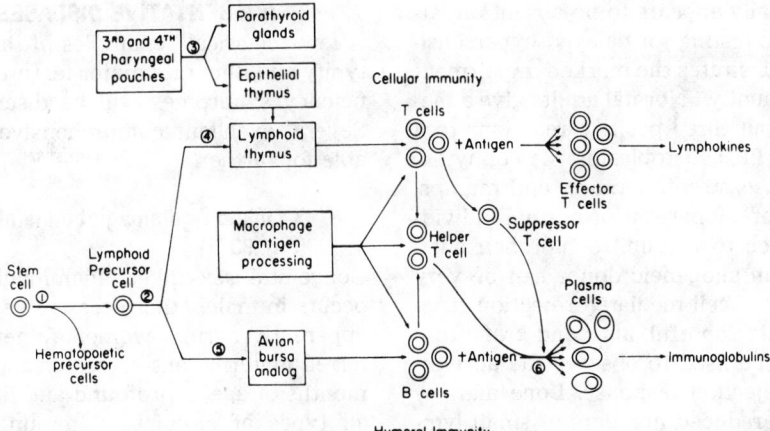

FIGURE 93-1. The development of the immune system is diagrammatically illustrated showing its separation into the T-cell mediated cellular and B-cell mediated humoral components. Also illustrated are some of the interactions between the various cell systems including antigen processing by macrophage, helper T-cell, and suppressor T-cell modulation of B-cell activity. Postulated sites of defects giving rise to the major (prototype) immunodeficiency syndromes are illustrated: 1) severe combined immunodeficiency with generalized hematopoietic hypoplasia (reticular dysgenesis); 2) severe combined immunodeficiency (Swiss-type lymphopenic agammaglobulinemia); 3) thymic hypoplasia (DiGeorge syndrome); 4) immunodeficiency with lymphopenia and "normal" immunoglobulins (Nezelof syndrome); 5) X-linked agammaglobulinemia (Bruton-type), and 6) common variable hypogammaglobulinemia.

HUMORAL IMMUNODEFICIENCY

Diagnostic Considerations

Humoral immunodeficiency is characterized by recurrent bacterial infections, such as pneumonitis, meningitis, otitis, often complicated by bacteremia or septicemia. The microorganisms responsible usually are encapsulated pyogenic bacteria such as pneumococcus, streptococcus, meningococcus, pseudomonas, and hemophilus. Eczema may be a prominent feature. Severe hepatitis may result from the transfusion of blood products. Family history may include other affected individuals (especially males, if sex-linked).

On physical examination, the affected individuals often appear wasted and chronically ill. In children, growth usually is retarded. Lymph nodes and tonsils are quite small. Serum immunoglobulin concentrations are very low or undetectable. Since low serum immunoglobulin concentrations do not preclude clinically useful antibody synthesis, responses to various antigens should be tested directly. The following tests are used because of their ready availability in most clinical settings: isohemagglutinin titers, Schick skin test (remains positive after DPT immunization), teta-

nus antitoxin titers, and absent response to typhoid-paratyphoid vaccination (febrile agglutinins). In addition, no plasma cells will be found on bone marrow aspiration or gut biopsy, and germinal centers and lymphoid follicles will be absent or poorly developed.

CELL-MEDIATED IMMUNODEFICIENCY

Diagnostic Considerations

In contrast, cell-mediated immunodeficiency is characterized by a propensity for severe viral and fungal infections. The microorganisms responsible include cytomegalovirus, rubeola, rubella, candida, and histoplasma. If vaccinated against smallpox, disseminated vaccinia may result, and this is also true for vaccination with BCG and other live attenuated organisms. In addition, the administration of live immunocompetent cells (e.g., blood or platelet transfusions) may result in graft versus host reactions if there are HLA differences between donor and recipient. Family history may be positive for similarly affected siblings or early infant deaths. On physical examination, growth may be retarded, lymph nodes and tonsils will be small, and the individuals may appear chronically ill. Routine laboratory studies reveal marked lymphopenia. The thymus usually appears to be absent on lateral chest x-ray. Skin testing for delayed hypersensitivity reactions demonstrates the marked impairment of cell-mediated immunity. (Normal adults give a median response of about three positive reactions to a battery that includes PPD, histoplasmin, Tricophyton, Candida, streptokinase/streptodornase, and mumps. In addition, more than 99 percent of normal individuals can be sensitized to 2,4-dinitrochlorobenzene.) Skin grafting from an allogeneic donor can be very helpful in assessing the cell-mediated rejection reaction. If the outcome is doubtful, a second graft from the same donor can be used to observe the accelerated "second set" rejection response. Bone marrow aspiration will show reduced numbers of small lymphocytes, and lymph node biopsy will show absent lymphocytes in the deep cortical areas.

Additional tests that have been used to define the impairment of these two parts of the immune system include: measurement of the percentage of T and B cells among circulating lymphocytes, in vitro immunoglobulin production after stimulation with lipopolysaccharide or pokeweed mitogen, or in vitro response (e.g., tritiated thymidine incorporation) to phytohemagglutinin (PHA) or after incubation with allogeneic cells (mixed lymphocyte culture or MLC). These laboratory tests are summarized in Table 93–1.

REPRESENTATIVE DISEASES

A few "classical" examples of the diseases that best typify and illustrate major features of the immunodeficiency syndromes will be discussed (Table 93–2). Several excellent comprehensive reviews are available for further study.[58,59,62,65,67]

X-Linked Agammaglobulinemia (Bruton-Type) (Fig. 93–1)

Congenital sex-linked agammaglobulinemia always occurs in males, the recessive gene being carried by apparently normal women. When placentally transferred maternal antibodies disappear at about 6 to 9 months of age, a profound and lifelong deficiency of all types of circulating immunoglobulins becomes manifest. Although minute amounts of IgG and sometimes IgM are identifiable by sensitive immunochemical methods, functional levels of antibody are absent. Antigenic stimulation by bacterial or viral infections or by injected soluble or particulate antigens produces no demonstrable antibody response. However, these patients are capable of developing delayed or cellular hypersensitivity and will display normal reactions to skin tests and can be sensitized with DNCB (Table 93–1). The lymph nodes, adenoids, and tonsils are small and hypoplastic and lack active germinal centers. Plasma cells are completely absent from

---

TABLE 93–1
Laboratory Evaluation of Immunocompetence

I. Humoral Immunity (B-Cell Function)

1. Immunoglobulin levels (IgG, IgA, IgM)

2. Isohemagglutinin titers (anti-A, anti-B)

3. Schick skin test (if positive, retest after DPT immunization)

4. Tetanus antitoxin titers (before and after DPT immunization)

5. Febrile agglutinins (before and after typhoid-paratyphoid immunization)

6. In vitro immunoglobulin production following antigen or nonspecific stimulation (e.g., pokeweed mitogen)

7. Biopsy bone marrow, lymph node, gut and examine for plasma cells and germinal centers

8. Enumerate B cells in peripheral blood (e.g., surface Ig)

II. Cellular Immunity (T-Cell Function)

1. Peripheral lymphocyte count and morphology

2. Delayed hypersensitivity skin tests (e.g., PPD, histoplasmin, Tricophyton, Candida, mumps, streptokinase/streptodornase)

3. DNCB skin sensitization (2,4-dinitrochlorobenzene)

4. Release of lymphokines (e.g., migratory inhibition factor [MIF], etc.)

5. In vitro lymphocyte transformation by phytohemagglutinin (PHA) or mixed lymphocyte culture (MLC)

6. Skin homograft survival

7. Biopsy lymph node and examine for lymphocytes in thymus dependent areas

8. Enumerate T cells in peripheral blood (e.g., sheep rbc rosette formation)

TABLE 93-2
Primary Immunodeficiency Disorders (Partial Listing)

Defect		Disease	Inheritance
I. **B Cells**	1.	X-linked agammaglobulinemia (Bruton-type) ⑤ in Fig. 93-1	X-linked
	2.	Selective immunoglobulin deficiency (e.g., IgA)	Variable or uncertain
	3.	X-linked immunoglobulin deficiency with increased IgM	X-linked or uncertain
	4.	Common variable hypogammaglobulinemia ⑥ in Fig. 93-1	Variable or uncertain
II. **T Cells**	1.	Thymic hypoplasia (DiGeorge syndrome) ③ in Fig. 93-1	Variable or uncertain
	2.	Immunodeficiency with lymphopenia and "normal" immunoglobulins (Nezelof syndrome) ④ in Fig. 93-1	Autosomal recessive
	3.	Immunodeficiency with cartilage-hair hypoplasia	Autosomal recessive
III. **Combined B and T Cells**	1.	Severe combined immunodeficiency (Swiss-type lymphopenic agammaglobulinemia) ② in Fig. 93-1	X-linked, autosomal recessive or sporadic
	2.	Severe combined immunodeficiency with generalized hematopoietic hypoplasia (reticular dysgenesis) ⑦ in Fig. 93-1	Autosomal recessive
	3.	Immunodeficiency with ataxia-telangiectasia	Autosomal recessive
	4.	Immunodeficiency with thymoma (Good syndrome)	Variable or uncertain
	5.	Immunodeficiency with short-limbed dwarfism	Autosomal recessive
	6.	Immunodeficiency with thrombocytopenia and eczema (Wiskott-Aldrich syndrome)	X-linked

lymph nodes, Peyer's patches, appendix, and bone marrow. The thymus is histologically normal. Clinically, these patients are susceptible to repeated life-threatening infections with hemophilus, pseudomonas, etc.; pneumonia, septicemia, meningitis, otitis, bronchitis, and sinusitis are a recurrent problem. Viral and fungal infections do not occur repeatedly, but exposure to hepatitis virus usually leads to fulminant hepatitis or chronic progressive hepatitis and is often fatal. Accordingly, transfusion with blood products should be avoided if at all possible.

Unlike the adult or "acquired" agammaglobulinemia these patients do not develop chronic diarrhea, but a malabsorption syndrome caused by *Giardia lamblia* has been recognized. This diagnosis is best made by biopsy of the small intestine. Giardiasis responds to treatment with metronidazole.

There is an unusual incidence of certain other conditions in patients with congenital sex-linked agammaglobulinemia. About one-third develop clinically typical rheumatoid arthritis, including rheumatoid nodules. Histologically, the lesions are also typical except for the absence of plasma cells. Tests for rheumatoid factor are invariably negative. This ar-

thritis will subside with replacement gamma globulin therapy. In other cases, dermatomyositis or scleroderma has been recognized. In a few instances, progressive demyelination of the central nervous system has been observed, perhaps due to a chronic echo virus infection.

Typical childhood eczema also occurs with increased frequency in patients with congenital sex-linked antibody deficiency. Skin tests to various allergens are negative and the wheal and flare reaction is absent.

A number of instances have been identified of pneumonia caused by *Pneumocystis carinii*, which is fatal in these patients unless treated promptly. There may be an increased incidence of granulomatous infections, such as tuberculosis and histoplasmosis, but these diseases also respond well to antibiotic therapy.

Treatment consists of prompt use of appropriate antimicrobials and chronic administration of gamma globulin.[64] The prophylactic use of antibiotics is not likely to prevent many infections but only to select antibiotic resistant ones. Long-term results are fairly good, but these patients often develop chronic lung disease due to destruction of lung parenchyma by repeated infections. They are also prone to develop leukemia.[63]

Thymic Hypoplasia (DiGeorge Syndrome) (Fig. 93-1)

Attention is drawn to these infants by the appearance of hypocalcemic tetany shortly after birth. This results from the failure of both the parathyroids and thymus to be formed from the third and fourth pharyngeal pouches during embryonic development. There are often a number of associated physical abnormalities including hyperteliorism, antimongoloid slant of the eyes, low set and notched ears, micrognathia, and cardiac and aortic arch anomalies (tetralogy of Fallot).

The absence of the epithelial portion of the thymus results in a failure to develop T cells and cell-mediated immunity. To the extent that it is T-cell independent, however, humoral-mediated immunity develops normally. The thymus is absent, and T lymphocytes are absent from blood and are not found in the thymus dependent areas of lymph nodes and spleen. These patients do not develop normal delayed hypersensitivity skin test reactions nor can they be sensitized with DNCB. These individuals are prone to develop infections with fungi and viruses. Vaccination with live attenuated organisms leads to generalized disseminated fatal disease, and all such agents should be avoided. In addition, the transfer of live immunocompetent cells (blood, platelet, fresh plasma, or white cell transfusions) will lead to a rapidly fatal graft versus host disease. Thus, these blood products should be irradiated prior to use.

Correction has been achieved by means of fetal thymus transplants, but with developing immunocompetence, these grafts have been rejected requiring repeated transplantation.[61]

Severe Combined Immunodeficiency (Swiss-Type Lymphopenic Agammaglobulinemia) (Fig. 93-1)

This disorder has several variants with different modes of inheritance and somewhat different severity. Basically, it can be thought of as a failure to develop lymphoid stem cells and so results in an absence of both the cellular and the humoral components of the immune response. Exposure to live vaccines or blood products (hepatitis virus) may lead to serious infections. Recurrent severe infections of all types are the rule and survival for more than a few months is unlikely. Successful treatment with correction of all of these abnormalities has been achieved using HLA compatible bone marrow transplantation.[61]

Severe Combined Immunodeficiency with Generalized Hematopoietic Hypoplasia (Reticular Dysgenesis) (Fig. 93-1)

This disorder is characterized by a severe deficiency of both T cells and B cells as well as a failure of development of granulocytes. There have been only a few reported cases, all of whom have died with overwhelming infection within a few days after birth. Marrow contains megakaryocytes and erythroid elements but granulocyte precursors are absent. It is thought to be inherited as an autosomal recessive but this is not established with certainty. Bone marrow transplantation would be the treatment of choice but would almost require an anticipation of the affected child in order to accomplish the procedure properly.

Immunodeficiency with Lymphopenia and "Normal" Immunoglobulins (Nezelof Syndrome) (Fig. 93-1)

In many ways, this disorder resembles the severe combined immunodeficiency, but immunoglobulin levels are normal and antibody response to some antigens can be demonstrated. The thymus is represented by epithelial remnants and T cells are absent. Thymus transplants have failed to correct this disorder and so it seems reasonable to postulate a defective stem cell that more seriously affects the cellular mediated than the humoral mediated compartment. Onset of symptoms is often in late infancy or childhood and some patients may survive for several years. Bone marrow transplantation from an HLA compatible donor may offer hope of complete reconstitution.[61]

Common Variable Hypogammaglobulinemia[65,66] (Fig. 93-1)

This is a markedly heterogeneous group of disorders that will undoubtedly be more appropriately classified as further knowledge is developed.

Altogether, these patients represent the commonest form of immunodeficiency. Often occurring in adults, with a history of previous good health, the presumption is that their immune system was previously normal and so it is an "acquired" disorder. Sometimes an antecedent infection or other illness is recognized, but in most instances no "etiology" can be identified. Bruton's original case was probably an example of the former type, although his name has since become associated with the X-linked form of agammaglobulinemia. Diagnostic and treatment implications are the same as discussed in the preceding sections, but when antibody deficiency is noted, particularly in the older age group, a search for underlying diseases such as chronic lymphocytic leukemia, lymphoma, and multiple myeloma is indicated.

Other conditions, such as collagen vascular disorders (rheumatoid arthritis, dermatomyositis), malabsorption, pernicious anemia, etc., have been associated with or observed to develop in these patients. The malabsorption with steatorrhea is not accompanied by easily demonstrable changes in intestinal flora nor is it relieved by antibiotics. *Giardia lamblia* infestation should be considered and intestinal biopsy performed to rule it out. There is also a high incidence of rheumatoid arthritis in the families of patients with hypogammaglobulinemia and in some families of systemic lupus erythematosus. Hemolytic anemia may occur, and several cases of megaloblastic anemia from vitamin B_{12} deficiency associated with defective absorption of vitamin B_{12} have been observed.

Frequent attacks of bronchitis and pneumonia lead to structural damage of the lungs, with lung abscess, empyema, diffuse fibrosis, or bronchiectasis. Nearly all affected individuals develop some degree of bronchiectasis if they live long enough. Also common are recurrent infections of the paranasal sinuses and middle ear. Repeated attacks of bacterial conjunctivitis may also occur. Episodes of acute pyoderma, meningitis, and urinary tract infections are noted with increased frequency but are less often a problem than respiratory, middle ear, and conjunctival infections. Bacterial infections respond well to treatment with the appropriate antibiotic, and the course run by a single infection under treatment is not unusual. It is the high frequency of recurrence that constitutes the problem.

Recent studies indicate that in some of these patients the defect lies with overactive suppressor T cells, and these observations may lead to new ways to treat or control the disorder.[66,68]

Currently, therapy consists of supportive care during the acute infection and prophylactic gamma globulin injections. Sometimes, enough of the immune response remains so that anaphylaxis is a problem with the gamma globulin treatments, and this requires very careful monitoring and observation during these injections. If this complication develops, an occasional patient can still be helped if a single related donor can be used for plasma transfer.

Selective Immunoglobulin Deficiencies

These occur in a variety of patterns and with varying degrees of completeness. The commonest of the specific immunodeficiency states is the syndrome of isolated IgA deficiency. The incidence in the general population is about one case per 500 to 700. Mode of inheritance is uncertain or seems to vary among families. Fortunately, most of these individuals are asymptomatic, but occasionally, sinopulmonary infections are troublesome. Other syndromes have been recognized, and this deficiency has been related to allergies, autoimmune disorders, various malignancies, malabsorption, and mental retardation. The etiologic connection, if any, in most of these situations is obscure.[57]

A serious difficulty for some of these patients is the presence of anti-IgA antibodies which can lead to gastrointestinal symptoms following milk ingestion. This also may lead to laboratory error if this reaction to ungulate IgA is not recognized and proper controls are not used when measuring IgA levels. Another hazard that these patients face is with the administration of blood or plasma. They can develop antibodies to human IgA encountered in this fashion, and life-threatening anaplylaxis may result later when more blood or plasma is administered.

Sinopulmonary hygiene and specific antibiotic therapy are currently the only available treatment. No commercial source of IgA is available for administration, and in addition, there would be serious reservations about its use (anaphylaxis, probable lack of transport to the mucous membrane surface, and hence no effectiveness at the major deficient site).

CHAPTER 94
Serum Sickness and Anaphylaxis
PHILIP S. NORMAN

Serum sickness[69] and anaphylaxis[72] are acute diseases of hypersensitivity that formerly were noted after the administration of antiserums from animal sources. Now they are most commonly precipitated by a variety of drugs, particularly penicillin. Serum sickness is an immune complex disease characterized by urticaria or other rashes, fever, lymphadenopathy, arthralgia, and facial edema. Anaphylaxis results from immune mediator release characterized by collapse, profound hypotension, wheezing, and cyanosis and may be followed by manifestations of serum sickness.

PATHOGENESIS OF SERUM SICKNESS

Serum sickness can readily be produced in rabbits, providing a thorough description of the pathophysiology of the disease. Figure 94–1 shows the course of events after a single intravenous dose of a large amount of a protein antigen, bovine serum albumin. After equilibration, the albumin circulates freely, being slowly metabolized at the same rate as the rabbit's own serum albumin. At about the sixth day, the rate of decline becomes greatly accelerated as antigen antibody complexes appear in the circulation. At antigen–antibody ratios, which are efficient at fixing complement, complexes including complement factors are predisposed to deposit in blood vessel walls. The IgE antibodies which are formed simultaneously may help to initiate deposition by local histamine release which increases vascular permeability. At the site of complex deposition, lesions include an acute arteritis and periarteritis, glomerulonephritis, and an intimal inflammatory reaction in large arteries. Splenic and lymph node enlargement, with activation of germinal centers and accumulations of plasma cells, also occurs. The albumin disappears entirely by the 12th to the 14th day, and circulating antibody begins to appear immediately thereafter. Lesions rapidly regress after circulating antibody appears. By the 28th day the animal is normal again.

Serum Sickness Caused by Heterologous Antisera

Serum sickness in man follows a similar course.[7,72] After one or several closely spaced injections of foreign serum, in 6 to 10 days, there is abrupt onset of skin eruption, fever, lymphadenopathy, edema, and arthralgia often accompanied by malaise, muscle pain, nausea, and vomiting. Urticaria is the most common eruption and usually appears first, often starting in the area of injection. Urticaria may be accompanied or followed by erythematous, morbilliform, or purpuric rashes or by erythema multiforme. Angioedema of the face, lips, eyelids, or glottis is also common. Lymphadenopathy often begins and is most prominent in the area draining the site of the injection of foreign serum but commonly is also generalized. There is leukocytosis but no eosinophilia. Arthralgia may be distressing but is not usually accompanied by true arthritis. There may be albuminuria and even temporary reduction of renal function. Unusual but serious manifestations are cardiac arrhythmias, meningismus, optic neuritis, and peripheral neuritis. The peripheral neuropathy is most commonly a unilateral mononeuritis involving the shoulder girdle or arm and characterized by weakness and sensory deficit. Any nerve, however, may be involved.

These manifestations peak within a few days and then subside somewhat less rapidly. There may be, however, one or more less severe recrudescences over several weeks. Except for the neuropathy, recovery is always complete, but *the patient retains a tendency to have the same reactions on subsequent administration of the same antigen. Such reactions are accelerated and often more severe, perhaps even fatal.*

The syndrome is associated with antibodies to the injected foreign protein. The antigens circulate freely in the individual during the incubation period. They tend to disappear shortly after the appearance of disease, and antibodies are detectable for the first time after the syndrome is well developed. Animal serums include a number of major antigens, hence relapses may be associated with the development of antibodies to different serum proteins at different times. The disease subsides rapidly when free antibody appears. Sensitization in human subjects is detected most readily by positive wheal and erythema skin reactions when minute amounts of serum are injected intradermally. Such skin reactivity persists for very long periods.

The incidence of symptoms is roughly related to the dose of serum administered, 10 ml of serum giving about 10 percent incidence of disease and 100 ml giving about 90 percent incidence of disease. The histologic lesion in the few human cases of serum sickness on which autopsies have been performed has been an acute arteritis and periarteritis in multiple organs, similar to that seen in animals used in serumsickness experiments.

The incidence of serum sickness from animal serum has been greatly reduced by the commercial development of immune human gamma globulin for the prophylaxis of tetanus. Animal sera, however, are

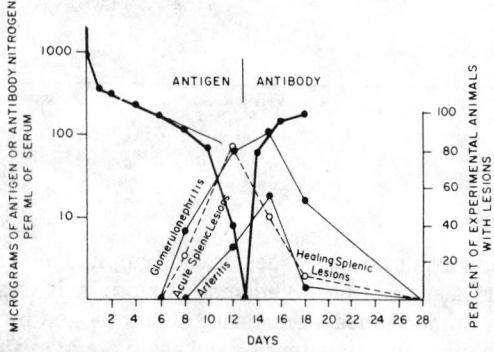

FIGURE 94–1. Serum sickness and anaphylaxis. (From Germuth. J. Exp. Med., 97:257, 1953.)

still employed as antilymphocyte globulin, as anti-venom for snake bites, in the treatment of gas gangrene and botulism, and in active–passive immunization against rabies.

Serum Sickness Caused by Drugs

Serum sickness caused by drugs was first described when sulfanilamide was introduced.[7,72] That drug is no longer used, and currently employed sulfonamides rarely cause the syndrome. *Penicillin has become the most common cause of serum sickness,* exceeding animal serums greatly as their use has declined. Penicillin is not ordinarily antigenic; being a simple chemical, it must conjugate with a body protein in order to become a complete antigen. Penicillin itself conjugates poorly, but penicillenic acid is capable of reacting with proteins to produce highly antigenic penicilloyl-protein conjugates. Penicillenic acid is formed in alkaline solutions of penicillin and readily sensitizes animals. Penicilloyl-protein or polylysine conjugates produce high rates of positive wheal and erythema skin reactions in patients who have had serum-sickness reactions to penicillin at times when many of these same patients do not have skin reactions to penicillin itself.[69]

Penicillin reactions are unlike serum sickness in that only a relatively small number of people are likely to develop sensitivity and the sensitivity is not clearly related to the dose of penicillin. These reactions can, however, reproduce all the phenomena of serum sickness caused by animal serums, although commonly they are comparatively mild and produce only urticaria. For unknown reasons, an occasional penicillin reaction gives prolonged symptoms over many months, a very rare occurrence with serum sickness from animal serums. Although full-blown serum sickness is relatively uncommon with other drugs (procainamide, salicylates, and streptomycin are the next most common causes), urticaria without other manifestations is well known to occur from a wide variety of drugs and has characteristics that resemble a mild serum-sickness reaction (Table 94–1). There is usually an incubation period of seven to ten days after the first administration of the drug before hives appear, and subsequent administration of the drug may provoke an accelerated reaction.

Management

When the manifestations of serum sickness are mild they may be suppressed with such antihistaminic drugs as tripellenamine hydrochloride (Pyribenzamine) 100 mg or diphenhydramine hydrochloride (Benadryl) 50 mg three to four times a day. Occasionally, however, these drugs will not be effective, and an adrenal corticosteroid, such as prednisone, may be required in a dose of 10 to 40 mg each day. Of crucial importance is the cessation of antigen administration, after which the reaction becomes self-limited.

ANAPHYLAXIS

As with serum sickness, an animal model (anaphylaxis in guinea pigs) reproduces many of the manifestations of the human disease.[5,7,70] A single injection of egg albumin sensitizes guinea pigs in 10 to 21 days so that a second intravenous dose causes sudden death 3 to 5 minutes later from bronchospasm. The principle mediator of the bronchospasm is histamine released from the granules of mast cells. Histamine is a potent bronchoconstrictor and capillary relaxant. Serotonin, slow-reacting substances (SRS-A), and plasma kinins may be released by the anaphylactic reaction. These substances have potent effects on smooth muscle and small blood vessels. Antibodies which do not fix complement but become fixed to mast cells mediate the reaction.

In man, specific IgE antibodies to the offending agent have been demonstrated in some instances in the serum or fixed to basophils. The systemic reaction occurs within minutes after introduction of the agent and is manifested by collapse, profound hypotension, wheezing, and cyanosis. Autopsy may show almost no anatomic alterations but often shows evidence of bronchoconstriction or edema of the upper airway to the point of closure. Anaphylaxis is particularly likely to occur with injected agents, but its occurrence has been well documented after oral doses of drugs. Anaphylactic sensitization to the venom of bees, yellow jackets, hornets, and wasps occurs at times and may cause sudden death after one or more stings. Anaphylaxis not only occurs with serum or drugs given therapeutically but also occurs after the use of injected diagnostic reagents (Table 94–2). Intradermal skin testing of atopic individuals with pollen, inhal-

---

TABLE 94-1
Agents Known To Cause Serum Sickness

Animal serums	Penicillins
Barbiturates	Phenylbutazone
Griseofulvin	Probenecid
Hydralazine	Procainamide
Insulin	Quinidine
Iodides	Quinine
Mercurial diuretics	Salicylates
Nitrofurantoin	Streptomycin
Oxphenbutazone	Sulfonamides
Para-aminosalicylic acid	

ant, or food extracts carries with it a definite but small hazard of anaphylaxis. Rarely, x-ray contrast media, bromsulfonphthalein, sodium dehydrocholate, and local anesthetics also cause sudden shock and death after their administration. *They should never be injected into a patient without the presence of facilities for resuscitation, since the syndrome is frequently fatal.* Some cases of anaphylactic reactions such as those induced by contrast media or local anesthetics do not appear to depend upon prior sensitization and may not have a true immunologic basis.

Anaphylaxis is best managed by prior detection of the tendency to react and avoiding the offending agent. The detection of preexisting sensitivity to serums or drugs, however, is difficult. Before serum or any drug known occasionally to cause anaphylaxis is administered to a patient, careful inquiry about previous use of the drug and hypersensitivity to it should be made. If there is a history of hypersensitivity to a drug, an appropriate substitute should be sought. If a patient has never received antiserum, skin testing with a high dilution of serum is indicated. The presence of a wheal and erythema reaction indicates the need for caution in proceeding with antiserum therapy. Skin testing for drugs, on the other hand, is highly unsatisfactory; *intracutaneous tests and patch tests with drugs are often negative when a patient has recently had a severe reaction to a drug.* The explanation for this phenomenon may be that the patient is sensitive not to the drug itself but to a protein conjugate or a metabolic product of the drug. In penicillin sensitivity skin testing with penicilloyl-polylysine will identify patients likely to develop serum sickness or urticaria but not all those in danger of anaphylaxis. Skin tests with both penicillin *and* penicilloyl-polylysine will detect most anaphylactically sensitive individuals. A history of prior reaction to penicillin is a poor predictor of future reactions; 75 percent of patients with a suggestive history will have negative skin tests and can take penicillin safely.[69]

Anaphylaxis to insect stings, on the other hand, is usually a straightforward IgE mediated reaction to venom proteins. Intradermal skin tests with diluted venom from one or more of the hymenoptera will produce a diagnostic wheal and erythema, and immunization with gradually increasing doses of the appropriate venom will induce IgE antibodies and solid immunity. Whole body extract of the insects is much less satisfactory than isolated venom for immunization. The immunity must be maintained by monthly booster injections.[71]

Management

Anaphylaxis requires emergency treatment to control circulation and respiration. Epinephrine hydrochloride, 0.5 ml to 1.0 ml of a 1:1000 solution, should be given subcutaneously or intramuscularly at once. If the patient is in shock with severe hypotension, the epinephrine may have to be given intravenously along with rapid intravenous fluid administration. The patient's head should be lowered. If he shows evidence of airway obstruction and cyanosis, tracheostomy is required. Antihistamines and corticosteroids are of no immediate value in treating anaphylaxis but may be required to control manifestations of serum sickness if they supervene. All medical personnel should be fully trained in the fundamental techniques of resuscitation (mouth-to-mouth breathing and closed-chest cardiac massage).

TABLE 94–2
Agents Known To Cause Anaphylaxis

ACTH	Liver extract
Allergenic extracts of pollens, molds, dusts, and foods	Local anesthetics
	Meprobamate
Aminopyrine	Mercurial diuretics
Amphotericin B	Para-aminosalicylic acid
Animal serums	Penicillins
Chymotrypsin	Procainamide
Heparin	Radiographic contrast media
Human gamma globulin	Salicylates
Indanedione derivatives	Sodium dehydrocholate
Insect stings (bees, yellow jackets, wasps, and hornets)	Streptomycin
	Succinylcholine
Insulin	Sulfobromophthalein
	Sulfonamides

CHAPTER 95
Hay Fever
PHILIP S. NORMAN

Hay fever is characterized by recurrent, usually seasonal, rhinitis, with watery nasal discharge, sneezing, edema of the nasal mucous membranes, nasal obstruction, conjunctivitis, pharyngeal itching, and cough. It is a classic allergic disease—one resulting from exposure to agents that clearly would be innocuous were it not for the individual's reaction to them.[5,75] The condition affects from 5 to 10 percent of the population.

INCITING AGENTS[74]

Hay fever results when sensitized individuals inhale pollens from certain plants among the relatively small number that propagate by producing large clouds of windborne pollen. Pollens range in size from 10 to 100 μ, the size most suitable for entrapment on the moist surfaces of the turbinates. Only particles as small as 5 μ will regularly pass the entrapment mechanisms of the nose and be inhaled into the lungs. Therefore, pollen allergy characteristically produces nasal symptoms and only occasionally causes asthma.

Most plants depend on insects or birds to transfer pollen, and only a few species depend on air currents. For this process to be successful, the plant must be widespread and must produce large quantities of light, dry pollen that is easily blown about by the wind. Not all such pollens, however, cause hay fever because some do not contain antigens capable of inciting the disease.

In the temperate zone of North America there are three principal seasons in which pollen is spread: the *early spring,* in which tree pollen is spread; the *early summer,* in which grass pollen is spread; and the *early fall,* in which weed pollen is spread. Ubiquitous outdoor molds, growing on decaying vegetation, also produce airborne spores in the fall of the year. Local exposure to animal danders, dust, insect detritus, and molds may cause symptoms like hay fever.

Ragweed is the most common cause of hay fever in the United States and may therefore be used as a general example. Ragweed plants are extremely widespread, springing up as annual weeds in fields or vacant lots, wherever the ground is not under cultivation. The plants mature in August and begin to produce pollen then. A single plant can produce 2 billion grains of pollen, and an acre of ragweed has been estimated to produce 16 tons. Pollen is characteristi-

cally shed in the early morning hours. The grains are about 20 μ in diameter and are easily blown about by air currents; they have been found in the atmosphere 400 miles out to sea and at elevations of 14,000 feet. The concentration of pollen ranges up to several thousand grains per cubic meter of air. On dry, windy days large clouds of pollen are spread, whereas on rainy days the air is often washed free of pollen. When the pollen grain is trapped in the nose of the sensitive individual, it releases its content on the nasal mucosa. Of the proteins contained in the pollen, only a few act as sensitizing antigens. The major one of these, antigen "E," has a molecular weight of 37,800 and represents only about 0.5 percent of the extractable solids of pollen. It is a simple globular protein whose properties do not explain its ability to sensitize. A second antigen, "K," has a molecular weight of 38,200 and represents about 0.3 percent of the solids. Several still smaller antigens sensitize an occasional individual in addition to the above antigens.

PATHOGENESIS[77]

The exposure of a sensitized person to pollen leads to the rapid development of hyperemia and edema of the nasal mucosa. The edema is at first unaccompanied by cellular infiltration, but after an hour the tissues become infiltrated with eosinophils. The swelling is accompanied by hypersecretion of mucus and obstruction of the nasal airway. There is intense itching, accompanied by frequent sneezing. Pollen antigen is also released in the eye and causes a reaction similar to that in the nose. *The severity of symptoms is closely related to the quantity of pollen inhaled,* as is shown by careful daily records of hay fever symptoms that correlate closely with pollen concentrations obtained by air sampling.

Antibodies[76]

Although the nose and eyes are the shock organs in hay fever, the sensitivity is general. A small amount of pollen extract introduced anywhere into the skin produces a prompt wheal and erythema reaction. These reactions are conferred by IgE antibodies, the least abundant of the known classes of immunoglobulins, being present in normal persons at levels of 5×10^{-6} mg/ml to 5×10^{-4} mg/ml of serum. IgE antibodies are distinguished from other antibodies biologically by their ability to fix to histamine-containing cells (basophils and mast cells) in skin and other tissues and chemically and immunologically by having ε heavy chains. ε chains are heavier (MW-ca. 75,000) than the heavy chains of other classes of antibodies and fixation to cells is a function of the Fc end of ε chains. The lymphoid cells which synthesize IgE antibodies are mostly associated with the respiratory and gastrointestinal tracts and the skin. The ability to synthesize IgE antibody is not confined to allergic individuals; nearly everyone will form these antibodies to intradermal injections of such antigens as ascaris extract and bovine ribonuclease. A recessive gene appears to confer elevated serum IgE levels on homozygotes, but other factors appear to be necessary for the development of specific IgE antibodies. Thus, some individuals with elevated IgE levels do not have clinical allergy, and occasional individuals with normal IgE levels are allergic. There is a strong familial tendency in allergies. From 5 to 15 percent of individuals develop allergy to inhaled agents.

Mediator Secretion[77]

The itching, swelling, and redness resulting from the union of pollen antigen and antibody are probably mediated by secretion of histamine and other mediators in basophils and tissue mast cells. The histamine of basophils or mast cells of pollen-sensitive individuals is readily released in vitro by minute amounts of pollen antigen in a reaction mediated by cell-fixed IgE antibody. The sensitivity of basophils from peripheral blood to specific antigen is related to clinical symptoms; individuals with the most severe hay fever have basophils that secrete histamine in the presence of the smallest amount of antigen. What intermediate steps lead from antigen–antibody union to histamine release is unknown, but the characteristics of the reaction suggest that enzymatic steps are involved. Complement, however, is not a factor. Histamine is released from living, intact cells, and the process does not injure or lyse the releasing cells. Substances which increase intracellular levels of cyclic AMP, such as catecholamines and methyl xanthines, inhibit histamine release, thus at least partially explaining the usefulness of these classes of drugs in allergic reactions.

Secondary Factors

In addition to the primary immunologic factors in the pathogenesis of hay fever just outlined, a variety of nonspecific secondary factors may influence the symptomatology. During prolonged allergic reactions, such as continuous pollen exposure during a "season," there is fragmentation of the basement membrane of the nasal mucosa. Under such circumstances the mucosa becomes "primed" for further reactions and less pollen is required to induce a reaction of given intensity than when the mucosa has gone unchallenged. Priming is nonspecific and individuals are more sensitive after priming to allergens other than the priming allergen. Nonspecific irritants, such as smoke, chemical, or cooking odors, and so on, may also become unusually noxious to the mucous membranes at such times. Atmospheric pollution in cities and days of high relative humidity may exacerbate symptoms. Emotional reactions involving disgust or hostility may increase the severity of symptoms. Exercise or excitement may cause temporary lessening of the manifestations of allergy followed by rebound increase in symptoms. The manifestations of ordinary respiratory infections may be unusually severe during the hay fever season, although there is little evidence that seasonal allergy predisposes the sensitized individual to develop such infections.

DIAGNOSIS

The diagnosis of hay fever depends on *relating the symptoms to exposure to an inciting agent.* A history of recurrent seasonal coryza and conjunctivitis is strongly suggestive of pollen or mold hay fever. Air sampling and the identification of pollens by their characteristic morphology is performed in many localities and has provided data on the average season of pollination of plants significant in hay fever. Such information is available in textbooks on allergy. In addition, allergy clinics in many localities perform air sampling as a guide to the current situation. Correlation of such information with the patient's symptoms may provide the clue to the responsible agent. Environmental exposure to dusts, danders, molds, and so on must also be discussed closely with the patient and sometimes local sampling of air in the home or place of work performed.[73,77]

Skin Tests

The suspected sensitivity can be confirmed by skin testing with extracts of pollen or other allergens or by direct application of extracts to the membranes of the eye or nose. Very dilute solutions of the allergen must be employed to avoid inducing systemic reactions in allergic persons. A positive response is the rapid development of allergic inflammation. Allergic individuals often have positive skin tests to a number of potential allergens that are unimportant in producing symptoms; thus, *a positive skin test alone is not enough to make an etiologic diagnosis.* It is essential to correlate symptoms with exposure to allergens. In vitro tests for specific IgE antibodies by the "radio allergosorbent technique" (RAST) correlate well with skin tests and are useful in diagnosis in patients who have skin diseases which make skin testing impractical.

A thorough search for inciting agents by history and skin testing will fail to reveal a satisfactory allergic cause in many patients with typically allergic symptoms. Sinus x-rays reveal structural abnormalities that will satisfactorily account for a few of such problems. There remains a group of patients, usually with nonseasonal perennial symptoms, some of whom develop nasal polyps and have eosinophils in the nasal secretions, in whom the search for external causes of disease is not productive. Whether these patients have allergic reactions to allergens that are as yet unrecognized, chronic low-grade infections, physiologic disturbances (vasomotor rhinitis), or psychophysiologic reactions to environmental stress is not readily determined. The existence of such patients serves to emphasize that there is nothing specific about the symptoms usually associated with allergic reactions and that the same symptoms may arise from nonallergic causes.

TREATMENT

Avoidance[77]

Treatment of allergic rhinitis is, first, avoidance of the inciting agent. Local contamination with dusts, molds, insects, and so on should be eliminated by appropriate cleanliness or extermination. Many patients choose to go to areas free of pollens to which they are sensitive, either permanently or temporarily during the pollen season. Air conditioners or filters can clean the air in rooms or buildings. When the offending agent cannot be avoided, symptomatic relief can be achieved by a number of measures.

Drugs[77]

Antihistamines taken orally (chlorpheniramine, 4 mg 3 to 4 times a day), vasoconstrictors applied locally (0.25 to 0.5 percent phenylephrine) or taken systemically, and anticholinergics to dry secretions are all helpful measures. Adrenal corticosteroids taken orally or applied locally will inhibit the edema and inflammation almost completely. Seasonal allergic rhinitis can usually be controlled by small doses (10 to 15 mg daily of prednisone or its equivalent) taken for a short period. Side effects are rare at such a limited dosage. A water-soluble steroid, such as dexamethasone, sprayed into the nose in small amounts, will control the symptoms in all but the most severe cases.

Immunotherapy[76]

The only method of treatment that may alter the patient's basic reactivity is so-called desensitization, better called *immunotherapy*. Weekly or twice weekly injections of gradually increasing amounts of extracts of the offending allergen are given before natural exposure to the allergen is expected. In many cases, the patient's reactivity is sufficiently reduced for exposure to result in less severe symptoms. The application of graded concentrations of specific allergen to mucous membranes after desensitization shows that more allergen is now required for a reaction than before desensitization. The mechanism by which the alteration is obtained involves several immunologic changes. Circulating antibodies of the IgG class that can inhibit reactions in sensitized skin or histamine release by sensitized leukocytes are increased by immunotherapy. Similar IgA and IgG antibodies in secretions are increased. The level of specific IgE antibodies also declines somewhat over several years of repeated injections, presumably because of stimulation of suppressor T cells. Cell sensitivity to histamine release by specific antigen may be decreased also in the patients with the most striking symptomatic response. IgG and IgA antibodies are immunologically specific for the antigen administered; decreases in cell sensitivity are not necessarily specific. The degree of symptomatic relief is related to the dose of allergen administered in groups of patients under careful study, better results being obtained with larger doses. Standardization of pollen extracts in order to express dosage in a universally applicable unitage has yet to be achieved, however. When injections are discontinued, IgG antibody declines in several months and at the next season of exposure IgE antibodies rise sharply.[73]

Immunotherapy may result in local or systemic allergic reactions, even anaphylaxis, as the dosage is increased. The amount of antigen needed to give adequate results is not predictable in the individual patient, and dosage must be increased cautiously until a satisfactory result is achieved or until adverse reactions cause the procedure to be abandoned.

REFERENCES

General References

1. Fudenberg, H.H., Pink, J.R.L., Wang, A.-C., and Douglas, S.D. Basic Immunogenetics, 2nd ed. New York, Oxford, 1978.
2. Fudenberg, H.H., Stites, D.P., Caldwell, J.L., and Wells, J.V., (eds.). Basic and Clinical Immunology, 2nd ed. Los Altos, Lange, 1978.

3. Gell, P.G.H., Coombs, R.R.A., and Lochman, P.J. (eds.). Clinical Aspects of Immunology, 3rd ed. Oxford, Blackwell, 1975.

4. Golub, E.S. The Cellular Basis of the Immune Response. Sunderland, Sinauer, 1977.

5. Middleton, E., Jr., Reed, C.E., and Ellis, E.F. (eds.). Allergy Principles and Practice, Vols. 1 and 2. St. Louis, Mosby, 1978.

6. Rose, N.R. and Friedman, H. (eds.). Manual of Clinical Immunology. Washington, American Society of Microbiology, 1976.

7. Samter, M. (ed.). Immunological Diseases, 3rd ed., Vols. 1 and 2. Boston, Little Brown, 1978

Immunoglobulins and the Plasma Cell Dyscrasias

8. Alexanian, R. Monoclonal gammopathy in lymphomas. Arch. Intern. Med., 135:62, 1975.

9. Alexanian, R., Balcerzak, S., Bonnet, J.D., Gehan, E., Haut, A., Hewlett, J.S., and Monto, R.W. Prognostic factors in multiple myeloma. Cancer, 36:1192, 1975.

10. Alexanian, R., Salmon, S., Bonnet, J. Gehan, E., Haut, A., and Weick, J. Combination therapy for multiple myeloma. Cancer, 40:2765, 1977.

11. Andrade, C., Araki, S., Block, W.D., Cohen, A.S., Jackson, C.E., Kuroiwa, Y., McKusick, V.A., Nissim, J., Sohar, E., and VanAllen, M.W. Hereditary amyloidosis. Arthritis Rheum., 13:902, 1970.

12. Bersagel, D.E. The treatment of plasma cell myeloma. Brit. J. Haematol., 33:443, 1976.

13. Bloch, K.J., Lee, L., Mills, J.A., and Haber, E. Gamma heavy chain disease: an expanding clinical and laboratory spectrum. Am. J. Med., 55:61, 1973.

14. Broder, S., Humphrey, R.L., Durm, M., Blackman, M., Meade, B., Goodman, C., Strober, W., and Waldmann, T.A. Impaired synthesis of polyclonal (non-paraprotein) immunoglobulins by circulating lymphocytes from patients with multiple myeloma. N. Engl. J. Med., 293:887, 1975.

15. Brouet, J.C. Biologic and clinical significance of cryoglobulins. Report of 86 cases. Am. J. Med., 57:775, 1974.

16. Capra, J.D., Winchester, R.J., and Kunkel, H.G. Hypergammaglobulinemic purpura: studies on the unusual anti γ globulins characteristic of the sera of these patients. Medicine, 50:125, 1971.

17. DeFronzo, R.A., Cooke, C.R., Wright, J.R., and Humphrey, R.L. Renal function in patients with multiple myeloma. Medicine, 57:151, 1978.

18. DeFronzo, R.A., Humphrey, R.L., Wright, J.R., and Cooke, C.R. Acute renal failure in multiple myeloma. Medicine, 54:209, 1975.

19. Eisen, H.N. Immunology: An Introduction to Molecular and Cellular Principles of the Immune Responses. Hagerstown, Md., Harper & Row, 1974.

20. Frangione, B. and Franklin, E.C. Heavy chain diseases: clinical features and molecular significance of the disordered immunoglobulin structure. Semin. Hematol., 10:53, 1973.

21. Franklin, E.C. μ-chain disease. Arch. Intern. Med., 135:71, 1975.

22. Franklin, E.C. and Buxbaum, J. Immunoglobulin structure, synthesis, secretion, and relation to neoplasms of B cells. Clin. Haematol., 6:503, 1977.

23. Gailani, S., Seon, B.K., and Henderson, E.S. Kappa light chain—myeloma associated with adult Fanconi syndrome: response of the nephropathy to treatment of myeloma. Med. Pediatr. Oncol., 4:141, 1978.

24. Glenner, G.G., Terry, W.D., and Isersky, C. Amyloidosis: its nature and pathogenesis. Semin. Hematol., 10:65, 1973.

25. Hood, L.E., Weissman, I.L., and Wood, W.B. Immunology. Menlo Park, Benjamin/Cummings, 1978.

26. Humphrey, R.L., Wright, J.R., Zachary, J.B., Sterioff, S., Jr., and DeFronzo, R.A. Renal transplantation in multiple myeloma. A case report. Ann. Intern. Med. 83:651, 1975.

27. Isobe, T., Ikeda, Y., Imura, H., and Ohta, H. Plasma cell leukemia. A clinical study of 13 cases, with a demonstration of small-sized plasma cells. Acta Haematol. Japan, 40:529, 1977.

28. Isobe, T. and Osserman, E.F. Pathologic conditions associated with plasma cell dyscrasias: a study of 806 cases. Ann. NY Acad. Sci., 190:507, 1971.

29. Jancelewicz, Z., Takatsuki, K., and Sugai, S. IgD multiple myeloma: review of 133 cases. Arch. Intern. Med., 135:87, 1975.

30. Krajny, M. and Pruzanski, W. Waldenström's macroglobulinemia: review of 45 cases. Can. Med. Assoc. J., 114:899, 1976.

31. Kyle, R.A. and Bayrd, E.D. Amyloidosis: review of 236 cases. Medicine, 54:271, 1975.

32. Kyle, R.A. and Bayrd, E.D. The Monoclonal Gammopathies. Multiple Myeloma and Related Plasma-cell Disorders. Springfield, Thomas, 1976.

33. Lackner, H. Hemostatic abnormalities associated with dysproteinemias. Semin. Hematol., 10:125, 1973.

34. Leb, L., Grimes, E.T., Baloug, K., and Merritt, J.A. Monoclonal macroglobulinemia with osteolytic lesions. A case report and review of the literature. Cancer, 39:227, 1977.

35. Lindstrom, F.D. and Dahlstrom, U. Multiple myeloma or benign monoclonal gammopathy? A study of differential diagnostic criteria in 44 cases. Clin. Immunol. Immunopathol., 10:168, 1978.

36. MacKenzie, M.R. and Lee, T.K. Blood viscosity in Waldenström's macroglobulinemia. Blood, 49:507, 1977.

37. Mancilla, R. and Davis, G.L. Nonsecretory multiple myeloma: immunohistologic and ultrastructural observations on two patients. Am. J. Med., 63:1015, 1977.

38. Matanoski, G.M., Seltser, R., Sartwell, P.E., Diamond, E.L., and Elliott, E.A. The current mortality rates of radiologists and other physician specialists: specific causes of death. Am. J. Epidemiol., 101:199, 1975.

39. Mellstedt, H., Ahre, A., Björkholm, M., Holm, G., Johansson, B., and Strander, H. Interferon therapy in myelomatosis. Lancet, 7:245, 1979.

40. Meltzer, M., Franklin, E.C., Elias, K., McCluskey, R.T., and Cooper, N. Cryoglobulinemia—a clinical and laboratory study. II. Cryoglobulins with rheumatoid factor activity. Am. J. Med., 40:837, 1966.

41. Meyers, B.R., Hirschman, S.Z., and Axelrod, J.A. Current patterns of infection in multiple myeloma. Am. J. Med., 52:87, 1972.

42. Mundy, G.R., Raisz, L.G., Cooper, R.A., Schichter, G.P., and Salmon, S.E. Evidence of the secretion of an osteo-

clast stimulating factor in myeloma. N. Engl. J. Med., 291:1041, 1974.

43. Natvig, J.B. and Kunkel, H.G. Human immunoglobulins: classes, subclasses, genetic variants, and idiotypes. Adv. Immunol., 16:1, 1973.

44. Poljak, R.J., Amzel, L.M., Avey, H.P., Chen, B.L., Phizachkerley, R.P., and Saul, F. Three-dimensional structure of the Fab fragment of a human immunoglobulin at 2.8A resolution. Proc. Natl. Acad. Sci. USA, 70:3305, 1973.

45. Pruzanski, W. Clinical manifestations of multiple myeloma: relation to class and type of M component. Can. Med. Assoc. J., 114:896, 1976.

46. Rogers, J.S., Spahr, J., Judge, D.M., Varano, L.A., and Eyster, M.E. IgE myeloma with osteoblastic lesions. Blood, 49:295, 1977.

47. Rousseau, J.J., Franck, G., Grisar, T., Reznik, M., Heyner, G., and Salmon, J. Osteosclerotic myeloma with polyneuropathy and ectopic secretion of calcitonin. Eur. J. Cancer, 14:133, 1978.

48. Salem, P.A., Nasser, V.H., Shahid, M.J., Hajj, A.A., Alami, S.Y., Balikian, J.B., and Salem, A.A. "Mediterranean abdominal lymphoma," or immunoproliferative small intestinal disease. Part I: clinical aspects. Cancer, 40:2941, 1977.

49. Shustik, C., Bergsagel, D.E., and Pruzanski, W. κ and λ light chain disease: survival rates and clinical manifestations. Blood, 48:41, 1976.

50. Sletten, K. and Husby G. The complete amino acid sequence of nonimmunoglobulin amyloid fibril protein AS in rheumatoid arthritis. Eur. J. Biochem., 41:117, 1974.

51. Snapper, I. and Kahn, A. Myelomatosis: Fundamentals and Clinical Features. Baltimore, University Park, 1971.

52. Waldenström, J.G. Monoclonal and Polyclonal Hypergammaglobulinemia: Clinical and Biolgical Significance. Nashville, Vanderbilt, 1969.

53. ———. Diagnosis and Treatment of Multiple Myeloma. New York, Grune & Stratton, 1970.

54. Westermark, P., Grimelius, L., Polak, J.M., Larson, L.I., Van Noorden, S., Wilander, O., and Pearse, A.G. Amyloid in polypeptide hormone-producing tumors. Lab. Invest., 37:212, 1977.

55. Wiltshaw, E. Chemotherapy in the management of extramedullary plasmacytoma. Cancer Chemotherapy and Pharmacology, 1:167, 1978.

The Immunodeficiency Diseases

56. Allen, J.C. Infection and the Compromised Host. Baltimore, Williams & Wilkins, 1976.

57. Atwater, J.S. and Tomasi, T.B., Jr. Suppressor cells and IgA deficiency. Clin. Immunol. Immunopathol., 9:379, 1978.

58. Benacerraf, B. Immunogenetics and Immunodeficiency. Baltimore, University Park, 1975.

59. Bergsma, D. and Good, R.A. (eds). Immunologic Deficiency Diseases in Man. Birth Defects Original Article Series, Vol. IV, No. 1. New York, National Foundation, 1968.

60. Dosch, H.M., Lee, J.W.W., Gelfand, E.W., and Falk, J.A. Severe combined immunodeficiency disease: model of T-cell dysfunction. Clin. Exp. Immunol., 34:260, 1978.

61. Good, R.A. and Bach, F.H. Bone Marrow and Thymus Transplants: Cellular Engineering to Correct Primary Immunodeficiency. In Bach, F.W. and Good, R.A. (eds.), Clinical Immunobiology, Vol. 2. New York, Academic, 1974, p. 63.

62. Kobayashi, N. (ed.). Immunodeficiency: Its Nature and Etiological Significance in Human Diseases. Baltimore, University Park, 1978.

63. Louite, S. and Schwartz, R.S. Immunodeficiency and pathogenesis of lymphoma and leukemia. Semin. Hematol., 15(2):117, 1978.

64. Magilavy, D.B., Cassidy, J.J., Tubergen, D.G., Petty, R.E., Chisholm, R., and McCall, K. Intravenous gammaglobulin in the management of patients with hypogammaglobulinemia. J. Allergy Clin. Immunol., 61:378, 1978.

65. Samter, M. (ed.) Immunological Diseases. 3rd ed., Vols. 1 and 2. Boston, Little, Brown, 1978.

66. Siegal, F.P., Siegal, M., and Good, R.A. Role of helper, suppressor and B-cell defects in the pathogenesis of the hypogammaglobulinemias. N. Engl. J. Med., 299:172, 1978.

67. Stiehm, E.R. and Fulginiti, V.A. (eds.). Immunologic Disorders in Infants and Children. Philadelphia, Saunders, 1973.

68. Waldmann, T.A., Blaese, R.M., Broder, S., and Krakaner, R.S. Disorders of suppressor immunoregulatory cells in the pathogenesis of immunodeficiency and autoimmunity. Ann. Intern. Med., 88:226, 1978.

Serum Sickness and Anaphylaxis

69. Adkinson, M.F., Jr. A guide to skin testing for penicillin allergy. Med. Times, 104:164, 1976.

70. Austen, K.F. Systemic anaphylaxis in man. JAMA, 192:116, 1965.

71. Hunt, K.J., Valentine, M.D., Sobotka, A.K., Benton, A.W., Amodio, F.J., and Lichtenstein, L.M. A controlled trial of immunotherapy in insect hypersensitivity. N. Engl. J. Med., 299:157, 1978.

72. Longcope, W.T. Serum sickness and analogous reactions from certain drugs, particularly the sulfonamides. Medicine, 22:251, 1943.

Hay Fever

73. Ishizaka, K. Human reaginic antibodies. Annu. Rev. Med., 21:187, 1970.

74. King, T.P. and Norman, P.S. Antigens that cause atopic disease. In Samter, M. (ed.), Immunological Diseases, 3rd ed. Boston, Little, Brown, 1978.

75. Lichtenstein, L.M. and Norman, P.S. Allergy. Clinical Immunobiology, 1:243, 1972.

76. Norman, P.S. A review of immunotherapy. Allergy, 33:62, 1978.

77. Norman, P.S. and Lichtenstein, L.M. Allergic Rhinitis. In Samter, M. (ed.), Immunological Diseases, 3rd ed. Boston, Little, Brown, 1978.

SECTION FOURTEEN
Rheumatic Disease
MARY BETTY STEVENS: SECTION EDITOR

Patients with rheumatic disorders seek specialized care for one of three reasons, namely, 1) musculoskeletal pain or dysfunction, 2) a multisystem illness, or 3) the incidental discovery of a seroprotein abnormality.

Most common is the development of arthritis or "rheumatism" which rank high on the list of major health problems in terms of prevalence as causes of temporary, even permanent, disability. Classification is difficult for the spectrum of disorders, ranging from minor trauma to complex systemic illness, that may cause rheumatic symptoms. The "tentative" classification by the American Rheumatism Association[9] based on etiology and pathogenesis emphasizes the paucity of knowledge of disease mechanisms in this area of medicine. A practical and functional classification, not encyclopedic, is presented in Table XIV-1, which also guides the physician in the approach to the patient with rheumatic complaints.

No attempt is made to present clinical descriptions of all the disorders that may give rise to rheumatic symptoms. Initial consideration is given to the special features of history, physical examination, and laboratory data that are important in evaluating the patient with rheumatic manifestations. Subsequent chapters emphasize the diagnostic features and management of the more frequently encountered disorders. Finally, the differential diagnosis of multisystem disease and arthritis is discussed.

TABLE XIV-1
Rheumatic Disorders

Type	Examples
I. Systemic Process	
Systemic features dominant	Systemic lupus erythematosus Progressive systemic sclerosis Polymyositis Polymyalgia rheumatica Sjögren syndrome Subacute infective endocarditis Sarcoidosis Leukemias
Arthritis dominant	Adult rheumatoid arthritis
II. Arthritis with Extra-articular Lesions	Ankylosing spondylitis Reiter syndrome Psoriatic arthritis Colitic arthropathy Gout Septic arthritis Hypertrophic osteoarthropathy
III. Arthropathy Alone	Degenerative joint disease Traumatic arthritis Pigmented villonodular synovitis Tumors of bone, cartilage, synovium
IV. Nonarticular Rheumatic Disease	Bursitis, tendinitis, fasciitis Myositis, neuritis

CHAPTER 96
Evaluation of the Patient
MARY BETTY STEVENS

In evaluating the patient with rheumatic complaints, an attempt is made to answer the following:

1. Is the problem, if rheumatic, localized to soft tissue, tendon, or joints?
2. What is the pattern of joint or periarticular involvement?
3. Is there evidence of past or present inflammation, locally or systemically?
4. Are multiple organ systems involved?

Only after a comprehensive history and physical examination can these key questions be resolved. The importance of the family history in suggesting genetic factors (e.g., gout, ankylosing spondylitis) and the social history in documenting exposures and occupational and emotional trauma cannot be overemphasized. The character, degree, and basis of disability must be precisely defined. All too often a patient is "crippled" by a diagnostic label, not a disease process. With thoughtful consideration of the total clinical array, the physician can arrive at the appropriate diagnosis in the majority of patients and develop support for that diagnosis through judicious use of ancillary studies.

Localization of Symptoms

Since rheumatic complaints may result from disorders involving joints (arthropathy) or periarticular soft tissues (bursitis, tendinitis) or tissue not directly related to joints (myositis, neuritis), the first step is to localize precisely the site of involvement. Pain caused by arthritis (i.e., joint inflammation) is usually confined to the joint(s) involved and is aggravated by movement or stretching of the joint. Symptoms of nonarticular rheumatism, such as tendinitis and bursitis, may mimic arthritic pain but can be distinguished on physical examination. Joint pain may occasionally be referred to other sites, as in disease of the hip, in which pain may be felt primarily in the groin or in the thigh just above the knee. However, moving the involved joint will aggravate the pain and examination will elicit signs referable to the joint itself. Pain unrelated to joint motion or not localized to the joint or periarticular tissues argues against an organic rheumatic condition.

Patients who complain of arthralgia or myalgia unaccompanied by physical signs pose a difficult problem. Sometimes these symptoms are indicative of systemic disease (infectious, neoplastic, connective-tissue disease, etc.). Rheumatoid arthritis in its early stages may present without objective signs. However, the most common causes of such rheumatic symptoms are simple fatigue, ill-defined nonarticular syndromes such as fibrositis, and psychological disorders, especially depressive reactions. The last are usually associated with a background of stress and emotional problems and, frequently, personal exposure to rheumatic disease. The failure of salicylates to provide relief and the persistence of complaints for prolonged periods without physical signs are characteristic of patients with psychological disorders (sometimes termed "psychogenic rheumatism").

Pattern of Joint Involvement

The characterization of an episode of arthritis according to onset, intensity of inflammation, location, progression of joint involvement, and duration is most valuable in establishing the diagnosis. Knowledge of prior episodes is helpful. A migratory pattern of arthritis, in which the arthritis leaves one joint as a new one is affected, is characteristic of acute rheumatic fever. In contrast, in rheumatoid arthritis new joint involvement is additive. The distribution of the arthritis is of major diagnostic import. For example, the large joints are particularly involved in rheumatic fever and the arthritis of inflammatory bowel disease, whereas in rheumatoid arthritis the small joints are affected in a bilaterally symmetric fashion.

Examination of Joints

The examination of joints should include all the peripheral joints and axial skeleton. Each joint is evaluated for pain on motion, signs of inflammation, structural deformity, and dysfunction.

Involvement of the joint itself is certain if there is an *effusion* sufficient to produce a soft, compressible distention of the joint capsule. A small effusion may be difficult to detect. In the knee a useful test of effusion is ballottement of the patella with the forefingers while the hands are compressing the lateral margins of the joint from above and below. Another useful maneuver is to produce the "bulge" or "fluid wave" sign. With the knee extended, fluid is displaced upward from the medial side of the joint by firm compression. Pressure then applied superiorly and laterally will cause the displaced fluid to flow back into the medial side of the joint in a wavelike motion. Although usually indicative of some joint disease, effusion may result from edema due to heart failure or other causes.

Enlargement of the joint may be due to soft-tissue swelling or to bony enlargement rather than to an effusion. The presence of a thickened synovial membrane can often be detected by palpation and is a certain sign of chronic arthritis.

Tenderness is best detected in patients with arthritis by direct pressure over the synovium, especially at sites where it is most superficial (for example, at the epicondyles of the humerus or adjacent to the malleoli). Pain or tenderness in the finger joints is elicited by firm compression of the joint, both in an anteroposterior position and in a mediolateral position. Compression of all of the metacarpophalangeal joints laterally, with a handshakelike grip, also demonstrates tenderness of these joints.

The determination of the *range of motion* should include an estimation of the degree of limitation and whether it is related to pain, soft-tissue swelling, contracture, or malalignment and bony deformity. A greater-than-normal range of motion is also important because it may suggest disruption of the normal supporting structures, either by trauma, by destructive inflammation, or by such hereditary disorders of connective tissue as Marfan syndrome. Crepitus on motion usually is indicative of irregularity of the cartilaginous joint surfaces or bony contours. It may also arise from the soft tissues—for example, from an inflamed tendon moving through a thickened, irregular sheath.

Nonarticular rheumatism is used to describe disorders involving the periarticular soft tissues, such as tendinitis and bursitis. In these conditions swelling and tenderness, when they occur, are confined to the affected periarticular structures. Pain can be elicited by direct pressure or by stretching or moving an involved tendon or muscle rather than the joint. For example, in acute tendonitis or bursitis of the shoulder, there commonly is a well-localized area of tenderness in the region of the subdeltoid bursa or supraspinatus tendon, with marked pain on abduction or internal rotation of the shoulder. In contrast to arthritis, direct pressure over the joint capsule of the shoulder does not cause pain.

Periarticular tissues may be affected by an arthritic disorder, but in most patients joint involvement will be evident as well. Periarticular pain, muscle spasm, or tenderness may result from the unusual stress placed on these structures by altered joint function. When examination fails to demonstrate abnormalities of the joints or periarticular tissues, one should look for lesions of the bones or periosteum and for evidence of neurogenic or vascular disorders.

Inflammation, Deformity, and Disability

The differentiation between inflammatory and noninflammatory joint disease is important. In many cases the distinction is obvious on the basis of local signs of redness, heat, and exquisite tenderness, such as occurs in acute gout or pyogenic infection. More subtle evidences of inflammation usually accompany such chronic disorders as rheumatoid arthritis in which an effusion and synovial-membrane thickening may continue despite the absence of local heat or marked tenderness.

The presence of deformity may be helpful in characterizing the nature of the rheumatic process. Deformity and disability are more likely to result from arthritis but can occasionally follow nonarticular processes (as in the contracted hand of the shoulder-hand syndrome or the swan-neck digital deformities of systemic lupus erythematosus).

Measurements of the degree of deformity are important in the overall assessment of the patient, in planning management, and in documenting progress. Recording the ranges of active and passive joint motion, noting fixed deformities, assessing muscle strength, and measuring the circumferences of enlarged joints at fixed reference points are all helpful. In evaluation of the hand, it may be useful to note the distance from the fingertips to the palm in the patient who cannot make a complete fist. Grip strength can be measured by having the patient grasp and squeeze the blood-pressure cuff inflated to 20 mm Hg and recording the rise in the mercury column. Some estimations of functional capacity can be made by asking the patient to perform a series of tasks that might be required in daily living, such as walking a measured distance, dressing himself, and placing objects on a shelf at various levels. If these tasks are standardized and repeated at intervals, some notion of progress can be obtained.

It must be remembered that *deformity* relates to structural alterations while *disability* is a failure of the patient to function in a normal life-style. Therefore, a patient with rheumatic complaints may be significantly disabled with or without an inflammatory or degenerative process affecting the articular structures and with little or no relationship to the degree of skeletal deformities. It is of therapeutic import to assess in every patient the deficit between normal function and performance and establish the basis for any disability.

Systemic Involvement

The evaluation of patients with rheumatic complaints should include a survey of all organ systems. Arthralgia may be an early or presenting symptom of a multisystem disease—for example, systemic lupus erythematosus (SLE) or sarcoidosis. Muscle pain and especially weakness dominate the spectrum of polymyositis. Peripheral neuropathy frequently accompanies polyarteritis, less frequently rheumatoid arthritis. Furthermore, extra-articular manifestations of the arthritides may be encountered that have diagnostic significance (e.g., the subcutaneous nodules of rheumatoid arthritis, tophaceous deposits of gout, the multisystem manifestations of connective tissue disease) or therapeutic implications (e.g., the iritis in Still's disease, the bowel lesion of Crohn's disease, the nephritis of SLE).

X-Ray Examination of the Joints

In general the changes noted on x-ray examination occur relatively late in the course of inflammatory joint disease. Therefore, a normal x-ray by no means excludes the diagnosis of arthritis. X-ray examinations are of value, especially in patients with chronic joint disease, both in supporting the clinical diagnosis and in evaluating the pattern and severity of articular changes. Early in the course of inflammatory joint disease, extra-articular x-rays are frequently of more diagnostic value than joint films (e.g., hilar nodes on chest x-ray or characteristic inflammatory changes in the small bowel).

Analysis of Synovial Fluid

Synovial fluid should be analyzed whenever there is an accessible effusion. The hazards of aspiration are negligible, and the information gained may prove invaluable. In some instances, such as in gout and infection, a diagnosis can be made from a few drops of fluid by the identification of crystals or organisms.

Synovial fluid analysis is particularly helpful in distinguishing the inflammatory from the noninflammatory causes of effusion (Table 96–1). Immediate indication of inflammation is obtained if the fluid is grossly turbid or purulent. Similarly, a bloody effusion suggests trauma, a bleeding disorder, or pig-

---

TABLE 96–1
Synovial Fluid Findings

Examination	Results in Most Noninflammatory Effusions	Results in Most Inflammatory Effusions	Diagnostic Features
Gross appearance	Clear yellow	Turbid	Grossly bloody effusions suggest trauma, pigmented villonodular synovitis, and, when fat droplets are present, a fracture communicating with the joint
Viscosity	Very viscid	Reduced viscosity	
Mucin clot	Firm, ropy clot	Clot forms poorly and fragments readily	
White cell count (WBC)	<2000 cells/μl	>2000 cells/μl	>50,000 cells strongly suggests infection
Glucose	Approximates blood glucose	May be reduced	Very low glucose strongly suggests infection
Protein	2–3.5 g/dl	>3 g/dl	
Complement	Normal	Normal or high	Reduced in rheumatoid arthritis, especially relative to protein concentration
Microscopic examination			
For crystals	None present	Cholesterol crystals found rarely in severely damaged joints	Urate crystals in gout; calcium pyrophosphate crystals in pseudogout Frequently intracellular in acute attacks
For cells	Predominantly mononuclear	Usually polymorphonuclear Phagocytic inclusions may be seen	Many phagocytic inclusions suggests rheumatoid arthritis (RA cells) Phagocytosis of leukocytes by macrophages in Reiter syndrome
For organisms	None	May be found in infection, intra- or extracellular	Infection
Culture	Sterile	Sterile except in infection	Microorganism isolated

mented villonodular synovitis. Normally, synovial fluid is very viscid, and a drop placed between the fingers or dropped from a needle will string out for two or more inches before breaking. *Viscosity* is reduced in many types of effusion, but is characteristically reduced in severe inflammatory processes. The *mucin clot test,* performed by the addition of a small amount of joint fluid to dilute acetic acid, normally and in most noninflammatory effusions produces a firm, tight, ropy clot of protein-bound hyaluronate which does not fragment. In many inflammatory effusions, the hyaluronate is depolymerized or diluted with other proteins so the clot fails to form or forms loosely and fragments readily.

The *white cell count* in synovial fluid is done as a blood white cell count, except that the usual diluents which contain weak acids may cause a mucin clot, trapping the cells and invalidating the count. Therefore, normal saline should be used as a diluent. A small amount of methylene blue or another nuclear stain can be added if desired. If there are many erythrocytes, 0.3 percent saline will lyse them, preserving the white cells. The white cell count usually reflects the degree of inflammation, being under 2000 cells/μl in most noninflammatory effusions.

Synovial fluid analysis should also include the microscopic examination of a fresh smear for crystals or phagocytic inclusions, a bacterial smear and culture, and determination of glucose, protein, and complement content. Further discussion of the diagnostic significance of these procedures is contained in subsequent chapters.

Synovial Biopsy[196]

Synovium, as a serous membrane, reacts in a limited way to insult. Most inflammatory disorders produce a nonspecific inflammatory response. However, a synovial biopsy can be diagnostic when granulomata, microcrystalline deposits, or neoplastic cells are present. Furthermore, the culture of synovial tissue may prove helpful even when synovial fluid is sterile.

Serum Protein Changes

Elevated levels of "acute-phase reactants" (erythrocyte sedimentation rate, C-reactive protein, serum glycoproteins) indicate the existence of an inflammatory condition. However, such elevations occur in a wide variety of conditions and are of little differential diagnostic value. Repeated determinations may be helpful in following the course of an inflammatory process. Serum gamma globulin elevations usually accompany a chronic inflammatory disorder, but they aid little in diagnosis unless marked in degree or monoclonal. The finding of serum antigammaglobulin rheumatoid factors or other "autoimmune" phenomena may support the diagnosis of rheumatoid arthritis or a connective tissue disorder. Furthermore, the presence of specific antibodies (e.g., antistreptolysin O, antiviral) may confirm host response to infection.

CHAPTER 97

Systemic Lupus Erythematosus

MARY BETTY STEVENS

Systemic lupus erythematosus (SLE) is a disease of unknown etiology that is characterized by inflammatory lesions involving multiple organ systems, especially the skin, joints, kidneys, and serous membranes. Equally characteristic are multiple immunologic abnormalities, especially the serum LE-cell factor, which have led to an increased appreciation of the varied manifestations of this disorder. Although it may be a fulminating illness, SLE more commonly is a chronic, recurrent disorder.[47]

The incidence of SLE approximates that of the lymphomas. Women are affected six to eight times more frequently than men. Blacks may be affected more often than whites.[31,51] Symptoms most commonly begin between the ages of 15 and 40 but have been noted at any age. Multiple cases have been reported in families and there may be a genetic predisposition to SLE.[24]

CLINICAL MANIFESTATIONS

The type and severity of the initial manifestations of SLE vary greatly.[31,36] Occasionally, patients present with a fulminant, febrile illness and functional derangement of many organ systems. There are also those relatively few individuals without clinical symptoms who are detected through abnormal laboratory tests (e.g., biologic false positive serologic test for syphilis). Most commonly, patients present with

TABLE 97-1
Initial Manifestations of SLE*

	Number of Patients
Arthritis or arthralgias	74
Skin rash	37
Fever	25
Pleurisy and/or pericarditis	16
Weight loss	9
Alopecia	6
Neuropsychiatric episode	5
Nephritis, thrombocytopenia, and BFP	3
Raynaud syndrome and anemia	2
Lymphadenopathy	1
Total	140

* Data from Johns Hopkins Rheumatic Disease Unit.[39]

constitutional symptoms such as fever and malaise, as well as evidence of the involvement of several organ systems, especially the skin, joints, and serous surfaces (Table 97-1).

The precise onset of SLE may be difficult to date. Frequently, over a period of months or years, a series of seemingly isolated illnesses may evolve into a pattern characteristic of SLE.

Systemic

Fever occurs in about 85 percent of patients during periods of disease activity. Shaking chills are noted rarely and most often relate to a complicating infection or to antipyretic therapy. Malaise, easy fatigability, anorexia, and weight loss are also commonly encountered.

Skin and Mucous Membranes

A wide variety of skin and mucous-membrane lesions have been noted in over 75 percent of patients. The most characteristic dermal abnormality is the butterfly erythema, which is distributed over the bridge of the nose and malar eminences in 30 percent of cases. Similar lesions, which at times become scaly and pruritic, may occur over the neck, upper chest, and extremities. Evanescent erythematous nodules on the digital pads and small, punctate, ulcerative lesions on the fingers and palms reflect an underlying vasculitis. Although uncommon, their presence should alert one to the existence of SLE. Similarly, characteristic but infrequent is the linear erythema along the margin of the eyelids. Ulcerative lesions may also be seen in the mucous membranes.

Many lesions occur which are less specifically related to SLE. Dermal atrophy, ulceration, and gangrene secondary to vascular insufficiency may develop in the setting of Raynaud's phenomenon, arteritis, or other evidences of vasomotor instability. The occasional episodes of urticaria and angioneurotic edema are reminiscent of histamine-mediated responses. A third group of mucocutaneous lesions (purpura, petechiae, ecchymoses) reflects either an underlying hemorrhagic tendency or vasculitis.

The erythematous, scaling, disc-like plaques characteristic of discoid lupus erythematosus may occur in SLE. Involvement of the face and scalp is seen most often, with infrequent extension to the trunk and extremities. Healing eventually occurs and results in atrophic, depigmented areas of skin. These discoid lesions may precede other systemic manifestations of SLE by months or years.

Photosensitive eruptions are noted in approximately one-third of cases. Frontal alopecia is frequent, especially in young women.

Musculoskeletal

Polyarthropathy is among the most commonly encountered manifestations of SLE, being present in 90 percent of individuals at some time during the course of their illnesses. Frequently, polyarthralgia is the dominant problem in the absence of objective joint abnormalities. Arthritis is apparent as a presenting feature in two-thirds of the cases.

An evanescent symmetric polyarthritis is observed most often. Any peripheral joint may be involved, especially interphalangeal and metacarpophalangeal. Mild deformities may develop in the digits, but the occurrence of contractures, ankylosis, and joint erosions on x-ray is unusual. As in rheumatoid arthritis, synovial (Baker) cysts can occur in the popliteal space and, with dissection or rupture, mimic thrombophlebitis.

Tenosynovitis occurs at times. A diffuse myopathy, especially one involving the pelvic and shoulder girdle musculature, is infrequent. Serum levels of muscle-cell enzymes usually are elevated in those with myositis in contrast to patients with steroid-related myopathy or disuse wasting.

Ischemic bone necrosis of the femoral heads[35,201] is a complication of SLE, especially in patients receiving corticosteroid therapy. Necrosis of humeral heads, knees, and carpal bones occurs less often.

Ocular

The most characteristic ocular lesions are the "cytoid bodies," which are found in 10 to 20 percent of patients. These small, oval, whitish opacities, which occur in the central portion of the fundus adjacent to blood vessels, represent foci of ischemic degeneration of the nerve-fiber layer of the retina. They may be difficult to distinguish from the lesions associated with diabetes mellitus, hypertension, bacteremia, macroglobulinemia, and increased intracranial pressure. Nonspecific conjunctivitis and retinal hemorrhages and exudates may also be encountered.

Pleuropulmonary

Episodes of pleuritic pain are common in patients with SLE. They may occur without other detectable evidence of pleuritis or in association with a pleural rub or effusion.

An atelectasizing pneumonitis is the most frequent pulmonary abnormality. Commonly, the development of pleural reaction and plate-like atelectasis at the lung bases are observed on serial chest films, unaccompanied by clinical findings. Widespread pulmonary lesions have been shown to impair alveolar-capillary diffusion, but marked respiratory insufficiency rarely develops.

Cardiovascular

Cardiac lesions are observed in 50 percent of patients. Pericarditis is encountered most commonly. Although frequently sufficient to cause enlargement of the cardiac silhouette (x-ray), pericardial effusions of large volume and tamponade are rare. Myocarditis, the most serious cardiac sign, occurs in less than 10 percent of patients but is especially found in those with skeletal muscle inflammation.

Endocarditis is often present on pathologic examination. The characteristic vegetations (Libman-Sacks) are usually found under the mitral valve leaflets. Mitral stenosis has been observed as a consequence of lupus valvulitis. However, functional deficits ascribable to Libman-Sacks endocarditis are rare.

Hypertension in individuals with SLE usually relates to renal involvement and/or steroid therapy.

Gastrointestinal

Nearly 40 percent of patients with SLE complain of abdominal pain which results from serositis or vasculitis. An acute abdomen, often difficult to interpret in the steroid-treated patient, may develop secondary to SLE, its therapy, or an intercurrent process.

Dysphagia is an occasional symptom. X-ray studies may reveal esophageal aperistalsis similar to that seen in systemic sclerosis. Similarly, segmental dilatation may be noted in one or more regions of the small bowel.

Hepatomegaly is present in about one-third of SLE cases. There is no distinctive hepatic functional abnormality or biopsy pattern characteristic of SLE. Severe functional impairment is rare.

Reticuloendothelial

Palpable splenomegaly, observed in 15 to 20 percent of patients, is less common than local or generalized lymphadenopathy, observed in over 50 percent of cases. Infrequently, these abnormalities are sufficiently impressive to suggest lymphoma, and, on occasion, lymph-node-biopsy findings have been thought to represent a lymphoid neoplasm.

Neurologic[34,38,39]

Mental or neurologic dysfunction is seen in 25 to 30 percent of patients with SLE. This usually relates to the central nervous system rather than to peripheral nerves.

A wide variety of behavioral disturbances, ranging from mild anxiety and minor memory defects to major psychoses, have been observed. Frequently, neuropsychiatric episodes of illness cannot be correlated with cerebrospinal-fluid abnormalities. However, evidence of disease activity in other organ systems is usually present.

Focal vascular lesions may result in seizures or frequently in multifocal neurologic deficits. Since antiepileptic drugs, such as trimethadione and the hydantoin derivatives, can induce or activate SLE in certain individuals, one should remain alert to this possibility in managing patients who present initially with seizures.

An "aseptic meningitis" may be seen in a small proportion of patients.

Lupus Nephritis[23,46]

Renal disease is present in most patients with SLE. Since progression to renal insufficiency and fatal outcome may occur, determination of the presence or absence of renal involvement and its severity is important in prognosis and therapy.

Lupus nephritis commonly develops early in the course of SLE and infrequently after 2 or more years of disease activity. Rarely is nephritis the sole manifestation of the disease. Proteinuria and abnormalities of urinary sediment including hematuria, cylinduria, and pyuria are commonly found, but may be minimal or transient early in the course of disease. At times, patients present with the nephrotic syndrome but features of an acute glomerulonephritis are more common. In general, active nephropathy may be correlated with disease activity in other organ systems. In some cases the renal disease is not progressive and remains mild throughout the illness. Hypertension often develops in patients with advanced renal disease.

Percutaneous renal biopsy is valuable in assessing the renal status of the patient with SLE both with respect to activity and severity of the nephritis. In some cases, renal biopsy may reveal involvement in patients with minimal or no abnormalities of their urinary sediments. In general, patients who have focal glomerulonephritis on biopsy have little functional impairment and a good prognosis. More severe disease is typically associated with diffuse proliferative or membranous glomerulonephritis.[25]

LABORATORY MANIFESTATIONS

Hematologic

A moderate normochromic anemia may be found in 80 percent of cases. A more severe anemia develops in relation to progressive renal insufficiency or superimposed infection. At times, an overt hemolytic anemia may develop. However, a positive Coombs' test may be seen in individuals without evidence of shortened red cell survival. The red cell agglutinins usually are of the warm type and lack specificity for known blood-group antigens.

A moderate leukopenia (1800 to 4000 white blood cell/μl) is seen in 70 percent of patients at some point in their courses and is often associated with lymphopenia. A significant leukocytosis, rare in uncomplicated, untreated SLE, usually represents a response to corticosteroids or intercurrent infection.

Thrombocytopenia occurs in 30 percent of individuals with SLE but infrequently is of sufficient severity to produce a hemorrhagic diathesis. However, thrombocytopenic purpura can be the dominant disease manifestation. Circulating anticoagulants (antibodies to clotting factors) are other rare causes of bleeding.

The erythrocyte sedimentation rate and other acute-phase reactants are elevated in patients with active SLE and may remain slightly elevated during periods of apparent clinical remission.

Immunologic[50]

Immunoglobulin abnormalities are present in most patients with SLE, many of which are relatively nonspecific. Serum globulin concentrations in excess of 4.0 g/dl are seen in over 50 percent of cases. On electrophoresis, broad-based gamma globulin elevations (heterogeneous globulin molecules) may be seen which contrast with the narrow-based peaks (homogeneous molecular species) of the monoclonal dysproteinemias. Cryoproteins are sometimes present, especially in patients with active nephritis.

One of the hallmarks of SLE is serologic autoreactivity. The autoantibodies that are directed against red cells (Coombs' test) may result in a hemolytic anemia, and autoantibodies that react with clotting factors (circulating anticoagulants) may cause a hemorrhagic diathesis. DNA/anti-DNA (native or double stranded) immune complexes are responsible, in part, for induction of the glomerular lesions.[29,40] Other immune complex systems have not been implicated in specific tissue injury, although patients with antibody to ribonucleoprotein (nRNP) have significantly more frequent sicca features and myositis.

Most patients with SLE develop positive LE-cell tests during their illness, but if they do not, the diagnosis is not excluded. The serum factor responsible for LE-cell formation is an antibody capable of reacting with desoxyribonucleoprotein.

Several antinuclear and anticytoplasmic antibodies, generally neither species nor organ specific, have been identified in patients with SLE. Probably the most widely used method for detecting antinuclear factors employs immunofluorescence. The interpretation of antinuclear-antibody (ANA) titers varies according to the methodology and reagents used. The immunofluorescent assay for ANA detects multiple autoantibodies (including the LE-cell factor) to nuclear constituents. In relation to the diagnosis of SLE, the test is more sensitive and, therefore, less specific than the LE-cell phenomenon. Nearly all patients with active SLE are ANA positive. Since titers may vary according to the intensity of disease activity, serial ANA determinations are of value in managing patients.

A persistent biologic false positive serologic test for syphilis (BFP) may precede overt manifestations of SLE by months or years.[128] Such reactions with cardiolipin antigen occur in individuals without histories of syphilitic infection and with negative *Treponema pallidum* immobilization (TPI) tests. False positive and atypical fluorescent treponemal antibody-absorption tests also occur in SLE.[41]

Serum complement is reduced in about three-fourths of patients with active SLE.[49] The observed reduction in complement levels may be correlated with the activity of the illness, especially in individuals with nephritis.[50,55] Serum complement usually varies inversely with ANA titers.[56] Since many disorders which simulate SLE, such as rheumatic fever, polyarteritis, rheumatoid arthritis, and various infections, are usually characterized by a normal or elevated serum complement level, a low serum complement would favor the diagnosis of SLE. However, reduced serum complement may also be encountered in patients with serum sickness, acute glomerulonephritis, the nephrotic syndrome, and occasionally, other disorders.[55] When hypocomplementemia is associated with ANA, especially in high titers, at least 85 percent of patients will have SLE.[44]

Rheumatoid factors are present in almost 50 percent of patients at some time during their course. Unlike rheumatoid arthritis, in SLE they are intermittently present and usually in low titer.

Biopsy

Many of the tissue abnormalities encountered in biopsy specimens are relatively nonspecific (Table 97-2). Most characteristic of SLE are hematoxylin bodies (swollen cell nuclei devoid of cytoplasm and coated with globulin), but these are rarely found.

DIAGNOSIS

The diagnosis of SLE is not a problem when the patient presents with several of the characteristic clinical and laboratory manifestations of a multisystem

---

TABLE 97-2
Biopsy Findings in Systemic Lupus Erythematosus

Skin

Edema of the cutis, dilatation of capillaries, liquefaction and degeneration of the basal layer, perivascular and subepidermal accumulation of cellular infiltrates with predominantly round cells
Hyperkeratosis without parakeratosis
Positive direct immunofluorescence for IgG immunoglobulin at dermal-epidermal junction (also in 60 percent of cases at uninvolved sites)[28,57]

Lymph Node

Reticulum and lymphoid cell hyperplasia
Occasionally necrobiosis with cell degeneration, pyknosis, and formation of hematoxylin bodies

Muscle

Nonspecific focal degeneration and perivascular round cell infiltration. Histology indistinguishable from polymyositis may be found

Kidney

Focal membranous, proliferative, and/or necrotizing glomerulonephritis
Karyorrhexis and fibrinoid change, often present with active disease
Hematoxylin bodies rare, but diagnostic when present
Diffuse membranous thickening with focal exaggeration (wire-loop lesions) is a fairly characteristic but late finding
Positive direct immunofluorescence for IgG immunoglobulin in renal glomeruli and β1C globulin in nodular deposits beneath basement membrane. Complexes containing DNA can be eluted from the glomeruli[32,40]

---

disorder. A febrile, young woman with a butterfly rash, arthritis, pleuritis, mild anemia, positive LE-cell test, high ANA titer and hypocomplementemia would be diagnosed promptly. Frequently, however, the course of the disease is chronic and evolves episodically over many years. In such cases, the relationship between seemingly isolated episodes of illness may not be appreciated. Therefore, one must interpret a patient's present complaint (e.g., arthritis) in the light of his past history. A prior attack of pleurisy, or a skin eruption following sun exposure, should give added meaning to the current complaint of arthritis.

Occasionally, the involvement of one organ system overshadows other features of SLE for prolonged periods. Since other clinical and laboratory features of the disorder may develop insidiously, they should be looked for repeatedly. Thus, idiopathic nephrosis, glomerulonephritis, hemolytic anemia, purpura, pleurisy, and pericarditis may eventually be recognized as components of a multisystem disorder.

There are no absolute criteria for the diagnosis of SLE although preliminary criteria for the classification of SLE have been proposed recently by the American Rheumatism Association.[30] Generally, definitive diagnosis rests on a combination of characteristic clinical and immunologic features, especially the LE-cell and ANA tests. While the presence of LE-cells and ANA titers do not themselves establish the diagnosis, the absence of these immunologic abnormalities in symptomatic individuals casts serious doubt on the presence of SLE.

It is of basic importance to remain aware of the various diseases that may produce symptoms similar to SLE, especially if specific therapy would alter their outcome (e.g., tuberculosis, subacute bacterial endocarditis, lymphoma). Furthermore, several manifestations of SLE overlap with those of the other collagen diseases, from which they should be distinguished (Chap. 103).

COURSE AND PROGNOSIS

In most instances the course of SLE is characterized by periods of remission and exacerbation, with the course protracted over many years.[34] Rarely, the illness is fulminant, resulting in death in a few weeks.

Commonly, the various manifestations of SLE become evident sequentially over a period of years. Most recurrent episodes of disease activity are spontaneous although in some instances intercurrent infection, drug administration, and severe emotional stress have been cited as precipitating factors. Remissions may occur spontaneously or in response to corticosteroid therapy and may last for months or even years.

There are no satisfactory data descriptive of the natural history of SLE. Recent survival rates at 5 (94 percent) and 10 (82 percent) years after diagnosis provide a basis for genuine optimism. Death results from renal failure, central nervous system involvement, acute abdominal catastrophes, or intercurrent infection. Severe disturbances, such as thrombocytopenia with bleeding, hemolytic anemia, fulminant arteritis, and lupus crises, are potentially fatal but frequently respond well to therapy.

Progressive nephritis with renal failure may continue despite satisfactory control of other disease manifestations. Individuals whose disease remains confined to the skin, joints, or serous surfaces, or in whom immunologic abnormalities are present without vital organ involvement, have good prognoses.

The effect of pregnancy on the course of SLE is variable and may be associated with either exacerbations or remissions of the disease.[33] There is no evidence that SLE affects the developing fetus, even though the LE-cell factor and other antibodies have been shown to enter the fetal circulation.

MANAGEMENT

The therapeutic management of patients with SLE depends on the nature and severity of their disease manifestations. In addition to treatment designed to suppress inflammation and relieve symptoms, careful attention must be directed toward the general care of each patient. Furthermore, failure to recognize and deal with the personal needs of patients and their families can nullify an otherwise sound therapeutic program.

Intercurrent Illness

It is important to remember that findings which develop during the course of SLE may be caused by intercurrent disorders. For example, infections caused by pyogenic bacteria,[45] mycobacteria, or fungi may produce symptoms and signs that could be confused with those of SLE. Therefore, the pathogenesis of each new disease manifestation should be evaluated promptly in order to provide a firm basis for therapy.

Precipitating Events

At times, excerbations of SLE seem to follow infections, drug administration, severe emotional turmoil, or surgical procedures. Similarly, exposure to the sun may result in worsening of dermal lesions. Such apparent precipitating events may be identified through the initial history or continued observation of each patient. It follows that sensible avoidance of these factors is in order. In general, nonessential surgical procedures and drug administration should be guarded against. However, care should be taken not to cripple patients with ritualistic prohibitions.

General Therapy

Multiple therapeutic problems arise during the course of SLE, depending on the organ system involved and the related physiologic consequences. For example, lupus nephritis may result in progressive renal failure and hypertension. Furthermore, congestive heart failure may develop in this setting. Each of these abnormalities should receive the same basic supportive treatment accorded similar physiologic deficits due to other causes.

Suppressive Therapy

There is no known curative therapy for SLE. Nor is there evidence that suppressing minor manifestations of SLE early in its course will prevent the emergence of more serious multisystem involvement. Therefore, decisions concerning suppressive therapy are based on the nature and intensity of the disease manifestations. When needed, the safest anti-inflammatory agents are employed in doses sufficient to allay clinical evidence of the disorder.

Thus, an asymptomatic individual with a positive LE-cell test but without other abnormality requires no drug therapy. A patient with recurrent dermal lesions, myalgia, and arthralgia will benefit from salicylates and antimalarials as well as from local therapy to the skin lesions. Patients with nephritis or involvement of the myocardium or central nervous system usually require corticosteroids in high doses.

SALICYLATES.   Salicylates are helpful in controlling musculoskeletal pain and should be prescribed so that adequate blood levels are maintained. In patients with polyarthritis the response is occasionally dramatic and may resemble that seen in rheumatic fever. Frequently, however, the response to salicylates is incomplete and other measures are required.

ADRENAL CORTICOSTEROIDS.   Corticosteroids are the most effective agents for suppressing inflammation. Steroids are reserved for those situations that will not yield to simpler measures. The prime indications for steroid therapy in SLE are active involvement of the kidneys, skeletal muscle and myocardium, or central nervous system, hemolytic anemia, and thrombocytopenic purpura. At times, corticosteroids are needed to control progressive skin lesions, fever, and the other constitutional features of the illness.

The dosage level, schedule, and even route of administration of corticosteroids vary with the pattern and intensity of SLE activity. For individuals with minor manifestations, 20 mg of prednisone (or equivalent) in a single morning dose may be sufficient. Those with major organ involvement and polymyositis usually require therapy with 50 mg or more, occasionally 100 to 200 mg daily, initially.

After successful suppression of disease activity for a few weeks, the dose of prednisone can be tapered slowly to levels of 20 to 30 mg daily. Below this level, reductions at a rate of 5 mg or less per month may be necessary to avoid exacerbation of the disease. In some instances, the drug can be withdrawn entirely. More often, prolonged maintenance at low dose levels is required to prevent recurrence of symptoms.

Development of the Cushing syndrome is common in patients treated with large doses of corticosteroids. If renal function permits, a high-protein diet may be given to compensate partially for the protein-wasting effect of steroids. Diabetes occasionally occurs and may be modified by diet therapy and the use of oral hypoglycemic agents or insulin as needed. Fluid retention, rarely a problem when compounds producing little mineralocorticoid effect are used, can be managed by salt restriction or the use of diuretic agents. Hypertension occasionally requires control with antihypertensive drugs.

Peptic ulceration occurs and may cause significant bleeding or perforation. It should be remembered that corticosteroids may mask the clinical findings which usually result from a perforated ulcer.

Myopathy due to steroid administration is encountered occasionally. Fluorinated derivatives of prednisone are of special concern in this regard. The girdle musculature usually is affected most severely. Return of strength follows reduction of steroid dosage.

Posterior subcapsular cataracts are a late complication of steroid therapy encountered chiefly in individuals who have taken 15 mg or more of prednisone daily (or equivalent amounts of other congeners) for two years or more. Aseptic bone necrosis is seen on occasion, especially in the heads of the femurs and humeri. It should be remembered that pain may be present weeks, even months, before bone lesions are evident on x-ray.

ANTIMALARIALS. Hydroxychloroquine (Plaquenil) may control the discoid and other skin lesions as well as the rheumatic manifestations of SLE after several weeks of treatment. However, the drug is generally ineffective in individuals with visceral involvement.

Gastrointestinal intolerance and dermatitis may occur in patients receiving an antimalarial. It should not be given to pregnant women, because fetal abnormalities may result. Rarely, individuals who have taken hydroxychloroquine for several months, especially those receiving more than 200 mg daily, may develop (pigmentary) retinal degeneration resulting in serious visual impairment. Deposits of the drug may also occur in the cornea.

CYTOTOXIC AGENTS.[37,42,52-54] Azathioprine, cyclophosphamide, 6-mercaptopurine, and chlorambucil have been shown to suppress the manifestations of SLE. At present, there is insufficient evidence to compare long-term effectiveness and toxicity of these agents with corticosteroids. Generally, an immunosuppressive agent is added when corticosteroids fail to control the inflammatory process in major organ-systems (i.e., kidney, CNS). Currently, any of these agents should be reserved for patients who are refractory to corticosteroids or who cannot tolerate the dosage level required.

SLE-LIKE SYNDROMES

There are four SLE-like syndromes—drug-related lupus, discoid lupus, rheumatoid arthritis with LE cells, and chronic active hepatitis—that should be differentiated from SLE because of their inherent differences in prognosis and management. In most instances, the clinical patterns of these syndromes may be readily recognized.

Drug-Induced SLE[26,27,132]

Drug responses may relate to SLE in one of several ways (Table 97-3). Prompt recognition of SLE or lupus-like syndromes caused by drug administration is important because withdrawal of the agent may result in eventual subsidence of the illness. There is no known chemical relationship among the drugs which activate or induce SLE. Drug-related SLE usually develops in individuals who have been given drugs over prolonged periods. For example, in hydralazine-induced cases, generally more than 400 mg had been taken daily for more than 6 months. However, similar

---

TABLE 97-3
Drug Reactions and SLE

Drug reactions may mimic SLE
  Serum sickness

Drugs may activate SLE or unmask a lupus diathesis
  Hydralazine (Apresoline)
  Hydantoins (Mesantoin, Dilantin)
  Trimethadione (Tridione)

Drugs may induce SLE de novo
  Procainamide (Pronestyl)

syndromes have also been seen following much smaller doses given for much briefer periods especially with procainamide.

The clinical features of drug-related SLE usually are mild and include fever, arthritis or arthralgia, and positive LE-cell and ANA tests. In rare cases, the more intense and full-blown features of SLE develop. In the majority of patients, the clinical syndrome will subside after the offending agent is withdrawn, but serologic abnormalities, especially the ANA, may persist.

In some instances, minor evidences of illness (e.g., hypergammaglobulinemia) have existed prior to drug administration and further manifestations of SLE evolved after drug withdrawal. Such observations have led to the hypothesis that there exists an abnormality which predisposes certain persons to such aberrant immunologic reactivity. However, the frequent development of antinuclear antibodies and clinical manifestations in patients, regardless of age and sex, receiving procainamide suggests that this reaction is truly drug-induced SLE and does not represent an unmasking of a lupus diathesis.[26,27]

Discoid Lupus

The typical skin lesions of discoid lupus are not common in patients with SLE, and they may recur or persist for many years in individuals who fail to develop evidences of a multisystem disorder.[48] Perhaps 10 percent of patients presenting with discoid lesions will develop clinical and laboratory abnormalities characteristic of SLE during the later course of their illnesses. Since there are no features which identify these persons at the outset, it is wise to evaluate such patients thoroughly at periodic intervals. In some cases, joint pains, mild anemia, and leukopenia may be encountered in the absence of other findings characteristic of SLE.

Rheumatoid Arthritis with LE Cells

LE cells occur in approximately 25 percent of patients with otherwise typical rheumatoid arthritis. These patients tend to have a deforming and erosive type of arthritis uncommonly seen in SLE. In general they have lower leukocyte counts, higher gamma globulin concentrations, and more variant syndromes (i.e., Felty, Sjögren) than do similar patients without LE cells, but no other features suggestive of SLE.[127]

Rarely, a patient with rheumatoid arthritis and LE cells will develop typical features of SLE including nephritis.

Chronic Active Hepatitis[43] (See Chap. 67)

A chronic active hepatitis has been described in young women which was formerly termed "lupoid" hepatitis because of the association with LE cells in some patients. In this syndrome, the major clinical manifestations are those of hepatic-cell dysfunction caused by a chronic active hepatitis. Several of the serologic abnormalities characteristically seen in SLE may be present, such as antinuclear antibodies, LE cells, and lowered serum complement levels. In a few patients clinical features suggestive of SLE also occur, predominantly skin rashes, arthritis, serositis, thrombocytopenia, leucopenia, and rarely hemolytic anemia. Nephritis is also rare.

In many instances the etiology of the chronic hepatitis is known (e.g., infectious hepatitis or alcoholic cirrhosis). Liver biopsy may reveal areas of necrosis and prominent plasma-cell infiltration (plasma-cell hepatitis), in contrast to the minimal nonspecific changes occasionally noted in SLE. The liver disease continues to dominate the course and usually determines the prognosis, even in those patients who have multisystem manifestations. There is no evidence to support chronic active hepatitis with LE cells as a unique entity.

—CHAPTER 98—
Progressive Systemic Sclerosis
MARY BETTY STEVENS AND ALEXANDER S. TOWNES

Progressive systemic sclerosis (PSS) is a chronic disease of unknown etiology characterized by peripheral vascular instability and sclerosis of the skin and subcutaneous tissue (scleroderma), as well as alterations in various internal organs, especially the lungs, heart, gastrointestinal tract, and kidneys.[65-67,69] Immunologic reactions involving cellular constituents occur but are not prominent features of the disease.

PSS is not a rare disease, being somewhat less frequent than SLE but more common than either polyarteritis or dermatomyositis. Females are affected twice as often as males, most commonly in the third to sixth decades of life.[61] Familial occurrence is rare, but an increased incidence of hyperglobulinemia and antinuclear antibodies in first-degree relatives has been reported.

CLINICAL MANIFESTATIONS

Presenting Complaints

Patients often present with Raynaud's phenomenon, which may antedate sclerodermatous skin changes by years. Other patients may first complain of thickening of the skin or pain and stiffness in and around the joints. Scleroderma usually persists for years, even decades, before visceral involvement becomes apparent.

Systemic

Weight loss is common and may be profound when associated with malabsorption. Fatigue and musculoskeletal aching or weakness, prominent early in the disorder, may be mistaken for psychogenic complaints. Fever is rare and, when present, more often reflects an intercurrent process or overlap syndrome.

Raynaud's Phenomenon

Raynaud's phenomenon is present in 80 percent of cases. It may produce ischemic changes in the digits, infrequently leading to gangrene.[62] The course of Raynaud's phenomenon is variable. In some patients it may persist for years as the only significant disease manifestation while in others gradual thickening and tightening of the skin of the fingers develops (sclerodactyly). In still others the complete picture of PSS or the CRST syndrome develops.

Skin and Mucous Membranes

The skin and subcutaneous tissues are affected in most patients although cases of PSS sine scleroderma are rarely seen.[64] Symmetrical changes usually first appear in the distal portions of the extremities (especially the upper) and progress centrally. Initially, the skin is shiny and edematous. Later it becomes waxy, taut, and atrophic, with elasticity, sweating, and hair growth diminished. The taut and thickened skin becomes bound to underlying structures and contractures develop which may limit skeletal movement. Facial involvement may result in a fixed expression and an inability to wrinkle the forehead, close the eyelids tightly, or fully open the mouth. A diffuse increase in skin pigmentation, as well as spotty areas of depigmentation, may characterize the involved sites. Telangiectases are common and may involve the mucous membranes of the mouth and lips. Calcific deposits are sometimes present in the digits or around joints but often escape detection except on x-ray examination. The CRST syndrome (calcinosis, Raynaud's, sclerodactyly, telangiectasia) has been emphasized because of its relatively benign prognosis in most patients. The frequency of esophageal dysfunction has led to the modified acronym CREST syndrome being now used more often.

Lungs and Pleura

Pulmonary involvement[60] is present in one-half to two-thirds of cases but is often asymptomatic and detected only by x-ray or tests of pulmonary function. Exertional dyspnea and a chronic cough occur late. Basilar end-inspiratory rales due to fibrosis are characteristic. With extensive sclerodermatous involvement of the trunk and, rarely, myositic involvement of the intercostals, the respiratory excursion may be impaired. Symptomatic pleurisy and effusion are rare. A rather nonspecific reticular or mottled infiltrate confined to the lower two-thirds of the lung fields is the usual x-ray finding.

Ventilatory dysfunction[66] results from pulmonary infiltration or fibrosis and far less frequently from impaired chest-wall motion. Gas diffusion impairment (alveolar-capillary block) results from diffuse thickening of the alveolar septa and basement membranes of the small vessels. Pulmonary hypertension may develop in this setting or as a result of direct involvement of the smaller pulmonary arteries (Chap. 26).

Such patients are prone to repeated pulmonary infections and may develop lung abscesses or bronchiectasis. Marked proliferation of the bronchial epithelium has been noted in some cases and has been related to the development of neoplasms.

Cardiac[66]

The heart is involved in a high proportion of fatal cases. Congestive heart failure, arrhythmias, and conduction defects may be encountered and related to patchy interstitial and perivascular fibrosis of the myocardium. Cor pulmonale may result from progressive pulmonary hypertension. Congestive heart failure resulting from pulmonary hypertension is more common than that resulting from myocardial involvement and in some instances is the primary manifestation of PSS. Pericarditis occurs occasionally and at times with effusion.

Gastrointestinal[68]

Involvement of the gastrointestinal tract is often asymptomatic and revealed by x-ray or physiologic studies. The symptoms most frequently encountered include dysphagia, a sense of substernal or epigastric fullness, heartburn, and indigestion. They result from esophageal aperistalsis and peptic esophagitis. Studies of motor function are most likely to reveal an absence of peristalsis in the lower two-thirds of the esophagus and an incompetence of the cardioesophageal sphincter which permits reflux of acid gastric contents. These abnormalities may be also shown by radiologic examination. In those with skeletal muscle inflammation and involvement of pharyngeal musculature, there may be difficulty in initiating the swallow.

Less often, intestinal involvement leads to intermittent distension, vomiting, diarrhea, constipation, or the development of the malabsorption syndrome. X-ray studies may demonstrate irregular dilatations in the second and third portions of the duodenum and hypersegmentation of the barium and delayed transit time throughout the jejunum and distal small bowel. When the colon is affected, diffuse dilatation and stasis or characteristic large saccular dilatations (pseudodiverticula) may be present.

The mechanism of altered esophageal and intestinal motility is not clear, but it is closely correlated with such neurovascular abnormalities as Raynaud's phenomenon.[68] Atrophic smooth muscle is the only pathologic finding that may be related to the observed dilatation of the esophagus and bowel.

Kidney[59]
Renal involvement, as evidenced by proteinuria, abnormalities of the urinary sediment, hypertension, and progressive renal failure, usually begins months or years after the onset of PSS. Biopsy reveals vascular lesions similar to those seen in malignant hypertension or allograft rejection. Occasionally, areas of cortical infarction are encountered.

Renal involvement carries a grave prognosis and contributes significantly to the death of nearly 50 percent of patients with PSS.

Musculoskeletal
Muscle weakness and atrophy are commonly seen in patients with PSS. Biopsy usually reveals a nodular interstitial myositis and a picture indistinguishable from polymyositis alone.

Polyarthralgia, stiffness, and occasionally a frank arthritis may occur, usually in the fingers, wrists, and knees.[63] Associated tenosynovitis gives rise to leathery friction rubs on motion.

LABORATORY MANIFESTATIONS
The formed elements of the peripheral blood are generally normal, as is the erythrocyte sedimentation rate. The anemia is usually mild unless the bacterial overgrowth in static bowel segments and malabsorption syndrome are severe. Hypergammaglobulinemia is present in about 50 percent of cases. Fewer patients have rheumatoid factor in their serum, but this does not correlate with the existence of joint disease. Antinuclear antibodies in low titer are detected in up to 50 percent of cases especially antibody to ribonucleoprotein. A positive LE-cell test is infrequent. The pattern of seroreactivity, however, is not of diagnostic value.

Skin biopsy often reveals the characteristic marked thickening of the dermis, caused by an absolute increase in dermal collagen. In advanced cases the collagen fibers may appear smudged and fragmented and there may be atrophy of the epidermis and skin appendages and occasional hyalinization of small arterioles. The view that disease of the capillaries and small blood vessels is the basis of all pathologic changes in PSS has been strengthened by ultrastructural studies.[59]

DIAGNOSIS
The diagnosis is based chiefly on the presence of scleroderma. The presence of Raynaud's phenomenon and visceral lesions materially strengthens the diagnosis, especially in instances where the skin changes may be early or atypical.

It is not possible to forecast the course of patients who present with Raynaud's phenomenon, with or without the esophageal changes described above. After months or years some may develop the typical features of scleroderma and PSS. Others may evolve features of SLE or dermatomyositis, while some develop only the sclerodactyly and ulcerative lesions of "primary" Raynaud's disease.

PSS shares many manifestations with other connective-tissue diseases, especially dermatomyositis, SLE, and rheumatoid arthritis. The existence of scleroderma, however, distinguishes PSS.

Scleroderma must be differentiated from *scleredema,* which occurs commonly in children and young adults and may follow beta-hemolytic streptococcal infections. Scleredema may also occur in older adults with diabetes mellitus. The skin over the face, neck, and upper trunk usually appears brawny and does not pit. The arms and hands are involved in only 10 percent of cases or fewer, in contrast to scleroderma. Skin biopsy reveals an accumulation of mucopolysaccharide between the collagen fibers of the dermis. Resolution of the skin lesions begins in several weeks, and most cases clear completely in 18 to 24 months. Raynaud's phenomenon does not occur.

A *diffuse fasciitis* may also mimic scleroderma although careful examination will show the skin to be delicate overlying dense inflammatory masses. Eosinophilia and hyperglobulinemia may be associated with this steroid-responsive process (Shulman syndrome). The diagnosis is established histologically.

COURSE AND PROGNOSIS
Progressive systemic sclerosis is a chronic disease with a variable but generally progressive course. The disease may improve or remain static for prolonged periods even in the absence of treatment.

Localized scleroderma, or morphea, may occur in patches about the neck and trunk or sometimes as linear streaks following nerves or blood vessels. The prognosis is generally excellent as these lesions tend to remain localized and visceral involvement seldom occurs.

The CREST (CRST) syndrome lies within the spectrum of manifestations of PSS. It may resemble hereditary telangiectasia because of the prominent telangiectases involving the skin and mucous membranes. In general, the course of the illness is prolonged and benign.

Death in PSS usually results from progressive renal involvement, cerebral hemorrhage, or cardiac or pulmonary failure.

MANAGEMENT

There is no therapy that effectively alters the course of PSS. General supportive measures include the avoidance of exposure to cold, the maintenance of strength and musculoskeletal function with physical therapy, and the judicious use of sedatives and analgesics. Neither vasodilators nor sympathectomy sig-nificantly alters skin changes and neither is of unpredictable benefit to the neurovascular problem of Raynaud's phenomenon in this setting. No drug relieves esophageal or intestinal dysfunction. The many other therapeutic problems that arise during the course of PSS (e.g., heart failure, renal failure, hypertension, peptic esophagitis, malabsorption) and that result from visceral involvement should receive the same basic therapy accorded similar physiologic deficits in other settings. For example, therapy with tetracycline may dramatically relieve intestinal malabsorption with response of the nutritional anemia and weight gain.[58]

Adrenal corticosteroids are clearly indicated only in the presence of an inflammatory myopathy. Although some think the daily administration of 15 to 20 mg of prednisone may slow the progress of the disorder and possibly improve the early edematous skin lesions, there is little to indicate that the eventual outcome is altered. Similarly, sodium versenate, relaxin, anticoagulants, and para-aminobenzoic acid and penicillamine are without proven therapeutic utility.

CHAPTER 99

Polymyositis

MARY BETTY STEVENS

Polymyositis, or dermatomyositis, is a disorder of unknown etiology, characterized primarily by an inflammatory myopathy. Recent studies[70,74,75] support an autoimmune hypothesis with tissue injury the consequence of cytotoxic lymphocytes specifically sensitized to antigens of skeletal muscle. Fever, skin lesions, arthritis, vasomotor instability, and other visceral manifestations may occur, but weakness of girdle and proximal muscles is the dominant feature of the disease.[9,17,71]

The major consideration in the patient with a polymyositis (Table 99–1) is whether the myopathy occurs alone, is associated with a neoplasm, or is one manifestation of a multisystem process (i.e., SLE, PSS).

CLINICAL MANIFESTATIONS

Presenting Complaints

Polymyositis commonly begins insidiously. Patients with pelvic-girdle involvement may note difficulty in rising from a reclining or sitting position or in climbing stairs. Weakness of the shoulder girdle usually begins with difficulty in raising and maintaining the arms overhead. Weakness of the neck flexors and pharyngeal weakness with dysphagia may also be early manifestations.

In some, the onset is acute, and fever, skin rash (especially facial), or arthritis may be associated with rapidly progressing muscle weakness, pain, and tenderness.

Skin and Mucous Membranes

Typical skin lesions occur in 40 percent of cases (Table 99–1). Dusky, erythematous lesions appear on the face, neck, upper trunk, and proximal portions of the extremities. Periorbital edema often accompanies the facial rash. A characteristic lilac-colored or heliotrope rash over the eyelids is occasionally seen. In 20 percent of patients, patchy, erythematous, sometimes scaling maculopapular lesions are present over the knuckles (Gottron sign), knees, elbows, or medial malleoli. Erythema around the nail margins and erythema and atrophy of the finger pads may also occur. Raynaud's phenomenon occurs in 30 percent of patients.

┌─TABLE 99–1───
Distinguishing Features of Types of Polymyositis

Type	Age and Sex Affected	Skin Lesions	Other Features
Polymyositis or dermatomyositis	Adults, especially fourth to sixth decades Female 3:1	Typical facial rash in one-third Extremity lesions more common	Insidious onset in those without skin lesions; occasional fever, muscle pain and tenderness Arthralgias 25% Raynaud's 15% ANA, rheumatoid factors uncommon Usually steroid responsive
Childhood dermatomyositis	From age 2 No sex dominance	Typical facial and extremity lesions present	Contractures, calcinosis of muscles Vasculitic lesions prominent on biopsy Usually steroid responsive
Polymyositis or, more often, dermatomyositis with malignancy	Over age 40 Males 3:1	Typical facial lesions and Gottron sign in most	Acute or subacute onset; malignancy can be occult Raynaud's not present Seronegative Poor response to steroids but may improve with treatment of tumor
Polymyositis with connective tissue disorders	Age determined by associated disorder Females	Skin lesions of SLE, PSS, etc., dominant	Acute or subacute onset except in Sjögren Major associations: SLE, PSS, MCTD, rarely Sjögren and rheumatoid arthritis Clinicolaboratory features of associated disorder dominant Usually a steroid responsive myopathy

Gastrointestinal

Dysphagia occurs in 60 percent of cases and may be associated with nasal regurgitation. Physiologic studies show impaired initiation of swallowing and diminished motor activity in the upper third of the esophagus (striated muscle). About 30 percent of patients with dysphagia show aperistalsis of the distal esophagus (smooth muscle), usually associated with Raynaud's phenomenon. Peptic esophagitis may result from gastric reflux resulting from an incompetent cardioesophageal sphincter. Motor dysfunction of the intestinal tract is rare. Abdominal pain and intestinal ulceration, perforation, and bleeding may be seen in childhood dermatomyositis (caused by vasculitis).[73]

Musculoskeletal

Weakness of the proximal and girdle musculature is a cardinal feature of polymyositis. Although muscular pain and tenderness are common in the more acute cases, these features are often absent.

Arthralgia or arthritis, especially of the fingers, wrists, and knees, occurs early in one-third of the cases, often in those patients who have experienced acute onset.[76] Muscular atrophy, contractures, and calcinosis are late features.

In the later stages of the disease the respiratory muscles may be severely weakened. Progressive respiratory insufficiency and repeated pulmonary infection and aspiration are frequently the causes of death.

Malignancies

Dermatomyositis may be associated with malignant tumors of many types (lung, breast, prostate, colon). In many instances the tumor is discovered only after a diligent search. The association of malignancies with dermatomyositis increases with age, especially in men. A man over 40 with dermatomyositis has a 50 percent chance of having a malignant tumor; if he is over 50, he has a 70 percent chance.

LABORATORY MANIFESTATIONS

The laboratory findings that characterize polymyositis are shown in Table 99–2. Serum enzymes, such as serum glutamic oxalacetic transaminase (SGOT), aldolase, lactic dehydrogenase (LDH), and creatine phosphokinase (CPK), are released from damaged muscle and reflect to some degree the activity and severity of the myositis.

The electromyographic findings (Table 99–2) are not specific. Abnormal action potentials at rest and pseudomyotonic discharges are rather characteristic of polymyositis.

The histologic patterns differ to some extent in the several types of polymyositis (Tables 99–1, 99–2). In childhood dermatomyositis, for example, vasculitis with endothelial proliferation, thrombosis, and infarction of muscle tissue is often prominent.[73] Extensive interstitial infiltration with lymphocytes and plasma cells is the chief feature of the myositis associated with Sjögren syndrome. When seeking diagnostic material, care should be taken that the muscle biopsy is performed on an actively involved muscle, usually in the proximal groups.

DIAGNOSIS

The diagnosis of polymyositis is based chiefly on the occurrence of muscular weakness, especially of the girdle and proximal musculature, which is often associated with skin lesions, arthralgia or arthritis, and other features suggestive of connective-tissue disorders (Table 99–1). The concentrations of serum enzymes are elevated in most patients with active polymyositis and, like electromyographic findings, help distinguish this disorder from other types of myopathy (Chap. 124). The histopathologic findings may serve to confirm the diagnosis.

COURSE AND PROGNOSIS

The natural course of polymyositis varies somewhat according to type (Table 99–1). In the more chronic varieties, remissions and exacerbations may be seen, but without treatment the general trend is toward increasing impairment. The course of the myopathy,

TABLE 99–2
Laboratory Manifestations of Polymyositis

Hematologic	Leukocytosis in some cases, mild anemia Elevated sedimentation rate
Serum proteins	Elevated α_2 and γ globulins in 50% of cases
Immunologic reactions	Rheumatoid factor (10% to 50%) Antinuclear antibodies, low titer, in some cases
Serum enzymes	Elevated transaminases (SGOT and SGPT), aldolase, creatine phosphokinase, LDH, etc., during active stages of the disease
Electromyography	Little or no reduction in total number of motor unit potentials on volitional contraction Individual potentials often of short duration, low amplitude, and polyphasic Spontaneous fibrillation and positive (sawtooth) potentials at rest Short bursts of rapidly repeating action potentials Abnormal intensity–duration curves
Muscle biopsy findings	Focal or segmental degeneration of muscle fibers, sometimes with vacuolization Regeneration of damaged muscle fibers as evidenced by sarcoplasmal basophilia, large nuclei, and prominent nucleoli Necrosis of part of or whole muscle fiber with phagocytosis of its substance Infiltration of inflammatory cells most often in the perimysium near blood vessels, but sometimes diffusely Extreme variation in size of muscle fibers Interstitial fibrosis Vasculitis in childhood type

except when associated with malignancies, can be altered beneficially by the administration of adrenal corticosteroids. Steroid refractory patients may respond dramatically to the addition of an immunosuppressive agent.[70]

MANAGEMENT

General supportive care is important to the management of patients with polymyositis. Rest is helpful during disease activity, and measures should be taken to preserve muscle strength and to prevent the development of contractures. All adult patients, especially men over 40, should be examined carefully for occult tumors. On occasion the removal of a tumor has been associated with remission of the myositis.

Most patients with typical polymyositis or dermatomyositis respond to adrenal corticosteroid therapy. Best results are obtained when treatment is instituted early. Although response to treatment is less dramatic in patients with advanced disease, most patients should nevertheless have a trial of corticosteroids. Such treatment is usually begun at high dose levels (40 to 80 mg of prednisone daily). When a maximal response has been achieved, the steroid dose should be reduced slowly (by 5 mg of prednisone every 2 to 4 weeks). Usually it is possible to reduce the dose to a small maintenance dose, and therapy may be discontinued after months or years. In patients refractory to steroid therapy or intolerant for the steroid dosage required for disease control, the addition of an immunosuppressive agent, especially methotrexate, has been beneficial.[70] Initially, methotrexate is administered intravenously, 35 to 50 mg each week, until clinical and chemical remission is achieved. Oral drug administration is associated with increased frequency and severity of toxic reaction (e.g., mucosal ulcerations, hepatotoxicity, interstitial pneumonitis).

CHAPTER 100
Polyarteritis
MARY BETTY STEVENS AND ALEXANDER S. TOWNES

Polyarteritis is a disease of unknown etiology characterized by widespread segmental inflammation of medium-sized and small blood vessels, especially arteries, which usually results in a systemic illness with multiple-organ involvement.[9,17,79,90] The clinical picture may vary considerably, depending on the organ(s) most critically damaged by ischemia and necrosis of tissue resulting from the vascular lesions.

Immunologic mechanisms have been implicated in the pathogenesis of polyarteritis on the basis of similarities to experimental hypersensitivity disease produced by antigen–antibody complexes[88] and on the basis of similarities of the clinical features to those of such other immunologic diseases as serum sickness and SLE. Furthermore, in many cases the onset of symptoms has followed closely upon serum sickness, sensitivity reactions to such drugs as sulfonamides, iodides, penicillin, and thiouracil, or in a significant number of cases in association with hepatitis B antigen.[84,93] Acute serous otitis media occasionally precedes necrotizing arteritis.[92]

Polyarteritis is a relatively uncommon disorder, being less frequent, for example, than SLE or progressive systemic sclerosis. In contrast to other disorders with immunologic features, it is two to three times more common in men than in women. It may occur at any age but is observed most frequently in the fourth through the sixth decades. There is no known racial or familial predisposition.

CLINICAL MANIFESTATIONS

Presenting Complaints

The initial manifestations of polyarteritis are variable. Symptoms sometimes appear abruptly in a healthy individual, but often the process appears to follow a recent illness such as a respiratory infection or a drug reaction. Although disease of a single organ, such as nephritis or neuritis, may be the first manifestation of polyarteritis, patients more often seem to be suffering from a subacute, febrile, systemic disease (Table 100–1). Fever, fatigability, myalgia, anorexia, and weight loss dominate the early symptomatology.

Skin and Mucous Membranes[94]

Rather characteristic small (0.5 to 1 cm) nodular lesions (arteritis) appear in the skin and subcutaneous tissues of a minority of patients. They may occur singly or in crops in any area of the body and may be distributed linearly along blood vessels. Splinter hemorrhages in the nails and small periungual infarcts are characteristic although not invariably present. Nonspecific lesions such as urticaria, petechiae, purpura, hemorrhagic bullae, and a variety of erythematous rashes are encountered more frequently. Livedo reticularis is an occasional finding. Localized edema about the face, trunk, or extremities may result from blood vessel involvement.

TABLE 100-1

Presenting Manifestations That Should Arouse Suspicion of Polyarteritis

1. A nonspecific subacute or chronic febrile illness with loss of weight and leukocytosis

2. An atypical abdominal illness which may simulate a condition requiring laparotomy

3. A primary renal disease frequently thought to be acute or subacute glomerulonephritis

4. Polyneuropathy, sometimes in combination with myositis

5. Bronchial asthma or focal pulmonary infiltrates suggesting infection

6. Myocardial infarction or coronary insufficiency especially in association with any of the above

7. Unexplained severe hypertension

Ocular

Four types of ocular manifestations are common in polyarteritis:

1. Direct involvement of retinal vessels, with exudations, hemorrhage, "cytoid" bodies, arterial occlusion, papilledema, and optic atrophy

2. Exudative lesions of mesenchymal elements leading to episcleritis or iridocyclitis

3. Cerebral arterial disease with extraocular palsy, pupillomotor disturbance, and visual-field defects

4. Hypertensive retinopathy associated with renal impairment

Lungs and Pleura

Pulmonary manifestations occur in about 25 percent of cases. Polyarteritis frequently begins with symptoms of pneumonia or bronchitis. Asthma may precede the appearance of other findings by months or years. Clinical symptomatology may be minimal despite extensive localized or diffuse changes on x-ray. Secondary infection may lead to pneumonia or abscess formation.

The diagnosis of polyarteritis as a cause of pulmonary lesions requires the careful exclusion of other causes, especially infection, and rests on the recognition of the typical clinical pattern in other organs. There is a group of patients with polyarteritis whose illness is primarily pulmonary (allergic granulomatous arteritis,[80] polyarteritis with pulmonary involvement).[90] Such an individual has asthma or chronic pulmonary disease. Following an apparent respiratory infection, he develops generalized arteritis, eosinophilia, and many focal necrotic or granulomatous lesions in the liver, spleen, kidneys, lymph nodes, and heart that are unrelated to blood vessels. The presence of such granulomatous lesions, often with dense eosinophilic infiltrations, is distinctly uncommon in the absence of pulmonary involvement.

Cardiovascular

Episodes of pericarditis with or without effusions may occur; a massive, bloody effusion with tamponade may result from a ruptured vessel. Patients may present with coronary insufficiency or myocardial infarction caused by arteritis of the coronary vessels. Cardiac arrhythmias are occasionally encountered. Congestive heart failure may result from diffuse myocardial damage from arteritis or from granulomatous myocarditis or may be secondary to hypertension and renal insufficiency.

Raynaud's phenomenon is encountered infrequently. Rarely lesions similar to thromboangiitis obliterans produce acrogangrene.

Gastrointestinal

Abdominal pain, nausea, vomiting, diarrhea, and intestinal bleeding are common manifestations of polyarteritis. Depending on the extent and localization of vascular disease, almost any intra-abdominal disease may be mimicked. Hematomas (especially retroperitoneal) caused by the rupture of an arteritic lesion may present as a mass, often accompanied by pain and, when massive, by symptoms of acute blood loss. Lesions of the bowel, accompanied by bleeding, perforation, or infarction, are common.

The liver is involved more frequently than has been recognized clinically. In those patients with polyarteritis associated with hepatitis B antigen, liver involvement inevitably develops although it may be late in appearance and mild in degree.[84] A moderate degree of hepatomegaly is usually present. Pain over the liver and a friction rub may accompany hepatic infarction, and jaundice may develop if the infarction is sufficiently extensive. Smaller, clinically silent infarctions may result in bromsulphalein retention and in increased alkaline phosphatase and serum transaminases. Liver biopsy only occasionally yields a diagnosis of arteritis.

Spleen and Lymph Nodes

Lymphadenopathy is not characteristic of polyarteritis. Slight splenic enlargement is present in about one-third of the cases. Rarely, splenic infarction or perisplenic hemorrhage has been observed.

Genitourinary

Renal involvement is present in 70 to 80 percent of patients with polyarteritis. Occasionally, patients present with manifestations resembling those of acute, subacute, or chronic glomerulonephritis. More commonly, renal disease becomes evident later as systemic involvement progresses. Hypertension in polyarteritis is generally secondary to renal disease. Hypertension may be mild and sustained, may fluctuate strikingly, suggesting pheochromocytoma; or may be severe, with a clinical picture of malignant hypertension. The last condition may result from segmental involvement of a single renal artery.

There are two types of renal lesions, which may occur simultaneously or independently: 1) a widespread focal or, occasionally, diffuse glomerulonephritis; and 2) arteritis involving the renal artery and its branches. Renal arteritis may lead to renal infarction or to a perirenal or retroperitoneal hematoma.

The vessels of the bladder may be affected, producing hemorrhagic cystitis. Testicular infarction with severe pain and subsequent atrophy is more frequent in polyarteritis nodosa than in any other single condition. Even in the absence of local symptoms, testicular biopsy shows arteritis as frequently as does the muscle biopsy.

Musculoskeletal

Myalgia and arthralgia are often prominent symptoms. Occasionally, trichinosis or primary myositis is suggested by the severity of the muscle pain. Later, profound weakness and atrophy may develop, affecting peripheral and truncal muscles alike. Frank arthritis is relatively unusual, although deformities indistinguishable from rheumatoid disease have been noted. Occasionally, typical rheumatoid arthritis may antedate the appearance of polyarteritis by many months or years.

Neurologic

The most common neurologic manifestation of polyarteritis is a mononeuritis caused by arteritis of the nutrient vessels of major nerve trunks, such as the radial nerve, causing wrist drop, and the peroneal nerve, causing foot drop. Sensory and motor deficits, which may be symmetric, usually accompany this type of neuritis. Whereas the occurrence of peripheral neuritis in any obscure illness should always suggest the possibility of polyarteritis, involvement of several major nerve trunks (mononeuritis multiplex) is virtually diagnostic.

Polyarteritis may also affect other components of the nervous system in a variable and confusing pattern. Involvement of carotid, vertebral, meningeal, or deep cerebral vessels can lead to hemiplegia, transverse myelitis, convulsions, cerebellar dysfunction, extrapyramidal disorders, optic atrophy, or subarachnoid hemorrhage. Cranial-nerve palsies are uncommon.

LABORATORY MANIFESTATIONS

Polyarteritis is usually associated with leukocytosis, often 15,000/μl or more. A mild to moderate eosinophilia may be present, especially in patients with pulmonary involvement. An increased platelet count (greater than 500,000/μl) is frequently found. Anemia is usually mild and may be absent in the early phases. The erythrocyte sedimentation rate is almost always increased and generally reflects the intensity of disease activity. Proteinuria and, often, microscopic hematuria, pyuria, and casts are found in patients with glomerular disease. With renal arterial involvement, mild proteinuria may be noted with little or no abnormality of the sediment.

Occasionally, serum gamma globulin levels are increased. Rheumatoid factor is present in some patients. Antinuclear antibodies are detected rarely. Serum complement is normal or increased, even in patients with renal involvement.

Biopsy

Typical lesions show segmental inflammation and necrosis of medium-sized or small arteries, usually extending throughout the vessel wall and disrupting the internal elastic lamina. Thrombosis, aneurysmal dilatation or rupture of the vessel and hemorrhage may be evident, as well as degeneration or infarction of the distal tissue. Lesions in all stages of development are encountered commonly.

If a skin nodule or tender muscle is apparent, it should be biopsied. If not, a generous biopsy of the skin, subcutaneous tissue, and muscle should be obtained in the area of the deltoid or pectoral muscle. In symptomatic patients, testicular or peripheral nerve biopsies may be helpful. A negative biopsy does not exclude the diagnosis.

Arteritis is a feature of many diseases, including SLE, rheumatoid arthritis, serum sickness, and rheumatic fever. Vascular changes similar to those of polyarteritis can also be found at the periphery of necrotizing or suppurative bacterial lesions. Therefore, arteritis must be interpreted in the light of the entire clinical picture. This is particularly true when an apparently isolated arteritis is unexpectedly found in tissue (e.g., the appendix or gallbladder) removed for other reasons.

DIAGNOSIS

The diagnosis rests on a compatible clinical picture in conjunction with biopsy demonstration of arteritic lesions. Leukocytosis and thrombocytosis are the most helpful laboratory features. The presence of fever, weight loss, and muscle or joint pain, combined with neural, pulmonary, or renal lesions, is the most common clinical pattern suggesting the diagnosis of polyarteritis. The coexistence of systemic symptoms and disorders in more than one organ system usually leads to the suspicion of polyarteritis and to appropriate tissue examinations (Table 100–1). Arteriography may be a useful diagnostic method, especially when biopsy material is negative for arteritis.[86]

Several attempts have been made to separate certain cases of polyarteritis from others on the basis of clinical or pathologic differences.[80,90,95] (Several variants of polyarteritis will be discussed later.) Since it is likely that multiple etiologic agents are operative in polyarteritis, these divisions have some merit. However, these distinctions are frequently difficult to make.

Differential Diagnosis

It is usually not difficult to distinguish polyarteritis from other connective-tissue disorders, even those in which arteritis is present. Childhood dermatomyositis is usually identified by its typical rash. SLE, which most often occurs in young women, can be recognized by the serologic autoreactivity, which is uncommon in polyarteritis. Goodpasture syndrome may be confused with polyarteritis because fever, systemic symptoms, and pulmonary and renal disease are features held in common. However, hemoptysis is a more prominent feature in the Goodpasture syndrome, and neither involvement of other organ systems nor necrotizing arteritis is encountered.

In some instances involvement of one organ system may dominate the clinical picture for a time. Thus, the renal, pulmonary, neuritic, or muscular involvement of polyarteritis may be confused with abnormalities of these organs due to other causes. Similarly, when fever, weakness, and systemic symptoms are prominent, polyarteritis must be separated from disorders capable of producing such symptoms (Chap. 103).

COURSE AND PROGNOSIS

The course of polyarteritis is variable,[89] but in most cases the disease progresses at a varying rate over a period of months or years. Spontaneous remissions have been described, and remissions may be induced with corticosteroid therapy. Complete recovery may also occur, especially in patients in whom the disease seems drug induced. Patients with only cutaneous vasculitis have better prognoses. Their courses may be prolonged, and at times their disease resolves completely.[94]

Although there may have been some improvement in prognosis since the advent of corticosteroid therapy, the overall outlook is not good and the disease is frequently fatal. Renal failure, massive retroperitoneal or gastrointestinal bleeding, perforation or infarction of the bowel, and central-nervous-system lesions are the major causes of death.

MANAGEMENT

The general principles of managing patients with polyarteritis are similar to those described for managing patients with SLE (p. 1120). Vigorous therapy with adrenal corticosteroids is required to control symptoms and to prevent progression of the disease. Prednisone, or its equivalent, is begun at a dose of 50 to 100 mg daily, and the patient is observed for evidence of disease regression (e.g., symptomatic improvement, lack of new lesions, and return of the erythrocyte sedimentation rate and platelet count to normal). Frequently, a higher dose may be required to control the disease. Sometimes there is a paradoxical transient worsening of the situation as occlusion of vessels occurs upon healing. High dosage should be continued until stabilization has been achieved (in weeks or months). Then the dose is gradually tapered, provided there is no recrudescence of the disease. Side effects of corticosteroid administration are commonly encountered. In most patients, prolonged treatment is required, and the disease frequently progresses despite continued therapy.

Immunosuppressive drugs, especially cyclophosphamide and azathioprine, have been used in combination with corticosteroids apparently with significant benefit in some cases. More long-term studies are required to assess the eventual role of these agents in management of patients with polyarteritis; but, because of the frequent fatal outcome of this disease, they can be justified in patients with serious vital organ involvement not responsive to steroid therapy.

VARIANTS OF POLYARTERITIS

There is a spectrum of clinical and pathologic syndromes, at one end of which is histologically pure necrotizing and granulomatous lesions without arteritis and at the other end of which is pure panarteritis without any granulomatous reaction. Certain reasonably defined syndromes have been identified on this continuum which are referred to as variants of polyarteritis. Each has distinguishing features in regard to the population involved, the distribution of the vascular lesions, the size of the vessels affected, and the histologic details of the lesions.

Hypersensitivity Angiitis

Hypersensitivity angiitis involves small vessels, both arteries and veins, especially in the skin, heart, and kidneys.[95] The lesions are all the same age, suggesting a single precipitating event. Women are affected more commonly than men, and there is often a history of allergy or drug administration. Dramatic recovery follows withdrawal of the drug that is playing a causative role and the administration of adrenal corticosteroids.

Cranial or Temporal Arteritis[85]

Cranial or temporal arteritis is part of a generalized vascular disease characterized by granulomatous inflammation of the vessels, but because the arteries of the carotid system are so prominently involved it deserves designation as a separate clinical entity. Involvement of the temporal vessels is most typical, but disease of the ophthalmic and retinal arteries is common. Other arteries may be affected, including the carotid, subclavian, coronary, renal, mesenteric, and pulmonary vessels, as well as those of the extremities. Both sexes are susceptible, but it is a disease of the elderly, infrequently seen before the sixth decade.

There are three stages in the clinical course of the disease, and the patient may first be seen by the physician in any of the three phases: headache, ocular complications, and systemic involvement.

The stage of headache is characterized by a pain that is boring in character, often more severe on one side, and frequently intractable. It is often preceded by prodromal symptoms of malaise, anorexia, loss of weight, and diffuse musculoskeletal discomfort. After two or three weeks of headache the temporal vessels become prominent and tender, and painful nodules may develop along their course.

The ocular complications include ophthalmoplegia or, more commonly, vascular lesions affecting the optic nerves and retinas. Complete blindness in one or both eyes may result. An episode of transient or partial visual loss may precede onset of blindness. These symptoms may also occur in the absence of headache or other signs of temporal artery disease.

The stage of systemic involvement is referred to as polymyalgia rheumatica.[77,85] Muscle pains especially in the shoulder and hip girdle, in some instances associated with a low grade fever, weight loss, and anemia, and invariably accompanied by a striking elevation of ESR are characteristic. Diminished or absent pulsations in the temporal artery may be found in the absence of any cranial symptoms, and a temporal artery biopsy may reveal typical lesions.[85] Among the widespread manifestations are skin and visceral lesions, polyneuropathy, generalized muscle tenderness and wasting, and joint involvement. Confusion, convulsions, hemiparesis, and coma have been noted.

The process is usually self-limited, with a course extending from 6 to 30 months. The most important complication is the visual impairment, which can be prevented by early diagnosis of the disease and prompt administration of adrenal corticosteroids.

Aortic-Arch Arteritis[91]

Aortic-arch arteritis, also referred to as pulseless disease and Takayasu disease, is characterized by a segmental panarteritis involving the elastic arteries originating from the aortic arch or thoracic aorta (Chap. 28). It is seen almost exclusively in young females, and is particularly frequent in Orientals. Headache, syncope, reduced visual acuity, mental confusion, and convulsions may result from reduced cerebral blood flow. Symptoms may also include those of coronary insufficiency, heart failure, and arterial insufficiency of the upper extremities. These manifestations are often precipitated or accentuated by physical activity.

Pulses may be absent in the neck, head, and upper extremities, and there may be evidence of collateral circulation about the shoulders or elsewhere. The blood pressure may be unobtainable in the arms and elevated in the legs. The funduscopic examination may reveal a crownlike collection of dilated vessels about the optic disk as the result of arteriovenous anastomoses. A high-pitched systolic or continuous murmur may be noted over the upper chest. Fever, weight loss, muscle atrophy, anemia, leukocytosis, increased erythrocyte sedimentation rate, and hypergammaglobulinemia may be present.

Differential diagnosis involves aortic aneurysm, syphilitic aortitis, congenital anomalies of the aorta, and various tumors and infections of the mediastinum. Early diagnosis and prompt institution of corticosteroid therapy are essential, for many patients develop cerebral and cardiac insufficiency before the diagnosis has been suspected or established. The outlook is generally favorable.

Wegener's Granulomatosis[81,87]

Wegener's granulomatosis is characterized histologically by:

1. Necrotizing granulomatous lesions in the upper air passages, lower respiratory tract, or both
2. Widespread focal necrotizing vasculitis, involving both arteries and veins, almost always in the lungs and widely disseminated in other sites
3. Glomerulitis

It affects young or middle-aged adults of either sex. The clinical course is characterized by two phases, frequently quite distinct. The onset is generally insidious, with manifestations suggesting chronic respiratory tract infection. Two-thirds of the cases exhibit purulent rhinorrhea, antral pain, and epistaxis. In the other third there is chronic cough, hemoptysis, or pleurisy at the onset. As the disease progresses, mucosal ulceration and cartilaginous or osseous destruction of the nose, palate, and orbit may develop, as well as widespread pulmonary consolidation. Later in the illness evidence of generalized involvement appears, including fever, skin lesions, musculoskeletal abnormalities, peripheral neuropathy, and severe renal disease. Anemia and leukocytosis are common, and eosinophilia is present in over half the cases. The diagnosis may be confirmed by biopsy of the respiratory tract or renal lesions. The cases referred to as polyarteritis with lung involvement[90] and as allergic granulomatous arteritis[80] may actually be Wegener's granulomatosis. A limited form of Wegener's with characteristic lesions in the respiratory tract but without renal involvement has been described.[78] Treatment with adrenal corticosteroids alone has been ineffective but the use of corticosteroids with an immunosuppressive agent, especially cyclophosphamide, constitutes effective therapy when initiated early.[82,83]

CHAPTER 101

The Sjögren Syndrome

ALEXANDER S. TOWNES AND MARY BETTY STEVENS

Sjögren syndrome is defined as a combination of two of the following features: 1) keratoconjunctivitis sicca (dry eyes); 2) sialadenitis (dry mouth); and 3) rheumatoid arthritis or, less frequently, one of the connective-tissue disorders (SLE, PSS, or polymyositis).[97,99] All three manifestations are present in about half the cases.

The hallmark of Sjögren syndrome is the ocular- and oral-membrane dryness (the sicca syndrome), which results from an insufficiency of lacrimal, salivary, and mucous-gland secretion. Equally characteristic is the variety of serum antibodies to autologous antigens, especially rheumatoid and antinuclear factors.[96,98]

The sicca syndrome has been found in from 9 to 34 percent of patients with rheumatoid arthritis and seems more prevalent in those with severe and long-standing disease. Females, especially those in the fourth to sixth decades, are affected nine times more often than males. No familial or racial predisposition has been recognized.

CLINICAL MANIFESTATIONS

Sicca Manifestations

Patients may present with the sicca syndrome, but more often the ocular and oral involvement develops during the course of rheumatoid arthritis or one of the connective-tissue disorders. The eyes are involved in 80 to 90 percent of cases. Patients usually complain of a foreign-body sensation or a feeling of grittiness but may also note burning and redness of the eyes or lids or pain from corneal ulceration. Decrease in visual acuity is uncommon. The eyes usually appear moist and without striking abnormality. The lacrimal glands may be enlarged. Deficiencies in tear formation are revealed by Schirmer's test (Chap. 154), and slit-lamp examination may reveal typical superficial filamentous erosions of the corneal epithelium and areas of punctate keratitis.

Dryness of the mouth and salivary-gland enlargement occur in about 90 percent of cases. Patients complain of soreness of the buccal lining, dry mouth, and difficulty in eating dry foods, because of impaired formation of saliva. Enlargement of the parotid glands (in 50 percent of cases) and submaxillary glands (in 20 percent) is usually bilaterally symmetric and painless. However, marked impairment of salivation may be seen in patients without obvious glandular enlargement.

Sicca manifestations are not always confined to the conjunctival and buccal membranes. Dryness and scaliness of the skin and decreased sweating may be noted. The entire respiratory tract may be involved, with dryness and crusting of the nose, dry throat, hoarseness, and a nonproductive cough being common symptoms. Gastrointestinal manifestations are uncommon, but achlorhydria is occasionally found and acute pancreatitis occurs rarely with morphologic changes similar to those found in the salivary glands. Dryness of the vagina is common. Polyuria is frequent and is usually related to excessive fluid intake (to relieve the dry mouth). In a few patients, hyposthenuria unresponsive to water deprivation or vasopressin has been encountered.

Systemic Manifestations

The systemic features of Sjögren syndrome are predominantly those of the associated rheumatoid or connective-tissue disease. The arthritis, present in over half the cases, is rheumatoid in type and may be severely deforming. Subcutaneous nodules occur in a high proportion of patients. A myopathy peculiar to Sjögren syndrome has been reported, but more often muscle weakness and atrophy are found in association with rheumatoid disease or polymyositis. Raynaud's phenomenon occurs in about 20 percent of cases and, like esophageal aperistalsis, may be encountered without the other features of systemic sclerosis. Lymphadenopathy and lymphoid infiltration of the lungs and other organs may occur infrequently and present the picture of pseudolymphoma.[100,101]

LABORATORY MANIFESTATIONS

A mild anemia is found in about half the cases and leukopenia in up to one-third. Occasionally, a marked neutropenia is encountered with the other features of Felty syndrome. The erythrocyte sedimentation rate is generally increased.

Hyperglobulinemia is present in most cases. Rheumatoid factor is usually present whether arthritis is present or not. The sheep-cell agglutination test is positive less frequently (75 percent of cases) than are the tests using human F II gamma globulin (95 percent).[97]

A variety of antibodies to tissue antigens that are not organ specific have been demonstrated. Antinuclear factors are present in about 60 percent (fluorescent technique) with LE cells usually found in those with rheumatoid arthritis or SLE. Antibodies to salivary or lacrimal-gland extracts are not organ specific. However, antibodies specific for ductal epithelium have been detected.

Parotid sialadenitis and sialectasis may be demonstrated by the injection of radiopaque material into Stensen's duct. Sicca symptoms are usually present before the radiologic changes are apparent. However, x-ray changes may be evident in glands that are not obviously enlarged, especially with isotopic scanning techniques.

Salivary gland biopsy reveals a typical picture. Normal acini are replaced by an extensive lymphoid infiltration. Myoepithelial hyperplasia of the interlobular ducts is associated with proximal ductal dilatation.

DIAGNOSIS

The diagnosis of Sjögren syndrome is based primarily on the association of keratoconjunctivitis sicca with sialadenitis or on one or both of these abnormalities occurring in conjunction with rheumatoid arthritis or a connective-tissue disorder. Slit-lamp examination with Rose Bengal staining of the corneal erosions may be necessary to confirm the presence of keratoconjunctivitis sicca. In some patients, especially those with asymmetrical lacrimal- or salivary-gland enlargement, biopsy may be needed to distinguish Sjögren syndrome from sarcoidosis, lymphoma, and other tumors. Although autoantibodies are often present, there is no diagnostic pattern of seroreactivity.

COURSE AND PROGNOSIS

In patients with rheumatoid arthritis or one of the connective-tissue disorders, the course and prognosis are determined by the underlying disease; the sicca symptoms usually remain mild. The ocular and oral involvement is usually more severe in individuals with the sicca syndrome alone. The late development of malignant lymphoma in patients with Sjögren syndrome has been noted but seems to be rare.

MANAGEMENT

Much can be accomplished with symptomatic measures to relieve ocular, oral, or mucous-membrane dryness. Methylcellulose eye drops ("artificial tears") will relieve conjunctival dryness and prevent corneal erosions, and lozenges of glycerine or gelatin may alleviate oral dryness.

No specific treatment is known to alter the course of the sicca syndrome. Adrenal corticosteroids do not prevent further progression of the disorder, and their use is rarely justified. Radiotherapy to enlarged parotid glands was given in the past, but this type of treatment seems unwise in view of the potential hazards of irradiation and the excellent prognosis for long-term survival in most of these patients. Surgical resection of grossly enlarged glands is rarely required.

CHAPTER 102
Rheumatoid Arthritis
THOMAS M. ZIZIC

Rheumatoid arthritis is a systemic disease of unknown etiology characterized by a chronic proliferative and inflammatory reaction in the synovial membrane which eventually results in erosion and destruction of joint cartilage and supporting structures, giving rise to typical joint deformities and characteristic radiologic abnormalities. Synovial inflammation is accompanied by proliferation of the lining cells, many of which are rich in hydrolytic enzymes.[126] Masses of the inflamed and hypertrophied tissue (pannus) extend into and erode the articular cartilages, especially at their margins, and weaken or destroy soft-tissue structures, such as ligaments and tendons.

Another characteristic but less constant feature of rheumatoid arthritis is the rheumatoid granuloma, or rheumatoid nodule. This lesion is most frequently situated in the subcutaneous tissue adjacent to joints but may also occur in the synovial membrane and viscera.

CLINICAL MANIFESTATIONS

Incidence

Rheumatoid arthritis has a worldwide distribution and affects approximately 2.5 percent of the adult population. The age of onset ranges from infancy to the ninth decade, with the peak being between the ages of 40 and 60. Females are affected twice as frequently as males. Over the age of 50 the sex incidence tends to equalize. Rheumatoid disease appears to be associated with HLA Dw4,[117] suggesting possible hereditary predisposition. Emotional stress has been implicated as one possible precipitating or predisposing factor.

Articular Manifestations

The *onset* of rheumatoid arthritis is highly variable, ranging from the abrupt appearance of acute polyarthritis to the gradual development of stiffness and joint changes over a period of months or years. Symptoms may be intermittent, especially during the early course, or may be continuous. In most cases some degree of joint damage and deformity eventually develops.

Joint symptoms usually dominate the clinical course. Pain, stiffness, joint swelling, limitation of motion, and loss of function are present in variable degree. During the acute phase of the inflammatory process, muscular weakness develops, and disuse muscle atrophy often occurs. With hand involvement, weakness of grip strength is a prominent feature and is one of the more reliable reflections of the intensity of the underlying inflammatory process. Another symptom is the so-called gel phenomenon, or stiffness after rest, which subsides after activity is resumed. Morning stiffness that persists for longer than 30 minutes after rising is highly suggestive of rheumatoid arthritis. This feeling of stiffness may be more related to muscle weakness and atrophy than to joint involvement per se. Eventually, displacement of normal alignment may add further weakness, resulting in more severe loss of function.

The pattern of joint involvement is also highly variable. It may begin as a monarticular arthritis (usually in a knee) and remain so for months. More commonly, patients present with symmetric involvement of the small joints of the hands, wrists, and feet. The elbows, shoulders, knees, hips, and ankles are also frequently involved, and the temporomandibular, sternoclavicular, and cricoarytenoid joints are occasionally affected, especially late in the course of the disease. Spine involvement is limited chiefly to the upper cervical segments. The symmetry of joint disease, in contrast to many other inflammatory joint disorders, is often complete. Involvement of the periarticular structures, including tendon sheaths, is also common.

The pattern of rheumatoid arthritis in the hands

is frequently characteristic, especially as the disease progresses. The distal interphalangeal (DIP) joints are usually spared. Swelling of the proximal interphalangeal (PIP) joints because of synovial and soft-tissue involvement frequently produces a fusiform enlargement of the fingers. Symmetric swelling of the metacarpophalangeal (MCP) joints (especially of the index and third fingers) and of the wrists is even more frequent than PIP involvement. Wrist involvement usually results in diffuse enlargement, soft-tissue swelling, and tenderness, particularly in the area of the ulnar styloid. A soft, boggy synovium with cyst-like prominences is often present over the dorsum of the hands and wrists due to a tenosynovitis of the extensor tendons. Frequently, synovial involvement at the wrist results in carpal tunnel entrapment of the median nerve which can lead to digital pain, paresthesias, and loss of muscle strength. Tinel's sign is helpful in suggesting the diagnosis which can be established with greater certainty by nerve conduction studies. Because of the limitation of motion in the MCP or PIP joints or both, the inability to make a tight fist is a common feature of rheumatoid hand involvement.

Although rheumatoid arthritis is basically an inflammatory process, frequently the local tissue signs of acute inflammation are minimal or absent. Thus, the continued presence of a thickened synovial membrane, effusion, tenderness on pressure, or pain on motion may be the only evidence of active synovitis.

In most instances, deformity is produced by destruction of the supporting structures of the joint, imbalance of muscle action through atrophy, and tendon disrupture contracture. Ulnar deviation at the MCP joints is highly suggestive of rheumatoid disease. The extensor tendon may slip off the metacarpal head into the ulnar valley as the deformity develops, followed by subluxation of the proximal phalanx toward the palmar surface and to the ulnar side. Also common is hyperextension at the PIP joints with slight flexion at the DIP joints, the so-called swan-neck deformity. Another frequent alteration is flexion of the PIP joints and hyperextension at the DIP joints (boutonnière deformity). Thumb involvement often occurs at the MCP joint, resulting in flexion and inability to extend this joint. Rheumatoid disease of the foot commonly produces hallux valgus and cock-up toes, with upward displacement of the proximal phalanx at the metatarsophalangeal joint and flexion at the PIP joint of the toes. As a result, weight is borne distally entirely by the metatarsal heads, a frequent cause of pain on walking. Flexion contractures may follow involvement of the knees, hips, and elbows.

Extra-Articular Manifestations[103,110]

Rheumatoid arthritis is a systemic disease and may be accompanied by weight loss, low-grade fever, and anemia, as well as a variety of visceral lesions. In some patients these features are striking, but in most, articular disease dominates the clinical picture.

The most characteristic extra-articular manifestation is the rheumatoid granuloma, or subcutaneous nodule. These nodules may be firmly attached to deeper structures or may be freely movable in the subcutaneous tissue. They are usually found over the extensor surfaces of the forearm along the ulnar ridge or in the ulnar bursa. They may be encountered over other pressure points, such as the ischial tuberosities or bony prominences of joints, and may develop along tendons or tendon sheaths. The rheumatoid nodule occurs in up to 35 percent of patients with rheumatoid arthritis and is almost pathognomonic. However, nodules, clinically and histologically identical to "rheumatoid" nodules, can occur in systemic lupus erythematosus.[111]

Lymphadenopathy is present in 25 percent of patients and extensive enough on occasion to suggest the diagnosis of lymphoma. Splenomegaly is present in 5 percent. Felty syndrome (rheumatoid arthritis, splenomegaly, and neutropenia) is occasionally associated with massive splenic enlargement. In these patients, vasculitic leg ulcers are especially common and recurrent infections pose a special problem in management.

Ocular involvement is not as common in adult rheumatoid arthritis as it is in the juvenile form. Dryness of the eyes accompanied by a foreign-body sensation may result from keratitis sicca or from Sjögren syndrome (Chap. 101). Episcleritis has been observed in cases of rheumatoid arthritis in which necrotizing arteritis has developed. Rarely, granulomatous involvement of the sclera results in thinning and perforation of the eye and loss of vitreous (scleromalacia perforans).

Cardiac involvement[108,125] with rheumatoid granulomas may rarely give rise to arrhythmias. Because of the frequency of other types of cardiac disease in the same age group, certain diagnosis is not possible. Aortitis resulting from similar lesions is a rare cause of aortic regurgitation. Pericarditis is observed in less than 10 percent of patients. Chronic constrictive pericarditis requiring surgical decortication of the heart develops in some patients.[113]

Pleuritis occurs occasionally and may produce an effusion characterized by a low glucose content in the absence of any evident infectious process. The complement is reduced in the rheumatoid effusion suggesting immune complex fixation at the local membrane level.

Pulmonary involvement[124] with rheumatoid granulomas is uncommon. Caplan described nodular pulmonary lesions in Welsh miners that in some instances preceded the onset of rheumatoid arthritis (Caplan syndrome).[106] Similar findings have been described in rheumatoid patients who are not miners. Pulmonary insufficiency rarely results. Pulmonary fibrosis has been reported to be a feature of rheumatoid arthritis, but this relationship remains to be clarified as does the frequent finding of a restrictive ventilatory defect on testing pulmonary function of asymptomatic patients with rheumatoid disease.

Leg ulcers, especially over the malleoli, may develop in long-standing and severe disease. There are probably multiple factors involved in their formation, including inflammatory involvement of the veins and arteries.

Vasculitis or arteritis is recognized in approximately 10 percent of patients with rheumatoid disease and has been shown to be an early event in the development of rheumatoid nodules.[122] The arteritis associated with rheumatoid arthritis may be necrotizing, disseminated, and indistinguishable from classical polyarteritis. More often it occurs in more isolated areas and tends to involve smaller vessels and to pursue a less progressive course.[120] An endarteritis involving the digital vessels occasionally produces small areas of necrosis adjacent to nail margins. More commonly, vasculitis of the nutrient vessels to peripheral nerves may result in a peripheral neuropathy, especially in the lower extremities.

LABORATORY MANIFESTATIONS

Hematologic

Mild anemia is common in rheumatoid arthritis, occurring in approximately 40 percent of cases. Typically, the anemia of chronic disease is found with a low serum iron and low serum iron-binding capacity. However, iron deficiency per se is seen frequently, often as a result of gastrointestinal blood loss. Anemia caused by chronic folic-acid deficiency has also been reported; thus, complete evaluation of any anemia is indicated, especially if the hematocrit is 30 percent or less.

Leukocytosis may occur and at times is striking. Leukopenia is also occasionally present and characteristically so in Felty syndrome in which granulocytes are depleted. However, most patients have normal white cell counts.[121] An elevated platelet count may accompany highly active disease. The erythro-

cyte sedimentation rate and other acute-phase reactants are widely used indices of activity. Elevation of serum globulin, especially the gamma and alpha-2 fractions, occurs in some 50 percent of all patients and in the majority with progressive chronic disease.

Serologic Tests

Serologic tests for rheumatoid factor[123] have proved useful in clinical diagnosis and have been instrumental in the clinical separation of syndromes formerly considered as variants of rheumatoid arthritis. The test is based upon the presence of gamma globulin (usually an IgM globulin) in rheumatoid serum which reacts specifically as an antibody to altered gamma globulin.[102] Various particles or cells are used as carriers of the aggregated globulin (antigen) from human or animal sources, and the endpoint is agglutination. The slide modification of the FII latex test (Hyland RA slide test), which is widely used in clinical practice, is useful as a screening test, since there are very few false negatives. Positive reactions, especially weak ones, occur in approximately 15 percent of hospitalized patients without rheumatoid arthritis, and thus a more definitive technique should be used if this slide test is positive.

The occurrence of rheumatoid factors is not limited to rheumatoid arthritis, although they occur most frequently and in highest titer in this disease. Rheumatoid factors are found in 2 and 10 percent of healthy individuals, depending on the test used, and this incidence increases appreciably with age. Positive tests may also be seen in the various connective-tissue diseases, liver disease, sarcoidosis, syphilis, tuberculosis, subacute infective endocarditis, leprosy, and other chronic illnesses. Titers are usually higher in rheumatoid arthritis than in these other disorders, but there is some overlap. Thus, a positive test is not diagnostic of rheumatoid arthritis but may be helpful when considered with other clinical information. Despite its lesser sensitivity, the sheep-cell agglutination test (SCAT) is useful because the anti-gammaglobulin factors in diseases other than rheumatoid arthritis usually do not give positive reactions, and thus, it is a more specific test for rheumatoid arthritis. All tests for rheumatoid factor are positive with few exceptions in patients with rheumatoid nodules, in those with variant syndromes (i.e., Felty, Sjögren, Caplan), and in most of those with extensive bony destruction by x-ray. If a patient has a positive test, it usually remains positive, but titers do not correlate with the activity of the disease. Twenty-five to 30 percent of patients with definite rheumatoid arthritis have negative tests.

LE-cell tests are positive in up to 25 percent of patients with rheumatoid arthritis. Typically, the number of LE cells seen in a preparation is less than in SLE. However, some patients may have strongly positive tests. Antinuclear antibody is also present in serum of 10 to 50 percent of patients with rheumatoid arthritis (depending on the technique used) but is also usually in low titer compared to that in SLE. High titers may occur, especially in patients with severe and long-standing destructive rheumatoid disease, and in the Felty syndrome.[129]

Hypocomplementemia is an infrequent finding and has been associated with severe systemic disease and arteritis.[112]

Synovial Fluid

Rheumatoid synovial fluid is characteristically turbid, with reduced viscosity, increased protein content, poor mucin clot, and slightly reduced glucose content.[16] The white cell count is elevated (3000 to 60,000/μl, with an average of around 10,000/μl), with predominantly a polymorphonuclear response at times of active disease. Phagocytes with cytoplasmic inclusions (the so-called RA cells) occur most frequently and abundantly in rheumatoid synovial fluids, although this finding is not specific. Cells with inclusions can be detected on examination of wet smears with high magnification in regular light, phase contrast microscopy, or with a supravital stain, such as 1 percent neutral red.[9] The inclusions have been shown to contain fibrin, cell debris, and in some instances complexes of rheumatoid factor and gamma globulin. Early reports of studies on the detection of rheumatoid factor in eluates from washed, disrupted synovial fluid leukocytes suggest that this test may be useful in diagnosis. The complement level in rheumatoid synovial fluid is low compared to that in other types of inflammatory joint effusions, especially in relation to the total protein concentration.[105,116,119]

Radiologic Abnormalities (Fig. 102–1)[19]

Early in the course of rheumatoid arthritis no abnormality may be discerned on x-ray other than soft-tissue swelling or the visualization of joint effusions (Fig. 102–1B). Periarticular osteoporosis is the earliest radiologic feature. The decrease in bone density is probably related to the remarkable increase in local blood flow in and around the inflamed joints and to disuse. In more advanced cases resorption of portions or even all of certain bones may occur. The carpal bones are particularly prone to undergo this change.

Juxta-articular erosions, sometimes having punched-out appearances, result from replacement of bone at the margins of the articular cartilage by the synovial pannus (Fig. 102–1C). They may appear in any joint but are particularly prominent in the metacarpal heads, at the PIP joints, in the carpal bones, in the distal radius, radioulnar joint, and ulnar styloid. Large cystic erosions are sometimes seen in more advanced disease. As the inflammatory process continues, the entire articular cartilage is destroyed, especially in weight-bearing joints. The joint space becomes narrowed and may eventually disappear altogether (Fig. 102–1D). Subchondral sclerosis and bony proliferation or secondary degenerative arthritis eventually results. In the late stages of rheumatoid arthritis, the deformities noted grossly may also be observed radiographically (Fig. 102–1E).

Biopsy

The histopathologic changes in the rheumatoid nodule are usually sufficiently characteristic to establish a diagnosis. Arteritis or vasculitis has been implicated in their production, but in the mature lesion vasculitis is seldom found. Generally, an area of central necrosis and fibrinoid degeneration is surrounded by epithelioid and chronic inflammatory cells in a palisading pattern.

Muscle biopsy may demonstrate arteritis. The presence of lymphorrhages in muscle and perivascular round-cell infiltration are common in rheumatoid arthritis but are nonspecific findings and not indicative of arteritis. Lymph nodes usually show nonspecific hyperplasia of varying degree. Synovial biopsy is seldom helpful, since the histologic picture is characteristic only in well-advanced cases. In the acute phase the synovial reaction consists of an inflammatory infiltration, an exudation of fibrin, and an intense proliferation of the superficial cell layers of the synovial membrane. Synovial hypertrophy may result in the formation of multiple villous projections. The lymphocytic and plasma-cell infiltration of the deeper layers of the synovium and in the regional lymph nodes has been related to the production of rheumatoid factor.

DIAGNOSIS

The diagnosis of rheumatoid arthritis depends upon a combination of clinical, laboratory, and radiologic features that may require weeks, even months, to evolve. The pattern of the arthropathy is most helpful: an additive, symmetric, peripheral, inflammatory joint involvement. Subcutaneous nodules, when present, are characteristic; and in all patients the gel phenomenon is prominent. Supportive laboratory findings include serum rheumatoid factor and an inflammatory synovial fluid with markedly reduced hemolytic complement. Radiologically, diagnostic

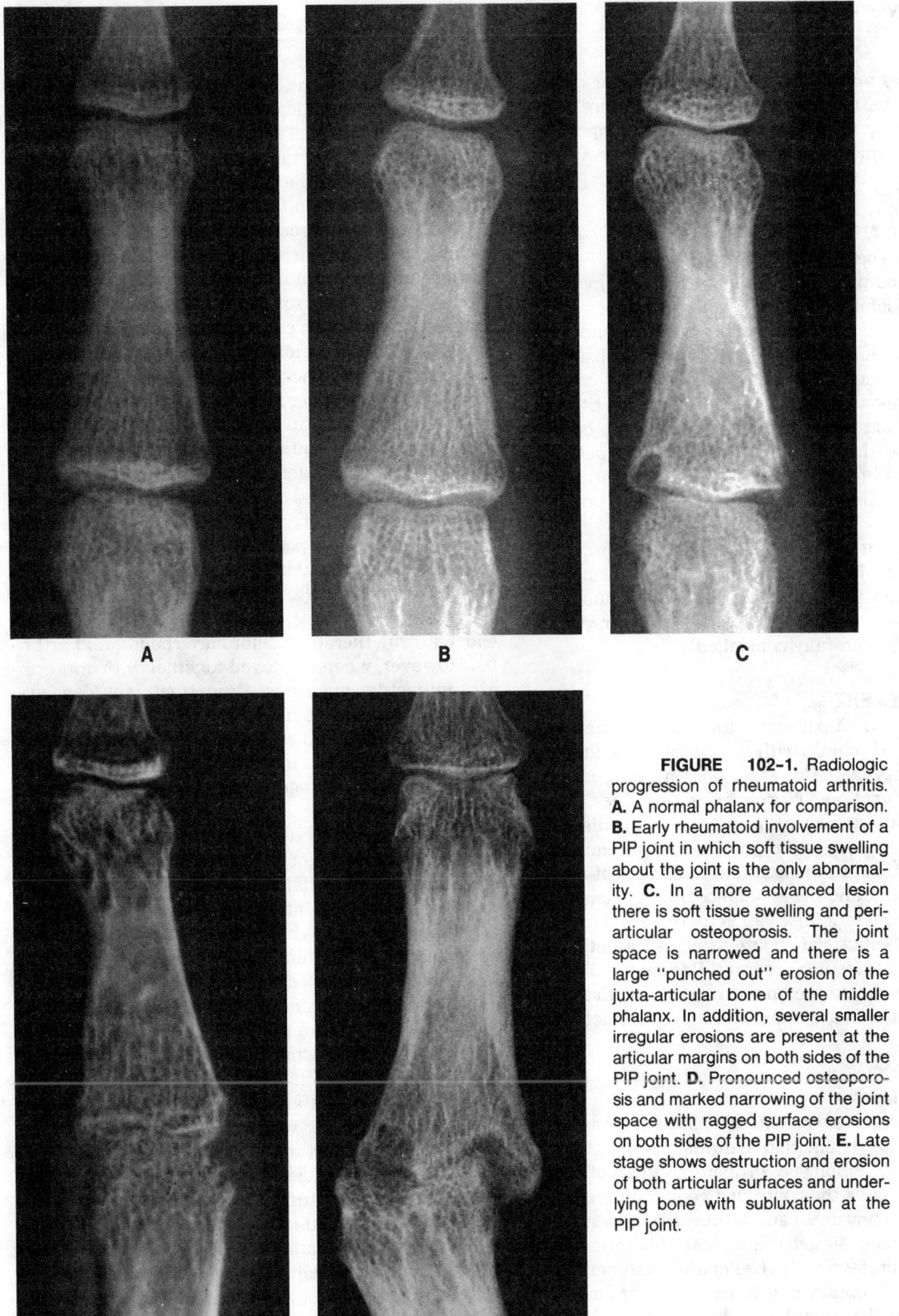

FIGURE 102-1. Radiologic progression of rheumatoid arthritis. **A.** A normal phalanx for comparison. **B.** Early rheumatoid involvement of a PIP joint in which soft tissue swelling about the joint is the only abnormality. **C.** In a more advanced lesion there is soft tissue swelling and periarticular osteoporosis. The joint space is narrowed and there is a large "punched out" erosion of the juxta-articular bone of the middle phalanx. In addition, several smaller irregular erosions are present at the articular margins on both sides of the PIP joint. **D.** Pronounced osteoporosis and marked narrowing of the joint space with ragged surface erosions on both sides of the PIP joint. **E.** Late stage shows destruction and erosion of both articular surfaces and underlying bone with subluxation at the PIP joint.

changes occur only late although periarticular osteo-porosis may be a striking early finding before joint space narrowing and erosions develop. It is important to recognize that time and continued observation may be essential for diagnostic certainty.

COURSE AND PROGNOSIS

The course of rheumatoid arthritis is variable, but ap-proximately 60 percent of patients suffer from some degree of disability. Patients whose diseases have acute onsets seem to have good prognoses and may experience prolonged remissions. Those whose dis-eases have chronic indolent courses have less chance of a spontaneous remission. Although the titer of rheumatoid factor does not closely reflect the course of the disease, there is some indication that patients with persistently positive tests (especially with high titers) early in their courses may have worse progno-ses.

Treatment will relieve the acute inflammatory manifestations of rheumatoid arthritis but cannot be considered curative. Since the course of rheumatoid arthritis is variable, the evaluation of therapeutic agents must be carefully controlled.

MANAGEMENT

The management of patients with rheumatoid arthri-tis is concerned mainly with suppressing the inflam-matory aspects of the disease, preventing musculo-skeletal dysfunction, correcting deformities, and controlling the extra-articular features of the disease. Of equal importance is the general care of each pa-tient, the prompt recognition and treatment of inter-current illnesses, and the avoidance of circumstances likely to precipitate disease activity. Similarly, a sound patient–physician relationship is essential to an effective therapeutic program. Patients and their families often equate rheumatoid arthritis with hope-less invalidism and are in need of sensible emotional support.

General Measures

A program of rest, exercise, and splinting is basic to the treatment of rheumatoid arthritis, irrespective of the drug therapy employed. Proper execution of such a program requires the continued cooperation of the patient and his physician and frequently the services of an orthopedic surgeon, physical therapist, and other skilled professionals. Generally, such services are most readily obtained at large treatment centers. It is important that they be made available to every patient early in the course of his disease in order to restore and preserve maximum functional capacity.

Rest is important, especially during more active phases of the disorder. Patients must be cautioned against strenuous and prolonged activity undertaken with the mistaken notion that it prevents crippling. A balance of rest and therapeutic (not aimless) exercise is needed to maintain function.

Therapeutic exercises are designed to prevent de-formities, to maintain and improve the range of joint motion, and to promote muscular coordination and performance. Both isotonic and isometric exercises are useful, the latter especially in enhancing muscle strength. The alleviation of pain and stiffness through the judicious use of heat and analgesic agents permits maximal participation in an exercise program.

Splinting is useful in the management of highly inflamed joints. Splinting also aids in the prevention of contractures and deformities and in the correction of these abnormalities once they are established. Fur-thermore, the use of supports and other orthopedic devices may permit patients partially to compensate for various functional impairments.

Drug Therapy

Current drug therapy cannot cure rheumatoid arthri-tis. However, when employed together with appropri-ate adjunctive measures, drug treatment can sup-press many of the inflammatory manifestations of the disorder and can aid in the prevention of musculo-skeletal dysfunction. In Table 102–1, currently used drugs with their dosage range and potential adverse effects are listed.

Salicylates (e.g., acetylsalicylic acid, or aspirin) have anti-inflammatory and analgesic effects and should be used in initial drug treatment. Aspirin alone may control disease manifestations and is the main drug used in treating rheumatoid patients. It may also be employed in combination with other drugs and in fact should be included in all multiple-drug regimens unless specific contraindications exist. Impaired renal excretion may require the use of a smaller dose.

Enteric-coated aspirin may be used to minimize the gastric side effects, but the physician should be certain that it is satisfactorily absorbed by finding se-rum salicylate levels which approximate 20 mg/dl. Other available anti-inflammatory agents seem to have greater tendencies than aspirin does to cause gastrointestinal irritation, ulceration, and bleeding.

Nonsteroidol anti-inflammatory drugs (*NSAIDs*), a new group of organic acid antagonists to prosta-glandin synthetase, emerged following the discovery that a major action of aspirin related to inhibition of prostaglandin synthesis. Chemically, they are deriva-tives of indole or propionic acid (Table 102-1). These may substitute for salicylates when aspirin is not effi-

TABLE 102-1
Drug Therapy in Rheumatoid Arthritis

Drug	Dosage (daily)		Adverse Effects
Salicylates			
Acetylsalicylic acid (Aspirin)	3.0–4.5 g	Salicylism	The salicylates and the nonsteroidol anti-inflammatory drugs are all associated with gastric irritation, even gastrointestinal ulceration and bleeding, in a significant number of patients. Except for the salicylates, headache may be a prominent, often transient, early symptom of drug intolerance. In all, dizziness and tinnitus may occur. Skin rashes and pruritis are infrequent and respond promptly to drug discontinuance
Indole derivatives			
Indomethacin (Indocin)	75–150 mg	Psychic change	
Tolmetin (Tolectin)	1200–1800 mg	Fluid retention	
Propionic acid derivatives			
Ibuprofen (Motrin)	900–2400 mg	Fluid retention	
Fenoprofen (Nalfon)	2400–3000 mg	Somnolence	
Naproxen (Naprosyn)	500–750 mg	Fluid retention	
Hydroxycholoroquine (Plaquenil)	200 mg	Gastric irritation with anorexia, nausea, and rarely diarrhea; skin rash; rarely, ocular toxicity at this dosage level	
Gold (Myochrysine, Thiomalate)	10 mg initially, increasing to 50 mg weekly; after response, maintenance at 50 mg q 3–4 weeks	Skin rash and rarely an exfoliative dermatitis; stomatitis; depression of granulocytes and platelets; hepatitis; neuritis; proteinuria, rarely nephrotic syndrome	
Penicillamine	250–750 mg	Skin rash; hepatic dysfunction; nephropathy with hematuria and proteinuria; hematologic depression	
Adrenal corticosteroids (Prednisone)	5–15 mg daily or on alternate days	Peptic ulceration, osteoporosis, muscle wasting, capillary purpura, cataracts, ischemic bone necrosis, suppression of adrenal function; cushingoid habitus	

cacious or not tolerated in adequate dosage. The advantages of this NSAID group over aspirin is yet to be fully determined in most instances, and most compete with salicylates so that they generally are not administered simultaneously. The longer half-life of naproxen, allowing dosage at 12-hour intervals, may increase patient compliance.

When salicylates or a NSAID alone fail to control the disease and additional therapy is required, the next step is usually the addition of either antimalarial drugs, gold salts, or, more recently, penicillamine.

Hydroxychloroquine, in conjunction with aspirin, may alleviate the inflammation of rheumatoid arthritis, but 2 to 6 months of therapy are often required to achieve maximal benefit. When hydroxychloroquine is administered for prolonged periods (years), a small proportion of patients develop retinal damage, but this is exceedingly rare. If adequate control is not achieved in 6 months, the drug should be discontinued.

Gold therapy (chrysotherapy) is used especially in early progressive rheumatoid disease. The use of gold has received new impetus from a controlled trial which showed a definite therapeutic effect.[107] Remission is seldom realized before a total dose of 500 mg has been received, and may require 1.0 g or more, hence, 10 to 20 weeks of therapy. Maintenance of monthly doses of 50 mg may prolong a remission once obtained.

The major disadvantage of gold therapy is its potential toxicity. Thus, patients receiving gold therapy should be closely watched, with careful examination of skin and mucous membranes, urinalysis, and white blood count performed before each dose of drug is administered.

D-Penicillamine is now under extensive use and study in rheumatoid arthritis as a second line drug. Its efficacy is comparable to that of chrysotherapy. With response now demonstrated at low dosage (less than 1 g), adverse reactions are less frequent and severe. Nonetheless, patients must be followed closely with blood counts and urinalyses when the drug is prescribed with initial 125 to 250 mg dosage, increasing bimonthly by 125 to 250 mg to a maximal 750 mg daily. At present, D-penicillamine is reserved for antimalarial and gold failures.

Adrenal corticosteroids are able to suppress the inflammatory aspects of rheumatoid disease more promptly than other agents now available. Despite this, they are not used as initial therapy because of the several undesirable biologic effects that result from long-term administration. Steroid therapy may be considered when an adequate trial of salicylates and physical measures has failed to produce satisfactory results, especially when the disease is intensely active and rapidly progressive. Prednisone, in doses not exceeding 5 to 15 mg daily or even on alternate days, may provide necessary symptomatic relief during the initial period of antimalarial, gold, or penicillamine therapy before maximal benefit from these agents can be expected. When suppression has been maintained for a few weeks, the dose of prednisone should be tapered slowly and steadily until minimal dose is achieved or the drug discontinued.

The injection of steroids into joints has limited utility. Relief of symptoms may persist for several weeks and permit initiation of physical therapy, but reliance on repeated intra-articular steroids is not advised. In some instances, pyogenic infections or further deterioration of joint have been observed following repeated intra-articular steroid injections.

Recent observations suggest that cyclophosphamide (Cytoxan) is effective in treating rheumatoid disease.[109,114] In some cases, hypertrophic synovium may regress and erosive changes may be halted. Azathioprine (Imuran), similarly, has been reported to suppress the rheumatoid process, in some cases with lasting remissions. Nonetheless, these agents are strictly reserved for life-threatening or crippling disease which has not responded to conventional therapy.

Orthopedic Surgery

Two types of surgical procedures may help patients with rheumatoid arthritis. Reconstructive surgery is an established adjunct to rehabilitation. Recent advances in technique with total joint replacements have enhanced the usefulness of these reconstructive procedures.[118] In addition, it has become clear that operative procedures can be employed while the disease is active to prevent major deformities. Synovectomy appears at times to produce lasting improvement despite continued disease in other joints. A recent 3-year study of synovectomy showed minimal clinical and no radiologic lasting benefit. Although synovectomy may be helpful in a single, refractory, painful joint with invasive synovial proliferation and in wrists with threatened extensor tendon rupture, it would not appear to be of major value in general patient management.

RHEUMATOID VARIANTS

The variants of rheumatoid arthritis include juvenile rheumatoid arthritis, systemic forms of primarily adult disease (i.e., rheumatoid arthritis with vasculitis and syndromes of Felty, Sjögren, and Caplan), and those with immunoprotein abnormalities other than rheumatoid factors (i.e., LE cells, hypocomplementemia, cryoglobulinemia). Only the frequently encountered rheumatoid arthritis of children and Felty syndrome will be discussed here.

Juvenile Rheumatoid Arthritis

Juvenile rheumatoid arthritis (JRA) is a chronic process that begins before the individual reaches the age of 16. This disease is thought by most to be the same process as adult rheumatoid arthritis because of some basic similarities and the fact that some patients continue to have typical rheumatoid disease into adult life. It is considered separately primarily because certain manifestations are peculiar to the childhood form.

Patients with JRA present in one of three ways, namely, 1) a systemic illness, 2) a polyarthritis, or 3) involvement of one or at most very few (oligoarticular) inflamed joints. Those whose disease begins in early childhood commonly have the clinical picture known as Still's disease.[9] In this syndrome, joint symptoms are often overshadowed by a high, spiking fever, erythematous rash, pleuropericarditis, splenomegaly, and generalized lymphadenopathy. There is often a delayed and incomplete response to aspirin. Renal disease is not present, and LE cells are not found. These features allow differentiation of the disorder from acute rheumatic fever and SLE, diagnoses often considered because of the marked systemic manifestations. Arthritis, which occurs in most cases, may appear only after several days or weeks, and thus the disease may present as an obscure febrile illness.[104] The rash and the high, spiking fever may suggest the correct diagnosis in these instances. A few patients develop rheumatoid nodules. Cervical-spine involvement is common. It is in the oligoarticular group that iridocyclitis occurs, a dreaded complication because of the visual loss that can result. The eye involvement may or may not coincide with active joint disease but is frequently associated with serum antinuclear antibody in moderate titer. Patients between the ages of 9 and 15 often present with a polyarthritis with some deformity in the absence of marked systemic symptoms. Some of those whose disease begins in adolescence will have monarticular arthritis or oligoarticular disease. The significant association of HLA B27 in boys with late onset oligoarticular disease emphasizes the heterogeneity of juvenile chronic arthritis. (See Chap. 104.) The overall prognosis in JRA is good, especially in patients with monarticular involvement. Prolonged remissions are common, and complete remission of active disease may occur. However, in some cases severely crippling deformities may result. At times, secondary degenerative joint disease may cause symptoms to continue after the active inflammatory process has ceased. Amyloidosis is occasionally encountered, especially in Still's disease.

Management[9] is similar to that described for adult rheumatoid arthritis. Salicylates alone or in combination with gold are the regimens of choice for most patients. Those with iridocyclitis should be promptly treated as well with corticosteroids to prevent blindness. The use of corticosteroids carries the additional hazard of disturbing normal growth in children. Preliminary studies with penicillamine suggest significant benefit.

The Felty Syndrome

Rheumatoid arthritis, splenomegaly, and leukopenia constitute the triad of Felty syndrome. There is general agreement that Felty syndrome is basically a rheumatoid process. However, the peculiar features of splenomegaly and severe leukopenia present a distinct clinical problem.

Felty syndrome occurs equally in males and females. It usually begins after age 50 and is rare before age 35. Typical rheumatoid arthritis usually precedes splenomegaly and leukopenia, frequently by many years. Generally, the arthritis may be severe and associated with significant deformity. At times it is relatively inactive and considered to be "burned out." The extra-articular manifestations of rheumatoid disease are frequently prominent in Felty syndrome. Severe weight loss is the rule. Fever, sometimes episodic, may occur. Rheumatoid nodules occur more often than in uncomplicated rheumatoid arthritis. Leg ulcers and keratitis sicca are common. The spleen, usually only slightly enlarged, may be very large and easily confused with the spleen of chronic leukemia.[115]

There is increased susceptibility to infection in some cases. Infections, when they occur, respond well to antibiotics if a sensitive organism is involved. Patients are able to mobilize granulocytes (although at a somewhat delayed rate) and to produce pus at local sites of infection despite the paucity of granulocytes in the circulation. There is leukopenia with a granulocytopenia (fewer than 1500 granulocytes/μl). In severe cases, mature granulocytes are virtually absent from the circulation and total white counts of fewer than 1000/μl are sometimes encountered. Anemia is generally only moderate and rarely hemolytic. Some degree of thrombocytopenia may occur, although it is seldom severe enough to cause purpura. The bone marrow is cellular and shows a maturation arrest in the granulocytic series. Rheumatoid-factor tests are invariably positive and occasionally reach very high titers. LE cells and antinuclear antibodies are also more common than in uncomplicated rheumatoid arthritis.

The management of patients with Felty syndrome is similar to that of patients with rheumatoid arthritis. The frequent occurrence of infection in certain patients poses an additional problem. Several reports have indicated striking improvement in severely ill patients following splenectomy. This improvement relates particularly to a reversal of the hematologic abnormalities, the healing of ankle ulcers, and a cessation of infection. These favorable results, however, often are not obtained and at best may be temporary. More recently, improvement in these features of Felty syndrome has been reported with chrysotherapy.

CHAPTER 103

The Differential Diagnosis of Multisystem Disease

MARY BETTY STEVENS

The protean nature of the clinical manifestations of diseases with immunologic features results in their many varied presentations.[127-130,132] The illness that appears at the onset may suggest that a single organ is principally involved, or there may be a confusing array of symptoms involving multiple organ systems. There are, however, certain patterns that occur repeatedly and that can alert the physician to the fact that one is dealing with one of these diseases. Some of the clinical manifestations, occurring singly or in combination, that should signal the possibility that the patient may have a multisystem connective tissue disease are listed in Table 103–1.

In evaluating the patient's presenting problem,

TABLE 103-1

Presenting Manifestations That May Suggest the Diagnosis of One of the Systemic Rheumatic Diseases

1. Fever of unexplained origin
2. Arthralgia or arthritis
3. Noninfectious pleuritis, pericarditis, or peritonitis
4. Skin lesions, in particular erythema, urticaria, nodules, purpura
5. Unexplained valvulitis or myocarditis
6. Pneumonitis or pulmonary infiltration unresponsive to antibiotics
7. Unexplained myositis or neuritis
8. Glomerulitis or glomerulonephritis
9. Central nervous system manifestations, often localized and transient, which may mimic almost any neurologic syndrome
10. Ocular involvement including keratitis, uveitis, etc.
11. Unexplained lymph node enlargement or splenomegaly
12. Unexplained acute hemolytic anemia, thrombocytopenic purpura, leukopenia, eosinophilia
13. Chronic false-positive serologic test for syphilis
14. Evidence on biopsy of skin, lymph node, muscle, kidney of
    A. Focal collagen degeneration or necrosis
    B. Necrosis and inflammation of arteries
    C. Myositis
    D. Lymphoid hyperplasia
    E. Glomerulonephritis, especially focal

---

one should keep in mind certain characteristic features of multisystem diseases with immunologic abnormalities, including:

1. Multiplicity of organ involvement
2. Chronicity of the illness combined with repeated failure to find a specific cause
3. Episodicity, with periods of activity interspersed with periods of spontaneous improvement
4. A multiplicity of previous diagnoses, since these disorders may mimic almost any type of illness
5. The tendency of some organs to be involved more than others and of this involvement to be the dominant feature of the disease for months or years

Additional problems are presented to the physician by the patient with a known collagen disease in whom an acute illness develops, a frequent event in the patient who is receiving one or more therapeutic

agents. In such a circumstance the physician must ask several specific questions:

1. Is the acute illness the result of an exacerbation of the underlying disease, for example, SLE? If so, is it a spontaneous event? Is it a result of inadequate treatment? Was it precipitated by an infection or some other antigenic exposure, such as to a drug?
2. Is the present episode caused by the concurrent development of another type of "autoimmune" disease, for example, the appearance of Hashimoto's disease in a patient with SLE or rheumatoid arthritis?
3. Is it a result of some complication of the underlying collagen disease, although not directly caused by it, for example, pulmonary or urinary tract infection in a patient who already has involvement of the lungs or kidneys as part of his basic disease?
4. Is it a complication of the treatment he is receiving, for example, vertebral collapse, aseptic necrosis, or diabetes in a patient on high doses of an adrenal corticosteroid?
5. Is it a completely new and unrelated event? The collagen diseases may mimic many other diseases, and it is easy mistakenly to attribute a new manifestation to the underlying chronic illness. For example, a patient with classical SLE who had been followed for many years developed Jacksonian fits that were found to be caused by a meningioma, not by SLE. Similarly, a pleural effusion can be tuberculous or a joint septic rather than expressions of activity of underlying SLE or rheumatoid arthritis.

One of the most important principles in the consideration of the patient with multiple system manifestations is to rule out other diseases that may present in a similar fashion, particularly those that can be effectively treated. Only then can the diagnosis of a connective tissue disease be accepted. Some of the particular illnesses that must be considered in the study of this type of problem are listed in Table 103–2.

DIFFERENTIAL DIAGNOSIS AMONG DISEASES WITH IMMUNOLOGIC FEATURES

In the majority of cases, differential diagnosis can be made on the basis of the dominant clinical disease pattern. Most helpful is the presence or absence of manifestations, especially in certain combinations, that have a high degree of association with a particu-

---

TABLE 103-2

Other Multisystem Diseases To Be Considered in the Differential Diagnosis of Systemic Rheumatic Disease

I. **Infections**

  A. Pyogenic with metastatic lesions
  B. Localized infection with multiple systemic manifestations
  C. Specific infection with multisystem involvement
    1. Tuberculosis
    2. Brucellosis
    3. Mycotic infections
    4. Syphilis
    5. Infectious mononucleosis
    6. Parasitic disease (e.g., trichinosis)
    7. Whipple's disease

II. **Granulomatous Diseases**

  A. Sarcoidosis

III. **Metabolic Diseases**

  A. Porphyria
  B. Amyloidosis
  C. Chemical or drug toxicity or hypersensitivity, e.g., lead poisoning

IV. **Neoplasms**

  A. Metastatic neoplastic disease
  B. Tumors which produce a physiologically active polypeptide: carcinoma of the lung, carcinoid
  C. Benign atrial myxoma with tumor emboli
  D. Acute leukemia
  E. Hodgkin's disease
  F. Lymphosarcoma
  G. Plasma cell disease, macroglobulinemia

V. **Cardiovascular Disease**

  A. Infective endocarditis with minimal systemic signs of infection
  B. Intramural thrombi with systemic embolization
  C. Multiple pulmonary embolization

---

lar clinical syndrome. For example, two young women are seen who have recently developed erythematous eruptions in a butterfly distribution, fever, diffuse muscle aching, and acute polyarthritis. In addition to these common symptoms, however, one patient has a history of several unexplained febrile episodes in the recent past with pleuritic pain, and laboratory investigations reveal microscopic hematuria, proteinuria, and LE cells. With this combination of findings there can be little doubt that the diagnosis is SLE. In the other patient, weakness of the proximal muscle groups is demonstrated on examination, and serum transaminase concentrations are found to be increased. This clinical pattern is most compatible with dermatomyositis, rather than with SLE. SLE can be excluded with a greater degree of certainty in the absence of LE cells or a high titer of antinuclear antibodies or hypocomplementemia. Thus, making a differential diagnosis of these disorders usually requires carefully assembling and analyzing clinical data, summarizing the features present, and adding significant negative information. A summary of some of the manifestations that may be useful in distinguishing these disorders is presented in Table 103-3.

TRANSITIONAL OR OVERLAP SYNDROMES

Cases are being described with increasing frequency that have been designated as "transitional" or "overlap" syndromes involving features of SLE, rheumatoid arthritis, progressive systemic sclerosis, dermatomyositis, Sjögren syndrome, polyarteritis nodosa, and thrombotic thrombocytopenic purpura. Some patients with "mixed connective tissue disease" have been found to have antibody to extractable nuclear antigens (ENA, especially RNP) which may favor a relatively benign prognosis.[131] In these cases the diagnosis of two or more of these diseases is suggested on the basis of the accumulated clinical, serologic, and histologic evidence. More study is required to reveal the significance of these clinical and serologic relationships. However, their existence presents frequent practical problems for the physician in regard to diagnosis and treatment.

These overlap syndromes involve many clinical, pathologic, and immunologic manifestations (Tables 103-4, 103-5, and 103-6). Moreover, these manifestations and the sequence in which they emerge present differing clinical problems which may be of prognostic import.

1. *Manifestations common to more than one of the connective tissue diseases may be present without a characteristic pattern to establish the diagnosis of any single disorder.* Such is often the case early in the course of one of these disorders. For example, a young female presented with clinical manifestations of Raynaud's phenomenon, mild polyarthritis, anemia, increased sedimentation rate, and hyperglobulinemia. The latex fixation test was positive in a titer of 1:640, but a sheep-cell agglutination test was negative. No LE cells were found, but antinuclear antibodies were demonstrated by the immunofluorescent technique in a titer of 1:10. Diagnoses of rheumatoid arthritis, progressive systemic sclerosis, and SLE were all suggested, but there was insufficient evidence to establish a definite diagnosis. Several months later this patient developed pleuritic pain, fever, skin lesions, and LE cells and undoubtedly had SLE, but the same presenting manifestations could have been observed with any of the other disorders initially considered. Only careful, continued observa-

TABLE 103-3

Summary of Manifestations That May Be Helpful in Distinguishing Systemic Rheumatic Diseases

Disease	Clinical	Laboratory
Systemic lupus erythematosus	Females 8:1 Most common age at onset 15–40 Combinations of manifestations, e.g., fever (85%), skin lesions (85%) especially butterfly rash (30%), arthritis or arthralgias (90%), nephritis (60%), pleurisy and/or pericarditis (50%), central nervous system lesions (25%) especially psychosis	LE cells (75–80%) Antinuclear antibodies (95%) usually in high titer especially anti-nDNA, anti-Sm antibodies Leukopenia (70%) Hemolytic anemia (10%) or positive Coombs test (25%), BFP reaction Low serum complement Basement membrane immuno-fluoresence on skin biopsy Hematoxylin bodies in lymph node or kidney biopsy (rare) Focal necrotizing and membranous glomerulonephritis on renal biopsy
Progressive systemic sclerosis	Females 2:1 Most common age at onset 20–50 Scleroderma present in almost all patients, Raynaud's phenomenon (80%), altered intestinal motility, pulmonary fibrosis, myocardial failure, renal failure, and hypertension	None distinctive Skin biopsy may show typical pattern of scleroderma
Polymyositis (dermatomyositis)	Females 2:1 Most common age at onset 20–50 Proximal muscle weakness Heliotrope eruption on face or erythematous rash on extremities especially overlying joints	Elevated serum enzymes, such as SGOT and CPK Muscle biopsy showing inflammatory myopathy Electromyographic findings
Polyarteritis	Males 3:1 Most common age at onset 30–50 Combination of manifestations including fever, weight loss, myalgia and weakness, pulmonary lesions, nephritis, hypertension, focal infarction of heart, central nervous system, liver, etc. Peripheral neuropathy, especially mononeuritis multiplex	Leukocytosis Thrombocytosis Eosinophilia Necrotizing arteritis on biopsy
Rheumatoid arthritis	Females 2:1 Most common age at onset 30–50 Deforming, additive polyarthritis with synovial thickening, typical x-ray changes, subcutaneous nodules, muscle weakness (especially grip strength) Systemic features include arteritis with leg ulcers and peripheral neuropathy, pericarditis and pleurisy, pulmonary fibrosis, splenomegaly and Felty syndrome, sicca manifestations of Sjögren syndrome	Rheumatoid factors (80%) LE cells (20%) ANA positivity (30%) but usually in low titer Neutropenia (Felty syndrome) Thrombocytosis Hypocomplementemia (rare)

TABLE 103-4
Some of the Overlapping Clinical Manifestations of Systemic Rheumatic Diseases*

Disease	Fever	Erythematous Skin Eruption	Muscle Weakness	Rheumatoid-like Arthritis	Sicca Syndrome	Pleurisy or Pericarditis	Pulmonary Fibrosis	Myocardial Disease	Hypertension	Raynaud's Phenomenon	Altered Esophageal or Intestinal Motility	Nephritis	Focal Brain Involvement	Leukopenia	Hemolytic Anemia	Thrombocytosis
SLE	++	++	+	+	±	++	−	+	+	+	±	++	+	++	+	−
Progressive systemic sclerosis	−	−	+	+	±	+	+	+	+	++	++	+	−	−	±	±
Polymyositis	+	++	++	+	±	−	±	−	−	±	+	−	−	−	−	±
Polyarteritis	++	±	+	+	±	±	±	±	+	±	±	++	+	−	−	++
Rheumatoid arthritis	±	−	+	++	+	+	±	±	−	+	±	−	−	±	−	+

* Estimations of approximate frequency: ++ = > 50%; + = > 10%; ± = < 10%; − = not present.

TABLE 103-5
Overlapping Pathologic Manifestations of Systemic Rheumatic Disease*

Disease	Myositis	Glomerulonephritis	Lymphocytic Infiltration of Solid Organs	Lymphoid Hyperplasia	Perivascular Inflammation	Vasculitis	Necrotizing Arteritis
SLE	+	++	+	++	+	+	+
Progressive systemic sclerosis	+	+	−	±	+	+	−
Polymyositis	++	−	±	−	+	+	±
Polyarteritis	+	+	−	±	++	++	++
Rheumatoid arthritis	+	−	±	+	+	+	±

* Estimations of approximate frequency: ++ = > 50%; + = > 10%; ± = < 10%; − = not present.

tion and reevaluation will provide the final answer in such instances.

2. *In the presence of a definite connective tissue disorder, manifestations may develop which are far more characteristic of a second disease process.* The occurrence of a rheumatoidlike arthritis in associ-

ation with several disorders has already been mentioned. Overlapping immunologic manifestations are the most frequently encountered. The hypothesis that autoantibodies are specific for a certain disease is not tenable (Table 103-6). For example, although the LE-cell factor is more common in classical SLE, and

TABLE 103-6

Overlapping Serologic Manifestations of Systemic Rheumatic Disease*

Disease	Hypergammaglobulinemia	LE Cells	ANA	Rheumatoid Factor	Positive Coombs Test	BFP Reaction	Reduced Serum Complement
SLE	+ +	+ +	+ +	+	+	+	+ +
Progressive systemic sclerosis	±	±	+	+	−	±	−
Polymyositis	+	±	±	±	−	−	−
Polyarteritis	±	−	−	+	−	−	−
Rheumatoid arthritis	+	+	+	+ +	−	±	±

* Estimation of approximate frequency: + + = > 50%; + = > 10%; ± = < 10%; − = not present.

rheumatoid factor in typical rheumatoid arthritis, these antibodies are found in other diseases with considerable frequency and even occasionally in supposedly normal individuals. Thus, an immunologic reaction commonly associated with one disorder does not necessarily alter the diagnosis when it is present in another.

Combinations of overlapping clinical, pathologic, or immunologic manifestations may also occur in patients without altering the basic diagnosis. Thus, a patient with classical rheumatoid arthritis and LE cells who develops leukopenia, anemia, and ankle ulcers would still be considered by most authorities to have rheumatoid arthritis, not SLE. Similarly, the diagnosis of progressive systemic sclerosis rather than SLE would be made in a patient with typical scleroderma who has a pericardial effusion and antinuclear antibodies.

3. *Occasionally, one connective tissue disease tends to evolve into another or, less frequently, a complex illness emerges with features entirely characteristic of more than one disorder.* The coexistence of two disorders in a single patient is not uncommon. For example, a patient initially had features of SLE, including fever, arthritis, Raynaud's phenomenon, pleurisy, and LE cells. Then the LE-cell test became negative, and sclerodactylia, intestinal motor dysfunction, and pulmonary fibrosis subsequently became the dominant manifestations. This may be interpreted in several ways. The patient may be considered to have one disease (either SLE or progressive systemic sclerosis) with overlapping mani-

festations, or both diagnoses may be considered applicable, or it may be held that the diagnostic pattern of neither is complete and that the patient should be put in some intermediate category of having the "overlap syndrome." The patients with anti-ENA antibody and the combined features of SLE, scleroderma, and polymyositis are of special interest in this regard.

Another example of a high degree of overlap is the development of a generalized necrotizing arteritis indistinguishable from polyarteritis, or of typical SLE, including nephritis, in a patient who has apparently had rheumatoid arthritis for many years.

Significance of Overlap in Diagnosis

Continued reevaluation of syndromes that are not clinically well defined is important, since in such situations the exclusion of disorders of known etiology is more difficult. In those patients who defy precise nosologic classification, broad descriptive terms (for example, "incomplete or atypical connective tissue disease syndrome characterized by nondeforming polyarthritis, Raynaud's phenomenon, and antinuclear antibody") or the use of multiple designations (for example, "rheumatoid arthritis and scleroderma") may be required.

Finally, it must be reemphasized that the therapeutic approach to the patient is not determined by a diagnostic label. Thus, in patients with overlap syndromes as in those with well-defined disease entities, management will depend on the type and the severity of clinical manifestations.

CHAPTER 104

Ankylosing Spondylitis and Related Disorders
FRANK C. ARNETT, Jr.

The interrelationships between ankylosing spondylitis, Reiter syndrome, and psoriatic and colitic arthropathies are uncertain.[140,141] However, spondylitis and sacroiliitis are prominent articular features in each. Furthermore, the recent demonstration of the histocompatibility antigen HLA B27 in ankylosing spondylitis and those patients with the other disorders in which the spine is involved lends support to their consideration as a group.[139]

ANKYLOSING SPONDYLITIS
Ankylosing spondylitis (Marie-Strumpell arthritis) is primarily an inflammatory disease of the spine that results in fusion of the joints and ligamentous calcification.[9] In addition to the familial frequency of ankylosing spondylitis, an increased incidence of sacroiliitis, Reiter syndrome, and juvenile chronic polyarthritis is also found in the families of spondylitics. Ankylosing spondylitis is predominantly a disease of males (occurring nine times as often as in women) and has its onset in young adult life.

Articular Manifestations
Typically, the onset of back symptoms is insidious. Pain often located in the lumbar or buttock areas may be severe but usually is not and may even be absent. Muscle spasm may be prominent, and tenderness over the sacroiliac joints is often encountered. Stiffness and limitation of motion develop rapidly and spread gradually to involve the entire spine in most patients. Characteristically, a dorsal kyphosis develops and may reach grotesque proportions. Involvement of the hips with the appearance of flexion contractures is also common. A convenient way to follow the progress of this deformity is to have the patient stand as straight as he can, with his heels to the wall, and to measure the distance from the wall to the occiput. Fusion of the costovertebral joints and the facet joints of the vertebrae limits expansion of the chest. Because of this, breathing becomes largely diaphragmatic, but ventilatory function is usually not significantly impaired.

Peripheral joint involvement occurs most commonly in the hips and shoulders, with limitation of motion rather than pain. The manubriosternal joint may also be affected. Involvement of other peripheral joints is encountered occasionally, but many patients with such involvement are found to have psoriasis or Reiter syndrome.

Extra-Articular Manifestations
Signs of systemic disease in ankylosing spondylitis are rare. An acute polyarthritis resembling rheumatic fever or juvenile chronic arthritis sometimes occurs several months or years before back symptoms appear. Iritis occurs in 15 to 25 percent of patients and may precede the development of back symptoms. Rheumatoid nodules do not occur. Fixation of the rib cage and dorsal kyphosis reduces the vital capacity. Pulmonary emphysema, fibrosis, infection, and progressive insufficiency may follow. Rarely, apical fibrosis with cavitary lesions resembling tuberculosis is found. Occasionally, aortic regurgitation results from an inflammatory lesion that produces thickening of the aortic root and valvular cusps. Heart block may occur and is sometimes associated with aortic involvement. Occasionally, an ankylosing spondylitis is seen in association with ulcerative colitis and Crohn's disease.[133]

Laboratory Findings
The sedimentation rate is usually elevated in the active phase of the disease, and a mild anemia may occur. Tests for rheumatoid factor are negative. The HLA B27 histocompatibility antigen is found in almost all patients.[145]

Radiologic Features
Fusion and marginal sclerosis or obliteration of the sacroiliac joints are constant findings and may be the earliest abnormality detected. Spine involvement is confined primarily to the facets and costovertebral joints. The disk spaces are well maintained. Marginal sclerosis, erosion, and periosteal reaction are characteristic features. Fusion is accompanied by calcification in the anterior spinal ligament and actual bony bridging of all the vertebral segments, creating the appearance of a "bamboo" spine. Periosteal reaction also occurs in the pelvis, especially in the ischium, and results in a striking radiologic abnormality.

Diagnosis
Ankylosing spondylitis is characterized primarily by pain, stiffness, and limitation of motion of the spine and by the associated radiologic abnormalities. Certain diagnosis may not be possible before bony ankylosis or typical x-ray findings develop. The occurrence of sacroiliitis in a young man or the association of back pain with iritis may suggest the diagnosis in

this early phase. A summary of features helpful in differentiating ankylosing spondylitis from other arthritides of the spine is presented in Table 104–1.

Course

The disease progresses to spinal fusion in most instances.[9] When fusion is complete, pain often subsides, and if functional position has been maintained, little disability results. Nerve-root compression may occur but is rarely a serious problem. Subluxation of the upper cervical segments, with a consequent compression of the cord, is an unusual but potentially fatal event. Secondary amyloidosis has been reported in a few cases. Aortic regurgitation and complete heart block are also potentially serious but fortunately rare complications.

Management[9]

The prevention of deformity and the relief of pain are the major goals of therapy. Deformity can usually be prevented by physical therapy, a simple program of exercises, a firm mattress, and a low pillow. Salicylates may be helpful in relieving pain and merit initial trial. However, phenylbutazone or indomethacin are usually required for satisfactory results. The iritis may respond to topical corticosteroid but occasionally requires systemic administration for control.

REITER SYNDROME

Reiter syndrome[137,146] is the most frequent cause of arthritis in young men. Although often considered a venereal disease, venereal transmission has never been proved. Moreover, epidemic Reiter syndrome may follow acute bacillary dysentery.[142,143] In the sporadic case, recent studies indicate that a *Chlamydia* infection (microorganisms of the psittacosis-lymphogranuloma venereum-trachoma group) may be one cause of the disease.[144] Genetic factors also play a major role since HLA B27 occurs in most patients.

Clinical Manifestations

Although Reiter syndrome classically constitutes the triad of urethritis, arthritis, and conjunctivitis, a diagnosis is also possible without the ocular or urethral findings when characteristic skin lesions are present. These lesions, known as keratodermia blenorrhagica, appear on the palms of the hands and the soles of the feet and occasionally are present on the extremities or trunk. They appear first as erythematous macules and later become hyperkeratotic. Recent surveys of patients with gonococcal arthritis have failed to show any instances of keratodermia, and it is assumed that the older literature attributing this lesion to gonor-

rhea was inaccurate. Other skin lesions include a circinate balanitis, painless superficial ulcers of the oral mucosa, a chronic erythematous lesion resembling pustular psoriasis with yellow, hyperkeratotic scales, and nail lesions. Ocular involvement may be only a conjunctivitis, but iritis may develop. Urethritis usually precedes the onset of arthritis by days or weeks and often fails to respond to antibiotic treatment. In some cases the urethral discharge may be overlooked unless examination is performed before urination in the morning. Usually, however, the discharge is quite evident and accompanied by dysuria. Identification of gonorrheal organisms in the urethral discharge does not indicate with certainty that the subsequent arthritis is due to gonorrhea unless the organism is also demonstrated in the joints and the arthritis responds promptly to penicillin.

The joint disease of Reiter syndrome is usually acute in onset and may be monarticular or polyarticular. The lower extremities are most often affected, especially the knees and the ankles. Pain in the heels is common. Small joints of the hands and feet may be involved also. The pattern of joint involvement is characteristically asymmetric. For example, a single PIP joint in one hand, one knee, and the opposite ankle may be affected. The arthritis usually persists for several weeks and then gradually subsides. Deformity may develop, with recurrent or residual chronic arthritis, but this is seldom as disabling as in rheumatoid arthritis. Chronic synovial thickening is less marked than in rheumatoid arthritis, and some deformity may result from periostitis and new bone formation rather than from joint destruction per se. Spinal involvement is spotty and asymmetric. The sacroiliac articulations are often affected. In contrast to ankylosing spondylitis, fusion and ligamentous calcification are uncommon.

Systemic signs are present to some degree in Reiter syndrome. Fever of 102 to 103°F, persisting for days or weeks, may be seen in acute cases. Prolongation of the PR interval and, rarely, heart block may occur. Aortic regurgitation similar to that seen in ankylosing spondylitis has also been described in Reiter syndrome with spondylitis.

Laboratory Studies

Leukocytosis and elevation of sedimentation rate are common. Mild anemia also occurs. Tests for rheumatoid factor and antinuclear factor are negative. Synovial fluid is typically inflammatory, with cell counts up to 60,000/μl. Wright-Giemsa stain of synovial-fluid cells may demonstrate a number of large macrophages containing one or more ingested polymorphonuclear leukocytes. More than half the patients will

TABLE 104–1
Distinguishing Features of Arthritis of the Spine*

Disease	Age at Onset	Sex	Systemic Symptoms	Peripheral Arthritis	Area of Spine Involved	X-Ray Changes	Other Features
Ankylosing spondylitis	12–40	Males 9:1	±	Hips and shoulders	Entire spine	Obliteration of sacroiliac joints Sclerosis apophyseal joints Dorsal kyphosis Extensive fusion and ligamentous calcification	Negative rheumatoid factor Iritis 15 percent HLA B27 (90%)
Reiter syndrome	Young adults	Males 9:1	+ +	+ +	Sacroiliac joints Usually spotty, asymptomatic apophyseal joint disease	Extensive fusion uncommon except in sacroiliac joints	Eye disease Skin lesions Urethritis Negative rheumatoid factor HLA B27 (75%)
Psoriatic arthropathy	20–60	Both sexes	+	+ +	Same as Reiter	Same as Reiter	Skin lesions Negative rheumatoid factor HLA B27 (50%)
Colitic arthropathy	Children and young adults	Both sexes	+	+ +	Same as Reiter	Same as ankylosing spondylitis	Bowel involvement often subtle clinically Erythema nodosum Negative rheumatoid factor HLA B27 (50%)
Rheumatoid arthritis	Any age	Females 2:1	+	+ +	Upper cervical segments	Erosion, fusion rare Subluxation, cervical spine, especially C1–C2	Rheumatoid factor Negative HLA B27 Nodules
Degenerative arthritis	Over 35	Both sexes	−	±	Cervical and lumbar segments No sacroiliitis	Sclerosis and spur formation Spondylosis	Nerve root compression
Tuberculosis	Usually young adults	Both sexes	+	−	Thoracic or lumbar segments	Destructive lesion in disc space with anterior collapse	Tuberculosis elsewhere
Ochronosis	Over 30	Both sexes	−	+	Diffuse	Disc degeneration and calcification. Secondary degenerative changes	Hereditary alkaptonuria
Other infections	Any age	Both sexes	+	±	Disc space Apophyseal joints Unilateral sacroiliac	No change, or destructive lesions of bone	All rare Brucellosis Syphilis Acute bacterial IV drug abuse

* + + = A frequent or characteristic manifestation; + = usually present but sometimes absent; ± = an occasional finding; − = no association.

have the HLA B27 histocompatibility antigen, especially those with chronic disease and spondylitis.[139]

Radiologic Findings

No abnormalities may be noted early in the disease, but periarticular joint erosion closely resembling that of rheumatoid arthritis may develop subsequently. Periosteal reaction is often prominent and may be followed by new bone formation. Periostitis of the os calcis with or without the formation of a calcaneal spur, apparent on lateral films of the foot, is sufficiently characteristic to be of some diagnostic value when present. X-ray evidence of sacroiliitis and asymmetric spondylitis in association with peripheral arthritis should also suggest the diagnosis of Reiter syndrome.

Course

The acute episode usually subsides spontaneously after several weeks. Recurrences involving previously unaffected joints may occur at varying intervals, occasionally after a decade or more. Mild chronic symptoms may persist. A report on patients followed for many years suggests that recurrence and some degree of chronic symptoms may be the rule rather than the exception.[146] The overall prognosis, however, is good, and extensive disability and deformity occur infrequently.

Although urethritis, ocular signs, skin lesions, and arthritis usually occur simultaneously in the initial episode, subsequent recurrence of these lesions may occur independently or in incomplete combinations.

Management

The major goal of treatment is the relief of inflammation. Splinting may be helpful. When patients fail to respond to salicylates, phenylbutazone or indomethacin can be used. Infrequently, moderate doses of adrenal corticosteroids are required. Exacerbations often occur on reduction of dosage. The iritis may respond to local application of steroids. The skin and nail lesions are resistant to therapy but eventually subside in most cases. Occasionally, lesions indistinguishable from psoriasis may persist.

PSORIATIC ARTHROPATHY

Arthritis associated with psoriasis may take one of three clinical forms.[147] Psoriasis may occur in a patient with typical rheumatoid arthritis with rheumatoid nodules and positive rheumatoid-factor tests. This association is infrequent and probably represents the coincidental occurrence of two rather common diseases.

The second type of joint disease seen has been designated as psoriatic arthropathy because of the distinctive deep punctate pitting of the nails associated with a chronic arthritis of the DIP joints. Nodules do not occur in these patients, and the tests for rheumatoid factor are negative. The arthritis tends to be spotty in distribution and may be severely destructive or may be very mild and minimally disabling. Spine involvement, especially sacroiliitis, is seen at times.

In the third type, psoriasis is associated with a mild rheumatoid-like arthritis. Patients with this type do not have nail involvement, DIP arthritis, rheumatoid nodules, or rheumatoid factor. There seems to be no definite correlation between the severity of the psoriasis and that of the arthritis.

Elevation of uric acid occurs in many patients with active psoriasis, and an association with gout has been reported in a few cases.

The approach to the management of psoriatic arthropathy is similar to that employed in rheumatoid arthritis. Antimalarials, because of their tendency to exacerbate psoriasis, are not given to these patients. If satisfactory results cannot be achieved with acetylsalicylic acid, phenylbutazone or indomethacin, adrenal corticosteroids may be used. An antimetabolite such as methotrexate may control both skin and joint symptoms but should be reserved for patients with severe disease.[9]

COLITIC ARTHROPATHY

The term colitic arthropathy has been applied to the arthritis associated with ulcerative colitis and Crohn's disease.[133,134,136,138] It is usually an acute process of mild to moderate intensity involving one or more joints. Its activity relates closely to that of the bowel disease.[148] For example, after colectomy this type of arthritis goes into remission and does not recur unless the parent disease develops in the small bowel. Patients with this disorder do not usually develop chronic proliferative synovitis, so residual deformities do not occur. Nodules and rheumatoid factors are absent. In childhood the arthritis may precede evidence of colitis. Erythema nodosum is an occasional extra-articular feature which, when present, is a useful aid in the diagnosis of arthritis with inflammatory bowel disease.

Ulcerative colitis may be associated with classical rheumatoid arthritis with nodules, and in the few cases in which this occurs the association is presumably coincidental. In these instances the arthritis follows a course independent of the bowel disease.[148]

Finally, the association of sacroiliitis or spondylitis occurs in nearly 10 percent of patients with colitis, especially in those with HLA B27 antigen.[135,139,145] When these diseases are associated, their courses seem to be independent.

Since colitic arthropathy is usually a relatively mild disorder, it does not often present a difficult therapeutic problem per se. Salicylates are sufficient to control the symptoms in most cases. When the underlying bowel disease is brought under control, the arthropathy usually subsides.

JUVENILE CHRONIC ARTHRITIS (JCA)

Chronic arthritis in childhood has previously been termed juvenile rheumatoid arthritis (JRA) despite the broad variability in onset, clinical features, and course. Recent studies have shown that HLA B27 is found in over one-third of these children. The characteristics of this subset include late-childhood onset, male predominance, oligoarticular joint involvement with subsequent development of sacroiliitis and spondylitis, and acute iritis. Rheumatoid factors and ANA are absent. Thus, this HLA B27 group of children stand apart from those with JRA and relates more closely to those with ankylosing spondylitis or Reiter syndrome than to adult rheumatoid arthritis.

Therapy consists primarily of salicylates, possibly other NSAIDs and physical therapy. Corticosteroids are rarely required and, when necessary, should be given on alternate days to minimize growth effects.

CHAPTER 105

Gout and Pseudogout

DAVID S. NEWCOMBE

GOUT

Gout is a derangement of purine metabolism that results in hyperuricemia, crystalline deposits of urate in tissues (tophi), and recurrent episodes of acute arthritis. There are two well-recognized forms of gout in which the acute arthritis is similar: primary gout, which is related to inborn metabolic errors, and secondary gout, in which hyperuricemia is produced by either an increased breakdown of nucleic acids in certain diseases or interference with renal excretion of urate.

CLINICAL MANIFESTATIONS

Incidence

Primary gout is largely a disease of males. Onset before puberty is rare, and the incidence rises appreciably in early middle age. Primary gout and tophi are rare in females before the menopause. In rare cases, primary gout is inherited as an X-linked recessive; but in most cases, the familial occurrence suggests either sex-influenced autosomal dominant or multifactorial inheritance. A positive family history of gouty arthritis was obtained in slightly more than 50 percent of patients with gout in one reported series, with other series reporting familial occurrence of as low as 11 percent.[166]

Articular Manifestations

THE ACUTE GOUTY ATTACK. The onset is abrupt and may follow trauma, illness, operation, fasting, or dietary indiscretion, or may have no discernible stimulus. Intense inflammation develops with surprising rapidity. The patient may report being well on retiring and being unable to walk on arising. The metatarsal-phalangeal joint of the great toe is a typical site of the acute attack (podagra). Involvement of other joints is also common, especially the ankle, knee, wrist, and elbow, and small joints of the hands or feet. Bursitis (especially olecranon) may occur with or without simultaneous joint involvement. The acute episode is generally monarticular but may affect several joints at once or in sequence.

Fever (101 to 103°F) is often present. The joint involved becomes painful and swollen and often red. Tenderness is so exquisite that the patient cannot move the affected joint or even bear the weight of the bedclothes. The inflammatory process often extends above and below the joint suggesting in some instances a cellulitis or superficial thrombophlebitis. Extensive effusions may occur in a large joint, such as the knee. If no treatment is given, the acute episode will subside in a period of days, leaving no residual changes. Recurrence, however, is characteristic, and the history of repeated episodes of acute arthritis, especially when monarticular or involving the great toe, should always suggest the possibility of gout. Recurrent attacks frequently involve the same joint; and once recurrence is established, there is wide variation in the frequency and severity of the acute attacks. Many patients with recurrent gout (especially women and those whose gout began late in life) never develop chronic arthritis or tophaceous deposits, even if their disease is not treated. During the interval between attacks (intercritical gout) these patients may have no manifestations of the disease other than hyperuricemia.

CHRONIC GOUTY ARTHRITIS. Chronic gouty arthritis occurs primarily in patients who have tophaceous gout. In some patients, especially those in whom uricosuric drugs have been only partially effective, chronic arthritis may occur in the absence of visible or palpable tophi. These patients often have x-ray evidence of urate deposition in bone adjacent to the joints.

Chronic gouty arthritis may cause morning stiffness, aching in various joints (especially in bad weather), as well as swelling, and pain on motion of joints, even during the intercritical period. Acute attacks of arthritis continue to occur and are commonly polyarticular. Effusions and synovial thickening may persist after the acute attack subsides. Deformity may result from the deposit of urate, with the displacement of soft tissue or bony substance. In its chronic and polyarticular form, gout may closely resemble rheumatoid arthritis, and one is sometimes tempted to make a dual diagnosis. However, these disorders rarely occur together.

Extra-Articular Manifestations

TOPHI. The formation of soft tissue deposits of sodium urate increases with the severity of hyperuricemia and its duration. Tophaceous deposits are commonly found in bursae, especially the olecranon and prepatellar bursae; in the cartilage of the ear; in tendon sheaths; in articular cartilage and bone; and in soft tissue immediately adjacent to joints, especially in the fingers and toes.

Tophi may be confused with rheumatoid nodules, especially when they occur in the olecranon bursa or on the extensor surface of the forearm in association with polyarticular gout. The gouty nodule is more gritty and irregular in consistency than the rheumatoid nodule, but biopsy may be required for differentiation. Superficial deposits form small, whitish plaques or nodules having hard, irregular, gritty surfaces. These may break through the overlying skin and discharge a chalklike material which contains urate crystals.

Deposits of urate in tissue sites may result in damage or dysfunction. A tophus on a heart valve causing a heart murmur, and in the vocal cord producing hoarseness and obstruction are examples of this rare clinical event.

RENAL CALCULI. About 10 to 20 percent of gout patients eventually develop urate stones. These are radiolucent unless mixed with calcium salts. Since asymptomatic hyperuricemia may precede acute gouty arthritis, urate stones may be the presenting manifestation of gout. Urate stones may also occur in patients with hyperuricemia who never develop arthritis and in a few patients without hyperuricemia who have persistently low urine pHs. Urate renal calculi are more likely to occur in patients with secondary gout because of their very high serum and urine concentrations of uric acid. Following therapy for the primary disorder (e.g., leukemia), a massive precipitation of urate may occur and cause acute renal failure.

RENAL DISEASE AND HYPERTENSION. Chronic renal disease, as evidenced by hyposthenuria, mild proteinuria, and mild azotemia, is often associated with severe gout. Severe renal insufficiency rarely develops in the absence of hypertension.[166] Multiple factors contribute to gouty nephropathy. The deposit of urates in the renal tubules may cause local obstruction and may predispose to infection. Hypertension and vascular disease may add to the tissue damage.

The relation of hypertension to the renal disease is complex. It is often not clear whether hypertension is a primary event or one secondary to the renal disease. There is a high incidence and earlier than usual onset of hypertension in gouty subjects. The study of family members of patients with hyperuricemia and gout suggests that primary gout and hypertension are inherited by separate though perhaps related genetic factors.

LABORATORY MANIFESTATIONS

Hematologic Findings

Acute gout is usually accompanied by leukocytosis and elevation of the erythrocyte sedimentation rate, and other acute-phase reactants. These findings may be present to a variable degree in chronic gouty arthritis.

Hyperuricemia is helpful but does not establish the diagnosis of gout. It may be observed in asymptomatic individuals and in those with renal insufficiency and as the result of the administration of a drug such as chlorothiazide (Table 105-1). It is also seen in other disorders that may cause joint symptoms, such as psoriasis and sarcoidosis.

TABLE 105-1
Drugs That Affect Serum and Urinary Uric Acid Concentration*

Drugs That May Increase Serum Uric Acid Concentrations
1. Small doses of salicylate (<2 g per 24 hours)
2. Thiazide diuretics
3. Acetazolamide
4. Pyrazinamide
5. Ethambutal

Drugs That May Decrease Serum Uric Acid Concentrations
1. Large doses of salicylates (4-6 g per 24 hours)
2. Phenylbutazone, oxyphenylbutazone
3. Probenecid
4. Sulfinpyrazone
5. Allopurinol
6. Corticosteroids and ACTH
7. Coumarin compounds
8. Estrogens
9. Glyceryl guaiacolate (Robitussin)
10. Organic iodides (contrast dyes)

* Colchicine has no effect on serum uric acid.

Analysis of Synovial Fluid

The synovial fluid in acute gout is typical of inflammatory reactions, showing decreased viscosity, poor mucin clot, polymorphonuclear leukocytosis (5000 to 50,000/μl), an increase in protein content, and sometimes a slight reduction in glucose. Urate crystals can be identified in at least 90 percent of cases and provide the absolute diagnostic criterion.[160] They are not as uniformly needlelike as in tissue tophi but can be identified within white cells or extracellularly by polarized light microscopy. Urates stand out brightly when the Nicol prisms are crossed and the field is almost completely dark. Furthermore, with select filters, urate crystals demonstrate characteristic negative birefringence in compensated polarized light. Urate crystals are difficult to detect with regular light microscopy.

Biopsy

Identification of typical crystalline deposits may be made in a soft-tissue mass or synovial membrane removed by biopsy. The solubility of urates in aqueous solutions requires that absolute alcohol be used as a fixative for their preservation for histologic identification.

Radiologic Abnormalities

There are no x-ray findings in early gout except possible soft tissue swelling. With continued urate deposition, punched-out, radiolucent areas of varying size develop in the bone adjacent to involved joints. The defects are often larger than those of rheumatoid ar-

thritis and have irregular margins (Fig. 105-1). Furthermore, periarticular osteoporosis is not usually present, but marginal erosions are occasionally seen in gout.

DIAGNOSIS

The diagnosis of gout is strongly suggested in a male by the typical attack of acute arthritis frequently involving the great toe and by the history of recurrent attacks. A positive family history of primary gout and a history of renal calculi are also important diagnostic leads. The presence of tophi is diagnostic. In most patients the diagnosis rests on the clinical history and physical findings in conjunction with hyperuricemia, and the presence of urate crystals in the synovial fluid or tissues.

PATHOGENESIS

Mechanisms of Hyperuricemia[151,153,165]

Hyperuricemia represents an imbalance between endogenous production of uric acid (de novo biosynthesis or nucleic acid turnover), dietary intake, and renal or gastrointestinal urate excretion. In man, only abnormalities of endogenous production and/or renal excretion are significant pathogenic factors. Primary gout is characterized, at least in a substantial number of gouty subjects, by an overproduction of uric acid. A deficiency in a purine biosynthetic enzyme, hypoxanthine-guanine phosphoribosyltransferase (HGPRT), has been established as one mechanism of uric acid overproduction.[154] An X-linked partial HGPRT deficiency has been associated with especially severe gouty arthritis of early onset.[150] A glutaminase deficiency has also been postulated, but the evidence is incomplete. There appears to be more than one mechanism of production of hyperuricemia in primary gout. A renal defect has been suggested in some gouty subjects who are not obvious overproducers of uric acid.[163]

In secondary gout the excessive uric acid is derived from the breakdown of purine. Thus, secondary gout occurs with a variety of diseases associated with an overproduction and destruction of cells, especially blood cells (Table 105-2). Serum urates in patients with secondary gout are generally higher than in those with primary gout. Secondary gout more often arises as a result of the administration of drugs that interfere with the excretion of urate. It may occur in patients with chronic renal failure and in obese subjects on starvation diets. The hyperuricemia in the last situation may partly result from the competition of ketones and organic acids with urate in the tubular secretion of uric acid.

The renal mechanism for the secretion of urate seems to be important in the pathogenesis of gout, as

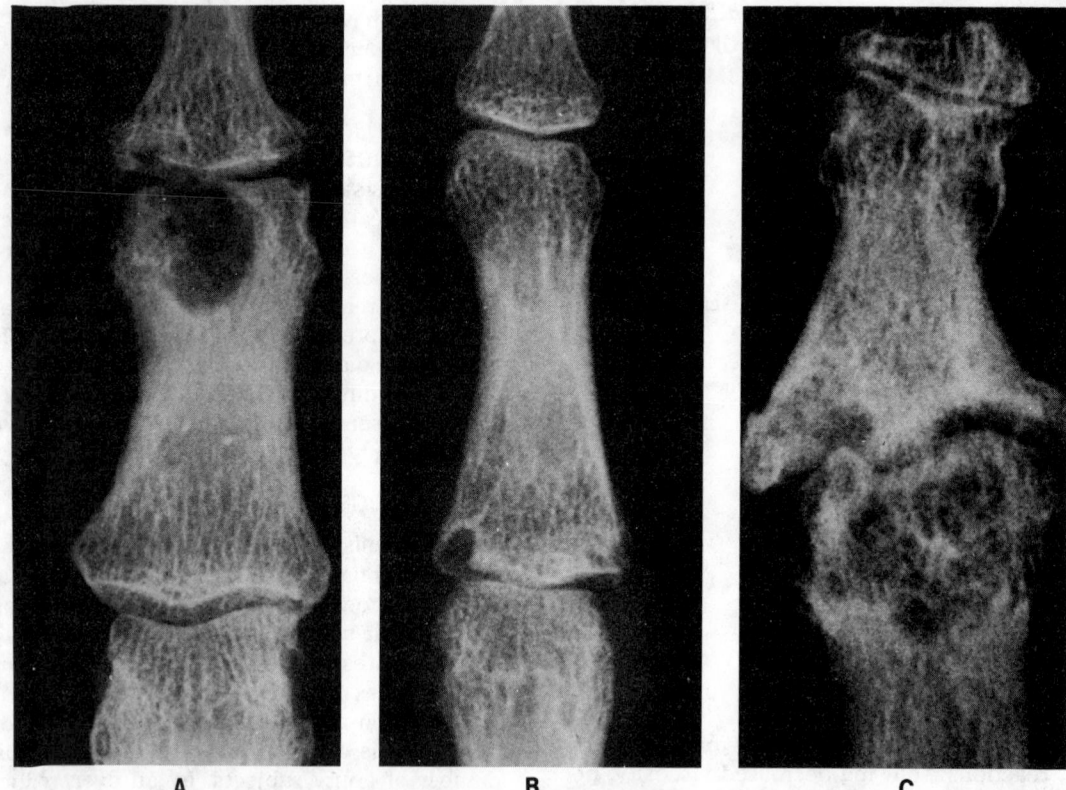

A   **B**   **C**

FIGURE 105–1. Comparison of punched-out lesions of gout, rheumatoid arthritis, and degenerative joint disease. **A.** A large punched-out lesion in the phalanx adjacent to and communicating with the distal interphalangeal joint (DIP) in a patient with tophaceous gout. There is no bony reaction around the defect or at the margin of the joint, no osteoporosis, and the joint space is not narrowed. There is a tophus in the adjacent soft tissue which accounts for the soft tissue enlargement. **B.** "Punched-out" erosion at the proximal interphalangeal (PIP) joint of a patient with rheumatoid arthritis. Note also the soft tissue swelling, osteoporosis, narrowing of the joint space, and smaller irregular erosions on both sides of the PIP joint. The DIP joint is not affected. **C.** Lesion of severe degenerative joint disease. There are many punched-out defects or pseudocysts in the bone adjacent to the PIP joint. There is narrowing and irregular destruction of the joint space. There is also marked bony proliferation at both margins of the joint with overhanging edges. Soft tissue enlargement corresponds to the bony prominences. Note also similar involvement at the DIP joint.

is the effect of various drugs on serum urate concentration.[152,152a,163] Normally, serum urate is completely filtered at the glomerulus and nearly completely reabsorbed in the proximal tubule. An active secretory mechanism in the distal tubule is responsible for the total urinary urate. This is also a site at which drugs may block urate secretion and promote the retention of urate in the serum. Drugs that are uricosuric act by blocking the reabsorption of urate in the proximal tubule. These drugs also often block tubular secretion but so overwhelm the reabsorption mechanism that the net effect is increased loss of uric acid in the urine. This accounts for the paradoxic effect of such drugs as salicylates, which may cause urate retention

at low doses by blocking the tubular secretion mechanism and which are uricosuric at high doses because of their effect on reabsorption.

Mechanism of Acute Attack

With acute gout, leukocytosis and phagocytosis of crystals by synovial-fluid leukocytes and sometimes synovial membrane cells occur.[161,167] Furthermore, the injection of microcrystalline urate into normal or gouty joints produces leukocytosis, phagocytosis of crystals, and acute inflammation.[164] The exact mechanism by which phagocytosis is stimulated, however, has not been elucidated. As a sequel to phagocytosis, leukocytes release their lysosomal enzymes, which

TABLE 105–2
**Causes of Secondary Gout
and Hyperuricemia**

Increased Nucleic Acid Turnover

Myeloid metaplasia

Polycythemia

Chronic leukemia (especially myelogenous)

Lymphosarcoma and Hodgkin's disease (especially
  under treatment)

Chronic hemolytic anemia

Acute leukemia (rare)

Psoriasis

Decreased Renal Excretion

Drug administration (especially thiazides,
  pyrazinamide)

Renal failure (including lead nephropathy, toxemia)

Ketoacidosis (diabetic, starvation)

Acute ethanol ingestion

apparently cause tissue injury and intensify inflammation. The metabolic activity that accompanies phagocytosis of urate crystals may cause a lowering of the pH of the joint fluid, and in the patient with hyperuricemia this may result in further crystallization of urates, further phagocytosis, and so on, in a perpetuating cycle.[151,164] Colchicine can inhibit the metabolic activity of leukocytes and their release of lysosomal enzymes and possibly in this way may interrupt the cycle.[162]

MANAGEMENT

The Acute Attack

Phenylbutazone is the drug of choice in managing acute gouty arthritis. The administration of 600 to 800 mg during the first 24 hours and 300 mg for three or four succeeding days is usually effective. Indomethacin also provides prompt relief in most patients. Reliance on oral colchicine as the sole agent for treating acute gout (0.5 mg given every 2 hours until response or gastrointestinal toxicity supervene) has lost favor in view of the severe nausea and diarrhea which frequently occur. Intravenous colchicine, 1 mg initially and 0.5 mg 6 to 12 hours later (not exceeding a total dose of 2 mg), is also effective and may avoid the gastrointestinal effects. Uricosuric drugs should never be used in the treatment of the acute attack. Once the acute attack is resolved, if it is the first attack, no other therapy may be indicated. If there is a history of recurrent attacks, the chronic administration of colchicine, 1.0 to 1.5 mg daily is effective and safe prophylaxis.

Diet is no longer severely restricted in patients with gout, because of the difficulty of maintaining a truly low purine intake, the relatively small effect that normal dietary intake of purine has on urate levels, and the greater efficacy of prophylactic colchicine and uricosuric drugs in controlling the disease. Only foods very high in purine, such as glandular meats, should be avoided. If a patient must lose weight, gradual loss is advisable because of the decreased urate secretion by the kidney resulting from severe caloric restriction.

Adequate fluid intake is important in the prevention of urate renal calculi. If uricosuric therapy is given, forcing fluids is essential. Alkalinization of the urine to maintain a pH above 7.0 by the administration of sodium bicarbonate or citrate may also be helpful in preventing urate stones.

Measures To Lower Serum Uric Acid

There is no general agreement concerning the indications for the administration of drugs to lower serum uric acid. The presence of tophi is a definite reason for their use. In the patient without tophi, a history of recurrent episodes, despite the prophylactic administration of colchicine, is also an indication. A persistent serum uric-acid level of 9 mg/dl or higher may be the basis for their administration, as may evidence of developing impairment of renal function. These drugs, when they are effective in lowering serum uric acid, can promote the slow resolution of tophi and, in the long run, may appreciably reduce the incidence of acute gout. Thus, in general, they should be administered in all except the mild cases of gout, which can be maintained with a minimal number of acute attacks on prophylaxis with colchicine alone for many years. The decision to administer uricosuric drugs does not alter the necessity for the administration of prophylactic colchicine until the patient has been free from acute attacks for many months or years.

Probenecid is the oldest and the safest uricosuric agent. The initial dose should be 0.5 g every 12 hours. This may be increased up to 3 g daily if necessary. Some patients, especially those with some renal dysfunction, will not respond adequately to this agent, and sulfinpyrazone (Anturane) may be effective as an alternative. This drug is relatively short-acting and has to be given at 6-hour intervals in divided doses ranging from 0.3 to 1.0 g daily. The serum uric acid must be monitored and the dosage of uricosuric agents adjusted to achieve the therapeutic objective of reducing the serum uric-acid level to 6 mg/dl or less whenever possible. Once initiated, uricosuric drugs should probably be continued indefinitely.

Allopurinol causes a profound reduction of serum uric acid by blocking the metabolic pathway of uric-acid production, specifically inhibiting xanthine oxidase.[155] Since this agent does not produce its effect through the kidney and actually reduces renal urate load, it is particularly useful in patients who have renal disease or renal calculi and in those with severe secondary hyperuricemia, such as occurs during the treatment of leukemia and lymphomas. The initial dose of 100 mg of allopurinol twice daily may be gradually increased to 600 mg daily to achieve the desired effect. It may be used in conjunction with uricosuric agents.

Surgery to remove large tophi, especially those which are draining, causing deformity, or interfering with normal function, is occasionally indicated.

The most common cause of failure of therapy in gout is inadequate follow-up and continuation of therapy. If treatment is managed wisely and begun early enough, it should be possible to prevent the occurrence of tophi and chronic gouty arthritis.

PSEUDOGOUT

Pseudogout is a microcrystalline synovitis induced by crystals of calcium pyrophosphate dihydrate[158] and associated with calcification of hyaline and fibrocartilage (chondrocalcinosis). More properly, this disorder is now named *calcium pyrophosphate dihydrate (CPPD) crystal deposition disease*. While the mechanism of cartilage calcification is poorly understood, the association of chondrocalcinosis and pseudogout with an array of disease processes suggest that multiple factors play a role. Although no cause and effect relationships have been established certain genetic (e.g., hemochromatosis, Wilson's disease) and metabolic (e.g., hyperparathyroidism, acromegaly, hypothyroidism) disorders have been observed with unusual frequency.[159] Moreover, there is a familial form of chondrocalcinosis.

Pseudogout is rare before the fifth decade and increases in frequency with advancing age, which may help to explain an apparent association with degenerative osteoarthropathy.

CLINICAL MANIFESTATIONS

The term pseudogout was coined to emphasize the acute, episodic, goutlike attacks of synovial inflammation which are so characteristic of the disorder. Unlike gout, the large joints are preferentially involved in CPPD crystal deposition disease, especially the knee which is the most frequent site of arthritis found in over half the cases. Involvement of the shoulder, hip, wrist, elbow and, rarely, small joints of the hands (MCP joints) also occurs, and acute inflammation of the first metatarsophalangeal joint can mimic gouty podagra. Generally, episodes of pseudogout are less intense and more protracted than those of gout. In both disorders, surgery and trauma are common precipitating events. The only extra-articular feature of illness is the low grade fever which frequently accompanies the acute attack.

In more than half the patients with chondrocalcinosis, multiple joint involvement occurs with a chronic and progressive arthritis in some cases mimicking rheumatoid arthritis and in others leading to articular changes indistinguishable from degenerative osteoarthropathy.[157] Flexion contractures, especially of the knees, commonly develop.

LABORATORY MANIFESTATIONS

Hematologic findings are nonspecific. The sedimentation rate is elevated during acute attacks, and a mild polymorphonuclear leukocytosis may occur. Serum studies are normal except as related to associated diseases. The finding of hyperuricemia or, in the elderly, rheumatoid factor may confuse the picture and often delays diagnosis.

Synovial Fluid

The synovial fluid in acute pseudogout is typical of an inflammatory process except that a good mucin clot forms on exposure to dilute acetic acid in most instances, indicating a normal or near normal hyaluronate concentration. A leukocytosis (2000 to 50,000 cells/μl), predominantly polymorphonuclear, is present, the degree of white cell response relating to the duration and intensity of the acute attack. Intra- and extracellular crystals of calcium pyrophosphate can be identified in over 95 percent of effusions with careful examination.[156] In ordinary light microscopy, the needle forms are difficult to distinguish from urate crystals and even the more characteristic rodlike and rhomboid forms can be easily overlooked. With polarized light, calcium pyrophosphate crystals are not as highly refractive as urates and with select filters, calcium pyrophosphate crystals demonstrate weakly positive birefringence.

As in gout, microcrystalline deposits are found in the synovial membrane.[149]

Radiologic Abnormalities

Chondrocalcinosis is the characteristic finding with linear, sometimes punctate or stippled, calcifications in the fibrocartilagenous menisci of the knees most frequently seen. Additional common sites of calcification include the radioulnar joint, the symphysis pubis, the articular discs of the sternoclavicular joints and,

treatment if the organism is sensitive and if the dosage employed is adequate. In gonococcal or pneumococcal arthritis, for example, parenteral procaine penicillin in a dose of 600,000 units every 6 hours is generally rapidly effective. Organisms resistant to penicillin were isolated from military personnel in Southeast Asia. In patients with penicillin-resistant gonococcal arthritis or known allergy to penicillin, tetracycline, 500 mg every 6 hours, should be given. If a relatively resistant organism such as staphylococcus is suspected, larger doses of antibiotics should be employed (e.g., 12 million units of penicillin daily). The use of a penicillinase-resistant compound such as methacillin is advisable until sensitivities are known. The intrasynovial injection of antibiotics is not necessary in most infections. Of course, treatment of the primary focus of infection should not be neglected.

TUBERCULOUS ARTHRITIS

The incidence of tuberculous arthritis has declined markedly with the availability of antituberculosis drugs and with improved early case-finding. However, tuberculous joint disease is still seen with some frequency, and early recognition is important because prompt treatment may prevent severe destruction of the involved joint.[169,170]

Clinical Manifestations

Tuberculous arthritis arises through hematogenous spread from an active focus of tuberculous activity elsewhere than in the joints. Some patients present mainly with arthritic complaints, their primary tuberculous foci being quiescent. In an equal number, the evidences of disseminated tuberculosis may dominate the clinical presentation.

The spinal joints are commonly affected, especially in children and young adults (Pott's disease). Pain, tenderness, and muscle spasm are usually present in the area involved but may not be noticed in children until an abnormality of gait or posture develops. Progressive destruction of the disc space and vertebral body produces a kyphotic deformity. Adjacent soft-tissue abscesses often form and may impinge on nerve roots or may cause cord compression.

In peripheral joints, the disease is generally monarticular, involving a large joint, especially the hip or knee. Pain, limitation of motion, and swelling are usually observed. The swelling is commonly unaccompanied by heat and is sometimes described as "doughy" because the synovial enlargement is accompanied by a relatively small effusion. A tenosynovitis at the wrist, especially on its volar aspect, may be encountered. Grating or creaking may be observed as the tendons move within their irregular, thickened sheaths. Remissions and exacerbations of symptoms are not uncommon, and the course of the disorder may be surprisingly indolent.

Laboratory Findings

The synovial-fluid white cell count is elevated, and the glucose content is markedly reduced. Organisms are occasionally found on smear, but culture of the fluid is more likely to yield positive results. Synovial biopsy should be performed if other tests have not confirmed the diagnosis.

X-rays early in the course may be negative or may show only localized osteoporosis and soft-tissue swelling. As the lesion progresses, marginal erosions and decreased bone density are seen. Bone necrosis producing radiodensities on either side of the joint is a late finding. Eventually, extensive narrowing and destruction of the joint space and subchondral bone become evident. In the spine, the disc space is involved first and the body of the vertebra soon after, causing partial collapse or erosion of the vertebra anteriorly.

Management

If begun early in the disease, prolonged treatment with antituberculosis drugs and immobilization of the involved joint may be sufficient therapy.[170] However, surgical intervention is generally required to drain abscesses or remove necrotic debris. If the joint surface or bone has been extensively involved, fusion of the joint may be necessary. At times, when the diagnosis is strongly suspected, therapy may be initiated prior to bacteriologic confirmation to avoid joint destruction.

VIRAL ARTHRITIS

Several viral infections including mumps, infectious hepatitis, smallpox, erythema infectiosum, and rubella may be associated with acute polyarthritis.[168,172,180,183] Because of the benign course of the viral arthritides, it is important to recognize and differentiate these disorders from the more serious forms of acute arthritis which they may mimic. Best characterized is rubella arthritis which has an abrupt onset, usually beginning a few days after the morbilliform rash is first evident but occasionally appearing only after the rash has completely faded. Malaise, fever, and posterior cervical lymphadenopathy are characteristically present. The most commonly affected joints are the small joints of the hands, wrists, knees, and ankles. A migratory pattern of arthritis may occur with joint effusions often present. Tenosynovitis is common.

Leukopenia is sometimes found. Joint fluid may show a mononuclear-cell or polymorphonuclear reaction with 10,000 to 30,000 cells/μl and an abnormal mucin clot. The rheumatoid-factor test is positive on occasion. A rise in rubella antibody titer in convalescent serum allows a specific diagnosis.

The arthritis responds well to salicylates in most cases with prompt relief of symptoms although effusions may persist for several days. All symptoms and signs usually subside within one week, and there is no recurrence or residual joint abnormality.[183]

ARTHRITIS CAUSED BY SYPHILIS

Arthritis caused by syphilis is relatively uncommon.[171] Arthralgia and a transient polyarthritis are seen as manifestations of secondary syphilis. Gum-matous involvement may occur in tertiary infections. Congenital syphilis[171] is characterized by two types of joint lesions. One variety, seen in children in the first weeks of life, results from an osteochondritis occurring just below the epiphysis. Periarticular swelling and periosteal thickening may be demonstrated on x-ray. The second type, Clutton joints, is the more common. Symmetric involvement of the knees or elbows may result in persistent, painless effusions that eventually resolve and recur. Spirochetes are not present in the joint fluid or synovial tissues. This late manifestation of congenital syphilis may continue into young adult life. Interstitial keratitis may be present at the same time. The serologic test for syphilis is usually positive in patients with Clutton joints. Treatment may not alter the course of the disorder.

CHAPTER 107

Degenerative Joint Disease

MARY BETTY STEVENS AND ALEXANDER S. TOWNES

Degenerative joint disease, or osteoarthropathy, is a noninflammatory disorder that affects the joint cartilage primarily and, to a lesser extent, the synovial membrane.[184,186,190,191] Degeneration of the superficial layers of the articular cartilage results in fragmentation and shedding of fibrils into the joint spaces. This change is followed by proliferation of subchondral bone, resulting in marginal spur formation. There are no systemic manifestations characteristic of this disease. Although the terms *degenerative joint disease*, *osteoarthritis*, *osteoarthrosis*, and *hypertrophic arthritis*, are used synonymously, the term *degenerative joint disease* is best because it emphasizes the essential nature of the disorder.

CLINICAL MANIFESTATIONS

Incidence

Degenerative joint disease is the most prevalent form of arthropathy. Its incidence increases with age, the majority of those over 60 being affected. Many individuals are asymptomatic or nearly so. In others, the onset and severity of the disorder have been related to several factors. The presence of Heberden's nodes (marginal bony proliferation at the DIP joints) and Bouchard's nodes (similar bony lesions at the PIP joints) follows a hereditary pattern with female preponderance.[185] When related to trauma, postural defects, obesity, or prior inflammatory arthritis, degen-erative arthritis is often referred to as secondary in type. When no precipitating factors save heredity can be identified, the disorder is called primary.

Articular Manifestations

The gradual onset of pain, stiffness, or aching in one or more joints is frequently first noted in middle life or beyond. Occasionally, minor trauma may precipitate symptoms. Pain in weight-bearing joints may be greatest after activity and may subside on rest. The stiffness after rest that is often noted is generally not so prolonged as it is in rheumatoid arthritis. Major disability rarely results, except when the knees or hips are involved.

On examination, signs of inflammation of the joint or surrounding soft tissues are rarely encountered. Swelling is minimal or absent and effusions infrequently detected, except in the knees. Inflammation and effusion may be related to superimposed trauma, to the stress of continual weight bearing, to loose bodies within the joint, or to an intercurrent condition. Deformities result largely from marginal bony overgrowth (osteophytes) and from the loss of articular cartilage, rather than from soft-tissue abnormalities. Crepitus is frequently felt.

The pattern of joint involvement is of some importance in differential diagnosis. Weight-bearing joints are the most common sites of symptoms. In the hands, involvement of the DIP joints (Heberden's nodes) is commonly asymptomatic, whereas PIP involvement (Bouchard's nodes) may cause stiffness. The MCP joints of the hands and wrists are rarely involved.

Involvement of the knee joint may affect the patella also. Symptoms on walking or stair climbing result from the sliding of the uneven surface of the patella over the femur. Degeneration of cartilage on both sides of the tibiofemoral joint, especially on the medial aspect of the tibial plateau, produces some distortion of the joint space, so motion may be limited and lateral instability may result. New bone formation or a loose body occasionally produces a mechanical block to motion of the joint, limiting flexion more commonly than extension.

Involvement of the hip joint may result in pain which is referred to the thigh, knee, or groin and which is usually greatest upon bearing weight. Pain and limitation of motion of the hip (internal rotation, extension, and/or abduction) are frequent associated findings.

Primary generalized osteoarthritis is a syndrome to be differentiated from rheumatoid arthritis. Most patients are females, who are affected 10 times as often as males, and are of menopausal age. Involvement of the DIP and PIP joints and the carpal-metacarpal joints of the thumbs, as well as the knees, hips, and spine, is common. The polyarticular nature of the disorder, and the occasional occurrence of mild inflammatory changes in the joints, may be suggestive of rheumatoid arthritis. However, the presence of bony (not soft-tissue) enlargement of the finger joints, the sparing of MCP joints and wrists, the absence of systemic signs, and the radiologic findings permit ready differentiation of this disorder from the inflammatory arthritides.

Erosive osteoarthritis is a variant more difficult at times to distinguish from rheumatoid arthritis because of recurrent inflammatory episodes and a proliferative synovitis which leads to cartilage destruction and occasionally bony ankylosis. This process, affecting the DIP, PIP, and occasionally, MCP joints of middle-aged women, is felt to be distinct from either classical osteoarthropathy or seronegative rheumatoid arthritis. The sedimentation rate is normal or only minimally elevated and tests for rheumatoid factor are negative. X-ray examination is most helpful in supporting the diagnosis.[189]

Involvement of the spine is asymptomatic in the vast majority of patients. The lower cervical and lumbar segments are most prone to the development of symptoms and associated degenerative disc disease. Bony spurs may compress nerve roots leading to characteristic pain and neurologic deficits.[188] Tenderness over the segment affected or pain on extremes of motion of that segment may aid in determining its location. Forced hyperextension (pressure applied downward on the forehead when the neck is extended) may reproduce symptoms when the lower cervical segments are involved. Marked flexion is likely to cause discomfort in upper-cervical disease.

LABORATORY AND RADIOLOGIC MANIFESTATIONS

Laboratory Findings

There are evidences neither of local inflammation nor of systemic disease. The synovial fluid is viscid, has few white cells, and usually has a good mucin clot.[16] Cartilage fibrils may be found in the joint fluid, but their finding cannot be considered specific.

Radiologic Abnormalities

Narrowing of the joint space secondary to the loss of radiolucent cartilage occurs early. Subchondral sclerosis and marginal spur formation then develop and are the radiologic hallmarks of the disease. Osteoporosis is not a feature of degenerative joint disease. Erosions are also uncommon. Subchondral cysts are often seen and can be differentiated from erosions of rheumatoid arthritis, since the bony cortex overlying the cyst remains intact. (See Fig. 105–1C.) In the spine, narrowing of the disc space is seen early, followed by bony proliferation at the anterior margins of the vertebral body. Spur formation also occurs posteriorly, tending to encroach on the neural foramina. Oblique views of the spine are helpful in demonstrating this latter finding. Views in flexion and extension are also useful, especially in the cervical spine.

DIAGNOSIS

Degenerative joint disease is characterized by its noninflammatory nature and by the lack of systemic involvement. Symptomatic disease, which infrequently results in marked disability, is most likely to develop in weight-bearing joints. The typical physical and radiologic findings result from the degeneration of articular cartilage and overgrowth of subchondral bone.

A major problem in diagnosis results from the prevalence of degenerative joint disease, especially in older individuals. Degenerative arthritis is asymptomatic in most individuals so affected. Thus, one must evaluate all complaints carefully if one is to avoid the common error of ascribing them to easily demonstrable degenerative joint lesions.

MANAGEMENT

An important initial step to take in the management of symptomatic degenerative joint disease is to reassure patients about the nature of the disorder, its usual indolent course, and good prognosis. When weight-bearing joints are involved, rest from bearing weight is advisable. With spine involvement, immobilization may be helpful. Postural defects, obesity, occupational trauma, and other predisposing factors should be looked for and eliminated when possible. Muscle-strengthening exercises may enhance stability and minimize the likelihood of exacerbation by minor trauma.

Aspirin in moderate dosage is frequently beneficial. Indomethacin in doses of 50 to 100 mg daily may help in the management of more painful lesions (e.g., those of the hips). Corticosteroids systemically should not be administered but the injection of corticosteroid into a joint may provide relief, particularly following trauma. Repeated injections should be avoided.

Surgical measures[187] are of benefit in lesions of the knee, hip, and spine. Patellectomy often provides relief from symptoms related to chondromalacia of the patella. In severe lesions of the hip and knee, surgical procedures, including joint replacements, may provide relief of pain and improve ambulation. In spine disease, spontaneous fusion of the joint may occur and relieve symptoms. Operative fusion is employed in selected cases when symptoms persist despite conservative measures.

CHAPTER 108
The Differential Diagnosis of Arthritis
MARY BETTY STEVENS

This chapter offers an approach to the diagnosis of the patient who presents with arthritis, emphasizing the clinical features pertinent to the differential diagnosis of the more common syndromes encountered. The character and pattern of articular involvement, especially whether one or multiple joints are affected by the disease process, is a primary diagnostic consideration in the majority of patients. While it must be emphasized that the patient who presents with a monarthritis may represent the initial stage of a process which, with time, will involve multiple joints, there are certain disorders which remain predominantly monarticular and merit separate discussion.

POLYARTHRITIS

Patients with polyarthritis constitute a difficult group to diagnose properly, especially early in the course of disease. Despite differences in the underlying cause of the acute and chronic arthritides (Table 108-1), the patterns of arthritis and joint findings are often similar. In addition, arthritis is frequently but one aspect of some generalized disease process. Thus, one has to rely on a detailed analysis of historical data, careful physical examination, and selective laboratory studies to arrive at the correct diagnosis. Even so, in the early and acute phase, there are patients in whom the cause remains uncertain.

The clinical problems associated with acute and with chronic polyarthritis differ in several respects. Many of the disorders that produce an acute polyarthritis can be eliminated or given only minor consideration as possible causes of chronic arthritis, for example, pyogenic infections and acute rheumatic fever. Other disorders that do not present acutely must be considered when evaluating patients with chronic arthropathy—for example, degenerative joint disease. Finally, those arthritides, such as rheumatoid arthritis and gout, which may present as either acute or chronic disorders offer different diagnostic problems depending upon the stage of disease when the patient seeks evaluation.

Personal Factors

The age, sex, family, and social histories of the patient are important in considering the possible causes of polyarthritis. In the absence of rheumatic heart disease or a history of previous attacks, acute rheumatic fever is infrequent after the age of 21. Primary gout and ankylosing spondylitis are predominantly diseases of young men, and in both disorders a positive family history may be obtained. Reiter syndrome is almost exclusively a disease of men in the younger age groups, although the chronic arthritis of Reiter may extend into the fifth and sixth decades. Gonococcal arthritis is largely found in women. Chronic arthritis and tumor syndromes are more common in the older age groups. Degenerative joint disease (osteoarthropathy) is unusual before the age of 35 unless there is some predisposing cause, and its incidence increases with advancing age.

---TABLE 108-1---
Causes of Polyarthritis

	Acute	Chronic
Infection	Acute bacterial, especially gonococcus and meningococcus Haverhill fever Subacute infective endocarditis Lyme arthritis[181] Viral infection, rubella, other Syphilis (especially congenital)	 Viral infection, especially lymphogranuloma venereum Syphilis (especially congenital)
Sequel to infection	Acute rheumatic fever Whipple's disease[202]	Jaccoud arthritis[125] Whipple's disease
Allergic or hypersensitivity disease	Drug reaction, serum sickness Henoch–Schönlein purpura Erythema nodosum[193,207] Erythema multiforme	 Erythema nodosum
Connective tissue disease	Systemic lupus erythematosus Polyarteritis Progressive systemic sclerosis Dermatomyositis Sjögren syndrome Relapsing polychondritis[205]	Systemic lupus erythematosus Polyarteritis Progressive systemic sclerosis Sjögren syndrome Relapsing polychondritis
Inflammatory joint disease, cause unknown	Rheumatoid arthritis Juvenile rheumatoid arthritis Reiter syndrome Behçet's disease[209]	Rheumatoid arthritis Juvenile rheumatoid arthritis Agammaglobulinemia[9] Reiter syndrome Psoriatic arthropathy Ankylosing spondylitis Behçet's disease
Arthritis with disease of the intestinal tract	Ulcerative colitis Regional enteritis	 Regional enteritis
Metabolic disease	Gout	Gout Ochronosis[204] Type IV hyperlipoproteinemia[197]
Malignant disease	Multiple myeloma Lymphoma Leukemia[194]	Multiple myeloma
Degenerative		Degenerative joint disease Primary generalized osteoarthropathy
Miscellaneous	Hypertrophic pulmonary osteoarthropathy Sarcoidosis[198,206] Amyloidosis Familial Mediterranean fever[200] Sickle cell anemia[9] Pseudogout[157]	Hypertrophic pulmonary osteoarthropathy Sarcoidosis Hemochromatosis[192,199] Acromegaly[203] Hemophilia[9] Neurogenic[9] Reticulohistiocytosis[195]

Information about exposure to infections, antecedent procedures, and any history of drug or serum administration should be specifically sought in those with acute polyarthritis. Occupational demands and exposures are similarly important.

General Manifestations

Most patients with acute polyarthritis have fever. In a child with polyarthritis, a very high fever (104°F or higher) with marked diurnal peaks suggests the possibility of juvenile rheumatoid arthritis. Rheumatic fever is less likely to cause fever of this magnitude and its fever usually shows less diurnal variation. Because bacteremia and viremia are mechanisms by which multiple joints are involved in an infectious process, the history of shaking chills and fever in a patient with acute polyarthritis should strongly suggest these possibilities. However, shaking chills may occasionally occur in the absence of infection, especially when salicylates have been administered to reduce fever.

Weight loss, fatigue, malaise, or myalgia that precedes the onset of polyarthritis suggests an underlying systemic disorder, such as one of the connective-tissue disorders, infectious process such as subacute infective endocarditis, or tumor syndrome. Weight loss which is occasionally profound is evident in many patients during the course of rheumatoid arthritis. In contrast, degenerative joint disease is characterized by the absence of any systemic signs.

Articular Manifestations

The pattern of articular involvement is particularly valuable in differential diagnosis. It is essential to determine in detail, by history and physical examination, the character and distribution of joint symptoms, their intensity, and progression. For example, gout frequently involves the great toe, but in its polyarticular form it commonly does not affect that joint and instead involves knees, ankles, elbows, wrists, or small joints of the hands. Frequently, gonococcal arthritis begins as a polyarthritis and then settles predominantly in one or two joints. In both gout and gonococcal arthritis, tenosynovitis is common, which helps to distinguish them from rheumatoid arthritis or rheumatic fever. Furthermore, the intensity of joint inflammation in microcrystalline and septic arthritides is usually more intense than in other disorders, reflecting the phagocytic response to crystals and organisms in the synovial space.

The occurrence of similar attacks in the past is an important feature in the diagnosis of acute rheumatic fever, gout, Reiter syndrome, or systemic lupus erythematosus. In the majority of patients, rheumatoid arthritis is less episodic and, without therapy, additive and progressive.

The symmetry of the joints affected in rheumatoid arthritis is also characteristic and contrasts with the usual pattern of psoriatic arthropathy and Reiter syndrome. In the hand, the DIP joints are commonly spared in rheumatoid arthritis but are characteristically involved in the psoriatic and are also the sites of Heberden's nodes. The PIP joints typically are involved in rheumatoid arthritis but also may be affected in degenerative osteoarthropathy (Bouchard's nodes). In contrast, the MCP joints are rarely affected

in primary degenerative joint disease but are almost always involved in rheumatoid arthritis of the hands.

Reiter syndrome is most common in the lower extremities but may involve any joint. Hips and shoulders are the most frequently affected peripheral joints in ankylosing spondylitis which rarely, if ever, involves interphalangeal joints. Other disorders which affect the lumbar spine and sacroiliac joints include psoriatic arthropathy, the arthritis of inflammatory bowel disease, and Reiter syndrome but not rheumatoid arthritis. When the axial skeleton is involved by the rheumatoid process, the cervical segments are affected and usually late in the course of the disease. Degenerative joint disease is more likely to become symptomatic when present in weight-bearing joints; hence, complaints referable to knees or hips are most common.

Helpful in distinguishing degenerative from inflammatory joint disease is the relationship between physical activity and joint symptoms. Stiffness after rest (gel phenomenon) which tends to subside with activity is commonly present in patients with polyarthritis, especially rheumatoid arthritis. In contrast, the pain and stiffness of degenerative joint disease is intensified by activity and weight bearing. Thus, the early morning hours are the most difficult for patients with rheumatoid arthritis as compared to the end of the day for those with degenerative osteoarthropathy.

Extra-Articular Manifestations

The extra-articular manifestations are often of more specific value in the differential diagnosis than the arthritis itself (Table 108–2). When certain of these manifestations occur concomitantly with arthritis, they may lead directly to the diagnosis. However, the arthritis may precede the obvious expression of the extra-articular abnormalities, and thus a careful initial evaluation and a continued search for new developments are required.

Since iritis may come and go independent of the arthritis, a history of iritis as well as the demonstration of synechiae or scars of an old process are also important. The uveitis of sarcoidosis which is granulomatous can usually be distinguished from other types. Sarcoidal lesions of the conjunctiva are usually without symptomatic inflammation.

The type of skin involvement may be virtually diagnostic in some instances, for example, erythema marginatum in rheumatic fever, the typical butterfly rash of SLE, the circinate balanitis, and keratodermia in Reiter syndrome, and the transient rash of Still's disease. In psoriatic arthropathy, deep pitting of the nails is a common feature leading one to suspect the correct diagnosis in patients whose skin lesions are quiescent or atypical. The diagnosis of serum sick-

TABLE 108-2
Extra-Articular Manifestations of Acute and Chronic Polyarthritis

System	Manifestation	Disease Association
Ocular	Conjunctivitis	Reiter syndrome
	Episcleritis	Rheumatoid arthritis, polyarteritis
	Keratitis sicca	Sjögren syndrome
	Visual changes, band keratopathy	Juvenile rheumatoid arthritis
	Uveitis	Juvenile rheumatoid arthritis, Reiter syndrome, ulcerative colitis, regional enteritis, ankylosing spondylitis, sarcoid
Skin	Butterfly rash	Systemic lupus erythematosus
	Erythema marginatum	Rheumatic fever
	Urticaria, erythema multiforme	Drug reaction, systemic lupus erythematosus, serum sickness
	Keratodermia and circinate balanitis	Reiter syndrome
	Psoriatic lesions	Psoriatic arthropathy
	Transient red rash	Juvenile rheumatoid arthritis (Still's disease)
	Small, red, nonblanching spots especially on upper extremities or adjacent to joints	Gonococcal arthritis Rubella
	Petechiae and purpura	Henoch–Schönlein, systemic lupus erythematosus, subacute infective endocarditis
	Infiltrative lesions	Sarcoid, amyloid, reticulohistiocytosis
	Nail lesions	Psoriatic arthropathy, Reiter syndrome, systemic lupus erythematosus
Tendon	Tendonitis	Gonococcal arthritis, gout, psoriatic arthritis
	Tendon sheath effusions	Rheumatoid arthritis
Muscle	Myositis	Systemic lupus erythematosus, progressive systemic sclerosis, dermatomyositis, Sjögren syndrome, sarcoidosis
	Nodules: extensor surfaces of forearms over joints, pressure points	Rheumatoid arthritis, rheumatic fever, gout (tophi)
	Ulcers, especially ankles	Rheumatoid arthritis
Hematopoietic	Lymphadenopathy, splenomegaly	Rheumatoid arthritis, Still's disease, systemic lupus erythematosus, sarcoid, rubella, leukemia, lymphoma
	Bleeding disorders	Hemophilia, systemic lupus erythematosus
Pulmonary	Pleuritis	Systemic lupus erythematosus, rheumatoid arthritis, juvenile rheumatoid arthritis
	Parenchymal infiltrates	Sarcoid, rheumatoid arthritis, polyarteritis, systemic lupus erythematosus
	Hilar adenopathy	Erythema nodosum, sarcoid, lymphoma
Cardiovascular	Pericarditis	Rheumatic fever, systemic lupus erythematosus, Still's disease, rare rheumatoid arthritis
	Myocarditis (including conduction defects)	Rheumatic fever, systemic lupus erythematosus
	Endocarditis (including murmurs)	Rheumatic fever, systemic lupus erythematosus, subacute infective endocarditis
	Aortitis (aortic regurgitation)	Ankylosing spondylitis, Reiter syndrome, rarely rheumatoid arthritis
	Raynaud's phenomenon	Systemic sclerosis, systemic lupus erythematosus, rheumatoid arthritis
Gastrointestinal	Malabsorption	Whipple's disease (arthritis usually precedes gastrointestinal signs)
	Enteritis, colitis	Colitic arthropathy, arthritis with regional enteritis, Reiter syndrome, rheumatoid arthritis
Genitourinary	Urethritis, prostatitis, vaginitis, cervicitis, pelvic inflammation	Gonococcal arthritis, Reiter syndrome
	Calculi, nephropathy	Gout
	Proteinuria, abnormal sediment	Polyarteritis, systemic lupus erythematosus, subacute infective endocarditis, serum sickness, progressive systemic sclerosis
Neurologic	Loss of proprioception, deep pain, e.g., tabes dorsalis, syringomyelia, diabetes mellitus	Neurogenic arthropathy

ness or a drug hypersensitivity reaction may be suggested by the presence of urticaria or erythema multiforme. Erythema nodosum may be associated with arthritis when there is no other evident systemic disorder. However, polyarthritis with erythema nodosum is often an early, sometimes presenting manifestation of sarcoidosis as well as a late manifestation of inflammatory bowel disease, commonly occurring after the peak of the bowel inflammation has been reached.

Pleurisy and pericarditis are common in SLE and Still's disease and occur infrequently in adult rheumatoid arthritis. Moreover, serositis usually occurs early and may be an initial feature of SLE and juvenile rheumatoid arthritis, in contrast to the usual appearance late in the course of adult rheumatoid disease. Pulmonary hypertrophic osteoarthropathy is most often related to the presence of a pulmonary or pleural tumor and may be the initial manifestation of carcinoma of the lung. Clubbing of the fingers is invariably present in the patient with this condition.

The presence of a diastolic heart murmur in a young patient with acute polyarthritis immediately suggests acute rheumatic fever or subacute infective endocarditis (SIE). The presence of Libman-Sachs endocarditis in SLE correlates poorly with the presence or absence of cardiac murmurs on physical examination.

In contrast to the usual sequence of events in ulcerative colitis and Crohn's disease, the arthritis of Whipple's disease may precede overt evidence of gastrointestinal tract involvement by months or even years. Reiter syndrome, in its epidemic form, has been described in association with acute bacillary dysentery but the sporadic cases are more commonly associated with venereal exposure and urethritis. The onset of gonococcal arthritis in females frequently occurs in association with menses or pregnancy.

Evidence of nephritis in a patient with acute polyarthritis points toward the diagnosis of a multisystem disorder, especially SLE or polyarteritis. However, careful search for infection (SIE) and detailed history of drug administration (serum sickness) are indicated in all patients with such a symptom complex.

Laboratory Findings

Routine blood counts are seldom of diagnostic value although a modest degree of anemia is frequent in patients with rheumatoid arthritis, chronic infection (SIE), and the connective tissue disorders. When the anemia is hemolytic, especially Coombs' test positive, SLE is likely. Similarly, leukopenia and less frequently thrombocytopenia in patients with polyar-

thritis favor the diagnosis of SLE or rheumatoid disease.

Although acute-phase reactants lack diagnostic specificity, the sedimentation rate is almost always elevated in patients with active inflammatory joint diseases but rarely in degenerative osteoarthropathy. Similarly, serum globulin elevations are found in many disorders causing polyarthritis, but determination of specific antibody levels is more valuable than total globulin determinations. For example, serologic evidence of a recent streptococcal infection is the principal support for the diagnosis of acute rheumatic fever in the absence of carditis.

Antinuclear antibodies (ANA), as demonstrated by the indirect immunofluorescent method, are present in all but 5 percent of patients with active SLE, usually in high titer, but may be found also in other disorders (e.g., rheumatoid arthritis and variants, progressive systemic sclerosis, chronic active hepatitis). A strongly positive LE cell test correlates more closely with the diagnosis of SLE but, even so, is not specific.

Rheumatoid factors (demonstrated by the latex fixation test) are present in 75 percent of patients with adult rheumatoid arthritis and nearly all with the variants of Felty and Sjögren. In children with rheumatoid arthritis, rheumatoid factors are seldom found and they are characteristically absent in Reiter syndrome, psoriatic arthropathy, and ankylosing spondylitis. However, rheumatoid factors commonly occur in disorders other than rheumatoid disease, including approximately half the patients with SLE and SIE, less frequently in other connective tissue disorders, sarcoidosis, chronic infections, and hepatocellular disease. Furthermore, circulating rheumatoid factors seem to represent a phenomenon of aging independent of disease.

Reduction of serum complement is characteristic of SLE, especially when concomitant with antinuclear antibodies in high titer. Hypocomplementemia also occurs in serum sickness (usually only a transient fall) and occasionally in SIE. When hypocomplementemia occurs in rheumatoid arthritis, it has been associated with the presence of peripheral vasculitis, circulating cryoprecipitable complexes, or other systemic features of rheumatoid disease.

Synovial fluid findings often provide the most useful information, especially in infection (high white blood count, low glucose, and organisms on culture or smear) and microcrystalline synovitis (urate crystals in gout, calcium pyrophosphate crystals in pseudogout). The presence of noncrystalline inclusions in phagocytes is a common finding in rheumatoid arthritis (protein complexes) and Reiter syndrome (white blood cells). Most helpful in rheumatoid arthritis is the demonstration of a reduced synovial fluid complement, especially relative to the protein concentration, which reflects intrasynovial utilization by immune complexes. The complement level is normal or elevated in most inflammatory synovial fluids such as infection, gout, and Reiter syndrome. Even in the absence of such diagnostic findings as organisms or crystals, careful examination of synovial fluid is useful in discriminating between inflammatory (poor mucin clot, reduced viscosity, leukocytosis, and often increased protein) and typically noninflammatory fluid of degenerative joint disease. Of interest in this regard is the usual finding, difficult to explain, of a good mucin clot and marginal leukocytosis (less than 5000 cells/μl) in SLE and rheumatic fever.

Joint x-rays are least helpful early in the course of polyarthritis except in the negative sense to exclude such infrequent disorders as pulmonary osteoarthropathy, leukemia, or myeloma. Even with septic processes, it may require weeks, even months, for characteristic radiologic lesions to become evident. Occasionally, findings of gout or rheumatoid arthritis may be present early, but these are commonly absent until more chronic symptoms are evident. X-ray findings of particular value are the periarticular osteoporosis and juxta-articular erosions characteristic of rheumatoid arthritis and the marginal sclerosis and bony spurs and bridges of degenerative joint disease. Patients with chronic gout often have punched-out defects in bone adjacent to joints (urate deposits) and the presence of chondrocalcinosis, especially knees, wrists, or symphysis, alerts one to possible pseudogout. Destructive and asymmetric lesions in the distal phalangeal joints are characteristic of psoriatic arthropathy. Periostitis, so frequent in pulmonary osteoarthropathy, is also a feature of Reiter syndrome and the juvenile form of rheumatoid arthritis. X-rays of the sacroiliac joints and lumbar spine are helpful early in those with low back syndromes (with or without peripheral arthritis) to distinguish the group of spondylitic disorders from degenerative joint and intervertebral disc disease.

Biopsy of the synovial membrane is infrequently essential in acute and chronic polyarthritis. While diagnostic synovial membrane features include the granulomata of tuberculosis and sarcoid, crystalline deposits, and abnormal cell types, these diagnoses can usually be established more readily on other grounds. Otherwise, the histology is seldom indicative of more than reactive synovium. In contrast, biopsy of the subcutaneous nodules or skin lesions may yield information of diagnostic value.

A summary of the distinguishing features of the

major forms of acute and chronic polyarthritis is presented in Table 108–3.

Course

A significant number of patients with acute polyarthritis seen within the first 1 or 2 weeks of illness will have a self-limited process which subsides in a period of days or weeks, even without treatment. Many patients never have recurrences of arthritis. Some of these individuals may have unrecognized acute infections (possibly viral), and population surveys have shown that such single episodes of acute polyarthritis are rather common.

Recurrent episodes of arthritis suggest rheumatic fever, gout, Reiter syndrome, or a multisystem disease such as SLE. Similar bouts of synovitis with symptom-free intervals may be associated with inflammatory bowel disease, often in relationship to exacerbations of the intestinal lesions. Rheumatoid arthritis, psoriatic arthritis, and ankylosing spondylitis, after presenting acutely, usually persist and progress in the absence of therapeutic intervention. Finally, some patients with "undiagnosed polyarthritis" continue to have recurrent and unexplained synovitis. Even after months or years they fail to develop the articular features which allow further categorization or the extra-articular manifestations of the multisystem connective-tissue disorders. Such patients require continued, long-term observation and anti-inflammatory therapy with constant reevaluation in search for specific cause.

It is important to recognize the development of residual joint damage with continued inflammation, whatever the cause. Infection, if not adequately treated in its early stages, may cause significant joint destruction within a few weeks. Residual changes are apt to follow closely the polyarticular onset of rheumatoid arthritis, and are also common in Reiter syndrome, but fewer joints are usually affected in the latter.

Diagnostic Value of Therapeutic Trials

Information can be obtained occasionally in some types of acute polyarthritis. If one suspects gout but the diagnosis is uncertain, the administration of colchicine (especially intravenously) may be followed by a prompt response which helps to confirm the diagnosis. In infectious arthritis, a rapid response may be obtained to appropriate antibiotics when a sensitive organism is involved. Careful collection of material for cultures is mandatory, of course, before a trial of antibiotics is undertaken.

Obviously, in conducting a therapeutic trial, only one agent should be administered. Placing a patient

TABLE 108-3
Distinguishing Features of Acute and Chronic Polyarthritis

Disease	Important Differential Diagnostic Features
Gonococcal arthritis	Young adults, especially females
	History of exposure
	Associated with menses or pregnancy
	After polyarticular onset, often settles in one or two joints; tenosynovitis prominent
	Association with skin lesions
	Frequent history of shaking chills, genitourinary symptoms (urethritis, salpingitis)
	Isolation of organism from genitourinary tract and joints
	Response to penicillin
Viral	History of exposure, frequently during an epidemic
	Rise in serologic titer
	Leukopenia
	Spontaneous remission without sequelae in acute forms
	In lymphogranuloma venereum: chronic synovitis of large joints, hyperglobulinemia, positive Frei test
Acute rheumatic fever	Child or young adult
	Evidence of recent beta streptococcal infection
	Migratory involvement of large joints; often previous attacks
	Association with carditis
	Response to aspirin
Serum sickness or drug hypersensitivity	History of drug administration, especially horse serum, penicillin, but also patent medicines
	Migratory involvement large and small joints
	Frequent association with rash (urticaria, erythema multiforme, others)
	Decreased serum complement level in serum sickness
	Response to drug withdrawal, antihistamines, or corticosteroid therapy
Connective tissue diseases	Females predominate except in polyarteritis
	Joint involvement infrequently progresses to deformity
	Systemic signs and multisystem organ involvement, especially nephritis, in systemic lupus erythematosus and polyarteritis
	LE cells, ANA, and decreased serum complement level in systemic lupus erythematosus

TABLE 108-3 (cont.)

Disease	Important Differential Diagnostic Features
Rheumatoid arthritis	Women 2:1
	Initial frequent involvement hands (PIP, MCP joints) and wrists
	Symmetrical, additive involvement; chronically, all peripheral joints may be involved
	Morning stiffness prominent
	Subcutaneous nodules
	Tendon sheath effusions
	Characteristic deformities and erosive changes on x-ray in chronic stage
	Rheumatoid factor in up to 75% with time
	LE cells occasionally
	Moderate anemia common
Juvenile rheumatoid arthritis	Onset before age 16
	Cervical spine involvement in 25%
	Growth impairment variable, age-dependent
	Still's disease associated with rash, serositis, lymphadenopathy, splenomegaly
	Subcutaneous nodules and rheumatoid factor uncommon
	Tends to remission at adolescence
Ankylosing spondylitis	Young men 9:1
	Spine disease with extensive fusion principal manifestation
	Hips and shoulders frequently involved; small joints hands and feet, rarely
	Association with iritis, aortitis
	Subcutaneous nodules and rheumatoid factor not present
Reiter syndrome	Young men
	Genitourinary symptoms, signs (urethritis, prostatitis)
	Often asymmetrical arthritis; most commonly lower extremities
	Association with skin (keratodermia), membrane (oral, balanitis), and ocular lesions
	ECG changes may be present (heart block)
	Tends to recur; knees, ankles, spine most often involved in chronic form

┌─ **TABLE 108–3 (cont.)** ─┐

Disease	Important Differential Diagnostic Features
Psoriatic arthropathy	Typical skin lesions and nail involvement Asymmetrical arthritis; frequent DIP joint involvement Spine disease, especially sacroiliitis Subcutaneous nodules and rheumatoid factor not present Hyperuricemia may be found
Colitic arthropathy	Active ulcerative colitis, regional enteritis Large joints predominate Parallels course of intestinal disorder Negative rheumatoid factor tests
Erythema nodosum	Typical skin lesions Hilar adenopathy Arthritis usually lower extremities, especially ankles; usually evanescent May be associated with sarcoid, tuberculosis, regional enteritis, drug hypersensitivity, others
Sarcoidosis	Arthritis usually occurs early in disease course, rarely progressive Hilar adenopathy and other systemic features Lesions demonstrable on biopsy of node or liver Hypergammaglobulinemia Elevated serum calcium or uric acid may occur
Gout	Males or postmenopausal females Familial occurrence Podagra and prominent periarticular inflammation in acute attacks Precipitating factors (drugs, trauma, etc.) Tophi, clinically and on x-ray, in chronic stage Increased serum uric acid and urate crystals in synovial fluid Response of acute attack to colchincine
Pseudogout	Males predominate Mimics gout, with intense inflammation, especially knees Chondrocalcinosis on x-ray Calcium pyrophosphate crystals in synovial fluid

┌─ **TABLE 108–3 (cont.)** ─┐

Disease	Important Differential Diagnostic Features
Hypertrophic osteoarthropathy	Clubbing of fingers Knees, wrists, ankles, fingers may be involved; rheumatoidlike Periostitis, especially at distal ends of long bones Association with pulmonary, mediastinal, other lesions—often malignant Course determined by underlying disease
Degenerative joint disease	Lower extremities predominate DIP (Heberden's nodes) and PIP (Bouchard's nodes) involvement Absence of MCP and wrist disease Pain after activity, improved with rest Absence of inflammatory signs Bony proliferation with spur formation

on salicylates and penicillin simultaneously, for example, may obscure a therapeutic response of some diagnostic value. Moreover, it must be remembered that spontaneous and rapid resolution of polyarthritis may occur in many patients placed at bed rest alone, so the results of therapeutic trials demand cautious interpretation.

MONARTICULAR ARTHRITIS

Processes capable of involving multiple joints may be encountered initially as monarthritides. Hence, many of the diseases discussed as causes of polyarthritis are listed again in relation to monarticular arthritis (Table 108–4). Several disorders, however, remain predominantly monarticular and are emphasized here. The most immediate concern of the physician dealing with the problem of acute monarthritis is the recognition of septic arthritis and mechanical derangement of a joint both of which can lead to unnecessary, sometimes permanent disability if appropriate therapy is not promptly instituted.

Articular Manifestations

The abrupt onset of monarticular arthritis with intense local inflammation, fever, peripheral and synovial fluid leukocytosis should suggest infection or microcrystalline synovitis (gout, pseudogout) as the

---TABLE 108-4---
Causes of Monarticular Arthritis*

Infection

Acute bacterial (gonococcus, pneumococcus, streptococcus, staphylococcus, meningococcus, gram-negative)

Tuberculosis

Fungus

Inflammatory Joint Disease

Rheumatoid arthritis (especially teen-age juvenile onset)

Reiter syndrome

Ulcerative colitis

Regional enteritis

Metabolic

Gout

Trauma

Hemarthrosis

Tear of ligament or cartilage

Degenerative Joint Disease

Primary

Secondary (postinflammatory, posttrauma, neuropathic)

Neoplasms

Pigmented villonodular synovitis (inflammatory granuloma or true neoplasm?)

Primary (osteochondromatosis, lipoma, angioma, synovioma)

Metastatic

Miscellaneous

Intermittent hydrarthrosis

Osteochondritis dissecans

Bleeding disorders (hemophilia) with hemarthrosis

* Any form of polyarthritis may present initially with monarticular involvement.

leading etiologic possibility. Since infection usually occurs via the bloodstream, a history of chills is common and a focus from which the bacteremia originated may be evident (e.g., pneumococcal pneumonia, acute salpingitis, or soft-tissue abscess). Although large joints are most commonly involved in infection, one of the small joints of the hands or feet may occasionally be involved (especially with gonococci, meningococci, or SIE). An acute arthritis caused by gout or pseudogout may closely resemble infection, especially with regard to the intensity of articular inflammation. The metatarsophalangeal joint of the great toe (podagra) is frequently involved in acute gouty attacks early in the course of the disease and is seldom affected by other arthritides unrelated to trauma. Inflammation of the surrounding soft tissue resembling cellulitis or thrombophlebitis is common in acute gout. Trauma (e.g., a recent operation or local physical injury) often precedes an acute gouty attack.

Trauma is also a frequent precipitating factor in pseudogout. Pseudogout commonly affects the knees and, less frequently, elbows, hips, and wrists. Only occasionally is pseudogout polyarticular. This syndrome of chondrocalcinosis and acute arthritis secondary to the presence of calcium pyrophosphate microcrystals in synovial fluid has been called pseudogout because of the clinical resemblance to gout which results from the fact that, in both disorders, microcrystals are responsible for inducing inflammation.

Trauma may result directly in an acute painful swelling of a joint, especially when the injury involves rupture of a ligament or damage to cartilage. A history of significant trauma may be obtained in these patients but not infrequently the injury may have been so minor an event that it is forgotten, or it may not be recalled for other reasons such as alcoholism, seizures, or disorientation (especially in the elderly). Low grade fever (occasionally as high as 101°F) is sometimes associated with a traumatic effusion but rarely persists longer than 24 to 48 hours.

Acute painful swelling of a joint may be produced occasionally by a loose fragment of cartilage that is trapped or wedged between the articulating surfaces of a joint. Such loose bodies are common in degenerative joint disease or osteochondromatosis and, especially in the knee, osteochondritis dissecans. A meniscus injury as well as a loose body may result in locking of the knee in addition to painful swelling.

Acute arthritis of colitic arthropathy is frequently a monarticular process. In most patients, active ulcerative colitis or regional enteritis is evident and the rheumatologic diagnosis is not difficult. The major consideration is acute infection secondary to a frequent complication of inflammatory bowel disease.

Rheumatoid arthritis may remain localized to a single joint, especially the knee, for months and even years before other joints become involved. Rheumatoid arthritis with onset in the early teens may remain monarticular throughout its course. Intermittent swelling of one or both knees, independently or simultaneously, in a young woman without marked articular symptoms or evident systemic features, suggests the diagnosis of intermittent hydrarthrosis. Exacerbation of joint swelling with menses is often observed with this condition.

Tuberculous arthritis is usually a subacute or chronic monarticular process. It may be produced by *Mycobacterium tuberculosis* and atypical chromogenic strains. Early recognition is imperative since specific therapy is available which will minimize otherwise inevitable joint destruction. The peripheral joint most frequently affected in adults is the knee in contrast to more common hip involvement in children. Spinal involvement (Pott's disease) is rarely associated with peripheral tuberculous arthritis.

Tumors involving joints are uncommon. The most frequently encountered tumor is benign osteochondroma, commonly multiple (multiple exostoses). Metastasis of tumors in the joint is rare although extension to the joint of an adjacent bony tumor focus is occasionally seen.

The most common cause of chronic monarticular arthropathy is degenerative joint disease. Knees or hips are the most frequently affected joints. Effusions may be encountered, especially in the knee, usually without evidence of significant inflammation.

Traumatic insult to a joint may produce recurrent or chronic symptoms which relate to the development of secondary degenerative change. Such may be the basis of neurogenic arthropathy which is more often monarticular. Loss of proprioception in such disorders as tabes dorsalis, syringomyelia, and diabetes mellitus leads to repeated joint trauma, relaxation of supporting structures with marked instability and, finally, severe degenerative changes and bony proliferation. The knees are most frequently affected in tabes dorsalis, the shoulders and elbows in syringomyelia, and the ankles, tarsal, and metatarsal joints in diabetic neuropathy. Examination usually reveals an effusion, hypermobility of the joint, and remarkable bony overgrowth and crepitation in the advanced cases. Pain, when present, seems less in degree than the deformity and effusion should produce.

Extra-Articular Features

The same concern for the patient's personal characteristics, environmental exposures, and general health status applies to those with monarticular arthritis as has been stressed for patients with multiple inflamed joints. Particularly important here is care in the documentation of exposure to infection and episodes of possible physical injury to the joint. It must be remembered that trauma, in addition to direct alteration of joint integrity, provides a frequent precipitating factor for acute microcrystalline synovitis. Similarly, a detailed history of drug administration

may reveal agents (e.g., thiazides) which alter uric acid metabolism and favor gouty attacks.

Laboratory Findings

Leukocytosis and elevation of the erythrocyte sedimentation rate are frequently found in acute infection, gout, and pseudogout but are usually absent in traumatic, degenerative, and neuropathic joint disease. Elevation of the serum uric acid favors the diagnosis of gout. A negative tuberculin skin test is substantial evidence against the diagnosis of tuberculosis.

Aspiration of synovial fluid is particularly useful in the diagnosis of monarticular arthritis. The mucin clot test is usually normal and the white cell count is usually less than 2000/μl in trauma, osteochondritis dissecans, neurogenic arthropathy, and degenerative joint disease. Sanguinous effusions are characteristic of acute trauma but may also occur in pigmented villonodular synovitis, osteochondritis dissecans, and bleeding disorders. A white cell count higher than 50,000 cells/μl and a low glucose level strongly implicate an acute bacterial infection even though microorganisms may not be seen on smear or cultured. A low synovial fluid glucose in a chronic monarthritis is highly suggestive of tuberculosis.

The recognition and identification of crystals in synovial fluid allow the diagnosis of gout or pseudogout to be made with certainty. The abundance of crystals varies with the time of synovial fluid examination relative to onset of the joint inflammation. During the first 12 hours or after the second day, crystals may be few in number and require careful search. In the acute inflammatory reaction they are predominantly intracellular but in the interval or chronic phase are extracellular.

Tests for rheumatoid factor in synovial fluid usually parallel those of serum, but a few cases with positive tests in the synovial fluid and negative serum reactions have been reported in patients with adult monarticular rheumatoid arthritis. In such patients, a low synovial fluid complement is expected.

X-ray changes are helpful in distinguishing rheumatoid arthritis, gout, and degenerative joint disease. However, it must be recalled that degenerative changes are commonly encountered and may be unrelated to the clinical problem. Chondrocalcinosis may be overlooked unless it is specifically considered. It usually occurs as a stippled, linear calcification of the meniscal, or articular cartilage of the knee joint, in the wrist, hip, pubic symphysis, or intervertebral discs. Osteochondritis dissecans also presents a characteristic x-ray picture which is best seen in a tunnel view of the knee. The lesion is usually seen as

TABLE 108–5
Distinguishing Features of Monarticular Arthritis

Disease	Important Differential Diagnostic Features
Bacterial infection	Acute onset Focus of infection elsewhere Fever, occasionally chills Large joints primarily; intense inflammation Inflammatory synovial fluid with white blood cells often > 50,000, low glucose, organisms on smear or culture Response to antibiotics
Tuberculous arthritis	Usually active tuberculosis elsewhere Tuberculin-positive Large joints (knee, hip) or tenosynovitis at wrist Cold inflammation clinically, but inflammatory synovial fluid Frequently bony involvement on x-ray Synovial biopsy characteristic Response to antituberculous therapy
Gout	Acute onset Family history Men, postmenopausal women Often recurrent attacks in single joint, especially podagra Intense inflammation with uric acid crystals in synovial fluid Elevated serum uric acid Response to colchicine
Pseudogout (chondrocalcinosis)	Middle-aged, elderly men predominantly Mimics gout in acuteness and intensity of inflammation Calcium pyrophosphate crystals in synovial fluid Calcification joint cartilage knee, wrist, symphysis pubis
Trauma	Abrupt onset Frequent history of significant direct trauma Lack of systemic signs Normal sedimentation rate Noninflammatory synovial fluid with red blood cells
Degenerative joint disease	Pain with weight-bearing and exercise Minimal or absent inflammation Characteristic x-ray changes with subchondral sclerosis, marginal spur formation Chronic inflammation, recurrent trauma, and neuropathic (Charcot) joints predisposing factors

TABLE 108–5 (cont.)

Disease	Important Differential Diagnostic Features
Osteochondritis dissecans	Acute and chronic symptoms Adolescents, young adults Knee joint predominantly involved Noninflammatory effusions related to extrusion of cartilage fragment into joint X-ray characteristic with density or defect on articular surface of femoral condyle
Intermittent hydrarthrosis	Young women primarily One or both knees Effusion exacerbated with menses Synovial fluid nonspecific No systemic features Negative x-rays Rheumatoid arthritis develops subsequently in a few
Pigmented villonodular synovitis	Knee joint primarily Recurrent bloody effusions and synovial hypertrophy Tumor versus granulomatous synovitis Characteristic biopsy Surgical removal necessary

a defect or density in the non-weight-bearing articular surface of the femoral condyle. Neurotrophic arthropathy is associated with an extreme degree of bony proliferation.

Acute infection has no radiologic manifestations unless it originates from a juxta-articular focus of osteomyelitis. Several weeks after an acute infection, a narrowing of the joint space may be evident because of the destruction of articular cartilage. Tuberculosis causes early narrowing of the joint space.

Biopsy of the synovium either by open exploration or by closed needle techniques is of greatest usefulness in the patient with obscure monarticular arthritis. Confirmation of the diagnosis of tuberculous arthritis, sarcoidosis, pigmented villonodular synovitis and, occasionally, gout can be made on the basis of characteristic alteration of the synovial membrane. Open exploration is particularly applicable when traumatic injury is suspected, since the defect can often be corrected at the same time. Such defects (especially meniscal tears) can often be visualized preoperatively by arthrography and arthroscopy.

A summary of the distinguishing features of various disorders producing monarthritis is presented in Table 108–5.

REFERENCES

General References

1. American Rheumatism Association. Index of Rheumatology, Vol. 1, 1965–Vol. 10, 1974.

    A current monthly worldwide compilation of journal articles pertaining to rheumatic disease.

2. Arthritis Foundation Rheumatism Reviews. Reviews of the American and English literature in rheumatic disease. Fifteenth, Ann. Intern. Med., 59, Suppl. 4, 1963; Sixteenth, Ann. Intern. Med., 61, Suppl. 6, 1964; Seventeenth, Arthritis Rheum. 9:93, 1966; Eighteenth, Arthritis Rheum. 11:523, 1968; Nineteenth, Arthritis Rheum. 13:457, 1970; Twentieth, New York, The Arthritis Foundation, 1973; Twenty-first, Arthritis Rheum. 17:651, 1974; Twenty-second, Arthritis Rheum., 19:973, 1976; Twenty-third, Arthritis Rheum., 21 Suppl. 8, 1978.

3. Burnet, F.M. The Integrity of the Body. Cambridge, Harvard University Press, 1962.

4. Clinics in Rheumatic Diseases. Vols. 1–5, Philadelphia, Saunders, 1975–1979.

5. Cohen, A.S. (ed.). Laboratory Diagnostic Procedure in the Rheumatic Diseases. Boston, Little, Brown, 1967.

6. Dumonde, D.C. (ed.). Infection and Immunology in the Rheumatic Diseases. Philadelphia, Lippincott, 1976.

7. Ferguson, R.H. and Worthington, J.W. Recent advances in rheumatic disease: 1967 through 1969. Ann. Intern. Med., 73:109, 1970.

8. Gardner, D.L. Pathology of the Connective Tissue Diseases. Baltimore, Williams & Wilkins, 1965.

9. Jaffe, H.L. Metabolic, Degenerative and Inflammatory Diseases of Bones and Joints. Philadelphia, Lea & Febiger, 1972.

10. Katz, W.A. (ed.). Rheumatic Diseases: Diagnosis and Management. Philadelphia, Lippincott, 1977.

11. Kunkel, H.G. and Tan, E.M. Autoantibodies and disease. In Dixon, F.J., Jr. and Humphrey, J.H. (eds.), Advances in Immunology. New York, Academic, 1964.

12. Landsteiner, K. The Specificity of Serological Reactions. New York, Dover (A36), 1962.

13. McCarty, D.J. (ed.). Arthritis and Allied Conditions, 9th ed. Philadelphia, Lea & Febiger, 1979.

14. Moskowitz, R.M. Clinical Rheumatology. Philadelphia, Lea & Febiger, 1975.

15. Miescher, P.A. and Muller-Eberhard, E.J. (eds.). Textbook of Immunopathology. New York, Grune & Stratton, 1968.

16. Ropes, M.W. and Bauer, W. Synovial Fluid Changes in Joint Disease. Cambridge, Harvard University, 1956.

17. Samter, M. and Alexander, H.L. (eds.). Immunological Diseases, 2nd ed. Boston, Little, Brown, 1971.

18. Schur, P.H. and Austen, K.F. Complement in human disease. Annu. Rev. Med., 19:1, 1968.

19. Scott, J.T. (ed.) Copeman's Textbook of the Rheumatic Diseases, 5th ed. Edinburgh, Churchill Livingston, 1978.

20. Sokoloff, L. (ed.). The Joints and Synovial Fluid. New York, Academic, 1978.

21. Talmage, D.W. and Cann, J.R. The Chemistry of Immunity in Health and Disease. Springfield, Ill., Thomas, 1961.

22. Waksman, B.H. Autoimmunization and the lesions of autoimmunity. Medicine, 41:93, 1962.

Systemic Lupus Erythematosus

23. Appel, G.P., Silva, F.G., Pirani, C.L., Meltzer, J.I., and Estes, D. Renal involvement in systemic lupus erythematosus. Medicine, 57:371, 1978.

24. Arnett, F.C. and Shulman, L.E. Studies in familial systemic lupus erythematosus. Medicine, 55:313, 1976.

25. Baldwin, D.S., Lowenstein, J., Rothfield, N.F., Galio, G., and McCluskey, R.T. The clinical course of the proliferative and membranous forms of lupus nephritis. Ann. Intern. Med., 73:929, 1970.

26. Blomgren, S.E., Condemi, J.J., Bignal, M.C., and Vaughan, J.H. Antinuclear antibody induced by procaine amide: a prospective study. N. Engl. J. Med., 281:64, 1969.

27. ———, ———, and Vaughan, J.H. Procainamide-induced lupus erythematosus. Am. J. Med., 52:338, 1972.

28. Burnham, T.K. and Fine, G. The immunofluorescent "band" test for lupus erythematosus. Arch. Dermatol., 103:24, 1971.

29. Christian, C.L. Immune complex disease. N. Engl. J. Med., 280:878, 1969.

30. Cohen, A.S., Reynolds, W.E., Franklin, E.C., Kulka, J.P., Ropes, M.W., Shulman, L.E., and Wallace, S.L. Preliminary criteria for the classification of systemic lupus erythematosus. Bull. Rheum. Dis., 21:643, 1971.

31. Dubois, E.L. Lupus Erythematosus. A Review of the Current Status of Discord and Systemic Lupus Erythematosus and Their Variants, 2nd ed. New York, McGraw-Hill, 1974.

    Contains an extensive bibliography.

32. Dujorne, L., Pollak, V.E., Pirani, C.L., and Dillard, M.G. The distribution and character of glomerular deposits in systemic lupus erythematosus. Kidney Int., 2:33, 1972.

33. Estes, D. and Larsen, D.L. Systemic lupus erythematosus and pregnancy. Clin. Obstet. Gynecol., 8:307, 1965.

34. ——— and Christian, C.L. The natural history of systemic lupus erythematosus by prospective analysis. Medicine, 50:85, 1971.

35. Klipper, A.R., Stevens, M.B., Zizic, T.M., and Hungerford, D.S. Ischemic necrosis of bone in systemic lupus erythematosus. Medicine, 55:251, 1976.

36. Harvey, A.M., Shulman, L.E., Tumulty, P.A., Conley, C.L., and Schoenrich, E.H. Systemic lupus erythematosus. A review of the literature and clinical analysis of 138 cases. Medicine, 33:291, 1954.

37. Hayslett, J.P., Kashgarian, M., Cook, C.D., and Spargo, B.H. The effect of azathioprine on lupus glomerulonephritis. Medicine, 51:393, 1972.

38. Johnson, R.T. and Richardson, E.P. The neurological manifestations of systemic lupus erythematosus. Medicine, 47:337, 1968.

39. Feinglass, E.J., Arnett, F.C., Dorsch, C.A., Zizic, T.M., and Stevens, M.B. Neuropsychiatric manifestations of systemic lupus erythematosus: diagnosis, clinical spectrum and relationship to other features of the disease. Medicine, 55:323, 1976.

40. Koffler, D., Schur, P.H., and Kunkel, H.G. Immunologic studies concerning the nephritis of systemic lupus erythematosus. J. Exp. Med., 126:607, 1967.

41. Kraus, S.J., Haserick, J.R., and Lantz, M.A. Fluorescent treponemal antibody absorption test in lupus erythematosus. N. Engl. J. Med., 282:1287, 1970.

42. Maher, J.F. and Schreiner, G.E. Treatment of lupus nephritis with azathioprine. Arch. Intern. Med., 125:293, 1970.

43. Maclachlan, M.J., Rodnan, G.P., Cooper, W.M., and Fennell, R.H., Jr. Chronic active ("lupoid") hepatitis. A clinical, serological and pathological study of 20 patients. Ann. Intern. Med., 62:425, 1965.

44. Morris, J.L., Zizic, T.M., and Stevens, M.B. Clinical significance of antinuclear antibodies with hypocomplementemia. Johns Hopkins Med. J., 133:321, 1973.

45. ———. Proteus polyarthritis complicating systemic lupus erythematosus. Johns Hopkins Med. J., 133:262, 1973.

46. Muehrcke, R.C., Kark, R.M., Pirani, C.L., and Pollak, V.E. Lupus nephritis. A clinical and pathologic study based on renal biopsies. Medicine, 36:1, 1957.

47. Ropes, M.W. Systemic Lupus Erythematosus. Cambridge, Harvard University, 1976.

48. Rothfield, N.F., March, C., Miescher, P., and McEwen, C. Discoid lupus erythematosus. A study of 65 patients and 65 controls. N. Engl. J. Med., 269:1155, 1963.

49. Schur, P.H. Complement in lupus. Clinics in Rheumatic Disease, 1:519, 1975.

50. ——— and Sandson, J. Immunologic factors and clinical activity in systemic lupus erythematosus. N. Engl. J. Med., 278:533, 1968.

51. Siegel, H. and Seelenfreund, M. Racial and social factors in systemic lupus erythematosus. JAMA, 191:77, 1965.

52. Steinberg, A.D., Kaltreider, H.B., Stiples, P.J., Goetzl, E.J., Talal, N., and Decker, J.L. Controlled trial of cyclophosphamide in systemic lupus erythematosus nephritis. Arthritis Rheum., 13:351, 1970.

53. Swanson, M.A. and Schwartz, R. Immunosuppressive therapy. The relation between clinical response and immunologic competence. N. Engl. J. Med., 277:163, 1967.

54. Sztejnbok, M., Stewart, A., Diamond, H., and Kaplan, D. Azathioprine in the treatment of systemic lupus erythematosus. A controlled study. Arthritis Rheum., 14:639, 1971.

55. Townes, A.S. Complement levels in disease. Johns Hopkins Med. J., 5:337, 1967.

56. ———, Stewart, C.R., Jr., and Osler, A.G. Immunologic studies of systemic lupus erythematosus. II. Variations of nucleoprotein-reactive gamma globulin and hemolytic serum complement with disease activity. Johns Hopkins Med. J., 112:202, 1963.

57. Tuffanelli, D.C., Kay, D., and Fukuyama, K. Dermal-epidermal junction in lupus erythematosus. Arch. Dermatol., 99:652, 1969.

Progressive Systemic Sclerosis

58. Alpert, L.I. and Warner, R.P. Systemic sclerosis. Case presenting with tetracycline-responsive malabsorption syndrome. Am. J. Med., 45:468, 1968.

59. Cannon, P.J., Hessar, M., Case, D.B., Casarella, W.J., Sommers, S.C., and LeRoy, E.C. The relationship of hypertension and renal failure in scleroderma (progressive systemic sclerosis) to structural and functional abnormalities of the renal cortical circulation. Medicine, 53:1, 1974.

60. Guttadauria, M., Ellman, H., Emmanuel, G., Kaplan, D., and Diamond, H. Pulmonary function in scleroderma. Arthritis Rheum., 20:1071, 1977.

61. Medsger, T.A. and Masi, A.T. Epidemiology of systemic sclerosis. Ann. Intern. Med., 74:714, 1971.

62. Norton, W.L. and Nardo, J.M. Vascular disease in progressive systemic sclerosis (scleroderma). Ann. Intern. Med., 73:317, 1970.

63. Rodnan, G.P. The nature of joint involvement in progressive systemic sclerosis (diffuse scleroderma), clinical study and pathological examination of synovium in 29 patients. Ann. Intern. Med., 56:422, 1962.

64. ——— and Fennell, R.N., Jr. Progressive systemic sclerosis sine scleroderma. JAMA, 180:665, 1962.

65. Sackner, M.A. Scleroderma. New York, Grune & Stratton, 1966.

66. ———, Akgun, N., Kimbel, P., and Lewis, D.H. The pathophysiology of scleroderma involving the heart and respiratory systems. Ann. Intern. Med., 60:611, 1964.

67. Siegel, R.C. Scleroderma. Med. Clin. North Am., 61:283, 1977.

68. Stevens, M.B., Hookman, P., Siegal, C., Esterly, J., Shulman, L.E., and Hendrix, T.R. Aperistalsis of the esophagus in connective tissue disorders and Raynaud's phenomenon. N. Engl. J. Med., 270:1218, 1964.

69. Tufanelli, D.L. and Winkelmann, R.K. Systemic scleroderma: a clinical study of 727 cases. Arch. Dermatol., 84:359, 1961.

Polymyositis

70. Arnett, F.C., Jr., Whelton, J.C., Zizic, T.M., and Stevens, M.B. Methotrexate therapy in polymyositis. Ann. Rheum. Dis., 32:536, 1973.

71. Barwick, D.D. and Walton, J.N. Polymyositis. Am. J. Med., 35:646, 1963.

72. Bohan, A., Peter, J.B., Bowman, R.L., and Pearson, C.M. A computer-assisted analysis of 153 patients with polymyositis and dermatomyositis. Medicine, 56:255, 1977.

73. Cook, C.D., Rosen, F.S., and Banker, B.Q. Dermatomyositis and focal scleroderma. Pediatr. Clin. North Am., 10:879, 1963.

    A large pediatric series with description of pathology.

74. Currie, S., Saunders, M., Knowles, M., and Brown, A.E. Immunologic aspects of polymyositis: the in vitro activity of lymphocytes on incubation with muscle antigen and with muscle cultures. Q. J. Med., 157:63, 1971.

75. Johnson, R.L., Fink, C.W., and Ziff, M. Lymphotoxin formation by lymphocytes and muscle in polymyositis. J. Clin. Invest., 51:2435, 1972.

76. Pearson, C.M. Rheumatic manifestations of polymyositis and dermatomyositis. Arthritis Rheum., 2:127, 1959.

Polyarteritis

77. Bell, N.R. and Klinefelter, H.F. Polymyalgia rheumatica. Johns Hopkins Med. J., 121:175, 1967.

78. Cassan, S.M., Coles, D.T., and Harrison, E.G., Jr. The concept of limited forms of Wegener's granulomatosis. Am. J. Med., 49:366, 1970.

79. Christian, C.L. and Sergent, J.S. Vasculitis syndromes: clinical and experimental models. Am. J. Med., 61:385, 1976.

80. Churg, J. Granulomatosis and granulomatous-vascular syndromes. Ann. Allergy, 21:619, 1963.

81. Fahey, J.L., Leonard, E., Churg, J., and Godman, G. Wegener's granulomatosis. Am. J. Med., 17:168, 1954.

82. Fauci, A.S. The spectrum of vasculitis. Clinical, pathologic, immunologic and therapeutic considerations. Ann. Intern. Med., 89:660, 1978.

83. ———— and Wolff, S.M. Wegener's granulomatosis: studies in eighteen patients and a review of the literature. Medicine, 52:535, 1973.

84. Gocke, D.J., Morgan, C., Lockshin, M., Hsu, M., Bombardier, S., and Christian, C.L. Association between polyarteritis and Australia antigen. Lancet, 2:1149, 1970.

85. Hamilton, C.R., Jr. and Tumulty, P.A. Giant cell arteritis including temporal arteritis and polymyalgia rheumatica. Medicine, 50:1, 1971.

86. Leonhardt, E.T.G., Jakobson, H., and Ringqvist, O.T.A. Angiography and clinico-physiologic investigations of a case of polyarteritis nodosa. Am. J. Med., 53:242, 1972.

87. Reza, M.J., Dornfeld, L., Goldberg, L.S., Bluestone, R., and Pearson, C.M. Wegener's granulomatosis: long-term follow-up of patients treated with cyclophosphamide. Arthritis Rheum., 18:501, 1975.

88. Rich, A.R. and Gregory, J.C. The experimental demonstration that periarteritis nodosa is a manifestation of hypersensitivity. Johns Hopkins Med. J., 72:65, 1943.

89. Rose, G.A. The natural history of polyarteritis. Br. Med. J., 2:1148, 1957.

90. ———— and Spencer, H. Polyarteritis nodosa. Q. J. Med., 26:43, 1957.

91. Schrire, V. and Asherson, R.A. Arteritis of the aorta and its major branches. Q. J. Med., 33:439, 1964.

92. Sergent, J.S. and Christian, C.L. Necrotizing vasculitis after acute serous otitis media. Ann. Intern. Med., 56:412, 1974.

93. ————, Lockshin, M.D., Gocke, D.J., and Christian, C.L. Polyarteritis nodosa with and without persistent hepatitis-associated antigen. Long-term course in 21 patients. Arthritis Rheum., 16:568, 1973.

94. Winkelmann, R.K. and Winkelmann, W.B. Cutaneous and visceral syndromes of necrotizing or "allergic" angiitis. Medicine, 43:59, 1964.

95. Zeek, P.M. Periarteritis nodosa and other forms of necrotizing arteritis. N. Engl. J. Med., 248:764, 1953.

The Sjögren Syndrome

96. Anderson, L.G., Cummings, N.A., Asofsky, R., Hylton, M.B., Tarpley, T.M., Jr., Tomasi, T.B., Jr., Wolf, R.O., Schall, G.L., and Talal, N. Salivary gland immunoglobulin and rheumatoid factor synthesis in Sjögren's syndrome. Natural history and response to treatment. Am. J. Med., 53:456, 1972.

97. Block, K.J., Buchanan, W.W., Wohl, M.J., and Bunim, J.J. Sjögren's syndrome, a clinical, pathological and serologic study of 62 cases. Medicine, 44:187, 1965.

98. Cummings, N.A., Schall, G.L., Asofsky, R., et al. Sjögren's syndrome. Newer aspects of research, diagnosis and treatment. Ann. Intern. Med., 75:937, 1971.

99. Shearn, M.A. Sjögren's Syndrome. Philadelphia, Saunders, 1971.

100. Talal, N. and Bunim, J.J. The development of malignant lymphoma in the course of Sjögren's syndrome. Am. J. Med., 36:529, 1964.

101. ————, Sokoloff, L., and Barth, W. Extra-salivary lymphoid abnormalities in Sjögren's syndrome (reticulum cell sarcoma, "pseudolymphoma," macroglobulinemia). Am. J. Med., 43:50, 1967.

Rheumatoid Arthritis

102. Bartfield, H. and Epstein, W. (eds.). Rheumatoid factors and their biological significance. Ann. N.Y. Acad. Sci., 168:1, 1969.

103. Bluestone, R. and Bacon, P.A. (eds.). Extra-articular manifestations of rheumatoid arthritis. Clinics in Rheumatic Diseases, Vol. 3(3). Philadelphia, Saunders, 1977.

104. Bujak, J.S., Aptekar, R.G., Decker, J.L., and Wolff, S.M. Juvenile rheumatoid arthritis presenting in the adult as fever of unknown origin. Medicine, 52:431, 1973.

105. Bunch, T.W., Hunder, G.G., Offord, K., and McDuffie, F.C. Synovial fluid complement: usefulness in diagnosis and classification of rheumatoid arthritis. Ann. Intern. Med., 81:32, 1974.

106. Caplan, A. Certain unusual radiological appearances in the chest of coal miners suffering from rheumatoid arthritis. Thorax, 8:29, 1953.

107. The Cooperating Clinics Committee of the American Rheumatism Association. A controlled trial of gold salt therapy in rheumatoid arthritis. Arthritis Rheum., 16:353, 1973.

108. Cruickshank, B. Heart lesions in rheumatoid disease. J. Pathol., 76:223, 1958.

109. Fosdick, W.M., Parsons, J.L., and Hill, D.F. Long-term cyclophosphamide therapy in rheumatoid arthritis. Arthritis Rheum., 11:151, 1968.

110. Gordon, D.A., Stein, J.L., and Broder, I. The extra-articular features of rheumatoid arthritis. A systematic analysis of 127 cases. Am. J. Med., 54:445, 1973.

111. Hahn, B.H., Yardley, J.H., and Stevens, M.B. "Rheumatoid" nodules in systemic lupus erythematosus. Ann. Intern. Med., 72:49, 1970.

112. Hunder, G.G. and McDuffie, F.C. Hypocomplementemia in rheumatoid arthritis. Am. J. Med., 54:461, 1973.

113. John, J.T., Jr., Hough, A., and Sergent, J.S. Pericardial disease in rheumatoid arthritis. Am. J. Med., 66:385, 1979.

114. Mainland, D.M. and Decker, J.L. Cooperating Clinics Committee of the American Rheumatism Association. A controlled trial of cyclophosphamide in rheumatoid arthritis. N. Engl. J. Med., 283:883, 1970.

115. Mason, D.T. and Morris, J.J. The variable features of Felty's syndrome. Review of the literature and report of a case with massive splenomegaly. Am. J. Med., 36:463, 1964.

116. Marcus, R.L. and Townes, A.S. The occurrence of cryoproteins in synovial fluid: the association of a complement-fixing activity in rheumatoid synovial fluid with cold-precipitable protein. J. Clin. Invest., 50:282, 1971.

117. McMichael, A.J., Sasazuki, T., McDevitt, H.O., and Payne, R.O. Increased frequency of HLA–Cw3 and HLA–Dw4 in rheumatoid arthritis. Arthritis Rheum., 20:1037, 1977.

118. Mowat, A.G. (ed.). Surgical management of rheumatoid arthritis. Clinics in Rheumatic Diseases, Vol. 4 (2). Philadelphia, Saunders, 1978.

119. Ruddy, S. and Austin, K.F. The complement system in rheumatoid synovitis. Arthritis Rheum., 13:713, 1970.

120. Schmid, R.F., Cooper, N.S., Ziff, M., and McEwen, C. Arteritis in rheumatoid arthritis. Am. J. Med., 30:56, 1961.

121. Short, C.L., Bauer, W., and Reynolds, W.E. Rheumatoid Arthritis. Cambridge, Harvard University, 1957.

122. Sokoloff, C., McCluskey, R.T., and Bunim, J.J. Vascularity of the early subcutaneous nodule in rheumatoid arthritis. Arch. Pathol., 55:475, 1953.

123. Stage, D.E. and Mannik, M. Rheumatoid factors in rheumatoid arthritis. Bull. Rheum. Dis., 23:720, 1972–73.

124. Walker, W.C. and Wright, V. Pulmonary lesions and rheumatoid arthritis. Medicine, 47:501, 1968.

125. Weintraub, A.M. and Zwaifler, N.J. The occurrence of valvular and myocardial disease in patients with chronic joint deformity. A spectrum. Am. J. Med., 35:145, 1963.

126. Weissmann, G. Lysosomal mechanisms of tissue injury in arthritis. N. Engl. J. Med., 286:141, 1972.

The Differential Diagnosis of Multisystem Disease

127. Goldfine, L.J., Stevens, M.B., Masi, A.T., and Shulman, L.E. Clinical significance of the LE cell phenomenon in rheumatoid arthritis. Ann. Rheum. Dis., 24:153, 1965.

128. Harvey, A.M. Auto-immune disease and the chronic biologic false-positive test for syphilis. JAMA, 182:516, 1962.

129. Hijmans, W., Doniach, D., Roitt, I.M., and Holborow, E.J. Serologic overlap between lupus erythematosus, rheumatoid arthritis and thyroid autoimmune disease. Br. Med. J., 2:909, 1961.

130. Peterson, R.D.A. and Good, R.A. Interrelationships of the mesenchymal diseases with consideration of possible genetic mechanisms. Annu. Rev. Med., 14:1, 1963.

131. Sharp, G.C., Irvin, W.S., Tan, E.M., Gould, R.G., and Holman, H.R. Mixed Connective Tissue Disease—An apparently distinct rheumatic disease syndrome associated with a specific antibody to an extractable nuclear antigen (ENA). Am. J. Med., 52:148, 1972.

132. Shulman, L.E. Inducing agents and relationship to other diseases. Arthritis Rheum., 6:559, 1963.

Ankylosing Spondylitis and Related Disorders

133. Acheson, E.D. An association between ulcerative colitis, regional enteritis and ankylosing spondylitis. Q. J. Med., 29:489, 1960.

134. Ansell, B.M. and Wigley, R.A.D. Arthritic manifestations in regional enteritis. Ann. Rheum. Dis., 23:64, 1964.

135. Arnett, F.C., Schacter, B.Z., Hochberg, M.C., Hsu, S.H., and Bias, W.B. Homozygosity for HLA–B27: impact on rheumatic disease expression in two families. Arthritis Rheum., 20:797, 1977.

136. Fernandez-Herlihy, L. The articular manifestations of chronic ulcerative colitis. An analysis of 555 cases. N. Engl. J. Med., 261:259, 1959.

137. Ford, D.K. Reiter's syndrome. Bull. Rheum. Dis., 20:588, 1970.

138. Haslock, I. and Wright, V. The musculoskeletal complications of Crohn's disease. Medicine, 52:217, 1973.

139. McClusky, O.E., Lordon, R.E., and Arnett, F.C., Jr. HL-A 27 in Reiter's syndrome and psoriatic arthritis. A genetic factor in disease susceptibility and expression. J. Rheumatol., 1:263, 1974.

140. McEwen, C., DiTata, D., Lingg, C., Pozini, A., Good, A., and Rankin, T. Ankylosing spondylitis and spondylitis accompanying ulcerative colitis, regional enteritis, psoriasis and Reiter's disease. Arthritis Rheum., 14:291, 1971.

141. Moll, J.M.H., Haslock, I., Macrae, I.F., and Wright, V. Associations between ankylosing spondylitis, psoriatic arthritis, Reiter's disease, and intestinal arthropathies and Behçet's syndrome. Medicine, 53:343, 1974.

142. Noer, H.R. An "experimental" epidemic of Reiter's syndrome. JAMA, 198:693, 1966.

143. Sairanen, C., Paronen, K., and Mahonen, H. Reiter's syndrome: a follow-up study. Acta Med. Scand., 185:57, 1969.

144. Schachter, J., Barnes, M.G., Jones, J.P., Jr., Engleman, E.P., and Meyer, K.T. Isolation of Bedsonia from joints of patients with Reiter's syndrome. Proc. Soc. Exp. Biol. Med., 122:283, 1966.

145. Schlosstein, L., Terasaki, P., Bluestone, R., and Pearson, C.M. High association of an HL-A antigen, W27, with ankylosing spondylitis. N. Engl. J. Med., 288:704, 1973.

146. Weinberger, H.W., Ropes, M.W., Kulka, J.P., and Bauer, W. Reiter's syndrome, clinical and pathological observations. Medicine, 41:35, 1962.

147. Wright, V. Rheumatism and psoriasis, a reevaluation. Am. J. Med., 27:454, 1959.

148. ——— and Watkinson, G. The arthritis of ulcerative colitis. Medicine, 38:243, 1959.

Gout and Pseudogout

149. Bywaters, E.G.L. Calcium pyrophosphate crystal deposits in synovial membrane. Ann. Rheum. Dis., 31:219, 1972.

149a. Dieppe, P.A., Huskisson, E.C., Crocker, P., and Willoughby, D.A. Apatite deposition disease. Lancet, 1:266, 1976.

150. Green, M.L. Clinical features of patients with "partial" deficiency of the X-linked uricaciduria enzyme. Arch. Intern. Med., 130:193, 1972.

151. Gutman, A.B. (ed.). Proceedings of the conference on gout and purine metabolism. Arthritis Rheum., 8:598, 1965.

152. ———. Significance of the renal clearance of uric acid in normal and gouty man. Am. J. Med., 37:833, 1964.

152a. Halverson, P.B. and McCarty, D.J. Identification of hydroxyapatite crystals in synovial fluid. Arthritis Rheum., 22:389, 1979.

153. Kelley, W.N. (ed.). Crystal-induced arthropathies. Clinics in Rheumatic Diseases, Vol. 3 (1). Philadelphia, Saunders, 1977.

154. Kelley, W.N., Greene, M.L., Rosenbloom, F.M., et al. Hypoxanthinequanine phosphoribosyl transferase deficiency in gout. Ann. Intern. Med., 70:155, 1969.

155. Klinenberg, J.R., Goldfinger, S.E., and Seegmiller, J.E. The effectiveness of the xanthine oxidase inhibitor, allopurinol, in the treatment of gout. Ann. Intern. Med., 62:639, 1965.

156. Kohn, N.N., Hughes, R.E., McCarty, D.J., and Faires, J.S. The significance of calcium phosphate crystals in the synovial fluid of arthritic patients. II. Identification of crystals. Ann. Intern. Med., 56:738, 1962.

157. McCarty, D.J. Diagnostic mimicry in arthritis-patterns of joint involvement associated with calcium pyrophosphate dihydrate crystal deposits. Bull. Rheum. Dis., 25:804, 1974–75.

158. ———, Kohn, N.N., and Faires, J.S. The significance of calcium phosphate crystals in the synovial fluid of arthritic patients: the pseudogout syndrome. I. Clinical aspects. Ann. Intern. Med., 36:71, 1962.

159. ———, Silcox, D.C., Coe, F., et al. Diseases associated with calcium pyrophosphate dihydrate crystal deposition. A controlled study. Am. J. Med., 56:704, 1974.

160. ——— and Hollander, J.L. Identification of urate crystals in gouty synovial fluid. Ann. Intern. Med., 54:542, 1961.

161. Phelps, P. Polymorphonuclear leucocyte mobility in vitro. III. Possible release of a chemotactic substance after phagocytosis of urate crystals by polymorphonuclear leucocytes. Arthritis Rheum., 12:197, 1969.

162. ———. Polymorphonuclear leucocyte mobility in vitro. IV. Colchicine inhibition of chemotactic activity formation after phagocytosis of urate crystals. Arthritis Rheum., 13:1, 1970.

163. Reiselbach, R.E., Sorensen, L.B., Shelp, W.D., and Steele, T.H. Diminished urate secretion per nephron as a basis for primary gout. Ann. Intern. Med., 73:359, 1970.

163a. Schumacher, H.R., Smolyo, A.P., Tse, R.L., and Maurer, K. Arthritis associated with apatite crystals. Ann. Intern. Med., 87:411, 1977.

164. Seegmiller, J.E., Howell, R.R., and Malawista, S.E. The inflammatory reaction to sodium urate. JAMA, 180:469, 1962.

165. ———, Laster, I., and Howell, R.R. Biochemistry of uric acid and its relation to gout. N. Engl. J. Med., 268:712, 764, 821, 1963.

166. Talbott, J.H. Gout, 3rd ed. New York, Grune & Stratton, 1967.

167. Tse, R.L. and Phelps, P. Polymorphonuclear leucocyte motility in vitro. V. Release of chemotactic activity following phagocytosis of calcium pyrophosphate crystals, diamond dust and urate crystals. J. Lab. Clin. Med., 76:403, 1970.

Arthritis Caused by Infection

168. Alpert, E., Isselbacher, K.J., and Schur, P.H. The pathogenesis of arthritis associated with viral hepatitis: complement-component studies. N. Engl. J. Med., 285:185, 1971.

169. Berney, S., Goldstein, M., and Bishko, F. Clinical and diagnostic features of tuberculous arthritis. Am. J. Med., 53:36, 1972.

170. Davidson, P.T. and Horowitz, I. Skeletal tuberculosis: a review with patient presentations and discussion. Am. J. Med., 48:77, 1970.

171. Gray, M. and Philip, T. Syphilitic arthritis: diagnostic problems with special reference to congenital syphilis. Ann. Rheum. Dis., 22:19, 1963.

172. Hyer, F.H. and Gottlieb, N.L. Rheumatic disorders associated with viral infections. Semin. Arthritis Rheum., 8:17, 1978.

173. Karten, I. Septic arthritis complicating rheumatoid arthritis. Ann. Intern. Med., 70:1147, 1969.

174. Keiser, H., Ruben, F.L., Wolinsky, E., and Kushner, I. Clinical forms of gonococcal arthritis. N. Engl. J. Med., 279:234, 1968.

175. Kelly, P.J., Martin, W.J., Schirger, A., and Weed, L.A. Brucellosis of the bones and joints, experience with thirty-six patients. JAMA, 174:347, 1960.

176. ———, ———, and Coventry, M.B. Bacterial (suppurative) arthritis in the adult. J. Bone Joint Surg., 52A:1595, 1970.

177. Morris, J.L., Zizic, T.M., and Stevens, M.B. Proteus polyarthritis complicating systemic lupus erythematosus. Johns Hopkins Med. J., 133:262, 1973.

   The literature is reviewed relating to implications of corticosteroid therapy and septic arthritis.

178. Pinals, R.S. and Ropes, M.W. Meningococcal arthritis. Arthritis Rheum., 7:241, 1964.

179. Russell, A.S. and Ansel, B.M. Septic arthritis. Ann. Rheum. Dis., 31:40, 1972.

180. Smith, J.W. and Sanford, J.P. Viral arthritis. Ann. Intern. Med., 67:651, 1967.

181. Steere, A.C., Malawista, S.E., Syndman, D.R., Shope, R.E., Andiman, W.A., Ross, M.R., and Steele, F.M. Lyme arthritis. Arthritis Rheum., 20:7, 1977.

182. Warren, C.P.W. Arthritis associated with Salmonella infection. Ann. Rheum. Dis., 29:483, 1970.

183. Yancy, J.E., Thompson, G.R., Mikkelson, W.M., and Bartholomew, L.E. Rubella arthritis. Ann. Intern. Med., 64:772, 1966.

Degenerative Joint Disease

184. Bollet, A.J. An essay on the biology of osteoarthritis. Arthritis Rheum., 12:152, 1969.

185. Kellgren, J.H., Lawrence, J.S., and Bies, F. Genetic factors in generalized osteoarthritis. Ann. Rheum. Dis., 22:237, 1963.

186. Mankin, H.J. Biochemical and metabolic aspects of osteoarthritis. Orthop. Clin. North Am., 2:19, 1971.

187. Marmor, L. Surgery of osteoarthritis. Semin. Arthritis Rheum., 2:117, 1972.

188. Nugent, G.R. Clinicopathologic correlations in cervical spondylosis. Neurology, 9:273, 1955.

189. Peter, J.B., Pearson, C.M., and Marmor, L. Erosive osteoarthritis of the hands. Arthritis Rheum., 9:365, 1966.

190. Weiss, C. and Mirow, S. An ultrastructural study of osteoarthritic changes in the articular cartilage of human knees. J. Bone Joint Surg., 54A:954, 1972.

191. Wright, V. (ed.). Osteoarthrosis. Clinics in Rheumatic Diseases, Vol. 2 (3). Philadelphia, Saunders, 1976.

The Differential Diagnosis of Arthritis

192. Atkins, C.J., McIvor, J., Smith, P.M., et al. Chondrocalcinosis and arthropathy: studies in haemochromatosis and in idiopathic chondrocalcinosis. Q. J. Med., 39:71, 1970.

193. Blomgren, S.E. Conditions associated with erythema nodosum. N.Y. State J. Med., 72:2302, 1972.

194. Dressner, E. The bone and joint lesions of acute leukemia and their response to folic acid antagonists. Q. J. Med., 19:339, 1950.

195. Ehrlich, G.E., Young, I., Nosheny, S.Z., et al. Multicentric reticulohistiocytosis (lipoid dermatoarthritis): a multisystem disorder. Am. J. Med., 52:830, 1972.

196. Goldenberg, D.L. and Cohen, A.S. Synovial membrane histopathology in the differential diagnosis of rheumatoid arthritis, gout, pseudogout, systemic lupus erythematosus, infectious arthritis and degenerative joint disease. Medicine, 57:239, 1978.

197. Goldman, J.A., Glueck, C.J., Abrams, N.R., et al. Musculoskeletal disorders associated with Type IV hyperlipoproteinemia. Lancet, 1:449, 1972.

198. Gumpel, J.M., Johns, C.J., and Shulman, L.E. The joint disease of sarcoidosis. Ann. Rheum. Dis., 26:194, 1967.

199. Hamilton, E., Williams, R., Barlow, K.A., and Smith, P.M. The arthropathy of idiopathic hemochromatosis. Q. J. Med., 37:171, 1968.

200. Heller, H., Gafni, J., Michaeli, D., Shakin, N., Sohar, G.E., Karten, I., and Sokoloff, L. The arthritis of familial Mediterranean fever (FMF). Arthritis Rheum., 9:1, 1966.

201. Herndon, J.H. and Aufranc, O.E. Avascular necrosis of the femoral head in the adult. A review of the incidence in a variety of conditions. Clin. Orthop., 86:43, 1972.

202. Kelley, J.J. and Weisiger, B.B. The arthritis of Whipple's disease. Arthritis Rheum., 6:615, 1963.

203. Kellgren, J.H., Bau, J., and Tutton, G.K. The arthritis and other limb changes in acromegaly: a clinical and pathological study of 25 cases. Q. J. Med., 21:405, 1952.

204. O'Brien, W.M., LaDuc, B.N., and Bunim, J.J. Biochemical, pathologic and clinical aspects of alkaptonuria, ochronosis and ochronotic arthritis. Am. J. Med., 34:813, 1963.

205. Pearson, C.M., Kline, H.M., and Newcomer, V.D. Relapsing polychondritis. N. Engl. J. Med., 263:51, 1960.

206. Spilberg, I., Siltzbach, L.E., and McEwen, C. The arthritis of sarcoidosis. Arthritis Rheum., 12:126, 1969.

207. Truelove, L.H. Articular manifestations of erythema nodosum. Ann. Rheum. Dis., 19:174, 1960.

208. Whelton, M.J. Arthropathy and liver disease. Ir. Med. J., 65:456, 1972.

209. Zizic, T.M. and Stevens, M.B. The arthritis of Behçet's disease. Johns Hopkins Med. J., 136:243, 1975.

Disorders of the Nervous System
GUY M. McKHANN: SECTION EDITOR

CHAPTER 109
Introduction to Disorders of the Nervous System
GUY M. McKHANN

An increasing number of people are or will be afflicted with disorders of the nervous system. As the age distribution of the United States shifts toward an older range, the incidence of common neurologic afflictions of the elderly, such as stroke, dementia, parkinsonism, and osteoarthritis of the spine will continue to increase.

These disorders do not represent what the average physician sees in practice: the large number of patients with headache, dizziness, chronic back pain, weakness, or insomnia, symptom complexes which may or may not be associated with a significant abnormality of the nervous system. Most of these patients will be seen first by nonneurologists; thus, it is essential that practicing physicians: 1) learn to do a rapid screening examination of the nervous system; and 2) know how to focus their efforts on the area of dysfunction.

There are many approaches to the analysis and management of disorders of the nervous system and muscles. In many instances, the *clinical manifestations* are clear, e.g., seizures, dementia, headaches. We have taken this approach (the management of well-recognized symptom complexes) in chapters dealing with disorders of higher cortical function, disorders of movement, disorders of sensation, seizures, dizziness, increased intracranial pressure, and disorders of aging.

On other occasions, the patient presents with a *recognized diagnostic entity,* such as a stroke or peripheral neuropathy. We have presented material relating to these conditions in chapters on stroke, demyelinating disease, mass lesions, trauma, spinal cord disorders, myopathies, peripheral neuropathies, and disorders of the neuromuscular junction.

CHAPTER 110
The Neurologic History and Examination
GUY M. McKHANN

THE HISTORY

The history of neurologic symptoms is elicited as part of the general history taking (see Chaps. 1, 2, and 3). However, there are certain aspects to be emphasized.

1. What is the *pattern of disease?* Many disease processes may result in similar disabilities, in part because dysfunction of a particular region of the nervous system will lead to predictable symptoms. However, the rate and pattern of progression may be quite diagnostic. Several examples of patterns of disease are given in Figure 110–1.

2. Can we *bracket the lesion?* By that we mean what is the highest and what is the lowest point in the nervous system that can account for the dysfunction. Do the symptoms suggest a single lesion or multiple lesions?

3. Where should we *concentrate our efforts?* A detailed examination of all possible neurologic functions is lengthy, dull, and unrewarding. Proper interpretation of the history should steer the physician to the parts of the neurologic examination requiring greater attention.

4. Is the *patient aware* of his dysfunction? In many instances of acute disease, such as strokes or seizures, the patient is totally un-

1181

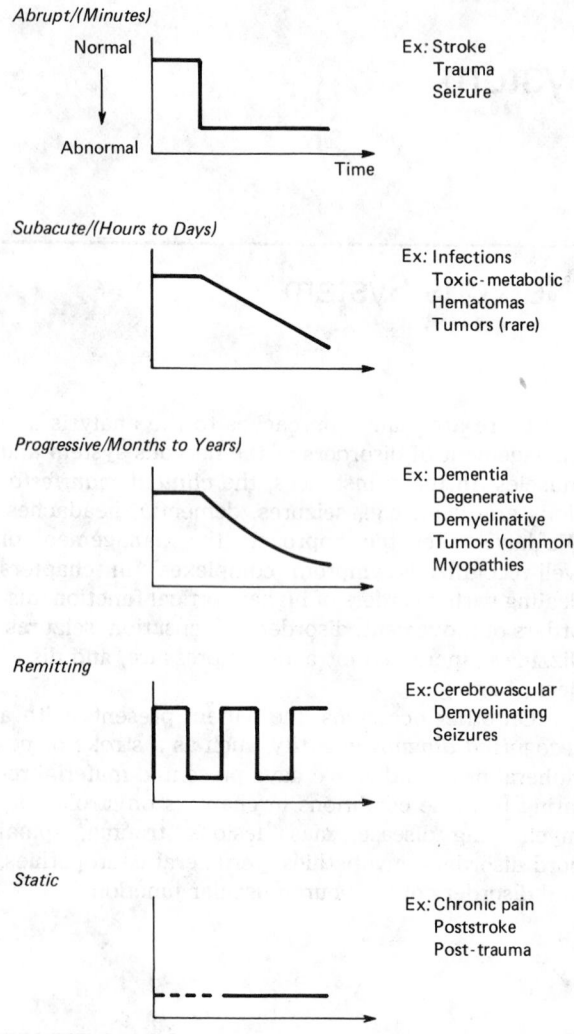

FIGURE 110–1. Patterns of progression of neurologic illness.

able to report what has happened. In these circumstances, important observations about the onset and pattern require another person. In eliciting this outside information, one should be aware that sudden disruption of neurologic function can be an extremely frightening event for witnesses. Thus, comments on subjects such as the duration or degree of unresponsiveness should be interpreted cautiously.

5. Is there an *underlying disease?* Many treatable conditions affecting the nervous system are manifestations of systemic diseases. Thinking of the nervous system in isolation from the rest of the body can lead to serious errors in diagnosis and management.

PHYSICAL EXAMINATION

Examination of the nervous system starts the moment the patient is first seen and should be, as much as possible, integrated into the general physical examination. Thus, cranial nerve function is tested when other features of the head are being examined; motor performance and sensory integrity of the limbs are best judged when the pulses, joints, and skin of the extremities are also under examination. Used in this regional manner, neurologic testing loses its artificiality and serves as a natural and functional challenge. The monotony and fatigue of special perceptive studies, e.g., visual and sensory testing, are reduced by variety, and, finally, through diversion of attention, artifacts that may be engendered by tension or malingering are avoided.

There are a number of guides to examination of the nervous system.[8,10–12]

The guide presented here serves two purposes:

1. It presents the strategy for a screening examination.
2. It provides a format for the description of neurologic findings and serves as a reminder to the examiner of the aspects of the nervous system he wishes to assess.

In appropriate chapters, more detailed aspects of the examination are presented.

A Guide to Neurologic Examination

I. Mental and Emotional State

State of consciousness: alert, slow, confused, stuporous, comatose

Mood: depressed, manic, labile

Orientation: to time, place, and person

Memory: recent and remote; specific tests of recall

Hallucinations or delusions: describe

Comprehension: spoken and written words, familiar objects; simple interpretation; calculation

Verbal expression: spoken, written

Purposeful motor activity: in absence of paralysis or receptive defect

II. Head and Neck

Scalp tenderness

Neck stiffness

Carotid pulsations

Bruits: carotids, heart, head

Vision: acuity*

Hearing: gentle whisper; air and bone conduction*

* These items may be obtained, in part, by history.

Cranial nerves
  I: test sense of smell†
  III, IV, VI: pupils—size, symmetry, reaction to light and convergence; ophthalmoscopy without mydriatics
      External ocular movements: ptosis; range of movement of eyes
  V: deviation of lower jaw on opening; sensibility of face; corneal reflex†
  VII: facial symmetry, palpebral fissures; voluntary and expressional movements
  IX, X: palate and gag responses, nasal voice, regurgitation swallowing†
  XII: movements and size of tongue

III. Motor System
Atrophy: local or generalized
Tone
Voluntary power: fine movements; rate of movement
Automatic movements: arm swinging, blinking
Coordination and repetition of movements: finger-nose, heel-shin
Involuntary movements: fasciculations; tremor
Posture: sitting, standing (Romberg's sign)
Gait

IV. Sensory System
Spontaneous: subjective pain, paresthesias, and their distribution*

† These items are not routinely tested.

Cutaneous sensibility: pin, touch, localization of stimuli, two–point discrimination, presence of sensory level
Proprioceptive sensibility: position sense, vibration

V. Reflexes
Stretch
  Biceps (C5,C6) musculocutaneous nerve
  Brachioradial (C5,C6) radial nerve
  Triceps (C6,C7,C8) radial nerve
  Finger (C7,C8) median nerve, ulnar nerve
  Knee (L2,L3,L4) femoral nerve
  Hamstring (L5,S1) sciatic nerve
  Ankle (L5,S1) sciatic nerve
Cutaneous
  Upper abdominal (T6,T7,T8,T9)
  Lower abdominal (T10,T11,T12)
Other
  Corneal (V, VII) trigeminal nerve, facial nerve†
  Jaw (V) trigeminal nerve
  Gag (IX, X) vagus nerve†
  Plantar response (Babinski)

VI. Bladder and Rectum
  Hesitancy
  Retention
  Urgency
  Incontinence
  Conscious sensation*

VII. Sexual Function*

CHAPTER 111
The Use of Ancillary Diagnostic Tests
GUY M. McKHANN

The functional or morphologic derangement of the nervous system may be demonstrated by a number of different diagnostic procedures.[19,20] The physician should know what each procedure can and cannot do, the relative risks of each procedure, and the most effective and efficient sequence of tests for a particular problem. In addition, the physician should be clear about what questions he is asking. For example, the technique of electroencephalography or angiography is varied depending on the type of information being sought.

When possible, one proceeds from the simpler tests, which have little attendant risk or discomfort, to more complex tests, ones which may, for example, upset intracranial dynamics. Certain test procedures make performance or interpretation of other procedures more difficult. For this reason, a lumbar puncture should be deferred in a patient being considered for myelography or pneumoencephalography, because a tear in the arachnoidal membrane may allow the air or dye to escape from the subarachnoid to the subdural space.

NEURORADIOLOGY

The usefulness of various neuroradiographic procedures is indicated in Table 111-1.

Skull Films[19,20]

Skull films may indicate disruption or distortion of the bony structures of the skull, the location of normally calcified structures such as the pineal or choroid plexus, and the presence of abnormal calcifications. Skull films are indicated in cases of trauma and suspected intracranial tumor. They are part of the investigation of seizures, headaches, disturbances of consciousness, and focal neurologic signs. In certain instances, special views of the base of the skull, sinuses, optic foramina, internal auditory meati, and sella turcica are indicated.

Spine Films[19,20]

Roentgenograms of the vertebral column are indicated in patients with symptoms and signs suggesting involvement of the spinal cord, nerve roots, meninges, or vertebral bodies. Routine films of the appropriate region include anterior–posterior and lateral projections and, in the cervical region, oblique views to demonstrate the intervertebral foramina. More precise information may be obtained by localized spot films and tomograms. Cervical spine films should also be obtained in cases of head trauma, because partial as well as impending cervical dislocations can often be detected before cord compression occurs.

Computerized Axial Tomography (CAT Scanning)[14,15]

This noninvasive procedure provides a rapid, safe analysis of the radiographic density of the skull and its contents. The procedure demonstrates the morphology of brain substance, ventricular cavities, orbits, the subarachnoid space, and the surrounding bone. Areas of altered permeability and vascularity can be demonstrated by an "enhanced scan" which is obtained by repeating the scan after intravenous injection of an iodinated dye.

AREAS OF USEFULNESS. The CAT scan has replaced pneumoencephalography, arteriography, and isotopic brain scanning as the primary diagnostic procedure for detection of intracranial masses, cerebral atrophy, hydrocephalus, areas of cortical infarction, and delineation of developmental defects of the nervous system.

RISKS. The procedure is safe. The patient is exposed to a dosage of x-irradiation equivalent to that

TABLE 111-1
Usefulness of Neuroradiographic Procedures

	Skull X-Ray	CAT Scan	Angio-gram	Isotopic Scan
Skull				
Fracture	+			
Bone density	+	+		
Bone erosion	+	±		
Intracranial calcification	+	±		
Ventricular system				
Size		+	+	
Displacement		+	±	
CSF dynamics				+
Brain substance				
Atrophy		+	±	
Masses		+	±	+
Infarction		+		
Hematoma		+	±	±
Vascular pattern				
Patency			+	
Displacement			+	
Malformation	±		+	±
Aneurysm			+	

of a skull series. With increasing availability of CAT scanning, overinterpretation of CAT scans has become a common problem. The physician should be cautious of reported abnormalities which do not correspond to the patient's neurologic signs and symptoms. Artifacts do occur on CAT scans, and are best checked by repeating the procedure.

Angiography[18,20]

The technique of cranial angiography has changed in recent years, so that direct injection of radiopaque material into the carotid and vertebral arteries is often replaced by retrograde brachial injection or selective catheterization approaches in which a catheter is passed up the femoral artery to the arch of the aorta. These advances have made angiography a considerably safer, faster, and more pleasant procedure than previously.

AREAS OF USEFULNESS. Angiography indicates processes which obstruct, disrupt, or displace the normal intracranial vascular patterns. Thus, local obstruction secondary to *arteriosclerotic disease* can be demonstrated. In these cases, selective catheterization studies may be required to demonstrate the takeoff of the major vessels from the aortic arch. A block in the extracranial vessels may be amenable to surgery (Chap. 129).

In *subarachnoid bleeding*, careful angiography is essential for demonstrating the site of bleeding, either aneurysm or arteriovenous malformation. In these cases, it is extremely important that careful coordination between the neurologic, neurosurgical, and neuroradiologic personnel be achieved so that the correct assessment of surgical feasibility be reached. Special views are often required to demonstrate the exact shape and position of an aneurysm. Vascular malformations may also involve the spinal cord. In these cases it may be necessary to catheterize intercostal arteries selectively to identify the blood supply of the malformation.

Angiography is of assistance in delineating the size and position of the ventricular system in patients with *increased intracranial pressure*. Symmetrical enlargement of the lateral ventricles is indicated by an increased sweep of the pericallosal branches of the anterior cerebral arteries as they pass around the anterior horn of the lateral ventricles and a widened curve of the thalamostriate veins, situated in the floor of the lateral ventricles. In patients with increased intracranial pressure, it is reassuring to find the posterior inferior cerebellar arteries in their normal position, indicating no preexisting herniation through the foramen magnum.

Intracranial mass lesions may be extramedullary, such as *meningiomas, epidural* or *subdural hematomas,* or intramedullary, such as *glial tumors, abscesses,* or *hematomas.* In both locations, masses declare themselves by displacement of major vessels. In some cases, particularly *malignant neoplasms,* their abnormal small vessels or capillaries appear as a "tumor blush."

RISKS. The change to retrograde and catheter injections has decreased the rate of complications. However, complications do occur. In most large series, there is a 0.5 percent risk of serious neurologic complication and a 5 to 7 percent risk of transient, reversible neurologic signs or symptoms. Hematoma or vascular spasm at the site of injection are usually self-limited. The more serious problems are emboli, either from the end of the catheter or dislodged from a vessel wall, and hypersensitivity reactions to the dye. In elderly patients with known arteriosclerotic vascular disease the increased risks of arteriography should be weighed against whether the physician is prepared to take any therapeutic steps, i.e., vascular surgery, on the basis of the information obtained.

Air Encephalography[20]

In air encephalography, the ventricular system and subarachnoid space are delineated radiographically by the partial displacement of CSF with air. In pneumoencephalography, air is injected into the lumbar subarachnoid space, whereas in ventriculography, air is placed directly into a lateral ventricle through an opening in the skull. Pneumoencephalography demonstrates not only the ventricular system but also the basal cisterns and the subarachnoid space overlying the cerebral hemispheres. Ventriculography is reserved for patients with increased intracranial pressure in whom an air study from below could upset intracranial pressure relationships. Occasionally, it is necessary to outline intraventricular masses by the intraventricular injections of a radiopaque material such as Pantopaque.

AREAS OF USEFULNESS. Air encephalography has been largely displaced by CAT scanning. It may still be useful in determining the site of CSF obstruction in hydrocephalus or demonstrating structural abnormalities of the posterior fossa.

RISKS. Many patients have some degree of headache following air encephalography. Some have fever and hypotension. Patients with increased intracranial pressure or occult hydrocephalus may have signs of increased intracranial pressure or foraminal herniation. For this reason, air encephalography is a procedure for which the physician should have clearcut indications and be ready to proceed immediately with definitive surgical correction when indicated.

Myelography[19,20]

Myelography is performed to demonstrate mass lesions within the spinal canal. Radiopaque material is injected into the lumbar subarachnoid space, the dye column is followed by fluoroscopy, and x-ray films are taken of the suspected regions.

AREAS OF USEFULNESS. Myelography is useful for demonstrating external compression of the spinal cord and roots by masses such as *protruded intervertebral discs, osteoarthritic bone, tumors,* or *abscesses.* In addition, the size of the cord can be determined; an increase indicating an intramedullary process such as *syringomyelia* or an *intramedullary tumor.* In certain instances, the cord can be outlined to a greater degree by air myelography rather than by the use of an opaque contrast material.

RISKS. If care is taken to avoid injection of the contrast material into a subdural or epidural spaces, myelography is a safe procedure. Occasionally, patients with a mass impinging on the spinal cord will develop further compression following myelography.

Brain Scan[16]

Scintillation scanning of the head is carried out after intravenous injection of appropriate radioactive substances, such as [99m] Technetium. Normally, the blood-borne isotope is excluded by brain parenchyma. Uptake by brain indicates either a breakdown of the blood–brain barrier or formation of new, permeable vessels. The procedure is particularly useful for detection of tumors, abscesses, and hematomas. However, areas of recent infarction or contusion will also give a positive uptake as will the normal extracranial soft tissues at the base of the skull.

Cisternal scans are used to demonstrate ventricular size and patency of pathways of CSF flow and reabsorption. Radioactive material is injected in the subarachnoid space and serial scans of the head are performed for up to 72 hours. Normally, little isotope enters the ventricles, the majority going over the cortical surface as CSF is reabsorbed. With a communicating hydrocephalus, secondary to a block in paths of reabsorption of CSF, isotope enters the ventricular system to an abnormal degree, and may remain for 24 to 72 hours (ventricular stasis). Cisternography may also be useful for detecting the site of a CSF leak in a patient with recurrent meningitis.

CEREBROSPINAL FLUID EXAMINATION

Cerebrospinal fluid (CSF) is formed within the ventricular system, primarily from the choroid plexus. There is a circulation through the ventricular foramina, down over the surface of the spinal cord and roots, and up through the basal cisterns to the sites of reabsorption over the surface of the brain. Ordinarily, one samples the spinal subarachnoid fluid by lumbar puncture in order to obtain information about intracranial pressure, composition of CSF, and evidence of infection or cellular reaction of meningeal membranes.

Areas of Usefulness

Changes in the CSF may be diagnostic of intracranial infections or subarachnoid hemorrhages. Unless there is clear contraindication, the CSF should be examined in anyone suspected of having meningitis (that is, anyone with headaches and fever, stiff neck, or altered mental state). The CSF should be examined in all patients with a positive serologic test for syphilis and in patients suspected of having neurosyphilis. The presence of red blood cells or xanthochromic fluid is an indication of intracranial bleeding. It should be remembered, however, that normal find-

ings do not exclude *thrombosis, embolism, intracranial hemorrhage,* or *epidural* or *subdural hematoma.*

The CSF protein may be elevated in *polyneuropathy.* This finding can be helpful in differentiating polyneuropathy from other conditions producing weakness. The diagnosis of *intracranial masses* can be aided by the finding of either elevated protein or increase in pressure. Similarly, the protein may be elevated or abnormal in degenerative or demyelinative diseases. Manometrics are not routinely done but are useful when a block in CSF circulation at the spinal level is suspected (Queckenstedt test).

Technique

Many lumbar punctures have to be repeated needlessly because of poor technique. Proper positioning of the patient is essential for easy entry into the lumbar subarachnoid space. The patient should lie on his side with his neck flexed and his head supported by a pillow. The thighs should be flexed on the abdomen with the plane of the back perpendicular to the bed. The L2–L3 interspace may be identified by an imaginary line connecting the iliac crests. After the skin is cleaned and the skin and intraspinous ligament are infiltrated with local anesthetic, the lumbar puncture needle is advanced. It should be kept parallel to the bed, with the bevel turned to pass through the longitudinally running fibers of the dura. There is often a distinct "pop" as the dura is penetrated. The stylet should be withdrawn periodically as the needle is advanced.

After the needle has entered the subarachnoid space, particularly with an anxious or uncooperative patient, it is wise to remove a few drops of fluid for cell count before moving the patient. The patient is then allowed to extend his neck and thighs slowly to avoid a spurious increase in intracranial pressure. The manometer is attached and the initial pressure measured. At this point, jugular compression may be performed if spinal disease is suspected. It should be emphasized, however, that *jugular compression is contraindicated* if there is any increase in CSF pressure. After removal of appropriate fluid for studies, a final pressure is determined, and the needle withdrawn.

If the pressure is unexpectedly high, there will be enough fluid within the manometer for cell count, bacterial studies, and protein. It is important that no excess fluid be removed.

The most common problem is the distinction between a "bloody tap" and true subarachnoid bleeding. The major factor is whether the amount of blood decreases in successive samples of CSF. Serial observations of the fluid with blood counts are essential. The presence of xanthochromia after the CSF has been centrifuged is indicative of previous subarachnoid bleeding under these circumstances.

Risks

The major risk of lumbar puncture is that intracranial dynamics will be upset and the brain will shift downward through the tentorial notch or foramen magnum. This is particularly likely to happen when there is a large, asymmetrical, supratentorial mass, or a mass in the posterior fossa. In contrast, tentorial or foraminal herniation are seldom seen with diffuse increases in intracranial volume, as occurs in infections, subarachnoid bleeding, or meningeal involvement with neoplasm. Each patient requires a judgment decision. If CNS infection or bleeding is suspected, lumbar puncture cannot be deferred. If the probable diagnosis is a localized intracranial mass, other procedures, such as CAT scan, brain scan, or angiography will provide more information without the risk of upsetting intracranial pressure relationships.

Examinations

Certain examinations should always be performed on the CSF. These include gross description of its appearance, cell count, protein determination, and Wasserman. CSF should be collected for culture and glucose determinations when an increased white cell count is found or infection is suspected. A simultaneous blood sugar should be obtained for comparison with the CSF sugar. There is a tendency to send CSF to the laboratory for analysis. However, in certain conditions, particularly infection and possible meningeal tumor, the physician should do the cell count personally.

In performing the cell count the physician should proceed along the logical path listed in Table 111–2 until the cells are identified with certainty. In certain situations, special tests may be of help. An increase in gamma globulin, with particular patterns of oligoclonal bands demonstrated by *spinal fluid electrophoresis* is found in chronic infections (syphilis or inclusion body encephalitis) or demyelination diseases. *Cytology* is of help in cases with possible meningeal involvement with neoplasm.

ELECTROENCEPHALOGRAPHY[17]

The electroencephalogram (EEG) records electrical activity generated from the surface of the brain. One can find a variety of patterns ranging from absence of all activity, as in "cerebral death," to excessive, synchronous activity as occurs in seizures.

TABLE 111–2
Steps in Evaluation of Cells in Cerebrospinal Fluid

I. **Perform Chamber Count and Differential**
   Count the number of cells in all 9 ruled squares (0.9 μl) of a hemocytometer filled with undiluted CSF. Multiply by 1.1 to obtain count per μl. Identify each cell under high power

   A. If there are too many white cells:
      Dilute CSF 1 to 11 with Turck's solution in WBC pipette. Count the number of cells in all nine ruled squares (0.9 μl) of a hemocytometer. Multiply by 10 to obtain count per μl. Identify each cell or up to 100 cells under high power

   B. If there are too many red cells:
      1. Evaluate red cells by hematocrit
      2. Perform chamber count and differential after acid hemolysis
         Dilute glacial (28 percent) acetic acid 1 to 11 with CSF in a WBC pipette. The acid hemolyses the red cells without much dilution of the white cells.
         Count the number of cells in the nine ruled squares. (0.9 μl) of a hemocytometer. This is the number of cells per μl. Identify each cell or up to 100 cells under high power

II. **If There Are Increased Polymorphonuclear Cells, Obtain:**

   A. Cultures:
      For bacteria (including warmed chocolate agar in carbon dioxide for meningococci), fungi, and tubercle bacilli

   B. Glucose
   C. Gram stain of centrifuged sediment
   D. Acid-fast stain of centrifuged sediment

III. **If There Are Increased Mononuclear Cells, Obtain:**

   A.
   B. } As above
   C.
   D.

   E. India ink preparation:
      Cover a drop of CSF (or spun sediment) containing the cells with a coverslip. Put a split drop of India ink at the edge of the coverslip. Look for a clear halo around the cell indicating the capsule of cryptococcus

IV. **If There Are Bizarre or Unidentified Cells, Obtain:**

   A.
   B.
   C. } As above
   D.
   E.

   F. Wright's stain of sediment (lymphoma)
   G. Cytopathologic examination of sediment (tumor)

Areas of Usefulness

The EEG is useful in determining the overall activity of the brain and in detecting focal slowing and focal or generalized seizure activity. Discrete sharp waves and spikes are seen with focal seizure discharges; three-per-second spike and wave activity suggests subcortical discharges. It is possible, however, for seizure activity, particularly from temporal lobe, not to be reflected as an abnormality on scalp recording.

The EEG may be helpful in detecting *intracranial masses* (slow, delta waves) or *subdural hematoma* (locally decreased amplitude). Although in these circumstances, abnormal findings are meaningful, negative findings do not exclude a mass lesion.

Finally, the EEG can be used to determine the overall functional activity of the brain. This assessment can be useful in cases of *drug intoxication, metabolic encephalopathies, diffuse infections,* or *severe trauma.* An electrically silent, or flat, EEG has become a requirement for the diagnosis of "cerebral death."[21]

Technique

It is important that the electroencephalographer know what medications the patient is taking and the nature of the diagnostic problem. For example, if temporal lobe seizures are suspected, recording during sleep or recording with specially placed electrodes will be required.

BIOPSY

Biopsies can be obtained from brain, peripheral nerve, or muscle. *Brain biopsy* is used for diagnostic purposes in cases of suspected tumor and certain types of degenerative diseases or chronic infections. *Peripheral nerve biopsy* is usually of a sensory nerve, such as the sural nerve, and is of limited value except in certain metabolic disorders which specifically affect nerve, i.e., metachromatic leukodystrophy or amyloidosis. *Muscle biopsy* is an essential part of the workup of neuromyopathies (see Chap. 124).

CHAPTER 112
Disorders of Consciousness
GUY M. McKHANN

The term *conscious* implies that a patient is awake, alert, aware of himself and of his environment. Some authors have divided this concept further to include a state of *arousal* and a state of being aware of the *content* of what is going on. At the other extreme, is the comatose patient, responding to no outside stimulus. Some of the terms used to define altered states of consciousness are indicated in Table 112–1.

Consciousness requires two parts of the brain to be functionally intact and interrelated: the cerebral hemispheres and the ascending reticular activating systems from the brain stem. Thus, disorders of consciousness are seen with two types of central nervous system disease

1. Diffuse involvement of cerebral hemispheres, as occurs with abnormal metabolic states
2. Specific lesions which involve brain stem activating mechanisms

Brain stem involvement can occur with either supratentorial lesions which compress the brain stem, as occurs with tentorial herniation secondary to a mass, or by infratentorial lesions which specifically involve the central portions of the brain stem, as in a brain stem infarction or hemorrhage.

Patients can move through various stages of consciousness quite quickly. However, there are two stages with which the physician commonly has to deal, confusion and coma.

CONFUSION

The confused patient is often disoriented in time and place, with a decreased attention span and altered short-term memory. In addition, he may be irritable or drowsy. The causes of confusion are indicated in Table 112–2. The pattern of onset and duration is important in distinguishing the various causes. In a general hospital, the most common causes of acute confusion are drugs and intercurrent illnesses, e.g., pneumonia, cardiac failure, fever. In the elderly, confusion is often superimposed on dementia.

TABLE 112-1
Altered States of Consciousness[22]

Term	Characteristics
Conscious	Alert, awake Aware of one's self and environment
Confusion	Disorientation in time Irritability and/or drowsiness Misjudgment of sensory input Shortened attention span Decrease in memory
Delirium	Disorientation, fear Misperception of sensory stimuli Visual and auditory hallucinations Loss of contact with environment
Stupor	Unresponsive, but can be aroused back to a near normal state
Coma	Unresponsive to external stimuli
Akinetic mutism	Alert-appearing Immobile Mental activity absent
Locked-in syndrome	No effective verbal or motor communication Consciousness may be intact EEG indicates a preservation of cerebral activity Secondary to bilateral supranuclear paralysis at the level of the brain stem
Chronic vegetative state	Secondary to severe brain damage Often follows a period of coma Vital functions preserved with no evidence of active mental processes EEG indicates absence of cerebral activity

TABLE 112-2
Causes of Confusion

Primary CNS	Systemic (See Chap. 147)
Trauma	Infection
Cerebral contusion	Pneumonia
Cerebral concussion	Septicemia
Subdural and epidural hematoma	Fever
Cerebrovascular	Cardiovascular
Transient ischemic attack	Congestive heart failure
	Hypotension
Cerebral infarction	Hypertension
Cerebral hemorrhage	Drug intoxication
Subarachnoid hemorrhage	Drug withdrawal
Infection	Metabolic
Meningitis	Hypoglycemia
Encephalitis	Hypoxia
Tumor	Hypercapnia
Increased intracranial pressure	Uremia
	Hepatic failure
Dementia	Hyperviscosity
Seizures and postictal states	Hyponatremia
	Hypernatremia
	Myxedema
	Hyperthyroidism

The confused patient should be kept quiet, with a minimum of external stimuli. One should resist the temptation to add even more medications, until sure of the etiology.

COMA

This term implies that a patient is unresponsive to external stimuli. There are various stages of coma ranging from "deep coma" (unresponsive to all stimuli) to "semicoma" (partial response to noxious stimuli). Rather than use descriptive terms, it is preferable for the physician to describe exactly what the patient can and cannot do. Thus, it is possible for a subsequent observer to determine if the patient's condition is deteriorating or improving.

As the patient's neurologic function decompensates in a cephalad to caudal direction, functions such as respirations, eye movements, and reflexes deteriorate in predictable ways. To a certain extent, recovery follows the reverse of this pattern. However, many patients change rapidly and progress through various stages very quickly. The variables one follows are respirations, pupillary responses, extraocular movements, and motor function. The changes in motor function are discussed in Chapter 116 and extraocular movements in Chapter 119. Progressive changes in respiration and pupillary response are indicated in Table 112-3.

The acute confusional state is a diagnosable condition. However, modern diagnostic techniques such as CAT scans or multiple blood analyses are not of help. Rather, a systematic search for an underlying cause, particularly drug ingestion, is required. In this age of specialization it is common for patients to receive drugs from different specialists, so that a total of 10 or 12 different preparations are taken. Systematic removal of drugs is often an essential step in both diagnosis and cure.

TABLE 112–3
Neurologic Variables in Coma

Respirations

Location	Pattern	Description
Cerebral hemi-spheres (Bilateral deep lesions, metabolic en-cephalopathies	Cheyne-Stokes	Alternating hypercapnia and apnea
Low midbrain and middle one-third of pons	Central hyperventila-tion	Sustained, rapid hyperpnea
Mid- and caudal pons	Apneustic	Prolonged inspiratory pause
Medulla	Ataxic	Completely irregular pattern

Pupillary Responses

Location	Finding
Cerebral hemispheres Structural Metabolic	Normal Often small
Unilateral hemispheric	Ipsilateral dilation (Third-nerve paresis)
Hypothalamus	Ipsilateral constriction with ptosis and anhydrosis on ipsilateral body (central Horner syndrome)
Tectal midbrain	Large, fixed to light, ciliospinal reflex intact, spontaneous hippus may occur
Midbrain	Midposition, fixed, irregular
Pons	Small, may be pin-point, light reflex present, but hard to detect

TABLE 112–4
Neurologic Distinction Between Coma of Structural Versus Metabolic Causes[22]

	Structural	Metabolic-Toxic
Respirations	Predictable pattern of respiratory dysfunction with other brain stem signs (Table 112–3).	Respiration selectively depressed Distinctive patterns in diabetic acidosis
Extraocular move-ments	Paralysis a late sign	Drugs may give paresis of movement with normal pupillary responses
	Nystagmus on lateral gaze suggests cerebellar hemorrhage	Nystagmus in all directions of gaze suggests drug ingestion
Pupils	Predictable findings with specific levels of brain stem dysfunction (Table 112–3)	Specific drugs give small or large pupils

When faced with a patient in coma, the physician must think, almost simultaneously, of both diagnosis and management. The approach to management is outlined in Chapter 147. A crucial distinction is between coma secondary to a structural lesion and coma secondary to toxic-metabolic causes (Table 112–4).

Prognosis

Patients do not remain in deep coma. They either die, recover to various degrees, or plateau at a level described as a *chronic vegetative state*. In this condi-tion, patients have no meaningful higher cortical function. Brain stem function, however, may be pre-served with maintenance of cardiac and respiratory functions, and primitive reflex withdrawal from nox-ious stimuli. The EEG is helpful in establishing this diagnosis, the pattern being marked diffuse, low-volt-age slowing. In severe cases there may be little evi-dence of cerebral electrical activity. At later stages, the CAT scan may show cortical atrophy and second-ary enlargement of the ventricles.

LOCKED-IN SYNDROME

In contrast to the patients with irreversible cortical damage are the patients who have damaged the ven-tral brain stem so that corticobulbar and corticospi-nal impulses from cerebral cortex are disconnected. These patients, referred to as being "locked-in," have

are 1) progressive multifocal leukoencephalopathy, 2) subacute sclerosing panencephalitis, 3) Creutzfeldt-Jakob disease, and 4) Kuru. These processes are rare, but may serve as models of a disease mechanism which may apply to other degenerative conditions of the nervous system.

Progressive multifocal leukoencephalopathy[23,31] usually occurs in patients who have some other debilitating disease, particularly lymphomas. JC virus, a new papovavirus, has been isolated from most cases. In two cases viruses antigenically similar to simian virus 40 (SV 40) have been obtained. The initial symptom is usually dementia, followed by evidence of visual field or motor impairment. There is no reliable laboratory test short of brain biopsy. Pathologically, there are numerous small patches of demyelination and many cells, particularly oligodendroglia, containing intranuclear inclusions which have the ultrastructural appearance of papovavirus virions.

Subacute sclerosing panencephalitis[23,24] is a progressive, dementing disease of children and young adults. The dementia is rapid and usually associated with myoclonic jerks or seizures. The disease is apparently related to chronic infection with the measles virus.[23,24] The diagnosis can be established by a rise in gamma globulin in cerebrospinal fluid, a first zone rise in the colloidal gold curve, and an elevation of antibodies to measles virus in cerebrospinal fluid or serum.

Creutzfeldt-Jakob disease[25,26] is a well-defined clinical entity which was formerly classed as a presenile dementia of unknown etiology. Pathologically, there are widespread spongiform changes with associated neuronal loss. Although the agent has not been isolated, the disease has been successfully passed, by intracerebral inoculation of affected brain, to chimpanzees. Clinically, the onset is more rapid than in other dementias, and progression is such that day-to-day deterioration may be noted. Two-thirds of patients are dead within five months of onset. Myoclonic jerks are a constant feature and may be brought out by any sudden stimulus, such as switching on the light or making a sudden noise. Extrapyramidal signs (particularly rigidity) and fasciculations caused by lower motor neuron involvement are common.

Knowledge of the existence of this disease is of particular importance to pathologists and neurosurgeons because of the potential for man-to-man transmission. This concern is based on the transmission through corneal transplantation from a donor with Cretzfeldt-Jakob disease and by the use of stereotactic electrodes which had been previously used in a patient with the disease. Guidelines for medical care and handling of tissues have recently been proposed.[26]

Kuru is a disease limited to the natives of eastern New Guinea and is characterized by ataxia and dementia. This endemic disease was spread by human cannabalism. It is of importance because it was the first "slow" virus infection of man to be transmitted to laboratory animals.

Therapeutic Management of the Patient with Progressive Dementia

The first step, as already mentioned, is to be sure that treatable causes have been ruled out. Second, the patient's current status should be carefully evaluated. It is important that the patient's family or associates know his limitations.

The presenile and senile dementias are progressive processes. If the patient is not becoming progressively worse, the diagnosis should be reconsidered. When progression is not occurring, the possibility that the basic process is depression and not dementia should be seriously considered. Many patients with dementia do become depressed and withdrawn so that this differential can be quite difficult.

As the process progresses, the patient needs a stable, nonstressful environment. The memory deficit can be helped by developing a strict routine for the patient, and providing the patient with written reminders of what is to be done. Some patients can become agitated, especially at night ("sun-downing" is a colloquial term for this phenemonon). In these patients, haloperidol, 0.5 mg twice a day, may be of help. The dose may be increased to 1 to 2 mg three times a day. Chloral hydrate, 500 mg, is useful for sleep. Barbiturates are to be avoided because many patients will become confused and agitated on these drugs.

CHAPTER 114

Disorders of Communication
BARRY GORDON AND GUY M. McKHANN

NORMAL LANGUAGE PROCESSING

In order to understand what happens in disease, it is important to understand how the brain normally processes language.

Speech and language depend upon the left cerebral hemisphere in almost all right-handers and most left-handers (Fig. 114–1). Specific areas of the cortex (centers) have more or less specific functions. The cortical auditory areas 41 and 42 (on the dorsal aspect of the temporal lobe, hidden in the figure) receive the acoustic input and pass it on to Wernicke's area and the adjacent cortical areas (the supramarginal and angular gyri). There the raw sounds are transformed into meaningful speech sounds and then into their actual meanings. The angular gyrus is probably also where visual symbols (written words) are translated into their meanings. It is not understood where our own inner speech comes from, but it is probably also channeled through these centers. In order to speak, language information is transmitted by the arcuate fasciculus (and possibly other paths) to Broca's area (roughly area 44) in the inferior frontal lobe, where it is converted into motor commands. The commands are sent from Broca's area to nearby areas in the motor strip, which are the cortical areas for control of the speech musculature. These areas, in turn, control the brain stem nuclei of the cranial nerves and the centers of respiration to orchestrate the speech act. Overall, we can think of these processes as the input (receptive), central, and output (expressive) functions that are necessary for normal speech.

DYSARTHRIAS

This outline will help the physician diagnose the site and nature of the lesion responsible for many disorders of speech and communication, even though many of the details are vague or unknown. An important distinction to make when first seeing the patient is between dysarthria and aphasia. Dysarthria is difficulty with the motor control of the tongue, lips, palate, pharynx, larynx, and respiratory muscles. Dysarthria can, therefore, be caused by a wide variety of lesions of either or both cerebral hemispheres, the basal ganglia, the brain stem, or even the muscles themselves (Table 114–1).

APHASIAS

Aphasia (dysphasia) is a true disturbance of language and, therefore, implies a cerebral lesion, usually on the left, and usually cortical. There are two common patterns of aphasic disorder corresponding to the receptive/expressive processes, which have rough correlations with the sites of the lesions (Table 114–2).

Receptive Aphasia (Wernicke's Asphasia)
These patients have very poor comprehension of speech as well as language. Often their inner speech or thought appears to be impaired as well. Their speech is usually of normal speed and rhythm (fluent), and there is usually no expressive motor deficit. Yet the words they produce are often distorted (paraphasic) or even completely unrecognizable (neologisms). In extreme cases there may be so many neologisms that the speech sounds like a foreign language ("jargon aphasia"). The lesion is posterior, damaging the primary auditory areas, Wernicke's area, and the other surrounding speech reception areas. The etiology is frequently infarction in the territory supplied by the inferior division of the middle cerebral artery.

Expressive Aphasia (Broca's Aphasia)
The patient's remaining speech is produced with great effort, often slow and halting, with loss of the normal rhythms and flow of speech (nonfluent aphasia). The speech is often poorly articulated (dysarthric). Relatively few words can be spoken, but the ones produced are usually nouns or verbs so that the patient's intended meaning can often be understood ("telegraphic speech"). Clinically, comprehension of spoken and written speech is fairly good. It is important to realize that despite their poor speech performance, their inner speech and thought is usually quite good. This type of aphasia is associated with anterior lesions damaging Broca's area and the nearby expressive motor areas. Often the lesion is quite extensive. The most common cause is infarction in the territory supplied by the upper main division of the middle cerebral artery, which often results from embolism from more proximal vessels.

TABLE 114-1
Dysarthria: Disordered Articulation

Type	Site/Nature of Lesion	Associated Features	Common Causes
Inarticulate/slurred	Paralysis or incoordination of tongue, pharynx		Brain stem or hemispheral lesion (either side); local lesions of tongue, mouth; intoxication by drug, alcohol
Nasal	Soft palate: IX or X cranial N. or nuclei	Nasal regurgitation; dysphagia	Local myopathy; myasthenia gravis; polyneuritis; motor neuron disease; brain stem lesions
Hoarse	Larynx; unilateral X or recurrent laryngeal N. damage	Dysphagia and discomfort only with local lesions; otherwise none	Laryngitis and regional tumor; surgical trauma; mitral stenosis; aortic aneurysm; mediastinal lesions
Weak	Larynx; bilateral X or recurrent laryngeal N. damage; intercostal, diaphragmatic weakness	Dysphagia; pharyngeal regurgitation; dyspnea; weak cough; stridor; may extend to aphonia	Surgical trauma; polyneuritis, motor neuron disease; local laryngeal disease, e.g., cancer of esophagus, larynx; mediastinal, cervical adenopathy
Hesitant	Bilateral pyramidal tract damage above mid-pons; pseudobulbar palsy	Indistinct: aphonic if severe; dysphagia; emotional lability; faulty tongue movement; brisk jaw jerk	Motor neuron disease; vascular lesions; tumor; encephalitis
Slow	Corpus striatum; substantia nigra	Monotonous; weak; slurred; other features of parkinsonism	Parkinson's disease; Wilson's disease; rigid Huntington's chorea
Slurred	Cerebellum and brain stem connections; other basal ganglia	Explosive; scanning; other signs of cerebellar damage, chorea, athetosis	Heredofamilial cerebellar disorders; demyelinating disease; brain stem vascular disease; chorea; athetosis

---

Other Disorders

There are many other types of language disruption, such as conduction aphasia and the disconnections. In *conduction aphasia*, spontaneous speech and comprehension are relatively well preserved, but the patient is strikingly unable to repeat items such as digits or sentences. The classic explanation is a block between the receptive and expressive centers (a lesion of the arcuate fasciculus), but some cases seem to be caused by an impaired memory for the material. In the *disconnection syndromes*, major functional areas are cut off from each other. For example, both the visual and language centers may be intact, but visual information can be blocked from getting to the language areas. Although such a patient is able to speak normally and to write normally, he is completely unable to read at all, and is unable even to read his own writing (alexia without agraphia). The many different varieties of aphasia are discussed more completely in the references.[33-35]

DIAGNOSTIC AND THERAPEUTIC MANAGEMENT

Clinical and Laboratory Examination

One function of the clinical examination of these patients (Tables 114-2, 114-3) is to determine which language processes are disrupted and which are intact, and thereby localize where the disturbance might be in the brain. In practice, relatively few patients correspond exactly to the prototypes given in the table and most textbooks. One reason for these

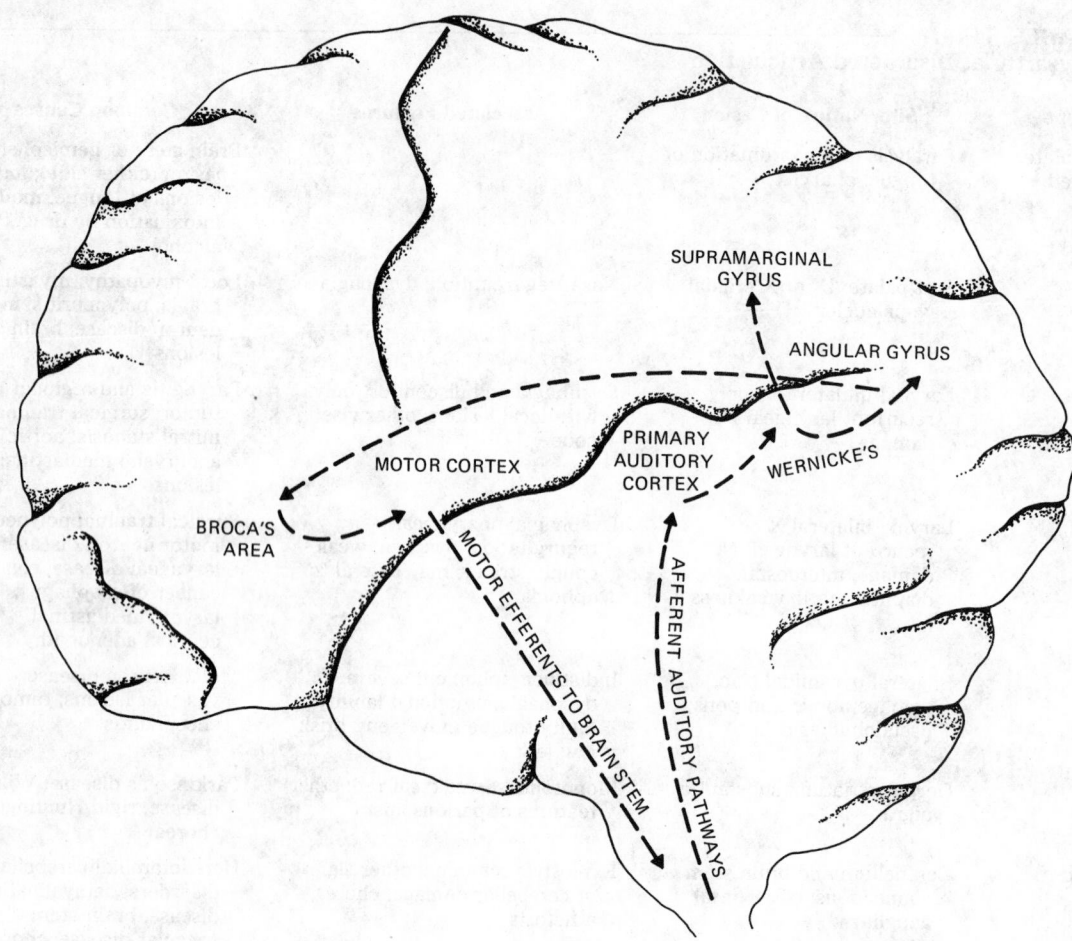

FIGURE 114-1. Language and language-related areas of the left hemisphere.

differences in presentation are differences in the size and location of the lesions (see below). Another reason for the diversity is that the mechanism—whether infarction, tumor, trauma, or other lesion—frequently involves several functional areas. Yet another reason is that people probably differ somewhat in how language is represented in their brain.[35] For these reasons, there is wide range of severity of impairment, with some patients having only a mild, transient speech disorder whereas others have a massive global, permanent aphasia. Furthermore, different types of aphasic symptoms can present at different times in the same patient with variability caused by stresses (both mental and physical, such as fever) and poorly understood healing processes. This may, however, be due to the fact that the underlying lesion is getting worse. The important point in localization is to use

the patient's pattern of impairments initially as a guide to understanding where the lesion can be and then as an aide for determining how to communicate with the patient and for planning his therapy (see below).

Etiologic Diagnosis

The clinical examination will help define how language is being disrupted, and to some extent determine the location of the disturbance. Other features of the history and examination will help define the etiology. Aphasia of sudden onset is usually vascular, i.e., infarction. Slowly progressive deficits may be vascular (hours to days) or caused by mass lesions (days to weeks or longer). The nature of the disturbance may be suggested by associated signs or symptoms. A hemianopsia helps to support the diagnosis

TABLE 114-2
Aphasia: Disturbance of Language

	Name(s)		
	Expressive Aphasia	**Receptive Aphasia**	**Conduction Aphasia**
	Broca's aphasia Motor aphasia Nonfluent aphasia	Wernicke's aphasia Posterior aphasia Fluent aphasia Jargon aphasia—when severe	Auditory, verbal, short-term memory disorder
	Characteristics		
Spontaneous speech	Nonfluent, effortful, dropping of small, grammatical words, retaining meaningful words, may be poor pronunciation, dysarthria	Fluent, little effort, high output of words, often poor in meaningful words with many circumlocutions, often paraphasias (substitutions of different sounds or words) or neologisms (completely uninterpretable sounds), pronunciation normal, no dysarthria	Spontaneous speech, fluent, often with paraphasic errors
Comprehension	Usually fairly good, or normal	Poor	Usually good, or normal
Repetition	Poor (consistent with spontaneous speech)	Poor	Very poor
Naming	Better than spontaneous speech	Poor, often paraphasic	Often paraphasic
Reading	Poor reading aloud, often good reading comprehension	Poor reading aloud, little or no comprehension	Poor reading aloud, good reading comprehension
Writing	When possible, often poorly formed letters and words	Letters well-formed, but poorly combined into words, words often jumbled	Spelling errors
	Localization		
	Anterior: inferior frontal lobe (often extensive and more posterior as well)	Posterior, superior temporal gyrus (Wernicke's area) and inferior parietal lobe	Posterior temporal and/or inferior parietal regions (arcuate fasciculus)

of a localized cerebral lesion. Conversely, disturbances occurring with global confusional states or dementia do not necessarily represent focal lesions.

Brain scanning, CAT scanning, and other tests can then be used where appropriate to define further the location and nature of the lesion(s) (Table 114–3).[34]

Treatment and Prognosis

Specific treatment for the basic cause, if possible, is the best form of treatment for aphasia (such as anticoagulation or vascular surgery for certain types of stroke). Once the brain damage causing the aphasia

has been established, prognosis depends upon the patient's age (the younger the patient, the better; children often recover full function even after severe aphasia), the location of the lesion (anterior lesions are less disabling and are more likely to recover), the size of the lesion (based on other neurologic signs or the brain or CAT scan), and the patient's handedness and sex (left-handed persons and women have a somewhat better prognosis). However, prediction on an individual basis is hazardous. Much of the potential improvement occurs in the first 6 to 8 weeks, but the ultimate degree of recovery may not occur for 12 to 18 months or more.

TABLE 114-3
Clinical and Laboratory Investigation

Clinical Task	Observation

Spontaneous speech	Rate (fast, slow, or normal)
	Effort
	Rhythm (prosody)
	Pronunciation/dysarthria
	Content:
	    phonemic (literal)
	        paraphasias: sound
	        substitutions
	    semantic (verbal)
	        paraphasias: word
	        substitutions
	    neologisms
	    types of words
	        preserved/omitted

Comprehension of
    spoken language:
    yes-no questions
    simple commands
    pointing to objects
	Kinds of difficulty and types
	of errors (controlling for
	expressive difficulties)

Repetition:
    digits
    words
    sentences
	Abilities/inabilities and
	types of errors

Naming
    objects
    body parts
	Abilities/inabilities and
	types of errors

Reading
    out loud
    comprehension:
        written commands
        questions, etc.
	Reading out loud may be
	impaired by both
	receptive and expressive
	problems
	Reading comprehension
	requires only receptive
	abilities

Writing	Difficulty with letter production Difficulty spelling Neologisms Omission of words Disorganization of words

TABLE 114-3 (cont.)

Laboratory Test	Findings/Usefulness
EEG	Focal slowing will help confirm localization

Brain scan
    flow study
    static scan
	Suggest carotid disease
	Localize lesion (not usually
	positive until 2–3 weeks
	after ischemic infarct;
	may not show hemorrhage
	or small lesion)

CAT scan	Localize lesion and suggest nature of lesion, particularly good for hemorrhage; may not show early or very small infarctions
Arteriography	Directly visualize arterial disease; help determine whether lesion is operable

Speech Therapy

Although it is not certain that speech therapy can actually improve language ability by itself, it serves a number of important functions and is usually indicated. A speech therapist can best determine what are the patient's remaining capabilities, and show the patient how to optimize his use of those abilities to communicate. The speech therapist can concentrate on trying to improve borderline abilities, which could make a great difference in the patient's performance. For the severely aphasic patient, the speech therapist can try to set up new forms of communication. Finally, the speech therapist can provide invaluable emotional support for a patient and a family who have suffered a devastating illness.

CHAPTER 115

Disorders of Aging

GUY M. McKHANN

Faced with an elderly patient with a neurologic dysfunction, the physician needs to distinguish between these neurologic signs and symptoms which are the effects of age and those which may be indicative of logic diseases commonly occurring in the elderly. Changes which can be considered a normal part of the aging process are indicated in Table 115-1.

The weight of the brain decreases with age. In addition, neurofibrillary tangles and senile plaques, pathologic changes that are characteristic of malig-

TABLE 115-1
Changes Normally Occurring with Age

Function	Change
Vision	Presbyopia
Hearing	Presbycusis
Motor	Decreased rate and amount of movement
	Decreased reaction time
	Flexed posture of trunk
	Loss of fine motor coordination
	Decreased ankle jerks
Sensory	Decreased vibratory sense in feet
EOM	Limitation of upward gaze
	Small pupils
Benign senescent forgetfulness	Intermittent forgetfulness, often for names, dates, and places, but not events (see Chap. 113)

nant forms of dementia (Alzheimer's disease), occur with increasing frequency with age. These changes, however, do not necessarily correlate with the degree of the benign forgetfulness syndrome.[29,32]

The incidence of atherosclerotic vascular disease increases with age; thus, there has been a tendency to ascribe not only the milder changes in mentation and behavior but also the severe changes of dementia to cerebrovascular disease. However, the lesions in the aged brain are entirely different from the recognized lesions of vascular disease. Thus, it appears much more likely that two conditions, atherosclerosis and involution, are going on simultaneously in the aged without a causal relationship between the two.

NEUROLOGIC ABNORMALITIES IN THE AGED

A number of neurologic conditions increase in frequency or first appear in the older age group. These include dementia (Chap. 113), stroke (Chap. 129), parkinsonism (Chap. 117), osteoarthritis of the spine (Chap. 120), tumors and secondary effects of metabolic disease such as diabetes (Chap. 71). These conditions have all been described in other sections.

MANAGEMENT OF THE AGED WITH NEUROLOGIC PROBLEMS

Our society has tended to discard its elderly. Functioning people are forced to retire from jobs, move from lifelong homes, and enter impersonal or marginal facilities for custodial care. Few younger families have the space, money, time, or motivation to care for an elder relative. It is not surprising that feelings of rejection, overconcern with personal health, and depression become common in this age group. Thus, dealing with neurologic problems of the elderly is at once a social, a familial, and a medical problem. Nor are these problems going to disappear; they are going to increase as the population becomes older.

The physician, in dealing with the elderly, acts as a pediatrician, working through a relative to interpret the patient's needs and care. Hospitalization of elderly patients is often necessary. From a neurologic point of view, several points about hospitalization should be made:

1. Elderly patients, particularly those with various degrees of dementia, do not do well in the hospital. The change from their regulated home environment, the large number of new faces and experiences, and the unfamiliar surroundings at night can all add to the patient's confusion.

2. When hospitalization is required, the pace of workup should be altered and made flexible. Often the patient needs a day of rest after a complex study or a period of fasting.

3. The incidence of complications from diagnostic tests goes up with age. It is important to ask how one will use information obtained before performing a test. For example, in the 80-year-old woman complaining of dizziness with both generalized and cerebrovascular disease, in whom vascular surgery is extremely unlikely, knowledge obtained by arteriography is of little help in medical management.

4. Elderly persons react bizarrely to drugs, particularly barbiturates and other sedatives. For agitated patients, 0.5 to 2.0 mg of haloperidol (Haldol), and for sleep, 500 mg of chloral hydrate may be useful.

5. The hospital setting provides an unreliable environment for tests of higher cortical function. One should balance the results of these tests against the description of how the patient does in his home setting.

6. Difficult ethical questions arise in relation to severely brain-damaged patients. Whether or not to treat actively the pneumonia of a severely demented person or whether to maintain or institute support measures for the patient who has suffered massive cerebral damage from a stroke are examples of the types of decisions that have to be made. There

are no easy answers. It is helpful if the physician and the patient's family can discuss alternatives and reach an accord on overall strategy. After that, the physician must make day-to-day decisions, recognizing that not all illnesses can be cured, that actively prolonging the life of a patient with irreversible severe brain damage may not be the best course, and that death of a patient is not some kind of personal defeat for the physician.

CHAPTER 116
Disorders of Movement
MAHLON R. DeLONG

Several areas of the brain, e.g., brain stem, basal ganglia, cerebellum, and motor and premotor cortex, have long been recognized as playing an important role in the control of movement and posture. Normally, the net output from these several control systems results in a highly coordinated smooth performance. When portions of the motor system are damaged through disease, however, there occur certain highly characteristic abnormalities of movement and posture.

ORGANIZATION OF THE MOTOR SYSTEM

The major components of the motor system and their more prominent anatomic relationships as understood at the present time are shown in Figure 116–1. Certain simplifications and omissions have been made in order to emphasize the major features and the overall organization of the motor system.

At the outset it should be emphasized that all supraspinal motor systems ultimately exert their influence upon a limited number of spinal circuits which link each muscle with the spinal cord (segmental motor apparatus). Although these spinal circuits are capable of mediating simple reflexes, their activity is largely controlled by descending motor pathways. One major pathway originates from the sensorimotor cortex and descends directly to spinal levels. This is the *pyramidal* or *corticospinal tract*. All other descending tracts take origin from nuclei located in the brain stem. These *brain stem motor nuclei* constitute a major prespinal integrating center, regulated in part by higher centers including the cerebellum, basal ganglia, and motor cortex. As seen in Figure 116–1, both the cerebellum and the basal ganglia exert a direct influence on the brain stem, yet a major portion of their output is directed to the motor cortex via the thalamus. These *ascending pathways* from the cerebellum and basal ganglia constitute the major input to the motor cortex from these subcortical motor systems. Figure 116–1 also emphasizes the fact that both the cerebellum and the basal ganglia receive a major input from the entire cortex. This input is especially rich from the association areas in the frontal and parietal regions and from the motor cortex itself. From the foregoing it can be seen that the motor cortex, rather than being located at the highest level of the motor system seems to be at a rather low level in the sequence of events from sensory input to motor output. The motor cortex is, in fact, situated quite close to the final output stage of the system and would appear to be influenced largely by activity in the cerebral cortex, cerebellum, and basal ganglia, rather than being the major controller itself.

CLINICAL MANIFESTATIONS

Upper Motor Neuron Lesions
Lesions of the motor cortex, subcortical white matter, internal capsule, or brain stem produce shock, paralysis, release phenomena, and reflex changes. These effects are caused in part by damage to the pyramidal tracts and in part by damage to other motor pathways. The term *upper motor neuron* is used to refer to the signs resulting from such combined damage.

Shock
With lesions of rapid onset, regardless of the level, some degree of shock occurs. Shock means the widespread depression of neuronal activity as evidenced by profound paralysis and decreased or absent muscle tone and tendon reflexes. Shock results largely from the removal of pyramidal tract influence, and it is generally commensurate with the severity and rate of onset of the noxious process. It is usually deep and

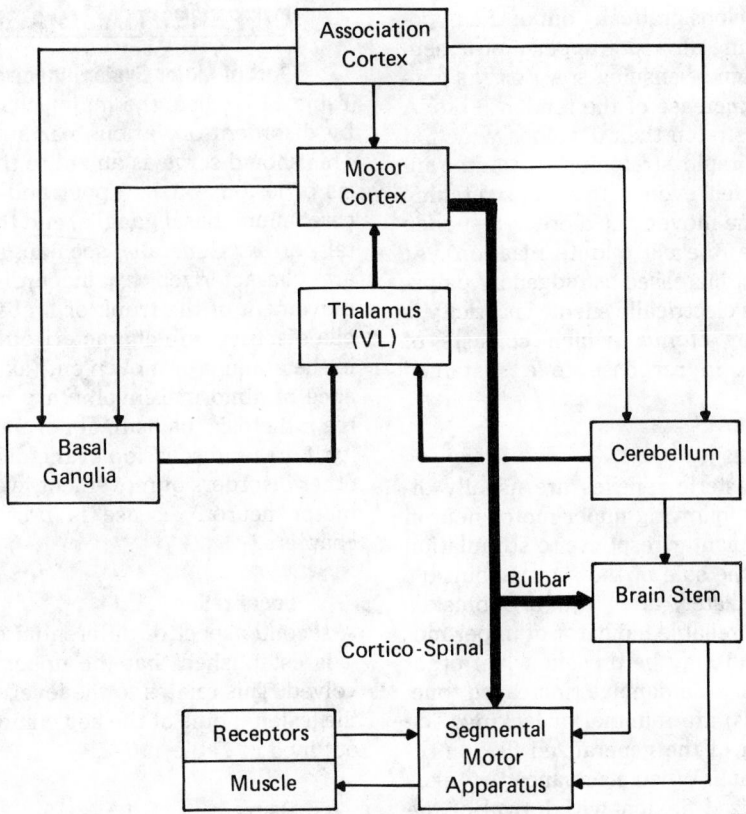

FIGURE 116–1. Schematic diagram of the motor system showing the current concepts of the interactions between the elements. See text for details.

long-lasting with severe sudden physical trauma or a massive stroke, whereas it may be minimal or absent when the damage results from a slowly growing tumor or other mass lesion.

Paralysis

The paralysis or weakness that remains after recovery from an upper motor neuron lesion has certain characteristic features which are largely caused by loss of pyramidal tracts. The functional deficit is greatest in isolated, finely coordinated, delicate acts, particularly those involving the distal musculature of the hands and feet. The impairment is disproportionate to the degree of weakness. Thus, individual movements of the fingers may be greatly impaired even though arm movements are well preserved. Certain movements may be impaired on volition, yet be present in certain reflex behaviors or in associated movements mediated by the spared subcortical motor mechanisms (such as the movement of an hemiparetic limb during yawning). Movements which are generally bilateral and symmetrical involving eyes, jaw, pharynx, larynx, thorax, and abdomen are spared in unilateral upper motor neuron lesions. As one might expect, with unilateral lesions the contralateral hand musculature is most severely affected, the leg next, and, of the cranial musculature, only the lower face and to variable extent the tongue are involved. When the weakness extends to the more proximal musculature it preferentially involves the extensors of the upper extremity and physiologic flexors of the lower extremity.

Release Phenomena

Following upper motor neuron lesions *spasticity* gradually develops. It is characterized by increased resistance to passive muscle stretch and increased tendon reflexes in the antigravity muscles, i.e., the flexors of the upper limbs and the physiologic extensors and adductors of the lower limbs. Characteristically, the arm is held in a posture of flexion and adduction and the leg in extension and adduction.

Spasticity usually develops gradually out of the hypotonic paralysis following an acute upper motor neuron lesion. The first sign of ensuing spasticity is generally the return and increase of the tendon jerks. A resistance to passive stretch then develops which at first is felt only with rapid stretching. Later the increased resistance is felt even with slow stretching and near the end of the movement there is a sudden decrease in resistance (the clasp-knife reaction). At rest, muscle tone is not increased as judged by palpation, and the muscle is electrically silent. Spasticity is often accompanied by *clonus,* which consists of rhythmic contractions in response to a sustained stretch of the muscle.

Cutaneous Reflexes

Abdominal and cremasteric reflexes are usually diminished or abolished following upper motor neuron damage. An extensor plantar response to stimulation of the lateral part of the sole of the foot (Babinski's sign) is present immediately after injury. Babinski's sign is by far the most reliable indicator of upper motor neuron damage and may be present when other signs of upper motor neuron damage (increased tone, reflexes, and weakness) are minimal or lacking. The reflex is basically part of the generalized flexion response to noxious stimuli. When pronounced, it takes the form of a generalized flexion–withdrawal of the entire limb and may be triggered by stimulation from a wide area of the foot. Generally speaking, only the Babinski (stroking of the outer sole of the foot) sign is of use clinically.

DIFFERENTIAL DIAGNOSIS

Part of Motor System Involved

Table 116–1 lists the major characteristics produced by disorders of various parts of the motor system. This should serve as an aid to the differential diagnosis of lesions of the upper and lower motor neuron, cerebellum, basal ganglia, and the premotor and frontal cortex. Generally speaking, cerebellar disorders are characterized by incoordination of attempted movement of the trunk or limbs, whereas basal ganglia disorders are characterized by either a reduction in the amount of movement (akinesia) or the appearance of abnormal involuntary movements, e.g., chorea, athetosis, ballism, abnormal postures, and rigidity. Further discussion of the differential diagnosis of other disorders of movement, weakness, and of lower motor neuron disease is presented in subsequent chapters.

Localization

A second aspect of differential diagnosis arises once it is established that the upper motor neuron is involved. This relates to the level, or the localization of the lesion. Some of the key clinical characteristics are outlined in Table 116–2.

Cause

Once the lesion has been localized, the various causes should be considered. The common causes are also listed in Table 116–2 together with references to the chapters which discuss the entities in more detail.

TABLE 116–1
Localization of Lesions of the Motor System

Lesion	Weakness	Tone	Tendon Reflexes	Movement Abnormalities	Atrophy
Lower motor neuron (anterior horn cell, root, peripheral nerve)	+ +	Flaccid	Decreased	Paresis or paralysis	+ +
Upper motor neuron (motor cortex) internal capsule, brain stem, and spinal cord)	+ +	Spastic	Increased	Paresis or paralysis	± (disuse)
Cerebellum	±	Hypotonia	Decreased	Action tremor Ataxia	0
Basal ganglia	0	Rigidity or hypotonia	Normal	Tremor at rest Chorea Athetosis Akinesia Hemiballismus	0
Premotor and frontal cortex	0	Normal	Normal	Apraxia	0

┌───┐
TABLE 116-2
Localization of Upper Motor Neuron Lesions

Region	Findings	Cause (Chapter References)
Motor cortex	Restricted lesions proportional to motor homunculus Focal seizures with Jacksonian march Hemiparesis indicates widespread lesion	Acute: stroke (129), trauma (132), anoxia (146), hypoglycemia (72), post-ictal (128) Chronic: tumor (131), degenerations (113), repetitive seizures (128)
Motor and parietal cortex	Cortical sensory loss Receptive aphasia Homonymous hemianopsia	Same as above
Motor and frontal cortex	Expressive aphasia Transient gaze paresis Grasp reflex	Same as above
Internal capsule	Contralateral hemiparesis Pure motor hemiparesis	Acute: stroke (129), demyelinations (130), hemorrhage (128) Chronic: tumor (131)
Brain stem	Hemiparesis and cranial nerve dysfunction Damage to brain stem regulatory mechanisms	Acute: stroke (129) demyelinations (130) Chronic: tumor (131), syringobulbia (120)
└───┘

┌───┐
TABLE 116-2 (cont.)

Region	Findings	Cause (Chapter References)
Spinal cord	Often bilateral Greater involvement of lower extremities	Acute: vascular (129), trauma (132), demyelinations (130) Chronic: tumor (131), osteoarthritis (120), meningeal infiltrations (120), abscess (120)
└───┘

MANAGEMENT OF A PATIENT WITH AN UPPER MOTOR LESION[36-38]

Acute Phase

In the acute phase, weakness and shock cannot be altered. The therapy is aimed at avoiding factors that will limit recovery. Contractures can be avoided by passive motion and the use of a foot board. There is no evidence, however, that any form of physical therapy actually speeds the recovery process.

Recovery Phase

In the recovery phase, the strength of proximal, large bulk muscles returns first. Thus, standing and movements around the shoulder and around the hip can be encouraged. In most patients, spasticity is not a disabling symptom and may be of value in aiding standing. However, when spasticity is bilateral, it may disrupt locomotion and other movements. There is no drug which specifically alters spasticity. Diazepam (Valium) 5 mg three times daily, dantrolene sodium (Dantrium), given in gradually increasing dosage to 100 mg four times daily, may be of value in some patients. Physical therapy can be of benefit in gait training, instructing patients in the use of slow, bulk movements to compensate for the loss of fine, distal movements, and to avoid disuse of a limb and subsequent contractures.

CHAPTER 117

Parkinsonism and Other Disorders of Extrapyramidal Function

GUY M. McKHANN AND THOMAS J. PREZIOSI

In general the most prominent symptoms of extrapyramidal disorders are *positive* symptoms characterized by involuntary movements such as chorea, athetosis, dystonia, hemiballismus, tremor, and rigidity. These movement disorders characteristically disappear with sleep and are made worse by emotional stress. The *negative* symptoms resulting from loss of neural function, however, may be seriously disabling as in the case of akinesia in parkinsonism and the associated loss of postural fixation and reflexes. In contrast to upper motor neuron lesions, weakness per se is not a prominent feature. Unless the process is clearly focal, trauma or neoplasm do not have to be considered seriously as diagnostic possibilities.

The characteristics of these and other movement disorders requiring differentiation are indicated in Table 117–1.

PARKINSONISM AND RELATED DISORDERS

PARKINSONISM

The terms "parkinsonism," "Parkinson's disease," and "paralysis agitans" all refer to a progressive neurologic disease whose essential features are tremor, bradykinesia, rigidity, and disturbances of postural reflexes. One manifestation may precede the others by months. At the outset the disease is most frequently asymmetrical and may be unilateral or truncal. In addition, there are other patients who have one or more of the characteristic symptoms of parkinsonism but are distinguished by having other additional neurologic findings, a different clinical course, or a different mechanism as outlined in Table 117–2.

Clinical Features

Idiopathic parkinsonism is a disease of the elderly, affecting 1 percent of the population over 50. The *tremor* of parkinsonism often starts distally, in one hand. The rhythmic opposition of the thumb and forefinger, at a frequency of four to eight per second, has been called a "pill-rolling tremor." The tremor may remain localized for months, or spread to involve all four limbs. Characteristically, the tremor is present at rest, decreased but not absent with intention, disappears during sleep, and is made worse by emotional stress.

In contrast, the tremor present in the elderly (benign essential tremor or senile tremor) is more rapid, is not present at rest, is made worse by intention, is associated with decreased tone, and is improved on ingestion of ethanol.

The *rigidity* of parkinsonism is the most common symptom, often presenting as a failure of associated movement of the arms during walking. The rigidity usually involves the proximal musculature first, particularly the shoulders and neck. Involvement of the face results in mask-like facies, with infrequent blinking. As the limbs become involved, the cog-wheeling nature of the rigidity is noted. In this phenomenon, there is free passive movement around a joint for 5 to 10 degrees and then a sudden catch, as a contraction of the stretched muscles takes place. As the movement progresses, there is repetitive relaxation and contraction of the stretched muscles.

The *bradykinesia,* or inability to initiate and plan the execution of a movement, is the most disabling symptom of parkinsonism. It affects both fine motor movements such as writing or buttoning one's shirt, as well as gross movements such as walking, standing, and sitting.

The *gait* is characterized by small, shuffling steps with increasing speed, as if chasing one's center of gravity (festinating gait). In addition there is a lack of associated movements, and a stooped, rigid posture. In advanced cases, the gait is distinctive. In early cases there can be confusion with patients with spastic paraparesis, which may be associated with cervical spondylosis or occult hydrocephalus. In these spastic patients there is often evidence of long-tract involvement including hyperreflexia and extensor plantar responses. There may also be confusion with truncal ataxia, as found in cerebellar disease.

Etiology

Parkinsonism is a syndrome with a number of etiologies (Table 117–3). However, the idiopathic and postencephalitic forms account for the majority of cases.

The major lesion in parkinsonism is degeneration of the pigmented neurons of the substantia nigra. These neurons project to the striatal regions of the basal ganglia and utilize dopamine as transmitter. Thus, the chemical lesion of parkinsonism is decreased dopamine in regions of the caudate, putamen,

TABLE 117-1

Extrapyramidal and Other Disorders of Movement

Disorder	Character	Cause	Distinguishing Features
Bradykinesia (akinesia)	Slowness and poverty of all movements Maintenance of fixed postures Decreased associated movements	Parkinsonism (dopamine, deficiency in the striatum)	
Rigidity	Increased tone in all muscle groups throughout full range of passive movement, ("leadpipe" or "plastic" quality)	Parkinsonism Huntington's disease Phenothiazines Reserpine	
Chorea	Frequent, varied, irregular involuntary movements of the extremities, trunk, and face	Acute infectious (Sydenham's)	Often (but not always) follows streptococcal infection Females: males (2:1) Early sign is irregular jerky pronation of arms extended overhead Onset insidious or acute Duration 4-6 weeks May recur
		Gravidarum	Associated with pregnancy Often previous history of infectious chorea Reversible
		Vascular	Acute onset Usually unilateral May merge with ballismic movements Remission over several months May be manifestation of systemic vasculitis
		Huntington's	Organic mental change common (early or late) Dominant inheritance Males = females
Athetosis	Extension and flexion of limbs with grimacing of the face	Perinatal insult (hypoxia)	Usually bilateral Associated with mental retardation and signs of cerebral diplegia
Ballism	Wild, involuntary movements of arm or leg or both Unilateral	Hemorrhage or softening in subthalamic nucleus	Sudden onset Usually subsides in a few weeks Rarely death may result from exhaustion
Dystonia	Slow twisting and posturing of body parts—limb and trunk may become extremely grotesque	Dystonia musculorum deformans	Slowly progressive May start with torticollis Sometimes caused by birth injury, neonatal jaundice, or other condition causing nonfatal cerebral anoxia
		Hepatolenticular degeneration (childhood variety of Wilson's disease)	Insidious onset with gaping mouth, minor abnormal posturing Rapidly progressive course Progressive dementia Other features similar to adult variety Onset age 10-20
		Drug-induced	Phenothiazines L-Dopa toxicity

(Continued)

TABLE 117–1 (cont.)

Disorder	Character	Cause	Distinguishing Features
Myoclonus	Very rapid, irregular movements of single fasiculus to entire limb	Viral infections acute and subacute inclusion body encephalitis Creutzfeldt-Jakob disease Postanoxia Metabolic uremia Hepatic insufficiency Progressive myoclonic epilepsy Lafora body group System degenerations (Ramsey-Hunt) Benign essential myoclonus Nocturnal myoclonus	
Asterixis	Periodic, brisk, repetitive flapping of outstretched arms and hands	Chronic cerebral hypoxia (in liver failure, chronic lung disease) Cerebral metabolic derangement (with liver or renal disease) Cerebral degenerations or diffuse infections	Sudden loss of tone in antigravity muscles
Tics	Rapid, stereotyped movements	Unknown	Usually involves facial or neck musculature

and globus pallidus. The rationale for the use of L-dopa is the replacement of endogenous transmitter by exogenous transmitter. The precursor, levo-dihydroxyphenylalanine (L-dopa), is decarboxylated in the brain to the active transmitter, dopamine. Exogenously administered dopamine is not effective because it is excluded from the brain by the blood–brain barrier.

Parkinsonism has a variable rate of progression. There is little to suggest that L-dopa alters the basic process. Patients who stop taking L-dopa return quickly to their pretreatment level of disability.

Management of Parkinsonism

L-Dopa is the drug of choice, usually given in combination with an inhibitor of peripheral L-dopa decarboxylase (Sinemet). The initial effects of therapy can be dramatic, with 50 to 75 percent of patients showing dramatic improvement.[45] The degree of responsiveness of the three major expressions of the disease—tremor, rigidity, and bradykinesia—are individually variable. Usually the bradykinesia responds first, followed by the rigidity and, finally, the tremor.[41]

The side effects of L-dopa are both peripheral and central. The peripheral side effects are primarily gastrointestinal and cardiac. The most frequent are anorexia, constipation, and nausea. Cardiac arrhythmias may be precipitated. The use of Sinemet has greatly reduced the incidence of peripheral side effects.

The central side effects are not influenced by the peripheral inhibitor, and are usually dose related. Insomnia, restlessness, and agitation are common. At higher dosages, confusion and hallucinations may occur.[39]

The beneficial effects which are likely to persist are improvement in rigidity and in bradykinesia. On the other hand, postural dysequilibrium, gait disturbances, and dementia are more likely to progress.

The long-term outcome of therapy with L-dopa is unpredictable. It is clear that L-dopa is therapeutic, but does not alter the progressive nature of the disease. L-Dopa prolongs the life of patients with Parkinsonism.[43] However, in some patients the effectiveness of therapy will decrease after 3 to 5 years. The symptoms likely to return or appear de novo are indicated in Table 117–4.[46]

─TABLE 117–2─
System Degenerations Associated with Parkinson Syndrome

1. Familial Parkinson's disease
2. Parkinson dementia
3. Striatonigral degeneration
4. Hereditary essential tremor
5. Hallevorden-Spatz disease
6. Cerebral hemosiderosis
7. Huntington's chorea
8. Shy-Drager syndrome (idiopathic postural hypotension)
9. Progressive supranuclear palsy
10. Creutzfeldt-Jakob disease
11. Olivopontocerebellar atrophy
12. Familial basal ganglia calcification
13. Normal pressure hydrocephalus

─TABLE 117–4─
Symptoms Appearing in Patients Treated with Sinemet

	Symptom	Remarks
Early	Facial dyskinesias Anxiety Hallucinations Delusions	Usually dose related
Late	Dyskinesias Hallucinations	May be dose related
	Abrupt changes in therapeutic benefit ("on-off" phenomenon)	Usually not dose related Probably related to progression of disease
	Postural dysequilibrium Gait disturbances Dementia	Probably related to progression of disease

It should be emphasized, however, that there is no way of predicting the outcome for the individual patient.

The medical management of parkinsonism is indicated in Table 117–5. In addition to L-dopa, benztropine (Cogentin) and amantadine (Symmetrel) may be helpful for the relief of tremor. Trihexyphenidyl HCl (Artane) may also be useful for alleviating rigidity.

PARKINSON-LIKE SYSTEM DEGENERATIONS

There are a number of system degenerations which may have symptoms of parkinsonism at some stage of their evolution (Table 117–2). These syndromes are distinguished by often being hereditary in nature and by associated nonparkinsonian features such as dementia, ophthalmoplegia, or autonomic disturbances.

Progressive Supranuclear Palsy[42,48]

This is a parkinson-like disorder whose conspicuous feature is a progressive decrease in conjugate ocular

─TABLE 117–3─
Basic Etiologies of Parkinson's Disease

Idiopathic
Postencephalitic
Manganese poisoning
Hypoxia
Carbon monoxide poisoning
Drug intoxication
  1. Reserpine (usually reversible)
  2. Phenothiazines
Iron intoxication
Familial

movement. Characteristically, downward conjugate movement of the eyes is affected first and remains the most impaired. Disturbance of upward movement follows and finally lateral conjugate movements are restricted. Rigidity is most prominent in the neck musculature. Rigidity and hypokinesia are more prominent and tremor is rarely conspicuous. Mild mental changes and progressive bulbar palsy with disturbances in speech, swallowing, and palatal movements complete the clinical picture. This disease affects the same age group as parkinsonism and has no particular sex preference. It is not ordinarily a familial disorder. It is probably not modified by L-dopa.

The Shy-Drager Syndrome[47,51]

This is another disorder with conspicuous parkinson-like features. Here a major manifestation is intractable postural hypotension. This is often associated

─TABLE 117–5─
Medical Therapy of Parkinsonism

Primary Drugs	Average Daily Dose
L-Dopa (Dopar and Larodopa)	3–6 g
L-Dopa and carbidopa (Sinemet)	0.75–1.5 g
Adjunctive Drugs (Primarily To Alleviate Tremor)	
Benztropine (Cogentin)	2–6 mg
Trihexyphenidyl HCl (Artane)	6–15 mg
Procyclidine HCl (Kemadrin)	15 mg
Bipiriden (Akineton)	6 mg
Amantadine HCl (Symmetrel)	200–300 mg

with other evidences of dysautonomia, such as segmental losses in sweating patterns, Horner syndrome, fixed cardiac rate, reduced bowel motility, impotence, and bladder dysfunction. The parkinsonian symptoms (rigidity and bradykinesia) may respond to L-dopa. Postural hypotension does not and may require the use of mineralocorticoids (Florinef) and ephedrine. Tremor is an inconspicuous feature, but pseudobulbar features, particularly emotional lability, are often prominent.

Pathologically, the process is a diffuse neuronal loss and gliosis involving the substantia nigra, striatum, cerebral cortex and, most conspicuously, the intermediolateral column of the spinal cord.

HYPERKINESIAS

THE CHOREAS

Rheumatic Chorea (Sydenham's Chorea)

This is an acute, benign disorder characterized by involuntary, rapid, nonrepetitive movements occurring in a focal or multifocal fashion often associated with disturbances of behavior and mood. The movement disorder may be unilateral. Face, extremities, and trunk are variably involved. It may be associated with other evidences of acute rheumatic fever. The disease occurs in the peak-age period of acute rheumatic fever, namely, in the second half of the first and during the second decade.

The disorder is characteristically benign and reversible over a period of several weeks. However, behavioral manifestations, such as withdrawal, irritability, and emotional instability, frequently continue beyond the period of disordered movement. About one-third of patients eventually show evidence of rheumatic fever or rheumatic carditis.

The chorea can be modified in the acute phase by small doses of phenobarbital. Sydenham's chorea is considered to be an indication for long-term prophylactic therapy with penicillin.

Chorea Gravidarum

The chorea of pregnancy is now considered to be a modified form of rheumatic chorea occurring during pregnancy. Many such episodes occur in a background of previous episodes of rheumatic chorea during adolescence.

Huntington's Chorea

This is a form of chronic chorea which in contrast to the infectious type tends to occur in the latter half of life usually in the third to fifth decades. It is an he-

reditary disorder with clear-cut autosomal dominant characteristics. Unfortunately, there is no way to detect the affected individual prior to the onset of neurologic symptoms. The disorder is slowly progressive, appearing as bizarre movements and postures and mental deterioration. Either of these expressions may dominate. The disordered behavior presents the more serious problem in management and is the reason for custodial care of many patients. In each kindred the disease may be expressed to varying degrees, rarely with a varying rate of progression. An extrapyramidal component may appear giving a parkinson-like picture.[40] This form with rigidity appears more commonly in the juvenile cases which can appear in the second decade.

The pathologic changes are a severe atrophy of caudate and putamen with marked loss of neurons. This atrophy is demonstrable by pneumoencephalography. Similar changes are present to a lesser extent in the thalamus, cerebrum, and cerebellum. Other portions of the nervous system appear to be spared and there are no characteristic visceral changes. At present there is no effective form of therapy. Haloperidol, reserpine, and the phenothiazines may reduce the severity of the movement disorder. L-Dopa worsens the involuntary movements.

HEPATOLENTICULAR DEGENERATION (WILSON'S DISEASE)[49,52]

This process, related to an abnormality in copper metabolism, has a characteristic triad of cirrhosis of the liver, signs of basal ganglia disease, and brownish green deposits of copper at the corneoscleral junctions of the eyes (Kayser-Fleischer rings).

The onset is usually during adolescence, but may be before age 10 years or after age 35 or 40 years. A few patients begin with symptoms of liver dysfunction such as jaundice or ascites. The majority of patients, however, begin with abnormal movements, usually a tremor. Initially the tremor is brought out by movement or by attempts to maintain posture. Athetoid or dystonic contortions and myoclonic jerks may appear. As the disease progresses, transition from one pattern of involuntary movement to another may occur. In the late stages, generalized rigidity with contractures occurs. Speech becomes indistinct or even unintelligible. Dementia is a late manifestation, associated with emotional lability.

Evidences of liver damage, hepatomegaly, and aminoaciduria are variable. The Kayser-Fleischer ring is best demonstrated by tangential illumination of the cornea and most easily seen by slit-lamp examination.

The pathologic features are nodular cirrhosis of

the liver and gliosis of the putamen and globus pallidus, often with cavitation. Nerve cell loss is widespread, including the basal ganglia, caudate nuclei, and cerebral cortex.

The disease is thought to be caused by an impaired ability to incorporate copper into a number of proteins, particularly ceruloplasmin, the protein to which copper is normally bound in serum. Unbound copper is subsequently deposited in tissues throughout the body.[44]

With the full clinical picture, the diagnosis of hepatolenticular degeneration is generally easy. Variations, however, make it important to consider this entity whenever abnormal tone and postures, or involuntary movements, are encountered. Low serum ceruloplasmin levels and elevated serum copper, when present, are confirmatory. Copper deposits can be demonstrated in liver biopsy material. Untreated, the course is progressive.

The objectives of therapy are to diminish the absorption and to increase the excretion of copper. Absorption is decreased by avoiding foods rich in copper (such as liver) and by precipitating copper in the gastrointestinal tract with potassium sulfide in doses of 0.2 g, taken with each meal. Renal excretion is enhanced by chelating the copper with penicillamine, in a dose of 0.5 to 1.0 g taken three times daily. A gauge of the effectiveness of mobilization is the disappearance of the Kayser-Fleischer ring.[49] Ideally, therapy should begin before there is much neural change, thus the importance of recognizing early cases. For some reason, treatment is less helpful in the juvenile variety, which progresses rapidly.

MYOCLONUS AND MYOCLONIC JERKS

This movement disorder is characterized by irregular, rapid, and asynchronous jerks. The disorder has diverse etiologies and can arise at multiple levels within the nervous system.[50] It is important to distinguish between 1) patients with a benign, nonprogressive myoclonus, 2) those with myoclonus secondary to an acute insult to the nervous system, such as anoxia, and 3) those in which myoclonic jerks are an indication of a diffuse, progressive disease of the nervous system, such as inclusion body encephalitis or a lipidosis.

TREMORS

A tremor is a rhythmic oscillation of a body part resulting from alternating contractions of opposing muscle groups. It is convenient to classify tremors according to their relationship to movement and posture (Table 117–6). Thus, a tremor which is present when the limb is at complete rest is termed a *static* tremor. Tremors which are present only during movement or during sustained maintenance of posture are referred to as *action tremors.* Two types of action tremors are recognized: 1) *postural tremor,* which is present during sustained posture (such as holding the arms outstretched) and throughout the course of movement and 2) *intention tremor,* which is absent during steady maintenance of posture but develops during movement of the limb, especially as the object is approached.

Physiologic Tremor

It should be recognized that in all normal individuals there is a physiologic action tremor which is present both during maintained posture and during movement. Although normally of low amplitude it may be greatly heightened during states of anxiety, thyrotoxicosis, and fatigue.

Static Tremor

Static tremor is almost always caused by parkinsonism of one etiology or another. Parkinsonian tremor is most often confused with essential tremor which may in some cases be present at rest.

Action Tremors

ESSENTIAL TREMOR. Essential tremor is generally an inherited disorder (autosomal dominant). It is sometimes termed familial tremor. Occasionally, a family history is lacking. Typically the tremor develops in middle age but may come on in late life, when it is termed senile tremor. The onset is gradual over many years.

Essential tremor is a coarse tremor whose frequency is similar to that of physiologic tremor (9 to 11 per second). It is most noticeable in the distal upper extremities, usually sparing the lower extremities. While completely absent at rest, it is best brought out by having the patient extend his arms forward. With movements of the arm the tremor may increase somewhat in amplitude, i.e., there may be in addition an intentional component. When severe, the tremor seriously interferes with writing, feeding, and fine movements. This form of tremor may also appear in the lips, tongue, face, and head and cause tremulous speech. Patients with essential tremor often find that the tremor is controlled by one or two drinks of alcohol. The tremor is exacerbated by emotional stress and often is a source of considerable embarrassment to patients.

TABLE 117-6
Tremors—Classification

Type	Character	Cause	Age of Onset	Distinguishing Features
Static				
"Parkinsonian"	Present at rest 4-6/sec	Parkinsonism Reserpine CO poisoning Mn poisoning	40+	Rigidity or akinesia usually present Responds to antiparkinson drugs, thalamotomy
"Rubral"	Present at rest but with action components 3-5/sec at rest	Damage to multiple pathways in the midbrain tegmentum incl. brachium conjunctivum	Any	Looks parkinsonian at rest but with intention component
Postural				
Physiologic	Present normally Adults: 9-11/sec Children and aged: 6-8/sec		All ages	Increased with anxiety, effort, fatigue, thyrotoxicosis, and epinephrine
Essential "Familial" "Senile"	9-11/sec	Unknown	Middle age or late life ("senile")	Coarse, best seen when hands are outstretched Not seen in legs Usually bilateral Usually no intentional component Increased by stress Decreased by alcohol Responds to sedatives, Propranolol, thalamotomy if severe
Intention	Absent during maintained posture and first part of movement Worse with precise movements	Cerebellar damage: cortex or "outflow" (brachium conjunctivum) tumors, vascular disease, multiple sclerosis, Dilantin toxicity	Any age	When severe, the target may never be attained and has "wingbeating" character

The treatment of essential tremor has until recently been largely restricted to tranquilizers and sedatives, which have at best an ameliorating effect. More recently, the beta-adrenergic blocker, propranalol, has been used with better results. In the most severe cases thalamotomy has been performed with good results.

INTENTION TREMOR. Intention tremor is distinguished from postural tremor in that the tremor does not appear unless the limb is used in goal-directed activity, such as reaching for an object or bringing an object to the mouth as in eating and drinking. The tremor is absent at the onset of the movement but increases rapidly as the target is reached and greater

precision is required. After reaching the target, the tremor ceases. In the most severe instances the target may never be attained. The tremor is frequently accompanied by ataxia and is sometimes referred to as ataxic tremor. This type of tremor nearly always indicates disease of the cerebellum, and is most often caused by lesions of the cerebellar outflow, i.e., the brachium conjunctivum or the lateral cerebellar hemisphere. It is seen most often in multiple sclerosis, but may also be a manifestation of tumors, vascular, and degenerative diseases of the cerebellum. Intention tremor is also seen in dilantin toxicity. If severe and incapacitating, thalamotomy may greatly ameliorate tremor in the contralateral limbs.

RUBRAL TREMOR.   Although rubral tremor is often present at rest, it is greatly intensified with the maintenance of posture and movement. It is usually of low frequency (3 to 5 per second). It is termed "rubral" tremor because of the presumed localization of the pathologic lesion in the red nucleus. However, it is now believed that this tremor is caused by the interruption of several pathways in this region (including the brachium conjunctivum which passes through the red nucleus) and other pathways crossing the midbrain tegmentum. The tremor at rest is often associated with an intention tremor which reflects involvement of the cerebellar outflow (brachium conjunctivum).

CHAPTER 118
Ataxia and Other Abnormalities of Cerebellar Function
MAHLON R. DeLONG AND GUY M. McKHANN

MANIFESTATIONS
Lesions of the cerebellum interfere with the programming of movements and important feedback mechanisms involved in motor control. They are marked by a disorder of the rate, rhythm, force, and sequence of movements with little associated weakness (see Chap. 116).

Hemisphere
With acute lesions of a cerebellar hemisphere, there is disordered motor control of the ipsilateral extremities. This consists of a generalized *decrease in muscle tone, dysmetria* (inability to move to a given point precisely), *intention tremor* (tremor absent at rest which appears with movement), and *dysdiadochokinesia* (inability to make repetitive movements in a normal rhythmic fashion).

Vermis
Lesions of the cerebellar vermis result in *truncal ataxia* with an unsteady staggering wide based gait, difficulty sitting unsupported, and often *dysarthric,* "scanning" speech which is an explosive speech that results from inability to coordinate the expulsion of air and movement of the larynx, palate, tongue, and lips.

DIAGNOSTIC EVALUATION
The evaluation of a patient with ataxia is indicated in Table 118-1. Unfortunately, we do not know enough about the neurophysiology and neurochemistry of ataxia to have a rational pharmacologic approach to its management. In severe cases, particularly where tremor is the disabling symptom, a stereotactically placed lesion in the ventrolateral nucleus of the thalamus or dentate nucleus may be of help.

ACUTE CEREBELLAR ATAXIA
Causes of acute ataxia and their distinguishing features are indicated in Table 118-2. The involvement is usually diffuse with the exception of cerebellar hemorrhage and multiple sclerosis which are often quite asymmetrical in their involvement. Cerebellar hemorrhage is important to recognize since prompt diagnosis permits surgical evacuation in this condition that otherwise may be fatal.

CHRONIC AND PROGRESSIVE ATAXIA
The causes and characteristics of chronic ataxia of cerebellar origin are indicated in Table 118-3. In the United States, the most common causes in adults are alcoholism, cerebellar degeneration secondary to neoplasm, multiple sclerosis, and a large number of patients in whom no etiology is found.

CEREBELLAR AND SPINOCEREBELLAR DEGENERATIONS[54,55]
This group of processes is often called "system degenerations" because specific groups of neurons degenerate. The different entities are distinguished by age of onset, pattern of progression, and degree of involvement of the nervous system and other organs (Table 118-4). Many of the conditions are genetically determined. Unfortunately, there is neither information about the basic mechanisms of these diseases nor effective therapy.

Friedreich's ataxia is the best known and one of the more common of the spinocerebellar degenerations. The pattern of inheritance appears to be recessive. Partial or incomplete forms of the disease are fairly common. Symptoms start in childhood, usually in the first decade of life. Patients commonly give a history that they have never been able to run well or

TABLE 118-1
Evaluation of Ataxia

Procedure	Findings	Significance
History	Pattern of progression Drug usage Symptoms of systemic illness Other neurologic dysfunctions Family history	Acute *vs.* chronic (Tables 118–2 and 118–3) Toxic (Tables 118–2 and 118–3) Metabolic, malignancy, infection, toxic Multiple sclerosis, brain stem tumor Wilson's disease, degenerative diseases (Table 118–4)
Physical examination	Truncal or limb involvement Symmetry, other neurologic signs Evidence of underlying systemic illness Papilledema	Hemisphere *vs.* vermis Diffuse or focal disease Metabolic, malignancy, infection, toxic Mass lesion (tumor, abscess, hemorrhage)
Skull x-ray	Increased intracranial pressure (chronic)	Mass lesion
CAT scan	Mass, atrophy, hydrocephalus Ventricular size and position	
Brain scan	Abscess or tumor	
Arteriography	Ventricular size and position Herniation of tonsils Cerebellar mass	Mass lesion
Lumbar puncture (deferred if intracranial pressure is possibly elevated)	Elevated protein Elevated gamma globulin CSF pressure Pleocytosis	Multiple sclerosis or tumor Multiple sclerosis Stop, if elevated Evidence of infection
Air study	Mass or atrophy	

keep up in athletic activities. A progressive ataxia with muscle wasting and weakness and a profound loss of proprioception develops by the middle of the second decade. Pes cavus and kyphoscoliosis are usually present. The deep tendon reflexes are depressed or absent, but the plantars are extensor, indicating pyramidal tract involvement.

A cardiomyopathy is often present and may show up on ECG well before clinical evidence of heart failure is noted. Many patients with Friedreich's ataxia die from cardiac complications. Cases within a family usually run a similar course, though in some families minor manifestations such as pes cavus or absent tendon jerks will appear in members of the family who escape the full-blown disorder.

A number of cases clinically indistinguishable from the milder forms of Friedreich's ataxia have been described in which there are decreased or absent beta-lipoproteins. Steatorrhea may be seen as an early manifestation, and in the recessively transmitted a-beta-lipoproteinemic cases acanthocytosis of erythrocytes and retinitis pigmentosa are usually present. There is no effective treatment and slow progression is usual.

Ataxia telangiectasia is a progressive degenerative disease of the cerebellum which is probably recessively transmitted. It begins in early childhood with ataxia and increased susceptibility to infections followed by the appearance of conjunctival and cutaneous telangiectasia between 3 and 6 years of age. The serum gamma globulin may be decreased, perhaps accounting for the increased susceptibility to infection and the resulting decreased life span.

Olivopontocerebellar degeneration includes a number of closely related disorders which have in common degeneration of the inferior olivary nuclei, nuclei pontis, and cerebellum with variable involvement of dorsal columns, spinocerebellar pathways, and other neuronal systems. Most of these appear to be transmitted as an autosomal dominant trait, but a few families display a recessive pattern, and sporadic cases also occur. The age of onset ranges from infancy to advanced age; it may even vary widely within a given family.

The clinical characteristics are progressive ataxia, dysarthria, and clumsiness in the hands with a variable degree of spasticity. In some families other neurologic signs, such as progressive visual loss, ri-

TABLE 118-2
Ataxias of Acute Onset

Etiology	Characteristics	Therapy	Remarks
Toxic			

Ethanol
Anticonvulsants
  (diphenylhydantoin)
Sedatives
  (barbiturates)
	Acute, truncal
	May have rapid, pendular
	  nystagmus
	Dose related, reversible
		Withdrawal of toxin	Chronic toxicity may be
			  irreversible
			Underlying lesion, such as
			  Wernicke's may be
			  missed

Organomercurials	Subacute, irreversible Associated with dementia	Withdrawal of mercurial	
Nutritional			

Wernicke's encephalopathy	Truncal ataxia
	Paresis of extraocular
	  muscles
	Confusion
	Defects in recent memory
	Peripheral neuropathy
		Thiamine, 100 mg	Underlying Korsakoff
			  syndrome may be missed
			May not be reversible
			  (Chaps. 128 and 161)

Cerebrovascular			

Cerebellar hemorrhage	Nausea and vomiting,
	  headache
	Unsteadiness of gait limb
	  ataxia
	Long tract findings
	Nystagmus
	Gaze paresis
	Progressive obtundation
		Surgical evacuation on
		  emergency basis
			History of hypertension,
			  anticoagulation
			CAT scans and
			  arteriography are
			  diagnostic
			Xanthochromic CSF

Vertebral-basilar artery
  ischemia
	Asymmetrical ataxia
	Associated brain stem signs
	  (Chap. 128)
	Progressive deterioration in
	  some patients
		Anticoagulation in some
		  patients
			Demonstrable by vertebral
			  angiography

Parainfections			

Acute ataxia of childhood	Truncal and limb ataxia
	Nystagmus
	Lymphocytosis of CSF
	Self-limited
		None	Associated with varicella,
			  Coxsackie, polio, and
			  echo viruses

Landry-Guillain-Barré	Ascending motor weakness
	Areflexia
	Gait ataxia
	Decreasing respiratory
	  function
		Supportive (Chap. 130)	CSF protein elevated
			Often preceded by
			  nonspecific respiratory
			  infection

Demyelinating			

Multiple sclerosis	May be either part of first
	  attack or of
	  exacerbations
	CSF gamma globulin
	  elevated in 70% of cases
		ACTH or corticosteroids
		  may shorten acute
		  attacks (Chap. 133)
			Neurologic lesions spread
			  topographically and
			  temporally

TABLE 118-3
Chronic and Progressive Ataxia

Etiology	Characteristics	Therapy	Remarks
Toxic			
Alcohol	Superior vermis involved Gait ataxia Slowly progressive	Abstinence	(see Chap. 153)
Phenytoin	Gait ataxia Nystagmus	Decrease dosage	Associated with lethargy May be irreversible
Organomercurials	Limb and gait ataxia Dementia Visual loss	Stop exposure	
Metabolic			
Wilson's disease	Dyskinesia Choreoathetosis Kayser-Fleischer rings Elevated serum copper Decreased ceruloplasmin	Decrease copper (penicillamine)	Similar picture after portocaval shunt
Hypothyroidism	Ataxia Thickened, dry skin Cold intolerance Low T_4	Thyroid replacement	(see Chap. 76)
Metachromatic leukodystrophy	Ataxia Dementia Dystonia Peripheral neuropathy Decreased arylsulfatase A	None	Occurs as a juvenile and adult form
Associated with Malignancy			
Metastasis	Asymmetrical headache May be increased intracranial pressure Abnormal brain scan or arteriogram	Surgery if single metastasis May be helped by steroids	Lung and breast common primaries
Cerebellar degeneration	Truncal ataxia (early) May be associated brain stem involvement	Removal of primary	May improve after removal of pituitary tumor
Primary Tumor astrocytoma medulloblastoma hemangioblastoma ependymoma	Usually asymmetrical	Surgical removal	More common in children
Infection			
Abscess	Asymmetrical headache Increased intracranial pressure Abnormal brain scan or arteriogram	Surgical removal	Follows chronic otitis media, septicemia, SBE, or lung abscess
Kuru	Ataxia Tremor Dementia Slowly progressive	None	Confined to New Guinea Transmissable
Demyelination			
Multiple sclerosis	CSF gamma globulin elevated in 70%	Stereotactic surgery for tremor in some patients	(Chap. 130)
Genetic			(see Table 118-4)
Idiopathic			
	No distinguishing features	None	Probably a spectrum of disorders Diagnosis by exclusion

TABLE 118-4
Cerebellar and Spinocerebellar Degenerations

Disease	Age of Onset	Progression	Life Expectancy	Neurologic Findings	Non-Neurologic Findings	Inheritance	Eponym and Remarks
Ataxia telangiectasia	1–5 yrs	Ataxia Mental retardation Pulmonary infections	25 yrs	Ataxia Choreoathetosis	Sino-pulmonary infections Telangiectasia of sclera and skin Decreased IgG	Recessive	
Friedreich's ataxia	5–15 yrs	Ataxia Scoliosis Cardiomyopathy	10–15 yrs from onset	Ataxia Nystagmus Areflexia Extensor plantars	Scoliosis Cardiac failure Pes cavus	Recessive	Form fruste common
A-beta lipoproteinemia	Childhood to early adult	Ataxia Visual loss	May be normal	Ataxia Areflexia Extensor plantars Retinitis pigmentosa	Steatorrhea Acanthocytosis Absent beta lipoproteins	Recessive	Bassen-Kornzweig disease
Hypo-beta lipoproteinemia		Ataxia	May be normal	Ataxia Areflexia Extensor plantars	Decrease beta lipoproteins	Probably dominant with incomplete penetrance	
Familial ataxia	Adult	Ataxia	May be normal	Ataxia	None	Mixed	Multiple forms
Olivoponto-cerebellar degenerations	Childhood and adult	Ataxia Visual loss Dementia	20+ yrs from onset	Ataxia Bulbar dysfunction Posterior column dysfunction Parkinsonian features Retinitis pigmentosa Dementia		Mixed	Multiple forms

gidity, or dementia are regular features of the condition. The condition is slowly progressive with many patients surviving 10 to 20 years.

Late cortical cerebellar atrophy is a heterogeneous group of degenerations of insidious onset usually beginning in the fifties or sixties. It is occasionally familial, and usually has a rather prolonged course.

SENSORY AND FRONTAL ATAXIA

Not all ataxia is on the basis of cerebellar dysfunction. Sensory ataxia occurs when there is inappropri-ate sensory feedback relative to limb position and movement. The pathologic bases for sensory ataxia are lesions of posterior roots (tabes dorsalis or polyneuropathies) or of the posterior columns (pernicious anemia). In these patients the ataxia is much worse in the absence of visual cues (eyes closed), and the defect in position sense is clearly demonstrable.

Frontal ataxia occurs with lesions of the frontal lobe such as tumors, occult hydrocephalus, or presenile dementia (Pick's disease). Ataxia of frontal origin may be difficult to distinguish from ataxia of cerebellar origin. The presence of dysmetria and dysdiadochokinesia are indicative of cerebellar dysfunction.

CHAPTER 119

Brain Stem Dysfunction

DAVID S. ZEE AND GUY M. McKHANN

The brain stem of an adult is in essence a cylinder 2 to 4 cm in diameter and 8 cm long (Fig. 119–1). Ascending and descending sensory and motor fiber tracts course through it longitudinally and cranial nerve nuclei and reticular formation (tegmental) nuclei are arranged within it. Lesions can be precisely localized since the combined manifestations of nuclear involvement and tract involvement give information about the axial and lateral location of the lesion, respectively. Furthermore, some kinds of lesions, e.g., occlusion of the vertebral artery with infarction of the lateral medulla, (p. 1280) produce highly characteristic clinical patterns.

CRANIAL NERVE SIGNS[58]

Although cranial nerve dysfunction per se does not localize lesions to the brain stem, certain patterns of involvement suggest intrinsic involvement of either the cranial nerve nuclei or their intramedullary nerve fibers. In general, either multiple or bilateral cranial nerve involvement points to a proximal and often intrinsic lesion. This is especially true if the affected cranial nerves exit the skull through different bony foramina. For example, isolated involvement of cranial nerves IX, X, and XI usually reflects a lesion at the level of the jugular foramen while a combined VI and VII nerve paresis usually indicates a lesion within the pons (Fig. 119–1).

A dissociated loss of cranial nerve function is of even more localizing value. Dissociated sensory loss (loss of pain and temperature, preservation of touch) on the face suggests a lesion of the descending tract and nucleus of the trigeminal nerve within the pons or medulla for these structures subserve only pain and temperature modalities (see Table 119–1B). Similarly, an onion skin pattern of sensory loss (loss of sensation around the nose and mouth with preservation of sensation more peripherally on the face) points to a brain stem lesion (often a syringobulbia). Loss of taste over both anterior and posterior portions of one side of the tongue (the anterior two-thirds is usually innervated by VII and the posterior one-third by IX) with preservation of the function of other structures innervated by the facial and glossopharyngeal nerves indicates an intrinsic lesion involving the tractus solitarius in the upper medulla (see Table 119–1C).

The combination of signs of cranial nerve involvement with signs of a motor or sensory deficit in the trunk or limbs suggests that the lesion is in the brain stem involving both the cranial nerve nucleus and the long ascending or descending fiber tracts. For example, a single lesion in the midbrain can involve the intramedullary portion of the III nerve and the cerebral peduncle on the same side causing an ipsilateral III nerve paresis and contralateral hemiparesis, Weber syndrome (see Table 119–1A). This pattern can occur with any of the cranial nerves. Although various eponyms have been attached to each of these syndromes, they all illustrate the same phenomenon at different levels within the brain stem. That is, the cranial nerve is involved on one side and the hemiplegic manifestations are on the opposite side (crossed hemiplegia, contralateral hemiplegia, hemiplegia alterna).

Hemisensory loss (either complete or dissoci-

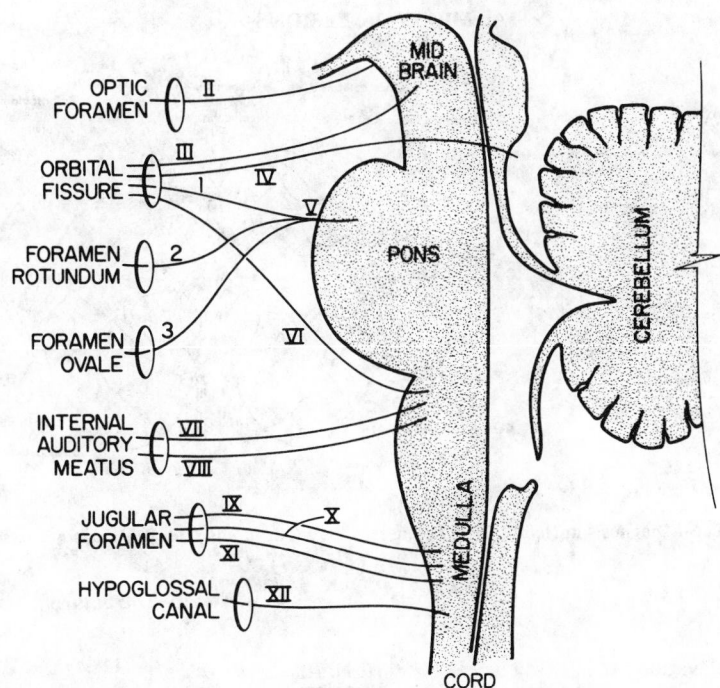

FIGURE 119–1. Diagram showing the different adjacencies of the cranial nerves in the brain stem and as they exit the skull. This provides useful information about the site of lesions. See text.

ated) with cranial nerve signs has the same localizing significance as crossed hemiplegia. However, since the intramedullary portions of the motor cranial nerves do not course as close to the ascending sensory fiber tracts as they do to the pyramidal tracts, an isolated cranial nerve motor loss with a contralateral hemisensory loss occurs infrequently. In contrast, a single lesion interrupting the descending tract of the trigeminal nerve and the ascending spinothalamic tract on the same side does occur frequently (see Table 119–1A). It causes loss of pain and temperature sensation on the ipsilateral face and contralateral trunk and extremities.

Descending sympathetic fibers also course through the brain stem and ipsilateral Horner syndrome (ptosis, miosis, enophthalmos, with hypohydrosis) often occurs with brain stem lesions.

EYE SIGNS[56]
Disorders of ocular motility frequently provide the best clues to precise brain stem localization. The first step in diagnosis is to localize the lesion either to the peripheral ocular motor apparatus (nucleus, nerve, or muscle) or to the intramedullary structures mediating supranuclear eye movement control. Peripheral involvement can usually be recognized by the pattern of extraocular muscle involvement. For example, a III

nerve paralysis causes paresis of adduction and elevation of the globe often with associated ptosis and pupillary mydriasis. Depression (IV cranial nerve) and abduction (VI cranial nerve) of the globe are spared. Special causes of peripheral ocular motor palsies are considered in Chapter 154. On the other hand if the pattern of involvement does not conform to a peripheral ocular motor paralysis, and especially if the peripheral apparatus can be shown to be intact for some, but not other types of eye movements, a supranuclear disorder is suggested.

There are four major types of eye movements; saccadic, smooth pursuit, vestibular, and vergence. *Saccades* are rapid refix eye movements that bring the images of objects seen in the periphery onto the fovea. They may be more or less automatic (quick phases of nystagmus) or under voluntary control (saccades). *Smooth pursuit* movements are lower-velocity, smooth, following, eye movements that enable one to track moving targets. *Vestibular* movements function to stabilize images upon the retina during head movements. The *vestibuloocular reflex* smoothly moves the eye in the orbit (slow phase of vestibular nystagmus) an amount exactly equal and opposite to a head movement in order to maintain clear vision. Quick phases of *vestibular nystagmus* are rapid resetting movements that keep the eye from

TABLE 119-1
Brain Stem Lesions

A: MIDBRAIN LESIONS

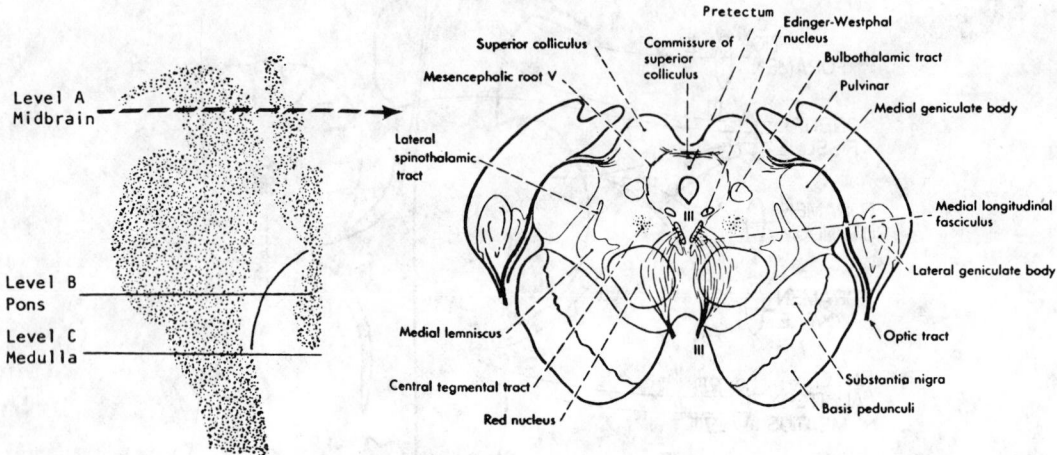

(From Haymaker, W. Bing's Local Diagnosis in Neurological Diseases, 15th ed. St. Louis, The C. V. Mosby Co., 1969)

Neurologic Sign	Affected Structure
Ipsilateral	
Paresis eye adduction, elevation	C.N. III
Paresis depression	C.N. IV
Ptosis, unreactive pupil	Descending sympathetic
Paresis upward gaze	Pretectum
Paresis downward gaze	Ventral periaquaductal gray
Ataxia and tremor	Superior cerebellar peduncle
Contralateral	
Ataxia and tremor	Red nucleus
Hemiparesis	Corticobulbar and spinal tracts
Hemihypesthesia	Medial lemniscus, spinothalamic, and quintothalamic tracts

B: PONTINE LESIONS

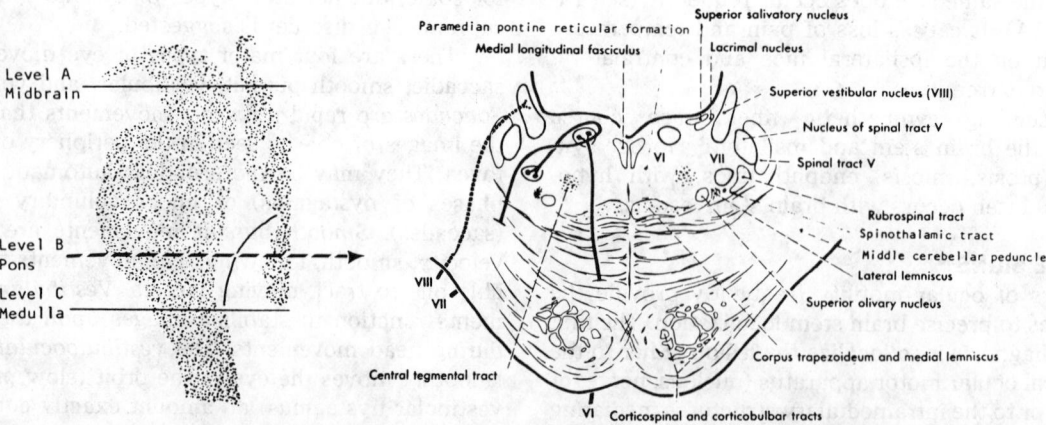

(From Haymaker, W. Bing's Local Diagnosis in Neurological Diseases, 15th ed. St. Louis, The C. V. Mosby Co., 1969.)

Neurologic Sign	Affected Structure
Ipsilateral	
Paresis eye abduction	C.N. VI
Paresis conjugate gaze	Paramedian pontine reticular formation (PPRF)
Internuclear ophthalmoplegia	Medial longitudinal fasciculus
Nystagmus	Vestibular nuclei, PPRF
Facial paresis	C.N. VII
Deafness	C.N. VIII
Ataxia	Middle cerebellar peduncle
Facial hypesthesia	C.N. V
Paresis chewing	C.N. V
Horner syndrome	Descending sympathetic
Contralateral	
Hemiparesis	Corticobulbar and spinal tract
Hemihypesthesia	Medial lemniscus, spinothalamic tract

C: MEDULLARY LESIONS

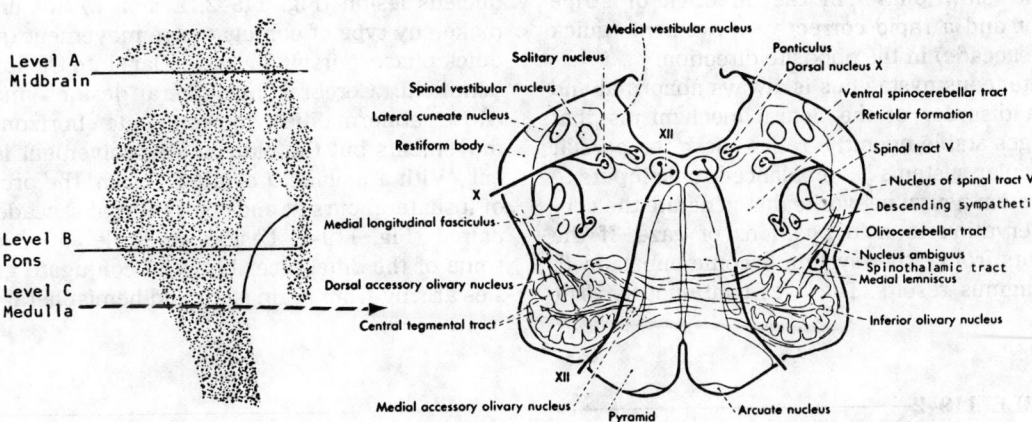

(From Haymaker, W. Bing's Local Diagnosis in Neurological Diseases, 15th ed. St. Louis, The C. V. Mosby Co., 1969.)

Neurologic Sign	Affected Structure
Ipsilateral	
Paresis of tongue	C.N. XII
Facial hypalgesia	Spinal tract C.N. V
Ataxia	Inferior cerebellar peduncle
Nystagmus	Vestibular nuclei
Horner syndrome	Descending sympathetic
Loss of taste	Tractus solitarius
Dysphagia, dysarthria	Nucleus ambiguus, C.N. IX and X
Contralateral	
Hemiparesis, arm, leg	Corticospinal tract
Hemihypesthesia, arm, leg	Medial lemniscus, spinothalamic tract
Crossed monoplegia	
Paresis of one upper extremity and opposite lower extremity	Decussation of pyramids

reaching extreme degrees of deviation in the orbit. *Vergence* movements are slow dysjunctive movements that keep images of the target on the fovea of each eye as the object approaches the face.

DISORDERS OF EYE MOVEMENTS

Nystagmus

Nystagmus is an involuntary rhythmic movement of the eyes. It may consist of a slow drift in one direction (slow phase) followed by a rapid corrective move in the other (quick phase) in which case it is called jerk nystagmus. If oscillations are of approximately equal velocity in each direction it is designated pendular nystagmus. Jerk nystagmus can be induced in normal individuals by rotating them in a chair and then suddenly stopping the chair (postrotatory vestibular nystagmus) or by passing a band of stripes across the patient's visual field (optokinetic nystagmus). The latter consists of a smooth following eye movement (slow phase) in the direction of stripe movement and a rapid corrective movement (quick phase or saccade) in the opposite direction.

Spontaneous nystagmus is always abnormal and reflects a disorder of the neural mechanisms that keep images stable upon the retina. Both the pursuit and vestibular systems have balanced tonic inputs to the brain stem neural networks that generate the constant innervation to hold positions of gaze. If the tonic inputs from either system become unbalanced, jerk nystagmus results. The eyes continuously drift off fixation (slow phase) and saccades are required to bring back images to the fovea (quick phase). However, if the neural network itself that holds positions of gaze becomes defective, the patient will not be able to hold eccentric positions of gaze. The eyes will drift back toward the primary position and the patient must repeatedly make saccades to look eccentrically. The continuous centripetal drift with repetitive corrective saccades is called gaze-paretic nystagmus. Table 119-2 summarizes some of the distinguishing features of different types of nystagmus.

Paresis of Horizontal Gaze

The portion of the reticular formation lying just ventral to the medial longitudinal fasiculus between the IV and VI cranial nerve nuclei (paramedian pontine reticular formation, or PPRF), and the abducens nucleus region itself are important for production of ipsilateral horizontal conjugate eye movements (Fig. 119-2). Patients with a unilateral PPRF or abducens nucleus lesion (Fig. 119-2, Lesion 2) are unable to make any type of conjugate eye movement (saccade, quick phase, pursuit, or vestibular) into the ipsilateral hemifield. Cerebral hemipheral lesions may also cause abnormalities in conjugate horizontal eye movements but the pattern of involvement is different. With a unilateral cerebral lesion, the production of ipsilateral pursuit and contralateral saccades is impaired (Fig. 119-2, Lesion 1). Table 119-2 outlines some of the differences between conjugate gaze palsies arising from brain stem and hemispheral lesions.

TABLE 119-2
Common Forms of Nystagmus

Type	Wave Form	Special Features
Congenital	Usually pendular Occasionally jerk component on lateral gaze	Usually horizontal Persists on up and down gaze Often associated with visual defect, strabismus or head turn
Vestibular	Jerk	Decreased by fixation If purely vertical or purely rotatory, it indicates central vestibular involvement
Pursuit	Pendular or jerk	Increased or not affected by fixation Associated with defects in smooth pursuit eye movements (smooth tracking) If pendular, it suggests lesion in dentato-rubro-olivo pathway If jerk, it suggests lesion in lower brain stem or inferior cerebellum
Gaze-paretic (inability to hold eccentric gaze)	Jerk	Small amount may be observed in normal subjects on far lateral gaze May occur with lesions in brain stem or cerebellum Most common cause is drug side effects (sedatives, anticonvulsants)

TABLE 119-3
Horizontal Conjugate Gaze Palsies

	Location of Lesion	
	Brain Stem	**Cerebral Hemisphere**
Motor signs	Eyes deviate toward side of hemiparesis	Eyes deviate away from side of hemiparesis
Defect	All ipsilateral conjugate movements (Vestibular, saccades, and pursuit) Lesion 2, Fig. 119-2	Contralateral saccades, Ipsilateral pursuit Vestibular spared Lesion 1, Fig. 119-2
Duration	Permanent	Temporary

Internuclear Ophthalmoplegia

The medial longitudinal fasciculus (MLF) carries fibers that mediate impulses from the abducens nucleus region to the contralateral oculomotor nucleus for adduction of the eye during conjugate horizontal gaze.

A lesion interrupting the MLF (Fig. 119-2, Lesion 3) causes

1. Paresis of adduction of the eye ipsilateral to the side of the lesion during all types of conjugate movements
2. Sparing of adduction during convergence
3. Jerk nystagmus in the abducting eye

This syndrome is called internuclear ophthalmoplegia and is pathognomonic for a lesion of the MLF in the

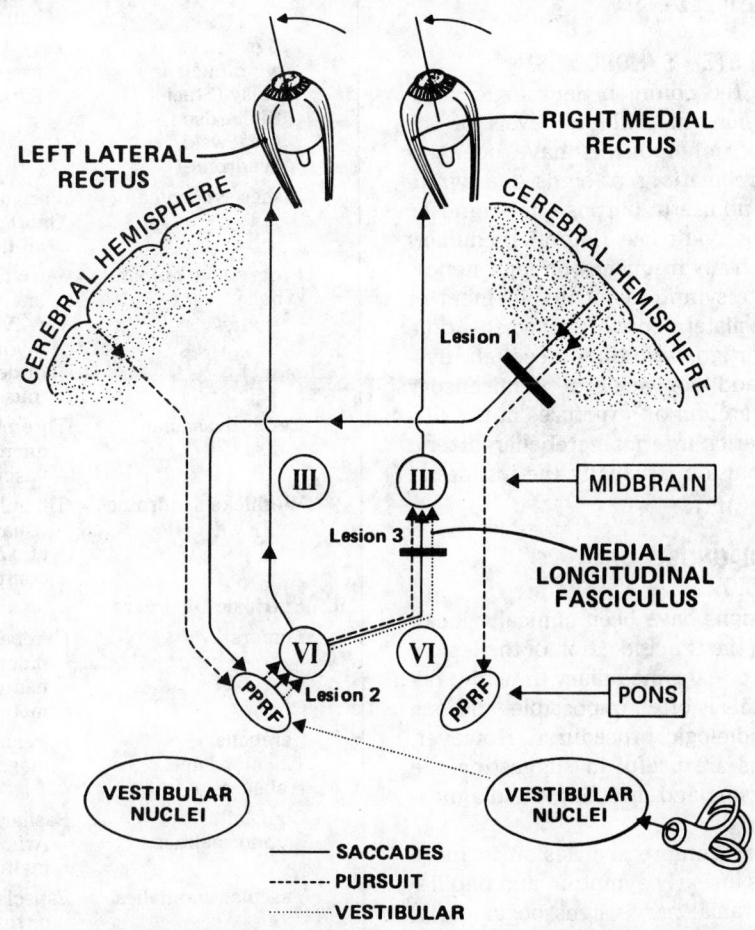

FIGURE 119-2. The control of conjugate eye movements. This explains the manifestations of hemispheral lesions (Lesion 1), pontine lesions involving the paramedian pontine reticular formation, PPRF or abduceus nucleus (Lesion 2), and lesions involving the medial longitudinal fasciculus (Lesion 3). See text for full description.

caudal midbrain or pons. When bilateral, it is often associated with multiple sclerosis; if unilateral, vascular disease.

Paresis of Vertical Gaze

Vertical eye movements are primarily controlled by midbrain structures. Lesions in the region of the pretectum and posterior commissure cause a loss of upward gaze (Parinaud syndrome). Associated signs in Parinaud syndrome are retractory and convergence nystagmus, lid retraction, and loss of pupillary reactions. Downward eye movements are more diffusely represented in the midbrain, and bilateral lesions at the ventral midbrain–thalamic junction are required to cause paresis of downward gaze. Vertical gaze disorders frequently are the earliest signs of compressive lesions arising in the region of the pineal gland (pinealoma, teratoma). Hemispheral lesions rarely cause defects in vertical gaze.

SPECIFIC BRAIN STEM SYNDROMES[57,58]

Table 119–1 outlines the common neurologic signs and symptoms of lesions at different levels of the brain stem. A number of eponyms have been attached to various combinations of signs and symptoms, but they serve no useful purpose in diagnosis. Only one, Wallenberg syndrome (lateral medullary infarction), occurs with any frequency or consistency. Patients develop acute symptoms of involvement of the lateral medulla (ipsilateral loss of facial sensation, ataxia, nystagmus, vertigo, vomiting, hiccough, dysphagia, dysarthria, and contralateral hemisensory loss) secondary to infarction of structures in the distribution of the posterior inferior cerebellar artery. The actual site of occlusion is usually the ipsilateral vertebral artery.

DIFFERENTIAL DIAGNOSIS OF BRAIN STEM LESIONS

Once the neurologic signs have been clinically localized to the brain stem, the exact location of the lesion, either intramedullary or extramedullary, must be determined. Clinically, this is often impossible, and one must rely on neuroradiologic procedures. However, certain generalizations are useful in suggesting the probable site of the lesion and directing the diagnostic evaluation accordingly.

An *extramedullary* compressive lesion is more likely if 1) headache is an early symptom and papilledema is present; 2) cranial nerve signs occur early; and 3) brain stem signs occur late.

An *intramedullary* lesion is likely if 1) headache is not present or is a late symptom and papilledema is absent; 2) brain stem signs occur early and are suggestive of intrinsic involvement, e.g., internuclear

---

TABLE 119–4
Common Brain Stem Lesions

Lesion	Characteristics
I. Intrinsic Disorders	
Primary tumors	Glioma common in childhood
Metastatic tumors	Carcinoma of lung, breast, melanoma frequent
Brain stem encephalitis	Etiology obscure, may cause transient enlargement of brain stem on pneumoencephalogram, occasionally paraneoplastic
Multiple sclerosis	Internuclear ophthalmoplegia, nystagmus, ataxia, elevated CSF gamma globulin, positive myelin basic protein, oligoclonal bands
Progressive supranuclear palsy (Steele-Richardson—Olszewski syndrome)	Paresis of downward gaze frequently first sign, Parkinson's syndrome
Fisher syndrome	Variant of Guillain-Barré Ophthalmoplegia, ataxia, areflexia
Progressive bulbar palsy	Variant of amyotrophic lateral sclerosis C.N. VII–XII primarily involved, often with signs of denervation in limb muscles
Cerebrovascular disease	Thrombosis, hemorrhage, aneurysms, vasculitis, vascular malformations
Wernicke syndrome	Thiamine deficiency, usually in alcoholics, ataxia, C.N. VI paresis, confusion
II. Extrinsic Disorders	
Tumors	Cerebellum, IV ventricle, pinealoma, acoustic neuroma, chordoma, metastatic
Cerebellar hemorrhage, abscess	Surgically remediable if diagnosed early
Congenital abnormalities	Basilar invagination, Arnold-Chiari malformation
Vascular anomalies	Especially basilar aneurysm or tortuous, dilated basilar artery
Basilar meningitis	Especially listeria, tuberculosis, fungus, syphilis, sarcoidosis, meningeal carcinomatosis

ophthalmoplegia, dissociated sensory loss, Horner syndrome; and 3) cranial nerve signs are not prominent or occur late. Table 119–4 outlines some common causes of brain stem lesions and their characteristic features.

DIAGNOSTIC EVALUATION

In general, lumbar punctures should not be done initially in patients with papilledema or whose neurologic signs suggest an extramedullary compressive lesion. A CAT scan should be done first to look for a mass lesion or hydrocephalus. If these tests are negative, papilledema is absent, and a compressive lesion is not suspected, a lumbar puncture can then be safely performed. In patients where the site of the lesion is unclear, arteriography should be performed. If tests are still inconclusive, pneumoencephalography may be indicated, since the CAT scan does not always adequately delineate the structures of the posterior fossa.

CHAPTER 120
Spinal Cord Diseases
GUY M. McKHANN

The spinal cord and spinal roots are extremely intolerant of compression, displacement, or ischemia. There are a number of conditions which can affect the spinal cord and roots. Some act acutely (Table 120–1) and some subacutely (Table 120–2). When the cord is displaced, compressed, or rendered ischemic, the reversibility of the process depends in large measure on how quickly the proper therapy is instituted. This time factor, together with the dire consequences of permanent cord damage, make it essential that physicians

1. Correctly recognize spinal cord lesions
2. Identify the location and mechanism of the lesion
3. Institute appropriate therapy *promptly*

MANIFESTATIONS OF CORD TRANSECTION

When the spinal cord is transected, *spinal shock* ensues. In this condition the cord, below the level of the lesion, is physiologically inert. Thus, below the lesion the patient is without motor, sensory, or autonomic function, is areflexic and hypotonic. After 3 to 6 weeks, physiologic function returns to the isolated section of cord as evidenced by an increase in tone and reflexes, evolving into a spastic paralysis with increased deep tendon reflexes, clonus, and extensor plantar responses. There may be involuntary spasms of the limbs to minor stimuli (flexor or extensor spasms). There is no evidence that the spinal cord can functionally regenerate.

MANIFESTATIONS OF INCOMPLETE CORD LESIONS

Incomplete lesions are identified by evaluating the 1) pattern, 2) level (cephalad-caudad), 3) progression, and 4) site (intramedullary or extramedullary) of the process. These factors and their clinical interpretation will be discussed in turn.

Pattern

An *upper motor neuron* pattern with hyperreflexia, increased tone, and minimal atrophy suggests cord involvement. A *lower motor neuron* pattern with hyporeflexia, decreased tone, and atrophy indicates anterior horn cell, root, or peripheral nerve involvement.

Level of the Lesion

The spinal cord may be involved at a single or at multiple levels. The level is determined by sensory, motor, and autonomic findings.

Sensory manifestations are produced *at* the level of the lesion by involvement of the posterior roots. These radicular symptoms occur in the form of radiating pain corresponding to one or more dermatomes at the level of the lesion. The pain is often aggravated by coughing and straining and by movement of the vertebral column. In addition, cutaneous sensory impairment may be detected in these dermatomes.

Other sensory manifestations are produced *at and below* the lesion by interruption of the tracts subserving the various sensory modalities. Of these modalities *pain* is the most reliably tested. Since fibers conveying pain ascend before crossing to the opposite side of the spinal cord, the observed level of response to pinprick is usually a few segments below the actual lesion.

Motor manifestations are produced at the level of the lesion by involvement of anterior horn cells or ventral roots. Thus, lower motor neuron signs such as wasting, weakness of muscles, and depressed or absent deep tendon reflexes have definite localizing significance.

TABLE 120-1
Acute Spinal Cord Injuries and Diseases

Trauma
Penetrating wounds
Vertebral dislocations
Herniation of intervertebral discs
Whiplash injuries

Infection
Epidural abscess
Viral infection
  Poliomyelitis, Coxsackie, herpes
Meningitis
  Bacterial

Vascular
Occlusion of feeding arteries
  Anterior spinal artery occlusion
  Dissecting aortic aneurism
Arteriovenous malformation
Hematomyelia

Demyelinative and Inflammatory
Transverse myelitis
Multiple sclerosis
Chemical meningitis

Neoplastic
Metastatic
  Extradural
  Intradural

TABLE 120-2
Subacute Spinal Cord Diseases

Trauma or Compression
Cervical spondylosis
Herniation of intervertebral discs
Syringomyelia

Infections
Chronic meningitis
  Syphilis, tuberculosis or fungal
Epidural abscess (usually acute)

Inflammatory
Arachnoiditis

Vascular
Arteriovenous malformations
Arteritis

Demyelination
Multiple sclerosis

Neoplastic
Meningioma
Neurinoma
Lymphoma or leukemia
Metastatic
Seeding from brain tumor

Metabolic
Pernicious anemia

Degenerations
Spinocerebellar
Amyotrophic lateral sclerosis
Peroneal muscular atrophy

Autonomic findings, such as decreased or absent sweating, may be detected below the level of the lesion, but usually do not provide precise localizing information.

Pattern of Progression

In lesions of *acute* onset, particularly traumatic ones, the initial features are those of spinal shock. Although this condition may persist for an indefinite period, pyramidal tract manifestations (spasticity, hyperreflexia, extensor plantar responses, and urgency of urination) usually supervene. In the more *slowly evolving* forms of cord compression, pyramidal tract manifestations may be apparent from the onset.

Site of the Lesion

Intraspinal mass lesions are conveniently divided into two groups. Those situated within the spinal cord are *intramedullary,* and those lesions outside the cord, originating from vertebrae, meninges, or nerve roots, are *extramedullary.* The various extramedullary and intramedullary forms of cord compression are presented in Table 120-3, and in Table 120-4 the differentiating features are shown.

COMPRESSION OF SPINAL CORD AND ROOTS

Differential Diagnosis

It is essential that spinal cord compression be differentiated from other lesions of the cord that may cause paraplegia, namely, transverse myelitis, ischemic myelomalacia, syphilis, multiple sclerosis, subacute combined degeneration of the cord, and motor neuron disease. The extremities may also be involved in a hysterical paralysis, which may be accompanied by sensory loss but no involvement of bladder or bowel control and no alteration in the reflexes. Flaccid paraplegia may occur with lesions of anterior horn cells of the lumbosacral region, e.g., poliomyelitis, with lesions of the cauda equina or the peripheral nerves, e.g., polyneuritis, or as the result of primary muscle disease. Bilateral leg weakness may also result from a parasagittal meningioma if the pyramidal fibers from both leg areas of the motor cortex are involved. On occasion an early symptom of spinal compression is root pain, which may be confused

TABLE 120-3
Intraspinal Mass Lesions

	Extra-Medullary	Intra-Medullary
Neoplastic		
	Meningioma	Glioma
	Neurinoma	ependymoma
	Metastatic (common)	Metastatic (rare)
	Congenital epidermoid, dermoid, teratoma, chordoma, cyst, angioma, lipoma	Congenital syringomyelia, angioma, lipoma
	Lymphoma, leukemia, myeloma, sarcoma	
Non-Neoplastic		
	Degenerative cervical spondylosis (common)	Trauma hematomyelia
	Inflammatory epidural abscess Pott's disease, osteomyelitis arachnoiditis granuloma	Inflammatory abscess (rare)
	Trauma epidural hematoma herniated intervertebral disc dislocation, compression fracture	

with that caused by such visceral disorders as pleurisy, angina, cholecystitis, or peptic ulcer. Furthermore, these radicular pains may be mistaken for local joint disease.

Usually the distinction between a mass lesion and these other conditions can be made clinically. Whenever there is doubt, myelography is carried out to exclude cord compression, especially the more treatable forms.

Diagnostic Studies

Roentgenograms of the spine may reveal loss of mobility, bony erosion, bony overgrowth, or narrowing of the intervertebral space. *Lumbar puncture* may reveal CSF abnormalities, such as increased protein concentration and xanthochromia (Froin syndrome). Queckenstedt's test may reveal obstructed flow of spinal fluid. All these studies, however, may be normal despite the presence of a mass lesion.

Myelography (Chap. 141) provides a definitive answer to the question of the presence or absence of a mass lesion and its location. Myelograms should be performed for *all* patients seriously considered to have cord compression.

Treatment

In general, mass lesions of undetermined nature which are of acute onset or rapid progression warrant prompt surgical exploration, as do epidural abscesses and epidural hematomas.

Compression caused by lymphomatous or carcinomatous involvement of meninges or vertebral bodies should probably be treated by irradiation or chemotherapy if the tumor is thought to be responsive to these forms of therapy. In some instances surgical decompression is warranted.

The treatment of meningioma, neurofibroma, and other benign extramedullary neoplasms is surgical excision. Irradiation alone is indicated in intramedullary neoplasms.

SPECIFIC DISEASE ENTITIES

Of the many causes of spinal cord compression, some syndromes have distinguishing clinical features and are sufficiently important to warrant further consideration.

Spinal Epidural Abscess[60]

Spinal epidural abscess is not common, but is eminently treatable and is often misdiagnosed. The infection usually results from hematogenous spread, but the cord signs appear days or weeks after the bacteremia, and the usual signs of infection may be minimal or even absent. The abscess commonly arises from the vertebral body, but, as is often the case with early osteomyelitis, there may be no roentgenographic abnormalities.

Signs and symptoms of cord compression usually appear abruptly and progress over the course of hours or days. Often there is prodromal local pain, and there may be local tenderness on palpation or motion, but the absence of these features should not deter one from making this diagnosis. Indeed, it should be suspected whenever there is abrupt or progressive cord compression.

Cord damage is produced in part by impairment of the arterial supply of the cord. It is, therefore, essential that the abscess be drained promptly if perma-

TABLE 120-4
Intraspinal Mass Lesions

	Extramedullary	Intramedullary
Incidence	95%	5%
Presence of associated systemic disease	Frequent	Nil
Duration of symptoms	Short	Long
Pain Local or radicular, overlying tenderness	Frequent	Infrequent
Sphincter involvement	Late	Early
Cerebrospinal fluid block Positive queckenstedt, Froin syndrome	Early	Late
Radiologic findings Spine films—spondylosis, erosion, destruction of vertebra, widening of spinal canal, narrowed disc space	Frequent	Infrequent
Myelogram	Positive	May be negative
Prognosis with treatment	Poor (metastatic carcinoma) Good (meningioma, neurinoma, epidural abscess)	Poor

nent ischemic damage is to be prevented. The definitive diagnostic test is myelography.

Cervical Spondylosis[59,63,64,65]

Spondylosis in the cervical region is a relatively common cause of spinal cord compression occurring after middle life. The degeneration of one or more intervertebral discs, with the development of osteoarthritic changes, leads to compression of not only cord but also spinal roots. The onset is usually insidious, but acute protrusions do occur. There is some limitation of both active and passive movements of the head, and pain may radiate to the shoulders, upper extremities, and to the scapular region.

The clinical picture depends on the level or levels at which cord compression occurs and on the extent of the damage. There is often a mixture of symptoms, owing to upper and lower motor neuron involvement in the upper extremities, and to upper motor neuron dysfunction in the lower limbs. There may be no sensory loss, but often there is diminished appreciation of light touch and of pinprick over the fingers, with or without loss of position sense. Similar sensory alteration may be noted in the legs. The deep tendon reflexes may be diminished or increased in the arms, and there is often an inverted brachioradialis reflex (tapping the radius results only in flexion of the fingers). CSF dynamics are usually normal.

Since the radiologic features of cervical spondylosis are commonly detected in asymptomatic older

individuals, some caution should be used in attributing spinal cord compression to this condition.

The first step in treatment is immobilization with a supportive collar. The indications for further evaluation, e.g., myelography and surgery, are

1. Intractable pain
2. Progressive weakness and atrophy in the musculature of the arms or hands
3. Progressive gait disorder secondary to a spastic paraparesis

In such patients, an anterior fusion is the preferred operation.[63,64] Seventy percent of patients can expect significant long-term benefit from this procedure.

Herniated Intervertebral Disc

In contrast to the slowly progressing compression of the spinal cord or cervical roots in cervical spondylosis, there may be acute symptoms from herniated intervertebral discs. These occur most commonly in the lumbar and cervical areas. Thoracic discs are rare, and are usually associated with direct trauma.

Herniated cervical discs usually occur at the C5-C6 and C6-C7 levels. The first symptom is usually radicular pain, made worse by moving of the neck, coughing, or straining. Weakness in the affected muscles (C5, rhomboid, supraspinatus, deltoid; C6, biceps, brachioradialis; C7, triceps) appears next. Depression of the biceps jerk (C6) or triceps jerk (C7) may often be useful in localizing the level of herniation. Occasionally, a midline protrusion of a cervical disc occurs, with direct cord compression resulting in long-tract findings.

Treatment involves immobilization of the neck by cervical traction or a supportive collar and relief of muscle spasm and pain. If a patient does not respond to cervical traction, or develops signs of cord compression, myelography and surgical removal of the protruded disc material are indicated.

Herniated lumbar discs are often preceded by an injury or strain to the back accompanied by a feeling of a "snap" in the lower back. Nonlocalized pain appears in the lower back which makes it difficult for the patient to stand erect or walk. The pain then becomes more localized to the buttock, posterior thigh, and leg. Exacerbations of pain occur with bending, coughing, or lifting objects. Muscle weakness and absent knee jerk (L4-L5) or ankle jerk (L5-S1) may occur.

Treatment is bed rest and analgesics. Surgery may be required, but is appropriate only after at least a 3 week trial of bed rest. Myelography is indicated only in patients in whom the diagnosis is not certain or for whom surgery is intended.

Syringomyelia[62]

In syringomyelia an elongated cavity lined with ependymal cells develops in close relationship to the central canal of the spinal cord, particularly in the cervicothoracic region, and on occasion in the medulla (syringobulbia). The cavitation destroys decussating pain and temperature fibers and compresses adjacent motor neurons as well as the long ascending and descending tracts. Although it is considered a congenital abnormality, clinical manifestations do not appear until early adult life.

The initial signs are usually confined to one hand and consist of wasting and weakness, together with deficits of pain and temperature sensation. Scars resulting from painless burns or other traumas are frequently seen. Perception of light touch and position are usually spared; this dissociated sensory loss is characteristic. As the lesion progresses, the contralateral upper extremity becomes similarly afflicted, and upper motor neuron signs and sensory disturbances appear in the lower limbs. Horner syndrome, dysarthria, dysphagia, and nystagmus may also occur. With involvement of the spinal nucleus and tract of the trigeminal nerve, dissociated sensory loss may occur on the face in an onionskin pattern; the involvement is not in order of the sensory divisions but from behind forward, converging on the nose and upper lip. Spontaneous pain is not encountered. Arthropath-

ies in the upper limbs (Charcot's joint), kyphoscoliosis, and congenital abnormalities of the vertebral column (Klippel-Feil and Arnold-Chiari syndromes) are also seen. In addition, there is an increased incidence of gliomas. The course is slowly progressive, but spontaneous arrest may occur. Rarely, an acute exacerbation, caused by a spontaneous or traumatic hemorrhage into the cavity occurs.

Other extramedullary conditions, including cervical spondylosis, cervical rib, and various compressive syndromes of peripheral nerves, may also produce wasting of muscle and sensory impairment in upper limbs, but pain is usually conspicuous, and dissociated sensory loss is not encountered. Differentiating syringomyelia from other intraspinal lesions may be more difficult, and myelography may be necessary. Spinal block rarely occurs in syringomyelia and the CSF is normal. Motor neuron disease (amyotrophic lateral sclerosis) commonly presents with wasting of small hand muscles, but this disease is more rapidly progressive, and the sensory deficits are never encountered.

BACKACHE[61]

So far we have emphasized well-delineated entities involving the spine, spinal cord, or their membranes. The problem the physician encounters most commonly is the patient complaining of backache. It is convenient to divide patients into those with an acute onset and those with a more chronic course.

Acute Backache

Acute backache often comes on after an injury or strain, such as a fall, lifting a heavy object or twisting suddenly. However, many patients "throw their back out" without any apparent preceding event. The symptoms are usually in the lower back and consist of pain, spasm of the paravertebral muscles, and inability to bend. Coughing, straining, or bending make the symptoms worse. When lying down, the patient may feel almost paralyzed, with the slightest flexion or extension movement bringing on pain. In the cervical region, there is more commonly a preceding event, such as a whiplash (sudden extension-flexion movement of the neck). The pain is usually over the lower portion of the neck, with palpable spasm of the posterior cervical musculature.

Many patients with the syndrome of a herniated cervical or lumbar disc will report previous minor problems with their back. In some instances the pain is radicular, down an arm or the posterior aspect of a leg, minimizing the full blown syndrome of the herniated disc.

The management of a patient with an acute backache is symptomatic. It is not clear what the exact mechanism of the pain is. Patients appear to set up a cycle of pain, muscle spasm, and more pain. In addition, radicular symptoms indicate irritation or compression of nerve roots. The acute therapy is bed rest, analgesics, and agents, such as a diazepam (Valium), which may relieve the muscle spasm. In many cases the acute pain subsides after a few days of rest. In others it may take weeks, with a gradual increase of physical activity. Traction is of little help for lumbar pain but may be quite helpful for pain in the cervical area.

Chronic Backache

Chronic backache is often a symptom of depression. In addition, the industrial compensation aspects of many cases makes it difficult to sort out what is functional and what is not. There remain, however, a number of patients with "weak backs." These people have repeated episodes of acute pain, superimposed on chronic pain, usually of the lower back. The pain is usually across the back, not radiating into the legs, and not associated with significant muscle spasm. Varying degrees of osteoarthritis may be demonstrated by x-ray examination. Therapy with these patients is difficult. Improvement of posture and exercises to strengthen back musculature aid some patients. A supporting corset, sleeping with a firm mattress, and avoiding lifting and bending are also of help. Surgery is usually not of help and should be considered only after one is convinced that medical management has failed, and that emotional or compensation factors are not dominant influences. Myelography is done as a preparation for surgery, but is of little aid in the medical management.

CHAPTER 121
Weakness
DANIEL B. DRACHMAN

Any disturbance of the power to act may be reported by a patient as "weakness." However, motor impairment may represent the outward manifestation of a wide variety of disorders, only some of which involve the motor system. Underlying the patient's complaint of weakness may be

1. A disorder of the central nervous system, particularly the corticospinal pathways
2. Damage to the motor neurons in the spinal cord
3. A disorder of the nerve roots or peripheral nerves
4. A defect of neuromuscular transmission
5. A disorder of muscles
6. A painful affection of the musculoskeletal system
7. An unrelated systemic disease
8. A purely psychogenic cause

It is the purpose of this section to present an orderly approach to the problem of weakness, so that the physician can quickly sort out these possibilities.

From the standpoint of diagnosis, it is useful to distinguish three separate entities: *weakness, fatigue,* and *tiredness,* which are defined as follows:

Weakness is a reduction in the maximum force of muscle contraction. Clinical testing of muscles evaluates the maximum muscle force. True weakness always indicates an organic disorder.

Fatigue is a reduction in muscular force on repeated contraction. To some extent, muscle fatigue is a normal phenomenon. A normal person may fatigue after 15 or 20 push-ups, and be unable to resume until he has rested the exercised muscles. In the presence of weakness, fatigue may occur more rapidly than normal. Muscular fatigue is especially prominent in myasthenia gravis.

Tiredness is a subjective sensation of listlessness and lethargy which follows muscular exertion. Like fatigue, it is experienced by normal individuals. As a presenting complaint, it is most often psychogenic, but may accompany systemic disease.

APPROACH TO THE PATIENT

HISTORY

Weakness should be assessed against the background of the patient's usual activities. The interviewer should determine whether there has been a specific *change* in the patient's motor abilities. Often a direct question is useful, such as, "What can't you do now that you previously were able to do?" For a construction worker, the inability to lift a 200-pound sack of cement may represent a real change. Obviously, the same criterion could hardly apply to a high school girl. The *earliest manifestation* of weakness should be sought, since it may give an important clue to the true course of the disorder. A housewife may first have noticed difficulty in lifting the baby, or in placing grocery packages on high shelves. A school boy may have had trouble in throwing a baseball or in carrying out exercises in gymnasium. If the patient has had no change in motor performance, has he merely noted a sensation of *tiredness,* or an unwillingness to undertake physical activity? If so, the problem is more likely not organic.

The *distribution* of weakness may often be ascertained from the history. The interviewer should determine which extremities are involved, and whether the weakness is *symmetrical* or *asymmetrical.* Does it involve the *proximal* or the *distal* musculature? Proximal weakness of the lower limbs may first be noticed as difficulty in getting out of the bathtub or arising from a low chair. Proximal weakness of the upper limbs interferes with any heavy manual labor, and may make shaving in men or brushing the hair in women difficult. Distal weakness results in foot drop, or in "clumsiness" in the use of the hands.

If the "weakness" is universal and uniform, it is more likely to be psychogenic or systemic in cause, rather than to be a disorder of the motor system. Proximal, symmetrical weakness suggests myopathy. A distal symmetrical distribution of weakness is often seen in neuropathic disorders.

Associated symptoms may provide important clues to the nature of the problem. If sensory loss or other neurologic symptoms are present, a disorder of the peripheral or central nervous system should be considered. Fever or weight loss would point to an underlying systemic disease. Local pain in the weak limb may be an important symptom. The patient's emotional status must be evaluated critically. Has depression or apathy preceded the onset of symptoms?

PHYSICAL EXAMINATION

Coordinated Actions

A great deal can be learned from observing the patient closely as he performs natural coordinated movements. For example, the patient's gait may be very revealing. A waddling gait, in which the pelvis tilts from side to side, suggests proximal muscle weakness. Weakness of the ankle extensors may be seen as a tendency to overlift the leg, so as to compensate for a slight degree of foot drop. In testing the proximal musculature, it is useful to watch the patient as he arises from a chair, or from a seated posi-

tion on the floor. Patients with proximal weakness may boost themselves by using the upper limbs for added support. In patients with minimal weakness, deep-knee bends or push-ups may reveal a minor degree of impairment.

Formal Testing[9]

When weakness is present, it should be evaluated as objectively as practicable by testing the function of individual muscles and rating the results according to a quantitative scale. This requires that the examiner know the action of each muscle tested. An illustrated manual on muscle testing published by the British Medical Research Council is available. Muscle strength is graded according to standardized criteria:

No muscle contraction	0
Flicker of muscle contraction	1
Full range of motion, with gravity excluded	2
Full range of motion against gravity only	3
Full range of motion, against gravity and some external resistance	4
Normal power	5

With this method of grading many weak muscles will fall in the range 4 to 5. Although this is not sensitive to detecting minor degrees of weakness, further refinements of grading are not reliable, since they depend too heavily on subjective impressions.

It must be emphasized that the purpose of individual muscle testing is to obtain an objective assessment of the degree and pattern of weakness. Beginners must be cautioned to avoid bogging down in the testing ritual; try to determine *patterns* of weakness if possible.

Hysteria and Malingering

When the examiner suspects that the patient may not be cooperating fully, he must try to distinguish between organic weakness and apparent weakness caused by hysteria or malingering. The following points are often helpful: 1) When the examiner overcomes the force of a genuinely weak muscle, he will notice that it yields smoothly to pressure. By contrast, the malingering or hysterical patient releases the muscle contraction in a step-wise or *jerky* manner. 2) When the muscle strength demonstrated in coordinated actions (especially when the patient is not aware that he is being observed) is greater than that found on formal muscle testing, the *disparity* may suggest that real weakness is not present. 3) The examiner may use *subterfuge* to elicit maximal effort from the patient. For example, some patients may pretend to be weak when moving the limb through a range of motion, but will exert full power when directed to maintain a fixed posture.

Muscle Bulk

This may be evaluated by inspection or measurement of the muscles. In cachectic patients one must avoid confusing loss of subcutaneous fatty tissue with muscle atrophy. When measuring the circumference of a limb, it is necessary to specify the point at which the measurement is made. For example, the calf circumference may be measured at a level 8 to 12 cm below the tibial tubercle.

Muscle Fasciculations

These should be sought when denervation atrophy is suspected. The patient must be at complete rest, and comfortably warm. Good lighting is essential. Fasciculations are spontaneous twitching of *motor units* or parts of motor units. They are seen more commonly in disorders of the anterior horn cells or nerve roots than in the more distal peripheral neuropathies. It should be emphasized that fasciculations also occur occasionally in well over 90 percent of the normal population. They are particularly common in times of stress and fatigue, and are aggravated by smoking and drinking coffee.

Fibrillations, or the spontaneous contraction of single muscle fibers, cannot be seen through the skin. They are visible only through the thin mucosa of the tongue, and can best be seen with the tongue at rest within the mouth.

Reflexes

The deep tendon reflexes should be tested in all patients with weakness. Weakness associated with absent reflexes is usually suggestive of neuropathy rather than myopathy.

SPECIAL EXAMINATIONS

In most cases of neuromuscular disorders, muscle biopsy, electromyography (EMG), and determination of serum enzymes released from muscle are essential to establish a correct diagnosis.

Muscle Biopsy

This procedure discloses the histopathology of the affected muscle directly. However, only one or at the most two muscles may be sampled in this way, and of necessity, only a small fragment of muscle is studied. It is important for the clinician to know what kind of information can be provided by proper interpretation of a muscle biopsy:

1. It can confirm the clinical diagnosis of myopathy. Usually the biopsy findings do not permit any

further statement about the specific kind of myopathy present. The severity and acuteness of the disease process in the muscle from which the specimen was taken can also be estimated.

2. It can occasionally provide a definitive diagnosis of a specific type of myopathy on the basis of pathognomonic histologic, histochemical, or electron microscopic findings. Polyarteritis, sarcoidosis, and some of the "rare" myopathies may be identified by biopsy.

3. It can identify neurogenic atrophy caused by lesions of motor nerve cells or peripheral nerves, and reliably distinguish it from myopathy.

A negative muscle biopsy is much less helpful. It may mean that

1. The clinical diagnosis of neuropathy or myopathy is incorrect.
2. The portion of muscle selected for the biopsy is not yet involved, although changes may be present elsewhere.
3. The disorder is one which does not produce histologic lesions in muscles (metabolic myopathies, upper motor neuron lesions, psychogenic disorders, or systemic disease).

A detailed discussion of the histopathology of muscle is not possible here. However, the principles of diagnosis are very simple. In the *myopathies,* muscle fibers are attacked *at random,* and show typical *destructive* changes. Thus, degenerative changes in muscle fibers scattered randomly throughout the biopsy specimen are typical of myopathy. Reactive changes, such as phagocytosis, fibrosis, and fatty infiltration are also seen (Fig. 121–1).

By contrast, *denervation* produces a shrinkage of muscle fibers, without destructive changes. Neighboring *groups* of muscle fibers formerly supplied by the damaged nerves (motor units) are affected (Fig. 121–2).

Electrophysiology

Electromyography (EMG) and nerve conduction studies provide information about the function, rather than the structure, of muscle and nerve.

By the use of needle electrodes, the electrical activity of muscle fibers is sampled and displayed on an oscilloscopic screen for viewing and photographic recording. Several different muscles can be tested at a single examination.

EMG patterns which are characteristic of myopathy, peripheral neuropathy, and anterior horn cell destruction can be identified. In the *neuropathies,* two defects are apparent: 1) Whole motor units are lost,

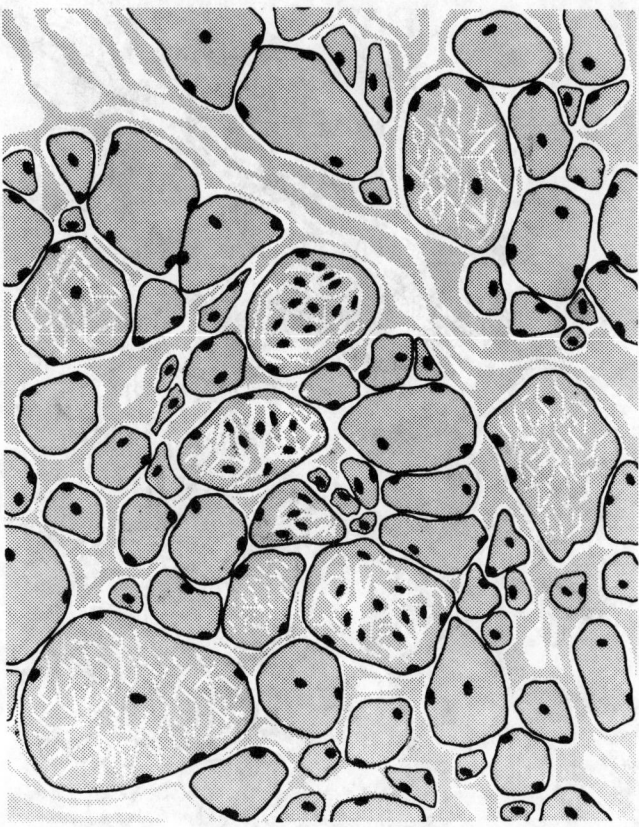

FIGURE 121-1. Drawing of myopathic changes in muscle biopsy (transverse section). There is random variation in muscle fiber size. The sarcolemmal nuclei are placed centrally rather than in their normal position immediately under the sarcolemmal membrane. Several fibers are undergoing floccular degenerative changes. There is an increase in endomysial connective tissue.

and 2) denervated muscle fibers show spontaneous electrical discharges called fibrillations and positive denervation potentials (Fig. 121-3). In the *myopathies,* the total number of motor units available is not substantially decreased, but destruction of individual muscle fibers within the remaining motor units results in a diminution in the amplitude and duration of action potentials and a ragged (polyphasic) appearance to the action potentials (Fig. 121-3).

In most peripheral neuropathies, damage to the nerve fibers results in slowing of their electrical conductivity. It is a simple matter to measure the speed of electrical conduction in certain superficial nerves, as outlined in Figure 121-4.

Serum Enzymes

The enzymes contained within the muscle fiber leak out when the muscle membrane is damaged and eventually reach the bloodstream. In the destructive myopathies the serum levels of certain enzymes may be elevated. These values are highest at a time when the destructive process is most active. In contrast, disorders of the motor neurons or peripheral nerves seldom cause elevation of serum enzymes levels. Those enzymes which have been used in the diagnosis of muscle diseases are serum glutamic oxaloacetic transaminase (SGOT), serum glutamic pyruvic transaminase (SGPT), lactic dehydrogenase (LDH), and creatine phosphokinase (CPK).

Elevation of the serum creatine phosphokinase appears to be most specific for myopathy. This enzyme is not present to any appreciable extent in liver or red blood cells, and its serum levels are unaffected by malignancy, hepatic disease, or in vitro hemolysis. Although the CPK concentration may be raised in the acute stages of myocardial infarction, this rarely presents a problem in interpretation. The chief value of serum enzyme determination is to confirm the di-

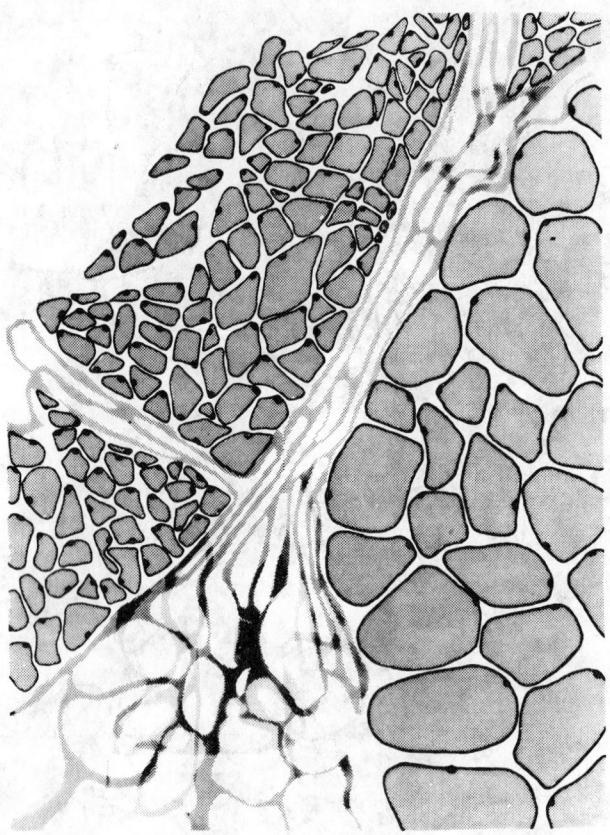

FIGURE 121–2. Neurogenic atrophy in muscle biopsy (transverse section). Groups of atrophic (small) muscle fibers are shown above to the left. The group of muscle fibers to the right is of normal size. The muscle nuclei remain peripheral in position. Degenerative changes are absent.

agnosis of myopathy. The enzyme levels should also be followed in assessing the efficacy of treatment (see Chap. 124).

CHARACTERISTICS OF WEAKNESS DUE TO VARIOUS CAUSES

Although a detailed description of the findings in each of the following conditions is beyond the scope of this section, the characteristics of the weakness and certain associated findings may be helpful.

Central Nervous System

Lesions of the corticospinal (pyramidal) system usually produce spasticity, with hyperactive deep tendon reflexes, and extensor plantar responses. However, the motor weakness may overshadow the other signs. The weakness is often most pronounced in the "physiologic flexor muscles," while there is relative sparing of the "antigravity" muscles. In the lower extremities, the iliopsoas, hamstring, and anterior tibial groups are physiologic flexors, while the glutei, quadriceps, and gastrocnemius groups are antigravity muscles. The finding of this distribution of weakness often confirms the diagnosis. Corticospinal involvement may be unilateral or bilateral. It may affect only the lower extremities if the lesion is at the level of the spinal cord, or may affect the upper extremities and face as well if the lesion is at a higher level.

Other disorders of the central nervous system involving the extrapyramidal system or cerebellum may be interpreted as "weakness" by the patient. However, careful examination will reveal that muscle power is intact, and will disclose the typical neurologic deficit secondary to dysfunction of these systems.

Anterior Horn Cells

The anterior horn cells are involved in amyotrophic lateral sclerosis, poliomyelitis, and other disorders. Typically, muscle weakness is scattered and asymmetrical. Muscle wasting and fasciculations are prominent. The deep tendon reflexes are lost early when weakness is caused by anterior horn cell damage.

A. FIBRILLATIONS

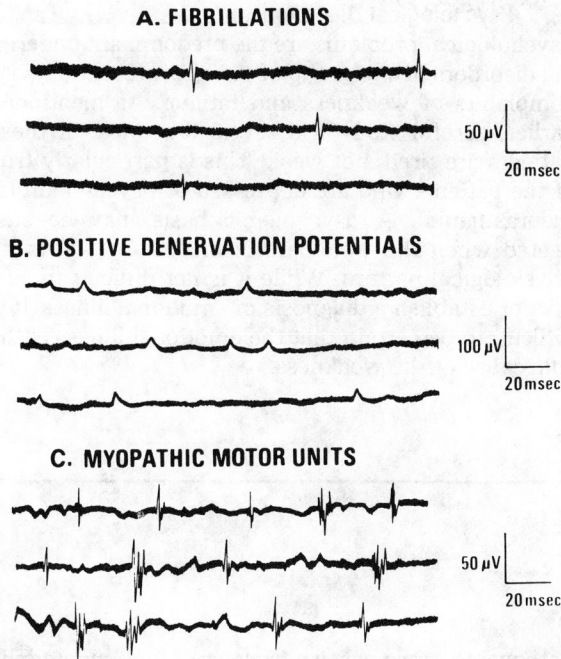

50 µV

20 msec

B. POSITIVE DENERVATION POTENTIALS

100 µV

20 msec

C. MYOPATHIC MOTOR UNITS

50 µV

20 msec

FIGURE 121-3. Electromyographic features. **A.** Fibrillations consist of spontaneous depolarization of single muscle fibers which have been denervated. They appear as short duration di- or triphasic potentials of low amplitude. **B.** Positive denervation potentials also occur spontaneously in denervated muscle fibers. They are larger in amplitude and longer in duration than fibrillations. There is an initial rapid upward phase followed by a slower return to the baseline. **C.** Myopathic action potentials are low in amplitude and short in duration. They have a characteristic ragged, polyphasic appearance.

Peripheral Neuropathies and Myopathies

These are discussed fully in Chapters 123 and 124. In the neuropathies, weakness is often distal. Sensory changes, when present, exclude myopathy as the cause of weakness. Electrodiagnostic testing, muscle biopsy, and serum muscle enzyme determinations are helpful in distinguishing among these conditions.

Disorders of Neuromuscular Transmission

A defect of neuromuscular transmission produces weakness and easy fatigability, but no other manifestations. Since psychological disorders are associated with tiredness and asthenic manifestations, these two groups of disorders may be confused. Many patients with myasthenia gravis are initially diagnosed as being "neurasthenic." Conversely, some patients with psychogenic weakness are treated as though they had myasthenia gravis. An important differentiating feature is that objective weakness can be dem-

onstrated in virtually all patients with impaired neuromuscular transmission. Electrodiagnostic and pharmacologic tests may be helpful in distinguishing between the two.

Pain

Disorders that produce pain in the joints, bones, or muscles may limit the patient's ability to exert maximum muscle force. The apparent weakness may be beyond the patient's voluntary control. The finding of local tenderness in the affected part supports this diagnosis.

Systemic Disease

Any serious illness may cause weakness. The weakness is usually not localized, but involves all muscle

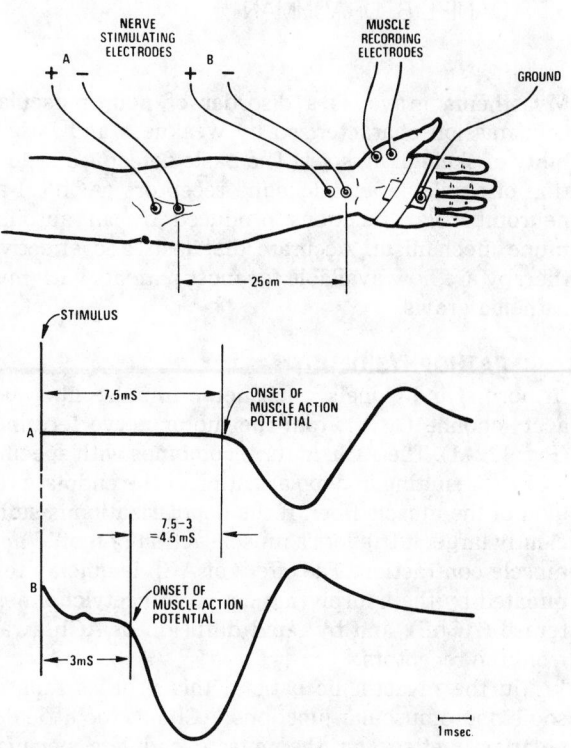

FIGURE 121-4. Median nerve conduction velocity. The recording electrodes are placed over the thenar muscles. Two pairs of nerve stimulating electrodes are represented in A and B. In lower panel tracing A represents the muscle action potential evoked by nerve stimulation at the elbow, while tracing B represents the action potential evoked by stimulation of the median nerve at the wrist. The velocity of conduction in the median nerve from point A to point B equals the distance from A to B (25 cm or 0.25 m) divided by the time it takes the impulse to travel from A to B (7.5 msec − 3 msec = 4.5 msec). In this case the velocity is normal, 55.6 m per second.

groups. There may be loss of muscle bulk, as well as loss of subcutaneous fat. Those patients who present with weakness as the sole complaint, present difficult diagnostic problems. In most of these patients other manifestations of their disease can be found upon careful questioning or examination. In some, however, general weakness is the only evidence of disease on initial appraisal. This may be true in the weakness associated with endocrinopathies (hyperthyroidism, Addison's disease, and hypopituitarism), in indolent infections (tuberculosis, subacute bacterial endocarditis), and in various neoplastic and metabolic diseases.

Psychological Disorders

Psychological problems are the predominant underlying disorders in any group of patients presenting with complaints of weakness and fatigue. As mentioned earlier, careful study will reveal that most of these patients are tired, not weak. This is particularly true of the patients who are depressed or psychoneurotic (neurasthenic). A psychogenic basis may be suspected when the weakness is inconstant or fits no physiological pattern. While it is not difficult to suspect or establish a diagnosis of emotional illness, it is difficult to be certain that the emotional illness is the *sole* cause of the weakness.

CHAPTER 122
Myasthenia Gravis
DANIEL B. DRACHMAN

Myasthenia gravis is a disorder of neuromuscular transmission characterized by weakness and fatigability of skeletal muscles. The basic defect is a reduction of available acetylcholine receptors (AChRs) at neuromuscular junctions produced by an autoimmune mechanism. Accurate diagnosis and effective therapy are now available for most patients with myasthenia gravis.

PATHOPHYSIOLOGY[68]

In normal individuals, each nerve impulse liberates acetylcholine (ACh) from the motor nerve terminal (Fig. 122-1). The ACh, in turn, combines with specific AChRs, resulting in depolarization of the endplate region of the muscle fiber. If the depolarization is sufficiently large, it triggers a muscle action potential and muscle contraction. The effect of ACh is quickly terminated by the hydrolyzing action of acetylcholinesterase (AChE), and by rapid diffusion of ACh away from the receptors.

In the myasthenic patient, this process fails at some neuromuscular junctions. ACh has too little depolarizing effect on the muscle endplate because there is a marked reduction of available AChRs.[68] This reduction of receptors accounts for the abnormalities in myasthenia, since experimental blockade of AChRs in animals has been shown to reproduce all the physiologic effects found in the disease.

There is extensive evidence that autoimmune mechanisms are involved in the pathogenesis of myasthenia gravis. Antibodies directed against AChRs are found in the serum of 75 to 80 percent of patients.[70] These antibodies have been shown to be pathogenic, since passive transfer of immunoglobulin G from myasthenic patients to mice reproduces the basic features of the disease in the recipient.[68] The antibody molecules bind to AChRs to the neuromuscular junction and decrease the number of available AChRs by several different mechanisms:

1. AChRs with bound antibody are degraded at a more rapid rate than normal.[69]
2. The active site of the AChR molecule, i.e., the site that normally accepts ACh, may be blocked by the antibody.
3. The postjunctional portion of the endplate may be damaged by the antibody, possibly by complement-mediated mechanisms.

CLINICAL FEATURES[68]

Myasthenia gravis may affect individuals in any age group, but there are peaks of incidence in young women in their 20s and 30s and older males in their 50s and 60s. The cardinal features are weakness and fatigability of muscles. The weakness increases during repeated use of the muscle, and may improve after rest. The course of myasthenia gravis is often variable. Exacerbations and remissions occur in some patients, but the remissions are rarely complete or permanent. Intercurrent infections or systemic disorders may aggravate the weakness.

Distribution of Muscle Weakness

Myasthenia gravis usually affects bulbar musculature. Involvement of limb muscles only is rare. Involvement of the ocular muscles, resulting in diplopia

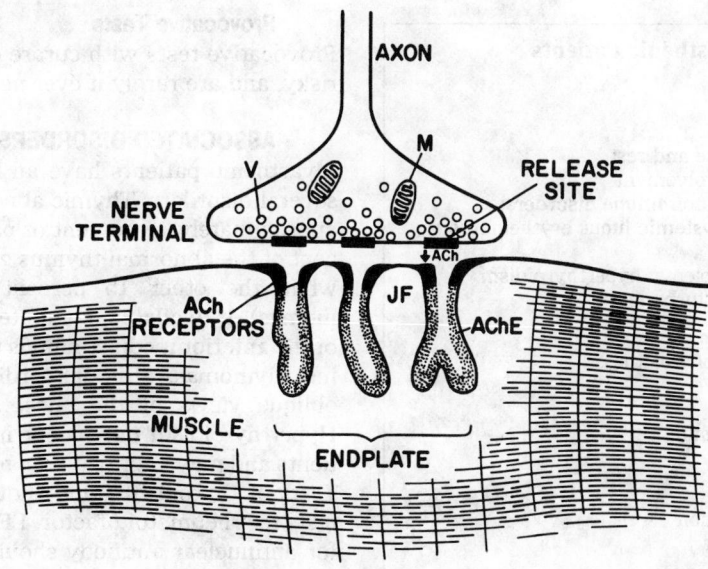

FIGURE 122-1. Diagram of the neuromuscular junction. Vesicles (V) release their acetylcholine (ACh) contents at specialized release sites. After crossing the narrow synaptic space (path indicated by arrow) ACh reaches the ACh receptors, which are most densely situated at the peaks of the junctional folds (JF). Acetylcholinesterase (AChE) in the clefts rapidly hydrolyzes the ACh. M denotes mitochondia. (Reprinted by permission of New England Journal of Medicine 298:136, 1978.)

and ptosis, is a common initial complaint. Many patients may have symptoms restricted to ocular muscles during the early stages of their disease. Facial weakness leads to the "myasthenic snarl" upon attempting to smile. Weakness in chewing is most noticeable after prolonged effort, as in chewing meat. Difficulty in swallowing may be secondary to weakness of the palate, tongue, or pharynx. Speech may have a nasal quality caused by palatal weakness, or a dysarthric quality caused by tongue weakness. The limb weakness in myasthenia is often proximal and may be asymmetrical. The deep tendon reflexes are almost invariably preserved.

DIAGNOSIS AND EVALUATION (Table 122-1)

The diagnosis is suspected on the basis of weakness and fatigability as described above. The suspected diagnosis should always be confirmed by one or more of the following diagnostic tests.

Trial of Anticholinesterase Drugs

The simplest and most frequently used method is the edrophonium (Tensilon) test. This test is based on the fact that Tensilon, an inhibitor of AChE, produces an improvement in the strength of myasthenic muscles. The beneficial effect begins within 30 seconds, and is

over in about 5 minutes. It is essential that an objective endpoint be used to evaluate the effect of edrophonium. The examiner should select an unequivocally weak muscle group, and evaluate its strength in an objective manner. For example, it is often useful to determine how long the patient is able to maintain upward gaze before the lids become ptotic. Similarly, the time that the patient is able to maintain his arms in forward abduction is a useful measure. Weakness of extraocular muscles, impairment of speech, or other objective signs may also be followed. Two milligrams of edrophonium are administered intravenously. The patient is then asked to repeat the test maneuver. If objective improvement occurs, the test is considered positive and is terminated. If there is no change, the patient is given an additional 8 mg intravenously. The dose is administered in two parts, because some patients react to a small dose of edrophonium with unpleasant side effects such as nausea, diarrhea, excessive salivation, fasciculations, and rarely, syncope. Atropine (0.6 mg) should be at hand for administration by vein, should these symptoms be troublesome.

False positive tests occur in placebo-reactors and in rare patients with other neurologic disorders such as amyotrophic lateral sclerosis. False negative or equivocal tests may also occur. In some cases, it is helpful to give a trial of a longer acting drug, such as

┌───┐
TABLE 122-1
Work-Up for Myasthenic Patients

I. History
Distribution of weakness
Fluctuations with exercise and rest
Respiratory or bulbar involvement
Association with other autoimmune disorders:
    rheumatoid arthritis, systemic lupus erythematosus,
    thyroiditis, pemphigus
Intercurrent medical problems: hyperthyroidism,
    infection, endocrine disturbance, etc.

II. Physical Examination
Distribution and degree of weakness:
    Arm abduction time
    Vital capacity
    Quantitative muscle testing

III. Diagnostic Tests
Tensilon test
Repetitive nerve stimulation
Anti-AChR antibody titer

IV. Tests for Associated Conditions
Thyroid function tests
Rheumatoid factor, L.E. cell preparations, ANA
Quantitative immunoglobulins
Pulmonary function studies
CAT scan of anterior mediastinum (or radiographs of
    chest PA, lateral, obliques)
└───┘

pyridostigmine (Mestinon) or neostigmine (Prostigmine) orally. They permit more time for detailed strength evaluation.

Electrodiagnostic Tests

It is sometimes helpful to carry out electrodiagnostic tests, especially in doubtful cases. Electric shocks are delivered repetitively at rates of 3 to 5 per second to the ulnar, median, or axillary nerves, and action potentials are recorded from the appropriate muscles. In normal individuals the amplitude of the evoked muscle action potentials will not change at these rates of stimulation. However, in myasthenic patients there is a rapid reduction in the amplitude of the evoked response. A single dose of edrophonium prevents or diminishes this myasthenic reaction.

Antiacetylcholine Receptor Antibody

As noted above, anti-AChR antibody is detectable in the serum of up to 87 percent of myasthenic patients. The antibody titer corresponds only approximately to the patient's state, but the presence of anti-AChR antibodies is useful in the diagnosis. The test is a radioimmunoassay which was developed as a research tool, but is becoming more widely available clinically. A negative test does not exclude the disease.

Provocative Tests

Provocative tests with curare or decamathonium are risky, and are rarely if ever necessary.

ASSOCIATED DISORDERS

Myasthenic patients have an increased incidence of several disorders. Thymic abnormalities are found in approximately 75 percent of patients.[67] Some 85 percent of the abnormal thymus glands are hyperplastic, while the other 15 percent are neoplastic (thymomas). If available, computer assisted tomography of the anterior mediastinum is the best test for detecting thymomas, although ordinary PA, lateral, and oblique views of the chest are usually sufficient. Hyperthyroidism may occur in 3 to 8 percent of patients and may aggravate the myasthenic weakness.[73] Tests of thyroid function should be obtained. Blood tests for rheumatoid factor, LE preparations, and test for antinuclear antibody should be carried out in all patients. Abnormalities of immunoglobulin levels should be determined by quantitative immunoglobulin measurements (not paper electrophoresis). Finally, measurements of ventilatory function are valuable because of the frequency and seriousness of respiratory impairment in myasthenic patients.

MEDICAL AND SURGICAL THERAPY
(Tables 122-2 and 122-3)

The prognosis has improved markedly in the past few years as a result of improved therapy. In general, patients with myasthenia limited to ocular involvement have the most favorable prognosis, and those with severe bulbar or generalized myasthenia the poorest.

Anticholinesterase Medications

The most important medications used in the treatment of myasthenia gravis are the anticholinesterase (anti-ChE) agents and adrenal corticosteroids (Table 122-3). Most myasthenics can be improved, but very few can be brought completely to normal by anti-ChE medication. In general, there is no difference in efficacy among the various anti-ChE drugs, but oral pyridostigmine bromide (Mestinon) seems to have the optimum duration of action for most circumstances. As a rule, the beneficial action of oral Mestinon begins within 15 to 30 minutes, and lasts for 3 to 4 hours, but the individual patient's response may vary greatly from the average. Therapy is begun with a moderate dose, e.g., 60 mg at 4-hour intervals, five times daily. The dose is then increased until optimum strength is achieved (Fig. 122-2). Adjustment of the dosage should be tailored to the patient's individual requirements throughout the day, based on carefully

TABLE 122-2
Treatment Plan

I. Initial Treatment
   A. Establish definite diagnosis
   B. Treat with anticholinesterase medication (pyridostigmine bromide), adjust dosage to obtain optimal effect
   C. If results are not satisfactory, consider thymectomy or corticosteroids

II. Thymectomy
   A. Indications:
      1. Thymoma
      2. Generalized myasthenia gravis not satisfactorily controlled with anticholinesterase drugs
         a. Patients younger than 50 years
         b. Wait long enough to exclude early spontaneous remission (usually 6–12 months after onset of myasthenia)
   B. Preoperative preparation: If operation would pose risk because of patient's state of weakness, give course of corticosteroids until condition is satisfactory
   C. Surgical approach—median sternotomy, must be done in institution with facilities and experience for postoperative management of thymectomy patient

III. Corticosteroid Therapy
   A. Indications:
      1. After thymectomy for *invasive thymoma*
      2. Any of the following in a patient not satisfactorily controlled by anticholinesterase drugs
         a. Older age group (older than 50 years of age)
         b. Declines to have thymectomy
         c. Status postthymectomy
         d. Purely ocular involvement when disability outweighs risks
   B. Method:
      1. Optimal adjustment of anticholinesterase drugs
      2. Begin with daily administration of small dose (e.g., 12.5–20 mg of prednisone) and increase gradually to optimal response or as tolerated (maximum usually 50–60 mg of prednisone/day)
      3. Gradually switch to alternate-day schedule
      4. Maintain dose until improvement reaches plateau (usually 6–12 months)
      5. Decrease *very* gradually: establish minimal maintenance dose
      6. Observe full precautions for side effects
      7. Anticholinesterase dosage may be cautiously decreased, as tolerated

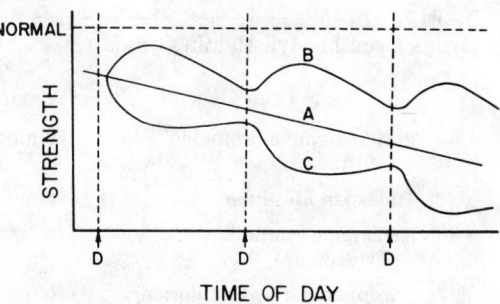

FIGURE 122-2. Relationship between the time of day and strength during no treatment **(A)**, optimal treatment **(B)**, and overtreatment **(C)**. Doses are given at times marked **D**. It is apparent that in going from optimal **(B)** to excessive medication the patient may pass through a state similar to no treatment **(A)**. (From Johns, R.J. Drug therapy in myasthenia gravis. Mod. Med., 33:286, 1965.)

culties are often benefited by adjusting the time of medication to precede meals by 45 minutes, so that optimal strength coincides with mealtime. Mestinon Timespan tablets which have prolonged effect, may be helpful at night, but should not be used for daytime medication. The dose of these drugs should not be revised more frequently than every 2 days to permit the full effect of a given regimen to be seen.

Atropine

Atropine or atropine-like drugs are sometimes necessary to block the unpleasant "muscarinic" side effect produced by the anti-ChE medication (diarrhea, abdominal cramps, excessive salivation, nausea). Atropine blocks the autonomic effects without influencing the beneficial effects on skeletal muscle. However, it is preferable to avoid masking these side effects, since they may provide important clues to anti-ChE overdosage. The use of atropine should therefore be limited to those patients who would overwise be unable to tolerate the optimum dose of anti-ChE drugs.

Ephedrine

Ephedrine benefits some patients. The usual dose is 25 mg, three times daily. It occasionally causes excitement or nervousness, but insomnia can be avoided by giving the last dose before 6 P.M.

Steroid Therapy

During the past decade adrenal corticosteroids in various dosage regimens have been used with beneficial effect in some patients with myasthenia gravis who do not respond fully to anticholinesterases. Early weakening seen with the abrupt onset of high dose

kept records of strength and motor abilities. For example, many patients are strongest in the morning and weakest in the late afternoon. They may, therefore, require a larger dose of Mestinon at 4 P.M. then at 8 A.M. Patients with chewing and swallowing diffi-

TABLE 122–3
Drugs Used in Myasthenia Gravis

Drug	Preparation	Usual Dose	Comment
Pyridostigmine bromide (Mestinon)	60 mg tablet	60–120 mg/4 hours	Adjust dosage, as needed
Timespan Mestinon	180 mg tablet	180 mg	Only at night
Neostigmine bromide (Prostigmin)	15 mg tablet	15–30 mg/4 hours	Not in general use
Edrophonium hydrochloride (Tensilon)	10 mg/ml	0.2 ml + 0.8 ml	For diagnosis
Prednisone	5 mg, 20 mg, 50 mg	100 mg qod	Regimen in text
Azathioprine (Imuran)	50 mg	2–3 mg/kg	See cautions, in text

prednisone regimens can usually be avoided by beginning treatment with 25 mg per day, and increasing the dose in steps of 2.5 mg at 3-day intervals, until the dose of 50 mg per day is reached.[74] This dose is maintained for a month or more, and then is gradually changed to an alternate day regimen, over the course of an additional month, until the dosage of 100 mg on alternate days is reached. Some patients experience weakness on the "off day," and require 5 to 15 mg. The prednisone may eventually be reduced to levels of 30 to 60 mg every other day in most patients, but this usually takes many months or years to accomplish, and must be monitored closely by both patient and doctor. Few patients are able to do without prednisone entirely.

Immunosuppressive Drugs

Recently, immunosuppressive drugs such as azathioprine (Imuran) or cyclophosphamide (Cytoxan) have been found effective in some patients who are refractory to other medical therapy or thymectomy.[71] The full beneficial effect of these drugs may not be present for many months. These immunosuppressive agents are used only in refractory cases because of the adverse side effects which include bone marrow depression and the uncertain risk of late development of malignancies.

Thymectomy

Two separate problems should be distinguished: thymectomy as a treatment for myasthenia gravis and thymectomy for thymoma. Thymectomy has for many years been proposed as a therapuetic measure. The available evidence suggests that up to 85 percent of patients may benefit from thymectomy, regardless of age or sex.[66] However, the improvement is usually partial, and may not occur for 1 to 10 years after surgery. The advantage of thymectomy is that it offers the possibility of long-term benefit, in some cases diminishing or eliminating the need for continuing medical treatment. We therefore recommend thymectomy in young adult patients with generalized disease of moderate to severe degree.

Thymectomy is the preferred method of treatment of thymoma in whom the operative risk is acceptable, because of the possibility of local tumor spread.

Plasmapheresis

In view of the antibody-mediated pathogenesis of myasthenia gravis, plasma exchange or plasmapheresis have been used therapeutically.[71,72] Modern plasmapheresis machines separate the plasma from blood cells. The plasma, containing the pathogenic antibodies is removed, and the blood cells are returned to the patient in a suitable fluid medium. Plasmapheresis produces a short-term reduction in anti-AChR antibody levels accompanied by clinical improvement in many patients. It is useful as a temporary expedient in seriously affected patients. The long-term treatment of myasthenic patients requires other methods of therapy outlined in this chapter.

Management of Myasthenic Crisis

Myasthenic crisis may be defined as an exacerbation of weakness of sufficient severity to endanger life. The common serious threats to life are respiratory failure caused by intercostal or diaphragmatic weakness and aspiration secondary to pharyngeal weakness. The possibility that the deterioration is the result of excessive administration of anticholinesterases ("cholinergic crisis") should be excluded. This is best accomplished by the temporary stopping of anticholinesterase drugs. Physicians experienced in the management of myasthenia gravis, respiratory problems, infectious disease, and fluid management are necessary for the effective treatment of a patient in myasthenic crisis. Often an intensive care unit is required. Pulmonary infection occurs commonly and

should be treated promptly, because the mechanical and immunologic defenses of the patient may be impaired. Early and effective antibiotic therapy, respiratory assistance, and pulmonary physiotherapy are essentials of the treatment program.

CHAPTER 123
Peripheral Neuropathies
JOHN W. GRIFFIN

The peripheral nerves provide the major interface between the central nervous system and the environment. In addition to somatic motor and sensory functions, the peripheral nervous system (PNS), through the autonomic nerves, is intimately involved in cardiovascular, thermoregulatory, and sexual function, and in control of micturition and defecation. The peripheral nerves are susceptible to injury by a variety of known metabolic, toxic, inflammatory, vascular, physical, and infectious insults, and are undoubtedly vulnerable to other agents yet to be identified.

The pathologic responses of the PNS in disease are limited, so that specific etiologies usually do not produce distinctive pathologic changes. Normal function depends on the integrity of both the nerve fiber (axon) and its supporting elements, the Schwann cells with their myelin sheaths. Some processes selectively affect the Schwann cells or myelin resulting in *demyelination;* examples are diphtheria and the Guillain-Barré syndrome. Other disorders primarily affect the nerve cell body or axon, resulting in *axonal degeneration,* as seen in the toxic neuropathies induced by vincristine or isoniazid, for example. Many of the most common metabolic and heritable neuropathies show evidence of both axonal degeneration and demyelination. This presumably reflects the mutual interdependence between cellular elements of the peripheral nervous system.[75,76]

CLASSIFICATION
A basic and clinically useful distinction is among mononeuropathies, multiple mononeuropathies, and polyneuropathies (Table 123-1).

SYMPTOMS AND SIGNS OF NEUROPATHIES[77]

Alterations in Sensibility
Patients with alterations in sensibility caused by peripheral nerve disease may use a remarkable variety of descriptions to communicate their subjective

symptoms. It is helpful to encourage the patient to describe his symptoms in his own words: "numbness" may cover a host of meanings, but phrases such as "it feels as if I were walking on cotton wool" or "it's like walking on coals" cannot be misunderstood. Common types of complaints include: *paresthesias*—subjective tingling, "pins and needles"; *dysesthesias*—unpleasant perceptions of normally innocuous stimuli; and *hyperpathia*—a markedly painful experience of tactile or thermal stimuli. *Hypesthesia* describes an elevated threshold to perception of a stimulus; for example, a patient may appreciate the sharpness or painful quality of a pinprick only with considerable pressure. *Hyperesthesia* is a seemingly heightened sensibility, in that light stimuli will be experienced intensely. Careful testing will reveal that the threshold stimulus is actually elevated above normal, but when the threshold is reached, an unusually intense perception is experienced. Finally, it should be added that occasional patients will show profound deficits in sensibility on examination with few subjective sensory symptoms and little functional deficit.

Many patients have loss of all sensory modalities—pain, temperature, light touch, vibration, and joint movement (proprioception). It is helpful to look for selective loss which often occurs in one or two patterns: selective loss of pain and temperature sensibility, or selective loss of joint position sense and vibratory sensibility. The significance of these selective functional deficits in differential diagnosis is discussed later (see Table 123-3).

Motor Changes
Flaccid weakness or paralysis of muscles results from involvement of motor fibers in the nerves. If denervated for more than a few weeks, atrophy of the muscles will be apparent. The distribution of weakness is of major importance in accurate diagnosis, and often detailed individual muscle testing is required. In asymmetrical processes, particularly involving only

TABLE 123-1

Classification of Peripheral Neuropathies

Form	Characteristics	Mechanism
Mononeuropathy	Involves a single nerve, e.g., ulnar, median, or peroneal	Trauma, pressure, compression
Multiple mononeuropathies	Involves two or more nerves, assymmetrical, step-wise progression	Involvement of small blood vessels (e.g., diabetes, vasculitis)
Polyneuropathy	Symmetrical, distal involvement, usually of feet and legs first	Multiple (see Table 123–2)

one extremity, it is necessary to distinguish between lesions of a nerve root (radiculopathy), nerve plexus (brachial or lumbosacral), or nerve. For example, injury to the C5 root may produce marked weakness of the deltoid, supraspinatus, infraspinatus, and some weakness of the biceps. On the other hand, weakness of the opponens, short abductor, and short flexors of the thumb would suggest median nerve damage, rather than a nerve root lesion. When weakness in such processes is mild, comparison of strength (and bulk) with the contralateral limb is helpful. A convenient guide to individual muscle testing and the innervation patters of muscle is the "Aid to the Investigation of Peripheral Nerve Injuries."[9]

In polyneuropathies, weakness is usually greatest distally. Early manifestations often include weakness of dorsiflexion of the toes and ankles. Atrophy may be seen in the short extensor of toes and in the anterior tibials. In the hands, the intrinsic muscles are often involved first; atrophy may be found in the thenar and hypothenar eminences and first dorsal interosseus muscles.

Autonomic Abnormalities

Autonomic dysfunction is frequently overlooked but is of considerable importance in differential diagnosis and management. Screening for autonomic involvement can quickly be accomplished at the bedside. *Cardiovascular* responses can be screened by testing for orthostatic hypotension and for slowing of pulse rate during the Valsalva maneuver. Abnormal patterns of *sweating* should be sought; often patients will have anhidrosis over large areas of the body. They may complain, however, of *excessive* sweating in those areas that are uninvolved. In a warm room, the pattern of sweating can be determined by rubbing the

dorsum of the examiner's hand over the skin. *Pupillary reactions* are easily examined; symptomatically, abnormalities may be associated with loss of accommodation or photophobia (caused by loss of the light reflex). *Gastrointestinal* symptoms may include constipation or diarrhea. *Bladder involvement* should be sought by specific questioning. Finally, it is essential to inquire for impotence in men; this is often an early manifestation of autonomic neuropathy and is rarely volunteered by the patient.

Laboratory Findings

Determination of nerve conduction velocities is useful in evaluation of neuropathies. Conduction velocities can be measured in both motor and sensory nerves. The values obtained represent the velocities of the most rapidly conducting fibers only; in general, the test is more sensitive to slowing of conduction than to loss of axons. Partly for this reason, there may be differences between the severity of the clinical disease and the degree of abnormality in the conduction velocities.

Electromyography can aid in confirming that weakness is caused by denervation and in demonstrating the distribution of involvement.

Muscle biopsy can also confirm the presence of a denervating process, if this is in question.

The usefulness of nerve biopsy is limited by several factors. Only a sensory nerve (usually the sural) can be biopsied. Even then, a minor but sometimes irritating patch of sensory loss and paresthesias may result. The biopsy must be specially processed to provide maximum information. The major limitation is that few neuropathies produce specific lesions; this lack of specificity reflects the limited pathologic responses mentioned previously. Specific diagnosis, including amyloidosis, sarcoidosis, vasculitis, leprosy, or some inherited metabolic disorders, such as metachromatic leukodystrophy, may be made by nerve biopsy, but often laboratory tests or biopsy of other tissues would more easily establish the diagnosis. On the other hand, in selected patients determination of the type of lesion (acute demyelination, recurrent demyelination, axonal degeneration with large fiber or small fiber loss) can orient further diagnostic evaluation.

DIFFERENTIAL DIAGNOSIS OF POLYNEUROPATHIES

When faced with a peripheral neuropathy, especially one of the polyneuropathies, the physician may find himself overwhelmed by the large number of possible underlying causes. It is useful to have a simple scheme available for remembering some of these conditions. As a convenient mnemonic device, one may use the words "Dang Therapist." Table 123–2 indicates the meaning of each initial.

The approach to an individual patient with an undiagnosed polyneuropathy is often best begun by asking, "What is unusual or distinctive about this patient's neuropathy?" The unusual features may provide clues to orient further evaluation. In particular, the age of onset, rate of progression, selectivity of functional involvement, distribution, and presence of associated neurologic disease should be sought. Table 123–3 presents polyneuropathies typically associated with the various features that may provide clues. The most common etiologies are given in italic type. Less common disorders are also listed for completeness; details of their clinical presentation may be found in neurology texts or specialized references.[75,76]

The *rate of progression* may be difficult to ascertain in long-standing neuropathies, since neither the patient nor his family may have been aware of mild neuropathy in childhood. Often such patients will recall never having kept up with their peers in races and sports or always having been chosen last for teams. Often they have never engaged in sports of any sort for recreation. High-arched feet (pes cavus) with hammer-toe deformities are important indicators of childhood onset, since they are the consequence of long-standing muscle imbalances. Such patients usually have a form of heritable predominantly motor neuropathy (Charcot-Marie-Tooth).

Selective functional involvement is often particularly helpful. Some neuropathies are typically predominantly *motor* (see Table 123–3); of these, the Guillain-Barré syndrome (acute inflammatory polyneuropathy; postinfectious polyneuropathy) requires emphasis, because prompt diagnosis and hospitalization may be life saving. Often preceded by a nonspecific viral illness or by surgery or pregnancy, this disorder is characterized by rapidly progressive weakness. Although vague discomfort or aching in the limbs may be an early complaint, objective sensory findings are mild. Tendon reflexes are usually lost early. The weakness may progress with alarming rapidity, so that occasional patients may present with minor findings and within hours require respiratory assistance. The diagnosis is aided by findings of slowed nerve conduction velocities and elevated spinal fluid protein without an increase in cells (albumino-cytologic-dissociation). The differential diagnosis of the Guillain-Barré syndrome often includes porphyric and diphtheritic neuropathies and botulism.

Development of a progressive *sensory* neurop-

TABLE 123-2

Mnemonic for Peripheral Polyneuropathies: "Dang Therapist"

Diabetic	Polyneuropathy: mild to moderate, predominantly sensory, paresthesias, absent ankle jerks, may occur even with good diabetic control
	Severe polyneuropathy: diabetic "pseudotabes," occurs in severe diabetics, sensorimotor and autonomic
	Mononeuropathy: femoral or oculomotor nerves commonly affected
Alcoholic	Sensorimotor neuropathy with multiple nutritional deficiencies
Nutritional	Individual B-complex vitamins: thiamine, niacin, B_6, B_{12}
Guillain-Barré	May follow infection, ascending, chiefly motor neuropathy, respiratory and facial muscles may be involved, rise in CSF protein, but no pleocytosis
Toxic	Lead: radial nerve commonly affected producing wrist drop
	Other heavy metals: may be found in blood, urine, hair, nails
	Drugs: Furadantin, Vinblastine, Thalidomide
	Organophosphorus compounds: triorthocresylphosphate
Hereditary	Charcot-Marie-Tooth neuropathy (peroneal palsy): very slowly progressive, distal motor-sensory neuropathy, high arches, stork legs, dominant inheritance
	Interstitial hypertrophic neuropathy (Dejerine-Sottas): palpably enlarged nerves
	Refsum's disease: ataxia, retinitis pigmentosa, enlarged nerves, deafness, elevated serum phytanic acid
Recurrent	Responds to steroids, elevated CSF protein
Amyloidosis	Hereditary amyloidosis primarily, slowly progressive, may be painful, involves sensory, motor, and autonomic nerves
Porphyric	Chiefly motor neuropathy, may progress rapidly, younger patients, with acute intermittent form of porphyria
Infectious	Diphtheria, mononucleosis
Systemic	Associated with collagen diseases, uremia, sarcoidosis
Tumor	Carcinomatous neuropathies: pure sensory or sensorimotor neuropathy, may be combined with myopathy

TABLE 123-3
Differential Diagnosis of Polyneuropathies*

I. Course

    A.   Acute (days)
        Guillain-Barré syndrome
        Porphyric neuropathy
        Diphtheritic neuropathy
        Some toxins (e.g., tri-orthocresyl phosphate)
    B.   Subacute (weeks)
        Many toxins
        Nutritional neuropathies
        Carcinomatous neuropathies
        Uremic neuropathy
    C.   Relapsing
        Relapsing inflammatory neuropathy
        Refsum's disease
    D.   Chronic (many months or years)
        Diabetic motor-sensory neuropathy
        Chronic inflammatory neuropathies
    E.   Very chronic (childhood onset)
        Heritable motor-sensory neuropathies (e.g.,
           Charcot-Marie-Tooth disease)

II. Selective Functional Involvement†

    A.   Predominately motor
        Guillain-Barré syndrome
        Relapsing and chronic inflammatory
           neuropathy
        Acute intermittent porphyria
        Lead neuropathy
        Heritable motor-sensory neuropathies
           (Charcot-Marie-Tooth)
        Diphtheritic neuropathy
    B.   Predominately sensory
        Diabetes
        Carcinomatous sensory neuropathy
           (ganglioradiculitis)
        Paraproteinemic and cryoglobulinemic
           neuropathy
        Tabes dorsalis

        Dissociated loss of pain sensibility

        Diabetes (small fiber type)
        Amyloidosis
        Hereditary sensory neuropathies
        Lepromatous leprosy

        Dissociated loss of joint position and
          vibration sensibility

        Subacute combined degeneration
        Friedreich's ataxia
    C.   Autonomic neuropathy
        Diabetes
        Amyloid
        Acute, chronic, and relapsing
          pandysautonomia
        Dysautonomia (Riley-Day)

* The most common etiologies are set in italic.
† Most polyneuropathies produce sensory and motor disturbances.

TABLE 123-3 (cont.)

III. Distribution‡

    A.   Proximal weakness
        Guillain-Barré
        Porphyria
        Carcinomatous neuropathy with proximal
          weakness ("carcinomatous
          neuromyopathy")
        Spinal muscular atrophies
    B.   Proximal sensory loss
        Porphyria
        Tangier disease (analphalipoproteinemia)
    C.   Temperature-related distribution
        Lepromatous leprosy

IV. Age

    A.   Childhood
        "Steroid dependent" inflammatory
          neuropathies
        Giant axonal neuropathy
        Krabbe's disease
        Metachromatic leukodystrophy
        Neuroaxonal dystrophy
        Heritable sensorimotor neuropathy
          (Dejerine-Sottas)

‡Most polyneuropathies produce distal involvement.

athy in adult life may be a remote manifestation of underlying malignancy. The responsible lesion is an inflammatory destruction of dorsal root ganglion cells (ganglioradiculitis). This syndrome is among the most distinctive of the malignancy-related neurologic syndromes; thorough search for tumor and long-term observation are indicated.

Neuropathies with prominent *autonomic* involvement may present with complaints of impotence, urinary hesitancy, constipation, or symptoms of orthostatic hypotension. Often autonomic neuropathies are associated with spontaneous pain and loss of pain and temperature sensibility. Strength, vibration, and proprioceptive sensibilities, and tendon reflexes may be preserved. This picture represents a "small fiber" polyneuropathy and is seen as one of the manifold syndromes of diabetic neuropathy as well as in systemic amyloidosis and, occasionally, in association with paraproteinemia or cryoglobulinemia.

The various manifestations of *diabetic neuropathies* cover in themselves nearly the full spectrum of peripheral nerve disease (Table 123-3).[78] Diabetic mononeuropathies and multiple mononeuropathies represent vascular insufficiency or infarction in nerve, presumably caused by small vessel disease. Their onset is typically abrupt and often painful.

Cranial nerves III and VI, the femoral nerve, or other major nerves of the extremities may be involved. Occasionally, lumbosacral plexus involvement occurs, producing a picture often confused with intraspinal disease. There is often asymmetrical weakness of the hip girdles with little sensory loss. Although the initial manifestations may be incapacitating, the prognosis for eventual recovery in diabetic multiple mononeuropathies is usually good. Diabetic polyneuropathies include distal sensorimotor neuropathy and severe sensory neuropathy which may be of the "large fiber" or "small fiber" types, the latter often associated with autonomic involvement. Diabetic polyneuropathies may be mild and asymptomatic; they are often progressive and are major causes of morbidity and disability in diabetes.

Finally, the *toxic neuropathies* require emphasis, both because of the increasing list of pharmaceutical, industrial, and environmental agents which can injure peripheral nerves and also because of the therapeutic importance of proper diagnosis. They may be subacute in evolution as in vincristine or Furadantin neuropathy, or may be insidious and progressive as often seen in industrial exposure (for example, to solvents such as methy-n-butyl ketone). In the vast majority of toxic neuropathies, the lesion is degeneration of the distal regions of the longest or largest axons (dying back), so that early clinical involvement may involve blunting of sensation in the toes, loss of the Achilles tendon reflex, and weakness of the intrinsic muscles of the feet. Such a distal axonal degeneration may occur in the central nervous system as well, and produce degeneration of the corticospinal tracts in the lumbrosacral cord and of the gracile tract of the dorsal columns in the cervical cord. Such central involvement may be "masked" by the peripheral neuropathy when the patient is first seen, and becomes apparent as a spastic paraparesis only when the neuropathy has recovered. Careful occupational and recreational history, and in some instances visits to home or place of work, may suggest the possibility of toxic exposure.

TREATMENT

This section has emphasized diagnosis, because the best treatment is directed toward the etiologic disorder. Unfortunately, of patients referred for evaluation of neuropathy a substantial proportion remain without etiologic diagnosis after initial screening. Nonspecific therapeutic measures include maintenance of optimal nutritional status (with supplemental B vitamin preparations if the diet is suspect) and avoidance of potential neurotoxins, particularly alcohol, which might have a synergistic effect.

For neuropathic weakness, appropriate bracing is helpful. Daily activities such as eating, writing, or buttoning are often made easier by "built up" (large) utensils.

The sensory deficits are often more bothersome. The small-fiber neuropathies are particularly difficult medical and psychological problems. The diminished pain sensibility can lead to painless injuries (e.g., Charcot joints caused by traumatic arthropathy) and contribute to "trophic" ulcers, osteomyelitis, and ultimately spontaneous or surgical amputation. Prevention through education is paramount. Foot care, avoidance of trauma and pressure on anesthetic extremities, and prompt attention to early lesions are mandatory. The spontaneous pain that often accompanies the small-fiber neuropathies may respond to anticonvulsants such as phenytoin or carbamazepine; opiates are contraindicated because of the potential for addiction. Although neurogenic impotence cannot be satisfactorily corrected, understanding the neurologic cause of the impaired function may relieve considerable anxiety.

CHAPTER 124
Myopathies
DANIEL B. DRACHMAN

The term *myopathy* is used for those conditions which produce weakness by affecting muscle fibers without interfering with their nerve supply. By contrast, we speak of *neurogenic atrophy* or *neuropathy* when describing the changes in muscle which follow denervation, as for example, in poliomyelitis or peripheral neuropathy. The myopathies include conditions with or without known biochemical abnormalities, and with or without any hereditary tendency.

It is useful to discuss this heterogeneous group of diseases together because of similarities in the clinical manifestations of weakness, the diagnostic methods used, and the management of patients. Other members of the heterogeneous group must often be considered in the differential diagnosis. This chapter discusses these aspects of the clinical management.

CLINICAL RECOGNITION

The cardinal feature of myopathy is weakness. The weakness usually involves the proximal musculature in a symmetric pattern. Proximal weakness of the upper limbs may interfere with the patient's ability to maintain the arms abducted, as in shaving, brushing the hair, or placing objects on high shelves. Proximal weakness in the lower extremities may produce a waddling gait, and results in difficulty climbing stairs and getting out of a bathtub or low chair. As a rule, pain and tenderness of the muscles are *not* prominent features, even in the inflammatory myopathies. If pain and tenderness are the only or the most prominent symptoms, one may suspect that myopathy is not the problem. Disorders such as polymyalgia rheumatica or polyarteritis more commonly produce severe pain.

On physical examination, the outstanding finding is weakness usually in the proximal muscles. If the patient is asked to arise from a seated position on the floor, he may "climb up himself" in a characteristic fashion (Gower's sign). The gait should be observed with the patient wearing only undergarments, to determine whether the pelvis tilts from side to side. Individual muscle testing (as described in Chap. 121) is important in determining the distribution of weakness.

Apart from the muscle weakness, the remainder of the neuromuscular examination is normal. The tendon reflexes are usually obtainable until weakness is advanced (the Duchenne form of muscular dystrophy is an exception to this rule). Fasciculations are not present. The plantar responses are flexor. Sensation is normal. These negative findings are important in distinguishing myopathy from diseases of the central or peripheral nervous system.

Once it is recognized that a patient's weakness is probably myopathic in origin, attention turns to determining *which* myopathy afflicts the patient. As has been indicated, the similarity of the weakness seen in all these conditions renders weakness per se a poor feature for distinguishing one myopathy from another. Other clinical and laboratory features of the myopathies must be used. This evaluation should be done in an orderly and systematic fashion.

CLASSIFICATION

The myopathies have been classified in many different ways. From the clinical point of view, the separation into four groups, the muscular dystrophies, inflammatory myopathies, metabolic myopathies, and rare myopathies, has the virtue of combining simplicity with suggesting a rational approach to diagnosis (Table 124–1).

Diagnostic Approach

As indicated in Table 124–1, some myopathies have distinctive clinical characteristics which permit the knowledgeable physician to recognize the constellation of manifestations—syndrome recognition. Other disorders have nondescript manifestations, but have distinctive histopathologic lesions. Still others, especially those associated with systemic diseases, have neither unique muscle manifestations nor unique lesions; these are diagnosed by demonstrating the underlying disease.

The remainder of the chapter is devoted to a description of the entities listed in Table 124–1 with emphasis on 1) those which are recognized by their clinical manifestations; and 2) those which are amenable to therapy.

THE MUSCULAR DYSTROPHIES

The dystrophies are a group of myopathies which are classified together largely for historical reasons. In general, they are characterized by

1. A strong hereditary predisposition
2. Onset of weakness in the first to third decade, with varying rates of progression
3. Fairly consistent clinical patterns

There are exceptions to all of these criteria, and cases without a clear family history, and with uncommon patterns of muscular involvement, may defy classification. The etiology is as yet unknown for any of the dystrophies. There is a growing body of evidence to suggest that abnormalities of the cell membrane of muscle and other tissues may be present at least in some of the dystrophies.[83] At present there is no curative treatment for any of the dystrophies, and the efforts of the physician must be directed toward supportive measures. Nevertheless, it is of great importance to identify the dystrophy accurately so that the physician is able to give an accurate prognosis, and undertake genetic counseling for the other members of the family. The forms of dystrophy are outlined in Table 124–2. Two forms, the pseudohyper-

┌───┐

TABLE 124-1

Classification and Diagnostic Approach to the Myopathies

Classification and Examples	Approach to Diagnosis
I. Dystrophies	
1. Pseudohypertrophic (Duchenne)	1. Syndrome recognition (see Table 124–2)
2. Facio-scapulo-humeral (Landouzy-Dejerine)	2. Genetic history
3. Limb-girdle (Erb)	3. Biopsy and serum enzyme confirmation
4. Distal (Gower)	
5. Myotonic	Same plus demonstrable myotonia
6. Ocular Myopathy	Syndrome recognition
Inflammatory (Polymyositis, Dermatomyositis)	
1. With malignancy	
2. With connective tissue disease (lupus, rheumatoid arthritis, systemic sclerosis, Sjögren syndrome)	1. Demonstrable confirmation on biopsy 2. Demonstration of underlying disease
3. With sarcoidosis	Diagnostic lesions in biopsy
4. Without associated disease	Diagnosis of exclusion in an inflammatory myopathy
II. Metabolic	
1. Adrenal steroid myopathy (iatrogenic and spontaneous)	
2. Dysthyroid myopathy	Demonstration of the metabolic disorder
3. Hyperparathyroid myopathy	
4. Hypoadrenal Myopathy (Addison's)	
5. Periodic paralysis	Syndrome recognition
6. Glycogen storage diseases (McArdle's, Pompe's, phosphofructokinase deficiency)	Demonstration of metabolic disorder
III. Miscellaneous Rarer Causes	
1. Congenital myopathies (central core disease, rod or nemaline myopathy, mitochondrial and myotubular myopathies)	Distinctive histopathology
2. Trichinosis	
3. Myositis ossificans	Same plus calcification on x-ray
4. Myotonia congenita (Thompsen)	1. Syndrome recognition 2. Myotonia
5. Paroxysmal rhabdomyolysis (myoglobinuria)	1. Syndrome recognition 2. Myoglobinuria
6. Drug-induced (chloroquin)	History

└───┘

trophic form and myotonic dystrophy are discussed in greater detail.

Pseudohypertrophic (Duchenne) Form of Muscular Dystrophy

This is the most common and the most devastating form of muscular dystrophy. It is inherited as a sex-linked recessive trait, and therefore affects only males, while being carried by the females. It begins in childhood, often within the first few years of life. The earliest symptoms may be a tendency to walk on the toes, to be a slower runner than other boys of the same age, or to fall easily. The parents may first notice enlargement of the calves, or of other muscles. Later, the child has difficulty in walking upstairs, develops lordosis, and has great difficulty in arising from a seated position on the floor. Eventually, the patients are reduced to a bed and wheelchair existence. Fortunately, the distal musculature is relatively spared until late in the disease and the patients are able to feed themselves and perform other useful tasks with their hands. The cardiac musculature is

TABLE 124-2
Clinical Features of the Muscular Dystrophies

Name	Distribution	Age of Onset	Progression	Inheritance	Remarks or Associated Conditions
Pseudohypertrophic (Duchenne)	Generalized	Under age 8	Rapid	Sex-linked recessive	Pseudohypertrophic cardiac involvement Mental retardation Death by adulthood
Benign pseudohypertrophic	Generalized	8–20 yrs	Slow	Sex-linked recessive	Possible normal life expectancy
Facio-scapulo-humeral	Face, shoulders	10–20 yrs	Slow	Dominant or recessive (rare)	May "burn-out" in adult life
Limb-girdle	Shoulder and pelvic musculature	10–30 yrs	Slow (varies)	Varies	Heterogeneous group
Ocular myopathy[82]	Eyelids and extra-ocular muscles	30+ yrs	Slow	Varies	Retinal abnormalities dysphagia
Distal dystrophy (Gowers)	Distal limb musculature	20+ yrs	Slow	Dominant or sporadic	Heterogeneous group

affected in some patients, with the development of a wide variety of arrhythmias and electrocardiographic changes. Approximately 30 percent of patients with the Duchenne form of muscular dystrophy have associated mental retardation.[84]

The *diagnosis* of the Duchenne form of muscular dystrophy is not difficult, because of the remarkably consistent pattern of muscular involvement, exclusive affection of males and uniformly rapid progression of weakness. The serum CPK levels are usually very high in this disorder. The muscle biopsy shows severe changes of myopathy.

Myotonic Dystrophy

Myotonic dystrophy is characterized by difficulty in relaxing muscles after contraction, and progressive weakness and wasting of muscles. The muscles of the face and jaw, and the distal muscles of the limbs are affected first and involved most severely. Inheritance is as an autosomal dominant trait. The rate of progression varies, even among members of a given family. Some individuals may be able to live essentially normal lives, while others are severely disabled by the third or fourth decade. When the clinical manifestations of myotonic dystrophy are present at birth, a poor prognosis is the rule. In addition to the muscular defects, abnormalities of several other systems may be present. Cataracts, frontal baldness, testicular atrophy, and myocardial abnormalities are common. Some patients suffer from intellectual impairment

which may progress, and may constitute the major disability.

The diagnosis of myotonia may be made by percussion of the thenar eminence. Patients with myotonia show a delayed relaxation of the contraction. Myotonia may also prevent prompt relaxation of a firm hand grip. If troublesome, the myotonia may be treated with quinine, dilantin, or procainamide. When the distal weakness causes foot drop, braces are useful.

Treatment of the Dystrophies

At present there is no curative treatment for any of the forms of muscular dystrophy. From time to time various forms of empirical therapy have been proposed, such as vitamin E, androgenic steroids, coenzyme Q, and extracts of safflower oil, although without definite benefit. The treatment of these conditions must therefore be symptomatic at present.

Patients with muscular dystrophy have a tendency to develop muscular contractures when immobilized for even short periods of time. Therefore, it is essential that they remain active as consistently as possible. Once put in a wheelchair, a child with muscular dystrophy may never get out. If confined to bed while recuperating from an orthopedic operation, the child may never resume his former level of activity. Physiotherapy, with passive and active stretching of muscles and tendons is useful in preventing the development of contractures, but rigorous exercise is unnecessary. Bracing of limbs and various mechanical devices are often helpful in prolonging the patient's ability to ambulate or care for himself.

GENETIC COUNSELING. One of the most important developments in the management of muscular dystrophy has been achieved through a greater understanding of the genetics of the dystrophies. With knowledge of the mode of inheritance, the physician can advise the patient or his relatives accurately as to the likelihood of future offspring being affected by the disease (see Section 6).

THE INFLAMMATORY MYOPATHIES [79-81,85]

This group of disorders is known by a number of synonyms, including polymyositis, polymyopathy, late-onset myopathy, and dermatomyositis (when the skin is also involved). (See Chap. 99.) It occurs predominantly in adults. The childhood form of dermatomyositis, which has been shown to be due to vasculitis, is a separate disorder which will not be considered here.

Clinical Manifestations
The outstanding symptom of the inflammatory myopathies is *weakness,* which is usually symmetrical and proximal. In a minority of cases pain and tenderness may be present in the affected muscles, but they are not prominent symptoms. If untreated, the weakness is progressive, but the rate of progression varies widely. In some cases progression may be very gradual over the course of years, while in others it may be explosive. In some cases the myositis is accompanied by an erythematous, scaly *dermatitis* of the face (especially eyelids), upper chest, arms, and knuckles. *Laboratory* tests are helpful in making the diagnosis. The serum creatine phosphokinase (CPK) is elevated, except in the most slowly progressive forms of the disorder. Muscle biopsy reveals "myopathic changes." In some instances, the appearance is indistinguishable from that of dystrophy. In others, destruction may be more severe, and inflammatory changes more important. Similarly, electromyography reveals the findings characteristic of myopathy in affected muscles.

Associated Diseases [85]
In many adults with inflammatory myopathy, a link exists with another disease. The most commonly associated conditions are malignancies and the connective tissue disorders. A careful search must be made for clinical and laboratory evidence of these conditions.

The incidence of *malignancy* in adults with inflammatory myopathy is 18 to 24 percent. This percentage increases with advancing age, and is somewhat higher in males than in females. More than 70 percent of males over 50 years with myopathy proved to have a malignancy in one series. Almost every type of neoplasm has been reported in association with myopathy. The most common sites of origin are lung, uterus, ovary, breast, prostate, and gastrointestinal tract. The manifestations of myopathy may precede detection of the neoplasm by as long as 3 years, so in every adult with myopathy or dermatomyositis, especially those in the older age group, a thorough survey must be made to unearth an occult malignancy. In addition to a scrupulous physical examination, the following screening tests are recommended: chest x-ray, sedimentation rate, stool guaiac, alkaline phosphatase, proctoscopy, barium enema, upper gastrointestinal series, intravenous pyelogram, metastatic bone series; in females a Papanicolaou smear, and in males an acid phosphatase determination. When no tumor is found on the initial workup, follow-up examinations should be made at intervals of 6 months.

Inflammatory myopathies may also occur in company with each of the *connective tissue diseases.* In patients under the age of 50 a careful search should be made for a related connective tissue disease. The clinical manifestations of the associated disease may or may not be prominent. Frequently, minor signs of more than one of the connective tissue diseases may coexist in the patient with inflammatory myopathy. The typical eruption of dermatomyositis may be present. More often, however, the skin is thin and shiny, especially over the dorsum of the hand. The butterfly rash of lupus erythematosus or the cutaneous thickening of scleroderma are sometimes present. Raynaud's phenomenon may be noted on exposure to cold. Arthritis commonly occurs in association with inflammatory myopathies in the adult. Joint swelling and pain may be mild and transient, or typical of rheumatoid arthritis. When extreme tenderness of the limbs is found, polyarteritis should be considered. Sjögren syndrome includes the classical triad of keratoconjunctivitis sicca (dry, crusting eyes with redness of the conjunctiva), rheumatoid arthritis, and diminished salivary secretion. Late onset myopathy has been reported in association with this disorder.

The diagnosis of an associated connective tissue disease depends upon a systematic search for its physical and laboratory manifestations. Particular attention should be paid to the skin and joints. The investigation should routinely include repeated laboratory tests for lupus erythematosus and rheumatoid arthritis. A skin biopsy may be helpful in the diagnosis of dermatomyositis or scleroderma and the barium swallow is a useful test when the latter condition is suspected. In cases associated with polyarteritis nodosa, the muscle biopsy itself may contain blood vessels with pathognomonic lesions.

Boeck's sarcoid occasionally presents with proximal symmetrical muscle weakness. In such cases, the manifestations of sarcoidosis in other systems may be obscure or absent. The diagnosis is established by the finding of typical noncaseating granulomas on muscle biopsy.

Treatment (See Chap. 99)

The agents which have had the most consistently favorable effects on the course of the inflammatory myopathies are the adrenal corticosteroids. Immunosuppressive drugs are also helpful in some cases.[85] Treatment should be started as soon as possible, since the clinical response is best before muscle destruction has become far advanced. The majority of cases can be expected to show some improvement. However, steroids are most effective when the myopathy occurs alone or in association with one of the connective tissue diseases. Less favorable responses are seen in those cases associated with neoplastic disease or Sjögren syndrome. Many of the glucocorticoids have been used, including cortisone, prednisone, prednisolone, triamcinolone, and dexamethasone. The latter two are best avoided because of their greater tendency to produce "steroid myopathy" (see below). The initial dose should be equivalent to 50 or 60 mg of prednisone per day. This is continued until improvement is apparent. It may require 4 weeks to observe significant improvement. Then, very gradually, over the course of weeks or months, the dose may be reduced to maintenance levels. Muscle strength, skin and joint symptoms, and especially serum enzyme levels should be monitored closely while the dosage is being adjusted. The maintenance dosage must be tailored to the needs of the individual patient, but averages 7.5 to 22 mg of prednisone per day. As in other instances where steroid therapy is used, antacids and potassium supplements must be given. The patients should be observed carefully for the development of hypertension or diabetes.

Recently, immunosuppressive agents, such as azathioprine and methotrexate, have been used successfully in inflammatory myopathy, alone or in conjunction with adrenal corticosteroids. The risks of adverse side effects limit the use of these drugs to steroid-resistant cases.

When an underlying neoplasm is detected, it must be treated appropriately, for its own sake. Although the course of the myopathy is usually independent of the course of the malignant disease, cure of the malignancy is occasionally followed by a dramatic remission in muscle weakness.

METABOLIC MYOPATHIES

Clinical Manifestations

Like the other myopathies, these disorders present with proximal weakness. However, the serum muscle enzymes and the muscle biopsy are usually normal in these conditions. The electromyogram may be normal as well. The *absence* of confirmatory laboratory evidence in a patient with proximal weakness may first suggest a diagnosis of a metabolic myopathy.

Steroid Myopathy

Steroid myopathy is one of the most common endocrine-metabolic causes of muscle disease in the adult. The steroids may have been secreted by a hyperfunctioning adrenal cortex, or more often prescribed by a physician for the treatment of some other condition. In either case, the patient develops proximal weakness which closely resembles that found in the other myopathies. The halogenated steroids (triamcinolone and dexamethasone) are most likely to produce this syndrome. The differential diagnosis is especially difficult when a patient develops weakness in the course of a connective tissue disease for which he is receiving steroid therapy. It may be necessary to discontinue the steroids temporarily or to switch from triamcinolone or dexamethasone to prednisone.

Thyrotoxic Myopathy

Chronic thyrotoxicosis is often accompanied by weakness of the proximal limb muscles. Although the manifestations of the hyperthyroid state are usually obvious by the time myopathy is manifest, they may be masked, especially in older patients. Tachycardia, fasciculations, and a fine tremor of the outstretched fingers may provide clues to the diagnosis. Biopsy and electromyography show relatively minor abnormalities. Serum thyroxin and radioactive iodine uptake tests establish the diagnosis. The BMR is not reliable, as it may be elevated in myopathy of any etiology.

Hyperparathyroidism

Hyperparathyroidism and Milkman syndrome are occasional causes of proximal muscle weakness in the adult. Although these conditions are uncommon, the symptoms they produce may be clinically indistinguishable from those of the inflammatory myopathies. The diagnosis is made on the basis of the characteristic abnormalities of calcium and phosphorus metabolism. X-rays of the bones may be helpful.

Hypopituitarism

In Addison's disease muscular weakness is usually present, but does not dominate the picture. The characteristic endocrine abnormalities readily identify this condition.

McArdle's Disease. [83,86]

This rare myopathy is so distinctive that its clinical recognition is simple once the physician considers the diagnosis. The underlying biochemical defect is a lack of the muscle enzyme, phosphorylase. As a result, glycogen cannot be broken down, and the muscle is without a source of quick energy. However, since the pathways of oxidative metabolism are intact, energy for muscle contraction can still be supplied at a slower rate.

In clinical terms, this metabolic defect results in the patient's inability to perform vigorous exercise for more than a brief period. Muscle strength may be normal or only slightly diminished and the patient is able to carry out mild or moderate exercise normally. However, when he attempts to sustain a greater degree of muscular activity for a more prolonged period, he develops cramps and paralysis. If the cramps are particularly severe, there may be some muscle damage, with myoglobinuria (dark urine).

Laboratory studies provide definitive confirmation of the diagnosis. Because of the lack of myophosphorylase, the patient with McArdle's disease is unable to break glycogen down to lactate under anaerobic conditions. The ischemic exercise test is carried out by inflating a cuff around the patient's arm above systolic pressure, and instructing him to clench his fist repeatedly for 40 seconds. The cuff is released and blood samples are drawn at intervals after the exercise. Normal individuals show a marked rise in serum lactate concentration, while patients with McArdle's disease show a flat curve. Other laboratory aids are now available, including histochemical and chemical measurements of the phosphorylase activity in muscle biopsy material.

The treatment of McArdle's disease is the avoidance of excessive exercise.

CHAPTER 125

Disorders of Sensation: Pain and Headache

GUY M. McKHANN AND WILLIAM G. SPEED III

ORGANIZATION OF THE SENSORY SYSTEM

Within the dorsal roots there is an incomplete lamination of sensory fibers into two broad groups. The large fibers tend to lie dorsally and medially. They include high-velocity afferents, not only from muscle, tendon, and joints, but also proprioceptive fibers from other deep structures. These sensory fibers enter the dorsal columns and bend cranially almost immediately. Some end in the adjacent gray matter of Clarke's column, from which secondary spinocerebellar relays arise. The majority, however, are uninterrupted and run upward in the dorsal columns to end in the gracile and cuneate nuclei in the lower medulla (Fig. 125–1). The primary afferents of each successively higher root displace medially those of the lower levels. The gracile nucleus, therefore, receives impulses coming predominantly from the legs, whereas the upper parts of the body are represented more in the cuneate nucleus. Secondary neurons activated in these dorsal column nuclei immediately cross the midline, just above the pyramidal decussation in the lower brain stem, to become the medial lemniscus of the opposite side.

The more laterally placed afferent fibers in the dorsal roots, including many of smaller size and slower conduction rates, end on cells at the base of the ipsilateral dorsal horn. Some form synapses at the level of entry, whereas others divide and run up or down for several segments before forming synapses. The axons of the dorsal horn cells, as secondary sensory neurons, cross the midline to the opposite side and form the ventral and lateral spinothalamic tracts. These run upward, maintaining a lateral position throughout the lower brain stem (Fig. 125–2).

Impulses conveyed in the dorsal columns are responsible for appreciation of movement and altered posture, localization of stimuli, spatial discrimination of points, recognition of texture and weight, and vibratory sensibility, as well as simple tactile sensation. Fibers in the lateral spinothalamic tract convey sen-

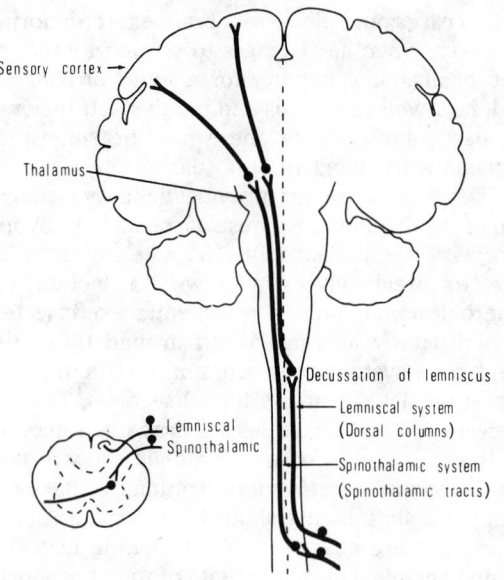

FIGURE 125–1. Diagram to show the principal somatic sensory pathways within the central nervous system—lemniscal (proprioceptive); spinothalamic (pain and temperature).

sations of pain and temperature, and those in the ventral spinothalamic tract mediate, in common with dorsal columns, tactile sensibility.

In the pons there is little spatial separation of the lateral spinothalamic tract and the medial lemniscus. The systems then run together to the ventrolateral nucleus of the thalamus, from which final neurons project to the sensory cortex. Functionally, however, these two systems retain their distinctive features at the upper brain stem, thalamic, and cortical levels. There is good reason, therefore, to refer to them as the lemniscal and spinothalamic systems.

Sensory fibers from the face and cranial structures are similarly distinctive. Cutaneous impulses enter the brain stem predominantly through the fifth and ninth nerves and terminate in their nuclei. Trigeminal tactile impulses end in the main sensory nucleus in the pons, those of pain and temperature in the descending nucleus that extends into the upper cervical spinal cord (Fig. 125–2). Glossopharyngeal fibers end in the nucleus solitarius. Proprioceptive impulses, in contrast, enter the brain stem with the appropriate motor cranial nerves and form synapses with nuclei there. All secondary fibers cross the midline and join the lemniscal and spinothalamic systems on the opposite side.

Central cortical recognition and interpretation of

the various modalities of sensation are not understood, and our concepts of them are based only on defects accompanying cerebral lesions. With extensive cortical sensory damage, crude appreciation of pain persists, gross differences in temperature are still perceived, heavy tactile stimuli felt, and even strong tuning-fork vibrations detected. It seems probable, therefore, that some conscious recognition of sensation takes place at the thalamic level. Fine discriminations, however, require the integrity of the sensory cortex.

The clinical features of sensory disturbances, therefore, depend not only on the general system involved but also on the level at which they occur. Extensive disruption of the spinothalamic pathways may be compatible with satisfactory performance. All but slight impairment in the lemniscal system, on the other hand, generally leads to disastrous ataxia. Sensory testing with crude stimuli that would be perfectly suitable for outlining boundaries of analgesia caused by a complete peripheral nerve lesion may not detect deficits resulting from sensory cortical damage.

PERIPHERAL NERVE OR ROOT. Sensory interruption at a peripheral nerve or root level generally affects all modalities. The areas of impaired skin sensibility are fairly uniform, although the boundaries in response to painful stimuli extend farther than those in response to light touch. It is only in marking out these zones, or in search of cord sensory levels, that the detailed use of a pin and cotton wool is really necessary in the neurologic examination. Accurate contours are important in differentiating root from peripheral nerve damage (Figs. 125–3 and 125–4). It should be stressed, however, that in both instances appropriate lower motor neuron signs are generally also present and less difficult to assess objectively.

SPINAL CORD. Within the spinal cord, damage to sensory systems and pathways can, in all but complete transection, be relatively selective. Predominant, or exclusive, damage to the dorsal columns leads to impaired recognition of postural change, joint movement, tactile discrimination, and vibration caudal to the lesion. If the damage is unilateral, the deficit is on the same side as the cord lesion. Simple touch sensibility is preserved. With interruption of the spinothalamic pathways the faulty recognition of pain and temperature is on the side of the body opposite to the site of spinal cord damage and tactile appreciation is preserved. The level can be detected most easily by testing upward from affected regions to a level of normal sensation. Sometimes, because of concomitant damage to descending autonomic path-

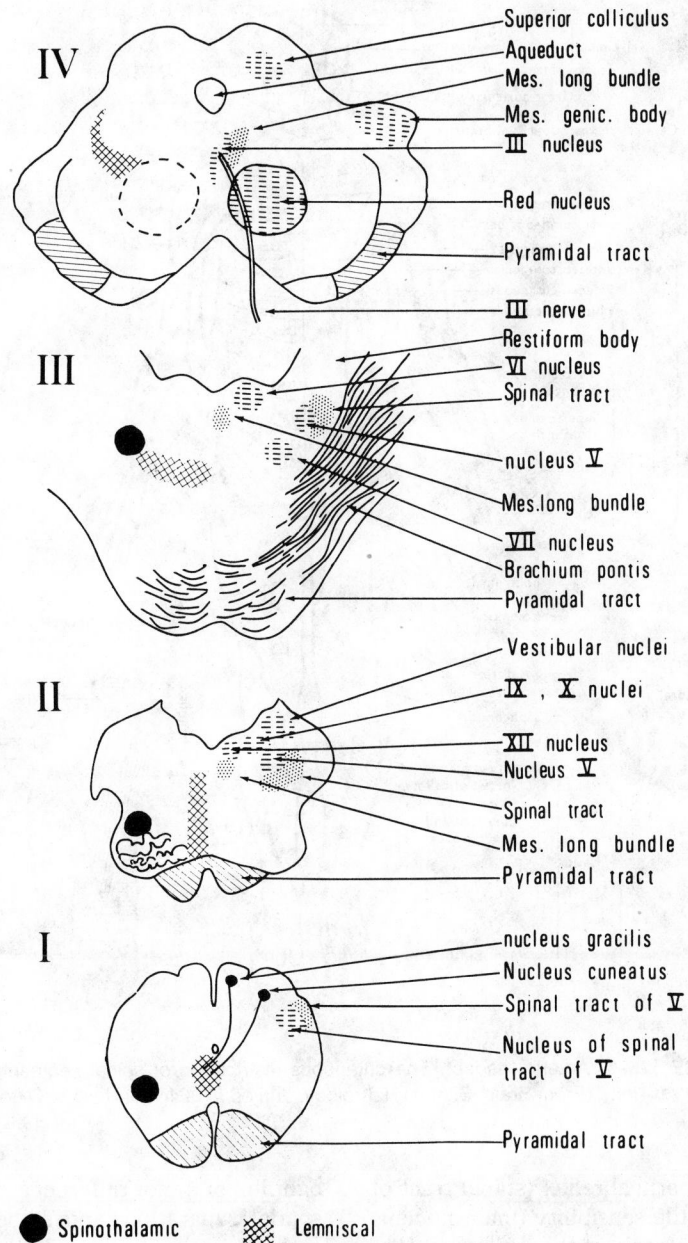

IV

- Superior colliculus
- Aqueduct
- Mes. long bundle
- Mes. genic. body
- III nucleus
- Red nucleus
- Pyramidal tract
- III nerve

III

- Restiform body
- VI nucleus
- Spinal tract
- nucleus V
- Mes. long bundle
- VII nucleus
- Brachium pontis
- Pyramidal tract

II

- Vestibular nuclei
- IX , X nuclei
- XII nucleus
- Nucleus V
- Spinal tract
- Mes. long bundle
- Pyramidal tract

I

- nucleus gracilis
- Nucleus cuneatus
- Spinal tract of V
- Nucleus of spinal tract of V
- Pyramidal tract

● Spinothalamic   ▨ Lemniscal

FIGURE 125-2. Principal pathways of somatic sensation, with some identifying adjacent structures, at successively higher levels of the brain stem. I—medulla, just above the pyramidal decussation; II—rostral medulla; III—pons; IV—midbrain.

ways, corresponding sweat levels on the trunk may be palpated. At the segmental level of the lesion, appropriate evidence of lower motor neuron damage (ventral root or motor nerve cell), or evident dorsal root sensory impairment (Figs. 125-3 and 125-4),

may be present. These may be accompanied by a transitional zone of dysesthesia or pain.

BRAIN STEM. In the lower brain stem, dissociated sensory loss may also result from local lesions. Defective recognition of pinprick over the face, some-

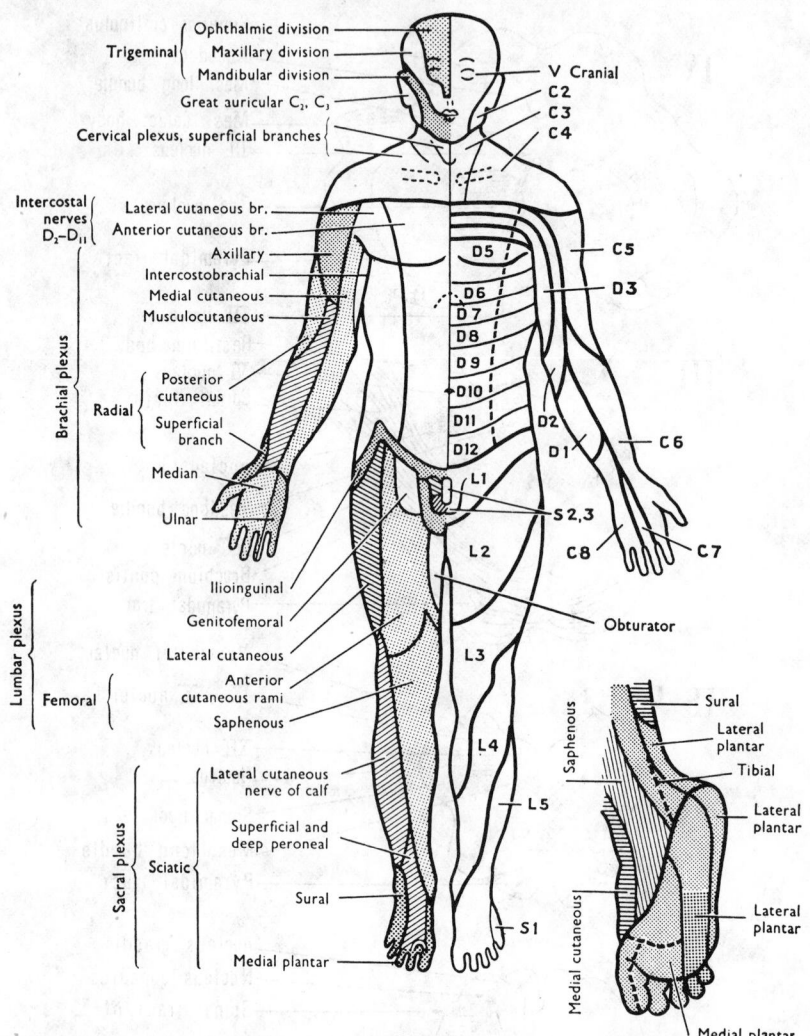

FIGURE 125–3. Anterior aspect. The cutaneous distribution of spinal segments (right) and peripheral nerves (left). (From Brain. Clinical Neurology, 2nd ed., 1964. Courtesy of Oxford University Press.)

times with an impaired corneal reflex (spinal tract of V), may occur when tactile sensibility (main nucleus of V) is intact. Also hypalgesia of the ipsilateral face and of regions of the body below that level on the opposite side may occur with preservation of facial proprioceptive function.

THALAMUS. Severe thalamic damage causes profound crossed hemianesthesia in which all forms of sensation suffer. When incomplete, the distortion of afferent inflow may be painful and apparently spontaneous.

CORTEX. When sensory impairment occurs solely at the level of the sensory cortex, or parietal lobe, the functional loss is in fine discrimination. Rec-

ognition of minor differences in texture, weight, form, spatial separation, and sidedness is, in varying degrees, impaired. When both sides of the body are stimulated simultaneously, the side opposite to the affected parietal cortex may be disregarded. Inconsistency of response may be prominent and falsely interpreted as willful.

MANAGEMENT OF PAIN

It is now clear that the brain contains endogenous systems for the regulation of pain.[87] These systems are probably dependent on both endogenous endor-

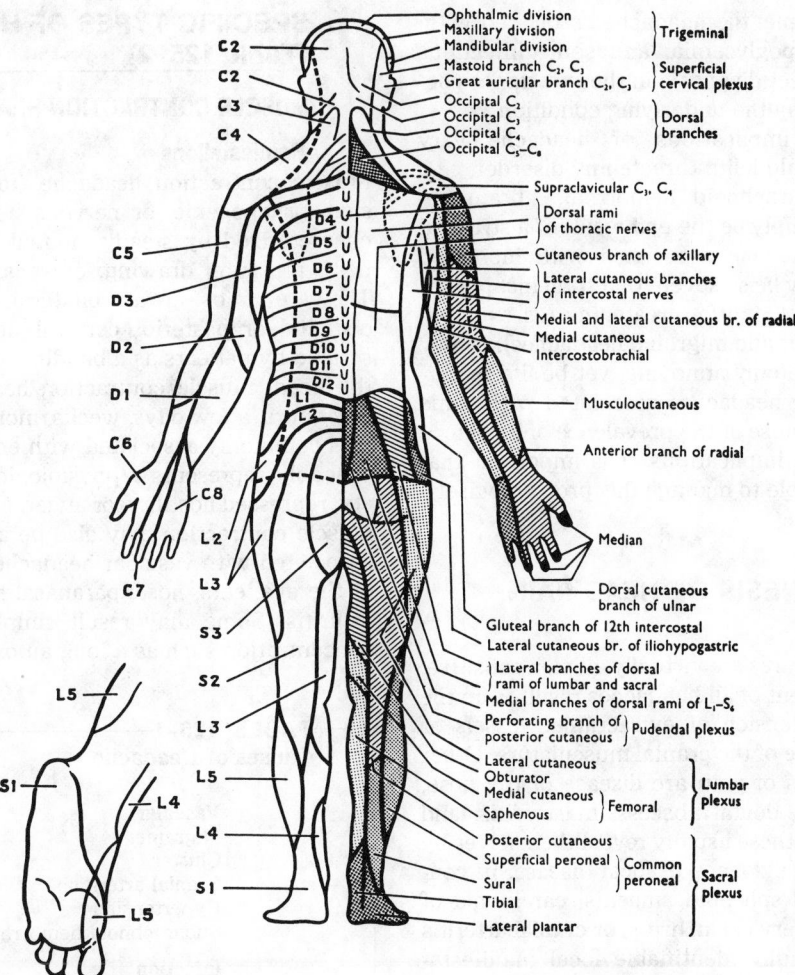

FIGURE 125-4. Posterior aspect. The cutaneous distribution of spinal segments (left) and peripheral nerves (right). (From Brain. Clinical Neurology, 2nd ed., 1964. Courtesy of Oxford University Press.)

phins and on levels of serotonin. Advances in knowledge of these systems may lead to newer therapeutic approaches to chronic pain. At the present time, opiates and opiate derivatives are most successful for acute pain. In chronic pain, drugs which alter levels of serotonin and catecholamines, such as the tricyclic antidepressants alone or in combination with phenothiazines, may be effective. Opiates should be avoided in these patients because of the risk of addiction.

There are a number of neurosurgical procedures utilized for control of pain. Of the destructive, or lytic lesions, percutaneous anterolateral cordotomy is useful, particularly for unilateral pain associated with cancer. Similarly, percutaneous radiofrequency lesions of the gasserian ganglion may be helpful for relief of trigeminal neuralgia. Neuroaugmentation procedures have a role in selected patients; peripheral neuron stimulators can relieve the pain of peripheral nerve injuries. The role of spinal cord and deep brain stimulators remains to be established.

HEADACHES[88-90,93]

Many types of headache must be differentiated solely on the basis of history. Others are diffuse and nondescript and must be differentiated by their associated findings, for example, the headache associated with, anemia, fever, hypoglycemia, and some infectious diseases. The correct diagnosis in these instances depends on identifying the underlying condition.

The clinical implications of headache vary widely. It may herald a life-threatening disorder, e.g., brain tumor, subarachnoid hemorrhage, brain abscess, or it may simply be the end result of a stressful day, e.g., the headache associated with increased muscle tone. It may be so severe that total incapacitation occurs, yet not be life-threatening (as exemplified by some cluster and migraine headaches). It may be so mild as to be only annoying, yet be life-threatening (such as the headaches associated with some brain tumors). Because of the prevalence of headache and these variable implications, it is important that all physicians be able to manage this problem wisely.

PATHOGENESIS OF HEAD PAIN[88]

Extracranial

Extracranial structures are virtually all pain sensitive. More than 90 percent of all headaches result from the dilatation and distension of extracranial vessels or from increased tone of the cranial musculature. Other extracranial causes of pain are disease of the nose, sinuses, glaucoma, dental abscess, mastoiditis, and otitis media. All of these usually reveal themselves by readily identifiable evidence of local disease. In contrast, ethmoid and sphenoid sinusitis, carcinoma of the nasopharynx, cervical arthritis, or cranial arteritis may cause no readily identifiable local manifestations.

Intracranial

The intracranial structures that are pain sensitive include the venous sinuses and their tributaries, parts of the dura at the base of the brain, the fifth, seventh, ninth, and tenth cranial nerves, and the first three cervical nerves. The skull itself, the brain parenchyma, most of the dura, most of the pia-arachnoid, and the ependymal linings of the ventricles, and the choroid plexuses are not sensitive to pain.

There are several mechanisms involved in the production of pain from an intracranial source. These include traction or displacement of the venous sinuses and their tributaries, and the large arteries at the base of the brain and their main branches; dilatation and distension of the intracranial arteries; inflammation in or about any of the pain sensitive structures of the cranial vault; and direct pressure by tumors on the pain sensitive cranial and cervical nerves (Table 125–1).

SPECIFIC TYPES OF HEADACHE (Table 125–2)

MUSCLE CONTRACTION HEADACHE

Manifestations

Muscle contraction headache (formerly called tension, psychogenic, or nervous headache) is usually characterized by steady, nonpulsatile aching, tightness, pressure, drawing, or sensations of soreness. They are almost always bilateral, and commonly are occipital or posterior cervical. It is sometimes described by patients as a bandlike constriction around the head. Muscle contraction headache may last a few hours, a few days, weeks, months, or even years. It is commonly associated with emotional stress and probably represents a physiologic response to anxiety, repressed hostility, or anger. Moreover, sustained muscle contraction may also be a factor in the pain associated with vascular headache, and with disease of the eye, ears, nose, paranasal sinuses, or cervical arthritis. Some may result simply from prolonged concentration such as a long automobile drive, or in-

---

TABLE 125–1
Causes of Headache

Vascular
Migraine
Cluster
Cranial arteritis
Hypertension
Subarachnoid hemorrhage

Infection
Meningitis
Encephalitis
Brain abscess
Systemic infection

Mass Lesions (Chap. 131)
Brain tumors
Brain abscess
Subdural hematoma

Neural Dysfunction
Trigeminal neuralgia
Glossopharyngeal neuralgia
Atypical facial pain

Muscle
Muscle contraction

Trauma
Posttraumatic headache

Focal Structural Disease
Sinusitis
Eye disease
Ear disease
Dental disease
Cervical spine disease

TABLE 125-2
Common Forms of Headache

	Location	Duration	Onset	Associations
Muscle contraction	Occipital Posterior cervical	Hours to days	Gradual	Emotional stress Head and neck position
Migraine	Any area May be unilateral and repetitive	Hours	Gradual	Positive family history Aura secondary to vasoconstrictive events
Cluster	Temporal-ocular areas	Hours Groups of attacks	Abrupt	Homolateral vasocongestion and lacrimation Often nocturnal
Lumbar puncture	Occipital to frontal	Hours	Abrupt on standing	Relieved by lying down
Trigeminal neuralgia	One or more diseases of 5th nerve (Unilateral)	Minutes to hours	Abrupt	"Trigger" areas often present Occur in attacks
Subarachnoid hemorrhage	Postcervical Occipital Frontal	Hours to days	Abrupt	Very severe Nausea, vomiting, Lethargy Localizing signs (Partial III nerve paresis)
Meningitis and encephalitis	Postcervical Frontal	Days	Gradual	Fever, lethargy, seizures
Cranial arteritis	Temporal areas	Weeks	Gradual	Painful vessels Systemic symptoms Increased E.S.R. Retinal arteritis Anterior optic neuritis
Hypertension	Occipital Frontal	Weeks	Gradual	Worse in A.M.

tense studying with the neck held in a limited position.

There are no characteristic physical findings, and diagnosis is based on the clinical description.

Management

The milder varieties respond to simple heat or massage or the use of common analgesics such as aspirin, or to correction of the underlying associated disturbance. Those related to emotional factors may respond to a straightforward explanation, reassurance, aspirin, or moderate doses of a tranquilizer such as diazepam (Valium). Those that fail to respond to such measures should be referred for psychiatric management. The physician, however, should always understand that these patients are neither hysterical nor malingering. This should be made clear to the patient, who otherwise may conclude that the physician believes his headache to be imaginary or feigned.

The diagnosis is not difficult when the relationship between the headache and emotional stress factors is clear. When this relationship is not definite or there is some concern about more serious causes of the head pain, a skull x-ray and CAT scan or brain scan are indicated.

MIGRAINE[91,95]

Migraine is a constitutional, genetically determined, and psychologically influenced, recurrent disorder of the cranial vasculature. Its headache ranges from the mildest discomfort, easily tolerated or controlled by simple analgesics, to the most severe incapacitating, excruciating headache. Its diagnosis is based upon the characteristic manifestations and sequence of manifestations. While repetitive episodes of classical migraine are readily diagnosed, the wide variability of manifestations from patient to patient may confuse the physician unless he is familiar with the full spectrum. The physician must also be skilled in the nuances of therapeutic management, for inept management may lead to incapacitation of the patient or even narcotic addiction.

Manifestations

The attacks usually begin with some degree of cranial arterial vasoconstriction. This phase may be asymptomatic. However, if the vasoconstriction of the branches of the internal carotid artery or basilar artery are of sufficient degree to produce ischemia, various transient neurologic deficits may occur such as visual impairment, dysarthria, dysphasia, hemiparesis, hemianesthesia, disturbed consciousness, vertigo, or ataxia. These manifestations usually subside as the vasoconstriction is supplanted by dilatation.

Vasodilatation is the painful phase of migraine and predominantly relates to the external carotid system. Pain may be expressed unilaterally or bilaterally in any area of the head including the eye, ear, neck, and face (sometimes including the teeth) either alone, in any combination, or involving the entire head, face, or neck in a generalized fashion. It is frequently pounding and throbbing in nature, but may be described as dull, boring, or expanding. Sudden movements of the head, bending over, coughing, sneezing, straining, and exposure to bright lights or loud noises may aggravate the pain. Nausea and vomiting commonly occur. Neurologic disturbances, similar to those associated with vasoconstriction, may also occur during the height of the more intense pain, possibly as a result of focal cerebral edema. Disturbed consciousness, ataxia, and vertigo are also more likely to occur at this time. This phase and its attendant disability may last for one or many hours before subsiding.

The vascular malfunction of migraine is often triggered by emotional stress. Although the emotional state does not cause migraine in the absence of the inherited vascular dysfunction, when the two conditions coexist in the same person a vicious circle of events occurs—the emotional trigger stimulates the migraine process which then in turn aggravates the emotional mechanism until a state of complete invalidism may be induced.

Differential Diagnosis

Many of the neurologic manifestations of migraine may also be seen in older individuals with structural disease of the carotid or cerebral vessels (Chap. 129). The symptoms include unilateral weakness, sensory changes, or visual deficits lasting for several minutes to several hours, clearing completely or almost completely. When these symptoms occur spontaneously without an antecedent history compatible with the diagnosis of migraine, ischemia secondary to cerebrovascular disease is the more likely diagnosis, and angiographic studies are indicated.

Diagnosis

A clear understanding of the migraine process, a detailed history, and physical examination are usually sufficient to make the appropriate diagnosis.

In the unusual headache which is thought to be migraine a *provocative histamine test* may be useful in confirming the diagnosis. This test is useful in provoking the vascular component of any headache caused by vasodilatation, e.g., tension, cluster, posttraumatic, and is, therefore, not specific for migraine. It simply establishes the vascular basis for the headache being tested. Histamine base 0.35 mg is given subcutaneously, preferably in the headache-free state. If no headache is produced or the intensity of the existing headache is not increased in 15 or 20 minutes, then 0.15 mg of the base is given subcutaneously and the patient observed for about one-half hour. Most patients who have a vascular component to their headache will be triggered by this method. If one is able to reproduce or exacerbate the type of pain and the location of pain, this is a positive provocative test and indicates a vascular component in that particular patient's complaint of headache.

Management

Migraine lends itself to a rational approach to management. The vasoconstrictive phase seldom needs to be considered in treatment; although the symptoms may be alarming to the patient and sometimes to the physician, they are transient and permanent sequellae are rare. It is the pain produced by the vasodilating component of migraine that forces the migraine victim to seek help. The question whether vasodilatation alone is capable of producing the painful state has led to a search for factors associated with the vasodilatation which may play a role in the production of pain (Table 125–3).[95]

Treatment may be divided into two phases, management of the individual attack and prophylaxis.

INDIVIDUAL ATTACK. *Ergotamine tartrate* is the treatment of choice. It has a direct vasoconstrictive effect on the smooth muscles of arteries. It may be given by mouth, oral inhalation, sublingually, rectally, subcutaneously, or intravenously. For best results the minimal effective dose must be given immediately at the onset of headache. Vasovasorum of the involved vessels also participate in the migraine syndrome, and dilatation of these vessels tends to produce edema of the wall of the vessel they are supply-

TABLE 125-3
Management of Migraine

Preparations	Indications and Use
I. Individual Attacks	

Cafergot
ergotamine
  tartrate—1 mg
caffeine alkaloid—
  100 mg
	2 tablets at onset of
	  headache
	2 tablets each ½ hour, to
	  a maximum of 6 in 24
	  hours

Cafergot-PB
ergotamine
  tartrate—2 mg
caffeine—100 mg
Bellafoline—0.125
  mg
pentobarbital—30
  mg
	Useful in patients with
	  nausea

Cafergot Rectal
Suppositories
ergotamine
  tartrate—2 mg
caffeine—1 mg
	Useful in patients with
	  nausea

Medihaler Ergotamine
ergotamine tartrate
  0.36 mg per
  compression
	1 inhalation at start of
	  headache. Repeat at 5
	  minute intervals to a
	  maximum of 6 times

Ergotamine Tartrate Ampoules 0.5 mg per ml	0.25 to 0.50 mg subcutaneously Total dose 1.0 mg
II. Prophylaxis	

Bellergal
ergotamine
  tartrate—0.3 mg
belladonna—0.1 mg
phenobarbital—20
  mg
	1 tablet, 4 times per day

Gynergen ergotamine tartrate—1 mg	1 tablet, 4 times per day

Sansert
methysergide
  maleate—2 mg
	1 tablet, 3 times per day
	  (see text for
	  precautions)

Periactin cyproheptadine—4 mg	1 tablet, 3 times per day
Inderal propranolol	Up to 160 mg per day
Nardil phenylzine sulfate—15 mg	1 tablet, 3 times per day
Steroids (see text)	
Low tyramine diet (see text)	

ing. Ergotamine is less effective in constricting an edematous vessel, hence the necessity to insist that patients take this medication at the first sign of headache. Some patients may tolerate ergotamine on a daily basis for weeks or months, although it is not generally recommended. It is essential to discontinue it if there is aching of the extremities, intermittent claudication, cold, numb, tingling feelings in the fingers or toes, decreased peripheral vascular pulsations, or elevation of blood pressure. Tolerance may rarely develop with prolonged use of ergot or a headache rebound phenomenon may result; ergotamine withdrawal is indicated in these instances.

Ergot alkaloids are contraindicated in peripheral vascular disease, coronary artery disease, hypertension, impaired hepatic or renal function, sepsis, and pregnancy.

A particularly severe attack, unresponsive to ergotamine, may require the use of a strong analgesic and antiemetic such as meperidine (Demerol) 100 mg and promethazine (Phenergan) 25 mg intramuscularly. More than infrequent use of such medications is to be condemned since the potential for narcotic addiction in this nonlethal pain syndrome is high.

PROPHYLACTIC MANAGEMENT. Prophylactic therapy of migraine is indicated in those patients whose pains are chronic or are recurring at such frequency that they will readily comply to the nuisance of taking prophylactic medication several times a day on a regular basis. *Methysergide maleate* (Sansert), an antiserotonin compound, is of considerable benefit in the management of some, but not all, chronic or recurring migraine. It potentiates the action of circulating catecholamines, potentiates the action of ergot derivatives, moderates central vasomotor function, and interferes with histamine liberators. It is a competitive antagonist of serotonin. It is contraindicated in hypertension, peripheral vascular disease, coronary artery disease, in the presence of cardiac murmurs, vascular bruits, impaired liver or renal function, and pregnancy. Long-term use may produce various fibroproliferative phenomena which if recognized early usually, but not always, subside with discontinuation of Sansert. Fibroproliferation may produce cardiac murmurs, arterial stenosis, pleural and pulmonary fibrosis, and retroperitoneal fibrosis. It has been suggested by some that therapy should be interrupted for one month out of every six. There has been a decrease in the number of reported instances of fibroproliferative disorders caused by Sansert since this has been advocated. Whether this is caused by this suggestion or by closer physician supervision of patients has not been proven.

Cyproheptadine (Periactin) is an antihistaminic

with antiserotonin properties. It is not as effective as Sansert but there are no known fibroproliferative phenomena. It may produce sleepiness or weight gain.

Propranolol is a beta-adrenergic blocker and, therefore, permits an increase in alpha-adrenergic response (vasoconstriction). It should not be used in those patients with an asthmatic history or poor ventricular function.

Tricyclic compounds (Elavil, Tofranil) are antidepressant agents. Depression occurs in frequently recurring or chronic migraine and the use of antidepressant medications may be of some value.

Monoamine oxidase (MAO) inhibitors, e.g., phenylzine sulfate (Nardil), increase levels of serotonin. Serotonin levels are decreased at the onset of migraine and it is reasonable to consider these agents in the therapeutic management of migraine. Such medication should be reserved for those unresponsive to the conventional and less complex forms of therapy. Hypertensive crises have resulted from tyramine–MAO inhibitor interaction. Patients, therefore, must be warned to avoid the use of cheese, alcoholic beverages, pickled herring, chicken livers, canned figs, yeast extract, and pods of broad beans. Since MAO inhibitors may potentiate the action of sympathomimetic substances, medications containing such substances are contraindicated. *Corticosteroids,* among other actions, reduce inflammation and stabilize cell membrane, and through these actions may be beneficial in chronic migraine. A few patients do respond to high dose prednisone (60 mg a day), but not many will maintain a satisfactory response on doses low enough to be reasonably safe over a long period. The use of prednisone should be considered only in those cases of migraine that are chronic, severe, and unresponsive to the more usual form of treatment.

Tyramine is a vasoactive monamine which undergoes deamination by monamine oxidase enzymes. A small group of migraineurs may have their headache attacks precipitated by the ingestion of tyramine-containing foods. These patients conjugate less tyramine than others both on normal diets and diets containing additional tyramine. There is no specific test to identify those who have this difficulty. When dealing with frequent attacks of migraine, therefore, it is worthwhile to try a *low tyramine diet* for a month.

Psychotherapy plays an important, but limited, role in the management of migraine. As previously noted, migraine is an inherited disorder, influenced by the autonomic nervous system, and possibly related to disturbances in vasoactive substances. It is not fundamentally a disorder of the psyche, but the defective mechanism is quite vulnerable to emotional stress factors. At times such stimuli are so intense that pharmacotherapy may have very little influence. Psychotherapy then becomes the treatment of choice. Not all such patients need intensive psychotherapy and some may benefit by a simple explanation of the role of the autonomic nervous system and the ease with which it may malfunction in a setting of anxiety, stress, pressures, worry, guilt, hostility, and depression. Reassurance in the form of an explanation of the nature of migraine and emphasizing that no permanent damage results from either the intensity of the pain or the alarming neurologic phenomena may be helpful.

CLUSTER HEADACHES

Cluster headaches represent a distinct clinical syndrome of headaches which were originally described by Romberg in 1840 as ciliary neuralgia. It appears in the literature under various names such as sphenopalatine neuralgia, hemicephalic vasodilatation of sympathetic origin, periodic migrainous neuralgia, vidian nerve neuralgia, erythromyalgia of the head, histaminic cephalgia, petrosal neuralgia, migraine variant, and Horton syndrome. Now this syndrome is usually called cluster headache because of its tendency to occur in clusters.

Manifestations

The clusters occur frequently in the spring or fall, but not limited to these times. Clusters vary in duration from weeks to months and occasionally may be of a noncluster variety occurring over a period of years. The individual attacks of pain are usually of short duration, lasting from 10 to 120 minutes, rarely longer. One to 3 attacks in 24 hours are common and they often occur with clock-like predictability for a particular patient in a particular cluster. There may be as few as two attacks in a week or up to eight or more in 24 hours. The remission between clusters may last for weeks, months, or years. The pain is probably caused by vasodilatation of branches of both the external and internal carotid artery systems. The role of vasoactive amines in this disorder, if any, has not been established, although histamine blood levels appear to be elevated.

The pains predominantly involve the temporal ocular regions. They are often supraorbital, frontal, facial (including the teeth), and occasionally spread to the parietal, occipital or cervical regions. The pain is usually extremely severe, and its peak is likely to be reached within a few minutes of the onset. It is described as burning, boring, gnawing, throbbing, pounding, stabbing, or any combination of these.

Homolateral rhinorrhea, nasal congestion, lacrimation, and conjunctival injection frequently accompany the pains. Nausea is quite infrequent and vomiting is rare. Homolateral ocular sympathetic paralysis occurs occasionally and is usually transient. The attacks may be nocturnal, awakening the patient a couple of hours after going to sleep, and may be precipitated by vasodilating drugs, including the ingestion of alcohol, or by lying down to take a nap.

Cluster headache differs from migraine in that:

1. There is no vomiting and rarely nausea.
2. There is no significant family history.
3. It involves many more men than women.
4. There is no menstrual relationship.
5. There are no neurologic deficits except for ocular sympathetic paralysis.
6. The average frequency of attacks is greater than that of migraine.
7. The average duration of attacks is shorter than that of migraine.
8. Nocturnal attacks are more frequent than in migraine.
9. There is no demonstrable fall of serotonin at the onset of an attack as there is in migraine.

These features permit cluster headaches to be distinguished from migraine.

Management

Ergotamine tartrate is the medication of choice in this syndrome. In many cases the attacks in a particular cluster occur at a predictable time which makes it possible to give an effective dose of ergotamine shortly before the anticipated onset. For example, if most attacks are occurring 2 hours after going to sleep, an appropriate dose can be given at bedtime. If more than one attack occurs predictably at different times of the day, the permissible dose per 24 hours can be divided accordingly. With proper supervision 4 mg (or in some patients up to 6 mg) can be used orally per 24 hours. In particularly difficult clusters the patient can be taught the self-administration of Gynergen or DHE-45 subcutaneously. The appropriate amount can be given once or twice a day within the limits and precautions previously described in the management of migraine. Careful monitoring of the patient is essential if ergotamine is required over long periods of time.

Methysergide (Sansert) is occasionally useful because it seems to potentiate the action of ergotamine. A 2-mg tablet (not to exceed three tablets a day) may be given with each dose of ergotamine, again with careful observation of the patient.

Adrenal corticosteroids may control some clusters, but if response does not occur within 2 or 3 days this medication should be promptly discontinued. Prednisone may be given at an initial dose of 60 mg daily with gradual appropriate reduction to a reasonable maintenance level. Since there may be an increased incidence of peptic ulcer in these patients, antacid therapy is indicated with the use of prednisone.

Antihistaminics are of little value.

Histamine intravenously or subcutaneously as previously described under migraine may be tried. The response is not predictable.

It is unlikely that psychogenic factors play a primary role in this syndrome and psychotherapy does not produce improvement.

LUMBAR PUNCTURE HEADACHE

The headache that follows lumbar puncture is caused by lowering of the cerebral spinal fluid pressure and results from traction on pain-sensitive intracranial venous structures. The headache is usually throbbing and principally occipital in location, but may become generalized and include the neck. It usually begins a few hours after the puncture, comes on in the erect position, and subsides when the patient lies down. It usually lasts 24 to 72 hours, but an occasional patient develops more severe symptoms that sometimes last as long as 10 to 14 days. For the most part the patient is helped by maintaining a flat position and using ordinary analgesics.

The lowered spinal fluid pressure probably results from leakage through the dura at the site of puncture. The number of postlumbar puncture headaches can be kept at a minimum by using a sharp number 20 spinal puncture needle.

TRIGEMINAL NEURALGIA

Manifestations

The cause of trigeminal neuralgia (tic douloureux) is unknown. Pain occurs in brief lancinating jabs of great severity; the patient may wince, and hence the name "tic." The pain is unilateral and localized to one or another division of the nerve (usually maxillary or mandibular) but may spread to other divisions when severe. Pain may be precipitated by touch, cold, or motion of a certain spot innervated by that division—a trigger area. Pain may recur over a matter of several seconds in episodes that can occur once or many times a day. Exacerbations during which pain recurs frequently tend to last for weeks and may be separated by long periods free of pain.

Diagnosis depends on the physician's recognition of these characteristics. On examination there are usually no abnormalities; rarely there is some tenderness of the skin or over the nerves in the involved area. Cerebellar pontine angle tumor and other mass lesions may produce trigeminal pain, but the pain is apt to be constant and the pattern rarely resembles that of a tic.

Management
Carbamazepine (Tegretol) 200 mg 2 to 4 times daily may be effective. Phenytoin (Dilantin) 100 mg 3 times a day appears to be helpful to some patients. Those patients who are not helped by these medications may require surgical intervention.

PAROXYSMAL GLOSSOPHARYNGEAL NEURALGIA
Although it is less common than trigeminal neuralgia, paroxysmal glossopharyngeal neuralgia is otherwise quite similar and may occur with trigeminal neuralgia. Pain occurs in the pharynx or auditory canal, and

swallowing is usually the trigger. Intracranial division of the ninth nerve provides relief.

ATYPICAL FACIAL PAIN
Atypical neuralgias involving the head and face may be seen in multiple sclerosis, angina pectoris, myocardial infarction, apical petrositis (Gradenigo syndrome), Raeder's paratrigeminal neuralgia, intra- or extracervical spinal abnormalities (usually in the area of C1 to C3 but occasionally from lower spinal areas), postherpetic neuralgia, central pain from brain stem or thalamic area, temporal mandibular joint dysfunction, lethal midline granuloma, intracranial aneurysm, inflammation of the teeth or gums, glaucoma, iritis, retrobulbar neuralgia, or cranial arteritis. Some are psychogenic and some are caused by vasodilatation. The diagnosis and treatment depend entirely on identifying the underlying source of pain by way of a detailed history, physical examination, and appropriate ancillary studies.

CHAPTER 126
Disturbances of Sleep
GUY M. McKHANN AND ERNST F. L. NIEDERMEYER

NORMAL SLEEP MECHANISMS[96,97,101]
In recent years it has become apparent that sleep is not a passive period for the nervous system, but is an active process. There are two forms of sleep: desynchronized sleep or rapid-eye-movement sleep (REM sleep), and slow-wave or non-REM sleep. The differences between the two forms of sleep are summarized in Table 126–1.

The initiation of sleep follows a sequence of stages from drowsiness (Stage 1), to light (Stage 2), deep (Stage 3), and very deep (Stage 4) sleep; all of these stages fall into the category of non-REM sleep. About 60 to 90 minutes following sleep onset, the first REM sleep period is usually noted. Dreaming is facilitated during REM sleep, but it may also occur in non-REM stages. In the further course of nocturnal sleep, several REM stages occur and become most prominent in the early morning hours.

During development there is a decreasing need for sleep by human beings, and the time occupied by REM sleep decreases from approximately 50 percent in the newborn to 20 percent in the adult. In addition, there is a spectrum in the amount of sleep normal individuals require. Some persons do well with only 4 to 5 hours sleep per night, with or without a brief

daytime nap. At the other extreme are people who regularly sleep 12 to 14 hours per day.

DISTURBANCES OF SLEEP[99,100]
Sleep may be altered by phenomena that occur so commonly, such as nocturnal myoclonus, that they are considered normal phenomena. At the other extreme are true disorders of sleep mechanisms such as narcolepsy or Undine's curse. The disturbances of sleep are outlined in Table 126–2.

Sleep Deprivation
Even though we do not know the mechanisms of the restorative function of sleep, sleep deprivation leads to intolerable sleepiness and tiredness. Normal volunteers are virtually unable to remain awake after 60 hours without sleep. Associated with sleepiness are such symptoms as irritability, a gritty feeling of the eyes, slowing of motor and mental functions, inability to learn and retain new information, and difficulties in accurately recalling past events. With prolonged sleep deprivation, physical symptoms similar to drunkenness (diplopia, staggering, and visual or auditory hallucinations) will appear.

Recovery from sleep deprivation requires a

TABLE 126-1
Principal Differences Between Non-REM and REM Sleep

	Non-REM Sleep	REM Sleep
EEG	Slow (delta) activity of considerable voltage, sleep spindles, vertex waves	Mixed activity, mostly of low to medium voltage with enhanced medium and fast frequencies (alpha and beta range)
Eye movement (electro-oculogram)	Unremarkable, usually very slow	Rapid eye movements (REM) of irregular and jerky character
Muscle tone (EMG)	A constantly demonstrable moderate degree of EMG activity (best demonstrable from the hyoid muscle)	Marked hypotonia or atonia evidenced by considerably diminished EMG activity
Respiration	Regular	Moderate irregularities changes in rate
Cardiac rhythm	Normal	Arrhythmias may occur
Body movements	Absent	Often present (despite pronounced muscular hypotonia probably occurring between stretches of REM activity)
Dreaming	Sometimes	Very frequently
Neurochemical mechanism	Serotonergic brain stem (mainly pontine raphe nuclei and midbrain structures)	Noradrenergic pontine (locus coeruleus) and possibly brain stem structures

TABLE 126-2
Disturbances of Sleep[99,100]

Sleep deprivation
Hypnogogic phenomena
Insomnia
Narcolepsy
Nightmares
Nocturnal seizures
Sleepwalking and sleeptalking
Enuresis
Sleep apneas

Hypnogogic Phenomena

As a person first falls asleep, a number of normal phenomena may occur. The most common of these are sudden *jerks* (nocturnal myoclonus), often associated with a feeling of falling. These jerks often awaken the patient quite suddenly. It is important to recognize that these movements are not seizures, or associated with epilepsy.

There may be separate or associated *sensory illusions* such as hearing a loud noise, or one's name being called, or the visual experience of a sudden flash of light or more formed visual pictures.

Upon awakening some persons experience transient *sleep paralysis*. For a few moments they are conscious, but are unable to initiate voluntary movement.

Insomnia

The inability to fall asleep or to remain asleep for the accustomed six to eight hours is a common complaint. It is estimated that 25 percent of the adult population of the United States regularly takes some drug to aid sleep. This may, in part, reflect the overprescribing of sedatives coupled with sedative dependence.

The management of insomnia requires that the basis for the symptom be understood. The most common cause is emotional tension, but other physical and emotional illnesses must be considered (Table 126-3). In these conditions sedative drugs may only delay the correct diagnosis.

It is important to determine if inability to go to sleep or subsequent awakening is the problem. In the former instance tranquilizers, such as diazepam or short-acting sedatives are effective, while a longer-acting drug is needed for those who awaken during the night. Finally, the prudent physician is aware of

catch-up, or rebound, phenomenon. First, there are prolonged periods of stage 4 (non-REM) sleep; later there is a catch-up of REM sleep. If different phases of sleep are selectively deprived, as when an individual is awakened every time REM sleep occurs, there is a selective catch-up.

TABLE 126–3
Insomnia

Cause	Characteristic
Emotional Disturbances	
Anxiety	Sporadic, difficulty falling asleep, early awakening
Depression	Early awakening with morbid or ruminative thoughts
Mania	Early awakening with excess physical activity
Physical Ailments	
Pain	Usually associated with
Hunger	difficulty falling asleep and
Coldness or warmth	subsequent fitful or restless
Cough	sleep
Hyperthyroidism	
Uremia	
Pruritis	
Nocturia	
Chronic brain syndrome	
Orthopnea	
Changes in Environment	
New surroundings	Difficulty falling asleep
Different times for sleep	
"Jet lag"	
Toxins and Drugs	
Coffee	Difficulty falling asleep
Tea	Loss of sleep rhythm
Alcohol	Decreased total sleep
Amphetamines	
Withdrawal of drugs (barbiturates amphetamines)	
Lesions of Hypothalamus and Midbrain	
Encephalitis	No diurnal rhythm
Trauma	Associated disturbances of
Tumors	temperature regulation or appetite
	Hypersomnia in some cases

the pitfalls of sedation which include the risk of disorientation in the elderly, hypercapnia in the patient with even mild chronic obstructive pulmonary disease, depression in the alcoholic, and drug dependence in all patients.

Narcolepsy[102,103]

In this condition, patients have an overwhelming urge to fall asleep, particularly during times of boredom and decreased physical activity. The onset is between ages 10 and 30 years, and some cases are familial. The onset of sleep is quite abrupt and the duration

brief, for about 10 to 15 minutes. Patients can be kept awake by increasing environmental stimuli, but if kept awake may show the symptoms of sleep deprivation. There may be three associated symptoms: *hypnogogic hallucinations, sleep paralysis* (described earlier), and *cataplexy*. Sleep paralysis occurs at both the beginning and at the end of a narcoleptic attack. Cataplexy refers to the sudden loss of muscle tone associated with emotional responses such as laughing, crying, anger, or fear. In some patients there is a sagging of the jaw; in stress there may be a sudden collapse to the floor with no movement for a few minutes.

During sleep paralysis and cataplexy, the patient apparently has the abrupt onset of REM sleep. This may also be what occurs in some, but not all, patients with narcolepsy.

The therapy of narcolepsy and its associated symptoms is difficult, and the overall prognosis is poor. Patients should be encouraged to sleep at night, using tranquilizers or mild sedatives if necessary. During the daytime, cataplexy and sleep paralysis may be helped by imipramine (Tofranil). The narcolepsy may respond to amphetamines, dextroamphetamine (Dexedrine), or methylphenidate (Ritalin). Some patients take massive doses of amphetamines (50 to 80 mg per day), and a drug-induced paranoid psychosis may supervene. Many patients will become refractory to the continued use of amphetamines, and have to reserve the drug for special occasions when they must not fall asleep.

Other Forms of Hypersomnia

The *Pickwickian syndrome* includes hypersomnia and hypoventilation and is seen in patients with extreme obesity.

Patients with *hypersomnia with sleep drunkenness* are confused and disoriented on awakening from sleep and may exhibit some gait ataxia. These symptoms may improve as the day progresses but may return at random intervals during the day. It has been presumed that this disorder is caused by an increase of the stages of deep non-REM sleep (Stages 3 and 4).

The *Kleine-Levin syndrome* consists of prolonged episodes of hypersomnia and bulimia (ravenous appetite) and is encountered mainly in adolescents and young adults. The nature of the rare disorder is obscure.

Sleep Apneas[98]

Variations in the rate and rhythm of respiration are common during sleep. The extreme form of this variation is sleep apnea. In this condition the patient ceases breathing during sleep. The condition may be secondary to a defect in the brain stem reticular activating system. Identifiable etiologies are a brain stem stroke or cervical syringomyelia. It has been suggested that sleep apnea may play a role in the sudden-death syndrome of infants and young children, "crib death."

In older adults, sleep apnea may interfere with the nocturnal pattern of sleep. In some instances, the apnea may be related to intermittent upper airway obstruction.

Nightmares, Sleepwalking, and Sleeptalking

Nightmares usually occur during REM sleep, and consist of terrifying dreams which are often associated with a feeling of helplessness and inability to move. Nightmares are particularly common during withdrawal from barbiturates or alcohol, when the

patient may be in REM sleep almost 100 percent of the time.

Sleepwalking and sleeptalking occur during non-REM sleep and are often associated with thrashing movements. The episodes usually occur during the first few hours of sleep, and the patient has total amnesia for what occurred or what he may have done.

Enuresis

Persistent bed-wetting may have organic causes such as urinary tract infection, dysfunction of the neural control of the bladder, or polyuria. However, most cases are on a psychogenic basis. Enuresis occurs during non-REM sleep, particularly when the patient arouses from deep (stage 4) sleep. The therapy is difficult. Various forms of "conditioning" such as alarms which ring at particular times or upon bed-wetting have had some success. Imiprimine (Tofranil), 25 to 50 mg at night is helpful in some cases.

CHAPTER 127

Dizziness, Vertigo, and Hearing Loss
DAVID S. ZEE

INTRODUCTION

Patients may use a variety of words such as dizziness, giddiness, lightheadedness, swaying, or vertigo to describe a sensation of imbalance or dysequilibrium. Most of those patients do not have a primary disorder of vestibular function, but have their symptoms secondary to a number of nonneurologic causes. However, dizziness and vertigo may be important symptoms of a number of neurologic conditions. Three sensations—vertigo, oscillopsia, and impulsion—should be explicitly defined and distinguished from vague giddiness since they are suggestive of a primary disorder of the vestibular system, either peripherally or centrally. *Vertigo* is the illusion that either the patient or his environment is rotating. *Oscillopsia* is the visual illusion that the environment is moving back and forth. *Impulsion* is the sensation that one is being forcibly propelled. Precipitation or exacerbation of these sensations by head movements is further evidence of vestibular system involvement.

The assessment of hearing is essential in the evaluation of patients with vestibular dysfunction so that any associated disturbances of hearing or tinnitus may be explicitly defined and evaluated.

PATHOPHYSIOLOGY OF VESTIBULAR DISORDERS

The vestibular system functions through two phylogenetically old responses, the vestibulospinal and vestibulo-ocular reflexes. The vestibulospinal reflex uses information from both the semicircular canals and the otolith organs (utricle and saccule) to determine the orientation of the head with respect to the ground, and to promote appropriate postural adjustments to keep the body upright. The vestibulo-ocular reflex uses information from the semicircular canals to detect rotational movements of the head, and to generate appropriate compensatory eye movements which are exactly equal and opposite to head movements. This reflex permits one to maintain ocular fixation during head movements.

For both systems there is a tonic discharge from each vestibular end organ that is perfectly balanced in the central nervous system. When the head is tilted or rotated in one direction the labyrinthine output from one side increases while the other decreases, and it is this temporary imbalance of sensory input that elicits the compensatory motor commands for vestibulospinal and vestibulo-ocular reflexes. If, for some reason, the input from the peripheral labyrinths becomes imbalanced or its central processing disordered, inappropriate motor responses are elicited.

Vestibulospinal disorders are manifest by a tendency to fall or by the sensation of impulsion. With acute unilateral loss of labyrinthine function the patient will fall or feel propelled towards the side of the lesion. In the vestibulo-ocular system inappropriate oculomotor responses are manifest as oscillopsia during head movements, vertigo, and spontaneous nystagmus. Since the tonic input from each labyrinth tends to drive the eyes in the opposite direction, removal of one labyrinth causes jerk nystagmus with a slow drift off fixation (slow phase) towards the affected ear and a rapid corrective movement (quick phase) towards the intact ear. Nystagmus arising from the peripheral vestibular apparatus must be distinguished both from nystagmus of central vestibular origin (Table 127–1) and from nystagmus caused by other central nervous system lesions (Chap. 119).

Positional nystagmus is a special form of vestibular nystagmus and is often associated with positional vertigo. It can be elicited by rapidly moving the patient from the sitting to the lying position and turning the head towards one side. Positional nystagmus can be caused by either peripheral or central lesions. If of peripheral origin, it usually occurs in only one head position, and begins after a short delay (2 to 10 seconds) after assuming the recumbent position. It dies out within a minute and it becomes more difficult to elicit with repeated testing. In contrast, positional nystagmus of central origin usually occurs in more than one head position, begins with no delay, and does not fatigue upon repeated testing.

APPROACH TO THE PATIENT WITH VERTIGO[104,105]

On the basis of the history and physical examination, it is necessary to establish whether the patient's symptoms are of vestibular origin. In a patient whose history reveals vague giddiness or dizziness without vertigo, oscillopsia, or impulsion, and whose neurologic and auditory review of systems and examination are completely normal, further neurologic workup is not initially indicated, and a careful search for nonneurologic causes of dizziness (Table 127–2) should be made. However, if either the history or examination suggest auditory, vestibular, or neurologic involvement, special tests of vestibular and auditory function should be performed in order to localize the site of origin of the patient's symptoms to the labyrinth, eighth cranial nerve, or central nervous system (Table 127–1).

TABLE 127–1

Approach to the Patient with Dizziness and Vertigo

Variable	Observation
History	Establish presence or absence of vertigo, oscillopsia, impulsion, decreased hearing or tinnitus
Physical Examination	
Vestibulospinal reflex (with eyes closed patient stands with feet together or tandem walks)	Falling or veering to one side
	Patient falls to side of acute peripheral lesion
Vestibulo-ocular reflex (head rotation)	Presence and characteristics of spontaneous nystagmus, positional nystagmus
	Patient will develop oscillopsia during head movement
Hearing	Weber, Rinne tests
Localization of the Defect	
Labyrinth	Associated auditory dysfunction. No other neurological findings
Eighth nerve	Auditory and vestibular dysfunction
	Brain stem compression with large masses
Brain stem	Auditory function normal, other neurological findings, pure vertical or rotatory nystagmus indicates central lesion
Ancillary Tests	
Caloric stimulation	See Table 127–3
Audiometry	See Table 127–4
Skull x-rays Tomograms	Erosion of internal auditory meatus with acoustic neuroma
CAT scan	Demonstration of mass in cerebellar-pontine angle
Angle myelogram	Demonstration of eighth nerve tumor
Lumbar puncture	Protein may be elevated with acoustic neuroma

---

TABLE 127-2
Common Nonneurologic Causes of Dizziness

Hyperventilation, anxiety

Syncope

Anemia

Postural hypotension

Hypoglycemia

Cardiac arrhythmia

Hypothroidism

Drug side effects

Hypertension

Emphysema

ANCILLARY DIAGNOSTIC TESTS[104]

Caloric Test (Table 127-3)

The most important test of peripheral vestibular function is the caloric examination. When an external auditory canal is irrigated with water above or below, body temperature convection currents are induced in the endolymph of the semicircular canals. The movements of the fluid mimic labyrinthine stimulation by head rotation with the exception (and the advantage) that each labyrinth can be tested individually. If cold water is used and the head positioned such that the horizontal canal is in the vertical plane (with the patient recumbent and the head elevated 30° above the horizontal), horizontal nystagmus is induced with the slow phase directed towards the stimulated ear. Hot water induces nystagmus with the slow phase directed away from the stimulated ear. The caloric test can be standardized by carefully controlling water temperature and volume and duration of irrigation. Responses can be quantified by measuring the frequency and duration of nystagmus under direct observation. The effect of fixation upon the induced nystagmus should be determined by using Fresnel's

---

TABLE 127-3
Caloric Tests

Lesion	Response
Peripheral	Decreased on side of lesion
	Fixation decreases nystagmus
Central	Relatively normal
	Fixation may not decrease nystagmus

---

glasses which, by blurring the patient's vision, eliminate the patient's ability to use fixation to suppress nystagmus. For more precise measurements eye movements can be recorded with electronystagmography.

Audiometry

Audiometric tests are used primarily to localize lesions peripheral to the brain stem. Sensorineural (cochlear or retrocochlear) deafness can be easily distinguished from conductive (middle ear) deafness by preservation of bone-conducted hearing in the latter. Clinically this is detected by the Rinne test in which a vibrating tuning fork is held against the mastoid process until the sound fades, then is placed near the ear. Normal subjects hear the sound about twice as long by air as by bone. The Weber test compares bone-conducted hearing between the two ears. A vibrating tuning fork is placed at the center of the head. In conductive hearing losses the sound lateralizes to the abnormal ear, in sensorineural hearing losses, to the normal ear. Table 127-4 outlines common causes of disorders of hearing and Table 127-5 outlines the basic patterns of hearing loss in cochlear and retrocochlear lesions.

PERIPHERAL VESTIBULAR DISORDERS

With the exception of acoustic neuromas, disorders of the peripheral vestibular system usually present acutely. The common causes are indicated in Table 127-6. Patients are usually severely ill with incapacitating vertigo, impulsion, nausea, vomiting, and prostration. Nystagmus is usually present at the onset of illness and is usually horizontal, but varying degrees of rotatory or vertical components may be present. The direction of the horizontal component of nystagmus in peripheral disorders depends upon whether the lesion is paralytic or irritative. In the former, as in vestibular neuronitis, slow phases of nystagmus are directed towards the side of the involved labyrinth; in the latter (as in the Menière syndrome), the slow phase is away from the side of the involved labyrinth. In peripheral disorders, auditory symptoms and signs may be present, but other evidence of neurologic involvement is absent. Caloric tests usually show decreased responses in the involved ear.

CENTRAL VESTIBULAR DISORDERS

Vertigo of central origin may arise from lesions anywhere in the vestibular nuclei or its cerebellar connections (Table 127-7). Hence, pontine, medullary, or

TABLE 127-4
Common Disorders of Hearing

Type	Examples	Distinguishing Characteristics
Conductive	Obstruction in external canal (cerumen) Damage to tympanic membrane Middle ear infection or fluid accumulation Otosclerosis	Hearing loss usually spares high frequencies Sounds are muffled with paracusis (hear better in loud room) and a low pitched, fluctuating tinnitus. With otosclerosis tinnitus is usually whistling and constant
Sensorineural	Hereditary Congenital (rubella, erythroblastosis) Presbycusis Trauma (occupational, skull fractures)	
	Infections: postmeningitic (*H. influenzae*, meningococcal), viral (mumps, measles, *H. zoster*); rickettsial (murine typhus) Drug toxicity (quinine, salicylate, dihydrostreptomycin, gentamycin, kanamycin, arsenic)	Hearing loss usually affects high frequencies. Must differentiate retrocochlear from cochlear pattern (Table 127-5) Acoustic trauma usually gives a specific loss of hearing at 4000 Hz Facial palsy often occurs with *H. zoster*
	Menierès syndrome	Menieres syndrome may be mimicked by hypothyroidism and neurosyphilis
	Lesions of the eighth nerve	See Table 127-8

TABLE 127-5
Evaluation of Hearing Loss

Cochlear	Retrocochlear
1. Pure tone loss proportional to speech discrimination loss	1. Pure tone loss much less than speech discrimination loss
2. Recruitment (sudden abnormal loudness growth as sound intensity is slowly increased)	2. No recruitment
3. High SISI (short increment sensitivity index, ability to detect slight increases in loudness)	3. Low SISI
4. Minimal tone decay	4. Pronounced tone decay
5. Interrupted *vs.* continuous tone thresholds nearly equal (Bekesy Type II)	5. Interrupted tone thresholds lower than continuous (Bekesy Type III or IV)

cerebellar lesions all may cause vertigo, but patients usually have additional neurologic symptoms or signs pointing to the location of the lesions. Occasionally, vertigo is part of temporal lobe seizures or is associated with a migraine syndrome. Patients with recent onset of an extraocular muscle paresis may also complain of mild degrees of vertigo.

Acute, severe vertigo occurs with brain stem lesions such as multiple sclerosis or brain stem infarction. Positional vertigo and nystagmus are more characteristic of chronic processes such as posterior fossa neoplasms, spinocerebellar degenerations, or malformations.

The distinction between acute attacks of vertigo and transient ischemic attacks of the brain stem may be difficult. Persistent vertigo, without other neurologic signs or symptoms, is seldom secondary to brain stem ischemia.

EIGHTH NERVE TUMORS

Early diagnosis of acoustic nerve tumors has become increasingly important because of the comparatively low morbidity and mortality of surgical removal if the tumor is small. Every patient with unexplained unilateral hearing loss or vague dizziness and imbalance must be considered a tumor suspect and evaluated accordingly.

Although acoustic neuroma is the most common lesion of the eighth nerve, a number of other lesions may have a similar clinical presentation (Table 127-8). Patients usually complain first of insidious hearing loss or tinnitus, and, if specifically asked, they may describe a vague feeling of unsteadiness. Attacks of vertigo may occur but are unusual. As the tumor enlarges patients may have headache, retroau-

TABLE 127-6
Peripheral Vestibular Disorders

Disorder	Characteristics	Auditory	Caloric	Nystagmus	Neurologic Symptoms and Signs
Menière syndrome	Paroxysmal vertigo, tinnitus, fluctuating but eventually progressive permanent hearing loss Recurrent attacks	Cochlear pattern of hearing loss (occasionally bilateral)	Minimally abnormal	Only at peak attack Usually horizontal often with slow phase towards good ear	None
Benign paroxysmal positional vertigo	Only positional vertigo Severe, usually self-limited, often secondary to trauma	Normal	Usually normal	Positional nystagmus is of peripheral type Mixture of vertical and rotatory Elicited with affected ear down	None
Vestibular neuronitis	Acute onset, nonpositional vertigo, usually self-limited, etiology unknown	Normal	Marked hypoactivity	Horizontal-rotatory Slow phase towards bad ear	None
Drug toxicity					
Streptomycin Kanamycin Gentamycin	Insidious onset Often irreversible Bilateral	Usually not affected	Decreased bilaterally	Often absent	None
Blood dyscrasias (hemorrhage into labyrinth)	Acute	Normal	Absent on side of lesion	Horizontal rotatory Slow phase toward bad ear	None
Acoustic neuroma	Insidious onset Vertigo unusual Commonly imbalance, vague dizziness with unilateral hearing loss or tinnitus	Retrocochlear pattern of hearing loss	Hypoactive responses	If present, usually horizontal with slow phase in either direction	Decreased corneal response Trigeminal sensory loss Gait ataxic Mild facial nerve involvement

ral discomfort, facial numbness, pain, or paresthesia, ataxia, loss of taste, dysphagia, or dysarthria. Early in the course of the condition neurologic examination may be normal except for hearing loss, but eventually patients show signs of involvement of other cranial nerves, the cerebellum, and brain stem. Papilledema and lower cranial nerve dysfunction are late signs and indicate a large tumor.

If the neurologic examination shows any abnormality, or caloric or audiometric tests reveal an abnormality suggestive of an eighth nerve tumor, the patient should have a CAT scan and polytomograms

TABLE 127-7
CNS Disorders in Which Vertigo May Be a Prominent Feature

Disease	Comment
Multiple sclerosis	Acute vertiginous episode may be first manifestation; oscillopsia frequent
Syringobulbia	Pure rotatory nystagmus common
Lateral medullary infarction (Wallenberg syndrome)	Severe lateropulsion to side of lesion, nystagmus, and vertigo
Cerebellar hemorrhage	Severe nausea and vomiting, gait ataxia, surgically remediable
Transient ischemic attacks	Usually associated with brain stem symptoms and signs
Posterior fossa tumors	Positional nystagmus of central type, gaze-paretic nystagmus
Arnold-Chiari malformation	Vertical oscillopsia, downbeat nystagmus Postional nystagmus of central type
Basilar migraine	Other signs of brain stem involvement, headache
Temporal lobe epilepsy	Usually with loss of consciousness and other automatisms suggestive of a seizure

TABLE 127-8
Eighth Nerve Lesions

Acoustic neuroma (if bilateral, von Recklinghausen's disease)

Cholesteatoma

Meningioma

Teratoma

Metastatic carcinoma (especially lung and breast)

Arachnoid cysts

Vascular malformations and aneurysms

Paget's disease

Glomus jugulare tumors

Mononeuropathy (meningeal carcinomatosis, diabetes, vasculitis, sarcoidosis)

TABLE 127-9
Drugs Used in the Treatment of Vertigo

Sedatives	
Phenobarbital	32 mg p.o. t.i.d.
Diazepam (Valium)	2–5 mg p.o. t.i.d.
Anticholinergics	
Atropine	0.4 mg sublingual prn
Scopalamine	0.1 mg p.o.
Antiemetics	
Trimethobenzamide (Tigan)	200 mg p.o. or p.r.
Prochlorperazine (Compazine)	5–25 mg p.o. or p.r.
Antihistamines	
Dimenhydrinate (Dramamine)	50 mg p.o. t.i.d.
Meclizine (Bonine Antivert)	25–50 mg p.o. t.i.d.

of the internal auditory meatus. If the CAT scan is negative, a cisternal (cerebellopontine angle) myelogram with tomography should be performed and, at the same time, the CSF protein level determined since it may be elevated in acoustic tumors. If all tests are negative careful follow-up examination is still indicated with audiograms, caloric tests, CAT scans, and tomograms as necessary.

Treatment is surgical. For small tumors, translabyrinthine removal is possible with minimal risk. For larger tumors, posterior fossa exploration is indicated but, with microsurgical techniques, the outlook is much improved.

TREATMENT

Symptomatic treatment of vertigo is often unsatisfactory and therapy aimed at the underlying cause is most effective. Fortunately, most peripheral disorders are self-limited and reassurance of the patient along with judicious use of sedatives, antiemetics, and antivertiginous agents (Table 127-9) is indicated. These agents are more effective when used prophylactically between attacks than in an attempt to abort an attack already in progress.

Patients with intractable, incapacitating vertigo occasionally require destruction of either the labyrinth or portions of the vestibular nerve.

CHAPTER 128

Seizures and Syncope

GUY M. McKHANN

It is estimated that 3 to 5 percent of the population will have at least one seizure during their lifetime and that 0.5 percent have a significant problem with recurrent seizures.[113]

A seizure represents the uncontrolled, synchronous firing of a group of cerebral neurons. The spread of the seizure involves the recruitment of surrounding or closely interconnected groups of neurons in similar activity. Any abnormal motor, sensory, or psychic phenomenon which is abrupt in onset, of short duration, and followed by a return to normal, could represent a seizure. The specific clinical features depend largely on the regions of the brain initially involved and the rate and pattern of spread of the abnormal discharge.

Several investigators have suggested that the basic pathophysiology involves abnormal "epileptic neurons," with lower thresholds for firing. Other investigators have suggested that the neurons are responding to an abnormal or excessive input. It is entirely possible that there are different cellular mechanisms depending on the etiology of the seizure disorder or the type of model system being studied.[108]

At present, there are many unanswered questions about seizures, such as how they start, what governs their pattern of spread, and why they stop. Management of seizures is based primarily on empirical observations regarding how certain types of seizures behave in patients of various ages and the response of these seizures to various modes of therapy.

CLINICAL MANIFESTATIONS

CLASSIFICATION

Seizures may be considered in two broad categories: 1) focal seizures including temporal lobe seizures; and 2) generalized seizures (Table 128–1). This categorization has both diagnostic and therapeutic implications. Diagnostically, if a patient has focal or temporal lobe seizures, the physician is obliged to investigate the nature of the lesion thoroughly, for in certain age groups a treatable mass (neoplasm or abscess) is the most likely etiology (Tables 128–2 and 128–3). Generalized seizures, on the other hand, rarely have a definable, remediable etiology. Therapeutically, as indicated in Table 128–4, drug treatment differs with different types of seizures. However, more than half of patients with epilepsy will have more than one type of seizure.

Focal Seizures

This type of seizure arises from a single focus, or multiple foci, in the gray matter of the cerebral cortex. Certain areas, particularly the primary motor and sensory areas of the cortex, are more frequently involved than others, such as the occipital cortex. In a typical seizure there is an *aura* or warning, the onset of motor activity, often with tonic-clonic movements, and a *spread* from one involved area to another, followed by a *postictal phase,* during which lethargy, confusion, headache, or focal weakness may last for many hours. The exact pattern of the seizure depends on the area of cortex involved. Thus, seizures may be sharply focal in onset with a characteristic march, dictated by the sequence of recruitment of neighboring motor cortex, as in so-called *Jacksonian epilepsy.* Conversely, the primary manifestations may be sensory, such as numbness, a tingling in the leg or hand, followed closely by motor phenomena.

TEMPORAL LOBE (PSYCHOMOTOR) SEIZURES. Temporal lobe seizures can be considered a subcategory of focal seizures, but the clinical manifestations may be divided into the four categories outlined in Table 128–1.

Some cortical foci fire downstream, to deeper, central structures of the brain which then discharge simultaneously back up to the cortex. This phenomenon, known as *secondary bilateral synchrony,* often arises from foci in the temporal or mesial frontal cortex, and may present as staring spells in association with some lateralizing phenomena. This form of seizure is difficult to distinguish from the less common petit mal attack of primary subcortical origin and requires careful electroencephalographic analysis. The distinction is important, because the patient with secondary bilateral synchrony should be evaluated in a fashion similar to a patient with more classical cortical seizures.

Generalized Seizures

TONIC-CLONIC. Discharges from an abnormal focus may remain localized or lead abruptly to generalized seizures. In the latter case, consciousness is suddenly lost, the patient falls, stiffens out, may stop

1271

┌───┐

TABLE 128-1
Seizure Classification

Type	Characteristics	Electroencephalographic Localization
I. Focal		
A. Motor		
Focal motor	Aura → lateralized motor	Cortical foci of spikes and slow waves
Jacksonian	March of motor events	Same as above
Aversive	Turning of head and eyes to opposite side	Often of frontal lobe origin
B. Sensory		
Somatosensory	Tingling, numbness	Parietal lobe
Visual	Flashing lights and color, postictal blindness (rare)	Occipital lobe
C. Temporal Lobe		
Psychomotor and emotional states	Automatisms, dream states, fear and other emotional responses, lip smacking, and chewing	Anterior temporal lobe foci
Visceral and autonomic	Epigastric distress, nausea, vomiting, sweating, tachycardia	Mesial temporal foci (may require sleep activation)
Illusory and hallucinatory	Olfactory (unicinate fits), sense of familiarity (déjà vu), feeling of unreality, memory flashbacks, formed visual hallucinations	Mesial and anterior temporal foci
Auditory and vertiginous	Unformed and formed auditory sensations, dizziness	Lateral temporal foci
II. Generalized		
A. Generalized tonic-clonic	Aura → unconsciousness → tonic + clonic movements → postictal drowsiness	Single or multiple coritcal foci of spikes in any area of cortex
B. Absence		
Minor motor (petit mal)	Brief lapses in contact with staring and speech arrest	Synchronous, symmetrical 3/second spike and wave discharges. No cortical localization
Temporal lobe	Staring spells plus motor movements	2° bilateral synchrony
C. Other		
Akinetic	Sudden loss of consciousness	Synchronous firing from deep lesions (often frontal)
Myclonic	Quick repetitive jerks	Multifocal spikes

└───┘

breathing and become cyanotic, bite his tongue, and empty his bladder and rectum. This tonic phase may last for 30 to 60 seconds (to the observer it seems forever), and is followed by a clonic phase consisting of rhythmic jerking of all parts of the body, labored respirations, frothing at the mouth, and then complete flaccidity. There is then a gradual return to consciousness, often blending into a period of confusion, lethargy, or of sleep of varying duration.

Many variations of the above-described sequence can occur. Commonly, the aura is poorly described or absent, as in an akinetic seizure, or "drop" attack, in which a patient suddenly crashes to the ground. Anticonvulsant drugs can alter the pattern of seizures in a particular patient. For example, inadequate therapy may remove the aura or warning, but leave a patient with uncontrolled major motor attacks.

ABSENCE SEIZURES (PETIT MAL, MINOR MOTOR SEIZURES). These attacks commonly begin in childhood or adolescence, and have a self-limited course. In a typical episode, the patient has a sudden loss of contact with his environment of short duration, during which he will develop a dazed expression, pause in what he is doing, or have a transient arrest of speech.

---TABLE 128-2---
Causes of Seizures

Severe birth trauma	Anoxia, contusion
Congenital	Maldevelopment
Metabolic	Hypoglycemia, hypocalcemia, hyponatremia, uremia, disorders of amino acid and vitamin metabolism, lipidoses
Infection	Encephalitis, meningitis
Perinatal injury	Temporal lobe sclerosis
Neoplastic	Primary and metastatic tumors
Vascular	Postinfarction, arteriovenous malformations, sickle cell disease, hematomas, arteritis
Postnatal trauma	Penetrating head wounds, contusion, anoxia
Toxins and withdrawal	Lead, alcohol, barbiturates, steroids, organic phosphates, change in anticonvulsants

Often, the episodes are so brief that only a close observer can detect them at all. The frequency may be strikingly high, with over 100 attacks per day. When attacks occur very frequently, each attack may not be recognized because the patient may have hours or days of confusion or impaired memory (petit mal status).

This type of seizure may have a classical electro-encephalographic representation: synchronous, symmetrical spike and wave discharges at three-per-second.

The distinction of petit mal from seizures resulting from bilateral secondary discharge from a cortical focus is important because this latter type of seizure continues into adult life, may change in its clinical manifestations with the appearance of more motor phenomena, and requires a different therapeutic approach (Table 128-4). This distinction requires careful electroencephalography.

Status Epilepticus
When attacks of any sort occur so frequently that there is incomplete recovery, the patient is in status epilepticus. The diagnosis is not always easy. Repeated tonic-clonic attacks are obvious. Other patients present in coma, without movements or perhaps only sustained deviation of the eyes. Other patients may have focal manifestations, such as occurs in *epilepsia partialis continua,* in which focal seizure activity may persist for weeks.

Status epilepticus may be precipitated by a number of factors, such as the abrupt withdrawal of anticonvulsant medications, particularly barbiturates. Chronic alcoholics who stop drinking may have seizures ("rum fits") within 12 to 48 hours. These seizures are sometimes induced by photic stimulation and may be related to hypomagnesemia and respiratory alkalosis (see Chapter 153).

---TABLE 128-3---
Causes of Seizures at Various Ages of Onset

	Newborn	Infant	Child	Adolescent	Young Adult	Old Adult
Severe birth trauma	+ + + +*	+ + +	+	+	±	−
Congenital defect	+ + +	+ + +	+	±	−	−
Metabolic defect	+ +	+ / + / + +	+ +	+	+	±
Infection	+ + +	+ + +	+ +	+	+	+
Perinatal injury	+	+	+	+ + +	+ +	−
Postnatal trauma	−	−	+	+ +	+ + +	+ + +
Brain tumor	−	−	±	+	+ + +	+ +
Vascular disease	−	−	±	±	+	+ + +
Toxins and withdrawal	+	±	±	+	+ + +	+ +

*(+ + + + = most likely; − = unlikely).

TABLE 128-4
Characteristics of Common Anticonvulsants

Drug	Dosage (mg/day)	Responsive Seizure Type	Serum Half-life (hrs)	Effective Blood Level ($\mu g/ml$)	Toxic Level ($\mu g/ml$)	Toxicity Dose-Related	Toxicity Non-Dose-Related
Phenytoin (Dilantin)	300–400	Focal Generalized Temporal lobe	24 ± 12	10–20	>20	Nystagmus, ataxia, drowsiness	Gingival hyperplasia, skin eruptions, lymphadenopathy, blood dyscrasias, SLE
Phenobarbital	45–180	Focal Generalized Temporal lobe	96 ± 12	15–40	>40	Slowness, ataxia, coma	Sedatation, hyperactivity, blood dyscrasias, rash
Primidone (Mysoline)	125–750	Temporal lobe	12 ± 6	8–12	>12	Same as for phenobarbital	
Ethosuximide (Zarontin)	500–1500	Absence seizures	30 ± 6	40–100	>100	Nausea, vomiting, anorexia, dizziness	Skin rash, blood dyscrasias, SLE
Carbamazepine (Tegretol)	600–1200	Temporal lobe	12 ± 3	4	>8	Vertigo, dizziness, drowsiness, diplopia, water intoxication	Blood dyscrasias, gastrointestinal disturbances
Valproic acid (Depakene)	15–45* kg.	Absence seizures Myoclonic seizures	Varies 8–20	50	?	Nausea, vomiting, cramps	Increase in phenobarbital levels from 30–200%, ? hepatic toxicity

* mg/kg.

DIAGNOSTIC MANAGEMENT

The approach to the patient may be divided into 1) the recognition that the symptoms are caused by seizures; 2) the categorization of the seizures; 3) a search for an underlying cause; and 4) the institution of therapy. The order in which these steps are performed depends on the clinical circumstances. For example, with status epilepticus, primary attention is given to controlling the seizures.

RECOGNITION OF SEIZURES
The recognition of seizures depends on the correct interpretation of the clinical features, which vary widely. Essential to the evaluation is first-hand observation of the seizure or a detailed description by a competent witness. Particular attention should be paid to the *onset* of the seizure. It should be noted that the aura is part of the seizure and often an indi-

cation of the focus of initial discharge. Also of importance are the *sequence of spread*, either motor or sensory, and any indication of *lateralizing signs* during or after the seizure.

Several misleading presentations are worthy of mention. Generalized seizures may be confused with hysteria. Akinetic seizures may be confused with syncope. Temporal lobe seizures may be difficult to separate from acute psychotic episodes. Focal motor seizures may be confused with other movement disorders such as myoclonus or chorea. Recognition of the fact that seizures are one of the few motor disturbances which occur in sleep can be helpful in distinguishing seizures from other movement disorders.

SEARCH FOR CAUSE
The search for an underlying cause is aided by recognizing that different processes deserve greater emphasis for patients of different ages (Tables 128–2 and

---

TABLE 128-5
Diagnostic Studies in Seizures

Hemogram and sedimentation rate
Urinalysis
Serologic test for syphilis
Fasting blood glucose
Serum urea nitrogen
Serum calcium and phosphorus
Carbon dioxide combining power
Chest x-ray
Skull x-ray
Electroencephalogram
Cerebral scintiscan or CAT scan
Lumbar puncture ⎫
Cerebral arteriogram ⎬ if indicated

128–3). It is desirable to limit investigations to likely conditions, emphasizing treatable possibilities. A common error is the failure to realize that a generalized metabolic state, such as hypoglycemia or hypocalcemia may present as focal or lateralizing seizures. Thus, one is ill advised to take any shortcuts in the initial metabolic screening. The electroencephalogram is useful for establishing the pattern, degree, and location of electrical abnormality (Table 128–5).

In the age group where neoplasm is likely, one should proceed in a logical, step-wise fashion in a search for a mass lesion, as outlined in Chapter 131. The decision whether to include invasive studies such as angiography requires careful judgment. If there is any suggestion of a progressive process in a patient between 20 to 50 years of age, then a thorough search for an underlying tumor should be undertaken.

THERAPEUTIC MANAGEMENT

DRUG TREATMENT

The goal of drug treatment is optimal seizure control without significant side effects from medication. It is wise for the physician to learn how to use a few anticonvulsant drugs properly rather than be in a confused state regarding the large number of potential anticonvulsants.[112] The choice of anticonvulsant medication is dictated, in part, by the pattern of electrical and clinical seizures, as outlined in Table 128–4.

Phenobarbital is an effective anticonvulsant, whose primary pharmacological effect may be to suppress the primary epileptogenic foci.[112] In many instances, this drug is used in conjunction with *phenyt-*

oin (Dilantin), which may have as its primary effect the suppression of spread, of propagation, of the abnormal activity.[110] These drugs are most effective in modifying seizures of cortical origin.

Absence seizures may respond to succinimides, such as *ethosuximide* (Zarontin) or *valproate* (Depakene). In patients with secondary bilateral synchrony, the combination of cortical drugs (phenobarbital and Dilantin) and a subcortical drug (Zarontin) may be quite effective.

Seizures of temporal lobe origin are the most difficult to treat. A certain percentage of patients will respond to the combination of phenobarbital and Dilantin. Others require *primidone* (Mysoline) or *carbamazepine* (Tegretol).

Surgical Therapy

Surgical therapy is considered for patients with focal, cortical seizures who have failed to respond to adequate medical therapy. This therapy requires careful delineation of the epileptogenic focus and a weighing of the possibility of postsurgical defects against the disability of continuing seizures. For this reason, the usefulness of surgical therapy has been limited primarily to patients with temporal lobe and frontal lobe foci.

MANAGEMENT OF STATUS EPILEPTICUS

Status epilepticus, with generalized seizures, is a medical emergency with a significant mortality. Death or brain damage may occur from the continuing seizures and accompanying anoxia, or the underlying cerebral trauma or disease, or from injudicious medical management.

Patients with status epilepticus should be managed as described for coma (Chap. 147). The physician should be constantly concerned about the maintenance of an adequate airway. Other intercurrent problems besides aspiration are dehydration and electrolyte imbalance (Chap. 9), hyperthermia (Chap. 149), cardiac arrhythmias (Chap. 21), shock (Chap. 145), and respiratory depression (Chap. 144). A tabular chronologic account of the patient's clinical state and therapy greatly aids proper management.

In a patient not previously known to have seizures, the treatable causes of seizures should be excluded. In a patient with known seizures it is helpful to ascertain if the clinical state is related to the omission of therapy, alcohol withdrawal, infection, or trauma.

A physician should develop a logical plan for management of status epilepticus, become familiar with the effects and side effects of anticonvulsant drugs in adequate dosage, and be prepared to relieve respiratory depression. Probably the most common error in the treatment of status epilepticus is the use of inadequate amounts of too many drugs (Table 128–6).

Certain principles of therapy of status epilepticus with generalized seizures may be listed.

1. Recognize that there are two phases to drug therapy. The stopping of seizures, acutely, and the prevention of recurrence, with longer-acting drugs.
2. Use drugs in adequate amounts.
3. Administer drugs by a reliable route. Slow, intravenous administration is preferred.
4. Assess central depression carefully; between seizures, if possible.
5. Keep in mind that potentially lethal amounts of drugs are being administered and that deep coma with respiratory depression and hypotension may result. It should be recognized that in some patients the depressant effects of the drugs are more threatening than the continuation of the seizures.

TABLE 128–6
Treatment of Status Epilepticus in Adults

Step	Remarks
1. Maintain adequate airway and oxygenation	Patient may require O$_2$ by mask
2. Obtain blood glucose and anticonvulsant levels	
3. Thiamine, 100 mg intravenously	May be omitted in known seizure patient
4. Glucose, 25–50 g intravenously	May be omitted in known seizure patient
5. Initial anticonvulsant therapy	
A. Diazepam,[107,113] 5–10 mg intravenously or	May be repeated 2–3 times at 10-minute intervals
B. Phenytoin, 250 mg intravenously or	May be repeated 2–3 times at 20–30-minute intervals
C. Phenobarbital, 100 g intravenously	May be repeated 2–3 times at 20–30-minute intervals
6. If seizures continue after Step 5, then administer	
A. Paraldehyde, 4–6 ml intravenously	Administer slowly, may be repeated 2–3 times
B. Sodium amytal, 500 mg intravenously or	Administer slowly, patient may require respiratory assistance
7. If seizures still continue, use	
A. General anesthesia	Only as a last resort, very rarely required
8. Maintenance anticonvulsants	Depends on previous treatment, phenobarbital or phenytoin required after use of diazepam

---

LONG-TERM MANAGEMENT OF SEIZURES

It is incorrect to emphasize the acute therapy of seizures and to disregard the problems associated with continuing management. For a given patient, questions about how to adjust medications for proper seizure control, when to stop medications, when to reevaluate the patient for an underlying, progressive lesion, and what to tell the patient in terms of his pattern of living are more common and more important than how to treat status.

USE OF ANTICONVULSANTS

In adjusting anticonvulsants, two principles should be kept in mind. 1) Before abandoning a particular drug, increase the dosage to the maximum amount the patient can tolerate; and 2) change only one medication at a time. If a new medication is to be tried, it is preferable to add it to existing medications. A previous medication can be removed after seizure control is achieved. Measurement of blood levels of anticonvulsant drugs can be helpful in adjusting dosages, confirming toxicity, or confirming compliance with the prescribed therapy. Often the use of blood levels provides objective data about lack of compliance.

INDICATIONS FOR REEVALUATION

If the physician is going to follow a patient with seizures in whom a progressive, mass lesion is a possibility, he should have a clear set of criteria for reevaluation. These criteria include: 1) a failure to respond to medication or a recurrence of previously controlled seizures, 2) a changing clinical pattern of seizures, 3) the appearance of previously absent neurologic symptoms and signs, including behavioral changes, and 4) changing laboratory data such as a more focal electroencephalographic abnormality, a positive CAT scan, or the appearance of intracranial calcification on skull x-ray.

COUNSELING

A seizure is a frightening experience for a patient, his family, and his colleagues. There are still many misconceptions and superstitions regarding seizures. It is important to explore with the patient his ideas and concerns about seizures and the need for continuing medications. Patients will have many questions regarding restrictions on their pattern of living, such as driving, riding a bicycle, working conditions, swimming, pregnancy, or long-term effects of medications. It is difficult to generalize, because seizures are a symptom rather than a specific disease. However, guidelines can be offered.

The answer to common questions about seizures are as follows:

1. *Do I have epilepsy?*

Epilepsy is not a disease entity. It is another term for seizures. The term implies an active seizure process requiring medication for control.

2. *Are seizures hereditary?*

Except for certain well-characterized conditions, such as tuberous sclerosis or disorders of amino acid, carbohydrate, or lipid metabolism, seizures are not genetically determined.

3. *Do anticonvulsants provide an increased risk to a fetus?*

If there is a teratogenic effect of anticonvulsants it is early in pregnancy. Thus, in the woman who wants to become pregnant and is taking anticonvulsants, certain guidelines can be suggested.

a. Review the patient's seizure history carefully to be sure anticonvulsants are needed.

b. Trimethadione is associated with fetal malformations and should not be used during pregnancy.[106]

c. Phenytoin is associated with a 4 to 5 percent risk of abnormalities; a poorly defined "fetal hydantoin syndrome" has been suggested.[106] If possible, an other anticonvulsant, such as phenobarbital, should be used.

d. Phenobarbital does not appear to be teratogenic.[106,112] There are insufficient data to make statements about other anticonvulsants.

4. *Will anticonvulsants interfere with my intellectual performance?*

There is no evidence that anticonvulsant drugs, maintained at therapeutic blood levels, significantly impair a person's ability to function. If such seems to be the case, blood levels should be monitored to determine if the patient is metabolizing an anticonvulsant in an aberrant way.

5. *May I drive?*

Legal restrictions on driving by patients with seizures vary from state to state. A guideline can be that a patient should be seizure-free for one year, with or without medications, before driving. The duration and pattern of seizures in an individual patient, however, might lead the physician to modify this advice.

6. *How should I lead my life?*

The guideline for general living is common sense. The goal is for the patient to live as normal a life as possible. The physician must balance the disrupting effects of restrictions against potential risk to the patient. For example, it is as needlessly restrictive to a patient to prohibit swimming regardless of the degree of supervision, as it is foolhardy to allow such a patient to swim alone.

7. *I am free of seizures. Can I stop my anticonvulsants?*

There are very little data with which to answer this question. Patients who have a history of multiple seizures prior to therapy, or a persistently abnormal EEG are advised to continue medication despite being clinically free of seizures.

FAINTING AND SYNCOPE

Many patients will have transient feelings of lightheadedness, faintness, or dizziness. Some will go on to frank syncope, in which the patient will become pale, pulseless, collapse to the ground, and remain unconscious for a brief period. Usually after lying flat, or sitting with his head lowered between his knees, the patient will recover to his normal state. There are distinguishing features between syncope and a seizure as outlined in Table 128–7.

The cause of lightheadedness and syncope is a lack of proper perfusion or nutrition of the brain. There are a variety of causes (Table 128–8), most of which are self-evident. However, there are a large number of people who faint in a combination of conditions such as prolonged standing, a stuffy atmosphere, and anxiety, for whom the exact mechanism is not clear. The term "vasovagal" has been applied to this group without any clear idea of the mechanism.

---TABLE 128–7---
Seizures Versus Syncope

	Seizure	Syncope
Premonitory symptoms	May have aura	Tinnitus, dim vision
Onset	Sudden	Gradual
Position	Any	Usually standing
Color	Normal	Pale
Duration	Varied	Brief
Blood pressure	Varied	Low
Recovery	Delayed	Prompt
Postictal state	Confused	Normal
Tonic-clonic movements	Common	Rare
Incontinence	Common	Rare
EEG	Seizure discharge	Slowing

---TABLE 128–8---
Causes of Syncope

I. **Decreased Cerebral Perfusion**
  A. Postural hypotension
    1. Primary autonomic neuropathy
      a. diabetic, amyloid, Shy-Drager syndrome
    2. Postsympathectomy
    3. Pharmacologic sympathectomy
    4. End-organ insensitivity
    5. Hypovolemia
      a. Blood loss
      b. Excess diuretics or sweating
    6. Vasovagel syncope
  B. Decreased cardiac output (Chap. 16)
  C. Cardiac arrythmias (Chap. 21)

II. **Decreased Venous Return**
  A. Micturition
  B. Valsalva
  C. Cough

III. **Altered Metabolism**
  A. Hypoglycemia
  B. Anemia
  C. Hypoxia
  D. Decreased CO_2 (Hyperventilation)

IV. **Emotional**
  A. Anxiety
  B. Hysteria

---CHAPTER 129---
Stroke Syndromes and Cerebrovascular Disorders
THOMAS J. PREZIOSI

Strokes are caused by impaired cerebral circulation and are manifest by an abrupt deficit in neurologic function. This impairment may be in motor, sensory, or mental function; the dysfunction may be major or minor, transient or permanent. Although the term "stroke" does not give precise indications of etiology or pathogenesis, it does convey an image of abrupt onset, the most characteristic feature of the syndrome. It is at least as acceptable as the pseudoscientific terms "cerebral apoplexy" or "cerebrovascular accident."

It is important that all physicians be competent in the management of strokes for several reasons:

1. Strokes are the most common disorder affecting the central nervous system.
2. Other disorders may mimic strokes and vice versa.

3. In many instances proper diagnostic and therapeutic management has a profound influence on the outcome.[115]

Therapeutic management obviously rests upon optimal diagnostic definition. Diagnosis, in turn, depends upon several factors:

1. Syndrome recognition: The physician must be familiar with the common constellations of symptoms and signs which are associated with various clinical entities.
2. Analysis of time course: Strokes of various etiologies often have distinctive temporal patterns.
3. Anatomic localization: The site of the lesion, as determined by interpretation of the neurologic findings, may provide information re-

garding the probable cause. Furthermore, a single, precisely localized lesion suggests a different etiology from that which causes multiple lesions.

4. Ancillary tests: The wise use of additional studies may reveal the diagnosis, while an unwise strategy can subject the patient to unnecessary risk and expense.

This chapter presents an approach to the management of the patient with a stroke or who appears to have sustained a stroke. Topics include: 1) a description of the clinical entities which cause strokes (with emphasis on the distinguishing clinical features); 2) a strategy for approaching the common modes of presentation (including differential diagnosis); 3) comments on the situations which lead to incorrect management; and finally 4) the principles of therapeutic management. These aspects will be discussed in order.

CLINICAL ENTITIES

These conditions include occlusions and hemorrhages involving arteries or veins. They should properly be regarded as clinical entities rather than diseases in the etiologic sense. For example, there is no essential difference between the clinical manifestations of a cerebral arterial embolus whether the etiology is infective endocarditis or mural thrombosis following myocardial infarction. As mentioned earlier, many of these entities can be sufficiently distinctive that the clinician can be reasonably certain of the diagnosis on clinical findings alone. At other times diligent investigation may fail to reveal the precise cause of the disorder. This section emphasizes the distinctive clinical features of each entity and lists the etiologic causes that must be considered.

OCCLUSION

Arterial Occlusion

Occlusion of a vessel may produce effects that range from disastrous to undetectable. The outcome depends upon the availability of the collateral flow into the involved territory from neighboring vessels, the size and position in the vascular tree of the occluded vessel, the duration of the occlusion, and the nature of the occluding agent. The clinical effects reflect the locus and extent of the damaged tissue, not the exact vessels occluded, or the etiology of the occlusions. Accordingly, even the major etiologic categories of

embolus and thrombus are frequently difficult to separate from one another. What follows is a description of clinical features which, although not invariably present, can be helpful in distinguishing the differing etiologies.

Clinical features which are found with occlusion of individual major intracranial vessels are found in Table 129-1.

EMBOLISM. Cerebral emboli may arise from mural cardiac thrombi[122] in atrial fibrillation or myocardial infarction, vegetations in infective endocarditis, calcific plaques in the major extracranial arteries, thrombi from leg veins via a patent foramen ovale, fat, air, tumor, foreign bodies, and from various other sources. No neurologic symptoms occur prior to the arrival of emboli to the brain. Accordingly, embolic strokes appear as a sudden surprise, frequently occurring shortly after the patient arises in the morning, or during periods of activity. Little is known of the physical means by which emboli make their way into the brain circulation, but they appear to be arrested at bifurcations, after which they may fragment, passing into single or multiple vessels further along in the circulation. These events are reflected in the occasional spectacular improvement in the clinical picture in which a large neurologic deficit caused by occlusion of a large artery becomes reduced to that of a smaller cortical artery's territory. Since individual cortical arteries may be the point of final embolic occlusion, isolated cortical deficits, such as pure sensory aphasia[135] or alexia, are most easily attributable to emboli.

Emboli are frequently difficult to find at autopsy, and an arteriogram done immediately after an embolic episode may occasionally demonstrate an embolus which is then no longer seen on a repeat arteriogram a day or more later. Emboli almost invariably occur in showers. Therefore, the clinical picture is frequently that of multifocal neurologic deficits which shift with time. However, other causes, including thrombocytopenic purpura, thrombotic thrombocytopenic purpura, and systemic lupus erythematosus must be considered.

THROMBOSIS. An enormous variety of etiologies can set the stage for thrombosis (see Table 129-2). Those detailed here are the more common. Like embolism, thrombosis may appear in a sudden, surprising fashion. However, a number of features of thrombosis, when present, help to separate it from embolism.

Atheromatous thrombosis is often characterized by a stepwise increment of deficits in the same vascular territory.[128] The deficits may be minor in the first attack, but grow steadily in severity and number with

---
TABLE 129–1

Major Symptoms and Signs of Cerebral Arterial Occlusions

Artery	Motor and Sensory Signs	Speech/Language Deficits

1. Middle cerebral
upper division
	Contralateral hemiplegia, hemisensory loss
	Paresis of conjugate gaze to opposite side
	Occasional contralateral homonymous
	   hemianopia
		Dominant hemisphere
		   Motor speech dyspraxia (Broca's
		      aphasia)
		   Dysgraphia
		   Dyspraxia of nondominant extremities

Lower division	Contralateral homonymous hemianopia	Dominant hemisphere
		   Central (sensory) aphasia (Wernicke's)
		   Dyslexia with dysgraphia
		   Gerstmann syndrome
		   Global dyspraxia
		Nondominant hemisphere
		   Contralateral hemisphere
		   Dyspraxias for constructions, dressing

Lenticulostriates	Contralateral "pure" motor hemiplegia,
	   without sensory loss, hemianopia,
	   language deficits
		None

2. Posterior cerebral
central regions
	Contralateral hemisensory loss,
	   occasionally with "thalamic syndrome"
	   of pain, dysesthesias
	Contralateral ataxic tremor
	Paresis of upward gaze (Parinaud
	   syndrome)
		Possible dysnomic aphasia

Peripheral regions	Contralateral homonymous hemianopia,
	   occasionally upper quadrantic
		Korsakoff memory deficit
		Wide variety of complex visual deficits
		   including dyslexia, inability to name
		   objects, estimate depth, direction
		Unawareness of deficits

3. Anterior cerebral central regions	Contralateral hemiplegia, leg predominating Grasp, suck reflexes, gegenhalten	Akinetic mutism Apraxia of nondominant limbs
Peripheral regions	Urinary incontinence Contralateral paresis foot, ankle, leg Contralateral sensory deficit foot, ankle, leg	

4. Internal carotid	Any combination of the above
	Frequently disproportionate motor and
	   sensory deficits referable to fingers,
	   hand, arm	

5. Vertebro-basilar	Ipsilateral cranial nerve deficits Contralateral (or bilateral) motor, sensory, or cerebellar signs	Dysarthria without aphasia

succeeding attacks. A frequent additional feature is the tendency for atherothrombosis to involve the larger arteries, especially the extracranial carotid arteries, and to spare the individual cortical surface arteries. Symptoms and signs of *carotid artery disease*[118] may include transient monocular blindness (from involvement of the ophthalmic artery); a reduced carotid artery pulse in the neck (common carotid artery), or in front of the ear (external carotid, reflecting involvement of the common carotid artery),

or low central retinal artery pressure (internal carotid artery via ophthalmic artery) as revealed by ophthalmodynamometry; a bruit heard over the carotid bifurcation or over the orbit (indicating flow through a stenotic vessel, flow over a plaque, or murmur from the heart); occasionally a bruit is heard over the carotid artery opposite the one occluded (caused by augmented flow through the open carotid artery). Neurologic symptoms referable to carotid artery involvement vary considerably.[134] Most commonly, they are

TABLE 129–2
Causes of Cerebral Arterial Thrombosis

I. Disease of the Arterial Wall

    A. Atherosclerosis
    B. Inflammation
        1. Infectious: Meningovascular syphilis; septic embolism, arteritis secondary to pyogenic or granulomatous meningitis
        2. Noninfectious: Lupus erythematosus, rheumatic arteritis, polyarteritis nodosa, granulomatous arteritis, giant-cell (temporal) arteritis

II. Mechanical Constriction of Arteries

    A. Cervical spondylosis, involving vertebral arteries
    B. Compression against bony prominences or dural folds caused by increased intracranial pressure, especially the posterior cerebral artery compressed against the tentorium

III. Prolonged Vasoconstriction

    A. Subarachnoid hemorrhage, especially in the territory of the involved artery
    B. Migraine
    C. Malignant hypertension (small arteries only)

IV. Inadequate Cerebral Perfusion

    A. Systemic hypotension from any cause

V. Hematologic Disorders with Hypercoagulability

    A. Sickle cell disease
    B. Polycythemia, vera or secondary
    C. Dysproteinemias

VI. Miscellaneous

    A. Carotid artery trauma in the neck or pharynx
    B. Radiotherapy with radiation necrosis
    C. Dissecting aortic aneurysm

Causes of Intracranial Venous and Sinus Thrombosis

I. Septic Thrombosis

    A. Secondary to ear, mastoid, and paranasal infections
    B. Secondary to pyogenic or granulomatous meningitis, brain abscess, or subdural empyema

II. Aseptic Thrombosis

    A. Secondary to ear or mastoid infection (lateral sinus thrombosis)
    B. Secondary to dehydration
    C. Hematologic disorders with hypercoagulability
        1. Sickle cell disease
        2. Polycythemia, vera or secondary
    D. Congenital heart disease
    E. Postpartum and postoperative (with high platelet counts and fibrinogen levels)

predominantly those of the middle cerebral artery, with frequent coexistence of those referable to the anterior cerebral artery, and occasionally of the posterior cerebral artery (see Table 129–1). Collateral inflow across the Circle of Willis from the opposite carotid artery frequently spares the more proximal territories of the dependent arteries. Consequently, the distal territories, especially those shared by the middle and the anterior cerebral arteries, are the more commonly involved. In most cases, such involvement encompasses the superior central and frontal regions of the cerebrum, with prominent symptoms referable to the fingers, thumb, hand, and forearm. Atherothrombosis also frequently involves the *vertebral and basilar arteries* (see Table 129–1). Here the neurologic involvement is characterized by ipsilateral cranial nerve findings and contralateral or bilateral motor, sensory, or cerebellar findings. Less frequently, the stem of the posterior cerebral artery is involved.

Selective involvement of the middle or anterior cerebral arteries is rare. Hence, the diagnosis of middle cerebral artery thrombosis is usually in error. Either atherothrombosis of the internal carotid artery or embolus into the internal carotid or middle cerebral artery is usually responsible.

Small arterial thrombosis may result from hypertension. These lesions commonly involve the small arteries which penetrate the deep white matter of the frontal lobes, the basal ganglia, internal capsule, and thalamus in the cerebrum, and the pons in the brain stem. When such vessels are individually occluded, the late result of the infarct is a small cavity or lacuna.[119] Occlusion of these vessels gives rise to specific syndromes only rarely observed in occlusion of the large vessels. These include pure motor hemiplegia, pure hemisensory deficit, dysarthria with a clumsy hand, or homolateral ataxia with leg paresis. In cases with multiple frontal white matter infarcts, a syndrome of spastic gait, and pseudobulbar palsy with emotional lability is seen. Such cases are worthy of clinical delineation since arteriography is rarely helpful in their diagnosis, anticoagulants may be contraindicated in their management, and the outlook for improvement is generally good. Lacunae may also occur as a consequence of emboli arising from more proximal stenosis of larger extracranial arteries, e.g., the internal carotid or basilar. If other evidence of extracranial arterial stenosis exists further studies may be indicated.

Systemic hypotension from whatever cause reduces cerebral arterial perfusion and has its first effects in the territories most distal from the heart.[126] These are the dorsal, parietal, and lateral occipital regions of the cerebrum. With increasing severity and duration of hypotension, superior frontal, orbital, temporal, and precuneal regions are involved simultaneously with a proximal spread of involvement from superior parietal and lateral occipital regions toward the more central sylvian region. In the severe cases, virtually the entire brain may become involved. Initially the patient has difficulties with visual recognition and sensory perception. With increasing cortical involvement, the patient develops frontal lobe signs (grasping, sucking), receptive aphasia, and fluctuating levels of consciousness. In severe cases, coma, which may be irreversible, appears. Clinical and laboratory diagnosis of the functional state of the brain by electroencephalography may be indicated at that time to determine the presence or absence of cerebral death.

Venous Occlusion (Thrombosis)

Disease in the venous system is restricted to thrombosis. Its occurrence is directly related to a change in the coagulable state of the blood, inflammation of the vein, or obstruction of the venous drainage system. The potential for collateral drainage is extremely good, and the resultant neurologic deficit is usually mild and frequently reversible. An exception to this statement is disease arising in the deep venous system where occlusion is usually catastrophic.

Occlusion of venous outflow, following thrombosis of the *internal jugular vein* or the *lateral sinus* may simply produce increased intracranial pressure, which will frequently resolve after an effective collateral drainage system develops. This type of occlusion may be one of the mechanisms of pseudotumor cerebri (Chap. 131). On the other hand, if the occlusion begins or extends from the region of the *Torcula Herophile* into the *superior sagittal sinus* and superficial collecting veins, then a specific syndrome develops, consisting of multifocal neurologic signs with convulsions, severe headache, nuchal rigidity, and fever. The cerebrospinal fluid is usually bloody and the pressure may be elevated. Jugular compression may demonstrate a manometric block. The course of such occlusion may be benign as patients recover when the collateral drainage system becomes effective.

HEMORRHAGE

Hemorrhage can occur in a large number of settings (Table 129–3), but ruptured congenital aneurysm, intracerebral hemorrhage associated with hypertension, and hemorrhage from arteriovenous malformations (AVM) account for the vast majority. Their clinical syndromes are frequently sufficiently characteristic to permit a clear differential diagnosis.

TABLE 129–3
Causes of Intracranial Hemorrhage

1. Hypertensive cerebral hemorrhage
2. Ruptured congenital aneurysm
3. Ruptured arteriovenous malformation
4. Trauma
5. Hemorrhagic disorders
   A. Leukemia
   B. Hemophilia, sickle cell disease, aplastic anemia
   C. Bleeding diathesis, including excessive anticoagulant therapy
6. Hemorrhage into primary or secondary brain tumor
7. Ruptured mycotic aneurysm, secondary to septic embolism
8. Hemorrhagic (red) infarction, arterial or venous
9. Secondary brain stem hemorrhage from temporal lobe herniation

---

Aneurysm

ANATOMY. Most congenital aneurysms are saccular, and arise at the bifurcations of the arteries forming the circle of Willis (Fig. 129–1). These include the junction of the internal carotid with the middle cerebral and posterior communicating arteries, the region of the anterior communicating artery, and the first bifurcation of the middle cerebral artery. The basilar artery and its branches occasionally show aneurysm. Aneurysms are frequently multiple.

CLINICAL FEATURES. Prior to rupture, few aneurysms give evidence of their presence. It is said that recurrent unilateral migraine headaches may be a sign of aneurysm. Occasionally, an aneurysm of the posterior communicating artery, as it enlarges prior to rupture, will press against the subarachnoid course of the oculomotor nerve causing ptosis, mydriasis, and oculomotor ophthalmoplegia. In most instances, however, the first evidence of an aneurysm is its rupture.[133]

Ruptures occur frequently during strenuous physical activity, including intercourse. Virtually every case has excruciating headache. Approximately half the patients are rendered unconscious at the onset, and awakened minutes or hours later. On examination, preretinal hemorrhages are occasionally observed. The clinical profile just described is virtually diagnostic of ruptured aneurysm. Since aneurysms rupture into the subarachnoid space directly, and only incidentally and infrequently directly into the brain substance, it is common for the patient to show surprisingly few focal or lateralizing neurologic signs. The occurrence of such signs may represent rupture

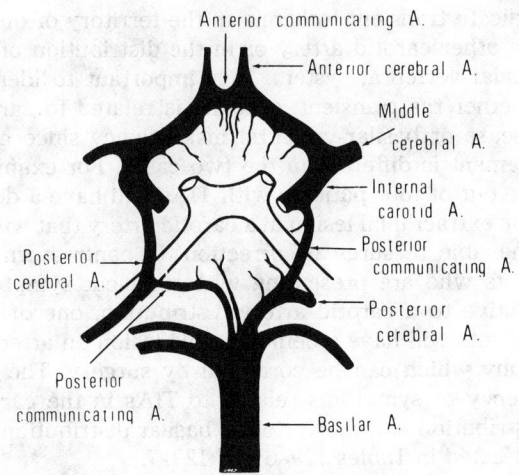

Anterior communicating A.

Anterior cerebral A.

Middle cerebral A.

Internal carotid A.

Posterior cerebral A.

Posterior communicating A.

Posterior cerebral A.

Posterior communicating A.

Basilar A.

FIGURE 129-1. Drawing of circle of Willis. (Modified from Peele. The Neuroanatomical Basis for Clinical Neurology. Courtesy of McGraw-Hill Book Company.)

into the brain substance or vasospasm following the rupture.[132] Such vasospasm need not invariably be in the territory of the involved artery.

For reasons which are not completely understood, patients often develop increased intracranial pressure after a subarachnoid hemorrhage. This may appear within hours, but usually is most severe 24 to 48 hours after the bleed, and may produce headache and altered consciousness. Bleeding occurs again in about half of cases and is most likely to occur during the first week. The differentiation of increased intracranial pressure from a rebleed may be difficult, and require repeated lumbar punctures. When present, increased intracranial pressure may be relieved by steroids or osmotic agents (Chap. 131).

LABORATORY FINDINGS. Another consequence of rupture into the subarachnoid space is the invariable presence of blood on lumbar puncture. The number of red cells remain constant on serial samples. By contrast, in a "traumatic tap" lumbar puncture, the number of red cells diminish in serial samples taken on the same puncture, and there is no xanthochromia. Arteriograms frequently reveal the aneurysm. When multiple aneurysms are seen, the larger is usually the one that ruptured. Since multiple aneurysms occur, it is essential for arteriography to give complete views of all intracranial vascular territories.

PROGNOSIS. Aneurysms have an unfortunate tendency to rerupture. Approximately half the patients die within 24 to 48 hours of the first rupture. Of those surviving, approximately half die of rerupture

within 6 months, with the greatest period of vulnerability in the first 24 to 48 hours, declining steadily thereafter.

Hypertensive Hemorrhage

ANATOMY. In contrast to ruptured aneurysm, hypertensive hemorrhage arises in small penetrating arteries deep in the brain substance. The artery involved can be regarded as "springing a leak," the resultant hemorrhage continuing in a steady fashion to enlarge over time to a mass of varying size. The hemorrhage then either ceases spontaneously or continues to thrust aside brain tissue until the mass causes death.

CLINICAL FEATURES. Clinically, the patients are usually elderly, hypertensive, and show not an explosive syndrome as in aneurysm, but one that evolves smoothly over time. Admittedly, the time may be very brief—a matter of minutes before the patient loses consciousness—but sufficiently long that a careful history reveals the smooth progress of symptoms. Patients with hypertensive hemorrhage show findings of local involvement, including disorders of ocular motility (see Table 129–8).[120]

Of significance in differentiation from occlusion, hypertensive hemorrhage is never rapidly reversible. As a rule, surviving patients show an unchanging deficit at least 10 to 14 days before improvements begin. Headache, so invariable with ruptured aneurysms, is not always seen in hypertensive hemorrhage, even with a bloody cerebrospinal fluid. Subhyloid or preretinal hemorrhage occur much less frequently.

LABORATORY FINDINGS. Since blood reaches the cerebrospinal fluid via seepage into the ventricle, occasionally a patient undergoes lumbar puncture before blood has reached the lumbar space, and, in small hypertensive hemorrhages wholly confined to the brain substance, the cerebrospinal fluid may remain clear. However, if the patient is comatose from a hypertensive hemorrhage, bloody cerebrospinal fluid is to be expected. Arteriograms usually show a localized mass lesion or are normal. Hypertensive hemorrhage occurs in the putamen in the majority of cases, less commonly in the thalamus, cerebellum, and pons, and the subcortical white matter of the temporo-parieto-occipital region. By contrast, intracerebral hematoma from hemorrhagic diathesis, as in poorly controlled cases on anticoagulant therapy, may occur virtually anywhere.

PROGNOSIS. Approximately 75 percent of symptomatic cases die with the original hemorrhage. As a clinical rule, a patient who continues to deteriorate after arrival at the hospital will probably die unless some form of intervention is undertaken. Those surviving probably never bleed again from the same site.

Arteriovenous Malformation (AVM)

These vascular malformations are congenital defects consisting of tangled masses of arteriovenous shunts. They can "leak," sometimes repeatedly in patients of any age, and should be suspected as the source of intracerebral bleeding in the younger, nonhypertensive patient. Since malformations lie within the substance of brain, there is always some form of focal neurologic deficit, including focal seizures, associated with their rupture. However, in contrast to hemorrhages from aneurysms or hypertensive vessels, the seepage of blood in arteriovenous malformations is from low pressure shunts. Thus there is not an explosive destruction of brain tissue. Many patients have repeated bleeds from an arteriovascular malformation with amazingly little neurologic residue. Giant arteriovenous malformations may involve the blood supply to the major portion of a cerebral hemisphere and produce a murmur that the patient can hear. Rupture of a giant arteriovenous malformation is often catastrophic and rarely amenable to therapy.[139]

THE APPROACH TO DIAGNOSTIC MANAGEMENT

In this section, the emphasis is on how the patient with an acute stroke presents to the physician. The factors to be considered are the condition of the patient, the history of previous similar or different episodes, and the symptoms associated with the stroke, as summarized in Table 129–4. The sequence of diagnostic studies is indicated in Table 129–5.

Asymptomatic Patient

One common mode of presentation is an asymptomatic patient who gives a history of one or more episodes of transient neurologic symptoms. These episodes in which the onset is abrupt, the duration is 12 to 24 hours, and recovery is complete are known as *transient ischemic attacks* (TIA).[115,124,131] A single such episode may be either embolic or thrombotic in origin. When attacks are multiple and repetitive, the patient has a 30 percent probability of developing a stroke. Therefore, it is of extreme importance that the underlying cause be defined and managed before such a stroke occurs. With multiple attacks, recurrence of the *same* symptoms suggests a thrombotic origin while the appearance of *different* symptoms implies an embolic origin. Rarely, a patient with arteritis will have similar transient episodes.

TIAs are varied and multiple; usually the signs

indicate transient ischemia in the territory of one or the other carotid artery or in the distribution of the basilar-vertebral system. It is important to identify whether the transient ischemia is related to carotid disease or basilar-vertebral insufficiency since management is different in the two cases. For example, one out of four patients with TIAs will have a definable extracranial lesion in a carotid artery that will be amenable to surgical correction. In contrast, in patients who are presenting with clear-cut symptoms relative to a carotid artery distribution, one of two patients will have a demonstrable lesion on arteriography which can be corrected by surgery. The frequency of symptoms related to TIAs in the carotid distribution and the vertebral basilar distribution are indicated in Tables 129–6 and 129–7.

INVESTIGATION. The currently asymptomatic patient can be investigated with some leisure. However, if the TIAs are occurring with increasing frequency, severity, and duration, the investigation should be undertaken promptly. The investigation is aimed at a search for evidence of stenotic or occluded vessels by such means as palpation for diminished carotid or preauricular pulses, auscultation of the neck for bruits, ophthalmodynamometry and ocular pulse studies. Doppler ultrasound flow studies of the external carotids and thermography of the face may suggest reduced flow or the presence of collaterals. Abrupt, transient cardiac arrhythmias may seriously reduce cerebral blood flow and be manifest primarily as transient, focal neurologic signs. In addition, a source for emboli is sought by evaluation of cardiac rhythm and evidence of a previous myocardial infarction or cardiac valvular disease. Arteriography is performed to define the locus of occlusion or stenosis. Extracranial sites are particularly important since they are amenable to surgical correction.[127,131] Lumbar puncture is performed to rule out the possibility of an intracerebral or subarachnoid bleed. This procedure is essential if anticoagulation is contemplated.

First Known Stroke

Strokes without premonitory TIAs may be either occlusive or hemorrhagic in origin. With a clear cerebrospinal fluid, onset during sleep favors thrombosis, while that shortly after arising or during activity favors embolus. With a bloody cerebrospinal fluid, abrupt onset favors aneurysm, less often arteriovenous malformation, while some history of a smooth increment of deficit favors hypertensive hemorrhage. Occasionally, an embolus may result in hemorrhagic infarction with moderate numbers of red cells in the cerebrospinal fluid. Such cases may be almost impossible to differentiate from small hypertensive hemorrhages.

TABLE 129-4
Common Presentations of Strokes

Condition When Seen	History	Mechanism	Differential Diagnosis and Features
A. Asymptomatic	1. First episode of transient neurologic deficit (TIA)	Embolus Thrombosis	Seizures Syncope Vertiginous states (migraine) Migraine Demyelinating disease Arteritis Hypoglycemia
	2. Repeated identical transient deficits (TIA's)	Thrombosis Emboli (rarely) Arteriovenous malformations	Seizures Migraine Vertiginous states
	3. Repeated, different transient deficits	Emboli Thrombosis (rarely)	Seizures Arteritis Demyelinating disease
B. Symptomatic, not progressing	1. Sudden onset Headache No localizing findings	Subarachnoid hemorrhage	Bloody cerebrospinal fluid
	2. Sudden onset No headache Lateralizing findings	Embolus Thrombosis	Clear cerebrospinal fluid
	3. Previous TIAs in same area	Thrombosis Arteriovenous malformation	Tumor with seizures
	4. Previous TIAs in different areas	Emboli	Arteritis
C. Symptomatic, progressing	1. Headache Smooth progression Localizing signs (Table 129-1)	Hypertensive hemorrhage Arteriovenous malformation	Migraine
	2. Step-wise progression or signs from same area	Thrombosis	Migraine Seizures with postictal paralysis
	3. Progression, with different areas of involvement	Emboli	
	4. Step-wise progression with headache and altered consciousness	Repeated subarachnoid bleeds	

INVESTIGATION. How aggressive the physician is in investigation is dictated by whether the patient has the potential to progress to further neurologic deficit. If the deficit is submaximal for the territory of the artery or arteries in question, further progression is possible. Such a patient is considered as a progressing stroke.

Symptomatic Patient with Previous Episodes

The nature of the previous episodes is of diagnostic importance. When the patient has a history of previous TIA, with step-wise increment in severity leading to the present deficit, the diagnosis of thrombosis is virtually certain. Previous deficits different from the current one suggest embolism. Arteriovenous malformations may recur with similar deficits, but the finding of bloody cerebrospinal fluid serves to separate them from thrombosis. Ruptured aneurysm or hypertensive hemorrhage rarely present with a previous deficit.

Progressing Deficit

The patient with continuing evolution of neurologic symptoms and signs requires prompt evaluation. Determination of such progression requires establishment of a baseline by careful examination. All forms of submaximal stroke from vascular occlusion may show progression. Progression of a thrombosis in a

TABLE 129–5
Diagnostic Evaluation of Strokes

Procedure	Findings
History	Previous episodes
	Pattern of progression
	Associated symptoms
	Underlying disease
Examination	Baseline
	Location of lesion
	Completeness of lesion
	Meningeal irritation
	Cardiac dysfunction
	Vital signs
	Evidence of brain stem dysfunction
	Decreased carotid pulsations
	Vascular bruits
Examination-repeat	Evidence of progression or regression
Blood and urine examination	Evidence of underlying systemic disease
Lumbar puncture	Evidence of intracranial bleed, or increased pressure
Ophthalmo-dynamometry Ocular pulse studies	Stenosis central to ophthalmic artery
Dynamic brain scan	Regional flow of isotope
Electroencephalography	Regional cerebral dysfunction
Doppler flow studies of carotid	Abnormal external carotid flow with reversal indicates serious stenosis
Thermography	Reduced hemifacial temperature may indicate carotid stenosis
Arteriography[127]	Location of occluded vessel(s)
	Evidence of hematoma
	Evidence of increased intracranial pressure

TABLE 129–6
TIAs in the Carotid Distribution*

Symptoms	Percent of Patients
Paresis (mono-, hemi-)	61
Paresthesias (mono-, hemi-)	57
Monocular visual disturbance	32
Paresthesiae (facial)	30
Paresis (facial)	22
Dysphasia	17
Dysarthria	16
Headache	12
Lightheadedness Dizziness Convulsion (focal) Convulsion (generalized) Binocular visual (hemianopsia) Visual hallucinations Mental changes	3

* Presenting symptoms in 133 patients.

TABLE 129–7
TIAs in the Vertebral Basilar Distribution*

Symptoms	Percent of Patients
Binocular visual disturbances	57
Vertigo	50
Paresthesias	40
Diplopia	38
Ataxia	33
Paresis	33
Dizziness	20
Headache	18
Nausea and vomiting	14
Dysarthria	14
Loss of consciousness	14
Visual hallucinations	7
Tinnitus	5
Mental change	5
Drop attacks	3
Drowsiness Lightheadedness Hearing loss Hyperacusis Dysphasia Weakness	>3

* Presenting symptoms in 54 patients.

step-wise fashion may result in an instantaneous change from a seemingly trivial to a disastrous deficit. Continuous progression is common in cases of hypertensive hemorrhage, and often indicates the hemorrhage will not arrest spontaneously. The physician should be particularly alert in the patient with signs or symptoms suggestive of cerebellar hemorrhage (Table 129–8). Such patients may require immediate computerized axial tomography (Chap. 111) or arteriography to detect the hemorrhagic mass and subsequent exploration of the posterior fossa.

TABLE 129-8
Symptoms and Signs of Hypertensive Hemorrhage

Site	Ocular Signs	Other Signs
Putamen	Conjugate horizontal deviation of eyes toward side of lesion	Contralateral hemiplegia, hemisensory loss, hemianopia Aphasia in dominant hemisphere Contralateral neglect, unawareness of deficit in nondominant hemisphere
Thalmus	Conjugate downward deviation of eyes	Contralateral hemisensory deficit, later hemiplegia, transient hemianopia Transient aphasia in dominant hemisphere
Pons	Dysconjugate ocular deviations Pinpoint, reactive pupils	Abrupt onset Coma Bilateral motor, sensory signs
Cerebellum[123]	Occasionally conjugate deviation of eyes away from side of lesion Small, reactive pupils	No motor, sensory, visual field deficit Vomiting, ataxia, inability to stand and walk

COMMON PROBLEMS IN MANAGEMENT

The most serious error is to assume the patient has a stroke when the underlying process is some other, treatable condition. When the history is inadequate or the patient may have fallen, as occurs in the alcoholic, a *subdural hematoma* must always be suspected. Here, arteriography is the definitive diagnostic procedure. Another common differential problem is the distinction between strokes and *seizures*. The electroencephalographic findings are often needed to make this decision.

A variety of episodic deficits can be confused with transient ischemic episodes. *Stokes-Adams* attacks and *seizures* often involve loss of consciousness, a symptom rarely associated with TIA. Isolated *dizziness* is often associated with vertebrobasilar artery disease. However, as an isolated symptom it is usually not an indication of TIA unless other neurological symptoms or signs appear. Episodic *behavioral abnormalities* are seldom vascular in origin.

The conditions most likely to mimic a progressing stroke are migraine (Chap. 125), epidural or subdural hematoma (Chap. 131), brain tumor with or without a bleed, and repeated seizures. These conditions can usually be differentiated by history and diagnostic studies.

In this discussion, involvement of large vessels in occlusive disease has been emphasized. Small vessel occlusion occurs in a number of conditions such as arteritis, syphilis, thrombotic thrombocytopenia purpura, or hypercoagulable states. These conditions are usually diagnosed on the basis of their systemic involvement. However, in some patients the differentiation from repeated embolic infarction, involving different areas of the brain, may be impossible until systemic manifestations appear.

THERAPY

OCCLUSIVE DISEASE

Antiplatelet Therapy[116,117]

Recent studies have shown that the frequency of embolization from arterial sites of arterial thrombosis into the distal circulation is significantly reduced by the use of a series of pharmacologic agents that inhibit platelet aggregation. Since platelet aggregation is believed to be one of the most common pathogenic mechanisms for transient focal cerebral ischemia, treatment with these agents has become an important addition to medical management. The most effective agents include acetylsalicylic acid (1200 mg/day), dipyridamole (150 to 200 mg/day), or sulfinpyrazone (400 mg/day). Control studies have indicated that these agents are efficient in reducing the frequency of transient ischemic attacks, particularly in males.

Anticoagulation

Anticoagulation is used only in cases in which an accurate diagnosis of occlusive disease has been established. In the case of *completed stroke*, there is no indication for anticoagulation. In the *progressing stroke*, particularly involving the vertebrobasilar system, anticoagulation is often used. However, the evidence that it effects the outcome is controversial.

Transient ischemic attacks are altered by anticoagulation in terms of frequency, and in those due to emboli, in terms of long-term morbidity. Anticoagulation is usually carried out with heparin, followed by an antiprothrombin compound (Chap. 30).

Arterial Surgery

There are two phases to extracranial surgery for occlusive cerebrovascular disease. The acute phase is removal of an acute embolism to the carotid bifurcation by carotid embolectomy. Precise arteriography is required and a surgical team which can be mobilized very quickly. There is little reason to operate if the occlusion has been present for more than 30 minutes. Even under ideal circumstances, there is a question whether hemorrhagic infarction occurs when the previously ischemic area is suddenly reperfused following successful embolectomy.

Prophylactic carotid surgery is a controversial issue for which there are little hard data. Removal of a thrombotic plaque from a carotid artery which is seeding emboli to the cerebral circulation is of value. Although controlled studies raise some question, it is generally accepted that symptomatic extracranial stenoses (particularly of the carotid artery) should be surgically corrected. In centers where there is close collaboration between neurologists and experienced neurovascular surgeons, the optimal treatment for symptomatic carotid artery stenosis is surgical correction. Experience in the past several years at the Johns Hopkins Hospital indicates that patients treated surgically have little significant surgical morbidity and fare better in terms of stroke prevention over several years of careful follow-up than patients who do not have surgical intervention. For stenoses (other than those at the carotid bifurcation) bypass procedures appear to be more beneficial than removal of the atherosclerotic plaque by endarterectomy. Although the clinical efficacy has not been proven, surgical anastamosis between distal branches of the external and internal carotid have been shown to improve intracranial blood flow and may prove beneficial to symptomatically deficient hemispheral circulation. The beneficial effects of opening stenotic vessels which cannot be directly related to the patient's symptoms remain to be demonstrated.

HEMORRHAGE[123]

A patient with an intracerebral hemorrhage may be considered a candidate for surgery if the hemorrhage is in the cerebellum or, less commonly, in the nondominant putamen. At the present time there is no surgical therapy available for patients with pontine or thalamic hemorrhage. Immediate management for the patient with intracerebral hematoma or subarachnoid hemorrhage is to maintain the patient at bed rest and to relieve agitation. This may require large amounts of sedatives and analgesics which should not be withheld after the diagnosis is established. A comatose patient will require the general management of this state as outlined in Chapter 147. Attempts should be instituted to lower the diastolic pressure, especially if it is excessively high and it should be maintained at a range of 100 to 110 mm of Hg. Increased intracranial pressure may be helped by steroids or osmotic agents such as glycerol or mannitol as outlined in Chapter 15. Surgical intervention for ruptured aneurysm requires accurate diagnosis and detailed definition of the lesion and its surrounding circulation (Fig. 129–1). The continuing evolution of surgical techniques for direct and indirect attack on aneurysms prevents any definite statement at the present time about the best surgical procedures.

REHABILITATION

The goals of management during the acute phase of stroke are to prevent decubiti, contractures, hypostatic pneumonia, thrombophlebitis, and bladder dysfunction.

CHAPTER 130
Multiple Sclerosis and Other Demyelinating Diseases
GUY M. McKHANN

INTRODUCTION

Myelin sheaths are multilayered lamellae formed by apposition of the plasma membranes of processes of satellite cells that wind around axons. In the peripheral nervous system, the processes extend from Schwann cells, and in the central nervous system from oligodendroglia. Myelin serves as a high resistance insulator acting to increase conduction velocity along the axon of a nerve cell.

┌───┐
TABLE 130–1
Disorders of the Myelin Sheath

Acquired disorders—etiology unknown
    Multiple sclerosis
    Neuromyelitis optica (Devic's disease)

Acquired disorders—possible immune mechanism[152]
    Acute disseminated encephalomyelitis
    Acute hemorrhagic leukoencephalitis
    Postinfectious polyneuritis (Landry-Guillain-Barré
      syndrome)

Acquired disorders—secondary to generalized diseases
    Postanoxia
    Aminoacidurias
    Nutritional deprivation
    Hypothyroidism

Acquired disorders—viral infection
    Progressive multifocal leukoencephalopathy
    Subacute sclerosing panencephalitis
      (inclusion body encephalitis)

Disorders of myelin metabolism[153]
    Metachromatic leukodystrophy
    Globoid cell leukodystrophy
    Sudanophilic leukodystrophy
    Alexander's disease
    Pelizaeus-Merzbacher disease
    Adrenoleukodystrophy[147,158]
└───┘

Destruction of myelin is associated with a number of processes which damage all components of the nervous system such as ischemia, tumors, or infections. The term *demyelinating* disease is reserved for disorders in which myelin breakdown is the primary abnormality and neural elements, particularly axons, are relatively spared. It is helpful to divide the breakdown of myelin into two broad categories, *acquired disorders* of myelin destruction and *metabolic disorders* involving myelin breakdown. In the former, myelin is synthesized normally and maintained until some acquired process results in subsequent breakdown. In the latter, there is an inherited defect in the metabolism of myelin, involving either the synthesis or maintenance of myelin lipids or proteins. A further classification of disorders of myelin is presented in Table 130–1.

ACQUIRED DISORDERS— ETIOLOGY UNKNOWN

MULTIPLE SCLEROSIS[140]

Multiple sclerosis is a disease of young adults. The peak age is 30, and one hesitates to make the diagnosis with an onset under age 10 or over age 50. The disease is more prevalent in northern latitudes. The prevalence in northern Europe and the northern United States is 30 to 80 per 100,000, in southern Europe and the southern United States 6 to 14 per 100,000, and in the tropics probably less than 1 per 100,000. Although there are no obvious predisposing factors, patients have histocompatability antigens HLA-A3, B7, and Dw2 more frequently than the general population.[142,151]

There are two characteristic clinical features: 1) an episodic, intermittent course with *remissions* and *exacerbations* and 2) the presence of multiple *topographically spread lesions*. In many patients the frequency of exacerbations, or attacks, decreases, and the disease process evolves into a static or slowly progressive process. The clinical features relate to the anatomic location and multiplicity of the lesions.

Clinical Description

In the most common type, there is an acute onset of focal neurologic deficit followed by a complete or nearly complete recovery over a period of weeks or months. This period of recovery is followed, at unpredictable intervals, by another acute episode. With each episode, the residual symptoms may increase.

Probably sensory disturbances and localized weakness are the commonest first signs. However, unilateral retrobulbar neuritis is often the initial event. Approximately 30 percent of patients with retrobulbar neuritis will go on to develop other manifestations of multiple sclerosis. The patient complains of pain in the eye with loss of visual acuity. There is frequently a normal appearing optic disc or, in the case of optic neuritis, a swollen optic nerve head with blurred disc margins. After a period of time the disc may become atrophic and a central scotomata may persist.

Other signs of the initial attack are ataxia, thick speech, or diplopia, particularly the dysconjugate gaze of internuclear ophthalmoplegia (Chap. 119). This phenomenon of limitation of adduction in one eye and nystagmus of the abducting eye on lateral gaze is rarely caused in young adults by anything but multiple sclerosis. Objective signs may be meager or lacking, and in many cases, the differential diagnosis of a functional disorder is raised. Pain is uncommon except for the electric sensation of Lhermitte's sign, that is, transient shocks that spread down the body into the arms and legs when the patient flexes his head forward. Facial pain similar to tic douloureaux may, on rare occasions, also be present. Spinal cord problems may not occur early, but eventually most patients are affected, with signs emerging over a long period of time. Bladder dysfunction with frequent urinary tract infections is common late in the disease. Seizures occur in less than 5 percent of patients. Unilateral facial twitching called facial myokymia may also occur. Emotional lability with euphoria or depression is often present, but dementia may develop.

There are variations in the clinical course which should be noted. Some patients have a chronic insidious course, with primary involvement of the spinal cord. A slowly developing paraplegia, with bladder involvement, is characteristic. The differential diagnosis includes treatable causes of myelopathy such as compressive lesions or vascular malformations. A second group of patients have a fulminant course with brain stem involvement consisting of ophthalmoplegia, dysphagia, marked ataxia, paraplegia, and respiratory distress. This form of the disease may be unremitting.

Diagnosis

At the present time, there is no specific laboratory test for multiple sclerosis. The diagnosis depends on the history of multiple attacks with characteristic exacerbations and remissions, and multifocal involvement of the central nervous system. Supporting evidence may be obtained from ancillary laboratory data, particularly the examination of cerebrospinal fluid (Table 130–2).

About 50 percent of patients have mononuclear cells in the CSF during an acute episode in the range of 10 to 50 cells. In all forms of multiple sclerosis approximately 90 percent of patients have abnormalities of CSF proteins. An elevated protein may be present, but more often there is an increase in total immunoglobulin G (IgG). On spinal fluid electrophoresis there are oligoclonal bands of IgG. It is not clear to what antigens these antibodies are directed. An individual patient may have increased antibodies in cerebrospinal fluid to three or four common viruses, e.g., measles, rubella, mumps, and varicella. The current interpretation is that the MS patient reacts in a hyperimmune fashion to a variety of antigens.[148]

Myelin basic protein, a component of myelin, appears in cerebrospinal fluid during acute exacerbations and may be a useful indication of disease activity.[143]

Prognosis

The prognosis is highly variable. Statistical studies are dependent on the thoroughness of case finding, particularly on the inclusion of benign forms of disease. Longitudinal studies indicate that over the past 25 years there has been no increased incidence in disease and that the 25 year survival of the multiple sclerosis population was 74 percent as compared to 86 percent for the control group. Two-thirds of the surviving patients were ambulatory 25 years after onset.[154]

Therapy

In acute cases, general supportive care is essential, particularly respiratory support. Results of a collaborative study indicate ACTH has some transient beneficial effects in acute exacerbations.[157] The regimen used is 80 units per day for 7 days, 40 units per day for 4 days, and 20 units for 3 days. There is little evidence to support long-term steroid therapy in multiple sclerosis. Immunosuppressive agents have been tried in a number of cases but have not been thoroughly evaluated.

In chronic cases, supportive care should deal with the emotional state of the patient, infections, bladder care, decubitus ulcers, and painful flexor spasms. Bladder problems are foremost, and proper irrigation and changing of catheters are important.

TABLE 130–2
Diagnosis of Multiple Sclerosis

Test	Finding
1. History	a. Recurrent attacks
	b. Recurrent attacks followed by progression
	c. Progression without clear-cut remissions
2. Examination	Evidence of scattered involvement of the nervous system
3. Evoked potential studies[145,146,156] a. Visual b. Brain stem	Evidence of delayed conduction in the visual or auditory systems
4. Cerebrospinal fluid[148] a. Cells	50% of patients may have increased mononuclears during an attack
b. Protein	Protein may be elevated
c. Immunoglobulin G (IgG)	Elevated in 70% of patients; does not correlate with disease activity
d. Oligoclonal bands of IgG	Present in 90% of patients; does not correlate with disease activity
e. Myelin basic protein[143]	Present in patients having an acute attack

Atropine can reduce urgency. Diazepam (Valium) in doses of 15 to 60 mg per day can reduce the intensity of flexor spasms.

Differential Diagnosis

The differential diagnosis varies with the form and stage of the disease. Thus, in the chronic relapsing form, the distinction between the early manifestations of multiple sclerosis and a functional disorder may be extremely difficult. If a patient's symptoms can be explained by a single lesion, questions should be constantly raised about the diagnosis. There are many other progressive disorders of the nervous system which may have a stuttering course, such as tumors, vascular disease, degenerative diseases, and infections. The astute physician is constantly on the lookout for more treatable entities in a patient who has been diagnosed as having multiple sclerosis.

ACQUIRED DISORDERS— POSSIBLE IMMUNE MECHANISM

ACUTE DISSEMINATED ENCEPHALOMYELITIS[152]

This disease of rapid onset is usually associated with an antecedent infection (measles, mumps, and chicken pox), vaccinations (smallpox and rabies vaccination), or antiserum administration. Pathologically, there is edema, perivascular cellular infiltration, and patchy areas of demyelination about veins in the white matter of brain and spinal cord. Because of the temporal relationship of antecedent infection or immunization and the pathologic similarity to the animal model, experimental allergic encephalomyelitis, it is suggested that these disorders may have an immunologic basis.

Clinically, the picture is quite varied from a mild malaise and headache occurring 10 to 15 days after vaccination to a fulminant illness with severe headache, confusion, stupor, coma, fever, and vomiting, and in patients with antecedent measles, the mortality is about 20 percent. Stiffness of the neck, focal cerebral signs, and myoclonic jerks are common. Cerebellar signs, optic neuritis, brain stem signs, and evidence of myelitis, such as incontinence and paraplegia, may also be present. The CSF protein is elevated with increased γ-globulin and mononuclear cells. The mortality rate may be high as in measles or rare as in mumps. Neurologic residua are common in survivors. Efficacy of treatment is uncertain. ACTH in doses similar to those used in acute attacks of multiple sclerosis may be of benefit.

POSTINFECTIOUS POLYNEURITIS (Landry-Guillain-Barré Syndrome)

Clinical Features

This process can occur at any age. A nonspecific infection, usually an upper respiratory infection, is often present a week or 10 days prior to onset. The patient initially complains of weakness of feet, hands, or face with occasional nondescript paresthesias in the extremities. These initial signs may occur for days or weeks before progression occurs. There is then an ascending or descending flaccid paralysis. Fever may be absent or low grade, the pulse rapid, and occasionally the neck stiff. Deep tendon reflexes are lost. The major threats to life are respiratory failure and cardiac arrhythmias. The latter are secondary to involvement of the autonomic nervous system.

Pathogenesis

Experimentally, a similar picture of inflammation and demyelination of nerve roots can be produced in experimental animals by sensitization to peripheral nerve myelin proteins. In man, antibodies to peripheral nerve myelin have been demonstrated in a number of patients, and immunoglobulin levels are elevated in the CSF. Thus, this syndrome may have an immunologic basis.[141]

Clinical Variants

There are some variants of the clinical presentation and course which should be recognized. The course may not be a smooth but a stuttering progression with rapid ascension of paralysis after a patient has appeared to be stable or even improving. The disease process may also skip areas of the nervous system. Thus, it is not uncommon for a patient to have marked involvement of the lower extremities and cranial nerves, with little involvement of the arms. Another clinical variant is that reported by Fisher,[144] in which the patient has cerebellar ataxia, ophthalmoplegia, or pareses of extraocular muscles, and mild peripheral sensory loss or weakness.

Diagnosis

Diagnosis is made by the presence of a diffuse symmetrical flaccid paralysis with bilateral facial paresis, minimal sensory findings, loss of reflexes, and, in many cases, a preceding infectious process. The spinal fluid shows a gradual increase in protein, almost all of which is albumin, with few, if any, cells. Those that are present are mononuclear cells. Peripheral white count is normal or low, and occasionally atypical lymphocytes may be seen. Other laboratory studies are normal unless there is an underlying disorder such as infectious mononucleosis, or hepatitis.

Prognosis

The prognosis is excellent except in the elderly. Most patients make a full functional recovery within 6 months. A small number of patients do, however, have significant deficits and may need braces and other mechanical assistance to walk. In a disease with such a favorable prognosis, attention must center on the dangers during the acute illness. Respiratory and cardiac function should be monitored closely in patients with ascending disease. In older patients, measures such as passive movement of the extremities, leg wrappings and elevation of the feet, should be taken to prevent pulmonary emboli. Careful cardiac and respiratory monitoring are an essential part of the management.

Differential Diagnosis

Consideration includes other entities that can acutely affect spinal cord, anterior horn cells, nerve roots, or peripheral nerves. Thus, a patient with an acute myelopathy may be confused with a patient with Guillain-Barré syndrome, the differences in myelopathy being the presence of a motor and sensory level, the early involvement of bowel and bladder, and if incomplete, the presence of long-tract findings. Patients with viral infections, such as poliomyelitis or Coxsackie disease, often present with asymmetrical, flaccid paralysis which may progress rather rapidly. The asymmetry, lack of sensory findings, associated fever, meningismus, and spinal cord findings all favor the diagnosis of poliomyelitis. Peripheral neuropathies can be confused with Guillain-Barré syndrome. The course of the disease, pattern of involvement, and spinal fluid findings may be of help in distinguishing between the proximal involvement in Guillain-Barré and the distal involvement of most neuropathies.

ACQUIRED DISORDERS— SECONDARY TO GENERALIZED DISEASES

POSTANOXIC ENCEPHALOPATHY[155]

Seven to twenty-one days following any acute hypoxic episode a small number of patients show signs and symptoms of a progressive encephalopathy. Pathologically, the brain shows diffuse, widespread demyelination in the hemispheres with intact neurons in both the hemispheres and brain stem. The basal ganglia are sometimes infarcted.

The clinical picture is that of a patient who is initially comatose from the anoxic insult, but usually awakens within 24 hours. Some patients, with lesser degrees of anoxia are initially only dazed. Following the hypoxia, the patient is quite normal from 7 to 21 days, and then develops irritability and confusion, diffuse spasticity, and rigidity. Some patients have a progression to coma and death, while others make a full recovery. The mechanism is not known, but cerebral edema may play a role.

ACQUIRED DISORDERS— VIRAL INFECTIONS[149]

There are two human demyelinating diseases in which viruses play a role. *Progressive multifocal leukoencephalopathy* occurs in patients with other diseases which interfere with cell-mediated immunity such as sarcoidosis, tuberculosis, neoplasms, or in the presence of immunosuppressive drugs. The disease is secondary to a papovavirus, usually the Jc virus, a virus antigenically related to SV 40. *Subacute sclerosing panencephalitis* occurs more commonly in children and appears to be a persistent infection with measles virus. Both diseases are subacute problems with a clinical course lasting for months in the former, and for months to years in the latter.

CHAPTER 131

Increased Intracranial Pressure and Intracranial Masses

GUY M. McKHANN

Except in the infant and very young child, the skull acts as a nonexpansible box. Thus, any increase in the volume of any of the three intracranial components,

brain, blood, or cerebrospinal fluid will result in increased intracranial pressure. See Table 131–1 for the mechanisms of increased intracranial pressure.

┌───┐
TABLE 131-1
Mechanisms of Increased
Intracranial Pressure

Mechanism	Example
1. Mass effect	
Acute	Intracranial hematomas
Chronic	Slow-growing tumors (e.g., meningioma)
2. Obstruction of flow of cerebrospinal fluid	
a. Obstruction of Foramen of Munro	Hemispheric tumor (glioblastoma)
b. Obstruction of aqueduct and outlets of fourth ventricle	Posterior fossa tumors
c. Obstruction of subarachnoid space	Chronic meningitis Meningeal carcinomatosis
3. Overproduction of cerebrospinal fluid	Choroid plexus papilloma
4. Brain edema	Anoxia Acute meningitis Tumors
└───┘

MECHANISMS OF DYSFUNCTION

The neurologic dysfunction may be related to a diffuse increase in intracranial pressure as occurs in brain edema, acute meningitis, anoxia, and in acute obstructions of cerebrospinal fluid dynamics (as when a shunt blocks). Such patients may present with an altered state of consciousness (lethargy and obtundation), headache, vomiting, and a minimum of localizing neurologic signs (Table 131-2).

More commonly, the pressure is asymetrically distributed within the compartments of the skull defined by the rigid tentorium. In these instances, brain substance shifts through holes in the tentorium and under the falx, through the tentorium, or through the foramen magnum.

There is a definite pattern of events which occur with temporal lobe herniation (Table 131-3).

The sequence of neurologic findings with herniation through the foramen magnum is less well-defined. In children with posterior fossa tumors, stiff neck and head-tilt may suggest chronic herniation. Acute herniation may present as respiratory arrest.

DIFFERENTIAL DIAGNOSIS

The crucial question is whether the patient has a potentially treatable *intracranial mass*. This subject is covered later in this chapter.

There are a number of conditions that are associated with diffuse increases in intracranial pressure (Table 131-4).

Cerebral Edema[160]

This term implies an abnormal accumulation of fluid by brain substance. The fluid may be either within cells or in the interstitial (extracellular) space. Attempts have been made to divide edema into *vasogenic,* in which there is abnormal vascular permeability as occurs around tumors or after certain toxins, e.g., lead, and *cytotoxic,* in which there is interference with cellular membranous functions, as occurs with anoxia of various types. This distinction may have some clinical relevance, because vasogenic edema is more responsive to corticosteroids.

Pseudotumor Cerebri[159,161]

Benign intracranial hypertension is associated with an elevated CSF pressure, the cause of which is obscure. This condition is most commonly encountered in young, obese females often with accompanying menstrual irregularities. Papilledema, headache, and drowsiness are conspicuous features. No other abnormal neurologic findings are usually detected, although third- and sixth-nerve palsies may develop secondary to increased intracranial pressure. On CAT scans, there is no evidence of a mass lesion and the ventricles are smaller than normal. Other than an increased pressure, the findings on lumbar puncture are normal. This process is usually self-limited, with resolution over a period of months. The most serious complication is episodes of cloudy vision which in rare instances lead to blindness. In such patients, the increased intracranial pressure may be relieved by repeated (daily) lumbar punctures, corticosteroids, acetazolamide, or oral osmotic agents such as glycerol. The efficacy of these agents is unpredictable in an individual case. The availability of devices for continuous monitoring of intracranial pressure may clarify the dynamics of this process.

The headache associated with increased intracranial pressure or intracranial masses is important to distinguish from the headaches of many other causes. It may not be clear whether increased intracranial

┌─ **TABLE 131–2** ─────────────────────────────────
Manifestations of Increasing Intracranial Pressure[162]

Symptoms	Early	Late	Severe
Headache	Nocturnal or on awakening, worse with cough and head motion	Constant, dull	Constant, dull
Mental state	Lethargy Slowness of response	Stupor	Coma
Vomiting	May occur without nausea	Projectile	May be projectile
Signs			
Pupils	Unilateral irregularity or dilation	Unilateral dilation	Unilateral dilation
Fundi	Blurring of disc margins Loss of venous pulsations	Disc hyperemia Flame-shaped hemorrhages at disc margin	Disc margins obscured Hemorrhages in retina
Extraocular movements	Ptosis, unilateral	Unilateral third and sixth nerve	Ophthalmoplegia Loss of vestibular-ocular reflexes
Motor	Normal	Hemiparesis (may be false localizing, see Table 131–2)	Bilateral hemiparesis
Arterial pressure	Normal	Normal	Systemic elevation Widening of pulse pressure
Pulse	Normal	Normal	Slow, irregular

┌─ **TABLE 131–3** ─────────────
Manifestations of Herniation of the Right Temporal Lobe

Clinical Symptoms and Signs	Mechanism
Pupils (findings on right, left normal) Unilateral dilatation Ptosis Ophthalmoplegia (late)	Pressure on the outer fibers of the oculomotor nerve between herniating tissue and the medial petroclinoid ligament
Motor function Hemiplegia on right side (a false localizing sign)	Pressure of the brain stem against the opposite tentorium
Progressive coma with involvement of respirations, pupils (bilaterally), and extraocular movements (Chap. 112)	Flattening of midbrain against tentorium with secondary vascular occlusions
Increasing coma Rising blood pressure Bradycardia	Flattening of aqueduct and blockage of perimesencephalic subarachnoid space

pressure or a direct effect of the mass is causal. There are certain features that should warn the physician that this particular patient may have one of these problems:

1. Nocturnal headaches or headaches present on arising are characteristic of increased intracranial pressure.
2. A patient of middle age, who previously has not had headaches and has a different type of headache
3. The evolution of the headache to a dull ache, present all the time, made worse by coughing and straining
4. Headache in a child under age 10, unless there is a strong family history of headaches

The changes in mental state are also distinctive. The early changes may be quite subtle and consist of lethargy, slowness of action or decision, irritability, and some loss of normal social behavior. These symptoms may be falsely attributed to depression or the effects of chronic headache. In later stages, more significant disorders of consciousness occur with stupor and finally coma. Some patients may go through a stage of irrational hyperactivity.

There is a marked difference in presentation between the patient with an acute onset of increased intracranial pressure and that with a slowly progressive increase. With slowly growing tumors, patients may have papilledema, headache, early changes in mental state, and no other neurologic findings, de-

---

TABLE 131-4
Increased Intracranial Pressure Without Localizing Signs

Cerebral edema
  Vasogenic (increased permeability of blood vessels)
    Tumors in "silent" area, e.g., frontal lobe
    Toxins, e.g., lead
  Cytotoxic (increased uptake of fluid by cells)
    Anoxia
    Hypoglycemia
Pseudotumor cerebri
Hypertensive encephalopathy
Chronic obstructive lung disease with hypercapnia
Chronic meningitis; e.g., tuberculous, fungal
Addison's disease
Corticosteroid withdrawal
Vitamin A intoxication
Tetracycline (in children)
Tumors
  Tumors that block CSF flow
  Posterior fossa tumors
  Frontal lobe tumors

---

spite having a large tumor and significantly elevated intracranial pressure.

It should be stressed that the "classical signs" of increasing intracranial pressure, e.g., rising blood pressure, bradycardia, and florid papilledema, are late manifestations. Thus, their presence reflects an urgent problem. Their absence in no way excludes increased intracranial pressure.

Hypertension
Papilledema, headache, focal neurologic signs, and seizures may be encountered in patients with severe hypertension. In hypertension the papilledema is usually minimal compared to the exudative changes in the fundi, and visual acuity is appreciably impaired. Renal dysfunction is usually apparent (Chap. 25).

Chronic Meningitis
A difficult diagnostic problem is represented by the patient who presents with papilledema, increased intracranial pressure, and an increase in protein and mononuclear cells in the cerebrospinal fluid. The differential diagnosis is between tuberculosis, fungus (cryptococcus), syphilis, tumor, sarcoid, or one of the ill-defined meningitides which may be of viral origin. In these patients, repeated cultures for tubercle bacilli and fungi are necessary.

Optic Neuritis
Edema of the optic disc is frequently present during the acute stage of optic neuritis. In addition, there is profound visual loss. However, the other ophthalmos-

copic findings may be minimal, the retinal veins are not distended, and hemorrhages and exudates are uncommon. In patients with choked discs from increased intracranial pressure, central vision is usually preserved despite prominent ophthalmoscopic findings. Myelinated nerve fibers may be confused with the blurred disc margin of papilledema. These abnormalities are usually confined to one eye and may be detected in other members of the patient's family (Chap. 154).

MANAGEMENT OF INCREASED INTRACRANIAL PRESSURE

It is of utmost importance to recognize the premonitory signs which indicate increasing intracranial pressure and possible tentorial or foraminal herniation (Tables 131-2, 131-3). In patients with a chronic elevation of intracranial pressure, as may occur in pseudotumor cerebri or hydrocephalus, visual acuity may decrease. This symptom is an indication for active medical or surgical intervention.

Intracranial pressure may be decreased by allowing more room (surgically) or by decreasing brain or cerebrospinal fluid volume. Brain volume, particularly if cerebral edema is present, may be decreased by hyperventilation (hypocapnia), osmotic agents, such as urea, mannitol or glycerol, or corticosteroids (Table 131-5). There is little evidence that the rate of secretion or volume of cerebrospinal fluid can be pharmacologically altered. However, repeated lum-

---

TABLE 131-5
Medical Management of Increased Intracranial Pressure

Agent	Dose	Comment
Mannitol	1-2 g/kg body wt. (25% solution)	Given intravenously over 30 minutes
Glycerol	25 ml in 25 ml of fluid	Given orally or by tube. Orange juice will disguise the taste
Dexamethasone (Decadron)	10 mg initially 2 mg q 4 hr	Particularly effective for the cerebral edema around brain tumors
Methylprednisolone	600-2000 mg/day	

bar punctures or continuous drainage of cerebrospinal fluid may be useful in acute situations. There are a number of implantable devices for monitoring intracranial pressure continuously. The objective data obtained can be very useful in management of increased intracranial pressure.

The surgical approach depends on the mechanism of increased intracranial pressure. Accumulation of cerebrospinal fluid may be relieved by some form of shunting procedure. Increased brain volume may require decompression by removal of subtemporal bone.

INTRACRANIAL MASS LESIONS[162]

The term *intracranial mass lesion* is often used to mean primary and metastatic neoplasms of the central nervous system. However, it is of clinical importance to include inflammatory lesions and hematomas in considering mass lesions. These lesions may present in the same manner as neoplasms, are generally more amenable to treatment, and progress more rapidly if neglected.

Intracranial mass lesions produce their symptoms by two mechanisms: 1) increased intracranial pressure; and 2) local dysfunction of the nervous system. The clinical manifestation of increased intracranial pressure is discussed in the previous section. The approach to the patient is indicated in Table 131–6.

PRIMARY BRAIN TUMORS (Table 131–7)

Glioblastoma

This is a rapidly growing tumor, occurring in the cerebral hemispheres. Thus, it presents with seizures, mentation changes, and increased intracranial pressure. The effect of the tumor is greatly augmented by the surrounding edema. This edema may respond dramatically to corticosteroids. The overall prognosis is poor with average survival in treated patients being 12 to 18 months from clinical onset.[164,166,167]

Astrocytoma

This is a slower growing tumor, usually occurring in the cerebral hemispheres, but may occur in the cerebellum or spinal cord. In its most common form, it presents much as a glioblastoma, which progresses at a slower pace. The duration may be years rather than months. The distinction between astrocytoma and glioblastoma is not clear histologically; many tumors on biopsy or autopsy have elements of both. Nevertheless, the average survival is 4 to 5 years.

TABLE 131–6	
Evaluation of Possible Intracranial Masses	
Procedure	**Possible Findings**
1. No evidence of increased intracranial pressure	
A. Neurologic examination	Evidence of localizing or lateralizing findings
B. Skull x-ray	See Table 111–1
C. CAT scanning	Ventricular size and position Hemispheric mass Cerebral atrophy
D. Brain scan	Abnormal uptake
E. Electroencephalogram	Focal slowing or seizure activity
F. Lumbar puncture	Increased pressure Elevated protein Evidence of infection, pleocytosis, low sugar, positive STS
G. Angiography	Ventricular size and position Position of cerebral vessels Abnormal vessels Evidence of herniation
H. Pneumoencephalography (replaced by CAT scanning)	Ventricular size Displacement of ventricles Cerebral atrophy
2. Known increased intracranial pressure	
A. Neurologic examination	Evidence of localizing or lateralizing findings
B. Skull x-ray	See Table 111–1
C. CAT scanning	Ventricular size and position Hemispheric mass Cerebral atrophy
D. Brain Scan	Abnormal uptake
E. Electroencephalography	May provide localization
F. Angiography	Ventricular size and position Position of cerebral vessels Abnormal vessels Evidence of herniation
G. Air encephalography	Performed with knowledge that patient may require immediate surgery

Oligodendroglioma

These are rare tumors that grow very slowly. They usually present with seizures or intracranial calcification on skull x-ray. The average survival is 10 to 15 years.

```
┌─TABLE 131-7─────────────────────┐
│   The Frequency of Common Brain Tumors │
│                                  │
│                                  │
│ Supratentorial                   │
│   Glioma—40%                     │
│     Glioblastoma                 │
│     Astrocytoma                  │
│     Oligodendroglioma            │
│   Meningioma—15%                 │
│   Metastatic carcinoma—20%       │
│     Lung                         │
│     Breast                       │
│     Gastrointestinal             │
│     Kidney                       │
│                                  │
│ Infratentorial                   │
│   Metastatic carcinoma—5%        │
│   Glioma—5%                      │
│     Medulloblastoma              │
│     Astrocytoma                  │
│     Ependynoma                   │
│   Cranial nerve neuromas—5%      │
│                                  │
│ Suprasellar                      │
│   Craniopharyngioma—3%           │
│   Pituitary tumors—7%            │
│     Chromophobe adenoma          │
│     Acidophilic                  │
│     Basophilic                   │
└──────────────────────────────────┘
```

Meningioma

These tumors occur over the surface of the brain, arising from the dura. The most common sites are the sylvian region, parasagittal area, olfactory grooves, and the wing of the sphenoid. These are benign tumors and very slow growing, and can reach enormous size (5 to 10 cm) before producing symptoms. The supratentorial tumors usually present with seizures or focal motor deficits. These tumors are potentially curable with surgery.

Metastatic Carcinoma

Certain cancers, particularly lung, breast, gastrointestinal, and kidney, metastasize to brain; others, such as melanoma or thyroid do so less frequently. Interestingly, cancers of the prostate, ovaries, and skin (except melanoma) almost never go to brain. Brain metastases are often multiple. Sometimes matastases go to the meninges rather than brain substance, appearing as a form of chronic meningitis. The prognosis in patients with brain metastases is very poor, with survival 6 to 12 months at best.

Craniopharyngioma

These are suprasellar tumors, which are slow growing and may be cystic. They present with visual dysfunction, because of pressure on the optic chiasm, nerves, or tracts, or because of endocrine dysfunction. They are potentially removable.

Cranial Nerve Neuromas

These are tumors of the sheaths of the Vth or VIIth cranial nerves. The most common is the *acoustic neuroma* which presents with hearing loss, tinnitus, vertigo, facial weakness, and sensory loss over the face (Chap. 127). These are slow growing tumors, and the patient may disregard the early symptom of hearing loss. Large tumors may press on the cerebellum to give unilateral ataxia, or compress the fourth ventricle and aqueduct to give hydrocephalus and increased intracranial pressure.

For unknown reasons, the cerebrospinal fluid protein may be quite elevated, above 100 mg/dl, in these tumors. These tumors can be successfully removed surgically.

MANAGEMENT OF INTRACRANIAL NEOPLASMS

These tumors can be divided into three categories:

1. Tumors that are benign, surgically approachable, and potentially curable.
2. Tumors that are benign and slow growing, but cannot be totally removed or surgically approached because of their location.
3. Tumors that are malignant, rapidly growing, and not altered by partial removal.

Meningiomas, neurinomas of the eighth or fifth cranial nerves, cystic juvenile astrocytomas and hemangioglastomas of the cerebellum, and craniopharyngiomas are all in the first category. All of these tumors are relatively slow growing, but can reach enormous size before being detected. Early diagnosis and surgical removal are associated with an excellent prognosis.

Oligodendrogliomas and low-grade astrocytomas are slow growing tumors that are probably not completely removed at surgery. They tend to recur, sometimes in a more malignant form than the original tumor.

Malignant gliomas (glioblastomas), medulloblastomas, and metastatic tumors are highly malignant and quite refractory to definitive surgical or radiation therapy. When such a tumor is suspected, the physician must make a decision whether intracranial surgery, beyond establishing a diagnosis, is indicated. The prognosis for patients with glioblastomas is still poor, but the combination of radiation and chemotherapy has lengthened median survival from 17 weeks in those with no therapy to 52 weeks in those receiving combination therapy.

At the present time the recommended therapy is corticosteriods (Decadron) or methylprednisolone for cerebral edema, 6000 rads to the tumor area, and BCNU (carmustine [1,3-bis (2-chloroethyl-1-nitrosourea)] or CCNU (lomustine [1-(2-chloroethyl)3-cyclohexyl-1-nitrosourea]) at 6 to 8 week intervals. On this regimen, 25 percent of patients are alive at 18 months.[164,166]

OTHER INTRACRANIAL MASSES

Intracranial Hematomas

The primary factors in determining the prognosis of intracranial hematomas are their location, size, and speed of development. Those on the surface (epidural and subdural hematomas) are potentially curable. The clinical features of these entities are covered in the chapter on head injury (Chap. 132). Hematomas or hemorrhages within brain substance always destroy tissue. A hemispheric hemorrhage, cerebellar hemorrhage, or putaminal hemorrhage, may be tolerated by the patient, or successfully evacuated without damaging vital structures or leaving significant residual dysfunction. Conversely, thalamic or pontine hemorrhages are usually fatal and not amenable to surgical therapy.

Brain Abscesses

A brain abscess is potentially treatable. One of the reasons for making a definitive surgical diagnosis in a patient for whom the suspicion of a neoplasm is high, is the possibility that the mass is a treatable abscess.

In some parts of the world parasitic cysts (cysticercosis cellulosae in South American and hydatid cysts in South America and Africa) have a high incidence. Their presentation can be identical to brain tumors.

Common Pitfalls in Management

Certain errors in recognition of intracranial masses occur with sufficient frequency to deserve special comment.

In *elderly patients,* mental and neurologic symptoms may be ascribed to senility or strokes. Papilledema, although present, is often not appreciated. Subdural hematomas may easily go unrecognized in this setting.

In *alcoholics,* manifestations of subdural and epidural hematomas may be mistakenly attributed to alcoholic intoxication, delirium tremens, ataxia, or peripheral neuropathies.

Gradual changes in mental status are, in the absence of focal signs, often attributed to depression, agitation, or other nonorganic mental illness. This is most common when the mass produces bizarre behavior rather than stupor, e.g., frontal lobe mass. The administration of sedative, tranquilizing, or stimulant drugs often further obscures the clinical problem.

Abrupt changes in status are often taken as evidence that the lesion is a vascular lesion rather than a mass. Abrupt changes occur in both neoplastic and nonneoplastic mass lesions usually because of local hemorrhage. Indeed, sudden worsening makes rapid diagnosis mandatory.

The *absence of history of trauma* may be erroneously used to exclude subdural hematoma. More than half the patients with proven chronic subdural hematoma give no elicitable histories of head trauma.

Similarly, the *absence of fever or of leukocytosis* may be wrongly used to exclude a brain abscess. A well-encapsulated brain abscess may present solely as a mass lesion without any systemic manifestations of infection.

INVESTIGATION

In general, the simpler and safer procedures are performed first. Since some of these studies are associated with morbidity and complications, e.g., arteriography and pneumoencephalography, the question soon arises of how far studies should be pursued in a given instance. The clinical situation for each patient will determine whether the potential gain outweighs the risk of the study.

Patients with seizures developing in adulthood and patients with increased intracranial pressure deserve full investigation, for the possibility of a mass lesion is great. Occipital headache appearing de novo and made worse by coughing and straining similarly warrants thorough study despite the risks involved. In patients with deepening coma or increasing hemiparesis, studies are often performed even when a mass lesion appears unlikely, because it is feared that the patient may not survive unless a remediable lesion is found. Similarly, these studies may be done when the most likely diagnosis offers no therapeutic possibilities.

The ancillary diagnostic procedures are outlined in Chapter 142 and Table 131–6. However, in relation to intracranial masses, three studies are of particular value: 1) computerized axial tomography; 2) plain skull x-rays; and 3) isotopic brain scanning. In certain instances the lumbar puncture will reveal indirect evidence, such as increased pressure or protein, as will the electroencephalogram (focal slowing).

Lumbar puncture is indicated when an infectious process is suspected. However, in the presence of focal neurologic signs or signs of increased intracranial pressure, a CAT scan should be performed prior to lumbar puncture unless the patient is thought to have bacterial meningitis.

CHAPTER 132

Trauma to the Head and Neck

GUY M. McKHANN

HEAD INJURY

Somewhere between 1 and 3 million people have significant head trauma each year in the United States. While it is true that the inpatient management of these patients is handled by the surgeon or neurosurgeon, the general physician should be familiar enough with the entity to be able to answer such questions as: When should the patient be hospitalized? What are indications of a progressive disorder? What factors influence prognosis? What symptoms can be related to trauma?

The clinical symptoms associated with head injury are outlined in Table 132–1.

ACUTE EFFECTS

Skull Fracture

About 70 percent of skull fractures are *linear*. These fractures may indicate at what site the underlying brain injury is centered. More importantly, if they cross the middle meningeal artery or a dural sinus, the physician should be alerted to the possibility of a subsequent epidural or subdural hematoma. Fractures of the cribiform plate or base of the skull may lead to cerebrospinal fluid rhinorrhea or otorrhea, and to subsequent intracranial infection.

Depressed skull fractures are associated with direct contusion and laceration of brain and should be elevated.

Trauma to the head takes three forms: *blunt trauma,* such as occurs in falls or blows to the head; *penetrating head wounds,* as occur with bullets; and *indirect trauma,* as occurs in blast injuries or in sudden flexion–extension movements of the neck (whiplash). In all instances, forces of deformation, acceleration, and deceleration are inflicted on a relatively movable brain which is limited by the fixed skull, dura, cranial nerves, blood vessels, and brain stem. In addition, with penetrating head wounds, the missile will impart a shock wave through the brain that will cause tearing of tissue some distance from the path of the object. A review of the possible underlying stresses associated with these forces has been provided by Walker.[170]

Epidural Hematoma

This entity results from the rapid accumulation of blood between the skull and the dura, usually secondary to a linear skull fracture that tears the middle meningeal artery. The classical clinical presentation is a brief period of unconsciousness at the time of the injury followed by an interval of lucidity, and then progressive drowsiness, stupor, and localizing neurologic signs. Evidence of brain stem compression and coma are late manifestations. However, only 50 percent of patients follow this course. Many patients have just the second phase of the classical biphasic course.

The diagnosis can be suspected on the basis of clinical history and physical examination and the presence of a skull fracture. The definitive tests are CAT scanning or arteriography. The epidural hematoma is seen as an avascular mass displacing the brain away from the inner table of the skull. The only therapy is prompt surgical evacuation of the hematoma. In patients who are rapidly deteriorating, exploration without arteriography may be necessary. Following evacuation of the epidural hematoma, it is advisable to open the dura to exclude the possibility of a concomitant subdural hematoma.

TABLE 132-1
Sequellae of Head Trauma

Acute

Skull fracture
Epidural hematoma
Subdural hematoma
Concussion
Contusion and laceration of brain
Subararchnoid hemorrhage
Headache

Subacute

Amnesia and personality changes
Cranial nerve dysfunction
Focal neurologic deficit including aphasias
Subdural hematoma
Prolonged coma
Seizures
Headache

Chronic

Seizures
Focal neurologic deficits
Defects in memory, judgement, and personality
Psychoneurosis
Headache

Subdural Hematoma

Subdural hematomas can be either acute or chronic. The mode of presentation of the two types is quite different.

Acute subdural hematomas are acute venous hemorrhages into the subdural space, usually from a torn dural sinus or bridging meningeal vein. The clinical presentation may be similar to an epidural hematoma, but over a longer period of time.

The diagnosis is aided by the finding of a fracture on skull x-rays with shift of the calcified pineal gland away from the hematoma. As with epidural hematoma, the definitive diagnostic tests are CAT scanning or arteriography. The treatment is evacuation, often on an emergency basis.

Chronic subdural hematomas are frequently missed and should be suspected in any patient with a history of even minor head trauma. Some patients have a clear history of head trauma, unconsciousness, recovery and the persistence of confusion, lethargy, and neurologic findings. Such patients are not difficult to diagnose. More commonly the patient or his family consider the preceding trauma so minor that they do not report it. The clinical presentation is often headache, dementia, localizing neurologic deficit, such as an hemiparesis, and eventually signs of brain stem compression.

In certain groups of patients, such as the alcoholic, the elderly demented patient, or the patient receiving anticoagulant therapy, the presence of progressive local neurologic signs and symptoms should be considered to be secondary to a subdural hematoma until proven otherwise.

The diagnosis depends primarily on a high index of suspicion. The approach to diagnostic management and results of diagnostic tests are indicated in Table 132-2.

TABLE 132-2
Approach to the Patient with Suspected Subdural Hematoma

Test	Findings	Pitfalls
History	Previous trauma	May be minimal or forgotten
	Dementia	May be ascribed to other causes
Examination	Hemiparesis	May be ascribed to vascular disease
	Aphasia	
	Papilledema	May be missed
	Third-nerve paresis	Difficult to elicit in an uncooperative patient
Skull x-rays	Shift of pineal	25–30% do not have calcified pineal
	Previous fracture	
Lumbar puncture	Increased pressure	All of these may be absent
	Xanthochromia	
	Increased protein	
Electroencephalographs	Decreased voltage and slowing on the side of the hematoma	May be normal
Computer assisted tomography	Abnormal absorbance	May be normal
Arteriography	Displacement of brain away from the inner table	Definitive test Should be done bilaterally

The therapy for most subdural hematomas is evacuation. Occasionally, small hematomas are found which do not adequately explain the patients' symptoms and do not require removal. Such patients must be followed closely for signs of progression.

Concussion and Contusion

A *concussion* refers to the acute loss of neurologic function following a head injury. Some authors limit this term to describe patients who have had a loss of consciousness, no matter how brief. The associated symptoms are amnesia, both retrograde and anterograde, dizziness, diplopia, and headache.

Contusion and *laceration* are terms used to describe the patient with a longer period of unconsciousness, slow recovery, and focal neurologic signs. Regardless of the terms used, unconsciousness and amnesia are indicative of significant brain injury. The prognosis is related to the age of the patient (children recovering to a much greater extent than adults), the duration of unconsciousness, and the persistence of amnesia.

Management of Acute Head Injuries

The key to management is careful *observation*. Any patient with a period of unconsciousness must be watched closely for at least 12 hours for evidence of progressive deterioration. Skull x-rays should be obtained to rule out a possible fracture which could lead to an epidural or subdural hematoma.

The clinical variables which one monitors are indicated in Table 132–3.

During the period of observation, medications that might alter the variables being followed should be avoided. Thus, one is ill-advised to use sedatives or mydriatics unless absolutely necessary. The patient should be kept quiet and given reassurance. The sleeping patient should be aroused at least hourly until the physician is convinced that the patient's condition is stable or improving.

The severely injured patient, in a comatose or semicomatose state, should be observed as outlined in Table 132–3. In addition, attention should be paid to proper position and turning of the patient with the supine position avoided.

Seizures may occur in approximately 10 percent of patients. In such cases, diazepam (Valium) or paraldehyde are less likely to depress respirations than high doses of barbiturates. Phenytoin (Dilantin) is the drug of choice for maintenance.

Cerebral edema is usually generalized, and may become the most life-threatening factor. The management is similar to that outlined in Chapter 131.

TABLE 132–3
Observations To Make in a Patient with Head Injury

Variable	Evidence of Deterioration
Mental State	
Arousal	Persistence of defect or
Awareness	inability to perform at
Orientation	previously tested level
Speech	
Comprehension	
Abstract thinking	
Pupillary Responses	
Diameter at rest	Asymmetrical dilatation at
Response to light	rest or after exposure to
	light
Extraocular movements	
	Evidence of a N III or N VI
	paresis
Motor System	
Strength	Asymmetry of response
Tone	Increase in tone
Sensory System	
Pain	Asymmetry of response
Position	Presence of a sensory level
Reflexes	
Corneal	Asymmetry of response
Tendon jerks	Changing response
Babinski	Present
Vital Signs	
Blood Pressure	Changes indicate brain
Pulse	stem compression
Respiration	

SUBACUTE AND CHRONIC EFFECTS[171]

Seizures[168]

The occurrence of seizures is related to the severity and location of the trauma. In patients with closed head injuries without prolonged coma, the incidence is around 5 percent. Conversely, in patients with penetrating wounds, particularly those involving the precentral and postcentral gyri and temporal lobes, the incidence may be well over 50 percent. There may be a lag of months to years between the time of the injury and the subsequent appearance of seizures.

The chances of posttraumatic seizures may be minimized by avoiding anoxia, cerebral edema, and repetitive seizures at the time of injury. Potential epileptogenic cicatrixes may be prevented by decompression, debridement of grossly damaged brain tissue, and closure of dural lacerations. There is no convincing evidence that anticonvulsant drugs, particularly phenytoin (Dilantin), given prophylactically will prevent the subsequent appearance of posttraumatic seizures. The management of posttraumatic seizures is similar to that for seizures from other causes (Chap. 128). There is evidence that patients with focal seizures from a discrete focus should be considered for surgery, if the focus can be removed without leaving significant neurological deficit.

Defects in Memory, Judgment, and Personality

Patients who have had a significant head injury may take a long time to recover. Ultimate prognosis is hard to judge until 12 to 18 months after the injury, particularly in the younger patient. Severity of the initial injury; presence of specific neurologic deficits; e.g., hemiparesis, aphasia; duration of coma; and agitated behavior during coma or during the transition to alertness are all associated with an increased incidence of residual behavioral sequelae, particularly conceptual disorganization, motor retardation, and emotional withdrawal.[169] Initially, the patient may complain of headaches, dizziness, and various psychogenic symptoms. As the headache and dizziness recover, the psychogenic complaints may be the limiting factor. Such patients are irritable, have a short span of attention, have lost confidence in their ability to perform, and may be emotionally quite labile. They should not be pushed into stressful situations in which they cannot perform adequately. The patients' recovery can be judged by their behavior in nonstressful situations and by serial psychological testing. Patients may require mild tranquilizers to handle reactions of anxiety and depression. The physician must recognize that many of the patients' complaints are real, regardless of the compensation aspects of the case, and that continuing reassurance, job retraining, and physical therapy are all helpful.

CERVICAL SPINE INJURIES

This section is included here to remind the physician that many patients with head injuries also have injuries to the cervical spine. When there is any question of spine injury, the head and neck should be immobilized until proper x-rays can be obtained. While these x-rays are being obtained, attention should be directed to maintaining respiratory function and excluding injuries to somatic organs which could lead to circulatory failure. The management of cervical cord injury is beyond the scope of this chapter but is well outlined by White and Yashon.[172]

Despite the serious neurologic disability associated with spinal cord trauma, the large majority of patients survive. Of those with paraplegia who survive the first three months, 86 percent are alive 10 years later; of those with quadriplegia, 80 percent are alive 10 years later.

REFERENCES

General References

1. Adams, R.D. and Victor, M. Principles of Neurology. New York, McGraw-Hill, 1977.
2. Baker, A.B. and Baker, L.H. Clinical Neurology, Vols. 1–3. Hagerstown, Md., Harper & Row, 1977.
3. Gilroy, J. and Meyer, J.S. Medical Neurology, 3rd ed. New York, Macmillan, 1979.
4. Merritt, H.H. Textbook of Neurology, 6th ed. Philadelphia, Lea & Febiger, 1979.
5. Tyler, H.R. and Dawson, D.M. Current Neurology, Vol. 1. Boston, Houghton Mifflin, 1978.
6. Youmans, S.R. Neurological Surgery, Vols. 1–3. Philadelphia, Saunders, 1973.
7. Vinken, P.J. and Bruyn, G.W. Handbook of Clinical Neurology, Vols. 1–35. Amsterdam, North Holland, 1969–1979.

The Neurologic History and Examination

8. Denny-Brown, D. Handbook of Neurological Examination and Case Recording. Cambridge, Ma., Harvard University, 1957.
9. Medical Research Council, War Memorandum No. 7. Aids to the Investigation of Peripheral Nerve Injuries. London, Her Majesty's Stationary Office, reprinted 1978.
10. Ross, R.T. How to Examine the Nervous System. Springfield, Ill., Thomas, 1978.
11. Samuels, M.A. (ed.). Manual of Neurologic Therapeutics. Boston, Little, Brown, 1978.
12. Strub, R. and Black, F.W. The Mental Status Examination in Neurology. Philadelphia, F.A. Davis, 1977.
13. Walsh, F.B. and Hoyt, W.F. Clinical Neuro-ophthalmology (3 vols.), 3rd ed. Baltimore, Williams & Wilkins, 1969.

The Use of Ancillary Diagnostic Tests

14. Abrams, H.L. and McNeil, B.J. Medical implications of computed tomography ("CAT Scanning"). N. Engl. J. Med., 198:255, 1978.
15. Bradac, G.B., Simon, R.S., Grumme, T., and Schramm, J. Limitations of computed tomography for diagnostic neuroradiology. Neuroradiology, 13:243, 1977.
16. Deland, F.H. and Wagner, H.N. Atlas of Nuclear Medicine, Vol. 1. Brain. Philadelphia, Saunders, 1969.
17. Kiloh, L.G., McComas, A.J., and Osselton, J.W. Clinical Electroencephalography, 3rd ed. London, Butterworth, 1972.

18. Krayenbühl, H.A. and Yasargil, M.G. Cerebral Angiography, 2nd ed. London, Butterworth, 1968.
19. Taveras, J.M. and Wood, E.H. Diagnostic Neuroradiology, 2nd ed. Baltimore, Williams & Wilkins, 1976.
20. Toole, J.F. Special Techniques for Neurologic Diagnosis. Philadelphia, F.A. Davis, 1969.
21. Walker, A.E. Cerebral Death. Dallas, Professional Informational Library, 1977.

Disorders of Consciousness

22. Plum, F. and Posner, J.B. The Diagnosis of Stupor and Coma, 2nd ed. Philadelphia, Davis, 1972.

Disorders of Memory

23. Brooks, B.R., Jubelt, B., Swarz, J.R., and Johnson, R.T. Slow virus infections. Annu. Rev. Neurosci., 2:309, 1979.
24. Freeman, J.M. The clinical spectrum and early diagnosis of Dawson's encephalitis. J. Pediatr., 75:590, 1969.
25. Gadjusek, D.C. and Gibbs, C.J., Jr. Kuru, Creutzfeldt-Jakob disease, and transmissible presenile dementias. In ter Meulen, V. and Katz, M. (eds.), Slow Virus Infections of the Central Nervous System. New York, Springer-Verlag, 1977.
26. Gadjusek, D.C., Gibbs, C.J. Jr., Asher, D.M., Brown, P., Diwan, A., Hoffman, P., Nemo, G., Rohwer, R., and White, L. Precautions in medical care of, and in handling materials from, patients with transmissible virus dementia (Creutzfeldt-Jakob Disease). N. Engl. J. Med., 297:1253, 1977.
27. Gibbs, C.J. Jr. and Gadjusek, D.C. Atypical viruses as the cause of sporodic, epidemic and familial chronic diseases in man: slow viruses and human diseases. Perspect. in Virol. 10:161, 1978.
28. Katzman, R., Terry, R.D., and Bick, K.L. (eds.). Alzheimer's Disease: Senile Dementia and Related Disorders. New York, Raven, 1978.
29. Kral, V.A. Benign senescent forgetfulness. In Katzman, R., Terry, R.D., and Bick, K.L. (eds.), Alzheimer's Disease: Senile Dementia and Related Disorders. New York, Raven, 1978.
30. Litjmaer, H., Field, P.A., and Katzman, R. Prevalence and malignancy of Alzheimer's disease. Arch. Neurol., 39:304, 1976.
31. Richardson, E.P. Jr. Progressive multifocal leukoencephalopathy. N. Engl. J. Med., 265:815, 1961.
32. Selkoe, D.J. Cerebral aging and dementia. In Tyler, H.R. and Dawson, D.M. (eds.), Current Neurology, Vol. 1. Boston, Houghton Mifflin, 1978.

Disorders of Communication

33. Benson, D.F. and Geschwind, N. The aphasias and related disturbances. In A.B. Baker and L.H. Baker (eds.), Clinical Neurology, Vol. 1. Hagerstown, Md., Harper & Row, 1976.
34. Naeser, M.A. and Hayward, R.W. Lesion localization in aphasia with cranial computed tomography and the Boston Diagnostic Aphasia Exam. Neurology, 28:545, 1978.
35. Ojemann, G.A. and Whitaker, H.A. Language localization and variability. Brain and Language, 6:239, 1978.

Disorders of Movement

36. Hurwitz, L.J. and Adams, G.F. Rehabilitation of hemiplegia: indices of assessment and prognosis. Br. Med. J., 1:94, 1972.
37. Marshall, J., Crawford, T., and Crompton, M.F. The Management of Cerebrovascular Disease. Boston, Little, Brown, 1968.
38. Toole, J.F. and Patel, A.N. Cerebrovascular Disorders. New York, McGraw-Hill, 1967.

Parkinsonism and Other Disorders of Extrapyramidal Function

39. Biachine, J.R., Messiha, F.S., and Preziosi, T.J. Carbidopa. In Parkinsonism: Inhibition of the Metabolism of $L-[2-^{14}C]=DOPA$. In Melvin Yahr (ed.), Advances in Neurology: Treatment of Parkinsonism, Vol. 2. New York, Raven, 1973.
40. Campbell, A.M.G., Corner, B., Norman, R.M., and Urish, H. The rigid form of Huntington's disease. J. Neurol. Neurosurg. Psychiatry, 27:71, 1961.
41. Cotzias, G.C., Papavasiliou, P.S., and Gellene, R. Modification of parkinsonism: chronic treatment with L-dopa. N. Engl. J. Med., 280:337, 1969.
42. David, N.J., Mackey, E.A., and Smith, J.L. Further observations in progressive supranuclear palsy. Neurology, 18:349, 1968.
43. Diamond, S.G. and Markham, Ch.H. Present mortality in Parkinson's disease: the ratio of observed to expected deaths with a method to calculate expected deaths. J. Neurol. Transmission, 38:259, 1976.
44. Holtzman, N.A., Naughton, M.A., Iber, F.L., and Gaumnitz, B.M. Ceruloplasmin in Wilson's disease. J. Clin. Invest., 46:993, 1967.
45. Horneykiewicz, O.D. Physiologic, biochemical and pathological backgrounds of levodopa and possibilities for the future. Neurology, 20:1, 1970.
46. Mardsen, C.D. and Parkes, J.D. Success and problems of long-term levodopa therapy in Parkinson's Disease. Lancet, 1:345, 1977.
47. Shy, G.M. and Drager, G.A. A neurological syndrome associated with orthostatic hypotension: a clinical-pathologic study. Arch. Neurol., 2:511, 1960.
48. Steele, J.C., Richardson, J.C., and Olszewski, J. Progressive supranuclear palsy, a heterogeneous degeneration involving the brain stem, basal ganglia, and cerebellum with vertical gaze and pseudobulbar palsy, nuchal dystonia and dementia. Arch. Neurol., 10:333, 1964.
49. Sternleib, J. and Scheinberg, I.H. Penicillamine therapy for hepatolenticular degeneration. JAMA, 189:748, 1964.
50. Swanson, P.D., Luttrell, C.N., and Magladery, J.W. Myoclonus: a report of 67 cases and review of the literature. Medicine, 41:339, 1962.
51. Vanderhaeghan, J.-J., Perier, O., and Sternon, J.E. Pathological findings in idiopathic orthostatic hypotension. Arch. Neurol., 22:207, 1970.
52. Wilson, S.A.K. Progressive lenticular degeneration: a familial nervous disease associated with cirrhosis of the liver. Brain, 34:295, 1912.

Ataxia and Other Abnormalities of Cerebellar Function

53. Kark, R.A.P., Rosenberg, R.N., and Schut, L.J. (eds.). The Inherited Ataxias. Advances in Neurology, Vol. 21. New York, Raven, 1978.
54. Konigsmark, B.W. and Weiner, L.P. The olivopontocerebellar atrophies: a review. Medicine, 49:227, 1970.
55. Stumpf, D.A. Freidreich's ataxia and other hereditary ataxias. In Tyler, H.R. and Dawson, D.M. (eds.), Current Neurology, Vol. 1. Boston, Houghton Mifflin, 1978, p. 86.

Brain Stem Dysfunction

56. Daroff, R.B. and Hoyt, W.F. Supranuclear disorders of the ocular control system in man. In Bach-y-Rita, P. and Collins, C.C. (eds.), The Control of Eye Movements. New York, Academic Press, 1971, pp. 175–235.
57. Haymaker, W. and Kuhlenbeck, H. Disorders of the brainstem and its cranial nerves. In Baker, A.B. and Baker, L.N. (eds.), Clinical Neurology, Vol. III. Hagerstown, Md., Harper & Row, 1974.
58. Vinken, P.J. and Bruyn, G.W. Localization in clinical neurology. In Vinken, P.J. and Bruyn, G.W. (eds.), Handbook of Clinical Neurology, Vol. 2. Amsterdam, North-Holland, 1969.

Spinal Cord Disease

59. Brain, W.R. and Wilkinson, M. (eds.). Cervical Spondylosis and Other Disorders of the Cervical Spine. Philadelphia, Saunders, 1967.
60. Keener, E.B. Abscess formation in the spinal cord. Brain, 78:394, 1955.
61. McNabb, I. Backache. Toronto, Workmen's Compensation Board of Ontario, 1973.
62. Netsky, M.G. Syringomyelia. A clinicopathological study. Arch. Neurol., 70:741, 1953.
63. Riley, L.H., Jr., Robinson, R.A., Johnson, K.A., and Walker, A.E. The results of anterior interbody fusion of the cervical spine. Review of ninety-three consecutive cases. J. Neurosurg., 30:127, 1969.
64. Robinson, R.A. Approaches to the cervical spine C1–T1. In Schmidek, H.H. and Sweet, W.H. (eds.), Current Techniques in Operative Neurosurgery. New York, Grune & Stratton, 1977.
65. Wilkinson, M. Morbid anatomy of cervical spondylosis and myelopathy. Brain, 83:589, 1960.

Myasthenia Gravis

66. Buckingham, J.M., Howard, F.M., Bernatz, P.E. The value of thymectomy in myasthenia gravis. Ann. Surg., 184:453, 1976.
67. Castleman, B. The pathology of the thymus gland in myasthenia gravis. Ann. N.Y. Acad. Sci., 135:496, 1966.
68. Drachman, D.B. Myasthenia gravis. N. Engl. J. Med., 298:136, 1978.
69. Kao, I., Drachman, D.B. Myasthenic immunoglobulin accelerates acetylcholine receptor degradation. Science, 196:527, 1977.
70. Lindstrom, J.M., Seybold, M.E., Lennon, V.A., Whittingham, S., and Duane, D.D. Antibody to acetylcholine receptor in myasthenia gravis: prevalence, clinical correlates, and diagnostic value. Neurology, 26:1054, 1976.
71. Matell, G., Bergstrom, K., Franksson, C., Hammarstrom, L., Lefvert, A.K., Moller, E., von Reis, G., and Smith, E. Effect of some immunosuppressive procedures on myasthenia gravis. Ann. N.Y. Acad. Sci., 274:659, 1976.
72. Pinching, A.J., Peters, D.K., and Newsom-Davis, J. Remission of myasthenia gravis following plasma-exchange. Lancet, 2:1373, 1976.
73. Sahay, B.M., Blendis, L.M., and Green, R. Relation between myasthenia gravis and thyroid disease. Br. Med. J., 1:762, 1965.
74. Seybold, M.E. and Drachman, D.B. Gradually increasing doses of prednisone in myasthenia gravis. Reducing the hazards of treatment. N. Engl. J. Med., 290:81, 1974.

Peripheral Neuropathies

75. Asbury, A. and Johnston, P. Pathology of Peripheral Nerve. Philadelphia, Saunders, 1978.
76. Dyck, P., Thomas, P.K., and Lambert, E.H. (eds.). Peripheral Neuropathy. Philadelphia, Saunders, 1975.
77. Haymaker, W. and Woodhall, B. Peripheral Nerve Injuries: Principles of Diagnosis. Philadelphia, Saunders, 1953.
78. Raff, M. and Asbury, A. Ischemic mononeuropathy and mononeuropathy multiplex in diabetes mellitus. N. Engl. J. Med., 279:17, 1968.

Myopathies

79. Bohan, A. and Peter, J.B. Polymyositis and dermatomyositis. N. Engl. J. Med., 292:344, 1975.
80. Bonan, A., Peter, J.B., Bowman, R.L., and Pearson, C.M. A computer-assisted analysis of 153 patients with polymyositis and dermatomyositis. Medicine, 56:255, 1977.
81. DeVere, R., Bradley, W.G. Polymyositis: its presentation, morbidity and mortality. Brain, 98:637, 1975.
82. Drachman, D.A. Ophthalmoplegia plus. Arch. Neurol., 18:654, 1968.
83. Moxley, R.T. Myopathies. In Tyler, R.T. and Dawson, D.A. (eds.), Current Neurology, Vol. 1. Boston, Houghton Mifflin, 1978.
84. Prosser, E.J., Murphy, E.G., and Thompson, M.W. Intelligence and the gene for Duchenne muscular dystrophy. Arch. Dis. Child., 44:221, 1969.
85. Rowland, L.P., Clark, C., and Olarte, M. Therapy for dermatomyositis and polymyositis. In Griggs, R.L. and Moxley, R.T. (eds.), Advances in Neurology, Vol. 17. New York, Raven, 1977.
86. Rowland, L.P., Fahn, S., and Schotland, D. McArdle's disease. Arch. Neurol., 9:325, 1963.

Disorders of Sensation: Pain and Headache

87. Basbaum, A.I. and Fields, H.L. Endogenous pain control mechanisms: review and hypothesis. Ann. Neurol., 4:451, 1979.
88. Dalessio, D.J. (ed.). Wolf's Headache and Other Head Pain, 2nd ed. New York, Oxford, 1972.

89. Friedman, A.P. Research and Clinical Studies in Headache, Vol. 1. Baltimore, Williams & Wilkins, 1967.
90. ———. Research and Clinical Studies in Headache, Vol. II. Baltimore, Williams & Wilkins, 1969.
91. ———. Migraine headaches. JAMA, 222:1399. 1972.
92. Hamilton, C.R., Shelley, W.M., and Tumulty, P.A. Giant cell arteritis: including temporal arteritis and polymyalgia rheumatica. Medicine, 50:1, 1971.
93. Lance, J.W. Mechanism and Management of Headache. London, Butterworth, 1973.
94. Robinson, B.C. Histaminic cephalgia. Medicine, 37:161, 1968.
95. Speed, W.G. III. Migraine and other vascular headaches. In Harvey, J.C. (ed.), Practice of Medicine, Chap. 5., Vol. 10. New York, Harper & Row, 1967.

Disturbances of Sleep

96. Aserinsky, E. and Kleitman, N. Regularly occurring periods of eye motility and concomitant phenomena during sleep. Science, 118:273, 1953.
97. Chase, M.H. (ed.). The Sleeping Brain. Los Angeles, Brain Information Service, 1972.
98. Guilleminault, C., Eldridge, F., and Dement, W. Sleep apnea: a syndrome associated with several sleep disorders. Neurology (Minneap.), 23:389, 1973.
99. Kales, A. and Kales, T.K. Sleep disorders: recent findings in the diagnosis and treatment of disturbed sleep. N. Engl. J. Med., 290:487, 1974.
100. Oswald, I. Sleep and its disorders. In Vinken, P.J. and Bruyn, G.W. (eds.), Handbook of Clinical Neurology, Vol. 3. Amsterdam, North-Holland, 1969, pp. 80–111.
101. Weizman, E.D. (ed.). Advances in Sleep Research, Vol. 1. Flushing, N.Y., Spectrum, 1974.
102. Yoss, R.E. and Daly, D.D. Criteria for the diagnosis of the narcoleptic syndrome. Mayo Clin. Proc., 32:320, 1957.
103. Zarcone, V. Narcolepsy. N. Engl. J. Med., 288:1156, 1973.

Dizziness, Vertigo, and Hearing Loss

104. Baloh, R.W. and Honrubia, U. Clinical Neurophysiology of the Vestibular System. Philadelphia, F.A. Davis, 1978.
105. Dix, M.R. The vestibular acoustic system. In Vinken, P.J. and Bruyn, G.W. (eds.), Handbook of Clinical Neurology, Vol. 16. Amsterdam, Elsevier, 1974, p. 301.

Seizures and Syncope

106. American Academy of Pediatrics Committee on Drugs. Anticonvulsants in pregnancy. Pediatrics, 6:331, 1979.
107. Gastaut, H., Naquet, R., Poire, R., and Tassinari, C.A. Treatment of status epilepticus with diazepam (Valium). Epilepsia (Amsterdam), 6:167, 1965.
108. Jasper, H.H., Ward, A.A., and Pope, A. Basic Mechanisms of the Epilepsies, Boston, Little, Brown, 1969.
109. Kutt, H. and Penry, I.K. Usefulness of blood levels of antiepileptic drugs. Arch. Neurol., 31:283, 1974.
110. Morrell, F., Bradley, W., and Ptashne, M. Effects of drugs on discharge characteristics of chronic-epileptogenic lesions. Neurology, 9:492, 1959.
111. Niedermeyer, E. Compendium of the Epilepsies. Springfield, Ill., Thomas, 1974.
112. Penry, I.K. and Newmark, M.E. The use of antiepileptic drugs. Ann. Intern Med., 90:207, 1979.
113. Prensky, A.L., Raff M.D., Moore, M.J., and Schwab, R. Intravenous diazepam in the treatment of prolonged seizure activity. N. Engl. J. Med., 276:779, 1967.

Stroke Syndromes and Cerebrovascular Disorders

114. Ad hoc committee of NINDB. A classification and outline of cerebrovascular diseases. Neurology, 8:395, 1958.
115. Baker, R.B. Prospective study of transient ischemic attacks. In Moosy, J. and Janeway, R. (eds.), Seventh Princeton Conference on Cerebrovascular Disease. New York, Grune & Stratton, 1971, pp. 166–169.
116. Canadian Cooperative Study Group. A randomized trial of aspirin and sulfinpyrazone in threatened stroke. N. Engl. J. Med., 299:53, 1978.
117. Fields, W.S., Lemak, N.A., Frankowski, R.F., and Hardy, R.J. Controlled trial of aspirin in cerebral ischemia. Stroke, 8:301, 1977.
118. Fisher, C.M. Occlusion of the carotid arteries: further experiences. A.M.A. Arch. Neurol. Psychiat., 72:187, 1954.
119. Fisher, C.M. Lacunes: small, deep, cerebral infarcts. Neurology (Minneap.), 15:774, 1965.
120. ———, et al. Atherosclerosis of the carotid and vertebral arteries: extra- and intra-cranial. J. Neuropathol. Exp. Neurol., 24:455, 1965.
121. ———, Mohr, J.P., and Adams, R.D. Cerebrovascular diseases. In Wintrobe, M.M., Thorn, G.W., et al. (eds.), Harrison's Principles of Internal Medicine, 7th ed. New York, McGraw-Hill, 1974. Chap. 26, pp.1743–1779.
122. ———. and Pearlman, A. Non-sudden onset of cerebral embolism. Neurology, 17:1025, 1967.
123. ———, et al. Acute hypertensive cerebellar hemorrhage: diagnosis and surgical treatment. J. Nerv. Ment. Dis., 140:38, 1965.
124. Heyman, H., et al. Transient focal cerebral ischemia epidemiological and clinical aspects. Stroke, 5:277, 1974.
125. Lhermitte, F., Gautier, J.C., and Derouesne, C. Nature of occlusions of the middle cerebral artery. Neurology (Minneap.), 20:82, 1970.
126. Lindenberg, R. Patterns of CNS vulnerability in acute hypoxia, including anaesthetic accidents. In Schade, J.P. and McMenemy, W.H. (eds.), Selective Vulnerability of the Brain to Hypoxemia. Oxford, Blackwell, 1963, pp. 189–210.
127. Marshall, J. Angiography in the investigation of ischemic episodes in the territory of the internal carotid artery. Lancet, 1:719, 1971.
128. ———. The natural history of transient ischemic attacks. Q. J. Med., 33:309, 1964.
129. McDonald, W.I. Recurrent cholesterol emboli as a cause of fluctuating cerebral symptoms. J. Neurol. Neurosurg. Psychiatry, 30:489, 1967.
130. Mohr, J.P. Distal field infarction. Neurology (Minneap.), 19:279, 1969.
131. ———. Transient ischemic attacks and the prevention of strokes. N. Engl. J. Med., 299:93, 1978.

132. Sahs, A.L., et al. (eds.). Intracranial Aneurysms and Subarachnoid Hemmorrhage: a Cooperative Study. Philadelphia, Lippincott, 1969.

133. Sarner, M. and Rose, F.C. Clinical presentation of ruptured intracranial aneurysm. J. Neurol. Neurosurg. Psychiatry, 30:67, 1967.

134. Sindermann, F., Bechinger, D., and Dichagans, J. Occlusions of the internal carotid artery compared with those of the middle cerebral artery. Brain, 93:199, 1970.

135. Starr, M.A. The pathology of sensory aphasia. Brain, 12:82, 1889.

136. Thomas, J.E. and Reagan, T.J. Nonhemorrhagic complications of intracranial aneurysms of the internal carotid artery. Neurology (Minneap.), 20:1043, 1970.

137. Toole, J.F. Medical and surgical management of stroke. Stroke, 4:273, 1973.

138. ———. and Patel, A.N. Cerebrovascular Disorders, 2nd ed. New York, McGraw-Hill, 1974.

139. Troupp, H. Arteriovenous anomalies of the brain: prognosis without operation. Acta Neurol. Scand., 41:39, 1965.

Multiple Sclerosis and Other Demyelinating Diseases

140. Adams, R.D. and Kubik, C.S. The morbid anatomy of the demyelinative diseases. Am. J. Med., 12:510, 1952.

141. Arnason, B.G.W. Idiopathic polyneuritis (Landry-Guillain-Barre-Strohl Syndrome) and experimental allergic neuritis: A comparison. In Immunological Disorders of the Nervous System, A.R.N.M.D., Vol. 49. Baltimore, Williams & Wilkins, 1971, p. 156.

142. Batchelor, I.R., Compston, A., and McDonald, W.I. The significance of the association between HLA and multiple sclerosis. Br. Med. Bull., 34:279, 1978.

143. Cohen, S.R., Herndon, R.M., and McKhann, G.M. Radioimmunoassay of myelin basic protein in spinal fluid. N. Engl. J. Med., 295:1455, 1976.

144. Fisher, M. Unusual variant of acute idiopathic polyneuritis (syndrome of ophthalmoplegia, ataxia and areflexia). N. Engl. J. Med., 255:57, 1956.

145. Halliday, A.M., McDonald, W.I., and Mushin, J. Visual evoked potentials in patients with demyelinating disease. In Desmedt, J.E. (ed.), Visual Evoked Potentials in Man: New Developments. Oxford, Clarendon Press, 1977.

146. Hoeppner, T. and Lolas, F. Visual evoked responses and visual symptoms in multiple sclerosis. J. Neurol., Neruosurg. Psychiatry, 41:493, 1978.

147. Igarashi, M., Schaumberg, H.H., Powers, J., Kishimoto, Y., Kolodney, E., and Suzuki, K. Fatty acid abnormality in adrenoleukodystrophy. J. Neurochem., 26:851, 1976.

148. Johnson, K.P. and Nelson, B.J. Multiple sclerosis: diagnostic usefulness of cerebrospinal fluid. Ann. Neurol., 2:425, 1977.

149. Johnson, R.T. Slow viral diseases of the central nervous system: transmissibility vs. communicability. Clin. Neurosurg., 24:590, 1977.

150. McAlpine, D., Lumsden, C.E., and Acheson, E.D. Multiple Sclerosis: A Reappraisal, 2nd ed. Edinburgh and London, Churchill Livingstone, 1972.

151. McFarlin, D. and McFarland, H. Histocompatibility studies and multiple sclerosis. Arch. Neurol., 33:395, 1976.

152. Miller, H.G., Stanton, J.B., and Gibbons, J.L. Parainfectious encephalomyelitis and related syndromes: a critical review of the neurological complications of certain specific fevers. Q. J. Med., 25:427, 1956.

153. Percy, A.K. and McKhann, G.M. The biochemistry of myelin and the leukodystrophies. In Vinken, P.J. and Bruyn, G.W. (eds.), Handbook of Clinical Neurology, Vol. 10. Amsterdam, Elsevier, 1970.

154. Percy, A.K., Nobrega, F.T., Okazaki, H., Glattre, E., and Kurland, L.T. Multiple sclerosis in Rochester, Minn. Arch. Neurol., 25:105, 1971.

155. Plum, F., Posner, J.B., and Hain, R.F. Delayed neurological deterioration after anoxia. Arch. Intern. Med., 110:18, 1962.

156. Robinson, K. and Rudge, P. Auditory evoked responses in multiple sclerosis. Lancet, 1:1164, 1975.

157. Rose, A.S., Kuzma, J.W., Kurtzeke, J.F., Namerow, N.S., Sibley, W.A., and Tourtellotte, W.W. Cooperative study in the evaluation of therapy in multiple sclerosis: ACTH vs. placebo (Pt. 2). Neurology, 20:1, 1970.

158. Schaumburg, H.H., Powers, J.M., Suzuki, K., and Raine, C.S. Adreno-leukodystrophy (sex-linked Schilder Disease). Arch. Neurol., 31:210, 1974.

Increased Intercranial Pressure and Intracranial Masses

159. Boddie, H.G., Banna, M., and Bradley, W.G. "Benign" intracranial hypertension: a survey of the clinical and radiological features, and long-term prognosis. Brain, 97:313, 1974.

160. Fishman, R.A. Brain edema. N. Engl. J. Med., 293:706, 1975.

161. Foley, J. Benign forms of intracranial hypertension—"Toxic" and "otitic" hydrocephalus. Brain, 78:1, 1965.

162. Mertens, H.G. and Schimrigk, K. Differential diagnosis of intracranial space-occupying lesions. In Vinken, P.J. and Bruyn, G.W. (eds.), Handbook of Clinical Neurology, Vol. 16. Amsterdam, North Holland, 1974, pp. 209–253.

163. Ojemann, R.G., Fisher, C.M., Adams, R.D., Sweet, W.H., and New, P.F.J. Further experience with the syndrome of "normal" pressure hydrocephalus. J. Neurosurg., 31:279, 1969.

164. Posner, J.B. and Shapiro, W.R. Brain tumor: current status of therapy and its complications. Arch. Neurol. 32:781, 1975.

165. Plum, F. and Posner, J.B. The Diagnosis of Stupor and Coma, 2nd ed. Philadelphia, Davis, 1972.

166. Shapiro, W.R. and Young, D.F. Treatment of malignant glioma: a controlled study of chemotherapy and irradiation. Arch. Neurol. 33:494, 1976.

167. Walker, M.D. and Strike, T.A. An evaluation of methyl CCNU, BCNU, and radiotherapy in the treatment of malignant glioma. Proc. Am. Assoc. Cancer Res., 17:163, 1970.

Trauma to the Head and Neck

168. Branch, C.L. Post-traumatic epilepsy. In Youmans, J.R. (ed.), Neurological Surgery, Vol. II. Philadelphia, Saunders, 1973.

169. Levin, H.S. and Grossman, R.G. Behavioral sequelae of closed head injuries. Arch. Neurol. 35:720, 1978.

170. Walker, A.E. Mechanisms of cerebral trauma and the impairment of consciousness. In Youmans, J.R. (ed.), Neurological Surgery, Vol. II. Philadelphia, Saunders, 1973, pp. 936–949.

171. Walker, A.E., Caveness, W.F., and Critchley, M. The Late Effects of Head Injury. Springfield, Ill., Thomas, 1969.

172. White, R.J. and Yashon, D. General care of cervical spine injuries. In Youmans, J.R. (ed.), Neurological Surgery, Vol. II. Philadelphia, Saunders, 1973.

SECTION SIXTEEN
Psychiatry in Medicine
JOHN B. IMBODEN: SECTION EDITOR

——CHAPTER 133——
The Place of Psychiatry in Medicine
JOHN B. IMBODEN

The nature of medical practice is such that physicians are inescapably involved in the practice of psychiatry. The facts which support this assertion are discussed below.

It is a general principle in medicine that many of the signs and symptoms of disease are manifestations of physiologic responses that represent attempts to cope with noxious agents or with alterations in the organism which may themselves be consequences of adaptive processes. The tachypnea, leukocytosis, and fever of pneumonia; the ventricular hypertrophy of long-standing hypertension; and the general malaise and weakness that lead to energy-conserving rest are commonplace examples of physiologic coping responses that comprise an important part of many clinical syndromes. Equally important, although often receiving only lip-service recognition, are the psychological adaptations to serious illness and concurrent life stresses; these coping reactions also constitute an important part of the whole clinical picture.

The critical nature of psychological coping responses to illness is apparent when one reflects upon the importance of the patient's initial registration of discomfort, his ability to make a judgment that help is needed, his efforts to reduce intolerable uncertainty by developing his own theories about what is wrong with himself, his feelings about those persons to whom he has entrusted his care, and his reaction to the separations and disruptions occasioned by illness and treatment. On occasion the emotional and behavioral accompaniments of psychological coping processes may even dominate the clinical situation and require just as careful diagnostic evaluation and management as do other aspects of the illness.

With this in mind, it behooves the physician to be aware that he himself, apart from any drugs or procedures which he may administer, is potentially a therapeutic agent, an agent that is not without the possibility of adverse side effects. In fact, the physician to whom the seriously ill or worried patient comes for help is in a unique position to form an influential relationship with the patient. Doctors since antiquity have known this, and the quotation from Peabody's classic essay on the first page of this book is a particularly eloquent reminder of the critical significance of the doctor–patient relationship. Traditionally, the physician has recognized that he must conduct himself in a way that will inspire "confidence," i.e., he must not only possess competence and integrity, but convey these attributes to the patient in the thoughtfulness and thoroughness of his approach. He must be capable of warmth and compassion, but without losing analytical objectivity. These and other time-honored qualities are so obviously essential to the art of medicine that no one has deemed it necessary to do a controlled study to establish their value. It is possible, however, for the physician to go beyond the utilization of these rather general and "nonspecific" aspects of his relationship with the patient in using that relationship as part of his diagnostic and therapeutic armamentarium. There are occasions when he may quite deliberately alter his approach in a given clinical situation in order to attain specific objectives or to help the patient to do so. To do this, he must have some understanding of the principles of human behavior and of the application of them in forging diagnostic and therapeutic approaches to specific emotional or behavioral components of the clinical problem.

The importance of the development of substantial psychiatric competence by the physician is further buttressed by the simple fact that he probably sees far more patients with primarily emotional disorders than any other specialist, including the psychiatrist. In 1939, a distinguished diagnostician reported the results of a review of 500 consecutive patients who consulted him.[3] He found that 33 percent of these patients "suffered solely or predominantly from functional disorders" by which the author meant that no "organic cause" at all was found or only "minor organic lesions" not related to the symptoms. In reviewing various reports on the frequency of psychiatric morbidity in nonpsychiatric divisions of general hospitals, Lipowski[4] concluded that there is evidence that "30 to 60 percent of inpatients and 50 to 80 percent of outpatients suffer from psychic distress or psychiatric illness" of a clinically significant degree. These are sobering figures even if one accepts only the lower end of the range of estimates. One cannot conclude from these data that every practicing physician must be able to engage his patients in intensive psychotherapy, but one can conclude that substantial diagnostic and therapeutic skill in relation to emotional disorders is as important as it is in other kinds of illness.

These observations support Hamman's[3] comment: "The physician studies and practices psychiatry continuously, even when he protests that he has not the least knowledge of formal psychiatry. It is the chief instrument of his success, even though he may practice it unconsciously."

Finally, an intriguing and controversial series of investigations has led to the development of the theory that in ways not yet understood, certain kinds of psychic stress contribute importantly to the etiology of various organic diseases, the psychophysiologic or psychosomatic disorders. Historically prominent among these disorders are duodenal ulcer and ulcerative colitis. Methodologic difficulties in proving the role of psychological factors in the causation and alleviation of these and other diseases postulated to be psychosomatic are enormous but in the interests of science and of the individual patient, it is important to be aware of the psychosomatic point of view. It is conceivable that further development of our knowledge of psychological influences upon human physiology may ultimately prove to have a considerable and possibly radical impact upon our understanding and management of certain organic disorders.

In summary, psychiatry has an integral relationship with internal medicine for several reasons:

1. Psychological responses to physical illness are as invariably a part of the clinical syndrome as are physiologic responses.
2. The therapeutic potential of the physician–patient relationship can be more fully realized if the physician deliberately cultivates an understanding of human behavior and of fundamental principles of psychiatric treatment.
3. Repeated surveys have shown that a substantial percentage of medical inpatients and outpatients suffer primarily from emotional disorders.
4. The study of the influence of psychological factors on physiology, while controversial, may prove to be of profound significance in the future of medicine.

In view of the above considerations, the remainder of this section will deal with general principles that are basic to an understanding of human behavior, the illustration of some of these principles in the various ways in which people react to physical illness and treatment, some common psychiatric problems encountered by the physician, a brief discussion of the major psychiatric disorders and psychosomatic illnesses, and a review of basic principles and techniques of psychiatric treatment.

CHAPTER 134

Human Behavior: Some Basic Considerations

JOHN B. IMBODEN

It is the purpose of this chapter to discuss certain general principles of human behavior which may be useful to the physician in his approach to understanding the patient. It is impossible to treat this complex subject in a truly comprehensive way in a single chapter, and even if unlimited space were available, limitations are imposed by the incompleteness of our knowledge.

STIMULUS AND RESPONSE

All living organisms respond to stimuli, but the human being differs from lower animals in the enormous complexity of variables that intervenes between stimulus and response. As a consequence, the repertoire of human responses is incomparably larger than that of the next most highly evolved species. Human behavior is much less dominated by inborn, stereotyped patterns of behavior or instincts than is that of lower animals and, therefore, is less predictable. Further, the human being compensates for the relative lack of instincts and of other adaptive advantages that lower animals have (a coat of fur, climbing agility, claws, and speed) by his advanced ability to use tools and language, by the transmission of knowledge from previous generations, and by his utilization of social organization for the attainment of common objectives.

What is meant by the "complexity of variables" that is situated between stimulus and response? From a neurophysiologic point of view, one could attempt to describe these variables in terms of that portion of the neuronal network of the central nervous system that is interposed, in any given instance, between the involved afferent and efferent peripheral nerve fibers. As important as this is, however, one cannot at this time give a useful account of the varieties of human responses in neurophysiologic terms, and it is doubtful that this will ever be possible. While the findings of neurophysiology and neurochemistry are becoming increasingly relevant to the practice of clinical psychiatry, it is nonetheless evident that to approach the subjective and behavior responses of human beings from a strictly neurophysiologic point of view would be comparable to evaluating the "answers" of a computer by examining its circuitry rather than by scrutinizing the way in which it has been programmed.

Approach and Avoidance

Perhaps a commonplace example will illustrate the preceding point. Mrs. Smith discovers a nodule in her right breast. Her first response is one of alarm, but not panic. She immediately mentions the discovery to her husband, and the next morning, after a night of fitful sleep, telephones her physician, explains the situation to him, and is given an appointment.

Her neighbor, Mrs. Jones, makes a similar discovery. She, too, responds with a feeling of concern, but says nothing to anyone. In the ensuing 2 months, her husband observes that she is more moody than usual and seems a bit distant and preoccupied. One evening he, too, discovers the lump in her breast and, over her protestations that it is "nothing," insists that she see the family doctor.

In general terms, one could say that Mrs. Smith coped with the disturbing "stimulus" by the response of "approach" while her neighbor's response to the same stimulus was one of "avoidance." It is of interest that Aitken-Swan and Paterson[5,11] in reviewing the histories of 2700 patients with carcinoma of the breast, cervix, skin, and mouth found that in 45 percent, 3 months or more elapsed between the initial appearance of symptoms and reporting to the physician. Many of the patients who delayed going to the physician apparently did so to avoid having their fears of cancer confirmed.

To understand fully the differences in response to the discovery of a nodule of the breast shown by these two patients would probably require an in-depth study of both individuals. It is likely, however, that a not so extensive study would enable one to gain partial comprehension of their behavior. Let us confine our attention to Mrs. Jones. Her history reveals that she has a tendency to respond to all threatening situations by putting her head in the sand and hoping they will somehow go away. Therefore, her response to the discovery of a nodule in her breast turns out to be characteristic of her, i.e., it is a feature of her character if one defines the latter as being composed of relatively enduring attitudes and patterns of behavior. Further, it is learned that at the age of 12, Mrs. Jones lost her mother who died of cancer, and at the time of this tragedy, she overheard some veiled criticisms of the doctors. As a consequence, Mrs. Jones developed a rather fatalistic notion about the treatability of cancer and was distrustful of physicians. She may even have felt destined to suffer the same fate as her mother, because she had felt inexplicably guilty following her mother's death, as if she may have been to blame in some way. This earlier family experience had reinforced her tendency to disregard anything having to do with cancer, including televised admonitions concerning early detection and treatment.

It should be noted that our limited knowledge of Mrs. Jones does not enable us to say that she has a psychiatric illness. It is true that her tendency to avoid facing unpleasant realities can be labeled as "neurotic behavior" yet she may not be afflicted with a constellation of symptoms that would warrant the diagnosis of a specific neurosis.

Further Elaboration of Coping Responses

The term "coping" usually connotes a type of response by which the individual successfully deals with a problem or adapts himself to a situation. If, however, one includes in this term behavior that is partially successful in allaying or preventing the emergence of an unbearable feeling, such as anxiety, the well-known defense mechanisms can be regarded as a category of coping responses.

In the normal paradigm, the individual "copes" with his environment (internal and external) by being alert to relevant cues. Perception of a problem is followed by actively seeking more information about it and by assessing its significance through comparison of the present situation with related past experiences. This, in turn, arouses the person to adopt a course of action that he believes suitable both to his ability and his needs or goals. It is unlikely that anyone always responds to the manifold situations of life in this ideal manner. Defensive behavior, in which some aspect of reality is avoided, is used to some extent by all human beings at various times in their lives. There are a variety of ways by which people may avoid painful aspects of the world around them or minimize anxiety engendered by intrapsychic conflict.

The following is a list of some of the more common defense mechanisms.

1. *Repression*—The exclusion from conscious awareness of feelings and ideas.
2. *Denial*—A process in which one avoids becoming aware of some aspect of reality, such as a severe loss or bodily illness, or associated feelings.
3. *Rationalization*—Behavior is often the outcome of more than one motivation. In rationalization, there is selective awareness of an acceptable motivation and unawareness of less acceptable ones.
4. *Projection*—An attribute of one's self, such as a feeling or impulse, is ascribed to someone else. Externalization is a form of projection illustrated by the person who avoids recognition of his own contribution to his problems by "blaming them" on some aspect of the environment.
5. *Displacement*—Feelings and attitudes toward one individual are directed to another. Displacement from early parental figures to current substitutes is transference.
6. *Reaction formation*—The repression of a feeling is bolstered by replacing it in conscious awareness with its opposite.
7. *Regression*—The individual adapts to a current situation by retreating to a mode of behavior characteristic of an earlier period of his life.

The reader is referred to the classical monograph by Anna Freud for further discussion of psychological defenses.[8]

PERSONALITY DEVELOPMENT

Students of human behavior have long been intrigued not only by the variability of human responses to nearly identical "stimuli" but also by the fact that a given individual tends to repeat patterns of behavior as he goes through life. This is one of the observations that has led to extensive examination of early childhood experiences, since detailed study of behavior patterns often reveals that they are traceable to the earliest periods of life that the subject can recall.

Early Dependency

There is little doubt that the long period of relative helplessness and dependency of the human infant is of profound psychological significance. In the first months of life, the baby is utterly dependent for life-support upon the mother or her substitute. It is impossible to know what is going on in the mind of the preverbal infant, but it is known that all infants are by no means alike at birth. Some are relatively placid, sleep a lot, cry little, and get on an eating and sleeping schedule with ease; others are noisy, very active, sleep less, and are more demanding; still others are in between. These differences are among the innate, perhaps hereditary, features that play a role in personality development and which doubtlessly influence the way the mother responds to the infant.

At the beginning, the mother characteristically becomes involved with the infant in a love relationship which has a rather "narcissistic" coloring; the baby, which not so long ago, was a part of her own body continues to be felt as an extension of herself for awhile. She is exquisitely aware of when her baby is hungry, wet, or in pain. The initial relationship of the mother and infant is such an intimate and interdependent one that some authors have referred to it as "symbiotic" in that the well-being of both mother and child depend (in different ways) on their relationship with each other.

Separation and Individuation

As the infant develops and learns to sit up, crawl, walk, and acquires language, he slowly separates himself from the mother. This process of separation and individuation begins in the first year of life, and under normal circumstances progresses rapidly during the remainder of childhood.[10] During this period, the child can be described as incorporating countless experiences of being cared for and as drawing upon these experiences in learning to care for himself. With this in mind, it is apparent that normal maturation is thwarted by severe maternal neglect on the one hand and by excessive indulgence on the other. Most mothers seem naturally to be attuned to their child's increasing autonomy and experience an intermingling of sadness and joy in fostering it.

Gratification

To return to the very early stage of development, it may be noted that the infant demands and usually gets quick gratification of his needs. It is not surprising that as he becomes aware of the existence of persons (parents) who meet these needs, he perceives them as godlike, i.e., omniscient, omnipotent, and good. It is also inevitable that he will, for awhile, believe in the magic power of his own thoughts and wishes, because at one time in his life he had but to cry and his needs would be met. Further, in the normal course of events in which the child has repeatedly had the experience that "being good" brings rewards and the opposite brings punishment, he will come to feel that when something good or bad (such as illness) happens to him, it is because he has done or thought something to deserve it; and, in varying degrees, this feeling persists throughout life.

In addition to having acquired the ability to tolerate the postponement of gratification, to relinquish unfulfillable wishes, and increasingly to take care of himself, the child develops a conscience, i.e., he internalizes parental standards and, henceforth, does not look exclusively to others for approval and disapproval.

Early School Years

The span of years from about age 6 to puberty is a time which Freud referred to as the "latency" period in which sexual drives and interests, though by no means absent, are *comparatively* dormant. During this period, the child continues to be free of conflict with parental values and regulations. He identifies himself primarily with his family and is home-centered, while at the same time he is progressively exposed to more experiences outside the home: in the classroom, the playground, and the neighborhood.

Boys and girls of this period tend to form friendships mainly with peers of their own sex, often having special friends or chums, forming clubs, and having secrets. All of this usually occurs without preoccupation with the defiance of authority that is so common at a later stage.

During these years there is a remarkable display of interest in a wide variety of subjects. Hobbies are cultivated, sometimes several at a time, and are often pursued to considerable length and with much industry before being dropped. As Erikson has noted, the child of this period becomes acquainted with the technology of his culture.

If the individual has successful experiences in the grade school period, his self-confidence is enhanced. On the other hand, if the youngster encounters serious learning difficulties that interfere with school work and hobbies; encounters a tense, conflict-laden, or confusing home environment; or is not given the freedom to socialize with peers, he is apt to emerge from this developmental stage with feelings of inferiority, possibly even cynicism, and with impaired ability to face the crucial challenges of adolescence.

Adolescence[7]

In this period, the individual makes the biologic and psychological transition from childhood to adulthood. Adolescence begins with puberty. Its beginning, thus, has relatively clear biologic markers: onset of menses, development of secondary sexual characteristics, and genital growth. The end of adolescence is more difficult to define since it refers to the attainment of adult status in a psychological as well as a physical sense. The psychological completion of adolescence implies that the individual has achieved independence from parents, the ability to incorporate sexual drives in his or her relationships with the opposite sex, and a realistic awareness of his own attributes, interests, and goals, including career goals.

Although normal development during adolescence is not invariably accompanied by marked turbulence, it frequently is. For this reason the assessment of adolescent behavior as normal or pathologic may be quite difficult, requiring considerable experience on the part of the observer and sometimes requiring repeated observations over a period of time. This is an important point, because unwarranted labeling of the adolescent may, in itself, have undesirable consequences.

It is to be expected that with the "awakening" of genital sexuality at puberty, the adolescent will begin to shift his emotional and libidinal investments to persons other than members of his own family, i.e., to teachers, coaches, youthful leaders at school, and to peers of the same and opposite sex. This move away from parents to persons outside the family is typically motivated on the one hand by the adolescent's need to guard himself from the possible intrusion of sexuality into his affectionate ties to his family and, on the other hand, by his incorporation of cultural expectations that he become more independent or "grown-up." The adolescent usually feels ambivalent about leaving his childhood. Feelings of sadness or mild depression in this period are common. From time to time, especially during stress, the adolescent may experience a regressive pull, a desire to be a child again, which in turn may evoke a compensatory reaction of exaggerated independence.

The adolescent, especially in the early teenage

years, may reinforce his psychological move away from his parents by developing an attitude of indifference toward them, by developing an oppositional attitude toward them, or by "dethroning" his parents through assessing their values and ideas as old-fashioned or as lacking any validity. During this early phase the adolescent begins to spend more and more time away from home, and this trend continues throughout this developmental period. Prior to the achievement of a comfortable acceptance of his own sexual urges, the adolescent may occasionally utilize his expanding intellectual abilities defensively, i.e., he may become transiently engrossed in abstract philosophical, artistic, or religious subjects, or various forms of idealism to the temporary exclusion of more earthy preoccupations.

During adolescence the individual becomes increasingly able to form lasting relationships outside the home. Peer relationships, both individual and group, more or less replace the parents as a source of guidance and acceptance. This new peer dependence is reflected in the intense need of the adolescent not to be too different from the others in his circle of friends, or to risk alienation from them in any other way. The adolescent eventually integrates sexual feelings in his relationships with others, and as he approaches adulthood, he develops enough confidence in his own ideas and ideals that he can once more relate to his parents without feeling threatened. Concomitantly with this, he develops a relatively stable set of values and goals, a sense of who he is and of what he wants to do with his life (at least in general terms). That is, he has developed an "identity" of his own. This normal development is facilitated by giving the adolescent recognition, in the sense of encouraging him to accept an appropriate degree of responsibility and independence, tempered by the judicious proffering of support and tolerance when he yields to the "regressive pull" and temporarily reverts to childish behavior.

SOME PROBLEMS OF ADOLESCENCE. In making the critically important move away from the parents in the early teenage years, the adolescent will be hampered if, for any reason, he anticipates rejection by his peers. Because of the rapid physical changes associated with puberty and accelerated growth, the adolescent is particularly sensitive about his physical status and appearance. Anything which makes him "too different" may arouse concern, such as being too bright, too dull, too fat, too skinny, or having some physical blemish such as acne. Therefore, the physician does well to take seriously the possible psychological problems of the teenager who is struggling with physical difficulties such as acne, obesity, or dia-

betes. Not only may these physical problems be felt as threatening to the adolescent's position with peers, but their medical management requires continuing compliance with a treatment plan. This situation calls for considerable understanding, tact, and flexibility on the part of the physician. Rebellion against the treatment plan is less apt to occur if

1. The adolescent understands the rationale of treatment and what he has to gain from compliance with the treatment plan.
2. He is given a chance to express his own feelings about his condition.
3. His suggestion about one or another aspect of the treatment plan is invited and taken seriously.

The adolescent will also have difficulty in achieving independent values and goals if he has sensed that one or both of his parents do not want him to grow up. In this instance he may be hampered more by guilt than by fear. Failure to achieve independent values, goals, and vocational or career direction (autonomy) by the early twenties is called identify diffusion or identity crisis. Many patients with anorexia nervosa seem to be unusually well-behaved, dependent, conforming adolescents, relatively lacking in self-directedness except for their stubborn insistence on self-starvation which understandably makes their parents frantic. Also in schizophrenic illness which may first become manifest during adolescence, the patient often seems not to have resolved basic issues concerning autonomy versus conformity.

Adulthood[6,9]

In adulthood, people continue to learn, change, and grow, although usually not as rapidly or as dramatically as during childhood or adolescence.

With the successful completion of adolescence, the young adult settles into or is clearly on a path toward careers of vocation, marriage, parenthood, or all three. In making his career choice, the young person attempts to match his own interests and aptitudes, as he assesses them, with the opportunities for training and for obtaining work which he believes are available to him. He must attain the technical competence required by his chosen field and must have the interpersonal skills necessary to form relatively lasting and productive relationships with superiors and peers. It is not at all uncommon for the young adult to feel a certain amount of insecurity or anxiety at this stage of life, because he has not yet had enough experience to be confident that his own abilities (as he assesses them) are sufficient for him to "make it" out in the world. The anxiety arising from a sense of disparity between his self-image, or what he is, with his image of what he ought to be may at times lead the young adult to withdraw or retreat from challenging situations on the one hand or, at the other extreme, to develop a defensive exaggeration of his abilities. Usually, however, these swings in attitudes are not as marked as those of adolescence. This type of concern is one of the factors related to the observation that the neuroses, which are characterized by anxiety or symptomatic defenses against anxiety, often have their onset in young adulthood.

Most young adults get married and have children. Successful marriage requires the individual to have a capacity for intimacy with another person. Persons involved in an intimate relationship have enough trust in each other and enough confidence in themselves to reveal their feelings and needs while at the same time respecting the other's autonomy and privacy. Conflicts between the demands of work and those of the family are common, and when they occur both parties of the marriage are called upon to order their priorities in a practical and flexible way.

Those young adults who marry and raise children have the enlightening experience of piloting someone else through the channels they themselves have traversed in the not-so-distant past. In doing so, the young parents are apt to encounter issues, problems, and conflicts in their children which are reminiscent of their own experiences at various stages of development.

Most young adults have, to some degree, an illusion of indestructibility and an understandable feeling of having an abundance of time in which to live and to accomplish their plans. Typically, the young person looks upon illness, disability, and death as rather abstract or remote possibilities if, indeed, he thinks about them at all. This, of course, changes markedly as the person gets into middle age.

Middle age bears some resemblance to adolescence in that it, too, is a period of life in which significant biologic changes occur in the individual. The male observes that he has less hair on his head and more on his chest; the torso may become more rounded, especially the lower abdomen; and the legs may become thinner and less strong. Various health problems, some minor and others more major, often develop. There is usually a perceptible, slow decline in resilience or endurance. While intellectual functions are usually well preserved there may, nonetheless, be a decrease in the person's inclination to learn new concepts. The menopause occurs signaling to the woman that the childbearing period of her life has come to a close.

If the middle-aged person anticipates (correctly or not) a diminution or termination of sexual activity he or she may defensively show a recrudescence of sexual interest. This may, in part, arise from a feeling, common among middle-aged persons, that life is passing them by. Thus, it is as if certain gratifications must be achieved "now or never." This is an especially pressing issue if the individual feels cheated by life either as a result of his or her own constrictedness, or because of a too-early marriage that deprived the person of sufficient experimentation, or for some other reason. The "cheated" person, feeling that his sexual drives or abilities are on the wane or soon will be, may try to make up for lost time. This is the so-called "dangerous age" for both sexes and may be accompanied by an adolescent-like striking out from home base, getting involved in affairs, or perhaps divorce and a new marriage. This may be an occasion of profound pathos, a frenetic search for new beginnings, new experiences, a flowering of pseudo-youthful behavior which may mask underlying despair.

Middle age is also a time when the individual may, in a healthy and constructive way, take stock of himself and his situation. Sometimes this stocktaking results in the appropriate relinquishment of long-held but unrealizable ambitions. This relinquishment, which usually occurs piecemeal, is often accompanied by sadness or depression but it may also result in a less burdened life, one in which the individual feels "settled," as though he has hit his stride and is continuing to be productive while released from the strain of burdensome ambitions and is thus freer to enjoy the fruits of his labor. As this occurs, the individual often begins to devote a somewhat larger share of his or her time and energy to the welfare of the community at large, including the needs of the older and younger generations.

Relinquishment, arising from a different source, may also occur in middle life. For example, the giving up of old roles and satisfactions and the search for new ones may be necessitated by the departure of the youngest child for college, career, or marriage, or by other environmental circumstances that disrupt or terminate important roles and relationships. It is in this period of life that the individual may experience the death of parents, and it is not rare for a sibling or a peer to become seriously ill or to die. These experiences, in combination with the biologic changes taking place in the person, help to reduce or abolish the youthful illusion of indestructibility. The middle-aged person experiences time very differently from youth: Time seems to pass ever more quickly, and he becomes increasingly aware of the essential transience of the human condition. With this change in his *Wel-*

tanschaunng, the middle-aged person often develops a more peaceful and keen appreciation of experiences in the "here and now." All of these and other changes of middle life may result in a reordering of priorities, and a focusing on the things "that really matter" in life.

Occupational retirement is a built-in eventuality for most persons in our society who are employed and who reach the mid-sixties in age. There are many people who, upon retirement, find great satisfaction in not working and in being free to pursue interests for which they had never had enough time. There are others, however, for whom retirement turns into a period of emptiness and boredom. This is especially apt to be the case for those persons who have centered their lives on their work to the exclusion of other activities and interests. Abrupt or total retirement for such persons is usually ill-advised. A period of part-time employment, in lieu of full-time retirement, can be helpful in giving the person a continuing feeling of being useful, something interesting to do, and time in which to develop non-work-related, satisfying interests. With these considerations in mind, it is apparent that retirement should be thoughtfully planned for some time in advance of its occurrence. The primary physician often has an opportunity to encourage such planning by his patient.

Eventually, the diminishments of old age result in a narrowing of functions, varying degrees of disability, and, in conjunction with a decreasing circle of friends and family from sickness and death, there ensues a progressive restriction of activities and increased dependence on surviving relatives and institutions. In some ways, of course, the increased dependence upon others for life support in old age, can be looked upon, as it classically has been, as a "second childhood." Nevertheless, the comparison of old age with childhood is quite superficial. The elderly person, dependent though he may be, is often called upon to make adjustments to new and bewildering situations, to deal somehow with the inevitable multiple losses that impinge upon him including the near-term prospect of final separation from all he has ever known. It is little wonder that regressive behavior and depression are so commonly seen from middle age to the end of the life span. As with the adolescent, a most vital factor in helping the elderly person to live out his life with a sense of wholeness and dignity is that of continuing to recognize him or her as a person who still counts, who is loved, and who is useful and needed.

THE MATURE PERSONALITY

In view of the enormous variability in hereditary endowment and life experiences, it is to be expected that each individual personality is unique. Nevertheless, it is possible to describe in a general way some characteristics which are associated with the attainment of health and maturity.

The mature person, while interested and responsive to the reactions of others, has an inwardly derived feeling of self-respect. He is able realistically to appraise his own abilities and limitations and develops life goals in accordance with them. He is capable of forsaking the immediate gratification of a wish in the interest of a more distant objective. He can place his trust in others when this is appropriate and is able to form lasting, important relationships in which he exhibits empathy and love.

He will not, of course, be free of problems, but responds to them by recognizing their existence and actively attempting to cope with them. His coping responses are not rigidly stereotyped but reflect his ability correctly to assess present reality and to learn from past experience. When he experiences a failure, as he inevitably will, he is disappointed, but not devastated.

He is not totally conflict-free, is quite capable of being anxious or frightened and, therefore, has developed his own repertoire of defenses. He may also at times have minor fluctuations in mood for no apparent reason, but they are generally brief and not incapacitating.

CHAPTER 135
Coping with the Stresses of Serious Physical Illness
JOHN B. IMBODEN AND THOMAS N. WISE

the preceding chapter, we discussed some of the ways in which people respond to the stresses of life in general. In this chapter, we will consider emotional and behavioral responses to a specific type of stress in which the physician has a special interest, namely, that posed by serious physical illness, i.e., illness which requires hospitalization but from which partial or complete recovery is expected. (The management of the dying patient was discussed in Chap. 4.)

The prospective patient initially has the tasks of:

1. Recognizing the existence of a problem.
2. Taking the necessary steps to obtain appropriate medical help.
3. Relinquishing his customary social role upon entering the hospital.
4. Adapting to the complexities and uncertainties of life in a modern hospital, and, during convalescence.
5. Relinquishing the role of patient (the "sick role").
6. Returning to his preillness position in society to the extent that his recovery allows.[17]

Usually this entire process goes smoothly, although some degree of apprehension and depression are almost inevitable at one time or another in the course of illness. Occasionally, serious emotional disturbance occurs and requires careful evaluation and management.

THE ONSET OF ILLNESS

Usually an individual whose illness produces serious discomfort, functional impairment, or a perceptible change in his body will seek medical attention unless the initial awareness of becoming ill is accompanied by overwhelming fear or a sense of hopelessness. It should be noted, however, that certain kinds of symptoms and signs are frequently not observed by the patient even though they are readily apparent to relatives and close associates. This occurs particularly when a slowly progressive disease process adversely affects higher cerebral functions or organs of perception. The patient with slowly progressive deafness may be annoyed at others for mumbling while remaining unaware of his own difficulty in hearing. Bitemporal hemianopsia, unilateral blindness, blunting of affect, and gradual intellectual deterioration are among the functional disabilities which may either remain unnoticed or be denied by the patient though readily apparent to the physician on examination.

Assuming that the patient has been able to observe initial signs of illness, his subsequent response is determined in part by what these signs of illness mean to him as well as by his habitual mode of responding to stress.

The Meanings of Illness

Illness is almost always perceived as a threat, but in some circumstances it can also be seen as a promise.

ILLNESS AS A THREAT. The patient usually views serious physical illness as a potential loss. The most basic fear is loss of life, but the patient may also fear that he will be left crippled, disfigured, or in some way less of a person and, therefore, less valued and loved. The primacy of the threat of loss helps explain the depressive reactions frequently seen in the physically ill.

If the illness or its treatment threatens to deprive the patient of a characteristic mode of behavior, or life-style, which has served important defensive purposes in the preservation of self-esteem, he may react with extreme anxiety, followed by depression. For example, a person who is compelled to be very independent will react differently to the limitations imposed by myocardial infarction than will the person whose approach to life is not "driven" but is flexibly related to the everchanging demands of reality. The adolescent with his age-appropriate need to defy authority and gain peer approval will be more distressed at having diabetes with its never ending treatment regimen than the mature adult for whom the issues of independence and peer acceptance are no longer emotionally charged.

In families with limited finances or inadequate health insurance, serious illness may present the threat of economic catastrophe.

At times, a patient perceives his illness as something shameful. This attitude is reminiscent of the pariah status conferred by disease in ancient times when illness was regarded as a sign of punishment.

ILLNESS AS A PROMISE. Illness may be welcomed by the individual for whom it provides an avenue of escape from a difficult situation. The prospect of being free of responsibilities and of being cared for may be viewed very positively by a person who has intense dependency needs.

The shades and nuances of the meaning of being seriously ill are by no means exhausted by the brief list given above. The sensitive physician will always want to ascertain the context in which the patient's illness developed, and through the establishment of rapport and trust, encourage the patient to communicate his feelings and expectations.

Habitual Mode of Response to Stress

Deeply engrained attitudes, needs, and habitual modes of responding to life, all of which reflect the sum total of the person's past experiences, are important determinants of how an individual behaves when he becomes ill. While there is no really satisfactory scheme for typing personality or character, one may conceive of people as being distributed along a continuum. At one end of this continuum is the person who confronts reality squarely, reacts to any problem situation by getting more information about it, and in a calm, emotionally controlled manner makes and executes his plans accordingly. At the other extreme is the individual who, upon meeting any sort of threat, becomes excited, tends to retreat from the situation, denies unpleasant facts, plans poorly, is scattered and acts more on the basis of feeling than reason.[22] Between these extremes reside the majority of patients.

There are other personality characteristics that also have an important influence on the patient's initial and subsequent adaptation to illness. For example, the paranoid personality may be sufficiently distrustful and suspicious so that it is difficult for him to place his welfare in the hands of others. The schizoid individual tends to keep his distance from others and his feelings to himself. The passive-dependent person may welcome the legitimized dependency gratification afforded by illness or he may be extremely threatened by the possibility of regression and deny his dependency needs by overcompensation, i.e., by displaying exaggerated attitudes of independence which may seriously complicate management in certain clinical situations.

HOSPITALIZATION

It is a rare person who does not experience some degree of both fear and depression upon entering the hospital. The reasons for this are numerous:

1. Separation from the important "others" in the patient's life and from customary sources of satisfaction in recreation and work.
2. The peculiarities of hospital life. The hospitalized patient is confronted with the prospect of placing himself almost totally in the care of people who, with the exception of his personal physician, are apt to be complete strangers. Further, he is subjected to a number of procedures which have a "leveling" effect: certain personal belongings are removed for safekeeping, he is tagged with a wristband and clothed in a short white gown more or less open in the back, he endures repeated history taking and physical examination by house staff and students, has various body orifices inspected and probed, is carted around by wheelchair or stretcher for x-rays or tests, and in general is in a relatively passive position of having things done to him which he does not understand by people who are often in a hurry and who may seem to him to be concerned with patients who are more ill than he.
3. Uncertainty. There is always some degree of uncertainty in the patient's mind regarding the danger to life and limb, duration of hospital stay, the likelihood of suffering, and the ultimate outcome of his hospital experience. During the course of hospitalization, the seriously ill patient almost invariably undergoes some degree of *regression* and develops a relationship with the physician that is heavily colored by *transference*.[20]

Transference

By transference is meant the displacement of feelings and attitudes from important relationships in childhood to someone in the present. In terms of the degree to which the patient is utterly dependent upon others, the experience of hospitalization more closely resembles that of infancy or childhood than almost any other situation of adult life. Further, it is to be expected that being unusually dependent upon others for comfort and survival evokes some measure of anxiety, more in some people than in others. This anxiety is allayed considerably by the development of a strongly positive transference in which the patient imputes to the physician the omniscient and omnipotent qualities which his parents *seemed* to possess when he was a small child. The hospitalized patient's situation is such that he *needs* to feel that *his* doctor is the best and is totally committed to his welfare. The early successes with the internal mammary implantation can be viewed in part as a result of the patient's trust in his surgeon rather than myocardial revascularization.[21] (In Chapter 2 it was noted that "what the physician says is regarded as infallible, even though the patient may actually know very little about his physician's qualifications.") This type of transference, so commonly seen, is therefore useful to the patient, and the physician does well simply to accept it.

There may, however, be transference reactions of a negative nature. Warning clues to this type of transference are obtained when the patient, in relating his history, is excessively critical of other physicians who have cared for him in the past. It may not be possible to prevent the development of negative transference. If the patient becomes resentful and critical it is important to assess the possibly realistic justification for his feelings. If such an assessment leads one to the conclusion that the patient's negative criticisms are overdone, it is likely that one is observing transference distortion. Recognition of this fact helps the physician to be more tolerant of the patient's feelings and to engage him in discussion of them. As a rule, however, it is not helpful to attempt to interpret the origins of transference feelings to the patient.

Regression

In the course of hospitalization many individuals revert to forms of behavior, feelings, and modes of thinking that were characteristic of them at a much earlier stage of life. Regression is clearly demonstrated when a cooperative, sensible patient becomes excessively dependent, demanding, seems constantly to need someone to do something for him, and is unduly upset by minor provocations. The actual dependency inherent in hospitalization combined with intense anxiety promotes regression. The development of an organic brain syndrome is often accompanied by severe anxiety and regression, since the patient does not have his usual cognitive ability to cope with unfamiliar surroundings.

SPECIAL SITUATIONS IN THE HOSPITAL

The Intensive Care Unit

Advances in medical technology have allowed the development of intensive care units, specifically equipped and staffed to provide life-saving care for patients with acute myocardial infarctions and other acute, life-threatening conditions. As invaluable as these units are, they nevertheless may present significant psychological hazards to the patient. Frequently, the patient is surrounded by complicated, sometimes frightening equipment; he may be immobilized, isolated from other people, and endure long periods of sleep deprivation. He may hear other patients moaning or rambling incoherently and he may observe or infer that a fellow patient has died. It is relatively rare for patients in the intensive care unit to complain of anxiety or depression, but it is not rare for them to experience it.[15] Tremulousness, restlessness, palmar sweating, and pressure of speech should alert the physician to the likely presence of an anxiety reaction. Depression may be manifested by sad facies, disinterest, pessimism, slow speech, and tearfulness. Delirium demonstrated by fear, disorientation, incoherent speech, memory impairment, and sometimes visual hallucinations frequently develops in an intensive care unit.

Hemodialysis

The psychological stresses involved in chronic renal insufficiency requiring hemodialysis include:

1. The individual's forced dependence upon the dialysis machine
2. The restrictive treatment schedule and strict dietary limitations
3. The experience of chronic fatigability or weakness

Feelings of depression, resentment, and intolerance of treatment may occur.

As in other conditions, an individual's past history of coping will frequently indicate how well he will tolerate this difficult form of treatment. A sensible past dietary pattern, good work history, family support, and religious convictions all appear to be factors that are positively correlated with successful adaptation to the treatment regimen.[23]

Surgery

Various surgical procedures can create psychological distress. Cosmetic surgery such as rhinoplasty can result in difficult psychological reactions if the individual's expectations are not met.[19] Therefore, it is imperative, prior to deciding upon such surgery, to evaluate fully the patient's reasons for the procedure so that unrealistic expectations, if present, may be discovered.

Other surgical procedures, particularly those involving sexual organs or disfigurement, can also create psychological distress. Hysterectomies can precipitate depressive reactions in women who have precarious self-esteem. Mastectomies also necessitate readjustment to an altered body image. It has been noted that men frequently report sexual dysfunction following colostomy. This is usually on an organic basis in operations for carcinoma but may be on a purely psychological basis in individuals with ulcerative colitis or regional ileitis where surgery does not interrupt nerve pathways to the genital system.[12]

CONVALESCENCE

During convalescence, the patient is expected to relinquish the "sick role" and to return to normal duties and responsibilities. It is comparable to the transitional period of adolescence in that the patient is expected to remain cooperative with the treatment team while at the same time becoming more independent of them. Among the factors influencing the convalescent process are: 1) the presence of "secondary gains;" 2) emotional illness, and 3) the life situation to which the patient is returning.

Secondary Gains

This term refers to psychological or material gains associated with illness. In general, the longer and more incapacitated the patient has been, the more difficult it is to give up the gratification of regression and dependency. Further, prolonged illness and incapacity allow illness-associated defenses to develop. The "sick role" protects the person who feels inadequate from anxiety-provoking situations. More obvious gains associated with illness may result from financial compensation, pending litigation, and excessive attention from solicitous relatives.

Emotional Illness

Specific psychiatric syndromes may retard symptomatic recovery: patients with conversion reactions unconsciously simulate physical illness; the depressed patient may complain of fatigue, weakness, and symptoms which may resemble those of the illness from which he is recovering.[17,18,24]

Life Situation

The patient's attitudes toward recovery are strongly influenced by his perception of the situations in his life to which he is returning. Stormy marital relationship, indebtedness, difficulties at work, and other troublesome situations may arouse considerable dread and anxiety in the convalescent patient.

SOME COMMENTS ON MANAGEMENT

From a psychological viewpoint, an immediate tactical objective of management is to achieve a relationship with the patient in which he not only feels trust and confidence in the technical skill of the physician, but also feels free to reveal feelings, fears, worries, and problems to him.

When confronted with denial of illness or one of its features, the physician should proceed cautiously. If the denial is interfering with compliance to essential treatment it may be necessary to point out tactfully those aspects of the situation which are essential for the patient to understand. It may also be necessary to modify the treatment regimen to conform with the patient's ability to accept his situation. Hamburg has pointed out that, when a human being is first confronted with adversity, some degree of denial may serve the useful purpose of giving him time to muster his resources and to prepare himself for what lies ahead.[16]

The observation of certain personality features in the patient gives the physician a basis for tailoring his approach in accordance with individual needs.[6] The controlled, intellectual, obsessive individual generally responds well to being given facts and explanations. He should be allowed the opportunity to ask questions or to settle various possibilities and doubts that may have arisen in his mind. On the other hand, the excited "hysterical" individual responds to an opportunity to ventilate his feelings, yet needs supportive, matter-of-fact reassurance. He, too, needs to be informed, but at his own pace. In dealing with suspicious or paranoid persons, it is important to avoid incomplete or ambiguous messages; clear communication is essential. If one observes some overt evidence of distress it may be necessary to engage the patient in open discussion of this matter. The schizoid individual is not particularly apt to pose a problem in management, but one should respect his need for privacy. The independent individual who is threatened by the prospect of immobilization and dependency may require discussion of his conflict with the treatment regimen; it is often best to settle for a modification or compromise plan of treatment.

The individual who fulfills the criteria for a "borderline personality disorder" can create particular havoc on a medical or surgical unit.[13,14] These individuals may exhibit severe denial, intense feelings, especially of a hostile sort, and impulsive behavior. Under the stress of illness and hospitalization they may regress to transient psychotic episodes. These patients tend to react to staff members as though they were divided into "good" and "bad" groups and may stimulate disagreement among members of the treating team through manipulative behavior. Thus, open communication among the ward personnel must be maintained so that the patient receives clear and unconflicted information. Firm, nonpunitive limits must also be set by the staff to control impulsive and hostile behavior. Making the patient aware that you acknowledge his distress because of his illness can help him to moderate his emotional reactions. The staff, however, should not attempt to gratify the patient's wish for dependency but should be aware that these individuals often feel that they are entitled to special treatment, which may try the patience of the treating staff. Recognition of these dependent and manipulative behaviors and understanding the style of the borderline patient can help the physician to deal with these individuals early in treatment and to prevent complicated emotional difficulties.

If the patient's life situation is a complicating issue, one that is worrisome to the patient, it is often helpful not only to encourage the patient to discuss it, but also to consult with members of the family who may be of help. The medical social worker is often of considerable assistance when the patient is apprehensive and feels helpless or guilty about family, financial, or occupational problems.

In the convalescent period, particularly when the illness has been prolonged, the patient requires support, encouragement, and approval, particularly when he makes a step forward in rehabilitation. Individuals who cling to the sick role despite physical recovery can be understood by viewing their behavior as a communication to the significant people in their environment. The physician can promote recovery by attempting to help the patient define and resolve the problems fostering invalidism.

The management of specific psychiatric problems and disorders is discussed in subsequent chapters.

CHAPTER 136

Psychiatric Evaluation of the Patient

JOHN B. IMBODEN

Psychiatric evaluation of a patient differs in no essential way from other types of clinical evaluation. It is based upon history taking, examination, and assessment of special tests, when appropriate. These data are used to formulate a diagnosis or understanding of the problem. This, in turn, permits the development of a rational plan for treatment.

The general principles and techniques discussed in Chapter 2 are as applicable to the patient with a psychiatric disorder as to those with other types of illness. These points will not be reiterated here. However, the psychiatric interview is one of the major tools used in evaluation. The salient features of this technique will be discussed in some detail.

PSYCHIATRIC DIAGNOSIS

Psychiatric illness can be defined as being any condition in which there is suffering and disability resulting primarily from a disorder of thinking, feeling, or behavior. This definition clearly encompasses 1) the organic brain syndromes, 2) the psychoses, and 3) the neuroses. We also include 4) the personality disorders, for these enduring maladaptive attitudes and behavior patterns commonly produce disability and suffering.

DIAGNOSTIC ENTITIES

Table 136–1 lists the major categories of psychiatric disorders; each (with the exception of mental retardation) is discussed elsewhere. In arriving at a diagnosis, the clinician will find it practical to approach diagnostic categorization by proceeding from the broad categories to more restricted ones, and finally to specific entities.

Categories

The first categorization is to distinguish *organic disorders* from *functional disorders*. Here the clinician must be alert not only to evidences of the organic brain syndromes (Chap. 140), but also to the organic diseases that can simulate emotional disorders. Organic disease can never be ruled out with certainty (proof of a negative universal), but all reasonable efforts should be made to exclude organic disorders, especially when intellect, memory, and other higher cortical functions are impaired, for these are the hallmarks of organic disease.

If organic causes seem unlikely, the next step is to distinguish between the functional *psychoses* (schizophrenic and affective disorders) and the *nonpsychotic disorders* (neuroses, personality disorders, or situational reactions). This requires understanding of the manifestations and dynamics which characterize these disorders (Chaps. 137 to 142). These insights are gained primarily through interviews with the patient and the family.

It should be noted that these categories of illness are not mutually exclusive. A schizophrenic patient may also be an alcoholic, and personality disorders frequently antedate the development of neurosis. Organic illness and the attendant stresses can exacerbate a preexisting emotional disorder.

Urgency

Quite apart from the diagnostic categorization of the psychiatric illness, the physician must determine if the patient's problem constitutes a psychiatric emergency. These problems and their management are discussed in Chapter 137. It is quite possible to assess the urgency of the situation even in the absence of a specific psychiatric diagnosis.

Management Responsibility

An important aspect of the initial evaluation is the determination of whether the problem is to be managed by the general physician, by the general physician with psychiatric consultation, or by a psychiatrist. The basis for these decisions depends upon urgency (Chap. 137), and the probable diagnosis and severity of the condition (Chap. 140). Psychiatric consultation is warranted to help resolve diagnostic problems and to assist in planning management. The decision regarding continuing responsibilities can be determined after consultation.

THE PSYCHIATRIC INTERVIEW

In conducting an interview the physician is in the roles of both participant and observer.[27,28] In practice, these two activities of participation and observation are so interrelated as to be virtually inseparable. On

---
TABLE 136-1
Major Categories of Psychiatric Disorders

1. Mental retardation[1,2]
2. Organic brain syndromes (Chaps. 112, 113, 137, 140)
3. Psychoses (potential or actual) without known organic etiology (Chaps. 137 and 140)
   Schizophrenic disorders
   Affective disorders
4. Neuroses (Chap. 140)
5. Personality disorders (Chaps. 134, 135, 140)
6. Alcohol and drug dependence (Chaps. 138 and 153)
7. Psychophysiologic disorders (Chap. 141)
8. Transient situational disturbances (Chaps. 135 and 140)

---

the one hand, what the physician observes will influence his approach to the patient and the particular areas of inquiry he chooses to emphasize. On the other hand, his attitudes, manner, and phraseology have an effect on how the patient feels, on what he chooses to reveal spontaneously or in answer to questions and nonverbal behavior.

PRINCIPLES AND TECHNIQUES

Patients with emotional problems or illnesses tend in general to suffer from loss of self-esteem. This, in part, stems from the notion that mental illness is in itself indicative of personal failure or inadequacy. Further, the illness is sometimes the surface manifestation of underlying inter- and intrapersonal problems and conflicts which give rise to painful feelings that are partially allayed and revealed by specific symptoms. In developing rapport with the patient, the physician needs to be mindful of these two related issues of self-esteem and defensiveness.

Respect and Collaboration

The interviewer proceeds in a manner that conveys respect, interest, and, if possible, intellectual and empathic understanding. He conducts the interview with an attitude that he and the patient are engaged in a collaborative undertaking which has as its goal 1) a better understanding of the patient's problems, 2) an understanding of the patient himself, and 3) assistance in returning him to a state of well-being. The deliberate adoption of this attitude carries the implication that the patient's role is an active one in which he works with the physician and not a merely passive one of receiving advice and pills.

DEFENSE

A common defense is that of somatization in which the patient avoids emotional problems by focusing on one or more physical complaints. The depressed patient, for example, may complain of insomnia, fatigue, or of some bodily pain for which no organic basis can be found. He may, thus, tend to minimize feelings of depression or dismiss them as secondary to one or another physical symptom. It is a useful technique to respect the patient's somatization of his problem by encouraging him to recount his complaints and their chronological development fully. During this phase of the interview, the physician listens for spontaneous references to feelings and experiences which may provide openings for inquiry into personal and emotional issues.[25] In proceeding in this fashion, the interviewer is taking advantage of the patient's associative processes to get clues to feelings, fantasies, and experiences relevant to the present illness. If the pursuit of a given line of inquiry arouses discomfort, the patient may temporarily return to somatic symptoms or some other psychologically safe area. The physician should be attuned to these defensive shifts in the conversation for they enable the interviewer to develop hypotheses about what may be troubling the patient. These may be confirmed or refuted as he gets more data.

Tact

Most people are uncomfortable if they feel they are being asked questions to test their mental functioning. It is, therefore, helpful to soften the impact of an otherwise jarring question by tactfully giving it a rationale in the context of the interview. For example, one may comment to the patient that, in view of certain symptoms or problems with which he has been suffering, it would seem likely that he has been preoccupied and perhaps has found it difficult to concentrate and keep track of the details of daily life. This can be followed by stating that the examiner would, therefore, like to ask several questions that will help him to assess these aspects of the patient's functioning.

Demeanor

During the interview, the physician is interested not only in what the patient says but in how he says it: the structure or form of his speech and accompanying affect as well as its content. He will also take note of nonverbal aspects of behavior implied by the patient's general appearance and revealed in motor activity such as posture and gestures.

ORGANIZATION

Although the actual order in which data are collected depends upon a number of factors, it is well for the clinician to have a mental outline of key areas to be covered in carrying out a psychiatric evaluation.

History

The organization of historical information does not differ essentially from that described for the general medical patient. In the case of psychiatric illness, somewhat more emphasis is placed upon a detailed psychosocial history which is often crucial to understanding the development of the presenting problem, present illness, previous episodes of illness, the patient's personality and development. It is convenient to classify psychosocial data temporally and topically.

Temporally, psychosocial data can be organized as follows: 1) present life situation, 2) life situation concurrent with the present illness, and 3) psychosocial history prior to the present illness.

Within these temporal groups, psychosocial data can be further organized *topically:* 1) present family and household, 2) family of origin, 3) occupational and educational history, 4) psychosexual history, 5) drug and alcohol ingestion, etc.

Present Mental Status

The mental status examination is carried out while one is interviewing the patient and is continued during the physical examination.

The psychobiological processes illustrated in Figure 136–1 should be carefully evaluated in the course of the examination: 1) integrity of the sensory and motor apparatuses, 2) cognitive processes, 3) affective processes, and 4) functional concomitants of emotional states. This diagram represents a schematic attempt to depict human responses to internal and external stimuli as a psychobiologic system. This method of illustration carries the danger of oversimplification and of representing human behavior as a mechanical thing. While the schema does not explicitly depict psychological defense mechanisms and unconscious motivation, it does not preclude these aspects of psychic functioning. Its purpose is to represent important functional categories which should be evaluated in examining the patient. The nu-

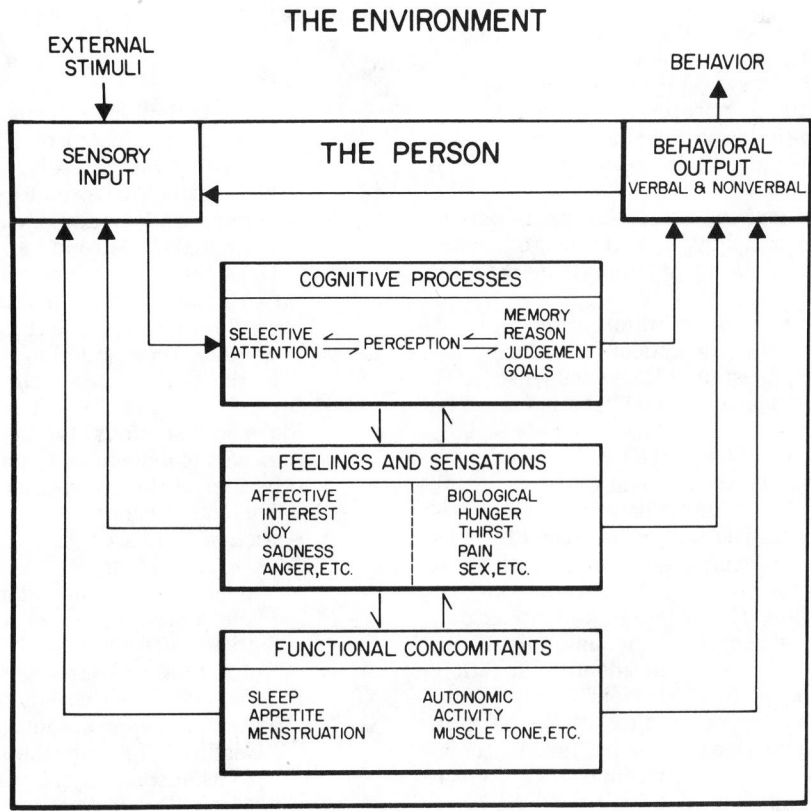

FIGURE 136-1.

merous two-way arrows in the figure signify the impressive way in which psychic processes influence each other.

These functions, illustrated in Figure 136–1, are evaluated by observing the patient's general appearance, the content and form of his speech, and nonverbal behavior. In conducting the mental status examination, the experienced physician will be guided by his own associations just as he is in any medical examination. For example, if the patient appears to have undergone recent weight loss the experienced physician will keep in mind the various features of severe depression as he proceeds with the mental status examination. A grossly unkempt or disheveled appearance in a middle-aged, successful businessman immediately raises the possibility of recent personality change secondary to organic brain damage or severe depression with accompanying retardation and loss of interest. These and other hypotheses are tested as the examination proceeds.

OUTLINE OF THE MENTAL STATUS EXAMINATION

1. *Integrity of Sensory and Motor Apparatus.* (Chap. 110.) Is there sensory deficit or motor weakness that does not conform to known anatomic and physiologic requirements?
2. *Cognitive Processes.* The term cognition refers to all those psychic processes by which knowledge of any kind is obtained and it includes all aspects of perceiving, remembering, and thinking.
   A. *General level of consciousness.* Is patient stuporous, sleepy, dull, or alert to his surroundings? Is he hyperalert, easily startled?
   B. *Attention, Concentration and Comprehension.* Does the patient listen to and understand questions? Is he easily distracted or preoccupied? Can he keep his mind on simple arithmetical tasks such as serially subtracting 7 from 100?
   C. *Memory.* Is the patient able to recall events in the immediate recent and remote past? The immediate recall of a series of numbers tests concentration as well as memory.
   D. *Perception.* This refers to a complex process by which one is meaningfully aware of objects, i.e., their identity, location, size, and state of motion. Gross abnormalities of perception may take the form of hallucinations, illusions, misidentification of persons, abnormal body sensations, and apparent failure to perceive with one or another sensory modality.
   E. *Orientation in time, place, person, and present situation.* Correct orientation depends upon conscious awareness, perception, comprehension, and memory.
   F. *Thinking and Speech.* In these categories are included all those remaining cognitive functions essential to successful adaptation to life: reasoning, ability to express oneself coherently, the accurate interpretation of reality, insight, judgment, and content of thought.

   In expressing himself does the patient communicate the goal idea of his statement? Does he become lost in circumstantial details, or does his line of thought become derailed by tangential associations? Does the patient talk rapidly and excessively? Does he appear to be experiencing a flight of ideas? Is his speech occasionally blocked so that he suddenly becomes silent and cannot remember what he was about to say?

   To some degree, everyone's conception of reality is influenced by wishes, fears, other feelings, and mood. Is the patient's thinking so vulnerable to such influence that he has delusional concepts of the world around him, of himself, of the future? Is he suspicious of others? Does he feel persecuted, watched, controlled by outside influence? Is he grandiose or self-demeaning? Does he have delusions involving his body? What is his concept of the future?

   Is the patient able to engage in abstract reasoning as manifested by his interpretation of proverbs? Can he solve simple arithmetic problems? Is his store of general information, grammar, and vocabulary in keeping with his educational background and station in life?

   Does the patient have an understanding of his own condition and situation? In discussing recent activities and future plans does he appear to exercise sound judgment?

   Is the patient preoccupied with particular topics? Does he have persistently recurrent ideas or obsessions? Is he compelled to engage in rituals to allay anxiety or to prevent harm to others even though recognizing the absurdity of the compulsions?
3. *Affective Processes*
   A. *Display of affect or feelings.* Does the patient show feelings that are appropriate to the content of his speech? Does he appear to be "affectively flat?" Does he tend to be dramatic or histrionic?
   B. *Anxiety.* Are there moments when the patient appears anxious, fearful, tense, or restless? If so, are there autonomic symptoms accompanying the anxiety state?
   C. *Mood.* This term refers to a prevailing and relatively enduring emotional state. There

are many varieties and shades of mood. Among the important abnormal states of mood are depression and elation which may be associated with a variety of behavioral manifestations. These are described in Chapter 140.
   D. *Depersonalization.* Does the patient have a feeling of unreality? Does he feel estranged from himself, his body, or his surroundings?
4. *Functional Concomitants of Emotional States*
   A. *Autonomic concomitants of anxiety,* such as dilated pupils, tachycardia, pallor, sweaty palms, and tremor are not uncommon.
   B. *Hyperventilation* and its sequelae, paresthesias and tetany.
   C. *Eating behavior.* Is there a history of undereating or excessive eating with corresponding effect on body weight?
   D. *Sleeping.* Does patient have difficulty in falling asleep? Does he awaken early? Does he sleep fitfully? Does he sleep more than is customary for him? Is there a history of irresistible urge to sleep at inappropriate times?
   E. *Miscellaneous.* Fatigue, diarrhea, constipation, sexual dysfunction, amenorrhea, urinary frequency, urinary retention, muscular tension, aching, and the like.

OTHER SOURCES OF INFORMATION

Family and Associates

In some cases, interviewing members of the immediate family or close associates can be a vital part of the examination. This is true, for example, when the patient's illness has adversely affected his memory or ability to observe, or when the patient's defenses grossly interfere with factual reporting, as is so often true in alcoholism. In addition, in the process of interviewing the family, the clinician may become aware of serious problems and tensions existing between family members which may be contributing to the patient's emotional condition. Occasionally, one finds that another member of the family, or the entire family, needs assistance and that the patient's illness is reflective of family problems.

Physical Examination

The general physical and neurologic examinations afford the clinician an excellent opportunity to observe the patient and to make casual inquiries pertaining to the "mental status." Observations of weight loss, a fine tremor, and skin excoriations provide important clues to further investigation.

Psychological Testing[26]

Psychological testing is a valuable adjunct to the psychiatric examination in several circumstances.

1. Determination of intelligence level may be useful in cases of school failure, apparent inadequacy at work, or when one suspects that the patient is seriously underchallenged by his occupation.
2. Psychological testing may be helpful when the clinical picture is equivocal. For example, standardized tests of higher cerebral function are useful when one suspects organic brain damage resulting in changes too slight or subtle to be detected by the conventional mental status examination.
3. Certain psychological tests may reveal psychodynamic themes or personality traits which were not discerned during the interview.

There are a variety of psychological tests available. Some, such as the Rorschach, Wechsler Adult Intelligence Scale, and the Thematic Apperception Test are administered by trained psychologists. Others, such as the Minnesota Multiphasic Personality Inventory and a variety of clinical "scales" to assess symptomatic states are self-administered.

Continued Observation

More often than not, thorough evaluation and comprehension of the patient's problems require a number of contacts over a period of time. Occasionally, a brief period of hospitalization, in which the patient can be observed by trained professionals, is necessary for adequate diagnostic evaluation.

Psychiatric Emergencies
JOHN B. IMBODEN

Psychiatric emergency means any serious mental or emotional disorder that requires prompt intervention. Most psychiatric emergencies have one or both of the following characteristics: 1) alarming behavior, and 2) acute, intense suffering.

Alarming Behavior

A wide variety of conditions may give rise to behavior that arouses alarm in the patient or in others. One of the most common emergencies is that posed by the patient who has made a suicidal attempt or who is judged to be in danger of doing so. Other forms of actual or potentially destructive behavior are not uncommon: violent or homicidal behavior, and behavior associated with delirious or other psychotic states which have unintended, accidental, or indirect destructive consequences. Occasionally, an acute behavioral disturbance of very low destructive potential, such as an acute conversion reaction, manifested, for example, by paralysis, may be extremely alarming to the patient or family and, therefore, require immediate attention.

Acute, Intense Suffering

Excruciating pain constitutes an emergency even if it is not associated with a life-threatening condition. One of the most "painful" of human conditions is acute anxiety which, in its most severe form, is often referred to as panic. Severe depression also may constitute an emergency, particularly if accompanied by despair and hopelessness.

For purposes of further discussion, it is convenient to consider the problem of suicidal behavior separately and to lump together other forms of alarming behavior arbitrarily under the rubric of "acute behavioral disturbances." The emergency situation sometimes posed by severe depression will be included in the section dealing with suicide while that of severe anxiety or panic will be discussed separately.

SUICIDAL BEHAVIOR

There are few occurrences in life that evoke a more intense welter of emotions in relatives and physicians than suicide. In fact, the physician, as a person dedicated to the alleviation of suffering and the preservation of life, often must come to grips with the intense ambivalence aroused in himself by a suicide attempt

if he is to approach the patient with the same compassion and objectivity that he exercises in other medical emergencies.

Definitions

It will be useful to define three terms as they are used in this chapter.

Completed suicide means an act by which an individual has intentionally killed himself.

Attempted suicide refers to an act deliberately carried out by an individual against himself, by which he intends to endanger or end his life, or to give the appearance of such an intent but which does not result in death. In many attempted suicides, the patient has conflicting feelings, simultaneously having a wish to live and a wish to die. In some instances, the death wish appears to be minimal, there being some other primary motivation, such as the manipulation of a spouse or the seeking of help. These have sometimes been referred to as *suicidal gestures* but are included here in the category of attempted suicide.

Potential suicide refers to the individual who, while not having made an attempt on his life, is thought to be in danger of doing so.

The Physician's Task

While it is true that there are cultures in which suicide is considered acceptable behavior, there is convincing evidence that, in this country, the overwhelming majority of persons who have died by suicide were afflicted with a psychiatric illness for some time prior to death.[36] Further, many of them had consulted a physician for one or another symptom of their illness within a year prior to death. In most instances, the physician consulted was not a psychiatrist.

Not only do most completed suicides have a recent history of medical consultation, but most attempted suicides are also seen initially by nonpsychiatrist physicians. It is apparent, therefore, that all physicians bear a heavy responsibility in the detection and management of suicidal behavior and associated psychiatric illness.

In potential suicide and attempted suicide, it is the physician's difficult task to determine the seriousness and immediacy of the current danger to the patient's life. Evaluation of suicidal risk and the associated psychiatric illness include the assessment of a variety of personal, interpersonal, and circumstantial variables. This process usually necessitates interviews with relatives and friends as well as the patient.

The assessment of suicidal risk can in certain instances be relatively easy and in others it can be all but impossible. A number of statistical studies have revealed that certain variables are consistently correlated with the rate of completed suicides in the general population.[31,33]

Completed Suicides

In the United States, the rate of recorded suicides is about 10.5 per 100,000 persons per year. An unknown number of suicides go unrecorded, death being wrongly attributed to other causes. The ratio of men to women is between 2 to 1 and 4 to 1 throughout the industrialized world. In men, the suicide rate increases with age until the mid-80s and in women it peaks between ages 55 and 65. The suicide rate is substantially higher among single persons, particularly the widowed and divorced, than among the married. The rate is higher among whites than blacks and somewhat higher among Protestants than Jews and Catholics.

Approximately 60 percent of completed suicides have made one or more previous attempts. As already indicated, retrospective studies indicate that most completed suicides occur in people who have a psychiatric illness. Persons afflicted with incurable or fatal physical illness account for a small fraction of completed suicides.

The above data are of rather limited use to the clinician who is dealing with an individual patient but are of some value if used in conjunction with the total clinical picture. For example, the diagnosis of depression in a 70-year-old white, divorced male who lives alone generally (but not always) carries a more ominous implication than the same diagnosis in a young married woman who lives at home with husband and children.

The Potential Suicidal Risk

Among both completed and attempted suicides, the most commonly made diagnosis is depression. Therefore, it is important to be alert to the presence of depressive illness in any patient and if found, to assess the suicidal risk.

Affective disorders will be discussed in Chapter 140. As previously noted, it is not uncommon for a depressed patient to focus primarily on physical symptoms and to rationalize his depressed mood as being secondary to them. In such cases, the diagnosis may be easily missed.

Once the diagnosis of depression is made, the assessment of suicidal danger is based upon: 1) the severity of the depression, 2) the presence of hopelessness, 3) a prior history of suicide attempts and death wishes, and 4) suicidal thoughts and suicidal intentions.[30,35]

SEVERITY OF DEPRESSION. In the general adult population, the incidence of relatively mild, transient periods of depressed mood is extremely high, perhaps universal. If, however, the degree of mood change is moderately severe, relatively long-lasting, and accompanied by other symptoms such as somatic complaints, insomnia, psychomotor retardation, decrease in interest, and decreased ability to experience pleasure, the patient can be regarded as suffering from a depressive condition of significant severity.

In persons suffering from affective disorders, the lifetime risk of suicide has been estimated to be 15 percent.[32] Although there are numerous exceptions, there is some correlation between severity of depression and suicidal risk. Paradoxically, however, apparent symptomatic improvement in the course of the illness does not necessarily mean that the risk of suicide has decreased. Some patients may seem to have improved because they have secretly made a decision to kill themselves while others, who had been functionally incapacitated by severe depression, may become better able to carry out a suicide plan as their depression begins to lift.

HOPELESSNESS. The patient who feels that his future is bleak, his problems insoluble, his illness incurable, he is not worthy of relief, or worthy of any other good fortune represents a greater suicidal risk than a person who, although depressed, has a hopeful outlook regarding his future. A hopeful, but nonetheless depressed patient, may make casual reference to future plans thus implying that he intends to be around.

PRIOR HISTORY OF SUICIDE ATTEMPTS. A history of previous suicide attempts increases the probability of another attempt being made.

VERBALIZATION OF SUICIDAL THOUGHTS AND INTENT. A common error in dealing with a suspected suicidal patient is that of failing to ask him directly about his wishes and intentions regarding death and suicide. It is likely that all depressed patients, at one time or another, feel a wish to die and have thoughts of suicide. It is important, however, to directly ask the patient if he has been *preoccupied* with death and suicidal thoughts and if he has, in the present or recently, actually *intended* to commit suicide. If the response to this inquiry is in the affirmative, the patient should also be asked to describe the method contemplated, whether he has procured the means to carry out the act, and other details.

The potentially suicidal patient may have an illness other than primary depression. In fact, any condition or situation that has resulted in a feeling of hopelessness may be associated with the danger of suicide. For example, persons confronted with public exposure of unethical behavior or evidence of incompetence, or individuals with progressive, incurable disease may choose death in preference to a future that is perceived as laden with unbearable misery. The schizophrenic patient may attempt suicide in a moment of despair or in response to an hallucinated command. The delirious patient, while not necessarily intending suicide, may seriously or fatally injure himself in a variety of ways such as leaving the room via a window. The presence of alcoholism, especially if associated with depressive illness, increases the risk of suicide.

In the event that the physician has made a judgment that the suicidal risk is grave, this should be discussed openly with the patient and his next of kin. Psychiatric consultation should be obtained without delay. There may be circumstances in which the physician decides upon immediate hospitalization and institution of suicidal observation while awaiting psychiatric consultation. In any event, precautions should be taken to prevent suicide until definitive therapy has taken effect. Management of associated illness, such as depression, schizophrenic illness, delirium, or alcoholism should be initiated immediately.

The Suicide Attempt

In addition to the immediate medical or surgical management necessitated by the attempt itself, the physician must assess the seriousness of suicidal intent. To assist him in carrying out this assessment, it is advisable, for both clinical and legal reasons, to obtain the assistance of a psychiatric consultant.

It would be impractical and probably unwise routinely to advise psychiatric hospitalization in every case of attempted suicide. The incidence of attempted suicides is conservatively estimated to be more than ten times that of completed suicides.[37] In contrast to the latter group, the rate of attempted suicides is higher among women than men and reaches its peak in the third decade of life. These statistical differences, coupled with the fact that most completed suicides have made previous attempts, suggest that the attempted suicide group is a heterogeneous one that partially contains those who will eventually comprise the completed group, i.e., as the attempted suicide group grows older it contributes substantially to those who complete suicide. It has been estimated that the risk of suicide in the attempted group is approximately 1 to 2 percent per year.

In assessing the seriousness of intent, the same principles apply that were discussed regarding the depressed patient. In addition, it is helpful to take into account: 1) the lethality of the attempt, 2) the circumstances surrounding the attempt, 3) precipitating factors, and 4) consequences.

LETHALITY OF THE ATTEMPT. This refers to the danger to life posed by the act itself regardless of any mitigating circumstances. For example, the ingestion of a large number of barbiturate capsules and self-inflicted gunshot wounds to the head or chest are highly lethal acts, whereas an overdose of chlordiazepoxide and superficial lacerations are not. If the attempt is judged to be highly lethal, that is, if death probably would have ensued in the absence of timely intervention, it is best to presume that the suicidal intent was extremely serious and remains so in the immediate postattempt period. This is a practical policy even though it is recognized that an occasional patient may not be aware of the relative dangerousness of one type of attempt as opposed to another, e.g., the lethality of barbiturate versus chlordiazepoxide overdosage. Obviously, the converse is not true. Low lethality does not necessarily point to low seriousness of intent.

SURROUNDING CIRCUMSTANCES. The following circumstances are positively correlated with seriousness of intent:

1. Being alone at time of attempt
2. Actively taking precautions against being discovered
3. The rescue of the patient could not reasonably have been foreseen by the patient
4. Evidence of premeditation, such as a suicide note, recent increase in life insurance, recently written will, acquisition of material or equipment specifically needed for the attempt

PRECIPITATING FACTORS. The attempt may have arisen out of hopelessness and despair as part of a depressive illness or in association with some other illness or life-situation. Not infrequently, however, the patient makes a suicide attempt, even a dangerous one, in order to bring about a change in his life-situation. For example, the attempt may well be a "cry for help," an effort to arouse sympathetic concern by others or to change the direction in which an important relationship has been going. The attempt may be designed to punish someone, symbolically or actually, by evoking guilt. It may be an attempt to punish oneself.

It is, therefore, important to review with the patient what was going on in his life and in his mind at the time of the attempt. The patient should be asked if he had felt that the attempt would result in death. Had he thought that he might live, but that his life would be different? If so, how? Had he been angry and wanting to "get even" with someone? Had he felt guilty and that he deserved to be punished? Had he wanted to die?

CONSEQUENCES. A key question is: does it appear that the suicide attempt will be followed by significant changes in the patient or in his circumstances? If the physician has been able to gauge the patient's original purposes, feelings, and expectations prior to the attempt, he may be able to ascertain the psychological and interpersonal results of the attempt. For example, if one infers that the patient had sought to be less isolated, to be more accepted by family, to get help for his problems or his depression, does the attempt promise to succeed in his substantially achieving these goals? Does the patient seem unsurprised, perhaps even glad, that he is still alive? Does he seem to feel less guilty than before the attempt? Did the suicide attempt achieve nothing as far as the patient is concerned? Does he now feel even less adequate and more isolated than before? Did he "wake up" to find a sullen, resentful spouse and an emergency room staff too harried with "real" emergencies to be very concerned with him?

All of the above categories of factors have to be weighed in forming a decision as to the seriousness of intent and the continuing danger of suicide.

MANAGEMENT. It is often and properly decided that the patient who has made a suicide attempt does not require psychiatric hospitalization. In that event, it is mandatory to recommend outpatient psychiatric observation and treatment. Unfortunately, a substantial percentage of suicide attempters for whom psychiatric treatment has been arranged fail to keep their appointments or drop out of treatment prematurely. This fact underscores the importance of thoroughly discussing the need for treatment with the patient and with important members of his family.

ACUTE BEHAVIORAL DISTURBANCES

More often than not, the patient who engages in aggressive, inappropriate, bizarre, or otherwise disturbing behavior does not seek medical attention on his own initiative because he is either unaware of the pathology of his behavior or is unconcerned about it, or both. Therefore, he frequently comes to medical attention at the behest of a concerned member of the family or a friend. Because of the patient's own lack of insight into his condition, the concerned relative may be perplexed as to "how to get him to the doctor" and may decide upon some sort of deceptive ruse such as telling the patient that he himself needs to see

the physician and wishes to have the patient accompany him. It is unwise for the physician to go along with any subterfuge designed to trick the patient into going to the doctor's office, for the loss of trust resulting from such a deception will often make further work with the patient impossible. The family should be advised to discuss the patient's condition directly, but gently, with him and firmly to insist upon the necessity of medical examination.

These kinds of behavior may be characterized by one or more of the following:

1. Recent development of impulsive behavior or behavior that is "out of character" for the patient
2. Aggressive or violent behavior
3. Excessive activity, verbal or nonverbal
4. Inactivity, withdrawal
5. Bizarre, silly, or "crazy" behavior
6. Behavior characterized by evidence of confusion

It is essential to have the best informed and most responsible members of the family accompany the patient to the place of examination. If the preexamination contact with the family indicates that there may be a problem in controlling the patient's behavior, it is wise to arrange for the examination to be in the hospital emergency room or other suitable location rather than in one's private office. The examination of the patient should in general follow that outlined in Chapter 2 and should include a careful physical and neurologic examination.

The Violent Patient

Although the diagnostic considerations that arise in the evaluation of violent behavior do not essentially differ from those of other kinds of disturbing behavior, the violent patient does require that certain immediate steps be taken. As with acute anxiety or panic, diagnosis and therapeutic management go hand in hand.

The excited, threatening, or combative patient instills fear in everyone in contact with him, including the physician. As Lion pointed out, it is useful to assume that the violent patient is afraid of losing control of his own aggressive impulses.[34] Thus, the physician has two immediate objectives: First, he should establish verbal contact with the patient and reassure him that he will be effectively helped to control his aggression, that he will not be allowed to translate his feelings into destructive behavior. Second, he should encourage the patient to talk freely about his current feelings including his fears and anger. This is done with the objective of helping the patient to substitute verbalization for action.

An excited, belligerent patient will often begin to grow calmer as the physician quietly explains that he would like to talk with him about his feelings and problems and offers the patient an opportunity to be interviewed alone. If the physician is fearful for his own safety, however, he should not make such an offer but instead talk with the patient in the presence of two or three attendants or in a room with the door open and with assistants standing nearby.

The focus of the interview should be primarily upon the patient's current feelings and thoughts. It is important to avoid promising the patient not to hospitalize him. The physician should simply indicate that the objective is to try to understand the patient's feelings and that the interviewer and his staff will help him to avoid loss of control of his impulses or angry feelings. In the initial stages of the evaluation, it is wise not to probe into the circumstances or issues which may have precipitated the rage, since this may provoke exacerbation. Such exploration, while important, can be done later. For example, if one suspects that the rage is covering homosexual panic, it would be unwise to "fish" for material to support that hypothesis.

Occasionally, the excited, violent patient will not respond to the approach described above or will be too disturbed to allow the physician to attempt such an approach. In this event, physical constraints are necessary. The application of them, such as devices to immobilize the patient's arms and legs, should be done by several attendants under the supervision of the physician. Once the patient is restrained on a stretcher or bed, the administration of a suitable drug is often indicated. The administration of 5 mg of haloperidol intramuscularly every 20 to 60 minutes may result in a marked reduction of psychotic behavior after three or four injections. Vital signs, including blood pressure, should be frequently monitored.

Diagnostic Evaluation of Acute Behavioral Disturbance

As enumerated above, from a descriptive viewpoint, there are a variety of behavior patterns which may alarm the family and prompt them to seek immediate medical attention. A useful diagnostic approach is to determine if the acute behavioral disturbance is organic or functional and then to proceed toward a more specific diagnostic entity.

In general, acute disturbances of behavior in which organic factors play a major etiologic role, such as delirium or toxic psychosis, are associated with evidence of impaired intellectual functions:

memory impairment, disorientation, rambling and incoherent speech, difficulty in comprehension, and abstract thinking. In the hallucinating patient, a predominance of visual hallucinations favors an organic basis although it may be a feature in early, acutely developing schizophrenic decompensation. A history of "spells" or repeated, discreet episodes of behavioral disturbance, with or without amnesia, should arouse suspicion of a seizure disorder. The medical history should be carefully reviewed. Insulin-induced hypoglycemic reactions, for example, can be associated with confusional states and bizarre behavior. Careful review of the alcohol and drug history is important to determine the possibility of intoxication or withdrawal syndrome.

Evidence in favor of an organic condition may indicate prompt chemical determinations of blood and urine, skull x-ray, EEG, repeated neurological examination, and other diagnostic procedures described in Chapter 111.

The diagnostic characteristics of functional disorders, namely schizophrenic illness, and manic states, will be discussed in Chapter 140. In general, functional disturbances are not associated with the type of intellectual impairment that produces defective recent memory and disorientation. Careful examination and judgment, however, may be required in order to determine that the patient has a clear sensorium. For example, the schizophrenic patient may give a bizarre response when asked to state where he is. Later in the interview, he may indicate, in response to a more oblique inquiry, that he is clearly aware of his location. The severely depressed patient, or any patient who is self-absorbed and preoccupied, may appear to have a poor memory for recent events. For example, he may not recall what he had for breakfast because he was too preoccupied to have noticed.

Management

It is wise to obtain prompt psychiatric consultation in all cases of acute behavioral disturbance, including those in which an organic component is strongly suspected.

If the acute behavioral disturbance is based upon an organic condition, hospitalization is mandatory in order to manage the patient safely while the specific nature of the organic or toxic factors is being determined. The patient's behavior may necessitate the temporary use of chemotherapeutic agents in order to allow further examination to proceed. Delirious patients must be carefully observed. Confusion and the likelihood of panic can be reduced, especially at night, by keeping the room well lighted, having a trained person in constant attendance, addressing the patient in clear, simple terms and otherwise avoiding ambiguous environmental cues.

Usually it is also wise to hospitalize the patient with acute functional psychosis. However, if such a patient is not suicidal or homicidal, responds well to the intramuscular administration of antipsychotic agents while under observation for a period of several hours, and has one or more responsible relatives to care for him, it may be feasible to offer psychiatric treatment in an outpatient setting in which he is seen initially on a daily basis.[29]

Special Cases

We have discussed emergency situations arising from acute behavioral disturbances. Occasionally, however, a chronically ill patient may present a type of emergency because of the particular life circumstances in which his illness developed. For example, the patient with an organic brain syndrome, even in the absence of an acute disturbance of behavior, requires immediate, active management if he is a practicing physician or is in any other position in which the welfare of others is gravely jeopardized by the effects of his illness.

SEVERE ANXIETY OR PANIC

Regardless of their cause, all states of acute, severe anxiety are characterized by intense fear, restlessness, and various other symptoms and signs such as palpitations, a feeling of suffocating, blurring of vision, tachycardia, pallor, and sweating. Commonly, the patient's fear becomes localized or specific such as fear of death through suffocation or cardiac arrest, or of going crazy. Sometimes the source of danger is projected onto the external world.

The most common conditions associated with severe acute anxiety or panic are: 1) anxiety neurosis; 2) a "bad trip" with an hallucinogenic agent; 3) acute phase of a schizophrenic illness (including homosexual panic); 4) amphetamine intoxication; and 5) delirium.

Diagnostic and therapeutic management of the acute attack must be done in parallel. Having established the presence of acute anxiety, the physician should matter-of-factly discuss that fact with the patient. While acknowledging the patient's extreme discomfort, he should reassure him about specific fears, e.g., that his condition will not cause his heart to stop and that his fearfulness itself has momentarily affected his judgment. Usually, a neurotic patient will respond to sympathetic attention, reassurance, and opportunity to discuss his feelings with the physician; in the process of symptomatic abatement, it becomes evident that he manifests no evidence of psychosis. In anxiety neurosis, the patient may have a history of previous attacks.

If the panic state is part of a psychotic condition, the patient does not usually respond to psychological support as readily as does the neurotic patient. As a general rule, acute schizophrenic illness and amphetamine intoxication are associated with a clear sensorium. The latter closely simulates paranoid schizophrenia and can only be diagnosed with confidence by obtaining a history of excessive amphetamine ingestion. The "bad trip" resulting from ingestion of an hallucinogen may be associated with extreme anxiety. The patient will often reveal his drug history, particularly if the importance of doing so is explained to him. He may or may not be disoriented. Delirium may be associated with extreme fear.

Management

Psychiatric consultation should be obtained. Chemotherapeutic intervention is often necessary in panic associated with psychosis whether functional or toxic. The choice of drug is based upon the considerations mentioned in management of the violent patient and will be discussed further in Chapters 138, 140, and 142. Phenothiazines are usually not employed in treating intoxication with hallucinogenic substances. If the anxiety state is associated with an organic or toxic psychosis, hospitalization is indicated. In the event of functional psychosis, the decision to hospitalize is based upon the same factors discussed in the management of acute behavioral disturbances.

CHAPTER 138

Drug Dependence

JOHN C. URBAITIS

The World Health Organization has defined drug dependence as "a state arising from repeated administration of a drug on a periodic or continuous basis." Drug dependence syndromes include the behavior of taking a drug, experiencing intoxication of some degree, and placing drug use at a higher priority than many other routine activities. An important further distinction is that various classes of drugs are associated with characteristic patterns of drug dependence, each with particular physical and psychological findings, both during the development of drug dependence, and during acute abstinence. For example, one properly refers to drug dependence of the sedative–alcohol type, drug dependence of the opiate type, and drug dependence of the cocaine type. We shall first discuss features common to all types of drug dependence, and then consider the specific types of drug dependence.

GENERAL INTRODUCTION

All drug dependence involves some desire or need on the part of the drug taker to use the drug repeatedly. This in itself constitutes *psychic dependence.* The drugs causing dependence are all active in the central nervous system (CNS), generally altering mood, thought, or feeling. More specifically, it appears that those CNS-active drugs most likely to cause dependence have such effects as relief of tension or anxiety, production of sleep, production of elation or euphoria, alteration of sensory perception, reduction of inhibitions in social situations, and change of sexual drives and sensation.

Some classes of drugs, notably opiates and sedatives, also cause *physical dependence* when taken in large enough doses for a sufficient length of time. A person who has developed physical dependence will have a withdrawal or *abstinence* syndrome, a predictable series of physiologic changes which ensue on abrupt cessation of drug taking. The abstinence syndrome of sedative drug dependence is particularly important to recognize, as it can proceed to delirium, or fatal seizures. The development of physical dependence is accompanied by the development of *tolerance,* the same dose of drug causing a lesser effect after repeated use. Tolerance occurs by two mechanisms, a change in the rate of metabolism of the drug, and an alteration in the cellular receptor site at which the drug acts.

Etiology

There are three categories of etiologic factors in drug dependence: physiologic, psychological, and social.

PHYSIOLOGIC FACTORS. The analgesic or sedative effect of drugs, the development of tolerance, and the occurrence of an abstinence syndrome upon discontinuance of drug use are important physiologic factors. It must be stressed, however, that these alone rarely can account for the development of drug dependence, and that medically supervised use of opiate analgesics for painful, acute illnesses does not lead to drug dependence. As for chronic illnesses, physicians may well decide that a patient's need for relief from severe discomfort outweighs the risks of developing dependence. In fact, studies have indicated that patients are more likely to receive too little rather than too much analgesia in usual hospital practice.[44]

SOCIAL FACTORS. Association with groups of drug-taking people, lack of opportunities for success, and lack of satisfying recreational outlets contribute to the development of drug dependence in many people. Family and community settings in which adults use and come to depend on such drugs as caffeine, nicotine, alcohol, or prescription medications may influence some children to experiment with drug use. Differences in the incidence of alcoholism in English, French, Irish, and Jewish populations have been observed; reasons for these differences include family attitudes and practices in the use of alcohol.

PSYCHOLOGICAL FACTORS. People who have various psychiatric disorders manifested by feelings of inadequacy, insecurity, or anxiety, chronic malaise, or frank psychotic disorganization, may find such relief in the effects of some self-administered drugs that they become drug dependent.

Wikler[49] has noted a conditioning effect; after months of documented abstinence, a former heroin user may experience the physical sensations of withdrawal and drug craving when he walks down a street where he was usually walking while beginning to suffer acute abstinence, on the way to purchase his fresh supply of heroin.

Effects

The various classes of drugs produce distinct signs and symptoms, to be described in subsequent sections. Nonetheless, there are certain general effects common in most drug-dependent persons. Foremost is drug-seeking behavior; this often takes precedence over any other activity. The alcoholic may take a drink first thing in the morning; the heroin user may spend rent or grocery money on heroin. Preoccupation with drug taking, as well as mind-altering effects of the drugs taken commonly result in impairment in social functioning; the drug dependent person may not be able to fulfill responsibilities at work or at home. The tension and anxiety from this impairment may be added to the anxiety associated with the psychological problems which originally led to the drug use; a vicious circle is, thus, established.

Diagnosis

Making the diagnosis of drug dependence is, of course, the first step in treatment planning. The general physician is often in an excellent position to find the early signs of the drug dependence. Patients may either come for care of some aspect or result of their drug taking, or they may present with other illnesses and the physician will diagnose drug dependence as a related or complicating condition. It is necessary to maintain an appropriate level of curiosity and suspicion without becoming a policeman or inquisitor.

The physician should be alert to patients who come requesting specific remedies, especially sedatives or strong analgesics; he should keep careful records of prescriptions to prevent premature refilling. Patients who have recently consulted a number of other physicians, or who are taking a variety of previously prescribed drugs from several sources, may be drug-dependent persons looking for a new supply of medications, or they may have genuinely difficult medical conditions which have not responded to treatment. A few patients may present with simulated conditions in an attempt to obtain analgesics; the patient who claims to have intractable pain of uncertain origin may be wanting drugs. In other instances, the drug-dependent patient may present with minimal intoxication.

Management

A matter-of-fact, nonjudgmental approach to the patient is essential. He or she needs treatment, and needs sound information on the risks of continuing drug dependence. Only by establishing a professional doctor–patient relationship, showing concern for the patient's condition, and gathering a thorough medical history, can the physician keep the drug-dependent patient under his care and offer definitive treatment either directly or by referral.

OPIATE DEPENDENCE

The most notorious but not the most common type of drug dependence is to the opiate class of drugs. Opiate dependence is an important condition because of the personal and family anguish and the medical complications associated with heroin use, and the social and economic effects of drug traffic in the community.

Opiates and other synthetic analgesics which can cause opiate-type drug dependence include morphine, heroin (diacetyl morphine), Dilaudid, codeine, opium (a mixture including morphine and codeine), meperidine, methadone, propoxyphene (Darvon), and diphenoxylate (Lomotil). The latter two are listed here because they can produce mild but definite opiate dependence syndromes. All of these medications have a combination of inhibitory and excitant effects in the central nervous system. Important pharmacologic properties which contribute to the development of drug dependence include antianxiety effects, the development of tolerance, and the development of physical dependence.

Etiology

PHARMACOLOGIC FACTORS. Intravenous injection of heroin or morphine produces sensations commonly described by users as pleasurable. First, they experience a "rush" or "flash," of explosive intensity, analogous to sexual orgasm. This is followed by a more gradual feeling of warmth and relaxation pervading the body, with a sense of tranquility. The pleasurable aspects of these sensations are sufficient to offset the experience of nausea and vomiting accompanying the first several experiences with intravenous opiates.

After tolerance develops (and it develops rapidly to the analgesic and antianxiety effects of opiates), the major factor responsible for drug dependence is physical dependence and the drug taker's desire to avoid the discomforts of the abstinence syndrome.

In the regions within the brain where specific receptors for opiates have been found, are also found endogenous compounds with opioid activities called endorphins. These polypeptides modulate neurotransmission of pain. If a person receives morphine or another opioid in large doses over several weeks, the brain's internal levels of endorphins are reduced; endorphins are thus probably involved in tolerance and the abstinence syndrome.[48]

PSYCHOLOGICAL FACTORS. There is no single psychiatric illness that is strongly associated with the production of opiate dependence. It does appear that many urban heroin users have suffered childhood deprivation which makes them vulnerable to emotional stresses and losses. Anxiety or any kind of dysphoria may lead the drug user to seek relief by continuing drug-taking. Immaturity and inability to tolerate frustration or to delay gratification are psychological traits found in many opiate-dependent persons.

SOCIAL FACTORS. Association with other users of heroin is an important determinant of urban patterns of opiate dependence. Membership in or contact with a group who use heroin generally provides the introduction to this pattern. Curiosity or thrill-seeking is the commonest explanation offered for starting drug use.

The small group of people who have medically related opiate dependence have generally suffered from a combination of chronic pain and anxiety and apprehension which is related to issues beyond the simple worries directly associated with their illnesses. The psychological factors are thought to include low self-esteem, depression, and some immaturity. Such patients can often be helped by coordinated medical and psychiatric care.

Recognition of the Patient

A patient may volunteer the fact of his drug dependence in giving medical history, or the physician may have to inquire diligently before finding this out. Some variables in the patient which may increase the physician's index of suspicion, include presenting conditions such as serum hepatitis, subacute infective endocarditis, or acute respiratory depression.[46] Also, the patient's social background, including who his friends and visitors are and how they behave may contribute to making the diagnosis. On physical examination, the findings of needle punctures, scarring and darkening over veins, and possible skin abscesses, are common in users of illicit narcotics.

The appearance of the opiate abstinence syndrome is a confirmatory phenomenon. This may occur naturally, in the patient who is away from his customary supply of drug, or the physician may elect to precipitate the abstinence syndrome by administering a narcotic antagonist. After obtaining the patient's consent, one can give 0.1 mg naloxone intravenously in order to precipitate the acute abstinence syndrome.

Intoxication

Acute intoxication with a usual dose of an opiate causes the patient to have constricted pupils, lowered respiratory rate, and spasm of smooth muscle sphincters (See Chap. 147 for management). The duration of these effects depends on the drug used, route of administration, and existence of tolerance. Psychic ef-

fects seem quite dependent upon the person's expectations and the drug-taking setting. The person in acute pain who receives morphine in the hospital, experiences relief of pain, with possible mild euphoria. Conversely, the person who injects an unknown but very small amount of heroin into himself, believing it to be a potent solution, obtains what he expects, namely the "rush" followed by relaxation, although after tolerance develops the occurrence of euphoria is minimal.

Abstinence

Severity and duration of the opiate abstinence syndrome vary according to the amount, frequency, and duration of drug intake, and according to the substance used. The syndrome following abrupt cessation of morphine or heroin use, after at least three weeks of daily use, is the prototypical opiate abstinence syndrome. About 16 hours after the last dose, the patient begins to have rhinorrhea, goose flesh, lacrimation, sweating, and yawning; these increase in severity over the next several hours. Sluggish pupillary response to light is an important objective finding. Next, restlessness, insomnia, and muscular twitching and cramping develop, and the patient experiences hot and cold flashes and abdominal cramping. By the end of 36 hours of abstinence, nausea, vomiting, and diarrhea generally have developed. The peak intensity of symptoms is at 48 to 72 hours after withdrawal, and within 7 to 10 days all objective signs of abstinence have declined. Patients may still complain of malaise, restlessness, and weakness for several weeks.

The important feature of this abstinence syndrome is that, while causing genuine discomfort, it is not life-threatening. Only a severely debilitated patient suffering from some condition such as chronic cardiac or pulmonary disease, might have medical difficulty during untreated withdrawal.

Management

Acute opiate withdrawal can be treated best with substitution of methadone given orally and slowly reduced. When the patient exhibits rhinorrhea, goose flesh, and slow pupillary responses to light, the physician can begin treatment by prescribing 10 mg of oral methadone, to be repeated when the patient next has the objective signs of beginning withdrawal. This therapy is, of course, best carried out in an inpatient hospital setting, so control can be maintained over the patient's access to other drugs.

The patient who has been taking an average amount of heroin in most United States cities, will be maintained without signs of withdrawal on 30 to 40 mg of methadone daily. This dose can be reduced to zero over 1 to 3 weeks. Although oral methadone treats the abstinence syndrome, it produces little or no euphoria, especially when given under medical supervision, since it is given orally, and since tolerance to euphoric effects has already developed. Accomplishing withdrawal with a reasonable minimum of discomfort may be the first step in the opiate dependent person's gaining enough trust in the people treating him, to continue in longer-term rehabilitation.

A wide range of services is necessary to provide treatment programs for opiate dependent persons.[45] Each person may have a different background and a different current situation, so the elements of a treatment plan must be chosen to meet individual needs. Psychotherapy, family therapy, educational and vocational services, legal aid, ongoing medical care, and social services, including possible provision of housing or income support, are all components of a complete treatment program. The staff in a program need to know enough about the behavior of drug users in general, and especially about those they are treating, to stay ahead of the client's attempts to avoid surveillance or abstinence. Urine checks to determine evidence of unauthorized drug use, and ongoing evaluation of the program to monitor the objective results with patients (employment, participation in family) are necessary to ensure the establishment of effective treatment programs.

The newer treatment approaches for opiate users are the methadone maintenance technique, and drug-free therapeutic communities. Methadone maintenance appears to be helpful for the person who has adopted heroin use as a life career, and who can benefit from additional vocational training and the rewards of placement in a steady job. Patients are given 40 to 120 mg methadone daily, which prevents them from getting any acute subjective pleasurable sensation if they should take an intravenous dose of heroin. Getting no "kick" from heroin, and being protected from withdrawal symptoms by methadone, they may discontinue seeking and using it. As part of a program providing counseling, training, and social services, methadone maintenance has been a help for many heroin users who had not been successfully treated in other programs.[40]

Communities of former heroin users, with strict enforcement of a complicated, comprehensive set of social rules, provide a new total life career for the person who enters and stays. Members begin by a long and demanding application procedure, often having to appear for appointments several days in a row before being accepted. They then are assigned to menial tasks in the house, and gradually may work their way up to positions of some responsibility. Programs in public speaking, education, and peer-group therapy are the usual added components of treatment. Many people drop out early in treatment, and reliable statistics are not published. It does appear that a few persons who stay on in the program find a new kind of involvement and do not return to drug use.

Studies to determine which kind of treatment program is more effective for different types of drug-dependent people have been instituted but no definitive results are yet reported. A typology of drug users, and a matching typology of treatment approaches, would be a significant advance in our knowledge. To date, it is clear that any treatment program which leads to recovery for opiate dependent patients involves several years of continuous outpatient care, with contact intensive enough to detect early relapse, and services comprehensive enough to provide new opportunities for those who want to change.

SEDATIVE-HYPNOTIC DEPENDENCE

While most abused opiates are obtained illegally, and alcohol is generally purchased over the counter, many people dependent upon sedatives can obtain their supplies by prescription. Despite the small percentage of people taking sedatives who have become dependent upon them, it has been estimated that in absolute numbers, as many as 2,000,000 Americans annually are taking more medications of the barbiturate class than is medically indicated. For these reasons, and because the withdrawal syndrome can be quite severe, the physician needs to be alert to this condition.

Etiology

All barbiturates, all potent nonbarbiturate hypnotics (with the possible exception of flurazepam) and all minor tranquilizers, including meprobamate and the benzodiazepines can, when a person ingests them in large quantities over a period of time, cause the development of drug dependence of the sedative–hypnotic class. These medications have acute effects similar to alcohol, and the chronic effects including drug dependence are not dissimilar. However, sedative drug dependence is not associated with the kinds of nervous system or hepatic damage seen in alcoholism (Chaps. 66, 67, and 153).

Development of physical dependence is a function of the variables of drug dosage and duration of continued intake. Daily doses of 400 mg of pentobarbital do not result in a state of physical dependence which leads to withdrawal convulsions or delirium. Doses above 800 mg daily, over 90 days, are highly likely to be followed by convulsions or delirium on abrupt withdrawal.[39] Even single hypnotic doses of glutethimide, methprylon, or pentobarbital do cause distinct changes in REM sleep; this is a subtle but definite indication of physiologic changes which might be the earliest stage of development of physical dependence.[42]

Social and psychological factors are the other major variables determining who may develop sedative drug dependence. People who do not tolerate anxiety or discouragement easily, and who find relief in the effects of sedatives or antianxiety medications, may well begin to use these in larger doses than their physician intends. Such people may have psychiatric syndromes of several varieties, including neuroses with much perceived anxiety, character, or personality disorders with immaturity, low self-esteem and difficulty in assertive behavior, or chronic depressions. The feature of relative passivity and inability to be assertive without being aggressive, is common to many patients. In addition, the social sanction of prescription medication, "if a doctor prescribed it, it must be all right," may be used by the patient to rationalize his or her increasing use of the medication.

Some patients seek the sedation or antianxiety effect of these substances, trying to escape the discomforts of emotional stress. Others may prefer the "high" which may ensue either as a paradoxical reaction after tolerance is established, or as a release of usual social–psychological inhibitions due to the CNS-depressant effects of sedatives. Still another group use the sedatives in combination with other substances, for instance to counteract or temper the stimulant effects of amphetamines, or to self-treat the discomforts of abstinence from some other substance such as opiates or alcohol. This latter combination is particularly dangerous because the substances potentiate each other and the drug taker can unintentionally take a lethal amount.

Recognition of the Patient

The physician should consider the possibility of sedative drug dependence in patients who complain of insomnia, show no evidence of sleep deprivation, and insist upon a specific potent medication being prescribed. Also, a patient who requests medication for anxiety or tension, but who declines a skillful inquiry into the possible psychological or social sources of, and remedies for, the tension, may be more interested in the effects of the medication than in any resolution of the underlying problems.

With the patient who has an unexpected and un-explained major seizure or delirium, the physician should investigate whether sedative use has been a contributing factor. A person who is known to be dependent upon opiates should be asked if he or she is also using sedatives; this combination is not uncommon in either street heroin users or medically-supplied opiate users. Patients who report that they see several physicians currently, or who have a large supply of many medications, may well be taking enough medications in the sedative class to have physical dependence.

Intoxication

The signs and symptoms of intoxication may also lead the physician to inquire about sedative use. The mildest intoxication syndrome includes nystagmus on vertical gaze, slight dysarthria, and mild ataxia or unsteadiness. With greater intake of sedatives, this may progress to marked ataxia, drowsiness, or somnolence. In brief, the signs and symptoms are quite similar to those of alcohol intoxication.[41] The major distinction is that the person using sedative medications will have none of the medical conditions associated with alcoholism, such as liver or brain disease.

Abstinence

Abstinence phenomena can be divided into minor (early) and major (later-appearing). The minor phenomena begin appearing within 24 hours of abrupt withdrawal and include apprehension, muscle weakness, tremors, postural faintness, anorexia, and twitches. The major, serious withdrawal phenomena in sedative dependence are seizures and delirium which develop in the second to eighth day after withdrawal. Sleep disturbance, with less than 4 hours of continuous sleep at night, is often a precursor of major withdrawal phenomena. Paroxysmal discharges may be seen on EEG after the second day of abstinence. These last two phenomena provide some objective measures for diagnosis.

Management

When a patient is suspected of having physical dependence to sedatives, withdrawal in a drug-free inpatient setting is the preferred treatment. Such a patient needs the close supervision and medical and nursing care afforded on a hospital unit, where the responsible physician can control the amount and kind of medication the patient receives. This can be the first step in the usually long treatment of this chronic and relapsing condition.

To determine the amount of medication necessary to safely treat the patient for withdrawal, a test dose of pentobarbital, 200 mg, should be given when there are no signs of intoxication. An hour after this dose, examine the patient for evidence of intoxication, looking first for nystagmus on upward gaze. A patient who is intoxicated on that first dose has no physical dependence and can be managed without further sedatives. A patient who is not intoxicated, should have further doses of pentobarbital 200 mg orally every 2 hours until intoxicated. This total amount of pentobarbital necessary to reach intoxication, is 100 mg over the patient's level of tolerance. Since there is cross tolerance with all drugs of the sedative–hypnotic class, pentobarbital will substitute for any one substance or for any combination.

After finding how much pentobarbital is required to mildly intoxicate the patient, the physician can begin a schedule of medication reduction, decreasing the daily dosage by 100 mg each day. The pentobarbital should be given in four to six divided doses, to provide a steady tissue level of the medication; a bedtime dose is not necessary in addition to an evening dose. If any signs of abstinence recur, the dosage should be temporarily increased by 100 mg, and the reduction continued the next day.

A patient who is already showing signs of abstinence on admission to hospital can be given the test dose then; ordinarily the test dose is given the first morning in the hospital, before breakfast.

While withdrawal is being medically managed, the longer-range treatment including psychotherapy and rehabilitation, should be planned and begun. As with other drug dependence problems, only a combination of good medical management and long range therapy designed to offer changes in the person's abilities to cope with life problems, can lead to recovery. Often the drug use is symptomatic of personal or family difficulties which must be recognized and dealt with before the patient can give up drug dependence. In some instances the primary physician will choose to carry out the long–term therapy; for other patients he will choose consultation with and referral to a psychiatrist.

OTHER TYPES OF DRUG DEPENDENCE[38]

Amphetamines

Amphetamines, useful in treatment of narcolepsy and minimal brain damage syndromes, are misused by some people. The effects include elation and euphoria, appetite suppression, and insomnia. Although tolerance develops rather rapidly, and strong psychic dependence is a feature, little physical dependence occurs. Withdrawal is characterized by increased sleep, increased appetite, and sometimes by severe depression. For this reason, the person who suddenly stops taking large doses of amphetamines needs close supervision during withdrawal.

People who take high doses over a protracted period may develop a paranoid psychosis indistinguishable from acute paranoid schizophrenia. They commonly have auditory hallucinations and may also experience tactile hallucinations or formication. This condition can be treated by hospitalization and chlorpromazine and responds within a few days.

Cocaine

This is another stimulant or activating drug, and intoxication results in euphoria and jitteriness. A toxic psychosis can occur, with paranoid features and occasional outbursts of violence. As with amphetamines, strong psychic dependence but no physical dependence develops. Withdrawal often leads to profound but transitory depression. The toxic psychosis can be treated with antipsychotic medications.

Cannabis

The resin of *Cannabis sativa* contains tetrahydrocannabinol, a psychoactive substance. When smoked or ingested, this results in a loss of time perception, alteration of visual and auditory perception with possible hallucinations, disorientation, and occasional tremors, ataxia, and drowsiness. This substance is usually taken socially, in a group, and the effects related to euphoria are dependent on the activities of the group and the person's expectations. Larger doses may result in dysphoria or depression.

No physical dependence is known to develop, but people who experience euphoria while using cannabis do often develop strong psychic dependence. Research into the possible desirable and undesirable effects of this drug is far from complete.

Hallucinogens

Mescaline (derived from peyote cactus), psilocybin (from several mushroom species), and such synthetic substances as lysergic acid diethylamide (LSD) and N,N-dimethyl tryptamine can induce psychic experiences including changes in visual perceptions, hallucinations, and feelings of omnipotence. There may be a loss of contact with reality, or psychosis, but this is a variable feature depending on dosage and user expectation, as well as the social setting of drug use. Carefully planned and supervised LSD experiences have been used experimentally as part of treatment of terminally ill patients.

The patient who presents for medical care during a "bad trip" may have been taking a mixture of these substances, and physicians are properly wary of using additional medications for treatment because of problems of drug effect interaction. Support, assurance, and "talking the person down," especially with friends he knows, can be helpful. If sedation is needed, diazepam, chloral hydrate, or short-acting barbiturates are useful adjuncts. Constant supervision in a quiet well-lighted room is the mainstay of emergency treatment.

Pentazocine (Talwin)

This analgesic has opiate-like effects as well as being an opiate antagonist. Patients taking the medication for long periods develop tolerance, and a mild but definite abstinence syndrome occurs, with nervousness, insomnia, muscle aches, and pains. This can lead to further use of the medication, especially in chronically ill patients who have difficulty tolerating further discomfort. Medically supervised withdrawal is helpful in these patients, and drug dependence of this type may be prevented by judicious prescribing practices.

Phencyclidine[43,47]

Phencyclidine (Sernylan) is a veterinary anesthetic which can produce alterations in state of consciousness and psychotic symptoms in man. It is marketed on the street as powder, pills, or capsules, and is called PCP, angel dust, and flakes, among other names. People take it by inhaling, smoking, or ingesting it alone or in combination with other substances such as cannabis.

Acute effects include a toxic delirium and other acute psychotic states mimicking manic or schizophrenic illnesses. Larger doses can produce seizures or coma. Chronic effects reportedly include dementia. Some patients are also said to have poor impulse control, but this may antedate their use of PCP. PCP's effects on the autonomic and cerebellar areas of the nervous system give some signs leading to diagnosis. Patients who have taken PCP will have tachycardia with hypertension, and sweating and flushing of the skin. They may have ataxia, dysarthria, muscle rigidity, and nystagmus. These signs, in combination with the psychological changes of cognitive and emotional disorganization, should lead the physician to suspect PCP use.

Management of acute effects includes good general medical and psychiatric care. Seizures will probably respond to diazepam, which may also be used for severe agitation. As with other "bad trips" minimal medication and the use of calm, constant companionship in a quiet room, are the best approach.

CHAPTER 139
Sexual Problems
JON K. MEYER

Since sexual problems may be associated with a wide variety of organic and emotional illnesses, they are frequently encountered in medical practice. Conversely, functional sexual disorder may mimic organic disability. In either case, impairment of sexual function affects adversely many aspects of the patient's life.

Thorough evaluation of sexual dysfunction requires

1. An understanding of the physiology and psychology of sexual function
2. An awareness of those organic conditions and emotional disorders commonly associated with impairment of sexual function
3. An appreciation of the patient's feelings about having a sexual problem
4. An ability to approach the evaluation comfortably and matter-of-factly

Depending upon his assessment, the physician may undertake treatment and management or refer the patient to a specialist.

THE PRESENTATION OF SEXUAL DISORDERS

Sexual problems present in a variety of ways, which may be categorized as direct or indirect.

Indirect Presentation

Headache, being "out of sorts," fatigability, back pain, being "run down," dysmenorrhea, and a gamut of other complaints may represent the calling cards of sexual disturbance. A detailed history defining the time of occurrence of the most severe symptomatology (for example, at bedtime, or when the spouse comes home in the evening) will often give a clue to the sexual underpinning of the complaint.

Willful dissimulation of the sexual nature of a complaint presents serious difficulties. Out of embarrassment, concern about physician reaction, or for other reasons, the dissimulating patient will confuse, deny, or camouflage to mislead the physician into dealing with nonsexual complaints as a means of avoiding the sexual nature of the disability. Only the passage of time or multiple consultations will gradually clarify the problem. Often, little can be done to hurry this process except to maintain regard for and interest in the patient.

Indirect presentation of sexual disorders may also occur in the context of disease processes. For example, diabetes not only has effects upon the retina, renal function, and blood pressure, but may also affect the capacity to achieve or maintain an erection. This symptom, occasionally the first manifestation of diabetes, may not be spontaneously mentioned by the patient. Sexual dysfunction may also be a silent companion of cardiac disease, not necessarily through decrease in functional capacity, but out of concern about angina or infarction. While sexual performance may be contraindicated in cardiac disease, in many patients the anxiety and tension generated by loss of sexual functioning is more stressful than reasonable indulgence.

Direct Presentation

In contrast to indirect presentation of sexual disabilities, some patients come forthrightly to the sexual nature of their complaints. It is tempting in this situation to focus on the sexual disability as an isolated and clearly demarcated phenomenon. Care must be taken, however, to evaluate the interpersonal, social, medical, surgical, and psychiatric context in which the disability presents.

ASSESSMENT OF SEXUAL DISABILITIES

The basic tools in the assessment of sexual disability are the history and physical examination. The physical examination is beyond the scope of this section. Several essential features of the history, however, are outlined below:

Allow Sufficient Time for the History

Since sexuality involves intimacy, is imbued with moral restraints and social mores, and involves others and their privacy, the sexual history will often

come haltingly, with gaps in the presentation. Set aside time to hear the patient out, even if it means rescheduling.

Determine the Nature of the Problem, as Perceived by the Patient

The introductory statement, "I don't enjoy sex!" may represent fear of pregnancy, primary anorgasmia, severe neurosis, or a sexual problem in the spouse. Women are often more willing than men to come forward with a complaint of sexual dysfunction and will occasionally attempt to bring a disabled husband into treatment by accepting responsibility for the disorder herself.

Elicit the Duration of the Problem

Was impotency, for example, intermittently present from the beginning of coital activity, or did it develop after previously satisfactory performance? Has the problem been constantly present or intermittent?

Explore the Concurrent Events

Birth of children, debts, affairs, career failures, drinking, physical illness, and emotional disorders may be concurrent events not recognized by the patient as precipitating factors. It will often be profitable to go over seemingly unrelated events coinciding with disability onset.

Investigate Factors Related to Temporarily Improved Functioning

Temporary improvements may be occasioned after a fight with the husband, getting the children away, being taken out for dinner, or using a tranquilizer. Events associated with improvement may provide clues to the nature of the pathogenic agents or circumstances.

Explore the Patient's Ideas About the Cause of the Problem, Its Seriousness, and Possible Treatment

Patients may have a clear perception of the etiology and seriousness of their difficulty. Treatment suggestions will run from hormones, to counseling, to psychotherapy. While the patient's preference should not outweigh medical judgment, knowledge of it may be helpful when the treatment plan is discussed.

Whenever possible, *see the spouse or partner.* The advantages of including the spouse or sexual partner are as follows:

Additional Valuable History

The sexual partner possesses 50 percent of the information regarding the sexual relationship and its dissatisfactions.

Minimization of the "Paranoid Position"

When sex is being discussed solely with one member of a sexual partnership, the other may feel excluded or, worse, suspicious. Even if the partner declines to come, he or she has at least been invited.

Contact with the More Dysfunctional Partner

Often the less dysfunctional partner, being less embarrassed, may seek consultation first, the more dysfunctional person requiring a specific invitation to participate.

Collaboration and Cooperation with Counseling or Referral

Whether direct counseling or referral is planned, cooperation of the partner is essential to its success.

THE PHYSIOLOGY AND EMOTIONALITY OF SEXUAL EXPERIENCE

For practical purposes, sexual adequacy is defined by the individual and his partner; if a complaint exists, the sexual partnership is inadequate by their definition. What is adequate performance for one individual with one partner, or in one set of circumstances, however, may be inadequate with another.

Variations in sex drive and arousal speed occur on both constitutional and experiential bases. Hormones are often invoked to explain variations; except in obvious deficiency states, a cause and effect relationship is seldom clear.

Physiology

On the physical side, the sexual response is divisible into four phases: excitement, plateau, orgasm, and resolution. The male excitement phase is indicated by erection, the female by vaginal lubrication. Male plateau phase arousal is indicated by additional penile tumescence, testicular approximation to the perineum, and the appearance of Cowper's gland secretions. Female plateau levels are indicated by increased pelvic vascular engorgement, development of a vaginal orgasmic platform, and further reddening of the labia minora.

The first hint of impending male orgasm and ejaculation comes with the feeling of heightened tension or activity deep to the symphysis related to contraction of the seminal vesicles. This is followed by prostatic and urethral contraction and the sensation of semen bulk moving along the urethra toward discharge. Discharge is followed by muscular relaxation and a refractoriness to further stimulation, erection, and ejaculation.

Female orgasm has its onset with a momentary cessation in arousal followed by sensual radiation from the clitoris into the pelvis. This is followed, in turn, by vaginal and pelvic muscular contraction and then by release of tension. In the female, as distinct from the male, there is no obligatory refractory period and further stimulation may lead to further orgasm. In the usual situation, however, there is dysesthesia to further touch so that contact may be avoided.

Psychology

Mature sexuality requires normal maturation of physical apparatus, freedom from disease, and progression through the stages of psychological development without too much residual conflict. Mature sexuality is built on a capacity for intimate assertiveness and receptivity, and the recognition of the sexual partner as a real person (with actual personal needs, desires, and responses) rather than a substitute for childhood figures. Maturity in the sexual sphere assumes that early experiences with intimacy have been satisfactory, that foreplay fantasies are not burdened with leftover anger or fear, that gender is secure, that conflicts growing out of the family relationships have mellowed, and that peers have provided sufficient opportunity for sexual experimentation. Mature sexuality comes with the realization that sensual and orgasmic satisfaction, as against mere discharge of sexual tension, requires mutual cooperation and involvement.

COMMON SEXUAL DISORDERS

The common disorders for males are premature ejaculation, impotence, and retarded ejaculation; for females, dyspareunia, anorgasmia (frigidity), and vaginismus. In general, sexual disorders in men involve performance failures, while disabilities in women usually relate to failures of satisfaction. Both sexes may exhibit a nonspecific sexual withdrawal defined as a decrease in sexual interest, frequency, or enjoyment without other specific symptoms. These disorders are outlined in Table 139–1.

These definitions do not adequately represent clinical complexity. For example, a man who ejaculates prematurely may be paired with a woman who doesn't experience orgasm. It may not be clear at first whether she has a primary disorder or whether her difficulty is secondary to the premature ejaculation.

---**TABLE 139-1**---

Male Disorders

Premature Ejaculation
Ejaculation during a process of foreplay understood by
both partners to be leading toward intercourse
Ejaculation just before or during the act of penetration
Ejaculation any time during the first 15 penile thrusts
after intromission

Impotence
Inability to achieve or maintain an erection—prior to
ejaculation—sufficient for penetration and completion
of the sexual act. This definition includes loss of
erection during coitus but prior to ejaculation

Retarded Ejaculation
Very slow ejaculation or virtual inability to ejaculate.
This condition is usually limited to an inability to
ejaculate intravaginally, with ejaculation by
masturbation being spared

Female Disorders

Dyspareunia
Vaginal or pelvic pain associated with penetration and
coitus, very often leading to termination of the sexual
encounter

Anorgasmia
Episodic or relatively continuous inability to reach
orgasm in situations judged to be appropriately
stimulating. There may be anorgasmia with both
coitus and masturbation or just with coitus

Vaginismus
Spasm of the perivaginal musculature rendering
penetration difficult or virtually impossible to
accomplish

Male and Female Disorders

Nonspecific Sexual Withdrawal
Withdrawal from sexual activities or decrease in sexual
frequency by either or both partners without evidence
of one of the specific disorders listed above. It is
nonspecific in that sense only; psychologically the
causes of withdrawal may be quite specific.

DIFFERENTIAL DIAGNOSIS OF ORGANIC AND FUNCTIONAL DISORDERS

Definition of the common disorders provides a framework for the differential diagnosis of organic *versus*
functional etiologies.

In the Male

Premature ejaculation is seldom primarily organic in
etiology. It is usually related to sexual anxiety which,
in turn, may be related to strife between partners, unreasonable performance expectations, or unconscious
emotional conflict. Anxiety about physical conditions
may contribute to the development of premature

ejaculation, for example, in patients with cardiac insufficiency. There are few physical problems directly
related to premature ejaculation, but irritation of the
glans or prepuce and inflammations of the urethra or
prostate are occasionally cited.

Impotence may be secondary to a number of
physical disorders. Organic disorders, however, usually affect erectile capacity differently from functional ones. An organic disorder will often produce
absolute or progressive interference with erection
while functional disorders will show intermittent, periodic, or situational potency disturbances. A functionally impotent man may be impotent with one
woman, but not another, or impotent in heterosexual
but not in homosexual relationships. Organically impotent men may attempt masturbation or relations
with various partners with no better results. When
awakening at night, or before voiding in the morning,
functionally impotent men will have full and firm
erections while organically impotent men will continue to show compromised function. The presence of
nocturnal or full-bladder erections with complete tumescence indicates the capacity for physiologic response and makes the diagnosis of organic impotence
less likely.

Retarded ejaculation, like premature ejaculation,
is seldom based on organic pathology. The absence of
or reduced ejaculate, which may at times mimic retarded ejaculation, is associated with urologic procedures giving rise to retrograde ejaculation and occasionally with psychotropic agents such as Mellaril.

In the Female

Anorgasmia in the female is seldom associated with
organic conditions as a primary etiology; rather,
physical illness or compromised function may establish the preconditions of anxiety or withdrawal sufficient for psychological anorgasmia. The functional
etiologies range through unwillingness to experiment
with more effective techniques, interpersonal dishar-
mony with the partner, and unresolved intrapsychic
conflicts.

Dyspareunia is commonly associated with physical etiology and a careful screening for such conditions as vulvovaginitis, endometriosis, or uterine ligament tear is indicated. Organic dyspareunia tends to
be consistent, being present with gynecologic examination and any and all partners, as contrasted with
episodic or situational functional dyspareunia.

Nonspecific

Nonspecific sexual withdrawal is "nonspecific" only
in the sense that there is no apparent primary sexual
dysfunction. The psychological causes for the with-

drawal are quite specific and may be deep-seated. Physical illness may also contribute to the withdrawal.

Diagnosis

The differential diagnosis of organic *versus* functional sexual disorders is, in the final analysis, dependent upon thorough history, physical examination, and laboratory studies. In general, however, organic disorders will show an unremitting consistency or progressive decline in function that is not found in the more situationally related, intermittent functional disorders.

SPECIAL SEXUAL PROBLEMS: THE PARAPHILIAS

The emphasis so far has been on the common sexual disorders, such as impotence and frigidity, which are manifest symptoms and specific complaints encountered with some regularity in the consultation room. There is another large group of disorders, which occur at a lesser frequency in the population and are seen even less frequently as a specific complaint. These include the sexual orientation disturbances: male and female *obligate homosexuality, preferential homosexuality, bisexuality,* and *latent homosexuality.* Also included are the deviations such as *transvestism, sadomasochism, fetishism, exhibitionism, pedophilia,* and *voyeurism.* A less frequent, but related group of problems are the *gender dysphoria syndromes* (transsexuals). These syndromes include the various categories of applicants for sex reassignment surgery.

Etiology

The sexual deviations (sadomasochism, pedophilia, fetishism), sexual orientation disturbances (homosexuality and lesbianism), and gender dysphoria syndromes (so-called transsexualism and its variants) are functional sexual problems rooted in individual psychological development. They are collectively called *paraphilias.* In man there is no convincing evidence for developmental or other abnormality in the central nervous system or for hormonal or endocrine dysfunction sufficient to account for these sexual patterns.

Mode of Presentation

COVERT.   Despite their lesser frequency as specific complaints, homosexuality or one of the sexual deviations may be behind other sexual dissatisfactions. For example, a married man whose interest and passion are largely committed to a homosexual partner may well experience impotence with his wife. This couple, seen in consultation, may complain of impotence, and the wife may be unaware of her husband's homosexuality.

INCIDENTAL.   There are several other common modes of presentation of these disorders in medical practice. First of all, they are not usually revealed. If some disclosure is made, more often than not it is incidental to an unusual disease presentation or requirement for treatment occasioned by the sexual practice. For example, syphilis may present with oropharangeal or anal manifestations in male homosexuals. When the aberrant sexual practices are disclosed incidentally, the patient usually considers them to be a behavior variant rather than an illness, sickness, or emotional problem. The legal, social, or health consequences of his practices may be considered undesirable by the patient, but he will usually be more adamant about changing society than changing himself. In these situations, psychiatric referral may be suggested appropriately enough, but in the absence of motivation the patient will seldom follow through.

URGENT.   There are certain situations, however, requiring more attention and psychological attunement if these sexual disorders are to receive good medical management. These include situations of homosexual panic, spouse or family discovery of the sexual deviancy, potential or actual public exposure, and encounters with the law.

PANIC.   Occasional attraction to the same sex is the rule rather than the exception in all individuals. In most circumstances the attraction is either not very strong or fleeting, presenting little actual difficulty. The attractions are strong and continuous among latent homosexuals, however, even though operating out of their awareness. Sudden eruption of these feelings into awareness or into action may result in high anxiety states or frank panic. Such a situation constitutes a medical and psychiatric emergency since suicidal or other destructive behavior may be the outcome. There should be immediate psychiatric referral. When that is not possible, and panic is present, the patient should be hospitalized and sedated until referral can be made.

FAMILY EXPOSURE.   Another crisis situation concerns the involvement of family members in the sexual deviancy, either when the spouse discovers the activities or is asked to participate in them (such as aiding a transvestite in his cross-dressing or being either degraded or degrading in a sadomasochistic perversion). Children of the family or of others may become involved bringing the deviancy into bold relief. Such a situation requires psychiatric evaluation and consultation for both man and wife, and occasionally, for the children. Advice leading to separation and divorce is often not useful. Such advice usually expresses the physician's moral outrage and ignores the factors that are positive in the marriage, underestimates the possibility that the sexual deviancy has had some utility in the marriage (for example, by providing vicarious satisfaction or avoiding coitus), and steers the couple away from potentially useful psychiatric consultation.

PUBLIC EXPOSURE. The risk of public exposure and entanglement with the law are often, though not necessarily, related. Public exposure may come through careless or incidental publicity without the law being involved. Public exposure and legal entanglements are constant hazards for the established individual. This is particularly the case when part of the fantasy motivating the homosexuality or transvestism involves being apprehended and punished; there is then a constant temptation to take unnecessary risks. When a patient has the sense of flirting with apprehension, psychiatric referral may be quite opportune. If he has already been apprehended or exposed, responsibility shifts to collaboration with the courts in securing consultation and providing understanding and counsel, or even psychiatric referral, for the spouse and family. As is true in panic states, public exposure or arrest may provide the occasion for suicide or other ruinous action. This risk should be recognized as contributing to a need for rapid action.

OFFICE AND SPECIAL TECHNIQUES FOR THE TREATMENT OF SEXUAL DISORDERS

Among the functional disorders, it is useful for treatment purposes to distinguish between ingrained neurotic and characterologic sexual problems and sexual problems related more to interpersonal problems or unfortunate life circumstances. *Neurotic* sexual disorders are accompanied by symptomatology such as unreasonable fears or dysphoric mood. *Characterologic* disorders are associated with alcoholism, drug abuse, chronic career failures, sexual deviancies, and other dysfunctional behavior of a subtle or gross sort. Sexual disorders that are *interpersonally based* or the product of life circumstances show clear evidence of time-limited difficulty between partners (such as surrounding the illness of a child) or extraordinary life events (job loss) in the absence of long-standing symptomatology.

Certain sexual disorders may conveniently be handled in office practice, i.e., those related to lack of information, lack of experience, or uncomplicated relationship issues. More long-standing relationship problems, severe character disorders, neurotic and psychotic disorders, or paraphilias are best handled by psychiatric referral.

Every medical specialist has a variety of medicinal or surgical techniques customarily used in dealing with the usual sexual problems seen in his practice. These familiar techniques may be complemented or expanded by the psychological measures that follow.

Provision of Information

Misinformation about sexual functioning is extreme in some couples and contributes to the sexual disability in many. In such cases, it may be useful to provide information on genital anatomy, the physiology of arousal and orgasm, techniques of foreplay, coital positions, and the broad range of sexual practice. Patients may be selected for this brief intervention when history indicates lack of information, inexperience, and factual misconceptions together with an interest in having more data. The primary effect of providing information in an understanding, matter-of-fact way is to take sexual functioning out of the realm of the mysterious and forbidden.

Counseling

To embark on a course of brief counseling implies not only the provision of factual information, as above, but also several consultations during which ongoing sexual activity can be verbally explored. At issue are when and how the sexual approach is made, whether arousal is experienced, how coitus is practiced, and what satisfactions are achieved. Suggestions may be made for practicing: for example, if arousal seems insufficient during foreplay the couple may be advised to share their individual preferences and to practice foreplay, relegating coitus for the moment to the background. If one partner has difficulty achieving adequate arousal, this partner may be made responsible for determining when coitus is to occur. If failure to achieve orgasm is the difficulty, instruction in afterplay techniques to achieve orgasm may be indicated.

The primary goal in brief counseling is to enable the individual, or couple, to be more aware of needs and to communicate them freely, giving nature an opportunity to take its course. Individuals or couples are selected for brief counseling when there is a problem of some standing, but not ingrained, where neurotic or characterologic aspects of the sexual difficulty are not apparent, and where simple lack of information is not primary.

Behavior Modification

Formal behavioral modification work is most frequently carried out with couples with more longstanding or complete disability. This technique requires participation by the couple in 10 to 20 sessions in which there is detailed attention to the sexual history, and a series of graded exercises gradually leading up to coital activity. This technique is selected for couples for whom there are more long-standing, ingrained, and serious relationship problems but without readily apparent, significant neurotic or characterologic dysfunctions. In general, this formal technique should not be attempted without previous training and experience.

Psychotherapy

Patients are selected for this program when there is overriding anxiety regarding a more direct approach to sexual functioning, or high levels of neurotic, affective, character, or psychotic problems. The paraphilias also should be referred for psychotherapy.

Psychotherapy of sexual disabilities may be undertaken either with a couple or individuals. The primary goal is to elucidate the historical roots of the difficulty, together with the associated fantasies, emotions, conflicts, and inhibitions. This technique requires experience and training and implies an openended time commitment to the treatment program. Extended time is required since the pathogenic elements are sealed off from conscious knowledge and volition, and the elapsed time required to reach and then rework such material is not under the physician's direct control.

CHAPTER 140

Major Psychiatric Disorders
JOHN B. IMBODEN

ORGANIC BRAIN SYNDROMES

Organic brain syndrome (OBS) refers to any condition in which there is evidence of diffuse impairment of higher cerebral function. In Chapters 112, 113, and 147 are listed some of the organic conditions and toxic agents commonly associated with OBS.

The various forms of OBS have in common significant impairment of cognitive functions, especially memory, orientation, and judgment. Other cognitive functions also may be affected. There is frequently noticeable change in affect and often the clinical picture is strongly colored by emotional reactions to the condition itself or to concurrent problems in the patient's life.

OBS may develop in a slowly progressive manner or it may present as a rapidly developing, confusional state.

SLOWLY DEVELOPING, SUBACUTE, OR CHRONIC ORGANIC BRAIN SYNDROME

The illness may be manifested by: 1) change in personality; 2) other evidence of impairment of intellectual and affective functions; 3) psychological reactions to the illness; and 4) neurologic signs.

Change in Personality

It is not unusual for slowly progressive OBS to be first manifested by a change in the patient's personality. This change may be related to the development of shallowness or blunting of affect so that, much to the family's consternation, the patient is no longer as responsive to others as is normal for him. Concomitantly, he may show a deterioration in personal habits of cleanliness, grooming, punctuality; he may display poor judgment or lack of caring in daily tasks at home and work. There may be disinhibition or diminished control of impulses as reflected in *uncharacteristic* vulgarity of speech, irritability, outbursts of anger, and indiscreet sexual behavior.

The patient is often unaware of the changes in himself and is brought to the physician by a relative.

Impairment of Cognitive and Affective Function

Typically, the mental status examination reveals impairment of memory, especially for recent events, disorientation in time and place, faulty comprehension, difficulty in concentrating and in other intellectual functions such as understanding and solving arithmetical problems. Concrete, literal interpretation of proverbs is often seen. The patient's speech may be circumstantial or, in advanced conditions, rambling and incoherent. Blunting or shallowness of affect may be apparent during the examination.

Psychological Reactions

Many patients with OBS are unaware of impaired intellectual functions. There is evidence that this lack of awareness is often the product of a psychological defense, denial. Denial of memory deficit may be unconsciously supported by confabulations which "fill in" gaps in memory. It is not rare, however, for the patient to be partially aware of his condition and, therefore, to react with painful distress when asked to answer questions or perform tasks which reveal intellectual deficit. Occasionally, severe emotional disturbances, such as reactive depression and paranoid states, develop early in the illness as the patient experiences progressive diminishment of intellectual abilities in the course of daily living.

Neurologic Signs

Dysarthric speech is not rare. There may or may not be localizing neurologic signs, depending upon the areas of the brain involved in the underlying disease process.

ACUTE ORGANIC BRAIN SYNDROME

A rapidly developing confusional state, often accompanied by frank psychosis, is commonly termed "delirium" or "toxic psychosis." The basic features of impaired cognition are typically present, namely, defective memory, disorientation, faulty judgment, difficulties in concentration, comprehension, and reasoning. Occasionally, these basic features of mental confusion dominate the clinical picture, the patient being relatively quiet and unperturbed. Not infrequently, however, delirium is accompanied by marked anxiety, excitement, agitation, fragmentary paranoid delusions, frightening visual and auditory hallucinations, and voluble, incoherent speech. Seizures may occur particularly in delirium associated with drug or alcohol withdrawal.[63]

In both chronic and acute forms of OBS, there is apt to be marked fluctuation in the sensorium, confusion tending to be worse at night and when the patient is placed in unfamiliar surroundings.

DIAGNOSIS

Diagnostic evaluation includes the determination that an organic brain syndrome exists and identification of the responsible, underlying condition. A history of recent personality change should always arouse suspicion of an organic process. Generally, evidence of impaired cognitive function is apparent on mental status examination. In instances of early or mild impairment, however, psychological testing is useful.

Determination of the associated condition requires general medical evaluation (see Chaps. 113, 114, and 147). A careful history of alcohol and drug ingestion or withdrawal should be obtained from the patient (if possible) and from the member of the family who knows the patient best.

MANAGEMENT

Specific treatment of the responsible, associated medical condition is obviously of the utmost importance. General management of the patient with OBS aims to 1) prevent the patient from harming himself; 2) provide an environment designed to reduce confusion; and 3) prevent exhaustion and dehydration.

The measures required to accomplish these goals vary considerably depending upon the condition of the individual patient, such as the presence of excitement, fear, or restlessness. The presence of a trained attendant at the bedside is often helpful and is essential if the patient is acutely disturbed. Often, the presence of a relative or someone familiar to the patient has a calming effect. The environment should be one that is well-lighted (when the patient is awake) and the staff should address the patient in clear, readily comprehensible terms; ambiguities of any sort should be reduced to a minimum. Active encouragement to maintain adequate food and fluid intake, with daily monitoring, is necessary because the patient's normal awareness of hunger and thirst is apt to be obtunded. The use of sedatives and tranquilizers depends to some degree upon the specific associated organic or toxic condition. The use of barbiturates (except in specific instances such as the management of addiction to hypnotics) should usually be avoided. Chlordiazepoxide, orally or intramuscularly, in sufficient dose may be useful in calming the patient and promoting sleep.

SCHIZOPHRENIC ILLNESSES

The term *schizophrenia* refers to a group of syndromes characterized by disturbances of thought, affect, and behavior which lead eventually to a wide variety of signs and symptoms including difficulty in forming and communicating concepts, social and emotional withdrawal, disturbances of mood, neurosis-like symptoms, periods of excitement and immobility, misinterpretations of reality, delusions and hallucinations. Although the constellation of manifestations is characteristic, there is no sign or symptom that is pathognomonic of schizophrenic illness. In making the diagnosis it is necessary to exclude other conditions such as organic brain syndromes and primary affective disorders which may be associated with any of the above symptoms.

Schizophrenic disorders occur in all races and socioeconomic groups, but the prevalence is higher among the poor.

Mode of Onset

Schizophrenic illness usually begins in adolescence or young adulthood. In some patients, there is a previous history of schizoid personality traits: shyness, oversensitivity, seclusiveness, avoidance of competitive relationships, tendency to daydream, and inability to express hostile or aggressive feelings. The onset may be insidious, sometimes consisting initially of an accentuation of schizoid personality traits, progressive withdrawal from friends and family, decline in academic interest and achievement, hypochondriacal preoccupations, and multiple somatic complaints or other neurotic symptoms, such as obsessions and compulsions. Months may go by before the family realizes that something serious is going on, and this realization may not occur until some bizarre, disturbing behavior develops.

In other patients, the illness develops rapidly and dramatically, the patient exhibiting such unmistakable evidences of profound disturbance as psychomotor excitement, marked alteration of mood, delusions, and hallucinations.

The initial development and subsequent exacerbations of schizophrenic illness may or may not be associated with stressful events or situations. Often the illness tends to develop or worsen around transitional periods of youth: puberty, adolescence, graduation from high school or college, leaving home or facing the prospects of going out into the world.

Disturbance of Affect

In schizophrenic illness, there is often a progressive diminution or narrowing of interests, loss of ability to experience pleasure, affective "flatness" and withdrawal, sometimes to the point that the patient becomes exasperatingly indifferent to everything and everybody. The patient may also display inappropriate affect, have periods of melancholy, elation, or become angrily excited and fearful without reasons that are apparent to others.

Disturbance of Cognitive Functions

Evidence of cognitive disorder may be revealed in difficulties in communication, and in the development of delusions and hallucinations. In normal communication, one attempts to convey a concept to the listener. In doing this, one must often relate background material or subordinate concepts in order to get the main idea across. This requires the speaker to be in touch with relevant associations and to screen out those which are irrelevant.

In schizophrenic thought disorder, the associative processes may be severely constricted, sometimes "blocked," so that the patient loses his train of thought. Abnormal constriction of associations may result in paucity of thought or in a tendency to concrete thinking (as manifested by very literal, narrow interpretations of simple proverbs). On the other hand, failure to screen out irrelevant, or tangential associations often occurs and may result in the patient's not getting to the point in conversation. The patient's associations may be so loosely connected that the listener cannot follow him; he may be strikingly overinclusive when asked straightforward questions or when confronted with simple tasks or problems.

Other disturbances of communication include the idiosyncratic use of words, creating new words (neologisms), repeating words or phrases in a stereotyped fashion, and negativism.

The patient's thought processes may be excessively influenced by his feelings so that beliefs and judgments become based on wishes and fears to the exclusion of evidence and logic. He may develop delusions of grandiosity, of being followed, persecuted, covertly referred to in newspapers and television, of having his thoughts, feelings, and behavior controlled by an external agency. Somatic delusions and feelings of unreality are common.

Hallucinations involving any sensory modality occur but often are predominantly auditory. The "voices" may call the patient's name, discuss him, describe his present activity, give him commands, praise him, insult him, or they may consist of his own thoughts in audible form.

Psychomotor Activity

Catatonic excitement, psychomotor inhibition, and various manifestations of severe regression may dominate the clinical picture.

Subtypes

Various types of schizophrenic illness have been described including the classical delineation of simple, hebephrenic, paranoid, and catatonic forms. These are still useful descriptive terms and the reader is referred to the works of Kraepelin, Bleuler, and current textbooks for detailed discussion of them.[1,2,58,59]

Currently, it has been found useful to classify schizophrenic illness into two types: one characterized by features associated with a relatively good prognosis and the other by features associated with a relatively poor prognosis. The good prognosis type, sometimes referred to as schizophreniform illness, reactive or remitting schizophrenia, and schizoaffective disorder is characterized by the following: relatively good preillness level of adjustment, presence of stress at time of onset, rapid development of the illness, symptoms of excitement, and affective symptoms. The group with relatively poor prognosis is sometimes referred to as "true" schizophrenia or process schizophrenia. The characteristics are: poor preillness adjustment, slow and insidious onset, absence of precipitating stress, relative lack of affective symptoms, and relatively high incidence of schizophrenic illness in the family.[65]

Diagnosis

In its florid form, the diagnosis of schizophrenic illness usually presents no difficulty. It should be kept in mind, however, that a variety of conditions can be associated with delusions, hallucinations, and other symptoms common in schizophrenia; among them are the organic brain syndromes and affective disorders. Typically, in schizophrenic illness, the sensorium is clear. In delirium, in addition to clouded sensorium, it is common for visual hallucinations to predominate. Hallucinations and delusions can occur in severe depressive and manic states; their content usually reflects a depressive or expansive attitude toward the self and the future. Other manifestations of primary affective illness should be sought including a family history of affective illness. Amphetamine intoxication can closely simulate schizophrenic illness; the diagnosis is made by a history of amphetamine ingestion and by marked clinical improvement within two weeks of separation from the drug. In schizophrenic illness, regardless of the obviousness of the diagnosis, careful neurologic and general medical evaluation are indicated.

Etiology

The causes and pathogenesis of schizophrenic disorders are not known. Numerous studies of the incidence of schizophrenic illness in close relatives of patients, including those comparing the concordance rates of monozygotic and dizygotic twins, strongly support the view that there is an hereditary predisposition. These same studies also indicate that hereditary factors alone are not enough to account for the development of the disorder. Current investigations have focused upon psychological and neurochemical (or neurophysiologic) variables that may be implicated in the development of schizophrenic illness.[60,64] It is entirely possible that both groups of factors are necessary in the development of at least some forms of schizophrenic illness.

Management

The patient with schizophrenic illness should be referred to the psychiatrist for continued evaluation and treatment. One of the antipsychotic drugs, usually a phenothiazine or haloperidol, is frequently administered, particularly if the patient is severely disturbed or during an acute episode. Often it is necessary to maintain the patient on a drug for an indefinite period. In recent years, it has often been found possible to avoid prolonged hospitalization and to utilize relatively brief periods in the hospital when symptomatic exacerbation requires them. The establishment of a psychotherapeutic relationship with the patient is of critical importance. More often than not, it is also important for the therapist to work with key members of the family.

PRIMARY AFFECTIVE DISORDERS

Every human being experiences some degree of fluctuation of mood in the course of his life. Affective disorders, however, are characterized by one or more relatively severe and enduring deviations in mood which may be associated with a variety of symptoms and signs.

Classification

Serious disturbances of mood may develop in the course of other psychiatric illnesses, such as organic brain syndromes, schizophrenic illness, and the neuroses. It has been suggested that in these instances, the preexisting psychiatric illness be considered the primary disorder and the associated affective disturbance, usually depression, secondary. Affective disturbances occurring in the absence of preexisting psychiatric illness are then considered manifestations of a primary affective disorder. There are two syndromes of affective disorder: depression and mania. Both are seen in all degrees of severity.

Primary affective disorders are *bipolar* if the mood disturbance consists of one or more manic episodes with or without episodes of depression. The term *unipolar* refers to a primary affective disorder characterized by one or more episodes of depression only.[65]

DEPRESSION

In addition to the unipolar–bipolar classification, other dichotomies have been proposed for depressive illness based on degree of severity and presence or absence of apparently precipitating events: neurotic *vs.* psychotic and reactive *vs.* endogenous depressions. The term "involutional melancholia" is sometimes used to refer to serious depression first occurring in late-middle life although it has not been established that involutional changes are responsible for the disorder.

Clinical Features

Depression may occur at all ages but tends to be more frequent in middle age or later. The incidence is higher among women than men. It may develop in the apparent absence of any precipitating event or it may seem to develop as a reaction to adversity, particularly one which involves "loss" of some type, such as death of a loved one, separation or divorce, loss of job, money, physical health, professional or social standing.

The clinical manifestations of depression may be grouped as follows: 1) subjective change in mood; 2) attitudes toward one's self; 3) attitudes toward the future; 4) psychomotor changes; and 5) physiologic symptoms and somatic complaints.

SUBJECTIVE CHANGE IN MOOD. Typically, the patient complains of feeling "down," "sad," "low," "blue," "despondent," or simply "depressed." This feeling may be worse in the morning than at night, but the reverse is also seen. The patient may state that nothing interests him or gives him pleasure. Of particular importance diagnostically is the fact that these subjective aspects of depression are sometimes minimized or denied by the patient or they may be dismissed as merely secondary to some other symptoms such as unexplained physical pain.

ATTITUDES TOWARD THE SELF. To some degree, the depressed patient is self-deprecatory, indicating that he sees himself as inadequate or "bad" or both. In severe depression, the debased self-concept may be expressed directly or metaphorically in somatic delusions, and in auditory hallucinations and paranoid delusions in which derision and accusations are leveled at the patient. The patient may attempt to justify his feeling of inadequacy and guilt by focusing upon past failures and misdeeds.

PSYCHOMOTOR SYMPTOMS. Depending upon the severity of the depression, the patient feels mentally and physically sluggish and "slowed down." He finds it difficult to concentrate, small tasks seem to require great effort, and he may withdraw from social and occupational activities. In severe psychomotor retardation, the patient may be silent, immobile, and seemingly unresponsive to his surroundings. However, restlessness and agitation also occur.

ATTITUDES TOWARD THE FUTURE. The patient's view of the future may vary from that of moderate pessimism to one of utter hopelessness. A businessman may be mistakenly convinced that he is on the verge of bankruptcy. He may feel unworthy of ever feeling happy again. Hopelessness is usually accompanied by a wish to die and sometimes by suicidal intentions.

SOMATIC COMPLAINTS AND PHYSIOLOGIC ACCOMPANIMENTS OF DEPRESSION. Among the most common somatic complaints in depression are: tiredness, a heavy or oppressive feeling over the chest, aches or pains of any part of the body, and symptoms related to functional changes discussed below.

Several bodily functions are affected, especially in severe depression. Anorexia with substantial weight loss is common. Occasionally the depressed patient eats excessively, especially at night. Hypersomnia may occur but insomnia is more common; awakening early is typical in severe depression although it is not unusual for the patient also to have difficulty in falling asleep and to sleep fitfully. Decrease in sexual interest, impotence, and constipation are not uncommon.

Diagnosis

When the above described constellation of symptoms and signs is present, the diagnosis is apparent. As previously noted, however, the depression is sometimes obscured by the dominance of physical symptoms. Unexplained pain, anorexia, weight loss, insomnia, loss of libido, and fatigue or loss of energy should arouse suspicion of depression. It is helpful to keep in mind that it is rare that a physical symptom or "depressive equivalent" will completely replace or "contain" other features of depression. Careful inquiry will usually reveal feelings of sadness, discouragement, subtle or indirect self-deprecation, decline in interests. Diagnosis of depression is further supported by a history of significant loss or adversity prior to or concomitant with the onset of the present illness. In the elderly patient with mild intellectual impairment, the development of depression may be accompanied by worsening of memory difficulties and confusion, giving the false impression of advanced senility. In these patients, it is important to be alert to symptomatic evidence of depression, and if the latter is suspected to test the diagnosis by a trial of treatment.

We have noted that depression may occur in the course of any psychiatric illness. Depressed states may also be associated with medical illnesses or treatment such as the administration of reserpine, carcinoma of the pancreas, porphyria, and debilitating conditions such as chronic renal insufficiency.

Etiology

Studies of close relatives of patients with primary affective illness, including concordance rates among monozygotic and dizygotic twins, point to an hereditary predisposition. Psychological factors have been studied intensively. There is suggestive evidence that the experience of traumatic loss early in life and the development of more than usual need for approval from others increase the likelihood of reacting to current losses and disappointments with depression. The "turning inward" of hostile feelings has also been implicated as a factor in developing depression[61.] Recent studies have pointed to a possible biochemical abnormality, perhaps a decrease in biogenic amines (serotonin and the catecholamines) in the brain of depressed patients.[57]

Management

Patients who are severely depressed or manifest evidence of hopelessness and suicidal danger should be referred to the psychiatrist and may require hospitalization. In those patients whose depression is not severe, has not resulted in gross misinterpretation of reality, and in whom the suicidal risk does not appear to be great, the primary physician may well undertake treatment and management. The patient should be seen once or twice a week initially for brief sessions in which the initial aim is to establish rapport and a supportive relationship. Depressions are usually self-limited, and the statement of this to the patient may be helpful. It is wise to avoid excessive reassurance. The use of antidepressant medications and other aspects of management are further discussed in Chapter 142.

MANIA

Bipolar affective illness, characterized by one or more manic episodes with or without episodes of depression, is much less common than affective illness characterized by depression alone (unipolar). The age of onset varies but the first attack is often in the 20s or early 30s.

Clinical Features

The manic or hypomanic (mildly manic) patient often has a history of having been an ambitious person who seems to need praise and approval more than the average individual. When the manic episode begins, the patient frequently has no insight into his condition. The principal features of the manic state are:

1. The patient experiences an alteration in mood. The patient feels "high" or euphoric but also may be irritable and quite intolerant if his wishes are not met.
2. The patient is typically hypertalkative. His speech is incessant, rapid and, in extreme cases, he exhibits flight of ideas.
3. The manic patient is hyperactive and usually has grand and unrealistic projects and plans. He may have delusions of grandeur and sometimes experiences hallucinations, paranoid delusions and feelings of depersonalization.

Diagnosis

The differentiation from schizophrenic illness is usually possible on the basis of the features of elevated mood or irritability, hyperactivity, and rapid speech even in the presence of symptoms suggestive of schizophrenia such as hallucinations and delusions. The sensorium is usually clear in manic states. A careful review of the history of drug ingestion is important in any patient who is euphoric or psychotic.

Management

The patient should be referred to a psychiatrist. Hospitalization is often indicated until the patient's condition has been brought under control with one of the antipsychotic drugs or lithium carbonate.

NEUROSES

Neurosis refers to a group of syndromes in which there is some degree of anxiety, often accompanied by other symptoms, such as phobias, obsessions, compulsions, conversion reactions, and hypochondriacal complaints. The name given a particular neurotic syndrome is determined by those symptoms which are predominant. While the patient with a severe neurosis may endure much suffering and be gravely incapacitated, his ability to comprehend reality is not grossly disturbed as it is in psychotic states. The neurotic patient may engage in inappropriate or irrational behavior but, unlike the psychotic person, be clearly aware that the behavior is inappropriate or irrational. For example, a phobic patient may be compelled to avoid elevators even though he knows they are safe; that is to say, the phobic avoidance of situations is not based upon delusions concerning them but upon a desire to avoid anxiety. Many neurotic symptoms *partially* protect the individual from the anxiety generated by emotional conflict while, at the same time, they express directly and symbolically the patient's unresolved emotional problems.[62]

NEUROTIC SYNDROMES

Anxiety Neurosis

This condition is characterized by one or both of the following:

1. A chronic or recurrent state of feeling tense, vaguely apprehensive or worried, and somatic symptoms which often accompany chronic tension such as occipital headaches, backache, and fatigue.
2. Acute attacks of anxiety, characterized by a feeling of fear, restlessness, tremor, and various autonomic symptoms such as tachycardia, pallor, sweating, dry mouth, pupillary dilatation, and blurring of vision; hyperventilation with paresthesias and a sense of suffocation may also occur.

While feelings of tension and acute attacks of anxiety often occur without the patient's awareness of a precipitating event, it is common for the patient, once he has developed severe anxiety, to focus his apprehension upon something specific. For example, in acute anxiety the patient may fear that his heart will stop beating, that "something terrible" is about to happen or that he might "go crazy." In chronic tension states, the apprehension may center upon a fear of cancer, some other dreaded disease, or upon some family or social problem. The content of these fears is not without significance, but it is important to bear in mind that it is characteristic of the human being to develop a rationale for any strong feeling that he experiences, including anxiety. Therefore, the psychic conflict actually precipitating the anxiety may be only remotely related to specific fears or worries expressed by the patient.

Phobic Neurosis

Once a patient has had an acute attack of anxiety, he may subsequently live in dread of having another one and may carefully avoid the places or situations similar to that in which the attack occurred; the patient has developed a fear of fear. In phobic neurosis, the patient has intense fear of one or more specific objects or situations even though usually there is no clear history of an initial anxiety attack experienced in conjunction with the feared object. The patient may be quite mystified by his own phobia, knowing that the avoided object or situation poses no real danger.

There are many phobias. A common one is a fear of going out of the house alone, the patient often expressing concern that he may become ill or disabled in a strange environment where no help is available. Other phobias include fear of closed places, heights, certain animals, and a wide variety of situations.

Hysterical Neurosis

There are two types of hysterical neurosis, conversion and dissociation, both of which are characterized by unconsciously produced loss or disorder of function.

CONVERSION TYPE. Conversion refers to an unconscious process in which the patient reduces the anxiety or dysphoria associated with an emotional problem by developing one or more physical symptoms which mainly involve the sensory and voluntary motor systems. Conversion symptoms may be seen in a variety of psychiatric disorders including schizophrenic illness and depression.[66] The diagnosis of conversion hysteria is reserved for those patients, the majority of whom are women, in whom the conversion symptoms dominate the clinical picture and are not secondary to some other condition. In this disorder, there is often a history of chronic symptoms or of recurrent episodes of a variety of physical symptoms for which no organic basis can be found.

Patients with conversion hysteria tend to be histrionic, suggestible, dependent persons who have a rather marked tendency to avoid or repress painful feelings and problems. The avoidance of feelings and problems is buttressed by "converting" or transforming the psychological problem into a physical one. The conversion serves the additional purpose of giving the patient an acceptable basis for seeking help as a physically sick person. The patient unconsciously simulates a physical illness and, if his concept of the illness is accurate, the conversion syndrome may pose a difficult diagnostic problem. The success of hysterical patients in simulating organic disease is unfortunately reflected in the frequency of a history of multiple surgical procedures. The unconscious choice of symptoms is, in part, determined by the patient's past experience with physical illness in himself or others and by the suitability of a particular symptom to symbolize the underlying conflict. Commonly seen hysterical symptoms include blindness, deafness, anesthesias, paresthesias, pain, weakness, seizure-like episodes, aphonia, and paralysis. No organic basis for the symptoms can be found and often it can be demonstrated that the disability does not conform to anatomic or physiologic requirements, such as paralysis in which the reflexes are preserved in the absence of upper motor neuron signs. Sometimes the patient seems anomalously unconcerned about her disability, *la belle indifference.*

It has been noted that in conversion hysteria, the patient *unconsciously* simulates physical illness. In *factitious disease,* on the other hand, the patient *knowingly* and *willfully* induces symptoms in himself by such means as self-administration of insulin, inducing vomiting, or feigning fever by warming the thermometer. The willful feigning or exaggeration of illness may serve some purpose such as to avoid court trial or to support litigation. More often than not, patients who feign illness or have factitious disease are emotionally disturbed and should be referred for psychiatric evaluation.

DISSOCIATIVE TYPE. Dissociative state refers to functional disorders characterized by amnesia or altered states of consciousness. Fugue is a condition in which the patient flees or travels, often considerable distances, during a period of amnesia. In the extremely rare "multiple personality," the patient assumes a different identity for which he has no memory when he "returns" to himself.

Obsessive-Compulsive Neurosis

Obsessions are persistently recurrent, unwanted thoughts that are often described by the patient as being alien to his own values and sense of propriety. Disturbing obsessive thoughts may contain ideas of destruction, mutilation, death, blasphemy, while others may seem superficially to be psychologically neutral such as the recurrent title of a song. Compulsions refer to acts or rituals, such as counting, hand washing, long prayers, which the patient must carry out in order to avoid anxiety. The anxiety in turn may be related to fear that an obsessive thought might, in some magical way, bring harm to someone.

Hypochondriacal Neurosis

In this condition, the patient is preoccupied with bodily functions and tends to interpret minor symptoms and physical feelings as being indicative of disease. He constantly worries about himself in spite of reassurance. Unlike conversion hysteria, there is no loss or disorder of function.

Other Neurotic States

Neurasthenia refers to neurosis in which the predominant symptoms are tiredness, feelings of weakness, and exhaustion. In depersonalization, the patient experiences feelings of unreality and estrangement from the self, body, or his surroundings.

DIAGNOSIS

The diagnosis is usually apparent from the presence of symptom constellations characteristic of the neuroses as described above. In making the diagnosis, however, two points deserve emphasis:

1. Any or all of the above-described neurotic symptoms can occur in the early or later stages of schizophrenia or affective disorders.
2. Careful medical evaluation is necessary to rule out coincident physical illness or an illness which may simulate neurosis such as hyperthyroidism, multiple sclerosis, brain tumor, or myasthenia gravis.

MANAGEMENT

The results of the medical evaluation should be openly discussed with the patient and it should be made clear that failure to find an organic basis for the patient's complaints do not make the symptoms any less real. An attitude of interest and tactful inquiry into the patient's life situation concurrent with the initial and most recent exacerbation may be enlightening and therapeutically beneficial. Antianxiety drugs may be indicated, but it is wise, if feasible, to use them for brief periods and in carefully regulated dosage to avoid psychological and physical dependence. Patients with moderately severe or incapacitating neurosis should be referred for psychiatric consultation.

PERSONALITY DISORDERS

Personality disorders are characterized by constellations of character traits, attitudes, and patterns of behavior that are deeply engrained, usually having been present since adolescence or earlier, and which interfere, to some degree, with the individual's adaptation to life. The diagnosis of a personality disorder *alone* implies that at the time of the diagnostic evaluation, symptoms indicative of other psychiatric disorders, such as anxiety neurosis, are minimal or absent. It is not unusual however, for the physician to discern the presence of a personality disorder in a patient who has developed symptoms of neurosis or other illness.

Classification and Diagnosis

The classification of personality disorders is not entirely satisfactory because individuals often do not fit neatly into any given category, sometimes exhibiting character traits of more than one type of personality disorder or traits that do not clearly belong to any of the types in the classification scheme. Nevertheless, the basis for diagnostic classification is similar to that of the neuroses, that is, the diagnosis of personality disorder is determined by those features which are predominant.

Some of the more common personality disorders and their distinguishing features are listed in Table 140-1. It will be noted that many of the manifestations of character disorders are present in minor form in healthy personalities. Therefore, the diagnosis of personality disorder requires that these features be somewhat pronounced and associated with impairment of adaptation. Under conditions of stress or with organic brain damage, features of personality disorder often become accentuated. However, per-

sonality disorders generally do not appear to be on a continuum with neurotic or psychotic illnesses. For example, most individuals with schizoid personality do *not* eventually become afflicted with schizophrenic illness. Further, when a patient with a given personality disorder decompensates the resulting neurotic or psychotic illness may or may not appear to be an outgrowth of the preexisting personality. For example, an obsessive-compulsive person who decompensates may develop an obsessive-compulsive neurosis, or a depression or, more rarely, a schizophrenic illness.

Management

The patient with personality disorder of serious degree should be referred to the psychiatrist for evaluation even though psychiatric treatment of certain character disorders (in particular the antisocial personality) may not be effective. The best response to psychiatric treatment occurs in those individuals who are capable of feeling anxiety and guilt and whose

---

TABLE 140-1
Personality Disorders

Personality Disorder Type	Salient Features
Antisocial personality	Has history of poor adjustment in school: academic failure, truancy; frequent arguments and fights; poor job performance; undependable, quitting without notice, getting fired; frequent conflicts with the law: larceny, robbery, rape, etc.; social behavior dominated by hedonism, poor impulse control, lying, charming or "conning" people, defective sense of guilt, shallow relationships, and failure to learn from experience
Asthenic personality	Tires easily, is low in energy and enthusiasm, overly sensitive to physical or emotional stress
Cyclothymic personality	Has mood swings of depression, elation, or both, which are of moderate degree and short duration, usually occurring without apparent precipitating factors
Explosive personality	Tends to react with intense emotion, such as rage, to relatively minor provocation. Temper outbursts are often followed by remorse
Hysterical (histrionic) personality	Tends to be excitable, histrionic, self-centered, attention-seeking, and seductive
Inadequate personality	Tends to be inept, ineffective, has poor judgment, frequently fails socially and at work, in spite of average educational opportunity and intelligence as measured by psychological tests
Obsessive–compulsive personality	Tends to be unusually conscientious, dutiful, perfectionistic, inhibited. Is often ambivalent and tends to doubt his own opinions and decisions
Paranoid personality	Shows behavior characterized by tendency to be rigid, opinionated, jealous, resentful, suspicious. Is quick to blame others for his problems
Passive–aggressive personality	Tends to express aggression passively by procrastination, pouting, stubborn withholding, and obstructionism
Passive–dependent personality	Tends to lack self-confidence. Often feels indecisive and clings to others for guidance, reassurance, and support
Schizoid personality	Feels vulnerable and therefore avoids close or competitive relationships. Tends to be seclusive, aloof, does not display feelings readily, daydreams

maladaptive behavior represents an effort to mini-mize uncomfortable feelings associated with psychic conflict. The determination of treatability often requires intensive psychiatric evaluation over a period of time.

Antisocial persons may seek medical help for incidental illness or for medical complications associated with their antisocial behavior. Alcoholism and drug dependence with their associated organic complications, venereal disease, and physical trauma from fights and accidents may cause the antisocial person to feel a genuine need for medical help. However, he may also contact the physician in the guise of seeking medical help, while actually intending to use the physician or the hospital for some other purpose, such as the obtaining of drugs or evasion of legal prosecution. The recognition of antisocial personality is important so that the physician can avoid being manipulated (which helps neither the patient nor the doctor) while at the same time offering needed medical help for any somatic illness that may be present. The physician may refer the patient to a psychiatrist for evaluation but the patient may not cooperate with the referral if he sees no immediate gain for himself.

We have previously noted that personality type is correlated with the way patients feel and behave when they become physically ill and, as a corollary, that the physician tailors his approach to management in accordance with the personality of the patient. For example, in dealing with a paranoid personality the physician is careful to communicate clearly, to avoid ambiguities, to invite the patient to ask questions, and to avoid bedside staff conferences in which the conversation is sprinkled with mysterious medical terms (see Chap. 135).

TRANSIENT SITUATIONAL DISTURBANCES

Transient situational disturbances refer to emotional states, such as fear, grief, depression, and irritability, that occur as a reaction to severe environmental stress in persons in whom there is no evidence of underlying mental disorder. Symptoms recede as the stress diminishes. For example, a conscientious person with heavy responsibilities may react with considerable apprehension and despondency to being laid off from work particularly at a time when jobs are scarce. Finding work restores his sense of well-being. If such an individual were seen during the distraught period of unemployment, his condition would be considered an adjustment reaction of adult life.

—CHAPTER 141—
Psychosomatic Medicine
JOHN B. IMBODEN

Introduction

Psychosomatic medicine is a field which has been rife with controversy. This is related to a variety of factors, among which are:

1. Exaggerated claims and therapeutic expectations
2. Methodological problems which make the scientific validation of psychosomatic hypotheses difficult
3. Overdone skepticism even in the face of data from carefully controlled studies
4. Misapplication of psychoanalytic interpretations to organic processes
5. Misunderstandings as to what is meant by the term psychosomatic

Despite the problems and controversies associated with it, psychosomatic medicine (as defined below) has important implications for both the principles and practice of medicine and deserves open-minded study by the student and practitioner. Accordingly, this chapter will focus upon the following aspects of psychosomatic medicine: 1) definitions; 2) historical perspective; 3) functional disorders associated with psychic stress; 4) psychosomatic theories of certain organic diseases and their application to three specific disorders, namely, peptic ulcer, ulcerative colitis and coronary heart disease; and 5) implications of psychosomatic concepts for management with special reference to the three disorders just named.

Definitions

In its broadest sense, psychosomatic medicine refers to the study and treatment of those conditions which are related to the interaction of psychic and somatic phenomena. As thus defined, psychosomatic medicine includes the following:

1. PSYCHOLOGICAL REACTIONS TO PHYSICAL ILLNESS. This category includes the whole range of emotional and behavioral responses to physical illness, such as the development of depression in the patient who has been informed that he has cancer or acute apprehension associated with myocardial infarction (see Chap. 135).

2. PSYCHOLOGICAL DISTURBANCE RESULTING FROM DISORDERS AFFECTING BRAIN FUNCTION. In this category are included not only the acute and chronic brain syndromes (Chaps. 112, 113, and 140) but also those disorders whose effect on cerebral function may result in psychological disturbance with or without symptoms of mental confusion. For example, some endocrine disorders, particularly those affecting pituitary, thyroid, parathyroid, adrenal, and gonadal functions may present with symptoms such as mild depression, listlessness, tension, anxiety, irritability, suspiciousness as well as manifestations of severe disturbance such as delusions and confusional states.

3. MEDICAL COMPLICATIONS OF MALADAPTIVE BEHAVIOR. This group includes the numerous physical complications associated with alcohol or drug dependence, overeating, self-starving as in anorexia nervosa, and the physical trauma associated with suicide attempts, accident proneness, and antisocial behavior.

4. EMOTIONAL DISORDERS MANIFESTED BY SOMATIC SYMPTOMS WITH NO ORGANIC BASIS. This group includes the conversion reactions and hypochondriasis (Chap. 140).

5. PHYSIOLOGIC CONCOMITANTS OF EMOTIONAL STATES. This group includes the manifestations of autonomic activity associated with acute anxiety or fear and other conditions in which the predominant symptoms are the consequences of the physiologic concomitants of emotional disturbance. These conditions, in which structural change or tissue damage is minimal or absent, will be referred to as *functional disorders*.

6. PSYCHOSOMATIC DISEASES. In this chapter, psychosomatic disease refers to an organic disorder in which there *is* structural change or tissue damage and in which it is postulated that psychological factors contribute importantly to etiology.

Frequently, the term "psychosomatic" is used in a restricted sense to refer only to conditions characterized by bodily manifestations or consequences of emotional factors, namely the functional disorders and psychosomatic disease and in this chapter we will confine our discussion primarily to these two groups of disorders.

First, we will briefly comment on the history of psychosomatic medicine with the aim of elucidating certain trends that are of general interest and that are related to the back and forth shifting of medical attitudes toward this field.

A BRIEF HISTORICAL PERSPECTIVE

The interdependence of mind and body, or perhaps more accurately, a monistic concept of the human being, in health and disease, prevailed in the practice of medicine in antiquity. This was clearly the case in those cultures and eras in which the roles of priest and healer were combined, but a psychosomatic viewpoint was also evident in the theory and practice of medicine in the nonmystical, rationalistic approach espoused by Hippocrates.

In the nineteenth century, there appears to have been a tendency to turn away from serious consideration of the role of psychological variables in the pathogenesis of disease states. This may have been caused, in part, by the impressive advances getting underway in cellular pathology and bacteriology and, in part, it may have been a reaction against the medieval theories, repugnant to the scientific mind, by which various manifestations of disease were ascribed to sin, diabolical possession, and witchcraft.

In the early decades of the present century, a swing back toward the psychosomatic approach in medicine developed, mainly under the influence of Freud's psychoanalytic theories and, to a lesser extent, the psychobiology of Adolf Meyer which emphasized the importance of "treating the whole person."

The revival of psychosomatic medicine in this century has thus far been a biphasic one in the sense that by the 1950s it had probably reached a zenith of popularity among the laity and physicians, followed by a period of disappointment and skepticism which is now being replaced by a less dramatic but more solid, scientific development of the field.

There were several factors which brought about the period of disenchantment with psychosomatic medicine.

1. THE INAPPROPRIATE APPLICATION OF PSYCHOANALYTIC INTERPRETATION. Symptoms and signs, which were manifestations of altered physiology or tissue damage, were sometimes interpreted as having symbolic meaning and, further, their alleged symbolic content was postulated to be of primary, etiologic significance. Thus, fever might be interpreted as symbolizing sexual excitement; a swollen, infected finger as unconsciously representing a tumescent penis, and so on. Such ludicrous interpretations of somatic symptoms, reflecting a faulty grasp of both psychoanalysis and pathophysiology, may well have struck many physicians as a return of medieval mysticism in secular guise. Franz Alexander, whose work will be discussed further, was one of the pioneers in psychosomatic medicine who helped to differentiate those somatic symptoms, which, from the outset, do have symbolic meaning, from those which do not.

2. PSYCHOSOMATIC MEDICINE WAS INADVERTENTLY OVERSOLD. The new insights into human behavior that psychoanalysis offered seemed to promise a new, powerful therapeutic approach to those disorders which were considered to be psychosomatic. While psychotherapy has its rightful place in the management of psychosomatic illness, it is not a cure-all. The elucidation of psychological factors in the genesis of peptic ulcer, for example, did not suddenly lead to a curative psychological approach, applicable to all patients with peptic ulcer. The leading scientific investigators never made the claim that it would, but nevertheless, a high expectation of definitive therapy developed among many people who were, of course, disappointed.

3. METHODOLOGIC PROBLEMS IN PSYCHOSOMATIC RESEARCH. The methodologic problems encountered in the investigation of the relationship between psychological factors and the pathogenesis of disease are numerous and serious. We will mention only a few:

1. In studying a patient with a given disorder, it may be difficult to distinguish between those characteristics which are primary and those which develop as a reaction to the illness.
2. In assessing the significance of psychological variables in relation to a particular disease, it may be technically difficult to develop a suitable control group and even more difficult to devise controlled prospective studies to test an hypothesis.
3. It is difficult to test predictions of the effect of psychotherapy on psychosomatic disease for several reasons, two of them being the problem in collecting large treatment and control samples and the problem of ruling out observer bias.
4. Ethical considerations forbid the deliberate introduction of psychological stress in order to observe its effect on the health of human subjects; while animal experimentation is useful it is often risky to apply the results of animal experiments to human beings particularly when one is dealing with phenomena associated with higher cerebral function.

None of these methodologic problems is insurmountable as is evidenced by the number and variety of excellent investigations conducted in the last 25 years.

In the remainder of this chapter we will discuss functional disorders associated with emotional disturbance and certain diseases postulated to be psychosomatic. In general, the concept of functional psychophysiologic disorders tends to be relatively well accepted while the concept of psychosomatic disease, particularly in certain contexts, is considerably more controversial.

FUNCTIONAL DISORDERS

Functional disorders include those conditions in which the predominant symptoms are the expression or consequences of physiologic concomitants of emotional disturbance and in which structural damage is minimal or absent.

While the neurophysiology of emotion is far from completely understood, the limbic system, including the hypothalamus, does appear to play a central role in the generation of emotions as well as some basic behavioral drives including sexual activity, aggression, experiencing of pleasure, and eating. Through the hypothalamic–pituitary–endocrine system and the hypothalamic–autonomic nervous system connections, impulses arising in association with emotional arousal can potentially have physiologic effects anywhere in the body, in addition to gaining access to higher cerebral centers involving conscious awareness and motor activity.

In discussing anxiety neurosis (Chap. 140), it was noted that in acute anxiety the physiologic responses associated with *sympathetic* discharge are observed. These responses to anxiety or fear were referred to by Cannon as constituting preparation for fight or flight.

In some patients, when confronted with acute stress, compensatory *parasympathetic* discharge occurs and the vasovagal syndrome, characterized by hypotension, bradycardia, and fainting, may result.

It was also noted previously that in states of chronic tension a variety of other symptoms may develop. Some symptomatic manifestations of chronic tension seem to involve visceral functions which are under autonomic influence while others, such as those related to sustained tension of skeletal muscle, are not. Some of the more common functional disorders associated with tension states are listed in Table 141-1. (It is to be noted that psychosomatic diseases, as defined in this chapter, are not listed in Table 141-1.)

┌───┐
│ **TABLE 141–1**

Functional Disorders Associated with Psychological Stress

Physiologic System	Syndrome
Cardiovascular	Migraine headache Vasovagal syndrome (fainting) Tachycardia, palpitations
Gastrointestinal	Irritable colon The following symptoms may occur singly or together: anorexia, nausea, vomiting, abdominal cramps, diarrhea, constipation, aerophagia
Genitourinary	Menstrual disturbances Difficulties in micturition; frequency (in both sexes), hesitancy (in males) Dyspareunia Anorgasmia Impotence Delayed ejaculation; premature ejaculation
Muscular	Pain secondary to increased muscle tension: occipital or bitemporal headaches, backaches, myalgia in various muscle groups; fatigue Tremor
Respiratory	Hyperventilation syndrome Bronchospasm Dyspnea
Skin	Urticaria Hyperhidrosis Pruritis

└───┘

Diagnosis

The diagnosis of a specific functional disorder is made by: 1) the presence of characteristic symptoms; 2) the exclusion of organic disease through appropriate examination and laboratory procedures; and 3) evidence of chronic tension or anxiety. The diagnosis of functional disorder is supported (but not proved) by obtaining evidence that exacerbations and remissions are correlated with tension-producing and tension-relieving changes in the patient's life situation. Thorough examination to exclude organic disease should be carried out even when symptoms are correlated with waxing and waning of anxiety.

Management

Specific symptomatic treatment depends upon the particular functional disorder present. If antianxiety agents are used, it is advisable to prescribe them for brief periods of time to avoid psychological or physical dependence. Diazepam (Valium) may be preferred in treating those conditions associated with increased muscle tension. Careful attention should be paid to psychological aspects of management which include the establishment of a supportive relationship and the exploration of psychic and social factors which may be related to the illness (see Chap. 142). In severe functional disorders or those which do not respond to treatment, psychiatric consultation is advisable.

PSYCHOSOMATIC DISEASES

Basic Concepts and Theories

As previously noted, psychosomatic disease refers to those disorders in which there is structural damage and in which it is postulated that psychological factors importantly contribute to etiology. A variety of theories and investigative approaches have emerged in recent decades, only several of which will be reviewed in this brief discussion.

Most psychosomatic theories have the following postulates in common:

1. Multicausality of disease. Most organic diseases are the result of a number of factors, some related to the organism, others to the environment. In psychosomatic diseases, psychological factors are held to be important or necessary, but not sufficient, in the causation of disease.

2. Certain psychological reactions to life events are associated with physiologic changes that promote development of disease. Most theories stress the point that premorbid personality development is an essential consideration because an event that is stressful for one person may not be for another.

3. Which specific organ is affected may in part be determined by early life experiences but is also determined by constitutional, hereditary, or other factors which are unknown at this time.

We will briefly review the following proposals:

1. For every emotional state there is a specific physiologic concomitant which, if sustained, may, in the presence of other essential factors, lead to organ dysfunction and tissue damage, *Alexander's theory*. Following a general review of this theory, we will present the application of it to peptic ulcer.

2. Reaction to stressful events, especially those involving loss or failure, may lead to an affective state of *helplessness and hopelessness* which, in turn, has somatic consequences which influence the time of onset of disease. We will discuss this theory and its application to ulcerative colitis.

3. A number of investigations have resulted in *empirical observations* showing a correlation between psychosocial variables and incidence of organic disease. We will review studies which demonstrate a correlation between a behavior pattern and the incidence of coronary heart disease.

4. Evidence that glandular and visceral responses can be influenced by *operant conditioning* opens up the possibility that learning experiences may result in predisposition to psychosomatic disease and that some symptoms may be learned or reinforced visceral responses. Miller has pioneered investigations in this area and, in the laboratory animal, has demonstrated the effect of operant conditioning (instrumental learning) on salivation, intestinal contractions, heart rate, blood pressure, rate of urine formation, and other functions. His observations on the learning of visceral responses have led him to dispute the distinction made by Alexander and others between conversion symptoms mediated by the cerebrospinal nervous system and psychophysiologic symptoms mediated by the autonomic nervous system. In addition to laboratory work with animals, clinical studies on humans have also demonstrated the effect of conditioning on visceral function, such as ventricular rate in patients with atrial fibrillation.

While the application of learning theory to the study of psychosomatic disorders is promising, it should be noted that symptomatic response to learning, such as the alteration of ventricular rate in patients with atrial fibrillation associated with rheumatic heart disease, obviously does not necessarily mean that the development of the underlying disease was caused by conditioning experiences.

For further discussion of this important subject, the reader is referred to the reference list.[68,71]

Alexander's Theory[67]

Preparatory to the elaboration of his own concepts, Alexander cleared away much confusion by emphasizing that hysterical conversion symptoms involve "voluntary innervation, expressive movement, or sensory perceptions" and therefore can symbolically represent unconscious psychological content. In contrast, while the viscera under autonomic nervous system influence, do respond physiologically to emotional states, these responses do not represent direct, symbolic expression of unconscious feelings and ideas, although secondarily they may acquire symbolic significance.

Alexander believed that for every emotion there is a specific syndrome of physical changes and that when the emotion subsides the physiologic processes, such as those affecting heart rate and blood pressure,

return to their baseline levels. However, if the emotion, such as fear, anger, longing, cannot be expressed and relieved freely through voluntary activities but is repressed, the physiologic effects (mediated largely through the autonomic and neuroendocrine systems) are sustained, leading to chronic functional disturbance and eventually tissue damage. The disturbances of "vegetative functions" are divided into two categories corresponding to the emotional attitudes involved in: 1) emergency preparations for fight or flight (predominantly sympathetic); or 2) withdrawal from outwardly directed activity (predominantly parasympathetic). If autonomic activation of either type is not followed by appropriate action, a chronic state of physiologic response persists followed by functional disorder or disease.

Alexander suggested that emotions of anger or aggression were associated with sympathetic stimulation and that blocking of aggressive or competitive behavior could eventually contribute to the development of a variety of disorders such as hypertension, migraine, hyperthyroidism, arthritis, vasodepressor syncope, and possibly diabetes. On the other hand, passive-dependent longings were associated with parasympathetic activity and if need-satisfying behavior were blocked such disorders as peptic ulcer, constipation, diarrhea, colitis, and asthma might develop in some people. Alexander was careful to point out the fact that various factors, other than psychological, were also necessary in the production of these diseases, since many persons who develop conflicts involving aggression or passive longings do not become physically ill.

We will now consider some of the evidence concerning Alexander's concept of psychological factors in peptic ulcer.

PEPTIC (DUODENAL) ULCER. Intensive study of individuals with peptic ulcer led Alexander and others to the conclusion that what characterized these patients was the presence of a conflict situation in which the patient wished to be dependent, loved, and cared for and in which these wishes were unfulfilled either because the individual himself repudiated or repressed them or because of frustrating external circumstances. Noting that being loved and being fed are intimately associated from birth on, Alexander postulated that a frustrated, persistent longing for infantile dependence is associated with gastric hypersecretion, as if the individual is constantly preparing to be fed. The intensity of the conflict depends in part on external events. Severe sustained conflict eventually results in gastric dysfunction and peptic ulcer in some individuals.

This concept led to a now classical study of army

inductees by Weiner et al.[75] in which they hypothesized that three factors contribute to development of duodenal ulcer:

1. Sustained gastric hypersecretion (as reflected in high serum pepsinogen levels)
2. Presence of the psychic conflict described above
3. Exposure to an environmental event (induction into army) that mobilizes the conflict and induces psychic tension

The subjects of their study were 2073 young men who were drafted into the army, for each of whom serum pepsinogen level was determined. Sixty-three subjects with values in the upper 15 percent and 57 with values in the lower 9 percent of serum pepsinogen level were selected for special study. Psychological data were independently obtained and gastrointestinal x-ray examinations were done initially and later in basic training. Three subjects had healed duodenal ulcers and six subjects had active duodenal ulcers; all nine of these subjects were in the upper 15 percent of blood pepsinogen distribution. The psychological data revealed that evidence of strong dependency needs was positively correlated with high pepsinogen levels. On the basis of the psychological data, 10 men (of 120) were selected as most likely to develop an ulcer; the predictions were accurate in 7 out of the 10.

While the results of this study are compatible with predictions based on Alexander's theory, it nonetheless does not prove the theory. There is evidence that the characteristic of high serum pepsinogen levels tends to be present from very early in life and to persist throughout life. This observation raises the interesting possibility that infants with this characteristic may have unusually strong oral or nursing needs which, in turn, could predispose the individual to the kind of oral dependence conflict described by Alexander. Likelihood of the latter outcome is enhanced if the infant with strong nursing needs happens to have a mother whose nursing capacity is limited. It may also be noted that the above-cited investigation does not shed light on how psychological stress might affect gastroduodenal physiology in a way which leads to ulcer formation.

The Helplessness–Hopelessness Theory

Many investigators have noted the frequency with which experiences involving separation from important other people or other kinds of important losses or disappointments are observed in close temporal connection with the onset or exacerbation of a wide variety of diseases. Engel and his co-workers at Roch-

ester have been particularly active in clinical investigations designed to test the validity of this observation and in the development of a related theoretical conception of disease. The Rochester studies have included patients with ulcerative colitis, leukemia, lymphoma, and patients consecutively admitted to a medical inpatient service who were suffering from a variety of disorders. In 80 percent or more of patients interviewed, it was ascertained that an experience of loss or threatened loss had occurred shortly before the onset of illness or its exacerbation. Further, the experience of loss was highly significant to the patient in that it was followed by an affective state of helplessness and hopelessness.

Helplessness refers to a feeling of being deprived of an essential gratification as a result of a change in a relationship about which the patient feels powerless so that his only recourse is to wait for a return of that which he has lost. Hopelessness refers to a feeling of despair or futility resulting from a loss of satisfaction for which the patient assumes complete responsibility and about which he can do nothing. Schmale and Engel refer to the inability to let go of wished for gratifications or unachievable goals as the "giving-up complex." They interpret their data as indicating that, in some way, the giving-up complex acts as a *permissive setting* for factors present in the patient which predispose him to a particular somatic or psychic disorder, i.e., as "a final common pathway to changes in health."[74]

The scientific establishment of this important concept is fraught with methodologic problems, such as the difficulty in operationally defining the giving-up complex and in setting up blind, controlled studies. Indirect support for this theory has been obtained from studies of large groups of people in whom it was observed that morbidity and mortality rates are positively correlated with antecedent stress including that of bereavement.

We will now review the application of this theory to a specific disease, ulcerative colitis.

ULCERATIVE COLITIS. In a series of papers published in the 1950s Engel reviewed the psychosomatic hypotheses of ulcerative colitis, certain somatic aspects of the disease, and reported observations on 39 of his own patients.[69]

Many patients with ulcerative colitis have premorbid obsessive–compulsive character traits, tending to be neat, orderly, conscientious, stubborn. They frequently seem immature and tend to develop an ambivalent, dependent relationship with one or two persons who appear to be key figures in their lives. Except for these dependent relationships, these patients often appear to lack the capacity for close, warm friendships.

Onset of the illness and exacerbations were observed by Engel to be associated with a disturbance in the relationship with the key person in the patient's life and with the subsequent development of helplessness or despair. Further, it was found that the ulcerative colitis patient had a history of a symbiotic relationship with his mother which left the patient permanently dependent on her or on a substitute and that this accounts in part for the patient's vulnerability to separation. The question of why the patient becomes afflicted specifically with ulcerative colitis remains unanswered. It is clear that somatic factors, in addition to psychological ones, are necessary for the development of the disease.

EMPIRICAL OBSERVATIONS

CORONARY HEART DISEASE (CHD). Near the turn of the century, Osler reported his impressions that heredity, rich diet, and psychological stress contributed to the etiology of atherosclerosis. He also commented that the typical patient with coronary disease is a "keen and ambitious man, the indicator of whose engines is always set at 'full speed ahead'." In subsequent years, a number of clinical observers have reported similar observations.[73]

Not until the work of Rosenman, Friedman et al., was the accuracy of these clinical impressions tested by a controlled, blind, prospective study.[72] These investigators predicted that individuals who showed evidence of "behavior pattern type A" would have a higher incidence of CHD than persons who did not. Type A behavior pattern is characterized by excessive drive, aggressiveness, ambition, an enhanced sense of time urgency, and relatively great preoccupation with competitive activity, deadlines, and similar pressures. By means of an oral questionnaire, 3182 male subjects who were free of evidence of CHD were classified as exhibiting behavior pattern type A or as not exhibiting that pattern type (type B). Numerous other data were obtained at the outset of the study, including socioeconomic data, smoking habits, physiologic and biochemical measures. During a 2-year follow-up the subjects were reevaluated for evidence of CHD by a senior medical referee who was independent of the study. During the 2-year period, 54 cases of CHD developed among the 1584 subjects exhibiting pattern A as compared with 16 cases among the 1598 subjects exhibiting pattern B. For the group as a whole, the relative risk ratio type A/type B was 3:40; among younger subjects (ages 39 to 49 years) the relative risk ratio was 6:48 compared with 1:88 in older subjects (ages 50 to 59 years). Using a computer-scored test questionnaire, another prospective study of 2750 men by Jenkins et al, revealed that subjects with high scores of behavior pattern A char-

acteristics had twice the incidence of CHD as did low scorers over a 4-year period.[70]

Other studies have, in addition, provided evidence that the incidence of life stresses is positively correlated with subsequent development of CHD and with elevation of blood cholesterol, acceleration of blood clotting, and stimulation of the autonomic nervous system.[73]

Implications For Management

Comprehensive management of patients with psychosomatic diseases rests upon an understanding of the pathophysiology of the disorders and upon a grasp of psychological factors which have contributed to the development of illness. It is apparent that if psychological problems have contributed to the onset of an illness, their persistence or recurrence may impede recovery or contribute to relapse. In most cases of psychosomatic disease, the psychological aspects of management can best be incorporated into the total treatment approach by the general physician. In selected cases, the general physician may find psychiatric consultation useful and occasionally he may choose to refer the patient to a psychiatrist for psychotherapy.

In the paragraphs below, we will briefly discuss only the psychological aspects of management of patients with peptic ulcer, ulcerative colitis, and coronary heart disease. (For general medical management of these disorders, see Chaps. 23, 58, and 60.) The psychological principles of management of these disorders logically follow from an understanding of the emotional factors associated with them.

PEPTIC ULCER. In the management of peptic ulcer, it is important to:

1. Ascertain what kind of stress, if any, was associated with the onset or current exacerbation of the disease
2. Attempt to provide the patient with satisfaction of his dependency needs in a manner acceptable to him

If, for example, the precipitating stress involved dependency need-deprivation secondary to marital conflict, it will be necessary to help the patient cope with the marital problems. This may involve the physician in working directly with the spouse as well as the patient. In addition, the physician himself can provide acceptable means of dependency gratification by establishing a relationship that evokes a sense of security in the patient, by scheduling return visits, by prescribing periods of rest or vacations, and by careful attention to symptom-alleviation through dietary and drug treatment.

ULCERATIVE COLITIS. In this serious, sometimes life-threatening disorder, the role of the physician in instituting medical and/or surgical procedures of crucial importance to the patient's life results in the physician becoming a person of profound significance to the patient. That is to say, the patient–physician relationship itself may become the key relationship upon which the patient comes to depend. This is particularly apt to occur if the illness episode was precipitated by the loss of an important person in the patient's life. As is true of other important, dependent relationships in his life, the patient is apt eventually to exhibit evidence of ambivalent feelings toward the physician. The ambivalence may be manifested in many ways such as exhibiting mistrust or occasionally by testing the physician's competence or commitment to the patient's care.

It is important that the physician's relationship with the patient be a stable one. The physician should guard against being provoked by ambivalent behavior. The impact of separations from the patient can be lessened by explaining their necessity and duration to the patient and sometimes by giving him a prescription to keep and use as needed. As rapport is established, the patient is encouraged to discuss his life situation and to express feelings. Referral to the psychiatrist for consultation or psychotherapy may be indicated but should be done in such a way that it is felt by the patient to be an addition to his therapeutic regimen, not a substitute for his relationship with the primary physician.

CORONARY HEART DISEASE. We will confine our discussion to patients with myocardial infarction. In the first 2 or 3 days of the acute illness, virtually all patients are apprehensive, some severely so. Frequent contact with the patient, reassurance both explicit and implied by an attitude of confidence and optimism, and administration of a minor tranquilizer may be indicated. If the patient exhibits denial of his illness, it is generally wise not to disturb this defense unless the denial leads to behavior which seriously compromises treatment. It may be helpful to assess the patient's need to comprehend his condition and accordingly to give him an understandable explanation of his illness.

After the first 2 or 3 days, the patient may become depressed. This may occur in any patient with an acute myocardial infarction but is perhaps particularly frequent and severe in individuals who have a history of type A behavior. These patients may find the temporary immobilization necessitated by treatment very difficult to bear and, in some cases, it is wise to liberalize the treatment plan to allow the patient somewhat more mobility than is ordinarily done. The patient's depression may be related to his anticipation of not being able to return to his customary high level of activity. This should be discussed with the patient. Some patients exaggerate the degree of disability they face and need to be given a more realistic appraisal of their prospects for returning to a useful life.

In the convalescent period and thereafter, the patient, particularly if he has exhibited type A behavior characteristics, will need to be rehabilitated through carefully graded exercises and will need reeducation to modify his life-style. He will need much support and guidance in learning how to relax, to give himself rest periods, to keep his ambitions from ceaselessly driving him, and to learn to take his time in the accomplishment of tasks. This educative effort will require persistence and patience on the part of the physician, the family and the patient himself.

CHAPTER 142
Management of Psychiatric Disorders
JOSEPH T. COYLE AND JOHN B. IMBODEN

The concepts of medical management discussed in Chapter 4 apply to the management of psychiatric disorders. As was emphasized in that chapter, management implies not only the application of specific therapeutic measures and continuing evaluation but also the design and implementation of an effective, comprehensive program of care for the problems of the individual patient.

GENERAL CONSIDERATIONS

Collection and Analysis of Data
Careful gathering of pertinent facts by interviewing the patient and family members (when indicated), physical examination, and laboratory procedures along with thoughtful analysis of the data are prerequisites to comprehensive diagnosis and management.

Comprehensive Diagnosis

Collection and analysis of data lead to: 1) the delineation of symptomatic and behavioral problems, 2) the diagnosis of a specific psychiatric disorder, and 3) the discernment of personal issues such as current situational stress and intrapsychic conflict associated with the development of the present illness. The physician will take into account all three categories of diagnostic assessment in developing a plan of care and in deciding whether he will manage the problem himself, with or without psychiatric consultation, or refer the patient to a psychiatrist.

Psychiatric Referral

In referring the patient to a psychiatrist, whether for consultation or continued treatment, the physician must take care to: 1) avoid giving the patient a feeling of being rejected; and 2) ensure that the patient understands the reasons for the referral and has had an opportunity to ask questions and express his views about it. The patient whose emotional disturbance is manifested by somatic symptoms and who has little awareness of significant emotional problems is apt to resist going to the psychiatrist if the referral is made prematurely; such a patient may feel that the physician missed the diagnosis and he may seek help elsewhere. As discussed in other parts of this section, psychiatric referral is indicated if there is evidence of psychosis, serious behavioral problems including suicidal behavior, severe neuroses, and character disorders.

Plan of Care

The management of emotional illness includes psychotherapy (which may involve other members of the family and alteration of environment) and chemotherapy. In developing a treatment plan, the physician will set realistically attainable goals. For example, in treating depression or an acute symptomatic flare-up in a patient with hysterical neurosis, the physician may have the goal of symptomatic relief of the present episode. In the process of accomplishing this goal, he and the patient may discover attitudes, behavior patterns, marital and other interpersonal problems which predispose the patient to future recurrence of illness. The physician may then elect to continue to work with the patient or refer him to a psychiatrist.

PSYCHOTHERAPY

Psychotherapy refers to a procedure in which one deliberately utilizes his relationship with the patient for the purpose of assisting him to recover from the emotional illness, to gain an understanding of his attitudes and problems in order to live a more satisfactory life, and to reduce the likelihood of future episodes of illness.[76,85] We will present an overview of general principles and techniques which are useful for the general physician. Intensive, psychoanalytically-oriented psychotherapy and the details of other treatment approaches, such as behavior modification, will not be discussed. Although psychotherapy and pharmacotherapy are discussed separately, they are frequently used in combination.

The Doctor-Patient Relationship

The most important element in psychotherapy is the establishment of a doctor-patient relationship in which the patient feels that the physician respects him, listens to him, attempts to understand him, has a therapeutic intent, and is truthful with him. Such a relationship is in itself strongly supportive to a person who has low self-esteem, who feels apprehensive, discouraged, and whose behavior and complaints may have alienated him from others.

Pitfalls

There are pitfalls to be avoided. It is a serious tactical error to treat the psychiatric patient as merely a passive recipient of sympathy, advice, and pills. Such an approach promotes passivity and dependence in the patient who needs, instead, to be helped to face his feelings, to work with the physician in identifying and understanding problems, to make his own decisions regarding the solution of problems and the setting of life goals, to be responsible for his own behavior, in short, to attain further emotional growth. All of this implies that the physician and the patient are in a collaborative undertaking in which the patient, his feelings, thoughts, and problems remain the focal point of interest.

It is important to avoid excessive reassurance or reassurance that is not solidly based on fact. Inappropriate reassurance, no matter how well intended, can leave the patient feeling that the physician does not understand him.

In undertaking the management of emotional illness, the physician should give careful consideration to the regularity, length, and frequency of return visits. To arrange follow-up visits on an "as needed" basis may set up a situation in which symptom recurrence (or persistence) is *rewarded*. Regularly scheduled visits, on the other hand, take place independently of symptomatic status. The frequency and duration of interviews are determined by the clinical situation and by the realities of the physician's schedule. Weekly sessions are often useful, particularly at the beginning of treatment, in order to allow continuity of therapy to develop. Acutely disturbed patients, for example, depressed patients, initially may need to be seen more frequently than once a week. Much may be accomplished in relatively brief interviews, i.e., 20 to 30 minutes. When the physician has set up a schedule of appointments, he, as well as the patient, is expected to abide by it; to keep a patient, who has a regular weekly appointment, waiting for an hour is to invite resentment for it is a way of saying that the doctor's time is important but the patient's is not. If a delay occurs and was unavoidable the physician should inform the patient of that fact.

Psychotherapeutic Techniques

The physician usually begins an interview by encouraging the patient to talk about feelings or thoughts which are uppermost in the patient's mind. In Chapter 136 ("The Psychiatric Interview," see p. 1321), the example was given of the patient who begins by talking about somatic symptoms and it was suggested that the interviewer listen for spontaneous references to personal issues, feelings, and experiences and, when they occur, that he express an interest in hearing more about them. As therapy progresses and as the relationship deepens, the physician's display of interest in relevant personal feelings and problems becomes important to the patient and reinforces his tendency to delve into the important issues of his life. Occasionally, the patient's associations may lead him toward a topic which arouses anxiety. He will then shift the conversation to another topic. In most instances the physician will not comment upon defensive avoidance though he may do so if he feels that the patient is ready to hear such an observation and to make constructive use of it.

The following lists several techniques that the physician may find useful in the course of treatment:

SUGGESTION. The power of suggestion increases as the doctor–patient relationship solidifies, particularly if a positive transference develops. Some patients are more influenced by suggestion than others. The physician should use suggestion sincerely, sparingly, and with a degree of subtlety commensurate with the sophistication of the patient. The physician may use suggestion unconsciously as when he prescribes a medicine with an air of confidence. He may use it quite deliberately in managing a patient with acute conversion symptoms.

VENTILATION OF FEELINGS (ABREACTION). This refers to a process in which the patient verbally expresses pent up feelings by relating emotionally charged experiences in the recent or remote past. While abreaction may give the patient only a temporary feeling of relief from tension, it may also be edu-

cational in that it gives him increased awareness of how certain experiences can remain emotionally charged and have a continuing influence on one's sense of well-being.

CLARIFICATION. The physician asks the patient to express more clearly or completely his feelings and thoughts about a particular issue or encourages the patient to clarify the relationship between certain events in his life. If the physician has discerned the repetition of certain kinds of behavior in certain situations, he may point this out to the patient thus helping him to develop a clearer grasp of his own behavioral history. The physician may point out that a given somatic symptom developed at about the time a certain event occurred in the patient's life. Clarification, when done persistently and with due regard for the patient's sensitivity, can result in the patient himself becoming a self-observing partner in the therapeutic work.

MANIPULATION. This refers to a procedure in which the therapist takes advantage of emotions or values existing in the patient in order to promote the therapeutic process. For example, in dealing with a patient who resists psychotherapy and who takes great pride in being independent, the physician may quietly emphasize the point that in psychotherapy it is really the patient who does most of the work.

DESENSITIZATION. This refers to a process in which the patient becomes less sensitive to or fearful of a topic, object, or situation by means of gradually increased exposure to it. This technique is sometimes employed in a rigorously systematic way. It is particularly useful in the treatment of phobias.

CONDITIONAL REINFORCEMENT OF BEHAVIOR. Although the theory and technique of operant conditioning will not be discussed, it is apparent that in conducting therapy, the physician will reinforce healthy behavioral change (verbal and nonverbal) in ways which are suitable for the individual patient. An example of reinforcing undesirable behavior was given above in pointing out that scheduling the patient on an "as needed" basis may have the effect of rewarding the development of symptoms.

ALTERATION OF ENVIRONMENT. Stressful situations in the patient's life must be carefully assessed. Tensions and conflicts between members of the patient's family may be strong factors working against the patient's recovery. When this is the case, members of the family or the entire family may be in need of counseling or psychotherapy. Ministers trained in pastoral counseling and skilled social workers may be of considerable help in the handling of family problems and in other situational stresses such as those stemming from occupational and economic problems.

PHARMACOTHERAPY

Introduction

The development of drugs that reduce or eliminate the symptoms of major psychiatric disorders has been a significant advance in psychiatric treatment. It has resulted in a considerable reduction in the number of chronically hospitalized patients as well as a reduction in the duration of hospitalization of most severely affected patients. While serendipity played a major role in the initial discovery of the clinical efficacy of these drugs, careful clinical testing unbiased by nonspecific effects of treatment (placebo-control) or of vested interests of the investigators (double-blind evaluation) has unequivocally demonstrated the effectiveness of these agents. These clinical studies have been augmented by an intense investigation of the action of effective psychotropic medications in the central nervous system. The information based on both clinical and basic studies provide the basis for a rational approach toward the pharmacotherapy of major psychiatric disturbances.

Physiologic Actions of Psychotropic Medications

Our current understanding of the specific actions of psychotropic medications in the brain is based on the chemical basis of neuronal communication.[77] (Fig. 142–1). The transmittal of information from the re-

ceptive region of the neuron, the dendrites, down the axon to the nerve terminals occurs by means of a wave of electrical depolarization; however, the communication between neurons depends upon chemicals called neurotransmitters. Thus, when the depolarizing signal reaches the nerve terminal, it releases a chemical substance that diffuses across the gap between the nerve terminal and adjacent dendrite to interact with specific receptors on the neighboring neuron. The neurotransmitters exert specific effects on the adjacent neurons that alter their activity. Throughout its many synaptic contacts, an individual neuron uses one and only one type of chemical neurotransmitter. The neurotransmitter utilized confers a biochemical identity on the neuron; as a result, the neuron has specialized processes for synthesizing, storing, and inactivating the neurotransmitter. Groups of neurons utilizing the same neurotransmitter generally innervate discreet regions of the brain, thereby regulating the functions that are controlled by the particular region. Because the types of neurotransmitters are limited in number, the neurons utilizing a particular neurotransmitter may subserve several different functions in the brain, although one function may predominate.

Most psychopharmacologic drugs exert their primary therapeutic effects by altering specific biochemical processes that mediate action for a single

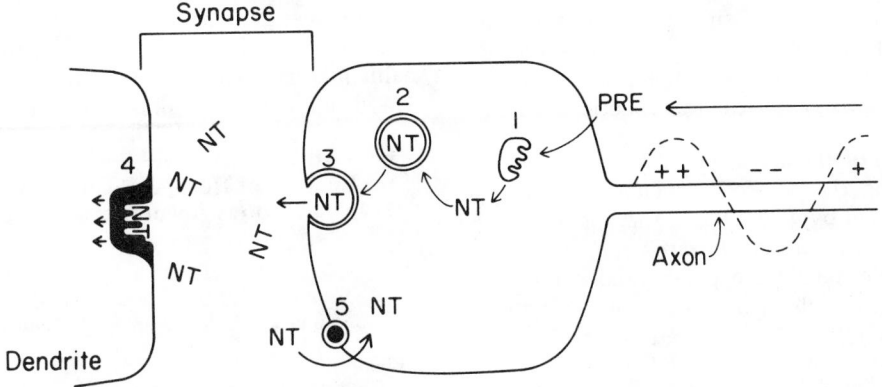

FIGURE 142–1. The major processes that mediate chemical neurotransmission at the synapse. **1.** Precursors (PRE) for the neurotransmitter are accumulated in the nerve terminal where specialized enzymes convert them to neurotransmitter (NT). **2.** The neurotransmitter is then sequestered in vesicles so that it can be released. **3.** When an action potential reaches the terminal, vesicles containing neurotransmitter expel their contents into the synaptic gap. **4.** The neurotransmitter diffuses across the intersynaptic space to activate specific receptors on the dendrite of the adjacent neuron. **5.** The action of the neurotransmitter is terminated by a high-affinity reuptake mechanism on the nerve terminal, which removes the neurotransmitter from the synaptic space for reutilization. Psychotropic medications exert their effects by altering one or more of these processes for certain types of neurotransmitters, thus augmenting or attenuating the influence of these neurons in the brain.

type of neurotransmitter. For example, in terms of the neurons that use dopamine or norepinephrine as their neurotransmitters a variety of drugs that are clinically relevant alter the disposition of these neurotransmitters at specific sites. The action of dopamine in the brain can be reduced

1. By inhibiting an enzyme in its synthetic pathway (α–methyl-dopa, Aldomet)
2. By interfering with the ability of the neuron to store dopamine (reserpine, Serpasil)
3. By blocking the receptors for dopamine on the adjacent neurons so that the chemical message cannot be transmitted (haloperidol, Haldol)

Conversely, other drugs have been shown to produce their effects through enhancing norepinephrine neurotransmission, by

1. Accelerating the release of norepinephrine (D-amphetamine, Dexadrine)
2. Inhibiting the process that inactivates the neurotransmitter (imipramine, Tofranil)
3. Directly stimulating the receptors for the neurotransmitter (clonidine, Catapres)

Because of the complex structure of psychotropic medications, they may interfere with the action of more than one neurotransmitter. Hence, the side effects that occur with treatment with psychotropic medications may reflect their interaction with another neurotransmitter system or their interference with the secondary function of the primary neurotransmitter responsible for the therapeutic action.

Limitations of Pharmacotherapy

As with any drug, the value of a psychotropic medication is determined by weighing its therapeutic effectiveness against the potential hazards of its use. All of the psychotropic agents are potent and carry with their use the threat of serious acute and potentially irreversible side effects. The indications for their use are relatively specific, as discussed below. Accordingly they should not be prescribed indiscriminately for "tranquilizing" patients. While the psychotropic drugs may be the single most effective treatment for major psychiatric disorders, their efficacy is generally limited to certain target symptoms. Consequently, psychotherapeutic intervention remains a keystone in treatment and plays a major role in resolution of psychic conflicts and reintegration of the patient into the social network.

NEUROLEPTICS

The neuroleptics are a class of drugs that have a spe-

cific action in reducing the symptoms of functional psychosis. Currently, nearly 20 different neuroleptics are available in the United States that represent five different structural classes including phenothiazines, thioxanthines, butyrophenones, dibenzoxazepines, and indolones (Table 142–1). In the literature, these drugs are also referred to as major tranquilizers (although their specific action is not due to tranquilization), antipsychotics, and ataractics. The neuroleptics are used primarily to treat psychotic symptoms in acute schizophrenic reactions and as prophylaxis in chronic schizophrenia to prevent the recurrence of psychotic symptoms. They are effective in reducing psychosis in the manic phase of manic-depressive illness and can be used as an adjunct to lithium treatment. In the management of chronic organic brain syndromes such as senile dementia, neuroleptics, when administered in small doses, may be effective in reducing secondary psychotic symptoms such as delusions and hallucinations. Neuroleptics should not be used in acute panic states resulting from ingestion of hallucinogenic drugs; they should also not be used as hypnotics or to relieve anxiety in less severe conditions where other drugs work equally well or better.

Mechanism of Action

Considerable clinical and basic evidence support the hypothesis that the primary mechanism of therapeutic action of neuroleptics is blockade of the receptors for the neurotransmitter dopamine.[78] The neuroleptics reduce the primary or core symptoms of the schizophrenic psychosis including thought disorder, hallucinatory experiences, and delusional thinking. The drugs have negligible effects on symptoms that

---

TABLE 142–1

Equivalent Dosage of Commonly Used Neuroleptics According to Chemical Class

Generic Name	Trade Name	Dose equivalent to 100 mg Chlorpromazine (mg)
Phenothiazines		
Chlorpromazine	Thorazine	100
Thioridazine	Mellaril	100
Trifluoperazine	Stelazine	5
Fluphenazine	Prolixin, Permitil	2
Thioxanthines		
Chlorprothixene	Taractan	65
Thiothixene	Navane	5
Dibenzazepines		
Loxapine	Loxitane	10
Butyrophenones		
Haloperidol	Haldol	2
Indolones		
Molindone	Moban	10

are not intrinsically involved in the funtinal psychosis and are ineffective in treating neurotic symptoms.

The likelihood that all neuroleptics exert their antipsychotic effects by the same mechanism has important therapeutic implications. First, no neuroleptic is specifically effective in ameliorating any particular subset of psychotic symptoms such as withdrawal or paranoid thinking; all are equally effective. Second, there is little justification for using more than one type of neuroleptic to treat a psychosis. A single neuroleptic is as effective as a combination. There is, however, a considerable range of potency among the neuroleptics that varies over a hundred-fold (Table 142–1). This variation in potency does not imply that one drug is inferior to another but rather that the less potent medications must be used in higher doses to achieve equivalent clinical responses. The major difference among the neuroleptics are the side effects associated with the various agents. For example, the less potent thioridazine and chlorpromazine may cause orthostatic hypotension because of their significant alpha-receptor-blocking activity whereas the potent fluphenazine and haloperidol exhibit a higher incidence of acute extrapyramidal side effects.

Use in Treatment

The goal of neuroleptic therapy is to achieve remission of psychotic symptoms through the attainment of adequate levels of neuroleptics. The dosage requirements and rate of remission vary among patients and are determined clinically by titration of symptoms with drug. Typically, therapy is initiated with a dose of 50 to 100 mg of chlorpromazine or its equivalent administered orally four times a day. The doses of neuroleptic are escalated progressively according to the response of the patient. Some patients may ultimately require the equivalent of 800 to 1500 mg of chlorpromazine per day before responding. In cases where behavior is extremely disruptive, more rapid control can be achieved with intramuscular injection of potent neuroleptics such as haloperidol. Clinical reports indicate that administration of 5 mg of haloperidol intramuscularly every 20 to 60 minutes will result in a marked reduction of psychotic behavior after three or four injections. Such aggressive, high-dose therapy, however, must be accompanied by careful monitoring of the patient's vital signs. Behavioral improvement precedes reduction in psychotic thought disturbances. As the psychotic process begins to resolve, sedating effects of the neuroleptic become much more prominent. At this point, the daily dosage of medication can be gradually and progressively reduced with careful monitoring of the patient for recurrence of symptoms.

In addition to their important role in reducing the symptoms of acute schizophrenic reactions, neuroleptics have proven to be quite effective when used prophylactically to prevent the recurrence of psychosis in chronic schizophrenics.[79] In patients in whom the chronicity of the disorder has been well established, discontinuation of neuroleptic treatment results in a three- to fourfold higher rate of relapse. For maintenance therapy, the lowest amount of neuroleptic that alleviates psychotic symptoms should be sought. The average dose is 200 to 300 mg of chlorpromazine or its equivalent per day. There is considerable variation among patients in terms of their drug requirements, however, and even with a particular patient, depending upon life events. Because of the prolonged half-life of neuroleptics, a single dose of medication is sufficient to maintain adequate blood levels throughout a 24-hour period. A single daily dose can reduce the expense of medication, simplifies the treatment schedule, and thus enhances compliance. When given at bedtime it focuses the sedating side effects at an appropriate time. For patients in whom compliance in taking medication is a serious problem, a long-acting, injectable form of neuroleptic, fluphenazine decanoate, can be used.[83] A single injection of this drug, which for the average patient is approximately 25 mg fluphenazine, provides neuroleptic coverage for a period of 2 to 4 weeks, without ancillary oral medication.

Side Effects

The most frequent serious side effects encountered with neuroleptic therapy resemble symptoms seen in disorders of the extrapyramidal system.[80] Pseudoparkinsonism is the most commonly encountered side effect and consists of rigidity, akinisia, mild tremor, masked faces, shuffling gait, and drooling. Dystonic reactions, more frequently seen in younger patients, involve episodic spasm of axial or facial muscles; typical symptoms include torticollis, oculogyric crisis (eyes fixed in an upward gaze), and opisthotonus. A diagnostically confusing side effect is akathisia in which the patient exhibits marked restlessness with pacing and constant shifting of bodily position. Akathisia can be distinguished from psychotic anxiety by the fact that the patient describes the discomfort as purely peripheral, and the symptom is increased with elevation of neuroleptic dosage. All three side effects are caused by the blockade of dopamine receptors in the corpus striatum by the neuroleptic. Thus the symptoms mimic those that occur in disorders in which the nigrostriatal dopaminergic pathway degenerates. The reduced dopamine receptor stimulation in the striatum results in disinhibition of striatal cholinergic neurons leading to overstimulation of their post-synaptic cholinergic muscarinic receptors. Accordingly, these side effects can be alleviated or markedly reduced by administration of antiparkinsonian anticholinergic drugs such as benztropine (Cogentin). Rapid relief of the symptoms can be achieved by intramuscular administration of diphenhydramine (25 to 50 mg). The potent anticholinergic drugs can produce serious side effects in their own right by inhibiting the peripheral parasympathetic nervous system resulting in urinary retention, blurred vision, and dry mouth as well as precipitating central toxic confusional states. Thus, these drugs should be prescribed only to patients exhibiting significant extrapyramidal side effects.

An irreversible or relatively irreversible neurologic side effect known as tardive dyskinesia may occur in patients who have received chronic, high-dose treatment. Tardive dyskinesia, however, has occasionally developed after a relatively brief period of neuroleptic treatment. The syndrome is characterized by adventitious movements, initially occurring in the facial region with vermiform movements of the tongue, repetitive protrusion of the tongue, lip smacking, and facial grimacing. It can progress to involve the extremities with motor restlessness and athetosis. The pathophysiologic basis for the disorder appears to be the development of dopamine-receptor supersensitivity in the striatum. Accordingly, increased doses of neuroleptics temporarily alleviate the symptoms whereas reduction in neuroleptic dose usually exacerbates the symptoms; in addition, anticholinergics or neuroleptics with prominent anticholinergic effects such as thioridazine can increase symptoms. Because of the seriousness of this side effect, neuroleptics should not be prescribed indiscriminately or in higher doses than necessary.

By blockade of the inhibitory influence of hypothalamic dopaminergic neurons, there is an increased release of prolactin from the pituitary; this can result in galactorrhea. The less potent neuroleptics such as thioridazine and chlorpromazine have prominent alpha-receptor-blocking activity which accounts for their greater tendency to cause sedation and orthostatic hypotension. Interference with peripheral autonomic function occasionally results in urinary retention, paralytic ileus, blurred vision, and, in males, inhibition of ejaculation. As with any drugs, allergic reactions, dermatitis, and hepatitis may occur. Fortunately, because of the marked structural heterogeneity among the different classes of neuroleptics, another neuroleptic which does not crossreact with the suspect agent can be substituted. A degenerative retinopathy may occur when thioridazine is administered in doses exceeding 800 mg per day.

ANTIDEPRESSANTS

Two classes of antidepressants are available for treatment: monoamine oxidase (MAO) inhibitors and tricyclic antidepressants (TCA). The MAO inhibitors are generally less effective than TCA and are accompanied by a significantly greater risk of adverse side effects. The use of MAO inhibitors is largely restricted to patients with depression refractory to TCA or certain atypical forms of depression. Since MAO inhibitors are not recommended for use by the general physician the present discussion will focus on TCA.

The tricyclic antidepressants have been shown to be effective in a variety of disorders in which depression is a prominent feature including psychotic depression, depressive neurosis, and involutional depression. Regardless of the diagnostic terminology, TCA are primarily effective in patients who are over the age of 30 with a clear-cut onset of their mood disturbance and who exhibit somatic symptoms thought to be indicative of endogenous depression. These somatic symptoms include insomnia especially with early morning awakening, anorexia, constipation, loss of libido, agitation, or retardation. A possible exception to this rule are patients with endogenous depression as part of manic-depressive disorder who may respond poorly to TCA but better to lithium treatment. If TCA are to be used in these patients it is advisable that lithium be administered concomitantly.

Mechanism of Action

The mechanism of therapeutic action of the tricyclic antidepressants remains unclear. As a class, these drugs are potent inhibitors of the high affinity uptake process on serotonergic and noradrenergic neurons that terminates the synaptic action of their neurotransmitters. Thus, they may potentiate and prolong the effects of synaptically released serotonin and norepinephrine in the CNS. Congruent with this hypothesis, amphetamine and related stimulants, which release central biogenic amines, can produce transient euphoria; however, serious problems with tachyphylaxis, dependency, and abuse liability contraindicate the use of stimulants for treatment of depression. The tricyclic antidepressants are also potent muscarinic-cholinergic receptor blockers with atropine-like effects. The combined anticholinergic and biogenic amine potentiating action of the drugs may contribute to their therapeutic efficacy.

Use in Treatment

Although the optimal daily dose for the tricyclic antidepressants has been established, this dose is at best an approximation (Table 142–2). Relatively low doses of drug should be administered initially (one-quarter

TABLE 142-2
Average Dosage for Tricyclic Antidepressants*

Generic Name	Trade Name	Average Dose (mg/day)
Amitriptyline	Elavil	150
Nortriptyline	Aventyl	100
Imipramine	Tofranil	150
Desipramine	Norpramin, Pertofane	125
Protriptyline	Vivactil	20
Doxepin	Sinequan, Adapin	150

* Studies of the relationship between plasma levels of parent drug and active metabolites and clinical response indicate that optimal dosage may vary by 50 percent or more from the recommended average dose.

of the therapeutic dose), and the dose should be increased at quarterly increments every few days as tolerated. Because of the long half-life of the drugs, the administration of the total dose once per day will maintain adequate plasma levels throughout a 24-hour period. The drug should be given at bedtime which focuses the sedating side effects at an appropriate time and often obviates the necessity of coprescription of sedatives.

The clinical response to TCA treatment is gradual, and the rate of improvement is inversely proportional to the severity of the depression. The somatic symptoms of endogenous depression generally respond more rapidly than the psychological symptoms. The early effects on insomnia and anorexia may be used as predictors of positive clinical outcome. The delay in improvement of cognitive symptoms such as impaired interests and pessimism may color the patient's appreciation of early remission in physiologic symptoms. Accordingly, it is useful to obtain corroborative information from family members or nursing staff on changes in activity, sleep pattern, and eating to document early signs of clinical response.

Recently a number of studies correlating clinical response with plasma levels of nortriptyline (Aventyl) indicate that there is a "therapeutic window" for this and possibly the other TCA.[84] Plasma levels of nortriptyline between 50 and 180 ng/ml are associated with improvement, whereas levels above or below are associated with a lack in clinical response. While the average daily dose recommended in Table 142-2 should result in appropriate plasma levels in the majority of patients, there is considerable variation among patients in their metabolism of the tricyclics which can result in plasma levels outside the therapeutic range. In particular, elderly patients tend

to attain higher steady-state plasma levels on a given dose of TCA. Accordingly, there is increasing emphasis on monitoring plasma tricyclic antidepressant levels in patients who exhibit poor response to treatment.

Side Effects

The potent atropine-like action of the tricyclic antidepressants is primarily responsible for the peripheral and occasional central side effects accompanying their use. By blocking peripheral muscarinic cholinergic receptors, the drugs interfere with parasympathetic tone which results in decreased salivary secretion, impaired visual accommodation, decreased gut motility, and difficulties in the initiation of micturition. In patients suffering from glaucoma, TCA may dangerously elevate intraocular pressure. The vagolytic action of tricyclics results in a consistent increase in heart rate. All the tricyclics, with the possible exception of doxapin, directly interfere with impulse conduction in the heart resulting in prolongation of the QRS interval and ST- and T-wave abnormalities. Although such cardiac effects generally occur with plasma levels well above the therapeutic range, they have been observed in patients with plasma levels within the therapeutic range. Thus, these drugs should be used cautiously in patients with preexisting cardiovascular disease. Although TCA potentiate the action of norepinephrine released from peripheral sympathetics, interaction at central sites often causes symptomatic orthostatic hypotension. Thus, they can enhance the action of certain antihypertensive agents, but interfere with the effectiveness of others, e.g., guanethedine and clonidine.

With regard to central side effects, the potent anticholinergic action of these drugs may produce delirious states, to which elderly patients are particularly susceptible. Behavioral deterioration and confusion herald this serious side effect, and physostigmine, a central acetylcholinesterase inhibitor, can transiently reverse the confusional state.

Tricyclic antidepressants can exacerbate schizophrenic psychosis or precipitate a fulminant psychosis in latent schizophrenics. They may also produce mania or hypomania in some depressed patients, especially those with an antecedent history of manic-depressive disorder. The potentially serious peripheral and central side effects of the tricyclics indicate the serious toxic potential of these drugs. As little as a 7-day prescription of tricyclic antidepressant when ingested acutely can be fatal. Only limited amounts of these drugs should be prescribed at any one time for the suicide-prone patient and appropriate care should be exercised to avoid accidental ingestion by children.

LITHIUM

The treatment of acute manic episodes is generally a psychiatric emergency, and is usually managed by a psychiatrist.[81] Nonetheless, because of the increasing prevalence of the prophylactic use of lithium salts for preventing recurrence of mood disturbances in manic-depressive illness, it is likely that the medical specialist will encounter patients receiving this agent who do not exhibit any psychiatric symptoms. Lithium, an alkaline earth metal, is administered in the form of a salt, usually lithium carbonate. It is effective in treating mania as well as depression in manic-depressive illness; more importantly, maintenance on lithium prevents the recurrence of mood disturbances in the majority of patients. While the mechanism of therapeutic action of lithium remains unknown, the ion selectively accumulates within neurons, altering their electrophysiologic characteristics and their ability to release, take up, and respond to neurotransmitters. As an ion, lithium is not metabolized but is eliminated by excretion via the kidneys. Accordingly, the half-life of lithium is directly related to renal function. Also, dietary sodium and diuretics can alter the rate of lithium excretion. Lithium is optimally effective in a rather narrow therapeutic window, between 0.9 and 1.5 mEq/L of plasma. Symptoms of toxicity generally appear at levels greater than 2.0 mEq/L, and potentially fatal toxicity occurs at twice this level (Table 142–3). For the average adult with normal renal function, therapeutic levels can be achieved with a dose of lithium carbonate of approximately 300 to 600 mg three times a day. Because of the narrow range between clinical effects and toxicity, lithium is administered in individual doses throughout the day to maintain the plasma levels within the therapeutic range. It is important that plasma levels of lithium be monitored at regular intervals and when there is a change in the medical status of the patient.

ANTIANXIETY DRUGS

Antianxiety agents are the most widely prescribed drugs in the United States today. While it is generally agreed that these drugs are effective in relieving anxiety, the physician must consider whether the use of these drugs will be advantageous for the patient. Anxiety is a part of the normal adaptation to stress and may serve a useful purpose in motivating a patient to make constructive changes in his life. Furthermore, many patients with anxiety respond well to a supportive relationship with the physician in which the patient is free not only to reveal the symptoms but also feelings and problems to which the anxiety is related. The premature or excessive use of anxiolytic drugs may divert the attention of such a patient away

---

TABLE 142–3
Side Effects of Lithium*

Plasma Level	Symptoms
≤1.5 mEq/L (therapeutic)	Nausea (limited to initial period of treatment) Fine tremor Mild polyuria
>1.5 <2.5 mEq/L	Vomiting and diarrhea Polyuria (concentration defect) Coarse tremor, ataxia Muscle weakness, fasciculations Sedation
>2.5 <4.0 mEq/L	Muscle hypertonia Choreiform movements Increased deep tendon reflexes Confusion and stupor Transient focal neurologic signs Seizures
>4.0 mEq/L	Coma Death

* The loss of sodium as a result of vomiting, diarrhea, polyuria, or the initiation of a sodium restricted diet with diuretics reduces the clearance of lithium. Thus, under these conditions, much higher plasma levels of lithium will occur on a fixed dose of lithium carbonate.

---

from the sources of distress. The use of anti-anxiety agents is, thus, indicated when anxiety is sufficiently severe that its manifestations interfere with the individual's overall functioning. However, treatment with these drugs should be time limited (less than 4 months); continued requests for anxiolytic agents by the patient merits further exploration of the basis of the anxiety preferably by a psychiatrist.

Drug Choice

A variety of psychotropic drugs have been recommended to treat anxiety, including phenothiazines, tricyclic antidepressants, barbiturates, meprobamate, and benzodiazepines. While tricyclics and neuroleptics may relieve anxiety in those disorders in which they are clinically effective (endogenous depression and schizophrenia, respectively), they are relatively ineffective in relieving situational anxiety. Barbiturates and meprobamate are relatively effective in reducing situational anxiety. These drugs bear serious limitations, however, since there is a high liability for tolerance, habituation, and physical dependence. Their abrupt withdrawal can result in life-threatening symptoms including seizures. Furthermore, they have a poor therapeutic:toxic ratio such that doses two- to threefold greater than the effective dose can result in respiratory depression and death. For treat-

TABLE 142-4

Dosage Range for Sedative and Anxiolytic Benzodiazepines

Generic Name	Trade Name	Dose Range (mg/day)
Chlordiazepoxide	Librium	15–100
Oxaxepam	Serax	30–120
Chlorazepate	Tranzene	15–60
Diazepam	Valium	5–40
Flurazepam*	Dalmane	15–30

* Flurazepam is used primarily as an hypnotic because of its greater sedative properties but shares with the other benzodiazepines the lesser liability for dependency and the better therapeutic:toxic ratio than barbiturates.

ment of situational anxiety, the benzodiazepines are clearly the drugs of choice;[82] they are anxiolytic at doses that do not produce serious sedation and have a relatively long duration of action. More importantly, the liability for tolerance, habituation, and physical dependence is less than with barbiturates and meprobamate. Some patients do become psychologically dependent on these agents. Finally, fatal overdosage with benzodiazepines is a rare occurrence.

Even with the benzodiazepines, sedation accompanies the anxiolytic effects. Thus, patients should be cautioned against driving or performing hazardous tasks while taking the drugs, and coadministration of other sedatives or ingestion of alcohol should be avoided. Clinical evidence suggests that anxiolytic drugs may accentuate mood swings and may reduce impulse control. The range of daily dosages for these commonly used benzodiazepines is shown in Table 142-4. Discontinuation of the drugs should be gradual, especially when high doses have been employed or administration has continued for longer than a month.

REFERENCES

General References

1. Freedman, A., Kaplan, H., and Sadock, B. (eds.). Comprehensive Textbook of Psychiatry, 2nd ed. Baltimore, Williams & Wilkins, 1975.

   A large volume, excellent as a reference book and as a guide to the literature.

2. Nicholi, A.M., Jr. (ed.). The Harvard Guide to Modern Psychiatry. Cambridge, Harvard University Press, 1978.

   An authoritative work, comprehensive in range and depth, an excellent introduction to the field.

The Place of Psychiatry in Medicine

3. Hamman, L. The relationship of psychiatry to internal medicine. Mental Hygiene, 23:177, 1939.
4. Lipowski, Z.J. Review of consultation psychiatry and psychosomatic medicine II. Clinical Aspects. Psychosom. Med., 29:201, 1967.

Human Behavior: Some Basic Considerations

5. Aitken-Swan, J. and Paterson, R. The cancer patient. Delay in seeking advice. Br. Med. J., 1:623, 1955.
6. Bibring, G.L. and Kahana, R.J. Lectures in Medical Psychology. New York, International Universities Press, 1968.
7. Blos, P. On Adolescence. New York, Free Press, 1968.
8. Freud, A. The Ego and the Mechanisms of Defense. New York, International Universities Press, 1946.
9. Levinson, D.J., Darrow, C.N., et al. The Seasons of a Man's Life. New York, Knopf, 1978.
10. Mahler, M.S. On human symbiosis and the vicissitudes of individuation. J. Am. Psychoanal. Assoc., 15:740, 1967.
11. Paterson, R. Why do cancer patients delay? Can. Med. Assoc. J., 73:931, 1955.

Coping with the Stresses of Serious Physical Illness

12. Druss, R.G., O'Connor, J.F., Prudden, J.F., et al. Psychological response to colectomy. Arch. Gen. Psychiatry, 18:53, 1968.
13. Groves, J.E. Management of the borderline patient on a medical or surgical ward. Int. J. Psychiatry Med., 6:337, 1975.
14. ———. Taking care of the hateful patient. N. Engl. J. Med., 298:883, 1978.
15. Hackett, T.P., Cassem, N.H., and Wishnie, H. Detection and treatment of anxiety in the coronary care unit. Am. Heart J., 78:727, 1969.
16. Hamburg, D.A. and Adams, J.E. A perspective on coping behavior. Seeking and utilizing information in major transitions. Arch. Gen. Psychiatry, 17:277, 1967.
17. Imboden, J.B. Psychosocial determinants of recovery. Adv. Psychosom. Med., 8:142, 1972.
18. ———, Canter, A., and Cluff, L.E. Convalescence from influenza. Arch. Intern. Med., 108:393, 1961.
19. Meyer, E., Jacobson, W.E., Edgerton, M.T., and Canter, A. Motivational patterns in patients seeking elective plastic surgery. Psychosom. Med., 22:193, 1960.
20. ——— and Mendelson, M. Psychiatric consultations with patients on medical and surgical wards: patterns and processes. Psychiatry, 24:197, 1961.
21. Ross, R.S. Surgery for coronary artery disease placed in perspective. Bull. N.Y. Acad. Med., 48:1163, 1972.
22. Wise, T.N. The emotional reactions of chronic illness. Primary Care, 1:373, 1974.
23. ———. Pitfalls of diagnosing depression in chronic renal disease. Psychosomatics, 15:83, 1974.
24. Ziegler, F.J. and Imboden, J.B. Contemporary conversion reactions II. A conceptual model. Arch. Gen. Psychiatry, 6:279, 1962.

Psychiatric Evaluation of the Patient

25. Lisansky, E.T. and Shochet, B.R. Comprehensive medical diagnosis for the internist. Med. Clin. North Am., 51:1381, 1967.
26. Schafer, R. Psychological tests in clinical psychiatry. In Redlich, F.C. and Freedman, D.X. (eds.), The Theory and Practice of Psychiatry. New York, Basic Books, 1966.
27. Sullivan, H.S. The Psychiatric Interview. New York, Norton, 1954.
28. Whitehorn, J.C. Guide to interviewing and clinical personality study. Arch. of Neur. and Psych., 52:197, 1944.

Psychiatric Emergencies

29. Anderson, W.H. and Kuehnic, J.C. Strategies for the treatment of acute psychosis. JAMA, 229:1884, 1974.
30. Beck, A.T., Resnik, H., Harvey, L.P., and Jettieri, D.H. The Prediction of Suicide. Bowie, Md., Charles Press Publishers, 1974.
31. Dublin, L.I. Suicide. A Sociological and Statistical Study. New York, Ronald Press, 1963.
32. Guze, S.B. and Robins, E. Suicide and primary affective disorders. Br. J. Psychiatry, 117:437, 1970.
33. Hendin, H. In Freedman, A.M. and Kaplan, H.I. (eds.), Comprehensive Textbook of Psychiatry. Baltimore, Williams & Wilkins, 1967, pp. 1170–1179.
34. Lion, J.R. Evaluation and Management of the Violent Patient. Springfield, Ill., Thomas, 1972.
35. Minkoff, M., Bergman, E., Beck, A.T., and Beck, R. Hopelessness, depression and attempted suicide. Am. J. Psychiatry, 130:455, 1973.
36. Robins, E., Gassner, S., Kayes, J., Wilkinson, R.H., Jr., and Murphy, G.E. The communication of suicidal intent: a study of 134 consecutive cases of successful (completed) suicide. Am. J. Psychiatry, 115:724, 1959.
37. Weissman, M.M. The epidemology of suicide attempts, 1960 to 1971. Arch. Gen. Psychiatry, 30:737, 1974.

Drug Dependence

38. Brecher, E. Licit and Illicit Drugs. Boston, Little, Brown, Co., 1972.
39. Essig, C. Clinical and experimental aspects of barbiturate withdrawal convulsions. Epilepsia, 8:21, 1967.
40. Goldstein, A. Heroin addiction and the role of methadone in its treatment. Arch. Gen. Psychiatry, 26:291, 1972.
41. Isbell, H., Altschul, S., Kornetsky, C., Eisenman, A., Flanary, H., and Fraser, H. Chronic barbiturate intoxication. Arch. Neurology and Psychiatry, 64:1, 1950.
42. Kales, A., Preston, T., Tan, T-L., and Allen, C. Hypnotics and altered sleep–dream patterns. Arch. Gen. Psychiatry, 23:211, 1970.
43. Luisada, P.V. and Brown, B.I. Clinical management of the phencyclidine psychosis. Clin. Toxicol., 9:539, 1976.
44. Marks, R. and Sachar, E. Undertreatment of medical inpatients with narcotic analgesics. Ann. Intern. Med., 78:173, 1973.
45. Meyer, R. Drug abuse rehabilitation. Curr. Psychiatr. Ther., 14:161, 1974.
46. Sapira, J. The narcotic addict as a medical patient. Am. J. Med., 45:555, 1968.

47. Showalter, C. and Thornton, W. Clinical pharmacology of phencyclidine toxicity. Am. J. Psychiatry, 134:1234, 1977.
48. Snyder, S., Opiate receptors in the brain. N. Engl. J. Med., 296:266, 1977.
49. Wikler, A. Conditioning factors in opiate addiction and relapse. In Wilner, D. and Kassebaum, G. (eds.), Narcotics. New York, McGraw-Hill, 1965.

Sexual Problems

50. Masters, W. and Johnson, V. Human Sexual Response. Boston, Little, Brown, 1966.
51. ———. Human Sexual Inadequacy. Boston, Little, Brown, 1970.
52. Meyer, J. (guest ed.). Sex assignment and reassignment: intersex and gender identity disorders. Clin. Plast. Surg., 1(2):199, 1974.
53. Meyer, J. Individual psychotherapy of sexual disabilities. In Freedman, A., Kaplan, H., and Sadock, B. (eds.), Comprehensive Textbook of Psychiatry, 2nd ed. Baltimore, Williams & Wilkins, 1975.
54. ———, Schmidt, C., Jr., Lucas, M., and Smith, E. Short-term treatment of sexual disorders: interim report. Am. J. Psychiatry, 132:172, 1975.
55. Money, J. Sex hormones and other variables in human eroticism. In Young, W. (ed.), Sex and Internal Secretions, Vol. II. Baltimore, Williams & Wilkins, 1961, pp. 1383–1400.
56. Schmidt, C., Jr., Meyer, J., and Lucas, M. Sexual deviations and personality disorders. In Lion, J. (ed.), Personality Disorders: Diagnosis and Management, Baltimore, Williams & Wilkins, 1974, pp. 154–177.

Major Psychiatric Disorders

57. Beck, A.T. Depression. New York, Hoeber Medical Division, Harper & Row, 1967.
58. Bleuler, E. Dementia Praecox or The Group of Schizophrenias. New York, International Universities Press, 1950.
59. Kraepelin, E. Dementia Praecox and Paraphrenia. (Trans. from 8th German ed.) Edinburgh, Livingstone, 1919.
60. Lidz, T., Fleck, S., and Cornelison, A.R. Schizophrenia and the Family. New York, International Universities Press, 1965.
61. Mendelson, M. Psychoanalytic Concepts of Depression. Springfield, Ill., Thomas, 1960.
62. Nemiah, J.C. Foundations of Psychopathology. New York, Oxford University, 1961.
63. Romano, J. and Engel, G. Physiologic and psychiatric considerations of delirium. Med. Clin. North Am., 28:629, 1944.
64. Snyder, S.H. Amphetamine psychosis: a "model" schizophrenia mediated by catecholamines. Am. J. Psychiatry, 130:61, 1973.
65. Woodruff, R.A., Jr., Goodwin, D.W., and Guze, S.B. Psychiatric Diagnosis. New York, Oxford University, 1974.
66. Ziegler, F.J., Imboden, J.B., and Meyer, E. Contemporary conversion reactions: clinical study. Am. J. Psychiatry, 116:901, 1960.

Psychosomatic Medicine

67. Alexander, F. Psychosomatic Medicine. New York, Norton, 1950.
68. Bleecker, E.R. and Engel, B.T. Learned control of ventricular rate in patients with atrial fibrillation. Psychosom. Med., 35:161, 1973.
69. Engel, G.L. Studies of ulcerative colitis III. The nature of the psychologic processes. Am. J. Med., 19:231, 1955.
70. Jenkins, D.C., Roseman, R.H., and Zyzanski, S.J. Prediction of clinical coronary heart disease by a test for the coronary-prone behavior pattern. N. Engl. J. Med., 290:1271, 1974.
71. Miller, N.E. Learning of visceral and glandular responses. Science, 163:434, 1969.
72. Roseman, R.H., Friedman, M., Straus, R., Wurm, M., Jenkins, C.D., and Messinger, H.B. Coronary heart disease in the western collaborative study group. JAMA, 195:130, 1966.
73. Russek, H.I. Role of emotional stress in the etiology of clinical coronary heart disease. Chest, 52:1, 1967.
74. Schmale, A.H. Giving up as a final common pathway to changes in health. In Lipowski, Z.J. (ed.), Psychosocial Aspects of Physical Illness. Adv. Psychosom. Med., 8:20, 1972.
75. Weiner, H., Thaler, M., Reiser, M.F., and Mirsky, I.A. Etiology of duodenal ulcer. Psychosom. Med., 19:1, 1957.

Management of Psychiatric Disorders

76. Castelnuovo-Tedesco, P. The Twenty-Minute Hour. Boston, Little, Brown, 1965.
77. Cooper, J.R., Bloom, F.E., and Roth, R.H. The Biochemical Basis of Neuropharmacology, 3rd ed. New York, Oxford University, 1978.
78. Creese, I., Burt, D.R., and Snyder, S.H. Dopamine receptor binding predicts clinical and pharmacologic potencies of antischizophrenic drugs. Science, 192:481, 1976.
79. Davis, J.M. Overview: maintenance therapy in psychiatry: I. Schizophrenia. Am. J. Psychiatry 133:1237, 1975.
80. Donlon, P.T. and Stetson, R.L. Neuroleptic induced extrapyramidal symptoms. Dis. Nerv. Syst., 37:629, 1976.
81. Gershon, J. and Shopsin, B. Lithium: Its Role in Psychiatric Research and Treatment. New York, Plenum Press, 1973.
82. Greenblatt, D.J. and Shrader, R.I. Benzodiazepines in Clinical Practice. New York, Rowen Press, 1974.
83. Groves, J.E. and Mandell, M.R. The long-acting phenothiazines. Arch. Gen. Psychiatry, 32:893, 1975.
84. Kragh-Sorensen, P., Hansen, C.E., Baastrup, P.C., and Hvidberg, E.F. Self-inhibiting action of nortriptyline's antidepressive effect at high plasma levels. Psychopharmacol. Bull, 45:305, 1976.
85. Whitehorn, J.C. Understanding psychotherapy. Am. J. Psychiatry, 112:328, 1955.

SECTION SEVENTEEN
Diseases of Medical Management

THOMAS P. DUFFY: SECTION EDITOR

Diseases of medical management are those that result from diagnostic or therapeutic procedures. Even a low incidence of such diseases is disturbing, as their occurrence conflicts with a basic principle of medical practice, *primum non nocere*, or "at least do no harm."[26] About 5 percent of hospital admissions are precipitated by such problems, and nearly 20 percent of hospitalized patients may expect to suffer from a disease of medical management.[11] A major part of this problem is adverse drug reactions, experienced by 10 to 18 percent of hospitalized patients and resulting in fatality rates up to 13 percent; drug-related deaths amount to about 1 per 1000 medical inpatients.[39]

Despite the alarming frequency of diseases of medical management, such illnesses may be no more numerous than previously. Patients today receive more potent drugs and diagnostic chemicals as well as undergo more complicated and rigorous diagnostic procedures than ever before. However, little more than a century ago the medical profession considered bloodletting appropriate therapy for sustained fever and relied on calomel in the treatment of cholera. Thus, physician-induced diseases are not unique to the modern era.

Since diseases of medical management are usually not predictable in the individual patient, they cannot be entirely eliminated. Every effort should be made, however, to minimize their incidence and severity. To achieve this goal the physician must 1) understand the potential complications of all diagnostic and therapeutic measures he uses and be prepared to treat them promptly; and 2) fully recognize that certain groups of individuals are unusually susceptible to the complications of specific medications or procedures and avoid using them on these patients. It is the purpose of this chapter to discuss representative examples of the more important types of diseases of medical management, including those resulting from diagnostic procedures, drug therapy, biologic products, mechanical therapeutic procedures, surgical treatment, and ionizing irradiation.

CHAPTER 143
Specific Complications of Medical Management

THOMAS P. DUFFY

HAZARDS OF DIAGNOSTIC PROCEDURES

Probably few diseases of medical management are more distressing to physician and patient alike than those that result from diagnostic procedures (Table 143-1). The physician must always ask: Is the information to be derived likely to benefit the patient? Do the potential benefits outweigh the risks (risk–benefit ratio)? Does the need to have such information clearly outweigh a mere desire to obtain it? Liver biopsy is certainly invaluable to diagnosis in many disorders, but not every alcoholic patient with hepatomegaly is a candidate for this invasive procedure.

Endoscopy has vastly improved the diagnosis of the Mallory-Weiss syndrome and esophageal variceal bleeding, but not every upper gastrointestinal bleed requires an invasive look.[27]

When diagnostic procedures involving significant hazard are considered, the physician should distinguish between the risk of the procedure in a moderately healthy individual, who might become worse if he develops a serious reaction, and the risk of the same procedure in an individual whose condition is deteriorating but who might improve if the results lead to more effective management of his illness. For example, pulmonary arteriography need not be used to establish the diagnosis of pulmonary embolism in a patient with stable vital signs, whose only complaints

┌───

TABLE 143-1

Complications of Diagnostic Procedures

Procedure	Complications	Precautions
I. Radiologic[4]		
Upper gastrointestinal series	Dehydration, hypovolemia, barium impaction	Maintain adequate hydration. Follow study with laxatives
Barium enema	Perforation, venous intravasation with pulmonary embolism, retroperitoneal emphysema, cardiac arrhythmias, bacteremia, water intoxication	Avoid routine use of balloon catheter; antibiotic prophylaxis with valvular disease; avoid tap water enemas with denuded surfaces
Oral cholecystography	50% incidence of nausea/vomiting/diarrhea or headache. Renal failure; alteration of thyroid function tests	Oral cholecystography is ineffective in the presence of jaundice (bilirubin >4). Liberal fluid intake
Intravenous cholangiography	Hypotension/bronchospasm, nephrotoxicity	Slow injection of dye
Bronchography	Anesthetic responsible for most fatalities; bronchospasm	Restrict the dose of local anesthetic
IVP[48]	Idiosyncratic reaction to dye; nausea and vomiting, urticaria; laryngeal edema, rigors; cardiac arrhythmias; nephrotoxicity, parotid swelling	Inquiry as to previous reactions; do not perform if renal function inadequate for visualization Avoid in multiple myeloma
Aortography	Thrombosis, embolization; bleeding, hematoma; artery dissection, spinal cord damage	Check pulse postprocedure Avoid unnecessary midstream aortograms
Cardiopulmonary angiography	Perforation, arrhythmias, neurologic complications, embolism	Morbidity related to skill of angiographer
Cerebral angiography	Death in 1:250 cerebral angiograms; intramural injection, atheromatous embolization, dye reactions	Well-trained neuroradiologist
Pneumoencephalogram	Seizures in epileptic patients; vomiting and severe headache; cardiac arrhythmias; foraminal crowding and coning	Diazepam control; be prepared to reduce intracranial pressure
Myelography	LP complications; spinal anesthetic reactions with hypotension; contrast media reactions— arachnoiditis	Neurosurgical intervention may be necessary if epidural block present
Lymphography	Allergic reactions, infection, pain; pulmonary microemboli, neurologic complications	Contraindicated in patients with R→L cardiac shunts, with borderline pulmonary function
Endoscopic retrograde cholangiopancreatography	Acute pancreatitis, rupture of bile duct with bile peritonitis, septicemia	Inject smallest amount of contrast material possible
II. Biopsy		
Lymph node	Paralysis of trapezius muscle, nondiagnostic pathology	Avoid posterior cervical nodes, do not biopsy inguinal nodes
Scalene node	Pneumothorax, air embolism	Perform in general operating room. Touch prep all biopsies
Liver	Hemorrhage, bile peritonitis, hepatic laceration	Avoid in presence of ascites. Perform only if clotting defenses are intact (PT, PTT, normal bleeding time)
Lung	Pneumothorax, air embolism	Perform only by physician experienced in technique. Monitor patient closely for 24 hours following the procedure

─── **TABLE 143-1 (cont.)** ───

Procedure	Complications	Precautions
II. Biopsy (cont.)		
Kidney	Hemorrhage (retroperitoneal or intracapsular); deterioration of renal function	
Intestinal (Crosby capsule)	Hemorrhage, perforation	
Sternal marrow aspiration	Mediastinitis, hemopericardium	Perform only if other sites (iliac) have been unproductive or irradiated
III. Endoscopy		
Bronchoscopy	Tracheal tear, vocal cord damage, arrhythmias, vagal syncope, hypoxemia	Be prepared to treat arrhythmias and/or cardiac arrest. Gentle passage of the instrument may lessen risk of perforation
Esophagoscopy	Esophageal tear, mediastinitis	
Gastroscopy	Arrhythmias, syncope	
Sigmoidoscopy	Bowel perforation, hemorrhage	
Colonoscopy		
Mediastinoscopy	Pneumothorax, tear of major blood vessel	Perform in GOR with equipment to perform thoracotomy if need arises
Peritonoscopy	Bowel perforation	
Cystoscopy	Infection, hemolysis with H_2O irrigation	Irrigate with isotonic solutions
IV. Special Tests		
Bromsulphalein (BSP) test	Anaphylactic reactions	Administer slowly
Cardiac catheterization	Vagal shock, arrhythmias, thrombosis, embolism	Observe limbs for ischemia
Lumbar puncture	Headache, brain herniation, hemorrhage	Avoid when cerebral mass lesion may be present
Schilling test	Inaccurate results	Faulty urine collections or renal insufficiency
Thoracentesis	Hypotension, pneumothorax, hemothorax, pulmonary edema	Premedicate with atropine; remove fluid slowly (not over 500 ml in 10 minutes), monitor vital signs closely, and terminate procedure if blood pressure falls. Remove no more than 1000 ml during a single thoracentesis

are dyspnea and pleuritic chest pain; a noninvasive ventilation–perfusion lung scan would be the appropriate means of evaluation.[46] In contrast, an arteriographic procedure might be exceedingly important in confirming this diagnosis in a patient presenting with the clinical picture of pulmonary embolism and symptoms of peptic ulcer disease; definitive diagnosis of embolism is essential if the risk–benefits of anticoagulation versus surgery are to be properly weighed.

In some situations, however, aggressive diagnostic studies are indicated even in a minimally ill patient because they may permit more accurate determination of the extent of disease and the initiation of curative therapy rather than merely palliation. For example, staging laparotomies in patients with Hodgkin's disease are associated with the morbidity of abdominal surgery as well as the long-term risk of asplenia; in selected patients, the morbidity is overshadowed, however, by the documented success of therapy based on staging.

Continued updating of the physician's knowledge constitutes "due care" in medical practice. Newer diagnostic procedures may substitute harmless, non-invasive techniques for studies with recognized dangers. Computerized axial tomography (CAT scanning) has revolutionized the approach to space-occupying lesions of the brain; it provides innocuously much of the information that arteriography and pneumoencephalograms previously afforded.[2] Ultrasound study of the retroperitoneal area is a reliable gauge of disease in this formerly silent area of the abdomen;[15] perinephric abscesses and hypernephroma no longer constitute a major dilemma for the internist.[38] Radionuclide cardiac imaging is not only facilitating diagnosis but is providing a tool to gauge efficacy of therapy in myocardial disorders.[35] Nevertheless all procedures should be examined critically with regard to the information obtained and the cost of such innovations in patient care. The physician can easily be misled by a loop of bowel masquerading on ultrasound as an abcess. Diagnostic agents may have unanticipated remote complications which retrospectively would forbid the use of such agents. Thorotrast, a radioactive contrast agent, is now unacceptable because of its proven role in causing hemangiosarcomas of the liver.

Improved knowledge of the pathophysiologic mechanisms of disease allows measurement of primary abnormalities rather than secondary manifestations. Measurement of urinary metanephrines in patients with possible pheochromocytomas has now completely superseded the potentially harmful provocative tests with histamine and tyramine.

Barium Enema

This is an example of a routine diagnostic study in which morbidity is much higher than generally realized. Even when barium enema is performed by an experienced radiologist, perforation may occur. In a mail survey of 100 hospitals, 50 cases of intraperitoneal perforation of the colon during barium enema were collected.[51] Only knowledge of the risks involved and of the types of patients in whom this study is particularly hazardous can minimize the complications.

Preparation for barium enema involves two potentially dangerous steps: stopping all oral intake and administering a cathartic on the night before the x-ray study. The situation is further compounded when the patient is blindly subjected to multiple gastrointestinal studies in a rapid sequence, or an antecedent upper gastrointestinal series has made visualization of the lower gastrointestinal tract impossible without several days of vigorous catharsis. Such rote investigation requires cessation of adequate food intake over a period of several days in addition to the cathar-

sis. Patients who frequently have difficulty with restriction of intake are diabetics and those with chronic renal disease. The diabetic patient may receive his usual morning dose of long-acting insulin, be placed on a "nothing-by-mouth" regimen after supper, fail to receive his usual late evening snack, and become severely hypoglycemic in the early morning hours. The patient with chronic renal disease and obligatory polyuria may become severely dehydrated during the period of no oral intake (which may extend to 20 hours if the procedures are delayed) with further deterioration of renal function. The administration of a cathartic may also cause serious damage. In the azotemic patient, for example, cathartic-induced fluid loss may seriously impair renal blood flow, especially when combined with restriction of oral fluids. In the patient with a large and friable colonic neoplasm, vigorous cathartic-induced peristalsis may precipitate serious hemorrhage. In the elderly or debilitated patient, the fluid and electrolyte loss by catharsis is often sufficient to cause postural syncope or even hypovolemic shock.

The barium enema is also hazardous for patients with significant cardiopulmonary disease. Arrhythmias, hypotension, or cardiac arrest may be precipitated by the colonic distension during barium administration in the patient with an irritable myocardium, whether due to arteriosclerotic disease, hypoxia, or drugs. Bacteremia induced by this procedure has led to recommendation of antibiotic prophylaxis in patients with rheumatic valvular disease or prosthetic valves undergoing barium enemas.[19] In patients with chronic pulmonary insufficiency, the abdominal distension caused by the barium, along with the taxing position required by the procedure, may cause hypoxia and increased hypercapnia. Whenever barium enema is required in situations such as these, the physician should be present and equipped to deal with complications.

Patients who are at greater risk of undesirable consequences from diagnostic procedures often derive little benefit from the information gained. For example, the patient whose pulmonary disease is so severe that barium enema precipitates significant hypoxia might not be a candidate for major colonic surgery even if the barium study were to reveal a sigmoid neoplasm.

Liver Biopsy

The liver biopsy is another diagnostic procedure that may be followed by serious complications, especially hemorrhage or bile peritonitis. Nevertheless, this procedure is generally regarded as relatively safe, and is frequently performed in patients with minimal indications, by inexperienced physicians, or without adequate evaluation of the patient's hemostatic function. The prothrombin activity and partial thromboplastin time should be measured as gauges of hemostatic function since many patients who require liver biopsy have hepatic functional impairment. However, the possibility of other abnormalities of the clotting mechanism should not be overlooked.

Near-fatal hemorrhage has been precipitated by performing percutaneous hepatic biopsy in patients with severe azotemia or myeloproliferative disorders; both conditions are associated with a qualitative defect in platelet functioning that can only be discovered by performance of a bleeding time. Although a low incidence of complications lowers the threshold for performing a diagnostic procedure, it does not justify its performance when there is little likelihood of obtaining useful diagnostic or therapeutic information.

Sternal Marrow Examination

This procedure may also be attended by serious complications. Because of the rarefaction of bone frequently associated with diseases in which marrow aspiration is indicated, penetration of the sternum, with resultant fatal mediastinitis or intrapericardial hemorrhage, may occur. Two guiding principles will reduce the incidence of such occurrences: First, sternal marrow aspiration should be attempted only after less hazardous aspiration sites, e.g., iliac crest or vertebral spine, have proved unsatisfactory; Second, sternal marrow aspiration should be performed only by or in the presence of a physician skilled in this technique.

Cardiac Catheterization

The overall risk of a major complication from cardiac catheterization is less than 1 percent, the risk of death is 0.5 percent. This risk varies with the state of compensation of the patient, the duration of the procedure, the level of experience of the laboratory, and the skill of the operator doing the particular study. The morbidity from catheterization in a laboratory doing one study a week may be greater than in one which does five or more each week. Even when a highly skilled and experienced laboratory is available, the physician should ask himself whether noninvasive methods, such as echocardiography or radionuclide imaging can provide the same information.

The complications of cardiac catheterization can be divided into those occurring during the procedure and those appearing later. Arrhythmias constitute the most important complication in the first group, and, although their appearance may necessitate stopping

the procedure, they have not been a frequent cause of death in recent years.

Hypotension sometimes develops during the manipulation of the catheter within the heart and great vessels. If associated with bradycardia, it is likely due to excessive vagal activity and should be treated with atropine, but hemorrhage and pericardial tamponade should be ruled out. Manipulation of catheters and needles within the central circulation occasionally results in perforation of the heart or great vessels, and bleeding may occur in the retroperitoneal tissues or pericardium. Reactions to the contrast medium used for angiography are rare but may be fatal.

Bleeding may start later and may not be evident until the patient returns to the ward. A drop in pressure, tachycardia, restlessness, and pallor may indicate that a retroperitoneal hematoma is developing. Arterial thrombosis is another late complication which should be recognized as soon as possible by vigilant observation of the pulses in the limb in which the arteriotomy has been made. Venous thrombosis may appear hours to days following a procedure and, in some instances, may be suspected only after pulmonary embolism has occurred. Venous thrombosis and pulmonary embolism are much more likely to develop in patients with cardiac decomposition.

Thoracentesis

Hemothorax, pneumothorax, splenic or hepatic lacerations, cardiac arrhythmias, and pulmonary edema may complicate thoracentesis. Inattention to the anatomic landmarks and ignorance of the location of the intercostal vessels on the inferior surface of the ribs have compromised precious breathing space with accumulation of blood. Vagal-induced bradycardia occurs in the absence of atropine premedication. Removal of greater than 1000 ml of pleural fluid has been followed by "reexpansion" unilateral pulmonary edema.

DRUG-INDUCED DISEASES

Introduction of many useful, often life-saving chemicals into modern therapeutics has been accompanied by a significant incidence of drug-induced diseases.[13] A cautious attitude and thoughtful consideration of specific indications and risks for each drug for each patient is mandatory. The clinician, therefore, must remain alert both to signs of progressive disease and to evidence of drug toxicity. Drug toxicities vary widely and may be clinically subtle or flagrant, minor or lethal, prompt in onset or delayed. Undoubtedly, certain important toxicities remain unrecognized. Some drug toxicities closely mimic progression of the disease under treatment (e.g., fever caused by penicillin during treatment of pneumonia).

No attempt will be made here to list even a small portion of the toxic effects of commonly used drugs. Well-documented compilations of drug-associated diseases are available.[18]

The mechanisms classically involved in such circumstances include overdosage, side effects, idiosyncrasy, and hypersensitivity (allergy). Certain commonly used drugs, e.g., penicillin, may produce iatrogenic illness by each of these four mechanisms. Other important drug-related diseases result from medication error (human error) and drug-induced alterations of the host defense mechanism.

In addition to these basic drug-induced diseases, two other more complex manifestations of drug toxicity are important. They are encountered when either the toxicity of a drug is potentiated by its administration in combination with one or more additional pharmacologic agents (drug interaction) or the toxicity of the drug is potentiated by underlying disease in the host. Formerly, the term *intolerance* was used to describe a lowered threshold to the normal pharmacologic action of a drug. Intolerance was considered merely to reflect one end of the normal distribution curve for drug dosage requirements. It is now clear that intolerance to certain drugs may represent significant variations in drug absorption, metabolism, and excretion as well as tissue susceptibility. While these variations in tolerance are at times genetically determined, acquired diseases, drug interactions, or bioavailability of drugs are clearly responsible in specific situations.[29]

Characteristic examples of each of the commonly encountered drug-induced diseases will be presented. Remember that the most important factor in reducing the incidence of such illnesses is strict adherence to the principles that no pharmacologic agent should be administered without a specific indication, that there are no harmless medications, and that some drugs, although safe and innocuous in solo, can be dangerous in concert with other drugs.

In a study on a large medical service of acutely ill patients, it was found that the average patient received 14 different drugs during his hospital course, and 14 percent of all patients developed reactions to at least one drug during the period of hospitalization.[34] It is unlikely that clear-cut indications for all components of such polypharmacy were present. Clearly the incidence of adverse drug reactions would have been less if fewer drugs had been administered to each patient.

Medication Errors

These may result from administration of the wrong medicine; from incorrect dilution, dosage, or specific formulation of a drug; and from adding incompatible compounds to intravenous solutions. Administration of the wrong medication has frequently occurred as the result of confusing similar-sounding names (e.g., administration of Kynex for Kantrex, vincristine for vinblastine, Myleran for Melphalan), of using abbreviations, or of preparing different medications in similar vials. An actual example of the last error was the use of 10 percent potassium chloride, bottled in the same type of vial as distilled water, as diluent for an intravenous medication. Errors of this sort can be minimized by preparing a distinctive label for each commonly used intravenous medication. Errors involving the wrong dilution, generally errors of decimal place, tend to occur with less commonly used medications or diagnostic agents. Such problems have proved serious, for example, when a 10- to 1000-fold dilutional error has been made in preparing the dose of intravenous lidocaine. Confusion of milligrams and milliequivalents in orders for additives to intravenous or peritoneal dialysis fluids, or confusion of "U" for a zero because of poor penmanship in an order for "insulin 15U" can obviously lead to serious difficulties.

The addition of incompatible compounds to intravenous solutions has become a problem of greater magnitude as use of intravenously administered therapeutic agents steadily increases. A still common error of this type is adding sodium bicarbonate and calcium gluconate to the same solution (with resultant precipitation of calcium carbonate) when treating patients with uremic acidosis. Carbenicillin and gentamicin are less potent when administered in the same intravenous mixture. To avoid such errors, the physician must know the compatibilities of compounds added to an intravenous solution; pharmacies are now equipped with listings of such incompatibilities.[28] If any doubt exists, the drugs should be administered by different routes.

Overdosage

A characteristic example of an insidious drug overdosage is salicylate intoxication. A patient may unwittingly take many aspirin-containing proprietary preparations over a relatively long period of time. The resultant lethargy and somnolence may pose a puzzling diagnostic problem unless the proprietary medications are suspected. The incidence of drug toxicity can be reduced by the physician's ascertaining that the patient is taking no other medications containing the same or analogous drugs, carefully explaining the dosage regimen of each prescribed drug, and clearly outlining to the patient the possible toxic effects of prescribed drugs. Acquainting patients with the necessity of bringing all current pills (not just medicines) to the hospital will frequently provide the answer to a difficult clinical problem.

Side Effects[18]

Only a few of the most commonly observed drug reactions will be discussed. Colchicine's side effects are prominent even with therapeutic doses. Although severe nausea, vomiting, and diarrhea often occur when amounts adequate to abort an acute gouty attack are ingested, these side effects are usually tolerated by the patient because of the effectiveness of the agent in relieving the gouty symptoms. Side effects may be abolished simply by decreasing the drug dose, or administering the drug via a different route. The discomfort and hazard of prominent side effects in the therapeutic dose range must be balanced against the desired therapeutic action of the drug. Side effects of drugs are especially important considerations when compliance is a problem. Impotence and ejaculatory dysfunction are unfortunate manifestations of many antihypertensive agents that alter sympathetic nervous function.[24] This by-product of the drug regimen may make an agent unacceptable to the patient. A disturbing side effect of drugs is the late appearance of other illnesses in patients treated with aggressive chemotherapeutic regimens of the cytotoxic variety. Prolonged survival in formerly fatal diseases has been purchased at the potential cost of significant immediate and delayed damage to the patient.[46] Second malignancies[10] and central nervous system damage are being increasingly recognized in patients cured of their initial neoplasm or other diseases. Controlled studies to determine the role of chemotherapeutic agents in nonmalignant disorders, and to establish the minimal curative dosage of drugs, are essential; use of in vitro techniques to predict differential sensitivity of human tumor cells to anticancer drugs may reduce the dose and number of drugs in such combination regimens.[44]

Allergic Reactions

Penicillin accounts for a relatively large proportion of drug allergic reactions encountered today. Its widespread use, as well as the incidence in the population of allergy to this antibiotic, are responsible. The allergic reactions may include local or generalized rash, urticaria, fever, arthralgia, erythema multiforme, hemolytic anemia, exfoliative dermatitis, and systemic anaphylaxis. Milder rashes and urticarial reactions generally respond satisfactorily to simple withdrawal

of the penicillin, whereas more severe reactions require epinephrine or relatively high dose glucocorticoid therapy. Once a patient has experienced an allergic reaction to penicillin, it is important that he be informed that he should never again (with exceptions described below) receive penicillin in any form. After a patient has had one mild penicillin reaction, it is entirely possible that, on subsequent exposure to penicillin, he may experience a potentially fatal anaphylactic reaction.

Penicillin components (polylysine and minor group determinants) will reliably predict those individuals who may develop a major immediate allergic reaction to penicillin administration.[36] A positive skin test with penicilloyl-polylysine component (Pre-Pen) is predictive of an allergic reaction, but a negative reaction does not exclude the possibility of anaphylaxis. Minor group determinants are correlated with anaphylaxis and very dilute solutions of aqueous penicillin are used for skin testing. In the absence of such testing, alternative drugs are available to combat almost every bacterial infection; however, penicillin derivatives must also be carefully avoided. Under certain exceedingly rare circumstances, e.g., infective endocarditis caused by enterococcus, it may be advisable to desensitize the patient; in such cases, high-dose glucocorticoid therapy (the equivalent of 40 to 60 mg prednisone daily) should be administered along with the antibiotic and maintained for several days after cessation of penicillin treatment. With such treatment, it is imperative that the physician be immediately available for several hours after the initial penicillin injection, so that he may deal with an anaphylactic reaction should it occur.

The most serious allergic reaction is anaphylaxis, most commonly observed after parenteral (especially intravenous) drug administration. The anaphylactic reaction may cause coma and death by one or more of the following mechanisms: 1) bronchospasm (severe dyspnea); 2) vasodilatation (profound shock); or 3) injury to capillary endothelium. The third mechanism may contribute to both airway obstruction (laryngeal edema) and shock (massive transudation of vascular fluid). Most of these manifestations usually respond dramatically to the intravenous injection of 1 ml of 1:1000 solution of aqueous epinephrine. This should be followed by intramuscular injection of 1 ml of 1:1000 epinephrine-in-oil. Maintenance of the airway, respiratory assistance, support of the circulation as needed, and close observation of the patient for at least 24 hours may be life saving. The immediate mortality from an untreated anaphylactic reaction is so great, and the response to appropriate therapy is generally so dramatic, that a physician should always have injectable aqueous epinephrine readily available when an antibiotic injection is given.

Idiosyncrasy and allergy to drugs are both commonly expressed as hematologic reactions.[14] For example, aplastic anemia is an infrequent, but serious and often fatal reaction which may follow the administration of chloramphenicol. Chloramphenicol also has a direct toxic marrow effect which is dose-related and which subsides when the drug is withdrawn. The idiosyncratic aplastic reaction is not related to the dose-dependent reversible inhibition of erythropoiesis.

In some instances, the specific characteristics of the immunologic reaction to the drug have been worked out in detail, e.g., the thrombocytopenic purpura which may follow administration of Sedormid or quinidine where the antibody is directed against the indicted drug. Metabolites of the parent drug have also been proven to be responsible for immunologically mediated thrombocytopenia.

Another serious hematologic complication of drug therapy is agranulocytosis,[43] which may follow treatment with such drugs as sulfonamides, aminopyrine, thiouracil, gold, immunosuppressive agents, and phenylbutazone. In most instances, the complication is probably immunologic. At present no way of predicting which patient will manifest an idiosyncratic reaction to a given drug exists. Treatment consists of withdrawal of the drug, enhancement of its elimination, and supportive therapy until the manifestations subside.

Any organ system may be involved in drug reactions; the respiratory system may be damaged in almost every aspect of its structure (Table 143–2).[42] Diffuse pulmonary fibrosis may mimic viral or fungal infections, glucocorticoids may enlarge mediastinal fat pads, the aminoglycoside drugs may cause respiratory muscle paralysis, and acetylsalicylic acid may cause bronchospasm in some individuals. The liver is especially sensitive to toxic drug reactions because of its central role in drug metabolism and its location at the port of entry for ingested substances (Table 143–3).[33] Such damage subsequently affects the metabolism of many other drugs. Similarly, the kidneys may be damaged by a particular drug, and elimination of that and other drugs may as a consequence be impaired. The drug-induced reduction of renal function necessitates close attention to drug doses to avert toxic accumulations.[7,8]

Alteration of Host Defense Mechanisms by Drug Therapy

This mechanism accounts for a number of serious diseases of medical progress (Table 143–4). Drugs most frequently responsible for such illnesses are glucocor-

---

TABLE 143–2

Roentgenologic, Histologic, and Clinical Patterns Associated with Drug-Induced Pulmonary Diseases*

Diffuse pulmonary disease
  Busulfan, cyclophosphamide
  Methotrexate
  Bleomycin
  Nitrofurantoin (acute and chronic)
  Methysergide
  Drug-induced systemic lupus erythematosus (SLE)
  Ganglionic blockers (hexamethonium, mecamylamine, pentolinium)
  Radiation
  Pituitary snuff
  Oxygen
  Corticosteroids
  Drug-induced pulmonary infiltration with eosinophila and polyarteritis
  Mineral oil (aspiration)
  Narcotics
  Blood (leukoagglutinins)

Mediastinal and hilar changes
  Phenytoin, methotrexate (adenopathy)
  Corticosteroids (lipomatosis)

Pleural effusion
  Nitrofurantoin (acute)
  Methysergide (chronic)
  Drug-induced SLE (acute and chronic)

Pulmonary calcification
  Vitamin D
  Inorganic phosphates

Bronchoconstriction
  Propranolol
  Aerosolized drugs
    Isoproterenol
    Polymyxin B
    Disodium cromoglycate
    Acetylcysteine
  Pituitary snuff
  Aspirin

Respiratory muscle paralysis
  Aminoglycoside antibiotics
  Quinidine

Fever (in presence of drug-induced pulmonary disease)
  Nitrofurantoin (acute)
  Busulfan, cyclophosphamide
  Methotrexate

* From Rosenow, E.C., III: Drug-induced pulmonary disease. Ann. Int. Med. 77:980, 1972.[42]

---

ticoids, broad-spectrum and combination antibiotics,[40] and antimetabolites.[47] A typical example of these illnesses is the serious gram-negative and fungal infections seen in the immunocompromised, leukoneutropenic patient receiving chemotherapy.

These diseases can be minimized by using as infrequently as possible those drugs which alter host

TABLE 143-3
Drug-Induced Liver Disease

I. **Toxic Reactions—Dose Related**

    Hepatitis
      Alcohol
      Barbiturates
      Phenylbutazone
      Ethchlorvynol
      Phenytoin
      Chloroform
      Acetaminophen
    Fibrosis and cirrhosis
      Methotrexate

II. **Sensitizing Reactions—Idiosyncratic**

    Cholestatic
      Chlorpromazine
      Chlorpropamide
      Contraceptives
      Erythromycin
      Anabolic steroids

    Hepatitic
      Anesthetics (halothane, methoxyflurane)
      Antituberculous drugs (isoniazid, rifampin)
      Antihypertensives (hydralazine, Aldomet)
      Anticonvulsants (phenytoin)
      Analgesics (ASA)

TABLE 143-4
Drugs Resulting in Impairment of Host Defense Mechanisms

Therapeutic Agent	Result of Altered Host Defenses
Corticosteroids	Mycobacterial, fungal, and *Pneumocystis carinii* infections
Oral neomycin	Staphylococcal enterocolitis
Tetracyclines and clindamycin	Pseudomembranous enterocolitis[6]
Antimetabolites	Bacterial and fungal infections
Antibiotic combinations	Bacterial overgrowth

defense mechanisms, by discontinuing them promptly when the therapeutic objective has been achieved, and by maintaining close surveillance for early signs of secondary disease when such drugs are being used.

Enhancement of Toxicity of One Drug by the Simultaneous Administration of a Second Agent

Probably the most common and the most serious example is the increased incidence of digitalis intoxication when this drug is administered in conjunction with a thiazide diuretic. The potent kaliuretic effect of the thiazides greatly increases the sensitivity of the myocardium to the digitalis glycosides, and the incidence of digitalis intoxication has increased dramatically since the introduction of thiazide diuretics. In one large general hospital, digitalis-induced arrhythmias occurred in about 20 percent of all patients receiving digitalis preparations.[41] Because the kaliuretic effect of thiazides varies in patients with congestive heart failure, the administration of a fixed dose of potassium chloride with each tablet of thiazide has given a false sense of security to the physician. If he is to reduce the incidence and severity of toxicity of this potent drug combination, the physician must not only administer supplementary potassium but also watch closely for early signs of digitalis intoxication, and for laboratory evidence of significant serum po-

tassium abnormalities. Measurement of digitalis blood levels now allows documentation of toxic states secondary to the drug; prevention of such levels can only be attained by knowledge of digitalis pharmacokinetics and interactions.[25]

The same general principle applies to the administration of other potentially hazardous drug combinations (Table 143-5). Since combinations of drugs are often necessary for optimal therapy, the physician must be aware of the potential toxic effects of any drug combinations which he may prescribe and be constantly alert to the development of early signs or symptoms of toxicity in all such situations. Extensive reviews and listings of confirmed or suspected interactions between drugs are available.[16]

A very practical example of drug interactions is the effect of phenobarbital on the hepatic microsomal enzyme responsible for the degradation of anticoagulants of the coumarin group. This sedative which is commonly used in hospitalized patients undergoing anticoagulant therapy stimulates the enzyme activity and thus increases the rate of degradation. As a result, larger doses of the anticoagulant are required to produce the desired anticoagulant effect. If the barbituate is discontinued, bleeding complications may ensue unless the maintenance dose of the anticoagulant is reduced. In contrast, hemorrhage due to decreased prothrombin activity may occur during the concomitant administration of phenytoins, which are drugs that inhibit the metabolism of coumarin drugs.

Still other mechanisms may be involved by which a drug may influence the anticoagulant effects of warfarin (Table 143-6). For example, salicylates or quinidine may depress the synthesis of clotting factors and thus potentiate the anticoagulant response. In contrast, a variety of estrogenic substances stimulate the synthesis of these clotting factors and hence

TABLE 143-5

Examples of Increase in Toxicity of One Drug by Concomitant Administration of Another Agent

Drug Combination	Toxicity
Digitalis and thiazide	Digitalis toxicity due to potassium depletion
Monamine oxidase inhibitors and sympathomimetic amines	Hyperpyrexia, coma, death, hypertensive crisis
Rauwolfia alkaloids and anesthetic agents	Prolonged hypotension
Sulfonamides and oral hypoglycemic agents	Hypoglycemia due to displacement of sulfonylurea from protein binding sites
Lithium and diuretics	Central nervous system depression, lithium intoxication
Allopurinol and 6-MP	Pancytopenia
Aminoglycoside antibiotics and cephalothin	Nephrotoxicity

TABLE 143-6

Drugs Reported to Potentiate and Inhibit the Effects of Oral Anticoagulants

Drug	Mechanism of Action
Drugs Reported To Potentiate the Effects of Oral Anticoagulants	
Alcohol (acute intoxication)	Decreased metabolism
Allopurinol Chloramphenicol Disulfiram Hypoglycemics Metronidazole Phenytoin	Inhibition of microsomal enzymes
Chloral hydrate Clofibrate Nalidixic acid Phenylbutazone, oxyphenbutazone Sulfonamides	Displacement from binding sites
Indomethicin Salicylates	Inhibition of platelet function Depress synthesis of clotting factors
Thyroid hormones	Increased clotting factor catabolism
Vitamin E Anabolic and androgenic steroids	Not established
Drugs Reported To Inhibit the Effects of Oral Anticoagulants	
Alcohol, chronic	Increased metabolism
Barbiturates Glutethimide Griseofulvin Rifampin	Induction of microsomal enzymes
Cholestyramine	Decreased anticoagulant absorption
Oral contraceptives	Increase in activity of clotting factors

estrogens may significantly diminish the anticoagulant effect of warfarin. Displacement of one acidic drug from binding sites on plasma albumin by another acidic binding drug may produce enhanced effectiveness or toxicity to the former drug. In man, drugs such as phenylbutazone, clofibrate, and tolbutamide may so displace warfarin and induce an increased anticoagulant response. On the other end of the spectrum, some patients (or kindreds) have altered drug receptor sites for coumadin and hence require enormous doses of the drug to achieve the desired pharmacologic effect. Fundamental differences in response to drugs by certain patients cannot be accurately predicted at present. However, we must always seriously consider the unusual course of a patient's illness to be related to the drug or drugs used in treatment. To anticipate drug interactions, dosages should always be reassessed each time a drug is added to or removed from a patient's regimen.

Increased Sensitivity to the Toxic Effects of a Given Drug as the Result of Underlying Disease

An example of this is the patient with right heart failure who is given coumarin drugs to prevent thromboembolic complications. In such patients, sensitivity to coumarin may be increased as the result of hepatic congestion, and such an increase may not parallel

other indices of impaired hepatic function. Furthermore, sensitivity to coumarins may vary with the degree of cardiac decompensation and may be enhanced by small pulmonary embolic episodes which increase the severity of the right heart failure. Hence in this setting the very situation which demands specific drug therapy may per se increase the hazard of such therapy.

Table 143-7 presents other situations in which drug toxicity is accentuated by an underlying disease. Several of these situations are similar to the above illustration in that the disease that demands treat-

┌─ **TABLE 143-7** ─

Examples of Increased Sensitivity to a Drug Caused by Underlying Disease

Drug and Setting	Toxicity
Coumarins plus right heart failure	Hemorrhage due to decreased prothrombin activity
Coumarins plus hepatic disease	Hemorrhage due to decreased prothrombin activity
Lidocaine and liver disease[50]	Seizures
Theophylline and liver disease[37]	Seizures
Hyperalimentation plus hepatic disease	Coma due to ammonia intoxication
Thiazide diuretics plus hepatic disease	Hepatic coma (?hypokalemia)
Thiazide diuretics plus hyperuricemia	Gouty exacerbations
Thiazide diuretics plus latent or known diabetes	Hyperglycemia or diabetic decompensation
Atropine-like drugs plus prostatism	Acute urinary retention
Atropine drugs plus glaucoma	Acute glaucoma attack
Narcotic analgesics with chronic ventilatory insufficiency, hypoadrenalism, or panhypopituitarism	Hypoventilation, respiratory arrest
Antihistamines in epileptics	Seizures
Phenothiazines in delirium tremens	Hypotension, collapse, death
Reserpine in early Parkinson's disease	Marked worsening of Parkinson's disease
Sedatives in elderly patients	Occasionally agitation and excitement
Neomycin, streptomycin or polymyxin in myasthenia gravis	Marked worsening of myasthenia
Quinidine or quinine in myasthenia gravis	Paralysis
Barbiturates in acute intermittent porphyria	Flare up of abdominal pain and/or psychic symptoms
Oxidant drugs plus glucose-6-phosphate dehydrogenase deficiency	Acute hemolytic reaction
Succinylcholine plus pseudocholinesterase deficiency	Prolonged, severe apnea

┌─ **TABLE 143-7 (cont.)** ─

Drug and Setting	Toxicity
Aspirin and systemic lupus erythematosus	Hepatitis
Penicillin and renal disease	Penicillin neurotoxicity
Digitalis in myxedema, old age, and potassium deficiency	Digitalis toxicity
Digoxin and renal disease	Digitalis toxicity
Tetracycline and renal disease	Azotemia
Aspirin and von Willebrand's disease, hemophilia, thrombopathy	Hemorrhage
Sedatives and hepatic disease[23]	Overdosage

ment heightens the toxicity of the indicated drug. Only by a thorough knowledge of the circumstances that enhance the toxicity of each drug administered and by continued surveillance for the development of early manifestations of toxicity can the morbidity from such reactions be decreased. Knowledge of drug kinetics and of the pathways of drug metabolism and excretion allows alteration of the amount of drug prescribed to compensate for underlying disease; substitution of drugs may also bypass this problem. Digoxin is mainly eliminated by the kidney, whereas digitoxin is metabolized mainly by the liver; presence of underlying hepatic or renal disease would, therefore, dictate alteration of the drug dose or substitution of a digitalis form not affected by the underlying condition.

Therapeutic agents may complicate medical management in still another important manner, i.e., by interfering with clinical laboratory tests. Drugs may simply introduce interfering chromogen in colorometric procedures (e.g., methocarbamol [Robaxin] in the 5-HIAA test), or interfere in spectrophotometric assays[5] (e.g., dilantin and phenobarbital, in theophylline assays) or further, drugs may alter the levels of blood elements measured (e.g., decreased serum uric acid after high-dose salicylates or increased serum amylase after morphine administration). The ubiquitous utilization of oral contraceptive hormones, for example, may result in a markedly increased serum level of a variety of important carrier proteins, such as thyroxin-binding globulins, ceruloplasmin, transferrin, and vitamin B_{12} binding globulins. The effect of iodinated radiopaque dyes used in diagnostic radiology on many thyroid function tests is now well known.

DISEASES RESULTING FROM ADMINISTRATION OF BIOLOGIC PRODUCTS

Diseases in this category include transfusion reactions, adverse reactions to plasma or plasma protein (IgA) factors,[3] blood components (WBC, platelets), and reactions to passive immunization techniques, e.g., serum sickness secondary to tetanus antitoxin administration. Whole blood transfusion reactions are the most common and serious of these diseases; all blood products may be vehicles for transmission of cytomegalovirus, Epstein-Barr virus, malaria, and syphilis. Concentrates of clotting factors (Factor VIII, Factor IX, vitamin K dependent factors) have introduced a very significant risk of hepatitis.[21,45]

White cell transfusions now constitute a cornerstone in support of the leukemic patient. Marked febrile reactions are commonplace because of HLA sensitizations. Frequently unrecognized is the volume expansion incurred with WBC transfusions; this arises because the suspending agent, hydroxyethyl starch, is a dextran-like plasma expander.

DISEASES RESULTING FROM MECHANICAL THERAPEUTIC PROCEDURES

Representative of the mechanical therapeutic procedures that may result in diseases of medical management (Table 143–8) is positive end-expiratory pressure (PEEP) breathing in acute respiratory failure.[30] This simple innovation in respirator support retards small airway closure during expiration, permitting a more efficient exchange of oxygen. Oxygen toxicity to the lung is averted because not so high oxygen tensions are necessary to maintain adequate oxygenation. But pneumothorax, subcutaneous or mediastinal emphysema, and bronchopleural fistulas may result from the mechanical trauma to the lungs. Paradoxically the improvement in blood gases attained with PEEP may be associated with decreased tissue O_2 delivery; the increased airway pressure with PEEP may be translated into a decreased cardiac output be-

cause of a decreased venous return. Measurement of mixed venous oxygen tensions allows assessment of this problem.

Transtracheal Aspiration

Mouth flora and upper airway contamination create misleading results when nasotracheal suctioning is used to obtain sputum cultures. Transtracheal aspiration with introduction of a needle catheter (Intercath) through the cricothyroid membrane provides access to lower respiratory tract secretions that are free of oropharyngeal contamination. But hemorrhage, hypoxemia, vasovagal reactions, and subcutaneous and mediastinal emphysema necessitate precautions in its performance. Paroxysmal coughing is a contraindication; the coagulation profile must be in order and high-risk patients should be monitored with electrocardiograms. Hypoxemic patients should not have their oxygen discontinued during the procedure.[49]

DISEASES RESULTING DIRECTLY FROM SURGICAL TREATMENT (Table 143-9)

The medical condition of any patient may introduce avoidable risk factors in the performance of surgical procedures; recognition and correction of these problems may simplify an otherwise disastrous postoperative course.[21]

Many complications resulting from surgical therapy are either so obvious, e.g., vocal cord paralysis after thyroidectomy, or so routinely anticipated, e.g., paralytic ileus after bowel surgery, that they are readily recognized and appropriately treated. With certain other complications, however, which have an insidious onset and are not distinguished by specific symptomatology, recognition may be delayed to the detriment of the patient. An example is the malabsorption resulting from inadequate intestinal absorptive surface. Such cases may result from one of several surgical procedures, including gastroenterostomy (with an unusually long afferent loop), gastrojejunocolic fistula (from perforation of marginal ulcer), or extensive small bowel resection in cases of regional enteritis or incarcerated hernia. The malabsorption is often least expected in the latter group of cases, because the surgeon may estimate that he has removed only 2 or 3 feet of small bowel and finds at subsequent laparotomy that only 3 to 4 feet of functioning small bowel remains. In such patients, the symptoms may be non-

TABLE 143-8
Diseases Resulting from Mechanical Therapeutic Procedures

Procedure	Complications	Precautions[1]
Peritoneal dialysis	Hypovolemic hypotension, pulmonary edema, peritonitis, perforation of bladder, perforation of intestine, hyperosmolality, arrhythmias, ketoacidosis	Record intake and output accurately, monitor vital signs closely, observe aseptic technique, empty bladder before inserting cannula, avoid in patient with prior extensive abdominal surgery
Hemodialysis	Hypovolemic hypotension, pulmonary edema, bacteremia, transfusion reactions, digitalis intoxication, hemorrhage, dysequilibrium syndrome, folate, iron deficiency, air embolism	Monitor vital signs closely, observe strict aseptic technique, cross-match blood carefully, avoid rapid lowering of serum potassium in digitalized patients, monitor clotting times closely if patient is anticoagulated
Urinary catheterization	Infection, bacteremia	Closed system; strict asepsis
Bladder catheterization in lower urinary obstruction	Hypotension, bladder wall hemorrhage	Remove fluid gradually, not over 500 ml/hour. Monitor and treat for postobstructive uropathy
Pericardiocentesis	Coronary arterial tear, rupture of ventricular or right atrial wall, air embolism, ventricular arrhythmias	Premedicate with atropine; perform only with ECG monitoring
Abdominal paracentesis	Hypotension, oliguria, hepatic coma in severe liver disease, hemorrhage, suprapubic catheterization	Empty bladder, remove fluid slowly (not over 500 ml in 10 minutes), taking no more than necessary for purpose of tap. Monitor vital signs closely, and begin saline (or albumin) infusion if pulse rises more than 20 beats/minute or BP falls more than 20 mm systolic. Avoid paracentesis whenever possible in presence of severe hepatic dysfunction. Avoid scar areas
Tracheostomy	Cellulitis, aspiration of blood, hemorrhage, pulmonary infection, tracheal stenosis	Observe aseptic technique. Tie off bleeders carefully. Suction thoroughly immediately after procedure. Use sterile catheter each time tracheal suction is performed
Insertion of indwelling intravenous catheters[32]	Bacteremia, endocarditis, thrombosis, hydrothorax	Observe aseptic technique in placing catheter. Never leave intravenous catheter in place over 48 hours. Apply antibiotic ointment around site of insertion of catheter
Subclavian line	Pneumothorax	
Internal jugular line	Pneumothorax	Never perform, unless forced, in patient with a single lung
Transtracheal aspiration	Mediastinal emphysema, hemorrhage, hypoxemia	Avoid in patient with paroxysmal coughing; check clotting parameters
PEEP (positive end expiratory pressure)	Pneumothorax, hypotension, respirator lung	Maintain intravascular volumes on high side; avoid $F_iO_2 > 50$ mm Hg

TABLE 143-9
Postsurgical Disease

Operation	Complication
Arterial or cardiac prosthesis	Hemolytic anemia, infective endarteritis or endocarditis
Cardiac bypass, open-heart surgery	Postpump mononucleosis-like illness, bacterial endarteritis, serum hepatitis
Gastrectomy, subtotal	Early and late dumping syndromes, malabsorption, iron-deficiency anemia
Gastrectomy, total	Above complications plus pernicious anemia
Inadvertent gastroileostomy	Severe malabsorption
Small bowel resection	Malabsorption, often initially unnoticed
Thyroidectomy	Hypothyroidism, hypoparathyroidism, vocal cord paralysis
Ureterosigmoidostomy	Hyperchloremic acidosis
Any major surgery	Foreign body retention and infection, vitamin deficiency
Any surgery, especially with catgut sutures	Tetanus in the nonimmunized patient
Splenectomy	Overwhelming sepsis
Anesthesia	Halothane, methoxyflurane hepatitis
Hyperalimentation	Hyperosmolality, hypophosphatemia, vitamin deficiency

specific, initially consisting of easy fatigability and vague malaise, often accompanied by mild anemia. Blood chemical tests, such as glucose and cholesterol, may be within normal limits. Only by recognizing that inadequate absorptive surface may occur from almost any bowel surgery and by carefully evaluating the absorptive function, e.g., by measurement of fecal fat excretion, can the diagnosis be established and appropriate corrective surgical or supplementary dietary therapy be initiated.

Purposeful induction of malabsorption by jejuno-ileal bypass (for treatment of obesity) has also resulted in major complications. Hepatic steatosis secondary to protein–calorie deficiencies, gallstones and oxalate renal stones, vitamin and electrolyte deficien-cies, polyarthritis and arthralgia have all complicated this surgical procedure.[9] Nutritional problems in general and those associated with a catabolic postoperative course are now being controlled with intravenous hyperalimentation. Assumption of responsibility for total nutritional support in this manner presupposes an understanding of the many problems (vascular access, infection, electrolyte imbalance, vitamin deficiency, hepatic failure) that such therapy may create.[17]

DISEASES SECONDARY TO IONIZING IRRADIATION

The illnesses caused by ionizing irradiation pose serious problems of medical management, especially since the subtle (mutagenic and carcinogenic) effects of irradiation are not immediately apparent. The inflammatory and cicatricial effects may be serious, but they can often be anticipated and surgically corrected. Excessive radiation to any tissue may induce destructive fibrous changes that include the pulmonary,[22] hepatic, and renal[31] parenchyma, and cardiac vessel involvement with premature atherosclerosis.

The mutagenic and carcinogenic effects of irradiation become evident only after many years (e.g., thyroid carcinoma after thymic irradiation) or after one or more generations (mutagenic effect on reproductive cells) following exposure to irradiation. For example, the unexpected carcinogenic effect is evident from an unfortunate group of patients who received spine irradiation for ankylosing spondylitis. In a follow-up, ranging from one to 15 years, of nearly 10,000 patients who received this treatment, the incidence of leukemia was at least five times that expected for a comparable age–sex group who received no irradiation.[12] The incidence of leukemia proved significantly greater in patients who received more than one course of spine irradiation.

The mutagenic risk of ionizing irradiation should prompt the physician to balance carefully the inherent risks against the potential benefits of irradiation. The balancing is, however, more difficult than with most procedures because of the unique nature of the radiation hazard. Attention to certain general principles can, however, minimize the risk. With diagnostic x-ray studies, the physician must consider the facts that the mutagenic effects of ionizing irradiation are cumulative, and that certain diagnostic procedures, e.g., gastrointestinal series, require relatively large doses of irradiation. Therefore, desirability of the procedure must be carefully considered in each case and every effort made to insure adequate preparation for the initial study so that the technical quality of the films will be satisfactory. Regarding x-ray therapy, the physician must make certain the diagnosis is correct before treatment is initiated. For example, patients with retroperitoneal fibrosis have mistakenly been treated with x-ray for nonexistent malignancy. Now that the potential risks of irradiation are well established, the need for accurate diagnosis prior to treatment with irradiation is obvious.

DISEASES RESULTING FROM HOSPITAL ADMISSION PER SE

With the increasing use of the hospital and its comprehensive diagnostic and treatment facilities, it has become obvious that problems resulting from hospital admission per se may cause increased morbidity and mortality. Certain types of patients, e.g., the elderly, those with inadequate host defense mechanisms, and those with chronic renal disease, are unusually susceptible to the hazards of hospital admission.

The patient with acute leukemia is a good example. The disease may have virtually eliminated functional granulocytes so that exposure to the hospital environment may result in the acquisition of a potentially fatal staphylococcal or gram-negative rod infection.

The acute leukemic patient should, especially when potent antimetabolites and glucocorticoids are administered, be hospitalized only where adequate facilities for protective isolation are available. This, however, poses a major therapeutic dilemma. There are often compelling reasons for admitting these patients to the hospital for treating major noninfectious complications, but few hospitals have isolation facilities adequate for the management of such patients. Carefully balanced judgment is, therefore, required to determine when the patient with acute leukemia should be hospitalized. Unless such a patient is in imminent danger from a potentially reversible problem, e.g., sepsis, hospitalization should generally be avoided. When hospitalization is necessary, discharge should be arranged as soon as the acute problem has been resolved. Even in cases in which the reason for admission is sound, (e.g., infection), the patient often remains in the hospital long after the specific problem has been adequately dealt with. Diseases of medical management are closely related to duration of stay. Thus, it is mandatory that patients unduly susceptible to the hazards of hospitalization be discharged as soon as possible.

The key question to be asked regarding the management of patients unusually susceptible to the hazards of hospitalization is whether admission will clearly benefit the patient, or whether it is arranged primarily for the convenience of the physician.

REFERENCES

1. Abrahams, P. and Webb, P. Clinical Anatomy of Practical Procedures. Philadelphia, Lippincott, 1975.
2. Abrams, H. and McNeil, B. Medical implications of computed tomography. N. Engl. J. Med., 298:255, 310, 1978.
3. Alving, B., Hojimo, Y., Pisano, J., et al. Hypotension associated with prekallikrein activator (Hageman-factor fragments) in plasma protein fraction. N. Engl. J. Med., 229:66, 1978.
4. Ansell, G. (ed.). Complications in Diagnostic Radiology. Oxford, England, Blackwell, 1976.
5. Banner, A., Berman, E., Sunderrajan, E., et al. Theophylline, drug interference with the spectrophotometric assay. N. Engl. J. Med., 297:170, 1977.
6. Bartlett, J., Chang, T., Gurwith, M., et al. Antibiotic-associated pseudomembranous colitis due to toxin producing clostridia. N. Engl. J. Med., 298:531, 1978.
7. Bennett, W., Plamp, C., and Porter, G.A. Drug related syndromes in clinical nephrology. Ann. Intern. Med., 87:582, 1977.
8. Bennett, W., Singer, I., Golper, T., et al. Guidelines for drug therapy in renal failure. Ann. Intern. Med., 86:754, 1977.
9. Bray, G., Barry, R., Benfield, J., et al. Intestinal bypass operation as a treatment for obesity. Ann. Intern. Med., 85:97, 1976.
10. Chabner, B.A. Second neoplasm—a complication of cancer chemotherapy. N. Engl. J. Med., 297:213, 1977.
11. Cluff, L.E., Thornton, G., Seidel, L., et al. Epidemiological study of adverse drug reactions. Trans. Assoc. Am. Physicians, 78:225, 1965.
12. Court-Brown, W.M. and Abbatt, J. The incidence of leukemia in ankylosing spondylitis treated with x-ray. Lancet, 268:1283, 1955.
13. Davies, D.M. (ed.). Textbook of Adverse Drug Reactions. New York, Oxford University, 1977.
14. deGruchy, G. Drug Induced Blood Disorders. Oxford, Blackwell, 1975.
15. DiMagno, E., Malagelada, J., Taylor, W., et al. A prospective comparison of current diagnostic tests for pancreatic cancer. N. Engl. J. Med., 297:737, 1977.
16. Drugs, adverse interactions of. Med. Lett. Drugs Ther., 19:5, 1977.
17. Dudrick, S. and Long, J. III. Application and hazards of total intravenous hyperalimentation. Annu. Rev. Med., 28:519, 1977.
18. Dukes, M.N.G. (ed.). Side Effects of Drugs: A Worldwide Yearly Survey of New Data and Trends. Amsterdam, Excerpta Medica, 1978.

19. Everett, E. and Hirschmann, J. Transient bacteremia and endocarditis prophylaxis. Medicine, 56:61, 1977.

20. Goldman, L., Caldera, D., and Southwick, F. Cardiac risk factors and complications in non-cardiac surgery. Medicine, 57:357, 1978.

21. Grady, G.F. Transfusions and hepatitis—update in '78. N. Engl. J. Med., 298:1413, 1978.

22. Gress, N.J. Pulmonary effect of radiation therapy. Ann. Intern. Med., 81:86, 1977.

23. Hoyumpa, A., Branch, R., and Schenker, S. The disposition and effects of sedatives and analgesics in liver disease. Annu. Rev. Med., 29:205, 1978.

24. Hypertension, drugs for. Med. Lett. Drugs Ther., 19:21, 1977.

25. Jelliffe, R.W. An improved method of digoxan therapy. Ann. Intern. Med., 69:703, 1968.

26. Jonsen, A. Do no harm. Ann. Intern. Med., 88:827, 1978.

27. Kern, F. Jr. Gastroenterology—1976: good news and bad news. Gastroenterology, 71:537, 1976.

28. King, J.C. Guide to Parenteral Admixtures. St. Louis, Cutter Laboratories, 1978.

29. Koch-Weser, J. Bioavailability of drugs. N. Engl. J. Med., 291:233, 1974.

30. Kumar, A., Falke, K., Geffin, B., et al. Continuous positive-pressure ventilation in acute respiratory failure: effects on hemodynamics and lung function. N. Engl. J. Med., 283:1430, 1970.

31. Madrazo, A., Schwartz, G., and Churg, J. Radiation nephritis: a review. J. Urol., 114:822, 1975.

32. Maki, D.G., Goldmann, D., and Rhame, F. Infection control in intravenous therapy. Ann. Intern. Med., 79:867, 1973.

33. Mitchell, J. and Lauterburg, B. Drug-induced liver injury. Hosp. Pract., 13:95, 1978.

34. Norman, P.S. and Cluff, L.E. Adverse drug reactions and alternative drugs of choice. In W.E. Modell (ed.), Drugs of Choice. St. Louis, Mosby, 1965.

35. Parisi, A., Tow, D., Felix, W., et al. Noninvasive cardiac diagnosis. N. Engl. J. Med., 296:316, 368, 427, 1977.

36. Penicillin allergy. Med. Lett. Drugs Ther., 20:14, 1978.

37. Piaksky, K., Sitar, D., Rangno, R., et al. Theophylline disposition in patients with hepatic cirrhosis. N. Engl. J. Med., 296:1495, 1977.

38. Pollack, H.M., Goldberg, B., Morales, J., et al. A systematized approach to the differential diagnosis of renal masses. Radiology, 113:653, 1974.

39. Porter, J. and Jick, H. Drug-related deaths among medical inpatients. JAMA, 237:879, 1977.

40. Rahal, J. Antibiotic combinations: the clinical relevance of synergy and antagonism. Medicine, 57:179, 1978.

41. Rodensky, P. and Wasserman, F. Observations on digitalis intoxication. Arch. Intern. Med., 108:171, 1961.

42. Rosenow, E.C. III. Drug-induced pulmonary disease. Ann. Intern. Med., 77:980, 1972.

43. Rosove, M.H. Agranulocytosis and antithyroid drugs. West. J. Med., 126:339, 1977.

44. Salmon, S., Hamburger, A., Soehulen, B., et al. Quantitation of differential sensitivity of human tumor stem cells to anticancer drugs. N. Engl. J. Med., 298:1321, 1978.

45. Seeff, L. and Hoofnage, J. Chronic hepatitis in hemophilia. Ann. Intern. Med., 86:818, 1977.

46. Sharma, G., Tow, D., Parisi, A., et al. Diagnosis of pulmonary embolism. Annu. Rev. Med., 28:159, 1977.

47. Sieber, S.M. and Adamson, R.H. Toxicity of antineoplastic agents in man. Adv. Cancer Res., 22:57, 1975.

48. Siegle, R. and Lieberman, P. A review of untoward reactions to iodinated contrast material. J. Urol., 119:581, 1978.

49. Spencer, C.D. and Beaty, H. Complications of transtracheal aspiration. N. Engl. J. Med., 286:304, 1972.

50. Zito, R. and Reid, P. Lidocaine kinetics predicted by indocyanine green clearance. N. Engl. J. Med., 298:116, 1978.

51. Zheutlin, N., Lasser, E.C., and Rigler, L.G. Clinical studies on effect of barium in the peritoneal cavity following rupture of the colon. Surgery, 32:967, 1952.

Medical Emergencies
JERRY L. SPIVAK: SECTION EDITOR

This section describes the management of medical disorders requiring immediate therapy. In the urgent situation, there is usually no time for a detailed history and examination before treatment is initiated. Although shock, coma, or cardiopulmonary arrest can be the presenting manifestation of a variety of diseases, in each instance, regardless of the underlying cause, the immediate goal is to restore and stabilize the patient's vital signs as quickly as possible.

Once that has been achieved, data gathering can be completed and definitive therapy administered. Therefore, the emphasis in this section will be on the critical initial phase of management of emergencies. No attempt has been made to provide a detailed approach to all medical emergencies since many of these are discussed elsewhere in this volume.

CHAPTER 144
Cardiorespiratory Arrest
JERRY L. SPIVAK

Cardiorespiratory arrest, the sudden, unexpected cessation of effective cardiac and respiratory function, can result from diverse causes ranging from pulmonary embolism to anaphylaxis. Regardless of the underlying etiology, treatment should initially be directed at restoring tissue oxygenation by the simple maneuvers of closed chest cardiac massage and artificial ventilation.[17] Once this is achieved, more definitive measures can be employed. Because cardiorespiratory arrest is an unexpected event and because the underlying disorder provoking the arrest is often reversible, it is important that all individuals participating in patient care be fully familiar with the basic life support techniques. Furthermore, because of the urgent nature of the situation and the large number of persons usually involved in the resuscitative effort, it is vital that an organized approach be employed and that one individual assume responsibility for directing resuscitation.

MANAGEMENT OF CARDIOPULMONARY RESUSCITATION (CPR)

Diagnosis of Cardiorespiratory Arrest
Irreversible brain damage develops after 4 to 6 minutes of circulatory arrest, a time interval which may be shortened in the presence of underlying disease.

Therefore, little time is available for diagnostic procedures. Immediate implementation of CPR is indicated when loss of consciousness does not respond rapidly to the recumbent position, when there is absence of a pulse in a major (carotid or femoral) artery, when heart sounds are absent, and when respiration is gasping or absent. In some patients, a convulsion signals cessation of effective cardiac output; respiration may continue for more than 30 seconds after cardiac arrest but not uncommonly, respiratory failure triggers the arrest of cardiac activity. Pupillary dilatation usually occurs within a minute of circulatory arrest. Although pupillary dilatation suggests that at least 25 percent of the period of potential reversibility has passed, in certain situations, such as lightning stroke, cold water immersion, and barbiturate overdose, resuscitation with good functional recovery has been achieved after a prolonged period of circulatory stasis.

Precordial Thump
When cardiorespiratory arrest is suspected, a sharp blow should be delivered to the mid-portion of the sternum with the fleshy side of the fist through a trajectory of no more than 12 inches. Such a blow can restore the heart beat when asystole has occurred secondary to heart block and can reverse ventricular tachycardia; it will not abort established ventricular fibrillation.[6] Although continued precordial blows can

function as an effective pacemaker in complete heart block, precious time must not be wasted in either assessing the effects of a single blow or delivering multiple blows if the initial one is not obviously successful.

Cardiopulmonary resuscitation must proceed in an orderly fashion if a successful outcome is to be achieved. The mnemonic A-airway, B-breathing, C-cardiac compression, D-definitive therapy, E-electrocardiogram is useful not only for codifying the necessary therapeutic maneuvers but also in defining a sequence in which these maneuvers are implemented.

A-Airway

A patent airway must be established since cardiac massage will benefit tissue respiration only if oxygenated blood is being circulated. An airway can be established rapidly, with the patient supine, by tilting the head backward while lifting the mandible upwards. This maneuver prevents the tongue from obstructing the pharynx and may be associated with the spontaneous return of respiration. Time should not be routinely devoted to examining the upper airway for foreign bodies. If, however, properly performed artificial ventilation does not result in chest expansion, the fingers should be used rapidly to explore and clear the pharynx. A classic instance in which this maneuver is indicated is the "café coronary" in which cardiorespiratory arrest is provoked by the impaction of a large bolus of food in the upper airway.[2] If the foreign body cannot be dislodged by the fingers, two other maneuvers can be employed. The Heimlich maneuver involves forcefully squeezing the patient's upper abdomen in a "bear hug" and thereby using the motion of the diaphragm to expel the obstructing object. Alternatively, the patient is rolled onto his side and is struck sharply between the shoulder blades. Tracheostomy should be performed if these maneuvers fail to clear the upper airway. (Large bore needles inserted into the trachea do not provide adequate airflow for ventilatory purposes.)

B-Breathing

Whether artificial ventilation is delivered initially by a mouth-to-mouth or mouth-to-nose route depends on the demands of the particular situation and the sensitivities of the rescuers. Whatever the route, ventilation cannot be considered adequate if there is no chest expansion since the pressure exerted by forceful expiration is more than sufficient to inflate normally compliant lungs. Chest wall motion associated with closed chest cardiac massage does not contribute significantly to effective gas exchange.

Oropharyngeal airways are esthetically pleasing and helpful in maintaining an open airway. Their use, however, does not assure that ventilation will be more efficient and when positioned they may precipitate vomiting with attendant pulmonary aspiration. Most airway and bag–mask devices also do not always provide a leak–proof seal, and specific training is required to use these devices successfully. Unless the trachea is intubated directly, any method of artificial ventilation can produce gastric distention and regurgitation. An esophageal obturator is an effective device for preventing this complication. Although endotracheal intubation is the most efficient method for delivering oxygen to the lungs, particularly when hyperventilation is desired, skill is required for this maneuver, and time must not be wasted in attempts to intubate the patient. The expired air of the rescuer will deliver approximately 17 percent oxygen to the patient, which is adequate if properly delivered. Taking up a position at the side of the patient, the rescuer should maintain extension of the patient's neck and after closing off either the mouth or nose, rapidly deliver four full breaths through the other orifice without allowing time for complete lung deflation. Both the mouth and the nose should be left unobstructed for expiration. Thereafter, artificial ventilation should be delivered at a rate of 12 to 15 cycles per minute. When one rescuer is performing artificial ventilation and another cardiac compression, one ventilation should be interposed after four to five chest compressions. *Chest compression should not be interrupted in order to deliver ventilation or to attempt synchronization between ventilation and compression* since such an interruption allows the blood pressure to fall to zero. When only one rescuer is performing CPR, the rescuer should deliver two rapid lung inflations after 15 cardiac compressions.

C-Cardiac Compression

Once ventilation is initiated, closed chest cardiac compression should be started with the patient in the horizontal position on a flat, solid surface. If in bed, a board or food tray should be placed between the patient and the mattress.

In order to avoid fatigue and minimize rib fractures and damage to abdominal viscera, the rescuer should be positioned at the patient's side and high enough for the arms to be straight when the shoulders are directly over the sternum. The heel of one hand should be placed on the lower third of the sternum (avoid the xiphoid process) and the heel of the other hand placed directly on the first. The fingers are not involved in the procedure. Chest compression is performed by exerting pressure on the sternum with the arms straight and using the weight of the rescuer's body. For effective closed chest cardiac massage, the lower sternum must be depressed at least 1.5 to 2 inches, at a rate of 60 times per minute. The compression stroke should be smooth and held for at least 50 percent of the cycle in order to maximize blood flow and mean arterial blood pressure.[8] Although the rescuer's hands should never leave the chest, the chest must be allowed to expand after each compression.

The adequacy of CPR can be evaluated by examining skin color, the carotid pulse (palpate gently), and the size and reactivity to light of the pupils. Pupillary size and reactivity may of course be altered by drug administration. Inadequate CPR may be the result of a blocked airway, inadequate depth, duration, or rate of cardiac compression, or profound hypovolemia. Open chest cardiac compression is indicated when there is pericardial tamponade, flail chest, tension pneumothorax with a mediastinal shift, or severe emphysema with a barrel chest deformity.

D-Definitive Therapy

Once basic CPR has been initiated, a secure intravenous route should be established for delivery of drugs using a large bore catheter, and electrocardiographic monitoring should be instituted. Definitive therapy is tailored to the specific situation. For example, for a patient who is already being monitored when cardiac arrest occurs, immediate countershock would be employed if ventricular fibrillation or ventricular tachycardia without a pulse is observed. Since ventricular fibrillation occurs in a large proportion of patients who arrest and since a prolonged duration of ventricular fibrillation lessens the chance for successful resuscitation, some authorities would extend the application of direct counter shock to all patients who arrest even if unmonitored. This is a reasonable approach as long as the application of direct countershock does not delay the initiation of artificial ventilation and closed chest compression.

Metabolic acidosis due to lactate accumulation is common after cardiac arrest. In patients with preexisting pulmonary disease or aspiration or when institution of adequate ventilation has been delayed, respiratory acidosis may be superimposed on the metabolic acidosis. In either case, adequate ventilation is the most important maneuver in correcting the acid–base disorder. Administration of small amounts of sodium bicarbonate may be beneficial if ventilation is adequate. When it is inadequate, administration of sodium bicarbonate will only lead to large increases in Pco_2, an accentuation of intracellular acidosis, and impairment of cardiac performance.[1] Administration of sodium bicarbonate in the doses currently advised (1 mEq/kg) may also lead to a substantial increase in

serum osmolality.[5] Consequently, control of ventilation (if possible by intubation) is the most important therapeutic maneuver in treating the acidosis of cardiac arrest. The use of sodium bicarbonate should be guided by blood gas determinations and avoided when there is a persistent, substantial elevation of the Pco_2.

Hypotension due to inadequate peripheral vasoconstriction should be corrected with infusions of either norepinephrine (16 mg in 500 ml of 5 percent dextrose in water (D_5W) with 5 mg of phentolamine to prevent tissue necrosis) or metaraminol (200 mg in 500 ml of D_5W). Maintenance of adequate blood pressure may protect the brain from ischemia.

E-Electrocardiogram

Definitive therapy of cardiac arrest is usually guided by the electrocardiogram.

ASYSTOLE. Epinephrine (5 ml of a 1:10,000 solution) may convert asystole to ventricular fibrillation. If an intravenous line is open, administration by this route is preferable. Otherwise, intracardiac injection (1 to 2 ml of 1:10,000 solution) should be used, avoiding intramyocardial injection which can result in irreversible ventricular fibrillation. Intracardiac injection is performed with a 3.5-inch No. 22 needle inserted 5 cm to the left of the sternum in the fourth or fifth left intercostal space. Injection of epinephrine can be repeated every 3 to 5 minutes if necessary to maintain pacemaker activity or it can be administered by intravenous infusion (4 to 8 μg/min). Transbronchial injection of epinephrine in the same schedule has advantages over intracardiac injection.

Other drugs that may enhance rhythmicity include calcium chloride (5 to 10 ml of a 10 percent solution administered every 10 minutes) if there is no suspicion of digitalis toxicity and isoproterenol (0.02 to 0.04 mg administered as described for epinephrine) particularly if ventricular fibrillation preceded the asystole.

If CPR and drug therapy are not successful in reversing asystole, electrical pacing by either an external or transvenous approach should be tried. Electromechanical dissociation is not uncommon in this situation.

VENTRICULAR FIBRILLATION. The only effective treatment for ventricular fibrillation is electrical defibrillation by direct countershock.[3,4] Direct countershock is most effective when delivered early in the course of ventricular fibrillation and should not be delayed for a confirmatory electrocardiogram. However, institution of CPR should also not be delayed by repeated countershocks if the initial one is unsuccessful since persistent fibrillation may be due to myocardial hypoxia. Regardless of body weight, 100 to 200 watt seconds (joules) should be delivered in the initial shock. A second shock should be higher in energy by 50 percent. Impedance to current flow can be reduced by using large paddles and electrode paste as the interface. If fibrillatory activity is weak, epinephrine (5 ml of a 1:10,000 solution) should be given in order to coarsen the fibrillation; calcium chloride can also be used for this purpose. If two shocks separated by a period of CPR are not successful in converting the fibrillation, intravenous lidocaine (50 to 100 mg) should also be given followed by a series of countershocks delivering maximal energy. If defibrillation is successful but fibrillation recurs, lidocaine should be infused at a rate of 200 to 300 mg per hour. Bretylium is a second drug useful in the management of ventricular fibrillation. It has been observed to revert fibrillation without shock. If repeated countershocks are necessary, the energy delivered should be reduced. The use of procainamide or quinidine to decrease ventricular irritability is less desirable since these agents depress myocardial contractility and atrioventricular conduction. Intravenous propranolol, up to a total of 5 to 10 mg in 1.0 mg boluses, may also be useful in treating recurrent ventricular fibrillation, particularly when large amounts of epinephrine have been employed, as well as in ischemic heart disease. Occasionally, electrical defibrillation will result in asystole which can be treated as outlined above.

HEART BLOCK.   Heart block associated with cardiac arrest may respond to atropine sulfate 0.4 to 2.0 mg intravenously, while isoproterenol can be employed to increase the rate of idioventricular pacemakers. In general, however, transvenous pacing is the best approach. Heart block is also one situation where repeated precordial thumps can temporarily maintain cardiac output.

Delivery of definitive therapy during CPR should be accompanied by continuing supportive therapy with attention to such details as decompressing the stomach by nasogastric tube, maintaining a clear airway by suction, and providing for delivery of 100 percent oxygen to the patient. Pneumothorax is a common complication of CPR and can be dealt with temporarily by insertion of a small bore needle attached to a syringe barrel filled with saline, into the pleural space.

CESSATION OF RESUSCITATION.   Once a strong spontaneous pulse has been restored, closed chest cardiac compression is discontinued. Artificial ventilation may be required for a longer period. Even if artificial ventilation is not required, one must not be too hasty in extubating the patient.

Failure to obtain ventricular electrical activity after 1 or 2 hours of CPR with appropriate definitive therapy constitutes sufficient indication for cessation of resuscitation.

Postresuscitation Care

Following successful resuscitation, the conditions responsible for the cardiac arrest must be sought and corrected if possible. The patient should also be carefully evaluated for the complications of the cardiac arrest and the resuscitative efforts. They include rib or sternal fractures, costochondral separations, pulmonary contusions, pneumothorax, aspiration, marrow emboli, lacerations of abdominal viscera, cortical blindness, renal tubular necrosis, myocardial lacerations, and disorders of acid–base balance. Particular attention should be paid to the presence of cerebral edema occurring as the result of cerebral anoxia during the period of cardiac arrest. Persistent coma, with lack of spontaneous respirations and fixed dilated pupils, suggests that brain death has occurred.

——CHAPTER 145——
Shock
HUBERT T. GURLEY

INTRODUCTION

"Shock," which has been called a rest-stop on the highway to death, is a clinical syndrome in which the common thread of inadequate organ perfusion runs through a myriad of clinical manifestations including anxiety, confusion, coma, hyperventilation, oliguria, anuria, hypotension, vasoconstriction, and vasodilatation. Shock and its varying features represent a dy-

namic state in which an initial derangement is followed by compensatory responses which are in turn altered by the effects of sustained ischemia to one or more organ systems. A rational approach to the patient presenting with the shock syndrome requires an understanding of the dynamic nature of shock and the specific actions of agents employed to combat the shock syndrome. The key to effective therapy of shock is constant reevaluation of the patient's status. Shock is always a consequence of some disorder such as myocardial infarction or infection; the underlying cause must be recognized and corrected in order to reverse the shock syndrome.

In assessing the patient in shock, frequent observations of pulse, temperature, and urine flow are as important as measurements of the arterial blood gases or determinations of the pulmonary capillary wedge pressure. Arterial blood pressure as measured by stethoscope and cuff is inadequate to diagnose shock or to follow the course of the patient and provides only an approximation of tissue perfusion. Patients with seemingly adequate cuff blood pressures may suffer irreversible organ damage if other signs of inadequate perfusion are ignored. Conversely, rigid insistence upon achieving a minimal cuff blood pressure through administration of a pressor agent may result in unnecessary renal, coronary, or splanchnic ischemia.

For purposes of discussion, the circulatory system may be likened to a three-component system of pump, vessels, and fluid. Disturbances of any component may lead to the shock syndrome. Treatment aims to maintain an adequate volume of fluid flowing through sufficiently open vessels under an adequate head of pressure. Often the primary cause of the shock syndrome may be readily apparent, e.g., massive hemorrhage following traumatic injury or cardiovascular collapse secondary to overwhelming bacterial infection. Frequently, however, the primary etiology of the shock syndrome is not apparent, especially when more than 24 hours have elapsed since the onset of shock, or when the patient is unable to provide a history. In those circumstances, methodical consideration of likely disturbances in each of the three components should lead to definition of the underlying disorder.

Electrical Disturbances of Pump Function

Disturbances of cardiac rate or rhythm can impair cardiac performance sufficiently to cause shock. The healthy heart can compensate for rate changes between 40 and 160 per minute. These limits may narrow to 50 to 120 in the patient with organic heart disease. Sinus bradycardia of less than 50 per minute occurs as a result of the increased vagal tone associated with vomiting or tissue manipulation (sigmoidoscopy, thoracentesis, or lumbar puncture), in association with hypothermia and myxedema, in the course of acute myocardial infarction, and with sinus node dysfunction.

Sinus tachycardia of greater than 140 per minute is generally in response to an abnormal physiologic state such as fever, hypoxia, hypovolemia, anemia, or hyperthyroidism. Therapy is directed at correction of the underlying disturbance.

Frequent ventricular premature beats may decrease the cerebral circulation by as much as 25 percent. The loss of atrial contraction in atrial fibrillation may reduce the cardiac output by 30 percent in patients with ischemic heart disease. Atrial flutter with a rapid ventricular response may also reduce the cardiac output. Ventricular tachycardia is usually associated with a marked reduction in cardiac output. Restoring tachy- or bradyarrhythmias to normal will reverse the symptoms resulting from inadequate tissue perfusion (Chap. 21).

Mechanical Disturbances of Pump Function

CARDIAC TAMPONADE. Cardiac tamponade occurs in patients with traumatic chest injury, uremia, neoplasm, bacterial pericarditis, tuberculous pericarditis, anticoagulant therapy, acute rheumatic fever, idiopathic pericarditis, and following cardiac catheterization or placement of a transvenous pacing wire. The patient may present with tachycardia, dyspnea, high venous pressure, and falling arterial blood pressure. High venous pressure is a key consequence of tamponade. The peripheral arteries usually manifest a paradoxic pulse, defined as an abnormal inspiratory fall in systolic blood pressure of greater than 10 mm Hg. However, a paradoxic pulse is not specific for tamponade and may be seen in a variety of low output states. Electrocardiographic changes may include S-T elevation of acute pericarditis, low voltage, nonspecific ST-T changes, or electrical alternans of the QRS complexes. The cardiac silhouette may be of normal size or only slightly increased. Lung fields are generally clear and pulmonary edema is absent. The presence of significant pericardial fluid can be documented by echocardiography or angiocardiography, but does not, per se, prove tamponade. The diagnosis of tamponade is best made by showing equalization of diastolic pressures in all cardiac chambers. The diagnosis is strongly supported by finding that the pulmonary capillary wedge pressure and central venous pressure are elevated to approximately the same level. Removal of a modest amount of fluid from the pericardial sac by needle aspiration under electrocardiographic monitoring can be life saving until more definitive treatment can be employed.

TENSION PNEUMOTHORAX. Tension pneumothorax occurs in patients with traumatic chest injury or chronic lung disease and in patients receiving assisted ventilation, especially those treated with continuous positive end expiratory pressure (PEEP). Accumulation of air within the pleural space can cause a shift of the mediastinal structures and interfere with cardiac filling and ejection. The systemic pressure may fall gradually or abruptly as the air accumulates. Contralateral distension of neck veins is present. Breath signs are absent on the affected side, and the area of mediastinal dullness to percussion is shifted to the opposite side. Treatment consists of introducing a small gauge needle under a water seal (e.g., attached to a water-filled large-barrel syringe) through the chest wall in the region of suspected air accumulation; air under pressure will escape into the syringe, with rapid increase in the arterial blood pressure, reappearance of breath sounds, and return of the mediastinum to its normal locations. If air reaccumulates, a chest tube will be required.

MASSIVE PULMONARY EMBOLUS. Massive pulmonary embolus results in mechanical obstruction of the circulation with acute cor pulmonale and shock or fatal rhythm disturbances. The diagnosis of pulmonary embolism is one of the most elusive in clinical medicine since the disorder can occur in any clinical setting. Massive pulmonary embolism is often accompanied by hyperventilation with decreased Po_2, decreased Pco_2, and mild alkalosis which may progress to severe acidosis following the onset of shock. Occlusion of more than 60 percent of the pulmonary circulation results in acute right ventricular strain and elevation of systemic venous pressure. Venous distension and hepatic enlargement and tenderness may follow. Tachycardia is the rule, and atrial or ventricular arrhythmias may be present. The sudden appearance of signs of right ventricular failure, distended neck veins, parasternal heave, and gallop rhythm in a patient without heart disease is suggestive of acute massive pulmonary embolism. The appearance of shock in association with pulmonary embolism is a grave prognostic sign. Death is most likely to occur in the first hour. Patients who survive begin to improve rapidly within 1 to 2 hours of the onset of symptoms. X-ray findings may include diminished or absent pulmonary vascular markings distal to the area of obstruction and enlargement of the cardiac silhouette due to dilation of the right ventricle, right atrium, or main pulmonary artery. EKG changes are variable and nondiagnostic.

Emergency therapy is directed at maintaining adequate oxygenation and supporting cardiac output with large volumes of intravenous fluids and pressor agents, if necessary. Intravenous heparin is administered to prevent the formation of additional clot. Thrombolytic agents may be considered. The use of vasodilators to reduce pulmonary arterial spasm is of undetermined benefit and is risky in patients in shock. Inability to combat shock effectively in the patient with a massive pulmonary embolism may be considered an indication for surgical intervention.

AORTIC VALVE DYSFUNCTION. Aortic valve dysfunction may occur in nonpenetrating trauma, infective endocarditis, prosthetic valve malfunction, or aortic dissection. Due to the regurgitation of ejected blood back into the left ventricle, there is marked reduction in effective cardiac output with an increased end-diastolic volume. The mitral valve closes prematurely, causing inadequate emptying of the left atrium and congestion within the pulmonary circulation. Right ventricular failure follows, and the patient may experience the sudden onset of dyspnea and rapid and forceful heart beat. The chest x-ray is consistent with congestive heart failure or pulmonary edema, and the clinical examination reveals the murmur of aortic regurgitation. Patients may respond to therapy for congestive heart failure while being prepared for surgical replacement of the aortic valve.

ACUTE MITRAL REGURGITATION. Acute mitral regurgitation usually occurs in the setting of acute myocardial infarction or infective endocarditis and may result from functional or anatomic lesions of the valve leaflets or of the chordae tendineae and papillary muscles. Increases in cardiac output, caused by exercise or excitement, may further augment mitral regurgitation, causing a sudden rise in left atrial pressure which in turn is responsible for paroxysmal pulmonary edema. Unexplained paroxysms of pulmonary edema in the patient with an acute myocardial infarction strongly suggest acute or intermittent mitral valve dysfunction. The clinical hallmark of mitral regurgitation is a blowing or harsh pansystolic murmur loudest at the apex and transmitted to the axilla. Rupture of a papillary muscle usually occurs in the first week after myocardial infarction but may occur later, and is then probably the result of silent reinfarction. Two-thirds of such patients die within 24 hours. However, with careful monitoring and treatment, these patients can sometimes be maintained for several months. The apical murmur is pansystolic, is transmitted to the axilla, and may be Grade III or IV, associated with a thrill. A loud S_3 and an S_4 may be present. The EKG generally shows an anterolateral or subendocardial infarction when the anterior papillary muscle is ruptured and an inferior or inferolateral infarction when the posterior muscle is involved. Treatment consists of conventional therapy for congestive heart failure and pulmonary edema until such time as angiography and mitral valve replacement can be performed. Vasodilators, such as nitroprusside, are useful in improving cardiac peformance and in achieving a balance between myocardial oxygen supply and demand.

Primary (nonarrhythmic) pump failure presenting as shock is most often due to acute myocardial infarction and loss of sufficient muscle mass to compromise cardiac performance significantly. The pathophysiology and treatment of congestive heart failure are described in Chapter 18.

Disturbances of Fluid Balance

SHOCK DUE TO FLUID LOSS. Hypovolemic shock may result from the loss of plasma or whole blood. Dehydration due to sweating, inadequate fluid intake, or losses resulting from vomiting or diarrhea can produce significant hypovolemia. Hemorrhage into body cavities, major muscle groups, or the intestine can lead to shock without visible blood loss. The physician must recognize the hypovolemic but compensated patient and he must detect occult blood loss occurring in the shock patient. The compensated patient with significant blood loss can be recognized by the presence of orthostatic changes in blood pressure. A decrease of 10 mm Hg systolic or more in the sitting as compared to the supine position indicates significant hypovolemia.

The location of inapparent bleeding must be aggressively sought. Percussion of the chest for dullness, palpation of the abdomen for rigidity, measurement of thigh girth, digital rectal examination, gastric aspiration, paracentesis with peritoneal lavage, and thoracentesis are used as circumstances dictate.

Initial hematocrit and hemoglobin determinations will be of little value in assessing the magnitude of blood loss in early shock since time is necessary for hemodilution to occur. Arterial blood gases will indicate the severity of acid–base disturbance, and serum lactate levels reflect the degree of anaerobic metabolism. Serum electrolyte and renal function tests provide useful baseline data.

Frequent vital signs, repeated physical examination and evaluation of the sensorium, hourly urinary output (via indwelling catheter), chest x-ray, EKG, and central venous pressure or pulmonary capillary wedge pressure serve as guides for fluid replacement. Replacement of fluid deficits takes precedence over the administration of vasopressor agents.

Choice of Fluids for Volume Replacement

Any fluid will improve perfusion at least transiently. The amount of fluid administered depends on the rate of ongoing loss and the magnitude or preexisting loss. Often, mild to moderate blood loss may be managed more safely and inexpensively with crystalloids or colloids than with blood itself. The most commonly employed solutions are crystalloids such as Ringer's lactate or normal saline. These are often referred to as "balanced" electrolyte solutions because their composition is approximately isotonic with the extracellular fluid. These fluids do not contain macromolecules and they do not contribute to the plasma oncotic pressure since they remain within the vascular space for only a brief period before escaping into the interstitium.

It is often said that crystalloids leave the circulation so rapidly that their administration is likely to cause pulmonary edema. There is evidence, however, that colloidal solutions also leak from pulmonary capillaries so that any fluid, if not given with appropriate monitoring, has the ability to produce interstitial pulmonary edema.

There is often reluctance to administer Ringer's lactate to a patient with lactic acidosis. The sodium lactate in this solution is not lactic acid, but rather a metabolic precursor of bicarbonate in the liver. As long as hepatic circulation is adequate, sodium lactate is metabolized to bicarbonate and serves an alkalinizing function.

Fluid Replacement

Generally, fluid replacement begins with infusion of a crystalloid. If the patient fails to stabilize, one must assume that either a major extracellular fluid deficit existed or blood loss is continuing.

Colloidal solutions contain higher molecular weight molecules that cannot readily diffuse across intact capillary membranes. Consequently, they remain within the vascular compartment for longer periods. By increasing plasma oncotic pressure, they delay loss of crystalloid into the interstitium. If capillary membranes are not damaged, they may attract interstitial fluid into the intravascular space.

Dextran is available in molecular weights of 40,000 and 70,000. These solutions are effective in volume expansion, but serious problems are associated with their use. They may cause anaphylactic reactions and renal failure, interfere with blood typing and cross matching, and produce a severe hemorrhagic diathesis.

Preparations of human plasma protein do not have the potential dangers of dextran. Human serum albumin is available as a 5 percent solution. A salt-poor 25 percent concentrate of human serum albumin is also available but is very expensive. Plasma protein fraction (Plasmanate) is essentially human plasma with fibrinogen and gamma globulins removed. Paradoxic hypotension has been observed following the administration of 5 percent plasma protein fraction. Hypotension may result from the presence of vasoactive amines or sodium acetate, a potent vasodilator. Albumin or crystalloid is preferred in the majority of clinical situations requiring volume expansion. The use of plasma protein fraction should be restricted to specific indications such as in association with transfusion of 5 or more units of packed red blood cells when whole blood is not available or in the rapid correction of severely low serum albumin levels. Both human serum albumin and plasma protein solutions are heat treated to kill hepatitis virus. Only blood is capable of transporting oxygen. With major blood loss, whole blood is required for replacement.

Shock Due to Fluid Maldistribution

There are a number of conditions in which shock is due to maldistribution of the intravascular fluid, the fluids ordinarily contained within the vascular tree having "leaked" to the interstitium or so-called "third space." Common to all such conditions is massive injury to capillary endothelium resulting in loss of integrity of this delicate layer and leakage of fluid. Relatively large volumes of fluids are usually required for correction of hypovolemia. Pharmacologic intervention aimed at redistributing body fluids is less effective.

In sensitive individuals, exposure to an allergen may be followed by an anaphylactic reaction with profound hypotension, wheezing, and cyanosis. Chemical mediators including histamine, slow-reacting substances, and plasma kinins play a role in producing increased vascular permeability and a critical reduction of plasma volume resulting in hemoconcentration and shock with or without angioedema of the upper respiratory tract. Epinephrine hydrochloride, 0.5 to 1.0 ml of a 1:1000 solution, should be given subcutaneously or intramuscularly immediately. In the presence of severe hypotension, epinephrine may be given intravenously along with large amounts of crystalloid and colloid solutions.

Massive fluid and protein losses occur in burn patients. Meticulous attention to maintenance of the circulating volume and electrolyte balance is essential for survival. Crush injuries in which there has been prolonged pressure to a limb may result in severe injury to muscle and other tissue. When the pressure is relieved, the limb swells from extravasation of red cells and plasma through damaged blood vessels. Myoglobin and other products of damaged tissue leak into the circulation. Hypotension, shock, and renal failure may follow. Treatment of these injuries includes restoration of the circulating volume with blood, plasma, or crystalloid solutions to maintain a urine flow of 75 to 100 ml/hr. Alkalinization of the urine may prevent precipitation of pigments within the renal tubules.

Drug overdose with a variety of sedative agents, most notably barbiturates, may result in capillary endothelial damage allowing volume loss from the central circulation. Treatment consists of supportive measures including volume restoration and pressor agents when hypotension is not reversed by volume restoration alone.

Spinal cord injury can produce a functional sympathectomy, which may be difficult to diagnose in the patient with multiple injuries. The presence of warm extremities in the patient with neurologic deficit and hypotension should alert the physician to the possibility of sympathetic injury. Treatment consists of intravenous fluids, vasopressors, and elastic support wraps to the limbs.

Perforation of a viscus, peritonitis, and acute pancreatitis may be accompanied by profound hypotension due to "third space" fluid losses. Expansion of the circulating volume is essential to patient survival.

Sepsis is the third most common cause of clinical shock, after hemorrhage and acute myocardial infarction. Shock associated with sepsis can be subdivided into two subgroups: 1) normal or high resistance shock; and 2) low resistance shock which is associated with inflammatory vasodilation and arteriovenous shunting.[14] Low resistance shock is more often observed in the early febrile stages of gram-negative shock, in gram-positive sepsis, and with peritonitis and pneumonitis. Arterial resistance is decreased and cardiac output is usually increased. High resistance shock is most commonly seen in the later stages of septic shock. The two types of septic shock are not mutually exclusive. Gram-negative sepsis in particular may initially present with increased cardiac output and low peripheral resistance only to progress to high resistance shock with low cardiac output and high total peripheral resistance.

The gram-negative bacteria are most commonly responsible for septic shock, although septic shock may follow infection with fungi, rickettsiae, viruses, and gram-positive bacteria. Bacteremia is rarely complicated by shock in persons under the age of 40, except in pregnant women and neonates. Manipulative procedures, diabetes, chronic liver disease, blood dyscrasias, and treatment with corticosteroids, immunosuppressive drugs, and antimetabolites predispose to bacteremia and shock.

Bacteremia typically begins with a shaking chill followed by fever between 2 and 24 hours after mechanical manipulation or surgery. Impaired mental status may result from reduced cerebral perfusion. Vomiting and diarrhea are frequent findings. Leukopenia and thrombocytopenia may precede leukocytosis. Abnormalities of the ST segment and T wave reflect a reduction in coronary perfusion. Sudden changes in behavior and personality, including organic psychosis, may be associated with decreased cerebral blood flow. The blood pressure will be found to be in the 80/50 range. The sensorium may be further clouded as the sequelae of hypoperfusion appear. The skin becomes pale, cool, and moist. Vomiting and diarrhea are common. Renal function is impaired and renal failure may follow.

Endotoxin, a lipopolysaccharide common to the cell wall of all gram-negative bacteria, effects a redistribution of blood within the vascular bed in such a way as to preclude the maintenance of an adequate circulating volume. Consequences of this pooling include poor tissue oxygenation resulting in anaerobic metabolism with lactic acidemia and eventually loss of cellular integrity.

Gram-negative infections are the most commonly encountered life-threatening infections in patients in general hospitals. The mortality in gram-negative bacteremia approximates 40 percent, while in patients in whom shock develops as a consequence of the bacteremia, the death rate ranges from 50 to 80 percent. Appropriate cultures of blood, urine, sputum, and wound exudates and prompt administration of appropriate antibiotics are essential for survival. When cultures and sensitivity studies are not yet available, antibiotics are administered on an empiric basis. The circulation is maintained by administration of fluids and pressor agents. Careful hemodynamic monitoring with central venous pulmonary capillary wedge pressure and intra-arterial pressures is essential to optimal management. The use of corticosteroids is discussed later.

Intravenous Lines

Access to the central circulation is imperative in the shock patient. Indwelling catheters within the external jugular vein, internal jugular vein, subclavian vein, or cephalic vein may be utilized for the measurement of central venous or pulmonary capillary wedge pressure, the passage of a temporary pacing wire, and the administration of blood products, intravenous fluids, and medications. Peripheral veins may be utilized for the administration of fluids. The number of intravenous lines required depends on the urgency of the situation and the type of fluids to be administered. The physician must be aware of the potential dangers of central line placement. Depending upon the entry site, complications may include pneumothorax, subcutaneous emphysema, hemothorax, arterial puncture, air embolus, catheter embolus, hemorrhage, cardiac irritability, or tamponade.

Strict asepsis of all intravenous lines and devices must be vigilantly maintained. It will not benefit a patient to survive an episode of shock if he is to be subjected to avoidable sepsis resulting from careless intravenous techniques.

The Central Venous Pressure

The central venous pressure (CVP) can guide fluid replacement in the hypovolemic patient. It is an indicator of the relationship between the volume of blood which enters the right heart and the effectiveness with which the heart ejects that volume. The CVP may, however, be paradoxically normal in the elderly patient with coronary artery disease and elevated left ventricular end diastolic pressure in the presence of significant blood loss. Nonetheless, when the CVP approaches zero, one may conclude that significant hypovolemia is present.

While single determinations of the CVP may not be of value in establishing a significant decrease in blood volume, serial measurements may reliably assist in the management of patients with fluid loss.

The method of Shubin and Weil[11] offers a practical guide to fluid replacement. CVP measurements are obtained during a 10-minute observation period. Fluid is then given intravenously. If the CVP is less than 12 cm H_2O, the fluid is infused at a rate of 20 ml/min for 10 minutes. If the CVP increases by more than 5 cm H_2O above the initial reading, the infusion is discontinued. If the CVP does not exceed the control pressure by more than 2 cm H_2O at the end of 10 minutes, an additional 200 ml of fluid is administered over 10 minutes. If the CVP increases by 2 to 5 cm H_2O over the initial pressure and continues to exceed the control pressure by more than 2 cm H_2O after the second 10-minute observation period, the subsequent aliquot of fluid is reduced to 100 ml over the next 10 minutes. The process is then repeated. A total of several liters of fluid may be required to restore fully effective circulation.

Progressive increase in the CVP indicates overloading and need for reduction in the rate of fluid infusion. If the initial pressure ranges from 12 to 20 cm H_2O, the rate of infusion is modified to deliver only 10 ml/min during each of the 10-minute challenge periods. Should the CVP increase by more than 5 cm H_2O, phlebotomy or diuretics may be indicated to prevent pulmonary edema.

With the awareness that the CVP is more appropriately considered as a trend indicator in the treatment of hypovolemia than an absolute indicator of the degrees of volume depletion, errors in fluid administration can be avoided. The tip of the CVP catheter must of course lie within the thorax. Measurements obtained from a catheter placed in a peripheral vein may be misleading and should never be used as a guide to volume replacement. If the catheter tip is within the thorax, respiratory changes in pressure should be observed. Documentation of the tip position should be obtained by x-ray. If blood cannot be easily withdrawn from the catheter, pressure measurements may be inaccurate. The venous pressure must be measured from a standard reference point on the patient's chest. The angle of Louis, which is situated between the corpus and manubrium sterni and is about 5 cm above the middle of the right atrium, is a convenient reference point. A sudden change in the CVP without an apparent change in clinical status strongly suggests a technical problem within the monitoring system. The catheter may have become clogged, advanced into the right ventricle, or withdrawn into a peripheral vein. Tricuspid regurgitation will give high pressure readings unrelated to the degree of volume expansion. Cannon "a" waves associated with atrioventricular dissociation and positive pressure ventilation will elevate CVP readings. CVP measurements should be obtained with the patient briefly disconnected from the respirator. Patients with severe pneumonia, chronic lung disease, or pulmonary emboli may also have spuriously high CVP readings relative to their volume status.

Pulmonary Artery Catheterization

In the face of myocardial failure, CVP measurements may be grossly misleading because of left ventricular dysfunction. Therefore, a flow-directed, balloon-tipped catheter may be introduced into a peripheral vein through a cutdown or into the external jugular or internal jugular vein percutaneously, and advanced to the level of the superior vena cava.[12] The balloon is then inflated and the catheter is advanced through the right atrium, across the tricuspid valve, and into the right ventricle. In most patients, the catheter can be floated into a peripheral pulmonary artery and the pulmonary capillary wedge pressure obtained. This measurement reflects the pressure in the left atrium. In diastole, the left atrial pressure is essentially equal to left ventricular pressure. Left ventricular end diastolic pressure (LVEDP) serves as an index of preload and helps delineate the relative position of the left ventricle on its Starling curve. If there is clinical evidence of inadequate tissue perfusion, and the pulmonary artery wedge pressure is borderline (12 to 20 mm Hg), patients may be challenged with fluid. If the pulmonary artery wedge pressure is elevated (20 mm Hg or greater), treatment with a diuretic or afterload reducing agent may be indicated. In those patients in whom the catheter cannot be floated into the wedge position, the pulmonary artery end diastolic pressure (PAEDP) may be used instead as an indicator of mean left atrial and left ventricular end diastolic pressure (LVEDP).

A comparison of the pulmonary artery wedge pressure with the pulmonary artery diastolic pressure is of value in determining the presence of obstructive pulmonary vascular disease or pulmonary embolus. A difference of 5 to 10 mm Hg in these two pressures strongly suggests the presence of one of these entities.

Pulmonary artery wedge pressures can be expected to be elevated in the presence of significant mitral stenosis. In this situation, left atrial end diastolic pressure may be higher than the LVEDP, thereby misleading the physician as to the degree of volume expansion and competence of the left ventricle.

Cardiac output may be obtained utilizing thermistor balloon-tipped, flow-directed catheters and the thermodilution technique of cardiac output. One may then measure the pulmonary artery wedge pressure, pulmonary artery systolic pressure, pulmonary artery diastolic pressure, central venous pressure, and cardiac output. The systemic and pulmonary vascular resistances may be calculated. With this information, the physician is more able to diagnose the underlying derangement in fluid balance or myocardial performance and to ascertain the effects of various pharmacologic interventions.

As is true with all monitoring devices, the physician must be aware of the limitations of the equipment and technique. The catheter position must be verified by fluoroscopy or A-P chest x-ray. Transducers must be accurately balanced and checked frequently. The catheter lumen must remain patent and free of small clots or pressures will be damped. The catheter must not be allowed to remain in the wedge position for more than the time required to obtain pressure readings, lest pulmonary infarction occur. Careful asepsis must be maintained. Pressure readings at variance with prior serial readings should lead the physician to suspect equipment malfunction and to validate its performance before proceeding with therapeutic intervention.

Drug Therapy of Shock

Tissue perfusion is the predominant concern in treating the clinical shock syndrome, and all pharmacologic manipulations must be directed to achieving this end with minimal drug-related toxicity.[13] Drug therapy begins where fluid therapy leaves off. Support of blood pressure is a major goal initially. The physician must understand that blood pressure alone is not a reliable indicator of tissue perfusion. However, once a blood pressure is obtained and maintained, attention can then be given to the reliability of the numerical reading and to the adequacy of vital organ perfusion as evidenced by the clinical correlates of level of consciousness, skin color and temperature, and urine flow. Once he has restored some level of blood pressure, the physician's work has only begun, and patient survival relates as much to subsequent therapy as it does to the initial effort.

Those functions amenable to manipulation include stroke volume, heart rate, and peripheral resistance which are closely interrelated as follows:

1. Cardiac output = stroke volume × heart rate
2. Systemic blood pressure = cardiac output × peripheral resistance

Combining these two relationships:

3. Systemic blood pressure = (stroke volume × heart rate) · (total peripheral resistance)

Pharmacologic intervention almost always affects more than one of these functions. Each drug affects them in its own particular fashion, and it is for this reason that the basic pharmacology of the commonly employed agents must be understood by the physician.

The stroke volume is dependent upon the filling pressure of the heart and the contractile force generated by the myocardium. To develop optimal contraction, the heart must have an adequate filling pressure. This phenomenon is described by the well-known Frank-Starling relationship. In the patient manifesting the shock syndrome, strict attention must be given to the adequacy of the circulating blood volume. Blood replacement or other means of volume expansion is therefore critical if the heart is to generate adequate pressure to achieve adequate flow through the vital coronary, cerebral, renal, and splanchnic circulations. The central venous pressure is valuable in assessing the degree of volume expansion. Catheterization of the pulmonary artery with a balloon-tipped, flow-directed catheter may be expected to give more reliable information in the patient with primary cardiac disease or injury. Drugs that increase the contractile state of the myocardium and hence increase the stroke volume include digitalis, ionized calcium, isoproterenol, and epinephrine.

Digitalis is useful in the patient who manifests signs of congestive heart failure, rapid atrial fibrillation, or sinus tachycardia resulting from congestive heart failure. Its effect on increasing myocardial contractility is, however, small compared to that of norepinephrine, dopamine, or isoproterenol (Table 145-1).

TABLE 145-1
Effects of Dopamine, Isoproterenol, and Norepinephrine

	Isopro-terenol	Norepine-phrine	Dopamine
Usual dose	1–5 µg/min	1–5 µg/min	5–50 µg/kg/min
Increases heart force	++++	+++	+++
Increases heart rate	++++	+	++
Causes arrhythmias	++++	++	+
Dilates bronchioles	++++	0	+
Constricts skin, renal, splanchnic vessels	0	++++	++ (Generally only in doses over 20 µg/kg/min)
Dilates skeletal muscle vessels	++++	0	++
Dilates renal, splanchnic, and coronary vessels	±	0	++++ (In doses 5–20 µg/kg/min)
Dilates the pupils	±	++	++++
Maintains central circulation during cardiac arrest	0	++++	++ (In doses above 100 µg/kg/min)
Extends myocardial infarct	++++	++	++

Each of these drugs has a half-life in the circulation of 3 minutes, so the dose can be adjusted rapidly for optimal effect. It is important to regulate the infusion with a pump or by very careful observation. It is especially important to connect the drug infusion directly at the central venous catheter so that extension tubing filled with potent drug will not be flushed into the circulation during determination of a venous pressure or administration of another drug.

All three drugs increase the oxygen utilization of the heart in proportion to the increase in heart force. For patients with myocardial infarction, norepinephrine or dopamine are preferred because they maintain a slow heart rate and high diastolic coronary perfusion pressure. Isoproterenol in these patients may cause a shift to anaerobic metabolism and extension of the infarct. Isoproterenol does not dilate the renal, splanchnic, or skin blood vessels; it produces high blood flow through skeletal muscles, and this may not be an appropriate distribution of blood flow in shock. Isoproterenol is advantageous because it lacks the potent vasoconstriction associated with norepinephrine, thereby avoiding ischemia of the kidney and gut. In some patients it does produce acceptable slow heart rates and near normal diastolic aortic pressures. The disadvantageous generalized vasoconstriction seen with norepinephrine can be antagonized by simultaneous infusion of phentolamine (Regitine, 5 to 30 mg/hr) or by chlorpromazine (Thorazine, 5 to 25 mg IV 2 to 4 hr). Dopamine, the immediate metabolic precursor of norepinephrine, has a unique direct effect of dilating the renal, splanchnic, and coronary vessels at low doses (2.5 to 10 μg/kg/min), increasing heart force without tachycardia or arrhythmias at medium doses (5 to 50 μg/kg/min), and causing generalized peripheral vasoconstriction (possibly due to metabolism to norepinephrine) at high doses (above 20 to 100 μg/kg/min).

The peripheral resistance can be dramatically increased by the administration of norepinephrine or high-dose dopamine, which act primarily as alpha-adrenergic agents (Table 145–2). Norepinephrine is the more potent of these agents and is the drug of choice in the patient in whom no blood pressure is obtainable in the face of an adequate cardiac rhythm. Norepinephrine is also a more toxic agent than dopamine, and its use must be limited to the briefest period possible to avoid the renal and splanchnic ischemia. Dopamine is the preferred agent when prolonged blood pressure support is anticipated. It has the additional theoretic benefit of protecting the renal, splanchnic, and coronary circulations by selectively increasing the circulation to these areas through stimulation of specific dopaminergic receptors. Dopamine increases urine flow, induces natriuresis, and may be of particular value in the patient with fluid overload, congestive heart failure, or myocardial infarction. Both norepinephrine and dopamine modestly increase heart rate and the force of myocardial contraction.

The peripheral resistance can be dramatically reduced by such agents as sublingual nitroglycerin, hydralazine, and sodium nitroprusside. These drugs are used in the pharmacologic management of patients in cardiogenic shock or after cardiac surgery to reduce the pressure against which the heart must eject a given stroke volume, thereby lowering the heart's work and oxygen requirements. The use of afterload reducing agents in the treatment of shock is both unproven and extremely hazardous, as these agents may produce profound and sustained hypotension even in normotensive patients. Their role in combating the vasoconstriction and depressed myocardial peformance which often accompany shock from all causes must await further study and evaluation.

Isoproterenol is the most potent agent for increasing the force of myocardial contraction (Table 145–2). It is also the most arrhythmogenic and the agent most likely to be inactivated by acidosis. Isoproterenol, a pure beta-adrenergic agent, increases

---

┌─ **TABLE 145–2** ─────────────────────────────
Use of Drugs in the Treatment of Shock

	Objective	Dilution	Dose (IV)	Toxicity	Comments
Atropine	Increase HR*	None	0.5 mg q 5 min 2.0 mg max	Tachycardia Ventricular fibrillation	Use only when bradycardia is accompanied by hypotension or rates below 40/min

* HR = heart rate.

───── **TABLE 145-2 (cont.)** ─────

	Objective	Dilution	Dose (IV)	Toxicity	Comments
Isoproterenol	Increase HR Increase HF†	1.0 mg in 500 ml D_5W = 2 $\mu g/ml$	2–20 $\mu g/min$	Tachycardia Tachyarrhythmias Ventricular fibrillation	Markedly increases myocardial O_2 consumption; contraindicated in acute MI except for control of rate while placing pacer
Calcium Cl or gluconate	Increase HF	10%	5.0 ml chloride 10 ml gluconate	Bradycardia Sinus arrest	May aggravate digitalis toxicity; will precipitate with $NaHCO_3$
Epinephrine	Increase BP Increase HR Increase HF Increase TPR‡	1:10,000	5 ml = 5 mg q 5 min	Tachycardia	Inactivated by $NaHCO_3$; may be given by intracardiac injection but with risks of tamponade, laceration of coronary artery, pneumothorax, interruption of CPR. Intramyocardial injection may produce intractable V-fib. May be given into endotracheal tube or sublingual if no IV available
Norepinephrine	Increase BP Increase TPR	8.0 mg base in 500 ml D_5W = 16 $\mu g/ml$	8–32 $\mu g/min$ to achieve 90 mm Hg systolic	Constricts skin, renal, splanchnic vessels	Always use large bore catheter in central vein. Infiltration produces sloughing which should be treated by local injection of phentolamine. Renal failure and mesenteric or hepatic infarction may follow prolonged administration

† HF = force of contraction.
‡ TPR = total peripheral resistance.

(Continued)

── **TABLE 145-2 (cont.)** ──────────────────────────

	Objective	Dilution	Dose (IV)	Toxicity	Comments
Dopamine	Increase BP Increase TPR Increase HR Increase renal blood flow	10 × wt in kg = mg to be added to 1 liter to achieve 10 μg/kg/ml	2.5–10 μg/kg/min to increase renal blood flow; 20–50 μg/kg/min to support BP	Vasoconstriction	Renal effects are dose related (2.5–10 μg/kg/min); less potent for BP support than norepinephrine
Sodium bicarbonate	Correct acidosis	—	1 mEq/kg initially, then ½ dose q 10 min	Alkalosis, hypernatremia, hyperosmolality, myocardial depression	May inactivate other drugs if mixed in same bottle or tubing. Adequate ventilation and frequent ABGs are essential to avoid elevated Pco_2 with myocardial depression and increased serum osmolality
Lidocaine	Suppress ventricular arrhythmias	1 g in 250 ml D_5W = 4 mg/ml	50–100 mg (or 1 mg/kg) IV bolus followed immediately by infusion of 1–4 mg/min	CNS depression, seizures, paresthesias, disorientation, agitation, heart block	CHF predisposes to high plasma levels and early toxicity. Total bolus injection in excess of 300 mg predisposes to toxicity. Repeat administration can produce complete heart block or abolish nodal rhythm
Propranolol	Control recurrent V-tach. or V-fib.	—	1.0 mg over 5 min not to exceed 10 mg total	Acute CHF, bronchospasm	Use only after lidocaine failure. May worsen bradyarrhythmias or heart block. Use with extreme caution in patients known to have bronchospasm
Morphine	Produce analgesia, decrease pulmonary congestion	As required to produce 1 mg/ml	Up to 4 mg initially, then 2 mg q 5 min	Respiratory depression, hypotension, vomiting	Titrate small doses at frequent intervals. Toxic effects antagonized by naloxone (0.4–0.8 mg IV)

blood flow through peripheral muscle and may thereby significantly decrease circulating blood volume. The resulting effect on blood pressure is dependent on the balance achieved between increased contractility, increased heart rate, and increased skeletal muscle blood flow. The blood pressure in a given patient receiving an infusion of isoproterenol may increase, remain unchanged, or decrease depending upon the overall effect of this agent. The physician must not be misled by the warm, pink appearance of the patient receiving isoproterenol. The vital perfusion pressures may be unacceptably low in spite of the patient's appearance.

Epinephrine has both alpha- and beta-adrenergic action. The drug has proven utility in the setting of cardiac arrest, although it may be less useful for long-term support of the circulation. Clinically, epinephrine elevates perfusion pressure generated during closed chest cardiac massage, improves myocardial contractility, stimulates spontaneous contractions, and facilitates conversion of fine fibrillation to a coarse one more amenable to termination by countershock.

While pressor agents, norepinephrine, epinephrine, isoproterenol, and dopamine are valuable for temporary support of the circulation, it must be remembered that no patient presents actually suffering from an acute deficiency of a pressor agent. That is to say, these agents are not curative. Each of them has significant toxicity, and it is incumbent upon the physician to initiate a plan for withdrawal of these drugs almost as soon as the patient has achieved some degree of cardiovascular stability. At best, these agents can be thought of as buying time for the basic physiologic derangements to be corrected. The optimal dose of each of these agents is the lowest one that will achieve the desired effect, administered over the briefest period possible. Mechanisms of action differ for each agent, and they are sometimes used in combination. If their therapeutic effects are additive, so are their toxicities.

Each of the pressor agents functions within a fairly narrow pH range. Hence, they cannot be expected to be of use in the patient who is severely acidotic and hypoxemic. Proper ventilatory support and the intermittent administration of sodium bicarbonate may facilitate the actions of these agents and decrease the occurrence of pressor-induced cardiac arrhythmias.

The patient in shock rapidly manifests metabolic and respiratory acidosis. Hypoperfusion and subsequent hypoxemia result in the generation of lactic acid, while ventilatory failure results in CO_2 retention and respiratory acidosis. Effective ventilation of the lungs is essential for the excretion of CO_2 as well as for oxygenation and is absolutely requisite for the management of the acidosis of shock. The importance of prompt and adequate ventilation cannot be overemphasized.

Administration of intravenous sodium bicarbonate can be a useful adjunct in managing the metabolic component of acidosis. Bicarbonate combines with excess hydrogen ion to produce water and carbon dioxide by the following reaction:

$$HCO_3{}^- + H^+ \rightleftharpoons H_2CO_3 \rightleftharpoons CO_2 + H_2O$$

However, bicarbonate administration raises the pH of the blood only if the CO_2 produced is excreted through the lung.[9] Administration of sodium bicarbonate in the absence of adequate ventilation does not result in a rise in arterial pH but only in substantial increases in arterial P_{CO_2} and serum osmolality.

Elevation of the P_{CO_2} may aggravate intracellular acidosis and result in further depression of myocardial performance. Therefore, sodium bicarbonate should be given in small amounts at appropriate intervals to allow recovery from an initial period of depressed myocardial function resulting from increased P_{CO_2} consequent to bicarbonate administration. Blood gas measurements should be made frequently. The adequacy of ventilation must be reassessed prior to the repeated administration of sodium bicarbonate.

Corticosteroids

The use of corticosteroids in the treatment of shock remains controversial. A recent study demonstrated a significant reduction in mortality in the group of patients with septic shock treated with steroids.[10] The suggested dose is 3 mg/kg of dexamethasone or 30 mg/kg of methylprednisolone. The dose may be repeated in 4 hours if shock persists. The evidence does not support the routine use of steroids in all patients in shock.

CHAPTER 146

Respiratory Emergencies
WARREN R. SUMMER

Acute respiratory failure is one of the most common problems encountered in the emergency room, intensive care unit, or acute hospital. It affects all age groups and is a major cause of mortality. Acute respiratory failure may be defined as any sudden condition producing a fall in Pa_{O_2} to 50 mm Hg or below or a rise in Pa_{CO_2} to 50 mm Hg or above. These are arbitrary levels and should be adjusted when chronic hypoxemia and hypercapnia are known to have been present.

The diagnosis of respiratory failure is made in two steps: 1) the recognition of acute respiratory distress or the presence of a condition which may predispose to respiratory failure; and 2) confirmation of respiratory failure by blood gas analysis. Clinical signs of hypoxemia (such as cyanosis) or hypercapnia (such as papilledema) are unreliable and are often such late indicators of respiratory failure that their presence should not be required before initiating emergency therapy.

Respiratory arrest, defined as complete cessation of respiratory function, is the most drastic form of acute respiratory failure. Fortunately, in adults the respiratory system, unlike the cardiovascular system, infrequently ceases effective function suddenly; status asthmaticus, neuromuscular diseases, upper airway obstruction, and severe glutethimide intoxication are exceptions.

Rapid diagnosis of acute respiratory failure depends in part on recognition of the conditions producing insufficient respiratory function (Table 146–l). The history and examination frequently provide the information most helpful for defining the pathogenesis of the respiratory failure. Known (or suspected) drug ingestion or grossly altered levels of consciousness point to a problem in the control of respiration, whereas neuromuscular abnormalities suggest an inability to reduce pleural pressure. Stridor, supraclavicular retraction, wheezing, and rales suggest disease of the airways.

Many causes of acute respiratory failure are due to small insults added to a background of severe musculoskeletal, neuromuscular, airway, parenchymal, or pulmonary vascular disease. An acute exacerbation of chronic obstructive pulmonary disease is an example and represents one of the most common causes of acute respiratory failure. Increasingly, however,

acute respiratory failure is being observed in patients with previously normal lungs. Many of these cases represent the adult respiratory distress syndrome.

Comprehensive management of respiratory failure secondary to chronic obstructive lung disease, cor pulmonale, drug overdose, neuromuscular disease, metabolic disease, and adult respiratory distress syndrome are discussed in Chapter 36. This section will be devoted to the initial recognition and emergency management of acute respiratory failure, stressing immediate life-support measures necessary to prevent hypoxic injury or death.

Clinical Recognition of Acute Respiratory Failure Secondary to Factors Affecting Respiratory Control or Neuromuscular Performance

The main causes of respiratory center depression are trauma, generalized intracranial disease, and drugs.[33] Isolated damage to the brain stem may result from vascular lesions or tumors. The absence of a gag or cough reflex and marked depression in the level of consciousness or coma is usually present when a patient has any degree of respiratory failure secondary to central nervous system (CNS) disease. Severe cerebral edema and herniation of the medulla through the foramen magnum usually result in sudden apnea. The latter patients rarely, if ever, recover neurologic function even when respiration is supported by artificial means.

Since the underlying lung is often normal in acute conditions depressing respiratory control or neuromuscular output, hypoxemia is usually not severe. Tachycardia, hypertension, and tachypnea are frequently present unless these functions have been influenced by cerebral edema or drug overdose. With severe respiratory failure, bradycardia and hypotension often occur.

The drugs most commonly associated with respiratory center depression are hypnotics and opiates. The diagnosis of drug intoxication is often facilitated by the history, the presence of empty medicine bottles or containers of commercial products found with the patient, and a history of previous suicide attempts. Further evidence of ingestion may be obtained by finding partially digested pills during gastric lavage. Barbiturates reduce the depth of respi-

┌─────────────────────────────────────┐
TABLE 146-1
Conditions Associated with Acute Respiratory Failure

A. Factors Affecting Control of Neuromuscular Function
I. Drugs and Toxins
Anesthetics and muscle relaxants
Antibiotics
Anticholinergics
Anticholinesterases
Botulism
Opiates
Sedatives
Tetanus

II. Endocrine and Metabolic Disorders
Acidosis
Alkalosis
Hypocalcemia
Hypokalemia
Hypophosphatemia
Hypothyroidism

III. Musculoskeletal Disease
Ankylosing spondylitis
Kyphoscoliosis (idiopathic, poliomyelitis, tuberculosis)
Marfan syndrome
Mucopolysaccharidoses

IV. Neuromuscular Disease
Anterior horn cell disease (poliomyelitis, amyotrophic lateral sclerosis)
Brain storm injury (infarct, tumor) diaphragmatic paralysis (usually bilateral)
Increased intracranial pressure (tumor, trauma, hypoxia, hemorrhage, thrombosis)
Multiple sclerosis
Muscular dystrophy
Myasthenia gravis
Parkinson's disease
Polymyositis
Polyneuritis
Porphyria
Rhabdomyolysis and myoglobinuria
Spinal cord injury (tumor, trauma, vascular, surgical)
Status epilepticus

B. Alteration in Pulmonary Mechanics
I. Airway Obstruction
Upper airway
    Allergic
    Chemical
    Foreign body
    Hemorrhage
    Infection—pharyngeal abscess, epiglottitis, infectious mononucleosis, diphtheria
    Hereditary angioneurotic edema

TABLE 146-1 (cont.)

B. Alteration in Pulmonary Mechanics (cont.)
I. Airway Obstruction (cont.)
    Obesity—hypoventilation syndrome (control of breathing may be important)
    Postintubation
    Rheumatoid arthritis
    Tracheal malacia or stenosis
    Trauma
    Tumor (intraluminal or extrinsic compression)
    Vocal cord paralysis
Lower airway
    Anaphylaxis
    Asthma
    Bronchiolitis
    Chronic obstructive pulmonary disease

II. Parenchymal Dysfunction
Extensive pneumonia
    Bacterial—tuberculosis (acute and chronic)
    Fungal
    Parasitic
    Viral
Pulmonary edema
    Chemical injury
        Aspiration of gastric contents
        Inhalation injury
        Immersion
        Oxygen toxicity
        Paraquat ingestion
    Hydrostatic
        Cardiogenic pulmonary edema (multiple causes; see Chapter 19)
    Increase capillary leak
        Nonspecific (adult respiratory distress syndrome; see Chapter 36)
Pulmonary fibrosis or interstitial pneumonitis
    Idiopathic (extrinsic allergic alveolitis, farmer's lung, etc.)
    Pneumoconiosis (multiple causes)
    Radiation therapy
    Sarcoidosis
    Tuberculosis
Intrapulmonary hemorrhage

III. Vascular
Pulmonary embolus
    Air
    Foreign body
    Parasitic
    Thrombosis
    Tumor

IV. Trauma
Flail chest
Postoperative
Pulmonary contusion

ration but have little effect on its rate. Often, moderate hypotension, hypothermia, and reduction in metabolic rate are present. As a result of the reduced CO_2 production, the patients may have only minor elevations in Pa_{CO_2} in spite of very small tidal volumes and markedly reduced minute ventilation. Opioid overdose usually results in the triad of coma, pinpoint pupils, and depressed respiration. A prompt response to naloxone is diagnostic. The respiratory depression is characterized by marked reduction in respiratory rate. The high Pa_{CO_2} and acute respiratory acidosis often make cyanosis more obvious in these patients. Fresh or old needle marks over the forearms or lower legs support the diagnosis of opiate overdose. A further discussion of physical signs suggesting the presence of specific poisons is given in Chapter 151.

Intracranial disease or trauma sufficient to produce respiratory failure is usually associated with gross neurologic changes in addition to altered levels of consciousness. Neuromuscular, metabolic, and endocrine disturbances associated with respiratory failure are usually identified by a relatively prolonged history of symptoms and abnormal physical findings. Electrocardiographic findings may be helpful in diagnosing gross metabolic derangements. The chest x-ray is helpful in ruling out underlying lung disease. A relatively clear chest x-ray with normal or elevated diaphragms (hypoinflation) suggests altered respiratory control or reduced neuromuscular strength as the mechanism of respiratory failure.

The ultimate diagnosis of acute respiratory failure secondary to altered respiratory control or ineffective chest cage function is determined by arterial blood gas measurements.

In an awake patient, diagnosis of respiratory muscle weakness may be confirmed by measuring the patient's ability to generate inspiratory force and the patient's ability to reduce the arterial P_{CO_2} upon command.[20] Most patients with severe parenchymal or airway abnormalities can reduce their P_{CO_2} to some extent upon request. In a patient with markedly altered consciousness and an elevated P_{CO_2}, it is sometimes difficult to tell whether the elevated P_{CO_2} resulted from the CNS depression or was the cause of it. However, the underlying CNS status will become apparent as the P_{CO_2} is corrected during appropriate respiratory therapy.

Drug overdose is the most common cause of respiratory failure due to altered control or neuromuscular function. There are few specific antidotes for drug overdosage. Therefore, except for certain drugs, such as opiates, it is more important to establish that one is dealing with an intoxication than initially to identify the specific drug or toxin. The essence of management is to anticipate and prevent complications. Morbidity and mortality result from excitation or depression of the nervous system leading to respiratory failure, aspiration of gastric contents, or cardiovascular collapse.

Principles of Management of Acute Respiratory Failure Secondary to Factors Affecting Control of Respiration or Neuromuscular Performance

The treatment of respiratory failure from central nervous system, neuromuscular, metabolic, and endocrine conditions depends on the severity and rapidity of development of the respiratory failure. There are certain general principles in the management of these patients. Immediate therapy should be directed toward reversal of hypoxemia and prevention of respiratory arrest. Initiation of emergency therapy should begin at the first suspicion of respiratory failure and should be continued until arterial blood gas levels establish the presence or absence of this diagnosis. Always, the first priority is securing a patent airway and maintaining adequate oxygenation.

As previously mentioned, the lung is usually not primarily affected under these circumstances and exchanges oxygen normally. However, potential anoxia from superimposed aspiration of gastric contents, pneumonia, or extremely high alveolar carbon dioxide tension may produce irreversible anoxic injury in minutes. Therefore, supplemental oxygen should be administered immediately. Initially, 3 to 4 liters per minute via nasal prongs or 30 to 40 percent oxygen via mask can be started. An arterial blood gas should be obtained as soon as the cardiopulmonary picture appears transiently stable. It is better to begin supplemental oxygen early than wait to be surprised by a dangerously low Pa_{CO_2}.

It is equally important to assure cardiovascular and CNS stability, as described elsewhere. The following discussion will outline a general approach to the patient with altered respiratory control or neuromuscular performance.

A superficial determination of the level of consciousness should be obtained immediately. If the patient is comatose and has a depressed gag reflex and shallow respiration, an endotracheal tube should be inserted. Before intubation, the oropharynx and nasopharynx should be carefully suctioned free of secretions, and loose teeth or dentures should be removed. Using an oral airway, mask, and manual recuscitor, several assisted ventilations with high concentrations of supplemental oxygen should be administered to guard against further hypoxemia during intubation. Once intubated, the patient should be slowly ventilated manually and arterial blood gases should be obtained immediately. The endotracheal tube must be securely taped in place after ensuring that *both* lungs are ventilated. Alveolar ventilation and the need for continued assisted ventilation are assessed by means of an arterial P_{CO_2} measurement. Again, it is better to err on the safe side rather than await a disastrously high P_{CO_2}. Respiratory arrest soon *after* the arrival of a patient to an emergency room, although infrequent, is an event that could be prevented by taking appropriate precautions rather than waiting for full documentation. Anticipation of potential respiratory failure from any condition noted in Table 146-1 is a critical aspect of good patient management.

The patient with documented respiratory failure should be transferred to an appropriate area for monitoring and continued respiratory support. If drug overdose is suspected and gastric lavage contemplated, all stuporous patients should be intubated to prevent aspiration, even if respiratory failure seems unlikely. The airway should also be protected before gastric lavage when large quantities of petroleum distillates, such as gasoline or kerosene, have been ingested, regardless of the level of consciousness. Following lavage, conscious patients may be extubated while stuporous patients should be allowed to breath via a "T" tube until serial blood gases remain normal and the patient is stabilized in an appropriate monitoring area. Extubation of a stuporous patient not significantly hypoventilating (Pa_{CO_2} about 40 mm Hg) requires close supervision. This is especially true if airway reflexes are blunted or absent. Because of the unpredictable nature of respiratory arrest following glutethimide overdose, these patients should not be extubated until they are fully alert. Once a patient with an altered level of consciousness has been extubated, he should be placed in a semiprone position with his head 30 to 40° lower than his hips to minimize aspiration of oral secretions. A supine posture is contraindicated. For easy suctioning, patients should have an oral or nasopharyngeal airway left in place until they are relatively alert.

Patients with pinpoint pupils suspected of opiate overdose should be treated with naloxone. Because this is a specific, safe, competitive antagonist, a prompt response is expected in narcotic overdose. Intubation should be performed before administering naloxone, since marked vomiting often follows and pulmonary aspiration may be extensive. If a diagnosis of narcotic overdosage is rather certain, large doses of naloxone may be administered initially. Some patients have required as much as 10 to 20 mg over 10 to 20 minutes.

Simultaneously with establishment of an airway and/or assisted ventilation, the circulation should be stabilized. Circulatory disturbance usually results from changes in vasomotor tone, depressed cardiac output, reduced intravascular volume, or arrhythmias. Orthostatic changes may be observed in patients with peripheral vascular dilatation or hypovolemia. In the presence of hypotension, a central venous catheter and measurement of central venous pressure are mandatory.[29] Following assisted ventilation, pleural pressure becomes more positive relative to atmospheric pressure and decreased venous return is common. Fall in cardiac output results. Careful monitoring of central venous pressure and its response to fluid administration are, therefore, helpful in preventing further circulatory embarrassment during the treatment of respiratory failure. Central venous pressure does not, however, necessarily reflect changes in left ventricular filling pressure. Correction of any electrolyte disturbance is important in preventing further respiratory insufficiency and cardiac arrhythmias.

Alert patients with severe respiratory distress thought to be secondary to neuromuscular or metabolic disease should be evaluated by measurement of forced vital capacity, inspiratory force, and arterial blood gases. Since the pulmonary parenchyma is usually normal under these conditions, arterial hypoxemia is not severe unless superimposed pneumonia, atelectasis, or aspiration has occurred. However, acute pneumonia often precipitates crisis in the patient with myasthenia gravis, and is not an uncommon superimposed event in any neuromuscular disorder or metabolic derangement. If the vital capacity is < 500 ml and inspiratory force is < 5 cm H_2O, apnea is imminent and elective intubation is warranted. If the vital capacity is between 1 and 1.5 liters or the neuromuscular disease appears unstable or progressive, the patient should be transferred to a medical intensive care unit. In patients with neuromuscular disease or with metabolic coma and arterial P_{CO_2} of greater than 55 mm Hg, intubation and assisted ventilation are warranted. An elevation of the arterial P_{CO_2} to between 45 and 55 mm Hg increases the possibility of sudden respiratory arrest. Depending on the vital capacity (near 1 liter) and the ability to monitor the patients carefully with frequent arterial blood gases, assisted ventilation may be held in reserve.

When assisted ventilation is begun as an emergency procedure, in drug overdoses, and in patients with neuromuscular, metabolic, or endocrine disorders, remember that the pulmonary mechanics are usually relatively normal and require only small inflation pressures from a manual recuscitator or pressure respirator (10 to 15 cm of water) or only small inflation volumes from a volume respirator (7 to 10 ml/

kg/breath). Overventilation with the production of acute respiratory alkalosis, seizures, and arrhythmias is common in these circumstances unless assisted ventilation is performed cautiously.

Traumatic Respiratory Failure

Patients with a flail chest and post-traumatic respiratory failure should be intubated immediately. These patients should be slightly hyperventilated so that they will not initiate respirations on their own. A small amount of end-expiratory pressure is helpful in preventing microatelectasis.[34] This form of assisted ventilation controls the patient's breathing pattern, stabilizes the chest for healing of fractured ribs, prevents laceration of the pulmonary parenchyma by displaced ribs, and usually corrects significant hypoxemia. If post-traumatic pulmonary insufficiency is associated with circulatory failure and decreased breath sounds in one or both chest cavities, with a shift of the trachea to either side, emergency thoracostomy must be performed. In extreme cases this can be accomplished initially with a needle and underwater seal. While it is preferable to wait for radiographic documentation of pneumothorax, this is not always possible with tension pneumothorax, significant hypotension, and respiratory failure that requires artificial positive pressure ventilation. Careful placement of a chest tube or a large intravenous catheter into the thoracic cage with an underwater seal may be life saving. False positive diagnosis of a tension pneumothorax and blind insertion of a chest tube during careful assisted ventilation rarely result in the production of a significant iatrogenic pneumothorax or worsening of the patient's condition. Spontaneous pneumothorax in an otherwise healthy individual rarely results in respiratory failure. Diagnosis and treatment of pneumothorax will be discussed later.

Emergency Management of Respiratory Failure Secondary to Alteration in Pulmonary Mechanics

Alteration in pulmonary mechanics is the most common cause of respiratory failure. The alterations are conveniently divided into conditions that result in airway obstruction and those that result in parenchymal dysfunction. The clinical presentation and treatment of these major categories are different. Of the two, airway obstruction is the more common. The pattern of respiratory failure depends on its etiology and whether the obstruction is located predominantly in the upper or lower airway.

UPPER AIRWAY OBSTRUCTION. Upper airway obstruction can result from a variety of conditions (Table 146–1). Marked increases in airway resistance due to supraglottal or laryngeal edema, laryngeal paralysis, tumor, or foreign body obstruction are often tolerated suprisingly well by both adults and children. Clinical evidence of obstruction does not occur until the upper airway is almost completely occluded, although moderate degrees of obstruction can be detected by measurement of airflow limitation. Measurements of forced inspiration are usually more sensitive than measurements of forced expiration in the detection of upper airway obstruction.[25]

Patients with upper airway obstruction usually complain of fatigue and shortness of breath. The shortness of breath is often more severe in the supine position (because of loss of mechanical advantage) and on exercise (because of the required increase in minute ventilation). Stridor with nasal flaring, marked accessory respiratory muscle activity, and suprasternal and intercostal retractions develops late in the course of upper airway obstruction and is often associated with pulsus paradoxus. Arterial Pa_{CO_2} may remain relatively normal in spite of the marked increased work of breathing until the patient tires or the obstruction become almost complete. Arterial Pco_2 then changes rapidly and death may quickly follow. The arterial Po_2 is often normal or only slightly reduced. Recognition of the illness is the key to avoiding catastrophe. Acute upper airway obstruction associated with swelling or paralysis of vocal cords is accompanied by hoarseness. Allergic or hereditary angioedema and hemorrhage almost always have associated swelling of the oropharynx or tongue. Ludwig's angina is a cellulitis of the submaxillary space which most commonly results from infections around the second and third molars. Airway obstruction results from edema of the floor of the mouth, which pushes the tongue posteriorly, and from cervical swelling. Dysphagia and a bull neck may occur, but hoarseness, adenopathy, or loculation of pus is usually absent. Involvement of the tonsils and pharynx is minimal. Fever and leukocytosis are common.

The symptoms of acute infectious epiglottitis in the adult are fever, chills, choking, drooling, dysphagia, and sore throat which usually precede evidence of respiratory insufficiency by several days.[22] Patients often appear toxic. Evidence of pharyngitis is minimal, but mild cervical swelling or adenopathy may be present. Hoarseness is uncommon. Inspiratory stridor may develop relatively abruptly and in hours progress to complete upper airway obstruction. The diagnosis can be determined only by indirect laryngoscopy, which shows edema and inflammation of the epiglottic and supraglottic tissue. Lateral neck x-rays with soft tissue technique provide evidence of supraglottic or cervical swelling in Ludwig's angina and epiglottic swelling in acute infectious epiglottitis.

The emergency management of acute upper airway obstruction resulting in respiratory failure revolves around the best means of bypassing or removing the obstruction. The upper airway should be examined and cleared, especially when acute respiratory distress occurs during food ingestion. In acute epiglottitis, upper airway examination should be performed in the operating room. Establishment of an adequate airway usually requires the insertion of an oral or nasal endotracheal tube. This is best performed under direct vision by an anesthesiologist. The exact timing of intubation is often debatable, but delay in establishing a safe airway may be disastrous. A Pa_{CO_2} above 50 mm Hg is a clear indication. Unlike lower airway obstruction, where we prefer not to intubate, early intubation is conservative therapy in upper airway obstruction. Acute infectious epiglottitis was originally thought to be a contraindication to endotracheal intubation. However, endotracheal intubation performed in the operating room is now the treatment of choice and tracheostomy can be avoided without increased morbidity or mortality.[16] Obstruction usually resolves in 2 to 5 days. Endotracheal intubation is dangerous and usually unsuccessful in Ludwig's angina, and tracheostomy should be performed immediately.

In most cases of acute upper airway obstruction, once a patent airway is established, respiratory embarrassment is relieved. Definitive therapy, such as tracheostomy, radiation therapy, or treatment of infection, can then proceed at a slower pace depending on the underlying etiology. If respiratory failure persists, bronchoscopy may be required to assess the trachea just below the endotracheal tube. If the airway is patent, respiratory failure must be due to factors other than upper respiratory obstruction. Since intubation often produces further laryngeal edema, severe upper airway obstruction from chemical injuries, such as smoke inhalation, requires early tracheostomy. Supplemental oxygen is required only if severe underlying or superimposed pulmonary disease exists. Once the upper airway is bypassed it is necessary to humidify all inspired air.

LOWER AIRWAY OBSTRUCTION. Acute respiratory failure from lower airway obstruction is usually secondary to asthma or chronic obstructive pulmonary disease (COPD). In both of these conditions acute deterioration is commonly precipitated by a chest infection, an operation, respiratory depressant drugs, or other illness.[30] Over hours or days, the patient experiences increasing dyspnea, wheezing, lethargy, insom-

nia, or somnolence. Cough with or without the production of secretions may be prominent. The obstruction must be severe and widespread in order to produce respiratory insufficiency. Since the degree of obstruction is not uniform throughout the lung, ventilation-perfusion inequalities occur. These result in an increase in dead space and venous admixture. The increased dead space or wasted ventilation can be compensated by an increase in total ventilation so that the arterial P_{CO_2} may remain near normal levels. However, the arterial P_{O_2} due to venous admixture is reduced early.

In *acute respiratory failure from COPD* the P_{CO_2} usually rises progressively over days. The diagnosis of acute hypercapnic respiratory failure requires both a change in the patient's respiratory symptoms and an elevation in arterial P_{CO_2} associated with an appropriate fall in arterial pH. The rate of rise in the P_{CO_2} dictates the acuteness of respiratory failure. In most instances of pure acute respiratory failure, there is a 0.008 decrease in arterial pH for every 1 mm Hg rise in arterial P_{CO_2}. In many cases of acute exacerbation of respiratory failure superimposed on chronic pulmonary insufficiency it is difficult to determine the exact degree of acute decompensation without knowledge of blood gas determinations in the recent past. Although elevated Pa_{CO_2} may cause narcosis, it is the hypoxemia which usually kills the patient. Death or permanent injury from hypoxemia may occur in minutes, while high-level Pa_{CO_2} may be well tolerated and result in no permanent tissue injury if oxygenation is well maintained.

The management of acute respiratory failure secondary to chronic obstructive pulmonary disease varies with the degree of respiratory failure.[18] Obtunded, confused, or comatose patients should immediately be ventilated manually with an oral airway, mask, and a recuscitator bag and then intubated. Patients who inadvertently receive excessive amounts of oxygen on the way to the hospital usually fall into this category. The method of intubation is not critical; both nasal and oral intubation have their proponents. If the patient appears critically ill and markedly cyanotic, but relatively alert, 24 percent oxygen via a venturi mask or 1 liter/min of oxygen via a nasal cannula should be administered.

In either of the above situations, intravenous infusion with dextrose 5 percent in water is begun to maintain a route for further therapy, and arterial blood gases are obtained for analysis. If the history suggests that dyspnea developed suddenly, an immediate chest film is mandatory to rule out pneumothorax. When the history is one of increasing dyspnea developing over hours to days, it is best to observe and monitor the patient closely until temporarily stable before obtaining a chest film. The patient should be promptly admitted to the hospital. In most cases, this should be a specialized area experienced in the treatment of acute respiratory failure and having the capability for continual electrocardiographic monitoring. If the arterial Pa_{CO_2} is above 55 mm Hg, admission to an intensive care unit is strongly suggested. On many occasions, a slightly elevated arterial Pco_2, in the presence of severe hypoxemia, rises rapidly as the Po_2 is partially corrected. If the Pa_{CO_2} increases following the addition of low flow oxygen, the oxygen cannot be withdrawn. Close monitoring is therefore desirable for all patients.

Patients with acute moderately severe respiratory distress should have arterial blood gases determined before initiating specific therapy. In most cases, hospital admission will be necessary but, occasionally, there may be only moderate hypoxemia or no change from previously determined arterial blood gas levels. In the absence of fever, chest pain, marked fatigue, acute roentgenographic changes, dehydration, hypotension, or altered consciousness, cautious administration of bronchodilators may be attempted. A moderate improvement in symptoms may allow the patient to be released as long as someone is available to supervise the patient closely and bring him back should there fail to be continued improvement. Disposition is greatly aided by a knowledge of previous pulmonary function measurements and comparison of current levels of pulmonary fuction before and immediately after administration of bronchodilators. A normal Pa_{CO_2} in the presence of severe tachypnea does not ensure against impending respiratory failure.

Bronchial Asthma. Bronchial asthma is one of the most common causes of acute respiratory distress. Although acute respiratory failure is uncommon in bronchial asthma, sudden death and severe pulmonary insufficiency occur.[31] Because of the frequency of this disease and the usual uneventful recovery with therapy, the potential seriousness of an asthmatic attack is often not appreciated. The approach to the acute asthmatic attack requires an assessment of early warnings of status asthmaticus and the appropriate administration of specific therapy known to reverse the majority of episodes of dyspnea.

Patients with acute asthma experience marked respiratory distress, diffuse expiratory and occasionally inspiratory wheezes, prolonged expiration, visable accessory respiratory muscle activity, and supra-clavicular and intercostal retractions. Occasionally, wheezes may be absent, and this is always associated with very poor air entry into the chest. Pulsus paradoxus is common in severe asthma. The early signals of the severe asthmatic attack are listed in Table 146-2. The patient with severe asthma is always at risk of sudden respiratory arrest and should be managed accordingly. The most significant early warning is the presence of severe airway obstruction which fails to respond to bronchodilator therapy. Documentation of the severity of the obstruction and lack of response requires a measurement of expiratory airflow before and after bronchodilators. In practice, one determines the FEV_1, vital capacity, or peak flow measurement initially and 15 minutes after 0.3 to 0.5 ml subcutaneous epinephrine 1:1000. Epinephrine may be given a total of three times before concluding that the patient is unresponsive. The significantly ill, markedly obstructed, unresponsive asthmatic should be admitted to hospital. Prolonged therapy and observation in an office or emergency room over 2 to 3 hours is unjustified. Patients with severe attacks of asthma are often restless, anxious, and apprehensive. However, the use of even mild sedatives has been associated with increased mortality and should not be administered unless a decision has been made to ventilate the patient artificially.

Therapy for acute and chronic asthma is discussed in Chapter 35. Emergency therapy usually requires intravenous hydration to loosen secretions, prevent mucus impaction, and maintain the circulation. Since patients are almost always significantly hypoxic, they should receive supplemental oxygen; 2 liters of oxygen per minute by nasal cannula is usually adequate. The administration of bronchodilators not infrequently worsens the arterial Pa_{O_2}. Except in

---

TABLE 146-2
Indicators of Severe Asthmatic Attack

Previous or current episodes of status asthmaticus

FEV_1 <0.5 liters; VC <1.0 liters; peak flow <100 liters/min

Little or no response to bronchodilator therapy within 15 min; repeated q 15–30 min × 3

Central cyanosis or Pa_{O_2} <55

Pa_{CO_2} >45

Pulsus paradoxus

Disturbances of consciousness and/or obvious exhaustion

Pneumothorax, pneumomediastinum

Electrocardiographic abnormalities

mild attacks, oxygen therapy should probably precede all bronchodilator therapy. Oxygen therapy usually does not suppress respiration in the asthmatic. In addition to subcutaneous epinephrine, other bronchodilators, such as intravenous aminophylline, may be administered depending on the patient's previous self-medication history. A full loading dose of 5.6 mg/kg of intravenous aminophylline administered over 20 minutes should be given only to a patient with no recent theophylline therapy. An aminophylline maintenance infusion of 0.9 mg/kg/hr may be started, but failure of the patient to improve in 30 to 60 minutes is an indication for admission to the hospital. Continued administration of intravenous aminophylline frequently requires an adjustment in maintenance dose based on the patient's age and liver function. Nebulized bronchodilators are thought to be less effective than subcutaneous or intravenous medication in the acute attack.

The administration of corticosteroids should not be expected to alter the course of an asthmatic attack for at least 6 hours. Therefore, steroids are not an emergency therapy for acute asthma, although they may ultimately save the patient's life in a severe, refractory case. Bicarbonate therapy in status asthmaticus, to correct superimposed metabolic acidosis, has not been well studied.

Anaphylaxis. Anaphylaxis may present with acute upper airway obstruction similar to angioedema or acute lower airway obstruction similar to status asthmaticus. In most cases, the predominant clinical emergency is circulatory collapse. Hypotension is secondary to marked reduction in peripheral vascular resistance. The usually recommended therapy includes repeated intravenous administration of a 1 ml bolus of epinephrine 1:1000 every 1 to 2 minutes and massive fluid replacement. As much as 5 to 10 mg of epinephrine and several liters of saline may be required. If the patient fails to respond to epinephrine, norepinephrine should be administered by continuous infusion to maintain a systolic blood pressure above 90 mm Hg. If there is hypotension with respiratory distress associated with upper airway swelling, stridor, generalized wheezing, or elevated Pa_{CO_2}, the patient should be intubated immediately and artificially ventilated with a high inspiratory oxygen mixture. This should allow appropriate attention to the patient's hypotension without concern over superimposed respiratory acidosis. If hypotension is mild, the patient should be treated with repeated subcutaneous injections of 0.5 ml epinephrine 1:1000 every 10 to 20 minutes and managed in general as outlined above for acute airway obstruction.

Respiratory Failure Secondary to Acute Parenchymal Dysfunction

CHEMICAL INJURY. Chemical injury to the lung from the inhalation of smoke or toxic gases, such as chlorine, nitrogen dioxide, and sulfuric acid, often produces acute respiratory distress.[32] Fire is a leading cause of accidental death in the United States, and respiratory tract injury from smoke inhalation is a major cause of death in fire victims. Early signs and symptoms of significant smoke inhalation are usually minimal, except for the finding of cough and carbon-tinted sputum. Most patients who develop respiratory symptoms have burns about the face. In exposed patients who feel relatively well, with or without carbon-tinted sputum, observation for periods of several hours is required because a lag period may precede respiratory distress. An abnormal spirogram is said to predict high-risk patients. If a spirogram shows little reduction in predicted vital capacity and no reduction of second forced expiratory volume (FEV_1) and the patient is reliable, he may be released with instructions to return immediately if new respiratory symptoms develop. Persistent respiratory distress, hoarseness, and inspiratory and expiratory wheezing suggest a poor prognosis. Stridor, secondary to upper airway obstruction from oropharyngeal or laryngeal edema, requires immediate intubation or tracheostomy. In hypoxic patients, inspired air or oxygen supersaturated with water should be started immediately regardless of the need for intubation. If the patient is obtunded or has a low arterial pH, he is likely to be suffering from carbon monoxide poisoning and should receive 100 percent oxygen. In the presence of documented airway obstruction or audible wheezes, aminophylline or other bronchodilators should be given. This therapy should not be continued without documentation of its effectiveness. The role of steroids in smoke inhalation for relief of acute symptoms or prevention of subsequent airways dysfunction is not clear.

PULMONARY EDEMA. Pulmonary edema may result from an increased capillary hydrostatic pressure, a decreased vascular oncotic pressure, or an alteration in capillary permeability. Obstruction to lymphatic flow may aggravate all of these conditions.

The *adult respiratory distress syndrome* is one of the most frequent causes of severe acute pulmonary edema. Patients usually present with acute dyspnea and refractory cyanosis several hours after being admitted to hospital with an apparently unrelated nonpulmonary illness such as sepsis, severe hemorrhage, nonthoracic trauma, or pancreatitis. Viral pneumonia and aspiration of gastric contents may also produce this syndrome. A number of different primary and secondary mechanisms may be responsible for the lung injury. The common factor of all these conditions is a leaky capillary endothelium resulting in severe high protein-containing pulmonary edema fluid which produces marked right to left intrapulmonary shunting not corrected by high concentrations of supplemental oxygen. These patients should immediately be placed on as much supplemental oxygen as possible and promptly transferred to an intensive care unit where 100 percent oxygen and methods to increase lung volume can be instituted. Clinical presentation and comprehensive treatment of these patients are discussed in Chapter 36.

Patients with Pulmonary Edema from Increased Hydrostatic Pressure. Although also initially very ill, patients with pulmonary edema from increased hydrostatic pressure usually present a rapidly reversible respiratory emergency.[23] Over 90 percent of these patients will respond to appropriate therapy. Before instituting therapy, it is important to establish the diagnosis of cardiogenic pulmonary edema and understand the mechanism for the sudden pulmonary congestion. Almost all these patients have a well-established history of heart disease and have recently altered their diet, stopped taking their medicines, or developed an infection. Occasionally, an arrhythmia or acute myocardial infarction has suddenly reduced myocardial function, producing elevated left ventricular end-diastolic pressure which results in acute pulmonary congestion. Patients with cardiogenic pulmonary edema present with acute shortness of breath, tachypnea, diaphoresis, and marked agitation. Blood pressure is usually elevated, diffuse rales are almost always present, and wheezes are occasionally audible. Arterial blood gases show moderate to severe hypoxemia and moderate hyperventilation. A mild to moderate metabolic acidosis is present in three-quarters of patients. Approximately 20 percent of patients with pulmonary edema have an elevated Pa_{CO_2} with respiratory or mixed respiratory-metabolic acidosis.[15] Exacerbations of chronic obstructive pulmonary disease may rarely mimic acute pulmonary edema and this fact should always be kept in mind since therapy for the latter is contraindicated in the former.

The primary concern in management of cardiogenic pulmonary edema is to reduce left ventricular and/or left atrial end-diastolic pressure and relieve pulmonary edema while not significantly decreasing cardiac output. An outline of recommended therapy for pulmonary edema is listed in Table 146–3. High-flow oxygen and assumption of a sitting position

should be instituted immediately. Morphine is an excellent agent in cardiogenic pulmonary edema. It decreases venous tone and reduces anxiety and respiratory rate.[35] A prompt improvement is seen in most patients several minutes after intravenous administration of 5 to 15 mg of morphine. Morphine appears to be safe in cardiogenic pulmonary edema even if the initial Pa_{CO_2} is elevated.[15] Potent diuretics are commonly administered to these patients. Diuretics, however, have not been shown to improve the rate of recovery from acute pulmonary edema, although they can be of value in preventing relapse.[26] Potent diuretics are more likely to be helpful and safe in the presence of cardiomegaly and peripheral edema. They may be harmful in patients with pulmonary edema secondary to an acute myocardial infarction, aortic stenosis, or asymmetric septal hypertrophy.[28] Intravenous furosemide, a potent diuretic, acutely reduces left ventricular end-diastolic pressure through venous pooling and produces improvement in symptoms before significant diuresis.[21] Vasodilatation followed by a marked diuresis reduces left ventricular end-diastolic pressure by producing venous pooling and acute reductions in intervascular blood volume. This may result in decreased cardiac output by shifting the heart to a lower point on its intrinsic diastolic filling curve. Recently, it has been demonstrated that 0.6 to 1.2 mg of sublingual nitroglycerine promptly relieves clinical pulmonary edema and results in an increased cardiac stroke work.[17] This is accomplished by venous pooling which reduces left ventricular end-diastolic pressure and pulmonary congestion combined

---

TABLE 146–3
Emergency Treatment of Acute Pulmonary Edema*

Initial therapy
    Elevate patient's head >45°
    Oxygen
    Morphine
    Vasodilators
Secondary therapy (for complicated or refractory cases)
    Diuretics
    Cardiac glycosides
    Phlebotomy
    Aminophylline
    Positive pressure respiration (IPPB, CPAP, CPPV)
    Inotropic agents
    Cardioversion
Extreme measures for treatment failures
    Peritoneal dialysis
    Intra-aortic balloon circulatory augmentation

* See text for discussion.

with reduction in arterial vascular resistance which allows for an increased stroke volume at any degree of ventricular distension.

Repeated administration of sublingual nitroglycerine or intravenous administration of nitroprusside may be resorted to in refractory cases. Other methods of therapy for cardiogenic pulmonary edema are usually not necessary. With wheezing or evidence of airway obstruction, aminophylline may be useful. Besides being a potent bronchodilator, aminophylline is a mild inotropic agent and a mild diuretic and reduces systemic and pulmonary vascular resistance. However, ventricular tachycardia and vomiting may occur. Cardiac glycosides are helpful in the presence of supraventricular tachyarrhythmias. In the absence of supraventricular tachyarrhythmias, rapid digitalization is of questionable value in acute pulmonary edema.

On rare occasions, pulmonary congestion persists in spite of the above therapy. Under these circumstances phlebotomy or intermittent positive pressure breathing (IPPB) with or without elevated end-expiratory pressure (CPPV) may be tried in order to relieve symptoms of pulmonary congestion. Both modes of therapy reduce venous return and should not be instituted simultaneously since a significantly decreased cardiac output may result. IPPB may also decrease the rate of fluid accumulation in the lung by decreasing pulmonary capillary transmural pressure and decreasing left ventricular afterload. Inotropic beta-agonists may reduce left ventricular end-diastolic pressure (LVEDP) while maintaining an increased cardiac output. Dopamine and debutamine have been the most effective agents in this regard. This form of therapy will also increase myocardial oxygen demand and may increase ischemia in patients with acute or chronic coronary artery disease. The combination of inotropic stimulants and afterload reduction may augment cardiac performance while further decreasing LVEDP without increasing myocardial oxygen demand.[27]

The use of rotating tourniquets has not been shown to hasten the relief of pulmonary edema and may actually elevate peripheral vascular resistance. Other methods of therapy (listed in Table 146-3) go beyond a discussion of emergency management of pulmonary edema.

Following relief of the acute dyspnea, the patient should be reevaluated. Decisions should be made concerning the possibility of an acute myocardial infarction and the need for digitalization or diuretic therapy. If a reliable history is not available from the patient or family, it is often better not to digitalize the patient. In the presence of long-standing congestive heart failure, serum electrolytes may be grossly abnormal. The administration of a potent diuretic usually can wait until serum electrolyte values are known.

DIFFUSE PULMONARY FIBROSIS. Diffuse pulmonary fibrosis from any cause may eventually result in death from respiratory failure. Episodes of acute respiratory failure frequently occur during the progression of this disorder secondary to superimposed respiratory infection, hemoptysis, pneumothorax, or pulmonary embolism. These patients should be seen by a physician at the first sign of increased respiratory distress and treated aggressively when objective evidence indicates deterioration in arterial blood gases or superimposed clinical problems. Treatment consists mainly of hospital observation and the administration of sufficient oxygen to relieve hypoxemia and related symptoms. Pa_{CO_2} usually does not rise in these patients until almost all their lung has been destroyed. Supplemental oxygen rarely elevates their arterial P_{CO_2} further.

Pulmonary vascular disease, such as acute thromboembolism to the lung, is a common respiratory emergency. However, it is a pulmonary emergency which predominantly results in cardiovascular symptoms just as cardiogenic pulmonary edema is a cardiac disease which results in predominantly pulmonary symptoms. Specific treatment for acute pulmonary embolus involves administration of oxygen and heparin. The Pa_{O_2} can usually be satisfactorily improved with 50 percent oxygen. Occasionally the Pa_{O_2} may remain extremely depressed even on 100 percent oxygen. Under these circumstances, elevating end-expiratory pressure will improve the P_{O_2} satisfactorily.

Other Respiratory Emergencies

PNEUMOTHORAX. Pneumothorax may occur "spontaneously" or be associated with a probable precipitating cause, such as tumor, diagnostic or therapeutic procedures, or assisted ventilation.

Spontaneous pneumothorax is most common in healthy young males and in patients with emphysema or cystic and cavitary lung disease. The majority of patients experience an abrupt onset of pain which is sharp, constant, and often intensified by breathing. The pain may radiate to the back, neck, mediastinum, or abdomen. There is no relationship between the severity of pain and degree of lung collapse. Dyspnea may begin abruptly or follow soon after the onset of pain. It is usually worse on exercise. The severity of the dyspnea is often related to the degree of collapse and the functional ability of the uncollapsed lung. However, in some young individuals, complete unilateral pneumothorax may be associated with vague chest discomfort and no dyspnea. Cough is frequent, and a small amount of blood-stained sputum, probably arising from the lung at the site of rupture, may be expectorated. Physical findings depend on the degree of collapse. The affected side may show decreased motion, diminished fremitus, hyperresonance, and diminished breath and voice sounds. Low-grade fever appears occasionally. With a large pneumothorax there may be tracheal shift away from the side of collapse. Subcutaneous emphysema may occur but is most often seen with traumatic pneumothorax. A small left pneumothorax can cause a clicking or crunching sound synchronized with the heart beat. A small serous or bloody effusion may accompany a pneumothorax.

Pneumothorax is usually quantified by a rough estimate of the percentage of lung collapse. In addition, spontaneous pneumothorax may be defined as 1) simple, or closed (when the opening that allowed the escape of air closes producing no further leak); or 2) open (when there is essentially a bronchopleural fistula). In the latter case, the pleural pressure is close to atmospheric. A tension pneumothorax occurs when a valve-like action is produced that allows air to enter the thorax during inspiration but obstructs its exit from the pleural cavity during expiration. This causes the intrapleural pressure to rise above atmospheric pressure. The positive pleural pressure may greatly shift the mediastinum toward the opposite side compressing the contralateral lung and decreasing the venous return to the heart. A tension pneumothorax is a true medical emergency. Bilateral, simultaneous, spontaneous pneumothoraces are fortunately rare, but sequential spontaneous pneumothoraces are not uncommon.

The treatment of a pneumothorax depends on its extent and cause, and on whether it is closed or open and producing positive intrathoracic pressure. In general, therapy is simple, although the roles of conservative therapy and surgery are not universally agreed upon.[24] In a young otherwise healthy individual a small (<20 percent) pneumothorax may be watched on an ambulatory basis with complete absorption usually requiring 10 days. Larger or symptomatic pneumothoraces are treated with closed tube thoracostomy and water-sealed drainage. This can be performed on an emergency basis in the presence of marked symptoms or later at the patient's bedside. Early reexpansion provides immediate relief of symptoms.

Traumatic pneumothorax and those occurring during assisted ventilation are always treated with immediate insertion of a chest tube. Pneumothorax following diagnostic or therapeutic procedures usually resolves spontaneously without requiring specific therapy. However, if the pneumothorax is greater than 50 percent or symptoms of shortness of breath develop, it is wise to evacuate most of the air from the chest cage. In most instances, this can be performed by inserting a catheter into the chest intended for intravenous fluid administration followed by manual evacuation of the air using a syringe and three-way stopcock. A cooperative patient may evacuate extrapulmonary intrathoracic air by performing several forced expirations following catheter insertion and underwater drainage. This therapy is usually satisfactory because the small hole placed in the lung usually seals spontaneously. Once all the air is removed, the small catheter should be sealed or placed for underwater drainage and a chest film obtained. If a 20 percent or less pneumothorax remains, the catheter should be removed and the patient given supplemental oxygen to breathe. Increasing the oxygen concentration in the blood increases the nitrogen gradient between the pneumothorax and capillary bed in the visceral and parietal pleura. Since nitrogen represents 80 percent of the free gas in the thorax, this speeds absorption of the pneumothorax.

ACUTE PLEURAL FLUID ACCUMULATION. Acute pleural fluid accumulation in the thorax or further enlargement of a subacute pleural effusion is not an uncommon cause of acute dyspnea. Diagnosis and therapy of pleural effusions are discussed in Chapter 38. In most instances, arterial blood gases are not severely deranged unless the effusion is associated with a significant pulmonary embolus, widespread pneumonia, or contralateral lung disease. In a large percentage of acute effusions, dyspnea is secondary to pleural pain and not the quantity of intrathoracic fluid. However, if the effusion is large, partial removal often results in symptomatic relief. In most patients, therapeutic thoracentesis should be delayed until a general medical evaluation has been completed. In that way, one may combine a diagnostic and therapeutic procedure. Atropine, 0.4 mg, given subcutaneously is often given prior to elective or emergency thoracentesis. Careful thoracentesis for large pleural effusions has few complications as long as no more than 1 liter of fluid is initially removed. Rarely, removal of larger amounts of fluid may result in hypotension. If the effusion has been present for several days, rapid removal may result in ipsilateral pulmonary edema.

MASSIVE HEMOPTYSIS. Massive hemoptysis is a very dramatic and frightening clinical event. Most authorities agree that expectoration of 200 ml at one time or 600 ml over 16 hours represents massive hemoptysis.[19] However, accurate measurement of expectorated blood is frequently impossible. Fortunately, massive hemoptysis is uncommon. The usual causes of massive hemoptysis are listed in Table 146–4. Death is from flooding of the tracheal bronchial tree with asphyxiation. As in all medical chest emergencies, history and examination combined with a chest film usually suggest the most likely diagnosis.

The management of massive hemoptysis includes prevention of airway obstruction and maintenance of adequate vital signs, hematocrit, and arterial oxygen tension while awaiting cessation of bleeding. The patient is immediately placed at bed rest in a slightly head-down, lateral decubitus position with the suspected site of hemoptysis dependent. This minimizes aspiration into the uninvolved lung and optimizes gravity-dependent postural drainage. Continuous monitoring in an intensive care unit with constant nursing care and immediate physician availability are recommended. Suction equipment with catheters, laryngoscope, endotracheal tube, manual recuscitator, or respirator should be available at the bedside. Patient fears and anxieties are best relieved by discourse with the physician and continual professional attention. Mild sedation may be helpful. If severe coughing is present, mild suppression should be initiated with codeine or other opiate derivatives.

Vital signs are supported by administration of adequate fluids and by blood transfusion. Supplemental oxygen is administered to maintain a Po_2 approximately 60 mm Hg. If a bleeding diathesis is present, it should be corrected. In the presence of acute bronchitis, broad spectrum antibiotic therapy is recommended.

Fortunately, most patients stop bleeding on their own. This allows conservative management in all but the few who continue to bleed and require repeated transfusions or suffer repeated compromise in pulmonary function. The most controversial aspect of management in massive hemoptysis involves the timing of bronchoscopy and the need for surgical intervention. Roentgenographic abnormalities seen at the time of hemoptysis are not always the cause of bleeding. Therefore, visualization of the bleeding site is essential for diagnosis.

Emergency bronchoscopy may irritate the tracheobronchial tree with increased coughing and exacerbation of hemoptysis. In addition, the presence of active bleeding compromising pulmonary function may increase the risk of bronchoscopy. Lastly, massive amounts of blood scattered around the trachea and bronchi make visual examination almost impossible. Most authorities now conclude that bronchoscopy may be deferred until the patient is stable and hemoptysis has subsided.[36] With the advent of fiberoptic bronchoscopy, visualization of peripheral lesions has become possible, and active bleeding as an indicator of the site of lesion is no longer necessary.

However, if massive hemoptysis persists, surgery offers the best prospect for survival unless there is far advanced bilateral disease. Immediate bronchoscopy with localization of the bleeding site, at least to right or left side, is a prerequisite to surgery. A device for control of bleeding during emergency pulmonary resection is crucial to prevent blood from entering the contralateral lung.

If a patient persists in bleeding and is not a candidate for surgery, attempts at packing the lobar bronchus on the side of the lesion have been successful. In the presence of respiratory failure, selective ventilation of the contralateral lung has also been successful in "waiting out" the bleeding. Recently, bronchial arteriography with selective vasopressin perfusion, gelfoam embolization, or balloon occlusion has been proposed as means of stopping massive inoperable bronchial bleeding.

┌─TABLE 146–4─────────────┐

Major Causes of Massive Hemoptysis

Infection (accounts for over half of all cases)
 Tuberculosis
 Bronchiectasis
 Lung abscess
 Necrotizing pneumonia
 Mycetoma (aspergilloma)

Neoplasm (primarily seen in <1 percent of lung
  tumors; much less frequent in metastatic disease)
 Bronchogenic carcinoma
 Metastatic carcinoma
 Endobronchial polyp

Cardiovascular disease
 Mitral stenosis
 Pulmonary arteriovenous malformation
 Pulmonary infarction (rare massive bleed)
 Primary pulmonary hypertension

Primary vascular and/or inflammatory conditions
 Goodpasture syndrome
 Idiopathic pulmonary hemosiderosis
 Wegener's granulomatosis
 Systemic lupus erythematosus

Unknown (in 2–15 percent, cause never found)
 Idiopathic hemoptysis

CHAPTER 147

Coma and Impaired Mentation
JERRY L. SPIVAK

Acute alterations in mentation or consciousness may be the presenting manifestation of disease, but the degree of change, be it mild confusion or deep coma, is not an accurate guide to either the severity of the underlying disease or its origin. Without familiarity with the patient's premorbid personality, minimal behavioral changes, such as irritability, short attention span, and impaired memory or judgment, may not be appreciated as disease-related or of diagnostic significance. More serious disturbances, such as delirium, stupor, or coma, of course, easily attract attention, but whatever the degree of mental impairment, a methodical approach to the problem is required if the diagnostic evaluation is to be accurate and therapy effective.

INITIAL MANAGEMENT

STUPOR AND COMA
These are the most profound disturbances of consciousness and require prompt action since the patient is unable to help himself or direct the attention of others to his particular problems. As in the case of cardiorespiratory arrest, a mnemonic is helpful in codifying the areas of major concern and the order in which they should be approached. For the comatose patient, the mnemonic ABCS, A-airway, B-Breathing, C-circulation, and S-Blood sugar, outlines the necessary first steps to take.

A—Airway
It is important that the upper airway be clear and aspiration prevented. The patient should be placed on his side with the head slightly dependent if possible. Periodically, the patient should be turned on the opposite side in order to promote drainage from all areas of the lung. Suctioning or passage of a nasogastric tube can precipitate vomiting, and endotracheal intubation should be performed before either of these maneuvers is attempted.

B—Breathing
Quantitative evaluation of respiration (rate, depth, rhythm) as well as blood gas measurements will serve to determine whether ventilatory assistance and oxygen therapy are required. Signs of airway obstruction, such as intercostal retraction or stridor

which is not relieved by proper positioning, are indications for endotracheal intubation. When this is achieved, the airway can be safely and effectively cleared by suctioning. The respiratory rhythm is also a valuable clue to the nature or location of the underlying disease.[43] For example, Cheyne-Stokes or periodic respiration suggests bilateral dysfunction of structures deep in the cerebral hemispheres. Hyperventilation suggests disease in the midbrain and pons (central neurogenic hyperventilation) but must be differentiated from hyperventilation due to metabolic acidosis, sepsis, hepatic coma, pulmonary disease, and salicylism. Apneustic breathing usually results from damage to the mid or lower pons, while ataxic respiration indicates medullary disease.

C—Circulation
A secure intravenous line must be established and hypotension corrected. Unless extreme, correction of hypertension should be deferred until the diagnostic evaluation is completed. Uremia, a cerebrovascular accident, CO_2 narcosis, pulmonary edema, or pseudotumor cerebri can mimic hypertensive encephalopathy, but rapid lowering of the blood pressure would have an adverse effect on cerebral blood flow in these disorders.

S—Blood Sugar
Hypoglycemia can result in irreversible brain damage. Therefore, as soon as blood is drawn for a glucose determination, 50 ml of 50 percent glucose should be administered intravenously.

Once these four initial steps (ABCS) have been taken, further diagnostic evaluation can be initiated. It is important to emphasize, however, that the ABCS approach can be life saving. For example, in barbiturate intoxication, respiratory arrest and hypotension occur at drug levels far below the level which is lethal. Also, in drug intoxication, the vital signs may change rapidly due either to continuing absorption of the drug from the intestine or, in the case of glutethimide, to reabsorption through the enterohepatic circulation.

DELIRIUM
The delirious patient represents a threat to himself as well as others. Disorientation, misperception of sensory stimuli, hallucinations, and loss of contact with

the environment promote restlessness, panic, and combativeness. A toxic psychosis can mask the underlying disease which gave rise to it and hinder diagnostic evaluation. Delirious patients should be closely attended in a quiet, enclosed environment which contains no potentially harmful objects or unsecured avenues of egress. Sedation is best reserved for the nocturnal hours since delirium is worse then; restraints should be avoided if possible.

DIAGNOSTIC EVALUATION

Disorders of consciousness can be separated into those that are potentially remediable with specific therapy, those that are of psychiatric origin, and those that are organic but not remediable by specific therapy (akinetic mutism and persistent vegetative state). The causes of potentially remediable states of altered consciousness are so many and varied that a thorough and methodical approach to diagnosis is mandatory. A mnemonic device employing the vowels A, E, I, O, U and the word "TIPS" as shown in Table 147-1 is helpful in remembering the major types of disorders that must be considered in evaluating the patient with a disturbance of consciousness.

HISTORY
Confusion, delirium, or coma render the patient useless as a source of information except for what can be gleaned from his appearance and clothing, the situation in which he was found, and the contents of his pockets. Useful facts may also be obtained from relatives, friends, police, ambulance attendants, bystanders, the patient's physician, the bathroom medicine cabinet, and old medical records. Alcoholism and drug abuse are two situations, however, where the information obtained can be misleading. Often, relatives are reluctant or refuse to divulge that the patient is an alcoholic; occasionally, they are totally unaware of the problem. This is also true for drug abuse, in which case the patient's friends, or at the very least, the size of their pupils may provide some clues. It is important, therefore, to remember that a negative history does not exclude the possibility of alcohol or drug abuse. Furthermore, evidence for either does not exclude another etiology for coma or impaired mentation.

PHYSICAL EXAMINATION
Although the patient's cooperation and comments are lacking, much can be learned from a meticulous physical examination. The vital signs have already been discussed with respect to respiration and blood pressure; they will also reveal hypothermia (Chapter 148) and hyperpyrexia (Chapter 149). The general examination may reveal evidence of liver disease, pulmonary disease, vitamin deficiency, endocrinopathy, plethora, cyanosis, anemia, hyperviscosity, dehydration, or hemorrhagic diathesis. Particular attention should be paid to the possibility of head trauma. Battle's sign (mastoid ecchymosis) or bilateral medial orbital ecchymosis suggest temporal or anterior basal skull fracture, respectively. The ears and nose should be examined for blood or leakage of cerebrospinal

---

TABLE 147-1
Causes of Coma and Disordered Mentation

Mnemonic	Mechanism	Comment
A—Alcoholism	Ethanol intoxication	Evidence of ethanol ingestion does not exclude other causes for coma
	Hypoglycemia	Hypoglycemia may cause hypothermia and muscular rigidity. Suspect insulin overdose in alcoholic diabetics[37]
	Hypothermia	Accidental exposure or hypoglycemia
	Delirium tremens	Can mask other disorders such as pneumonia or meningitis
	Thiamine deficiency (Wernicke's encephalopathy)	Administration of glucose without thiamine can exacerbate the encephalopathy
	Niacin deficiency (pellagra)	Insidious onset; dementia can be the most prominent manifestation[44]
	Intoxication with other agents	Simultaneous ingestion of barbiturates and alcohol is not uncommon
	Intoxication with alcohol substitutes	Methanol, isopropanol, ethylene glycol, moonshine (lead intoxication), paraldehyde
	Trauma	Subdural hematoma can be acute or chronic; if chronic, the initial trauma may be forgotten

(Continued)

TABLE 147-1 (cont.)

Mnemonic	Mechanism	Comment
E—Encephalopathy	Epilepsy	Status epilepticus can be mistaken for coma. Seizures may be due to a metabolic abnormality as opposed to a structural lesion. Postictal coma can mask an inciting neurologic disorder or drug intoxication
	Viral encephalitis	Focal neurologic signs in herpes simplex encephalitis are due to temporal lobe necrosis
	Intracranial hemorrhage	Must be considered as a cause of coma in patients taking anticoagulants. The EKG in subarachnoid hemorrhage can falsely suggest myocardial ischemia or infarction[45]
	Normal pressure hydrocephalus	A correctable cause of dementia[42]
	Intracranial mass lesions	Rostral-caudal neurologic deterioration distinguishes mass lesions from metabolic encephalopathies[43]
	Hypertensive encephalopathy	Can be confused clinically with intracranial mass lesions, CO_2 narcosis, pulmonary edema, and pseudotumor cerebri
	Hyperviscosity encephalopathy	Polycythemia, macroglobulemia, sickle cell anemia, leukemia, cerebral malaria
	Thrombotic thrombocytopenic purpura	Rapid fluctuation of neurologic signs is common. Diagnosis should be apparent from examination of the peripheral blood smear
	Heat stroke; hypothermia	Clinical thermometers usually do not register below 95.5°F or above 107.6°F
	Carcinoma	Hypoglycemia, multifocal leukoencephalopathy, metastases, marantic endocarditis, hypercalcemia, and progressive dementia
	Demyelinating and degenerative diseases	Postinfectious and posthypoxic encephalopathy, Marchiafava-Bignami disease, central pontine myelinosis, Jakob-Creuzfeldt disease, Alzheimer's disease
I—Insulin (excess or deficiency)	Hypoglycemia	Hypothermia is an important clue. Bizarre behavior can mask the diagnosis. The classic signs of anxiety, sweating, and tachycardia may be absent.[46] Hypoglycemia due to sulfonylureas may be prolonged
	Hyperosmolar coma	Often triggered by another disorder
	Diabetic coma	Precipitating cause must be identified and corrected. Ketoacidosis without profound hyperglycemia is occasionally seen in alcoholics[39]
O—Opiates and other drugs (and drug withdrawal)	Narcotics, hypnotics, tranquillizers, salicylates, poisons	Pupillary size and light reflex are altered by opiates, hypnotics, atropine, and scopolamine. Level of consciousness fluctuates with glutethimide intoxication
U—Uremia (and other metabolic abnormalities)	Uremia	Coma can be due to the uremia, water intoxication, postdialysis. dysequilibrium syndrome, or a subdural hematoma
	Hepatic coma	Identify correctable causes such as electrolyte imbalance, hypoglycemia, gastrointestinal hemorrhage, excessive dietary protein, or infection
	Hyponatremia	Often iatrogenic (diuretics, salt restriction, and volume overload) or as part of the syndrome of inappropriate ADH secretion. Seizures may be the initial manifestation

TABLE 147-1 (cont.)

Mnemonic	Mechanism	Comment
	Hypernatremia	Often iatrogenic (tube feeding, failure to hydrate adequately); rapid replacement of water can cause cerebral edema
	Hypoxia	Cyanosis is absent if the hemoglobin concentration is less than 5 g/dl%. Posthypoxic encephalopathy can occur 7–21 days after the initial insult. Carbon monoxide intoxication may present with coma and cerebral edema. Cyanosis may be due to methemoglobinemia (sulfonamides, acetophenetidin, aniline dyes, and nitrates)
	Hypercapnia	Carbon dioxide narcosis can mimic hypertensive encephalopathy and can be precipitated by sedative administration, oxygen administration, or infection
	Vasculitis	Systemic lupus erythematosus, polyarteritis, giant cell arteritis
	Addison's disease	Precipitating factor must be identified and corrected
	Panhypopituitarism	Presentation may be either as adrenal insufficiency or hypothyroidism
	Hypothyroidism	Can present as hypothermia or carbon dioxide narcosis
	Hyperthyroidism	Rarely may present with stupor or coma
	Porphyria	Urine may be colorless but will contain elevated levels of PBG
	Hypercalcemia	Mental changes may be the only manifestation
	Hypocalcemia	Cataracts and intracranial calcifications are important clues
	Lactic acidosis	Shock, leukemia, diabetes mellitus, phenformin therapy[40]
	Heavy metal intoxication	Lead, tetraethyl lead, arsenic, and mercury
T—Trauma	Head injury	Subdural hematoma and epidural hematoma, concussion, and cerebral laceration. Beware of associated cervical spine injuries
	Fat embolism	Hypoxemia, stupor, and petechiae over the upper portion of the body
I—Infection	Meningitis	Alteration in mentation may be the earliest sign; meningismus may be absent
	Subdural empyema	Severe unremitting headache is common
	Infective endocarditis	Toxic encephalopathy, meningitis, brain abscess, or mycotic aneurysm may develop
	Mass lesions	Many infections (tuberculosis, toxoplasmosis, brain abscess, cysticercosis) can present as intracranial mass lesions
	Pneumonia	Toxic delirium is common in the elderly
P—Psychiatric	Hysteria, schizophrenia, depression	Psychiatric abnormalities may be prominent with disorders such as systemic lupus erythematosus, Cushing syndrome, occult carcinoma, and porphyria
S—Syncope	Reduced cardiac output	Pulmonary embolism, Stokes-Adams attacks, atrial myxoma, pheochromocytoma, aortic stenosis, and subaortic stenosis

fluid. Occasionally, a local area of scalp edema is the only manifestation of head trauma.

The diagnostic information which can be gained from a careful evaluation of respiratory activity has been discussed above. Erythematous and bullous skin lesions occur in drug-induced coma and carbon monoxide intoxication, usually at sites of trauma or pressure.[41] When present, the possibility of underlying muscle necrosis and myoglobinuria should be considered.

The neurologic examination can provide assistance in distinguishing metabolic encephalopathies from intracranial disease and other forms of coma from psychogenic unresponsiveness. For example, preservation of the pupillary light reflex in the presence of decerebrate rigidity or flaccid paralysis suggests a metabolic encephalopathy as opposed to an intracranial structural lesion. The roving eye movements of coma cannot be duplicated voluntarily, and the ocular response to caloric stimulation in psychogenic unresponsiveness is nystagmus as opposed to tonic deviation (or lack of a response if coma is deep). Certain signs, such as papilledema, which can be produced by metabolic lesions (carbon dioxide narcosis, carbon monoxide intoxication, and pseudo-tumor cerebri), by hypertension, and by intracranial structural lesions have less specific diagnostic value. Furthermore, ingestion of atropine, scopolamine, or glutethimide can produce fixed dilated pupils. Hypothermia and severe barbiturate intoxication can also fix the pupils while opiates produce pinpoint but reactive pupils similar to those found with pontine lesions. In addition, while asterixis, tremor, and myoclonus are usually seen with metabolic encephalopathies, reversible focal abnormalities, such as hemipa-

resis, which are commonly associated with intracranial structural lesions, also may be observed in the same setting. Finally, lack of nuchal rigidity cannot be used to exclude the presence of meningitis, particularly in elderly individuals.

LABORATORY STUDIES

Judicious use of the laboratory can uncover many causes of coma. They include the metabolic encephalopathies, thrombotic thrombocytopenic purpura, sickle cell disease, porphyria, polycythemia, macroglobulinemia, leukemia, diabetic and hyperosmolar coma, and lactic acidosis. Toxicologic screening can be performed on body fluids but as emphasized in Chapter 151, screening procedures have limitations. Furthermore, the urine present in the bladder at initial catheterization may not accurately reflect the chemical abnormalities present in the blood. With subarachnoid hemorrhage, ST segment and T wave abnormalities may be present on the EKG in the absence of myocardial ischemia or infarction.[45] Skull x-rays may reveal metastatic lesions or intracranial calcifications or evidence of head trauma such as soft tissue edema or a fracture line. Characteristically, the EEG is diffusely slow in metabolic encephalopathies, normal in psychogenic unresponsiveness, and focally abnormal with structural lesions. Echoencephalography and computerized axial tomography are also useful, noninvasive diagnostic techniques. Invasive techniques, such as the lumbar puncture or arteriography, should be undertaken only in conjunction with neurosurgical consultation when there is suspicion of infection or to confirm and define a potentially remediable intracranial lesion.

CHAPTER 148

Hypothermia
JERRY L. SPIVAK

Hypothermia is defined as a body temperature below 96°F (35.5°C). Since temperature is one of the vital signs, the presence of hypothermia is easily established. However, because the lowest reading on the standard clinical thermometer is 95.5°F (35°C), the actual severity of the hypothermia can be underestimated. Hypothermia occurs in a variety of settings. Hypothermia resulting from accidental exposure is most common in alcoholics or senile individuals who

are unable to protect themselves from their environment. Drug intoxication can lead to hypothermia particularly with agents such as the phenothiazines and barbiturates, which impair shivering. Infusion of large volumes of cold fluid during blood transfusion, peritoneal dialysis, or gastric lavage can also produce hypothermia. Diseases causing hypothermia include myxedema, hypopituitarism, uremia, acute pancreatitis, starvation, diabetic ketoacidosis, bacterial sepsis, hypoglycemia, erythroderma, Wernicke's encephalopathy, parkinsonism, and cerebrovascular accidents.

As the body cools, a predictable sequence of events occurs. Initially, there is intense vasoconstriction and shivering accompanied by tachycardia and a diuresis. As the temperature falls below 89.6°F (32°C), bradycardia or atrial fibrillation may occur, and there is mental confusion and indifference to the cold environment and muscular rigidity replaces shivering. Below 84°F (29°C), the ventilatory rate falls, the patient becomes comatose, blood pressure and urine output falls, and the threshold for ventricular fibrillation is reduced. Below 79°F (26°C), ventricular fibrillation can occur spontaneously.

The chemical abnormalities which occur during hypothermia include an increase in serum transaminase levels, hyperglycemia, and alterations in the arterial pH and blood gases. The elevated transaminase levels are not associated with anatomic abnormalities in muscle, while hyperglycemia is due to an increase in glucose release from the liver associated with impairment of peripheral glucose utilization. Acidosis, either respiratory or metabolic, may develop. The arterial pH and the blood gases are also influenced by the fall in temperature.[49] Blood pH rises 0.014 units per 1°C fall in temperature while the Pco_2 falls 7 percent and the Po_2 falls 6 percent for each 1°C fall in temperature. Nomograms are available to correct for these temperature-related effects, but they will not usually obscure the actual status of the patient's acid–base balance.

Although the function of most organs is profoundly affected by hypothermia, the heart is the target organ in this disorder. Electrocardiographic abnormalities include prolongation of the P-R and Q-T intervals and the QRS complex. The T-wave vector may be shifted and, characteristically, the terminal vector of the QRS complex is altered producing the "J" or Osborn wave.[47] Although considered diagnostic for hypothermia, the "J" wave has been observed in normothermic individuals with subarachnoid hemorrhage or other central nervous system disorders and with myocardial ischemia. Arrhythmias are common in hypothermia and include sinus bradycardia, atrial fibrillation, idioventricular rhythms, ventricular fibrillation, and asystole. Since during hypothermia cardiac rhythmicity ceases before cardiac contractility, attempts at resuscitation are always worthwhile.

As soon as the diagnosis of hypothermia is established, rewarming should be initiated. Since hypoglycemia is an easily correctable cause of hypothermia, administration of glucose to patients whose medical history is unknown, after blood has been drawn for chemical studies, is also wise. Rewarming can be accomplished by either an external or core approach and in either an active or a passive fashion. Although there are advocates for each approach, there is no controlled prospective study to support the superiority of any of them. Furthermore, the prognosis of the hypothermic patient appears to depend more on the presence or absence of underlying disease than on the manner in which rewarming is carried out.[50] In developing rational guidelines for therapy, the following should be considered. First, the heart is the target organ in hypothermia, and ventricular fibrillation is usually refractory to treatment until the patient is rewarmed. Second, even after removal of the hypothermic patient from the cold environment, the temperature may continue to fall. Therefore, active rewarming is appropriate when the patient's temperature is 86°F (30°C) or less. Since procedures such as intubation or insertion of central lines can precipitate ventricular fibrillation, unnecessary manipulations should be avoided. External rewarming avoids the manipulations associated with core techniques. Although much emphasis has been placed on the possibility of hypovolemia, hypotension, and arrhythmias with rapid external rewarming, there is little to support these contentions. Rapid external rewarming is the most effective method for resuscitating profoundly hypothermic persons.[48] It seems reasonable, therefore, to apply this approach to all patients regardless of the cause of hypothermia.

Once the temperature is above the level at which ventricular fibrillation occurs, passive rewarming can be employed, diagnostic techniques can be initiated to determine the cause, and therapy that is specific for the underlying disorder can be employed. Ventricular fibrillation should be treated with lidocaine or quinidine but not with procainamide. As rewarming progresses, other arrhythmias, such as atrial fibrillation, may recur but they will disappear spontaneously.

CHAPTER 149

Hyperthermia
JERRY L. SPIVAK

Body temperature reflects the balance between heat production and heat dissipation. Evaporation, radiation, and convection are the major mechanisms by which heat dissipation occurs. The efficiency of radiation and convection depend on an adequate circulation, a gradient between body temperature and ambient temperature, and adequate exposure of the body surface. When the ambient temperature reaches 95°F (35°C) or there are significant barriers, such as layers of clothing or surgical drapes, radiation and convection become inefficient and evaporation becomes the major mechanism for heat exchange. However, if ambient humidity is high, heat dissipation by evaporation is ineffective and body temperature rises. Hyperthermia is arbitrarily defined as a temperature greater than 106°F (41°C). In most febrile illnesses, the body temperature seldom exceeds 106°F. Temperatures of 104 to 105° are not infrequent, however, suggesting that during fever the body's thermostat is reset to a higher but definite ceiling. The upper limit of body temperature which is compatible with life is 114.8°F (46°C), although lower temperatures are often fatal whether or not an underlying disease is present. The standard clinical thermometer does not register above 107.6°F. The rectal temperature, of course, is usually lower than the core temperature.

Hyperthermia is observed in five clinical settings: infection, delirium tremens, thyroid storm, intracerebral hemorrhage, and reactions to drugs (anticholinergic agents such as atropine and benztropine mesylate [Cogentin], antihistamines and phenothiazines which impair sweating, amphetamines and succinylcholine which promote excessive heat production, drug allergies, and the Jarisch-Herxheimer reaction). Illness due to heat may take a variety of forms of which the most important are heat cramps, heat exhaustion, and heat stroke.[52]

HEAT CRAMPS

These usually occur in highly acclimatized individuals who produce large quantities of sweat during strenuous exertion in a hot environment and who replace the water loss but not the salt deficit. Characteristically, the painful skeletal muscle cramps occur

after, not during, the period of exertion. Usually they subside spontaneously, but if unrelenting, they can be relieved by adminstration of sodium chloride, which is also effective in their prevention.

HEAT EXHAUSTION

This syndrome may be precipitated by either a predominant deficit of water due to inadequate hydration in a hot environment or a predominant deficit of salt due to replacement of water loss without replacement of the salt deficit. The symptoms of heat exhaustion due to inadequate hydration include thirst, weakness, restlessness, dizziness, dyspnea and hyperventilation, muscular incoordination, and delirium. When salt depletion predominates, there is weakness, dizziness, nausea, and vomiting; muscle cramps may also occur. Replacement of the deficit of water or salt will relieve the symptoms of heat exhaustion. If untreated, heat exhaustion due to water depletion will progress to heat stroke.

HEAT STROKE

This syndrome is characterized by high fever (usually but not always higher than 106°F (41°C)) and a profound disturbance of consciousness. Absence of sweating is a common but not invariable finding. Factors predisposing to heat stroke include age, obesity, underlying disorders (such as cardiac disease, diabetes mellitus, cerebrovascular disease), dermatologic or drug-induced compromise of sweat production, recent ingestion of alcohol, lack of acclimatization, or a prolonged continuous (day or night) period of heat exposure. High ambient humidity is not a prerequisite for heat stroke.

Elevation of the body temperature has a profound effect on metabolic processes. For each degree of temperature elevation, the basal metabolic rate increases about 7 percent. Thus, at a temperature of 106°F (41°C), the basal metabolic rate is increased by more than 50 percent. In response to this and the cutaneous vasodilatation required for heat dissipation, cardiac output increases correspondingly. However, the elevation of pulmonary vascular resistance that occurs with hyperthermia may lower cardiac output. Organ dysfunction is widespread with heat injury and is manifested by neurologic abnormalities (delirium, stupor, coma, seizures, ataxia, muscle weakness, or paralysis), circulatory abnormalities (tachycardia, hypotension), renal impairment (oliguria, hyposthenuria, acute tubular necrosis), hepatic abnormalities (hyperbilirubinemia, transaminase elevation), coagulation abnormalities (disseminated intravascular coagulation), abnormalities in water and electrolyte balance (dehydration, hypokalemia, hypophosphatemia, hypocalcemia), and metabolic (lactic) acidosis and muscle injury (rhabdomyolysis and myoglobinuria).

Although any illness causing hyperthermia can provoke heat stroke, it is most commonly seen in young unacclimatized individuals who perform strenuous exercise under conditions in which endogenous heat production exceeds heat dissipation and in elderly people living in an urban environment during prolonged periods of hot weather. Heat stroke may occur suddenly without prodrome or may be preceded by symptoms of heat exhaustion or psychotic behavior. In general, stupor or coma is common if the temperature is greater than 106°F (41°C).

Therapy in heat stroke is directed at rapidly lowering body temperature while maintaining the cardiac output at the required level.[51] Rapid reduction of body temperature can be achieved by removing the patient's clothing and either immersing the patient in an ice water bath and vigorously massaging the skin or massaging him with ice in the wake of a powerful fan. Vigorous cooling is mandatory if the temperature is above 106°F (41°C). Once the rectal temperature falls to 102°F (38.8°C), rapid cooling is stopped since the rectal temperature lags behind the core temperature. Hypotension often responds to cooling alone. In general, the central venous pressure in heat stroke is high and fluids must be administered cautiously. In a study of Marine recruits with heat stroke, an average of only 1200 ml of fluid was required during the first 4 hours.[53] Because of possible myocardial injury, overzealous fluid replacement may lead to pulmonary edema. Hypotension persisting after cooling and fluid administration can be treated with isoproterenol. Because of the common occurrence of hypokalemia and myocardial injury, digitalis should be administered with caution. A number of investigators have advocated use of phenothiazines to prevent thermogenesis due to shivering, but these agents can cause hypotension and may provoke seizures. Urine flow should be carefully monitored, and if there is initial oliguria, mannitol can be employed to initiate a diuresis. The urine should also be examined for myoglobin. Seizures, oliguria, and the hypercatabolic state promote hyperkalemia, and evidence of acute renal failure is an indication for early hemodialysis. The value of heparin in the coagulopathy of heat stroke is unsettled. Sweating is impaired for several days after correction of hyperthermia, and body temperature is labile during this period.

CHAPTER 150
Electrical Injury
JERRY L. SPIVAK

The skin provides the principal barrier to the flow of electricity through the body. In certain areas, such as the palms, skin resistance may be as high as 2 million ohms. Moistening of the skin or a break in its integrity can lower resistance to the extent that ordinary household current will be lethal. Skin resistance is also reduced by prolonged contact with an electrical current. When catheters or wires are inserted directly into the heart, bypassing the protective resistance and conductive effects of the surrounding tissues, a current too small to be perceived at the skin can be lethal.[56]

The type of injury produced by an electrical current depends on its magnitude and path. Respiratory arrest is usually the result of current passing through the medullary respiratory center as opposed to tetanic contraction of the respiratory muscles. The most common pathway for electrical current in accidental electrocution is, however, from limb to limb and consequently, cardiac rather than respiratory arrest is usually the fatal event. There is both an upper and a lower threshold for electrical induction of ventricular fibrillation. If current flow is prolonged, the threshold for triggering ventricular fibrillation falls. Extremely high voltage shocks, such as lightning, are not fibrillatory, and when cardiac activity is restored, it is usually with a sinus rhythm. Burns and tissue necrosis due to electricity occur when tissue resistance to current flow is sufficient to result in heat production.

Clinically, electric shock can produce severe pain due to tetanic muscle contraction. At currents above 6 milliamperes for women and 9 milliamperes for men, muscle contraction may be so intense that the victim is unable to release the object causing the electric shock. With severe shocks, such as occur with lightning, skeletal fractures and other blunt force injuries are common. Heat necrosis of muscle leads to myoglobinuria and hypovolemia; hypotension and oliguria due to extravascular fluid loss are not infrequent in this situation.[54] If consciousness is preserved, the victim may experience temporary deafness and visual disturbances. With high-voltage shock, consciousness is usually lost, and when the victim is revived, a variety of transitory neurologic and vascular disturbances may exist, including retrograde amnesia, aphasia, paraplegia with sensory deficit, and impairment of blood flow to the limbs. Transient hypertension is not uncommon. Permanent sequelae of high-voltage shock include deafness, cataracts, hemiplegia, spinal cord atrophy, and pe-

ripheral neuropathy. Many of the permanent neurologic sequelae are delayed in onset from weeks to months after the acute episode.[55]

Most electrical injuries are avoidable. In the hospital, this means careful maintenance of electrical equipment including attention to the adequacy of grounding arrangements. Electric beds and electrocardiographs are particularly suspect in this regard. Patients should, of course, always be completely isolated from ground. If an electric shock does occur, the victim must first be released from the current before other measures can be safely and effectively carried out. Cardiopulmonary resuscitation should be initiated in all apneic patients suffering from electrocution, even if the duration of apnea is unknown. This is particularly important with lightning shock since cardiac arrest in this instance is not associated with ventricular fibrillation.[57] Unfortunately, it is still a common practice to consider the apneic victim of a lightning stroke as dead without any attempt at resuscitation. Once revived, patients should be carefully evaluated for blunt force injuries, such as fractures, and for deep as well as superficial tissue injury. Adequate hydration should prevent renal failure due to hypovolemia and myoglobinuria.

CHAPTER 151

Poisoning
JAMES J. LIPSKY

Exposure to any chemical substance that can cause injury and/or death constitues a poisoning. The many problems associated with poisoning cut across all boundaries of medicine. Although the consequences of this fact may complicate the management of a poisoning, a logical systematic approach to all poisoned patients can still be undertaken. The management of the poisoned patient includes the general measures of supportive care as well as measures particular to the poison involved. In addition to medical problems, the poisoned patient may also have psychological problems which must not be neglected. Measures undertaken in the management of the poisoned patient are listed in Table 151–1.

Consider the Possibility
Failure to consider the possibility of poisoning is a common error. For example, in a study of acetylsalicylic acid ingestion, a common poisoning, it was found that in 20 of 73 ingestions the diagnosis was

initially missed.[58] The undiagnosed cases involved patients who initially gave no history of acetylsalicylic acid ingestion. Since this group of patients had an increased mortality, arriving at the diagnosis quickly is important. Poisoning should be considered even when a history of such is not obtained.

Maintain Vital Signs
The cornerstone of management of the poisoned patient is intensive supportive care to maintain vital functions.

Maintain Respiration
A patent airway must be established and maintained. The unconscious patient should be placed on his side to avoid aspiration. A cuffed endotracheal tube will assure a clear airway as well as prevent aspiration of the gastric contents. If respiration is inadequate, mechanical assistance of ventilation is indicated.

┌─────────────────────────────────────┐
TABLE 151-1
Measures in the Management of the Poisoned Patient

1. Consider the possibility
2. Maintain vital signs
3. Identify the poison
4. Prevent continued absorption of the poison
5. Hasten elimination of the poison
6. Correct or prevent toxic effects of the poison
└─────────────────────────────────────┘

Treat Shock

Maintenance of an adequate level of blood pressure may prove difficult. In general, shock should be treated initially with fluid replacement and, if possible, by elevation of the legs. If these simple measures fail to maintain tissue perfusion and urinary output, vasopressors are indicated (Chap. 145).

Watch the Temperature

The temperature of the severely poisoned patient should be carefully monitored and, if abnormal, corrected. Hypothermia may be present with overdoses of central nervous system depressants such as barbiturates. Hyperthermia may be associated with amphetamine or atropine poisoning.

Cardiac Arrhythmias

Treatment of cardiac arrhythmias is discussed in Chapter 21.

Identify the Poison

While supportive care alone is often adequate management, it is important to identify those poisons for which specific antidotes exist. In identifying the poison or poisons, history, physical examination, and laboratory tests may all be helpful.

In obtaining the history it is always important to consider its reliability. Patients or those with them are often incorrect concerning the number of pills ingested. Pill containers should be obtained if possible. Often the pharmacist who filled the prescription can give helpful information. Remember that an empty pill container may not have contained the medication described on the label. Furthermore, the possibility of multiple poisonings should be considered. For example, alcohol may accompany ingestion of other agents such as barbiturates.

Identification of the poison by the physical examination is usually difficult since most poisons do not produce pathognomonic signs. However, certain constellations of physical signs may be associated with certain poisons (Table 151-2).

┌─────────────────────────────────────┐
TABLE 151-2*
Common Poisons and Physical Signs of Ingestion

Poisons	Manifestations
Atropine-like agents— atropine, scopolamine, LSD, STP	Agitation, hallucinations, dilated pupils, beet-red color, dry skin, and fever
Amphetamines	Excessive activity, argumentativeness, tremors, headache, diarrhea, dry mouth with foul odor, sweating, tachycardia, arrhythmia, dilated pupils
Opiates	Slow respirations, pin-point pupils, euphoria, or coma
Organic phosphates or mushrooms (*Amanita muscaria*)	Salivation, lacrimation, urination, defecation, miosis, and pulmonary congestion
Barbiturates	Sleepy, slurred speech, nystagmus, staggering gait (ataxia) without alcohol odor to breath
Phenothiazines	Torsion head and neck syndrome, oculogyric crisis, and ataxia
Salicylates	Vomiting, hyperpnea, and fever

* From Mofenson, H.C., and Greensher, J.: Pediatrics 54:336–342, 1974.[66]
└─────────────────────────────────────┘

The laboratory is helpful in the identification of many substances. Blood, urine, and gastric contents can all be used. Many laboratories perform "toxicologic screens." The physician must know what is tested in these screens. A laboratory report of a negative toxicologic screen does not necessarily mean that the patient is not poisoned. It may only mean that the poison was not on the screen.

Although identification of the poison may be helpful, quantification is usually unnecessary. In most cases of poisoning, treatment would not be altered by knowledge of the blood level of the poison. Exceptions to this statement are few and include acetaminophen and acetylsalicylic acid. With these, a patient's initial physical examination may not indicate the severity of the poisoning and proper therapy may be unnecessarily delayed. In the case of acetaminophen, antidotes administered in time may interdict the toxic effects of the drug but are ineffective if administered 8 to 10 hours after the ingestion.

Prevent Continued Absorption

Emesis is an effective and rapid method to remove ingested poisons from the stomach. In the alert patient, emesis can be used in most poisonings with the exception of caustic alkali or small amounts of petroleum distillates. Emesis can be rapidly induced in some patients by mechanical stimulation of the oropharnx. Less rapid emesis can be induced pharmacologically by an emetic such as ipecac. Apomorphine has also been used; however, this drug produces undesirable central nervous system (CNS) depression.[63] Although emesis is generally considered to be the most effective way to empty the stomach, it does not always guarantee complete gastric emptying.[64]

Gastric lavage may also be employed to empty the stomach. However, a wide-bore orogastric tube is necessary if tablets and large particulate matter are to be aspirated. Most tablets cannot be aspirated through nasogastric tubes. If the patient is unconscious, gastric lavage may still be done. In this situation, a cuffed endotracheal tube should first be placed in order to prevent aspiration.

The earlier lavage is performed after an ingestion, the greater the benefit. However, since some poisons (such as acetylsalicylic acid), may cause pylorospasm and opioids (such as codeine) may cause ileus, lavage may still be worthwhile hours after the ingestion. In the case of acetylsalicylic acid, which does not rapidly leave the stomach, lavage should always be done. Lavage, like emesis, is not indicated for ingestions of caustic alkali or small amounts of petroleum products.

Following lavage or emesis, activated charcoal may be adminstered. Although activated charcoal adsorbs a wide range of poisons, it is not effective for all substances, e.g., paraquat (p. 1429). If activated charcoal is employed, it should be given before or shortly after oral antidotes or ipecac administration.

Following lavage or emesis, cathartics, such as magnesium citrate, may be given if ileus is not present.

Hasten Elimination of the Poison

Current methods for hastening elimination of some poisons are forced diuresis, dialysis, and charcoal or other hemoperfusion columns.[68] Before any of these procedures are undertaken, the physician should carefully consider whether it is indicated. The routine use of forced diuresis on poisoned patients is not recommended since this may result in the physician's having to treat fluid and electrolyte problems as well as the poisoning.

Drugs whose elimination may be hastened by a

TABLE 151-3
Antidotes

Acetaminophen	Methionine 2.5 g orally stat and q 4 hr × 3.
Anticholinesterases (Organophosphate insecticides)	Atropine 2.0 mg IV repeated as needed. Pralidoxime 1 g IV repeated as needed
Cyanide	Sodium nitrite 3%, 10 ml IV followed by sodium thiosulfate 25%, 50 ml IV
Ferrous sulfate	Desferoxamine 1 g IM initially followed by continuous intravenous infusion at a rate no more than 15 mg/kg/hr not to exceed 80 mg/kg/24 hr
Opioids (heroin, morphine, codeine, propoxyphene)	Naloxone 0.1 mg/kg IV as initial dose; repeat as needed
Phenothiazines	Benztropine 2 mg IV or diphenhydramine 25–50 mg IV
Tricyclic antidepressants (amitriptyline, doxepin, imipramine)	Physostigmine salicylate 1–2 mg IV

---

forced alkaline diuresis include lithium, salicylates, and long-acting barbiturates such as phenobarbital. Forced acid diuresis is helpful in the elimination of amphetamine. The use of peritoneal or hemodialysis may be of use in poisonings such as with alcohol, phenobarbital, bromide, lithium, chloral hydrate, and salicylates. The clinical course of the patient, such as the maintenence of vital signs, should be the major factor in deciding if dialysis is to be used.

Correct or Prevent Toxic Effects of the Poison

In some poisonings, administration of a specific antidote is indicated (Table 151–3). Since it is very difficult to be knowledgeable about every type of poisoning, one should not hesitate to seek sources of information on poisonings. Poison control centers are often helpful in providing information rapidly. Useful publications are listed in the references. The following sections in this chapter deal with some of the more common poisonings in adult.

SALICYLATES

Salicylate intoxication is common. Severe poisoning may be caused by acute ingestion as well as by chronic administration. The latter form of poisoning can result from accumulation of salicylates due to saturation of some of the metabolic processes in salicylate elimination. The severity of salicylate intoxication may initially be difficult to assess on clinical grounds. Patients can appear to be quite well or to have mild hyperventilation and tinnitus. Hyperpyrexia, nausea, and vomiting may also be present. Coma may not be an initial manifestation even in a heavy ingestion. However, in the absence of other causes, an altered state of consciousness indicates severe poisoning. The plasma salicylate level is the best way to assess severity. A nomogram has been devised by Done[60] which indicates the severity of an ingestion based on the serum level and time after ingestion. Any level greater than 50 mg/dl at 4 hours after the ingestion indicates a potentially serious ingestion. The nomogram should not be applied to chronic ingestions where the severity of the poisoning is not always related to the salicylate level. In adults, salicylate poisoning may produce respiratory alkalosis with metabolic acidosis, while young children usually present with metabolic acidosis. Dehydration, hypokalemia, and hypoglycemia may also be present.

Treatment is directed both at the removal of salicylate and the correction of the metabolic abnormalities. The gastric contents should be removed by emesis or lavage. Lavage may be effective as late as 4 hours after ingestion. Remember, "Don't procrastinate; it is never too late to aspirate salicylate." Alkalinization of the urine can enhance elimination of salicylate. However, in severe poisoning it may be difficult if not impossible to achieve an alkaline urine, particularly if hypokalemia is present. Therefore, one should not use the urinary pH to "titrate" the amount of bicarbonate administered. In cases of severe poisoning with profound acidosis, dialysis should be employed to remove the salicylates. Hypokalemia should be corrected with potassium administration and glucose given to correct hypoglycemia. In severe poisonings, glucose administration should be considered even in the presence of a normal blood sugar since experiments in animals have demonstrated decreased brain glucose under these conditions.[61]

ACETAMINOPHEN

Hepatic necrosis and subsequent death from liver failure are the most significant clinical problems following a large overdose of acetaminophen. The hepatic necrosis is the result of a toxic metabolite which is produced in increased amounts when large quantities of acetaminophen are ingested. The amount of acetaminophen necessary to produce liver damage is usually over 10 g in adults. Subsequent liver damage can be better predicted by a determination of the level of acetaminophen in the serum. Levels greater than 200 μg/ml at 4 hours after the ingestion may indicate eventual liver damage, and levels greater than 350 μg/ml may be associated with very severe liver necrosis and possible death. Nomograms for assessing the severity of an acetaminophen ingestion based on the serum level and the time following the ingestion have been published.[71]

Treatment of acetaminophen ingestion is directed at either inactivating the toxic metabolite or preventing its production. Although the exact mechanism of action of cysteamine, methionine, and n-acetylcysteine has not been proved, these compounds have been shown to prevent or lessen liver damage if they are given less than 10 hours after the ingestion. Their administration more than 10 hours after ingestion does not appear to be efficacious.

Thus, antidotes should be given as soon as possible, even before the acetaminophen level is known. Both methionine and n-acetylcysteine are commercially available and have no undesirable side effects of significance. Measures such as dialysis and forced diuresis are ineffective in acetaminophen ingestion.

LITHIUM

Lithium intoxication is usually associated with blood levels above 1.5 mEq/L. Lithium intoxication may result from acute ingestion as well as from chronic administration. Decreased tubular readsorption of sodium leads to increased readsorption of lithium. Consequently, elderly patients who are on salt-restricted diets and/or are on sodium-wasting diuretics are more susceptible to the development of toxicity from chronic administration. In mild cases of toxicity, there may be nausea and vomiting, polydipsia, and fine tremor of the hands as well as mental confusion. In more severe poisonings there is increased tremor, coma, and seizures. The EKG may show T-wave flattening or inversion. Treatment is directed toward removal of lithium from the body which may be accomplished by forced alkaline diuresis with careful monitoring of fluid and electrolyte status. If necessary, peritoneal or hemodialysis can be used; however, forced diuresis may be as effective as either form of dialysis.

OPIOIDS

The syndrome associated with opioid overdoses comprises coma, flaccid paralysis, miosis, and respiratory depression. Pulmonary edema may occur several hours after the first symptoms. In narcotic overdose patients, other causes of coma, such as trauma, must be considered. If narcotic overdose is suspected, then the specific narcotic antagonist, naloxone, should be administered immediately. The response to naloxone is both diagnostic and therapeutic. Since naloxone is a competitive antagonist of opioids, large doses may be required to reverse the effects of a large overdose of an opioid. Although the initial dose recommended is usually 0.4 mg intravenously, much larger doses may be needed. A total parenteral dose of 24 mg in a 70-kg patient has been given without adverse effect.[65] Since the effects of naloxone may last for only a few hours, one should carefully monitor the patient and readminister the antagonist if respiration and central nervous system depression redevelop. If pulmonary edema develops, it can be treated with oxygen and positive pressure ventilation.

TRICYCLIC ANTIDEPRESSANTS

Ingestion of excessive tricyclic antidepressants (amitriptyline, desipramine, doxepin, and imipramine) may result in central nervous system depression, anticholinergic manifestations, and cardiac arrhythmias. Although respiratory depression may be severe, patients are usually still responsive to painful stimuli. Cardiac arrhythmias may be life threatening, and prolongation of the QRS complex greater than 100 msec has been associated with serious intoxications.[70] Treatment of tricyclic poisoning is directed at reversing the anticholinergic manifestations. Physostigmine given intravenously may reverse the CNS effects. The reversal may be only of short duration and, thus, careful monitoring of the patient should continue. Whether physostigmine is able to reverse the cardiac arrhythmias is debatable. If hypotension is present, it may respond to volume expansion. Forced diuresis, hemodialysis, and charcoal perfusion are not effective measures in treating overdose of tricyclic antidepressants. Supportive care with physostigmine is usually sufficient.

ORGANOPHOSPHATES

Serious poisoning by organophosphates may be caused by exposure to commercial concentrates of insecticides. Exposure may occur via the skin, mucous membranes, respiratory tract, or gastrointestinal tract. The clinical features result from inhibition of acetylcholinesterase leading to excess acetylcholine. The clinical signs and symptoms of organophosphate poisoning are classified into muscarinic (including increased sweating, salivation, lacrimation, nausea, vomiting, increased bronchial secretion, and bronchoconstriction), nicotinic (including fasciculations, paralysis, and tachycardia), and CNS effects (including coma and respiratory depression). Low red cell or whole blood cholinesterase activity confirms the diagnosis.

Treatment of organophosphate poisoning involves several measures. Prevent continued exposure to the agent by washing the affected areas if necessary. Reverse muscarinic manifestations by administration of intravenous atropine in doses of 1 to 2 mg, repeating as often as necessary to maintain a mild degree of atropinization (dry mouth and mydriasis). Administer large amounts of atropine, even in excess of 100 mg per 24 hours, to accomplish this. Since atropine does not reverse the nicotinic effects, such as muscular weakness leading to respiratory paralysis, pralidoxine in a dose of 30 mg/kg intravenously should also be administered. This agent reactivates acetylcholinesterase in many types of organophosphate poisoning and may also reverse the CNS effects of the poisoning.[67] Repeat administration every 30 minutes and assist ventilation mechanically if necessary. Use measurements of FEV_1 and vital capacity as a guide to the degree of respiratory insufficiency. In cases of severe poisonings, administration of antidotes for several days or longer may be required.

BARBITURATES

The most serious effects of an overdose of a barbiturate are respiratory depression, coma, shock, and hypothermia. The degree of severity of the intoxication is best assessed by the clinical state of the patient rather than the blood level of the barbiturate. The cornerstone of management of barbiturate overdose is intensive supportive care. There are no specific antidotes, and neuroleptic agents have no place in the management. Respiration may have to be supported by mechanical ventilation. Shock associated with barbiturate ingestion appears to be due to an increase in the volume of the vascular bed with a relative decrease in intravascular volume.[69] Therefore, shock may be initially treated with plasma expanders and elevation of the feet. Vasopressors may be required when volume expansion might precipitate heart failure or is ineffective. Hypothermia should not be overlooked. Efforts to hasten the elimination of barbiturates are of limited value except for the long-acting drugs, such as phenobarbitol, for which forced alkaline diuresis may be effective. Hemodialysis may remove significant amounts of long-acting barbiturates but not the shorter acting ones. However, dialysis is needed only in severely poisoned patients with a deteriorating clinical status.

CARBON MONOXIDE

Although exposure to carbon monoxide is usually associated with obvious sources, such as exhaust fumes, it may occur in less evident situations such as inadequately ventilated indoor charcoal fires or space heaters. Furthermore, the cherry-red flush of the skin associated with carbon monoxide poisoning is not a common clinical occurrence. When the diagnosis is made, the patient should be immediately removed from the source of carbon monoxide and 100 percent oxygen administered. Administration of oxygen will usually promote the elimination of carboxyhemoglobin to safe levels by 4 hours. Five percent carbon dioxide should *not* be used as a respiratory stimulant, since hypoxia is the major problem and respiration can be supported by mechanical ventilation if necessary. After therapy is initiated, attention should be directed to the possible effects of hypoxic tissue damage. Cerebral edema must be vigorously treated with hypothermia or corticosteroids. Myocardial ischemia and/or infarction may occur even in young adults. Therefore, the EKG should be monitored for several days after severe intoxication.

PHENOTHIAZINES

Phenothiazine overdose may produce coma, respiratory depression, and shock as well as extrapyramidal manifestations such as muscle rigidity and torticollis. Respiratory depression and shock are relatively uncommon, although, when present, shock is profound. Cardiac arrhythmias which respond poorly to treatment may also be present. Shock should be treated with volume expansion and, if necessary, a vasopressor. Extrapyramidal effects can be abolished with the administration of diphenhydramine or benztropine. Forced diuresis or dialysis does not enhance the elimination of phenothiazines.

PARAQUAT

Paraquat is an herbicide which is available commercially as a 20 percent solution. Both paraquat and the vehicle in which it is dissolved may produce toxic effects. The vehicle has corrosive properties and may produce ulceration of the mouth as well as the esophagus. When taken orally, paraquat may produce damage to the kidneys, liver, and lungs. Lung damage in the form of a proliferative alveolitis may be delayed in appearance for up to a week. The mechanism of toxicity of paraquat is uncertain but may involve free radical formation. Treatment is directed at the rapid removal or inactivation of paraquat. Since activated charcoal does not adsorb paraquat, Fuller's earth should be used in gastric lavage and left in the stomach. Hemodialysis is not effective in removing large quantities of paraquat. Administration of oxygen may potentiate paraquat toxicity and, thus, it has been recommended that oxygen be used only when the arterial oxygen pressure is below 40 mm Hg.[59]

BROMIDE

Inorganic bromide intoxication has now become an uncommon disease as bromides have been removed from most over-the-counter preparations. Symptoms of bromide intoxication include drowsiness, slurred speech, confusion, and agitation. Coma may also occur. In 25 to 30 percent of cases, a rash occurs which is usually acneiform but may be nodular or bullous. Toxicity rarely occurs below serum bromide levels of 15 mEq/L. Treatment is directed at increasing renal elimination of bromide by saline loading.[72]

Organic bromide intoxication may occur by exposure to methylbromide. This compound is used as a refrigerant, delousing agent, and fire extinguishant.[62] Intoxication may produce CNS alterations including confusion, convulsions, and coma. Renal failure may also occur. Treatment consists of supportive care, removal of methylbromide from the skin, and avoidance of breathing the vapors.

REFERENCES

Cardiorespiratory Arrest

1. Bishop, R.L. and Weisfeldt, M.C. Sodium bicarbonate administration during cardiac arrest. JAMA, 235:506, 1976.
2. Eller, W.C. and Haugen, R.K. Food asphyxiation—restaurant rescue. N. Engl. J. Med., 289:81, 1973.
3. Ewy, G.A. Cardiopulmonary resuscitation. In Mason, D.J. (ed.), Cardiac Emergencies. Baltimore, Williams & Wilkins, 1978, pp. 15–42.
4. Lown, B., Crampton, R.S., DeSilva, R.A., and Gascho, H. The energy for ventricular defibrillation—too little or too much? N. Engl. J. Med., 298:1252, 1978.
5. Matter, J.A., Weil, M.H., Shubin, H., and Stein, L. Cardiac arrest in the critically ill. II. Hyperosmolal states following cardiac arrest. Am. J. Med., 56:162, 1974.
6. Pennington, J.E., Taylor, J., and Lown, B. Chest thump for reverting ventricular tachycardia. N. Engl. J. Med., 283:1192, 1970.
7. Standards for cardiopulmonary resuscitation (CPR) and emergency cardiac care (ECC). JAMA, 227 (Suppl.):833, 1974.
8. Taylor, G.J., Tucker, W.M., Green, H.L., et al. Prolonged compression during cardiopulmonary resuscitation in man. N. Engl. J. Med., 296:1555, 1977.

Shock

9. Bishop, R.L. and Weisfeldt M.L. Sodium bicarbonate administration during cardiac arrest—effect on arterial pH, Pco₂ and osmolality. JAMA, 235:506, 1976.
10. Schumen, W. Steroids in the treatment of clinical septic shock. Ann. Surg., 184:333, 1976.
11. Shubin, H. and Weil, M.H. Routine central venous catheterization for management of critically ill patients. In Ingelfinger, F., Ebert, R., Finland, M., and Relman, A.

(eds.), Controversies in Internal Medicine, Vol. 2. Philadelphia, Saunders, 1974, pp. 177–184.

12. Swan, H.J.C. The role of hemodynamic monitoring in the management of the critically ill. Crit. Care Med., 3:83, 1975.

13. Tarazi, R.C. Sympathomimetic agents in the treatment of shock. Ann. Intern. Med., 81:364, 1974.

14. Weil, M. Current understanding of mechanisms and treatment of circulatory shock caused by bacterial infections. Ann. Clin. Res., 9:181, 1977.

Acute Respiratory Failure

15. Aberman, A. and Fulop, M. The metabolic and respiratory acidosis of acute pulmonary edema. Ann. Intern. Med., 76:173, 1972.

16. Battaglia, J.D. and Lockhart, C.H. Management of acute epiglottitis by nasotracheal intubation. Am. J. Dis. Child., 129:334, 1975.

17. Bussmann, W.D. and Schupp, D. Effect of sublingual nitroglycerin in emergency treatment of severe pulmonary edema. Am. J. Cardiol., 41:931, 1978.

18. Campbell, E.J.M. The management of acute respiratory failure in chronic bronchitis and emphysema. Am. Rev. Respir. Dis., 96:626, 1967.

19. Crocco, J.A., Rooney, J.J., Fankushen, D.S., DiBenedetto, R.J., and Lyons, H.A. Massive hemoptysis. Arch. Intern. Med., 121:495, 1968.

20. Derenne, J., Macklem, P., and Roussos, C. The respiratory muscles: mechanics, control, and pathophysiology. Am. Rev. Respir. Dis., 118:119–133, 373–390, 581–601, 1978.

21. Dikshit, K., Vyden, J.K., Forrester, J.S., et al. Renal and extrarenal hemodynamic effects of furosemide in congestive heart failure after acute myocardial infarction. N. Engl. J. Med., 288:1087, 1973.

22. Garfinkel, J.H., Brown, R., and Kabins, S.A. Acute infectious epiglottitis in adults. Ann. Intern. Med., 70:289, 1969.

23. Gruiner, P.F. Treatment of acute pulmonary edema: conventional or intensive care? Ann. Intern. Med., 77:501, 1972.

24. Katz, S. Spontaneous pneumothorax. In Shibel, E.M. and Moser, K.M., (eds.), Respiratory Emergencies. St. Louis, Mosby, 1977. Chapter 10.

25. Kryger, M., Bode, F., Antic, R., and Anthenisen, N. Diagnosis of obstruction of the upper and central airways. Am. J. Med., 61:85, 1976.

26. Lesch, M., Caranasos, G.J., Mulholland, J.G., et al. Controlled study of ethacrynic acid and mercaptomerin in the treatment of acute pulmonary edema. N. Engl. J. Med., 279:115, 1968.

27. Mikulie, E., Cohn, J.W., and Franciosa, J.A. Comparative hemodynamic effects of inotropic and vasodilator drugs in severe heart failure. Circulation, 56:528, 1977.

28. Plumb, V.J. and James T.N. Clinical hazards of powerful diuretics. Mod. Concepts Cardiovasc. Dis., 48:91, 1978.

29. Shepherd, J.T. and Vanhoutte, P.M. Role of the venous system in circulatory control. Mayo Clin. Proc., 53:247, 1978.

30. Shibel, E.M. Acute respiratory failure with hypercapnia. In Shibel, E.M. and Moser, K.M. (eds.), Respiratory Emergencies. St. Louis, Mosby, 1977. Chapter 4.

31. Speizer, F.E. Epidemiology and mortality patterns in asthma. In Weiss, E.B. (ed.), Status Asthmaticus. Baltimore, University Park Press, 1978, p. 13.

32. Summer, W.R. Inhalation of noxious gases, fumes and vapors. In Shibel, E.M., and Moser, K.M., (eds.), Respiratory Emergencies. St. Louis, Mosby, 1977. Chapter 9.

33. Sykes, M.K., McNicol, M.W., and Campbell, E.J.M. Respiratory Failure, 2nd ed. Oxford, Blackwell, 1976.

34. Toung T.J.K., Saharia, P., Mitzner, W.A., Permutt, S., and Cameron, J.L. The beneficial and harmful effects of positive end-expiratory pressure. Surg. Gynecol. Obstet. 147:518, 1978.

35. Vasko, J.S., Henney, R.P., Oldham, H.N., et al. Mechanisms of action of morphine in the treatment of experimental pulmonary edema. Am. J. Cardiol., 18:876, 1966.

36. Wedel, M. Massive hemoptysis. In Shibel, E.M. and Moser, K.M. (eds.), Respiratory Emergencies. St. Louis, Mosby, 1977. Chapter 11.

Coma and Impaired Mentation

37. Arky, R.A., Veverbrants, E., and Abramson, E.A. Irreversible hypoglycemia: complication of alcohol and insulin. JAMA, 206:575, 1968.

38. Drenick, E.J., Joven, C.B., and Swenseid, M.E. Occurrence of acute Wernicke's encephalopathy during prolonged starvation for the treatment of obesity. N. Engl. J. Med., 274:937, 1966.

39. Jenkins, D.W., Eckel, R.E., and Craig, J.W. Alcoholic ketoacidosis. JAMA, 217:177, 1971.

40. Johnson, H.K. and Waterhouse, C. Lactic acidosis and phenformin. Arch. Intern. Med., 122:367, 1968.

41. Leavell, W.W., Farley, C.H., and McIntyre, J.S. Cutaneous changes in a patient with carbon monoxide poisoning. Arch. Dermatol., 99:429, 1969.

42. Messert, B. and Wannamaker, B.B. Reappraisal of the adult occult hydrocephalus syndrome. Neurology, 24:224, 1974.

43. Plum, F. and Posner, J.B. The Diagnosis of Stupor and Coma, 2nd ed. Philadelphia, Davis, 1972.

44. Spivak, J.L. and Jackson, D. Pellagra: an analysis of 18 patients and a review of the literature. Johns Hopkins Med. J., 140:295, 1977.

45. Srivastava, S.C. and Robson, A.O. Electrocardiographic abnormalities associated with subarachnoid hemorrhage. Lancet, 2:431, 1964.

46. Sussman, K.E., Crout, J.R., and Marble, A. Failure of warning in insulin-induced hypoglycemic reactions. Diabetes, 12:38, 1963.

Hypothermia

47. Clements, S.D., Jr. and Hurst, W. Diagnostic value of electrocardiographic abnormalities observed in subjects accidently exposed to cold. Am. J. Cardiol, 29:729, 1972.

48. Gagge, A.P. and Herrington, L.P. Physiological effects of heat and cold. Annu. Rev. Physiol., 9:409, 1947.

49. Severinghaus, J.W. Respiration and hypothermia. Ann. N.Y. Acad. Sci., 80:384, 1959.

50. Weyman, A.E., Greenbaum, D.M., and Grace, W.J. Accidental hypothermia in an alcoholic population. Am. J. Med., 56:13, 1974.

Hyperthermia

51. Clowes, G.H.A., Jr. and O'Donnell, T.F., Jr. Heat stroke. N. Engl. J. Med., 291:564, 1974.
52. Knochel, J.P. Environmental heat injury. Arch. Intern. Med., 133:841, 1974.
53. O'Donnell, T.F., Jr. and Clowes, G.H.A., Jr. The circulatory abnormalities of heat stroke. N. Engl. J. Med., 287:734, 1972.

Electrical Injury

54. Artz, C.P. Electrical injury simulates crush injury. Surg. Gynecol. Obstet., 125:1316, 1967.
55. Farrell, D.F. and Starr, D. Delayed neurological sequelae of electrical injuries. Neurology, 18:601, 1968.
56. Starmer, C.F., McIntosh, H.D., and Whalen, R.E. Electrical hazards and cardiovascular function. N. Engl. J. Med., 284:181, 1971.
57. Taussig, H.B. Death from lightning and the possibility of living again. Ann. Intern. Med., 68:1345, 1968.

Poisoning

58. Anderson, R.J., Potts, D.E., Gabow, P.A., Rumack, B.H., and Schrier, R.W. Unrecognized adult salicylate intoxication. Ann. Intern. Med., 85:745, 1976.
59. Dasta, J.F. Paraquat poisoning: a review. Am. J. Hosp. Pharm., 35:1368, 1978.
60. Done, A.K. Salicylate intoxication: significance of measurements of salicylate in blood in cases of acute ingestion. Pediatrics, 26:800, 1960.
61. Hill, J.B. Salicylate intoxication. N. Engl. J. Med., 288:1110, 1973.
62. Hine, C.H. Methyl bromide poisoning. JOM, 11:1, 1961.
63. MacLean, W.C. A comparison of ipecac syrup and apomorphine in the immediate treatment of ingestion of poisons. J. Pediatr., 82:121, 1973.
64. Matthew, H. Gastric aspiration and lavage. Clin. Toxicol., 3:179, 1970.
65. Matthew, H. and Lawson, A.A.N. Opium alkaloids and morphine derivatives. In Treatment of Common Acute Poisonings, 3rd ed. Edinburgh, Churchill Livingstone, 1975, pp. 138–145.
66. Mofenson, H.C. and Greensher, J. The unknown poison. Pediatrics, 54:336, 1974.
67. Namba, T., Nolte, C., Jackrel, J., and Grob, D. Poisonings due to organophosphate insecticides. Am. J. Med., 50:475, 1971.
68. Rosenbaum, J.L., Kramer, M.S., Raja, R., and Boreyko, C. Resin hemoperfusion: a new treatment for acute drug intoxication. N. Engl. J. Med., 284:874, 1971.
69. Shubin, H. and Weil, M.N. The mechanism of shock following suicidal doses of barbiturates, narcotics, and tranquilizer drugs, with observations on the effects of treatment. Am. J. Med., 38:853, 1965.
70. Spiker, D.G., Weiss, A.N., Chang, S.S., Ruwitch, J.F., and Biggs, J.T. Tricyclic antidepressant overdose: clinical presentation of plasma levels. Clin. Pharmacol. Ther., 18:539, 1975.
71. Symposium on paracetamol and the liver. J. Int. Med. Res., 4(Suppl. 4):, 1976.
72. Trump, D.L. and Hochberg, M.C. Bromide intoxication. Johns Hopkins Med. J., 138:119, 1976.

SECTION NINETEEN
Special Topics in Medicine
RICHARD J. JOHNS: SECTION EDITOR

CHAPTER 152
Special Aspects of Care for Adolescents and the Aged
PETER E. DANS AND CATHERINE DeANGELIS

INTRODUCTION

This new chapter devoted to the care of the adolescents and the aged has been developed because of the increasing realization that their care often requires special expertise beyond that necessary for other age groups. The purpose of the first section is to discuss some of the characteristics and problems of the teen years in order to enable the physician and other health care providers to function more effectively with teenagers. The second section will distinguish normal from pathologic aging and show how these changes affect the management of older persons.

MANAGEMENT OF THE ADOLESCENT PATIENT

Adolescence is the time and/or process of maturation from childhood to adulthood. It includes the period of life between puberty and maturity, usually ages 12 through 19. Over 30 million persons, 15 percent of the total population of the United States, are age 12 to 19. Differences in cultural, ethnic, geographic, and economic influences prevent teenagers from being an homogenous group. However, a number of characteristics common to all bind them together into a subculture with specific needs that require special understanding and management.

Mortality and Morbidity
It is interesting to contrast the leading causes of adolescent mortality and morbidity as perceived by health professionals working in a medical setting with those problems as perceived by the teenagers themselves.

The death rate in the age group from 12 to 19 years is 128 per 100,000 population. Neither physicians nor adolescents are usually aware that the four leading causes of death in this age group are accidents (58.1 percent), homicides (7.3 percent), malignant neoplasm (7.2 percent), and suicides (5.4 percent).[32]

From a medical viewpoint, the problems most often identified include: scoliosis, slipped epiphysis, acne, sports injuries, infectious mononucleosis, body image problems, drug abuse, venereal disease, goiter, sexual dysfunction, delinquency, tumors, anorexia nervosa, hepatitis, primary amenorrhea, and school-learning problems. The problems made worse by adolescence are tuberculosis, automotive injuries, unwed pregnancy, suicide, diabetes, inflammatory bowel disease, menstrual dysfunction, dental caries, abortion, gynecomastia, and mental retardation. The problems that often originate during adolescence are obesity, alcoholism, duodenal ulcer, hypercholesterolemia, labile hypertension, irritable colon syndrome, migraine headaches, and marital conflicts.[13]

This primarily disease-oriented list can be contrasted with those cited by teenagers. The problems and concerns ranked highest by adolescents were: school, drugs, how far to go with sex, getting along with parents and other adults, birth control, venereal disease, pregnancy, menstrual periods, sadness and depression, acne, and weight problems.[33]

This disparity emphasizes the importance of identifying what the adolescent feels his problem is and what his concerns are.

ADOLESCENT GROWTH AND DEVELOPMENT
Physical Development
Adolescence is associated with the second accelerated growth in height and weight; the first occurs in the first 2 years of life. The adolescent growth spurt is accompanied by the appearance of sexual characteristics. Physically, adolescence is terminated by fusion of the epiphyses and metaphyses of bone and by the ability to reproduce, thereby completing the transition from childhood to adulthood.

Essentially, the sooner puberty occurs, the sooner will the rate of growth decline and finally stop.[49] The onset of puberty is better correlated with the mean height and weight than with chronologic age.[19] Growth may proceed an average of 3 inches, with a range of 1 to 7 inches, after the onset of menses. The comparable measure in males is not known because a finite marker, like menses, does not exist in males.

A normal growth spurt may begin as early as 9.5 years in the female and 10.5 in the male or as late as 14.5 years in the female and 16.0 years in the male.[50] For both sexes the acceleration, peak, deceleration, and fusion of bone usually span a period of approxi-

mately 2 years; the gain in height equals about 20 percent of adult height.

In general, adolescent weight changes parallel those in height but the incremental changes and variabilities are greater. The weight gain is usually steady throughout puberty in the nonobese adolescent, and the total weight gain during this period is approximately half that of the ideal adult body weight. Figures 152–1 and 152–2 show the height and weight

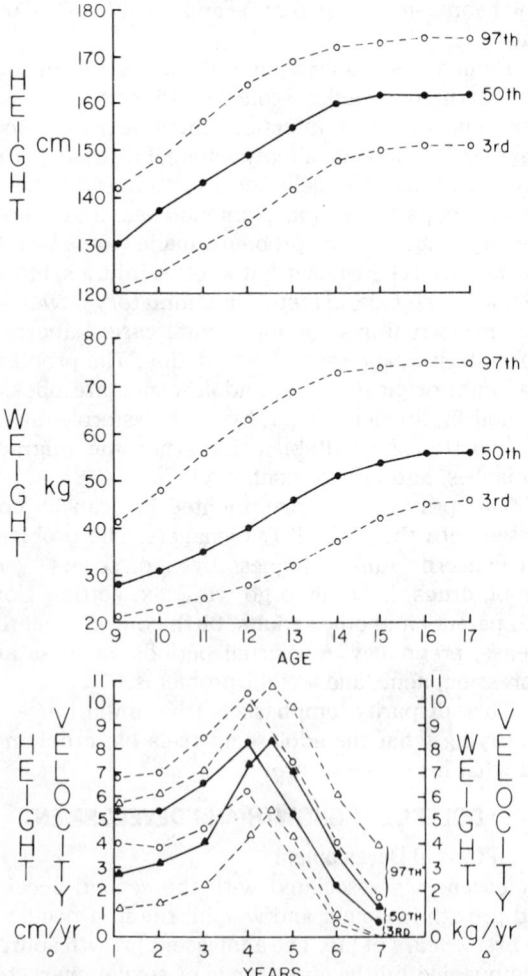

FIGURE 152–1. Cross-sectional female height and weight by chronologic age (3rd, 50th, 97th percentiles) and longitudinal values for height and weight during the year of peak height and weight velocity and the 3 years before and after PHV and PWV (3rd, 50th, 97th percentiles). (Adapted from Tanner.[50])

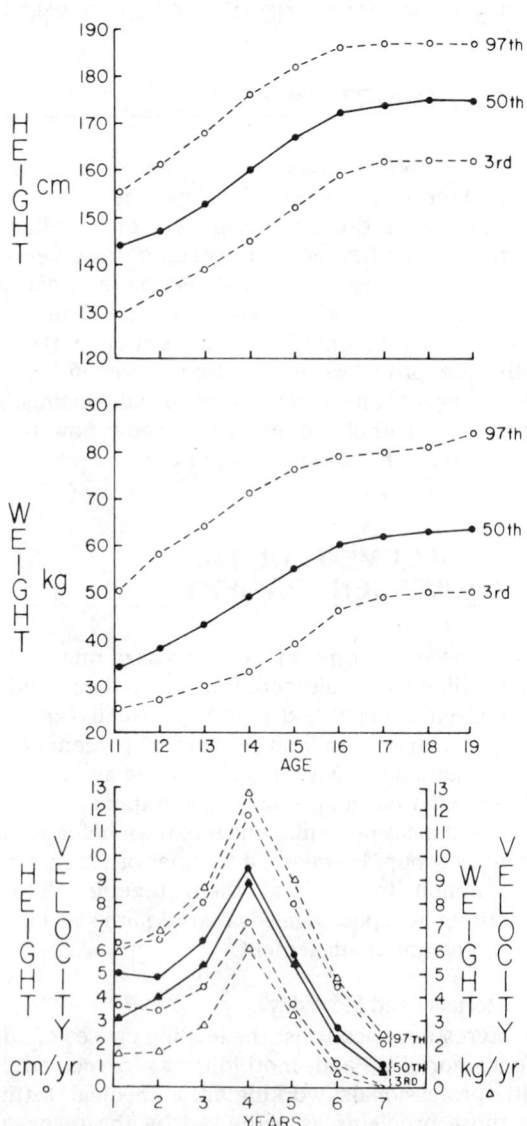

FIGURE 152–2. Cross-sectional male height and weight by chronologic age (3rd, 50th, 97th percentiles) and longitudinal values for height and weight during the year of peak height and weight velocity and the 3 years before and after PHV and PWV (3rd, 50th, 97th percentiles). (Adapted from Tanner.[50])

TABLE 152–1
Stages of Sexual Development in Females*

Age (years)		Stages
0–12	I.	Preadolescent. Female pelvic contour evident; breast flat; labia majora smooth and minora poorly developed; hymenal opening small or absent; mucous membranes dry and red; vaginal cells lack glycogen
8–13	II.	*Breasts:* Elevation of nipple; small mound beneath areola which is enlarging and begins pigmentation. *Labia majora:* become thickened, more prominent, and wrinkled. *Labia minora:* easily identified due to increased size along with clitoris; urethral opening more prominent, mucous membranes moist and pink; some glycogen present in vaginal cells *Hair:* First appears on mons and then on labia majora about time of menarche; still scanty, soft and straight *Skin:* Increased activity of sebaceous and merocrine sweat glands, and initial function of aprocrine glands in axilla and vulva begin
9–14	III.	Rapid growth peak is passed; menarche most often at this stage and invariably follows the peak of growth acceleration *Breasts:* Areola and nipple further enlarge and pigmentation more evident; continued increase in glandular size *Labia minora:* Well developed and vaginal cells have increased glycogen content; mucous membranes increasingly more pale *Hair:* In pubic region thicker, coarser, often curly (considerable normal variation including a few girls with early Stage II at menarche) *Skin:* Further increased activity of sebaceous and sweat glands with beginning of *acne* in some girls; adult body odor
12–15	IV.	*Breasts:* Projection of areola above breast plane and areolar (Montgomery) glands apparent (this development is absent in about 20% of normal girls); glands easily palpable *Labia:* Both majora and minora assume adult structure; glycogen content of vaginal cells begins cyclic characteristics *Hair:* In pubic area more abundant; axillary hair present (rarely present at Stage II, not uncommonly present at Stage III)

* From Lowrey.[30]

TABLE 152–1 (cont.)

Age (years)		Stages
12–17	V.	*Breasts:* Mature histologic morphology; nipple enlarged and erect; areolar (Montgomery) glands well developed; globular shape *Hair:* In pubic area more abundant and may spread to thighs (in about 10% of women it assumes "male" distribution with extension toward umbilicus); facial hair increased often in form of slight mustache *Skin:* Increased sebaceous gland activity and increased severity of *acne* if present before

growth curves for adolescent females and males. Change in the rate of growth from the beginning to the end of the growth spurt is relatively abrupt for the individual teenager and covers a period of months, rather than years. Hence, the individual growth curve is not nearly as smooth as those depicted in the figures.

There is variation in the age at which the various sequences of puberty begin and considerable differences in the rapidity with which each individual progresses from one stage to the next. However, the sequences themselves are the same for all individuals. Tables 152–1 and 152–2 list the stages of sexual development for females and males.

The exact causes of the onset of puberty are not clearly known. However, various hormonal assays have correlated the relationship of increased levels of pituitary luteinizing hormone and follicle stimulating hormone with 1) the advancing stages of adolescent psychological development, 2) gonadal growth and function, and 3) bony maturation.[9,38,46] Table 152–3 shows the hormones involved in puberty.

Over the past 140 years, menarche has occurred on the average of 3 months earlier each decade. Currently, menarche occurs at the average age of 12.5 years in the United States with a range of 6 to 17 years. It should be noted, however, that only 0.2 percent of girls are under 9 years at the onset of menses.[1]

Socioeconomic factors play an important role in the age of onset of puberty. Generally, menses occur earlier in young women from higher socioeconomic levels. Age of maternal menarche and race seem to have only minor influences. Factors such as malnutrition, blindness, and chronic illness tend to delay the onset of puberty in males and females.[53] Some other pathologic conditions associated with delayed or precocious sexual development are listed in Table 152–4.

Emotional Development

Generally, four major developmental tasks must be accomplished by the adolescent before emotional adulthood can be achieved. The first is to become emancipated from parents and other adults; the second is to acquire skills for future economic independence; the third is to learn to function in an adult, heterosexual role; and the fourth is to acquire a realistic, stable, and positive adult self-identity. Behavioral experimentation is the principal method used by adolescents to achieve these development tasks.

Early and mid-adolescence are times of strong peer group activities in what is commonly known as the adolescent subculture. During this phase, the adolescent has traded the safety of his childhood identification with his parents for the safety of a peer group identity. The individual identity of the adult is a phenomenon of the future, but behavioral experimentation with adult-like roles, such as dating, part-time jobs, and acquiring special educational interests, is common. Developmental conflicts frequently occur because emotional ties with the peer group are often superficial and the teenager's individuality may be compromised. Risk-taking behavior, such as high-speed driving with an automobile or motorcycle and experimentation with sexual activity and drug usage including alcohol and smoking, is common. For the most part, these are transient phases, but complications result when the adolescent has no friends, has poor peer-group ties, is multiply sexually active, becomes involved in drug abuse, or the initial experimentation with drugs ends in disaster.

The rebellion and withdrawal from adults, the heavy reliance on the group, and the constant, apparent changes in their value systems, which are reflections of their changing environment and behavioral experimentation are often confounding to even the most patient parents. Helping teenagers and their parents work through these times can be a very rewarding experience for the health professional.

In order to function as a sexually mature adult, an adolescent must concurrently integrate his personality with his developing biologic and physiologic capabilities. Bryt describes four distinct factors that influence psychosexual growth during adolescence.[8] First in importance, and becoming increasingly significant from early adolescence onward, is the irresistible urge for active expression of sexual impulses. Prior to puberty only anger is nearly so compelling. The second factor is the effect of prevailing social mores. The adolescent's need to express himself

---

TABLE 152–2

Stages of Sexual Development in Males*

Age (years)	Stages
0–14	I. Preadolescent
10–14	II. Increasing size of *testes* and *penis* is evident (testicle length reaches 2.0 cm or more). Scrotum integument is thinner and assumes an increased pendulous appearance *Hair:* First appearance of pubic hair in area at base of penis *Skin:* Increased activity of sebaceous and aprocrine sweat glands and initial function of apocrine glands of axilla and scrotal area begins
11–15	III. Rapid growth peak is passed; nocturnal emissions begin *Testes* and *penis:* Further increase in size and pigmentation apparent. Leydig cells (interstitial) first appear at Stage II; are now prominent in testes *Hair:* In pubic area more abundant and present on scrotum; still scanty and fine textured; axillary hair begins *Breasts:* Button-type hypertrophy in 70% of boys at Stages II and III *Larynx:* Changes in voice due to beginning of laryngeal growth *Skin:* Increasing activity of sebaceous and sweat glands with beginning of *acne;* adult body odor
12–16	IV. *Testes:* Further increase in size, length 4.0 cm or greater; increase in size of *penis* greatest at Stages III and IV *Hair:* Pubic hair thicker and coarser and in most ascends toward umbilicus in typical male pattern; axillary hair increases; facial hair increases over lip and upper cheeks *Larynx:* Voice deepens *Skin:* Increasing pigmentation of scrotum and penis; acne often more severe *Breasts:* Previous hypertrophy decreased or absent
13–17	V. *Testes:* Length greater than 4.5 cm *Hair:* Pubic hair thick, curly, heavily pigmented; extends to thighs and toward umbilicus. Adult distribution and increase in body hair (chest, shoulders, thighs, etc.) continues for more than another 10 years. Baldness, if present, may begin *Skin:* Acne may persist and increase *Larynx:* Adult character of voice

* From Lowrey.[30]

—TABLE 152–3—
Hormones Involved in Adolescent Development*

Luteinizing Hormone Release Factor

Activity	Stimulates pituitary to release gonadotropins (LH and FSH)
Source	Hypothalamus
Nature	Decapeptide

Luteinizing Hormone

Activity	Preparation and ripening of ovarian follicle, may stimulate release of progesterone, role not clear in prepubertal girl; in male stimulates interstitial (Leydig) cells of testes to secrete testosterone
Source	Pituitary
Name	LH, a glycoprotein

Follicle-Stimulating Hormone

Activity	In female, develops ovarian follicle to antrum stage, increases estrogen secretion from follicle; in male, matures sperm and may influence growth of seminiferous tubules
Source	Pituitary
Name	FSH, a glycoprotein

Estrogens

Activity	Feminizing; cause breast development, uterine growth, vaginal maturation, bone maturation; no effect on somatic growth
Source	Mainly ovarian but small and possibly significant amounts from adrenal cortex and testes
Names	Estrone, estradiol, estriol

Androgens

Activity	Virilizing; cause penile and prostatic development; promote hair growth of pubic, axillary, facial, and general body areas; bone maturation; laryngeal development; sebaceous and sweat gland development; stimulus to somatic growth
Source	Testicles, adrenal cortex, small amounts from ovary
Names	Dehydroepiandrosterone, testosterone, epitestosterone, androstenedione

Progesterones

Activity	Block estrogen effect on endometrium, stimulate endometrial gland secretion, stimulate lobule-alveolar breast formation and growth
Source	Mainly from ovarian corpus luteum, small amounts from testes and adrenal cortex (large amounts from placenta)
Names	Progesterone, pregnenolone

* From Lowrey.[30]

—TABLE 152–4—
Pathologic Conditions Associated with Abnormalities of Sexual Development*†

Conditions associated with *delayed onset* of puberty
  Pituitary dwarfism
  Hypothyroidism
  Hypogonadism (agenesis, atrophy, surgical or traumatic castration)
  Acromegaly (rare)
  Any severe chronic illness
  Hypothalamic lesions (Frölich syndrome)

Conditions associated with *precocious* sexual development
  Adrenal cortex tumors or hyperplasia
  Interstitial cell tumors of the testes
  Ovarian tumors (granulosa cell and thecoma)
  Pineal gland tumors (in males only)
  Third ventricle tumors of the brain
  Hydrocephalus (rare)
  Postencephalitis (rare)
  McCune-Albright syndrome (polyostotic fibrous dysplasia)

* From Lowrey.[30]
†Besides the endocrine glands, it will be noted that the central nervous system (hypothalamus) may also be involved.

sexually may or may not be at odds with the community's current morality. The chances of a significant confrontation with social mores increases in the later teens. Third is the unconscious influence of family ethics that have been an environmental factor since childhood. The adolescent's actual, rather than apparent, personal value system is an integral part of how he will respond to the later experiences that are essential for his psychosexual maturation. Fourth, the relationship between public and private morality may create and perpetuate internal conflicts and delay maturation in late adolescence. Gross discrepancies often exist between the two, and there is no readily available pattern after which the adolescent can model himself.

Should this developmental process be abbreviated or interrupted by pregnancy or marriage, the result is often catastrophic. Eighty percent of such teenage marriages result in divorce within 5 years. Many of the young mothers are without education or job training and have little choice other than to become welfare recipients. The effects on their infants are often even more catastrophic, since the parents are themselves children.

The availability of heterosexual peers is a necessary factor in the resolution of middle adolescent sexuality. Sociosexual experimentation such as dating, not sexual intercourse, is the vital ingredient. Currently, there seems to be inadequate limit-setting in this area for many teenagers, and pregnancy prevention has become a vital factor in allowing adolescents the time to work through the developmental tasks previously defined. Teenagers have had to develop new patterns to deal with the fact that sexual intercourse is an increasingly frequent part of midadolescence.

GENERAL APPROACHES TO THE TEENAGER

In addition to the concepts discussed in other sections of this textbook, certain key issues should be considered in the general approach to routine management of the adolescent patient.

History

A careful review of the *perinatal period* is essential. A teenage girl whose mother received diethylstibestrol during her pregnancy with the teenager should be examined and followed carefully to rule out vaginal adenocarcinoma.[24] Teenage boys with a similar history should be watched carefully for genitourinary anomalies.[23]

Immunization review is often neglected in teenagers. Consequently preventable, infectious disease often occurs in adolescents (see below).

Nutritional history is important because of the increased energy and protein demands of rapid growth and development and accelerated physical activity. Generally, teenage girls require about 2400 calories per day and boys about 2900 calories per day.

Teenagers eat according to habits and attitudes learned early in life which are very difficult to alter. The motivation to eat well-balanced meals does not come naturally. Foods are chosen primarily because they are pleasing to the senses and are convenient to obtain. Consequently, many teenagers are junk food enthusiasts. Further, the effects of good and bad nutrition are not easily demonstrated in the teen years, and the threat of illness from malnutrition seems so remote to an adolescent that the idea usually has little or no effect on him.

A recent study by Kelly has revealed that adolescents of both sexes, but especially girls, have inadequate intake of calcium, iron, and vitamins C and A.[27] These inadequacies in the diet are at least partially caused by the fad diets so frequently popular with adolescents.

About 10 to 15 percent of American adolescents are obese. In addition to the possible subsequent cardiovascular problems in later life, many overweight adolescents are not well adjusted emotionally. Physical appearance is a very important teenage socializing factor. Obese adolescents tend to be depressed, to have poor body images, to have difficulty making friends, to be very dependent on family approval, and to have severe psychiatric disturbances requiring treatment. Obese applicants to college are less likely to be accepted than the nonobese, even though academic achievement, social class, and motivation are essentially equivalent.[15]

A complete *sexual history* should include degree of sexual activity, use of contraception, possibility of venereal disease, and, in girls, menarche and menses. Questions should be asked directly, specifically, and in a nonjudgmental manner.

Inquiry should be made about the *use of alcohol, cigarettes, and other drugs.* About 25 percent of all teenagers smoke, and the number has increased by 50 percent between 1968 and 1974.[2] Teenagers who smoke can develop sputum production, cough, shortness of breath, and abnormally low expiratory flow rates that reflect small airway obstruction.[44]

Physical Examination

Special attention should be given to the examination of *breasts* in both males and females. This is an excellent time to teach teenage girls how to examine their breasts for masses and to reassure boys with gynecomastia that it is a normal variant that will regress.

Males should be taught self-examination of the *testes.* Most masses are benign varicoceles or hydroceles, but the incidence of malignant testicular tumors is highest during adolescence.

Pelvic examinations should be performed on all sexually active women. Significant abnormalities such as specific infection, smears with atypical inflammatory cells, and dysplasia can occur.[22,31]

It is especially important to *examine the spine* of teenagers to rule out scoliosis and kyphosis. Kyphosis, or "round shoulders" is found in up to 8 percent of adolescents of both sexes, typically in the early and mid-teen years. On x-ray, an irregularity of the vertebral end-plates is usually found early. Later, the anterior surface of one or more vertebrae is narrowed by at least 5°. Teenagers with this problem should be referred to an orthopedic surgeon for therapy.

Scoliosis is a lateral deviation or rotation of a series of vertebrae away from the normal spinal axis. It is usually first observed as a lowering of one scapula when the teenager is standing up straight with both feet close together. When he bends over and allows his arms and hands to hang down loosely, one side of the back is elevated over the other. Diagnosis is confirmed by x-ray, and treatment should be managed by an orthopedist.

It is essential to make the diagnosis in the early

teen years, before or early in the onset of rapid growth. By menarche, all girls will have begun the decelerating phase of growth, and nonsurgical correction is impossible. On the other hand, if only a slight deviation is found after the onset of menses, referral is probably not warranted.

Diagnostics

Routine tests should include:

1. Hemograms in menstruating females
2. Sickle cell screening in appropriate teenagers where genetic counseling is available
3. Tuberculin testing annually in tuberculin negative teenagers who live in endemic areas or who have traveled in such areas, and every 3 years in others
4. Rubella titers in sexually active women who are not certain of their immune status for that disease

Therapeutics

Diphtheria-tetanus vaccine (adult type) booster should be given every 10 years. Since most children receive their last childhood immunizations upon entering school, teenagers usually require the vaccine.

Mumps vaccine should be given to any teenager who has no history of receiving the vaccine or of having had the disease. Fifteen percent of mumps occurs after age 15 years, and 20 percent of these cases are associated with orchitis and a smaller percentage with salpingo-ophoritis.

Twenty-five percent of the cases of rubeola occur in teenagers. Anyone who has no history of having received the vaccine after 1 year of age or having had the disease should receive *rubeola vaccine*. It should be noted however, that rubeola is often confused with other viral illnesses. Rubeola is associated with fever, conjunctivitis, cough, coryza, Koplik spots, and a generalized maculo-papular rash that lasts 9 to 10 days.

As much as 20 to 30 percent of rubella infections occur during adolescence. Sexually active teenage girls with no history of rubella infection or immunization and with a low rubella titer should receive the *rubella vaccine*. Pregnancy should be prevented for at least 2 months following the administration of the vaccine because of the risk of transmission of live virus to the fetus.

Special Types of Health Facilities and Personnel

Management of the types of problems associated with the adolescent years requires something other than the traditional, one physician-to-one patient re-

lationship. The characteristics of a physician found to be most desirable by teenagers are a high degree of understanding, a good personality, and informality. Age, sex, and dress are of minor concern.[48]

Most teenagers consult a physician less than once a year, and these visits usually involve only a specific physical ailment. The vast majority of adolescents seek the help of other individuals such as nurses, teachers, school counselors, clergymen, social workers, community workers, and friends. In order to meet the health needs of teenagers better, care must be provided by the various types of health and other professionals and their assistants functioning as an integrated team. The team effort can help to alleviate gaps, prevent duplication, and decrease mixed and contradictory messages and advice.

The environment in which health care is provided should be designed especially for teenagers. The area does not require expensive decor, but the furniture, bulletin boards, magazines, and the like should be designed to appeal to teenagers. If at all possible, some clinic hours should be scheduled in the late afternoon or evening in order to prevent absence from school.

Consent and Confidentiality

Confidentiality is of utmost importance to ensure the trust of the adolescent, and his privacy and personal dignity must be preserved. Therefore, it is essential that guidelines be set and clearly explained regarding the involvement of parents and legal guardians in their care. Ideally, teenagers should be allowed to accept responsibility for their own care if they choose to do so. However, they must not be forced into accepting this responsibility if they have not yet reached that stage of emancipation. In crisis situations, teenagers should be encouraged to involve their parents.

Since 1967, almost every state has enacted legislation allowing at least specific groups of teenagers to consent to their own care.[7,25,34] In 1973, the American Academy of Pediatrics' Committee on Youth published a model minor consent act.[21] The goals of the proposed act are to ensure quality health services of all minors by granting them self-consent in instances where they might not seek care if parental consent were required and to encourage health professionals to provide quality care without incurring legal liability.

A recent survey of adolescent clinics revealed that 51 percent of respondents require parental consent for treatment and 67 percent of children's hospitals with teenage clinics require such consent.[32] These figures probably reflect the legal responsibilities and the financial realities of providing care.

The financial aspect of providing care for adolescents bears some discussion. As of 1971, 73 percent of medical bills for individuals under 19 were paid by private funds.[14] Currently, a number of federal programs provide funding for adolescent health services. However, most teenagers still must depend on their parents for support, and this makes it very difficult for them to receive care without their parents' permission or knowledge.

Compliance

One of the most exasperating areas of providing health care to teenagers involves poor compliance with suggested treatment and with follow-up appointments despite what appears to be elaborate individual and team counseling. The adolescent frequently misses appointments for no apparent reason and misuses or discontinues medications for what appear to be trivial reasons. For example, discontinuation of oral contraceptives may occur as a result of small, midcycle, vaginal spotting or because the teenager may suddenly decide it is not a "natural process."

When such situations occur frequently, there is a tendency for the health professional to retreat in despair and exasperation. However, it might be easier to maintain this important input if one considers two aspects of caring for adolescents. First, the teenager has the potential for over 50 more years of a healthy, happy life. Second, the behavior that often exasperates parents and health professionals is part of the normal developmental process toward adulthood and is self-limited.

SPECIAL PROBLEMS OF ADOLESCENCE

The three major problem areas in adolescent medicine are 1) sexuality, 2) drug abuse, including alcohol and nicotine, and 3) trauma including accidents, suicides, and homicides. The problems associated with drug abuse and trauma are discussed in Chapters 132 and 138, respectively.

Sexually transmitted infections (Chap. 88), sexual problems in general (Chap. 139), drug and alcohol dependence (Chaps. 138 and 153), and similar behavior are also discussed elsewhere in this text. Therefore, this discussion will be limited to teenage pregnancy and contraception.

Pregnancy and Contraception

A variety of birth control measures and programs have been available in the country for many years. However, the word has not yet reached much of the adolescent population. The birth rate and number of births for all ages have declined since 1966 except for the 12- to 17-year-old group. A nationwide study conducted in 1971 indicated that 80 percent of sexually experienced, never-married young women aged 15 to 19 had engaged in sexual intercourse without using contraception. About 10 percent of the 10 million female teenagers in this age group become pregnant and 6 percent give birth each year. In addition, approximately 30,000 youngsters under 15 years of age become pregnant each year. Stated another way, about one in six sexually active teenage women who do not practice birth control becomes pregnant.

Teenage pregnancy is a deadly serious problem. Maternal mortality is 13 percent higher for mothers from 15 to 19 and 60 percent higher for mothers under 15 than for mothers in their 20s. Infant mortality and low birth weight are twice as high for mothers under 15 years as for mothers in their 20s. Furthermore, the surviving infants do not fare as well intellectually or physically owing to prematurity and other factors.

The teenage mother is hampered in a number of respects. Physically, she is prone to iron deficiency anemia, cephalopelvic disproportion, and other problems of gestation and delivery. The teenage mother rarely has a chance to develop the normal independence that should be achieved during adolescence. She becomes emotionally and economically dependent. Her chance for social and economic advancement is hampered because her education is interrupted or ceases. In fact, pregnancy is the principal cause of school dropout for young women.

Very often, the father is also a teenager, and it is becoming more and more obvious that the emotional impact on the adolescent father is as serious as that on the mother. This is especially true as society moves away from placing the sole responsibility for contraception and unwanted pregnancy on women.

According to Lindemann,[29] the process whereby an adolescent moves from using no contraception to the consistent use of an effective contraceptive involves three stages: the natural, the peer, and the expert stages. During the *natural stage*, adolescents do nothing about contraception. Coitus is infrequent and unpredictable. There is a preference for the naturalness and spontaneity of sexual activity, and at this point, the adolescent is not willing to define herself as sexually active, capable of reproduction, or in need of contraception.

During the *peer stage*, adolescents acquire information from their peers and experiment with various methods of birth control. The longer a young woman remains in this stage, the more and various are the methods she uses. The variations in the use of contraception may increase the risk of pregnancy. Often pregnancy occurs as a result of a lack of skills and information, the boy–girl relationship changes, or because the use of peer prescription methods interrupt the spontaneity of the natural stage and are deemed to be unacceptable. The frequency and predictability of sexual intercourse continue to condition birth control behavior as does belief in the effectiveness of the methods being used and the lack of real commitment to nonmarital sexual intercourse.

A final and major step in the peer stage is the willingness of the adolescent to disclose his or her sexual activity if nothing more than by the need to purchase foam or condoms. This is often the psychosocial profile of the teenagers when they are identified as sexually active. During the peer prescription period, important psychological changes are occurring. The adolescent is moving from little to greater awareness, from noncommitment to commitment, from one self-concept to another, and from no birth control to planned birth control.

The *expert stage* involves the use of professionals for contraception advice. However, just because expert advice is sought, this does not imply that the teenager will comply with the advice.

Rapid psychological and physiologic change is the hallmark of midadolescence. By definition, therefore, it is the norm rather than the exception to have wide fluctuations in effective birth control use. However, it is the responsibility of the health professionals who care for teenagers to provide them with information and means for contraception either directly or by referral. The type of birth control used should be individualized according to the stage of psychological development and the environmental needs of the teenager. For example, condoms may be the best choice where there is a high risk of venereal disease and teenagers are accepting of this means of contraception. This aspect of care should be considered as vital as providing information and medication to a diabetic teenager.

CHRONIC DISEASE

The advent of modern therapy has made it possible for many children with illnesses, such as cystic fibrosis, to survive through adolescence. The problems of dealing with any chronic illness are compounded by the normal "developmental turmoil" of adolescence.

Diabetes mellitus can be used to illustrate this point. The adolescent characteristically has labile diabetes. Emotional stress may include temporary insulin insensitivity. Fluctuations in blood glucose levels may be caused by erratic eating habits, irregular hours, and bursts of physical activity.[28] Often, the teenager simply does not take his insulin as prescribed. Similar problems may be encountered with other chronic illnesses during adolescence.

It may be difficult or embarrassing for the adolescent to take medication or to explain signs or symp-

toms of a chronic illness to his peers. Whenever possible, medical regimens should be sufficiently flexible to allow for normal socialization to occur. Finally, emotional support must be an integral component to any treatment of chronic illness in a teenager.

MANAGEMENT OF THE AGED PATIENT

Age 65, although not necessarily demarcating biologic old age, has provided, until recently, a convenient benchmark for social, legislative, and statistical purposes. The group of patients age 65 and older represents one-third to one-half of an internist's practice, and this proportion is growing. In the United States, their number has increased from 3 to 23 million during this century and is expected to reach more than 50 million by the year 2030.[16] Advances in medical knowledge have increased the likelihood that people with chronic diseases will survive into old age. This has altered the balance between "hardy survivors" and the functionally dependent elderly, i.e., those whose illness or social problems reduce their ability to live independently.

Mortality And Morbidity

After the neonatal period, the death rate is very low until age 40 when it begins to double every 7 years (see Figure 152–3). The rate for women is lower than that for men, resulting in a relative increase in the survivorship of women over men, so that by age 85, the ratio is 2:1.

Most people, even those in their 80s, report themselves to be in good or excellent health. Although acute illnesses occur about half as often in those over 65 as in those under 65, the result is more days of restricted activity. For the most part, the complaints of the elderly are an amalgam of physiologic age-related changes and an accumulating burden of chronic

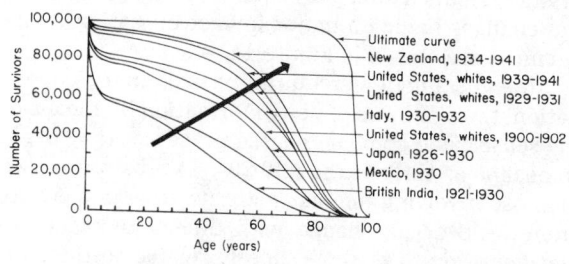

FIGURE 152–3. Life spans of various population groups. (Reprinted with permission from Hayflick, L. The cell biology of human aging. N. Engl. J. Med., 295:1302, 1976.)

illness. Arthritis, diabetes, hypertension, back pain, and visual impairment are more prevalent among elderly women than elderly men. Men have higher prevalence of asthma, chronic bronchitis, hernia, peptic ulcer, and hearing impairment.

Certain disease states occur more frequently in the aged such as coronary artery disease, senile dementia, osteoarthritis, Paget's disease, parkinsonism, cancer of the prostate, polymyalgia rheumatica, cerebrovascular accidents and transient ischemic attacks, decubitus ulcer, basal cell and squamous cell carcinoma of the skin, diverticulitis, parotitis, and chronic lymphatic leukemia. It is important to differentiate these diseases, whose attack rate increases with age, from normal aging.

Normal Aging[4,5,18]

Aging is time dependent; as we grow older, we age. Changes associated with aging result from the interaction of genetic, environmental, and life-style factors. Early life is dominated by incremental changes, i.e., growth and development. After sexual maturity, decremental changes predominate, and, for many processes, there is a linear decline in function. If one thinks teleologically, each species assures its continuity, and then with varying degrees of rapidity, individual members leave the stage. For the rat, the maximum life span is 3 years; for the elephant, 70 years; and for man, about 100 years.

Cells can be divided into three types, according to their proliferative capacity.[20] Continuously, mitotic cells in the blood, intestine, and skin are replaced at intervals of a few days to a few months. Intermittently mitotic cells in the kidney or liver have a potential for repair and replacement after injury. Postmitotic cells, such as in cardiac muscle or brain, cannot be replaced, making these organ systems particularly vulnerable.

Changes associated with aging in different organ systems are listed in Table 152-5. They are best characterized as losses, but their rate of occurrence varies not only for different individuals but also for specific organ systems within individuals.[45] Rates for some of the changes having a major impact on patient management are shown in Figure 152-4.

Mental functions requiring visual–motor coordination, the synthesis of new information by means of the senses, and some nonverbal processes may begin to decline as early as the mid 20s.[17] Verbal processes or those involving familiar patterns of response may show little or no change with time. The ability to learn appears to be more closely related to the pace and circumstances of learning than to any central nervous system deficit.

TABLE 152–5
Age-Related Changes

Organ Systems	Change with Age	Clinical Consequence
Skin	Atrophy, increased vascular fragility; changes in sebaceous and sweat glands, hair, nails	Wrinkling, susceptibility to trauma, decubitus ulcer, drying and pruritus of the skin and graying of the hair
Eyes	Changes in lens, vitreous, retina	Cataract, presbyopia, glaucoma, senile macular degeneration
Ears	Changes in hair cells	Decreased high-frequency hearing and discrimination of sound
Mouth	Decrease in taste buds and salivary gland secretion; changes in teeth, gums, and mandible	Decreased appreciation of food, dry mouth, loss of teeth, difficulty chewing
GI tract	Decreased pepsin and trypsin, achlorhydria; decrease in motility; changes in liver enzymes	Decreased absorption; increasing constipation, diverticulosis; decreased drug metabolism in liver
Respiratory tract	Decreased elasticity of lung	Decreased vital capacity, maximum breathing, fixed expiratory volume, and maximum diffusing capacity
Cardiovascular	Loss of myocardial cells, increased arterial stiffness	Decreased cardiac reserve, increased pulse pressure
Urinary tract	Loss of nephrons; basement membrane changes; decreased bladder tone and capacity, prostatic hypertrophy	Decreased glomerular filtration rate and tubular reabsorption; difficulty with urination
Endocrine	Hypogonadism	Change in secondary sex characteristics; atrophy of breasts, vagina, etc.

TABLE 152–5 (cont.)

Organ Systems	Change with Age	Clinical Consequence
	Decreased insulin response to glucose load; decreased thyroid and adrenal activity	Increase in 2-hour postprandial glucose, decreased basal metabolic rate, lesser response to stress
Musculo/skeletal	Decrease in muscle fiber number and diameter; decreased bone calcium and osteoid	Decreased strength; increased vulnerability to fracture; decreased height
Regulatory changes	Decreased homeostasis	Hypothermia, postural hypotension, dehydration
Immune system	Decreased cellular immunity; decreased primary antibody response; increase in abnormal immunoglobulin; increase in autoimmunity	Increased susceptibility to infection, neoplasms
Nervous system (see also Table 115-1)	Neuronal loss in cerebral cortex; basal ganglia changes; diminished dorsal column function; impaired righting reflex	Altered sleep patterns and memory; slowness of movement; falls

Decreased speed of performance as well as changes in vision, hearing, and other senses lead to a constriction of the older person's access to information and range of behavior. Increased support is necessary to counteract a tendency to withhold responses, especially in ambiguous circumstances. The elderly often need more reassurance as their fear of failure increases. The impact of cognitive deficits can be diminished by continued activity and social contact, or exaggerated by withdrawal and depression.

There are individual differences in the rate of aging, the ability to cope with the attendant physiologic changes, and in illness behavior. Some people are stoic and underreact to serious symptoms, or they ascribe disease symptoms to normal aging and do not seek care. Others with a higher bodily concern may overreact to minimal changes in bowel and bladder functions, sight, hearing, ambulation, and memory and view these changes as the harbingers of death. Although the latter group are in the minority, they are more familiar to physicians because they most often seek care. Such patients are often time consuming and demanding. They present a management challenge because of repetitive complaints about problems that cannot be "cured" and are often subjected to over testing and over treatment. An unsatisfactory relationship between doctor and patient can develop unless the physician approaches the patient with understanding. This is especially the case if the physician's manner produces agitation in the patient rather than calmness and reassurance.

Collection of Clinical Information

The validity of the history is directly related to the physician–patient rapport. We all carry with us our own attitudes and prejudices. We may mirror society's preference for the young and consider the elderly less attractive because they are often less vigorous and healthy.[11] On the other hand, if we have had relationships with elderly persons whom we have loved and respected, these feelings may carry over. Yet, even these can be eroded by peer pressure. A number of studies have shown that disparaging attitudes toward the aged by respected house officers or attending physicians can reinforce negative attitudes. "Gomer," "old crock," and other pejorative terms for the elderly are an ironic mocking of our future selves. Such negative attitudes will vitiate any communication and prejudice prudent management.

In addition to personal attitudinal barriers to communication, there are other practical barriers to history taking, including decreased hearing and vision, slower mentation, and recent memory loss. These may lead to confusion, embarrassment, or frustration on the part of the patient. In our haste, we may not establish the proper balance of direct and open-ended questions and may close off a line of inquiry prematurely. These factors may lead to misinformation and may alienate the patient as well. In some cases, we may have to communicate through a third party, which can adversely affect the quality of the history.

One major difference in history taking in older adults is the need to obtain information about the activies of daily life, which are crucial to maintenance of independence. These include the ability to feed and care for oneself; the quality of the diet in the face of decreased appetite, reduced income, or difficulty in shopping; fluid intake; bowel habits; sleep habits; and interactions with others. Katz has formulated an in-

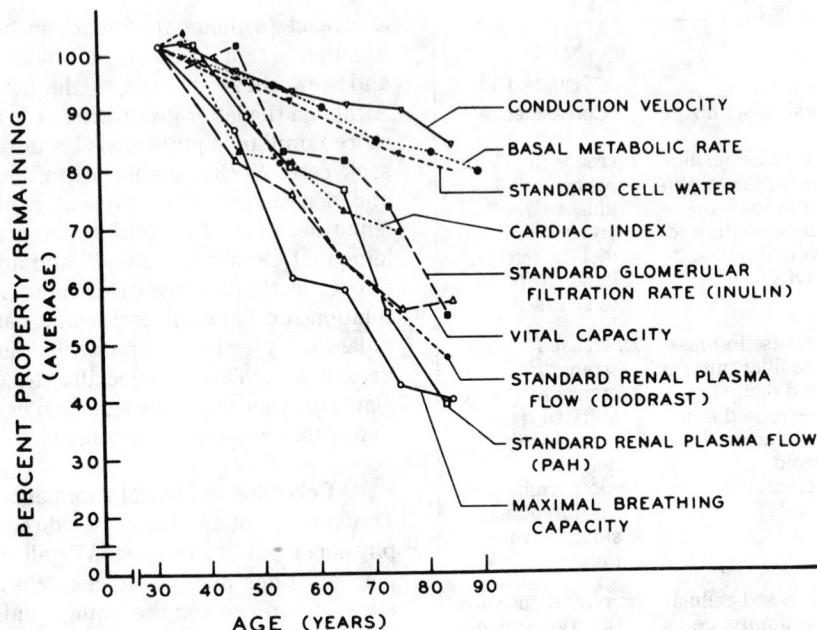

FIGURE 152–4. Age changes in various physiologic functions expressed as percent of mean value at age 30. (Reproduced with permission from Strehler, B.L. Origins and comparisons of the effects of time and high energy radiations on living systems. Q. Rev. Biol., 43:117, 1959.)

dex of independence in activities for daily living, which provides a useful check list (see Table 152–6).[26]

The physical examination must be conducted at a slower pace. The aged are not as nimble as young adults. They cannot hop on the examining table. They are more sensitive to rough handling and to cold. The examination itself should focus on specific areas where we can expect deficiency such as the senses, strength, foot care, postural effects, balance, and other areas with which we may not have been as concerned in younger adults.

Diagnostics

In dealing with the elderly, the best principle is that of minimal interference.[43] A test should not be done unless it will lead to something beneficial when balanced against the physical, social, and financial costs. These include travel time for the patients and others who bring them to care, the stress of the test, and the like. To conduct a costly, rigorous, and sometimes hazardous inquiry simply to verify a diagnosis is inappropriate unless it is likely to afford therapeutic benefit.[42]

Older patients do not rebound rapidly from diagnostic procedures. Preparations for such procedures can upset the patient's homeostasis because the mar-

gin of reserve is much lower. For example, withholding fluids for an intravenous pyelogram may lead to dehydration and renal failure. Vigorous bowel preparation for barium enemas can lead to exhaustion, dehydration, or exacerbation in bowel problems such as hemorrhoids or diverticulitis. When a test is judged to be indicated, it should be done under optimal conditions, not in haste, unless it is an emergency. Older patients are often apprehensive and easily confused. Hurried explanations will not suffice, and one should be sure that the patient understands what is to happen.

Another important consideration is knowing how normal values in the aged change. For example, the normal average blood glucose level 2 hours after a 75-g oral glucose load rises by approximately 10 mg/dl per decade.[3] It is important to approach blood sugar modification in the aged carefully, since most patients tolerate the increased glucose level well, but an abrupt decrease to hypoglycemic levels may produce permanent central nervous system deficits. Alkaline phosphatase levels increase with age for as yet unknown reasons.[47] Normal creatinine levels do not adequately reflect decreases in creatinine clearance because of decreases creatinine production from muscle.[40]

┌───┐
TABLE 152-6
**Index of Independence in Activities of
Daily Living*†**

Bathing (Sponge, Shower, or Tub)

Independent
Assistance only in bathing a single part (e.g. back
or disabled extremity) or bathes self completely

Dependent
Assistance in bathing more than one part of body;
assistance in getting in or out of tub or does not
bathe self

Dressing

Independent
Gets clothes from closets and drawers; puts on
clothes, outer garments, braces; manages
fasteners (excluding act of tying shoes)

Dependent
Does not dress self or remains partly undressed

Going to Toilet

Independent
Gets to toilet; gets on and off toilet; arranges
clothes, cleans organs of excretion (may manage
own bedpan used at night only and may or may
not be using mechanical supports)

Dependent
Uses bedpan or commode or receives assistance in
getting to and using toilet

Transfer

Independent
Moves in and out of bed independently and moves
in and out of chair independently (may or may
not be using mechanical supports)

Dependent
Assistance in moving in or out of bed and/or chair;
does not perform one or more transfers

Continence

Independent
Urination and defecation entirely self-controlled

Dependent
Partial or total incontinence in urination or
defecation; partial or total control by enemas,
catheters, or regulated use of urinals and/or
bedpans

---

* The Index of Independence in Activities of Daily Living is based
on an evaluation of the functional independence or dependence
of patients in bathing, dressing, going to toilet, transferring, continence, and feeding. Independence means without supervision,
direction, or active personal assistance, except as specifically
noted above. This is based on actual status and not on ability. A
patient who refuses to perform a function is considered as not
performing the function, even though he is deemed able.
† Reprinted with modification from Katz, Ford, and Moskowitz.
JAMA, 185:914–919, 1965. Copyright 1965, American Medical
Association.
└───┘

┌───┐
TABLE 152-6 (cont.)

Feeding

Independent
Gets food from plate or its equivalent into mouth;
(precutting of meat and preparation of food, as
buttering bread, are excluded from evaluation)

Dependent
Assistance in act of feeding (see above); does not
eat at all or parenteral feeding
└───┘

Therapeutics

One should set realistic treatment goals. Being overly
pessimistic may be just as harmful as being overly
optimistic. The considerations involved in the decision to perform surgery are particularly illustrative.
One should neither overuse surgery nor withhold a
potentially useful procedure. The decision must be individualized according to the potential effect on the
quality of life and life expectancy. The latter differs
from mean life expectancy for the patient's cohort. A
person who has survived to age 75 may live an additional 10 or more years, depending on his functional
status.

In one study, 80 percent of a group over 80 with
absent or minimal delayed hypersensitivity to specific
antigens were dead within 2 years as compared to 35
percent of those who had a good response.[36] Similarly, changes in other systems, such as the neurologic or cardiorespiratory, will also affect decision
making. Finally, while treatment goals should be
clearly defined, they should not be inflexible, but subject to reevaluation, since change in status can often
occur rapidly in the elderly.

There are other concerns incident to surgery in
the elderly. Mental and physical preparation appear
to be important determinants of outcome. Given the
potential fragility of neurologic and cardiorespiratory
systems, anesthesia must be carefully selected and
administered. In the postoperative period, the aged
require greater convalescence because of a lessened
recuperative power of individual tissues and the body
in general.

The problems encountered in pharmacotherapy
also deserve particular emphasis.[35,52] We are an
overmedicated society. In one study, healthy people
over 65 consumed regularly an average of more than
three over-the-counter drugs. The problem of excess
medication (polypharmacy) is compounded by the
existence of chronic illness and care by multiple physicians. When someone comes to a physician with a

problem, the pressures are enormous to write a prescription. Since most elderly have something identifiable as "wrong," although not necessarily causing a problem, they often get prescriptions. A longitudinal study of the aged in Sweden showed that only 30 percent of those treated with digitalis had definite cardiac disease for which digitalis was indicated. Antihypertensive drugs, psychotropic drugs, laxatives, sleeping pills, and hypoglycemic agents were also overprescribed. Similar results have been found in this country.

The issue of pharmacotherapy can be divided into drug handling, side effects, drug interactions, and compliance. Although gastrointestinal absorption is delayed, most drugs are well absorbed. The most common finding in the aged is increased active drug in the bloodstream caused by reduced catabolism; lowered binding by protein, tissue, or cells; and delayed excretion.

Induction of the enzymes necessary for metabolizing drugs in the liver is reduced in old age. This can affect the way the body handles such medications as barbiturates, tricyclic antidepressants, anticoagulants, phenothiazines, phenytoin, phenylbutazone, and diazepam. Drugs more than 80 percent bound to protein will have a greater degree of bioavailability in the presence of hypoproteinemia. Examples of such drugs are coumadin, phenylbutazone, aspirin, diazepam, chlorpromazine, and phenytoin. Red cell binding of meperidine is lowered in the aged, making more of the active drug available. Digoxin, penicillin, and methotrexate are excreted mainly by the kidney and have a longer half-life as creatinine clearance declines.

Excess active drugs combine with normal physiologic changes in the aged to produce a higher frequency of side effects.[12,35,52] Commonly implicated are: digitalis (arrhythmia, heart block, confusion); antihypertensives (orthostatic hypotension, falls, strokes); hypoglycemic agents (confusion); tranquilizers and sedatives (confusion, stupor); methyl-dopa (confusion, depression, augmentation of involuntary movements); and anticholinergics (urinary retention in males, anhidrosis, and heat stroke).

Old people undergoing treatment for various conditions may take six or more drugs per day. They also store medicines and even may swap them with friends. All of these make the potential for drug–drug interaction great.

As with other age groups, compliance is also a problem in the elderly, but often for different reasons. They may not purchase a drug because of financial problems or concern about toxicity. Pills prescribed three times a day with meals may not be taken in that manner if the person does not eat three meals a day. Confusion and memory loss may lead to taking more or less of a drug, or one drug for another. Declining vision may also lead to mixup of medication. Opening child-proof containers is more difficult as the older person's strength and dexterity diminish.

In order to deal with these issues, the following precepts are valuable whether the patient is aged or not:

1. Medications should not be prescribed unless they are essential.
2. The dose should be appropriate, given the physiologic status of the patient.
3. Consideration should be given to the possibility of drug interactions in those on multiple drugs; inquiry should be made regarding self-medication.
4. Drugs should be given as infrequently as possible. This allows patients not to have to alter their habits or to need to remember to take a medication.
5. Attention should be paid to the color and size of the pills to minimize confusion.
6. Directions written in large print should be used to supplement verbal instructions about medication.
7. Responsible family or friends should be instructed on the importance of medications and how they should be taken.
8. When assuming responsibility for patients' care, have them clean out their medicine cabinets and bring all their medicines at the initial visit. On the return visit, they should bring in all medicines that they are currently taking.

Prevention

A few examples may show why prevention is almost as important in the elderly as it is in the young. Falls, a very common problem in the aged, result from a combination of factors: 1) decreased muscular strength; 2) posterior column changes impairing position sense; 3) general decrease in vision and in adaptation to darkness; 4) lessened ability to maintain balance; and 5) impaired righting reflex. This tendency to fall is twice as great in older women than men. Falls can lead to fracture of the hip and ultimately result in depression and other side effects of immobilization such as pulmonary embolism, fecal impaction, and urinary retention.

Various preventive techniques can be directed against the truly accidental falls related to loose rugs, poor lighting, problems in negotiating steps, those related to wintry conditions, and those that occur with postural hypotension resulting from certain medications. Prevention might include cautioning people against rapid changes in position of the neck or head or quickly rising from a lying position; the use of railings in the bathroom and supports such as walking sticks; and attention to arrhythmias which predispose to complete heart block.

The aged must be protected from their decreased ability to respond to cold or to sense it. Accidental hypothermia in the elderly is increasingly being reported with mortality rates as high as 80 percent, depending on severity. Prevention involves awareness that the elderly require a warmer environment than the young, even in the face of an energy crisis.[51]

Other potentially useful preventive measures are immunizations against influenza, and in selected cases, the use of pneumococcal vaccine. Attention to the use of fiber in the diet and fluid intake can forestall constipation. In the hospital, care should be taken to prevent decubitus ulcers in the elderly who are immobile. Because of skin atrophy, decreased vascularity, and decreased sensation, low pressure over hours or high pressure for even minutes may start the process. Usually it begins with blistering, leading to ulceration and then, secondary infection, especially in those who are incontinent. Decubitus ulcers are much more difficult to handle once they have developed. Good nursing care, special mattresses, and support devices can help prevent this condition in those who are immobilized.

Often not considered is preventive mental health. Emotional support is essential for people at critical stages such as loss of a loved one, retirement, and change of home. The resulting depression may lead to withdrawal and loss of mobility, alcoholism, or drug abuse. The potential for drug abuse in enhanced by the increased prescribing of psychotropic drugs for the aged. In fact, the elderly account for about 25 percent of reported suicides, between 5000 and 8000 a year in the United States. Such suicides may be preventable by recognizing depression and helping the older person remain active.

Special Types of Health Facilities and Personnel

The care of the aged is a team effort. It is the premier illustration of the physician as manager. Physicians must be able to work with patients, their families, and community support services, as well as with other members of the health care team. They must be able to coordinate the use of a variety of facilities, ranging from geriatric day care centers, through acute care hospitals, to long-term care facilities of ascending order of complexity of care (domiciliary, intermediate care, and skilled nursing facilities.)

About 20 percent of those over 65 will pass through a long-term care facility before they die, and at any one time, 5 percent of those 65 and over are in long-term care facilities. This percentage increases to 19 percent for those 85 and over. Increasing functional disability with age and isolation after loss of spouse or family members are the major factors leading to institutionalization. Community support activities have been developed to help the elderly maintain independence. These include "meals on wheels," congregate dining facilities, special housing, and transportation. Current reimbursement mechanisms for care of the aged place physicians in a gatekeeper role for the provision of these services. Knowledge and skill are required to use them in a way that enhances a patient's independence and does not foster dependency.

Special Management Problems in the Elderly[6,12,35]

The elderly resemble other patients whose homeostatic and host defense mechanisms are compromised in that common diseases may present in an atypical manner. Pneumonia may present without fever, leukocytosis, or signs of consolidation because of alterations in thermoregulatory and inflammatory response. Nevertheless, such patients look sick and have respiratory distress or shallow breathing.

Similarly, one sometimes sees patients with acute subdural hematoma mistaken for stroke and chronic subdural hematoma mistaken for senility. Here the question arises, "Did a fall precipitate the confusion or did a cerebrovascular accident precipitate the fall?" Even in the case of the latter, one should be alert to superimposed head injury.

Myocardial infarction presents atypically with increasing frequency in the elderly. About one-quarter of those over 65 present without pain, and this increases to about half in those in their 80s.[37] Clues are dyspnea, sudden change in behavior or appearance, cyanosis, onset of "weak spells," or vomiting.

Urinary tract infection in the elderly does not usually present with hematuria or fever, but with slight burning, incontinence, and in males, urinary retention. Urinary tract infection with bacteremia should be suspected in the institutionalized elderly with indwelling catheters who become suddenly confused.

Appendicitis, diverticulitis, and other intra-abdominal emergencies often present without peritoneal signs or classic localizing findings. In one large series, 70 percent of elderly patients with appendicitis had early perforation.

A good example of the difference in problem identification in the elderly, as opposed to younger adults, is that of incontinence. Nothing is more embarrassing for the patient because of its social stigma and its implications for self-image. Often, physicians ignore this as "just a nursing problem." Certainly, it requires much more nursing or family time for cleaning and bathing, but physicians must be alert to this condition not only because of their role as managers of health resources, but also to make a diagnosis and institute an appropriate remedy. Differentiation should be made between the transient incontinence associated with acute urinary tract infection and the fixed incontinence produced by bladder outlet, neurogenic, or dementing causes.[6,12,35,39]

Certain presentations occur with such frequency that they are distinctly recognizable syndromes such as apathetic hyperthyroidism and hyperosmolar, nonketotic diabetic coma. As an example, in the former, the patient may complain of constipation rather than diarrhea, exhibit weight loss without polyphagia, and show no evidence of goiter in 40 percent of cases. Clues are congestive heart failure poorly responsive to digitalis plus increasing confusion or apathy. These conditions are covered more fully in Chapters 71 and 76.

Belief in the inevitability of senility and the consequent overdiagnosis of senile dementia are serious problems in the care of the aged. Transient episodes of confusion, to which the aged are subject, should be differentiated from senile dementia, a permanent pathologic state covered in Chapter 113. Disorientation in an unfamiliar environment is heightened by sensory deficits previously discussed, causing so called "sun-downing," a condition characterized by agitation and confusion toward nightfall. This can often be ameliorated by a night light and the provision of familiar objects at the bedside.

The differential diagnosis of confusion in the elderly is often difficult because of multiplicity and variability of etiologies (see Table 152–7).[12] Sudden occurrence of confusion suggests a definable and potentially reversible cause, such as drug side effect, infection, dehydration, or myocardial infarction. Examples of less acute but reversible causes are apathetic hyperthyroidism, anemias, and reactive depression.

Reactive depression is a major health problem of the aged. As one ages, one experiences losses in strength, mobility, job, friends, and relatives. The greatest trauma involves loss of spouse, a close relative, a succession of friends, or the abilities most prized, even simple ones like reading. Other factors contributing to depression are restricted or fixed income near poverty levels and fear of crime, especially in urban settings. Physicians must be aware of the increased vulnerability of the aged to loss or destruc-

---

TABLE 152–7
Causes of Acute Confusional States in Aged*

Causes	Examples
Drugs	Alcohol Hypnotic, tranquilizer Antihypertensive Antiparkinsonian Antidepressant and other drugs
Vascular accidents	Myocardial infarction Cerebral infarction Peripheral gangrene Pulmonary embolism
Infections	Pneumonia Urinary tract infection
Metabolic	Hypoglycemia Myxedema; hyperthyroidism Hepatic or renal failure
Circulatory	Congestive cardiac failure Tachyarrhythmia Heart block
Homeostatic failure	Postural hypotension Dehydration Electrolyte disturbance
Anemia	B_{12} or folate deficiency Occult hemorrhage
Trauma	Subdural hematoma
Surgery	Cataract enucleation
Depression	Bereavement; retirement
Environmental	Change of home; hospitalization

* Modified and reprinted with permission from Cape, R. Aging: Its Complex Management. New York, Harper & Row, 1978.

---

tion of home during prolonged hospitalization or fear of assault, which compounds their isolation.

Such stresses are additive, and when their clustering exceeds a given threshold, major medical or psychiatric disorders will result. Depression may be manifested as confusion or cognitive difficulty or masked by physical complaints. This potentially remediable condition must be carefully differentiated from senile dementia.

Lastly, there is the clinical syndrome which for want of a better term is called "the dwindles," or "predeath." This is a stage when one or more homeostatic mechanisms and organ systems have exhausted their reserves and operate routinely at subnormal levels. This period may last for a longer time than one would predict, i.e., months instead of days, before the individual dies. This raises ethical and social questions relating to quality of life and the dignity of death. These issues have been discussed in Chapters 4 and 135.

Conclusion

Care of the elderly can be a gratifying experience. Efforts should be directed toward helping them to lead active and productive lives by emphasizing prevention, being alert to common problems, and instituting prompt intervention. Physicians who are secure about their own aging can help the older person, as well as themselves, age gracefully. A good model might be Vannevar Bush, a scientist active until his death at 84, who said:

> We all know the troubles of old age. The bones creak; the eyes get dim, one forgets names. The joy of the battle is gone, for it is not proper to enter contest with an old man. But there is something to be said on the other side.
>
> It is pleasant to rise in the morning, look out at the snow, and remark, "I'm not going to go to the office today." It is a privilege to sit in the shade and watch the young men sweat out in the sun. One can find youths who genuinely like to sit and listen to old men's tales. The joys of youthful adventure are no greater than their recollection. The beauty of nature has lost none of its charm; the beauty of women none of its benediction. There is, after all, a possibility of growing old gracefully, and with content in one's heart. [10]

—CHAPTER 153—
Alcoholism and Associated Medical Problems
WILLIS C. MADDREY AND JOHN B. IMBODEN

DEFINITION

Alcoholism is characterized by the drinking of alcoholic beverages to the extent that one or more of the following occur:

1. There is psychological or physiologic dependence on alcohol.
2. There is impairment of physical or mental health.
3. There is impairment of the individual's functioning at home, school, work, or in any other sector of his life. [56]

With the attainment of physiologic dependence, the patient not only tends to increase the daily amount of alcohol consumed, but also drinks more frequently throughout his waking hours in an effort to allay the inexorably recurring discomfort of withdrawal. At this stage of the behavior disorder, alcoholism can be truly regarded as a disease, i.e., as a progressive morbid process with adverse physical and psychosocial consequences.

PREVALENCE AND CONSEQUENCE

Of the approximately 90,000,000 persons in the United States who drink, it is estimated that about 9,000,000 are alcoholics. The damaging consequences of this widespread disorder are enormous. Alcoholism not only affects the patient himself, but it also commonly has a severe impact upon the immediate family, especially upon those who are psychologically and economically dependent upon the patient. Divorce rates, suicide rates, and the incidence of serious physical illness are much higher among alcoholics than in the general adult population. Excessive drinking is frequently implicated in homicides and automobile accidents.

PHYSICIAN RESISTANCE TO RECOGNITION AND MANAGEMENT

Physicians, both generalists and specialists, encounter patients with alcoholism in all its states: Patients in whom the illness is incipient, patients who openly seek help for loss of control of their drinking, patients with physical illnesses frequently associated with alcoholism, and patients admitted to the hospital for an incidental medical or surgical illness who develop an alcohol withdrawal syndrome.

Despite the frequency and seriousness of alcoholism, physicians often feel a degree of reluctance to diagnose and manage alcoholism. There are several reasons for this:

1. Physicians who are not knowledgeable about alcoholism feel insecure about its management and may tend to avoid the diagnosis.

2. The physician may fear that he will alienate the patient if he confronts him with the diagnostic impression of alcoholism. The physician may even be reluctant to pursue a relevant line of inquiry.
3. The physician who moralistically condemns alcoholism as willfully destructive behavior is loathe to become involved in treating the alcoholic patient.
4. The physician who drinks may set his own drinking habit as the norm and thus regard drinking equal to or less than his own as clinically insignificant.

DIAGNOSIS OF ALCOHOLISM

In its early stages, alcoholism may pose a diagnostic challenge because the patient himself may not recognize that he has a drinking problem or he may tend to minimize his drinking. When the physician surmises that this is the case, he will usually find it helpful to include the patient's spouse or other close relative in an interview in which the patient is present.

One or more of the following characteristics points to the presence of alcoholism:

1. Poor control of drinking as manifested by repeated efforts to set limits on the amount of drinking, or persistence in drinking despite its obvious association with serious marital, social, and economic problems
2. Drinking to escape problems, to ameliorate feelings of nervousness or depression, or to "face the day," i.e., evidence of psychological dependence
3. Sneaking drinks
4. Tremulousness or other signs of withdrawal, i.e., physiologic dependence
5. Drinking in the morning
6. Amnesia ("blackouts") for events that occurred while drinking
7. Habitual excessive drinking such as drinking in excess of 5 ounces of whiskey per day, getting intoxicated frequently, or terminating periods of abstinence with "benders"

MANAGEMENT OF ALCOHOLISM

In managing the alcoholic patient, the physician increases his chance of success if he combines frankness with a factual, nonjudgmental approach. Fur-

ther, the physician is more likely to sustain his own interest in and respect for the patient if he does not expect the improbable of himself or the patient. That is to say, alcoholism is a chronic illness and, as with any chronic illness, there may be relapses after varying periods of remission. The occurrence of a relapse does not mean that the treatment plan has been a total failure, but it does mean that the patient's addiction to alcohol persists. A realistic attitude on the part of the physician may help the patient who has slipped back into drinking to continue treatment instead of being driven from treatment by his own shame or guilt.

The specific steps taken in management depend upon the severity of the drinking problem, the patient's attitudes, the presence or absence of physical dependence, associated psychological problems, and physical complications.

For example, if the physician feels that the patient's drinking behavior is cause for concern and may eventually lead to alcoholism but has not yet done so, he may state this opinion simply and clearly to the patient and solicit his thoughts on the matter. Candid discussions may lead to a plan acceptable to the patient whereby he modifies his drinking pattern. The individual may be strongly motivated to adhere to such a regimen if he realizes that progression to alcohol addiction would necessitate total abstinence. Follow-up visits with the patient who enters into such a plan are essential.

When the diagnosis of alcoholism is warranted, this fact should be stated to the patient. It is unwise to assume that the patient appreciates the real nature of his illness even if he has clearly revealed its presence by reporting his heavy drinking to the physician. Even in such an instance, the patient may not admit to himself that his drinking problem is serious and that he is an alcoholic.

Most authorities agree that the management of alcoholism requires that the patient totally and permanently abstain from drinking alcoholic beverages of any kind. When told this, the patient may react with dismay and disbelief. For this and other reasons, it is often essential to put the patient in contact with someone who himself has been an active alcoholic and who has achieved sustained sobriety. This may be done, in many communities, in one of two ways. The first and oldest method is by encouraging the patient to contact a local Alcoholics Anonymous group and to form a working relationship with one of its members. A second method, which may supplement the A.A. approach, is referral to an alcoholism clinic. The latter has on its staff trained counselors, some of whom may be former alcoholics. In the clinic setting, the patient has opportunities to participate in group sessions with patients who are at the same stage of treatment as himself as well as others who are further along.

In the initial phase of abstinence, the patient may experience withdrawal symptoms. The management of these will be discussed later. At this point, however, it is worth emphasizing that the alcoholic patient may easily transfer his dependence from alcohol to another substance such as minor tranquilizers. While the latter are often very useful they should be prescribed for a limited period, such as 3 or 4 weeks.

The administration of disulfiram (Antabuse) may be a useful adjunct in the management of the alcoholic patient who sincerely wants to stop drinking but who is prone to yield to an impulse to drink. Disulfiram impedes the intermediary step in alcohol metabolism in which acetaldehyde is oxidized in the tissues by the action of acetaldehyde dehydrogenase. In the presence of disulfiram, the ingestion of even a small amount of alcohol results in an uncomfortable and sometimes dangerous reaction: within 5 to 10 minutes there develops a sensation of warmth in the face followed by reddening of the face, chest, and arms, pulsating headache, nausea, vomiting, feelings of constriction in neck and chest, hypotension, marked apprehension, weakness, dizziness, and sweating. The initial flush may be replaced by pallor and orthostatic syncope may occur.

The initial dose of disulfiram is 0.5 g per day for the first week and 0.25 to 0.5 g per day thereafter. It is essential that the reaction to alcohol when taken in the presence of disulfiram be fully explained to the patient and that the possible danger to life of such a reaction be understood by him.

As indicated previously, evaluation of the patient with alcoholism includes the search for problems in the patient's life which may have contributed to or resulted from his drinking. In fact, in the presence of severe, prolonged drinking, serious problems in the patient's relationships with those in his immediate family practically always exist. For this reason as well as the alcoholic patient's well-known tendency to minimize or deny his difficulties, it is often essential to involve the close members of the family in the evaluation of the patient's condition and in the development of a plan of treatment. Persons trained in the counseling of alcoholic patients and their families can be of great assistance to the physician, particularly when the patient resists his therapeutic efforts.

It may be advisable for the patient to begin treatment in a hospital, "detoxification unit" of a general hospital, or a well-staffed sanatorium under the following circumstances:

1. There are current severe withdrawal symptoms or the likelihood of severe withdrawal as judged by the amount of alcohol recently consumed and/or a history of previous withdrawal syndromes.
2. The patient's general state of debilitation makes the assurance of adequate nutrition important.
3. The patient is without family or friends with whom to stay during the initial period of abstinence. It may be necessary to clarify for the patient that a brief stay in the hospital or other residential setting is in itself no more than a mere beginning of his treatment.

Depression or some other emotional disturbance sometimes becomes manifest either during the period of active drinking or during the early phase of abstinence. When emotional illness is present, active treatment of it is important and may require referral to a psychiatrist who is experienced in the treatment of emotionally ill, alcoholic patients.

MEDICAL PROBLEMS ASSOCIATED WITH ALCOHOLISM

In Table 153–1 are listed the major manifestations and probable pathogenesis of selected important alcohol-related medical disorders. The pathogenesis of many of these conditions includes both direct alcohol toxicity and the effects of poor nutrition.[58,59] Protein malnutrition and multiple vitamin deficiencies are usual in these patients. They are probably of importance in the susceptibility of the alcoholic to infection as are the alcoholic's likelihood to have increased exposure to extreme heat or cold and a general decrease in level of personal care.

In this section we shall emphasize effects of alcohol on the central nervous system with syndromes secondary to acute withdrawal, those associated with specific lesions in the nervous system, and commonly encountered alcohol-related nutritional deficiencies.

Effects of Alcohol on the Nervous System

Alcohol may affect the nervous system through direct toxicity or secondarily through associated vitamin deficiencies.[63] Alcohol has a direct depressant action on the central nervous system. The alteration in mood, coordination, reasoning, and judgment of the acutely intoxicated person is readily recognized. Management is discussed in Chapter 151.

Sudden cessation of drinking in the chronic alco-

┌─ TABLE 153-1 ─

Medical Problems Commonly Found in Alcoholics

Organ or System	Principle Manifestations	Probable Mechanism(s)	Discussion

Hematopoietic	Anemia
	Thrombocytopenia
	Leukopenia
		Direct suppression of bone marrow
		Interference with folate metabolism
		Dietary deficiency
		  Folic acid
		  Riboflavin
		  Other vitamins
			Chaps. 46, 48

Liver	Fatty liver Alcoholic hepatitis Cirrhosis	Direct toxin to hepatocyte ? Contribution of nutritional deficiency	Chaps. 63, 64, 67
Pancreas	Pancreatitis (acute and chronic)	Direct toxicity to pancreatic cell (probable)	Chap. 57
Gastrointestinal	Esophagitis Gastritis Duodenitis Peptic ulcer Mallory-Weiss syndrome Diarrhea	Direct irritative effect ? Effects on motility and secretion	Chaps. 56, 58–60
Endocrine	Hypoglycemia	Inhibition of gluconeogenesis	Chap. 72
Cardiac	Cardiomyopathy Cardiomegaly Congestive heart failure	? Direct toxicity to cardiac muscle ? Associated thiamine deficiency	Chap. 19
Muscle	Muscle weakness	? Direct toxicity	Chaps. 121, 124

Nervous system
  Withdrawal symptoms
    Tremors
    Hallucinations
    Seizures
    Delirium tremens
		? Direct CNS toxicity
		? Rapid decreases in blood alcohol levels
			Chaps. 112, 128

Specific lesions
  Cerebellar degeneration
  Cerebral atrophy
  Marchiafava-Bignami
  Pontine myelinolysis
  Polyneuropathy
  Alcohol amblyopia
	Ataxia, poor stance
	Cerebral function
	Emotional and thought disorders
	Pseudobulbar palsy
	Distal paresthesias, foot drop
	Blurred vision, scotomata
		? Contribution of nutritional deficits
		? Direct neural toxicity
			Chaps. 112–114, 118, 119, 123

Nutritional disorders (multisystem) Pellagra	Diarrhea Dermatitis Dementia	Niacin deficiency	
Wernicke's encephalopathy, Beriberi	VI Cranial nerve palsy, nystagmus, diplopia Circulatory collapse, high output heart failure	Thiamine deficiency	Chaps. 112, 113, 119
Riboflavin deficiency	Dermatitis, cheilosis, stomatitis	Riboflavin deficiency	
Pyridoxine deficiency	Anemia (sideroblastic)	Pyridoxine deficiency	Chap. 46
Folic acid deficiency	Anemia (macrocytic)	Folic acid deficiency	Chap. 46
Scurvy	Perifollicular hemorrhages Gingival hemorrhages	Vitamin C deficiency	Chap. 48

holic may produce withdrawal symptoms ranging from tremors to severe delirium tremens or seizures. The use of alcohol to prevent these unpleasant withdrawal symptoms is an integral part of the syndrome of progressively increasing alcohol intake. There are no specific pathologic alterations in alcohol withdrawal syndromes.

Tremulousness

The most frequent symptom of alcohol withdrawal is a tremulousness which appears 8 to 24 hours after cessation of drinking. The patient is generally irritable, excitable, and often has headache, nausea, and vomiting. Increased sweating and tachycardia are frequent, and the patient complains of excessive heat and often palpitations. Alcohol given at this time readily reverses the symptoms.

Alcohol Hallucinosis

Auditory and occasionally visual hallucinations may occur within 24 hours of cessation of alcohol.[61] Such hallucinations may last for days and be quite threatening to the patient. The hallucinations may resemble those found in schizophrenia. The hallucinating alcoholic during withdrawal generally differs from the schizophrenic in his response to the hallucinations, often talking back or becoming combative in response to supposed threats. These hallucinations may gradually disappear or be an early manifestation of delirium tremens. Administration of a mild tranquilizer is often helpful.

Alcohol-Induced Seizures

Grand mal seizures are frequent during alcohol withdrawal with an onset generally within the first 48 hours. Post-traumatic and hypoglycemic seizures must also be considered. Withdrawal seizures are often found in the delirium tremens syndrome and may be treated acutely with parenteral diazepam (Valium as described in Chap. 128.) Maintenance phenobarbital and phenytoin are usually not effective therapy for these acute seizures.

Delirium Tremens

Delirium tremens is the most serious alcohol withdrawal syndrome and is characterized by hyperactivity, gross tremulousness, combativeness, disorientation, and confusion. The syndrome may appear abruptly or as a gradual worsening in a patient who has been tremulous. Visual and auditory hallucinations are vivid and frightening to the patient. Autonomic hyperreactivity may be pronounced with dilated pupils, tachycardia, sweating, and tachypnea. Fever is common. Delirium tremens usually appears 1

to 3 days after cessation of alcohol intake but may have its onset as late as 7 to 10 days after withdrawal. The episode often lasts for 1 to 6 days and ends abruptly. Occasionally, episodes of delirium lasting several weeks recur. The fully established syndrome should be considered life-threatening. Associated conditions which may promote delirium tremens or occur during the agitated state include seizures, aspiration pneumonia, and dehydration.

The patient should be restrained for his and his attendants' protection. Sedation should be given to decrease the hyperactivity and to allow administration of other medications. In one controlled study, diazepam administered parenterally was found to be superior to paraldehyde in inducing and sustaining a tranquil state in these patients.[60] Intravenous fluid replacement should be determined on the basis of clinical evidence of dehydration and serum electrolytes. Glucose-containing solutions should be given with added thiamine since a large carbohydrate load may further deplete thiamine stores and induce Wernicke's encephalopathy. Magnesium replacement may be required, and parenteral vitamin B complex should be given.

Hepatic Encephalopathy

The neuropsychiatric abnormalities found in patients with chronic alcoholic liver disease and shunting of portal blood around the liver into the systemic circulation are described in Chapter 64.

ALCOHOL-RELATED CENTRAL NERVOUS SYSTEM SYNDROMES WITH PATHOLOGIC CHANGES

Alcoholic Cerebellar Degeneration

Progressive ataxia developing insidiously over several weeks to months may be observed in chronic alcoholics.[62] Characteristically, stance and gait are most affected; nystagmus and slurred speech are unusual. The pathologic changes in the cerebellar cortex are predominantly degeneration of Purkinje cells. Such cerebellar degeneration usually does not respond to abstinence or vitamin therapy.

Marchiafava-Bignami Syndrome

This unusual syndrome is associated with degenerative changes in the corpus callosum and was first described in Italian men drinking crude red wine. The symptoms are those of frontal lobe disease with emotional and thought disorders, seizures, delirium, tremors, and the occurrence of grasping, sucking, and snout reflexes. Recovery following abstinence is variable.

Cerebral Atrophy

Prolonged alcoholism may lead to a loss of cerebral cortex predominantly over the frontal lobes with diffuse enlargement of the ventricular system. A gradual deterioration in intellectual function is found in many such patients (Chaps. 112 and 140).

Pontine Myelinolysis

Development of pseudobulbar palsy and quadriplegia has been observed in chronic alcoholics associated with degenerative changes at the base of the pons. The role of nutritional deficiency in the pathogenesis of the syndrome is unknown.

Alcoholic Amblyopia

Progressive loss of vision with blurring developing over weeks to months may be the initial manifestation of alcohol damage. The decreased vision responds variably to abstinence and vitamin replacement.

ALCOHOL-RELATED NUTRITIONAL DEFICIENCIES

The diet of the alcoholic may be markedly unbalanced, and alcohol (7 cal per g) may be the major source of calories. Deficient intake of protein is especially frequent. Factors contributing to malnutrition are nausea and vomiting secondary to gastritis, diarrhea, and socioeconomic factors such as disrupted home situations with few facilities for storage and preparation of food and also the lack of funds. Clinically evident vitamin deficiencies in the United States are most commonly found in alcoholics.[57,59] Deficiencies of the B vitamins—niacin, thiamine, folic acid, ascorbic acid, and riboflavin—all lead to recognizable clinical syndromes. These deficits usually occur together making exact separation difficult. Only deficiencies of the B vitamins have been definitely associated with degenerative neurologic diseases. However, in patients with alcohol-induced cirrhosis with cholestasis, additional deficiencies of vitamins A, D, and K may be found.

Pellagra

Pellagra results from a deficiency in dietary niacin and its precursor, the essential amino acid, tryptophan. Pellagra is found in chronic alcoholics whose diets are poor in protein and relatively high in carbohydrates. In its advanced form pellagra presents with the classic triad of diarrhea, dermatitis, and dementia. Early manifestations are, however, quite nonspecific and include anorexia, insomnia, and headache. Sore, burning tongue and mouth are frequent, and the tongue borders are hyperemic. Chewing and swallowing are often painful. The dermatitis is erythematous and pruritic being more prominent over exposed areas and exacerbated by sunlight. The diarrhea consists of frequent small stools. Mental changes range from apathy to depression. Delirium occurs late in the illness. Paresthesias with severe burning of the distal extremities may be a major feature.

Therapy for pellagra includes administration of niacinamide 200 mg three times a day and dietary protein repletion. Since pellagra in alcoholics generally occurs in association with evidence of deficiencies of several B vitamins, other vitamins are administered as well.

Thiamine Deficiency (Beriberi)

Classical dietary deficiency of thiamine (beriberi) presents either as a neurologic syndrome characterized by fatigue, weakness, stiffness, and aching of the muscles, with anorexia and weight loss, or as a cardiac disease with cardiomegaly, chest pain, dyspnea, edema, and tachycardia. Cardiovascular collapse with sudden death may occur with high output heart failure. Both the major forms of beriberi may occur in alcoholics. Thiamine deficiency in alcoholics presents with an additional constellation of symptoms designated Wernicke's encephalopathy.[55] In these patients, bilateral paralysis of the external recti muscles (VI cranial nerve palsy) occurs in association with nystagmus, diplopia, dysconjugate gaze, and internal strabismus (Chap. 119). Wernicke's encephalopathy may appear acutely or develop over several weeks. Ataxia is usual, with difficulty in maintaining stance and in walking. Decreased mental function is initially characterized by a lack of awareness and general apathy. Such patients often are irrational with loss of recent memory and are suggestible and prone to confabulate (Korsakoff syndrome, Chaps. 112 and 113). Delirium is a late manifestation.

The lesions in Wernicke's encephalopathy are necrosis of cells in the mammillary bodies and paraventricular regions of the thalamus and hypothalamus. Similar changes may also be found in the cerebellar vermis. Thiamine plays an important role in glucose metabolism, and administration of glucose in a thiamine-depleted person may precipitate the syndrome.

In the initial therapy of alcoholic patients, 100 mg of thiamine should be given intravenously before administration of glucose. The treatment for Wernicke's encephalopathy and other forms of beriberi is 50 to 100 mg thiamine parenterally immediately and each day until a normal diet is restored. Such patients must be carefully evaluated for evidence of impending circulatory collapse.

Riboflavin Deficiency

The principal clinical manifestations of riboflavin deficiency are cheilosis, angular stomatitis, glossitis, and sore mouth. Photophobia is frequent and a diffuse dermatitis (especially over the face) may develop. Corneal vascularization may occur. Riboflavin deficiency usually occurs in a setting of multiple deficits. The treatment for presumed deficiency is riboflavin 10 mg a day.

Pyridoxine Deficiency

Deficiency of pyridoxine clinically is associated with the development of an anemia (sideroblastic anemia) which may respond only to large pharmacologic doses of pyridoxine, 50 mg per day (Chap. 46).

Folic Acid Deficiency

The development of macrocytic anemia in patients with chronic alcoholism is most frequently the result of a deficit of folic acid (Chap. 46). Alcoholics have decreased dietary intake of folic acid. In addition, alcohol interferes with folic acid metabolism. The usual therapeutic dose is 1 mg per day.

Scurvy

Vitamin C deficiency (scurvy) is often found in chronic alcoholics.[54] Hemorrhages around the base of hair follicles and along swollen gums are characteristic. The gum lesions are found only in the part of the gingiva surrounding teeth. Vitamin C (100 mg per day) plus an adequate diet is effective therapy.

Polyneuropathy

Polyneuropathy manifested by burning, numbness, and tenderness especially in the lower extremities is common in chronic alcoholics (Chap. 123). Foot drop may occur. Whether these manifestations are secondary to direct alcohol toxicity or result from B vitamin deficiency is not certain. The peripheral neuropathy is often associated with muscle atrophy (alcoholic myopathy). The polyneuropathy may respond to prolonged abstinence and vitamin B administration.

CHAPTER 154

Ophthalmology in Medicine

NEIL R. MILLER, LAWRENCE W. HIRST, AND ARNALL PATZ

INTRODUCTION

Ocular disorders are important to the general physician in three distinct ways:

1. Certain systemic diseases have important ocular manifestations, e.g., the retinopathy associated with diabetes mellitus. In these disorders the physician needs to know how to detect the ocular involvement and to understand how these findings may alter the diagnostic or therapeutic management of the patient. He also needs to know whether the management requires early collaboration with an ophthalmologist.

2. Certain patients may present themselves to the physician with specific ocular symptoms, e.g., pain or double vision. Here the physician needs to be able to assess the clinical symptom correctly and develop a rational diagnostic plan. Here, too, he must determine whether management requires referral to an ophthalmologist.

3. Finally, there are clinical signs referable to the eye that may or may not be associated with ocular symptoms, e.g., pupillary abnormalities or retinal hemorrhages. In these situations the clinician needs an approach to the differential diagnosis. This requires an understanding of the diseases or conditions that may produce such findings. This chapter is organized to reflect these aspects of ocular disorders.

OCULAR MANIFESTATIONS OF SYSTEMIC DISEASES

Many systemic diseases have ocular manifestations. Ocular motility may be disrupted by various systemic myopathies or neuropathies. In addition, the ocular fundus is the sole location in the body permitting observation of both arteries and veins. The retinal vessels may be affected by systemic diseases in the same way as the vasculature in other parts of the body.

Diabetes and Diabetic Retinopathy

Diabetic retinopathy is an important cause of blindness throughout the world, and it is the largest cause of blindness in patients under 60 years of age in the

United States. The incidence of diabetic retinopathy is directly correlated with the duration of the disease. After 10 years of diabetes, half the patients show some degree of retinopathy, and after 25 years 95 percent have retinopathy. Retinopathy is frequently associated with generalized microangiopathy involving small vessels throughout the body. Most noteworthy are the vascular lesions of the renal glomeruli consisting of diffuse and nodular glomerulosclerosis.

OPHTHALMOSCOPIC FINDINGS. Diabetic retinopathy is conveniently divided into a background stage where the vascular changes are contained within the retina and a proliferative stage where new vessels proliferate through the inner surface of the retina (Table 154–1; Fig. 154–1, Top). A more florid and advanced phase of *background* diabetic retinopathy is referred to as "preproliferative" retinopathy.

In *simple* background retinopathy, retinal edema particularly in the macula frequently occurs. The dot-and-blot hemorrhages are usually scattered at random throughout the posterior retina, and the hard exudates frequently take a ring or circinate pattern (Fig. 154–2A).

In *preproliferative* background retinopathy, cotton-wool, or soft exudates were previously thought to indicate an associated "hypertensive" component to the diabetic retinopathy. However, these areas representing local retinal infarcts occur commonly in normotensive diabetic patients with no history of hypertension. Venous beading consists of the irregular sausage-shaped changes in the appearance of the retinal veins. Intraretinal microvascular abnormalities—dilated capillary-shunt vessels in the retina—frequently develop around the focal areas of capillary

nonperfusion. The triad of preproliferative retinopathy (namely, soft exudates, venous beading, and microvascular abnormalities), especially when associated with noteworthy retinal hemorrhages, should alert the examiner to a more progressive and florid stage of retinopathy.

In *proliferative* retinopathy, the neovascularization may produce a major hemorrhage resulting from traction of the vitreous gel which is adherent to the new vessels (Fig. 154–2B). Organization of such a hemorrhage and formation of fibrous tissue frequently lead to a traction retinal detachment with severe visual loss.

THERAPY OF DIABETIC RETINOPATHY. Patients with *background* retinopathy do not generally require treatment unless significant macular edema is present. The therapeutic efficacy of photocoagulation and of aspirin and dipyridamole (Persantine) in *simple background* retinopathy and in *preproliferative* background retinopathy is under prospective study. Photocoagulation has proved beneficial in selected stages of proliferative retinopathy.

It is recommended that patients with any stage of diabetic retinopathy have routine ophthalmologic consultations. There is no urgency for patients with simple background retinopathy. Patients with preproliferative changes should be promptly referred, and the ophthalmologist will usually follow these cases at approximately 3-month intervals. All patients demonstrating any form of proliferative retinopathy (neovascularization at the optic disc or elsewhere in the retina) should be promptly referred for consideration of photocoagulation therapy.

In selected cases of advanced proliferative diabetic retinopathy where dense vitreous hemorrhages or fibrous tissue causing traction detachment of the retina are present, vitrectomy is often successful.

CONTROL OF DIABETES AND RETINOPATHY. Although clinical reports on small populations of patients and animal studies suggest that multiple insulin injections with improved control of diabetes reduce the occurrence of diabetic retinopathy, neither the experimental nor the human studies can be considered conclusive. Nevertheless, we recommend a strong effort to maintain good control of the diabetic patient.

OTHER OCULAR CHANGES OF DIABETES. *Cataracts* develop at an earlier age in diabetics than in the normal population. In children with very high blood sugars before the diabetes is regulated, a diffuse punctate opacification of the lens may occasionally occur causing poor vision. *Neovascularization of the iris* (rubeosis iridis) is a serious complication of proliferative diabetic retinopathy and frequently causes a severe type of glaucoma.

TABLE 154–1
Ophthalmoscopic Signs of Diabetic Retinopathy

Background Diabetic Retinopathy

Simple
  Microaneurysms
  Dot-and-blot hemorrhages
  Hard exudates
  Macular edema

Preproliferative
  Soft exudates (cotton-wool spots)
  Beaded veins
  Intraretinal microvascular abnormalities
  Extensive intraretinal hemorrhages frequently present

Proliferative Diabetic Retinopathy

Neovascularization emanating from disc area
Neovascularization emanating from elsewhere in
  fundus

Hypertensive and Atherosclerotic Retinopathy

Although mild retinal vascular abnormalities may occur in patients with atherosclerosis without associated systemic hypertension, the most severe vascular changes are seen with systemic hypertension. It is convenient to provide a general grade to the fundus changes using the broader category of *hypertensive arteriosclerotic* retinopathy (Table 154-2).

Retinal examination is especially reliable in accelerated hypertension where soft exudates (cotton-wool spots) and papilledema accurately reflect the hypertensive crisis. For lesser degrees of systemic atherosclerosis and arteriosclerosis, the retinal findings are a useful guide to the systemic vasculature but may not always reflect precisely the degree of generalized vascular disease.

Retinal changes associated with hypertension or atherosclerosis do not generally result in irreversible visual impairment; however, during hypertensive crises or as a result of atherosclerosis, the optic nerve may become ischemic, resulting in permanent visual loss. There is no specific treatment for hypertensive-atherosclerotic retinopathy, since it usually resolves once the underlying systemic disease is controlled.

In patients with either eclampsia or pheochromocytoma, fundus changes of severe hypertension may develop acutely. Generalized advanced arteriolar narrowing, soft (cottonwool) exudates, and diffuse retinal edema occur. In severe cases, bilateral retinal detachments result from fluid extravasation beneath the retina. Once the hypertension is controlled, the detachments subside, and the retinal vessels rapidly return to normal unless the hypertension has been long standing. In the latter cases, arteriolar narrowing and arteriovenous compressions persist.

Hematologic and Associated Disorders

The eye may become involved in various hematologic disorders as well as in all of the blood dyscrasias (Table 154-3).

GRAFT-VERSUS-HOST DISEASE. Both acute and chronic graft-versus-host disease occur in bone marrow transplant patients following aplastic anemia and may present with a dry eye syndrome in association with other dermatologic, hepatic, and respiratory manifestations of the disease. This may be treated with artificial tear solutions and ointments. In addition, the cornea and conjunctiva of such patients as well as patients who are immunosuppressed are frequently sites of infections caused by normally "nonpathogenic" organisms, fungi such as Candida or Aspergillus, and viruses such as *Herpes simplex* and cytomegalic inclusion virus. Such infections may be much more severe than in healthy patients and may rapidly progress to corneal perforation and loss of the eye. Any ocular infections that occur in debilitated or immunosuppressed patients should be seen for managment by an ophthalmologist as soon as possible.

Joint Disease

Ocular involvement in adult rheumatoid arthritis (Chap. 102) is characterized by the triad of scleritis, dry eye, and uveitis. The scleritis may be a florid, erythematous, and painful condition (nodular scleritis) or a quiet dissolution of the sclera with perforation (scleromalcia perforans). The cornea may be involved peripherally as part of a sclerokeratitis or may be secondarily involved. Sjögren syndrome, keratoconjunctivitis sicca, (Chap. 101) involves the lacrimal and salivary glands and produces a dry eye in approximately 50 percent of patients with rheumatoid arthritis. Such patients often complain of an irritated, scratchy sensation in their eyes or complain that the eyes feel tired. The diagnosis of a dry eye is made by testing basal tear secretion. After topical anesthetic has been placed in both eyes, a Schirmer's test strip (a small strip of filter paper) is folded approximately 5 mm from the end and hooked over the lateral third of both lower lids. The patient is asked to stare straight ahead with minimal blinking for 5 minutes, and the wetting of the strips beyond the fold is measured. Abnormal tear secretion under these circumstances is less than 5 mm. Such patients are best

---

TABLE 154-2
Grading of Hypertensive-Arteriosclerotic Retinopathy

Grade I
  Slight generalized arteriolar narrowing
  Increased arteriolar light reflexes
  Mild arteriovenous (A-V) compression (nicking)

Grade II
  Copper wire arterioles
  Moderate A-V nicking
  A-V crossings at right angles

Grade III
  Silver-wire arterioles
  Flame hemorrhages
  Occasional soft exudates (retinal infarcts)
  Prominent A-V nicking

Grade IV
  Optic disc edema
  Silver-wire arterioles, perivascular sheathing
  Numerous soft exudates
  Flame hemorrhages, especially around the disc
  Marked A-V nicking
  Macular exudates—star pattern

TABLE 154–3
The Eye in Hematologic Disorders

Disease	Cornea	Location				
		Conjunctiva	Anterior Chamber	Vitreous	Retina	Orbit
Anemia (Chap. 45)		Pallor			Hemorrhages	
Polycythemia (Chap. 50)		Tortuous vessels			Hemorrhages CRVO*	
Hemoglobinopathies (Chap. 46)						
S-C and S-thal		"C" sign		Hemorrhages	Hemorrhages, scarring, neovascularization, detachment	
S-S and S-A					Hemorrhages	
Leukemias (Chap. 50)	Peripheral infiltrates	Focal cellular accumulations	Uveitis Hemorrhages	Hemorrhages	Hemorrhages Roth spots	Chloroma
Lymphomas (Chap. 51)						
Lymphocytic						
Histiocytic			Uveitis	Cellular accumulation	Infiltration† Infiltration† hemorrhages	
Dysproteinemia (Chap. 92)	Crystalline deposits	Focal cellular accumulations			Hemorrhages, CRVO* infiltration†	

* CRVO-Central retinal vein occlusion.
† Usually in the form of specific masses, often involving the lacrimal gland.

treated with artificial tear solutions and ointments used as often as needed to eliminate the patient's symptoms. If this treatment fails, soft contact lenses or occlusion of tear drainage pathways may be of benefit.

Anterior uveitis also occurs in such patients and has a recurrent, chronic course. When this occurs, the patient should be referred to an ophthalmologist for management (see below).

Patients with juvenile rheumatoid arthritis (JRA) (Chap. 102) or ankylosing spondylitis (Chap. 104) commonly present with uveitis. Although the uveitis is generally manifested by pain, a red eye, and blurred vision, some patients with JRA develop uveitis without ocular symptoms. For this reason, patients with JRA should be examined by an ophthalmologist at regular intervals.

Reiter syndrome (Chap. 108) is a triad of arthritis, urethritis, and ocular inflammation. In most cases, the inflammation is simply a conjunctivitis; however, a severe uveitis may also occur.

Uveitis, whether idiopathic or part of a systemic process, requires treatment to prevent intraocular scarring with secondary cataract formation and glaucoma. Treatment relies on depressing the inflammatory response with topical and, if necessary, systemic corticosteroids. Mydriatics are also used to relieve pain.

Systemic Vasculitis

Loss of vision in the patient with *giant cell (temporal) arteritis* (Chaps. 100 and 129) is an ocular and medical emergency. Although systemic symptoms, such as fever, malaise, and migratory arthralgias, frequently precede the ocular involvement, these symptoms may be ignored, and sudden loss of visual acuity in one or both eyes may be the presenting symptom. The suspicion of giant cell arteritis by the internist demands immediate ocular assessment.

Although high-dose systemic corticosteroid administration may abort visual loss in the second eye, recovery of vision in the involved eye is rare. Ocular involvement includes ischemic optic neuropathy, central retinal artery occlusion, and retinal ischemia. Vision may be impaired from involvement of the intracranial vessels resulting in diplopia or cortical blindness.

Involvement of the eye by *systemic lupus erythematosus* (Chap. 97) and *Polyarteritis nodosa* (Chap. 100) may also occur as a primary retinal vasculitis or ischemic optic neuropathy.

Herpes zoster ophthalmicus may affect every structure of the eye, usually as a result of the associated vasculitis. The patient may present with a keratitis, anterior uveitis with cataracts and atrophic iris changes, a retinal vasculitis, or an optic neuritis. In addition, patients may also develop various ocular motor nerve palsies with and without pupillary abnormalities.

Other disorders such as *Wegener's granulomatosis* (Chaps. 34 and 100) with scleritis, ring ulcer, and perforation of the cornea, uveitis, and retinal vasculitis have been reported. The effects of scleroderma on the eye are generally related to lid contraction and secondary corneal changes.

All patients with systemic vasculitis and ocular involvement should be followed closely by both the ophthalmologist and internist. Treatment, usually a combination of topical and systemic corticosteroids or immunosuppresive agents, should be determined by the two physicians together.

Thyroid Disease

Patients with thyroid disease may develop ocular involvement at any time during the course of the disease. In many patients, systemic evidence of dysthyroidism has already appeared by the time ocular signs and symptoms begin; however, ocular involvement may begin when the disease appears to be under good control and may even occur in the absence of any other signs or symptoms of dysthyroidism. In some cases, it appears that ocular involvement begins or worsens after the patient with hyperthyroidism has been treated with radioactive iodine and is in a hypothyroid state.

Although the majority of patients with thyroid eye disease have abnormal thyroid function studies, approximately 20 percent of such patients have normal thyroid functions including the Werner suppression and TRH tests. The current status of thyroid eye disease and its relationship to exophthalmos producing substance (EPS) and long-acting thyroid stimulator (LATS) is discussed in the chapter on thyroid disease (Chap. 76).

The ocular lesion in thyroid eye disease is infiltration of orbital contents by mucopolysaccharide sub-

stances and chronic inflammatory cells, predominantly lymphocytes. Infiltration of orbital fat results in proptosis, while infiltration of ocular muscles results in motility restriction and subsequent double vision. In severe cases, infiltration of the ocular muscles at their origin at the orbital apex results in compression of the optic nerve leading to progressive visual loss.

As noted in Table 154–4, treatment is directed toward specific abnormalities as they arise. Patients with thyroid eye disease should be followed by an ophthalmologist at regular intervals. In addition to measurement of visual acuity and intraocular pressure, the amount of proptosis should be measured at each visit. Proptosis is measured using an exophthalmometer. This device uses prisms to measure the protrusion of the cornea beyond the lateral orbital rim. A difference of more than 2.5 mm between the two eyes is abnormal.

TABLE 154–4
Thyroid Eye Disease

Symptoms	Signs	Treatment
Tired, irritated eyes	Conjunctival redness	Tear substitutes
Lid swelling	Conjunctival and eyelid edema	Elevate head of bed at night
Prominent stare	Lid retraction and lag	Eyelid surgery
Prominent eyes	Proptosis	Depends on severity*
Double vision	Limitation of ocular motility	Prisms rarely of benefit; surgical correction usually required
Pain and blurred vision	Corneal ulceration from chronic exposure	Tarsorrhaphy; tear substitutes; orbital decompression
Blurred vision	Optic nerve dysfunction (from orbital compression)	Systemic steroids; orbital decompression; radiation to posterior orbit

* There is no specific treatment for proptosis alone, although some physicians consider the cosmetic deformity alone an indication for orbital decompression. Usually, treatment is directed toward the specific problems caused by the proptosis, e.g., corneal exposure, diplopia, or compressive optic neuropathy.

Myasthenia Gravis

Approximately 75 percent of patients with myasthenia gravis first complain of double vision or drooping of their eyelids, and 90 percent of patients with the disease will eventually develop ocular signs and symptoms. Typically, the onset of either ptosis or diplopia is insidious, intermittent, and fatigue related. Ptosis is usually incomplete and asymmetric but may be bilateral and severe. Diplopia may be vertical, horizontal, or skew. Differentiation from ocular motor nerve pareses is often extremely difficult unless other systemic signs and symptoms are present. As with other systemic manifestations of the disease, the diagnosis is based on a positive edrophonium (Tensilon) or neostigmine (Prostigmin) test (Chap. 122).

Although both the ptosis and diplopia may respond to medical treatment with either anticholinesterase agents or alternate day corticosteroids, the ocular signs of myasthenia gravis are notoriously refractory to treatment. Devices to elevate the eyelids may be affixed to the patient's glasses to alleviate residual ptosis (ptosis crutches); however, patients with severe, residual diplopia may need constant patching of one eye. Surgery of the ocular muscles is never indicated.

Approximately 10 percent of patients have a purely ocular form of myasthenia gravis. This diagnosis can only be made after the patient has been without systemic symptoms and signs for 18 months. It is important to remember, however, that the vast majority of patients in whom myasthenia gravis presents with ocular symptoms and signs will develop systemic myasthenia within 18 months. For this reason, such patients should be closely followed not only by the ophthalmologist but also by the internist or neurologist as well.

Commonly Used Systemic Drugs and Their Ocular Side Effects

Several commonly used systemic drugs have ocular side effects. In many cases, the effects are insignificant; however, in certain instances the ocular symptoms and signs are not only significant but also irreversible (Table 154–5).

COMMON OCULAR SYMPTOMS

Many patients with ocular disorders may first consult an internist with their symptoms. The physician should know which symptoms require immediate attention by an ophthalmologist and which symptoms are of minor significance.

Ocular Pain

Most pain that occurs in or around the eyes is associated with ocular inflammation or irritation. The etiology is usually within the eye or found on its surface. On rare occasions, diseases that affect the trigeminal nerve, such as migraine or aneurysm, cause severe pain that is referred to the eye and orbit. Patients with severe ocular pain should first be examined carefully by an ophthalmologist. If no ocular abnormality is found, a neurologic evaluation should be undertaken.

Diplopia

Although acquired diplopia may occur as a monocular phenomenon in rare patients with opacities of the ocular media, and as a functional disorder, most patients with acquired diplopia have a misalignment of the eye caused by abnormalities in the ocular muscles or in their innervation. The diagnosis of binocular diplopia is made by covering either eye and noting disappearance of the double vision. Binocular diplopia may be myopathic or neuropathic in origin. It has already been mentioned that two systemic diseases that may produce diplopia by affecting the extraocular muscles are thyroid disease and myasthenia gravis. These entities should always be considered in a patient who develops double vision without other symptoms of neurologic disease. Other myopathies may affect ocular motility; however, these are rare. In addition to myopathic disorders, diplopia is often caused by paralysis of one or more of the three oculomotor nerves (Table 154–6).

Visual Loss

Loss of visual acuity is always a significant symptom and usually indicates major ocular disease. In assessing the patient with visual loss, the physician should pay careful attention to whether the visual loss has been intermittent or permanent, how long it has lasted, and whether there are any associated symptoms.

Although some of the disorders mentioned in Tables 154–7 to 154–10 are manifestations of systemic diseases, most of them are purely ocular disorders. As such, some of the more important ocular disorders require further comment.

GLAUCOMA.   Glaucoma is defined as an elevation of intraocular pressure which damages the optic nerve and may ultimately result in loss of peripheral visual field and central visual acuity. There are two principal types of glaucoma that are determined by the anatomic configuration of the anterior chamber and should be considered as completely separate entities:

TABLE 154-5
Systemic Drugs and Their Ocular Toxicity

Drug	Condition	Comments
Atropine	Blurred vision	Caused by paralysis of accomodation; systemic administration of atropine had *never* been shown to cause glaucoma*
Chlor-amphenicol	Optic neuropathy	Rare; test visual acuity, color vision; usually reversible with withdrawal of drug
	Erythema multiforme bullosum (Stevens-Johnson syndrome)†	Variable scarring of conjunctiva causing dry eye syndrome. If mild, may respond to tear substitutes; however, if severe, irreversible blindness results
Chloroquine	Corneal deposits	Not clinically significant; disappear on withdrawal of drug
	Retinal degeneration	Visual function slowly lost; may be irreversible; regular testing of visual acuity, visual fields important
Corticosteroids	Cataracts	Related to length of use; irreversible; may progress despite steroid withdrawal; good prognosis with surgery
	Glaucoma	Dose and time-related; genetic predisposition; intraocular pressure returns to normal when drug is stopped. May require topical medication or surgery for control
Ethambutol	Optic neuropathy	Dose related; usually reversible if early withdrawal; not usually seen if dose kept at 15 mg/kg or less. Test visual acuity, color vision, and central visual field at 6-month intervals
Oxygen	Retrolental fibroplasia	In premature infants; related to incomplete development of retinal vasculature; monitor arterial blood gases
Phenothiazines	Eyelid skin pigmentation Blurred vision	After long-term therapy; caused by either temporary accomodative paralysis or induction of myopia; transient and reversible
	Corneal deposits	Not significant; reversibility uncertain
	Lens opacities	Not significant
	Chorio-retinopathy	Most significant side effect; almost exclusively with piperidines, e.g., Mellaril; dose and time-related; usually partially reversible with low total doses; check visual acuity, visual fields, and electroretinogram (if indicated)
Tetracycline	Papilledema (pseudotumor cerebri)	Also seen with vitamin A intoxication and nalidixic acid; syndrome resolves once drug withdrawn; loss of visual acuity or field may result depending on duration and severity of papilledema

* Similarly, the belladonna alkaloids used for various gastrointestinal disorders do not cause or exacerbate glaucoma.
† May also be caused by sulfonamides and penicillin.

Acute Narrow-Angle Glaucoma. In patients with narrow angles, the access of the aqueous humor to the outflow channels of the eye is partially blocked by the iris root. When the pupil dilates, either in sustained darkness or in response to drugs, the angle becomes completely blocked, and intraocular pressure rises. The patient may initially note blurred vision and halos around lights as the pressure begins to rise. As the pressure continues to rise, the patient develops severe, deep ocular pain, often with nausea and vomiting. Vision becomes extremely blurred and may be completely lost. The eye itself becomes red with a hazy cornea and a nonreactive pupil (Table 154–11). During an acute attack of narrow-angle glaucoma, the intraocular pressure will range between 40 and 90 mm Hg compared to the normal range of 10 to 20 mm Hg. When the pressure is increased to these levels, digital palpation reveals a firm, hard globe compared to the other eye.

Prompt referral to an ophthalmologist for immediate therapy is essential. If an ophthalmologist is not readily available, the physician should institute treatment with pilocarpine drops every 10 minutes. In addition, either oral glycerin or intravenous mannitol should be used to lower the intraocular pressure. Definitive therapy consists of an iridectomy performed surgically or with a laser.

Chronic Open-Angle Glaucoma. In open-angle

TABLE 154–6
Ocular Motor Nerve Palsies*

Type	Signs	Probable Etiology
Third nerve palsy	Ptosis Limitation of elevation Limitation of depression Limitation of adduction May or may not have pupillary involvement	With pupillary involvement: aneurysm; tumor; trauma Without pupillary involvement: diabetes mellitus
Fourth nerve palsy	Hypertropia on side of palsy Often have head tilt to opposite side May notice torsional diplopia	Trauma; rarely diabetes mellitus or hypertension
Sixth nerve palsy	Limitation of abduction	Vascular; trauma; tumor, especially nasopharyngeal or metastatic carcinoma

* What appears to be a partial ocular motor nerve palsy may actually represent the effects of a systemic myopathy, e.g., thyroid disease or myasthenia gravis.

glaucoma, the anterior chamber is of normal depth and the angle is open, allowing free access of aqueous humor to the drainage structures. A defect within the tissue of the drainage channels reduces the rate of drainage such that the intraocular pressure gradually rises to levels between 30 and 50 mm Hg. Unlike patients with acute narrow-angle glaucoma, patients with chronic open-angle glaucoma do not experience pain, discomfort, or acute visual loss. Rather, the sustained, moderately elevated intraocular pressure gradually results in loss of the peripheral visual field (Fig. 154-2E). The patient may, thus, be unaware of any visual difficulty until the disease is in an advanced state. For this reason, early detection by routine measurement of intraocular pressure in all patients undergoing ophthalmologic examination is essential. Because open-angle glaucoma is most common in the age group from 40 to 70 years, all patients over age 40 should have their intraocular pressure measured yearly.

Open-angle glaucoma is generally treated medically with both topical and oral agents. When these are ineffective, surgery is required.

SENILE MACULAR DEGENERATION. Senile macular degeneration is the greatest cause of legal blindness in patients over the age of 60 in the United States. It is most common in caucasians and is extremely rare in blacks. These patients usually show scattered dru-

TABLE 154–7
Abrupt (Seconds–Minutes) Intermittent Visual Loss

Cause	Clinical Findings	Management	Prognosis
Retinal emboli	Clear (platelets), white (calcific), or glistening yellow (cholesterol) Occlusive plug or plugs in retinal arterials Segmental retinal pallor sometimes	Seek cardiac or vascular (esp. carotid) source of emboli If macula affected, treat as central retinal artery occlusion Possible surgical treatment of carotid disease	Good
Papilledema	Elevated optic discs Blurred peripapillary nerve fiber layer Splinter hemorrhages Exudate and other vascular changes Associated with raised intracranial pressure, pseudotumor cerebri, or hypertension	Diagnosis and treatment of underlying condition; see Table 154–12 and Chapter 131	Depends on etiology and duration
Migraine	Often precedes headache, but can occur without headache Retinal arteries narrow often during attack	Treatment of migraine (Chap. 125)	Good

---

TABLE 154–8
Abrupt (Seconds–Minutes) Permanent Visual Loss

Cause	Clinical Findings	Management	Prognosis
Central retinal vein occlusion	"Blood and thunder" retinal appearance Optic disc edema Venous vascular tortusity and engorgement May be associated with hypertension, diabetes mellitus, or hyperviscosity states	Treat underlying systemic disease Anticoagulation or photocoagulation may be of value in selected cases	Poor 25% develop secondary glaucoma
Pituitary apoplexy	Severe headache Progressive lethargy Ocular motor nerve palsies Occasional endocrine crisis	Immediate neurosurgical decompression	Dependent on duration of visual loss Usually good
Occipital lobe vascular accident	Homonymous hemianopia, unilateral or bilateral Associated posterior cerebral artery insufficiency signs Hypertension	See Chapter 129	Poor
Vitreous hemorrhage	Hazy vitreous; no view of retina Associated hypertension and diabetes mellitus Ocular trauma	Ultrasound to exclude other retinal disease Bed rest Vitrectomy in selected cases	Dependent on etiology
Central retinal artery occlusion	Retinal edema Macular cherry-red spot Attenuated arterioles, eventual optic atrophy May be associated with carotid artery occlusive disease, hypertension, or giant cell arteritis	CO_2 inhalation Ocular massage Anterior chamber paracentesis	Poor

sen (yellowish-white spots) in the posterior fundus before developing more advanced changes. The pathogenesis consists of degeneration of Bruch's membrane, the layer between the retinal pigment epithelium and choriocapillaris, that allows ingrowth of choroidal vessels beneath the retina. Leakage of fluid and blood from these new vessels has a predilection for the macula producing serious visual impairment. Organization of the hemorrhages resulting in fibrous scar tissue is the final stage.

In some patients with senile macular degeneration, progressive atrophy of the outer layers of the retina and choriocapillaris leads to deterioration of central vision without hemorrhage and scar tissue formation. The macula shows a mottled atrophic appearance.

Treatment of senile macular degeneration by medical therapy is ineffective. Photocoagulation has been advocated for the choroidal neovascularization, but its role remains to be documented.

RETINAL VEIN OCCLUSION. *Branch vein occlusion* is the second most common cause, after diabetes, of retinal vascular disease observed in the United States. The obstruction occurs at an arteriovenous crossing where the artery and vein share a common adventitia. Distal to the obstruction, flame hemorrhages and retinal edema are common. In occasional cases, neovascularization develops several months

TABLE 154-9
Progressive (Hours–Days) Visual Loss

Cause	Clinical Findings	Management	Prognosis
Acute keratoconus	Opaque central cornea Frequently conical cornea on other side	Observation	Good
Acute angle-closure glaucoma	Raised intraocular pressure Red eye Semidilated pupil with shallow anterior chamber Severe pain	Pilocarpine drops Diamox and oral or intravenous hyperosmotic agents Surgery	Dependent on duration of angle closure glaucoma
Retinal detachment	Elevated retina Occasional vitreous hemorrhage	Surgical reattachment	Dependent upon duration and location of detachment
Optic neuritis (including ischemic)	Pale, swollen, or normal disc Afferent pupil defect Decreased color vision May be associated with demyelinating disease or giant cell arteritis	The use of systemic corticosteroids is controversial except in giant cell arteritis	Dependent on etiology

TABLE 154-10
Slowly Progressive (Months–Years) Visual Loss

Cause	Clinical Findings	Management	Prognosis
Corneal dystrophies	Corneal opacities bilaterally Frequent familial involvement	Corneal transplantation	Excellent
Chronic open-angle glaucoma	Quiet, nonpainful Characteristic visual field loss Raised intraocular pressure Optic nerve cupping	Parasympathomimetic or sympathic blocking agents topically Diamox Ocular surgery	Dependent on duration of glaucoma
Cataracts	Lens opacities	Ocular surgery	Excellent
Macular degeneration	Circumscribed fibrosis, hemorrhage, or pigmentary disturbances at maculae	Photocoagulation in selected cases	Poor for central vision but patients always maintain peripheral vision
Optic nerve compression	Optic atrophy Radiologic evidence of optic canal changes	Surgical exploration	Dependent on etiology and duration of compression

after the occlusion. Anticoagulant therapy is of no value, and the role of photocoagulation for macular edema is undergoing a clinical trial. Photocoagulation is frequently effective for treating the secondary neovascularization.

Systemic hypertension is found in the majority of patients; however, a medical evaluation should also include a work-up for diabetes.

Central vein occlusion produces the classic, vivid "blood-and-thunder" appearance to the entire poste-rior fundus (Fig. 154-2C). Extensive flame hemorrhages as well as dilatation and tortuosity of all the branch retinal veins are present. Soft (cotton-wool) exudates are frequently present and when extensive are a poor prognostic sign. In 1 to 3 months approximately 20 percent of patients will show iris neovascularization, which frequently leads to a severe form of glaucoma.

Medical evaluation should rule out diabetes and systemic hypertension. It should also include hemato-

TABLE 154-11
Red Eye: Differential Diagnosis

Sign	Conjunctivitis	Anterior Uveitis	Acute Glaucoma
Vision	Normal or intermittent blurring that clears with blinking	Slightly blurred	Marked blurring
Conjunctival injection	Diffuse	Circumcorneal (ciliary flush)	Diffuse and circumcorneal
Discharge	Significant, often with crusting of lashes	None	None
Pain	None or minimal	Moderately severe; stabbing or aching	Very severe; often nausea and vomiting
Pupil size	Normal	Normal or irregular	Mid-dilated and fixed
Pupillary response to light	Normal	Normal or irregular constriction	Minimal or no reaction
Intraocular pressure	Normal (sterilize tonometer after use)	Normal or slightly low	Elevated
Corneal appearance	Clear	Clear or slightly hazy	Steamy; opaque
Anterior chamber depth	Normal	Normal	Shallow
Comments*	If viral, spontaneous resolution; if bacterial, use topical bacteriocidal agent; if allergic or irritative, withdraw offending agent; all have good prognosis	Systemic workup indicated if recurrent; treat with topical steroids and cycloplegics	Immediate therapy with pilocarpine and osmotic agents; surgical or laser iridectomy is only definitive treatment; visual prognosis dependent on duration and severity of attack

* Topical steroid preparations should never be used to treat a red eye without a specific indication since they may cause the development of glaucoma, cataracts, or herpetic keratitis.

logic evaluation, since the occlusion may be a manifestation of such conditions as polycythemia, macroglobulinemia, blood dyscrasia, or dysproteinemia. Chronic simple glaucoma is a contributing factor in a substantial number of these patients and should be ruled out by the ophthalmologist.

The role of anticoagulant therapy is highly controversial and adequate studies are lacking. The possible therapeutic role of fibrinolytic agents in early cases is under investigation.

A milder form of central retinal vein occlusion, occurring usually in younger patients without systemic or hematologic abnormalities, is termed papillophlebitis and has a favorable prognosis.

RETINAL ARTERIAL OCCLUSION. The obstruction may involve either the entire central retinal artery or one of its branches. The area of retinal occlusion takes on a pale, milky-white appearance. In central retinal artery occlusion the entire posterior retina is pale except for the center of the macula which is not edematous and maintains its normal pinkish-red color to appear as a cherry-red spot (Fig. 154–2D).

Causes of central or branch retinal artery occlusion include emboli from carotid artery disease or valvular heart disease and giant cell arteritis. The condition also occurs in patients with hypertension.

Although some patients spontaneously improve, for the majority who do not, treatment is usually unsatisfactory. Systemic vasodilator drugs generally have no effect on the retinal vessels and may in fact be deleterious by reducing ocular perfusion through a reduction of systemic blood pressure. Because CO_2 dilates the retinal vessels, breathing into a bag or inhalation of a mixture of 95 percent O_2–5 percent CO_2 is advocated. Prompt referral to an ophthalmologist is advised for further management which may include ocular massage or paracentesis of the globe.

OCULAR HISTOPLASMOSIS (THE PRESUMED OCULAR HISTOPLASMOSIS SYNDROME). A significant part of the population throughout the Ohio River Valley (and to a lesser extent in the eastern and southern United States) has been exposed to histoplasma infection. The exact pathogenesis of the ocular lesion remains unclear, but during the active systemic infection, which may be mild or unnoticed, focal ocular lesions may develop which leave small atrophic spots in the fundus (histo-spots) or pigmented changes about the optic nerve. The histo-spots are of no visual significance per se except that years later choroidal neovascularization growing through a defect in Bruch's membrane about the histo-spot may produce hemorrhage and scar tissue in the retina similar to that seen in senile macular degeneration. The triad of atrophic spots scattered about the fundus, pigmented scars about the disc, and hemorrhage near the macula constitutes the presumed ocular histoplasmosis syndrome. In the endemic areas the presumed histo syndrome with macular hemorrhage is a significant cause of visual impairment. A positive histoplasmin skin test further supports the diagnosis but is of little practical value in endemic areas as the majority of the population are positive reactors.

No treatment is indicated for quiescent histospots. Corticosteroid therapy has been advocated for the active neovascularization by some investigators but the results have been variable and a controlled clinical trial has not been performed. Photocoagulation therapy has become increasingly popular in recent years.

COMMON OCULAR SIGNS

Certain ocular abnormalities that can be observed by the physician may or may not be associated with symptoms. The physician must, thus, be able to recognize the significance of these signs with respect to underlying ocular or systemic disease.

Red Eye
Disorders that irritate or inflame the eye result in redness of the conjunctiva (Table 154-11). See Figure 154-2H.

Optic Disc Abnormalities
OPTIC DISC EDEMA. Edema or swelling of the optic disc may be produced by a wide variety of neurologic or systemic diseases (Table 154-12).

Ophthalmoscopic findings of optic disc edema include hyperemia of the disc, blurred disc margins, blurring of the peripapillary retinal nerve fiber layer, small flame-shaped hemorrhages at the disc margin, and loss of venous pulsations (Fig. 154-2G).

Patients with optic disc edema should be referred to an ophthalmologist for evaluation unless systemic signs and symptoms suggest increased intracranial

TABLE 154-12
Optic Disc Edema

Type	Vision	Visual Field	Other Findings	Etiology
Papilledema	Normal	Full, enlarged blind spot	Headache, diplopia (sixth nerve palsy), nausea, vomiting	Intracranial mass pseudotumor cerebri, hypertension
Anterior ischemic optic neuropathy	Usually decreased	Altitudinal or arcuate defect	Sudden visual loss, (hours), painless, most patients over age 55	Giant cell arteritis, hypertension; diabetes mellitus, "idiopathic"
Anterior optic neuritis	Decreased	Central scotoma	Sudden visual loss (hours to days), often with pain on ocular movement, most often in ages 15-45	"Idiopathic," multiple sclerosis
Compressive optic neuropathy	Decreased	Peripheral defect, rarely central scotoma	Often proptosis and/or limited extraocular motion	Orbital or canal mass, e.g., meningioma or hemangioma
Toxic optic neuropathy	Decreased	Bilateral cecocentral scotomas	May have peripheral neuropathy or other evidence of toxicity	Nutritional, chloramphenicol, or ethambutal; lead
Hypotony	Decreased	Full	Low intraocular pressure	Intraocular surgery; trauma
Infiltrative optic neuropathy	Decreased	Variable	Other signs of inflammation or tumor, vitreous cells	Tumor, e.g., lymphoma, leukemia, Inflammation, e.g. sarcoid, tuberculosis

TABLE 154-13
Optic Atrophy

History of Visual Loss	Visual Field Defect	Probable Etiology	Other Findings
Rapid (hours to days)	Central scotoma	Optic neuritis	Most common in ages 15-45 Often with pain on ocular movement
Rapid (hours to days)	Altitudinal or arcuate scotoma	Ischemic optic neuropathy	Usually over age 55
Progressive (months)	Bilateral cecocentral scotomas	Toxic	May have peripheral neuropathy
Progressive (months to years)	Peripheral constriction	Compression	Headache, anosmia
	Bitemporal hemianopia	Optic chiasmal compression	May have pituitary insufficiency, may have pituitary over activity, e.g., acromegaly

pressure. In such cases, the patient should be immediately referred for neurologic evaluation (Chap. 131).

OPTIC ATROPHY. Optic atrophy results from damage to the fibers that comprise the optic nerve. The damage occurs to nerve fibers within the eye as in central retinal artery occlusion and glaucoma or to the fibers after they leave the eye as in compression from intracranial or intraorbital masses. The atrophic disc may appear yellow or grey-white and devoid of visible capillaries; however, the appearance of the disc generally does not indicate the nature of the process that caused the atrophy (Fig. 154-2F). In dealing with a patient who has optic atrophy, the history of visual loss with any associated symptoms is of primary importance. In general, optic atrophy associated with a history of sudden visual loss suggests either an inflammatory or ischemic process while the same picture associated with slowly progressive visual loss suggests a compressive lesion.

In addition to a history of visual loss, characteristic defects in the visual field may suggest a specific etiology in patients with optic atrophy. Optic atrophy after an attack of anterior or retrobulbar optic neuritis generally produces a defect in the central visual field, the central scotoma, while optic atrophy from anterior ischemic optic neuropathy is usually associated with an altitudinal visual field defect. Compression of the intracranial optic nerve may produce a variety of field defects; however, compression of the optic chiasm often produces a classic temporal defect in each eye with preservation of visual acuity. A bitemporal hemianopia, associated with optic atrophy, is indicative of compression of the optic chiasm, most often from a pituitary adenoma, meningioma, aneurysm, or craniopharyngioma (Table 154-13).

OPTIC DISC ANOMALIES. Various congenital anomalies of optic nerve development may mimic acquired optic nerve defects or may be associated with various systemic abnormalities. Drusen of the optic disc, concretions of material that stain positively for calcium and mucopolysaccharde, may be visible on the optic disc surface as small, glistening, refractile globules; however, they may also develop beneath the surface of the disc giving rise to a picture that is often confused with true optic disc edema. The differentiation between true and pseudo-optic disc edema may be extremely difficult and requires careful ophthalmoscopic examination. Other disc anomalies, such as optic disc tilting, dysplasia, and colobomas, may occur as isolated phenomena or may be associated with midline craniofacial abnormalities such as basal encephalocele. Optic nerve hypoplasia may occur as an isolated defect but is also found in children of diabetic mothers as well as in children whose mothers have taken various medications such as quinine and antiepileptic drugs. The observation of an optic disc anomaly should alert the examiner to consider the possibility of other developmental abnormalities.

Pupillary Abnormalities

Along with the appearance of the optic disc, pupillary abnormalities may be the only objective signs of neurologic dysfunction. For this reason, a knowledge of common pupillary abnormalities is essential. Iris movement is designed to control retinal illumination. Afferent impulses from the retina produce increased efferent impulses in the parasympathetic innervation of the iris and decreased activity in the sympathetic innervation. Both serve to constrict the pupil. A re-

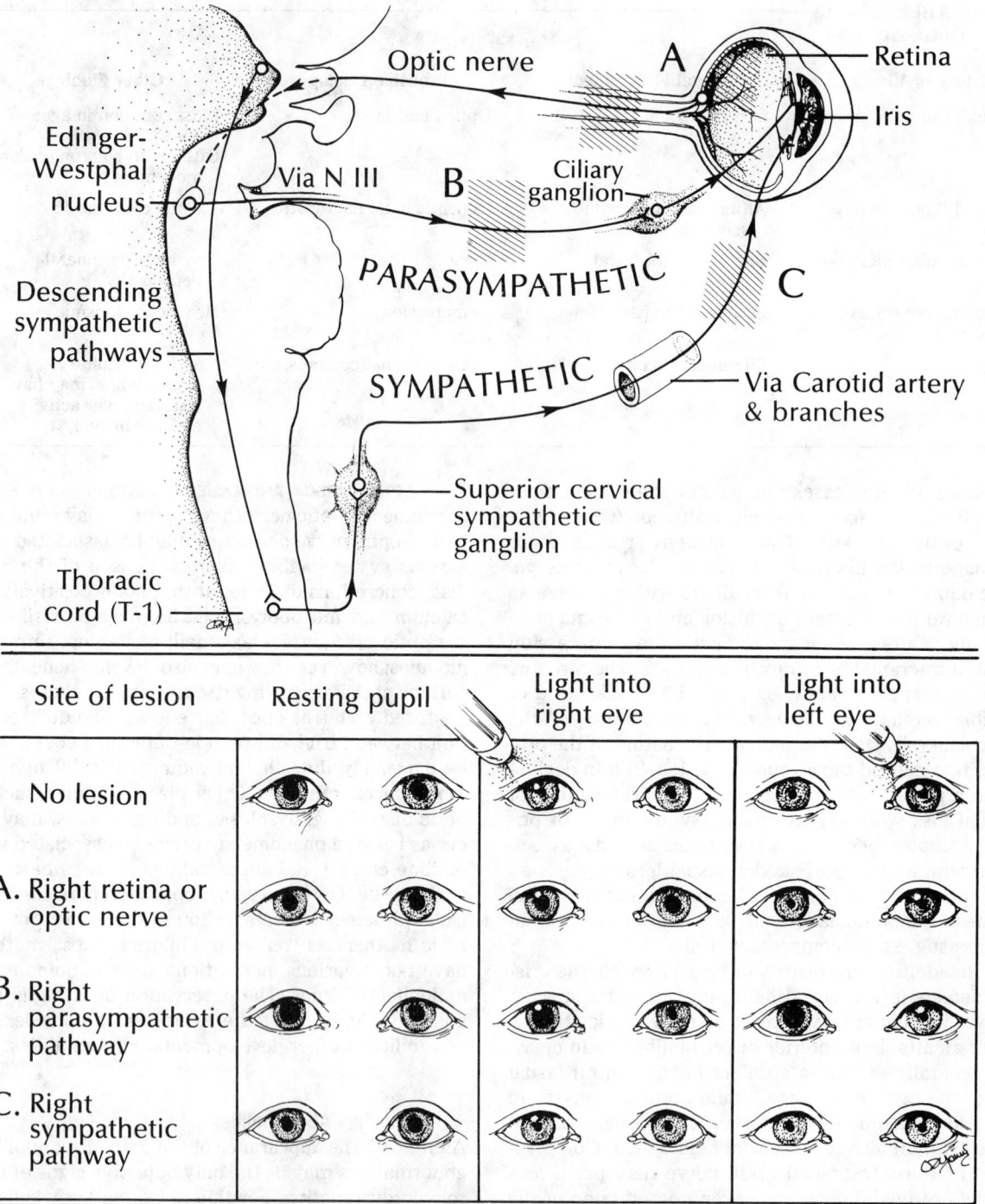

FIGURE 154–1. Pupillary reflex. The afferent pathway is from the retina via the optic nerve. The efferent parasympathetic pathway is from the Edinger-Westphal nucleus via the third nerve and the ciliary ganglion. The sympathetic efferent pathway is via the brainstem, thoracic cord, superior cervical ganglion and thence via the carotid and ophthalmic artery to the eye. The effect of a right-sided **(A)** lesion of retinal or optic nerve, **(B)** interruption of the parasympathetic pathway, and **(C)** interruption of the sympathetic pathway on the size of the resting pupil and the response to shining light into the right and left eye are illustrated.

duction in illumination reduces the afferent impulse, reduces parasympathetic activity, increases sympathetic activity, and causes dilatation of the pupil. Figure 154-1 shows the pathways which mediate this reflex control and the effect of lesions at different sites. These findings are helpful in defining isolated pupillary abnormalities and in localizing the level of more general neurologic deficits.

THE AFFERENT PUPILLARY DEFECT (MARCUS GUNN PUPIL). Damage to the afferent arc of the parasympathetic system, e.g., severe macular degeneration, optic neuritis, results in a characteristic pupillary abnormality commonly referred to as the Marcus Gunn or afferent pupillary defect. In such cases, shining a bright light in the normal eye produces a direct pupillary constriction in that eye as well as a consensual response in the opposite eye. When the light is shone into the abnormal eye, the total amount of light entering the system is reduced, and both pupils redilate to a resting state determined by the amount of ambient light in the room. The observer, looking at the pupil of the abnormal eye, sees what appears to be a paradoxical dilatation to light. Swinging the light back and forth between the two eyes results in the observation of pupillary constriction when the light is shined in the good eye and pupillary dilatation when the light is shined in the bad eye.

Observation of an afferent pupillary defect is objective evidence of a significant lesion of the anterior visual system. It is never seen with cataract or corneal disease. If the retina appears normal in a patient with an afferent pupillary defect, there is almost certainly an optic neuropathy present. Such patients should be referred to an ophthalmologist as soon as possible for evaluation and management.

THE FIXED, DILATED PUPIL. Interruption of the efferent arc of the parasympathetic pathway (the third nerve) results in a fixed, dilated pupil. When the third nerve is affected prior to the synapse of the pupillary fibers in the ciliary ganglion, other signs of third nerve palsy are apparent (Table 154-7). In such cases, the pupil is generally only mildly dilated. When a widely dilated, nonreactive pupil is the only ocular abnormality, postganglionic parasympathetic fibers have been damaged. The two most common causes for this ocular sign are damage to the ciliary ganglion (tonic or Adie pupil) and a pharmacologically dilated pupil due to the deliberate or inadvertent administration of a parasympatholytic agent, e.g., atropine, to the eye (Table 154-14). The diagnosis can usually be established through the use of gradually increasing solutions of pilocarpine, since the tonic pupil is generally hypersensitive to parasympathomimetic agents while the pharmacologically dilated pupil will not constrict to solutions that constrict the normal pupil.

TABLE 154-14
The Fixed, Dilated Pupil

Characteristics	Tonic (Adie) Pupil	Drug Induced
Age	Usually in middle-aged adults	Usually teenagers or young adults
Sex	Females predominate	Usually females; often hospital personnel
Neurologic signs	Diminished deep tendon reflexes in about 50%	None
Diagnosis	Constricts with 0.125% pilocarpine	Will not constrict to pilocarpine solutions strong enough to constrict the normal pupil (1 to 4%)
Treatment	None; accomodation usually returns within months to years; reassurance	If inadvertent, reassurance; if deliberate, consider psychiatric referral

THE ARGYLL ROBERTSON PUPIL. Bilateral, small pupils that are irregular and are nonreactive to light but normally reactive to a near target almost always represent a manifestation of syphilis (Table 154-15).

HORNER SYNDROME. Damage to the sympathetic system produces a characteristic picture known as Horner syndrome (Table 154-16). The diagnosis of a Horner syndrome and subsequent localization of the lesion are extremely important since lesions that affect the sympathetic fibers before their synapse at the superior cervical ganglion (preganglionic lesions) have a higher probability of being malignant than do lesions affecting the fibers after they synapse at the superior cervical ganglion (postganglionic lesions). The diagnosis of Horner syndrome and

TABLE 154-15
Argyll Robertson Pupil

Small irregular pupils
Nonreactive to light
React to near (accommodation) stimulus
Generally bilateral (occasionally unilateral)
Basic defect in dorsal midbrain
Always associated with neurosyphilis

TABLE 154–16
Horner Syndrome

Miotic pupil (more obvious in dim light)
Reacts normally to light
Variable ptosis
Facial anhydrosis on same side (preganglionic only)
Pupil fails to dilate with cocaine solution

its location is based on the inability of the Horner pupil to dilate upon instillation of a cocaine solution. In addition, hydroxy-amphetamine solution (which releases norepinephrine from the postganglionic nerve ending) can be used to differentiate between pre- and postganglionic lesions.

PHYSIOLOGIC (CENTRAL) ANISOCORIA. Approximately 20 percent of the normal population has a difference in size of the two pupils. This anisocoria is of no clinical significance. Differentiation from a Horner syndrome is made by the absence of other signs (ptosis, anhydrosis) and by the normal dilatation of both pupils to cocaine solution.

Retinal Exudates and Hemorrhages
The appearance of retinal exudates or hemorrhages suggests an abnormality in the systemic vasculature. This may be a hematologic disorder (Table 154–3) or a systemic vascular disease such as hypertension or diabetes mellitus (Tables 154–1 and 154–2). Such patients should undergo a complete medical and hematologic evaluation.

— PLATE 1 —

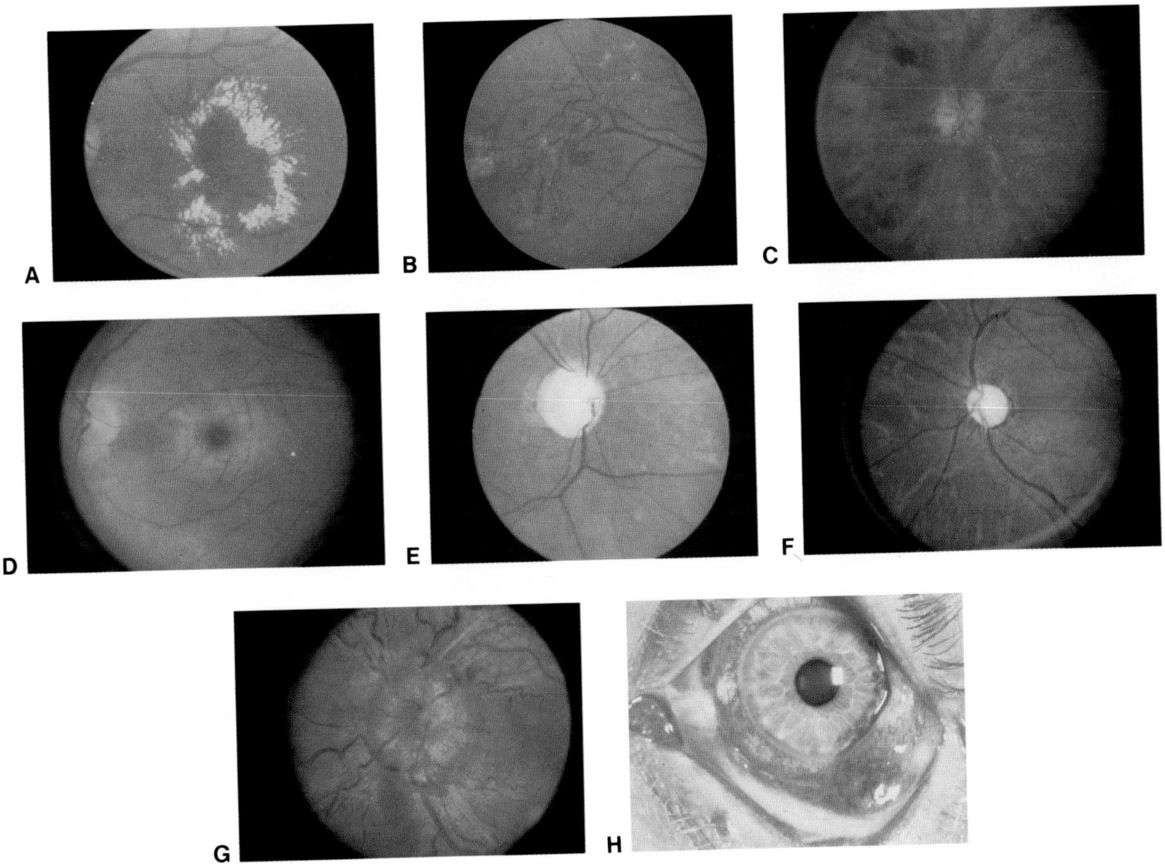

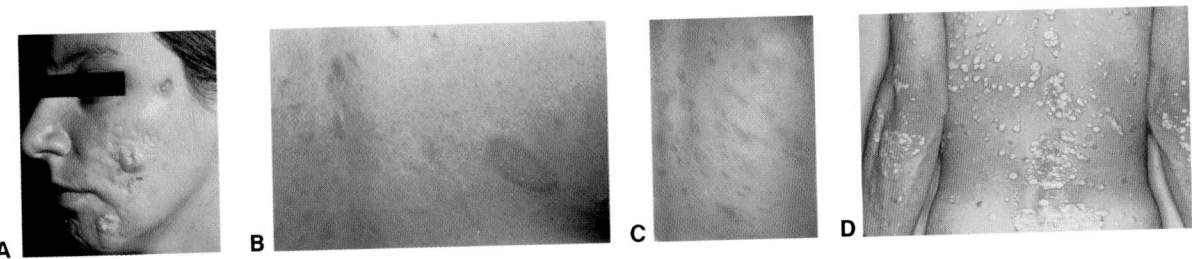

FIGURE 154–2. A. Background diabetic retinopathy with ring of hard exudates encircling macula. **B.** Proliferative diabetic retinopathy with extensive neovascularization. **C.** Central retinal vein occlusion showing extensive retinal hemorrhages. **D.** Central retinal artery occlusion. Macular cherry-red spot is evident. **E.** Chronic (open-angle) glaucoma with extensive cupping of the optic disc. **F.** Optic atrophy. Note diffuse pallor of the optic disc. **G.** Papilledema showing marked hyperemia and elevation of the optic disc, blurring of disc margin, and superficial peripapillary hemorrhages. **H.** Acute conjunctivitis. Note diffuse redness of conjunctiva and whitish exudate in the inferior conjunctival cul-de-sac.

FIGURE 155–1. The examples in this figure are either common skin diseases **(A–G)**, examples of characteristic morphology **(H–L)**, or lesions of general medical significance **(M–P). A.** Acne vulgaris with comedones, papules, pustules, and cysts. **B.** Pityriasis rosea in a white patient. The lesions are dark on a light background. **C.** Pityriasis rosea in a black patient. The lesions are light on a dark background. **D.** Psoriasis vulgaris characterized by erythematous papules and plaques with a mica-like scale on the surface. **(continued)**

— PLATE 2 —

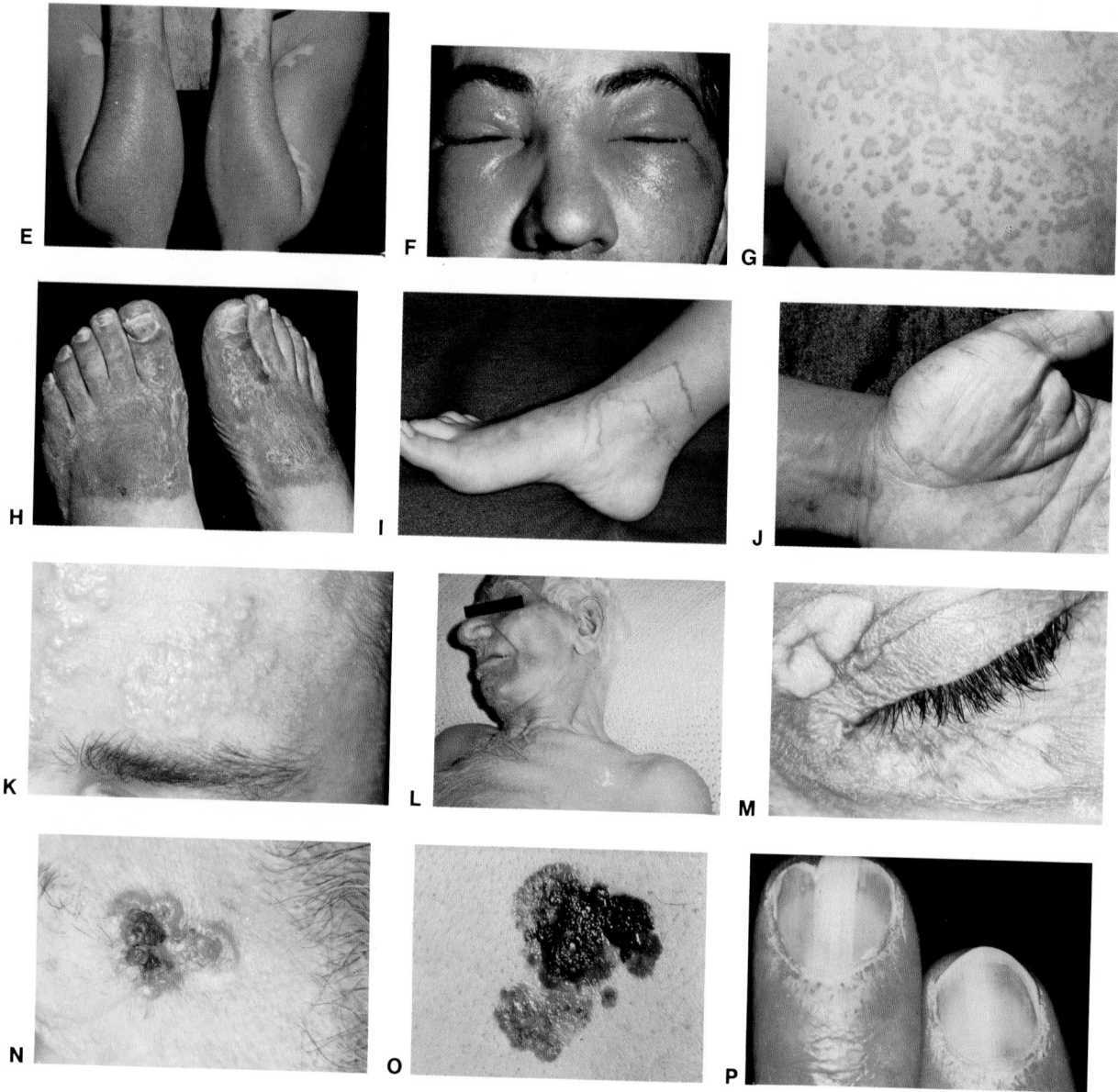

FIGURE 155–1 (cont.) E. Extensive psoriasis vulgaris, an example of a cutaneous problem which can affect a number of other organ systems. **F.** Contact dermatitis around the eyes, a common location since contactants may be carried to that area on the patient's hands. **G.** Drug reaction, which in this example is urticarial. **H.** Contact dermatitis from shoes, a pattern which is easily recognizable with its sharp proximal border. **I.** Portuguese man-of-war sting, an example of linear lesions obviously related to an external factor. **J.** Erythema multiforme with characteristic iris lesions. **K.** *Herpes simplex,* a viral infection characterized by grouped vesicles and pustules. **L.** Argyria, a process in which the blue color is striking but not harmful. **M.** Xanthelasma, a lesion in which the yellow–orange color may lead to the diagnosis of a significant abnormality of lipid metabolism. **N.** Basal cell carcinoma, a common skin tumor characterized by a translucent appearance, telangiectasia, a raised edge, and, ultimately, an ulcerated center. **O.** Superficial spreading melanoma, a lesion characterized by variegated colors and an irregular border. Early diagnosis is essential. **P.** Dermatomyositis with periungual telangiectasia which can also be seen in lupus erythematosis.

CHAPTER 155

Cutaneous Medicine

IRWIN M. FREEDBERG

INTRODUCTION

Skin diseases are common. A recent survey* showed that one-third of the population had a cutaneous problem of such significance that it required evaluation by a dermatologic health care provider at least once. One percent of the entire population had enough cutaneous disease to handicap them at work. The most prevalent skin diseases include (in order) acne, dermatophytosis, tumors, seborrheic dermatitis, atopic dermatitis or eczema, and ichthyosis or other keratoses.

The survey also proved that there could be a major impact of skin disease upon the patient and his life. As examples we may cite the surgeon with hand dermatitis, the farmer with skin cancer and actinic changes, or the theatrical performer with inflammatory disease of the face or other exposed areas. Each of these conditions can cause a major upset in the quality of life. Furthermore, many patients with skin lesions are extremely concerned about them. They are worried about their significance and are anxious or embarrassed about their appearance. Many believe they have malignancy, while others believe the skin lesions are punishment for evil deeds or thoughts. The entire feeling that patients have about skin disease is very different from the response to comparable problems in other organ systems. Health care providers must be aware of the seriousness with which patients regard skin disease and must avoid the error of discussing it lightly.

In this chapter we shall cover 1) the fundamental structure and function of skin; 2) the diagnostic approach to patients with skin lesions; 3) the management of the common skin disorders; 4) the cutaneous manifestations of systemic disorders; 5) the systemic manifestations of cutaneous disease, and finally 6) certain principles of therapeutic management.

* Johnson, M-LT, Roberts, J. Prevalence of dermatological disease among persons 1–74 years of age: United States Advance Data No. 4. U.S. Department of Health, Education, and Welfare.

STRUCTURE AND FUNCTION OF THE SKIN

Structure

The skin, the largest organ of the body ($\cong$ 17 kg; 2.O M²), is composed of three distinctly different types of tissue—epidermis, dermis, and subcutaneous tissue. (See Fig. 155–2.) It is a nonhomogeneous structure with marked regional differences in form, color, and consistency. Each of the tissue components contributes to the major function of the organ which is protection.

The deepest layer is the subcutaneous tissue, a fatty structure of variable thickness. It functions as a thermal barrier and protective cushion between the overlying cutaneous structures and the underlying bone prominences. More superficial is the dermis with collagen strands running from it through the subcutaneous tissue to the deep fascial planes. These strands limit lateral movement of the skin to various degrees in different body areas. Superficial to the dermis and interlocked with it by the undulating, PAS-positive basement membrane is the epidermis, a stratified squamous, keratinizing epithelial sheet.

EPIDERMIS. The major functions of epidermis are carried out primarily by two cell types of different embryologic origin—the melanocytes and the epithelial Malpighian cells, or keratinocytes. There are other, less well-studied cell types, such as the Langerhans cells, which may serve an immunologic function. Melanocytes from the neural crest invade the epidermis during fetal life and synthesize pigment. The Malpighian cells, derived from the embryonic ectodermal covering, show remarkable variations in function. Most produce a fibrous protein, keratin, which eventually fills the cell, replacing all organelles. Similar progenitor cells may develop into the intricate structures of eccrine and apocrine sweat glands, hair follicles, and sebaceous glands.

The epidermis is not a stagnant, inactive envelope but rather a dynamic, constantly proliferating stratified tissue. It is of relatively uniform thickness varying from 75 to 150 μm except over the palms and

1473

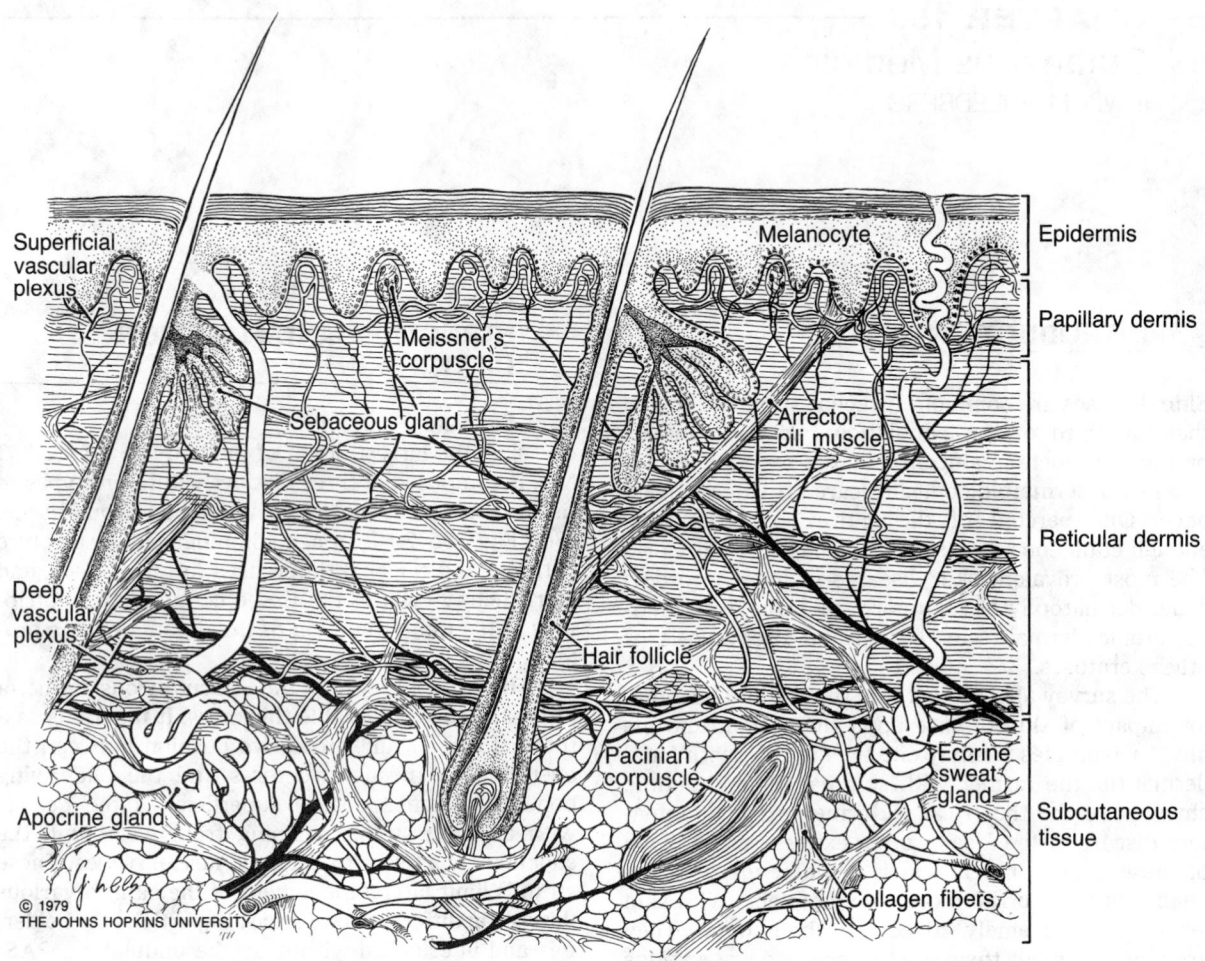

Superficial vascular plexus

Melanocyte

Epidermis

Papillary dermis

Meissner's corpuscle

Sebaceous gland

Arrector pili muscle

Reticular dermis

Deep vascular plexus

Hair follicle

Pacinian corpuscle

Eccrine sweat gland

Subcutaneous tissue

Apocrine gland

© 1979
THE JOHNS HOPKINS UNIVERSITY

Collagen fibers

FIGURE 155–2. Cross section of the skin.

soles where it attains a thickness of 400 to 600 μm. The inner layer (basal layer) contains intracellular keratin filaments and organelles typical for a cell which synthesizes and retains protein. Epidermis is a prime example of a steady-state proliferative system. Cell division takes place in the basal layers, and the cells biochemically and functionally mature as they ascend through the more superficial layers. The elapsed time from cell division to shedding is at least 4 weeks in normal human epidermis. New organelles, including keratohyaline granules and membrane-coating granules, appear during the maturation process, the end stage of which is production of the stratum corneum. This layer forms the outer surface of the epidermis containing as many as 25 cellular layers, all less than 1 μm thick. Relationships among cells in the normal stratum corneum remain highly ordered.

ECCRINE SWEAT GLANDS. Eccrine sweat glands are simple, coiled, tubular ectodermal derivatives found in the dermis or subcutaneous tissue several millimeters beneath the dermis. These cells produce most of the watery sweat which reaches the surface of the skin. Since sweat secretion under thermal stress reaches levels of 1 to 2 liters per hour, these minute glandular elements are well adapted to a high level of secretory activity.

APOCRINE SWEAT GLANDS. Apocrine sweat glands are found in the external auditory canal and in axillary, areolar, pubic, and perineal skin. They are tubular structures whose ducts lead in most cases to the pilosebaceous units and only occasionally directly onto the surface of the skin. The glands function only after puberty, and their secretory product is a thick, proteinaceous fluid that is of unknown function in man.

HAIR, SEBACEOUS GLANDS, AND NAILS. Hair arises from epithelial follicles distributed universally over the surface except for the palms and soles. Each follicle undergoes cycles of active growth (anagen), regression (catagen), and rest (telogen) (Fig. 155–3) which in man are dyssynchronous and independent. The duration of anagen on adult scalp hair varies from 2 to 6 years with telogen being approximately a tenth as long. Scalp hair grows 0.35 mm per day and hair on other parts of the body from 0.1 to 0.4 mm per day. During anagen, mitotic rates in the hair follicle cells are as high as in any tissue of the body.

Sebaceous glands are lipid producing, branched, acinar structures whose distribution is similar to that of the hair follicles which they usually accompany. The two are called pilosebaceous units. The glands are largest and most frequent on the face and forehead. They are also common on the vermillion border of the lip, the buccal mucosa, the genital region, the nipples, and the eyelids (meibomian glands). During differentiation, sebaceous gland cells accumulate lipid droplets which eventually fill the cells. Continuous proliferation of the peripheral cells displaces the differentiated structures toward the center of the acinus and eventually into the sebaceous duct. The secretory product (sebum) of these holocrine glands consists of fully differentiated sebaceous cells which are anucleate, membrane-enclosed masses of coalescent lipid droplets. The lipids of the skin surface include sebum and endogeneous epidermal lipid consisting of free as well as esterified fatty acids, wax and sterol esters, and squalene. These materials are modified by the resident surface bacterial flora and by industrial and atmospheric pollutants.

Androgens exert a major influence upon sebaceous gland size and, hence, upon sebum production. At birth the glands are large and well developed over the entire skin surface owing to natural androgens. Their size rapidly diminishes and their function is minimal until puberty when, in both male and females, a dramatic increase occurs. In old age sebum production decreases, especially in women.

Nails are cutaneous appendages whose function is much more important in lower species than in man. The nail plate is produced by the matrix, a keratin-producing zone which is represented by the white lunulae seen on thumb nails. The pink color of the nail bed is evidence of the amount of blood flow in this area. The rate of growth of nail depends upon the rate of cell division in the matrix. Fingernails grow approximately 0.7 mm/week in young adults; toenail growth is significantly slower. Growth decreases slowly with age and rapidly with severe illness.

DERMIS AND SUBCUTANEOUS TISSUE. The dermis accounts for 5 percent of the total body mass. It also varies significantly in different areas of the body. Directly below the epidermis is an undulating layer of loose connective tissue, rich in cells, vessels, and nerves, called the papillary dermis. Deeper is the more compact and less reactive reticular dermis.

There are three components to dermis. The fibrous component consists of collagen, which makes up the major bulk of the tissue, elastin, and reticulum fibers. The ground substance component forms the extracellular matrix between the fibers. It consists of a variety of complex macromolecules, predominantly glycosaminoglycans covalently linked to protein. The cellular component includes connective tissue cells and transient inflammatory cells such as mast cells, macrophages, histiocytes, and fibroblasts.

The dermis contains the cutaneous vascular network, a series of anastomotic channels which subserve critical thermoregulatory functions. There are lymphatic channels and several types of specialized nerve endings as well.

MELANIN AND MELANOCYTES. In addition to the keratin-synthesizing cells, the epidermis has a population of dendritic melanocytes with a copper-containing aerobic oxidase, tyrosinase. Melanocytes are located at the dermoepidermal junction and in hair bulbs. Melanin, a brown, insoluble, polymeric biochrome, is synthesized in melanocytes, and the pigmented granules are transferred by pinocytosis into keratinocytes. The epidermal-melanin unit is a functional entity composed of a single melanocyte and the pool of perhaps 35 to 50 keratinocytes which receive its pigmented product.

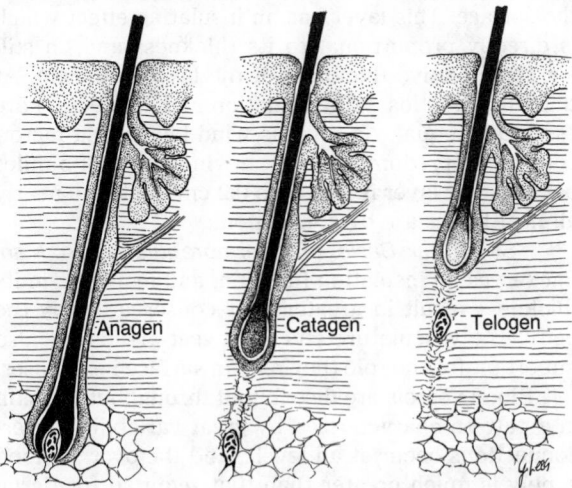

FIGURE 155–3. The hair cycle. The progressive changes from a growing hair (anagen) through catagen to the resting stage (telogen) affect the epithelial and connective tissue components.

The degree of pigmentation in man, although genetically and hormonally determined, is subject to major environmental influences, e.g., ultraviolet light. Comparison of skin from blacks and whites indicates equal numbers of melanocytes in both, although melanin granules in the latter are smaller, aggregated and membrane-bound compared to the larger, single, nonmembrane-bound granules in blacks.

Functions of the Skin

Although the structure of the skin is complex, its functions are simple. Serving as the interface between man and his environment, the skin is one of the prime organs of protection against the following:

1. The loss of essential host constituents
2. The entry into the host of toxic physical, chemical, and microbiologic agents
3. Significant temperature variation
4. Host damage which would be caused by interaction with environmental forces

In addition, there are nonprotective functions which, although critical, are usually ignored. Among these may be cited the synthesis of vitamin D and communication with the environment.

THE BARRIER AGAINST PENETRATION AND LOSS. This function is subserved by the stratum corneum, a composite, relatively thick membrane, less permeable to water than any other membrane in the body. One side is in equilibrium with relatively dry air and the other with the hydrated, viable cells of the epidermis. Since water loss through the intact stratum corneum is by passive diffusion, the rate of loss is directly proportional to the concentration gradient on the two sides of the membrane and inversely related to the membrane thickness (Fick's Law). In man at rest, in an environmental temperature of less than 30° C, the average water loss by the transepidermal route is 1.0 mg/cm²/hr (500 ml/day). Low molecular weight, water-soluble, nonelectrolytes (a category which includes most toxins, allergens, and topically applied drugs) penetrate the skin by a similar process of passive diffusion through the bound water in the stratum corneum, again proportional to the concentration gradient following Fick's Law. Since many substances reach the surface in a solvent, it must be remembered that relative solubility in the solvent and the skin are important factors in determining permeability. Lipid soluble, nonelectrolytes (nonpolar compounds) diffuse through a nonpolar pathway formed by the lipids of the stratum corneum. Electrolytes penetrate at a slower rate than nonelectrolytes owing to the forces of attraction between the penetrating ions and cell membranes.

In addition to this major pathway through the cells of the stratum corneum there are shunt pathways 1) between the cells, 2) into the sweat duct and gland, 3) into the hair follicle and through its walls, and 4) into the follicle, the sebaceous gland, and then into the dermis. The total cross-sectional area of these shunts is only about 1 percent of that of the stratum corneum, and thus, the major fluxes are still through the stratum corneum.

THERMOREGULATION. Man is homeothermic, able to function normally only if his core temperature remains within a very narrow range. To achieve this stability, sensitive mechanisms have developed to balance heat production, predominantly a consequence of intermediary metabolism, and heat loss. Although metabolic activity of the skin contributes to the sum of heat production, the integument is most important as a primary avenue of heat loss in man.

At rest and in the absence of solar radiation, the heat gain of the body, resulting primarily from oxidative reactions in various organs, is the basal metabolic rate (BMR). Its magnitude in man is 864 Kcal/M²/24 hr which means that daily, for a person of normal size, a minimum of 1500 Kcal must be dissipated. During normal activity this figure increases by a factor of two. Over 80 percent of the loss occurs from the skin.

Surface losses are primarily through radiation and convection except when the surface is in contact with a substance of high heat conductivity (the bare-bottomed boy sitting on a cool stone) or when the surface is moist and evaporation takes place. The losses through radiation and convection are markedly influenced by the thin layer of truly still air next to the surface. This layer has an insulating effect which is directly proportional to its thickness and, in still air, the effective thickness of the layer is 0.7 cm. At this thickness losses by radiation and convection are essentially equal. As soon as wind becomes a factor, convection predominates. At a wind speed of 5 miles per hour the layer is less than 0.2 cm thick and nearly all heat losses are by convection.

Structural Basis of Thermoregulation in Man. Fat serves an insulating function, and increases in its thickness result in greater heat conservation by the body. The vasculature and the sweat glands are also important for the role they play in surface heat losses.

Blood vessels are distributed throughout the skin in a pattern characterized by great variability. Interconnections occur at all levels, and the overall blood supply is much greater than that required for tissue nutrition. Only 0.8 ml of blood per minute are required to deliver nutrients to and remove wastes from 100 g of skin. This value is, in fact, the blood flow which can be measured in skin which has undergone intense vasoconstriction following exposure to cold. The mean and maximum skin blood flows are much higher. In the digits, mean flow is usually 25 ml of blood/min/100 g of tissue and in vasodilated skin, flow can reach 100 ml/min/100 g. This enormous range indicates that flow is governed not by the metabolic demands of the skin but by thermoregulatory requirements of the entire organism.

Tone in the cutaneous vessels is centrally determined in the hypothalamic temperature center where afferent impulses depend upon the central core temperature. In "acral" areas of the body (hands, feet, and central face) the active process is vasoconstriction, while in other areas, the active process is probably vasodilation mediated by acetylcholine. In addition, there are local effects of temperature upon cutaneous blood flow: cold causes direct vasoconstriction and heat results in vasodilation.

In man, the eccrine sweat glands also play a critical role in temperature control. The distribution of the 3 million eccrine glands varies greatly, there being 400/cm² on the palms and only 80/cm² on areas such as the thighs. In addition, their function varies. Those on palms and soles secrete in response to psychic stimuli while those over the lips, forehead, and nose respond in a reflex manner following the ingestion of hot or spicy foods (gustatory sweating). The remainder of the glands, which are predominantly found on the upper trunk or face, secrete hypotonic fluid in response to thermal stimuli. The glands are innervated by postganglionic cholinergic fibers, and thus, although sympathetically controlled, they secrete in response to transmitters such as acetylcholine.

The volume of sweat secreted varies widely to a maximum of 3 liters per hour which has been recorded from a group of acclimatized men working in severe heat. Heat loss only occurs when sweat evaporates from the surface, but the amount of loss by this route may be great in the appropriate environmental situation since each liter of water evaporated requires the dissipation of 580 Kcal.

Response of the Skin of Man to Cold. It can be calculated that naked man at rest in an environment without wind remains in thermal balance until the temperature falls below 29°C. Below this, cutaneous insulation is not sufficient, and other mechanisms must be called into play. Piloerection occurs ("gooseflesh"), although this method of increasing the still air layer above the skin is not effective in nonfurred species. Shivering increases metabolic activity and heat production, while vasoconstriction decreases blood flow and heat loss through the skin.

Response of Man to Heat. From 29° to 33°C, heat balance is maintained as losses through radiation and convection are adequate to dissipate metabolic heat. Through vasodilation the cutaneous blood flow and the surface temperature are increased so that the gradient for heat transfer to the environment is maintained. Above 33°C radiation and convection are inadequate as avenues of loss and sweat glands become active. The resulting evaporation can result in enormous heat losses reaching 12,000 Kcal/M²/24 hours, about 14 times the basal metabolic rate. To sustain such losses from the surface, the insulation of the skin must be reduced. This occurs as skin blood flow increases, but even at maximum the reduction is not perfect since the skin surface remains relatively cool even during maximum sweat evaporation. The limit of a viable environment is only reached when sweat cannot evaporate because the vapor concentration of ambient air approaches that of the skin surface.

APPROACH TO THE DIAGNOSTIC MANAGEMENT OF PATIENTS WITH SKIN LESIONS

The key to an effective approach to patients with cutaneous problems is related to an understanding of the skin and its pathophysiology coupled with an appreciation of the significance of the disease to the patient. Patients may present with lesions on their skin or they may complain of the one unique cutaneous symptom, pruritus. In each case the cutaneous signs and symptoms may represent disease which is primarily in the skin or, in a smaller number of patients, secondary to disease in an underlying organ.

HISTORY

At all times an appropriate history must be taken and a physical examination performed. The general history should be similar to that outlined in Chapter 2, with particular emphasis upon those components more directly related to cutaneous disease. Included in this category are family history, social and occupational history (toxic exposures), allergic manifestations, and medication review with emphasis upon topical medication either prescribed or otherwise obtained for the presenting problem. Seasonal variation, hobbies, and personal contacts are all important.

PHYSICAL EXAMINATION

The physical examination is the cornerstone of evaluation of patients with skin disease or with cutaneous manifestations of underlying systemic disease.

Patients should undress completely and be gowned or draped in such a manner that the entire cutaneous surface and all mucous membranes can be seen. Light should be adequate; natural daylight is the most desirable. An inexpensive hand lens of 3 to 10 power with a diameter of 2 to 5 cm is extremely useful in evaluating skin lesions. Inspection is not the sole method of examination. The added value of palpation to determine the texture and the degree and depth of infiltration of lesions is often not appreciated, and if lesions are not felt, clinical errors may result. Perhaps based upon the same ignorance and superstition which affects lay persons, health care providers are reluctant to touch patients with skin disease (or, as it has now been shown, patients with malignant disease).

Some cutaneous lesions are the site of microorganisms through which the specific disease, complication, or manifestation may be transmitted. Such lesions should be palpated with glove protection. The majority of skin lesions, however, are not contaminated, and there is no epidemiologic reason not to palpate them.

Examination of the skin lesions should address three specific elements: 1) their *distribution*, where they are; 2) their *configuration*, their relationship to one another; and finally 3) the *character or type* of the lesion. Each of these aspects will be discussed in turn.

Distribution

Distribution is the first thing to be determined when dealing with a patient with skin lesions. It is noted usually by "the view from afar." If the examiner does not determine the distribution initially, he may miss the forest for the trees.

LOCALIZED. Localized lesions are those which are limited to a single area such as the hand, face, cheek, or leg.

PATTERNED. Lesions are limited to a specific area with an obvious distribution pattern. The latter may be based upon a number of influences.

Anatomic Influences. Skin lesions may occur in areas based upon anatomic principles such as the *location of cutaneous appendages.* For example, acne, a disease of sebaceous glands, is most severe in places where sebaceous glands are in highest concentration (face, back). For reasons which are not clear, some processes present with lesions on *flexural* areas of the body (atopic dermatitis, lichen planus) while others are predominent in *extensor* areas (psoriasis, dermatitis herpetiformis). Some lesions occur on *dependent areas* of the body where hydrostatic pressure is highest. Stasis dermatitis is an excellent example.

External Influences. Because the skin serves as the interface between man and his environment, skin lesions are often caused by external events. For example, skin lesions may occur only where the skin is

exposed to wind or ultraviolet light. Lesions may occur only in areas in which the skin is *traumatized* by scratching or other physical forces or in areas where the skin comes into *contact* with a specific substance which causes an allergic or toxic reaction.

GENERALIZED. Certain skin diseases are neither localized nor patterned. They involve essentially the entire body surface and represent a *generalized distribution.*

Configuration

Once distribution is determined, the evaluation moves on to configuration, how the component parts of the lesion(s) are related (Fig. 155-4). The following

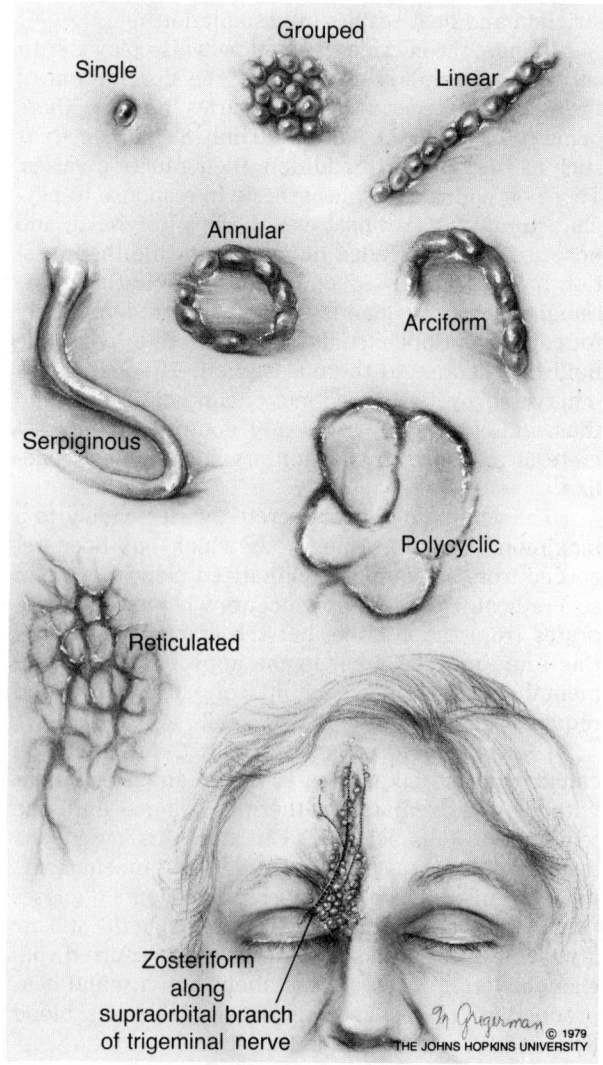

FIGURE 155–4. Configuration of skin lesions.

patterns of arrangement or configuration are generally accepted:

SINGLE. In a number of cases the lesions are single, unrelated to other lesions in the local area.

LINEAR. The lesions may form lines on the surface of the skin. Common examples of this configuration are the linear blisters seen in plant contact dermatitis.

SERPIGINOUS. Lesions may form an undulating, serpentine pattern on the surface. The configuration is seen when organisms burrow through the skin as in cutaneous larval migrans.

ARCIFORM. The pattern is one of single or multiple arcs but not complete circles. It is commonly seen on the skin of patients with drug reactions.

ANNULAR. As contrasted to the configuration noted above, annular lesions form complete circles. The configuration is typical of erythema multiforme.

POLYCYCLIC. A mixture of arciform and annular lesions leads to a pattern in which there are many complete or partial circles on the surface.

GROUPED. In this case there are multiple lesions which are not randomly scattered but are localized to apparently specific areas.

ZOSTERIFORM. Evolving from the typical configuration of lesions of herpes zoster, this pattern is one in which the lesions apparently are localized to the distribution of a superficial cutaneous nerve.

RETICULATED. Derived from the word "reticle" indicating that there is a net-like pattern, this configuration is commonly associated with the distribution of the superficial cutaneous vessels.

Type of Lesion

Once the determination of distribution and configuration has been made, the observer must next define the type of lesion of which the eruption is composed (Fig. 155–5). Lesions may be flat, elevated, or depressed below the surface of the skin. If elevated, they may contain solid material, liquid material, or a mixture of both. This scheme can be summarized as noted below.

FLAT LESIONS. *Macule.* A macule is a flat, circumscribed area of any size in which the skin texture is not changed. Typical macules cannot be localized by touch alone. They simply represent a color change. Macules may be hypopigmented, hyperpigmented, or erythematous. Pressure on the latter with a glass slide differentiates dilated blood vessels (fade) from extravasated blood (does not fade).

ELEVATED LESIONS FILLED WITH SOLID MATERIAL. *Papule.* A papule is a relatively small (< 0.5 to 1.0 cm by most conventions), elevated, superficial lesion. It may be firm or soft but by definition it does not contain loculated fluid.

Plaque. When papules enlarge and coalesce, they form plaques which are flat-topped, mesa-like lesions with a large surface area for the amount of elevation. Of variable size, some plaques may be 30 cm or more in diameter.

Nodule. Nodules are round or ellipsoidal lesions of greater diameter and particularly greater depth than papules. The dermis and subcutaneous tissue as well as the epidermis are involved in such lesions.

ELEVATED LESIONS FILLED WITH LOCULATED FLUID. *Vesicle.* This is a small (<0.5 cm) elevated lesion which can be opened and found to yield liquid, most usually serum, lymph, or blood. The vesicle may be in the epidermis, at the dermoepidermal junction, or in the dermis. The deeper lesions have thicker walls and do not rupture as easily as the superficial ones.

Pustules. These are simply vesicles which contain purulent material. The purulent exudate may be yellow, greenish yellow, or white. When pustules are localized to hair follicles, the lesion is called a *furun-*

Flat	Elevated			Depressed
	Solid	**Solid and Fluid**	**Fluid**	
Macule	Papule	Wheal	Vesicle	Atrophy
	Plaque	Iris	Pustule	Erosion
	Nodule		Bulla	Fissure
			Cyst	Ulcer
		Other		
		Scale		
		Crust		
		Lichenification		
		Vegetation		
Scar		Scar		Scar

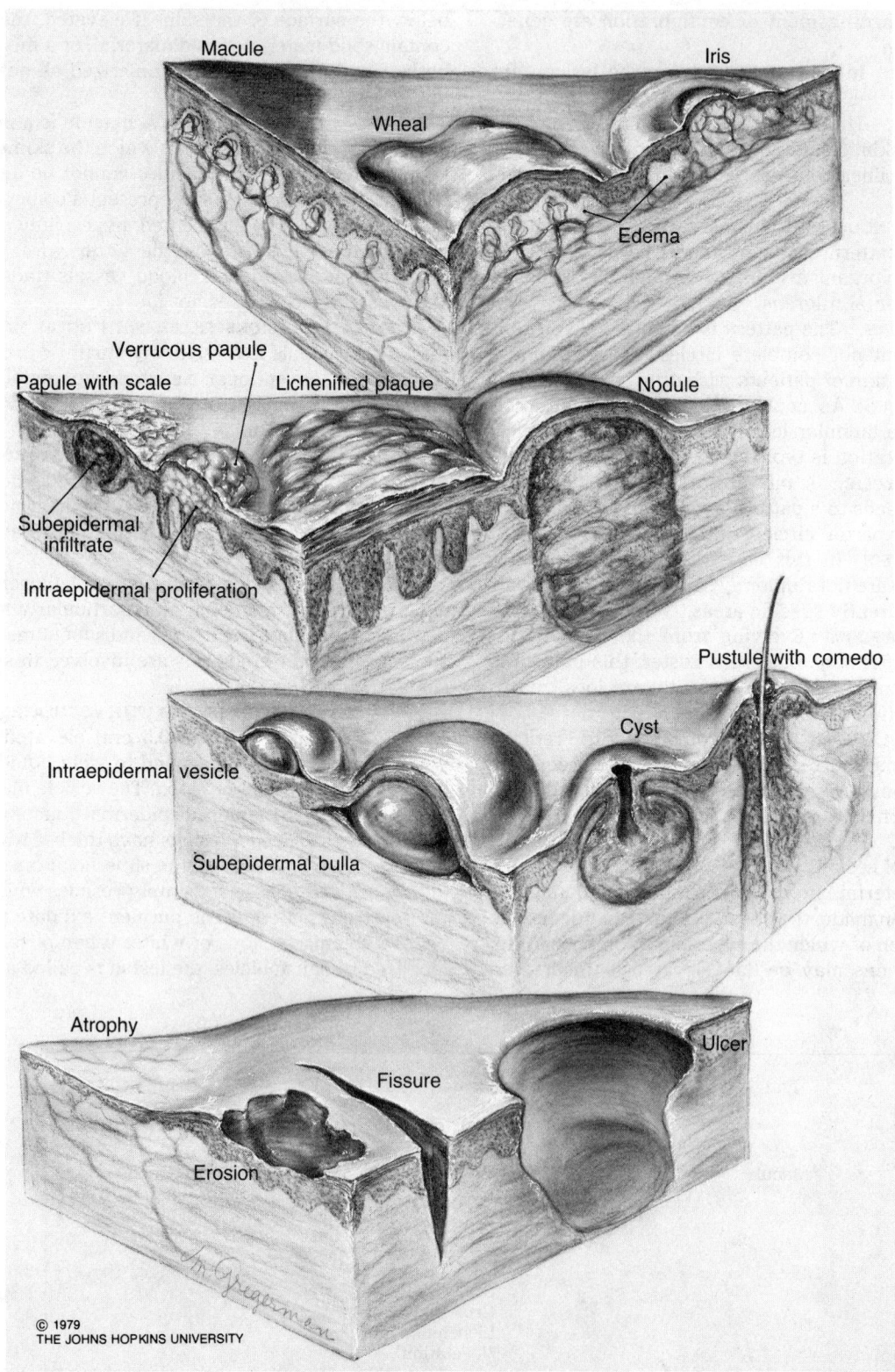

FIGURE 155–5. Types of skin lesions.

cle. Grouped furuncles are known as *carbuncles* and, if deep, they may form an abscess.

Bulla. Corresponding to a solid plaque, the bulla is merely an enlarged blister (>0.5 cm in diameter). Bullae may arise from confluency of smaller vesicles or from a nonconfluent increase in their size.

Cyst. This fluid-filled lesion corresponds to the nodule. It is a deep sac containing fluid or semisolid material.

OTHER RAISED LESIONS WHICH CONTAIN A MIXTURE OF SOLID MATERIAL AND LIQUID. These are not as easy to classify and are commonly classified separately.

Wheal. Also known as a hive, this lesion contains nonloculated edema fluid. It is round or flat-topped with an irregular outline. Wheals are commonly extremely pruritic and transient.

Iris. The typical lesion of erythema multiforme, the iris lesion, has the morphology of a target or a bull's eye. Most iris lesions are approximately 1 cm in diameter with a central vesicle surrounded by a white ring with a peripheral red rim.

OTHER RAISED LESIONS. There are also elevated lesions which are not primary but which represent something added to another type of lesion. Included in this category are:

Scale. Scales are the flakes of stratum corneum found commonly on top of macules, papules, or plaques.

Crust. Crust is dried serous or purulent exudate on the surface of what was originally a vesicle, bulla, erosion, or ulcerated area.

Lichenification. In response to rubbing or scratching in patients with atopy, the epidermis becomes thickened and the skin markings become more prominent. This complex change is known as lichenification.

Vegetation. This is a lesion composed of multiple grouped, closely packed papules. Such areas resemble the surface of a cauliflower.

Comedo. The primary lesion of acne, a comedo is a plug in a pilosebaceous orifice composed of protein and lipid. Oxidation of lipid may result in darkening of the plug at the end. These lesions are commonly referred to as blackheads or whiteheads in lay publications.

DEPRESSED LESIONS. These are divided into four easily recognizable and separable entities.

Atrophy. The loss of substance of epidermis, dermis, subcutaneous tissue, or a combination of these results in a depressed area in which the surface is intact.

Erosion. Superficial loss of epidermis leads to an open area, the base of which is the dermis.

Fissure. A fissure is the loss of skin in a cleft-like area.

Ulcer. Deep loss of portions of skin including epidermis and papillary dermis results in ulceration.

SCARS. Scars are categorized separately in this approach. They result from replacement of the normal tissue with fibrous tissue and may be flat, elevated, or depressed. Scarring skin diseases commonly result in a mixture of these types.

LABORATORY PROCEDURES

Although essentially all types of clinical laboratory procedures may be important in evaluating patients with cutaneous disease, there are a few procedures which are unique to the investigation of patients with skin problems. Among these are the trephine punch biopsy, examination of hair cuttings, nail cuttings, or skin scrapings for fungi, evaluation of the skin under ultraviolet light, and patch testing for contact allergies or photoallergies.

Skin Biopsy

Trephine skin biopsies are performed under local anesthesia. A 2- to 6-mm biopsy punch (usually 4 mm) is used to obtain a plug of skin including the epidermis, dermis, and subcutaneous tissue. The plug so formed is gently lifted with a toothed forceps or needle and the base is cut across as deeply as possible. In certain cases (subcutaneous lesions), excisional biopsies are more appropriate. In either case the tissue can be fixed for the required analysis (routine histology, electron microscopy, immunohistology) and the surface defect closed in a number of ways. A single suture, electrocoagulation, or chemical cautery are most common. Biopsy of a lesion in its early stages is most likely to assist in diagnosis.

Studies for Fungi

Fungal elements may be identified in fragments of tissue following alkaline hydrolysis of keratin (10 percent potassium hydroxide and gentle boiling). Staining is not required prior to microscopic examination of a wet preparation. Immunofluorescent analysis of such specimens may result in rapid identification of the responsible organisms.

Ultraviolet Light

The Wood's light filter removes all but 320 to 400 nm light from the incandescent spectrum. These wavelengths are useful in demonstrating the presence of certain fungal infections on the body and scalp and determining the extent of abnormalities of pigmentation. Both hypo- and hyperpigmentation are more prominent under Wood's light illumination. Descriptions of the techniques, significance, and indications for other tests, such as patch tests, are to be found in the major dermatologic texts (see References).

COMMON CUTANEOUS DISORDERS

This section describes the commonly encountered skin diseases which all physicians should be able to recognize and manage.

Acne Vulgaris

This problem affects almost all adolescents, and in most it clears without scarring. It may be seen in newborns, and in unusual cases it may persist through the third or fourth decades, especially in females. The fact that acne is extremely common and usually self-limited does not mean that treatment is unnecessary. It can and must be treated, for it can produce both physical and emotional scarring in young people at a particularly sensitive period in their lives.

The process begins with a keratin plug in a follicular orifice forming a comedone ("blackhead" or "whitehead"). The pathophysiology of acne has not been totally elucidated, but certain facts are clear. In the plugged pilosebaceous apparatus there is continued production of sebaceous gland material which consists, among other components, of esterified and free fatty acids. The saprophytic skin bacteria, such as the anaerobic pleomorphic *Propionibacterium acnes*, contain a lipase which can hydrolyze the esterified lipids produced by the sebaceous gland. These retained materials produce a lesion which may progress through erythematous, papular, and pustular stages to cystic lesions in some patients. If destruction is sufficient, there is loss of tissue, fibrous overgrowth, and scarring. Lesions of acne are localized to areas with the highest concentration of sebaceous glands including the face, back, chest, and shoulders. Sebaceous gland activity is under hormonal control, and the glands are extremely sensitive to androgen levels, hence the prevalence in adolescence.

THERAPY.   One of the cornerstones of acne management involves dispelling the multiple "old-wives' tales" involved in the disease. It must be emphasized that the disease is not related to poor hygiene. The blackheads are pigment and oxidized lipids, not dirt. Diet is not a major influence, although certain patients may develop lesions when they ingest chocolate, a lipid component of which can be excreted through the sebaceous glands. There is no evidence that seafood, sugar-containing beverages, or fatty foods have any influence on the course of the disease. Stress may adversely affect the process, but much of what has been written and passed on by oral tradition regarding effects of psyche and thoughts on acne has no factual basis.

Therapy consists of the use of commercially available abrasive agents (which contain several types of insoluble particles) and drying, peeling agents (containing sulfur, resorcinol, salicylic acid, benzoyl peroxide, vitamin A acid) several times each day in an attempt to eliminate the block at the sebaceous gland orifice, ultraviolet light (either natural sunlight or artificial UVB) which increases epidermal turnover and may decrease bacteria, and systemic and topical antibiotics. Tetracycline is the most commonly used systemic antibiotic (1 g per day is usual). It should not be used in children or pregnant women. When remission occurs, the dose can be decreased. Erythromycin is the second drug of choice for systemic therapy. Topical therapy with 1 percent clindamycin or tetracycline is currently being used commonly. In females with severe disease, the use of estrogens, usually in the form of an oral contraceptive, is effective. Progesterone can be metabolized to products with androgen activity, so oral contraceptives must be those with high estrogen and low progesterone content. Incision and drainage of lesions as well as injection of lesions with corticosteroid suspensions, e.g., triamcinolone acetonide, 2.5 mg/ml, to decrease inflammation are valuable in appropriate circumstances. Future developments may involve the use of topical antiandrogens and antikeratinizing agents which should affect the problem relatively specifically.

Certain drugs can cause an acneiform eruption (halogens, corticosteroids), and there are occupational exposures (cutting oils and other halogenated hydrocarbons) which can lead to a similar process.

Rosacea is an eruption occuring in middle and older aged patients, which is localized to the same regions as acne but is not based upon a keratin plug in a pilosebaceous orifice. This eruption is associated with vascular dilatation, papules, and pustules. It may progress to granuloma formation or to massive cutaneous overgrowth as is apparent in patients with rhinophyma. Although the pathophysiology is quite different, the management of rosacea is similar to that of acne vulgaris.

Dermatitis-Eczema Group

This group of clinical entities shares a common histopathologic alteration—*spongiosis*, which is edema fluid in the epidermis. The clinical manifestations form a spectrum from erythema and edema to the formation of vesicles which break, ooze, and crust in the acute types; to thickening of tissue or lichenification in more chronic examples. Among the acute types of eczema or dermatitis are contact and photocontact dermatitis while the more chronic, recurrent varieties include atopic dermatitis, localized neurodermatitis (the "itch and scratch" syndrome), statis dermatitis, and nummular ("coin-shaped") dermatitis.

Allergic contact dermatitis is localized to areas in which the specific agent comes in contact with the skin. History is very important in elucidating the etiologic agent. The patient must be carefully questioned specifically about environmental factors such as hobbies, new clothing, changes in work, etc. The distribution of the lesions is also of major significance. For example, one can easily recognize the pattern of a shoe contact dermatitis on the forefoot. A Sherlockian approach to problem solving is important in dealing with contact dermatitis. Patch tests are helpful in defining the process, but the cornerstone of management involves identification and elimination of the agent involved. In *photocontact dermatitis* the contactant alone is not enough to cause the problem—exposure of the skin or the contactant to ultraviolet light are required as well.

Atopic dermatitis is often associated with hay fever and asthma either in the same patient or in the same family. There may be seasonal exacerbations of the triad (hay fever, asthma, eczema). The dermatitis usually begins in infancy or childhood and by age 20 as many as one-half of all patients clear without specific therapy. In infancy the face, scalp, and extensor areas of the body are involved with pruritus, erythema, and small vesicles. In childhood there are generalized erythema, papules, thickening, and lichenification in addition. Flexural areas are usually involved by this time, and there is associated dry skin which may be of great enough severity to include ichthyosis in the differential diagnosis. The lesions may become secondarily infected leading to a number of systemic complications; in addition, cataracts may develop. Laboratory abnormalities include elevated IgE levels and incompletely defined T-cell abnormalities.

Nummular eczema is most commonly seen in patients in their fifth and sixth decades. It is characterized by coin-shaped lesions which are several centimeters in diameter, pruritic, and commonly more severe in winter than summer.

Stasis dermatitis may be either acute or chronic, is related to venous disease and dependency, and is commonly a recurrent problem.

In *lichen simplex chronicus* or the "itch-scratch syndrome" there are pruritic areas which are continually scratched or treated with agents which cause increased inflammation rather than remission. The process may resemble acute dermatitis, although most characteristic are the localized, lichenified, well-demarcated plaques.

THERAPY. Management of eczema in the acute state, once any contactants are removed, includes the use of compresses to remove any debris from the surface followed by the application of topical corticosteroid creams or ointments. Details concerning their use are found in the therapy section (p. 1491). The penetration of the steroid through inflamed, thickened skin to the site of the pathologic lesion is enhanced when occlusive therapy (see below) is used. In addition to topical corticosteroids, coal tar products (5 percent coal tar in cream or ointment base) may be used topically as anti-inflammatory and antipruritic agents. Systemic corticosteroids may be used when the problem is of major severity. The adult dose should be approximately 60 mg prednisone equivalents per day. Therapy should be continued for several weeks at a decreased, tapering dose once control is achieved. There are no specific antipruritic agents available, but sedatives, antihistamines, or ataractic agents are helpful in decreasing the sensation of itch. As examples, diphenhydramine hydrochloride, 50 mg orally, four times daily; tripelennamine hydrochloride, 50 mg four times daily, and hydroxyzine hydrochloride, 10 to 25 mg three times daily are effective drugs.

Viral Lesions

There are several types of *verrucae* including common warts (verrucae vulgaris), genital warts (condyloma accuminatum), plantar warts, and flat warts (verrucae plana), all of which are caused by the response of the affected tissue to viral multiplication. The interrelationships among the several types of wart virus are under active study, but it is already clear that the wart virus is an excellent example of an oncogenic virus causing proliferation of tissue. In this case, the proliferation is benign. Although warts do undergo spontaneous resolution, and although the literature is replete with therapeutic advice based upon hypnosis and suggestion, physical modalities of therapy based upon destruction are effective. Included among these and useful for management in most cases are the use of heat (electrocoagulation and fulguration), cold (liquid nitrogen), acids (low pH), and chemical blistering agents (cantharidin derivatives) or mitotic inhibitors (podophyllin derivatives). Condyloma accuminatum are among the most prevalent and bothersome of the sexually transmitted diseases at this time, and specific epidemiologic study is critical to prevent repeated recurrences. These lesions respond to application of podophyllin resin (25 percent in tincture of benzoin for 4 to 6 hours) or freezing.

Molluscum contagiosum is also a benign tumor caused by a large DNA virus. It was formerly most commonly a disease of childhood and it is now commonly a sexually transmitted disease in young people. The incubation period is variable (2 to 7 weeks), and the clinical presentation consists of discrete, pearly papules with an umbilicated center. Lesions, which may be on skin or mucous membranes, are treated by destructive methods including liquid nitrogen or curettage and desiccation.

Herpes simplex is a common viral infection of the skin. The primary problem occurs in children and young adults affecting the mouth and pharynx. There is a 3 to 10-day incubation period followed by the appearance of oral and pharyngeal vesicles associated with fever and lymphadenopathy. The primary problem lasts 2 to 6 weeks and is followed by a quiescent period. Recurrent herpes lasts 5 to 7 days and often follows trauma, sun exposure, emotional upsets, or menstrual periods, but it may occur without relationship to other events. The process presents as grouped, umbilicated vesicles which occur on an erythematous base; the overall diameter of the lesions usually is less than 1 cm. One of the most disturbing types of herpes simplex is that in the genital area. Lesions are the same as on other areas of the body, but the organism is different and there is much pain especially with vulvovaginitis in females.

There is no effective therapy for cutaneous herpes simplex save in the eye, where antiviral agents (topical 2'-deoxy-5-iodouridine and adenosine arabinoside) applied several times each day apparently are effective. Drying agents, such as alcohol, ether, and benzoyl peroxide, are used on lesions elsewhere, and they may shorten the course but do not limit the recurrences.

Herpes zoster, caused by the same virus which results in varicella (chicken pox), is usually a problem in adults, although children can be affected. It is commonly a self-limited disease with macules, papules, and grouped vesicles evident in a dermatomal distribution. The process is more common in immunosuppressed patients. If vesicles are unroofed and their bases scraped and stained with Wright's or Giemsa stain, multinucleated giant cells are evident. Therapy consists of cool compresses, analgesics as required, a topical antibiotic ointment (bacitracin, neomycin,

povidone—iodine), and protection of the lesion from further damage.

Papulosquamous Diseases

There is a group of cutaneous diseases in which the primary event is formation of a distinct papular lesion surmounted by scaling of various degrees. Included among these papulosquamous diseases are psoriasis, seborrheic dermatitis, pityriasis rosea, the secondary stage of syphilis, and other less common problems.

Psoriasis vulgaris is a chronic cutaneous disease, the pathophysiology of which involves loss of control of epidermal turnover. Cell division in the basal cell layer cells of epidermis is increased, and transit time of cells through the epidermis is speeded up 7 to 10 times. Cells on the surface of skin do not have time to complete their maturation processes. As a consequence, the stratum corneum is abnormal with residual nuclei and other intracellular organelles. The disease is chronic, beginning on occasion in infancy or childhood, but most commonly in the third or fourth decade. The primary lesion is an erythematous papule surmounted by a mica-like, silvery scale. The papules coalesce and enlarge to form plaques which may be quite widespread. The lesions may be reproduced on uninvolved skin of the psoriatic which is subjected to trauma (Koebner reaction). This phenomenon may cause the classical localization of disease to the elbows, knees, and buttocks. The scalp may be the site of dense plaques, but hair is usually not involved. Nails are pitted with subungual hyperkeratosis. Unusual developments during the life history of patients with psoriasis include the occurrence of pustular psoriasis and generalized erythroderma. A polyarticular arthritis is most apparent in the distal interphalangeal joints or the spine. This occurs usually between age 30 and 50.

Psoriasis is a treatable disease, and management should be vigorous. Topical corticosteroid creams and ointments (with or without occlusion) are effective as is the classical Goeckerman program involving the use of midrange ultraviolet light (UVB) with coal tar applications (1 to 5 percent creams, ointments, or liquids). Recent data have raised questions about the value of the tar in the program. Systemic antimetabolities, such as methotrexate, may be effective if other modalities fail, but there are major potential side effects associated with such drugs. Management capabilities have been broadened consequent to the observation that psoralen (P) and long-wave ultraviolet light (UVA) (PUVA photochemotherapy) effectively inhibit epidermal turnover.

Seborrheic dermatitis may present in infancy;

there is a postpubertal peak of incidence as well. The etiology is not known, but the problem begins in infancy as cradle cap or as a severe diaper dermatitis. Adults have a symmetrical, patchy, erythematous papular eruption with a yellow, greasy scale which affects the forehead, scalp, retroauricular, nasolabial, axillary, and groin areas as well as the central chest. Lesions in the anogenital and inframammary creases are common. There are no systemic manifestations, and arthritis or nail problems are not evident. Management includes the use of topical coal tar and/or corticosteroids. Other more classical anti-inflammatory agents include sulfur, salicylic acid, and iodohydroxychloroquine.

Pityriasis rosea, also a papulosquamous entity, is common between ages 10 and 35 and appears to have a seasonal variation, with many cases in spring and fall. The primary lesion (herald patch) is a erythematous, scaly plaque approximately 2 to 6 cm in diameter usually located on the truck or neck. Within several days there is an exacerbation of papules and scaly plaques which evolve to oval lesions following the lines of cleavage along the body. A fine collarette of scales exists, and the process is commonly asymptomatic, lasting up to 2 to 14 weeks. Recurrences are recorded, but are rare. There is no therapy for pityriasis rosea, although ultraviolet light may hasten remission.

Secondary syphilis can have a similar appearance and must be ruled out by either a negative VDRL or a negative darkfield examination of the lesion.

Vascular Reaction Group

There is a group of relatively common cutaneous problems in which the primary pathophysiologic event is related to the superficial dermal blood vessel. Included among these entities are urticaria, erythema multiforme, and many types of drug eruptions.

Urticaria is most commonly an acute problem, but there are examples of chronic urticaria lasting for months. Even in the latter circumstances, the individual hive-like lesions are transient, lasting less than 24 to 36 hours. Associated with IgE, the two cell types important in urticaria are mast cells and basophils. The causes include food and drug allergy as well as physical phenomena such as pressure, heat, and ultraviolet light. In many cases the primary etiology cannot be determined. The management includes avoidance of the cause, use of antihistaminic agents or epinephrine and, in cases in which the disease continues in a debilitating manner, use of systemic corticosteroids (40 to 60 mg of prednisone equivalents for

at least 1 week). Save for cool compresses to relieve pruritus, topical therapy is of no value.

Erythema multiforme is characterized by iris or target lesions of skin and mucosa which are not as transient or pruritic as urticarial wheals. Most common in the second and third decades, the process can also affect the pediatric age group and the elderly. There are multiple apparent etiologic relationships including *Herpes simplex*, mycoplasma infection preceeding the eruption, drug reactions, and neoplasia. In at least 50 percent of cases, the cause cannot be determined. The presentation may vary from relatively mild, limited involvement to a severe bullous disease with gastrointestinal, mucous membrane, and joint symptoms along with involvement of genitalia and eyes (Stevens-Johnson syndrome).

Topical therapy with compresses and nonsensitizing local anaesthetics, such as dyclonine hydrochloride, to mucous membranes is of help; systemic corticosteroids appear to halt progression of the lesions.

Drug reactions can present as erythema multiforme (especially sulfonamides), but a much more common presentation is as a diffuse macular and papular erythematous eruption (morbilliform). At the present time there are no adequate methods to determine the true cause of such reactions in patients who are taking multiple drugs. The relative risks have been determined statistically for a large number of agents but such a determination may not be directly helpful in a specific circumstance.

Hair Disease

Of the several cutaneous appendages, the hair follicle is the site of the most common problems. Hair has no functional significance in man, a homeothermic animal, but it is of great emotional significance. Abnormalities, be they too much or too little hair, are of great concern for affected patients.

ALOPECIA (HAIR LOSS). Evaluation of patients with complaints of hair loss must include examination of all hair-bearing areas and examination of the hairs themselves. There are rare congenital types of alopecia which may involve localized or generalized areas, but acquired problems are much more common. These have been subclassified into scarring and nonscarring alopecias—a differentiation based upon the amount and extent of the damage which has occurred. To be noticeable, approximately 50 percent of the normal amount of hair must be lost. Thus, most problems which are brought to the physician's attention are not of significant extent.

Nonscarring alopecia occurs in women several

months following delivery and it is seen in both sexes a month or so following a severe illness. This process, known as *telogen effluvium* is related to the fact that at these times hair cycles may become synchronized, an unusual situation in man but not other species which shed hair seasonally. The problem can be diagnosed by evaluating the number of telogen (club) or resting hairs in a random pluck of scalp hair. Normally only 10 percent of the scalp roots are in the telogen stage at any given time. During telogen effluvium this increases to 50 to 60 percent.

Male patterned baldness, a genetically determined loss which begins as frontal recession and occipital thinning, occurs in both men and women, although the progression is much greater in men. The prognosis for this problem is poor, since there is no effective therapy.

In contrast is the situation of *alopecia areata*, an acute problem which is most common in those under 25 years of age. Sometimes associated with acute emotional trauma, there is an increased frequency of vitiligo and autoimmune thyroid disease associated with alopecia areata. The disease presents as round, noninflammatory areas of complete hair loss which are several centimeters in diameter. At the periphery of an active area, hairs can easily be removed by traction, and many follicles throughout the area are filled with dark hairs broken off close to the skin surface. The management of alopecia areata has never been well defined. With small areas of short duration, the prognosis is excellent; with larger areas of longer duration, chance for regrowth decreases. Topical and systemic steroids have been used by some, and at the present time regular applications of irritating agents, such as dinitrochlorobenzene or psoralen and ultraviolet light, are being used in experimental groups.

Cicatricial or scarring alopecias are uncommon as are types of hair loss related to abnormalities of the hair shaft. These may represent genetic, acquired inflammatory, or neoplastic diseases. Details regarding these processes can be found in the major texts noted in the Reference section or in the treatises dealing specifically with hair.

HIRSUITISM (TOO MUCH HAIR). This is primarily a problem which presents in women, and it can be racially, ethnically (Mediterranean origin), or hormonally determined. The former two groups are constitutional, and therapy is limited to removal of unwanted hair by one of a variety of available techniques (wax, traction, or electric depilation). The pathologic, hormonally induced types of hirsuitism require evaluation of adrenal and ovarian function. (Chaps. 70 and 77).

The problems discussed above are the most common cutaneous disorders, but there are also diseases which are less common but of major importance to the host. Included are bullous or blistering diseases and cutaneous tumors.

Bullous Disorders (Table 155-1)

The unifying concept in a consideration of bullous disorders relates to impairment of skin coherence. This may occur between epidermal cells (intraepidermal bulla) or below the epidermis (subepidermal bulla). Epidermal cells are held together by desmosomes, and disease of these structures results in bulla formation. The epidermis and dermis are attached by the basal lamina with associated glycosaminoglycans and anchoring fibers. Diseases in this area also result in bullae. For effective management of patients with bullous lesions, a biopsy is central, for it yields the appropriate data to determine the nature of the problem and the subsequent therapeutic maneuvers. The following types of bullous disease must be discussed because of their relative frequency or significance.

Toxic epidermal necrolysis is caused by drug reactions and occasionally graft-versus-host disease. It is an acute problem in which sheets of epidermis can be removed from glabrous skin or mucous membranes. Patients are acutely ill and the problem is one in which the moult leads to death of epidermis. Patients require meticulous skin care similar to that given to those with significant burns. The epidermal barrier is lost, and the epidermis may easily become secondarily infected. Systemic corticosteroids are probably valuable in limiting the extent of the disease if they are used early enough in the course. Steroids are probably not effective in graft-versus-host disease.

Appearing to be similar to toxic epidermal necrolysis, but of a total different pathophysiology and requiring very different management, is the *scalded skin syndrome*, an acute problem which most commonly affects newborns but which may affect older children and adults. This problem is caused by an exotoxin produced by certain strains of *Staphylococcus aureus*. The toxin causes a split in the epidermis at the granular layer, and the problem must be treated with a penicillinase-resistant antibiotic appropriate to the organism causing the disease. The process is superficial enough so that the lesions heal without scar formation.

Pemphigus vulgaris is a rare disease which usually affects adults in the sixth, seventh, and eighth decades. The intraepidermal vesicles are associated with a circulating IgG antibody to the intercellular

---
TABLE 155-1
Bullous Diseases

Disease	Localization of Split	Characteristics	Treatment
Toxic epidermal necrolysis	Basal layer	Etiology: drug or idiopathic	Corticosteroids
Staphylococcal scalded skin syndrome	Granular layer	Etiology: proteolytic enzyme produced by staphyloccocus	Antibiotic
Pemphigus vulgaris	Basal layer	IgG directed at epidermal intercellular layer Flaccid bullae	Corticosteroids, immunosuppressives, gold
Bullous pemphigoid	Subepidermal	IgG and complement directed at basal lamina	Corticosteroids, immunosuppressives
Dermatitis herpetiformis	Subepidermal	Symmetrical, pruritic extensor areas IgA in dermal papillae Gluten-sensitive enteropathy	Sulfones
Epidermolysis bullosa	Subepidermal	Genetic Localized to areas of trauma	Protection
Erythema multiforme	Subepidermal	Iris—target lesions	Corticosteroids

---

area of epidermis. Bullae in pemphigus are flaccid, break easily, and mucous membrane involvement is common. Nikolsky's sign (the ability to form a bulla on normal skin with a shearing force) is positive when pemphigus is active. This disease, which is felt to represent autoimmunity, responds to systemic corticosteroids and/or immunosuppressive agents. Recent studies have indicated that gold may be an effective type of therapy, but its role in the care of patients with the disease has not yet been clarified.

Bullous pemphigoid also occurs in older patients, but it is a subepidermal process with fixation of IgG and complement to the basement membrane. The process responds relatively well to therapeutic doses of systemic corticosteroids.

Dermatitis herpetiformis is an unusual chronic bullous disease which affects patients in the second to fourth decades. The lesions begin as symmetrical papules on extensor areas and they are extremely pruritic. The primary pathologic event relates to IgA deposition in the dermal papillae followed by neutrophilic inflammation around the papillary vessels. The IgA is not limited to the site of the specific lesions but is seen in normal skin as well. Dermatitis herpetiformis is usually associated with gluten-sensitive enteropathy and the skin lesions respond to sulfones quite specifically. Patients must be screened for glucose-6-phosphate dehydrogenase activity before sulfone therapy.

In addition to these acquired bullous diseases, there are a group of genetically induced problems in which the attachment of epidermis and dermis is abnormal and blisters form wherever the skin is subjected to any shearing trauma (*epidermolysis bullosa*). Some types lead to scarring; many do not. In several types, specific defects of collagen structure and metabolism have been postulated but not proven.

Tumors (Fig. 155-1)

The skin is the site of premalignant and malignant tumors, most of which are found in sun-exposed areas. Among the *premalignant lesions* are Bowen's disease, actinic keratoses, arsenical keratoses, leukoplakia, and some cutaneous horns. Each of these can be diagnosed histologically, and clinically they are skin-colored to red, scaling papules or plaques up to 1

---TABLE 155–2---

Cutaneous Changes Indicating Disease in Other Organ Systems

Hair
Increase
  Porphyria
  Increased serum androgen
Loss
  Telogen effluvium
  Hypo- or hyperthyroidism
  Kwashiorkor
  Argininosuccinicaciduria
  Thallium intoxication
  Secondary syphilis

Nails
White distal half
  Cirrhosis—Terry's nails
Paired white lines
  Low serum albumin—Muchrcke's lines
White proximal half
  Renal disease—half-and-half nails
Yellow
  Edema
Blue lunulae
  Wilson's disease
Slate gray
  Argyria
Onycholysis
  Hyperthyroidism—Plummer's nails
Koilonychia—spoon nails
  Anemia
Clubbing
  Pulmonary disease
  Malignancy
  Biliary cirrhosis
  Chronic diarrhea
Splitting-ridging
  Raynaud's disease
Periungual telangiectasia
  Scleroderma
  Lupus erythematosus
  Dermatomyositis
Splinter hemorrhages
  Trauma
  Vasculitis
  Subacute infective endocarditis

Pigmentation
Hyperpigmentation
Diffuse
  Addison's disease
  Fanconi's anemia
  Liver disease
  Melanoma
  Hemochromatosis
  Uremia
  Pregnancy
  Silver intoxication

---TABLE 155–2 (cont.)---

Pigmentation (cont.)
Localized
  Acanthosis nigricans
    malignancy associated
    hormone associated
    idiopathic
  Lips and hands
    Peutz-Jeghers—gastrointestinal polyposis
  Neurofibromatosis
  Albright syndrome
Hypopigmentation
  Chediak–Higashi syndrome
  Kwashiorkor
  Tuberous sclerosis
  Phenylketonuria
  Vitiligo
  Albanism
  Hypopituitarism
Yellow-orange
  Carotenemia
  Jaundice
  Uremia

Diffuse Dermatitis (resembles atopic dermatitis)
Phenylketonuria
Histidinemia
Congenital anhydrotic
  ectodermal defect
Wiskott-Aldrich syndrome
Sex-linked agammaglobulinemia
Ataxia telangiectasia

Localized Dermatitis
Acral
  Acrodermatitis enteropathica
  Gluten-sensitive enteropathy
Exposed areas
  Pellagra
Perioroficial
  Zinc deficiency
  Glucagonoma
  Vitamin A therapy
  Acrodermatitis enteropathica
  Candida infection

Scaling
Refsum syndrome
Drug reactions
Kwashiorkor
Vitamin A deficiency
Essential fatty acid deficiency
Lymphoma

Seborrheic Dermatitis
Parkinson's disease
Letterer-Siewe disease

Hyperkeratosis of Palms and Soles
Tyrosinemia
Tylosis with esophageal cancer

──────TABLE 155-2 (cont.)──────

Follicular Hyperkeratosis
Nutritional deficiency
Scurvy

Leg Ulcers
Sickle cell disease or trait
Felty syndrome
Pyoderma gangrenosum
  Ulcerative colitis or Crohn's disease
Arteriovenous malformation

Papules and Nodules
Ear
  Gout
  Calcinosis cutis
Nose
  Adenoma sebaceum (tuberous sclerosis)
Diffuse
  Amyloid
  Xanthoma
  Juvenile xanthogranuloma
  Lipogranulomatosis (Farber syndrome)
  Neurofibroma

Elastosis Perforans Serpiginosa
(Elevated serpiginous plaques on neck, elbows, knees)
Down syndrome
Ehlers-Danlos syndrome
Pseudoxanthoma elasticum
Marfan syndrome
Osteogenesis imperfecta

Erythema Nodosum
Ulcerative colitis
Crohn's disease
Sarcoid
Drug reactions
Bacterial infections

Multiple Cysts
Gardner syndrome (colonic polyposis)

Petechiae
Subacute infective endocarditis
Vasculitis
Scurvy
Hematologic abnormalities

Cutaneous Hemorrhage and Bruising
Hematologic abnormalities
Amyloid
Sepsis
Wiskott-Aldrich syndrome
Kasabach-Merritt syndrome

Telangiectasia
Ataxia telangiectasia
Hepatic disease
Carcinoid
Dermatomyositis (adenocarcinoma association)

──────TABLE 155-2 (cont.)──────

Palmar Erythema
Diffuse—hepatic disease
Nodular—subacute infective endocarditis (Osler's nodes)

Flushing
Carcinoid syndrome

Eyes
Dryness
  Vitamin A deficiency
  Sjögren syndrome
Scleral pigment
  Grey-blue—alcaptonuria
Limbal pigment
  Wilson's disease

Perleche and Cheilitis
Riboflavin deficiency
Iron deficiency anemia

Infection–Superficial
Chronic granulomatous disease
Job syndrome
Hyperimmunoglobulin E syndrome

cm in diameter. They can be managed most effectively by destructive techniques including heat, cold, x-ray, surgery, or topical chemotherapeutic agents including 5-fluouracil.

Basal cell epitheliomata begin as flesh-colored papules with prominent telangiectasia. They grow to become plaques with an elevated rolled border and commonly a depressed, ulcerated center. There are several varieties including a sclerotic type which looks like a scar and a pigmented variety which must be differentiated from a nevus or melanoma. Basal cell tumors are locally destructive, potentially recurrent, but only rarely metastatic. They should be completely removed by surgery, radiotherapy, chemosurgery, or a similar destructive method.

Squamous cell carcinomas, in contrast to those we have already discussed, have the biologic capabilities of invasion and metastasis. They are irregular in size, commonly covered with thick scale, and up to several centimeters in diameter. The appropriate management involves adequate destruction by surgical, chemosurgical, or electrosurgical techniques.

Malignant melanoma is an extremely important cutaneous tumor, for early recognition by the health care provider can lead to therapy at a time when successful surgical excision is possible. Melanomata are most commonly found on sun-exposed surfaces and can be differentiated from benign nevi and other pigmented lesions by the irregularity of their borders and the heterogeneity of colors (red, white, blue, and black areas all in the same lesion). The prognosis for patients with melanoma is related to the size and depth of the lesion when it is excised. For this reason, patients should be carefully examined and all suspicious lesions should be excised (if possible) or biopsied.

Patients who have had one premalignant or malignant skin lesion must be watched especially carefully because they have an increased chance of developing a subsequent lesion.

CUTANEOUS MANIFESTATIONS OF SYSTEMIC DISEASE

Pruritus, as noted above, may be the clue to an underlying systemic disease. In addition, however, there are many cutaneous changes which should alert the health care provider to disease in other organ systems. A number of these clues are listed in Table 155–2.

SYSTEMIC MANIFESTATIONS OF CUTANEOUS DISEASE

Table 155–2 above indicates that many systemic diseases present with cutaneous manifestations. In addition, however, a number of cutaneous diseases affect the general body economy. The epitome of these processes is *generalized exfoliative dermatitis* or the "red man syndrome." This disease may be idiopathic or it may be a stage in a number of cutaneous diseases including psoriasis, atopic dermatitis, seborrheic dermatitis, contact dermatitis, mycosis fungoides, and drug eruptions. Normally, up to 1 g of scale may be lost from the surface of the skin each day, but in association with the diseases of rapid epidermal proliferation which are associated with this syndrome, up to 30 g of scale may be lost each day. If this loss is sufficiently great, patients can develop negative nitrogen balance with low serum albumin and edema. In addition, they may have significant vitamin and mineral loss. This negative balance can be reversed by forced feeding, so it is not as severe as the negative balance associated with extensive burns.

The general vasodilatation associated with the syndrome leads to increased blood flow as many shunt pathways through the skin are opened and cardiac output increases. In patients with borderline cardiac compensation, failure may result. Temperature control becomes a problem because of the excessive loss of heat (radiation and convection) to the environment through the widely dilated skin vessels. Patients shiver to make up the heat loss, and they often develop fever as their fine temperature control is lost. Many of these patients have anemia consequent to loss of iron, folate, and other nutrients in the scale. As their epidermal barrier is no longer intact, they have a vastly increased extrarenal water loss. They are constantly thirsty, excrete highly concentrated urine, and are subject to the development of renal stones. Finally, the increased epidermal turnover and shivering lead to elevations of the basal metabolic rate. Thus, generalized exfoliative erythroderma is one of the major causes of euthyroid hypermetabolism.

There is a close link between diseases of the skin and the gastrointestinal tract. This relationship is most commonly seen with *dermatitis herpetiformis*, a generalized vesicular and bullous skin disease which is associated with gluten-sensitive enteropathy manifest by steatorrhea and abnormal D-xylose absorption. The pathophysiology of the relationship between the skin lesions and the gastrointestinal manifestations has not been completely elucidated: skin may be primary, the gastrointestinal lesions may be primary, or both may be related to a change in some other organ system. English authors, in fact, have described an entity known as dermatogenic enteropathy in which there is steatorrhea associated with many types of generalized eczema or psoriasis. They have also noted the occurrence of gynecomastia in patients with extensive eczema. Again, the relationships among these manifestations have not yet been clarified.

PRINCIPLES OF TOPICAL DERMATOLOGIC THERAPY

Many of the systemic antibiotics, anti-inflammatory agents, and antimetabolites which have been described in other chapters are as valuable in treating diseases of the skin as in treating pathologic processes in other organ systems. What is unique about dermatologic therapy, however, is the availability of topical therapy—local therapy directed only at the diseased organ. This situation means that noncutaneous side effects can be minimized. However, the most important aspect of dermatologic therapy, which is not appreciated by an adequate number of health care providers, is that the majority of cutaneous problems for which patients seek care are readily treatable and, in many cases, curable. The reputation that most skin diseases are chronic and untreatable has not been true since effective antibiotic and anti-inflammatory agents became available. It is not even necessary in many circumstances to make an exact diagnosis in order to treat the process effectively. As long as the pathophysiologic basis of the problem or the reaction pattern (hyperplasia, acute inflammation, chronic inflammation, infection) can be determined, appropriate therapy can be recommended. In this section we shall review some of the more common ways to deliver medication to the skin and shall review the principles involved in topical corticosteroid therapy.

Topical medications are liquids, solids, or mixtures of each such as in lotions or pastes. Liquids are commonly used for wet dressings, soaks, or baths and as a component of lotions (suspensions of powder in liquid). They are particularly valuable for hair-bearing areas and for exudative lesions. Solids are used in powders, creams, or ointments. They can be used in all other areas and are lubricating and protective.

Wet Dressings

Water is the most important component of wet dressings or compresses which are prepared by soaking cloths in an appropriate solution. If left open to the air, the wet dressings cool the skin by evaporation. This is not the case if the dressings are occluded by an impermeable cover. Open wet dressings are used for acute, weeping, exudative areas, and as the dressings are changed, the crusts and exudates are removed. This removal may be even greater if the dressings are left to dry since some of the proteinaceous material sticks to the cloths and is physically debrided. A number of materials have been added to the basic water wet dressing (salt, aluminum acetate, acetic acid, potassium permanganate, silver nitrate) to increase bacteriostasis and form a thin crust of precipitated protein on the top of the area. During treatment of acute cutaneous inflammation, dressings should be used frequently (4 to 6 times each day) for 30 minutes each time. Nearly constant wet dressings (90 minutes each 2 hours) are used for extremely exudative problems during the first several days of therapy. Such dressings serve the same purpose as almost constant baths. Whirlpool therapy accomplishes the same type of physical debridement as is present when macerating wet dressings are used.

Baths or soaks are not as cooling as wet dressings but they effectively decrease pruritus and superficial exudate. Colloidal oatmeal or commercial bath oils may be added to the baths to prevent excessive drying of the skin.

Powders, Creams, and Ointments

Powders, which may be inert or may contain active ingredients, are used to absorb moisture and to decrease friction between opposing skin surfaces.

Creams are emulsions of oil in water-containing, emulsifying agents and preservatives. They can be removed easily by washing and are usually completely absorbed into the skin. Thus, they are cosmetically more acceptable and more drying than *ointments* which are more protective and less penetrable. There are several types of ointments including water-soluble, emulsifiable, and water-repellent varieties. The water-soluble (polyethylene glycol) ointments contain inert oils. The emulsifiable ointments are water-in-oil emulsions which will take up more water and are difficult to wash off as are the non-water-containing absorbent ointments. The latter can absorb water to become water-in-oil emulsions. The epitome of water repellent ointments is petrolatum, an inert hydrocarbon, which can be used as a lubricant for dry skin forming a protective barrier on the surface. An efficient way to rehydrate an area of skin is to soak the part in water and then apply a coating of a water repellent ointment. When powders are suspended in such ointments, a paste results.

How Much To Prescribe

It is important that adequate, but not excessive, amounts of topical medication be prescribed. With either creams or ointments, approximately 2 g are needed to cover the face or hands, 3 or 4 g are required for an arm or leg, and 30 to 60 g for the entire body. It has not yet been determined how frequent applications should be, but since tachyphylaxis (loss of effectiveness with continuing use) is known to occur, the rule "the more, the better" may not be correct. Absorption of topical agents is increased if the medication is applied under an airtight occlusive plastic dressing, but this method also increases potential side effects of the medications and it promotes infection, folliculitis, and miliaria.

Topical Corticosteroids

Among all of the topical agents utilized today, the most frequently prescribed are corticosteroid preparations. This is the case because such a large number of cutaneous problems are manifestations of inflammation. Although there is a correlation between the biochemical potency of a steroid molecule (induction of new protein synthesis and enzyme activity) and its anti-inflammatory effect, the actual basis of the molecule's effectiveness is not known. Three effects seem most closely related to the clinical results on skin: superficial vasoconstriction, reduction of leukocyte adherence with lysosomal stabilization, and the antimitotic effect. The vasoconstrictive effects are used as the standard assay for corticosteroid potency. The development of topical corticosteroids is in part more complicated than the development of systemic agents, since the compounds for topical use must be effective as anti-inflammatory agents, be stable on the skin surface, and have the ability to penetrate the stratum corneum. Agents which are more lipophilic are more effective and much effort has been used to produce better local agents via chemical modification.

The effect of the corticosteroids and other topical medications depends not only upon the active medication, but upon the vehicle. Most steroids are prepared as creams, gels, lotions, or ointments—the creams are cosmetically acceptable, but the ointments are usually more effective since they result in hydration of the stratum corneum and increase penetration of the steroid.

As noted, corticosteroids are extremely effective in many situations, but they are associated with potentially significant local and systemic side effects. The local side effects include hypopigmentation and atrophy of both epidermis and dermis, a problem which can be seen following several weeks of frequent applications of potent corticosteroids. An erythematous, telangiectatic, rosacea-like eruption can

be seen when potent steroids are used frequently on the face for a number of weeks. Such complications can be avoided if patients are educated not to overuse the agent.

Systemic side effects from topical corticosteroids are infrequent, but the agents can cause suppression of the hypothalamic–pituitary axis especially if they are used under occlusion (thereby enhancing penetration) for prolonged periods of time. These effects are more pronounced in young children and infants because of their thin skin and high surface area to volume ratio. Absorption is also much greater through areas of thin skin such as eyelids and scrotum.

Table 155–3 lists a number of topical corticosteroid preparations categorized by relative potency.

TABLE 155–3
Topical Corticosteroid Preparations*

Highest Potency

Group 1	Fluocinonide (0.05%) cream, ointment Halcinonide (0.1%) cream
Group 2	Betamethasone diproprionate (0.05%) cream Triamcinolone acetonide (0.5%) cream
Group 3	Triamcinolone acetonide (0.1%) cream, ointment Fluocinolone acetonide (0.025%) cream, ointment Betamethasone valerate (0.1%) cream, ointment Flurandronolide (0.025%) ointment, cream
Group 4	Flumethasone pivalate (0.03%) cream Desonide (0.05%) cream Hydrocortisone (1.0%) cream

Lowest Potency

* Since new agents are constantly being marketed by the pharmaceutical industry, the examples used are merely that—examples.

REFERENCES

Special Aspects of Care for Adolescents and the Aged

1. Age at Menarche, United States. Washington, D.C., U. S. Department of Health, Education, and Welfare, Public Health Service, 1973.
2. Adolescent Behavior and Health. Washington, D.C., Institute of Medicine, National Academy of Science, 1978.
3. Andres, R. Aging and diabetes. Med. Clin. North Am., 55:835, 1971.
4. Binstock, R. and Shanas, E. (eds.). Handbook of Aging and The Social Sciences. New York, Van Nostrand, 1976.
5. Birren, J.E. and Schaie, K.W. (eds.). Handbook of the Psychology of Aging. New York, Van Nostrand, 1977.
6. Brocklehurst, J. Textbook of Geriatric Medicine and Gerontology, 2nd ed. Edinburgh, Churchill Livingstone, 1979.
7. Brown, R.H. Consent. Pediatrics, 57:414, 1976.
8. Bryt, A. Adolescent sex causes. Med. Aspects Human Sexuality, 20:8, October 1978.
9. Burr, I.M., Sizon Enko, P.E., Kaplan, S.L., and Grumbach, M.M. Hormonal changes in puberty. I. Correlation of serum lutenizing hormone and follicle stimulating hormone with stages of puberty, testicular size and bone age in normal boys. Pediatr. Res., 4:25, 1970.
10. Bush, V. A Letter From Vannevar Bush. Bull. NY Acad. Med., 47:1274, 1971.
11. Butler, R.N. Why Survive? Being Old in America. New York, Harper & Row, 1973.
12. Cape, R. Aging: Its Complex Management. New York, Harper & Row, 1978.
13. Cohen, M.I. and Litt, I.F. Health care for adolescents in a traditional medical setting. Youth, Health and Social Systems Symposium, Washington, D.C., April 1974.
14. Cooper, B. and McGee, M. Medical care outlays for three age groups: young, intermediate and aged. Soc. Secur. Bull., 34:3, 1971.

15. Cunning, H. and Mayer, J. Obesity and its possible effects on college acceptance. N. Engl. J. Med., 275:1172, 1966.

16. Dans, P.E. and Kerr, M.R. Gerontology and geriatrics in medical education. N. Engl. J. Med., 300:228, 1979.

17. Eisdorfer, C. and Cohen, D. The cognitively impaired elderly: Differential diagnosis. In Storandt, M., Siegler, I.C., and Elias, M.F. (eds.), Clinical Phychology of Aging. New York, Plenum, 1978.

18. Finch, C.E. and Hayflick, L. (eds.). Handbook of the Biology of Aging. New York, Van Nostrand, 1977.

19. Frisch, R.E. A method of prediction of age of menarch from height and weight at ages 9 through 13 years. Pediatrics, 53:384, 1974.

20. Hayflick, L. The cell biology of human aging. N. Engl. J. Med., 295:1302, 1976.

21. Hazard, S.W., Allen R.V., and Eisner, V. A model act providing for consent of minors for health services. Pediatrics, 51:293, 1973.

22. Hein, K., Marks, A., and Cohen, M.I. Asymptomatic gonorrhea: prevalence in a population of urban adolescents. J. Pediatr., 90:634, 1971.

23. Henderson, B.E. Urogenital tract abnormalities in sons of women treated with diethyestilbesterol. Pediatrics, 58:505, 1976.

24. Herbst, A.L. Clear cell adenocarcinoma of the vagina and cervix in girls: analysis of 170 registry cases. Am. J. Obstet. Gynecol., 119:713, 1974.

25. Hormann, A. D. and Pilpel, H.F. The legal rights of minors. Pediatr. Clin. North Am., 20:989, 1973.

26. Katz, S., Ford, A.B., Moskowitz, R.W., Jackson, D.A., and Jaffe, M.A. Studies of illness in the aged. JAMA, 185:914, 1963.

27. Kelly, J. A compendium of nutritional status studies and dietary evaluations conducted in the U. S. for 1957–67. J. Nutr. (Suppl.), 1:99, 1967.

28. Laron, Z. Treatment of diabetes in children: revisited. Pediatr. Ann., 3:63, 1974.

29. Lindemann, C. Birth Control and Unmarried Women. New York, Springer, 1974.

30. Lowrey, G.H. Growth and Development of Children, 7th ed. Chicago, Year Book, 1978.

31. Marks, A. and Cohen, M.I. Health screening and assessment of adolescents. Pediatr. Ann., 49:177, 1978.

32. Millar, H.E. Approaches to Adolescent Health Care. Rockville, Md., U.S. Department of Health, Education, and Welfare, DHEW Pub. No. (HSA) 75-5014, 1975, p. 9.

33. Parcell, G.S., Nader, P.R., and Meyer, M.D. Adolescent health concerns, problems, and patterns of utilization in a triethnic urban population. Pediatrics, 60:157, 1977.

34. Raitt, G.E. The minor's right to consent to medical treatment: a corollary of the Constitutional right of privacy. S. Calif. Law. Rev., 48:1417, 1975.

35. Reichel, W. (ed.). The Geriatric Patient. New York, H P Publishing, 1978.

36. Roberts-Thomson, I.C., Whittingham, S., and Youngchaiyud, U. Aging, immune response, and mortality. Lancet, 2:368, 1974.

37. Rodstein, M. The characteristics of nonfatal myocardial infarction in the aged. Arch. Intern. Med., 98:84, 1956.

38. Root, A.W. Endocrinology of puberty. J. Pediatr., 83:1, 1973.

39. Rossman, I. (ed.). Clinical Geriatrics, 2nd ed. Philadelphia, Lippincott, 1979.

40. Rowe J., Andres, R., Tobin, J.D., Norris, A.H., and Shock, N.W. Age-adjusted standards for creatinine clearance. Ann. Intern. Med., 84:567, 1976.

41. Rush, D. Respiratory symptoms in a group of American secondary school students: the overwhelming association with cigarette smoking. Int. J. Epidemiol., 3:153, 1974.

42. Schimmel, E.M. The hazards of hospitalization. Ann. Intern. Med., 60:100, 1964.

43. Seegal, D. Some comments on the medical management of the older person. J. Chronic Dis., 3:101, 1956.

44. Seely, J., Zuskin, E., and Bouhays, A. Cigarette smoking: objective evidence for lung damage in teenagers. Science, 172:741, 1971.

45. Shock, N.W. The physiology of aging. Sci. Am., 206(1): 100, 1962.

46. Sizon Enko, P.C., Burr, I.M., Kaplan, S.L., and Grumbach, M.M. Hormonal changes in puberty. II. Correlation of serum lutenizing hormone and follicle stimulating hormone with stages of puberty and bone age in normal girls. Pediatr. Res., 4:36, 1970.

47. Steel, K., Williams, T.F., Fairbank, M., and Knox, K. Laboratory screening in the evaluation and placement of geriatric patients. J. Am. Geriatr. Soc., 22:538, 1974.

48. Sternlieb, J.J. and Munan, L. A survey of health problems, practices, and needs of youth. Pediatrics, 49:117, 1972.

49. Stuart, H.C. Physical growth during adolescence. Am. J. Dis. Child., 74:495, 1947.

50. Tanner, J.M. Growth at Adolescence, 2nd ed. Oxford, Blackwell, 1962.

51. Vaisrub, S. Accidental hypothermia in the elderly. JAMA, 239:1888, 1978.

52. Vestal, R.E. Drug use in the elderly: a review of problems and special considerations. Drugs, 16:358, 1978.

53. Zacharias, L. and Wurtman, R.J. Age at menarche. N. Engl. J. Med., 280:868, 1969.

Alcoholism and Associated Medical Problems

54. Chazan, J.A. and Mistilis, S.P. The pathophysiology of scurvy. Am. J. Med. 34:350, 1963.

55. Dreyfus, P.M. and Herbert, V. Effects of thiamine deficiency on the central nervous system. Am. J. Clin. Nutr., 9:414, 1961.

56. Imboden, J.B. and Urbaitis, J. Alcoholism. In Practical Psychiatry in Medicine. New York, Appleton-Century-Crofts, 1978, pp. 103–115.

57. Leevy, C.M., Thompson, A., and Baker, H. Vitamins and liver injury. Am. J. Clin. Nutr., 23:493, 1970.

58. Mendelson, J.H. Biologic concomitants of alcoholism. N. Engl. J. Med., 283:24, 71, 1970.

59. Mezey, E. Liver disease and nutrition. Gastroenterology, 74:770, 1978.

60. Thompson, W.L., Johnson, A.D., and Maddrey, W.C. Diazepam and paraldehyde for treatment of severe delirium tremens: a controlled trial. Ann. Intern. Med., 82:175, 1975

61. Victor, M. and Hope, J.M. The phenomenon of auditory hallucinations in chronic alcoholism. J. Nerv. Ment. Dis., 126:451, 1958.

62. Victor, M., Adams, R.D., and Mancall, E.L. A restricted form of cerebellar cortical degeneration occurring in alcoholic patients. Arch. Neurol., 1:579, 1959.

63. Victor, M. and Adams, R.D. On the etiology of the alcoholic neurologic diseases with special reference to the role of nutrition. Am. J. Clin. Nutr., 9:379, 1961.

Ophthalmology in Medicine

64. Glaser, J.S. Neuro-ophthalmology Symposium, Vol. 8. University of Miami and Bascom Palmer Eye Institute, 1977.

65. Newell, F.W. Ophthalmology: Principles and Concepts. St. Louis, Mosby, 1974.

66. Patz, A. Current concepts in ophthalmology, retinal vascular disease. N. Engl. J. Med., 298:1451, 1978.

67. Scheie, H.G. and Albert, D.M. Textbook of Ophthalmology. Philadelphia, Saunders, 1977.

68. Walsh, F.B. and Hoyt, W.F. Clinical Neuro-ophthalmology. Baltimore, Williams & Wilkins, 1969.

Cutaneous Medicine

69. Ackerman, A.B. Histologic Diagnosis of Inflammatory Skin Diseases. Philadelphia, Lea & Febiger, 1978.

70. Arndt, K.A. Manual of Dermatologic Therapeutics, 2nd ed. Boston, Little, Brown, 1978.

71. Demis, D.J., Dobson, R.L., and McGuire, J. Clinical Dermatology. Hagerstown, Harper & Row, 1979.

72. Epstein, E. and Epstein, E., Jr. Skin Surgery, 4th ed. Springfield, Ill., Thomas, 1977.

73. Fitzpatrick, T.B., Eisen, A.Z., Austen, K.F., Freedberg, I.M., and Wolff, K. Dermatology in General Medicine, 2nd ed. New York, McGraw-Hill, 1979.

74. Lever, W.F. and Schaumburg-Lever, G. Histopathology of the Skin, 5th ed. Philadelphia, Lippincott, 1975.

75. Moschella, S.L., Pillsbury, D.M., and Hurley, H.J. Dermatology. Philadelphia, Saunders, 1975.

76. Okun, M.R., and Edelstein, K.M. Gross and Microscopic Pathology of the Skin. Boston, Dermatopathology Foundation Press, 1976.

77. Rook, A., Wilkinson, D.S., and Ebling, F.I.G. Textbook of Dermatology, 3rd ed. Oxford, Blackwell, 1979.

APPENDIX
Laboratory Reference Values of Clinical Importance*
PREPARED BY REX B. CONN, M.D., EMORY UNIVERSITY SCHOOL OF MEDICINE, ATLANTA, GEORGIA

Physicians are accustomed to receiving laboratory reports with measurements expressed in metric units such as the gram, liter, or milliliter; however, an extensive modification of the metric system has been adopted by clinical laboratories in many countries, and plans are being formulated to make a similar change in the United States. This adaptation is the International System of Units (Le Système International d'Unités), usually abbreviated S.I. Units. Whereas the metric system utilizes the centimeter, the gram, and the second as basic units, the International System uses the meter, the kilogram, and the second as well as four other basic units.

The overriding consideration for adopting the International System is that it will provide a common language among the various scientific disciplines throughout the world for unambiguous communication regarding all types of measurements. In the medical field, the advantages of conversion are that chemical relationships between various substances will become more readily apparent and there will be an international uniformity in laboratory reporting. The most serious disadvantage in making this conversion is that physicians will have to become accustomed to a new set of figures for almost all laboratory measurements. Because of this inconvenience, as well as a potential for serious misinterpretation of laboratory data, the conversion must be undertaken cautiously and only after a logical plan has been formulated and discussed. There appears to be little question, however, that the International System will be adopted in this country. Clinical laboratories in most Western European countries, Canada, and Australia are already using S.I. Units, and American medical journals are adopting the practice of expressing measurements in both conventional and S.I. Units.

Tables accompanying this appendix indicate "normal values" for most of the commonly performed laboratory tests. The title of the tables has been changed from the "normal values" of previous editions to "reference values" to conform to current usage. The reference value is given in conventional units, the conversion factor is indicated when appropriate, and the value in S.I. Units is calculated from these figures. Notes (p. 1508) are used to provide additional information.

---

* Reprinted from *Current Diagnosis 5*. Howard F. Conn and Rex B. Conn (eds.), 1977, with permission of W. B. Saunders Company, Philadelphia, Pennsylvania.

Reference Values in Hematology

	Conventional Units*		Factor	S.I. Units†	Notes
Acid hemolysis test (Ham)	No hemolysis		—	No hemolysis	
Alkaline phosphatase, leukocyte	Total score 14–100		—	Total score 14–100	
Carboxyhemoglobin	Up to 5% of total		0.01	0.05 of total	
Cell counts					
Erythrocytes					
Males	4.6–6.2 million/μl		10^6	4.6–6.2 $\times$ 10^{12}/liter	
Females	4.2–5.4 million/μl			4.2–5.4 $\times$ 10^{12}/liter	
Children (varies with age)	4.5–5.1 million/μl			4.5–5.1 $\times$ 10^{12}/liter	
Leukocytes					
Total	4500–11,000/μl		10^6	4.5–11.0 $\times$ 10^9/liter	
Differential	**Percentage**	**Absolute**			
Myelocytes	0	0/μl	10^6	0/1	b
Band neutrophils	3–5	150–400/μl		150–400 $\times$ 10^6/liter	
Segmented neutrophils	54–62	3000–5800/μl		3000–5800 $\times$ 10^6/liter	
Lymphocytes	25–33	1500–3000/μl		1500–3000 $\times$ 10^6/liter	
Monocytes	3–7	300–500/μl		300–500 $\times$ 10^6/liter	
Eosinophils	1–3	50–250/μl		50–250 $\times$ 10^6/liter	
Basophils	0–0.75	15–50/μl		15–50 $\times$ 10^6/liter	
Platelets	150,000–350,000/μl		10^6	150–350 $\times$ 10^9/liter	
Reticulocytes	25,000–75,000/μl		10^6	25–75 $\times$ 10^9/liter	
	0.5–1.5% of erythrocytes				
Coagulation tests					
Bleeding time (Duke)	1–5 min		—	1–5 min	
Bleeding time (Ivy)	Less than 5 min		—	Less than 5 min	
Clot retraction, qualitative	Begins in 30–60 min		—	Begins in 30–60 min	
	Complete in 24 hr		—	Complete in 24 hr	
Coagulation time (Lee-White)	5–15 min (glass tubes)		—	5–15 min (glass tubes)	
	19–60 min (siliconized tubes)		—	19–60 min (siliconized tubes)	
Fibrinogen	200–400 mg/dl		0.0293	5.9–11.7 μmol/liter	c
Fibrinolysins	0		—	0	
Partial thromboplastin time, activated (APTT)	35–45 sec		—	35–45 sec	
Prothrombin consumption	Over 80% consumed in 1 hr		0.01	Over 80% consumed in 1 hr	
Prothrombin content	100% (calculated from prothrombin time)		0.01	1.0 (calculated from prothrombin time)	
Prothrombin time (one stage)	12.0–14.0 sec		—	12.0–14.0 sec	
Thromboplastin generation test	Compared to normal control		—	Compared to normal control	
Tourniquet test	Ten or fewer petechiae in a 2.5-cm circle after 5 min		—	Ten or fewer petechiae in a 2.5-cm circle after 5 min	

† Standard prefixes.

Prefix	Multiplication Factor	Symbol
atto	10^{-18}	a
femto	10^{-15}	f
pico	10^{-12}	p
nano	10^{-9}	n
micro	10^{-6}	μ
milli	10^{-3}	m
centi	10^{-2}	c
deci	10^{-1}	d
deca	10^1	da
hecto	10^2	h
kilo	10^3	k
mega	10^6	M
giga	10^9	G
tera	10^{12}	T

* Abbreviations:

kg	= kilogram	= 1000 g
mg	= milligram	= 0.001 g
μg	= microgram	= 0.000001 g
ng	= nanogram	= 0.000000001 g
pg	= picogram	= 0.000000000001 g
ml	= milliliter	= 0.001 liter
mm	= millimeter	= 0.001 meter
μ	= micron	= 0.000001 meter
mEq	= milliequivalent	
mOsm	= milliosmole	

	Conventional Units	Factor	S.I. Units	Notes
Cold hemolysin test (Donath-Landsteiner)	No hemolysis	—	No hemolysis	
Corpuscular values of erythrocytes (values for adults; in children, values vary with age)				
M.C.H. (mean corpuscular hemoglobin)	27–31 pg	0.0155	0.42–0.48 fmol	d
M.C.V. (mean corpuscular volume)	80–105 micra³	1.0	80–105 fl	
M.C.H.C. (mean corpuscular hemoglobin concentration)	32–36%	0.01	0.32–0.36	a
Haptoglobin (as hemoglobin binding capacity)	100–200 mg/dl	0.155	16–31 μmol/liter	d
Hematocrit				a
Males	40–54 ml/dl	0.01	0.40–0.54	
Females	37–47 ml/dl		0.37–0.47	
Newborn	49–54 ml/dl		0.49–0.54	
Children (varies with age)	35–49 ml/dl		0.35–0.49	
Hemoglobin				d
Males	14.0–18.0 g/dl	0.155	2.17–2.79 mmol/liter	
Females	12.0–16.0 g/dl		1.86–2.48 mmol/liter	
Newborn	16.5–19.5 g/dl		2.56–3.02 mmol/liter	
Children (varies with age)	11.2–16.5 g/dl		1.74–2.56 mmol/liter	
Hemoglobin, fetal	Less than 1% of total	0.01	Less than 0.01 of total	a
Hemoglobin A$_2$	1.5–3.0% of total	0.01	0.015–0.03 of total	a
Hemoglobin, plasma	0–5.0 mg/dl	0.155	0–0.8 μmol/liter	d
Methemoglobin	0–130 mg/dl	0.155	4.7–20 μmol/liter	e
Osmotic fragility of erythrocytes	Begins in 0.45–0.39% NaCl	171	Begins in 77–67 mmol/liter NaCl	
	Complete in 0.33–0.30% NaCl		Complete in 56–51 mmol/liter NaCl	
Sedimentation rate				
Wintrobe				
Males	0–5 mm in 1 hr	—	0–5 mm/hr	
Females	0–15 mm in 1 hr	—	0–15 mm/hr	
Westergren				
Males	0–15 mm in 1 hr	—	0–15 mm/hr	
Females	0–20 mm in 1 hr	—	0–20 mm/hr	
(May be slightly higher in children and during pregnancy)				
Bone marrow, differential cell count				

	Range (%)	Average (%)		Range	Average	
Myeloblasts	0.3–5.0	2.0	0.01	0.003–0.05	0.02	a
Promyelocytes	1.0–8.0	5.0		0.01–0.08	0.05	
Myelocytes						
Neutrophilic	5.0–19.0	12.0		0.05–0.19	0.12	
Eosinophilic	0.5–3.0	1.5		0.005–0.03	0.015	
Basophilic	0.0–0.5	0.3		0.00–0.005	0.003	
Metamyelocytes	13.0–32.0	22.0		0.13–0.32	0.22	
Polymorphonuclear neutrophils	7.0–30.0	20.0		0.07–0.30	0.20	
Polymorphonuclear eosinophils	0.5–4.0	2.0		0.005–0.04	0.02	
Polymorphonuclear basophils	0.0–0.7	0.2		0.00–0.007	0.002	
Lymphocytes	3.0–17.0	10.0		0.03–0.17	0.10	
Plasma cells	0.0–2.0	0.4		0.00–0.02	0.004	
Monocytes	0.5–5.0	2.0		0.005–0.05	0.02	
Reticulum cells	0.1–2.0	0.2		0.001–0.02	0.002	
Megakaryocytes	0.3–3.0	0.4		0.003–0.03	0.004	
Pronormoblasts	1.0–8.0	4.0		0.01–0.08	0.04	
Normoblasts	7.0–32.0	18.0		0.07–0.32	0.18	

Reference Values for Blood, Plasma, and Serum*

	Conventional Units	Factor	S.I. Units	Notes
Acetoacetate plus acetone, serum				
Qualitative	Negative	—	Negative	
Quantitative	0.3–2.0 mg/dl	10	3–20 mg/liter	
Aldolase, serum	0–11 milliunits/ml (I.U.) (30°)	1.0	0–11 units/liter (30 C)	f
Alpha amino nitrogen, serum	3.0–5.5 mg/dl	0.714	2.1–3.9 mmol/liter	
Ammonia, blood	80–100 μg/dl	0.587	47–65 μmol/liter	
Amylase, serum	Less than 160 Caraway units/dl	—	Less than 160 Caraway units/dl	f
Ascorbic acid, blood	0.4–1.5 mg/dl	56.8	23–85 μmol/liter	
Bilirubin, serum				
Direct	0.1–0.4 mg/dl	17.1	1.7–6.8 μmol/liter	
Indirect	0.2–0.7 mg/dl (Total minus direct)		3.4–12 μmol/liter (Total minus direct)	
Total	0.3–1.1 mg/dl		5.1–19 μmol/liter	
Bromsulphalein (BSP) (Inject 5 mg/kg body weight, draw sample at 45 min)	Less than 5%	0.01	Less than 0.05	a
Calcium, serum	4.5–5.5 mEq/L	0.50	2.25–2.75 mmol/liter	
	9.0–11.0 mg/dl	0.25	2.25–2.75 mmol/liter	
	(Slightly higher in children)		(Slightly higher in children)	
	(Varies with protein concentration)		(Varies with protein concentration)	
Calcium, ionized, serum	2.1–2.6 mEq/L	0.50	1.05–1.30 mmol/liter	
	4.25–5.25 mg/dl	0.25	1.05–1.30 mmol/liter	
Carbon dioxide content, serum				
Adults	24–30 mEq/L	1.0	24–30 mmol/liter	
Infants	20–28 mEq/L	1.0	20–28 mmol/liter	
Carbon dioxide tension (P_{CO_2}), blood	35–45 mm Hg	—	35–45 mm Hg	g
Carotene, serum	50–300 μg/dl	0.0186	0.93–5.58 μmol/liter	
Ceruloplasmin, serum	23–44 mg/dl	0.0662	1.5–2.9 μmol/liter	h
Chloride, serum	96–106 mEq/L	1.0	96–106 mmol/liter	
Chlolesterol, serum				
Total	150–250 mg/dl	0.0259	3.9–6.5 mmol/liter	
Esters	68–76% of total cholesterol	0.01	0.68–0.76 of total cholesterol	a
Cholinesterase				
Serum	0.5–1.3 pH units	—	0.5–1.3 pH units	f
Erythrocytes	0.5–1.0 pH unit	—	0.5–1.0 pH unit	f
Copper, serum				
Males	70–140 μg/dl	0.157	11–22 μmol/liter	
Females	85–155 μg/dl		13–24 μmol/liter	
Cortisol, plasma (8 A.M.)	6–16 μg/dl	27.6	170–440 nmol/liter	
Creatine, serum	0.2–0.8 mg/dl	76.3	15–61 μmol/liter	
Creatine phosphokinase, serum				
Males	0–50 milliunits/ml (I.U.) (30°)	1.0	0–50 units/liter (30 C)	f
Females	0–30 milliunits/ml (I.U.) (30°) (Oliver-Rosalki)		0–30 units/liter (30 C) (Oliver-Rosalki)	f
Creatine phosphokinase isoenzymes, serum				
CPK-MM	Present	—	Present	
CPK-MB	Absent	—	Absent	
CPK-BB	Absent	—	Absent	

* For some procedures, the reference values may vary depending upon the method used.

	Conventional Units	Factor	S.I. Units	Notes
Creatine, serum	0.7–1.5 mg/dl	88.4	62–133 μmol/liter	
Cryoglobulins, serum	0	—	0	
Fatty acids, total, serum	190–420 mg/dl	0.0352	7–15 mmol/liter	i
Fibrinogen, plasma	200–400 mg/dl	0.0293	5.9–11.7 μmol/liter	c
Folate, serum	5–21 ng/ml	2.27	11–48 nmol/liter	
Gastrin, serum	0–200 pg/ml	1.0	0–200 ng/liter	
Glucose (fasting)				
Blood	60–100 mg/dl	0.0555	3.33–5.55 mmol/liter	
Plasma or serum	70–115 mg/dl		3.89–6.38 mmol/liter	
Haptoglobin, serum	100–200 mg/dl (As hemoglobin binding capacity)	0.155	16–31 μmol/liter (As hemoglobin binding capacity)	d
Hydroxybutyric dehydrogenase, serum	0–180 milliunits/ml (I.U.) (30°) (Rosalki-Wilkinson)	1.0	0–180 units/liter (30 C) (Rosalki-Wilkinson)	f
	114–290 units/ml (Wroblewski)	—	114–290 units/ml (Wroblewski)	f
17-Hydroxycorticosteroids, plasma	8–18 μg/dl	0.0276	0.22–0.50 μmol/liter	j
Immunoglobins, serum				
IgG	550–1900 mg/dl	0.01	5.5–19.0 g/liter	
IgA	60–333 mg/dl	0.01	0.60–3.3 g/liter	
IgM	45–145 mg/dl (Varies with age in children)	0.01	0.45–1.5 g/liter (Varies with age in children)	
Insulin, plasma (fasting)	5–25 microunits/ml	1.0	5–25 milliunits/liter	
Iodine, protein bound, serum	3.5–8.0 μg/dl	0.0788	0.28–0.63 μmol/liter	k
Iron, serum	75–175 μg/dl	0.179	13–31 μmol/liter	
Iron binding capacity, serum				
Total	250–410 μg/dl	0.179	45–73 μmol/liter	
Saturation	20–55%	0.01	0.20–0.55	a
17-Ketosteroids, plasma	25–125 μg/dl	0.0347	0.87–4.34 μmol/liter	l
Lactate, blood, venous	0.6–1.8 mEq/L	1.0	0.6–1.8 mmol/liter	
Lactate dehydrogenase, serum	0–300 milliunits/ml (I.U.) (30°) (Wroblewski modified)	1.0	0–300 units/liter (30 C) (Wroblewski modified)	f
	150–450 units/ml (Wroblewski)	—	150–450 units/ml (Wroblewski)	
	80–120 units/ml (Wacker)	—	80–120 units/ml (Wacker)	
Lactate dehydrogenase isoenzymes, serum				
LDH_1	22–37% of total	0.01	0.22–0.37 of total	a
LDH_2	30–46% of total		0.30–0.46 of total	
LDH_3	14–29% of total		0.14–0.29 of total	
LDH_4	5–11% of total		0.05–0.11 of total	
LDH_5	2–11% of total		0.02–0.11 of total	
Leucine aminopeptidase, serum	14–40 milliunits/ml (I.U.) (30°)	1.0	14–40 units/liter (30 C)	f
Lipase, serum	0–1.5 units (Cherry-Crandall)	—	0–1.5 units (Cherry-Crandall)	f
Lipids, total, serum	450–850 mg/dl	0.01	4.5–8.5 g/liter	m
Magnesium, serum	1.5–2.5 mEq/L	0.50	0.75–1.25 mmol/liter	
	1.8–3.0 mg/dl	0.411	0.75–1.25 mmol/liter	
5′-Nucleotidase, serum	Less than 1.6 milliunits/ml (30°)	1.0	Less than 1.6 units/liter (30 C)	f
Nitrogen, nonprotein, serum	15–35 mg/dl	0.714	10.7–25.0 mmol/liter	
Osmolality, serum	285–295 mOsm/kg serum water	—	285–295 mmol/kg serum water	n

(Continued)

Reference Values for Blood, Plasma, and Serum (cont.)

	Conventional Units	Factor	S.I. Units	Notes
Oxygen, blood				
Capacity	16–24 vol.% (varies with hemoglobin)	0.446	7.14–10.7 mmol/liter (varies with hemoglobin)	o
Content				
Arterial	15–23 vol.%	0.446	6.69–10.3 mmol/liter	o
Venous	10–16 vol.%		4.46–7.14 mmol/liter	o
Saturation				
Arterial	94–100% of capacity	0.01	0.94–1.00 of capacity	a
Venous	60–85% of capacity		0.60–0.85 of capacity	a
Tension, Po_2				
Arterial	75–100 mm Hg	—	75–100 mm Hg	g
pH, arterial, blood	7.35–7.45	—	7.35–7.45	p
Phenylalanine, serum	Less than 3 mg/dl	0.0605	Less than 0.18 mmol/liter	
Phosphatase, acid, serum	0–7.0 milliunits/ml (I.U.) (30°)	1.0	0–7.0 units/liter (30 C)	f
	1.0–5.0 units (King-Armstrong)	—	1.0–5.0 units (King-Armstrong)	
Phosphatase, alkaline, serum	10–32 milliunits/ml (I.U.) (30°)	100	10–32 units/liter (30 C)	f
	5.0–13.0 units (King-Armstrong)	—	5.0–13.0 units (King-Armstrong)	
	(Values are higher in children)		(Values are higher in children)	
Phosphate, inorganic, serum				
Adults	3.0–4.5 mg/dl	0.323	1.0–1.5 mmol/liter	
Children	4.0–7.0 mg/dl		1.3–2.3 mmol/liter	
Phospholipids, serum	6–12 mg/dl (As lipid phosphorus)	0.323	1.9–3.9 mmol/liter (As lipid phosphorus)	
Potassium, serum	3.5–5.0 mEq/L	1.0	3.5–5.0 mmol/liter	
Protein, serum				
Total	6.0–8.0 g/dl	10	60–80 g/liter	m
Albumin	3.5–5.5 g/dl	10	35–55 g/liter	q
		0.154	0.54–0.85 mmol/liter	
Globulin	2.5–3.5 g/dl	10	25–35 g/liter	
Electrophoresis				
Albumin	3.5–5.5 g/dl	10	35–55 g/liter	q
	52–68% of total	0.01	0.52–0.68 of total	a
Globulin				
Alpha$_1$	0.2–0.4 g/dl	10	2–4 g/liter	m
	2–5% of total	0.01	0.02–0.05 of total	a
Alpha$_2$	0.5–0.9 g/dl	10	5–9 g/liter	m
	7–14% of total	0.01	0.07–0.14 of total	a
Beta	0.6–1.1 g/dl	10	6–11 g/liter	m
	9–15% of total	0.01	0.09–0.15 of total	a
Gamma	0.7–1.7 g/dl	10	7–17 g/liter	m
	11–21% of total	0.01	0.11–0.21 of total	a
Protoporphyrin, erythrocyte	27–61 μg/dl packed RBC	0.0178	0.48–1.09 μmol/liter packed RBC	
Pyruvate, blood	0.01–0.11 mEq/L	1.0	0.01–0.11 mmol/liter	
Sodium, serum	136–145 mEq/L	1.0	136–145 mmol/liter	
Sulfates, inorganic, serum	0.8–1.2 mg/dl	104	83–125 μmol/liter	
Testosterone, plasma				
Males	275–875 ng/dl	0.0347	9.5–30 nmol/liter	
Females	23–75 ng/dl		0.8–2.6 nmol/liter	
Pregnant	38–190 ng/dl		1.3–6.6 nmol/liter	
Thyroid stimulating hormone (TSH), serum	0–7 microunits/ml	1.0	0–7 milliunits/liter	
Thyroxin, free, serum	1.0–2.1 ng/dl	12.9	13–27 pmol/liter	
Thyroxine (T_4), serum	4.4–9.9 μg/dl	12.9	57–128 nmol/liter	

	Conventional Units	Factor	S.I. Units	Notes
Thyroxine binding globulin (TBG), serum (as thyroxine)	10–26 µg/dl	12.9	129–335 nmol/liter	
Tri-iodothyronine (T$_3$), serum	150–250 ng/dl	0.0154	2.3–3.9 nmol/liter	
Thyroxine iodine, serum	2.9–6.4 µg/dl	78.8	229–504 nmol/liter	k
Transaminase, serum				f
SGOT (aspartate aminotransferase)	0–19 milliunits/ml (I.U.) (30°) (Karmen modified)	1.0	0–19 units/liter (30 C) (Karmen modified)	
	15–40 units/ml (Karmen)		15–40 units/ml (Karmen)	
	18–40 units/ml (Reitman-Frankel)		18–40 units/ml (Reitman-Frankel)	
SGPT (alanine aminotransferase)	0–17 milliunits/ml (I.U.) (30°) (Karmen modified)	1.0	0–17 units/liter (30 C) (Karmen modified)	f
	6–35 units/ml (Karmen)		6–35 units/ml (Karmen)	
	5–35 units/ml (Reitman-Frankel)		5–35 units/ml (Reitman-Frankel)	
Triglycerides, serum	40–150 mg/dl	0.01	0.4–1.5 g/liter	r
		0.0114	0.45–1.71 mmol/liter	
Urate (serum)				
Males	2.5–8.0 mg/dl	0.0595	0.15–0.48 mmol/liter	
Females	1.5–7.0 mg/dl		0.09–0.42 mmol/liter	
Urea				
Blood	21–43 mg/dl	0.167	3.5–7.2 mmol/liter	
Plasma or serum	24–49 mg/dl		4.0–8.2 mmol/liter	
Urea nitrogen				
Blood	10–20 mg/dl	0.714	7.1–14.3 mmol/liter	k
Plasma or serum	11–23 mg/dl		7.9–16.4 mmol/liter	
Vitamin A, serum	20–80 µg/dl	0.0349	0.70–2.8 µmol/liter	
Vitamin B$_{12}$, serum	300–1000 pg/ml	0.738	220–740 pmol/liter	

Reference Values for Urine*

	Conventional Units	Factor	S.I. Units	Notes
Acetone and acetoacetate, qualitative	Negative	—	Negative	
Addis count				
Erythrocytes	0–130,000/24 hr	—	0–130,000/24 hr	
Leukocytes	0–650,000/24 hr	—	0–650,000/24 hr	
Casts (hyaline)	0–2000/24 hr	—	0–2000/24 hr	
Albumin				
Qualitative	Negative	—	Negative	
Quantitative	10–100 mg/24 hr	—	10–100 mg/24 hr	q
		0.0154	0.15–1.5 µmol/24 hr	
Aldosterone	3–20 µg/24 hr	2.77	8.3–55 nmol/24 hr	
Alpha amino nitrogen	50–200 mg/24 hr	0.0714	3.6–14.3 mmol/24 hr	
Ammonia nitrogen	20–70 mEq/24 hr	1.0	20–70 mmol/24 hr	
Amylase	35–260 Caraway units/hr	—	35–260 Caraway units/hr	f
Bilirubin, qualitative	Negative	—	Negative	
Calcium				
Low Ca diet	Less than 150 mg/24 hr	0.025	Less than 3.8 mmol/24 hr	
Usual diet	Less than 250 mg/24 hr		Less than 6.3 mmol/24 hr	
Catecholamines				
Epinephrine	Less than 10 µg/24 hr	5.46	Less than 55 nmol/24 hr	
Norepinephrine	Less than 100 µg/24 hr	5.91	Less than 590 nmol/24 hr	
Total free catecholamines	4–126 µg/24 hr	5.91	24–745 nmol/24 hr	s
Total metanephrines	0.1–1.6 mg/24 hr	5.07	0.5–8.1 µmol/24 hr	t
Chloride	110–250 mEq/24 hr (Varies with intake)	1.0	110–250 mmol/24 hr (Varies with intake)	

* For some procedures the reference values may vary depending upon the method used.

(Continued)

Reference Values for Urine (cont.)

	Conventional Units	Factor	S.I. Units	Notes
Chorionic gonadotropin	0	—	0	
Copper	0–50 μg/24 hr	0.0157	0–0.80 μmol/24 hr	
Creatine				
Males	0–40 mg/24 hr	0.00762	0–0.30 mmol/24 hr	
Females	0–100 mg/24 hr		0–0.76 mmol/24 hr	
	(Higher in children and during pregnancy)		(Higher in children and during pregnancy)	
Creatinine	15–25 mg/kg body weight/24 hr	0.00884	0.13–0.22 mmol kg^{-1} body weight/24 hr	
Creatinine clearance				
Males	110–150 ml/min	—	110–150 ml/min	
Females	105–132 ml/min (1.73 sq. meter surface area)	—	105–132 ml/min (1.73 m^2 surface area)	
Cystine or cysteine, qualitative	Negative	—	Negative	
Dehydroepiandrosterone	Less than 15% of total 17-ketosteroids	0.01	Less than 0.15 of total 17-ketosteroids	a
Delta aminolevulinic acid	1.3–7.0 mg/24 hr	7.63	10–53 μmol/24 hr	
Estrogens				
Males				
Estrone	3–8 μg/24 hr	3.70	11–30 nmol/24 hr	
Estradiol	0–6 μg/24 hr	3.67	1–22 nmol/24 hr	
Estriol	1–11 μg/24 hr	3.47	3–38 nmol/24 hr	
Total	4–25 μg/24 hr	3.60	14–90 nmol/24 hr	u
Females				
Estrone	4–31 μg/24 hr	3.70	15–115 nmol/24 hr	
Estradiol	0–14 μg/24 hr	3.67	0–51 nmol/24 hr	
Estriol	0–72 μg/24 hr	3.47	0–250 nmol/24 hr	
Total	5–100 μg/24 hr	3.60	18–360 nmol/24 hr	u
	(Markedly increased during pregnancy)		(Markedly increased during pregnancy)	
Glucose (as reducing substance)	Less than 250 mg/24 hr	—	Less than 250 mg/24 hr	
Gonadotropins, pituitary	10–50 mouse units/24 hr	—	10–50 mouse units/24 hr	
Hemoglobin and myoglobin, qualitative	Negative		Negative	
Hemogentisic acid, qualitative	Negative	—	Negative	
17-Hydroxycorticosteroids				
Males	3–9 mg/24 hr	2.76	8.3–25 μmol/24 hr	j
Females	2–8 mg/24 hr		5.5–22 μmol/24 hr	
5-Hydroxyindoleacetic acid				
Qualitative	Negative	—	Negative	
Quantitative	Less than 9 mg/24 hr	5.23	Less than 47 μmol/24 hr	
17-Ketosteroids				
Males	6–18 mg/24 hr	3.47	21–62 μmol/24 hr	l
Females	4–13 mg/24 hr		14–45 μmol/24 hr	
	(Varies with age)		(Varies with age)	
Magnesium	6.0–8.5 mEq/24 hr	0.5	3.0–4.3 mmol/24 hr	
Metanephrines (see Catecholamines)				
Osmolality	38–1400 mOsm/kg water	—	38–1400 mmol/kg water	n
pH	4.6–8.0, average 6.0	—	4.6–8.0, average 6.0	p
	(Depends on diet)		(Depends on diet)	
Phenosulfonphthalein excretion (PSP)				a
	25% or more in 15 min	0.01	0.25 or more in 15 min	
	40% or more in 30 min		0.40 or more in 30 min	
	55% or more in 2 hr		0.55 or more in 2 hr	
	(After injection of 1 ml PSP intravenously)		(After injection of 1 ml PSP intravenously)	

	Conventional Units	Factor	S.I. Units	Notes
Phenylpyruvic acid, qualitative	Negative	—	Negative	
Phosphorus	0.9–1.3 g/24 hr	32.3	29–42 mmol/24 hr	
Porphobilinogen				
Qualitative	Negative	—	Negative	
Quantitative	0–0.2 mg/dl	4.42	0–0.9 µmol/liter	
	Less than 2.0 mg/24 hr		Less than 9 µmol/24 hr	
Porphyrins				
Coproporphyrin	50–250 µg/24 hr	1.53	77–380 nmol/24 hr	
Uroporphyrin	10–30 µg/24 hr	1.20	12–36 nmol/24 hr	
Potassium	25–100 mEq/24 hr	1.0	25–100 mmol/24 hr	
	(Varies with intake)		(Varies with intake)	
Pregnanediol				
Males	0.4–1.4 mg/24 hr	3.12	1.2–4.4 µg/24 hr	
Females				
Proliferative phase	0.5–1.5 mg/24 hr		1.6–4.7 µmol/24 hr	
Luteal phase	2.0–7.0 mg/24 hr		6.2–22 µmol/24 hr	
Postmenopausal phase	0.2–1.0 mg/24 hr		0.6–3.1 µmol/24 hr	
Pregnant 16 weeks	5–21 mg/24 hr		16–66 µmol/24 hr	
Pregnant 20 weeks	6–26 mg/24 hr		19–81 µmol/24 hr	
Pregnant 24 weeks	12–32 mg/24 hr		37–100 µmol/24 hr	
Pregnant 28 weeks	19–51 mg/24 hr		59–159 µmol/24 hr	
Pregnant 32 weeks	22–66 mg/24 hr		69–206 µmol/24 hr	
Pregnant 36 weeks	23–77 mg/24 hr		72–240 µmol/24 hr	
Pregnant 40 weeks	23–63 mg/24 hr		72–197 µmol/24 hr	
Pregnanetriol	Less than 2.5 mg/24 hr in adults	2.97	Less than 7.4 µmol/24 hr in adults	
Protein				
Qualitative	Negative	—	Negative	
Quantitative	10–150 mg/24 hr		10–150 mg/24 hr	m
Sodium	130–260 mEq/24 hr	1.0	130–260 mmol/24 hr	
	(Varies with intake)		(Varies with intake)	
Specific gravity	1.003–1.030	—	1.003–1.030	
Titratable acidity	20–40 mEq/24 hr	1.0	20–40 mmol/24 hr	
Urate	200–500 mg/24 hr	0.00595	1.2–3.0 mmol/24 hr	
	(With normal diet)		(With normal diet)	
Urobilinogen	Up to 1.0 Ehrlich unit/2 hr	—	Up to 1.0 Ehrlich unit/2 hr	
	(1–3 P.M.)		(1–3 P.M.)	
	0–4.0 mg/24 hr	—	0–4.0 mg/24 hr	
Vanillymandelic acid (VMA) (4-hydroxy-3-methoxymandelic acid)	1–8 mg/24 hr	5.05	5–40 µmol/24 hr	

Reference Values for Therapeutic Drug Monitoring

	Conventional Units	Factor	S.I. Units	Notes
Carbamazepine, serum (Tegretol)	0	4.23	0	
	Therapeutic levels:		Therapeutic levels:	
	5.0–14.0 mg/liter		21–59 µmol/liter	
Digoxin, serum	0	1.28	0	
	Therapeutic levels:		Therapeutic levels:	
With dose of 0.25 mg per day	0.8–1.6 mg/liter		1.0–2.3 nmol/liter	
With dose of 0.5 mg per day	0.9–2.4 µg/liter		1.2–3.1 nmol/liter	
(Sample obtained 12 to 24 hr after last dose)				

(Continued)

Reference Values for Therapeutic Drug Monitoring (cont.)

	Conventional Units	Factor	S.I. Units	Notes
Diphenylhydantoin, serum (Dilantin)	0 Therapeutic levels: 10–20 mg/liter Toxic levels: Above 20 mg/liter	3.65	0 Therapeutic levels: 37–73 μmol/liter Toxic levels: Above 73 μmol/liter	
Ethosuximide, serum (Zarontin)	0 Therapeutic levels: 40–80 mg/liter	7.08	0 Therapeutic levels: 283–566 μmol/liter	
Lithium, serum	0 Therapeutic levels: 0.8–1.5 mEq/L Toxic level: Above 2 mEq/L	1.0	0 Therapeutic levels: 0.8–1.5 mmol/liter Toxic level: Above 2 mmol/liter	

Phenobarbital, serum	0
	Therapeutic levels:
	10.0–25.0 mg/liter
	Toxic levels:
	Vary widely because of
	   developed tolerance
		4.31	0
			Therapeutic levels:
			43–108 μmol/liter
			Toxic levels:
			Vary widely because of
			   developed tolerance	

Primidone, serum (Mysoline)	0 Therapeutic levels: 4.0–10.0 mg/liter	4.58	0 Therapeutic levels: 18–46 μmol/liter	
Procainamide, serum (Pronestyl)	0 Therapeutic levels: 4.0–8.0 mg/liter	4.24	0 Therapeutic levels: 17–34 μmol/liter	
Quinidine, serum	0 Therapeutic levels: 2.0–5.0 mg/liter Toxic levels: Over 10 mg/liter	3.08	0 Therapeutic levels: 6.2–15 μmol/liter Toxic levels: Over 31 μmol/liter	
Salicylate, plasma	0 Therapeutic levels: 20–25 mg/dl Toxic levels: Over 30 mg/dl Death 45–75 mg/dl	0.0555	0 Therapeutic levels: 1.0–1.4 mmol/liter Toxic levels: Over 1.7 mmol/liter Death 2.5–4.2 mmol/liter	
Theophylline, serum	0 Therapeutic levels: 5.0–20.0 mg/liter Toxic levels: Above 30.0 mg/liter	5.55	0 Therapeutic levels: 28–111 μmol/liter Toxic levels: Above 167 μmol/liter	
Thiocyanate, serum (Metabolite of sodium nitroprusside)	0 Therapeutic levels: 80–120 mg/liter	0.0169	0 Therapeutic levels: 1.4–2.0 mmol/liter	

Reference Values in Toxicology

	Conventional Units	Factor	S.I. Units	Notes
Arsenic, blood	3.5–7.2 μg/dl	0.133	0.47–0.96 μmol/liter	
Arsenic, urine	Less than 100 μg/24 hr	0.0133	Less than 1.3 μmol/24 hr	
Bromides, serum	0 Toxic levels: Above 17 mEq/L	1.0	0 Toxic levels: Above 17 mmol/liter	

	Conventional Units	Factor	S.I. Units	Notes
Carbon monoxide, blood	Up to 5% saturation	—	Up to 0.05 saturation	a
	Symptoms occur with 20% saturation		Symptoms occur with 0.20 saturation	
Ethanol, blood	Less than 0.005%	217	Less than 1 mmol/liter	
Marked intoxication	0.3–0.4%		65–87 mmol/liter	
Alcoholic stupor	0.4–0.5%		87–109 mmol/liter	
Coma	Above 0.5%		Above 109 mmol/liter	
Lead, blood	0–40 µg/dl	0.0483	0–2 µmol/liter	
Lead, urine	Less than 100 µg/24 hr	0.00483	Less than 0.48 µmol/24 hr	
Mercury, urine	Less than 10 µg/24 hr	4.98	Less than 50 nmol/24 hr	

Reference Values for Cerebrospinal Fluid

	Conventional Units	Factor	S.I. Units	Notes
Cells	Fewer than 5/µl; all mononuclear	—	Fewer than 5/µl; all mononuclear	
Chloride	120–130 mEq/L (20 mEq/L higher than serum)	1.0	120–130 mmol/liter (20 mmol/liter higher than serum)	
Electrophoresis	Predominantly albumin	—	Predominantly albumin	
Glucose	50–75 mg/dl (20 mg/dl less than serum)	0.0555	2.8–4.2 mmol/liter (1.1 mmol/liter less than serum)	
IgG				
Children under 14	Less than 8% of total protein	—	Less than 0.08 of total protein	a, m
Adults	Less than 14% of total protein		Less than 0.14 of total protein	
Pressure	70–180 mm water		70–180 mm water	g
Protein, total	15–45 mg/dl (Higher, up to 70 mg/dl, in elderly adults and children)	0.01	0.150–0.450 g/liter (Higher, up to 0.70 g/liter, in elderly adults and children)	m

Reference Values for Gastric Analysis

	Conventional Units	Factor	S.I. Units	Notes
Basal gastric secretion (1 hr)				
Concentration	(Mean ± 1 SD)		(Mean ± 1 SD)	
Males	25.8 ± 1.8 mEq/L	1.0	25.8 ± 1.8 mmol/liter	
Females	20.3 ± 3.0 mEq/L		20.3 ± 3.0 mmol/liter	
Output	(Mean ± 1 SD)		(Mean ± 1 SD)	
Males	2.57 ± 0.16 mEq/hr	1.0	2.57 ± 0.16 mmol/hr	
Females	1.61 ± 0.18 mEq/hr		1.61 ± 0.18 mmol/hr	
After histamine stimulation				
Normal	Mean output 11.8 mEq/hr	1.0	Mean output 11.8 mmol/hr	
Duodenal ulcer	Mean output 15.2 mEq/hr		Mean output 15.2 mmol/hr	
After maximal histamine stimulation				
Normal	Mean output 22.6 mEq/hr	1.0	Mean output 22.6 mmol/hr	
Duodenal ulcer	Mean output 44.6 mEq/hr		Mean output 44.6 mmol/hr	

(Continued)

Reference Values for Gastric Analysis (cont.)

	Conventional Units	Factor	S.I. Units	Notes
Diagnex blue (Squibb)				
Anacidity	0–0.3 mg in 2 hr	1.0	0–0.3 mg in 2 hr	
Doubtful	0.3–0.6 mg in 2 hr		0.3–0.6 mg in 2 hr	
Normal	Greater than 0.6 mg in 2 hr		Greater than 0.6 mg in 2 hr	
Volume, fasting stomach content	0.50–1 dl	—	0.05–0.1 liter	
Emptying time	3–6 hr	—	3–6 hr	
Color	Opalescent or colorless	—	Opalescent or colorless	
Specific gravity	1.006–1.009	—	1.006–1.009	
pH (adults)	0.9–1.5	—	0.9–1.5	p

Gastrointestinal Absorption Tests

	Conventional Units	Factor	S.I. Units	Notes
d-Xylose absorption test	After an 8-hr fast, 10 ml/kg body weight of a 0.05 solution of d-xylose is given by mouth. Nothing further by mouth is given until the test has been completed. All urine voided during the following 5 hr is pooled, and blood samples are taken at 0.60, and 120 min. Normally 0.26 (range 0.16–0.33) of ingested xylose is excreted within 5 hr, and the serum xylose reaches a level between 25 and 40 mg/dl after 1 hr and is maintained at this level for another 60 min.		No change	
Vitamin A absorption	A fasting blood specimen is obtained and 200,000 units of vitamin A in oil is given by mouth. Serum vitamin A level should rise to twice fasting level in 3 to 5 hr.		No change	

Reference Values for Feces

	Conventional Units	Factor	S.I. Units	Notes
Bulk	100–200 g/24 hr	—	100–200 g/24 hr	
Dry matter	23–32 g/24 hr	—	23–32 g/24 hr	
Fat, total	Less than 6.0 g/24 hr	—	Less than 6.0 g/24 hr	
Nitrogen, total	Less than 2.0 g/24 hr	—	Less than 2.0 g/24 hr	
Urobilinogen	40–280 mg/24 hr	—	40–280 mg/24 hr	
Water	Approximately 65%	0.01	Approximately 0.65	a

Reference Values for Semen Analysis

	Conventional Units	Factor	S.I. Units	Notes
Volume	2–5 ml; usually 3–4 ml	—	2–5 ml; usually 3–4 ml	
Liquefaction	Complete in 15 min	—	Complete in 15 min	
pH	7.2–8.0; average 7.8	—	7.2–8.0; average 7.8	p

	Conventional Units	Factor	S.I. Units	Notes
Leukocytes	Occasional or absent	—	Occasional or absent	
Count	60–150 million/ml	—	60–150 million/ml	
	Below 60 million/ml is abnormal	—	Below 60 million/ml is abnormal	
Motility	80% or more motile	—	0.80 or more motile	a
Morphology	80–90% normal forms	—	0.80–0.90 normal forms	a

Reference Values for Immunologic Procedures

	Conventional Units	Factor	S.I. Units	Notes
Syphilis serology (RPR and VDRL)	Negative		No change	
Mono screen				
R.A. test (latex)	Negative		No change	
	1:40 Negative		No change	
	1:80–1:160 Doubtful			
Rose test	1:320 Positive			
	1:10 Negative		No change	
	1:20–1:40 Doubtful			
	1:80 Positive			
Antistreptolysin O titer	Normal up to 1:128. Single test usually has little significance. Rise in titer or persistently elevated titer is significant.		No change	
Antihyaluronidase titer	Less than 1:200. Significant if rising titer can be demonstrated at weekly intervals.		No change	
C-reactive protein	Negative		No change	
Antinuclear antibody	One specimen is sufficient, unless the result is inconsistent with the clinical impression. Most patients with active lupus have high ANA titers (160 or greater); some have lower titers (20–40). Patients with inactive lupus may have a negative test. Antinuclear antibodies are occasionally present in patients with no evidence of systemic lupus, usually in lower titers (20–40).		No change	
Febrile agglutinins	Titers of 1:80 or greater may be significant, particularly if subsequent samples show rise in titer.		No change	
Tularemia agglutinins	1:80 Negative		No change	
	1:160 Doubtful			
	1:320 Positive			
Proteus OX-19 agglutinins	Titers of 1:80 or greater may be significant, particularly if subsequent samples show rise in titer.		No change	
Complement fixation tests	Titers of 1:8 or less are usually not significant. Paired sera showing rise in titer of more than two tubes are usually considered significant.		No change	
C3 test	80–140 mg/dl	0.01	0.80–1.40 g/liter	q
C4 test	11–75 mg/dl	0.01	0.11–0.75 g/liter	

NOTES

a. Percentage is expressed as a decimal fraction.

b. Percentage may be expressed as a decimal fraction; however, when the result expressed is itself a variable fraction of another variable, the absolute value is more meaningful. There is no reason, other than custom, for expressing reticulocyte counts and differential leukocyte counts in percentages or decimal fractions rather than in absolute numbers.

c. Molecular weight of fibrinogen = 341,000.

d. Molecular weight of hemoglobin = 64,500. Because of disagreement as to whether the monomer or tetramer of hemoglobin should be used in the conversion, it has been recommended that the conventional grams per deciliter be retained. The tetramer is used in the table; values given should be multiplied by 4 to obtain concentration of the monomer.

e. Molecular weight of methemoglobin = 64,500. See note "d" above.

f. Enzyme units have not been changed in these tables because the proposed enzyme unit, the katal, has not been universally adopted (1 International Unit = 16.7 nkat).

g. It has been proposed that pressure be expressed in the Pascal (1 mm Hg = 0.133 kPa); however, this convention has not been universally accepted.

h. Molecular weight of ceruloplasmin = 151,000.

i. "Fatty acids" include a mixture of different aliphatic acids of varying molecular weight. A mean molecular weight of 284 has been assumed in calculating the conversion factor.

j. Based upon molecular weight of cortisol, 362.47.

k. The practice of expressing concentration of an organic molecule in terms of one of its constituent elements originated when measurements included a heterogeneous class of compounds (nonprotein nitrogenous compounds, iodine-containing compounds bound to serum proteins). It was carried over to expressing measurements of specific substances (urea, thyroxine), but the practice should be discarded. For iodine and nitrogen, 1 mole is taken as the monoatomic form, although they occur as diatomic molecules.

l. Based upon molecular weight of dehydroepiandrosterone, 288.41.

m. Weight per volume is retained as the unit because of the heterogeneous nature of the material measured.

n. The proposal that osmolality be reported as freezing point depression using the millikelvin as the unit has not been received with universal enthusiasm. The milliosmole is not an S.I. unit, and the unit used here is the millimole.

o. Volumes percent might be converted to a decimal fraction; however, this would not permit direct correlation with hemoglobin content, which is possible when oxygen content and capacity are expressed in molar quantities. One millimole of hemoglobin combines with 4 millimoles of oxygen.

p. Hydrogen ion concentration in S.I. units would be expressed in nanomoles per liter; however, this change has not received general approval. Conversion can be calculated as antilog ($-$pH).

q. Albumin is expressed in grams per liter to be consistent with units used for other proteins. Concentration of albumin may be expressed im mmol per liter also, an expression that permits assessment of binding capacity of albumin for substances such as bilirubin. Molecular weight of albumin is 65,000.

r. Most techniques for quantitating triglycerides measure the glycerol moiety, and the total mass is calculated using an average molecular weight. The factor given assumes a mean molecular weight of 875 for triglycerides.

s. Calculated as norepinephrine, molecular weight 169.18.

t. Calculated as metanephrine, molecular weight 197.23.

u. Conversion factor calculated from molecular weights of estrone, estradiol, and estriol in proportions of 2:1:2.

BIBLIOGRAPHY

1. Baron, D.N., Broughton, P.M.G., Cohen, M., Lansley, T.S., Lewis, S.M., and Shinton, N.K. J. Clin. Pathol., 27:590, 1974.

2. Castleman, B. and McNeely, B.U. N. Engl. J. Med., 290:39, 1974.

3. Davidsohn, I. and Henry, J.B. Clinical Diagnosis by Laboratory Methods, 15th ed. Philadelphia, Saunders, 1974.

4. Dawson, R.M.C., Elliott, D.C., Elliott, W.H., and Jones, K.M. Data for Biochemical Research, 2nd ed. New York and Oxford, Oxford University, 1969.

5. Department of Laboratory Medicine, The Johns Hopkins Hospital: Clinical Laboratory Handbook. Baltimore, 1976.

6. Dybkaer, R. Am. J. Clin. Pathol., 52:637, 1969.

7. Henry, R.J., Cannon, D.C., and Winkleman, J.W. Clinical Chemistry—Principles and Techniques, 2nd ed. New York, Harper & Row, 1974.

8. International Committee for Standardization in Hematology, International Federation of Clinical Chemistry and World Association of Pathology Societies. Clin. Chem., 19:135, 1973.

9. Lehmann, H.P. Am. J. Clin. Pathol., 65:2, 1976.

10. Miale, J.B. Laboratory Medicine—Hematology, 4th ed. St. Louis, Mosby, 1972.

11. Page, C.H. and Vigoureux, P. The International System of Units (S.I.). U.S. Department of Commerce. National Bureau of Standards. Special Publication 330, 1974.

12. Tietz, N.W. Fundamentals of Clinical Chemistry, 2nd ed. Philadelphia, Saunders, 1976.

13. Wintrobe, M.D., Lee, G.R., Boggs, D.R., Bithell, T.C., Athens, J.W., and Foerster, J. Clinical Hematology, 7th ed. Philadelphia, Lea & Febiger, 1974.

14. Young, D.S. N. Engl. J. Med., 292:795, 1975.

Index

(Page numbers in **boldface type** indicate tables and illustrations.)